Present Knowledge in Nutrition

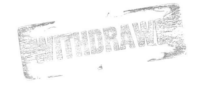

We dedicate this edition to our families who supported us during its creation, and to our scientific families (our mentors and colleagues) who make working in the field of nutritional sciences exciting, worthwhile, and a wonderful life's profession.

Present Knowledge in Nutrition

Tenth Edition

Edited by

John W. Erdman Jr.
PhD

Ian A. Macdonald
PhD

Steven H. Zeisel
MD, PhD

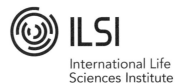

International Life
Sciences Institute

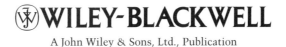

A John Wiley & Sons, Ltd., Publication

This edition first published 2012
© 1953, 1956, 1967, 1976, 1984, 1990, 1996, 2001, 2006, 2012 International Life Sciences Institute

Wiley-Blackwell is an imprint of John Wiley & Sons, formed by the merger of Wiley's global Scientific, Technical and Medical business with Blackwell Publishing.

Editorial offices: 2121 State Avenue, Ames, Iowa 50014-8300, USA
The Atrium, Southern Gate, Chichester, West Sussex, PO19 8SQ, UK
9600 Garsington Road, Oxford, OX4 2DQ, UK

For details of our global editorial offices, for customer services and for information about how to apply for permission to reuse the copyright material in this book please see our website at www.wiley.com/wiley-blackwell.

Library of Congress Cataloging-in-Publication Data

Present knowledge in nutrition. – 10th ed. / edited by John W. Erdman Jr., Ian A. Macdonald, Steven H. Zeisel.
p. ; cm.
Includes bibliographical references and index.
ISBN 978-0-470-95917-6 (pbk. : alk. paper)
I. Erdman, John W.   II. Macdonald, Ian A., 1952–   III. Zeisel, Steven H.   IV. International Life Sciences Institute.
[DNLM: 1. Nutritional Physiological Phenomena.   QU 145]

363.8–dc23
2012007483

A catalogue record for this book is available from the Library of Congress.

Cover images: iStockphoto.com
Cover design by Nicole Teut

Wiley also publishes its books in a variety of electronic formats. Some content that appears in print may not be available in electronic books.

Set in 11/13 pt Adobe Garamond by Toppan Best-set Premedia Limited, Hong Kong
Printed in Singapore by Ho Printing Singapore Pte Ltd

1   2012

Contents

Visit the supporting website for this book: www.pkn10.org

List of Contributors

Peter J. Aggett
School of Health and Medicine
Physics Building
Lancaster University
Lancaster LA1 4YD
UK

Janice Albert
Nutrition and Consumer Protection Division
Food and Agriculture Organization of the United
    Nations
Viale delle Terme di Caracalla
Rome 00153
Italy

Lindsay H. Allen
USDA-ARS Western Human Nutrition Research Center
University of California, Davis
430 W. Health Sciences Drive
Davis, CA 95616
USA

John J.B. Anderson
Department of Nutrition
Gillings School of Global Public Health
University of North Carolina
Chapel Hill, NC 27599-7461
USA

Arne Astrup
Faculty of Science
University of Copenhagen
Rolighedsvej 30
DK-1958 Frederiksberg
Denmark

Thiane G. Axelsson
Department of Clinical Science, Intervention and
    Technology
Divisions of Baxter Novum and Renal Medicine
Karolinska Institutet
Karolinska University Hospital
Huddinge
Stockholm 141 86
Sweden

Lynn B. Bailey
Department of Foods and Nutrition
University of Georgia
273 Dawson Hall
Athens, GA 30602
USA

Joseph L. Baumert
Department of Food Science and Technology
University of Nebraska
237 Food Industry Building
Lincoln, NE 68585-0919
USA

Prasad Bellur
Monsanto Research Centre
#44/2A, Vasants Business Park
Bellary Road NH 7, Hebbal
Bangalore 560092
India

Claire E. Berryman
Department of Nutritional Sciences
110 Chandlee Laboratory
The Pennsylvania State University
University Park, PA 16802
USA

Lucien Bettendorff
University of Liège–GIGA-Neurosciences
Av. de l'Hôpital 1 B36
Liège 4000
Belgium

Sekhar Boddupalli
Monsanto Vegetable Seeds
Woodland, CA 95695
USA

Annalies Borrel
UNICEF Office of Emergency Programmes-
    Humanitarian Policy and Advocacy
New York
USA

Jennie Brand-Miller
Boden Institute of Obesity, Nutrition, Exercise, and
    Eating Disorders
University of Sydney
Sydney, NSW 2006
Australia

Ronette R. Briefel
Mathematica Policy Research
1100 1st Street NE, 12th Floor
Washington, DC 20002-4221
USA

Alan L. Buchman
Department of Medicine
Feinberg School of Medicine
Northwestern University
Chicago, IL 60611
USA

Louise M. Burke
Australian Institute of Sport – Sports Nutrition
PO Box 176
Leverrier Crescent
Belconnen
ACT 2617
Australia

Leah E. Cahill
Department of Nutrition
Harvard School of Public Health
Building 2
655 Huntington Avenue
Boston, MA 02115
USA

Philip C. Calder
Institute of Human Nutrition
University of Southampton Faculty of Medicine
IDS Building MP887 Southampton General Hospital
Tremona Road
Southampton SO16 6YD
UK

Robert Carter, III
Military Nutrition Division
US Army Research Institute of Environmental Medicine
42 Kansas Street
Natick, MA 01760-5007
USA

Krista Casazza
Department of Nutrition Sciences
The University of Alabama at Birmingham
1675 University Blvd, WEBB 439
Birmingham, AL 35294-3360
USA

Marie A. Caudill
Division of Nutritional Sciences
Cornell University
228 Savage Hall
Ithaca, NY 14853
USA

Samuel N. Cheuvront
Military Nutrition Division
US Army Research Institute of Environmental Medicine
42 Kansas Street
Natick, MA 01760-5007
USA

Michal Chmielewski
Department of Nephrology, Transplantology and
    Internal Medicine
Medical University of Gdansk
ul. Debinki 7
20-811 Gdansk
Poland

Dallas L. Clouatre
Glykon Technologies Group, LLC
1112 Montana Avenue #541
Santa Monica, CA 90403
USA

Paul M. Coates
Office of Dietary Supplements
National Institutes of Health
6100 Executive Blvd, Room 3B01, MSC 7517
Bethesda, MD 20892-7517
USA

Stephen Colagiuri
Boden Institute of Obesity, Nutrition, Exercise, and
    Eating Disorders
University of Sydney
Sydney, NSW 2006
Australia

Karen D. Corbin
UNC Nutrition Research Institute
Department of Nutrition
University of North Carolina at Chapel Hill
500 Laureate Way, Rm 2218
Kannapolis, NC 28081
USA

Joseph Cornelius
Monsanto Company
800 North Lindbergh Blvd
St. Louis, MO 63167
USA

Vanessa R. da Silva
Department of Foods and Nutrition
University of Georgia
273 Dawson Hall
Athens, GA 30602
USA

Sai Krupa Das
Jean Mayer USDA Human Nutrition Research
    Center on Aging
Tufts University
711 Washington Street
Boston, MA 02111-1524
USA

Jeanne H.M. de Vries
Division of Human Nutrition
WU Agrotechnology & Food Sciences
Wageningen University
Bomenweg 2 # 307/214
6703HD Wageningen
The Netherlands

Alan M. Diamond
Department of Pathology
University of Illinois at Chicago
840 S. Wood Street, Suite 130 CSN
Chicago, IL 60612
USA

Kelly A. Dougherty
Department of Pediatrics
Gastroenterology, Hepatology, and Nutrition
The Children's Hospital of Philadelphia
University of Pennsylvania, Perelman School of Medicine
Philadelphia, PA 19104
USA

Adam Drewnowski
School of Public Health & Community Medicine
University of Washington
Box 353410
Seattle, WA 98195-3410
USA

Johanna T. Dwyer
Jean Meyer Human Nutrition Research
    Center on Aging
Tufts University
Box 783 Tufts Medical Center
800 Washington Street
Boston, MA 02111-1524
and Office of Dietary Supplements
National Institutes of Health
Bethesda, MD
USA

Ahmed El-Sohemy
Department of Nutritional Sciences
University of Toronto
150 College Street, Room 350
Toronto, Ontario M5S 3E2
Canada

Guylaine Ferland
Université de Montréal
Centre de recherche
Institut universitaire de gériatrie de Montréal
4565 chemin Queen-Mary
Montréal, Québec H3W 1W5
Canada

James C. Fleet
Department of Foods and Nutrition
Purdue University
700 West State Street
West Lafayette, IN 47906-2059
USA

Michael R. Flock
Department of Nutritional Sciences
110 Chandlee Laboratory
The Pennsylvania State University
University Park, PA 16802
USA

Edward A. Frongillo
Department of Health Promotion, Education, and
    Behavior
University of South Carolina, Columbia
800 Sumter Street
Columbia, SC 29208
USA

Amy Gorin
Department of Psychology
University of Connecticut
406 Babbidge Road, Unit 1020
Storrs, CT 06269-1020
USA

Jesse F. Gregory, III
Food Science and Human Nutrition Department
University of Florida
PO Box 110370
Gainesville, FL 32611-0370
USA

Kristina A. Harris
Department of Nutritional Sciences
110 Chandlee Laboratory
The Pennsylvania State University
University Park, PA 16802
USA

Robert P. Heaney
Creighton University Medical Center
601 North 30th Street – Suite 4841
Omaha, NE 68131
USA

William C. Heird
Department of Pediatrics
USDA-ARS Children's Nutrition Research Center
Baylor College of Medicine
1100 Bates Street
Houston, TX 77030-2600
USA

Helen L. Henry
Department of Biochemistry
University of California
Riverside, CA 92521
USA

Daniell B. Hill
Department of Medicine
Center for Translational Research
University of Louisville
505 South Hancock Street
Louisville, KY 40292
USA

Simone D. Holligan
Department of Nutritional Sciences
110 Chandlee Laboratory
The Pennsylvania State University
University Park, PA 16802
USA

Roberta R. Holt
Department of Nutrition
University of California, Davis
One Shields Avenue,
Davis, CA 95616
USA

Lindsay M. Jaacks
Department of Nutrition
UNC Gillings School of Global Public Health
2212 McGavran-Greenberg Hall
135 Dauer Drive
Chapel Hill, NC 27599
USA

Wei Jia
Department of Nutrition
University of North Carolina at Greensboro
North Carolina Research Campus
500 Laureate Way
Kannapolis, NC 28081
USA

Elizabeth J. Johnson
Jean Mayer USDA Human Nutrition Research
    Center on Aging
Tufts University
711 Washington Street
Boston, MA 02111-1524
USA

Ian T. Johnson
Institute of Food Research
Norwich Research Park
Colney, Norwich NR4 7UA
UK

Carol S. Johnston
Nutrition Program
College of Nursing and Health Innovation
Arizona State University
500 North 3rd Street
Phoenix, AZ 85004
USA

Alexandra M. Johnstone
Rowett Institute of Nutrition and Health
Greenburn Road
Bucksburn
Aberdeen AB21 9SB
UK

Peter J.H. Jones
Richardson Centre for Functional Foods
University of Manitoba
Smartpark Research and Technology Park
196 Innovation Drive
Winnipeg, Manitoba R3T 6C5
Canada

Jaya Joshi
Monsanto Research Centre
#44/2A, Vasants Business Park
Bellary Road NH 7, Hebbal
Bangalore 560092
India

Carl L. Keen
Department of Nutrition
University of California, Davis
One Shields Avenue
Davis, CA 95616
USA

Robert W. Kenefick
Military Nutrition Division
US Army Research Institute of Environmental Medicine
42 Kansas Street
Natick, MA 01760-5007
USA

James B. Kirkland
Department of Human Health and Nutritional Sciences
College of Biological Sciences
University of Guelph
Guelph, Ontario N1G 2W1
Canada

Penny M. Kris-Etherton
Department of Nutritional Sciences
110 Chandlee Laboratory
The Pennsylvania State University
University Park, PA 16802
USA

Toshinobu Kuroishi
Department of Nutrition and Health Sciences
University of Nebraska–Lincoln
316 Ruth Leverton Hall
Lincoln, NE 68583-0806
USA

Shantala Lakkanna
Monsanto Research Centre
#44/2A, Vasants Business Park
Bellary Road NH7, Hebbal
Bangalore 560092
India

Alice H. Lichtenstein
Jean Mayer USDA Human Nutrition Research
   Center on Aging
Tufts University
150 Harrison Avenue
Boston, MA 02111
USA

Bengt Lindholm
Department of Clinical Science, Intervention and
   Technology
Divisions of Baxter Novum and Renal Medicine
Karolinska Institutet
Karolinska University Hospital
Huddinge
Stockholm 141 86
Sweden

Brian L. Lindshield
Department of Human Nutrition
Kansas State University
208 Justin Hall
Manhattan, KS 66502
USA

Joanne R. Lupton
Department of Nutrition and Food Science
Texas A&M University, College Station
213 Kleberg Center
2253 TAMU
College Station, TX 77843-2253
USA

Asim Maqbool
Department of Pediatrics
Gastroenterology, Hepatology, and Nutrition
The Children's Hospital of Philadelphia
University of Pennsylvania, Perelman School of Medicine
Philadelphia, PA 19104
USA

Luis Marsano
Department of Medicine
Center for Translational Research
University of Louisville
505 South Hancock Street
Louisville, KY 40292
USA

Elizabeth J. Mayer-Davis
Department of Nutrition
UNC Gillings School of Global Public Health and
   School of Medicine
2212 McGavran-Greenberg Hall
135 Dauer Drive
Chapel Hill, NC 27599
USA

Craig J. McClain
Department of Medicine
Center for Translational Research
University of Louisville
505 South Hancock Street
Louisville, KY 40292
USA

Stephen A. McClave
University of Louisville School of Medicine
401 East Chestnut Street, Ste 310
Louisville, KY 40202
USA

Donald B. McCormick
Department of Biochemistry and Program in Nutrition
    and Health Science
Rollins Research Center
Emory University
Atlanta, GA 30322
USA

Margaret A. McDowell
National Institute of Health
Division of Nutrition Research Coordination
Two Democracy Plaza, Rm 629
6707 Democracy Blvd, MSC 5461
Bethesda, MD 20892-5461
USA

Joshua W. Miller
Department of Pathology and Laboratory Medicine
University of California Davis Medical Center
Research III
4645 2nd Avenue
Suite 3200A
Sacramento, CA 95817
USA

John A. Milner
Nutritional Sciences Research Group
National Cancer Institute
6130 Executive Blvd, Suite 3164 EPN
Rockville, MD 20852
USA

Pablo Monsivais
UKCRC Centre for Diet and Activity Research
Box 296
Cambridge Institute of Public Health
Forvie Site
Cambridge, CB2 0SR
UK

Scott J. Montain
Military Nutrition Division
US Army Research Institute of Environmental Medicine
42 Kansas Street
Natick, MA 01760-5007
USA

Tim R. Nagy
Department of Nutrition Sciences
The University of Alabama at Birmingham
1675 University Blvd, Webb 439
Birmingham, AL 35294-3360
USA

Marguerite A. Neill
The Warren Alpert Medical School
Brown University
Box G-A1
Providence, RI 02912
USA

Holly Nicastro
Nutritional Sciences Research Group
National Cancer Institute
6130 Executive Blvd, Suite 3164 EPN
Rockville, MD 20852
USA

Forrest H. Nielsen
Grand Forks Human Nutrition Research Center
USDA-ARS-NPA
2420 2 Avenue N, Stop 9034
Grand Forks, ND 58202-9034
USA

Anthony W. Norman
Department of Biochemistry and Division of Biomedical
    Sciences
University of California
Riverside, CA 92521
USA

Marga C. Ocké
The National Institute for Public Health and
    Environment
PO Box 1
3720 BA Bilthoven
The Netherlands

Thomas M. O'Connell
LipoScience Inc.
2500 Sumner Blvd
Raleigh, NC 27616
USA

Christine M. Olson
Division of Nutritional Sciences
Cornell University
376 Martha Van Rensselaer Hall
Ithaca, NY 14853
USA

Andrea A. Papamandjaris
Nestlé Inc.
Medical and Scientific Unit
North York, Ontario M2N 6S8
Canada

Elizabeth P. Parks
Department of Pediatrics
Gastroenterology, Hepatology, and Nutrition
The Children's Hospital of Philadelphia
University of Pennsylvania, Perelman School of Medicine
Philadelphia, PA 19104
USA

Sue D. Pedersen
LMC Endocrinology Centre
Suite 102
5940 MacLeod Tr SW
Calgary, Alberta T2H 2G4
Canada

David L. Pelletier
Division of Nutritional Sciences
Cornell University
212 Savage Hall
Ithaca, NY 14853
USA

W. Todd Penberthy
Department of Molecular Biology and Microbiology
University of Central Florida College of Medicine
Orlando, FL 32816
USA

Paul B. Pencharz
Departments of Paediatrics and Nutritional Sciences
Research Institute
The Hospital for Sick Children
University of Toronto
Toronto, Ontario M5G 1X8
Canada

Barry M. Popkin
Department of Nutrition
Carolina Population Center
University of North Carolina at Chapel Hill
University Square, CB# 8120
123 W. Franklin Street
Chapel Hill, NC 27516-3997
USA

Harry G. Preuss
Department of Biochemistry
Georgetown University Medical Center
Washington, DC 20057
USA

Joseph R. Prohaska
Department of Biomedical Sciences
University of Minnesota Medical School Duluth
1035 University Drive
Duluth, MN 55812
USA

Charles J. Rebouche (Retired)
Department of Pediatrics
University of Iowa
Iowa City, IA 52242
USA

Patrick Ritz
Gérontopôle de Toulouse
Unité de Nutrition
CHU Larrey
TS 30030
31059 Toulouse
France

Susan B. Roberts
Jean Mayer USDA Human Nutrition Research
   Center on Aging
Tufts University
711 Washington Street
Boston, MA 02111-1524
USA

Robert B. Rucker
Department of Nutrition
University of California, Davis
One Shields Avenue
3415 Meyer Hall
Davis, CA 95616-8575
USA

Katelyn A. Russell
Food Science and Human Nutrition Department
University of Florida
PO Box 110370
Gainesville, FL 32611-0370
USA

Kate Sadler
Friedman School of Nutrition Science and Policy
Feinstein International Center
Tufts University
200 Boston Avenue
Medford, MA 02155
USA

Lisa M. Sanders
Kellogg Company
Battle Creek, MI
USA

Thomas A.B. Sanders
Diabetes & Nutritional Sciences Division
School of Medicine
King's College London
4.43 Franklin-Wilkins Building
150 Stamford Street
London SE1 9NH
UK

Michael N. Sawka
Military Nutrition Division
US Army Research Institute of Environmental Medicine
42 Kansas Street
Natick, MA 01760-5007
USA

Marion Secher
Gérontopôle de Toulouse
Unité de Nutrition
CHU Larrey
TS 30030
31059 Toulouse
France

Anders Sjödin
Faculty of Science
University of Copenhagen
Rolighedsvej 30
DK-1958 Frederiksberg
Denmark

Noel W. Solomons
Center for Studies of Sensory Impairment
Sensory Impairment, Aging and Metabolism (CeSSIAM)
17a Avenida #16-89, Zona 11
Guatemala City 01011
Guatemala

Sally P. Stabler
Division of Hematology
University of Colorado School of Medicine
12700 E. 19th Avenue
Denver, CO 80045
USA

Virginia A. Stallings
Department of Pediatrics
Gastroenterology, Hepatology, and Nutrition
The Children's Hospital of Philadelphia
University of Pennsylvania, Perelman School of Medicine
Philadelphia, PA 19104
USA

Susan E. Steck
Department of Epidemiology and Biostatistics
University of South Carolina–Columbia
915 Greene Street, Rm 236
Columbia, SC 29208
USA

Paolo M. Suter
Clinic and Policlinic of Internal Medicine
University Hospital
Rämistrasse 100
8091 Zurich
Switzerland

Deborah F. Tate
Department of Health Behavior and Nutrition
Gillings School of Global Public Health
University of North Carolina at Chapel Hill
Chapel Hill, NC 27599
USA

Robert V. Tauxe
Division of Foodborne, Waterborne and Environmental
   Diseases
National Center for Emerging and Zoonotic Infectious
   Diseases
Centers for Disease Control and Prevention
Mailstop C-09
Atlanta, GA 30333
USA

Steve L. Taylor
Department of Food Science & Technology
University of Nebraska
255 Food Industry Bldg
Lincoln, NE 68585-0919
USA

Emily N. Terry
Department of Pathology
University of Illinois at Chicago
840 S. Wood St, Suite 130 CSN
Chicago, IL 60612
USA

Maret G. Traber
School of Biological and Population Health Sciences
Linus Pauling Institute
Oregon State University
307 Linus Pauling Science Center
Corvallis, OR 97331-6512
USA

Federico Tripodi
Monsanto Company
800 North Lindbergh Blvd
St. Louis, MO 63167
USA

Janet Y. Uriu-Adams
Department of Nutrition
University of California, Davis
One Shields Avenue
Davis, CA 95616
USA

Wija A. van Staveren
Division of Human Nutrition
WU Agrotechnology & Food Sciences
Wageningen University
Bomenweg 4 #309/2004
6703HD Wageningen
The Netherlands

Bruno Vellas
Gérontopôle de Toulouse
Unité de Nutrition
CHU Larrey
TS 30030
31059 Toulouse
France

Rohini Vishwanathan
Jean Mayer USDA Human Nutrition Research
   Center on Aging
Tufts University
711 Washington Street
Boston, MA 02111-1524
USA

Stella Lucia Volpe
Department of Nutrition Sciences
Drexel University College of Nursing and Health
  Professions
245 N. 15th Street
Bellet Building–Room 521
Mail Stop 1030
Philadelphia, PA 19102
USA

Li Wang
Department of Nutritional Sciences
110 Chandlee Laboratory
The Pennsylvania State University
University Park, PA 16802
USA

Robert A. Waterland
Departments of Pediatrics and Molecular & Human
  Genetics
USDA/ARS Children's Nutrition Research Center
Baylor College of Medicine
Houston, TX 77030-2600
USA

Connie M. Weaver
Department of Nutrition Science
Purdue University
1264 Stone Hall
700 W State Street
West Lafayette, IN 47907-2059
USA

Robert Weisell (Retired)
Food and Agriculture Organization of the United Nations
Viale delle Ginestre 8
Ariccia (RM) 00040
Italy

Subhashinee S.K. Wijeratne
Department of Nutrition and Health Sciences
University of Nebraska–Lincoln
316 Ruth Leverton Hall
Lincoln, NE 68586-0806
USA

Gary Williamson
School of Food Science and Nutrition
University of Leeds
Woodhouse Lane
Leeds, LS2 9JT
UK

Rena R. Wing
The Miriam Hospital
Alpert Medical School
Brown University
Providence, RI 02903
USA

Judith Wylie-Rosett
Department of Epidemiology and Population Health
Albert Einstein College of Medicine
Jack and Pearl Resnick Campus
1300 Morris Park Avenue
Belfer Building, Room 1307
Bronx, NY 10461
USA

Parveen Yaqoob
Food and Nutritional Sciences
University of Reading
2-55 Food Biosciences
Reading, RG6 6AH
UK

Helen Young
Friedman School of Nutrition Science and Policy
Feinstein International Center
Tufts University
200 Boston Avenue
Medford, MA 02155
USA

Steven H. Zeisel
UNC Nutrition Research Institute
Department of Nutrition
University of North Carolina at Chapel Hill
500 Laureate Way, Rm 2218
Kannapolis, NC 28081
USA

Janos Zempleni
Department of Nutrition and Health Sciences
University of Nebraska–Lincoln
316 Ruth Leverton Hall
Lincoln, NE 68583-0806
USA

Vivian M. Zhao
Nutrition and Metabolic Support Service and
    Department of Pharmaceutical Services
Emory University Hospital
1364 Clifton Road NE
Atlanta, GA 30322
USA

Thomas R. Ziegler
Emory University Hospital
Nutrition and Metabolic Support Service *and*
Emory University School of Medicine
1648 Pierce Drive NE
Atlanta, GA 30307
USA

Michael B. Zimmermann
Laboratory for Human Nutrition
Swiss Federal Institute of Technology Zürich
Schmelzbergstrasse 7
LFV E19
Zürich CH-8092
Switzerland

Preface

We are honored to have been asked to edit the tenth edition of *Present Knowledge in Nutrition*. The first edition was published in 1953, and throughout the book's history its authors have been a "Who's Who" of nutritional science. The current volume is no exception. With this edition, we aimed to find productive, knowledgeable, and well-known authors to help us provide integrated information on nutrition, physiology, health and disease, and public-health applications – all in one text. This ambitious goal was set for one purpose: to provide readers with the most comprehensive and current information covering the broad fields within the nutrition discipline. Reflecting the global relevance of nutrition, our authors come from a number of countries. It is hoped that this edition captures the current state of this vital and dynamic science from an international perspective.

New to this edition are chapters on topics such as epigenetics, metabolomics, and sports nutrition – areas that have developed significantly in recent years. The remaining chapters have all been thoroughly updated to reflect developments since the last edition. Suggested reading lists are now provided for readers wishing to delve further into specific subject areas.

To make this edition as accessible and continuously relevant as possible, it is available in both print and electronic formats. An accompanying website (visit **www. pkn10.org**) provides book owners with access to an Image Bank of tables and figures as well as to any updates the authors may post to their chapters in the future.

We hope this volume will be a valuable reference for researchers, health professionals, and policy experts, and a useful resource for educators and advanced nutrition students.

John W. Erdman Jr.
Urbana, Illinois
Ian A. Macdonald
Nottingham, England
Steven H. Zeisel
Chapel Hill, North Carolina

Acknowledgments

A great deal of work and dedication was involved in producing this extensive volume. First and foremost, we thank the authors of the 73 chapters who reviewed and condensed a vast amount of knowledge and literature. Their undertaking was significant, and our gratitude for their dedication cannot be overstated. The editors of the ninth edition, Barbara Bowman and Rob Russell, are thanked for the critical help they provided in the conceptualization of this edition as well as in the author selection. All of the chapters in this edition were externally reviewed by leaders in each chapter's field; their generous, voluntary assistance was invaluable. We thank the International Life Sciences Institute for continuing to foster the production of *Present Knowledge in Nutrition*, and we especially thank Allison Worden for her guidance and hundreds of hours of work, and for keeping everything on track.

1

SYSTEMS BIOLOGY APPROACHES TO NUTRITION

JAMES C. FLEET, PhD

Purdue University, West Lafayette, Indiana, USA

Summary

Systems biology is an integrative approach to the study of biology. It integrates information gathered from reductionist experiments and various high-density profiling tools to understand how the parts of the system interact with each other and with other external factors such as diet. The science of nutrition is well suited to a systems biology approach. The tools of systems biology can be applied to settings relevant to nutrition with the goal of better understanding the breadth and depth of the impact that changing nutrient status has on physiology and chronic disease risk. However, there are many challenges to appropriately applying the systems biology approach to nutritional science. Among the challenges are those related to cost, study design, statistical analysis, data visualization, data integration, and model building.

Introduction

Reductionism versus Systems Biology: A Changing Paradigm

Nutrition requires an understanding of disciplines such as physiology, cell biology, chemistry, biochemistry, and molecular biology among others. In contrast to this broad view, we apply reductionist experimental approaches to advance our understanding of specific nutrient functions. However, while these approaches have been useful, significant issues limit their utility. For example, it can be difficult to translate mechanism-focused research in cells into the complex physiology of a whole organism. As a result, biological models developed from reductionist experiments often fail to explain why gene knockout mice studies do not have the expected phenotype (e.g. the facilitated diffusion model used to describe intestinal calcium absorption

is being challenged by the results from calbindin D_{9k} and TRPV6 knockout mice (Benn *et al.*, 2008; Kutuzova *et al.*, 2008)). Even after extensive examination of a problem with reductionist approaches, we often find that gaps exist in our understanding. It is clear that re-applying the approaches we have traditionally used to investigate nutritional questions is unlikely to yield a different outcome. Because of this we need new approaches that complement traditional reductionist approaches but which give us a new, broader perspective of how nutrients are influencing human biology. Systems biology is such an approach.

Systems biology has been described as an approach to biological research that combines reductionist techniques with an "integrationist" approach to identify and characterize the components of a system, and then to evaluate how each of the components interacts with one another and with their environment. The goal of the systems

Present Knowledge in Nutrition, Tenth Edition. Edited by John W. Erdman Jr, Ian A. Macdonald and Steven H. Zeisel.
© 2012 International Life Sciences Institute. Published 2012 by John Wiley & Sons, Inc.

TABLE 1.1 Definitions related to systems biology

Term	Description
Genomics	The study of the genomes of organisms including influences of DNA sequence variation on biology and the impact of modifying DNA and histones on DNA function (i.e. epigenomics)
Transcriptomics	The study of transcripts from the genome including messenger RNA and non-coding RNA such as micro RNA
Proteomics	The study of proteins in a biological system including their level, location, physical properties, post-translational modifications, structures, and functions
Metabolomics	The study of the unique chemicals (metabolites) that are produced as a result of cellular processes, e.g. small molecules such as lipids, metabolites of intermediary metabolites
Ionomics	The study of the mineral nutrient and trace element composition of an organism
Next-generation sequencing	High-throughput DNA sequencing technologies that parallelize the sequencing process thereby producing millions of sequences at once
Cluster	A graphical representation of relationships between data based on similarities in their concentrations or changes in concentrations
Pathway	A graphical representation of biological data organized on the basis of accepted relationships (e.g. glycolysis; signaling through the insulin receptor; lipoprotein transport)
Network	A complex graphical representation of biological data that is developed from the experimental data. This will include known relationships (pathways) and new relationships linking pathways

biology approach is to integrate many types of information so that you get a more complete view of a system (Kohl *et al.*, 2010). This definition has a flexibility that is very attractive to nutrition. The notion of a "system" can be applied narrowly to a cell, where the parts are individual biochemical and signaling pathways and the "environment" is the growth factors and hormones that regulate these pathways. However, it can be applied more broadly to a person, where the integration relates to the physiologic systems and the "environment" is lifestyle variables such as diet. For example, we know that calcium influences bone metabolism *but* we know that this relies upon the efficiency of intestinal calcium absorption and renal calcium excretion as well as on hormones produced at various sites (e.g. PTH in the parathyroid gland, 1,25-dihydroxyvitamin D in the kidney). Thus, our understanding of how dietary calcium intake influences bone is enhanced by looking at the interactions between multiple tissues rather than just focusing only on bone.

Systems Biology as Discovery Tool

Systems biology is an approach but within this approach are also three classes of novel tools necessary for a success-

ful systems biology analysis. First, there are the high-density phenotyping platforms that allow simultaneous measurement of whole classes of biological compounds, i.e. omics methods such as genomics, transcriptomics, proteomics, metabolomics, and ionomics (Table 1.1). Next, the information from these platforms must be analyzed to identify the important changes resulting from a treatment. This requires the application of sophisticated statistics. Third, the information must be annotated and integrated with prior knowledge: this is the field of bioinformatics.

Systems Biology and Omics Tools for Biomarker Discovery

Omics analyses are often used to profile a biological state and then essential elements of the profile are used as a biomarker. Theoretically, the more independent traits one incorporates into a biomarker, the less likely it will be that the biomarker will be influenced by extraneous/confounding factors. To illustrate this point we can look to the field of iron metabolism. Nutritional iron status can be evaluated by measuring serum ferritin (high ferritin = high iron status) but this parameter is confounded by chronic inflammation (high inflammation = high ferritin) that can mask iron deficiency (Wang *et al.*, 2010). The serum levels of other proteins are also affected by the changes in iron status, e.g. hepcidin (high levels = high iron status) and soluble transferrin receptor (low levels = high iron status). Whereas hepcidin is affected negatively by inflammation (Nemeth and Ganz, 2009), transferrin receptor is not (Beguin, 2003). Thus, by simultaneously assessing the serum levels of ferritin, transferrin receptor, and a serum marker of chronic inflammation (e.g. C-reactive protein), one can assess iron status and remove the confounding caused by the inflammation associated with acute or chronic disease. The approach of using omics to identify measurements that can be combined to make an effective biomarker has been applied to the assessment of certain cancers (Sikaroodi *et al.*, 2010) and some argue that this approach may be useful for the assessment of nutrient status or of nutrition-related conditions that have proved resistant to the single marker approach (e.g. micronutrients such as zinc) (Lowe *et al.*, 2009).

Use of Systems Biology to Define New Modes of Regulation by a Nutrient or Metabolic State

A second way to use systems biology is to identify the groups of genes/transcripts/proteins/metabolites coordinately regulated under specific conditions. These groups could be organized within known biological pathways or as random groupings driven by statistical correlation, i.e. networks that expose new relationships not previously recognized from traditional reductionist research.

Understanding the Systems Biology Approach

It is an over-simplification to imply that there is just one way to do systems biology research but this section will attempt to provide a framework for approaching a nutritional research problem from the systems biology perspective (see Figure 1.1 for a summary of the steps in the framework).

Experimental Design

This is the single most important step of a systems biology research project for several reasons (Allison *et al.*, 2006). First, adequate experimental planning is necessary to focus the research and to use resources efficiently. One will likely need multiple time points to collect data on multiple phenotypes. For example, early time points may be more informative for measurement of direct transcriptional regulation (e.g. using transcriptomics or chromatin immunoprecipitation coupled to high-density DNA sequencing

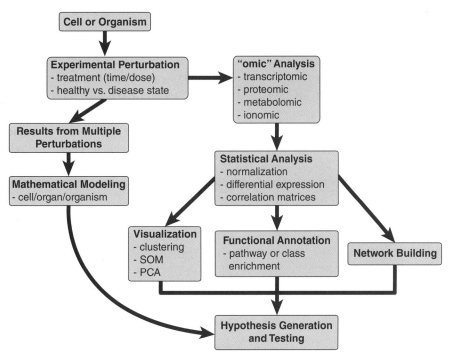

FIG. 1.1 An overview of the steps in a systems biology analysis.

[ChIP-seq]). However, later time points will be more informative for evaluating protein production or changes in metabolism. Second, the use of multiple conditions should be examined so that a broader, more representative view of the regulation can be determined. Work from model systems such as yeast, where a knockout line exists for each of the 6700 yeast genes, shows us that combining transcriptomic analysis for all of these lines permits computer modeling that can reveal new biological relationships and coordination of regulatory processes (Beer and Tavazoie, 2004). Third, sample replication is necessary so that the study has sufficient statistical power to detect biologically important differences between treatments. Finally, the experimental plan should control all extraneous variables so that any changes can be unambiguously attributed to the treatment of interest.

High-density Phenotyping Platforms
Genomics
Gene Promoter Analysis. Genetic regulation involves coordinated molecular regulation through transcription factor binding sites within groups of promoters (e.g. molecular regulation of cholesterol and lipid metabolism (Desvergne *et al.*, 2006)). A large number of computational methods are available to locate transcription factor binding sites in mammalian gene promoters (Elnitski *et al.*, 2006). Unfortunately, because transcription factor binding sites tolerate sequence heterogeneity, these computational methods have a high false-positive detection rate (Tompa *et al.*, 2005).

Recently a direct method has been developed to directly determine transcription factor binding sites throughout the genome. This approach starts with a chromatin immunoprecipitation (ChIP) assay where transcription factors are cross-linked to DNA at the site of their binding and the complex is isolated using antibodies to the transcription factor (Collas, 2010). The DNA from the ChIP assay is then used either to probe a genome-wide DNA tiling array (ChIP on chip) or sequenced directly using next-generation sequencing methods (ChIP-seq) (Park, 2009). This approach was recently used to identify 2776 genomic positions occupied by the vitamin D receptor (VDR) after treating lymphoblastoid cell lines with 1,25-dihydroxyvitamin D. These VDR binding sites were significantly enriched near autoimmune and cancer-associated genes identified from genome-wide association (GWA) studies (Ramagopalan *et al.*, 2010), suggesting this information will help us understand the relationship between transcriptional regulation and various disease states.

Genetic Mapping and Forward Genetics. Forward genetics, the measurement of phenotype and then determining the associations with variations in genotype, is an important approach that has been virtually untapped for the study of nutrient metabolism and function. The basic concept for this approach starts with the fact that natural sequence variations exist within the genome (e.g. single nucleotide polymorphisms or SNP, copy number variations or CNV), and that this variation is heritable. To be useful in forward genetics, these genetic variations must also influence phenotypes, e.g. tissue mineral levels or fatty acid oxidation rate. Finally, unlike the rare mutations that underlie various genetic diseases and cause extreme phenotypes (such as the mutations in copper transporting ATPases responsible for Wilson's and Menkes disease), the phenotypic changes resulting from the natural variation identified by forward genetics are not fatal but could result in extreme differences between individuals. The goal is to use variations in phenotypes that result from controlled breeding strategies or within pedigrees to map the location of the natural genetic variation that controls the phenotype. The forward genetics approach makes no assumptions about the genes that influence the trait. Rather, it lets variations in phenotype direct us to the regions of the genome containing genetic variants that have a significant biological impact. Forward genetics is particularly useful in instances where we don't know enough about the metabolism of a nutrient to justify making gene knockout or transgenic mice (i.e. use of reverse genetics) or when mice continue to have normal biology when a candidate gene is deleted (e.g. suggesting redundancies in the system that need to be revealed).

Relating nutritionally important phenotypes to natural variation can be accomplished in two ways: gene mapping and gene association. Linkage analysis within large families and quantitative trait loci (QTL) mapping in controlled crosses between genetically well-characterized inbred mouse lines have been traditionally used to correlate the variation in a phenotype to sequence variations in the genome (Flint *et al.*, 2005). More recently researchers have begun using the genome-wide association (GWA) study approach whereby a multitude of individual variants or haplotypes of variants are examined for their association with a nutritionally relevant trait within large populations of free-living individuals (Manolio, 2010). However, some are concerned that the GWAS approach is subject to false positives and that GWAS findings are difficult to replicate. Regardless of which approach one takes, once the genetic region or candidate polymorphism is identified, additional studies must be conducted to identify the genes that contain the variation controlling the trait, and traditional reductionist research must be done to learn how the genes identified are involved in the regulation of the trait. Because forward genetics approaches are unbiased and hypothesis free, they can lead to the identification of new biological roles for genes and their protein products (Flint et al., 2005).

The promise of forward genetics for nutrition was recently demonstrated for iron metabolism (Wang et al., 2007) where the genes controlling 30% of the variation in spleen iron levels between inbred mouse lines were mapped to chromosome 9. Within this locus, variation was identified in the Mon1a gene and this information was used to determine that Mon1a is a critical component of spleen iron uptake and recycling of red blood cell iron within macrophages. Thus, even though we have learned a tremendous amount about iron metabolism over the last 15 years from traditional approaches (Andrews, 2008), forward genetics permitted researchers to add another piece to this already complex picture.

Epigenomics. In addition to the regulation mediated through DNA sequences, DNA and histones can be modified and this will influence gene transcription (Mathers, 2008) (also, see Chapter 2). In humans, DNA is organized into a nucleosome complex with four histone proteins (H2A, H2B, H3, and H4). The amino terminal tails of the histones can be post-translationally modified in a variety of ways. Histone acetylation reduces histone association with DNA and is permissive for gene transcription whereas histone methylation is associated with both transcription repression and activation. DNA can also be methylated at the C5 position of cytosine in regions of DNA called CpG islands. Cytosine- and guanine-rich sequences are located near coding sequences in about 50% of mammalian genes. When the CpG islands are methylated, these regions become more compact and this prevents gene transcription (Attwood et al., 2002). DNA methylation is responsible for X chromosome inactivation, genomic imprinting, and tissue-specific gene transcription that occur during cellular differentiation.

Because of its importance in gene repression, researchers have developed DNA microarrays and next-generation DNA sequencing approaches for epigenetic profiling of CpG islands in the human genome (Fouse et al., 2010). Folate and other micronutrients are involved in the production of the universal methyl donor S-adenosyl methionine, so it has been proposed that dietary inadequacy may have a global influence on DNA methylation (Oommen et al., 2005). However, the evidence for this diet-induced regulatory paradigm is not yet secure.

Transcriptomics

It is now possible to simultaneously measure the primary transcripts and all of the alternatively spliced forms of transcripts produced from each gene in the genome of humans and several model organisms (i.e. the transcriptome). Transcript levels are a reflection of both primary regulation by a treatment and secondary regulation that follows from the initial regulatory events (Figure 1.2). There are many high quality options from assessing the transcriptome including spotted cDNA arrays, tiling oligonucleotide arrays, and even direct sequencing of RNA (Kirby et al., 2007; Forrest and Carninci, 2009). Many factors can influence the choice of a transcript profiling platform including cost, reproducibility of results, breadth of transcript coverage, and availability. Readers should consult other reviews for additional discussion of the strengths and weaknesses of various array platforms (Hoheisel, 2006; Kawasaki, 2006).

For some nutrients that are known to have a direct impact on gene transcription through the activation of a nuclear receptor (e.g. vitamin D and VDR, vitamin A and the retinoic acid receptor bioactive lipids and the peroxisome proliferator-activated receptor, [PPAR]), transcriptomics is a primary endpoint for understanding the impact of the nutrient on biology. A simple example of the value of transcriptomics comes from the area of lipid metabolism. The synthesis of fatty acids and cholesterol is regulated by the sterol regulatory element-binding proteins (SREBP)-1a, -1c, and -2. Horton et al. (2003) used transcriptomics to study transgenic mice overexpressing each SREBP isoform and mice lacking all three nuclear SREBPs (i.e. in SREBP cleavage activating protein (SCAP)-deficient mice). They found several hundred transcripts that were changed in the liver and from this data they defined a subset of 33 genes as SREBP targets that included 20 new SREBP target genes. Thus, in one short, directed set of experiments they dramatically expanded our understanding of how lipid metabolism is regulated.

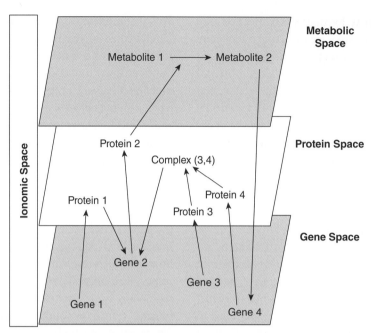

FIG. 1.2 A schematic demonstrating the interactions between the various levels of regulation within a cell. Regulatory events occur at the level of transcription (gene space), RNA translation (protein space), protein stability or interactions (protein space), and protein function (gene space, metabolic space). Inorganic elements are involved in all of these processes (ionomic space), and events occurring in one regulatory space can influence events occurring within another regulatory space (e.g. lipid metabolites bind to protein transcription factors with zinc finger DNA binding domains such as PPAR gamma and this interaction regulates gene transcription). Systems biology attempts to model these complex interactions. Reduced omic phenotyping (e.g. in just the gene space or the metabolic space) – combined with previously published research findings – can be used to infer regulatory interactions between these levels.

Proteomics

The proteome refers to all of the proteins expressed and functional in a system. Unfortunately, the methods to assess the proteome cannot measure the entire proteosome simultaneously. As a result, experiments usually measure one or more subproteomes, e.g. the phosphoproteome reflecting the proteins that are targets for protein kinases, proteins within subcellular compartments (e.g. mitochondrial proteome) or specific tissues (serum proteome), or proteins with specific physical properties (e.g. the membrane proteome).

There are two approaches to proteomics. The first is a "top-down" approach whereby whole proteins are studied using multidimensional separation techniques, e.g. separation by isoelectric point followed by size separation (2D polyacrylamide gel electrophoresis [PAGE]) or tandem mass spectrometry (Reid and McLuckey, 2002). In the top-down approach the proteins are isolated, then fragmented (e.g. through trypsin digestion), and the peptide

fragments are compared with a database to determine the identity of the protein. In contrast, the "bottom-up" approach digests proteins at the outset, isolates and identifies the peptide fragments using mass spectrometry methods, and then relates the peptide fragments to databases of known proteins to determine the identity of the proteins in a complex mixture.

The major challenge to proteomics is that the spectrometry methods are not standardized. This leads to problems of reproducibility across and within labs. In addition, there are some challenges to separating signal from noise that limit peak detection and quantification. Finally, some proteomic methods are not very sensitive. Specifically, 2D PAGE approaches are often used for serum proteomics and biomarker discovery. However, the ability of radioimmunoassay to detect proteins in serum is 100- to 1000-fold greater than 2D PAGE methods. Even with this weakness, 2D PAGE has been useful for identifying serum biomarkers of nutritional status. For example, Fuchs *et al.* (2007)

used this approach to identify biomarkers of a cardioprotective response to isoflavone supplementation in the peripheral blood mononuclear cells of postmenopausal women.

Metabolomics

Evaluating the metabolome gives a snapshot of the physiology of a cell or organism by simultaneously measuring the levels of metabolites within a biological space (also, see Chapter 4). Like proteomics, the metabolome is assessed by coupling separation techniques (e.g. electrophoresis, chromatography) with sophisticated detection methods (e.g. mass spectrometry, nuclear magnetic resonance imaging). As such, it suffers from the same problems as proteomics, namely the lack of method standardization and reproducibility. Also, like proteomics, the entire metabolome is too complex for one method to measure all possible metabolites simultaneously, and so submetabolomes based on location or chemical characteristics are commonly analyzed. While many studies use metabolomics for biomarker discovery, this approach can also be used to better understand the impact of physiologic conditions on the flow of information through specific metabolic pathways. For example, in a study of diet-induced insulin resistance, Li et al. (2010) identified many serum and liver metabolites as different between safflower-oil-fed wild-type and glycerol-3-phosphate acyltransferase deficient mice. Many of these were not previously known to be associated with insulin resistance and they point to the utility of metabolomics analysis for identifying biochemical pathways important in understanding the pathophysiology of diabetes. In addition to the standard metabolomic approach that measured changes in steady-state levels of metabolites, others have used radio- or stable isotopes to label compounds and trace their metabolic fate. This is a more dynamic approach that can give a picture of how physiologic states or treatments affect the flow of compounds through specific metabolic pathways (Hellerstein, 2004).

Ionomics

Mineral elements are involved at all levels of biological regulation, e.g. in transcription factors (zinc), in enzymes (zinc, iron, copper, calcium), and in establishing electrochemical gradients in cells (calcium, sodium, potassium). It is also well established that direct and indirect interactions exist between mineral elements that can affect biology (Hill and Matrone, 1970). Because the mineral elements are integrated into the overall biology of a cell (i.e. with

links to the metabolome, proteome, transcriptome, and ultimately the genome: Figure 1.2), examination of the entire elemental profile of a system (i.e. the ionome) may reflect broader, biologically relevant disturbances and may have the potential to capture information about the functional state of an organism under different environmental and physical conditions (Salt et al., 2008). Evaluating the ionome is accomplished using high-throughput elemental analysis technologies (e.g. inductively coupled plasma-atomic emission spectroscopy [ICP–AES] or ICP–mass spectroscopy [ICP–MS]).

An early example of ionomics was reported by Eide et al. (2005), who examined how gene deletions in budding yeast were linked to changes in the ionome. They conducted a 13-element profile for each of 4385 yeast gene deletion mutants and found that 212 mutants had significant disturbances in at least one member of the ionome. By using bioinformatic tools to identify clusters of functionally related genes within the list of the 212 mutants, they found that shifts in the ionome were a reflection of specific biological functions. For example, 27 of the 212 gene deletion mutants influenced mitochondrial function and these mutants were characterized by lower Se and Ni accumulation. This highlights the point that alterations in the ionome reflect changes in critical biological functions. Readers are encouraged to read one of several interesting reviews describing the use of ionomics in biology (e.g. Salt et al., 2008; Baxter, 2009).

How Important Is Validation of Results from High-Density Omic Tools?

A well-conducted omics experiment should be robust and reproducible. However, it is standard practice to confirm the changes in a subset of differentially expressed transcripts or proteins with traditional tools. While this raises confidence in the quality of the results from the omic platform, comprehensive validation is not feasible or desirable. Extensive re-evaluation of changes detected in omic analysis is conceptually the opposite approach to the systems biology approach where the breadth of changes is as important as any one specific change.

Balancing Cost and Content. By this time it should be obvious that the ideal collection of data for a systems biology experiment will be expensive. This is an unavoidable reality of the systems biology approach. While a time and dose response study in cells, animals, or people is not out of the ordinary, the costs of application of multiple

TABLE 1.2 Selected databases of omics data available for data mining

Name	Website	Description
Gene Expression Omnibus (GEO)	www.ncbi.nlm.nih.gov/ projects/geo/	National Center for Biotechnology Information (NCBI) database of microarray experiments
ArrayExpress	www.ebi.ac.uk/ arrayexpress	European Bioinformatics Institute of the EMBL database of microarray experiments
Human Metabolome Database (HMDB)	www.hmdb.ca/	Database containing detailed information about small molecule metabolites found in the human body
Cancer Biomedical Informatics Grid (caBIG)	cabig.nci.nih.gov/	National Cancer Institute site for cancer studies; includes data sets from genomic, transcriptomic, proteomic, and imaging analysis
Expert Protein Analysis System (ExPASy) Server	ca.expasy.org/	Database dedicated to the analysis of protein sequences and structures as well as 2D PAGE
Database of Genotype and Phenotype (dbGaP)	www.ncbi.nlm.nih.gov/ sites/entrez?Db=gap	National Institutes of Health database for studies on the interaction of genotype and phenotype
WebQTL	www.genenetwork.org/	Linked resources and analysis tools for systems genetics in mouse and some other models

"omic" tools, especially to multiple tissues, could become astronomical. For this reason, most scientists use two strategies for cost containment. First, individual investigators will focus on one "omic" tool that has the most relevance for their biological question. Researchers studying vitamin A or vitamin D may choose to examine the transcriptome because of the well-established understanding that metabolites of these compounds are direct regulators of gene expression. Researchers examining the effects of branched-chain amino acids on physical performance might choose to study the muscle proteome because of the anabolic effect mediated through mTOR signaling at the protein level. Others may examine the serum metabolome after feeding diets with changing macronutrient content. In these settings, the investigator will gain a great deal of insight into one aspect of the system but the full power of the systems biology approach may take a long time to be realized as an investigator slowly pieces together various "omic" views of their system over time. The second approach does not reduce the cost of these experiments but disperses the cost across many research groups. In this case, scientists will work as teams rather than individual labs. Each team member will take responsibility for a different aspect of the system where their interest and expertise are greatest. Related to this, researchers will pool related data from complementary experiments. This is proving fruitful for a number of integrative science projects and is the reason why many funding agencies now require a data sharing plan – so that people interested in integrating data have access to it (see Table 1.2 for a partial list of databases).

Identifying Significant Changes in a System after Perturbation

Statistical analysis is one of the unappreciated aspects of systems biology. Others have carefully reviewed the importance of statistical analysis for microarray experiments and other aspects of systems biology (Nadon and Shoemaker, 2002; Allison *et al.*, 2006) so here we will simply summarize a few crucial points.

First, in the absence of statistics one cannot assess the reliability of: a difference observed between treatment groups, the association of genetic variation with relevant phenotypes, or the enrichment of specific pathways or regulatory networks after a treatment or dietary intervention. Without statistics only a fold-change is available for assessing the "importance" of differences between groups. While large fold-changes may be biologically important, a collection of small fold-changes in the transcript levels for many of the components of a pathway or biological process is also important.

Second, a simple t-test with a significance level of $p < 0.05$ is inadequate to test statistical significance because it ignores the importance of type I error rates (false positives). For example, at $p < 0.05$ we would expect 5% of the t-tests to be false positives (i.e. 1000 targets on a 20 000 transcript array, 50 000 single nucleotide polymorphisms [SNPs] on a 1 million SNP chip). However, multiple test correction methods like Bonferroni (p-value/number of comparisons; e.g. $0.05/20 000 = 2.5 \times 10^{-6}$) are too conservative because they lead to a high type II error rate (false negative). As a result, statisticians have developed methods such as the false-discovery rate (FDR) approach to balance the type I and II error rate problems inherent when multiple independent comparisons are being conducted (Pounds and Cheng, 2006). Another way to reduce the multiple comparison problem is to filter out noise in the detection procedure. For example, although microarrays can measure all of the transcripts expressed in the human body, not all transcripts are expressed in every cell or tissue type. By removing "absent" transcripts from the dataset, one can reduce the number of independent comparisons to be conducted, reduce the multiple comparison problem that causes high type I error rates, and increase the power to detect differences between treatment groups.

Finally, the ability to detect significant differences is improved by sample replication. Replication is particularly useful when the biological variability in protein, metabolite, or transcript level is high.

Bioinformatics

The fundamental purpose of bioinformatics is to identify patterns within the complexity of the data from high-density omic analysis methods. In many ways, this is a problem of visualization (Gehlenborg et al., 2010). In the next several paragraphs some bioinformatic approaches that have been taken to reduce the complexity of omic data will be discussed.

Clustering

The large number of endpoints analyzed in an omic experiment (e.g. >20 000 transcripts) make it is impossible to see important patterns in the data even after filtering and statistical analysis (Tamayo et al., 1999). A number of clustering methods have been developed to overcome this problem. The most common methods are the tree-based methods such as hierarchical clustering and the graphical views based on self-organizing maps (SOM). These methods may require additional normalization so that important patterns are not lost due to issues of scale (i.e. combining data from metabolites that are present at high and low levels). In addition, mean values are used so prior filtering to eliminate low-fold change or non-significant changes is necessary. Ultimately functions of genes can be inferred from the patterns identified by clustering (e.g. genes whose transcripts cluster together may have similar functions (Iyer et al., 1999)).

Pathway Mapping

Functional annotation and pathway mapping identify changes in biological relationships that have previously been experimentally determined. Programs have been developed to permit grouping of omic data based upon gene ontology classes, e.g. gene set enrichment analysis (GSEA) (Subramanian et al., 2005) or on whether changes are accumulating in the proteins/transcripts of a known biological pathway or within the group of biological factors known to be important for a specific physiological or disease process (Werner, 2008). This sort of grouping can be represented easily in a graph or figure of a pathway. By relating omic data from an experiment to the known body of information in these ways, researchers can more easily find themes that describe the impact of a treatment on biology.

Network Analysis

The hope of systems biology is that it will identify relationships between molecules that represent new ways of understanding the complexity of biological regulation (Huang et al., 2007). These relationships can be between proteins (e.g. dimerization that activates a complex, kinases phosphorylating other proteins), proteins and DNA (e.g. transcription factor binding), nucleic acids (e.g. microRNA regulating expression of a specific mRNA), or proteins and metabolites (e.g. bioactive lipids regulating receptors). Some of these relationships are present in traditional pathway structures. However, other relationships are links between pathways. As a result, one can think of a network as a combination of interacting modules where each module is a regulatory pathway or process that is recognized by the scientific community. Conceptually, this is similar to what happened in the early days of biochemistry when metabolic pathways were studied independently and later joined as people recognized that metabolites in one pathway became substrates in other pathways (e.g. acetyl CoA joins pathways for glycolysis, the citric acid cycle, steroid synthesis, and fatty acid biosynthesis into a network). Finding these networks becomes a problem of identifying the connections, assessing their strength, and visualizing them. There are many network building algorithms that can be used on omic data. In these networks proteins or metabolites are visualized as nodes, and interactions between proteins or metabolites are viewed as lines (edges) (Aittokallio and Schwikowski, 2006). Readers interested in the procedure for building networks can refer to one of several reviews for more in-depth discussion of this topic (Alvarez-Buylla et al., 2006; Li et al., 2008).

Mathematical Modeling of Metabolic and Physiologic Processes

The relationship between variables in a biological system can be represented as a mathematical model. In a simple sense, this is what we do when we graph a dose response where the relationship between the dose and the outcome is expressed as a regression line. However, as the complexity of the system increases, simple graphical relationships between two parameters are insufficient to represent biology. Under these circumstances more elaborate mathematics can be applied to experimental observations to create a simplified model of the system. This approach is at the heart of kinetic modeling of nutrient metabolism (e.g. for calcium metabolism: Weaver, 1998) and was pioneered in nutrition by Dr R. Lee Baldwin in an attempt to develop predictive models for how nutrition regulates energy metabolism and performance of ruminants (Baldwin et al., 1994).

One of the barriers to effective mathematical modeling is the quality and depth of the data available for building the models (Klipp and Liebermeister, 2006). With the advances that have occurred in our data generation capabilities as a result of the omics era, researchers have begun to believe that comprehensive mathematical modeling of biological systems is possible. Nonetheless, reliable quantitative models are hard to develop. As a result, the first step in the process is to take existing experimental knowledge and use it to build a raw model. This process is not, however, implemented simply to reproduce all the parts of the system, but to direct researchers to areas where gaps exist in the model so that additional experimentation can be conducted. In other words, the raw model is improved over time by conducting additional experiments. In theory, by repeated cycles of developing and testing models followed by new hypothesis-based experiments, we have the potential to better understand the system and use the model for predictive purposes.

The Power of Public Databases

The expense of conducting a systems biology experiment using omics tools can be intimidating to many researchers. An alternative to conducting primary experiments is to re-analyze experiments that are available in public databases. Several useful databases for datamining are presented in Table 1.2. For example, a repository for genomic and transcriptomic datasets is the Gene Expression Omnibus (GEO) at NCBI. In the fall of 2010, a simple search using "intestine" as the keyword revealed 81 datasets and 440 data series (with some overlap in the lists). A search for "folate" identified 7 datasets and 34 data series. Of course, the value of data from public databases can be variable, e.g. in GEO some datasets provide replicates whereas others do not. In addition, there may be a substantial commitment for researchers to learn how to use the bioinformatic tools that allow one to make sense of these datasets (see Table 1.3 for a list of some tools that can be used for the analysis of omic data). However, the analysis of these datasets may allow an investigator to generate preliminary data for a hypothesis that could be used as a foundation for additional research or as preliminary data for a grant application.

Future Directions

Computer Infrastructure

Many of the steps in a systems biology approach are computationally intensive (Heath and Kavraki, 2009). While small studies can be analyzed on desktop computers, even these may challenge a computer unless it is set up appropriately in terms of RAM, operating system, and processor speed. For more sophisticated analysis, high-performance computing will be necessary to speed up the analysis. Finally, computer storage will become an issue for large integrative systems biology projects. This is particularly true if the project also includes an imaging component (e.g. histology or magnetic resonance imaging).

Integration of Data Types

The ultimate goal of systems biology is to generate a predictive model of the system. Most researchers work with only one type of data (e.g. metabolome or transcriptome)

TABLE 1.3 A Selection of Publicly Available Data Analysis Tools for Systems Biology[a]

Name	Website	Description
Bioconductor	www.bioconductor.org/	Open source and open development software project for the analysis and comprehension of omic data (based on R programming language)
Significance Analysis of Microarrays (SAM)	www-stat.stanford.edu/~tibs/SAM/	Excel-based tool for statistical analysis of omic data
GenePattern	www.broad.mit.edu/tools/software.html	A genomic analysis platform with access to more than 125 tools for analysis of omic data
Gene Set Enrichment Analysis (GSEA)	www.broad.mit.edu/tools/software.html	A computational method that determines if a set of genes with a common function (e.g. lipid metabolism) are significantly altered by treatment/condition
GenMAPP	www.GenMAPP.org	Tool for visualizing omic data on maps representing biological pathways and groupings of genes. Statistical analysis for enrichment of changes in maps can be determined
Cytoscape	www.cytoscape.org/	Tool for conducting network analysis and visualizing the results

[a]See Gehlenborg et al. (2010) for a comprehensive list of various omic analysis tools.

but the ideal is to use all types of data simultaneously. This not only includes the various omic data types but also clinical data on patients, image data from biological samples, text-based information from the literature, etc. Some methods already permit integration of multiple data types. For example, principal components analysis (PCA) is a mathematical procedure used to transform a number of correlated variables into a smaller number of uncorrelated variables called principal components. Each step in PCA attempts to account for as much of the variability in the data as possible. Jones et al. (2007) used PCA to integrate information from multiple iron-related phenotypes for use in QTL analysis and found that the combination of hemoglobin, hematocrit, and plasma total iron binding capacity were more useful for mapping than the individual traits. Bayesian statistics incorporate prior knowledge into an analysis of an experiment (see below) and can also be used to incorporate multiple data types into analysis. However, even these methods only scratch at the surface of what researchers believe can be done. This will be an active area of research in systems biology for the foreseeable future (Sullivan et al., 2010).

Application of Bayesian Statistical Approaches that Incorporate Prior Knowledge into the Analysis

There are several issues that limit the utility of traditional "frequentist" statistical approaches when applied to systems biology research, e.g. high false-positive detection rates due to the multiple comparison problem; violation of the assumption of independence between genetic markers; inability to incorporate environmental variables and multiple, related traits into models and analysis. In contrast to frequentist statistics, Bayesian inference is a statistical approach that accepts the reality that there is prior knowledge that can influence our evaluation of a hypothesis (Shoemaker et al., 1999; Beaumont and Rannala, 2004). By combining the inherent likelihood of a hypothesis with the compatibility of the observed evidence, one can better assess the likelihood that a particular hypothesis is true. There are many statisticians who use the Bayesian approach to test hypotheses. However, since most biologists are taught statistics from a frequentist perspective, approaching analysis from a Bayesian perspective will require more training. In addition, there are fewer packaged programs for Bayesian statistics, and the computational demands of Bayesian statistics are likely to be a barrier to most biologists.

Suggestions for Further Reading

De Graaf, A.A., Freidig, A.P., De Roos, B., *et al.* (2009) Nutritional systems biology modeling: from molecular mechanisms to physiology. *PLoS Comput Biol* **5**, e1000554.

Fu, W.J., Stromberg, A.J., Viele, K., *et al.* (2010) Statistics and bioinformatics in nutritional sciences: analysis of complex data in the era of systems biology. *J. Nutr Biochem* **21**, 561–572.

Gehlenborg, N., O'Donoghue, S.I., Baliga, N.S., *et al.* (2010) Visualization of omics data for systems biology. *Nat Methods* **7**, S56–S68.

Kohl, P., Crampin, E.J., Quinn, T.A., *et al.* (2010) Systems biology: an approach. *Clin Pharmacol Ther* **88**, 25–33.

References

Aittokallio, T. and Schwikowski, B. (2006) Graph-based methods for analysing networks in cell biology. *Brief Bioinform* **7**, 243–255.

Allison, D.B., Cui, X., Page, G.P., and Sabripour, M. (2006) Microarray data analysis: from disarray to consolidation and consensus. *Nat Rev Genet* **7**, 55–65.

Alvarez-Buylla, E.R., Benitez, M., Davila, E.B., *et al.* (2006) Gene regulatory network models for plant development. *Curr Opin Plant Biol* **10**, 83–91.

Andrews, N.C. (2008) Forging a field: the golden age of iron biology. *Blood* **112**, 219–230.

Attwood, J.T., Yung, R.L., and Richardson, B.C. (2002) DNA methylation and the regulation of gene transcription. *Cell Mol Life Sci* **59**, 241–257.

Baldwin, R.L., Emery, R.S., and McNamara, J.P. (1994) Metabolic relationships in the supply of nutrients for milk protein synthesis: integrative modeling. *J Dairy Sci* **77**, 2821–2836.

Baxter, I. (2009) Ionomics: studying the social network of mineral nutrients. *Curr Opin Plant Biol* **12**, 381–386.

Beaumont, M.A. and Rannala, B. (2004) The Bayesian revolution in genetics. *Nat Rev Genet* **5**, 251–261.

Beer, M.A. and Tavazoie, S. (2004) Predicting gene expression from sequence. *Cell* **117**, 185–198.

Beguin, Y. (2003) Soluble transferrin receptor for the evaluation of erythropoiesis and iron status. *Clin Chim Acta* **329**, 9–22.

Benn, B.S., Ajibade, D., Porta, A., *et al.* (2008) Active intestinal calcium transport in the absence of transient receptor potential vanilloid type 6 and calbindin-D9k. *Endocrinology* **149**, 3196–3205.

Collas, P. (2010) The current state of chromatin immunoprecipitation. *Mol Biotechnol* **45**, 87–100.

Desvergne, B., Michalik, L., and Wahli, W. (2006) Transcriptional regulation of metabolism. *Physiol Rev* **86**, 465–514.

Eide, D.J., Clark, S., Nair, T.M., *et al.* (2005) Characterization of the yeast ionome: a genome-wide analysis of nutrient mineral and trace element homeostasis in *Saccharomyces cerevisiae*. *Genome Biol* **6** (9), R77.

Elnitski, L., Jin, V.X., Farnham, P.J., *et al.* (2006) Locating mammalian transcription factor binding sites: a survey of computational and experimental techniques. *Genome Res* **16**, 1455–1464.

Flint, J., Valdar, W., Shifman, S., *et al.* (2005) Strategies for mapping and cloning quantitative trait genes in rodents. *Nat Rev Genet* **6**, 271–286.

Forrest, A.R. and Carninci, P. (2009) Whole genome transcriptome analysis. *RNA Biol* **6**, 107–112.

Fouse, S.D., Nagarajan, R.P., and Costello, J.F. (2010) Genome-scale DNA methylation analysis. *Epigenomics* **2**, 105–117.

Fuchs, D., Vafeiadou, K., Hall, W.L., *et al.* (2007) Proteomic biomarkers of peripheral blood mononuclear cells obtained from postmenopausal women undergoing an intervention with soy isoflavones. *Am J Clin Nutr* **86**, 1369–1375.

Gehlenborg, N., O'Donoghue, S.I., Baliga, N.S., *et al.* (2010) Visualization of omics data for systems biology. *Nat Methods* **7**, S56–S68.

Heath, A.P. and Kavraki, L.E. (2009) Computational challenges in systems biology. *Comput Sci Rev* **3**, 1–17.

Hellerstein, M.K. (2004) New stable isotope–mass spectrometric techniques for measuring fluxes through intact metabolic pathways in mammalian systems: introduction of moving pictures into functional genomics and biochemical phenotyping. *Metab Eng* **6**, 85–100.

Hill, C.H. and Matrone, G. (1970) Chemical parameters in the study of in vivo and in vitro interactions of transition elements. *Fed Proc* **29**, 1474–1481.

Hoheisel, J.D. (2006) Microarray technology: beyond transcript profiling and genotype analysis. *Nat Rev Genet* **7**, 200–210.

Horton, J.D., Shah, N.A., Warrington, J.A., *et al.* (2003) Combined analysis of oligonucleotide microarray data from transgenic and knockout mice identifies direct SREBP target genes. *Proc Natl Acad Sci USA* **100**, 12027–12032.

Huang, Z., Li, J., Su, H., *et al.* (2007). Large-scale regulatory network analysis from microarray data: modified Bayesian network learning and association rule mining. *Decis Supp Syst* **43**, 1207–1225.

Iyer, V.R., Eisen, M.B., Ross, D.T., *et al.* (1999) The transcriptional program in the response of human fibroblasts to serum. *Science* **283**, 83–87.

Jones, B.C., Beard, J.L., Gibson, J.N., *et al.* (2007) Systems genetic analysis of peripheral iron parameters in the mouse. *Am J Physiol Regul Integr Comp Physiol* **293**, R116–R124.

Kawasaki, E.S. (2006) The end of the microarray Tower of Babel: will universal standards lead the way? *J Biomol Tech* **17**, 200–206.

Kirby, J., Heath, P.R., Shaw, P.J., *et al.* (2007) Gene expression assays. *Adv Clin Chem* **44**, 247–292.

Klipp, E. and Liebermeister, W. (2006) Mathematical modeling of intracellular signaling pathways. *BMC Neurosci* **7** Suppl 1, S10.

Kohl, P., Crampin, E.J., Quinn, T.A., *et al.* (2010) Systems biology: an approach. *Clin Pharmacol Ther* **88**, 25–33.

Kutuzova, G.D., Sundersingh, F., Vaughan, J., *et al.* (2008) TRPV6 is not required for 1alpha,25-dihydroxyvitamin D3-induced intestinal calcium absorption in vivo. *Proc Natl Acad Sci USA* **105**, 19655–19659.

Li, H., Xuan, J., Wang, Y., *et al.* (2008) Inferring regulatory networks. *Front Biosci* **13**, 263–275.

Li, L.O., Hu, Y.F., Wang, L., *et al.* (2010) Early hepatic insulin resistance in mice: a metabolomics analysis. *Mol Endocrinol* **24**, 657–666.

Lowe, N.M., Fekete, K., and Decsi, T. (2009) Methods of assessment of zinc status in humans: a systematic review. *Am J Clin Nutr* **89**, 2040S–2051S.

Manolio, T.A. (2010) Genomewide association studies and assessment of the risk of disease. *N Engl J Med* **363**, 166–176.

Mathers, J.C. (2008) Session 2: Personalised nutrition. Epigenomics: a basis for understanding individual differences? *Proc Nutr Soc* **67**, 390–394.

Nadon, R. and Shoemaker, J. (2002) Statistical issue with microarrays: processing and analysis. *Trends Genet* **18**, 265–271.

Nemeth, E. and Ganz, T. (2009) The role of hepcidin in iron metabolism. *Acta Haematol* **122**, 78–86.

Oommen, A.M., Griffin, J.B., Sarath, G., *et al.* (2005) Roles for nutrients in epigenetic events. *J Nutr Biochem* **16**, 74–77.

Park, P.J. (2009) ChIP-seq: advantages and challenges of a maturing technology. *Nat Rev Genet* **10**, 669–680.

Pounds, S. and Cheng, C. (2006) Robust estimation of the false discovery rate. *Bioinformatics* **22**, 1979–1987.

Ramagopalan, S.V., Heger, A., Berlanga, A.J., *et al.* (2010) A ChIP-seq defined genome-wide map of vitamin D receptor binding: associations with disease and evolution. *Genome Res* **20**, 1352–1360.

Reid, G.E. and McLuckey, S.A. (2002) "Top down" protein characterization via tandem mass spectrometry. *J Mass Spectrom* **37**, 663–675.

Salt, D.E., Baxter, I., and Lahner, B. (2008) Ionomics and the study of the plant ionome. *Annu Rev Plant Biol* **59**, 709–733.

Shoemaker, J.S., Painter, I.S., and Weir, B.S. (1999) Bayesian statistics in genetics: a guide for the uninitiated. *Trends Genet* **15**, 354–358.

Sikaroodi, M., Galachiantz, Y., and Baranova, A. (2010) Tumor markers: the potential of "omics" approach. *Curr Mol Med* **10**, 249–257.

Subramanian, A., Tamayo, P., Mootha, V.K., *et al.* (2005) Gene set enrichment analysis: a knowledge-based approach for interpreting genome-wide expression profiles. *Proc Natl Acad Sci USA* **102**, 15545–15550.

Sullivan, D.E., Gabbard, J.L., Jr, Shukla, M., *et al.* (2010) Data integration for dynamic and sustainable systems biology resources: challenges and lessons learned. *Chem Biodivers* **7**, 1124–1141.

Tamayo, P., Slonim, D., Mesirov, J., *et al.* (1999) Interpreting patterns of gene expression with self-organizing maps: methods and application to hematopoietic differentiation. *Proc Natl Acad Sci USA* **96**, 2907–2912.

Tompa, M., Li, N., Bailey, T.L., *et al.* (2005) Assessing computational tools for the discovery of transcription factor binding sites. *Nat Biotechnol* **23**, 137–144.

Wang, F., Paradkar, P.N., Custodio, A.O., *et al.* (2007) Genetic variation in Mon1a affects protein trafficking and modifies macrophage iron loading in mice. *Nat Genet* **39**, 1025–1032.

Wang, W., Knovich, M.A., Coffman, L.G., *et al.* (2010) Serum ferritin: past, present and future. *Biochim Biophys Acta* **1800**, 760–769.

Weaver, C.M. (1998) Use of calcium tracers and biomarkers to determine calcium kinetics and bone turnover. *Bone* **22** (5 Suppl), 103S–104S.

Werner, T. (2008) Bioinformatics applications for pathway analysis of microarray data. *Curr Opin Biotechnol* **19**, 50–54.

2

NUTRITIONAL EPIGENETICS

ROBERT A. WATERLAND, PhD

Baylor College of Medicine, Houston, Texas, USA

Summary

This chapter is intended to provide a timely overview of the current state of research at the intersection of nutrition and epigenetics. I begin by describing epigenetics and molecular mechanisms of epigenetic regulation, then highlight four classes of nutritional exposures currently being investigated for their potential to induce epigenetic alterations: dietary perturbation of one-carbon metabolism, prenatal energy restriction/growth retardation, assisted reproductive technologies, and histone deacetylase inhibitors. The chapter concludes with a discussion of outstanding questions in the field, and an elaboration of epigenetic technologies available to nutrition scientists.

Introduction

The science of nutrigenomics seeks to improve human health by understanding how dietary constituents interact with the genome, and how individual genetic heterogeneity affects these interactions (Stover and Garza, 2002; Kaput, 2007). This complex field is further complicated by the growing recognition that nutrition, in addition to acutely affecting gene regulation, can influence epigenetic processes and thereby induce persistent changes in transcriptional regulation and associated phenotypes (Waterland and Jirtle, 2004; Jirtle and Skinner, 2007) (Figure 2.1). Epigenetic dysregulation, long recognized as playing a role in cancer and various developmental syndromes (Egger *et al.*, 2004), is increasingly being investigated as a potential factor in the etiology of a wide range of human diseases (Feinberg, 2008; Gluckman *et al.*, 2009). Given that epigenetic mechanisms are most susceptible to environmental perturbation when they are undergoing developmental changes (Waterland and Michels, 2007), nutritional influences on epigenetic processes must

be considered in a developmental perspective. Accordingly, a major goal of nutritional epigenetics is to understand the extent to which human nutrition affects developmental epigenetics to cause persistent changes in disease susceptibility (pathway g–e in Figure 2.1). This chapter will introduce the field of epigenetics and review data indicating nutritional influences on epigenetic regulation. Lastly, I will discuss outstanding questions in this field and important obstacles to research progress, and offer suggestions for nutrition scientists planning to examine epigenetic effects.

Epigenetic Mechanisms

The term "epigenetics" was proposed by Conrad Waddington several decades ago to describe the study of "the causal interactions between genes and their products which bring phenotype into being" (Waddington, 1968). Waddington coined a *double-entendre*, spanning and potentially unifying different disciplines of developmental

Present Knowledge in Nutrition, Tenth Edition. Edited by John W. Erdman Jr, Ian A. Macdonald and Steven H. Zeisel.
© 2012 International Life Sciences Institute. Published 2012 by John Wiley & Sons, Inc.

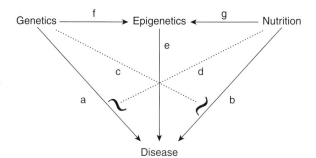

FIG. 2.1 Conceptual framework linking genetics, nutrition, epigenetics, and disease. Nutrigenomics has traditionally focused on the interactions between genetic susceptibility and nutrition in determining risk of disease (pathways a, b, c, d). Epigenetic mechanisms provide another pathway through which genetics and nutrition can affect risk of disease. While recognizing the potential influence of genetic variation on epigenetic processes (pathway f), nutritional epigenetics seeks to understand how nutrition affects epigenetic mechanisms, altering risk of disease (pathway g–e).

biology. As originally defined, epigenetics is the study of epigenesis, the process by which an animal develops from a single cell into an increasingly complex integrated system of differentiated cells and tissues. Additionally, however, "epigenetics" literally means "above genetics", evoking a system of gene regulatory mechanisms layered on top of the DNA sequence information. This latter connotation is more consistent with the currently accepted definition; epigenetics is the study of mitotically heritable alterations in gene expression potential that are not caused by changes in DNA sequence (Jaenisch and Bird, 2003). Hence, rather than encompassing all of developmental biology, modern epigenetics is focused on understanding the specific molecular mechanisms that convey cellular memory.

Within the nucleus, the mammalian genome is wrapped around nucleosomes, each comprised of an octamer of histone proteins; this complex of DNA and nucleosomes is called chromatin. The overall chromatin conformation of specific genomic regions – either more open and transcriptionally competent, or more condensed and transcriptionally down-regulated – is an integrated outcome of interacting epigenetic mechanisms (Cedar and Bergman, 2009; Margueron and Reinberg, 2010). Methylation of cytosines within CpG dinucleotides in DNA appears to be the most stable epigenetic mechanism. Once estab-

lished during development, cell-type specific patterns of CpG methylation are maintained during mitosis by the action of the "maintenance" DNA methyltransferase (Dnmt1). Regional patterns of CpG methylation regulate chromatin structure and gene expression by affecting the affinity of methylation-sensitive DNA binding proteins. The N-terminal tails of histone proteins protrude from the nucleosome and are subject to various post-translational modifications including acetylation, methylation, phosphorylation, and ubiquitination (Margueron and Reinberg, 2010). Regional patterns of specific histone modifications are associated with transcriptional activity, and may help regulate chromatin conformation. Cross-talk between DNA methylation and histone modifications serves to fine-tune establishment and reinforce maintenance of epigenomic states. During development, for example, histone modifications appear to guide regional de novo CpG methylation (Cedar and Bergman, 2009). Since DNA is believed to detach completely from nucleosomes during DNA replication, however, it remains unclear whether histone modifications can convey locus-specific information through mitosis (i.e. whether they are in fact epigenetic) (Ptashne, 2007). Hence, histone modifications are more dynamic and associated with establishment and modification of epigenetic states, whereas CpG methylation is a stable mark capable of conferring mitotic memory (Cedar and Bergman, 2009). The role of non-coding RNA in epigenetic regulation has been studied extensively in lower organisms such as yeast, and likely plays a role in regulating mammalian chromatin states (Aravin *et al.*, 2008).

Feed-forward autoregulation by proteins that can perpetuate alternate cellular states through mitosis comprises another level of epigenetic regulation. Such "stable feedback loops" were widely listed as key epigenetic mechanisms 15 years ago (Tilghman and Willard, 1995; Riggs and Porter, 1996), but now receive relatively little attention. Decades ago it was shown that *E. coli* can maintain alternate, mitotically heritable states of induction of the lac operon via a stable feedback loop (Novick, 1957). The lytic/lysogenic switch of the bacteriophage λ comprises a similar bistable epigenetic switch (Riggs and Porter, 1996). Epigenetic feed-forward autoregulation plays an important role in maintaining transcriptional states established during mammalian development. For example, in addition to regulating genes involved in muscle differentiation, the myogenic transcription factors MyoD and myogenin promote their own transcription, serving to perpetuate

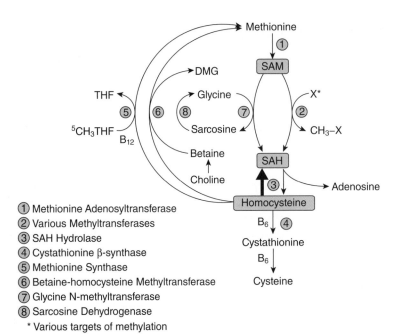

FIG. 2.2 The mammalian transmethylation pathway. Several nutrients including folate (shown here as 5-methyltetrahydrofolate), vitamin B$_{12}$, vitamin B$_6$, choline, betaine, and methionine serve as either methyl donors or cofactors in the transmethylation pathway. DNA is one of many biological substrates (indicated here as "X") for methyltransferase reactions which transfer methyl groups from S-adenosylmethionine (SAM). Glycine N-methyltransferase (reaction 7) is distinguished from other methyltransferases to emphasize its apparent role in regulating intracellular SAM concentrations.

their expression in committed muscle cells (Olson and Klein, 1994).

Most previous studies of nutritional epigenetics have focused on DNA methylation. This is highly stable, and only a small quantity of DNA is required for its measurement. DNA methylation in specific genomic regions is generally correlated with other epigenetic marks such as histone modifications, and our understanding of its association with gene expression is improving rapidly. It may therefore be logical in many cases to use DNA methylation as an integrative outcome by which to explore influences of nutritional exposures on epigenetic regulation.

Nutritional Influences on Epigenetics

Dietary Perturbation of One-carbon Metabolism

Methylation of DNA (and histones) is intimately dependent on nutrition. The methyl groups that are incorporated into DNA ultimately come from the diet (for example from methionine, choline, and betaine) and many nutrients, including folate, vitamin B$_{12}$, and vitamin B$_6$, are

critical cofactors in one-carbon metabolism (Figure 2.2). Extensive research in nutritional epigenetics has therefore focused on understanding how diet affects DNA methylation by influencing one-carbon metabolism (Van den Veyver, 2002; Ulrey *et al.*, 2005). Work in the agouti viable yellow (A^{vy}) mouse provided the first clear demonstration that a transient nutritional stimulus during a critical ontogenic period can cause a permanent phenotypic change via an epigenetic mechanism. The murine *agouti* gene regulates the production of a yellow pigment in fur; the A^{vy} mutation causes epigenetic dysregulation of *agouti*, and consequent interindividual variation in coat color among genetically identical A^{vy}/a mice. Supplementing the diet of female mice before and during pregnancy with folic acid, vitamin B$_{12}$, betaine, and choline caused a permanent change in the coat color distribution of A^{vy} heterozygous offspring (Wolff *et al.*, 1998) by increasing DNA methylation at A^{vy} (Waterland and Jirtle, 2003).

While it remains unclear which dietary components are the most potent modulators of DNA methylation capacity, effects of folate and folic acid intake on epigenetic regulation have been studied extensively. "Folate" describes various forms of polyglutaminated pteridine-p-aminoben-zoic acid, some of which (such as 5-methyltetrahydrofolate) are methyl donors. "Folic acid", on the other hand, is a synthetic form of folate that is not a dietary methyl donor (Smith *et al.*, 2008); ingested folic acid must be reduced and methylated (probably in the liver) before it can serve as a cofactor in the methionine synthase reaction (Figure 2.2) (also, see Chapter 21). An early study demonstrated that interindividual genetic variation interacts with folate status to determine DNA methylation. Healthy adults were assessed for plasma folate concentrations and periph-eral blood global DNA methylation, and genotyped for the C677T polymorphism in the gene encoding methyl-enetetrahydrofolate reductase (MTHFR). Plasma folate was positively correlated with global DNA methylation, but only in individuals homozygous for the T variant of *MTHFR* (which causes reduced enzymatic activity) (Friso *et al.*, 2002). This gene–nutrient–epigenome interaction was corroborated in a subsequent folate depletion–repletion study (Shelnutt *et al.*, 2004). Recent data indi-cate that maternal supplementation with folic acid before and during pregnancy may affect epigenetic regulation in the offspring. Methylation of Long Interspersed Elements (LINE-1) (an indicator of global DNA methylation) in cord blood DNA at delivery was slightly elevated in off-spring whose mothers took folic acid supplements (Steegers-Theunissen *et al.*, 2009).

Since folate is a critical cofactor in one-carbon metabo-lism, DNA methylation is generally expected to correlate positively with folate status. This is not always the case. In a large epidemiologic study, dietary folate intake was inversely correlated with LINE-1 methylation in colonic epithelium (Figueiredo *et al.*, 2009); the association was strongest in DNA from the ascending colon. Similarly, in a rat model, feeding a folate-free synthetic diet from age 21–56 days induced a persistent *increase* in hepatic global DNA methylation (Kotsopoulos *et al.*, 2008). One poten-tial explanation for this unexpected finding is that dietary methyl donor deficiency induces dramatic increases in expression of the DNA methyltransferases Dnmt1 and Dnmt3a in rat liver (Ghoshal *et al.*, 2006).

Elevated plasma homocysteine is associated with both nutritional and genetic factors, and is a risk factor for vascular disease (Selhub, 2006). Because homocysteine is a secondary product of biological methylation reactions (Figure 2.2), elevated homocysteine should impair DNA methylation. Indeed, in a small study of ~20 newborn infants (Fryer *et al.*, 2009), LINE-1 methylation in cord

blood DNA was inversely correlated with cord plasma homocysteine. The combined effects of dietary and genetic promotion of hyperhomocysteinemia by cystathione β-synthase (Cbs) haploinsufficiency (see Figure 2.2) were studied in mouse liver, kidney, brain, and testis (Caudill *et al.*, 2001). Despite dramatic differences in plasma total homocysteine concentrations, however, in most tissues global DNA methylation did not differ between wild type and $Cbs^{+/-}$ mice. Similarly, human patients with *CBS* defi-ciency showed no changes in either global or locus-specific DNA methylation (Heil *et al.*, 2007), despite exception-ally elevated plasma homocysteine concentrations. A small study of male patients with hyperhomocysteinemia and uremia, however, did find reduced genomic DNA meth-ylation in patients relative to controls (Ingrosso *et al.*, 2003); patients also displayed biallelic expression of *H19* in peripheral blood mononuclear cells. (*H19* is a genomi-cally imprinted gene, at which monoallelic expression is normally regulated by allele-specific methylation at a differentially methylated region [DMR]). Remarkably, in three patients who initially showed strong biallelic expression of *H19*, 60 days of treatment with oral 5-methyltetrahydrofolate (15 mg/day) restored normal monoallelic expression (Ingrosso *et al.*, 2003). The effects of hyperhomocysteinemia on epigenetic regulation of *H19* were subsequently examined in a mouse model; *Cbs* hap-loinsufficiency combined with a hyperhomocysteinemic diet resulted in a 20-fold elevation in plasma total homo-cysteine concentrations in adult mice (Devlin *et al.*, 2005). As expected, DNA methylation at the *H19* DMR was significantly reduced in the liver of hyperhomocysteinemic mice relative to controls. Paradoxically, however, in aorta and brain, *H19* DNA methylation was significantly ele-vated (dramatically so in brain).

Choline, required for the synthesis of phosphatidylcho-line and acetylcholine, is also an important methyl donor (Zeisel, 2006) (also, see Chapter 26). Choline appears to be particularly important for brain development (Zeisel, 2006); prenatal choline supplementation in rats leads to enhanced cognitive functioning in adulthood (Meck and Williams, 2003). In mice, maternal choline deficiency initi-ated in mid-pregnancy reduced DNA methylation at spe-cific genes in the fetal hippocampus at 17 days of fetal development (Niculescu *et al.*, 2006). It remains unclear, however, the extent to which the long-term cogni-tive benefits of choline supplementation are attributable to effects on epigenetic mechanisms such as DNA methy-lation. Following choline supplementation during fetal development, adult rats were found to have increased hippocampal neurogenesis (Glenn *et al.*, 2007), suggesting that early choline supplementation may induce persistent epigenetic changes in the neurogenic stem cell population.

The substantial body stores of creatine and phosphocreatine, which play central roles in energy metabolism, are spontaneously lost to creatinine and must be continuously synthesized (Brosnan and Brosnan, 2007). Creatine synthesis consumes about 40% of all S-adenosylmethionine in young adults (Brosnan and Brosnan, 2007), a huge methyl sink. Creatine supplementation therefore has the potential to facilitate DNA methylation by sparing S-adenosylmethionine. A recent study in adult rats, however, reported just the opposite. After just 14 days of supplementation with creatine monohydrate (2% wt/wt in diet), global DNA methylation in peripheral blood was significantly reduced (Taes *et al.*, 2007).

Prenatal Energy Restriction/Growth Retardation

Retrospective studies of individuals exposed to famine in early life have provided extensive insights into the potential for nutrition during critical periods of development to induce persistent changes in human metabolism and disease risk. A recent study of survivors of the Dutch famine of 1944–1945 tested the hypothesis that maternal exposure to famine leaves a permanent epigenetic mark on the offspring (Heijmans *et al.*, 2008). In peripheral blood from individuals almost 60 years old, bisulfite sequencing was used to measure DNA methylation at a DMR within the imprinted *IGF2* gene. Recognizing the potential for genetic variation to obscure induced epigenetic variation, *IGF2* DMR methylation in each periconceptionally exposed individual was compared with his or her same-sex unexposed sibling. The *IGF2* DMR was slightly but significantly less methylated in individuals exposed to famine periconceptionally, relative to unexposed siblings, providing the first convincing demonstration that an environmental exposure during early development can cause a persistent epigenetic alteration in humans (Heijmans *et al.*, 2008). Famine exposure during late fetal development was not associated with *IGF2* methylation, indicating that the period of susceptibility for this effect is limited to early embryonic development. The same group subsequently reported a study of DNA methylation at 15 candidate genes implicated in metabolic and cardiovascular disease (Tobi *et al.*, 2009). Periconceptional exposure was significantly associated with methylation at six of 15 genes meas-

ured; in most cases DNA methylation was higher in famine-exposed individuals (Tobi *et al.*, 2009).

The effects of maternal undernutrition before and during pregnancy have been studied extensively in rodents. Providing a low-protein diet (9% protein compared with 18% control) to mothers before and during pregnancy induces persistent physiological changes in the offspring. Effects of maternal low-protein diet on epigenetic regulation in the offspring are now being explored. Global DNA methylation in liver (but not heart or kidney) of day 21 fetal rats was reported to be elevated in response to maternal low-protein diet (Rees *et al.*, 2000). Focusing on the promoter of the Pparα gene, it was reported that specific CpG sites in hepatic DNA show reduced methylation in rat offspring of mothers fed a low-protein diet (Lillycrop *et al.*, 2008). Although the average methylation in this region was less than 10%, the epigenetic consequences of maternal diet were persistent; the same CpG sites showed reduced methylation in low-protein offspring at 34 and 80 days of age. Epigenetic effects of prenatal undernutrition have also been investigated in sheep (Stevens *et al.*, 2010). Ewes undernourished during the first month of pregnancy were subsequently allowed free access to feed until their fetuses were collected at fetal day 130. Despite the 100-day recuperation period, fetuses undernourished during early fetal development had increased expression of glucocorticoid receptor in the hypothalamus, associated with reduced DNA methylation and increased histone 3 lysine 9 (H3K9) acetylation of the *glucocorticoid receptor* promoter.

In a rat model, fetal growth restriction by intrauterine artery ligation cause permanent impairment of glucose tolerance. The developmental dynamics of epigenetic changes induced by intrauterine growth restriction were characterized at the *Pdx1* promoter in isolated pancreatic islets (Park *et al.*, 2008). Pdx1 is a homeobox transcription factor that regulates pancreas development and β cell differentiation. In pancreatic islets of 14-day-old rats that had been growth restricted *in utero*, reduced *Pdx1* expression was associated with lower density of several histone modifications at the *Pdx1* promoter, but no differences in DNA methylation. By age 6 months, however, extensive DNA methylation at the *Pdx1* promoter was found only in islets of previously growth-restricted rats (Park *et al.*, 2008), leading the authors to propose that aberrant epigenetic silencing at *Pdx1* is initiated by histone modification and subsequently stabilized by DNA methylation. Epigenetic changes associated with intrauterine growth retardation have also been explored in humans; genome-wide DNA methylation profiling identified epigenetic changes in hematopoietic stem and progenitor cells associated with intrauterine growth retardation (Einstein *et al.*, 2010).

Assisted Reproductive Technologies

Children conceived by assisted reproductive technologies (ART) have an elevated risk for rare developmental syndromes involving dysregulation of imprinted genes (Hansen *et al.*, 2002; DeBaun *et al.*, 2003). The synthetic medium bathing the cultured embryo essentially represents a nutritional exposure; the process of in vitro fertilization and subsequent embryo culture could therefore interfere with epigenetic reprogramming in the early embryo. Indeed, mouse studies have shown that embryo culture can affect epigenetic regulation at imprinted (Rivera *et al.*, 2008) and non-imprinted loci (Morgan *et al.*, 2008). A recent study (Katari *et al.*, 2009) used a methylation profiling technique to examine DNA methylation at over 700 genes in DNA isolated from cord blood and placenta of individuals conceived by ART, compared with those conceived naturally. Of 1536 CpG sites analyzed, hundreds showed differential methylation in either cord blood or placenta of in vitro compared with naturally conceived infants (Katari *et al.*, 2009). The methylation differences, though numerous, were slight in magnitude. It must be acknowledged that associations between in vitro conception and DNA methylation could be explained not only by an effect of early environment on epigenetic programming, but also by inheritance of genetic or epigenetic defects. For example, epigenetic aberrations in the sperm or egg could both contribute to infertility and be transmitted to the next generation following ART (Maher, 2005). This alternative explanation is supported by a recent study that compared DNA methylation profiles in both ART conceptuses and paternal sperm (Kobayashi *et al.*, 2009). In almost half of 17 cases showing abnormal DNA methylation in ART-conceived offspring, the identical epigenetic alteration was detected in the paternal sperm.

Histone Deacetylase Inhibitors

Locus-specific histone acetylation is dynamically regulated by histone acetyltransferases (which acetylate histones) and histone deacetylases (HDACs). Several diet-derived compounds are powerful HDAC inhibitors, and can therefore influence epigenetic regulation. One example is butyrate, a short-chain fatty acid. Although found in the diet (milk fat is a rich source), the principal source of butyrate in humans is from microbial digestion of dietary fiber in the colon (Wachtershauser and Stein, 2000); butyrate is the dominant energy source for colonic mucosal enterocytes. In rats fed diets of various wheat bran contents for 2 weeks, global histone H4 acetylation in colonic epithelial cells was directly correlated with butyrate concentration in the colonic lumen (Boffa *et al.*, 1992), providing an intriguing potential epigenetic link between dietary fiber intake and risk of colon cancer. Another dietary HDAC inhibitor, sulforaphane, an isothiocyanate found in cruciferous vegetables, is also implicated in cancer prevention (Ho *et al.*, 2009). A recent in vitro study (Meeran *et al.*, 2010) showed that sulforaphane inhibits the proliferation of breast cancer cells but not normal breast cells. Further, sulforaphane caused a dose-responsive increase in DNA methylation and epigenetic silencing of the gene encoding telomerase reverse transcriptase, offering a potential explanation for how sulforaphane specifically affects cancer cells.

Outstanding Questions in the Field

The preceding summary was not intended to be exhaustive but rather to indicate the breadth of research questions currently being pursued in nutritional epigenetics. Diet has important influences on epigenetic mechanisms, and epigenetic dysregulation is implicated in a broad range of human disease (Feinberg, 2008; Gluckman *et al.*, 2009). So far, however, there are no examples of nutritional exposures causing epigenetic changes that lead to human disease (pathway g–e in Figure 2.1). Elaboration of such causal pathways will pose numerous challenges. This section will summarize outstanding issues in this field, and provide guidance for nutrition investigators who wish to examine epigenetic effects.

By What Specific Mechanisms Does Nutrition Affect Epigenetic Regulation?

Nutritional influences on epigenetics have been studied most extensively from the perspective of dietary perturbation of one-carbon metabolism. Enhancing or impeding DNA methylation by nutritional manipulations affecting one-carbon metabolism seems straightforward, but many studies using various approaches have obtained paradoxical results (Devlin *et al.*, 2005; Ulrey *et al.*, 2005; Taes *et al.*, 2007). There are several potential explanations. Of central importance to so many biochemical functions, mammalian one-carbon metabolism is regulated at multiple levels. For example, attempts at dietary perturbation of the supply of S-adenosylmethionine may be trumped by the regulated expression of glycine-N-methyltransferase, which appears to exist primarily to regulate intracellular S-adenosylmethionine concentrations (Luka *et al.*, 2009) (Figure 2.2). Also, even if a dietary manipulation does alter transmethylation flux, DNA methylation represents such a small fraction of biological methylation reactions that the net impact on DNA methylation may be minor or unpredictable. For example, whereas DNA methylation at gene promoters is generally associated with gene repression, methylation of specific lysine residues on histone tails is associated with transcriptional activity (Margueron and Reinberg, 2010). Hence, dietary enhancement of transmethylation capacity could promote histone methylation at specific loci, with the secondary effect of impeding regional DNA methylation.

A much broader framework is envisaged if one acknowledges that any dietary stimulus that can affect transcriptional activity during a period of epigenetic development or maturation could have secondary effects on epigenetic regulation (Waterland and Michels, 2007). A vivid example was provided by the generation of induced pluripotent stem cells; simply by overexpressing four pluripotency-associated transcription factors, differentiated cells can undergo a dedifferentiation process involving genome-scale epigenetic reprogramming (Takahashi and Yamanaka, 2006). It is likely that myriad nutritional influences on epigenetic regulation, including many unrelated to one-carbon metabolism, are primarily mediated at the level of transcriptional activation during critical periods of epigenetic development.

During What Developmental Periods Are Epigenetic Mechanisms Most Susceptible to Nutrition?

Human and animal model data clearly indicate that, even in adulthood, epigenetic regulation can be influenced by nutrition. But what most clearly distinguishes epigenetic changes from other forms of transcriptional regulation is stability; the definitive mitotic stability of epigenetic mechanisms enables a transient environmental stimulus to have a lasting effect on transcriptional regulation. It appears that such persistent epigenetic effects can generally be induced only during developmental periods when epigenetic processes are undergoing developmental change or maturation. This is not so narrow a focus as it may seem; epigenetic development occurs over a wide range of life stages. Much emphasis has been placed on epigenetic

reprogramming that occurs in the early embryo (Santos and Dean, 2004; Reik, 2007) and during gametogenesis (Sasaki and Matsui, 2008). Indeed, the persistent effect of maternal nutrition on phenotype of A^{vy}/a mice occurs by affecting stochastic establishment of A^{vy} epigenotype during early embryonic development (Waterland and Jirtle, 2003). Additionally, however, epigenetic development continues in myriad cell types throughout fetal (Song *et al.*, 2009) and even early postnatal development (Waterland *et al.*, 2009; Kellermayer *et al.*, 2010), and may be influenced by environment. For example, maternal caregiving behavior was shown to affect postnatal developmental epigenetics in specific brain regions in the offspring (Weaver *et al.*, 2004; Champagne *et al.*, 2006), providing a plausible link between early postnatal environment and behavioral programming. Mouse studies indicate that epigenetic maturation of the gametes occurs during pre-adolescence (Janca *et al.*, 1986), suggesting another life stage during which nutrition might affect developmental epigenetics. To the extent that environmentally induced epigenetic information can be inherited transgenerationally (Whitelaw and Whitelaw, 2008), this offers a potential explanation for intriguing human epidemiologic observations in which nutritional status in pre-adolescence affects mortality in subsequent generations (Pembrey *et al.*, 2006). Lastly, even aging can be viewed as a developmental process. Extensive epigenetic changes occur with aging (Issa *et al.*, 1994), and may be affected by diet. In any case, investigators wishing to demonstrate that a transient nutritional exposure induces a persistent epigenetic effect must show that the specific epigenetic change is present both directly after the nutritional exposure, and later in life (Waterland and Garza, 1999).

What Genomic Regions Are Epigenetically Responsive to Nutrition?

The A^{vy} locus is characterized as a "metastable epiallele," meaning that in each individual the epigenetic state is established stochastically during early development, then maintained in all tissue lineages throughout life (Rakyan *et al.*, 2002). After it was demonstrated that early nutrition persistently affects epigenetic regulation in A^{vy} mice (Waterland and Jirtle, 2003), investigators studied effects of early environment on establishment of DNA methylation at the murine metastable epialleles $Axin^{Fused}$ and $Cabp^{IAP}$. Dietary methyl donor supplementation of female mice before and during pregnancy increased DNA methylation at $Axin^{Fused}$, reducing the incidence of tail kinking in $Axin^{Fused}$/+ offspring (Waterland *et al.*, 2006a). Conversely, maternal exposure to the environmental contaminant bisphenol-A (a key component of polycarbonate plastic) decreased DNA methylation at $Cabp^{IAP}$ in the offspring (Dolinoy *et al.*, 2007). Cumulatively, these data indicate that stochastic developmental establishment of DNA methylation at metastable epialleles is, in general, labile to maternal environment. Importantly, a recent study (Waterland *et al.*, 2010) indicates that human metastable epialleles exist and, as in the mouse, are epigenetically labile to the maternal periconceptional environment.

Metastable epialleles represent just one subset of genomic regions that may be epigenetically labile to nutritional stimuli during development. Over a decade ago (Pembrey, 1996) it was proposed that the unique epigenetic requirements for monoallelic expression may render genomically imprinted genes especially sensitive to epigenetic dysregulation. On this basis, genomically imprinted genes have been popular candidate genes in studies of environmental epigenetics (Biniszkiewicz *et al.*, 2002; Ingrosso *et al.*, 2003; Waterland *et al.*, 2006b). Recent data on humans exposed periconceptionally to famine (Tobi *et al.*, 2009) or conceived by ART (Turan *et al.*, 2010), however, while indicating that early environment can affect epigenetic regulation at genomically imprinted genes, do not support the hypothesis that genomically imprinted genes are especially susceptible to epigenetic dysregulation.

Most studies linking epigenetic modifications to transcriptional regulation have focused on gene promoters. In particular, many studies attempted to correlate developmental or tissue-specific differences in gene expression with DNA methylation at CpG-rich regions (CpG islands) in gene promoters (Ehrlich, 2003). Now, with the increasing sophistication of epigenomic studies that can map epigenetic marks and levels of associated transcripts in various cell and tissue types, it is clear that the focus on CpG island promoters has largely been misplaced. The majority of CpG island promoters are normally unmethylated in all tissues, regardless of tissue-specific expression; only about 4% of CpG island promoters regulate transcriptional activity via tissue-specific methylation (Shen *et al.*, 2007). Clearly, CpG islands are not the only important site of regulatory DNA methylation; developmental changes in DNA methylation at CpG-poor promoters correlate with developmental changes in gene expression (Waterland *et al.*, 2009). Human studies indicate that

DNA methylation in genomic regions up to 2 kilobases (kb) away from CpG islands (dubbed "CpG island shores") plays an important role in both cancer and normal development (Irizarry *et al.*, 2009). A recent epigenomic study showed that DNA methylation at intragenic CpG islands affects tissue-specific gene expression by regulating expression from alternate promoters (Maunakea *et al.*, 2010). A study of enhancer regions in various human cell types *in vitro* (Heintzman *et al.*, 2009) provided the broadest perspective of the complex distribution of epigenetic marks that regulate tissue-specific gene expression. Unlike gene promoters, at which histone modifications were largely invariant between different cell types, enhancer regions carried histone modification signatures that clearly distinguished different cell types (Heintzman *et al.*, 2009). Enhancers operate tissue-specifically and can be located up to 200 kb away from genes, underscoring the enormous challenge of linking nutritionally induced epigenetic changes to associated changes in gene expression.

A way forward is provided by the conjecture that epigenetic mechanisms are most susceptible to environmental influences during development or maturation; if this holds true, the genomic regions most susceptible to a specific exposure are those in flux during the exposure. Limited information is currently available on epigenetic ontogeny in various organs and cell types. But such information is rapidly being generated. For example, the NIH Roadmap Epigenomics Mapping Consortium is currently working to produce a public resource of human epigenomic data across various healthy cell and tissue types and developmental stages (Bernstein *et al.*, 2010). For those who wish to investigate potential epigenetic effects of nutrition but who do not have the resources or expertise to perform epigenomic assays, candidate gene regions may be selected by searching publicly available data sets to identify genomic regions at which epigenetic marks are changing in the tissue of interest during the time of the nutritional exposure.

How Can We Improve Our Understanding of the Role of Epigenetic Dysregulation in Disease?

The inherent tissue specificity of epigenetic regulation is arguably *the* major obstacle to studying epigenetics and human disease. In studies of genetic epidemiology, DNA from peripheral blood can be used to assay for a genetic variant present throughout the body. Conversely, epigenetic regulation (and dysregulation) will often be tissue- and cell-type specific (Waterland and Michels, 2007; Gluckman *et al.*, 2009); in most cases, therefore, epigenetic information present in easily obtainable biopsy samples will not provide insights into the epigenetic etiology of disease. Even within a given tissue, different cell types may have dramatically different epigenomes. This level of complexity was demonstrated in a recent study of genome-wide binding of the methyl-CpG binding protein MeCP2 in brain. Brain tissue is comprised generally of two cell types, neurons and glia. Taking advantage of the neuronal nuclear surface marker NeuN, fluorescence-activated cell sorting was used to separate neuronal and glial nuclei from mouse brain (Skene *et al.*, 2010). MeCP2 protein was highly enriched on neuronal compared with glial DNA, and appeared to play an important role in regulating chromatin architecture specifically in neurons. In studies of nutritional influences on epigenetic regulation, analysis of separated cell types will often be required to develop meaningful insights. Clearly, it will in many cases be highly advantageous to initially study nutritional epigenetics in animal models of human disease, in which tissues and cell types of interest can be readily obtained. The identification of human metastable epialleles (Waterland *et al.*, 2010) may enable investigators to circumvent the problem of epigenetic tissue specificity. As at murine metastable epialleles (Waterland and Jirtle, 2003; Waterland *et al.*, 2006a), the dramatic interindividual epigenetic variation at human metastable epialleles occurs systemically. Hence, at these loci, epigenetic regulation within cells and tissues of pathophysiologic relevance may be inferred from, say, a peripheral blood DNA sample (Waterland *et al.*, 2010). To the extent that human epigenetic metastability affects expression of genes implicated in human disease, currently archived peripheral blood DNA samples may be used to assess associations between nutrition, epigenetic regulation, and human disease (Waterland and Michels, 2007).

What New Epigenetic Technologies Are Available to Nutrition Scientists?

It has been common for investigators to assess effects of nutrition on global cytosine methylation or histone modifications. Global measurements are difficult to interpret, however, and will fail to detect important locus-specific epigenetic changes. Future studies should focus on candidate gene regions and/or apply genome-scale methods to screen for genomic regions of interest. Histone modifications in specific genomic regions are analyzed by chroma-

tin immunoprecipitation (ChIP); chromatin (genomic DNA still attached to nucleosomes) is cleaved into small fragments, then antibodies are used to isolate the fraction enriched for specific histone modifications. The DNA from this fraction is isolated, and quantitative PCR in genomic regions of interest is used to determine the relative enrichment of histone modifications across different samples. Genome-scale studies of histone modifications are becoming increasingly common. The ChIP "pulldown" can be labeled and hybridized to a tiling array (ChIP-microarray) (van Steensel and Henikoff, 2003), or shotgun sequenced (ChIP-seq) (Park, 2009). Shotgun sequencing – also called "short-read" or "next-generation" sequencing – offers several advantages over microarrays. Artifacts associated with non-linear hybridization dynamics are avoided; counting sequence reads potentially offers unbiased and highly sensitive quantitation of relative enrichment. Further, unlike microarrays, in which repetitive elements are not represented, shotgun sequencing offers the potential to "anchor" specific repetitive elements and thereby probe the nearly half of the genome that they comprise.

Most quantitative methods of DNA methylation analysis rely on bisulfite modification. Bisulfite modification followed by PCR converts unmethylated cytosines to thymines, while methylated cytosines remain cytosines (Frommer *et al.*, 1992), converting epigenetic information to genetic information. Post-bisulfite PCR products can then be sequenced by various methods. Coupling bisulfite modification with pyrosequencing (Shen and Waterland, 2007) is currently the "gold standard" technique for quantitative measurement of site-specific CpG methylation. Post-bisulfite PCR products can also be sub-cloned and sequenced. The molecule-specific data provided by this classic technique is often useful if analyzing DNA from mixtures of cells, for example, or in the study of genomic imprinting (Shen and Waterland, 2007). If a sufficient number of clones (~20 or more) from each sample are sequenced, quantitative results can be obtained. Genome-scale data on DNA methylation can be obtained in several ways. Methylated DNA immunoprecipitation (MeDIP) uses an antibody directed against 5-methylcytosine, and is generally analogous to ChIP. The MeDIP pulldown can be analyzed either on a tiling array (Weber *et al.*, 2005) or by shotgun sequencing (Maunakea *et al.*, 2010). One major caveat: MeDIP is not efficient in genomic regions of low CpG density (i.e. most of the genome). Various methods employ methylation-sensitive restriction endonucleases to generate genomic libraries representing methylated or unmethylated genomic regions; these can also be coupled with either microarray or shotgun sequencing to obtain genome-scale data (Khulan *et al.*, 2006; Shen *et al.*, 2007; Irizarry *et al.*, 2008). Although potentially quite sensitive, these methods provide low genomic coverage; methylation information is only obtained on the very small subset of CpG sites within the informative restriction enzyme sites. The only technique that currently offers the potential to provide truly genome-wide information on site-specific CpG methylation is shotgun sequencing of bisulfite-treated genomic DNA (Bisulfite-seq) (Lister *et al.*, 2009; Harris *et al.*, 2010). Although now prohibitively expensive for most applications, Bisulfite-seq will become more widespread as sequencing costs decline. Investigators planning to apply any of these epigenomic methods will need access to sophisticated bioinformatics infrastructure and personnel to effectively analyze the large and complex datasets.

Future Directions

The field of nutritional epigenetics faces extraordinary challenges: diverse nutritional exposures have the potential to influence epigenetic regulation in myriad genomic regions, potentially in a tissue-specific and cell-type-specific fashion. But this field also promises extraordinary opportunities to improve human health. Short-term nutrition interventions targeted to critical ontogenic periods could potentially optimize developmental epigenetics, conferring lifelong health benefits. Moreover, although characteristically stable, epigenetic mechanisms are inherently malleable, offering the promise of nutritional therapies designed to correct pathogenic epigenetic dysregulation. Such ambitious goals will become reality, however, only if we can improve dramatically our understanding of how diet affects the establishment and maintenance of epigenetic mechanisms, and how epigenetic dysregulation contributes to human disease. Controlled experiments in refined animal models are essential to identify the critical developmental periods, specific cell types, and genomic loci in which induced epigenetic alterations affect metabolic processes and disease susceptibility.

Acknowledgments

This work was supported by USDA CRIS 6250-51000-055. I thank Adam Gillum for assistance with the figures.

Suggestions for Further Reading

Jaenisch, R. and Bird, A. (2003) Epigenetic regulation of gene expression: how the genome integrates intrinsic and environmental signals. *Nat Genet* **33** Suppl, 245–254.

Jirtle, R.L. and Skinner, M.K. (2007) Environmental epigenomics and disease susceptibility. *Nat Rev Genet* **8**, 253–262.

Ptashne, M. (2007) On the use of the word "epigenetic". *Curr Biol* **17**, R233–236.

Ulrey, C.L., Liu, L., Andrews, L.G., and Tollefsbol, T.O. 2005. The impact of metabolism on DNA methylation. *Hum Mol Genet* **14** Spec No. 1, R139–147.

Waterland, R.A. and Michels, K.B. (2007) Epigenetic epidemiology of the developmental origins hypothesis. *Annu Rev Nutr* **27**, 363–388.

References

Aravin, A.A., Sachidanandam, R., Bourc'his, D., *et al.* (2008) A piRNA pathway primed by individual transposons is linked to de novo DNA methylation in mice. *Mol Cell* **31**, 785–799.

Bernstein, B.E., Stamatoyannopoulos, J.A., Costello, J.F., *et al.* (2010) The NIH Roadmap Epigenomics Mapping Consortium. *Nat Biotechnol* **28**, 1045–1048.

Bestor, T. and Hannon, G.J. (2008) A piRNA pathway primed by individual transposons is linked to de novo DNA methylation in mice. *Mol Cell* **31**, 785–799.

Biniszkiewicz, D., Gribnau, J., Ramsahoye, B., *et al.* (2002) Dnmt1 overexpression causes genomic hypermethylation, loss of imprinting, and embryonic lethality. *Mol Cell Biol* **22**, 2124–2135.

Boffa, L.C., Lupton, J.R., Mariani, M.R., *et al.* (1992) Modulation of colonic epithelial cell proliferation, histone acetylation, and luminal short chain fatty acids by variation of dietary fiber (wheat bran) in rats. *Cancer Res* **52**, 5906–5912.

Brosnan, J.T. and Brosnan, M.E. (2007) Creatine: endogenous metabolite, dietary, and therapeutic supplement. *Annu Rev Nutr* **27**, 241–261.

Caudill, M.A., Wang, J.C., Melnyk, S., *et al.* (2001) Intracellular S-adenosylhomocysteine concentrations predict global DNA hypomethylation in tissues of methyl-deficient cystathionine beta-synthase heterozygous mice. *J Nutr* **131**, 2811–2818.

Cedar, H. and Bergman, Y. (2009) Linking DNA methylation and histone modification: patterns and paradigms. *Nat Rev Genet* **10**, 295–304.

Champagne, F.A., Weaver, I.C., Diorio, J., *et al.* (2006) Maternal care associated with methylation of the estrogen receptor-alpha1b promoter and estrogen receptor-alpha expression in the medial preoptic area of female offspring. *Endocrinology* **147**, 2909–2915.

Debaun, M.R., Niemitz, E.L., and Feinberg, A.P. (2003) Association of in vitro fertilization with Beckwith-Wiedemann syndrome and epigenetic alterations of LIT1 and H19. *Am J Hum Genet* **72**, 156–160.

Devlin, A.M., Bottiglieri, T., Domann, F.E., *et al.* (2005) Tissue-specific changes in H19 methylation and expression in mice with hyperhomocysteinemia. *J Biol Chem* **280**, 25506–25511.

Dolinoy, D.C., Huang, D., and Jirtle, R.L. (2007) Maternal nutrient supplementation counteracts bisphenol A-induced DNA hypomethylation in early development. *Proc Natl Acad Sci USA* **104**, 13056–13061.

Egger, G., Liang, G., Aparicio, A. *et al.* (2004) Epigenetics in human disease and prospects for epigenetic therapy. *Nature* **429**, 457–463.

Ehrlich, M. (2003) Expression of various genes is controlled by DNA methylation during mammalian development. *J Cell Biochem* **88**, 899–910.

Einstein, F., Thompson, R.F., Bhagat, T.D., *et al.* (2010) Cytosine methylation dysregulation in neonates following intrauterine growth restriction. *PLoS One* **5**, e8887.

Feinberg, A.P. (2008) Epigenetics at the epicenter of modern medicine. *JAMA* **299**, 1345–1350.

Figueiredo, J.C., Grau, M.V., Wallace, K., *et al.* (2009) Global DNA hypomethylation (LINE-1) in the normal colon and lifestyle characteristics and dietary and genetic factors. *Cancer Epidemiol Biomarkers Prev* **18**, 1041–1049.

Friso, S., Choi, S.W., Girelli, D., *et al.* (2002) A common mutation in the 5,10-methylenetetrahydrofolate reductase gene affects genomic DNA methylation through an interaction with folate status. *Proc Natl Acad Sci USA* **99**, 5606–5611.

Frommer, M., McDonald, L.E., Millar, D.S., *et al.* (1992) A genomic sequencing protocol that yields a positive display of 5-methylcytosine residues in individual DNA strands. *Proc Natl Acad Sci USA* **89**, 1827–1831.

Fryer, A.A., Nafee, T.M., Ismail, K.M., *et al.* (2009) LINE-1 DNA methylation is inversely correlated with cord plasma homocysteine in man: a preliminary study. *Epigenetics* **4**, 394–398.

Ghoshal, K., Li, X., Datta, J., *et al.* (2006) A folate- and methyl-deficient diet alters the expression of DNA methyltransferases and methyl CpG binding proteins involved in epigenetic gene silencing in livers of F344 rats. *J Nutr* **136**, 1522–1527.

Glenn, M.J., Gibson, E.M., Kirby, E.D., *et al.* (2007) Prenatal choline availability modulates hippocampal neurogenesis and neurogenic responses to enriching experiences in adult female rats. *Eur J Neurosci* **25**, 2473–2482.

Gluckman, P.D., Hanson, M.A., Buklijas, T., *et al.* (2009) Epigenetic mechanisms that underpin metabolic and cardiovascular diseases. *Nat Rev Endocrinol* **5**, 401–408.

Hansen, M., Kurinczuk, J.J., Bower, C., *et al.* (2002) The risk of major birth defects after intracytoplasmic sperm injection and in vitro fertilization. *N Engl J Med* **346**, 725–730.

Harris, R.A., Wang, T., Coarfa, C., *et al.* (2010) Comparison of sequencing-based methods to profile DNA methylation and identification of monoallelic epigenetic modifications. *Nat Biotechnol* **28**, 1097–1105.

Heijmans, B.T., Tobi, E.W., Stein, A.D., *et al.* (2008) Persistent epigenetic differences associated with prenatal exposure to famine in humans. *Proc Natl Acad Sci USA* **105**, 17046–17049.

Heil, S.G., Riksen, N.P., Boers, G.H., *et al.* (2007) DNA methylation status is not impaired in treated cystathionine beta-synthase (CBS) deficient patients. *Mol Genet Metab* **91**, 55–60.

Heintzman, N.D., Hon, G.C., Hawkins, R.D., *et al.* (2009) Histone modifications at human enhancers reflect global cell-type-specific gene expression. *Nature* **459**, 108–112.

Ho, E., Clarke, J.D., and Dashwood, R.H. (2009) Dietary sulforaphane, a histone deacetylase inhibitor for cancer prevention. *J Nutr* **139**, 2393–2396.

Ingrosso, D., Cimmino, A., Perna, A.F., *et al.* (2003) Folate treatment and unbalanced methylation and changes of allelic expression induced by hyperhomocysteinaemia in patients with uraemia. *Lancet* **361**, 1693–1699.

Irizarry, R.A., Ladd-Acosta, C., Carvalho, B., *et al.* (2008) Comprehensive high-throughput arrays for relative methylation (CHARM). *Genome Res* **18**, 780–790.

Irizarry, R.A., Ladd-Acosta, C., Wen, B., *et al.* (2009) The human colon cancer methylome shows similar hypo- and hypermethylation at conserved tissue-specific CpG island shores. *Nat Genet* **41**, 178–186.

Issa, J.P., Ottaviano, Y.L., Celano, P., *et al.* (1994) Methylation of the oestrogen receptor CpG island links ageing and neoplasia in human colon. *Nat Genet* **7**, 536–540.

Jaenisch, R. and Bird, A. (2003) Epigenetic regulation of gene expression: how the genome integrates intrinsic and environmental signals. *Nat Genet* **33** Suppl, 245–254.

Janca, F.C., Jost, L.K., and Evenson, D.P. (1986) Mouse testicular and sperm cell development characterized from birth to adulthood by dual parameter flow cytometry. *Biol Reprod* **34**, 613–623.

Jirtle, R.L. and Skinner, M.K. (2007) Environmental epigenomics and disease susceptibility. *Nat Rev Genet* **8**, 253–262.

Kaput, J. (2007) Developing the promise of nutrigenomics through complete science and international collaborations. *Forum Nutr* **60**, 209–223.

Katari, S., Turan, N., Bibikova, M., *et al.* (2009) DNA methylation and gene expression differences in children conceived in vitro or in vivo. *Hum Mol Genet* **18**, 3769–3778.

Kellermayer, R., Balasa, A., Zhang, W., *et al.* (2010) Epigenetic maturation in colonic mucosa continues beyond infancy in mice. *Hum Mol Genet* **19**, 2168–2176.

Khulan, B., Thompson, R.F., Ye, K., *et al.* (2006) Comparative isoschizomer profiling of cytosine methylation: the HELP assay. *Genome Res* **16**, 1046–1055.

Kobayashi, H., Hiura, H., John, R.M., *et al.* (2009) DNA methylation errors at imprinted loci after assisted conception originate in the parental sperm. *Eur J Hum Genet* **17**, 1582–1591.

Kotsopoulos, J., Sohn, K.J., and Kim, Y.I. (2008) Postweaning dietary folate deficiency provided through childhood to puberty permanently increases genomic DNA methylation in adult rat liver. *J Nutr* **138**, 703–709.

Lillycrop, K.A., Phillips, E.S., Torrens, C., *et al.* (2008) Feeding pregnant rats a protein-restricted diet persistently alters the methylation of specific cytosines in the hepatic PPAR alpha promoter of the offspring. *Br J Nutr* **100**, 278–282.

Lister, R., Pelizzola, M., Dowen, R.H., *et al.* (2009) Human DNA methylomes at base resolution show widespread epigenomic differences. *Nature* **462**, 315–322.

Luka, Z., Mudd, S.H., and Wagner, C. (2009) Glycine N-methyltransferase and regulation of S-adenosylmethionine levels. *J Biol Chem* **284**, 22507–22511.

Maher, E.R. (2005) Imprinting and assisted reproductive technology. *Hum Mol Genet* **14**, Spec No. 1, R133–138.

Margueron, R. and Reinberg, D. (2010) Chromatin structure and the inheritance of epigenetic information. *Nat Rev Genet* **11**, 285–296.

Maunakea, A.K., Nagarajan, R.P., Bilenky, M., *et al.* (2010) Conserved role of intragenic DNA methylation in regulating alternative promoters. *Nature* **466**, 253–257.

Meck, W.H. and Williams, C.L. (2003) Metabolic imprinting of choline by its availability during gestation: implications for memory and attentional processing across the lifespan. *Neurosci Biobehav Rev* **27**, 385–399.

Meeran, S.M., Patel, S.N., and Tollefsbol, T.O. (2010) Sulforaphane causes epigenetic repression of hTERT expression in human breast cancer cell lines. *PLoS One* **5**, e11457.

Morgan, H.D., Jin, X.L., Li, A., *et al.* (2008) The culture of zygotes to the blastocyst stage changes the postnatal expression of an epigenetically labile allele, agouti viable yellow, in mice. *Biol Reprod* **79**, 618–623.

Niculescu, M.D., Craciunescu, C.N., and Zeisel, S.H. (2006) Dietary choline deficiency alters global and gene-specific DNA methylation in the developing hippocampus of mouse fetal brains. *FASEB J* **20**, 43–49.

Novick A.W.M. (1957) Enzyme induction as an all-or-none phenomenon. *Proc Natl Acad Sci USA* **43**, 553–566.

Olson, E.N. and Klein, W.H. (1994) bHLH factors in muscle development: dead lines and commitments, what to leave in and what to leave out. *Genes Dev* **8**, 1–8.

Park, J.H., Stoffers, D.A., Nicholls, R.D., *et al.* (2008) Development of type 2 diabetes following intrauterine growth retardation in rats is associated with progressive epigenetic silencing of Pdx1. *J Clin Invest* **118**, 2316–2324.

Park, P.J. (2009) ChIP-seq: advantages and challenges of a maturing technology. *Nat Rev Genet* **10**, 669–680.

Pembrey, M. (1996) Imprinting and transgenerational modulation of gene expression; human growth as a model. *Acta Genet Med Gemellol (Roma)* **45**, 111–125.

Pembrey, M.E., Bygren, L.O., Kaati, G., *et al.* (2006) Sex-specific, male-line transgenerational responses in humans. *Eur J Hum Genet* **14**, 159–166.

Ptashne, M. (2007) On the use of the word "epigenetic". *Curr Biol* **17**, R233–236.

Rakyan, V.K., Blewitt, M.E., Druker, R., *et al.* (2002) Metastable epialleles in mammals. *Trends Genet* **18**, 348–351.

Rees, W.D., Hay, S.M., Brown, D.S., *et al.* (2000) Maternal protein deficiency causes hypermethylation of DNA in the livers of rat fetuses. *J Nutr* **130**, 1821–1826.

Reik, W. (2007) Stability and flexibility of epigenetic gene regulation in mammalian development. *Nature* **447**, 425–432.

Riggs, A.D. and Porter, T.N. (1996) Overview of epigenetic mechanisms. In V.E. Russo, R.A. Martienssen, R.A. and A.D. Riggs (eds), *Epigenetic Mechanisms of Gene Regulation*. Cold Spring Harbor Laboratory Press, Plainview, pp. 29–46.

Rivera, R.M., Stein, P., Weaver, J.R., *et al.* (2008) Manipulations of mouse embryos prior to implantation result in aberrant expression of imprinted genes on day 9.5 of development. *Hum Mol Genet* **17**, 1–14.

Santos, F. and Dean, W. (2004) Epigenetic reprogramming during early development in mammals. *Reproduction* **127**, 643–651.

Sasaki, H. and Matsui, Y. (2008) Epigenetic events in mammalian germ-cell development: reprogramming and beyond. *Nat Rev Genet* **9**, 129–140.

Selhub, J. (2006) The many facets of hyperhomocysteinemia: studies from the Framingham cohorts. *J Nutr* **136**, 1726S–1730S.

Shelnutt, K.P., Kauwell, G.P., Gregory, J.F., 3rd, *et al.* (2004) Methylenetetrahydrofolate reductase 677C→T polymorphism affects DNA methylation in response to controlled folate intake in young women. *J Nutr Biochem* **15**, 554–560.

Shen, L., Kondo, Y., Guo, Y., *et al.* (2007) Genome-wide profiling of DNA methylation reveals a class of normally methylated CpG island promoters. *PLoS Genet* **3**, 2023–2036.

Shen, L. and Waterland, R.A. (2007) Methods of DNA methylation analysis. *Curr Opin Clin Nutr Metab Care* **10**, 576–581.

Skene, P.J., Illingworth, R.S., Webb, S., *et al.* (2010) Neuronal MeCP2 is expressed at near histone-octamer levels and globally alters the chromatin state. *Mol Cell* **37**, 457–468.

Smith, A.D., Kim, Y.-I., and Refsum, H. (2008) Is folic acid good for everyone? *Am J Clin Nutr* **87**, 517–533.

Song, F., Mahmood, S., Ghosh, S., *et al.* (2009) Tissue specific differentially methylated regions (TDMR): changes in DNA methylation during development. *Genomics* **93**, 130–139.

Steegers-Theunissen, R.P., Obermann-Borst, S.A., Kremer, D., *et al.* (2009) Periconceptional maternal folic acid use of 400 microg per day is related to increased methylation of the IGF2 gene in the very young child. *PLoS One* **4**, e7845.

Stevens, A., Begum, G., Cook, A., *et al.* (2010) Epigenetic changes in the hypothalamic proopiomelanocortin and glucocorticoid receptor genes in the ovine fetus after periconceptional undernutrition. *Endocrinology* **151**, 3652–3664.

Stover, P.J. and Garza, C. (2002) Bringing individuality to public health recommendations. *J Nutr* **132**, 2476S–2480S.

Taes, Y.E., Bruggeman, E., Bleys, J., *et al.* (2007) Lowering methylation demand by creatine supplementation paradoxically decreases DNA methylation. *Mol Genet Metab* **92**, 283–284.

Takahashi, K. and Yamanaka, S. (2006) Induction of pluripotent stem cells from mouse embryonic and adult fibroblast cultures by defined factors. *Cell* **126**, 663–676.

Tilghman, S.M. and Willard, H.F. (1995) Epigenetic regulation in mammals. In S.C. Elgin (ed.), *Chromatin Structure and Gene Expression*. IRL Press, Oxford, pp. 197–222.

Tobi, E.W., Lumey, L.H., Talens, R.P., *et al.* (2009) DNA methylation differences after exposure to prenatal famine are common and timing- and sex-specific. *Hum Mol Genet* **18**, 4046–4053.

Turan, N., Katari, S., Gerson, L.F., *et al.* (2010) Inter- and intra-individual variation in allele-specific DNA methylation and gene expression in children conceived using assisted reproductive technology. *PLoS Genet* **6**, e1001033.

Ulrey, C.L., Liu, L., Andrews, L.G., *et al.* (2005) The impact of metabolism on DNA methylation. *Hum Mol Genet* **14**, Spec No. 1, R139–147.

Van Den Veyver, I. (2002) Genetic effects of methylation diets. *Annu Rev Nutr* **22**, 255–282.

Van Steensel, B. and Henikoff, S. (2003) Epigenomic profiling using microarrays. *Biotechniques* **35**, 346–350, 352–354, 356–357.

Wachtershauser, A. and Stein, J. (2000) Rationale for the luminal provision of butyrate in intestinal diseases. *Eur J Nutr* **39**, 164–171.

Waddington, C.H. (1968) The basic ideas of biology. In C.H. Waddington (ed.), *Towards a Theoretical Biology*. Edinburgh University Press, Edinburgh, pp. 1–32.

Waterland, R.A. and Garza, C. (1999) Potential mechanisms of metabolic imprinting that lead to chronic disease. *Am J Clin Nutr* **69**, 179–197.

Waterland, R.A. and Jirtle, R.L. (2003) Transposable elements: targets for early nutritional effects on epigenetic gene regulation. *Mol Cell Biol* **23**, 5293–5300.

Waterland, R.A. and Jirtle, R.L. (2004) Early nutrition, epigenetic changes at transposons and imprinted genes, and enhanced susceptibility to adult chronic diseases. *Nutrition* **20**, 63–68.

Waterland, R.A. and Michels, K.B. (2007) Epigenetic epidemiology of the developmental origins hypothesis. *Annu Rev Nutr* **27**, 363–388.

Waterland, R.A., Dolinoy, D.C., Lin, J.R., *et al.* (2006a) Maternal methyl supplements increase offspring DNA methylation at Axin fused. *Genesis* **44**, 401–406.

Waterland, R.A., Kellermayer, R., Laritsky, E., *et al.* (2010) Season of conception in rural Gambia affects DNA methylation at putative human metastable epialleles. *PLoS Genet* **6**, e1001252.

Waterland, R.A., Kellermayer, R., Rached, M.T., *et al.* (2009) Epigenomic profiling indicates a role for DNA methylation in early postnatal liver development. *Hum Mol Genet* **18**, 3026–3038.

Waterland, R.A., Lin, J.R., Smith, C.A., *et al.* (2006b) Post-weaning diet affects genomic imprinting at the insulin-like growth factor 2 (Igf2) locus. *Hum Mol Genet* **15**, 705–716.

Weaver, I.C., Cervoni, N., Champagne, F.A., *et al.* (2004) Epigenetic programming by maternal behavior. *Nat Neurosci* **7**, 847–854.

Weber, M., Davies, J.J., Wittig, D., *et al.* (2005) Chromosome-wide and promoter-specific analyses identify sites of differential DNA methylation in normal and transformed human cells. *Nat Genet* **37**, 853–862.

Whitelaw, N.C. and Whitelaw, E. (2008) Transgenerational epigenetic inheritance in health and disease. *Curr Opin Genet Dev* **18**, 273–279.

Wolff, G.L., Kodell, R.L., Moore, S.R., *et al.* (1998) Maternal epigenetics and methyl supplements affect agouti gene expression in Avy/a mice. *FASEB J* **12**, 949–957.

Zeisel, S.H. (2006) Choline: critical role during fetal development and dietary requirements in adults. *Annu Rev Nutr* **26**, 229–250.

3

GENETIC VARIATION AND NUTRIENT METABOLISM

LEAH E. CAHILL[1], PhD, RD AND AHMED EL-SOHEMY[2], PhD

[1]*Harvard School of Public Health, Boston, Massachusetts, USA*
[2]*University of Toronto, Toronto, Ontario, Canada*

Summary

One of the continuing challenges of nutrition research is dealing with the variability in response to nutrients and other bioactive substances that are consumed. Response can be any phenotype such as blood levels of a nutrient, biomarker or disease. There is growing interest among researchers and health-care practitioners in utilizing genomic information to predict and manage the large interindividual differences in response to nutrient intakes. Recent advances in human genomics have uncovered extensive variations in genes affecting nutrient metabolism, but their full impact on nutrient requirements remains to be elucidated. Developments in high-throughput technologies have enabled cost-effective and rapid detection of genetic variants, which facilitates their incorporation into clinical and observational studies of nutrition. Differences in the rates of absorption, distribution, uptake, utilization, biotransformation, and excretion ultimately impact the concentration of a nutrient at a target site of interest. Variations in genes that code for target proteins such as receptors, enzymes, transporters or ion channels can also impact the response to a nutrient. Nutrigenomics describes the use of high-throughput "omics" technologies to study how nutrients interact with the genome at all levels of regulation, and nutrigenetics is sometimes used specifically to refer to the effect of genetic variations on nutrient response. The purpose of this chapter is to provide an overview of the current state of knowledge of the role of human genetic variation in nutrient metabolism, and to present some notable examples that illustrate particular developments in the field. Incorporating markers of genetic variation into studies of nutrition and health aims to benefit those seeking personalized dietary advice, and should also improve public health recommendations by providing sound scientific evidence linking diet and health.

Present Knowledge in Nutrition, Tenth Edition. Edited by John W. Erdman Jr, Ian A. Macdonald and Steven H. Zeisel.
© 2012 International Life Sciences Institute. Published 2012 by John Wiley & Sons, Inc.

Introduction

Nutrigenomics (or nutritional genomics) refers to the application of high-throughput "omics" technologies, together with systems biology and bioinformatics tools, to understand how nutrients interact with the flow of genetic information to impact various health outcomes (Ordovas *et al.*, 2007; Ordovas, 2008). Gene–nutrient interactions can be viewed as two sides of the same coin. On the one hand, nutrients can alter the expression or function of a gene (including epigenetic modifications), which is a topic that is discussed elsewhere in this book (Chapter 2). On the other hand, genetic polymorphisms can alter the response to a nutrient, which is sometimes referred to as *nutrigenetics* (El-Sohemy, 2007). This latter approach also includes the study of how genetic variations influence food intake and eating behaviors (Garcia-Bailo *et al.*, 2009; Eny and El-Sohemy, 2010), but this will not be elaborated on in this chapter. Although genetics can play a major role in the variable responses to nutrient intakes, it is also important to consider other factors such as age, sex, physical activity, smoking, and nutritional status.

The completion of the first draft sequence of the human genome about a decade ago ushered in a new era of nutrition research that began to focus more on understanding the variability in responses to nutrients and other dietary substances. Single nucleotide polymorphisms (SNPs) are the most abundant form of genetic variation with over 10 million SNPs cataloged in public databases such as dbSNP (Thorisson and Stein, 2003). Other types of genetic variations include nucleotide repeats, insertions, deletions, and copy number variants (CNVs). Depending on the region of the genome where the polymorphism occurs, the impact on nutrient metabolism can be negligible or profound. Early examples of how genetic variations have a severe effect on nutrient response are seen with inborn errors of metabolism such as phenylketonuria (PKU). This usually involves a mutation in a single gene along with the intake of a single nutrient to cause a specific disorder (Levy, 1989). The discovery that an essential amino acid such as phenylalanine could be toxic to some individuals has impacted labeling requirements in certain countries so that diet beverages containing aspartame, for example, must be labeled as containing phenylalanine. This is an example of a food product that is labeled primarily for individuals with a particular genotype. Lactose intolerance is another well known example of gene–nutrient interaction and demonstrates how food products can also be developed for specific genotypes, as in the case of lactose-free dairy products (Swallow, 2003). Individuals with lactose intolerance are unable to efficiently break down the primary milk sugar (lactose) from dairy products, and are consequently advised to limit lactose-containing foods or to use lactase supplements or lactose-free dairy products to prevent the acute gastrointestinal discomfort that can occur (Swagerty *et al.*, 2002). Unlike these examples, however, nutrition-related chronic diseases are polygenic, have complex etiologies and often take years or decades to develop. As such, a huge challenge has been to determine the role of specific dietary factors and gene variants in the development of complex chronic diseases such as diabetes, osteoporosis, cancer, and cardiovascular disease (CVD).

The daily ingestion, absorption, digestion, transport, uptake, utilization, biotransformation, and excretion of nutrients and food bioactives involve many proteins such as enzymes, receptors, transporters, ion channels, and hormones. Variations in genes encoding these proteins can alter both the amount of the protein produced as well as how efficiently that protein functions. If a genetic variation leads to altered production or function of a protein involved in the metabolism of a nutrient, then nutritional status could be affected. Studies that have incorporated markers of human genetic variation have traditionally relied on the candidate gene approach, which requires existing knowledge of the various metabolic processes that act on the nutrient of interest. Genome-wide association scans (GWAS) utilize more cutting-edge technologies and provide an *unbiased* approach to identifying genetic variants that modify a nutrient's response by examining the effect of large numbers of SNPs and CNVs; usually anywhere from 100 000 to ~2 million markers spread out across the genome. Rapid advances in sequencing technologies will continue to drive down the cost of genotyping and ultimately make whole genome sequencing of large numbers of individuals a reality (Levy *et al.*, 2007). In the meantime, the candidate gene approach remains the method of choice for most studies that include measures of both nutrition and genetics. Genes that are often selected as candidates tend be those that are the targets of a nutrient or food bioactive, or those that lie in the metabolic pathway of the bioactive compound (El-Sohemy, 2007). Since several SNPs can be inherited together in a single block (called haplotype), "tag" SNPs are typically used to capture most of the variation in a gene of interest. Studies to date have tended to focus on single SNPs or a few SNPs in a single gene, but there is growing interest in

TABLE 3.1 Links to useful databases and other resources for human genetics

Resource	Website
dbSNP	http://www.ncbi.nlm.nih.gov/projects/SNP/index.html
HapMap	www.hapmap.org
The Human Variome Project	http://www.humanvariomeproject.org/index.php/about
The Human Phenotype Ontology Website	http://www.human-phenotype-ontology.org/PhenExplorer/PhenExplorer.html
UCSC Genome Bioinformatics	http://genome.ucsc.edu/
P³G Observatory	http://www.p3gobservatory.org/
The Pharmacogenomics Knowledge Base	http://www.pharmgkb.org/index.jsp
HUGO Gene Nomenclature Committee	http://www.genenames.org/
The Gene Ontology	http://www.geneontology.org/
The Human Gene Compendium	http://www.genecards.org/
Online Mendelian Inheritance in Man	http://www.ncbi.nlm.nih.gov/omim
Broad Institute Software Page	http://www.broadinstitute.org//scientific-community/software
Reactome	http://www.reactome.org/ReactomeGWT/entrypoint.html
NHGRI	www.genome.gov
GWASCentral	www.gwascentral.org
The Centre for Applied Genomics	http://projects.tcag.ca/variation/

exploring multiple genetic variants along the metabolic pathway of a nutrient (van Ommen *et al.*, 2010). A number of resources are available to help select candidate genetic variants in candidate genes (Table 3.1).

Nutritional epidemiologic studies relating most nutrients to most health outcomes have often yielded inconsistent results. Although this is partly due to issues surrounding experimental study design such as inadequate control for confounders or misclassification of exposure, the genetic heterogeneity between studies certainly accounts for some of the discrepancies. As such, the incorporation of genetics into nutritional studies aims to improve their consistency (Figure 3.1). Genetic association studies that link gene variants to health outcomes have also yielded inconsistent results (Ioannidis *et al.*, 2001), even though genetic variants can be measured much more reliably and accurately than dietary exposures. Thus, not only can inconsistencies among nutrition studies be reconciled by the incorporation of genetic data, but conflicting and contradictory gene-association studies can also be explained by incorporating measures of environmental exposures such as diet (Luan *et al.*, 2001). Since the study of gene–diet interactions is a relatively young field with few laboratories conducting such research, there has been a paucity of studies

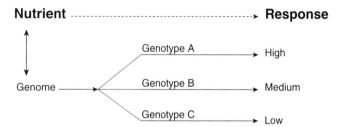

FIG. 3.1 Genetic variation modifies response to nutrient intake.

that have aimed to replicate previous findings. Evidence is beginning to emerge that some interactions can be replicated in diverse populations, but others have not been replicated, which could be due to genetic epistasis (i.e. gene–gene interactions) or other environmental or physiological differences between populations (Helgadottir *et al.*, 2006).

Dietary Fat

Some of the earliest work in this field was pioneered by Jose Ordovas and colleagues, and focused on identifying genetic variants that modified the blood lipid response to dietary fat and cholesterol (Ordovas, 2008). Genes involved in lipid metabolism along with dietary fat probably represent the most widely studied group of gene–diet interactions (also, see Chapters 9 and 10). Apolipoproteins (apo) A-I and A-II, coded by the *APOA1* and *APOA2* genes, respectively, play an important role in lipid metabolism. The interaction between a common functional *APOA2* polymorphism (-265T>C, rs5082) and saturated fat intake in relation to body mass index (BMI) was investigated using three populations in the United States: the Framingham Offspring Study (1454 Caucasians), the Genetics of Lipid Lowering Drugs and Diet Network Study (1078 Caucasians), and the Boston-Puerto Rican Centers on Population Health and Health Disparities Study (930 Hispanics of Caribbean origin) (Corella *et al.*, 2009). The prevalence of the CC genotype in the three populations ranged from about 10% to 16%. Statistically significant interactions between the *APOA2* -265T>C SNP and saturated fat intake in relation to BMI were identified in all three populations. Estimations of obesity for individuals with the CC genotype were approximately two-fold compared with carriers of the T allele among the subjects with high-saturated-fat intake, but no association was observed in the low-saturated-fat group. This study represented the first time that a diet–gene interaction influencing risk of obesity has been strongly and consistently replicated in three independent populations. The replication increases the robustness of the finding and is noted because few attempts have been made previously to replicate findings of diet–gene interactions. The finding that the results for the diet–*APOA2* polymorphism interaction effect was similar in genetically diverse populations (i.e. European Americans and Hispanic-Americans) suggests that this gene may interact directly with saturated fat intake to influence energy balance across distinct populations (Corella *et al.*, 2009). The same research group has since replicated this gene–diet interaction in two additional populations, providing further validation for this gene–diet interaction (Corella *et al.*, 2011).

Another notable example involving dietary fat is an interaction with the peroxisome proliferator-activated receptor-gamma (PPARγ) gene. PPARγ influences lipid metabolism, and common variations have been linked to metabolic disorders. PPARγ is a nuclear receptor that is involved in many processes, including lipid metabolism and adipocyte differentiation. Since the natural ligands for PPARγ include polyunsaturated fatty acids (PUFA), it has

been hypothesized that the effect of the common Pro12Ala variant of *PPARγ* may be altered by the type of dietary fat, especially the polyunsaturated to saturated fat ratio. Results of an earlier study showed that, when the dietary polyunsaturated fat to saturated fat ratio is low, the BMI of carriers of the Ala allele was greater than that of non-carriers, but when the dietary ratio is high, the opposite effect is observed (Luan *et al.*, 2001). This observation was made during a time when it became evident that genetic association studies, including those linking *PPARγ* to cardiometabolic diseases, were yielding inconsistent findings from one population to the next. The observation that the effect of *PPARγ* genotype is strongly influenced by the type of dietary fat suggested that genetic association studies needed to consider the dietary habits of the populations studied, a concept that has not yet been embraced fully by genetic epidemiologists.

Dietary PUFA can also alter HDL-cholesterol concentrations in humans (Wijendran and Hayes, 2004), although the effects of both n-3 and n-6 PUFA have not been consistent (Russo, 2009). For example, a common genetic polymorphism in the *APOA1* gene (-74G>A) modifies the association between dietary PUFA intake and plasma HDL-cholesterol concentrations among women in the Framingham Offspring Study (Ordovas *et al.*, 2002). Dietary PUFA has also been shown to interact with other genes to influence HDL-cholesterol concentrations. A common polymorphism in the nuclear factor kappa B (NF-κB) *NFKB1* gene (-94Ins/Del ATTG) interacts with PUFA intake to affect HDL-cholesterol (Fontaine-Bisson *et al.*, 2009). Among individuals with the Ins/Ins genotype, an increase in % energy from PUFA was associated with an increase in HDL-cholesterol whereas the inverse relationship was observed among those with the Del/Del genotype. This observation was made in two distinct populations, one consisting of young, healthy adults representing different ethnocultural groups, and the other an older population with type 2 diabetes (Fontaine-Bisson *et al.*, 2009).

Although most experiments that investigate potential gene–diet interactions have been observational studies, clinical studies that examine the difference in response to dietary treatment among genotypes have also started to be conducted. These are often based on initial findings from observational studies. For example, the plasma omega-3 fatty acid response to an omega-3 fatty acid supplement was found to be modulated by apoE ε4, but not by the common *PPAR-α* L162V polymorphism (Plourde *et al.*, 2009). After supplementation, only non-carriers of ε4 had increased omega-3 in their plasma (Plourde *et al.*, 2009). After 3 months of supplementation with 3.6 g of omega-3 fatty acids per day or placebo capsules containing olive oil, changes in serum cholesterol concentrations were similar among the *PPAR-α* L162V genotypes (Lindi *et al.*, 2003). Confirming gene–diet interactions from observational studies in a clinical setting is an important step towards personalized nutrition.

Vitamin B$_{12}$

Vitamin B$_{12}$ is necessary for important functions such as DNA synthesis during cell division, the formation of red blood cells, and the preservation of the myelin sheath around neurons (also, see Chapter 22). Clinically, vitamin B$_{12}$ deficiency is associated with conditions such as pernicious anemia, cardiovascular disease, cancer, and neurodegenerative disorders. It has been observed that vitamin B$_{12}$ deficiency is often related to altered intestinal vitamin B$_{12}$ absorption rather than inadequate intake of the vitamin (Watanabe, 2007). Furthermore, in some extreme cases, the ability to digest, absorb, and utilize vitamin B$_{12}$ has been linked to rare genetic mutations, resulting in diseases such as juvenile megaloblastic anemia (Tanner *et al.*, 2004). As such, there has been an interest in determining whether more common polymorphisms could be affecting vitamin B$_{12}$ status in the general population.

Hazra and co-workers were among the first to apply GWAS to identify genetic variants that influence nutrient metabolism (Hazra *et al.*, 2008). Using data from 1658 women, a GWAS was conducted to identify genetic loci that influence plasma vitamin B$_{12}$ concentrations. The associations between >500,000 SNPs and plasma vitamin B$_{12}$ levels were examined. A strong association between an SNP (rs492602) in *FUT2*, the gene that codes for fucosyltransferase 2, and plasma vitamin B$_{12}$ levels was observed. Women homozygous for the G allele had higher B$_{12}$ levels than carriers of the A allele. The rs492602 SNP is in strong linkage disequilibrium with another *FUT2* variant, which determines *FUT2* secretor status, suggesting a plausible mechanism for altered B$_{12}$ absorption and plasma levels. Absorption of vitamin B$_{12}$ requires the secretion of the glycoprotein intrinsic factor from the gastric cells and the binding of intrinsic factor to vitamin B$_{12}$. The *FUT2* secretor status has been associated with both *Helicobacter pylori* infection and gastritis, and can lead to reduced secretion of intrinsic factor (Carmel *et al.*, 1987). Insights gained from this GWAS of plasma vitamin B$_{12}$ are likely to have

implications for future research into complex diseases linked to inadequate intake such as cancer and CVD. Identifying genetic determinants of vitamin status opens the door for certain studies to explore hypotheses related to the vitamin when intake data are not available. Mendelian randomization refers to the concept of using a genetic variant associated with an environmental exposure, such as a specific nutrient, as a surrogate measure for the exposure itself when information on the exposure is lacking (Davey Smith, 2011). This may be the case with some of the large biobanks or genetic epidemiologic studies. Such a genetic marker could be viewed as more informative than assessing intake, which is often done at a single point in time whereas the gene variant would likely have influenced exposure over a lifetime.

Folate

Folate (folic acid, vitamin B$_9$) is important for a number of biological pathways, and inadequate levels have been implicated in the development of several chronic diseases (Jiang *et al.*, 2003) (also, see Chapter 21). For example, low levels of folate are associated with elevated blood homocysteine levels, which may increase risk of CVD (Boushey *et al.*, 1995). Deficient folate status can also lead to abnormal DNA synthesis, methylation, and repair, which may increase the risk of certain types of cancer (Blount *et al.*, 1997). Although higher total folate intake is inversely associated with the risk of some cancers such as colorectal cancer (Bailey, 2003), folate may actually increase the development of established tumors (Smith *et al.*, 2008). Thus, it is important to establish dietary recommendations that not only prevent deficiency, but also minimize the harmful effects of excess intake.

Methylenetetrahydrofolate reductase (MTHFR) is a key enzyme involved in the metabolism of folate. The *MTHFR* 677C/T (rs1801133) polymorphism is a non-synonymous SNP that results in impaired enzyme activity and is associated with a reduced risk of some forms of cancer (Frosst *et al.*, 1995). However, the protective effect of this folate-related polymorphism is dependent on adequate folate status (Bailey, 2003). Therefore, cancer risk may be increased in individuals with the homozygous genotype for the *MTHFR* 677C/T polymorphism who have low status of methyl-related nutrients such as folate (Bailey, 2003). Modeling analyses have recently been developed to project recommended dietary allowances (RDA) for nutrients based on genotype, as used in a study that assessed the effect of the *MTHFR* 677C/T polymorphism on the current folate RDA for American adults (400 μg/day) by race and ethnicity (Robitaille *et al.*, 2009). This assessment concluded that the *MTHFR* 677C/T variant, the most widely studied genotype affecting folate metabolism, may not necessarily affect individual requirements because the projected RDA for each genotype was similar to the current RDA (Robitaille *et al.*, 2009). Similar analyses could be conducted for determining upper limits for other nutrients since genetic variations can also impact the levels of nutrients that cause toxicity.

Choline

The normal function of all cells requires choline, which is particularly important for brain development and memory (also, see Chapter 26). Choline provides the first example of the integration of genetic polymorphisms in candidate genes into a classic depletion–repletion study of a nutrient. In addition to dietary sources, choline can also be synthesized endogenously. When fed a low-choline diet, some people deplete more quickly than others, potentially because of varying amounts of endogenous production of choline. A series of studies was carried out using a set study design in which adult men and women were fed diets containing adequate choline, followed by a diet containing almost no choline, until they were clinically determined to be choline-deficient. Organ dysfunction, a sign of choline deficiency, developed in 77% of men, 80% of postmenopausal women, and only 44% of premenopausal women (Fischer *et al.*, 2007). Higher circulating estrogen levels among premenopausal women were proposed to be the reason why this group is less prone to develop symptoms associated with deficiency because estrogen induces phosphatidylethanolamine N-methyltransferase (PEMT) gene expression, which contributes to increased endogenous choline synthesis. Polymorphisms in the *MTHFD1* gene were examined and shown to limit the availability of methyltetrahydrofolate, thereby increasing the use of choline as a methyl donor. Individuals with the common 5,10-methylenetetrahydrofolate dehydrogenase-1958A allele were seven times more likely than non-carriers to develop signs of choline deficiency (Kohlmeier *et al.*, 2005). Remarkably, premenopausal women with this allele had a 15-fold increased risk of developing organ dysfunction on a low-choline diet (Kohlmeier *et al.*, 2005). These findings indicate that nutrient needs can vary substantially

for different individuals and that gene variants could have different effects depending on age and sex.

Vitamin C

Vitamin C (ascorbic acid) is required for the synthesis of carnitine, collagen, norepinephrine, and epinephrine (also, see Chapter 16). Vitamin C functions to reduce oxidative damage, recycle other antioxidants, facilitate iron absorption, and aid in the conversion of cholesterol to bile acids. An inverse association has been observed between serum ascorbic acid concentrations and risk of chronic diseases such as CVD (Jacob and Sotoudeh, 2002; Boekholdt *et al.*, 2006) and diabetes (Paolisso *et al.*, 1994; Sinclair *et al.*, 1994). However, the findings remain inconsistent (Loria *et al.*, 1998). This discrepancy could be due to individual variability in serum ascorbic acid concentrations since studies report variable dose–response curves between dietary vitamin C and serum ascorbic acid (Levine *et al.*, 1996; Loria *et al.*, 1998). Although several nongenetic determinants of serum ascorbic acid have been identified, they only explain a small portion of the large individual variability (Block *et al.*, 1999).

Studies on the genetic determinants of serum ascorbic acid provide an example of how the effect of the gene variants is most pronounced among those with suboptimal intakes. Significant diet–gene interactions have been observed between dietary vitamin C and glutathione *S*-transferase (GST) (theta and mu classes) genotypes on blood concentrations of ascorbic acid (Cahill *et al.*, 2009). GSTs are a family of detoxifying enzymes that contribute to the glutathione–ascorbic acid antioxidant cycle in the human body. The omega class of GST is directly able to reduce dehydroascorbic acid back to ascorbic acid, but it is not known whether any of the other classes of GST can carry out this function as well. The mu and theta classes of GST each contain a common genetic polymorphism that results in a non-functional enzyme. The association between the GST genotype and serum ascorbic acid concentrations seems to depend on the amount of dietary vitamin C consumed. Individuals with the GST nonfunctional mu and theta genotypes were found to have an increased risk of serum ascorbic acid deficiency if they did not meet the RDA for vitamin C (Cahill *et al.*, 2009). For example, the odds ratio (95% confidence interval (CI)) for serum ascorbic acid deficiency (<11 μmol/L) was 2.17 (1.10, 4.28) for subjects with the functional *GSTT1*1* allele who did not meet the RDA of vitamin C compared with those who did. However, the odds ratio (95% CI) was 12.28 (4.26, 33.42) for individuals with the non-functional *GSTT1*0/*0* genotype. The corresponding odds ratios (95% CI) were 2.29 (0.96, 5.45) and 4.03 (2.01, 8.09) for the functional *GSTM1*1* allele and non-functional *GSTM1*0/*0* genotype, respectively. This study demonstrated that the RDA for vitamin C is protective against serum ascorbic acid deficiency, regardless of genotype. However, some individuals appear to be more vulnerable to deficiency if the RDA for vitamin C is not achieved. Moreover, because the functional version of the gene appears to protect against deficiency, these findings suggest a novel biological role for the GST theta and mu enzymes in sparing serum ascorbic acid, possibly by aiding in the reduction of dehydroascorbic acid to ascorbic acid. Variations in other genes that affect vitamin C transport (Cahill and El-Sohemy, 2009) and utilization (Cahill and El-Sohemy, 2010) have also affected circulating concentrations, and show that other pathways impacting ascorbic acid metabolism can modify the association between intake and plasma concentrations. Nevertheless, other genes remain to be identified since the polymorphisms identified to date still do not account for most of the variability in serum ascorbic acid concentrations.

Vitamin D

Vitamin D is essential for the maintenance of musculoskeletal health, but inadequate vitamin D has also been associated with an increased risk of several chronic diseases (also, see Chapter 13). The primary circulating form of vitamin D is 25-hydroxyvitamin D [25(OH)D], which can be influenced by both sun exposure and diet. The high heritability estimates from twin studies suggest that genetic factors are also important determinants of circulating 25(OH)D. Vitamin D provides another example of the use of GWAS, and in this case by more than one research group. One study assessed approximately 4500 individuals of European ancestry and found significant associations between 25(OH)D concentrations and SNPs in the following genes: *GC* (encoding vitamin D binding protein); *NADSYN1* (encoding nicotinamide adenine dinucleotide synthetase), and *CYP2R1* (encoding cytochrome P450, family 2, subfamily R, polypeptide 1, a C-25 hydroxylase that converts cholecalciferol to an active vitamin D receptor ligand) (Ahn *et al.*, 2010). A separate study evaluated serum levels of 25(OH)D and genetic variation in about 34,000 individuals of European descent (Wang *et al.*,

2010). That study also found significant associations between 25(OH)D levels and variants within or near *GC* and *CYP2R1*, as well as the *CYP24A1* gene, which encodes a cytochrome p450 hydroxylase (Wang *et al.*, 2010). Candidate gene studies have also found associations between common variations in some of these genes and circulating 25(OH)D concentrations (Fu *et al.*, 2009; Sinotte *et al.*, 2009). Taken together, these GWAS studies of circulating vitamin D demonstrate that several genetic variants affecting different aspects of a nutrient's metabolism can each influence nutrient status.

Caffeine

Caffeine is the most widely consumed stimulant in the world and is found primarily in coffee, tea, cola beverages, and energy drinks. Because of its widespread use there has been considerable interest in the health effects of caffeine. One of the challenges of studying the effects of caffeine is differentiating it from other bioactive substances found in the major dietary contributors of caffeine such as coffee or tea, each of which contain a diverse mixture of phytochemicals (Cornelis and El-Sohemy, 2007). Furthermore, those who consume large quantities of caffeine often have different lifestyles and attributes compared with moderate drinkers or abstainers. There is also evidence that polymorphisms in the primary target of caffeine action, the adenosine A_{2a} receptor, influence habitual consumption (Cornelis *et al.*, 2007). As such, it may be difficult to account for all potential confounders, and any associations could be a result of residual confounding.

Prior to the incorporation of genetic variants the association between coffee intake and CVD risk had been controversial. It was not clear whether it was caffeine, some other compound in coffee, or another environmental factor associated with coffee consumption that may have been responsible for the association between coffee and CVD, including hypertension and myocardial infarction (MI). Distinguishing between the effects of caffeine and other compounds found in coffee is a challenging task because of the strong co-linearity between caffeine and coffee intake in many populations. Caffeine is metabolized primarily by the cytochrome P450 1A2 (CYP1A2) enzyme, and a polymorphism in the *CYP1A2* gene influences the rate of caffeine metabolism. Individuals can be classified as either "fast" caffeine metabolizers (those who are homozygous for the -163 A allele) or "slow" caffeine metabolizers (carriers of the -163 C allele) based on the rs762551 SNP in *CYP1A2*. Knowledge of this genetic difference in caffeine metabolism led to the hypothesis that, if caffeine is involved in the development of CVD, then the *CYP1A2* genotype should modify the association between intake of caffeinated coffee and risk. The findings showed that, indeed, coffee consumption was associated with an increased risk of myocardial infarction (MI) only among individuals with slow caffeine metabolism (Cornelis *et al.*, 2006). This observation suggests that caffeine is the component in coffee that increases risk of MI because it is the only major compound that is known to be detoxified by CYP1A2. Furthermore, a protective effect of moderate coffee consumption was observed among the fast metabolizers, suggesting that other components of coffee might be protective and their effect was "unmasked" in those who eliminated caffeine efficiently. This coffee–*CYP1A2* genotype interaction with CVD risk has since been replicated in a prospective study investigating the effect of coffee intake on hypertension (Palatini *et al.*, 2009). That study found that the risk of hypertension associated with coffee intake varies according to *CYP1A2* genotype. Slow caffeine metabolizers were at increased risk of hypertension from drinking coffee, whereas individuals with the fast-caffeine-metabolizing genotype had no increased risk (Palatini *et al.*, 2009). This study also measured epinephrine and norepinephrine in the urine of the subjects because these catecholamines have been shown to increase after caffeine administration in humans. Urinary epinephrine was significantly higher in coffee drinkers than in abstainers, but only among slow caffeine metabolizers. This is particularly interesting because increased sympathetic activity is considered a main mechanism through which caffeine raises blood pressure.

A similar approach involving genetic variation in caffeine metabolism was used in an observational study of coffee and breast cancer (Kotsopoulos *et al.*, 2007). By grouping subjects into *CYP1A2* genotypes, this study aimed to determine if caffeine was the compound in coffee that explains the protective effect that had previously been observed between coffee and breast cancer risk (Baker *et al.*, 2006; Nkondjock *et al.*, 2006). Indeed, a gene–diet interaction was observed, but unlike the studies on risk of MI and hypertension, where slow caffeine metabolizers were at increased risk from drinking coffee, in this study coffee was associated with a lower risk of breast cancer among slow metabolizers (Kotsopoulos *et al.*, 2007). No protective effect was observed among fast metabolizers, suggesting that caffeine is likely the protective component

in coffee. This is consistent with findings from animal studies showing that caffeine inhibits the development of mammary tumors in rodents (Wolfrom *et al.*, 1991; Yang *et al.*, 2004).

Future Directions

As progress continues to be made in unravelling the complexities of human genetic variation, nutrition researchers will need to become proficient in applying state-of-the-art techniques in genotyping and sequencing along with the various databases and bioinformatics tools in order to advance knowledge of the variable response to nutrient intakes. Practitioners in the field of nutrition will need to understand how best to translate those findings into clinical practice (Zeisel, 2007). The knowledge gained from incorporating genetic variation into studies of nutrition and health should provide a more rational basis for giving personalized dietary advice while improving the quality of evidence used to make population-based dietary recommendations for the prevention of specific diseases. The application of nutrigenomics by health-care professionals for the prevention and treatment of complex chronic diseases has not yet been widely adopted. Whether such practice will be feasible for the population at large in the immediate future remains to be determined, but the principles and tools of nutrigenomics are expected soon to allow for earlier and more targeted interventions than currently exist (DeBusk, 2009). As the current research in nutrigenomics often focuses on how gene–diet interactions influence phenotypes that are predictive biomarkers of disease (Kaput *et al.*, 2007), it is likely that the path from research to applications will proceed into clinical practice using these markers of chronic disease as outcome measures.

Replication of current findings of gene–diet interactions and further research in the form of genotype-specific nutritional intervention studies are needed. The future of research involving human genetic variation should provide additional knowledge of biological function and individual response to diet. As GWAS studies and whole genome sequencing become more affordable and are integrated into studies with nutrition-related phenotypes, efforts will need to be made to account for differences in dietary intake levels, which is a limitation of the GWAS studies conducted to date. It is possible that different genetic loci influence a nutritional phenotype of interest, such as blood concentrations of a nutrient, depending on dietary intake

> **BOX 3.1   Benefits to using markers of genetic variation in nutritional epidemiology**
>
> - Minimize residual confounding
> - Eliminate recall bias
> - Address "reverse causation"
> - Identify specific bioactive or nutrient in a food/beverage
> - Improve measurement of biologically effective dose of nutrient
> - Elucidate molecular mechanisms
> - Identify potential responders and non-responders

levels. The application of genetic variation to nutrition research will help clarify the role of specific nutrients and food bioactives in health and disease, and will improve the quality of evidence from observational studies by addressing a number of issues that are often identified as limitations in nutritional epidemiology (Box 3.1). Research in this area is paving the way for personalized nutrition where dietary advice can ultimately be tailored to an individual's unique genetic profile in order to improve on the current one-size-fits-all approach to dietary guidance.

Suggestions for Further Reading

Davey Smith, G. (2011) Use of genetic markers and gene–diet interactions for interrogating population-level causal influences of diet on health. *Genes Nutr* **6**, 27–43.

Jenab, M., Slimani, N., Bictash, M., *et al*. (2009) Biomarkers in nutritional epidemiology: applications, needs and new horizons. *Hum Genet* **125**, 507–525.

Kaput, J., Noble, J., Hatipoglu, B., *et al*. (2007) Application of nutrigenomic concepts to type 2 diabetes mellitus. *Nutr Metab Cardiovasc Dis* **17**, 89–103.

Ordovas, J.M., Kaput, J., and Corella, D. (2007) Nutrition in the genomics era: cardiovascular disease risk and the Mediterranean diet. *Mol Nutr Food Res* **51**, 1293–1299.

van Ommen, B., El-Sohemy, A., Hesketh, J., *et al*. (2010) The Micronutrient Genomics Project: a community-driven knowledge base for micronutrient research. *Genes Nutr* **5**, 285–296.

References

Ahn, J., Yu, K., Stolzenberg-Solomon, R., *et al*. (2010) Genome-wide association study of circulating vitamin D levels. *Hum Mol Genet* **19**, 2739–2745.

Bailey, L.B. (2003) Folate, methyl-related nutrients, alcohol, and the MTHFR 677C→T polymorphism affect cancer risk: intake recommendations. *J Nutr* **133**(11 Suppl 1), 3748S–3753S.

Baker, J.A., Beehler, G.P., Sawant, A.C., *et al*. (2006) Consumption of coffee, but not black tea, is associated with decreased risk of premenopausal breast cancer. *J Nutr* **136**, 166–171.

Block, G., Mangels, A.R., Patterson, B.H., *et al*. (1999) Body weight and prior depletion affect plasma ascorbate levels attained on identical vitamin C intake: a controlled-diet study. *J Am Coll Nutr* **18**, 628–637.

Blount, B.C., Mack, M.M., Wehr, C.M., *et al*. (1997) Folate deficiency causes uracil misincorporation into human DNA and chromosome breakage: implications for cancer and neuronal damage. *Proc Natl Acad Sci USA* **94**, 3290–3295.

Boekholdt, S.M., Meuwese, M.C., Day, N.E., *et al*. (2006) Plasma concentrations of ascorbic acid and C-reactive protein, and risk of future coronary artery disease, in apparently healthy men and women: the EPIC-Norfolk prospective population study. *Br J Nutr* **96**, 516–522.

Boushey, C.J., Beresford, S.A., Omenn, G.S., *et al*. (1995) A quantitative assessment of plasma homocysteine as a risk factor for vascular disease. Probable benefits of increasing folic acid intakes. *JAMA* **274**, 1049–1057.

Cahill, L.E. and El-Sohemy, A. (2009) Vitamin C transporter gene polymorphisms, dietary vitamin C and serum ascorbic acid. *J Nutrigenet Nutrigenomics* **2**, 292–301.

Cahill, L.E. and El-Sohemy, A. (2010) Haptoglobin genotype modifies the association between dietary vitamin C and serum ascorbic acid deficiency. *Am J Clin Nutr* **92**, 1494–1500.

Cahill, L.E., Fontaine-Bisson, B., El-Sohemy, A., *et al*. (2009) Functional genetic variants of glutathione S-transferase protect against serum ascorbic acid deficiency. *Am J Clin Nutr* **90**, 1411–1417.

Carmel, R., Sinow, R.M., and Carnaze, D.S. (1987) Atypical cobalamin deficiency. Subtle biochemical evidence of deficiency is commonly demonstrable in patients without megaloblastic anemia and is often associated with protein-bound cobalamin malabsorption. *J Lab Clin Med* **109**, 454–463.

Corella, D., Peloso, G., Arnett, D.K., *et al*. (2009) APOA2, dietary fat, and body mass index: replication of a gene-diet interaction in 3 independent populations. *Arch Intern Med* **169**, 1897–1906.

Corella, D., Tai, E.S., Sorlí, J.V., *et al*. (2011) Association between the APOA2 promoter polymorphism and body weight in Mediterranean and Asian populations: replication of a gene-saturated fat interaction. *Int J Obes (Lond)* **35**, 666–675.

Cornelis, M.C. and El-Sohemy, A. (2007) Coffee, caffeine, and coronary heart disease. *Curr Opin Lipidol* **18**, 13–19.

Cornelis, M.C., El-Sohemy, A., and Campos, H. (2007) Genetic polymorphism of the adenosine A2A receptor is associated with habitual caffeine consumption. *Am J Clin Nutr* **86,** 240–244.

Cornelis, M.C., El-Sohemy, A., Kabagambe, E.K., *et al.* (2006) Coffee, CYP1A2 genotype, and risk of myocardial infarction. *JAMA* **295,** 1135–1141.

Davey Smith, G. (2011) Use of genetic markers and gene–diet interactions for interrogating population-level causal influences of diet on health. *Genes Nutr* **6,** 27–43.

DeBusk, R. (2009) Diet-related disease, nutritional genomics, and food and nutrition professionals. *J Am Diet Assoc* **109,** 410–413.

El-Sohemy, A. (2007) Nutrigenetics. *Forum Nutr* **60,** 25–30.

Eny, K.M. and El-Sohemy, A. (2010) Genetic determinants of ingestive behaviour: sensory, energy homeostasis and food reward aspects of ingestive behaviour. In L. Dube, A. Bechara, A. Dagher, *et al.* (eds), *Obesity Prevention: The Role of Brain and Society on Individual Behavior.* Elsevier, New York, pp. 149–160.

Fischer, L.M., daCosta, K.A., Kwock, L., *et al.* (2007) Sex and menopausal status influence human dietary requirements for the nutrient choline. *Am J Clin Nutr* **85,** 1275–1285.

Fontaine-Bisson, B., Wolever, T.M., Connelly, P.W., *et al.* (2009) NF-kappaB -94Ins/Del ATTG polymorphism modifies the association between dietary polyunsaturated fatty acids and HDL-cholesterol in two distinct populations. *Atherosclerosis* **204,** 465–470.

Frosst, P., Blom, H.J., Milos, R., *et al.* (1995) A candidate genetic risk factor for vascular disease: a common mutation in methylenetetrahydrofolate reductase. *Nat Genet* **10,** 111–113.

Fu, L., Yun, F., Oczak, M., *et al.* (2009) Common genetic variants of the vitamin D binding protein (DBP) predict differences in response of serum 25-hydroxyvitamin D [25(OH)D] to vitamin D supplementation. *Clin Biochem* **42,** 1174–1177.

Garcia-Bailo, B., Toguri, C., Eny, K.M., *et al.* (2009) Genetic variation in taste and its influence on food selection. *OMICS* **13,** 69–80.

Hazra, A., Kraft, P., Selhub, J., *et al.* (2008) Common variants of FUT2 are associated with plasma vitamin B12 levels. *Nat Genet* **40,** 1160–1162.

Helgadottir, A., Manolescu, A., Helgason, A., *et al.* (2006) A variant of the gene encoding leukotriene A4 hydrolase confers ethnicity-specific risk of myocardial infarction. *Nat Genet* **38,** 68–74.

Ioannidis, J.P., Ntzani, E.E., Trikalinos, T.K., *et al.* (2001) Replication validity of genetic association studies. *Nat Genet* **29,** 306–309.

Jacob, R.A. and Sotoudeh, G. (2002) Vitamin C function and status in chronic disease. *Nutr Clin Care* **5,** 66–74.

Jiang, R., Hu, F.B., Giovannucci, E.L., *et al.* (2003) Joint association of alcohol and folate intake with risk of major chronic disease in women. *Am J Epidemiol* **158,** 760–771.

Kaput, J., Noble, J., Hatipoglu, B., *et al.* (2007) Application of nutrigenomic concepts to type 2 diabetes mellitus. *Nutr Metab Cardiovasc Dis* **17,** 89–103.

Kohlmeier, M., da Costa, K.A., Fischer, L.M., *et al.* (2005) Genetic variation of folate-mediated one-carbon transfer pathway predicts susceptibility to choline deficiency in humans. *Proc Natl Acad Sci USA* **102,** 16025–16030.

Kotsopoulos, J., Ghadirian, P., El Sohemy, A., *et al.* (2007) The CYP1A2 genotype modifies the association between coffee consumption and breast cancer risk among BRCA1 mutation carriers. *Cancer Epidemiol Biomarkers Prev* **16,** 912–916.

Levine, M., Conry-Cantilena, C.,Wang, Y., *et al.* (1996) Vitamin C pharmacokinetics in healthy volunteers: evidence for a recommended dietary allowance. *Proc Natl Acad Sci USA* **93,** 3704–3709.

Levy, H.L. (1989) Nutritional therapy for selected inborn errors of metabolism. *J Am Coll Nutr* **8,** 54S–60S.

Levy, S., Sutton, G., Ng, P.C., *et al.* (2007) The diploid genome sequence of an individual human. *PLoS Biol* **5,** e254.

Lindi, V., Schwab, U., Louheranta, A., *et al.* (2003) Impact of the Pro12Ala polymorphism of the PPAR-gamma2 gene on serum triacylglycerol response to n-3 fatty acid supplementation. *Mol Genet Metab* **79,** 52–60.

Loria, C.M., Whelton, P.K., Caulfield, L.E., *et al.* (1998) Agreement among indicators of vitamin C status. *Am J Epidemiol* **147,** 587–596.

Luan, J., Browne, P.O., Harding, A.H., *et al.* (2001) Evidence for gene-nutrient interaction at the PPARgamma locus. *Diabetes* **50,** 686–689.

Nkondjock, A., Ghadirian, P., Kotsopoulos, J., *et al.* (2006) Coffee consumption and breast cancer risk among BRCA1 and BRCA2 mutation carriers. *Int J Cancer* **118,** 103–107.

Ordovas, J.M. (2008) Genotype–phenotype associations: modulation by diet and obesity. *Obesity (Silver Spring)* **16** Suppl 3, S40–46.

Ordovas, J.M., Corella, D., Cupples, L.A., *et al.* (2002) Polyunsaturated fatty acids modulate the effects of the APOA1 G-A polymorphism on HDL-cholesterol concentrations in a sex-specific manner: the Framingham Study. *Am J Clin Nutr* **75,** 38–46.

Ordovas, J.M., Kaput, J., and Corella, D. (2007) Nutrition in the genomics era: cardiovascular disease risk and the Mediterranean diet. *Mol Nutr Food Res* **51,** 1293–1299.

Palatini, P., Ceolotto, G., Ragazzo, F., *et al.* (2009) CYP1A2 genotype modifies the association between coffee intake and the risk of hypertension. *J Hypertens* **27,** 1594–1601.

Paolisso, G., D'Amore, A., Balbi, V., et al. (1994) Plasma vitamin C affects glucose homeostasis in healthy subjects and in non-insulin-dependent diabetics. *Am J Physiol* **266,** E261–E268.

Plourde, M., Vohl, M.C., Vandal, M., et al. (2009) Plasma n-3 fatty acid response to an n-3 fatty acid supplement is modulated by apoE epsilon4 but not by the common PPAR-alpha L162V polymorphism in men. *Br J Nutr* **102,** 1121–1124.

Robitaille, J., Hamner, H.C., Cogswell, M.E., et al. (2009) Does the MTHFR 677C→T variant affect the Recommended Dietary Allowance for folate in the US population? *Am J Clin Nutr* **89,** 1269–1273.

Russo, G.L. (2009) Dietary n-6 and n-3 polyunsaturated fatty acids: from biochemistry to clinical implications in cardiovascular prevention. *Biochem Pharmacol* **77,** 937–946.

Sinclair, A.J., Taylor, P.B., Lunec, J., et al. (1994) Low plasma ascorbate levels in patients with type 2 diabetes mellitus consuming adequate dietary vitamin C. *Diabet Med* **11,** 893–898.

Sinotte, M., Diorio, C., Bérubé, S., et al. (2009) Genetic polymorphisms of the vitamin D binding protein and plasma concentrations of 25-hydroxyvitamin D in premenopausal women. *Am J Clin Nutr* **89,** 634–640.

Smith, A.D., Kim, Y.I., and Refsum, H. (2008) Is folic acid good for everyone? *Am J Clin Nutr* **87,** 517–533.

Swagerty, D.L., Jr, Walling, A.D., and Klein, R.M. (2002) Lactose intolerance. *Am Fam Physician* **65,** 1845–1850.

Swallow, D.M. (2003) Genetics of lactase persistence and lactose intolerance. *Annu Rev Genet* **37,** 197–219.

Tanner, S.M., Li, Z., Bisson, R., et al. (2004) Genetically heterogeneous selective intestinal malabsorption of vitamin B12: founder effects, consanguinity, and high clinical awareness explain aggregations in Scandinavia and the Middle East. *Hum Mutat* **23,** 327–333.

Thorisson, G.A. and Stein, L.D. (2003) The SNP Consortium website: past, present and future. *Nucleic Acids Res* **31,** 124–127.

van Ommen, B., El-Sohemy, A., Hesketh, J., et al. (2010) The Micronutrient Genomics Project: a community-driven knowledge base for micronutrient research. *Genes Nutr* **5,** 285–296.

Wang, T.J., Zhang, F., Richards, J.B., et al. (2010) Common genetic determinants of vitamin D insufficiency: a genome-wide association study. *Lancet* **376,** 180–188.

Watanabe, F. (2007) Vitamin B12 sources and bioavailability. *Exp Biol Med (Maywood)* **232,** 1266–1274.

Wijendran, V. and Hayes, K.C. (2004) Dietary n-6 and n-3 fatty acid balance and cardiovascular health. *Annu Rev Nutr* **24,** 597–615.

Wolfrom, D.M., Rao, A.R., and Welsch, C.W. (1991) Caffeine inhibits development of benign mammary gland tumors in carcinogen-treated female Sprague-Dawley rats. *Breast Cancer Res Treat* **19,** 269–275.

Yang, H., Rouse, J., Lukes, L., et al. (2004) Caffeine suppresses metastasis in a transgenic mouse model: a prototype molecule for prophylaxis of metastasis. *Clin Exp Metastasis* **21,** 719–735.

Zeisel, S.H. (2007) Nutrigenomics and metabolomics will change clinical nutrition and public health practice: insights from studies on dietary requirements for choline. *Am J Clin Nutr* **86,** 542–548.

4

METABOLOMICS

THOMAS M. O'CONNELL[1], PhD AND WEI JIA[2], PhD

[1]*LiposScience Inc., Raleigh, North Carolina, USA*
[2]*University of North Carolina at Greensboro, Kannapolis, North Carolina, USA*

Summary

As the goal of genomics is to study all of our genes, the goal of metabolomics is to profile the entire complement of the small molecules that are involved in processes from signaling to transcription, from building proteins, to creating and shuttling energy. This chapter describes the challenges of nutritional metabolomics along with the current ways that nutrition scientists can overcome these challenges to gain more insights into the downstream metabolic effects of nutrition. Metabolomic applications in nutritional research are growing rapidly, primarily because metabolomics and nutrition address the same questions in metabolism, metabolic perturbations, oxidation, and inflammation as primary processes that maintain human health. Analytical and profiling techniques in metabolomics also are evolving rapidly, and the analytical platforms currently employed in metabolomic studies are summarized in this chapter along with the required data processing software. The examples provided in this chapter demonstrate that metabolomics is playing an increasingly important role in nutritional research, serving as a dietary assessment tool, a predictive tool for nutritional effects (nutrimetabonomics) and an epidemiological profiling tool, all of which involve gut microbial–mammalian co-metabolism.

Introduction

The genome is often referred to as the blueprint of what can happen in our bodies. Pushing this analogy further would suggest that the proteome describes the tools that make things happen and the metabolome would be the end result of that work. The interrelationships of these three components are shown in Figure 4.1. The small molecules that compose the metabolome do much of the work in our bodies from signaling transcription to building proteins to creating and shuttling energy. As the goal of genomics is to study all of our genes, so the goal of metabolomics is to profile the entire complement of the small-molecule metabolites in our bodies. Numerous definitions for metabolomics can be found in the literature, but one of the simplest and most succinct is "the comprehensive and quantitative analysis of all metabolites" (Fiehn, 2001). Note that this area of research is sometimes referred to as metabonomics and these terms have become interchangeable. There is a similarly large number of definitions of what constitutes a metabolite. In the broadest sense, total metabolite pool, or metabolome, includes the

Present Knowledge in Nutrition, Tenth Edition. Edited by John W. Erdman Jr, Ian A. Macdonald and Steven H. Zeisel.
© 2012 International Life Sciences Institute. Published 2012 by John Wiley & Sons, Inc.

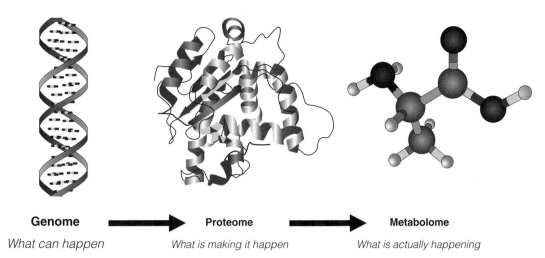

Genome	Proteome	Metabolome
What can happen	*What is making it happen*	*What is actually happening*

FIG. 4.1 Relationship between the genome, proteome, and metabolome.

complete complement of endogenous metabolites as well as metabolites derived from diet, medication, environmental exposures, and the gut microbiome (Dunn, 2008). Estimates of the size of the metabolome are also subject to debate, with estimates exceeding 10 000 if dietary components and all combinatorial possibilities of long chain fatty acids are considered. The Human Metabolome Database has been described as the blueprint of the human metabolome, in a fashion analogous to the Human Genome Project (Wishart *et al.*, 2009). This database currently consists of extensive clinical and chemical data for over 7900 compounds (HMDB version 2.5).

Being the newest of the post-genomics technologies, metabolomics is in a rapid growth phase. Figure 4.2 (left) shows the number of publications over the last 10 years in genomics, proteomics, and metabolomics. The earliest work in metabolomics focused heavily on toxicology studies. The development of metabolomics in this area is the subject of an excellent review by Robertson *et al.* (2011). Nutrition scientists realized the potential for metabolomics somewhat later. Figure 4.2 (right) compares the growth of the overall field of metabolomics with the applications specifically in the area of nutrition. Part of this delay may be due to the fact that nutritional interventions are almost always going to be more subtle, yielding smaller metabolic perturbations than pharmaceutical interventions. As the technologies used to profile the metabolome have matured, the ability to detect more subtle perturbations above the standard variability that is expected in the human population has increased. In this chapter the challenges of nutritional metabolomics will be described along with current ways in which nutritional scientists can overcome these challenges to gain more details of the downstream metabolic effects of nutrition.

Measuring the Metabolome

The vast chemical diversity of the metabolome presents a tremendous challenge when the goal is to provide an unbiased and quantitative measurement of all of it. The concentration ranges of metabolites span over a dozen orders of magnitude with compounds such as glucose in the millimolar range in blood, and compounds such as some eicosanoids down in the femtomolar range. The differences in size and polarity also present challenges for different platforms. No single analytical platform can measure the entire metabolome, so metabolomics studies need to select the optimal technology or combination of technologies to maximize the coverage.

The approaches to metabolomics can be broadly divided into three areas: fingerprinting, untargeted analysis, and targeted analysis. The selection of the approach depends upon the nature of the question and the goals of the study. The goal of metabolic fingerprinting is to look for spectroscopic signatures that distinguish one group from another. Insights into mechanisms of disease or toxicity are not sought in these studies. This is often the first step in metabolomics investigations, and ensures that the biological matrix being studied (e.g. plasma, urine, saliva, etc.) contains enough information to discriminate the different groups.

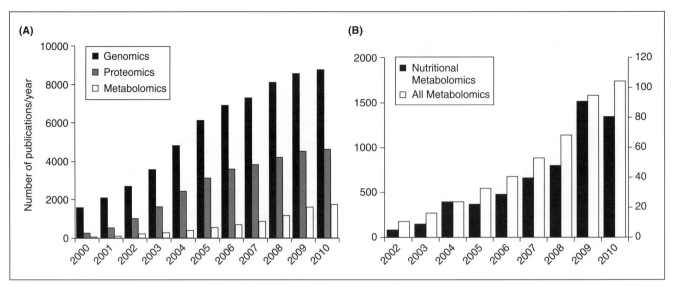

FIG. 4.2 Growth in omics publications. (A) The growth in genomics, proteomics, and metabolomics over the last decade. (B) Comparison of the growth of metabolomics and those metabolomics studies focusing on nutrition. These data were collected by PubMed searches by year using keywords: (genomics), (proteomics) and (metabolomics OR metabonomics OR metabolic profiling). The nutritional metabolomics studies were determined by appending (AND nutrition) to the last search term.

Untargeted metabolomics, sometimes called global metabolomics, seeks a comprehensive snapshot of as much of the metabolome as possible. This is a discovery approach in which new hypotheses on biochemical mechanisms of action are sought. It is critical in these studies to actually identify the metabolites that are perturbed in the study. Annotation of the spectra with specific metabolite names is a major emphasis for these studies. These metabolite changes can then be translated into perturbations in metabolic pathways. In this manner, untargeted metabolomics can confirm the involvement of metabolic pathways or suggest new ones.

Targeted metabolomics studies start with an initial hypothesis and focus on specific sets of metabolites that are quantitatively profiled. These studies typically contain panels of metabolites from selected chemical classes such as amino acids, acylcarnitines, or fatty acids. These panels are designed to reveal perturbations in suspected biochemical pathways. For example, acylcarnitine panels have been shown to correlate with changes in the extent of β-oxidation (Van Hove *et al.*, 1993). Panels of organic acids can reflect specific changes in tricarboxylic acid cycle functioning. Each of these approaches has its own value, and investigations can progress through each type as shown in Figure 4.3.

The workflow of a metabolomics investigation can be described as follows. The first step is to ensure that the groups (e.g. control and treated) can indeed be separated based on spectroscopic signatures. The next step is to annotate the signatures with specific metabolite names. Through this process specific metabolic pathways are implicated and new hypotheses may be generated. The untargeted approach may not yield enough detail on a specific pathway to make unequivocal conclusions about specific pathways, but may suggest specific metabolite classes that warrant further investigation. Targeted panels of metabolites are then specifically measured to test the new hypotheses generated in the untargeted approach. If the hypothesis is confirmed, then a set of mechanistically based biomarkers has been found. If not, the process can cycle back to the untargeted analysis state where the data can be re-interrogated or additional analyses with other analytical platforms to increase the metabolome coverage can be carried out.

Analytical Technologies

A wide variety of spectroscopic platforms have been applied to metabolomics including infrared (IR) spectroscopy, nuclear magnetic resonance (NMR) spectroscopy, and

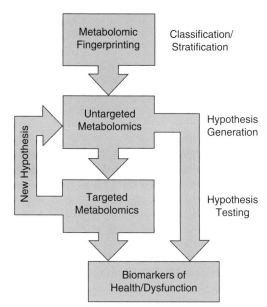

FIG. 4.3 Process of metabolomics investigations. Once the fingerprinting step has confirmed that a metabolic effect can be detected, the untargeted metabolomics approach is used to generate new hypotheses. The results can confirm this hypothesis or suggest a new one that may be further tested with a targeted metabolomics approach. The results of the targeted approach can confirm the hypothesis, or the process can cycle back to another round of untargeted metabolite analyses.

mass spectrometry (MS), often coupled with various chromatographic separation methods. Details on these methods are well described in numerous reviews and books (Robertson *et al.*, 2005; Vaidyanathan *et al.*, 2005). As the field has matured, two spectroscopic techniques, NMR and MS, have become the dominant platforms for metabolomics. Each of these platforms has its own set of advantages and disadvantages with the critical characteristics revolving around sensitivity, specificity, reproducibility, quantitation, and information content. Table 4.1 summarizes some of the key features of both technologies.

Nuclear Magnetic Resonance Spectroscopy

Most of the early work in metabolomics was based on NMR spectroscopy, and this work has been summarized in a number of excellent reviews (Reily and Lindon, 2005; Daykin and Wulfert, 2006; Ala-Korpela, 2008). NMR has long been a primary method for organic compound structure elucidation. When applied to complex mixtures, the

high information content, quantitative signal intensities, and very large linear dynamic range ($>10^5$) make it ideal for global metabolomics studies. High reproducibility, both inter- and intra-laboratory, make it well suited for large-scale metabolomics studies (Dumas *et al.*, 2006). The NMR instrumentation is highly stable, which ensures that spectra can be acquired over a long period of time with no instrumental batch effect. Samples for untargeted NMR analysis require minimal preparation. Urine and serum samples are typically prepared with the addition of a small amount of buffer containing a chemical shift and quantitation standard (Beckonert *et al.*, 2007). No chromatographic separation is required, which eliminates one source of potential metabolite loss and analytical variability. The non-destructive nature of NMR makes it possible to acquire spectra on samples and subsequently forward them on to mass spectrometry for further targeted or untargeted analyses.

The main drawback of NMR is the relatively low sensitivity. Metabolite concentrations must typically be at least in the low micromolar range in order to detect enough signal for structure elucidation and quantitation. Several avenues of development are improving the sensitivity of NMR. Increasing the magnetic field strength provides increases in sensitivity, and in 2010 the 1-GHz barrier was broken (Bhattacharya, 2010). Note that NMR spectroscopists refer to the strength of NMR magnets by the corresponding proton resonance frequency, rather than the actual unit of magnetic fields, the Tesla. A 14-Tesla magnet would be referred to as a 600-MHz magnet. Higher-field systems provide a linear increase in resolution but the sensitivity increases as $B_0^{3/2}$ (B_0 = field strength). Thus a 900-MHz magnet provides a less than two-fold increase in sensitivity over a more routine 600-MHz magnet, yet the cost of the ultra high field systems can be up to an order of magnitude greater. Ultra low temperature detection probes ("cryo-probes") can provide an increase of up to three- to four-fold in signal intensity by decreasing the noise from the electronic circuitry (Logan *et al.*, 1999). Micro-coil NMR probes in which samples can be concentrated down to volumes as low as 10 μL have been applied to metabolomics to provide added sensitivity (Grimes and O'Connell, 2011).

Most commonly, proton (^{1}H) NMR spectra are collected in metabolomics investigations due to the ubiquity of protons in metabolites and the high sensitivity.

An example of a ^{1}H NMR spectrum of healthy human urine and serum is shown in Figure 4.4. These spectra were

TABLE 4.1   Analytical features of NMR and mass spectrometry for metabolomics

	NMR	Mass spectrometry
Sample preparation	No sample preparation required Non-destructive	Extraction and deproteinization Chemical derivatization for GC–MS
Experiment time	^{1}H spectra in 5–20 minutes depending upon field strength and sample size	Typically ~ 30 minutes for GC–MS A few minutes with UPLC–MS; up to an hour with standard HPLC–MS methods
Sensitivity	m-molar to μ-molar	p-molar to f-molar
Sample requirements	Typically 100 μL for standard probe μ-coil probes allows for volumes of <10 μL	Typically 100 μL or more to allow for sample processing and preparation of replicates
Quantitation	Signals are inherently quantitative without the need for standards Highly reproducible within and across laboratories	Quantitation is achieved with reference standards Accurate, reproducible quantitation can be achieved with isotope-labeled chemical standards
Metabolome coverage	Thousands of metabolite signals detected No inherent compound bias although long-chain aliphatics (e.g. fatty acids) not well resolved Targeted approach can detect/ quantify higher concentration metabolites without standards	Thousands of metabolite signals detected High-polarity, differing ionization efficiencies and lack of volatility can hinder detection of various compounds Targeted approach detects/ quantifies specific sets of metabolites with chemical standards
Structure identification	Spectra have high structural information content Spectral libraries available for hundreds of compounds	Extensive GC–MS libraries available for structure identification (thousands of compounds) Fragmentation patterns aid in structure identification

collected on a typical "workhorse" 600-MHz NMR spectrometer in about 10 minutes. Unlike mass spectrometry, in which each peak represents a single chemical entity, e.g. a metabolite or metabolite adduct, in the NMR spectrum each peak represents a part of a metabolite, e.g. a methyl group or proton on an aromatic ring. Most metabolites are composed of several sets of peaks which, taken together, can provide structural information and unique evidence of identity. The drawback is that, with hundreds of metabolites each contributing multiple peaks, the spectra can be very crowded and overlapping, thereby hindering interpretation. As mentioned above, higher field magnets can reduce this spectral overlap, but this is an expensive solution that is often unavailable. Advanced experiments, including two-dimensional and multinuclear experiments,

spread the peaks out into a second dimension based on their ^{1}H or ^{13}C chemical shifts (Gronwald *et al.*, 2008; Xi *et al.*, 2008; Rai *et al.*, 2009; Ludwig and Viant, 2010). This orthogonal axis separates the signals in a manner analogous to two-dimensional chromatographic methods. These experiments can come at a significant cost in time and therefore are typically run on selected samples to aid in metabolite identification.

Mass Spectrometry

The use of mass spectrometry in metabolomics has increased dramatically in the last decade. Mass spectrometry measures the mass-to-charge ratio of charged particles and offers qualitative and quantitative analyses of metabolites with very high selectivity and sensitivity. The high

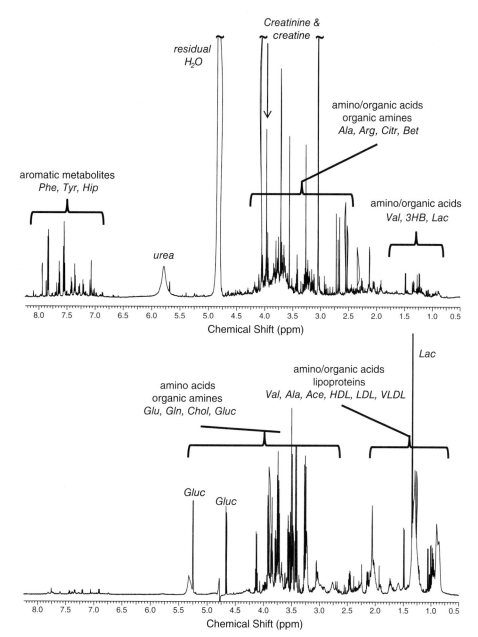

FIG. 4.4 The 600-MHz NMR spectrum of human urine (top) and serum (bottom) with some annotations of the metabolites that are seen in different spectral regions.

sensitivity enables the measurement of compounds at very low levels (down to femtomole) and can, with the right instrumentation and experiments, provide structural details (Want *et al.*, 2005). Although direct injection of complex mixtures into the MS has been carried out in metabolomics studies, various chromatographic methods are usually incorporated (Bedair and Sumner, 2008). Coupling of high resolution separations such as capillary

electrophoresis (CE), gas chromatography (GC), and liquid chromatography (LC) methods including high-performance liquid chromatography (HPLC) and ultra-performance liquid chromatography (UPLC) offers substantial enhancement in metabolome coverage.

Achieving fully quantitative results with mass spectrometry can be challenging due to the issue of ion suppression. The efficiency of generating a charge on a molecule is influenced by the other compounds in the source at that time. The chromatographic methods listed above greatly improve the problems of ion suppression by limiting the types of compound that are in the source at any given time. In this way, the efficiency of ionization of a compound will be much less variable over a large sample set. Fully quantitative results can be reliably achieved with the use of isotopically labeled standards as reviewed by Rychlik and Asam (2008).

GC–MS is one of the most widely used analytical techniques in metabolomics (Dettmer *et al.*, 2007). The typical GC–MS platforms used in metabolomics have very high analytical reproducibility and are relatively low cost compared with NMR or some of the other MS platforms. GC–MS is used to analyze volatile compounds or those compounds that can be made to be volatile through well established chemical derivatization protocols. A major prerequisite for GC–MS analysis is a sufficient vapor pressure and thermal stability of the analytes. The analysis of polar metabolites usually requires derivatization at the functional groups to reduce polarity and increase thermal stability and volatility. GC is traditionally coupled to quadrupole MS, which provides high sensitivity and large dynamic range, but relatively slow scan speeds. Recently, more advanced instrumentation such as GC time-of-flight MS (TOF–MS) and GC × GC TOF–MS are becoming more popular for metabolite profiling due to their higher mass accuracy and mass resolution relative to the quadrupole MS systems (Pasikanti *et al.*, 2008). With GC–MS,

universal electron ionization (EI) is most often used, providing a platform for the identification of characteristic and reproducible metabolite markers.

The application of LC–MS in metabolomics has been growing rapidly over the past few years. LC is a more universal separation technique that can be utilized in a non-targeted manner or tailored for the targeted analysis of specific metabolite groups. As mentioned earlier, LC can reduce the ion suppression that can occur with co-eluting compounds. The chromatographic retention time is a function of the polarity of the compound and can also yield useful structural information. For example, isobaric compounds (i.e. having the exact same molecular formula) may yield an identical mass spectrum, but the retention time can be taken into account to help decide which peak belongs to which isobaric metabolite.

MS-based metabolomics usually require a sample preparation or pretreatment step, which can be labor intensive and possibly cause metabolite losses (Bruce *et al.*, 2009). Metabolites of interest in different chemical classes may be discriminated depending on the analytical platforms used (Figure 4.5). Examples of GC–TOF–MS and UPLC–QTOF–MS spectra of healthy human urine are shown in Figure 4.6.

Statistical Analyses

Metabolomics datasets typically contain a large number of highly complex spectra, and the first step in deriving useful information from this abundance of data involves pattern

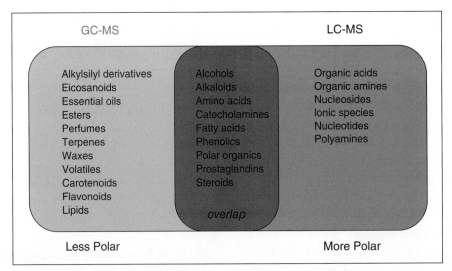

FIG. 4.5 Classes of chemicals and the analytical techniques with which they are most compatible (Agilent application note 5989-6328EN, 2007).

(A)

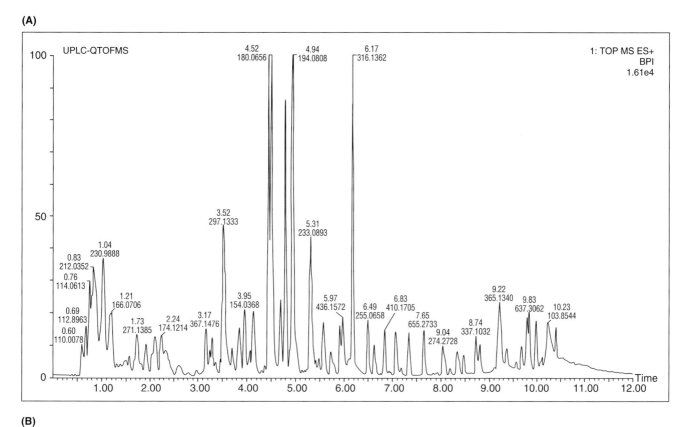

(B)

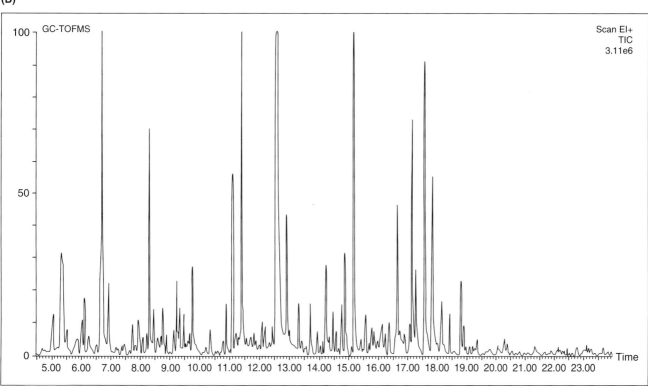

FIG. 4.6   GC–TOF–MS and UPLC–QTOF–MS spectra of human urine. (A) The total ion current (TIC) chromatogram of GC–TOF–MS collected on an Agilent 6890N gas chromatograph coupled with a Leco Pegasus HT
time-of-flight mass spectrometer. It represents the summed intensity across the entire range of masses (m/z
30–600) being detected in a 24-minute run. (B) The base peak intensity chromatogram (BPI) of UPLC–QTOF–
MS. This chromatogram was collected on a Waters ACQUITY Ultra performance liquid chromatograph coupled
with a Waters Q-TOF micro MS in about 12 minutes.

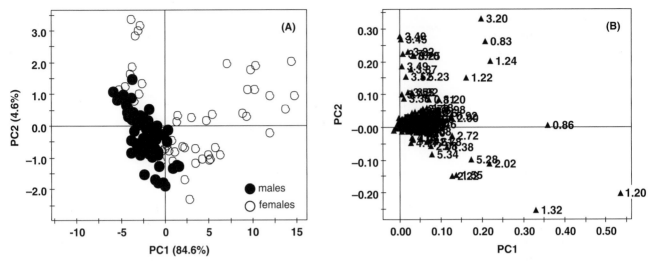

FIG. 4.7   Principal components analysis of serum from healthy adult males and females. (A) The scores plot maps the spectrum of each individual subject. The major axis of separation of the males and females is along the first principal component which explains 84.6% of the variation in the data. The second principal component accounts for only 4.6% of the remaining variation in the data and could be related to factors such as age, ethnicity or BMI. (B) The loadings plot indicates which spectral variables are most influential for each principal component. The features near the zero crossing are not related to the gender difference, but those peaks at the far right, e.g. 1.20, 1.323, and 0.86, are very influential in discriminating males from females. These peaks correspond to some of the major lipid/lipoprotein component in the serum.

recognition and multivariate statistical analysis. The simplest and most common statistical method is principal components analysis (PCA). This method aims to simplify the dataset by combining variables (such as spectral peaks from NMR or MS) that are correlated in order to reduce the dimensionality of the data. The end result is the reduction of the dataset from potentially thousands of spectral features to a small number (often less than 10) of linear combinations of variables that still explain the majority of the data.

Figure 4.7 shows a PCA analysis separating healthy males from females in a controlled dietary standardization study. Figure 4.7A is the scores plot in which each point represents a subject (actually the NMR spectrum of the serum of one subject). The separation of males and females is observed based on the entirety of their metabolic signatures. Figure 4.7B shows the corresponding loadings plot in which the critical features of the spectra which discriminate males from females are highlighted. The spectral features clustered around the zero crossing of the axes are those that are not significantly different between the groups, but the features at the edges of the plot, i.e. the "highly loaded" features, are significantly different. These

features comprise the unique spectroscopic features of males and females. In a typical metabolomics investigation, the next step after PCA analysis is to go back to the spectra and identify the metabolites corresponding to the highly loaded variables.

The PCA method is termed "unsupervised" as no information regarding the classification of the samples is input into the model. In this manner, all of the variation in the data is explained. Often the main source of variation may not be related to the focus of the study, e.g. nutritional intervention, but may be age, gender, or other such confounding factors. PCA is a valuable way to detect outliers in a sample set from biological or analytical variation, and is a routine, first-pass analysis in most metabolomics investigations.

A wide array of more advanced statistical methods have been developed and applied to extract information from rich metabolomics datasets (Waterman *et al.*, 2009; Madsen *et al.*, 2010). Methods such as partial least squares (PLS) analyses and orthogonal partial least squares discriminant analysis (OPLS–DA) methods are a frequent next step after PCA analysis. Note that PLS methods are also referred to as projection to latent structures with the same acronym. These methods are "supervised" in that the class membership (i.e. control versus treated) is input into the model. Unlike PCA, the goal is no longer to explain all of the variation in the data; with supervised analyses, the goal is to explain only the variation that is correlated to a classification. This is often a binary variable such as control versus treated or it can be a continuous variable such as a body mass index (BMI), age, or variable exposure to a food or toxin.

In the ever expanding arsenal of multivariate statistical methods, techniques such as linear discriminant analysis, support vector machines, and random forests are playing an increasing role. Recently the performance of these methods was compared with PLS in an untargeted GC–MS dataset. The performance characteristics, including accuracy, predictive capacity, stability, degree of over-fitting, and consistency in variable ranking were evaluated. In this study the performance of the random forests method was found to be superior. Currently the choice of which statistical method to employ in a metabolomics study is influenced by the sophistication of the bioinformatics group participating in the project and the availability and ease of use of statistical software packages to apply these methods. This recent comparison indicates that, as software packages mature, the statistical analyses available for routine use will continue to grow.

Stability of the Human Metabolome

When studying the potentially subtle effects of nutritional interventions, the stability of the human metabolome must be considered. Factors such as genetics, diet, age, gut microflora, and environmental factors can all contribute to the day-to-day as well as long-term stability in the human metabolome (Bictash et al., 2010). Numerous studies have been conducted to determine the metabolic signatures related to these potentially confounding influences. In a review by Bollard and co-workers, the intrinsic factors (species, strain, age, and hormonal effects) and extrinsic factors (diurnal effects, diet, stress, and gut microflora) were examined in animal models for their influence on the composition of the urinary metabolome (Bollard et al., 2005). In a study of healthy humans, Kochhar et al. (2006) demonstrated clear metabolic signatures that discriminated subjects based on age, gender, and BMI.

It is not surprising that each person's metabolome is different, but how distinct are our individual metabo-lomes? In a large-scale, longitudinal study, Assfalg et al. (2008) showed that a sophisticated statistical analysis of human urine samples contained an invariant part of the metabolome that is characteristic of each individual. A subsequent study by the same group demonstrated that these individual metabolic features were stable over the course of several years (Bernini et al., 2009). It was proposed that this metabolic phenotype be considered a metagenomic entity that is influenced by both the gut microbiome and the host metabolic phenotype.

Normalizing the Human Metabolome with Diet

Above the invariant core there still remain a large number of highly variable components of the metabolome so the challenge in clinical studies is to find ways to minimize these. The application of standardized diets has been investigated for their potential to normalize the metabolomes in subjects. In a study by Walsh et al. (2006), urine, serum, and saliva were collected from 30 healthy human subjects once per week over 4 weeks. For the first two study days, free food choice was allowed on the day before the visit. The third visit was meant to mimic the second visit and the subjects were instructed to eat as they had done on the day before the second visit. On the day before the last visit, all subjects consumed the same standardized meals. Above the considerable intra- and inter-subject variability, it was found that the standardized meal provided a detectable decrease in the variability of the urine samples. No normalization was observed with the plasma or saliva. The urine samples in this study were first void and evening collections. This study suggests that the urinary metabolome is a sensitive reflection of acute dietary intake whereas plasma and saliva are not.

In another study of the effects of an acute dietary intervention, Lenz et al. (2003) studied the urinary and plasma metabolome of subjects on two days, 14 days apart. In this study, serum samples were collected as well as first-void, 0–12 hours and 12–24 hours urine samples. The subjects were fed a standardized diet on the collection days. In the plasma there was relatively little variability between subjects and study days. Considerable inter-subject variability was found with the urine samples, but less intra-subject variability. This is consistent with the individuality of the urinary metabolome. The most significant finding of this study was that the first-void urines showed considerably greater diversity than the 0–12 hours and 12–24 hours collections. It seems that the first-void diversity may be more susceptible to variations from diet and lifestyle differences.

Acute dietary interventions appear to confer some normalizing effect on the urinary metabolome, but could this effect be enhanced with a more prolonged dietary intervention? In the study by Winnike et al. (2009) a group of 10 healthy human subjects was admitted to a clinical research center for 2 weeks and received a standardized whole-food diet. Pooled 24-hour urine samples were collected daily throughout the study. Daily overnight fasted serum samples were collected as well as on a single return visit 2 weeks after the study. The urinary metabolome of all of the subjects showed considerable inter-subject variability, consistent with the studies by Walsh et al. (2006) and Lenz et al. (2003). In contrast, the standardized diet appeared to provide no normalization over the course of the study. Each subject remained in their individual "metabolic space" for the 2-week period. The lack of an effect from the imposition of this standardized diet may be due to the fact that 24-hour urine samples were collected in this study. This would indicate that acute dietary interventions may be detectable in single collections such a first void, but that these differences are literally diluted out in the 24-hour collections.

The serum metabolome of the acute intervention studies indicated that no normalization could be detected. In the prolonged standardized diet, a distinct difference was observed in about half of the subjects in the first day and/ or the 2-week follow-up. There are two possible reasons why this effect was seen in this study and not in the others. First, by extending the dietary standardization, a clearer picture of each person's metabolic space was obtained and therefore the outlier days are more distinct. Secondly, the more stringent dietary and environmental controls in this inpatient clinical setting may have created a new homeostasis in the serum metabolome, giving rise to detectable differences from the free-living metabolome. Taken together, these studies indicate that a standardized meal prior to the start of a study may provide some detectable decrease in the urinary and serum metabolome, but extended normalization does not provide a progressive decrease in variation.

Metabolomics as a Dietary Assessment Tool

The accurate measurement of dietary intake is essential to understanding how diet relates to disease development and prevention. Conventional tools for collecting quantitative information on dietary intake include food frequency questionnaires (FFQ), dietary recalls, and diet diaries. These methods are subject to significant random and systematic errors. Bingham et al. (1994, 1997) investigated the accuracy of several dietary assessment methods by comparing weighed food records, FFQs, 24-hour recall, and a 7-day food diary. The results showed that the FFQ tended to overestimate almost all intake, the 24-hour recall underestimated carbohydrates, vitamin C, and alcohol intake, and the food diary over-estimated fat intake but underestimated carbohydrate and calcium intake. These errors clearly confound any comparison of results from nutritional studies utilizing different methods.

To overcome the problems associated with self-reporting methods, a number of targeted biomarkers have been developed which indicate consumption of particular foods or food groups. One such biomarker is urinary potassium to measure potassium intake (Bingham, 2002). The correlations between consumption and excretion have been demonstrated to be at least 0.7, but 24-hour urine collections are required which are more difficult to collect in a non-clinical setting. Total protein intake has been correlated with urinary nitrogen output, but again requiring 24-hour urine collections. The serum level of pentadecanoic acid (C15:0) has been shown to have a strong correlation with the intake of fats from milk or dairy products (Smedman et al., 1999). These individual markers for specific dietary components are very valuable, but less subjective and more comprehensive tools are needed to evaluate dietary exposures.

Metabolomics holds great promise as a tool to provide comprehensive assessments of the dietary intake in humans. When food is consumed, the chemical components of the food, i.e. the food metabolome, are absorbed either directly or after digestion, followed by biotransformations in the gastrointestinal tract (including the microbiome) and/or liver, and are then detectable either in the serum or urine. This interrelationship between the mammalian, microbial, and food metabolomics is diagrammed in Figure 4.8. The search for potential biomarkers of exposure has been described as "top-down" indicating that specific components of the food metabolome are sought in the biofluids (Mennen et al., 2006; Jenab et al., 2009). This targeted approach has been successfully applied to a number of foods, but kinetics of biological processing and excretion can make some specific biomarkers more challenging to detect (Fave et al., 2009; Manach et al., 2009; Scalbert

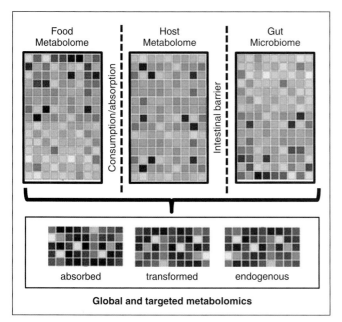

Food
Metabolome

Consumption/absorption

Host
Metabolome

Intestinal barrier

Gut
Microbiome

absorbed   transformed   endogenous

Global and targeted metabolomics

FIG. 4.8 Interactions of the host–food–microbial metabolomics to generate new metabolite signatures of consumption, absorption, transformation, and metabolism.

et al., 2009; Primrose *et al.*, 2011). The other approach, termed "bottom-up" involves the application of global metabolic profiling. The advantage of the latter approach is that no assumptions of the processing of the food metabolome are necessary. Experience in this area has shown that biomarkers found in the bottom-up approach are often unexpected, based on incomplete knowledge of the food metabolome and the subsequent absorption and biotransformation.

A large-scale study of the potential of global metabolomics to reveal biomarkers of food exposure is underway in the MEtabolomics to characterize Dietary Exposure (MEDE) study (Primrose *et al.*, 2011). In this study each subject received a standard dinner and subsequent breakfast on two occasions. In the test breakfast, one component of the standard breakfast (cornflakes and milk) was replaced with one of four foods of significant public health interest: broccoli (a cruciferous vegetable), smoked salmon (an oily fish), raspberries (berry fruit), and whole-wheat biscuit (whole-grain cereal). Fasting and postprandial changes in the urine were detected in all subjects. It was determined that urine and plasma samples collected 3 hours after test meals were the most informative about recent dietary intake. A consistent set of metabolites was

always highly ranked in the metabolome after the test breakfast, allowing these metabolites to be filtered from the data and enabling easier detection of the metabolites associated with the test foods. The results of this study identified putative biomarkers for several of the breakfast components including orange juice, raspberries, smoked salmon, and broccoli.

One finding of particular interest in this study involved the discrimination of which subjects consumed the cornflakes versus the whole-wheat biscuit. When all subjects were analyzed together, no robust discrimination from these two dietary components could be found. When a subset of subjects with similar overall metabolite profiles were examined, however, a good separation based on these two breakfast components could be achieved. It appears that the inter-subject differences initially overshadowed the more subtle dietary effect, but, by considering a more homogeneous subset of subjects based on their overall metabotype, this difference was revealed.

The search for dietary biomarkers is not limited to just acute exposure studies, but also includes biomarkers that indicate that the habitual intake patterns will also be very valuable. In a study by O'Sullivan *et al.* (2011), the urinary and serum metabolomes of 125 free-living subjects were analyzed. Dietary intakes were assessed by the use of 3-day estimated food records, completed at week 2 of the 3-week study. Individual foods and ingredients were aggregated into 33 groups based on cluster analysis of the dietary patterns in the Irish population in this study (Hearty and Gibney, 2009). Some food groups were comprised of single foods such as eggs, potatoes, and alcohol. Others were more general such as vegetables, poultry dishes, and confectionery. Cluster analysis of the data revealed three dietary patterns that distinctly influenced the total energy intake of each group. The first cluster was characterized by a high contribution from wholemeal bread, whole milk, fish, confectionery, and ice cream and desserts. This cluster had a lower contribution from low-energy beverages (e.g. water, tea, and sugar-free soft drinks). Cluster two had a high contribution from low-fat milk, yogurt, fruit, poultry, and sauces, and a low contribution from high-energy beverages (e.g. fruit-based concentrate drinks and soft drinks). Cluster three was considered the least healthy and contained higher concentrations of white bread, red meat and red-meat dishes, meat products, and alcohol, and had a lower contribution from vegetables. These dietary patterns were significantly different with respect to sex, but no discrimination could be made based on age or BMI.

In order to interrogate the specific metabolic differences between these groups, PLS–DA models were created for each pairing of the groups. The most significant model was the comparison of groups one and three. These clusters had the highest and lowest intakes of nine different food groups. The concentrations of glycine, phenylacetylglutamine, and acetoacetate were all higher in cluster one, whereas trimethylamine N-oxide (TMAO), O-acylcarnitine, and n,n-dimethylglycine were higher in cluster three. Further linear regression analysis revealed that the phenylacetylglutamine was positively correlated to vegetable consumption. A positive correlation between O-acylcarnitine and red-meat intake was found. This study demonstrated the ability of metabolomics to discriminate distinct dietary patterns in free-living adults and derive biomarkers for some critical components of those dietary patterns.

The controls imposed in a clinical setting can be very insightful, but the metabolic perturbations observed under those strictly controlled conditions may not be detectable in a free-living environment. Conversely, the large variation in the diets in free-living conditions may mask many important perturbations. One clever intermediate study design that can be implemented in long-term studies and mimics free-living conditions involves the "supermarket model" (Skov *et al.*, 1997; Rasmussen *et al.*, 2007; Bladbjerg *et al.*, 2010). In these studies, all participants obtained their food from a purpose-built shop stocked with all of the nutritional needs of the participants. Food items were selected by the participants *ad libitum* within the frame of the dietary design and the individual shopping selections were recorded in a specially designed computerized system. The supermarket method has been utilized in a number of long-term (up to 6 months) nutritional intervention studies to examine the effects of various fats and carbohydrates on weight loss, cardiovascular disease, and diabetes (Due *et al.*, 2008a,b). The model has significant potential to provide an intermediate level of control for large-scale, long-term metabolomics investigations.

Epidemiological Scale Metabolomics

Metabolomics will play an increasingly important role in responding to the challenges of population health and well being in the future. These epidemiological metabolomics studies are now possible with the advent of high-throughput, high-sensitivity methods that require minimal sample volumes and preparation. One of the critical challenges of metabolomics across populations is to understand the differences in the metabotypes that arise from cultural and environmental factors. One of the earliest untargeted metabolomics studies to examine the baseline metabolome differences in different countries was published by Zuppi *et al.* (1998). In this study, urine samples from 25 healthy subjects living in Rome were compared with an age- and gender-matched group living in Svaldbard in the Arctic region of northern Norway. The Rome group ate a typical Mediterranean diet of about 3000 kcal/day containing 50–55% carbohydrates, 25–30% lipids, and 20% proteins. The Svaldbard group ate a diet of about 4500 kcal/day with 30–33% carbohydrates, 47–50% lipids, and 20% protein. The lower levels of urinary alanine, lactate, and citrate in the Svaldbard group were ascribed to the lower carbohydrate portion of the diet. TMAO is a well established marker of fish consumption and was found to be higher in the Svaldbard group. The increased amounts of preservatives in the diet of that group led to higher exposure to benzoic acid. Lower glycine levels were also observed as glycine can conjugate to the benzoic acid resulting in the higher observed levels of hippurate. This type of controlled study to mimic the cultural and geographic preferences in different regions was a valuable demonstration of the ways in which the baseline metabolome must be considered in epidemiological metabolomics studies.

A metabolomic comparison of British and Swedish subjects was conducted without any dietary restrictions to look for culturally driven differences in the baseline metabolome under free-living conditions (Lenz *et al.*, 2004). In this study 20 healthy Swedish subjects and 10 healthy British subjects were enrolled. Each group contained males and females age 21 to 65 years. Principal components analysis revealed some distinction between the two countries based mainly on the levels of hippurate, TMAO, and creatinine. The higher TMAO concentrations in the Swedish subjects are concordant with the study by Zuppi *et al.* (1998), indicating that the Scandinavian diet is higher in fish consumption (Svensson *et al.*, 1994).

Interestingly, one British subject in this study had abnormally high levels of taurine. This particular metabolite has been reported to be an indicator of liver injury. Clinical follow-up with this subject found normal liver function, but examination of the dietary record indicated that she was on the Atkins diet which is very rich in meat. This high meat consumption can lead to elevated urinary taurine (Rana and Sanders, 1986; Laidlaw *et al.*, 1988). This is a good example of what can be learned from an examination of outliers and how diet must be considered in order to discern the difference between a biomarker of diet versus dysfunction.

After baseline metabolome differences are understood, metabolomics studies can be integrated into epidemiological studies to look for biomarkers of disease risk. The INTERSALT study is an example of a large-scale study in which relationship between salt intake and blood pressure was investigated (ICRG, 1988, 1989). In this study, 10 000+ men and women, age 20 to 59 years, from 32 countries with 52 discrete population groups, were studied to assess the role of salt in accounting for differences in blood pressure. A study of this magnitude requires rigorous protocols including standardization of blood pressure measurement techniques as well as assessment of salt intake and related data such as alcohol, potassium intake, and BMI. To minimize analytical variation, all analytical tests were conducted in a single laboratory. The results of this study demonstrated for the first time the positive correlation between salt, alcohol, and BMI with increased blood pressure.

An outgrowth of INTERSALT was the INTERMAP study, designed to evaluate the role of multiple dietary factors in accounting for interindividual differences in blood pressure (Beevers and Stamler, 2003; Stamler *et al.*, 2003). Comprehensive high-quality databases on the nutrient composition of foods were required for this study, therefore only four of the 32 countries in the INTERSALT study were included. Databases were available or could be created in these countries from existing national tables. Subjects from 17 population centers in China (*n*=832), Japan (*n*=1138), USA (*n*=2164), and UK (*n*=496) were included. Metabolomics was applied in order to develop a metabolic phenotyping approach to elucidate the mechanisms of the global cardiovascular disease epidemic. The study involved four 24-hour dietary recalls and two 24-hour urine collections. The aim was to identify a set of urinary metabolites that correlate with blood pressure across individuals and populations.

The results showed the unique metabolic patterns that distinguished the different populations. Geographic metabolic differences were greater than gender differences. The East Asian and western populations had well differentiated metabotypes. The metabotypes of southern (Guangzi) and northern (Beijing and Shanghai) China were also readily differentiated as were those of the USA and UK populations. Discriminatory metabolites were identified from pairwise comparisons across countries. The most significant metabolites included several that are predominantly of dietary origin such as amino acids, creatine, and TMAO. Significant differences in metabolic intermediates of energy metabolism included acetylcarnitine, tricarboxylic acid intermediates, and dicarboxylic acids. Gut microbial–mammalian co-metabolites such as hippurate, phenylacetylglutamine, and methylamines were also shown to be significant. Previous studies have shown that Chinese and American populations have structural differences in their gut microbial speciation, resulting in detectable differences in the metabolomes (Li *et al.*, 2008).

Four metabolites from this study were evaluated for correlations with systolic and diastolic blood pressure (SBP) and (DBP). These metabolites were alanine, formate, hippurate, and N-methylnicotinate. Multiple linear regression models of these metabolites were generated considering different adjustments for age, sex, supplement use, cardiovascular disease or diabetes or other confounding variables. Inverse associations of formate with both SBP and DBP were found in all eight models and similar associations were found with hippurate in six of the models. A direct association with alanine was found with five of the models.

The metabolic sources of each of these candidate biomarkers could reveal important mechanistic insights as to the coronary heart disease risks across different populations. Formate is mainly derived from the one-carbon metabolism from serine hydroxymethyltransferase activities and the tetrahydrofolate pathway. Formate is also generated from the fermentation of dietary fiber by the gut microbiome. The correlation of formate with urinary Na^+ excretion also points out the involvement with chlorine reabsorption in the kidney.

The inverse correlation with hippurate may further implicate the role of the gut microbiome in blood pressure. Polyphenols from many dietary plant sources such as black and green tea can be processed by gut bacteria into hippurate (Mulder *et al.*, 2005). Benzoic acid is commonly found in many berries and is also used as a preservative in many foods. Another action of the gut microbiome is to modulate availability of calories from the diet, which can influence the development of obesity which has a direct link with blood pressure (ICRG, 1988, 1989).

The positive correlation between urinary alanine levels and blood pressure could be related to differences in protein consumption. Dietary alanine levels are higher in those who consume higher animal-based protein rather than vegetable protein. Higher levels of the latter have been shown to have an inverse relationship with high blood pressure. Alanine also modulates cardiovascular responses to circulating catecholamines and increases blood pressure (Conlay *et al.*, 1990).

The cross-population metabolic differences revealed in the INTERMAP study confirm the role that metabolomics can play in epidemiological scale studies. The untargeted metabolomics data were effectively mined for culturally based dietary differences and disease risk. Global metabolite profiles will be a critical data component of epidemiological risk assessment as well as in the development of dietary recommendations.

Nutrimetabonomics and the Effects of Nutritional Challenges

Metabolomic Profiling as a Predictive Tool

The idea that the baseline metabolome of an individual contains information to predict the outcome of some physiological intervention was first demonstrated in the pharmacotherapy realm with acetaminophen. Clayton *et al.* (2006) demonstrated that the urinary metabolome of rats collected 24 hours prior to dosing with a toxic threshold dose of acetaminophen could discriminate those rats which would go on to develop moderate liver injury from those that would develop only mild liver injury. This approach, termed pharmaco-metabonomics, has been used in subsequent human clinical trials with some success. Pre-dose metabolite profiles in human subjects were found to be significantly correlated with the metabolism of both the anticoagulant ximelagatran (Andersson *et al.*, 2009) and the anti-rejection drug tacrolimus (Phapale *et al.*, 2010).

The nutrimetabolomic approach has been used to determine metabolic phenotypes which are correlated to dietary preferences. In a study by Rezzi *et al.* (2007) distinct metabotypes were found to correlate to predilection of a person to consume chocolate. Baseline urinary and plasma metabolic phenotypes were significantly correlated with the status of a person categorized as "chocolate desiring" or "chocolate indifferent". Plasma metabolic signatures were mainly different in their lipoprotein profiles while the urinary metabolomes were mainly distinguished by metabolites related to interactions with the gut microbiome. The ability to classify the dietary preferences of individuals and potentially of populations could have a significant impact in the development of dietary recommendations.

The nutrimetabolomic approach has been applied to predict the outcome of dietary choline deprivation in humans (Sha *et al.*, 2010). Choline is an essential nutrient, and deficiency can lead to liver and muscle dysfunction. In this study 53 subjects were fed a standard choline-containing diet for 10 days. A choline-deficient diet was then imposed for up to 42 days and subjects were monitored for signs of organ dysfunction. Finally subjects were given a 3-day choline repletion treatment. An untargeted analysis of the baseline metabolome was found to be strongly predictive of the outcome of the choline depletion phase. Distinct metabolic signatures were found for those who would develop liver dysfunction and those who would not. Choline deficiency is a common side-effect in patients treated with total parenteral nutrition (TPN), leading to a risk of liver dysfunction (Buchman *et al.*, 2001). This nutrimetabolomic approach may be useful in predicting the potential for liver dysfunction in patients on TPN treatment and in helping to develop more individualized therapy.

Metabolic Profiling of the Response to Nutritional Challenges

Some metabolic disorders may be difficult to detect above the noise inherent in the baseline metabolome. In order to detect some disorders, a dietary challenge may be required. For example, the oral glucose tolerance test (oGTT) is a common tool to use to provoke the metabolic processes that work to maintain glucose homeostasis. During an overnight fast, glucose levels are maintained through the action of glycogenolysis and gluconeogenesis. The large dose of glucose consumed in an oGTT triggers the rapid release of insulin, promoting glucose uptake and shifting the metabolism from a catabolic to an anabolic state. Currently, the time-dependent changes in glucose and insulin levels are used to draw conclusions on insulin sensitivity. The transition from fasting also leads to changes in a large number of metabolic pathways. Metabolomics offers a means to detect many of the suspected and unsuspected perturbations that may yield important biochemical insights into the processes that lead to insulin resistance.

An untargeted metabolomics study was undertaken by Zhao *et al.* (2009) to investigate the metabolic consequences of an oGTT. In this study a group of 16 individuals who were all classified as normal glucose tolerant were given an oGTT. Plasma was collected from all subjects over a 2-hour time window. Perturbations in four major metabolite groups were observed: free fatty acids (FFA), acylcarnitines, bile acids, and lysophosphatidylcholines (lyso-PC). The LC–MS platform used in this study utilized a reversed-phase-chromatography step so that polar metabolites (such as glucose) were not well detected. The nature of the lyso-PC and bile acid perturbations was not clear and warrants further investigation. The decrease in the plasma fatty acids is consistent with the expected decrease in lypolysis as the release of insulin inhibits the action of hormone-sensitive lipase. The decreases in acylcarnitines indicate a significant shift in energy metabolism. Acylcarnitines are generated from their respective acyl-CoA intermediates and are byproducts of mitochondrial β-oxidation. They can pass efficiently into the cytosol and then into the bloodstream so that plasma acylcarnitines are a reliable surrogate for the substrate flux through β-oxidation. The reduction in plasma levels therefore indicates a decreased reliance on β-oxidation after the glucose challenge. This untargeted metabolomics investigation resulted in a set of novel biomarkers to monitor the ability of a subject to regain metabolic homeostasis after an oGTT.

In a subsequent study, an untargeted metabolomics approach was used to investigate the ability of insulin-insensitive subjects to handle an oGTT (Shaham et al., 2008). In this manner, the metabolomics approach sought mechanistic as well as diagnostic biomarkers for the malfunctioning that occurs in insulin-insensitive individuals. This study also utilized an LC–MS analytical platform, but differences in the chromatography enabled the detection of more polar metabolites such as glucose, amino acids, and organic acids. This study identified 18 metabolites that implicated four distinct axes of insulin action. The metabolite markers indicate that, after an oGTT, glycolysis is up-regulated whereas lipolysis, ketogenesis and proteolysis are all down-regulated. Statistical analyses found that the blunted alterations in the levels of branched-chain amino acids plus the alteration in glycerol yielded a robust metabolic profile of insulin resistance. The branched-chain amino acid levels reflect perturbations in protein catabolism and the glycerol levels indicate changes in lipolysis. This result suggests that the same level of insulin resistance in two individuals could be the result of a different balance of these two insulin-sensitive pathways. This added detail from the metabolomics measurements could yield valuable insights into more individualized treatment for insulin resistance.

The Importance of the Gut Microbiota on Metabolic Profiles

The symbiotic relationships between microbes and the mammalian and plant hosts are an important factor in shaping our world. The gut microbiome tremendously increases the diversity of metabolic pathways accessible to mammalian hosts, enabling them to metabolize many things that they otherwise could not. As a result, gut microbes have been associated with various essential biological functions in humans through a "network" of microbial–host co-metabolism to process nutrients and drugs and modulate multiple pathways in a variety of organ systems (Martin et al., 2007, 2009; Claus et al., 2008). These studies by Nicholson and co-workers demonstrate that the metabolic variations in gastrointestinal compartments such as the duodenum, jejunum, and ileum, mammalian tissues such as kidney and liver, and biofluids such as blood and urine are directly related to the activities of the gut microbiota (Martin et al., 2008). Perhaps most importantly, gut microbes enable us to digest cellulose, the single largest nutritional energy source on the planet, and to survive on diets with low levels of particular nutrients and high levels of particular toxins. For example, gut microbes metabolize unabsorbed carbohydrates to short-chain fatty acids (SCFA), CO_2, and H_2 in the colon. SCFAs are monocarboxylic acids with a chain length up to six carbon atoms, i.e. acetic, propionic, butyric, isovaleric, valeric, isocaproic, and caproic acids. SCFAs function both as energy sources and as signaling molecules, and their abundance and type are directly related to the speciation of the microbiota and their syntrophic interactions. Other signaling pathways (such as through the SCFA receptor GPR43, for example) are similarly involved in host energy balance, and different microbial communities interact differently with these molecules (Ley et al., 2008). Most mammals can obtain essential amino acids, such as lysine, from their diet, but there is evidence that they also obtain them from their gut microbes (Metges et al., 2006). Many amino acids and perhaps other nitrogen-containing compounds may be cycling between humans and their microbiota, a process that could reduce dietary requirements for those nutrients (Metges et al., 2006). However, whether the fluxes of those amino acids or other essential nutrients between microbes and humans are great enough to contribute significantly to nutritional requirements is unresolved.

Diversity in gut microbial communities and function creates differences in nutrient milieux, digesta retention times, and temperatures that create diverse microbial environments. With the recent advances in molecular profiling technologies such as metagenomics and metabolomics, the direct correlation of global metabolic changes with the gut microbiome becomes increasingly important in the deciphering of the host–microbe relationships and in order to gain a mechanistic understanding of nutritional and drug interventions. Scientists from different disciplines are working together to determine the details of gut microbial diversity and to manipulate the complex interactions between the host metabolism and its symbionts for improved nutrition and disease treatment (Pang *et al.*, 2007; Li *et al.*, 2008, Wei *et al.*, 2010).

Future Directions

Gaining a better understanding of the nutritional status of individuals and populations is a major goal of metabolomics in the future. Generating databases of metabotypes could provide the means to detect variations that may signal disease risk at both individual and population levels. The analytical platforms are rapidly advancing so that a more sensitive and comprehensive coverage of the metabolome is generated. Biostatistical tools are also being developed so that critical metabolic features may be detected above the inherent noise from the confounding factors such as culture, age, BMI, etc. In the future, nutritional scientists will need to integrate into the network of scientists that includes analytical chemists, plant biologists, biostatisticians, and clinicians, to design and implement studies that generate a complete picture of the interaction of foods with our mammalian and microbial metabolism. These studies should enable the development of libraries containing metabolite biomarkers of food consumption as well as biomarkers of disease and dysfunction. The diagnostic and mechanistic knowledge that can be gained from metabolomics studies will have a tremendous impact on the development of personalized health in the future.

Suggestions for Further Reading

Kumar, M., Mohania, D., and Kumar, A. (2009) Metabolomics: an emerging tool for nutrition research. *Current Topics Nutr Res* 7, 97–104.
Oresic, M. (2009) Metabolomics, a novel tool for studies of nutrition, metabolism and lipid dysfunction. *Nutr Metab Cardiovasc Dis* 19, 816–824

References

Ala-Korpela, M. (2008) Critical evaluation of 1H NMR metabonomics of serum as a methodology for disease risk assessment and diagnostics. *Clin Chem Lab Med* **46**, 27–42.

Andersson, U., Lindberg, J., Wang, S., *et al.* (2009) A systems biology approach to understanding elevated serum alanine transaminase levels in a clinical trial with ximelagatran. *Biomarkers* **14**, 572–586.

Assfalg, M., Bertini, I., Colangiuli, D., *et al.* (2008) Evidence of different metabolic phenotypes in humans. *Proc Natl Acad Sci USA* **105**, 1420–1424.

Beckonert, O., Keun, H.C., Ebbels, T.M., *et al.* (2007) Metabolic profiling, metabolomic and metabonomic procedures for NMR spectroscopy of urine, plasma, serum and tissue extracts. *Nat Protoc* **2**, 2692–2703.

Bedair, M. and Sumner, L.W. (2008) Current and emerging mass-spectrometry technologies for metabolomics. *Trends Anal Chem* **27**, 238–248.

Beevers, D.G. and Stamler, J. (2003) Background to the INTERMAP study of nutrients and blood pressure. *J Hum Hypertens* **17**, 589–590.

Bernini, P., Bertini, I., Luchinat, C., *et al.* (2009) Individual human phenotypes in metabolic space and time. *J Proteome Res* **8**, 4264–4271.

Bhattacharya, A. (2010) Chemistry: Breaking the billion-Hertz barrier. *Nature* **463**, 605–606.

Bictash, M., Ebbels, T.M., Chan, Q., *et al.* (2010) Opening up the "Black Box": metabolic phenotyping and metabolome-wide association studies in epidemiology. *J Clin Epidemiol* **63**, 970–979.

Bingham, S.A. (2002) Biomarkers in nutritional epidemiology. *Public Health Nutr* **5**, 821–827.

Bingham, S.A., Gill, C., Welch, A., *et al.* (1994) Comparison of dietary assessment methods in nutritional epidemiology: weighed records v. 24 h recalls, food-frequency questionnaires and estimated-diet records. *Br J Nutr* **72**, 619–643.

Bingham, S.A., Gill, C., Welch, A., *et al.* (1997) Validation of dietary assessment methods in the UK arm of EPIC using weighed records, and 24-hour urinary nitrogen and potassium and serum vitamin C and carotenoids as biomarkers. *Int J Epidemiol* **26** Suppl 1, S137–151.

Bladbjerg, E.M., Larsen, T.M., Due, A., *et al.* (2010) Long-term effects on haemostatic variables of three ad libitum diets differing in type and amount of fat and carbohydrate: a 6-month randomised study in obese individuals. *Br J Nutr* **104**, 1824–1830.

Bollard, M.E., Stanley, E.G., Lindon, J.C., *et al.* (2005) NMR-based metabonomic approaches for evaluating physiological influences on biofluid composition. *NMR Biomed* **18**, 143–162.

Bruce, S.J., Tavazzi, I., Parisod, V., *et al.* (2009) Investigation of human blood plasma sample preparation for performing metabolomics using ultrahigh performance liquid chromatography/mass spectrometry. *Anal Chem* **81**, 3285–3296.

Buchman, A.L., Ament, M.E., Sohel, M., *et al.* (2001) Choline deficiency causes reversible hepatic abnormalities in patients receiving parenteral nutrition: proof of a human choline requirement: a placebo-controlled trial. *JPEN J Parenter Enteral Nutr* **25**, 260–268.

Claus, S.P., Tsang, T.M., Wang, Y., *et al.* (2008) Systemic multi-compartmental effects of the gut microbiome on mouse metabolic phenotypes. *Mol Syst Biol* **4**, 219.

Clayton, T.A., Lindon, J.C., Cloarec, O., *et al.* (2006) Pharmaco-metabonomic phenotyping and personalized drug treatment. *Nature* **440**, 1073–1077.

Conlay, L.A., Maher, T.J., and Wurtman, R.J. (1990) Alanine increases blood pressure during hypotension. *Pharmacol Toxicol* **66**, 415–416.

Daykin, C.A. and Wulfert, F. (2006) NMR spectroscopy based metabonomics: current technology and applications. In *Frontiers in Drug Design and Discovery*, Vol. 2. Bentham Science Publishers, Oak Park, IL, pp. 151–173.

Dettmer, K., Aronov, P.A., and Hammock, B.D. (2007) Mass spectrometry-based metabolomics. *Mass Spectrom Rev* **26**, 51–78.

Due, A., Larsen, T.M., Hermansen, K., *et al.* (2008a) Comparison of the effects on insulin resistance and glucose tolerance of 6-mo high-monounsaturated-fat, low-fat, and control diets. *Am J Clin Nutr* **87**, 855–862.

Due, A., Larsen, T.M., Mu, H., *et al.* (2008b) Comparison of 3 ad libitum diets for weight-loss maintenance, risk of cardiovascular disease, and diabetes: a 6-mo randomized, controlled trial. *Am J Clin Nutr* **88**, 1232–1241.

Dumas, M.E., Maibaum, E.C., Teague, C., *et al.* (2006) Assessment of analytical reproducibility of 1H NMR spectroscopy based metabonomics for large-scale epidemiological research: the INTERMAP Study. *Anal Chem* **78**, 2199–2208.

Dunn, W.B. (2008) Current trends and future requirements for the mass spectrometric investigation of microbial, mammalian and plant metabolomes. *Phys Biol* **5**, 011001.

Fave, G., Beckmann, M.E., Draper, J.H., *et al.* (2009) Measurement of dietary exposure: a challenging problem which may be overcome thanks to metabolomics? *Genes Nutr* **4**, 135–141.

Fiehn, O. (2001) Combining genomics, metabolome analysis, and biochemical modelling to understand metabolic networks. *Comp Funct Genomics* **2**, 155–168.

Grimes, J.H. and O'Connell, T.M. (2011) The application of micro-coil NMR probe technology to metabolomics of urine and serum. *J Biomol NMR* **49**, 297–305.

Gronwald, W., Klein, M.S., Kaspar, H., *et al.* (2008) Urinary metabolite quantification employing 2D NMR spectroscopy. *Anal Chem* **80**, 9288–9297.

Hearty, A.P. and Gibney, M.J. (2009) Comparison of cluster and principal component analysis techniques to derive dietary patterns in Irish adults. *Br J Nutr* **101**, 598–608.

ICRG (1988) Intersalt: an international study of electrolyte excretion and blood pressure. Results for 24 hour urinary sodium and potassium excretion. *BMJ* **297**, 319–328.

ICRG (1989) The INTERSALT study. An international co-operative study of electrolyte excretion and blood pressure: further results. *J Hum Hypertens* **3**, 279–407.

Jenab, M., Slimani, N., Bictash, M., *et al.* (2009) Biomarkers in nutritional epidemiology: applications, needs and new horizons. *Hum Genet* **125**, 507–525.

Kochhar, S., Jacobs, D.M., Ramadan, Z., *et al.* (2006) Probing gender-specific metabolism differences in humans by nuclear magnetic resonance-based metabonomics. *Anal Biochem* **352**, 274–281.

Laidlaw, S.A., Shultz, T.D., Cecchino, J.T., *et al.* (1988) Plasma and urine taurine levels in vegans. *Am J Clin Nutr* **47**, 660–663.

Lenz, E.M., Bright, J., Wilson, I.D., *et al.* (2003) A 1H NMR-based metabonomic study of urine and plasma samples obtained from healthy human subjects. *J Pharm Biomed Anal* **33**, 1103–1115.

Lenz, E.M., Bright, J., Wilson, I.D., *et al.* (2004) Metabonomics, dietary influences and cultural differences: a 1H NMR-based study of urine samples obtained from healthy British and Swedish subjects. *J Pharm Biomed Anal* **36**, 841–849.

Ley, R.E., Hamady, M., Lozupone, C., *et al.* (2008) Evolution of mammals and their gut microbes. *Science* **320**, 1647–1651.

Li, M., Wang, B., Zhang, M., *et al.* (2008) Symbiotic gut microbes modulate human metabolic phenotypes. *Proc Natl Acad Sci USA* **105**, 2117–2122.

Logan, T.M., Murali, N., Wang, G., *et al.* (1999) Application of a high-resolution superconducting NMR probe in natural product structure determination. *Magn Res Chem* **37**, 762–765.

Ludwig, C. and Viant, M.R. (2010) Two-dimensional J-resolved NMR spectroscopy: review of a key methodology in the metabolomics toolbox. *Phytochem Anal* **21**, 22–32.

Madsen, R., Lundstedt, T., and Trygg, J. (2010) Chemometrics in metabolomics – a review in human disease diagnosis. *Anal Chim Acta* **659**, 23–33.

Manach, C., Hubert, J., Llorach, R., *et al.* (2009) The complex links between dietary phytochemicals and human health deciphered by metabolomics. *Mol Nutr Food Res* **53**, 1303–1315.

Martin, F.P., Dumas, M.E., Wang, Y., *et al.* (2007) A top-down systems biology view of microbiome–mammalian metabolic interactions in a mouse model. *Mol Syst Biol* **3**, 112.

Martin, F.P., Wang, Y., Sprenger, N., *et al.* (2008) Top-down systems biology integration of conditional prebiotic modulated transgenomic interactions in a humanized microbiome mouse model. *Mol Syst Biol* **4**, 205.

Martin, F.P., Wang, Y., Yap, I.K., *et al.* (2009) Topographical variation in murine intestinal metabolic profiles in relation to microbiome speciation and functional ecological activity. *J Proteome Res* **8**, 3464–3474.

Mennen, L.I., Sapinho, D., Ito, H., *et al.* (2006) Urinary flavonoids and phenolic acids as biomarkers of intake for polyphenol-rich foods. *Br J Nutr* **96**, 191–198.

Metges, C.C., Eberhard, M., and Petzke, K.J. (2006) Synthesis and absorption of intestinal microbial lysine in humans and non-ruminant animals and impact on human estimated average requirement of dietary lysine. *Curr Opin Clin Nutr Metab Care* **9**, 37–41.

Mulder, T.P., Rietveld, A.G., and Van Amelsvoort, J.M. (2005) Consumption of both black tea and green tea results in an increase in the excretion of hippuric acid into urine. *Am J Clin Nutr* **81**, 256S–260S.

O'Sullivan, A., Gibney, M.J., and Brennan, L. (2011) Dietary intake patterns are reflected in metabolomic profiles: potential role in dietary assessment studies. *Am J Clin Nutr* **93**, 314–321.

Pang, X., Hua, X., Yang, Q., *et al.* (2007) Inter-species transplantation of gut microbiota from humans to pigs. *ISME J* **1**, 156–162.

Pasikanti, K.K., Ho, P.C., and Chan, E.C. (2008) Gas chromatography/mass spectrometry in metabolic profiling of biological fluids. *J Chromatogr B Analyt Technol Biomed Life Sci* **871**, 202–211.

Phapale, P.B., Kim, S.D., Lee, H.W., *et al.* (2010) An integrative approach for identifying a metabolic phenotype predictive of individualized pharmacokinetics of tacrolimus. *Clin Pharmacol Ther* **87**, 426–446.

Primrose, S., Draper, J., Elsom, R., *et al.* (2011) Metabolomics and human nutrition. *Br J Nutr* **105**, 1277–1283.

Rai, R.K., Tripathi, P., and Sinha, N. (2009) Quantification of metabolites from two-dimensional nuclear magnetic resonance spectroscopy: application to human urine samples. *Anal Chem* **81**, 10232–10238.

Rana, S.K. and Sanders, T.A. (1986) Taurine concentrations in the diet, plasma, urine and breast milk of vegans compared with omnivores. *Br J Nutr* **56**, 17–27.

Rasmussen, L.G., Larsen, T.M., Mortensen, P.K., *et al.* (2007) Effect on 24-h energy expenditure of a moderate-fat diet high in monounsaturated fatty acids compared with that of a low-fat, carbohydrate-rich diet: a 6-mo controlled dietary intervention trial. *Am J Clin Nutr* **85**, 1014–1022.

Reily, M.D. and Lindon, J.C. (2005) *NMR Spectroscopy: Principles and Instrumentation*. Taylor and Francis, New York.

Rezzi, S., Ramadan, Z., Martin, F.P., *et al.* (2007) Human metabolic phenotypes link directly to specific dietary preferences in healthy individuals. *J Proteome Res* **6**, 4469–4477.

Robertson, D., Lindon, J., Nicholson, J.K., *et al.* (2005) *Metabonomics in Toxicity Assessment*. CRC Press, Boca Raton, FL.

Robertson, D.G., Watkins, P.B., and Reily, M.D. (2011) Metabolomics in toxicology: preclinical and clinical applications. *Toxicol Sci* **120** Suppl 1, S146–170.

Rychlik, M. and Asam, S. (2008) Stable isotope dilution assays in mycotoxin analysis. *Anal Bioanal Chem* **390**, 617–628.

Scalbert, A., Brennan, L., Fiehn, O., *et al.* (2009) Mass-spectrometry-based metabolomics: limitations and recommendations for future progress with particular focus on nutrition research. *Metabolomics* **5**, 435–458.

Sha, W., Da Costa, K.A., Fischer, L.M., *et al.* (2010) Metabolomic profiling can predict which humans will develop liver dysfunction when deprived of dietary choline. *FASEB J* **24**, 2962–2975.

Shaham, O., Wei, R., Wang, T.J., *et al.* (2008) Metabolic profiling of the human response to a glucose challenge reveals distinct axes of insulin sensitivity. *Mol Syst Biol* **4**, 214.

Skov, A.R., Toubro, S., Raben, A., *et al.* (1997) A method to achieve control of dietary macronutrient composition in ad libitum diets consumed by free-living subjects. *Eur J Clin Nutr* **51**, 667–672.

Smedman, A.E., Gustafsson, I.B., Berglund, L.G., *et al.* (1999). Pentadecanoic acid in serum as a marker for intake of milk fat: relations between intake of milk fat and metabolic risk factors. *Am J Clin Nutr* **69**, 22–29.

Stamler, J., Elliott, P., Dennis, B., *et al.* (2003) INTERMAP: background, aims, design, methods, and descriptive statistics (non-dietary). *J Hum Hypertens* **17**, 591–608.

Svensson, B.G., Akesson, B., Nilsson, A., *et al.* (1994) Urinary excretion of methylamines in men with varying intake of fish from the Baltic Sea. *J Toxicol Environ Health* **41**, 411–420.

Vaidyanathan, S., Harrigan, G.G., and Goodacre, R. (2005) *Metabolome Analyses: Strategies for Systems Biology*. Springer, New York.

Van Hove, J.L., Zhang, W., Kahler, S.G., *et al.* (1993) Medium-chain acyl-CoA dehydrogenase (MCAD) deficiency: diagnosis by acylcarnitine analysis in blood. *Am J Hum Genet* **52**, 958–966.

Walsh, M.C., Brennan, L., Malthouse, J.P., *et al.* (2006) Effect of acute dietary standardization on the urinary, plasma, and salivary metabolomic profiles of healthy humans. *Am J Clin Nutr* **84,** 531–539.

Want, E.J., Cravatt, B.F., and Siuzdak, G. (2005) The expanding role of mass spectrometry in metabolite profiling and characterization. *Chembiochem* **6,** 1941–1951.

Waterman, D.S., Bonner, F.W., and Lindon, J.C. (2009) Spectroscopic and statistical methods in metabonomics. *Bioanalysis* **1,** 1559–1578.

Wei, H., Dong, L., Wang, T., *et al.* (2010) Structural shifts of gut microbiota as surrogate endpoints for monitoring host health changes induced by carcinogen exposure. *FEMS Microbiol Ecol* **73,** 577–586.

Winnike, J.H., Busby, M.G., Watkins, P.B., *et al.* (2009) Effects of a prolonged standardized diet on normalizing the human metabolome. *Am J Clin Nutr* **90,** 1496–1501.

Wishart, D.S., Knox, C., Guo, A.C., *et al.* (2009) HMDB: a knowledgebase for the human metabolome. *Nucleic Acids Res* **37,** D603–610.

Xi, Y., De Ropp, J.S., Viant, M.R., *et al.* (2008) Improved identification of metabolites in complex mixtures using HSQC NMR spectroscopy. *Anal Chim Acta* **614,** 127–133.

Zhao, X., Peter, A., Fritsche, J., *et al.* (2009) Changes of the plasma metabolome during an oral glucose tolerance test: is there more than glucose to look at? *Am J Physiol Endocrinol Metab* **296,** E384–393.

Zuppi, C., Messana, I., Forni, F., *et al.* (1998) Influence of feeding on metabolite excretion evidenced by urine 1H NMR spectral profiles: a comparison between subjects living in Rome and subjects living at arctic latitudes (Svaldbard). *Clin Chim Acta* **278,** 75–79.

5

ENERGY METABOLISM IN FASTING, FED, EXERCISE, AND RE-FEEDING STATES

SAI KRUPA DAS, PhD AND SUSAN B. ROBERTS, PhD

Tufts University, Boston, Massachusetts, USA

Summary

Energy balance is achieved when energy intake equals energy expenditure. Perturbations to this homeostatic model impact body weight regulation. A net energy surplus leads to weight gain and obesity and a net energy deficit results in weight loss and underweight. Energy metabolism in the fasted state is dependent on the duration of the fast, the type of meal ingested before the fast, and available body energy stores. Energy metabolism in the fed state is mediated by the cephalic phase response to a meal, meal size, meal type, structure and consistency, meal composition, and the metabolic processes required to digest, absorb, and store the ingested energy. Both energy intake and body energy stores affect activity-/exercise-related energy expenditure. Human beings, especially adults, do not maintain energy balance from one day to the next but do so over a period of several days with energy intake playing a stronger role in this regulatory process.

Introduction

Energy is expended by the body to maintain electrochemical gradients, transport molecules, support biosynthetic processes, produce the mechanical work required for respiration and blood circulation, and generate muscle contraction. Most of these biological processes cannot directly harness energy from the oxidation of energy-containing substrates (primarily carbohydrate and fat from food and body energy stores). Instead, the resulting energy from the oxidation of metabolic fuels is captured by adenosine triphosphate (ATP) in the form of high-energy bonds. ATP is the major energy carrier to body sites and releases the energy required for chemical and mechanical work. Use of that energy results in the production of heat, carbon dioxide, and water, which are all eliminated from the body. Definitions in energy metabolism, and relationships among oxygen consumption, carbon dioxide production and energy expenditure, and the stoichiometry of oxidation of different nutrients, are shown in Box 5.1 and Tables 5.1 and 5.2.

Nutrient degradation pathways (including the Krebs cycle and the β-oxidation of fatty acids) are linked to the formation of ATP from adenosine diphosphate (ADP) and inorganic phosphate (Pi) and are often referred to as ATP- or energy-generation pathways. Likewise, the term "energy

Present Knowledge in Nutrition, Tenth Edition. Edited by John W. Erdman Jr, Ian A. Macdonald and Steven H. Zeisel.

BOX 5.1 Definitions in energy metabolism

Calorie and Joule: A calorie is the amount of heat required to raise the temperature of 1 g of H_2O from 14.5 to 15.5°C. One kilocalorie (1 kcal) is 1000 times greater than 1 calorie (1 cal); 1 calorie is equivalent to 4.184 joules (J); and 1 kilocalorie to 4.184 kilojoules (kJ).

Energy balance: Attained when energy intake equals total energy expenditure (TEE) and body stores are stable. An individual is said to be in *positive energy balance* when energy intake exceeds TEE (and consequently body energy stores increase). *Negative energy balance* occurs when energy intake is less than TEE and body energy stores decrease.

Energy expenditure: The amount of energy used by the body, and equivalent to the heat released by hydrolysis of adenosine triphosphate (ATP) to adenosine diphosphate (ADP) or adenosine monophosphate (AMP) and inorganic phosphate (Pi).

Energy metabolism: The general term used to collectively describe the multiple biochemical pathways that govern the production and use of ATP and the reducing equivalents.

Energy regulation is the process by which energy intake and energy expenditure are balanced.

Malnutrition is the general term that denotes both undernutrition and overnutrition.

Overnutrition: Occurs when energy intake exceeds energy expenditure and results in excess body fat accumulation. Several levels of overnutrition are defined in adults using the body mass index (BMI, weight in kilograms divided by height in meters squared, kg/m^2) (Food and Agriculture Organization of the United Nations, 2001): Overweight BMI = 25–29.9, Class I Obesity BMI = 30–34.9, Class II Obesity BMI = 35–39.9, Class III Obesity BMI ≥40.0 kg/m^2. In children BMI changes with development; BMI definitions of overweight and obesity at different ages are now available (see Cole *et al.*, 2000; Roberts and Dallal, 2001).

Undernutrition: Occurs when energy intake is less than TEE over a considerable period of time, resulting in clinically significant weight loss. In adults undernutrition is classified using BMI (WHO, 1995). A BMI of 18.5–24.9 is considered normal, a BMI of 17–18.49 is mild undernutrition, a BMI of 16–16.99 is moderate undernutrition, and a BMI <16 is severe undernutrition. In children, undernutrition is classified using the weight-for-height (or length) index and height-for-age index with reference values derived from World Health Organization data (Food and Agriculture Organization of the United Nations, 2001).

Wasting is defined as low weight for height, with <–1SD (i.e. –1 z-score) being mild, <–2 SD being moderate, and <–3 SD being severely wasted relative to National Center for Health Statistics and the World Health Organization International Growth Reference. Similarly, *stunting* is associated with a low height for age with <–1 SD being mild, <–2 SD being moderate, and <–3 SD of the reference values being severely stunted.

TABLE 5.1 Substrate oxidation parameters. Relationships among VO_2, VCO_2, and energy expenditure for fat, protein, and carbohydrate[a]

Oxidation of 1 g	O_2 required (L)	CO_2 produced (L)	RQ	Energy expended, kJ (kcal)/g	Energy equivalent[1] L O_2, kJ (kcal)/L
Carbohydrate	827.7	827.7	1.000	17.5 (4.18)	21.1 (5.048)
Protein	1010.3	843.6	0.835	19.7 (4.70)	19.48 (4.655)
Fat	2018.9	1435.4	0.710	39.5 (9.45)	19.6 (5.682)
Ethanol	1459.4	977.8	0.670	29.7 (7.09)	20.3 (4.86)

[a]Carbohydrate is assumed to be starch; protein and fat are assumed to be mixed values found in typical human diets.
Data from Livesey and Elia (1988).

TABLE 5.2 Stoichiometry of oxidation of specific nutrients and high-energy bond production

$C_{16}H_{32}O_2 + 23\ O_2$	→	$16\ CO_2 + 16\ H_2O + 10{,}033\ kJ\ (2398\ kcal)$	[+131-2 ATP = 129 ATP] (Palmitate)
$C_{4.6}H_{8.4}O_{1.8}N_{1.25} + 9.6\ O_2$	→	$0.6\ UREA + 4.0\ CO_2 + 2.9\ H_2O + 2176\ kJ\ (520\ kcal)$	[29-6 ATP = +23 ATP] (Protein)
$C_6H_{12}O_6 + 6.0\ O_2$	→	$6.0\ CO_2 + 6.0\ H_2O + 2803\ kJ\ (670\ kcal)$	[+38-2 = +36 ATP] (Glucose)

Values are in moles.
Data from Kinney and Tucker (1992).

expenditure" is used to describe the degradation of ATP to ADP and Pi. In a resting adult ~25–35 g ATP is used every minute to drive the life-sustaining processes, and this is approximately the total amount contained in the body at any one time. Although ATP turnover at rest is relatively high, the enzymatic machinery in the body operates below its maximal capacity, and is poised to effectively maintain a high ratio of ATP to ADP. During vigorous exercise, when several hundred grams of ATP are required per minute, ATP levels fall because of increased use, the rate of ATP generation is adjusted rapidly to match ATP utilization, and synthesis of ATP is accelerated.

The circulating levels of energy substrates needed for ATP production are kept relatively constant despite wide variations in the availability of nutrients from the gastrointestinal tract by the balance of insulin and the counter-regulatory hormones, such as glucagon, glucocorticoids, adrenaline, and growth hormone. These hormones jointly serve to facilitate the rapid storage of incoming nutrients from the gastrointestinal tract (carbohydrate in the form of glycogen in the liver and muscle, and fat as triacylglycerol in adipose tissue) and maintain circulating levels in the fasting state by mobilization of body stores.

The close relationship between energy metabolism and oxygen consumption stems from the fact that oxygen is required to transform food to a usable source of energy. One liter of oxygen consumed generates approximately 5 kcal (20.92 kJ). Given that there is proportionality between VO_2 and ATP synthesis, and because each mole of ATP synthesized is accompanied by a given amount of heat, it would be possible to calculate heat production from VO_2 measurements alone. However, the heat produced by the utilization of 1 L oxygen varies somewhat with the foodstuff consumed (Tables 5.1 and 5.2). The combustion of 1 L oxygen during fat oxidation yields 4.682 kcal (19.60 kJ), whereas protein alone yields 4.655 kcal (19.48 kJ) and carbohydrate starch alone yields 5.048 kcal (21.12 kJ) (Livesey and Elia, 1988). Moreover, the amount of carbon dioxide produced also varies with nutrient type, with the amount produced per mole oxygen consumed during oxidation of fat, protein, and carbohydrate being 0.710, 0.835, and 1.00 mol, respectively. Thus, for precise conversion of oxygen utilization to energy expenditure, the balance of metabolic fuels being oxidized or carbon dioxide production must be known.

Because the ratio of carbon dioxide produced to oxygen consumed (i.e. the respiratory quotient) varies with nutri-

ent type, it can be used to predict the ratio of metabolic fuels being oxidized provided that additional information on urinary nitrogen excretion is also available. The first step in this calculation is to determine protein oxidation, with the assumption that urinary nitrogen reflects protein oxidation, and 1 g urinary nitrogen is equivalent to 6.25 g protein. VO_2 and VCO_2 not from protein (the non-protein VO_2 and VCO_2) are then calculated by subtracting the amount of oxygen and carbon dioxide equivalent to protein oxidation using the values in Table 5.1. After this, the non-protein respiratory quotient is used to calculate the ratio of fat to carbohydrate oxidation using values for the respiratory quotient of carbohydrate and fat.

Simple equations can also be used to predict energy expenditure from oxygen consumption and carbon dioxide production, of which de Weir's is probably most widely used today (de Weir, 1949). When 24-hour urine collections are made on the day of measurement of VO_2 and VCO_2, the complete de Weir equation, which includes an adjustment for energy expenditure for protein oxidation, is used. However, because of the difficulties obtaining complete 24-hour urine nitrogen measurements and because the difference between correcting for urinary N and not correcting for nitrogen is <2%, the abbreviated de Weir equation is often used. The complete de Weir equation is:

$$RMR\,(kcal/day) = 1.44\,(3.941 \cdot VO_2 + 1.106 \cdot VCO_2) - 2.17 \cdot UN$$

The abbreviated de Weir equation is:

$$RMR\,(kcal/day) = 1.44\,(3.941 \cdot VO_2 + 1.106 \cdot VCO_2)$$

Resting metabolic rate (RMR); VO_2 and VCO2 are measured in milliliters per minute and urinary nitrogen (UN) is measured in grams per day.

The following sections discuss the components of total energy expenditure in relation to the fasting state, namely basal metabolic rate (BMR) or resting metabolic rate (RMR); the fed state or the thermic effect of feeding (TEF); and the activity- and exercise-related energy expenditure which is termed activity energy expenditure (AEE) or physical activity energy expenditure (PAEE). Combined, these three components are equivalent to total energy expenditure (TEE), which in turn is equivalent to dietary energy requirements for non-growing individuals. In addition, the effects of changes in energy balance on energy expenditure are also considered.

Energy Expenditure in the Fasting State

Energy expenditure measured in the fasting state reflects energy use of the body for such basic functions as maintenance of electrochemical gradients, transporting of molecules around the body, and biosynthetic processes, and is an important measurement in energy expenditure research because it typically accounts for 60–70% of TEE. Basal metabolic rate is a standardized measurement of energy expenditure in the fasting state, defined as the rate of energy expenditure while lying supine in bed at physical and mental rest 12–14 hours after the last meal (i.e. in the postabsorptive state) and under thermoneutral conditions. Resting metabolic rate is another standardized measurement, which is similar to BMR except that the conditions are less rigid for the duration of the overnight fast, and that posture may differ (some measurements are performed in the semi-inclined rather than supine position) and thermoneutrality is not guaranteed. BMR and RMR are often used interchangeably. Both BMR and RMR are highly correlated with lean body mass, more commonly known as fat-free mass (FFM), and to a smaller extent with fat mass. Note that there is a positive intercept in the relationship between BMR/RMR and FFM, which is thought to result from the fact that organs have a high metabolic rate and sizes are relatively constant between adult individuals. One consequence of the non-zero intercept is that BMR per kilogram FFM is lower for higher levels of FFM than for lower ones. Thus, differences in BMR between groups of individuals should always be assessed using regression analysis to test the effect of a group in a model also incorporating FFM and fat mass; otherwise, heavy individuals (such as the obese) may falsely appear to have a low BMR relative to their body size.

There is also some variability in BMR because of age (elderly individuals have lower BMR after adjusting for differences in FFM between young and old groups [Roberts *et al.*, 1995]), and women may have lower adjusted BMR values than men (Ferraro *et al.*, 1992). Among young women, BMR variations of the order of 6–10% have been reported to occur in the course of the menstrual cycle, with values in the luteal phase tending to be higher than in the follicular phase (Solomon *et al.*, 1982). Factors such as exercise and conditions such as hyperthyroidism, catecholamine release, fever, stress, cold exposure, and burns increase BMR. There is also a hereditary component to BMR, seen in the fact that variations in FFM-adjusted metabolic rate are smaller among members of the same family than between unrelated individuals (Bogardus *et al.*, 1986).

Several equations have been developed to predict BMR from weight, height, and other simple measures. The Schofield equations (Schofield *et al.*, 1985) were derived from an analysis of the world literature on BMR. They consist of a series of simple linear regression equations predicting BMR for different gender and age categories from either weight alone or weight and height. These equations have an uncertainty of prediction of only ±7–10% for individual values, and are widely used. Although such equations may not be suitable for unusual populations such as the extremely obese or very old, they do provide a basis for predicting energy requirements in the general population (Table 5.3).

Energy Expenditure in the Fed State

The thermic effect of feeding, previously known as specific dynamic action, is the increase in energy expenditure above basal that is associated with consuming, digesting, and assimilating food. Some of the increase in energy expenditure associated with feeding can be directly attributed to the metabolic costs of eating and digestion and related processes (termed "obligatory thermogenesis"),

TABLE 5.3   Equations to predict BMR from body weight

Age range (years)	Basal metabolic rate	
	kcal/day	MJ/day
Males		
0–3	60.9 W − 54	0.255 W − 0.226
3–10	22.7 W + 495	0.0949 W + 2.07
10–18	17.5 W + 651	0.0732 W + 2.72
18–30	15.3 W + 679	0.0640 W + 2.84
30–60	11.6 W + 879	0.0485 W + 3.67
>60	13.5 W + 487	0.0565 W + 2.04
Females		
0–3	61.0 W − 51	0.255 W − 0.214
3–10	22.5 W + 499	0.0941 W + 2.09
10–18	12.2 W + 746	0.0510 W + 3.12
18–30	14.7 W + 496	0.0615 W + 2.08
30–60	8.7 W + 829	0.0364 W + 3.47
>60	10.5 W + 596	0.0439 W + 2.49

W, body weight in kg.
Data from WHO (1985).

while the other component of the increase appears to be due to concomitant activation of the sympathetic nervous system (termed "facultative thermogenesis") (Murgatroyd, 1984). A significant component of the TEF (estimated at 50–75%) is directed toward the obligatory thermogenesis component and is used for such work as regenerating the ATP used in the processing and storage of ingested nutrients (Flatt, 1978). Facultative thermogenesis (Major *et al.*, 2007) may include such factors as increased activity of the sympathetic nervous system resulting from the sensory and metabolic stimulation resulting from food. TEF typically accounts for 7–13% of energy intake over the 4-hour period after eating, and is directly proportional to the size of the meal consumed (Schutz *et al.*, 1984; Melanson *et al.*, 1998). TEF appears to be reduced in obese individuals (Segal *et al.*, 1990), but the question of whether this is a cause or consequence of excess weight gain has not been resolved (Golay *et al.*, 1989; Segal *et al.*, 1990). A separate estimate of the energy needed for TEF is not usually shown in predictions of energy requirements (see below), because measurements of total energy expenditure include energy expenditure attributable to the TEF.

Activity Energy Expenditure or Physical Activity Energy Expenditure

The final component of TEE is the AEE or PAEE, which is generally the second largest component of TEE and the most variable because to a large extent it is under voluntary control. This component will thus account for an increasing proportion of TEE as individuals become more physically active. In sedentary persons, AEE or PAEE may be only 15–20% of TEE, whereas it may be up to 50–60% in highly active individuals. In some individuals an important component of AEE or PAEE is subconscious (e.g. fidgeting, posture maintenance) and is referred to as spontaneous physical activity (SPA) (Levine *et al.*, 1999). The difficulty of measuring AEE or PAEE using traditional methods for determining energy expenditure has made this the least accurately measured component of TEE. Energy expenditure for different activities varies widely, and typical values are summarized in Table 5.4. These values are for the acute effects of exercise, and it is also recognized that chronic exercise may have effects on energy expenditure that extend beyond the period of exercise to influence RMR and TEF (Van Zant, 1992).

TABLE 5.4 Approximate energy expenditure for individual activities (expressed as multiple of resting metabolic rate)[a]

Activity category and activity examples	Activity factor X (RMR)
Resting Sleeping, reclining	1.0
Very light Seated and standing activities, painting trades, driving, laboratory work, typing, sewing, ironing, cooking, playing cards, playing a musical instrument	1.5
Light Walking on a level surface at 2.5 to 3 mph, garage work, electrical trades, carpentry, restaurant trades, housecleaning, child care, golf, sailing, table tennis	2.5
Moderate Walking 3.5 to 4 mph, weeding and hoeing, carrying a load, cycling, skiing, tennis, dancing	5.0
Heavy Walking with a load uphill, tree felling, heavy manual digging, basketball, climbing, football, soccer	7.0

[a]When reported as multiples of basal needs, the energy expenditures of males and females are similar.
Data from Durnin and Passamore (1967) and WHO (1985).

Energy Requirements

TEE is equivalent to energy requirements for non-growing individuals, and energy requirements can be defined as (WHO, 1985):

the level of energy intake that will balance energy expenditure when the individual has a body size and composition and a level of physical activity consistent with long-term good health; and that will allow for the maintenance of economically necessary and socially desirable physical activity. In children and pregnant or lactating women, the energy requirement includes the energy needs associated with the deposition of tissues or secretion of milk at rates consistent with good health.

Requirement refers to habitual or usual intake over a period of time, because many human beings (especially adults) do not maintain energy balance from one day to the next but do so over a period of several days or even over weeks. Energy requirements are equivalent to TEE when the individual is in "energy balance", i.e. neither gaining nor losing body fat, and in this case total energy intake will be equivalent to "metabolizable energy intake", which is energy metabolically available to the body after obligatory losses in urine and feces. Approximate metabolizable energy contents of fat, protein, and carbohydrate are 9 kcal (37.66 kJ/g), 4 kcal/g (16.74 kJ/g), and 4 kcal/g (16.74 kJ/g), respectively.

Currently, most estimations of energy requirement worldwide are based on estimates of components of energy expenditure summed together into 24-hour values in a "factorial" approach (WHO, 1985). However, while the factorial approach is recognized as relatively imprecise, it is preferred over measurement of energy intake during weight stability because energy intake is highly variable and most individuals under-report habitual intake by 25–50%, depending on their body fatness (Schoeller, 1990).

To avoid the pitfalls of the factorial method, substantial effort has been directed towards developing the doubly labeled water method as an alternative, longer-term, and more accurate technique for measurement of TEE. This method was originally developed for use in small animals (Lifson et al., 1955; Lifson and McClintock, 1966), based on the principle that if two isotopes of water ($H_2^{18}O$ and ^2H_2O) are administered and their disappearance rates from a body fluid such as urine are monitored, the disappearance rate of ^2H_2O reflects water flux and the disappearance rate of $H_2^{18}O$ reflects water flux plus carbon dioxide production rate (Lifson et al., 1949). The difference between the two disappearance rates can therefore be used to calculate carbon dioxide production rate over a period of 1–2 weeks, from which total energy expenditure can be calculated if information is available on respiratory quotient (RQ) (Surrao et al., 1998). Validation studies of the doubly labeled water method have been conducted in human infants and adults of different ages using respiratory gas exchange or dietary energy intake as the reference method (Schoeller, 1988; Roberts, 1989). All these studies showed a close agreement between total energy expenditure determined by doubly labeled water and total energy expenditure determined by a reference method, with a coefficient of variation for the new method of 2–6%. In consequence,

the doubly labeled water method is now widely recognized as an accurate and precise method for assessment of total energy expenditure in human subjects, and has recently been assessed as giving broadly comparable results to the factorial method (Shetty, 2005). Because the doubly labeled water method calculates the rate of carbon dioxide production, rather than the rate of energy expenditure, and because the heat equivalent of carbon dioxide varies with the substrates being oxidized (Schoeller, 1988; Roberts, 1989), it is necessary to have an estimate of the RQ of the subject during the measurement period. Usually, RQ is estimated from information on the subject's dietary intake – either their reported macronutrient intakes or normative data from population surveys – and errors from necessary assumptions and errors in dietary records are recognized to be small and usually <2% (Surrao et al., 1998).

A critical mass of doubly labeled water data has been accumulated, making it possible to evaluate typical changes in TEE and energy expenditure for physical activity (calculated as the difference between total energy expenditure and basal metabolic rate plus the thermic effect of feeding, or indicated by a physical activity level calculated as the ratio of total energy expenditure to basal metabolic rate). Equations predicting the energy requirements of humans throughout the lifespan were developed by the Institute of Medicine (2002) based on available doubly labeled water data, and are summarized in Table 5.5. Figure 5.1 shows

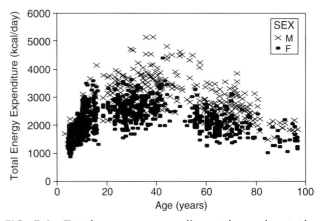

FIG. 5.1 Total energy expenditure throughout the lifecycle. Reprinted with permission from *Dietary Reference Intakes for Energy, Carbohydrate, Fiber, Fat, Acids, Cholesterol, Protein, and Amino Acids*, 2005, by the National Academy of Sciences, Courtesy of the National Academies Press, Washington, DC.

TABLE 5.5   Energy requirements (ER) for humans throughout the lifecycle

	Males	Females
Age group	ER	ER
0–3 months	(89W-100) + 175	(same)
4–6 months	(89W-100) + 56	(same)
7–12 months	(89W-100) + 22	(same)
13–25 months	(89W-100) + 20	(same)

Where W = weight in kg and the coefficients 20, 22, 56, 175 are estimated needs for energy deposition at these ages

3–8 years	88.5-61.9A + PA(26.7W + 903H) + 20	135.3-30.8A = PA(10.0W + 934H) + 20
Where PA =	*1.00 if activity level is sedentary (PAL is ≥1 <1.4)*	*1.00 if activity level is sedentary (PAL is ≥1 <1.4)*
	1.13 if activity level is low active (PAL is ≥1.4 <1.6)	*1.16 if activity level is low active (PAL is ≥1.4 <1.6)*
	1.26 if activity level is active (PAL is ≥1.6 <1.9)	*1.31 if activity level is active (PAL is ≥1.6 <1.9)*
	1.42 if activity level is very active (PAL is ≥1.9 <2.5)	*1.56 if activity level is very active (PAL is ≥1.9 <2.5)*
9–18 years	88.5-61.9A + PA(26.7W + 903H) + 25	135.3-30.8A = PA(10.0W + 934H) + 25
Where PA =	*1.00 if activity level is sedentary (PAL is ≥1 <1.4)*	*1.00 if activity level is sedentary (PAL is ≥1 <1.4)*
	1.13 if activity level is low active (PAL is ≥1.4 <1.6)	*1.16 if activity level is low active (PAL is ≥1.4 <1.6)*
	1.26 if activity level is active (PAL is ≥1.6 <1.9)	*1.31 if activity level is active (PAL is ≥1.6 <1.9)*
	1.42 if activity level is very active (PAL is ≥1.9 <2.5)	*1.56 if activity level is very active (PAL is ≥1.9 <2.5)*
19+ years	662-9.53A + PA(15.91W + 539.6H)	354-6.91A + PA(9.36W + 726H)
Where PA =	*1.00 if activity level is sedentary (PAL is ≥1.0 <1.4)*	*1.00 if activity level is sedentary (PAL is ≥1.0 <1.4)*
	1.11 if activity is low active (PAL is ≥1.4 <1.6)	*1.12 if activity is low active (PAL is ≥1.4 <1.6)*
	1.25 if activity level is active (PAL ≥1.6 <1.9)	*1.27 if activity level is active (PAL ≥1.6 <1.9)*
	1.48 if activity level is very active (PAL ≥ 1.9 < 2.5)	*1.45 if activity level is very active (PAL ≥1.9 <2.5)*

PAL, the physical activity level expressed as a ratio of total energy expenditure to basal or resting for the whole day.
W, weight, kg; H, height, inches; A, age, years; the coefficient 20 and 25 are the estimated energy needs for energy deposition at these ages (3–8 years, 9–18 years).

the data for TEE throughout the lifecycle used to generate the Institute of Medicine equations (Institute of Medicine, 2002).

A notable feature of Figure 5.1 is that there is a progressive increase in TEE throughout childhood, followed by a substantial decline in total energy expenditure with age after maturity, reflecting a modest decline in RMR and a greater decline in PAEE. The causes of declining physical activity with age are not well understood (Roberts and Dallal, 2005). The declines with age are reported to parallel an increase in body fat mass, suggesting that changes in body composition may be important (Roberts and Dallal, 1998). However, Westerterp and colleagues

(Meijer *et al.*, 2000; Westerterp and Meijer, 2001) have pointed out that the decline in energy requirements with age is most strongly predicted by age itself and not by body composition, indicating an effect of aging on expenditure independent of the quantity of lean tissue and fat mass. It is also noteworthy that maximal oxygen consumption is recognized to decline progressively with age, and very active individuals have declines of about 50% between 20 and 80 years that are a similar magnitude (albeit higher absolute values) to those experienced by sedentary individuals (DHHS, 1996). These observations suggest that some parallel changes in fitness, energy expenditure for physical activity, and body composition with age are an inevitable consequence of the aging process, probably due to underlying hormonal and biochemical changes in skeletal muscle and the cardiovascular system rather than a cumulative consequence of long-term inactivity. Further studies are needed to determine the extent to which energy expenditure for physical activity can be maintained in old age in the general population, since the potential specific effects of either low-intensity or high-intensity intentional exercise on energy balance will depend on compensatory changes in activity during other times of the day and this topic is currently controversial (Meijer *et al.*, 2000; Westerterp and Meijer, 2001; Westerterp, 2003; McLaughlin *et al.*, 2006). However small the effects on energy balance, additional effects of exercise include positive effects on cardiovascular and bone health, and prevention of falls and frailty (DiPietro, 2001).

Energy Expenditure During Refeeding and Energy Imbalance

Perturbations in energy balance underlie the most common public health nutrition problems today. In the United States, 68% of adults and 35% of children are now overweight or obese (Flegal *et al.*, 2010; Ogden *et al.*, 2006). The prevalence of obesity is also increasing in developing countries, where undernutrition has traditionally been the primary nutrition challenge and remains prevalent (Kurpad *et al.*, 2005). For example, the prevalence of obesity has increased recently in both Brazil and China, especially in urban areas but also in very low-income families such as those living in shantytowns (Sawaya *et al.*, 1995, 1998; Popkin *et al.*, 1996). In addition to being associated with increased risks of type 2 diabetes, osteoarthritis, angina, and hypertension, obesity is also associated with premature death and increased health-care costs (Uauy and Diaz, 2005). The estimated number of deaths attributable to obesity in the United States alone is ~300,000 per year.

The excess weight gain that accumulates in obesity results from energy intake exceeding energy expenditure over a considerable period of time and has both genetic and environmental origins. This positive energy balance can occur because energy expenditure is low or energy intake is high, or a combination of these two factors. The importance of energy expenditure is suggested by several (Ravussin *et al.*, 1988; Roberts *et al.*, 1988; DeLany, 1998; Goran *et al.*, 1998) though not all (Stunkard *et al.*, 1999) prospective studies showing that low energy expenditure

is a risk factor for excess weight gain, and mechanistically may result from the effects of energy expenditure on both energy requirements and insulin sensitivity (Ravussin *et al.*, 1988; Sigal *et al.*, 1997). In addition, the fact that excess energy intake is important, at least in the United States, is suggested by national survey statistics showing that per capita energy availability (adjusted for spoilage and waste) has increased over the past 20 years (Putnam, 1999; Economic Research Service, 2010).

Some studies suggest that humans possess a considerable capacity to increase energy expenditure (for RMR and TEF) during overfeeding with the result that in some individuals weight gain is less than expected for the magnitude of energy intake, and variability between individuals may be influenced by a genetic susceptibility or resistance to weight gain (Bouchard *et al.*, 1990; Levine *et al.*, 1999). However, even in studies that showed a significant capacity for energy dissipation during overeating, weight gain still occurred. Furthermore, other overfeeding studies suggest a substantially lower capacity for energy dissipation in normal volunteers (Ravussin *et al.*, 1985; Roberts *et al.*, 1990). Thus, although increased energy dissipation appears to occur during overeating, it is concomitant with positive energy balance and does not entirely prevent weight gain in most individuals.

Concerning negative energy balance, experimental underfeeding studies show a reduction in energy expenditure during weight loss (loss of both fat mass and FFM) that is disproportionate to the weight lost (Saltzman and Roberts, 1995). It is also important to note that the capacity for adaptive variations in energy expenditure appears to be greater in response to undereating than to overeating (Saltzman and Roberts, 1995). This implies that there is a greater metabolic priority in preventing weight loss than in preventing weight gain, a suggestion consistent with the presumption that food shortages were more common than food abundance during early human evolution. The question of whether energy expenditure remains depressed if weight is stabilized at a lower weight remains controversial (Leibel *et al.*, 1995; Saltzman and Roberts, 1995; Das *et al.*, 2003; Rosenbaum *et al.*, 2008), with different study approaches yielding different experimental findings. However, this issue has important implications in the formulation of refeeding energy requirements, for weight loss maintenance in individuals following dietary, pharmacological, or surgical weight loss, and for previously malnourished populations exposed to high-calorie low-nutrient-dense foods who may not be metabolically equipped to handle the caloric load and may be at risk of developing obesity.

Future Directions

Energy expenditure for resting metabolism, the thermic effect of feeding, and physical activity and arousal will balance energy intake in individuals maintaining energy balance, and are contributors to energy dysregulation in the obese state. Determinants of energy expenditure are the subject of considerable research but further studies are needed to accurately quantify the relative importance of genetic inheritance, early life influences, and current environmental factors in the prevention, development, and treatment of obesity.

Suggestions for Further Reading

Brooks, S.P.J. (2001) Fasting and refeeding: models of changes in metabolic efficiency. In K.B. Storey and J.M. Storey (eds), *Cell and Molecular Response to Stress*. Elsevier, Amsterdam, pp. 111–127.

Felber, J.-P. and Golay, A. (1995) Regulation of nutrient metabolism and energy expenditure. *Metabolism* **44**, 4–9.

Flatt, J.P. (1987) Dietary fat, carbohydrate balance, and weight maintenance: effects of exercise. *Am J Clin Nutr* **45**, 296–306.

Maughan, R.J., Fallah, J., and Coyle, E.F. (2010) The effects of fasting on metabolism and performance. *Br J Sports Med* **44**, 490–494.

References

Bogardus, C., Lillioja, S., Ravussin, E., *et al.* (1986) Familial dependence of the resting metabolic rate. *N Engl J Med* **315**, 96–100.

Bouchard, C., Tremblay, A., Despres, J.P., *et al.* (1990) The response to long-term overfeeding in identical twins. *N Engl J Med* **322**, 1477–1482.

Cole, T.J., Bellizzi, M.C., Flegal, K.M. and Dietz, W.H. (2000) Establishing a standard definition for child overweight and obesity worldwide: international survey. *Br Med J* **320**, 1240–1243.

Das, S.K., Roberts, S.B., McCrory, M.A., *et al.* (2003) Long-term changes in energy expenditure and body composition after massive weight loss induced by gastric bypass surgery. *Am J Clin Nutr* **78**, 22–30.

Delany, J.P. (1998) Role of energy expenditure in the development of pediatric obesity. *Am J Clin Nutr* **68**, 950S–955S.

de Weir, J.B. (1949) New methods for calculating metabolic rate with special reference to protein metabolism. *J Physiol* **109**, 1–9.

DHHS (1996) *Department of Health and Human Services. Physical Activity and Health: A Report of the Surgeon General.* USDHAA, Center for Disease Control and Prevention, Atlanta, GA.

DiPietro, L. (2001) Physical activity in aging: changes in patterns and their relationship to health and function. *J Gerontol A Biol Sci Med Sci* **56** Spec No 2, 13–22.

Durnin, J. and Passamore, R. (1967) *Energy, Work and Leisure.* Heinemann Educational Books, London.

Economic Research Service. U.S. per capita loss-adjusted food availability: Total calories. http://www.ers.usda.gov/Data/FoodConsumption/app/reports/displayCommodities.aspx?reportName=TotalCalories&id=36#startForm. Accessed June 30, 2010.

Ferraro, R., Lillioja, S., Fontvieille, A.M., *et al.* (1992) Lower sedentary metabolic rate in women compared with men. *J Clin Invest* **90**, 780–784.

Flatt, J. (1978) The biochemistry of energy expenditure. In G.A. Bray (ed.), *Recent Advances in Obesity Research. II. Proceedings of the 2nd International Congress on Obesity*. Food and Nutrition Press, Westport, CT, pp. 211–228.

Flegal, K.M., Carroll, M.D., Ogden, C.L., *et al.* (2010) Prevalence and trends in obesity among US adults, 1999–2008. *JAMA* **303** (3), 235–241.

Food and Agriculture Organization of the United Nations, WHO, and United Nations University (2001) *Report of a Joint FAO/WHO/UNU Expert Consultation. Human Energy Requirements.* World Health Organization, Geneva.

Golay, A., Schutz, Y., Felber, J.P., *et al.* (1989) Blunted glucose-induced thermogenesis in "overweight" patients: a factor contributing to relapse of obesity. *Int J Obes* **13**, 767–775.

Goran, M.I., Shewchuk, R., Gower, B.A., *et al.* (1998) Longitudinal changes in fatness in white children: no effect of childhood energy expenditure. *Am J Clin Nutr* **67**, 309–316.

Institute of Medicine (2002) *Dietary Reference Intakes for Macronutrients*. National Academy Press, Washington, DC.

Kinney, J. and Tucker, H. (1992) *Energy Metabolism: Tissue Determinants and Cellular Corollaries*. Raven Press, New York.

Kurpad, A.V., Muthayya, S., and Vaz, M. (2005) Consequences of inadequate food energy and negative energy balance in humans. *Public Health Nutr* **8**, 1053–1076.

Leibel, R.L., Rosenbaum, M., and Hirsch, J. (1995) Changes in energy expenditure resulting from altered body weight. *N Engl J Med* **332**, 621–628. [Erratum appears in *N Engl J Med* 1995; **333**, 399.]

Levine, J., Eberhardt, N., and Jensen, M. (1999) Role of non-exercise activity thermogenesis in resistance to fat gain in humans. *Science* **283**, 212–214.

Lifson, N. and McClintock, R. (1966) Theory of use of the turnover rates of body water for measuring energy and material balance. *J Theoret Biol* **12**, 46–74.

Lifson, N., Gordon, G.B., and McClintock, R. (1955) Measurement of total carbon dioxide production by means of D2O18. *J Appl Physiol* **7**, 704–710.

Lifson, N., Gordon, G.B., Visscher, M.B., *et al.* (1949) The fate of utilized molecular oxygen and the source of the oxygen of respiratory carbon dioxide, studied with the aid of heavy oxygen. *J Biol Chem* **180**, 803–811.

Livesey, G. and Elia, M. (1988) Estimation of energy expenditure, net carbohydrate utilization, and net fat oxidation and synthesis by indirect calorimetry: evaluation of errors with special reference to the detailed composition of fuels. *Am J Clin Nutr* **47**, 608–628.

Major, G.C., Doucet, E., Trayhurn, P., *et al.* (2007) Clinical significance of adaptive thermogenesis. *Int J Obesity* **31**, 204–212.

McLaughlin, R., Malkova, D., and Nimmo, M.A. (2006) Spontaneous activity responses to exercise in males and females. *Eur J Clin Nutr* **60**, 1055–1061.

Meijer, E.P., Westerterp, K.R., and Verstappen, F.T. (2000) Effect of exercise training on physical activity and substrate utilization in the elderly. *Int J Sports Med* **21**, 499–504.

Melanson, K.J., Saltzman, E., Vinken, A.G., *et al.* (1998) The effects of age on postprandial thermogenesis at four graded energetic challenges: findings in young and older women. *J Gerontol A Biol Sci Med Sci* **53A**, B409–B414.

Murgatroyd, P. (1984) A 30 m³ direct and indirect calorimeter. In A.J.H. Van Es (ed.), *Human Energy Metabolism: Physical Activity and Energy Expenditure Measurements in Epidemiological Research Based upon Direct and Indirect Calorimetry*. Euro-Nut, Wageningen, pp. 126–128.

Ogden, C.L., Carroll, M.D., Curtin, L.R., *et al.* (2006) Prevalence of overweight and obesity in the United States, 1999–2004. *JAMA* **295**, 1549–1555.

Popkin, B.M., Richards, M.K., and Montiero, C.A. (1996) Stunting is associated with overweight in children of four nations that are undergoing the nutrition transition. *J Nutr* **126**, 3009–3016.

Putnam, J. (1999) US food supply providing more food and calories. *Food Rev* **22**, 2–12.

Ravussin, E., Lillioja, S., Knowler, W.C., *et al.* (1988) Reduced rate of energy expenditure as a risk factor for body-weight gain. *N Engl J Med* **318**, 467–472.

Ravussin, E., Schutz, Y., Acheson, K.J., *et al.* (1985) Short-term, mixed-diet overfeeding in man: no evidence for "luxuskonsumption". *Am J Physiol Endocrinol Metab* **249**, E470–477.

Roberts, S.B. (1989) Use of the doubly labeled water method for measurement of energy expenditure, total body water, water intake, and metabolizable energy intake in humans and small animals. *Can J Physiol Pharmacol* **67**, 1190–1198.

Roberts, S.B. and Dallal, G.E. (1998) Effects of age on energy balance. *Am J Clin Nutr* **68**, 975S–979S.

Roberts, S.B. and Dallal, G.E. (2001) The new childhood growth charts. *Nutr Rev* **59**, 31–36.

Roberts, S.B. and Dallal, G.E. (2005) Energy requirements and aging. *Public Health Nutr* **8**, 1028–1036.

Roberts, S.B., Fuss, P., Heyman, M.B., *et al.* (1995) Influence of age on energy requirements. *Am J Clin Nutr* **62**, 1053S–1058S.

Roberts, S.B., Savage, J., Coward, W.A., *et al.* (1988) Energy expenditure and intake in infants born to lean and overweight mothers. *N Engl J Med* **318**, 461–466.

Roberts, S.B., Young, V.R., Fuss, P., *et al.* (1990) Energy expenditure and subsequent nutrient intakes in overfed young men. *Am J Physiol Regul Integr Comp Physiol* **259**, R461–469.

Rosenbaum, M., Hirsch, J., Gallagher, D.A., *et al.* (2008) Long-term persistence of adaptive thermogenesis in subjects who have maintained a reduced body weight. *Am J Clin Nutr* **88**, 906–912.

Saltzman, E. and Roberts, S.B. (1995) The role of energy expenditure in energy regulation: findings from a decade of research. *Nutr Rev* **53**, 209–220.

Sawaya, A.L., Dallal, G., Solymos, G., *et al.* (1995) Obesity and malnutrition in a shantytown population in the city of Sao Paulo, Brazil. *Obes Res* **3** Suppl 2, 107S–115S.

Sawaya, A.L., Grillo, L.P., Verreschi, I., *et al.* (1998) Mild stunting is associated with higher susceptibility to the effects of high fat diets: studies in a shantytown population in Sao Paulo, Brazil. *J Nutr* **128**, 415S–420S.

Schoeller, D.A. (1988) Measurement of energy expenditure in free-living humans by using doubly labeled water. *J Nutr* **118**, 1278–1289.

Schoeller, D.A. (1990) How accurate is self-reported dietary energy intake? *Nutr Rev* **48**, 373–379.

Schofield, W., Schofield, E., and James, W. (1985) Basal metabolic rate-review and prediction, together with an annotated bibliography of source material. *Hum Nutr Clin Nutr* **39C**, 1–96.

Schutz, Y., Bessard, T., and Jequier, E. (1984) Diet-induced thermogenesis measured over a whole day in obese and non-obese women. *Am J Clin Nutr* **40**, 542–552.

Segal, K.R., Edano, A., Blando, L., *et al.* (1990) Comparison of thermic effects of constant and relative caloric loads in lean and obese men. *Am J Clin Nutr* **51**, 14–21.

Shetty, P. (2005) Energy requirements of adults. *Public Health Nutr* **8**, 994–1009.

Sigal, R.J., El-Hashimy, M., Martin, B.C., *et al.* (1997) Acute postchallenge hyperinsulinemia predicts weight gain: a prospective study. *Diabetes* **46,** 1025–1029.

Solomon, S.J., Kurzer, M.S., and Calloway, D.H. (1982) Menstrual cycle and basal metabolic rate in women. *Am J Clin Nutr* **36,** 611–616.

Stunkard, A.J., Berkowitz, R.I., Stallings, V.A., *et al.* (1999) Energy intake, not energy output, is a determinant of body size in infants. *Am J Clin Nutr* **69,** 524–530.

Surrao, J., Sawaya, A.L., Dallal, G.E., *et al.* (1998) Use of food quotients in human doubly labeled water studies: comparable results obtained with four widely used food intake methods. *J Am Diet Assoc* **98,** 1015–1020.

Uauy, R. and Diaz, E. (2005) Consequences of food energy excess and positive energy balance. *Public Health Nutr* **8,** 1077–1099.

Van Zant, R.S. (1992) Influence of diet and exercise on energy expenditure–a review. *Int J Sport Nutr* **2,** 1–19.

Westerterp, K.R. (2003) Impacts of vigorous and non-vigorous activity on daily energy expenditure. *Proc Nutr Soc* **62,** 645–650.

Westerterp, K.R. and Meijer, E.P. (2001) Physical activity and parameters of aging: a physiological perspective. *J Gerontol A Biol Sci Med Sci* **56** Spec No 2, 7–12.

WHO (1985) *Energy and Protein Requirements. Report of a Joint FAO/WHO/UNU Expert* Consultation. WHO, Geneva.

WHO (1995) *Physical Status: The Use and Interpretation of Anthropometry. Report of a WHO Expert Committee.* Geneva, WHO.

6

PROTEIN AND AMINO ACIDS

PAUL B. PENCHARZ, MB, ChB, PhD, FRCP(C)

University of Toronto, Ontario, Canada

Summary

This chapter considers selected recent advances in amino acid function, and protein and amino acid utilization, during the prandial and postprandial period of amino acid metabolism. The importance of the gut and the splanchnic region as a whole in the regulation of whole-body amino acid metabolism has become better appreciated and understood. There remains uncertainty about quantitative aspects of amino acid nutrition, especially in healthy adults, but there is now a consensus that the current international requirement estimates for adults are far too low. This has potentially important implications for the evaluation of dietary protein quality and for the planning, now and in the future, of food protein supplies for population groups. Improved in vivo metabolic tools combined with molecular and cellular techniques appear to offer great promise for resolving some of the outstanding issues that limit our ability to predict precisely the effect of the dietary protein and amino acid component on function and the quantitative and qualitative character of the intake that optimizes development and health maintenance.

Introduction

Jac Berzelius invented the term "protein," which was accepted by the Dutch chemist, Gerardus J. Mulder, in the *Bulletin des Sciences Physiques et Naturelles en Neerlande* in 1838 (Korpes, 1970). A readable account of the history behind the development and understanding of protein and amino acid nutrition has appeared (Carpenter, 1994), and the earlier practical recommendations about dietary intakes for protein have been summarized by Munro (1985). This chapter will be confined to a discussion of selected, more recent developments in the general area of protein and amino acid metabolism and its nutritional corollaries, with particular emphasis on relevance to human protein and amino acid nutrition.

The Currency of Protein Metabolism and Nutrition – Amino Acid Functions

Proteins comprise one of the five classes of complex biomolecules found in cells and tissues, the others being DNA, RNA, polysaccharides, and lipids. The building blocks of proteins are amino acids and, as such, they are the currency of protein nutrition and metabolism.

Present Knowledge in Nutrition, Tenth Edition. Edited by John W. Erdman Jr, Ian A. Macdonald and Steven H. Zeisel.
© 2012 International Life Sciences Institute. Published 2012 by John Wiley & Sons, Inc.

Although there are hundreds of amino acids in nature, only ~20 of these commonly appear in proteins, via charging by their cognate tRNAs and subsequent recognition of a codon on the mRNA. In the special case of certain selenoproteins, such as glutathione peroxidase and type 2 iodothreonine 5'-deiodinase, there is formation and incorporation of selenocysteine into these proteins, which involves a complex process including conversion of a seryl-tRNA to selenocysteinyl-tRNA, which is then recognized by a UGA codon (Burke and Hill, 1993). Selenomethionine is also present in body proteins but this is derived from ingestion of this amino acid in plant foods or supplements such as yeasts (Schrauzer, 2000). Finally, other amino acids, such as hydroxyproline or N^τ-methylhistidine, are also present in proteins. These arise via a post-transitional modification of specific amino acid residues, which gives particular structural and functional properties to proteins; a good example of this relates to the vitamin K-dependent carboxylation of glutamic acid residues in a number of proteins involved in blood coagulation and bone matrix deposition (Ferland, 1998). However, the 20 common amino acids, along with a few others not in peptide-bound form, such as ornithine, citrulline, and taurine, are of more immediate interest in discussions of the nitrogen economy of the body and the protein and amino acid nutritional status of the human subject.

In addition to their role as substrates for polypeptide chain formation, amino acids serve multiple and diverse roles. Some of these are listed in Table 6.1. Many of these roles have been recognized for some time but an important new development relates to an increased understanding of the mechanisms that account for the stimulation of specific or global protein synthesis by amino acids. It is now clear that amino acids, especially the branched-chain amino acid leucine, can affect the initiation of mRNA translation (Pain, 1996; Jousse *et al.*, 1999; Vishwannath *et al.*, 1999; Anthony *et al.*, 2000; Lynch *et al.*, 2000).

Tissue and organ protein content is also determined by the rate at which proteins are degraded. This overall process of protein degradation or breakdown plays many essential roles in the functioning of organisms, including, for example, cell growth, adaptation to different physiological conditions, elimination of abnormal or damaged proteins, and normal functioning of the immune system (Lecker *et al.*, 1999). Multiple pathways for protein breakdown occur in all cells, with the bulk of intracellular protein being degraded via the energy-dependent, ubiquitin–proteasome pathway. Here the proteins are digested to small peptides and amino acids within a multisubunit 20S proteasome, which, in association with a large 19S regulatory particle, forms the 26S complex. The proteasome may account for up to 1% of cellular proteins. This powerful proteolytic enzyme system cleaves peptide bonds in a unique way involving an ordered cyclical bite–chew mechanism. The ubiquitin–proteasome pathway is activated under a number of conditions, including fasting (Lecker *et al.*, 1999). Studies of whole-body protein turnover have shown that protein degradation is inhibited with feeding

TABLE 6.1 Some functions of amino acids

Function	Example[a]
Substrates for protein synthesis	Those for which there is a codon
Regulators of protein turnover	Leucine, glutamine
Regulators of enzyme activity	Arginine and *N*-acetyl glutamate synthesis
	Phenylalanine and phenylalanine dehydroxylase activation
Precursor of signal transducer	Arginine, nitric oxide
Neurotransmitter	Tryptophan, glutamate
Ion fluxes	Taurine, glutamate, oxoproline
Precursor of nitrogen compounds	Nucleic acid, creatinine
Transporter of nitrogen	Glutamine, alanine, leucine (in the brain)
Translational regulator	Leucine (4E-BP1 and P70(s6k) via MTOR-dependent pathway)
Transcriptional regulator	Leucine limitation induces CHOP expression

[a]MTOR, Mammalian target of ripamycin; CHOP, CCAAT/enhancer binding protein (C/EBP) homologous protein.

and with increased protein intakes (Waterlow, 1995), although it remains unclear which organs and tissues contribute most to this decline, and the relative effect of the amino acids versus carbohydrate and other energy-yielding sources still is not entirely determined. For example, oral amino acids alone do not appear to alter the rate of protein breakdown in the vastus lateralis (Volpi *et al.*, 1999) whereas a mixed meal was shown to inhibit forearm muscle protein breakdown (Tessari *et al.*, 1996). Thus, it is possible, at least in muscle, that amino acids enhance the inhibitory effect of proteolysis because of a carbohydrate-induced rise in insulin availability (Flakoll *et al.*, 1989). In turn, insulin reduces proteolysis, possibly by decreasing ubiquitin-mediated proteasomal activity (Bennett *et al.*, 2000). The gut may be an important site of the meal-induced decline in whole-body protein breakdown (Tessari, 2000). In addition the balance of amino acids, or protein quality, may influence whole-body protein breakdown. In human low-birth-weight infants it has been shown that a higher quality amino acid mixture enhanced growth and amino nitrogen utilization by reducing whole-body protein breakdown and not by enhancing protein synthesis (Duffy *et al.*, 1981).

The other multiple functions of the different amino acids and their putative mechanisms of action will not be elaborated here because other accounts are available (Cynober, 1995; Fürst and Young, 2000). Two further points need to be made here. First, the functions of some of the amino acids can be varied and extensive, as indicated by the multiple functions played by glutamine (Box 6.1). These non-proteinogenic functions are relevant to dietary intake and requirement considerations, as suggested from the analysis made by Reeds (2000) and presented in Table 6.2. Some of the pathways of end-product production can substantially affect the overall utilization of the amino acid precursor (e.g. creatinine synthesis, glycine or glutathione synthesis, cysteine or glycine utilization). Second, from a nutritional perspective, in carrying out their roles as substrates in protein synthesis (e.g. for neurotransmitter signaling and detoxification functions) the amino acids turn over and part of their nitrogen and carbon is removed from the body via catabolic and excretory pathways. Thus, the maintenance of an adequate body protein and amino acid status requires a sufficient intake of some preformed amino acids together with a utilizable source of nitrogen for the synthesis of the other amino acids and for production of physiologically important nitrogen-containing compounds.

BOX 6.1 Functions of glutamine

Substrate of protein synthesis (codons; CAA, CAG)

Anabolic and trophic substance for muscle, intestine (competence factor)

Control for acid–base balance (renal ammoniagenesis)

Substrate for hepatic ureagenesis

Substrate for hepatic and renal gluconeogenesis

Fuel for intestinal enterocytes

Fuel and nucleic acid precursor and important for generation of cytotoxic products in immunocompetent cells

Ammonia scavenger

Possible substrate for citrulline and arginine synthesis, although in vivo proline appears to be used instead of glutamine/glutamate

Nitrogen donor (nucleotides, amino sugars, coenzymes)

Nitrogen transport (one-third circulating nitrogen) (muscle, lung)

Precursor of γ-aminobutyric acid (via glutamate)

Shuttle for glutamate (central nervous system)

Preferential substrate for glutathione peroxidase production?

Osmotic signaling mechanism in regulation of protein synthesis?

Stimulator of glycogen synthesis

Metabolism of L-arginine–nitric oxide

Nutritional Corollaries of the Amino Acids

It is no longer thought useful to classify the amino acids into two groups – those that are nutritionally indispensable (essential) or dispensable (non-essential) – as was done originally by Rose (1948) based on a series of now-classical qualitative nitrogen-balance experiments in adult men. Instead it is better to classify amino acids into three groups, the original two plus a third that is intermediate and is called conditionally indispensable (Table 6.3) (Pencharz *et al.*, 1996). An obligatory dietary requirement exists for tryptophan, leucine, isoleucine, valine, phenylalanine, methionine, lysine, threonine, and histidine, or more specifically, for the ketoacid derivatives of the first five of these. The last three of this indispensable group of amino acids cannot be transaminated and so must be supplied in the diet as such. The other common amino acids in proteins can be synthesized from carbon and nitrogen donors: transamination of α-ketoisocaproate, oxaloacetic acid, and

TABLE 6.2   Potential contribution of functionally important end-product synthesis to amino acid needs in adult humans[a]

	Glutamate	Glycine	Cysteine (μmol/kg/day)	Arginine	Methionine
Precursor kinetics					
Plasma flux	4200	3960	1320	1800	528
Net synthesis	358	2730	96	180	168
End-product production					
Creatine		170		170	170
Taurine			7		
Nitric oxide				15	
Glutathione	550	550	550		

[a]Modified from Table 7 in Reeds (2000), where original references for these values are given.

TABLE 6.3   Categorization of dietary amino acids[a]

Indispensable (Essential)	Conditionally indispensable (Conditionally essential)	Dispensable (Non-essential)
Histidine	Arginine	Alanine
Isoleucine	Cysteine	Aspartate
Leucine	Glutamine	Asparagine
Lysine	Glycine	Glutamate
Methionine	Proline	Serine
Phenylalanine	Tyrosine	
Threonine		
Tryptophan		
Valine		

[a]Modified from Pencharz et al. (1996).

pyruvate for glutamate, aspartic acid, and alanine, respectively; glycine from serine via serine hydroxymethyltransferase and serine from pyruvic acid; glycine from threonine; arginine from proline and glutamate; and asparagine from glutamine and aspartate. Tyrosine and cyst(e)ine are synthesized from their parent indispensable amino acids, phenylalanine and methionine, respectively. These two latter amino acids, tyrosine and cysteine, are included in the conditionally indispensable amino acid group together with glutamine, arginine, and perhaps glycine and proline, because each does not appear to be synthesized at a rate sufficient to meet cellular needs under certain physiological or pathological conditions (Jaksic et al., 1991; Reeds et al., 2000a). Thus, in severe burn injury, metabolic studies indicate that a dietary source of arginine is needed to maintain arginine homeostasis; low-birth-weight infants are unable to synthesize cysteine, proline, and possibly glycine, in sufficient quantities (Pencharz et al., 1996).

A more recent development concerns the possible need for a preformed source of α-amino nitrogen. Hitherto, it had been considered that, if intake of the indispensable amino acids was sufficient, only a source of non-specific nitrogen – which might be in the form of a simple mixture, such as urea and diammonium citrate – would be needed additionally (Williams et al., 1974). However, this may not be a sufficient description of what is actually required to sustain an adequate state of protein nutriture, for several reasons. The first relates to the utilization of urea nitrogen. Thus, recent emphasis has been given to a potentially key role played by the hydrolysis of urea nitrogen within the intestinal lumen (assumed to be largely a function of the activity of the microflora in the large bowel) and the significant contribution made by this liberated nitrogen to the nitrogen homeostasis of the host (Jackson, 2000). However, this concept has been questioned (Young et al., 2000a) because in other studies the production of urea has been shown to increase linearly with increased protein intake, and the nitrogen released from urea via hydrolysis appears to have been rechanneled into pathways of urea formation. Thus, the extent to which urea nitrogen might be a net source of utilizable nitrogen, even under conditions of a low protein intake, remains unclear. Furthermore, as clearly outlined by Waterlow (1999), a great deal of uncertainty still exists about in vivo mechanisms responsible for both short- and longer-term regulation of urea production and therefore about the mechanisms responsible for maintenance of body protein balance.

It has been suggested that glutamate is a key amino acid in making net amino nitrogen available to the mammalian organism; this glutamate would be derived ultimately from plant protein (Young and Ajami, 2000; Pencharz and Young, 2006). Despite the significant role of glutamate as a nitrogen portal, it remains unclear whether a specific dietary need for glutamate exists if a sufficient amount of α-amino nitrogen is supplied, for example, as alanine and for aspartate. This question cannot be answered unequivocally at present but it is clear that indispensable amino acids alone or in high concentration relative to the dispensable amino acids will not support adequate growth in experimental animals. In sum, a source of preformed α-amino nitrogen from other than the indispensable amino acids and glycine appears to be required, but whether glutamate is needed specifically or would be a more efficient source of this α-amino nitrogen than its homologues (Young and Ajami, 2000), for example, remains to be determined. Reeds (2000) reviewed a number of findings that revealed that diets completely devoid of glutamine and glutamate result in poorer growth in the otherwise healthy rat and pig, suggesting the possibility of a specific need for glutamate.

If the foregoing argument is correct, it introduces a new perspective on the nonspecific nitrogen component of the total protein requirement. In 1965, a Food and Agriculture Organization of the United Nations and the World Health Organization (FAO/WHO) Expert Group (1965) stated:

> The proportion of non essential amino acid nitrogen, and hence the E/T [g total essential amino acids to total nitrogen] ratio of the diet, has an obvious influence on essential amino acid requirements . . . To make the best use of the available food supplies there is an obvious need to determine the minimum E/T ratios for different physiological states . . . Finally, the question arises whether there is an optimal pattern of non-essential amino acids.

This statement can just as well be repeated today, but recent studies are beginning to provide deeper insight into the nature of the non-specific nitrogen needs of the human body. Not only is there an optimal E/T, as noted above, but it now seems likely that there is a desirable qualitative character to the non-specific nitrogen supply – which raises the issue of the optimal sources and levels of α-amino nitrogen compounds in enteral formulations. This issue, for example, includes considerations of glutamate–proline–arginine interrelations (Wu and Morris, 1998) not

only in terms of the nitrogen economy of the host but also with respect to specific functions such as capacity to maintain or stimulate the immune system and promote wound and tissue repair and the effect that non-specific nitrogen may have on polyamine and hormonal balance. The effect of a relatively high arginine intake in healthy subjects on arginine–citrulline–ornithine kinetics (Beaumier et al., 1995) has been examined; although changes were not observed in the activity of the whole-body L-arginine–nitric oxide pathway, the generous level of arginine supplementation reduced rates of urea production and excretion and increased circulating insulin concentrations. How this apparent protein anabolic effect of high arginine supplementation is brought about (perhaps enhanced by insulin action) and what significance it has for the immune system are not known. Also, in light of current interest in immune-enhancing diets and the role arginine plays in aggravating or attenuating renal injury (Narita et al., 1995; Reckelhoff et al., 1997), there are many unresolved questions about the quantitative role played by the non-specific nitrogen component in supporting protein metabolism and function in the host.

Postprandial Nitrogen and Amino Acid Utilization

The daily maintenance of body protein content is achieved through a complex set of integrated changes in rates of whole-body protein turnover, amino acid oxidation, urea production, and nitrogen excretion that occur at different rates during the postabsorptive, prandial, and postprandial periods of the 24-hour day (Millward and Pacy, 1995). Depending on diet composition, smaller or larger gains and losses of body proteins occur during the diurnal cycle of feeding and fasting. Amino acid and nitrogen requirements are met normally via ingestion of food proteins that undergo sequential metabolic and physiological processes. The processes include gastrointestinal digestion, peptide and amino acid absorption, transfer of amino acids into and among organs, and entry of the amino acids into metabolic pathways, quantitatively most notably into protein synthesis. We have termed this overall process the metabolic availability of dietary amino acids and have developed a method to determine the metabolic availability from protein in pigs (Moehn et al., 2005) and in humans (Humayun et al., 2007b; Elango et al., 2009).

Dietary Protein Nitrogen Distribution after Protein Ingestion

[15]N-labeled proteins have been used to follow the metabolic fate of dietary nitrogen after the ingestion of protein, and a number of these studies were summarized by Tomé and Bos (2000). As summarized in Figure 6.1, for ~100 g intake of well-balanced protein in the adult human, the fate of the dietary nitrogen is ~30–40% directed to anabolism, with a 17–25% loss via oxidative metabolism. A detailed model – based on data for [^{15}N] nitrogen kinetics determined in the intestine, blood and urine after ingestion of ^{15}N-labeled milk protein in humans – developed by Fouillet et al. (2000) predicted that, 8 hours after a meal, ~28% of the nitrogen is retained as free amino acids and 72% as protein. Approximately 30% of this protein retention occurred in the splanchnic region and 70% in peripheral tissues. This type of approach involving use of intrinsically labeled proteins will continue to help define the factors, the mechanisms, and their quantitative significance that affect the postprandial utilization of ingested protein.

The extent and regulation of postprandial protein utilization has also been studied by acute ^{13}C-leucine balance studies (Millward, 2000). Although postprandial protein utilization is not influenced by adult age in a healthy population, it is affected by the quality of protein and size of meals (Millward, 2000). This tracer-based approach also has the potential for assessing efficacy of enteral formulations (e.g. in the nutritional support of institutionalized subjects and sick patients).

Among the additional factors that can influence the postprandial utilization of proteins is the time course of release and absorption of peptides and amino acids. This has led to the concept of slow and fast dietary proteins based on studies using ^{13}C-leucine-labeled whey and caseins. Beaufrere et al. (2000) showed that postprandial whole-body leucine oxidation over 7 hours was lower with casein than with whey protein despite a similar leucine intake (i.e. the postprandial protein utilization for casein was higher than for whey). Both of these protein sources are of high quality in adult human nutrition. Hence, a difference in postprandial protein utilization under some circumstances might give a false indication of the comparative nutritional value of different formulations. Clearly, this new tracer-based metabolic paradigm requires further definition and standardization but in a general context it

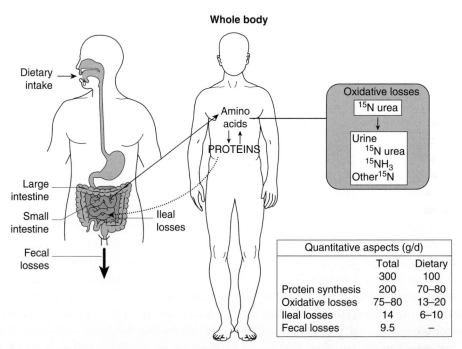

FIG. 6.1 Contribution of dietary protein to the principal pathways of protein metabolism.

promises to be a valuable tool for understanding the metabolic basis of the requirement for protein and amino acids.

The temporal nature of the amino acid supply or pattern of feeding influences the efficiency of nitrogen and amino acid utilization. Studies involving 24-hour [1-^{13}C]leucine tracer balance determinations showed that daily leucine oxidation is lower when three discrete meals versus ten small hourly meals are given over a 12-hour period (El-Khoury et al., 1995). This appears to be the case at both generous and limiting intakes of leucine, suggesting a better retention of oral amino acids with a less frequent meal intake. Whether this phenomenon might be explained by the so-called anabolic drive of amino acids (Millward and Pacy, 1995) cannot be determined yet, but it is evident that the pattern of protein and amino acid ingestion is a determinant of the efficiency of postprandial utilization. Furthermore, Arnal et al. (1999) showed in studies with elderly subjects that protein retention was higher when 80% of the daily intake was consumed at midday as compared with the daily protein supply given in four meals over 12 hours.

Amino Acid Utilization by the Splanchnic Bed and the Gut

The intestines and liver modify the profile and amount of amino acids that disappear from the intestinal lumen and enter the portal and peripheral blood circulation. Although this has been known for some time, in recent years a more elaborate account of the quantitative removal and metabolic transformations of amino acids by the splanchnic region after their uptake from the lumen has been developed in humans and animal models, particularly those involving the use of different isotope tracer paradigms. For example, the combined use of tracers given orally and intravenously showed that the extent of uptake by the splanchnic region in adults differs among amino acids (Table 6.4) (Young et al., 2000b) and that this might also depend on the level of amino acid intake. The uptake of cystine shown here is very high, which is consistent with the data obtained in the pig (Rerat et al., 1992). The high uptake might also explain why the concentration of cysteine in the circulation shows little postprandial response to a wide range of cystine intakes (Raguso et al., 1997).

Two important issues emerge from this rather global description of splanchnic amino acid metabolism, namely the relative importance of the gut versus the liver and the metabolic fate of the amino acids within these organ systems. This is a nutritionally important topic for several

TABLE 6.4 Dual isotope tracer model estimates of splanchnic uptake of amino acids: fed state in healthy adults[a]

Amino acid (intake)	Uptake (% of intake)
Leucine (adequate)	21 ± 6
Leucine (low)	37 ± 5
Leucine (adequate)	10 ± 6
Phenylalanine (adequate)	25
Phenylalanine (low)	58 ± 4
Tyrosine (adequate)	37
Arginine (adequate)	34 ± 8
Methionine (adequate)	23 ± 2
Cystine	>50

[a]Modified from Young et al. (2000b) where references to original studies are cited.

reasons. First, for example, Bertolo et al. (1998) have concluded that the threonine requirement of neonatal piglets during parenteral nutrition is 45% of the mean oral requirement. This could be a result of one or a combination of factors, including a lower rate of threonine oxidation by intestinal tissues when threonine is given intravenously and also reduced losses of threonine by the gastrointestinal tract because of reduced mucin production, these glycoproteins being rich in threonine. Second, Boirie et al. (1997) reported that the splanchnic extraction of dietary leucine was twice as high in elderly men (50 ± 11%) as it was in young men (23 ± 3%), although whole-body leucine oxidation was similar for the two age groups. These investigators concluded that this difference in splanchnic uptake might limit the availability of leucine for peripheral tissue metabolism. On the other hand, Volpi et al. (1999), while also observing that the splanchnic extraction of oral phenylalanine was significantly higher in the elderly (47 ± 3%) than in the young (29 ± 5%), found that, after an oral amino acid mixture, muscle protein synthesis was stimulated similarly in the young and the elderly.

Our understanding of the role of the gut and liver as the components of the splanchnic bed have been advanced by work from the laboratories of Reeds et al. (2000b) and Brunton et al. (2000). From this work it is now apparent that the small intestinal enterocyte plays an active role in amino acid metabolism, including the biosynthesis of arginine (Wilkinson et al., 2004). Arteriovenous differences and tracer studies have focused recently on the immediate fate of absorbed amino acids (Wu et al., 1998; Reeds et al., 2000b). From studies of the portal availability of amino acids in pigs, Reeds *et al.* (2000b) concluded that the portal outflow varies widely among amino acids, with the portal balance of dietary threonine being consistently lower than that of other essential amino acids; nutritionally significant quantities of dietary glutamate and aspartate rarely appear in the portal blood (also, a net extraction of glutamine occurs across the gut, and systemic glutamate, aspartate, and glutamine are derived almost exclusively from synthesis within the body); and some amino acids either appear in quantities similar to those ingested in dietary protein (arginine and tyrosine) or greatly exceed them (alanine).

Further details concerning the relative contributions of the arterial and dietary sources of amino acids to amino acid utilization by the intestine are given by Reeds *et al.* (2000b). Particularly important are the observations that the total utilization of lysine, leucine, and phenylalanine by the portal drained viscera might account for >40% of the whole-body flux; the utilization of dietary glutamate, aspartate, and glutamine is considerable and these amino acids contribute significantly to intestinal energy transformation; intestinal oxidation of leucine and lysine in milk-fed piglets accounts for around one-fifth to one-third of whole-body oxidation; with protein restriction the intestine continues to use a disproportionately large amount of indispensable amino acids (Van Goudoever *et al.*, 2000); the gut is an important site for synthesis of citrulline (Wu, 1998) that is then used for arginine synthesis, especially in the kidney (Young and El-Khoury, 1995); and mucosal glutathione is synthesized mainly from enteral precursor amino acids (Reeds *et al.*, 2000b).

In summary, beyond doubt the intestine plays a quantitatively and qualitatively crucial role in determining the amino acid needs of the individual and the availability of amino acids for the support of the body's physiological and organ systems.

Intestinal Amino Acid Synthesis

As reviewed recently by Metges (2000), the gastrointestinal microflora may make an important contribution to the status of nitrogen metabolism in the host. Tracer studies in animals and humans have shown a transfer of nonspecific nitrogen (ammonia, urea nitrogen, glutamate, etc.) into dispensable and indispensable amino acids (Metges *et al.*, 1999b). For most amino acids this input of ^{15}N from urea may reflect nitrogen exchange or reversible transamination. However, lysine and threonine do not undergo transamination in mammalian tissues, so the appearance of ^{15}N-labeled lysine or threonine in body proteins and plasma amino acids must reflect de novo synthesis of lysine and threonine by the intestinal microflora and the subsequent absorption of the labeled amino acids from the gastrointestinal tract. Comparative experiments with germ-free and conventional rats have confirmed that de novo synthesis of lysine is due to the activity of the indigenous microflora in the gastrointestinal tract.

However, a more cautious conclusion is possibly warranted. Although these recent studies (Metges *et al.*, 1999a) establish the significant presence of lysine and threonine of microbial origin in the plasma free amino acid pool, the quantitative significance of this source of amino acids is still unknown. Further, these new studies raise the question as to how various clinical states and diseases might affect the nutritional and metabolic interrelationships between the microbial flora of the intestine and the amino acid economy of host tissues.

Nitrogen (Protein) Requirements

Requirements for protein (and for amino acids) are determined by the change in physiological outcome to graduated intakes (Pencharz and Ball, 2003) (see Figure 6.2). As is detailed by Pencharz and Ball (2003) and by Elango *et al.* (2008a), it is important that each subject be studied across a full range from below the requirement level to

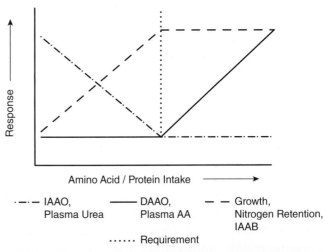

FIG. 6.2 Determination of amino acid (protein) requirements – patterns of response. DAAO, direct amino acid oxidation; IAAB, indicator amino acid balance; IAAO, indicator amino acid oxidation.

significantly above it. This approach was introduced by our group (Pencharz and Ball, 2003; Elango *et al.*, 2008a) but it has been adopted by others (Kurpad *et al.*, 2003, 2005, 2006). Further this response should be analyzed using non-linear regression. In practice we have found that two-phase linear regression crossover analysis is the best way of defining the average population requirement (Pencharz and Ball, 2003; Elango *et al.*, 2008b). Until recently the approach used to determine protein requirements was based on the nitrogen balance seen in response to graded intakes of protein (Institute of Medicine, 2002/2005; FAO/WHO, 2007; Humayun *et al.*, 2007a). Expert committees have reported recently from the National Academy of Sciences (Institute of Medicine, 2002/2005) and the United Nations Food and Agriculture Organization and World Health Organization (FAO/WHO, 2007) in which the relationship between protein intake and nitrogen balance was analyzed using monolinear regression. The author was a member of both expert committees but the closer I looked at the data the more reservations I had. Hence I and my colleagues recently reanalyzed this data using non-linear regression and published results that show that adult protein requirements have been underestimated by around 30% (Humayun *et al.*, 2007a; Elango *et al.*, 2010). In addition to this reanalysis of the nitrogen balance data, we introduced the use of indicator oxidation to determine protein requirements in humans (Humayun *et al.*, 2007a). The two independent approaches both showed that the mean adult population protein requirement was ~0.91 g/kg/day rather than the 0.66 g/kg/day reported by the expert committees (Institute of Medicine, 2002/2005; Campbell *et al.*, 2008). Our observations require confirmation from other groups, but the correspondence of the two independent methods is strong evidence that current protein recommendations are in error.

These observations raise the question as to whether protein requirements in other age groups are also in error. Except for the first 6 months of life when the intake of protein from human milk was used, protein requirements were based on nitrogen balance studies. Those in childhood were based on much more limited data than that available in adults (Institute of Medicine, 2002/2005; Campbell *et al.*, 2008). Because of the uncertainty, we have omitted a table of protein requirements that was in the previous version of this chapter (Pencharz and Young, 2006). The mean value of 0.91 g/kg/day using the same variance as used by the DRI and FAO of 12% would,

however, suggest an RDA or safe level of 1.0 g/kg/day. The protein intakes from human milk were estimated by the FAO/WHO (2007) report to range from 1.77 g/kg/day at 1 month to 1.14 g/kg/day at 6 months.

There are those who have written that the protein requirements in the elderly may be higher than in younger adults, approaching requirement values of 1 g/kg/day (Millward and Roberts, 1996; Millward *et al.*, 1997; Campbell *et al.*, 2008). However, when young adults and elderly subjects were studied using the same nitrogen balance techniques, no differences were seen (Campbell *et al.*, 2008). Hence, with our reappraisal of the mean protein requirements for young adults of 0.91 g/kg/day, we expect that future studies will show similar levels in the elderly.

Requirements for Indispensable Amino Acids

The expert committees at the National Academy of Sciences (Institute of Medicine, 2002/2005) and the United Nations (FAO/WHO, 2007) concluded that the indicator amino acid oxidation (IAAO) approach (Figure 6.2) should be the standard used, and the older nitrogen balance data was not used. At the time, a modification of IAAO, namely 24-hour indicator oxidation and balance, should be preferred over the fed-state IAAO, principally because the 24-hour studies had a week's adaptation to the changes in the test amino acid intake. It has subsequently been shown that the length of adaptation needed was only a matter of a few hours and hence that the fed-state IAAO model was valid (Elango *et al.*, 2008a, 2009). This opened the way to applying the IAAO model to children (Kuurpad *et al.*, 2003; Elango *et al.*, 2007; Hsu *et al.*, 2007; Pillai *et al.*, 2010). Table 6.5 summarizes the adult indispensable amino acid requirements. Currently there are no studies reported determining amino acid requirements in the elderly. Clearly, this matter requires attention.

Prior to the application of IAAO to the determination of the amino acid requirements of children there were studies that reported using nitrogen balance. These are reviewed in the expert committee reports (Institute of Medicine, 2002/2005; FAO/WHO, 2007). Since, in the view of the expert committees, the data were limited, the nitrogen balance data were not used and instead a factorial approach was employed, based on the adult requirement plus that required for growth. Our recent studies in children for lysine (Elango *et al.*, 2007; Pillai *et al.*, 2010),

TABLE 6.5 Amino acid requirements in healthy adults

Amino acid[a]	Indicator amino oxidation based[b]	Dietary reference intakes (2002/2005)	FAO/ WHO/ UNU (2007)
Histidine	–	11	10
Isoleucine	42	15	20
Leucine	55	34	39
Lysine	35	31	30
Methionine + cystine	13	15	15
Phenylalanine + tyrosine	42	27	25
Threonine	19	16	15
Tryptophan	4	4	4
Valine	47	19	26

[a]Values expressed as mg/kg/day.
[b]Modified from Elango et al. (2008b).

branched chain amino acids (Mager et al., 2003) and methionine (without cysteine) (Turner et al., 2006) provide confirmation of the factorial approach. As mentioned earlier in this chapter in the protein requirement section, sufficient levels need to be tested in order to apply two-phase linear regression analysis. In some cases the 24-hour IAAO studies did not have enough levels, and, as can be seen in Table 6.5, the DRI and FAO/WHO/UNU values are significantly lower than those derived by fed-state IAAO with a full range of intake values. The growth component of amino acid requirements is small so that except in infancy the maintenance level dominates (Mager et al., 2003; FAO/WHO, 2007).

Excessive Intakes of Protein and of Amino Acids

The upper limit of protein intake in adults has been set at no more than 30% of total energy intake (Institute of Medicine, 2002/2005, to which the reader is referred for full details). Briefly, consideration of maximal urea synthesis rates and observations of explorers who lived on exclusively animal-based diets provided the basis for this recommendation. For example, early American explorers suffered in the winter from "rabbit starvation" when they subsisted on a diet of rabbit meat which contains very little fat (Institute of Medicine, 2002/2005), resulting in protein intakes greater than 30% of total energy intake.

Data on excessive intakes of individual amino acids are limited except for phenylalanine where most of the data are centered on brain damage in persons with phenylketonuria. A recent review of available information on this topic, which systematically considers all amino acids, can be found in a report from the Institute of Medicine (2002/2005). An approach to the determination of the upper limits of amino acid intakes can be found in a previous report by Pencharz et al. (2008).

Protein Malnutrition

Protein is the fundamental component for cellular and organ function (Institute of Medicine, 2002/2005). The diet must contain not only enough protein and amino acids but also enough non-protein energy to permit optimal utilization of dietary protein (Duffy et al., 1981). Protein energy malnutrition (PEM) is quite common in the world as a whole and has been reported by the United Nations Food and Agriculture Organization in 2000 to be associated with 6 million deaths in children (FAO, 2000). In the industrialized world PEM is seen predominantly in hospitals and in association with disease (Bistrian, 1990; Wilson and Pencharz, 1997; Institute of Medicine, 2002/2005).

Protein deficiency has adverse effects on all organs (Cornish and Kennedy, 2000) and is of particular concern in infants and young children. PEM may have long-term adverse effects on brain function (Pollitt, 2000). Patients with PEM have reduced immune function and are hence more susceptible to infection (Bistrian, 1990). Total starvation will result in death in an initially normal-weight adult in 70 days (Allison, 1992); since these persons still had some adipose tissue reserves, their death can be regarded as primarily being due to protein deprivation. By way of contrast, protein and energy reserves are much lower in very-low-birth-weight premature infants, and with total starvation the survival of 1000-g neonates has been calculated to be only 5 days (Heird et al., 1992).

Conclusion

Knowledge continues to grow about the physiology of protein and amino acid metabolism in the mammalian organism and especially in relation to human protein and amino acid nutrition. This chapter has focused attention on selected recent advances in relation to amino acid function and protein and amino acid utilization during the prandial and postprandial period of amino acid metabolism. The importance of the gut and the splanchnic region as a whole in the regulation of whole-body amino acid metabolism has become better appreciated and understood. Now that the postgenome era has begun, the mechanisms underlying the effect of amino acids on physiological functions and metabolic processes – including transport, catabolism, and anabolic processes – will soon be more completely described. There remains uncertainty about quantitative aspects of amino acid nutrition, especially in healthy adults, but there is now a consensus that the current international requirement estimates for adults are far too low. This has potentially important implications for the evaluation of dietary protein quality and for the planning, now and in the future, of food protein supplies for population groups. Improved in vivo metabolic tools combined with molecular and cellular techniques appear to offer great promise for resolving some of the outstanding issues that limit our ability to predict precisely the effect of the dietary protein and amino acid component on function and the quantitative and qualitative character of the intake that optimizes development and health maintenance.

Future Directions

The issue of whether protein requirements have been significantly underestimated is important, especially since the underestimation of protein requirements of children in the developing world may be a key factor in stunting. There is a general consensus about this underestimation, but it is not universally accepted and more work is needed to confirm it. This will then lead to the need to evaluate protein requirements in a variety of conditions, including pregnancy and aging, taking into account the need for appropriate periods of adaptation to a new level of amino acid intake.

Another area of interest is the metabolic availability of amino acids from dietary protein, which was the focus of an FAO Expert Committee meeting in early 2011. The potential cause for concern is that defining protein requirements using crystalline amino acids may not be readily applicable to dietary protein without clear knowledge of the metabolic availability for protein synthesis of the amino acids within that protein.

Finally since health food stores are selling and promoting the ingestion of large doses of amino acid supplements, it is important that the safe upper limit of amino acid requirements be determined.

Acknowledgments

We are grateful to the late Dr Vernon Young (a former author of this chapter) for his stimulation and encouragement, and to the Canadian Institutes for Health Research for their support of our work in the areas of protein and amino acid metabolism and requirements.

Suggestions for Further Reading

Ball, R.O., Courtney-Martin, G., and Pencharz, P.B. (2006) The in vivo sparing effect of cysteine on methionine requirements in animal models and adult humans. *J Nutr* **136**, 1682S–1693S.

Elango, R., Ball, R.O., and Pencharz, P.B. (2008) Indicator amino acid oxidation: concept and application. *J Nutr* **138**, 243–246.

Elango, R., Ball, R.O., and Pencharz, P.B. (2008) Individual amino acid requirements in humans: an update. *Curr Opin Nutr Metab Care* **11**, 34–39.

Elango, R., Ball, R.O., and Pencharz, P.B. (2009) Amino acid requirements in humans: with a special emphasis on the metabolic availability of amino acids. *Amino Acids* **37**, 19–27.

Elango, R., Humayun, M.A., Ball, R.O., et al. (2010) Evidence that protein requirements have been significantly underestimated. *Curr Opin Clin Nutr* **13**, 52–57.

Pencharz, P.B., Elango, R., and Ball, R.O. (2008) An approach to defining the upper safe limits of amino acid intake. *J Nutr* **138**, 1996S–2002S.

References

Allison, S.P. (1992) The uses and limitations of nutrition support. *Clin Nutr* **11**, 319–330.

Anthony, J.C., Anthony, T.G., Kimball, S.R., et al. (2000) Orally administered leucine stimulates protein synthesis in skeletal muscle of postabsorptive rats in association with increased eIF4F formation. *J Nutr* **130**, 139–145.

Arnal, M.A., Mosoni, L., Boirie, Y., et al. (1999) Protein pulse feeding improves protein retention in elderly women. *Am J Clin Nutr* **69**, 1202–1208.

Ball, R.O., Courtney-Martin, G., and Pencharz, P.B. (2006) The in vivo sparing effect of cysteine on methionine requirements in animal models and adult humans. *J Nutr* **136**, 1682S–1693S.

Beaufrere, B., Dangin, M., and Boirie, Y. (2000) The "fast" and "slow" protein concept. In P. Fürst and V.R. Young (eds), *Proteins, Peptides and Amino Acids in Enteral Nutrition*. Nestec Ltd/Vevey and S. Karger AG, Basel, pp. 121–133.

Beaumier, L., Castillo, L., Ajami, A.M., *et al.* (1995) Urea cycle intermediate kinetics and nitrate excretion at normal and "therapeutic" intakes of arginine in humans. *Am J Physiol* **269**, E884–896.

Bennett, R.G., Hamel, F.G., and Duckworth, W.C. (2000) Insulin inhibits the ubiquitin-dependent degrading activity of the 26S proteasome. *Endocrinology* **141**, 2508–2517.

Bertolo, R.F.P., Chen, C.A.L., Law, G., *et al.* (1998) Threonine requirement of neonatal piglets receiving an identical diet intragastrically. *J Nutr* **122**, 1752–1759.

Bistrian, B.R. (1990) Recent advances in parenteral and enteral nutrition. A personal perspective. *JPEN J Parenter Enteral Nutr* **14**, 329–334.

Boirie, Y., Gachon, P., and Beaufrére, B. (1997) Splanchnic and whole body leucine kinetics in young and elderly men. *Am J Clin Nutr* **65**, 489–495.

Brunton, J.A., Ball, R.O., and Pencharz, P.B. (2000) Current total parenteral nutrition solutions for the neonate are inadequate. *Curr Opin Clin Nutr Metab Care* **3**, 299–304.

Burke, R.F. and Hill, K.E. (1993) Regulation of selenoproteins. *Annu Rev Nutr* **13**, 65–81.

Campbell, W.W., Johnson, C.A., McCabe, G.P., *et al.* (2008) Dietary protein requirements of younger and older adults. *Am J Clin Nutr* **88**, 1187–1188.

Carpenter, K.J. (1994) *Protein and Energy. A Study of Changing Ideas of Nutrition.* Cambridge University Press, Cambridge.

Cornish, C.A. and Kennedy, N.P. (2000) Protein-energy undernutrition in hospital in-patients. *Br J Nutr* **83**, 575–591.

Cynober, L.A. (1995) (ed.) *Amino Acid Metabolism and Therapy in Health and Nutritional Disease.* CRC Press, Boca Raton, FL.

Duffy, B., Gunn, T., Collinge, J., *et al.* (1981) The effect of varying protein quality and energy intake on the nitrogen metabolism of parenterally fed very low birthweight (<1600 g) infants. *Pediatr Res* **15**, 1040–1044.

Elango, R., Ball, R.O., and Pencharz, P.B. (2008a) Indicator amino acid oxidation: concept and application. *J Nutr* **138**, 243–246.

Elango, R., Ball, R.O., and Pencharz, P.B. (2008b) Individual amino acid requirements in humans: an update. *Curr Opin Nutr Metab Care* **11**, 34–39.

Elango, R., Ball, R.O., and Pencharz, P.B. (2009) Amino acid requirements in humans: with a special emphasis on the metabolic availability of amino acids. *Amino Acids* **37**, 19–27.

Elango, R., Humayun, M.A., Ball, R.O., *et al.* (2007) Lysine requirement of healthy school-age children determined by indicator amino acid oxidation method. *Am J Clin Nutr* **86**, 360–365.

Elango, R., Humayun, M.A., Ball, R.O., *et al.* (2009) Indicator amino acid oxidation is not affected by period of adaptation in response to a wide range of lysine intake in healthy young men. *J Nutr* **139**, 1082–1087.

Elango, R., Humayun, M.A., Ball, R.O., *et al.* (2010) Evidence that protein requirements have been significantly underestimated. *Curr Opin Clin Nutr* **13**, 52–57.

El-Khoury, A.E., Sánchez, M., Fukagawa, N.K., *et al.* (1995) The 24 hour kinetics of leucine oxidation in healthy adults receiving a generous leucine intake via three discrete meals. *Am J Clin Nutr* **62**, 579–590.

FAO (2000) *The State of Food and Agriculture.* Food and Agriculture Organization, Rome.

FAO/WHO (1965) *FAO/WHO Protein Requirements.* FAO Nutritional Studies No. 16. FAO, Rome.

FAO/WHO (2007) United Nations University. Protein and Amino Acid Requirements in Human Nutrition. Report of a Joint Expert Consultation. WHO Technical Report Series No. 935. WHO, Geneva.

Ferland, G. (1998) The vitamin K-dependent proteins: an update. *Nutr Rev* **56**, 223–230.

Flakoll, P.J., Kulaylot, M., Frexes-Steed, M., *et al.* (1989) Amino acids augment insulin's suppression of whole body proteolysis. *Am J Physiol* **257**, E839–847.

Fouillet, H., Gaudichon, C., Mariotti, F., *et al.* (2000) Compartmental modeling of postprandial dietary nitrogen distribution in humans. *Am J Physiol* **279**, E161–175.

Fürst, P. and Young, V. R. (2000) (eds) *Proteins, Peptides and Amino Acids in Enteral Nutrition.* Nestec Ltd/Vevey and S Karger AG, Basel.

Heird, W.C., Driscoll, J.M., Schullinger, J.N., *et al.* (1972) Intravenous alimentation in pediatric patients. *J Pediatr* **80**, 351–372.

Hsu, J.W.C., Ball, R.O., and Pencharz, P.B. (2007) Evidence that phenylalanine may not provide the full needs for aromatic amino acid needs in children. *Pediatr Res* **61**, 361–365.

Humayun, M.A., Elango, R., Ball, R.O., *et al.* (2007a) A reevaluation of protein requirement in young men using the indicator amino acid oxidation technique. *Am J Clin Nutr* **86**, 995–1002.

Humayun, M.A., Elango, R., Moehn, S., *et al.* (2007b) Application of the indicator amino acid oxidation technique for the determination of metabolic availability of sulphur amino acids from casein versus soy protein isolate in adult men. *J Nutr* **137**, 1874–1879.

Institute of Medicine (2002/2005) Panel on Macronutrients. *Dietary Reference Intakes for Energy, Carbohydrate, Fiber, Fat, Fatty Acids, Cholesterol, Protein and Amino Acids.* National Academies Press, Washington, DC.

Jackson, A.A. (2000) Nitrogen trafficking and recycling through the human bowel. In P. Fürst and V.R. Young (eds), *Proteins, Peptides and Amino Acids in Enteral Nutrition.* Nestec Ltd/Vevey and S. Karger AG, Basel, pp. 89–108.

Jaksic, T., Wagner, D.A., Burke, J.F., *et al.* (1991) Proline metabolism in adult male burned patients and healthy control subjects. *Am J Clin Nutr* **54,** 408–413.

Jousse, C., Bruhat, A., and Fafournoux, P. (1999) Amino acid regulation of gene expression. *Curr Opin Clin Nutr Metab Care* **2,** 297–301.

Korpes, J.E. (1970) *Jac Berzelius. His Life and Work.* Almqvist & Wiksell, Stockholm.

Kurpad, A.V., Regan, M.M., Varalkshmi, S., *et al.* (2003) Daily methionine requirements of healthy Indian men measured by 24-h indicator amino acid oxidation and balance technique. *Am J Clin Nutr* **77,** 1196–1205.

Kurpad, A.V., Regan, M.M., Raj, T.D., *et al.* (2005) The daily valine requirement of healthy adult Indians determined by 24-h indicator amino acid balance approach. *Am J Clin Nutr* **82,** 373–379.

Kurpad, A.V., Regan, M.M., Raj, T.D., *et al.* (2006) The daily phenylalanine requirement of healthy Indian adults. *Am J Clin Nutr* **83,** 1331–1336.

Law, G.K., Bertolo, R.F., Adiri-Awere, A., *et al.* (2007) Adequate oral threonine is critical for mucin production and gut function in neonatal piglets. *Am J Physiol* **292,** G1293–1301.

Lecker, S.H., Solomon, V., Mitch, W.E., *et al.* (1999) Muscle protein breakdown and the critical role of the ubiquitin–proteasome pathway in normal and diseased states. *J Nutr* **129,** 227S–237S.

Lynch, C.J., Fox, H.L., Vary, T.C., *et al.* (2000) Regulation of amino acid-sensitive TOR signaling by leucine analogues in adipocytes. *J Cell Biochem* **77,** 235–251.

Mager, D.R., Wykes, L.J., Ball, R.O., *et al.* (2003) Branched chain amino acid requirements in school aged children determined by Indicator Amino Acid Oxidation (IAAO). *J Nutr* **133,** 3540–3545.

Metges, C.C. (2000) Contribution of microbial amino acids to amino acid homeostasis of the host. *J Nutr* **130,** 1857S–1864S.

Metges, C.C., El-Khoury, A.E., Henneman, L., *et al.* (1999a) Availability of intestinal microbial lysine for whole-body lysine homeostasis in human subjects. *Am J Physiol* **277,** E597–607.

Metges, C.C., Petzke, K.J., El-Khoury, A.E., *et al.* (1999b) Incorporation of urea and ammonia nitrogen into ileal and fecal microbial proteins and plasma free amino acids in normal men and ileostomates. *Am J Clin Nutr* **70,** 1046–1058.

Millward, D.J. (2000) Postprandial protein utilization: implications for clinical nutrition. In P. Fürst and V.R. Young (eds), *Proteins, Peptides and Amino Acids in Enteral Nutrition.* Nestec Ltd/Vevey and S. Karger AG, Basel, pp. 135–155.

Millward, D.J. and Pacy, P.J. (1995) Postprandial protein utilization and protein quality assessment in man. *Clin Sci* **88,** 597–606.

Millward, D.J. and Roberts, S.B. (1996) Protein requirements of older individuals. *Nutr Res Rev* **9,** 67–87.

Millward, D.J., Fereday, A., Gibson, N., *et al.* (1997) Aging protein requirements and protein turnover. *Am J Clin Nutr* **66,** 774–786.

Moehn, S., Bertolo, R.F.P., Pencharz, P.B., *et al.* (2005) Development of the indicator amino acid oxidation technique to determine the availability of amino acids from dietary protein in pigs. *J Nutr* **135,** 2866–2870.

Munro, H.N. (1985) Historical perspective on protein requirements: objectives for the future. In K. Blaxter and J.C. Waterlow (eds), *Nutritional Adaptation in Man.* John Libbey, London, pp. 155–167.

Narita, I., Border, W.A., Ketteler, M., *et al.* (1995) L-Arginine may mediate the therapeutic effects of low protein diets. *Proc Natl Acad Sci USA* **92,** 4552–4556.

Pain, V.M. (1996) Initiation of protein synthesis in eukaryotic cells. *Eur J Biochem* **236,** 747–771.

Pencharz, P.B. and Ball, R.O. (2003) Different approaches to define individual amino acid requirements. *Annu Rev Nutr* **23,** 101–116.

Pencharz, P.B. and Young, V.R. (2006) Protein and amino acids. In B.A. Bowman and R.M. Russell (eds), *Present Knowledge in Nutrition,* 9th Edn. ILSI Press, Washington, DC, pp. 59–77.

Pencharz, P.B., Elango, R., and Ball, R.O. (2008) An approach to defining the upper safe limits of amino acid intake. *J Nutr* **138,** 1996S–2002S.

Pencharz, P.B., House, J.D., Wykes, L.J., *et al.* (1996) What are the essential amino acids for the preterm and term infant? *10th Nutricia Symposium, vol. 21.* Kluwer Academic Publishers, Dordrecht, pp. 278–296.

Pillai, R.R., Elango, R., Muthayya, S., *et al.* (2010) Lysine requirement of healthy Indian school-aged children determined by the indicator amino acid oxidation technique. *J Nutr* **140,** 54–59.

Pollitt, E. (2000) Developmental sequel from early nutritional deficiencies: Conclusive and probability judgments. *J Nutr* **130,** 350S–353S.

Raguso, C.A., Ajami, A.M., Gleason, R., *et al.* (1997) Effect of cystine intake on methionine kinetics and oxidation determined with oral tracers of methionine and cysteine in healthy adults. *Am J Clin Nutr* **66,** 283–292.

Reckelhoff, J.F., Kellum, J.A., Racusen, I., *et al.* (1997) Long-term dietary supplementation with L-arginine prevents age-related reduction in renal function. *Am J Physiol* **27,** R1768–1774.

Reeds, P.J. (2000) Dispensable and indispensable amino acids for humans. *J Nutr* **130,** 1835S–1840.

Reeds, P.J., Burrin, D.G., Davis, T.A., *et al.* (2000a) Protein nutrition of the neonate. *Proc Nutr Soc* **59,** 87–97.

Reeds, P.J., Burrin, D.G., Stoll, B., *et al.* (2000b) Role of the gut in the amino acid economy of the host. In P. Fürst and V.R. Young (eds), *Proteins, Peptides and Amino Acids in Enteral Nutrition.* Nestec Ltd/Vevey and S. Karger AG, Basel, pp. 25–46,

Rerat, A., Simoes-Nunes, C., Mendy, F., *et al.* (1992) Splanchnic fluxes of amino acids after duodenal infusion of carbohydrate solutions containing free amino acids or oligopeptides in the non-anaesthetized pig. *Br J Nutr* **68,** 111–138.

Rose, W.C. (1948) Amino acid requirements of man. *Fed Proc* **8,** 546–552.

Schrauzer, G.N. (2000) Selenomethionine: a review of its nutritional significance, metabolism and toxicity. *J Nutr* **130,** 1653–1656.

Tessari, P. (2000) Regulation of splanchnic protein synthesis by enteral feeding. In P. Fürst and V.R. Young (eds), *Proteins, Peptides and Amino Acids in Enteral Nutrition.* Nestec Ltd/Vevey and S. Karger AG, Basel, pp. 47–61.

Tessari, P., Zanetti, M., Barazzoni, R. *et al.* (1996) Mechanisms of postprandial protein accretion in human skeletal muscle. Insight from leucine and phenylalanine forearm kinetics. *J Clin Invest* **98,** 1361–1372.

Tomé, D. and Bos, C. (2000) Dietary protein and nitrogen utilization. *J Nutr* **130,** 18682–18673.

Turner, J.M., Humayun, A., Elango, R., *et al.* (2006). Total sulfur amino acid requirement of healthy school-aged children as determined by indicator amino acid oxidation technique. *Am J Clin Nutr* **83,** 619–623.

Van Goudoever, J.B., Stoll, B., Henry, J.F., *et al.* (2000) Adaptive regulation of intestinal lysine metabolism. *Proc Natl Acad Sci USA* **97,** 11620–11625.

Vishwannath, R.I., Eisen, M.B., Ross, D.T., *et al.* (1999) The transcriptional program in the response of human fibroblasts to serum. *Science* **283,** 83–87.

Volpi, E., Mittendorfer, B., Wolf, S.E., *et al.* (1999) Oral amino acids stimulate muscle protein anabolism in the elderly despite higher first-pass splanchnic extraction. *Am J Physiol* **277,** E513–520.

Waterlow, J.C. (1995) Whole-body protein turnover in humans – past, present and future. *Annu Rev Nutr* **15,** 57–92.

Waterlow, J.C. (1999) The mysteries of nitrogen balance. *Nutr Res Rev* **12,** 25–54.

Wilkinson, D.L., Bertolo, R.F.P., Brunton, J.A., *et al.* (2004) Arginine synthesis is regulated by dietary arginine intake in the enterally fed neonatal piglet. *Am J Physiol* **287,** E454–462.

Williams, H.H., Harper, A.E., Hegsted, D.M., *et al.* (1974) Nitrogen and amino acid requirements. In: *National Research Council. Improvement Protein Nutriture.* National Academy of Sciences, Washington, DC, pp. 23–63.

Wilson, D.C. and Pencharz, P.B. (1997) Nutritional care of the chronically ill. In R.C. Tsang, S.H. Zlotkin, B.L. Nichols, *et al.* (eds), *Nutrition During Infancy: Birth to 2 Years.* Digital Educational Publishing, Cincinnati, pp. 37–56.

Wu, G. (1998) Intestinal mucosal amino acid catabolism. *J Nutr* **128,** 1249–1252.

Wu, G. and Morris, S.M. (1998) Arginine metabolism: nitric oxide and beyond. *Biochem J* **336,** 1–17.

Young, V.R. and Ajami, A.M. (2000) Glutamate: an amino acid of particular distinction. *J Nutr* **130,** 892S–900S.

Young, V.R. and El-Khoury, A.E. (1995) The notion of the nutritional essentiality of amino acids, revisited, with a note on the indispensable amino acid requirements in adults. In L.A. Cynober (ed.), *Amino Acid Metabolism and Therapy in Health and Nutritional Disease.* CRC Press, Boca Raton, FL, pp. 191–232.

Young, V.R., El-Khoury, A.E., Raguso, C.A., *et al.* (2000a) Rates of urea production and hydrolysis and leucine oxidation change linearly over widely varying protein intakes in healthy adults. *J Nutr* **130,** 761–766.

Young, V.R., Yu, Y-M., and Borgonha, S. (2000b) Proteins, peptides and amino acids in enteral nutrition: overview and some research challenges. In P. Fürst and V.R. Young (eds), *Proteins, Peptides and Amino Acids in Enteral Nutrition.* Nestec Ltd/Vevey and S. Karger AG, Basel, pp. 1–23.

7

CARBOHYDRATES

LISA M. SANDERS[1], PhD, RD AND JOANNE R. LUPTON[2], PhD

[1]Kellogg Company, Battle Creek, Michigan, USA
[2]Texas A&M University, College Station, Texas, USA

Summary

Carbohydrates are the primary energy source for most people in the world. This makes carbohydrate *quality* a critical issue, since those who consume too few calories need nutrient-dense carbohydrate sources so that every calorie counts; and those who consume too many calories also need high-quality carbohydrates since they cannot afford to waste calories on less nutritious sources. This chapter reviews the primary classifications of carbohydrates (mono-, di- oligo-, and polysaccharides; glycemic and non-glycemic; and endogenous or added sugars). It tracks their digestion, absorption, and metabolism. It translates the biochemistry of carbohydrates into physiological effects and explains the most current recommendations for carbohydrate intake and the science behind those recommendations. Finally, intake of carbohydrates is related to key diseases including obesity, diabetes, cardiovascular disease, and cancer.

Introduction

Carbohydrates, which are found in fruits, vegetables, grains, and dairy products, are the major source of energy for most of the world's population. However, the role of carbohydrates in human health extends beyond their importance as an energy source. Carbohydrates vary tremendously in structure and physiological function, and much of the recent carbohydrate research has focused on these differences and their impact on chronic diseases such as diabetes and heart disease. Within the past several years, this research has led to the development of significant nutrition public-policy recommendations regarding carbohydrate intake for optimal health.

Carbohydrates in the Food Supply

Carbohydrates have traditionally been accepted as compounds containing carbon, hydrogen, and oxygen in a molar ratio of $1:2:1$. As this definition is not universal for all carbohydrates (e.g. sugar alcohols and some polysaccharides), it is more precise to define carbohydrates as polyhydroxy aldehydes, ketones, alcohols, and acids that exist as monomeric units or as polymers. The degree of polymerization is frequently used as a system by which to classify carbohydrates, with the major classes being monosaccharides and disaccharides (commonly referred to as sugars), oligosaccharides, and polysaccharides.

Present Knowledge in Nutrition, Tenth Edition. Edited by John W. Erdman Jr, Ian A. Macdonald and Steven H. Zeisel.
© 2012 International Life Sciences Institute. Published 2012 by John Wiley & Sons, Inc.

Sugars

Monosaccharides

According to the Food and Agriculture Organization of the World Health Organization (FAO/WHO, 1998) the term "sugars" refers collectively to monosaccharides, disaccharides, and sugar alcohols. Monosaccharides include glucose, fructose, and galactose, which are found naturally in small amounts in fruits, vegetables, and honey. However, over the past 30 years, corn syrups and high-fructose corn syrup (HFCS) have replaced refined sugars (such as sucrose) as a major source of monosaccharides in the American diet because of their increased use by the food industry as a low-cost sweetener (White, 1992). Corn syrups contain only individual glucose units. The term "high-fructose corn syrup" is accurate, but in some ways it is misleading since many interpret this to mean that there is more fructose than would be in an equivalent amount of table sugar (sucrose). The reason for the word "high" is that it contains more fructose than corn syrup, which is only glucose. However, compared with sucrose, which is 50% glucose and 50% fructose, it is not high. HFCS is made by hydrolyzing corn starch to individual glucose units and then using enzymes to convert glucose to fructose. The final corn syrup is made up of either 42% or 55% fructose, with the remaining sugars being glucose and higher sugars. HFCS-55 is predominant in carbonated soft drinks, whereas HFCS-42 is found in canned fruits, baked goods, flavored milks, yogurt, and ice cream (White, 1992; Hanover and White, 1993).

Disaccharides

Disaccharides consist of two monosaccharides covalently linked by a glycosidic bond. The major dietary disaccharides include sucrose (glucose + fructose) and lactose (glucose + galactose). Sucrose occurs naturally in plants, but most often is consumed as an extract of sugarcane or beet. Sucrose is widely used as a sweetener and preservative. Milk and other dairy products are the only source of lactose. Maltose and trehalose, both disaccharides of glucose (differing only in the configuration of the glycosidic bond), are also present in small amounts in the food supply. Maltose is found in wheat and barley, and is also a product of starch hydrolysis. Trehalose is found in yeast products, mushrooms, and crustacean seafood.

Sugar Alcohols

Also commonly referred to as polyols, sugar alcohols are derived from the hydrogenation of mono- and disaccharides, and include sorbitol, mannitol, xylitol, isomalt, lactitol, maltitol, and erythritol. Polyols are not as easily digested as other sugars, so they produce a lower glycemic response and a reduced caloric value. Additionally, sugar alcohols are less cariogenic than other carbohydrates (FDA, 1997). As a result, the food industry often uses sugar alcohols as bulk sweeteners to produce low-calorie or sugar-free candies, chewing gum, baked goods, sauces, jams, jellies, beverages, and frozen desserts.

Oligosaccharides

Carbohydrates with three to nine degrees of polymerization (i.e. three to nine monosaccharide units) are classified as oligosaccharides. Some oligosaccharides occur naturally in plants: stachyose and raffinose in soybeans and other legumes and fructooligosaccharides in fruits, vegetables, and grains (e.g. wheat, rye, onions, bananas, and garlic). However, because of their usefulness as food ingredients and their possible health benefits, an increasing number of oligosaccharides are now synthesized from sugars or obtained through extraction and/or partial hydrolysis of longer-chain plant polysaccharides. These manufactured oligosaccharides, such as inulin extracted from chicory root, can be found in a number of food items such as dairy products (e.g. yogurt), breads, beverages, and dessert foods. Being fairly resistant to digestion in the small intestine, oligosaccharides display physiological effects similar to fiber, and some appear to promote the growth of beneficial colonic microflora. Additionally, as a food additive, they do not change the texture or taste of the product significantly, making them ideal for creating healthier products with limited alteration in taste or mouth feel (Meyer, 2004).

Polysaccharides

The majority of carbohydrates consumed in the food supply are polysaccharides. As the name implies, these carbohydrates have a high degree of polymerization, ranging from 10 sugar units to several thousand. Polysaccharides can be subdivided into starch and nonstarch polysaccharides.

Starch

Starch is a polymer of glucose units covalently bound by either α-(1,4) or α-(1,6) linkages. Amylose contains only α-(1,4) bonds and thus maintains a constant linear form. Amylopectin contains α-(1,6) bonds in addition to α-(1,4) bonds, allowing for a highly branched structure.

Starch is the primary storage form of carbohydrate in plants, but is found primarily in grains and grain products (e.g. cereals, corn, flour, and rice) and in some root vegetables (e.g. potatoes and beets) and legumes. Most other vegetables and fruits contain very little starch.

Resistant Starch. While most starch is digested and absorbed in the small intestine, a small portion escapes digestive enzymes and passes into the colon, where it may be fermented. This is referred to as resistant starch. There are four types of resistant starch, which either occur naturally or are a consequence of food processing. Resistant starch-1 (RS1) is present in the cell walls of plants, but is physically inaccessible to digestive enzymes such as α-amylase. It is most frequently found in whole grains, whole-grain products (e.g. breads and cereals), seeds, and legumes. The amount of RS1 in a food is decreased by processing techniques such as milling and refining. Raw starch granules that are resistant to digestive enzymes due to their crystalline structure and size are classified as RS2. These can be found in raw potatoes and green bananas. Food processing, particularly gelatinization (making starch more soluble using heat, water, and/or enzymes), increases the accessibility of starch to digestive enzymes, thereby decreasing the amount of RS2. Because RS1 and RS2 occur naturally in plants, they are considered dietary fiber by some. RS3 and RS4 are both formed during food processing and do not occur naturally. RS3, also called retrograded starch, is formed during the cooking and cooling or extrusion process of starchy foods such as potatoes, rice, and cereals. RS4 is chemically modified starch, such as starch esters, starch ethers, and cross-linked starches, which are manufactured by the food industry to impart desired characteristics to food products such as color, temperature stability, and altered viscosity (Tungland and Meyer, 2002).

Non-Starch Polysaccharides

Similar to resistant starch, non-starch polysaccharides also escape digestion and absorption in the small intestine and are fermented in the colon. However, their resistance to digestion is due not to physical or structural barriers to digestive enzymes, but rather to the lack of enzymes capable of breaking the glycosidic bonds between the monomeric units. As a result of their indigestibility, non-starch polysaccharides are considered dietary fiber and include cellulose, hemicelluloses (e.g. β-glucans), gums and mucilages, and pectins. For more detailed information, see Chapter 8 on dietary fiber in this book.

Other Classifications of Carbohydrates

One of the difficulties in the classification of carbohydrates is reconciling their chemical composition with their physiological functions. Each of the chemical classes described above contains carbohydrates with varying physiological effects, some of which overlap among the categories (e.g. the indigestibility and colonic fermentation of oligosaccharides and non-starch polysaccharides). This can create confusion for the consumer and the food industry with regard to dietary guidelines, labeling guidelines, and health claims, and has therefore resulted in new terminology and classifications for dietary carbohydrates.

Added Sugars

Added sugars are sugars and syrups that are added to foods during processing or preparation (USDA, 2005). This does not include sugars that occur naturally in the food, such as lactose in milk or fructose in fruits. Added sugars are typically in the form of white table sugar, brown sugar, corn syrup, HFCS, molasses, honey, pancake syrups, fruit-juice concentrates, and dextrose. The major sources of these sugars include soft drinks, fruit beverages, candy, and sugar-sweetened grain-based dessert items, which account for 72% of the US added sugar intake (Figure 7.1) (Marriott *et al.*, 2010). Non-diet soft drinks account for 33% of added sugars in the American diet (Marriott *et al.*, 2010). Most of these food items also have lower micronutrient densities than foods and beverages with naturally occurring sugars. Therefore, beginning in 2000, the Dietary Guidelines for Americans included the term "added sugars" to assist consumers in identifying foods that are high in added sugars. Currently, US food labels are not required to distinguish between naturally occurring sugars and those that are added to the food. This is because there is a lack of methods for differentiating between naturally occurring and added sugars. Thus it is difficult for the consumer to identify the amount of added sugars they are getting in their foods.

Glycemic and Non-Glycemic Carbohydrates

This classification system is based on the digestibility of carbohydrates and thus their ability to provide glucose to the body for metabolism. Glycemic carbohydrates are digested and absorbed in the small intestine, thereby increasing blood glucose for metabolism by tissues, whereas

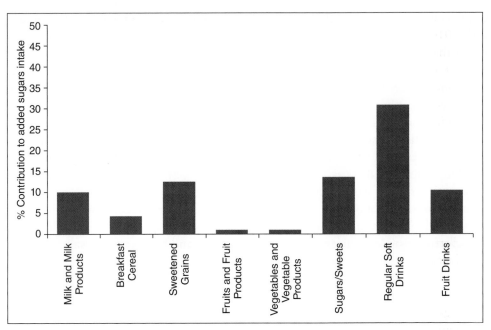

FIG. 7.1   Percent contribution of different food categories to added sugar intake. Data from Marriott *et al.* (2010).

non-glycemic carbohydrates remain undigested and pass into the colon where they can be fermented. Non-glycemic carbohydrates may still provide energy through fermentation; however, this energy is not in carbohydrate form such that it would alter blood glucose levels. Sugars and starches make up most of the glycemic carbohydrates, and oligosaccharides, resistant starches, and non-digestible polysaccharides (fiber) constitute the non-glycemic carbohydrates. The rate at which different glycemic carbohydrates are absorbed can also be measured and will be discussed further in the following section.

Digestion and Absorption of Carbohydrates

Digestion

Enzymatic digestion of carbohydrates begins immediately when food is placed in the mouth. Salivary α-amylase hydrolyzes the glycosidic bonds between glucose moieties in starches to yield glucose, maltose, and other starch fragments. Once food enters the stomach, salivary amylase is inactivated and carbohydrate digestion pauses. In the small intestine, pancreatic α-amylase completes the digestion of starch to glucose, maltose, maltotriose (a trisaccharide), and dextrins, oligosaccharide units containing one or more

α-(1,6) linkages. All carbohydrates must be broken down to individual monosaccharide units before absorption is possible. Therefore, bound to the brush border of the small intestine are enzymes that hydrolyze dextrins, trisaccharides, and disaccharides to their respective monosaccharides for absorption. These enzymes include glucoamylase, maltase, lactase, and sucrase, which hydrolyze dextrins, maltose, lactose, and sucrose, respectively. A deficiency of disaccharidases in the intestine can occur in rare genetic disorders such as sucrase–maltase deficiency and alactasia (absence of lactase). These deficiencies typically result in diarrhea, abdominal pain, and/or gas following the consumption of sucrose or lactose, and the condition can generally be controlled by removing the indigestible disaccharides from the diet or by predigestion of the sugars with commercially available enzymes (e.g. lactase). Additionally, the expression of the lactase enzyme decreases in most humans following weaning, allowing undigested lactose to reach the colon where it is fermented. This fermentation can result in the generation of gases, causing abdominal discomfort and possibly diarrhea. However, not all lactase activity is lost, as in the case of alactasia, and small amounts of milk products can be tolerated without adverse side effects according to the 2010 National Institutes of Health (NIH) Consensus

Development Conference on lactose intolerance and health (Suchy *et al.*, 2010).

Any carbohydrates that are not digested (e.g. resistant starches and fiber) pass into the colon, where they can be fermented by the colonic microflora to short-chain fatty acids and gases such as hydrogen, carbon dioxide, and methane. Again, more information can be found on this process in Chapter 8 on dietary fiber.

Absorption

Monosaccharide absorption occurs in the small intestine by one of two mechanisms: active transport and facilitated diffusion. At the brush-border surface, glucose and galactose are actively transported from the lumen into the enterocyte by a sodium/glucose co-transporter, SGLT1. In this process, glucose and galactose move against a concentration gradient, while sodium moves down a concentration gradient. The sodium gradient is maintained by pumping sodium out of the enterocyte at the basolateral membrane, a process requiring energy in the form of ATP. Fructose absorption at the brush border occurs passively and is facilitated by one of the GLUT family of glucose transporters, GLUT5. The GLUT5 uniporter has a high affinity for fructose and appears to move glucose very poorly. Once inside the enterocyte, movement of monosaccharides across the basolateral membrane and into the bloodstream is a passive process and is facilitated by GLUT2 and GLUT5 uniporters (Wright *et al.*, 2003). GLUT2 facilitates the movement of all three monosaccharides into the bloodstream, while GLUT5 appears to again be specific to fructose.

Mutations in these monosaccharide transporters, while rare, can lead to clinical disorders such as glucose–galactose malabsorption and Fanconi-Bickel syndrome. Glucose–galactose malabsorption, a congenital disorder, occurs when a defective SGLT1 transporter prevents the absorption of glucose and galactose, resulting in severe diarrhea when sugars and starches containing these monosaccharides are consumed. Treatment of this condition requires the removal of glucose and galactose from the diet, but fructose consumption may continue because there is no impairment of fructose absorption in this disorder. Fanconi-Bickel syndrome results from a congenital defect in the GLUT2 transporter. In addition to the intestine, GLUT2 is also expressed in the liver, kidney, and pancreas. Therefore, loss of function of this transporter results not only in monosaccharide malabsorption, but also in widespread systemic effects such as tubular nephropathy, hepatomegaly, and rickets (Wright *et al.*, 2003).

Glycemic Index and Response

As mentioned previously, glycemic carbohydrates are those that stimulate an increase in blood glucose levels after their digestion and absorption. This change in blood glucose over time is called the "glycemic response." A number of factors can influence the glycemic response to foods, including the nature of the carbohydrate consumed, the rate of digestion and absorption, the rate of clearance from the bloodstream, and the presence of other food components (e.g. fiber, fat, and protein). In an effort to better understand how different foods impact the glycemic response, Jenkins *et al.* (1981) proposed the use of the glycemic index (GI) as a relative indicator of blood glucose response to the carbohydrate contained in a particular food. The GI is determined by comparing the blood glucose response (area under the curve) of a test food containing a specified amount of available carbohydrate to a standard food containing the same amount of carbohydrate. The response to the test food is then expressed as a percentage of the response to the standard to give the GI. Originally, glucose or white bread was the traditional reference standard, but over time other standards have been used, such as rice and potato. Many of these foods can have different glycemic responses due to differing factors, including variety of the grain used and cooking conditions. As a result, GI values have become more difficult to interpret and compare as the same food may have a different GI based on what reference standard is used.

Foods are sometimes categorized into "high" and "low" GI foods based on their glycemic response. Typically, high-GI foods would include items with easily digested starches (e.g. refined grains and potatoes), free glucose, or large amounts of disaccharides rapidly hydrolyzed to glucose. Alternatively, low-GI foods (e.g. unprocessed grains, nonstarchy fruits, and vegetables) would contain more slowly digested or resistant starches or higher fiber content, or are rich in free fructose. Low-GI foods may also be high in fat, which slows carbohydrate digestion and absorption. A limitation of classifying foods by GI is that human subjects can have highly variable glycemic responses to the same food. Even the same person can vary in their glycemic response from day to day (FAO/WHO, 1998). This variation is often large enough that a food could transition from a "low" GI food to a "high" GI food if tested in different people or in the same subject on different days.

TABLE 7.1 Glycemic index based on glucose as index food. Glycemic load is calculated as the glycemic index multiplied by the grams of carbohydrate per serving and divided by 100.

Food	Glycemic index	Glycemic load
Apple	36 ± 3	5
Banana	48 ± 3	11
Cake, chocolate with frosting	38 ± 3	20
Carrot	92 ± 20	6
Kidney beans	34 ± 6	9
Lentils, red	26 ± 4	5
Macaroni and cheese	64	33
Oatmeal	55 ± 7	14
Orange juice	50 ± 2	12
Peaches, canned in light syrup	52	9
Peanuts	7 ± 4	0
Popcorn, plain	65 ± 5	7
Potato, baked	76	23
Raisin bran	61 ± 5	12
Rice, long grain	75 ± 7	28
Soda, non-diet	63	16
Spaghetti	38 ± 3	18
White bread	70	10
Whole milk	40	4

Data from Atkinson et al. (2008).

Considering some of the limitations in the measurement of GI, its utility and accuracy as a marker of carbohydrate quality are highly debated. Nevertheless, the GI has been determined for a number of foods (Atkinson et al., 2008; see Table 7.1) and has become more frequently used with limited success in studies relating carbohydrate intake to chronic disease, as will be discussed later in this chapter.

Metabolism of Carbohydrates

Energy Value of Carbohydrates

Traditionally, carbohydrates have been assigned an energy value of 4 kcal/g (17 kJ/g). This value is derived from Atwater's calculations of the heat of combustion of carbohydrates from various food commodities (Merrill and Watt, 1973). However, the actual caloric values of carbohydrates can vary from practically zero in the case of some fibers (e.g. gums and cellulose) to 4.2 kcal/g for most digestible starches. Most sugars have a lower caloric value than starches, ranging from 3.75 to 3.95 kcal/g. The greatest difficulty has come in assigning caloric values to non-digestible polysaccharides and oligosaccharides, which are primarily fermented in the colon. Short-chain fatty acids produced by fermentation (e.g. acetate, propionate, and butyrate) are quickly metabolized and therefore provide a source of energy. However, the amount of energy varies with the degree of fermentability. Smith et al. (1998) determined metabolizable energy values for several non-starch polysaccharides with values ranging from 0 to 2.3 kcal/g. The FAO/WHO consultation on carbohydrates recommended that the energy value for carbohydrates that enter the colon be set at 2 kcal/g (FAO/WHO, 1998). Polyols are also incompletely absorbed and thus provide fewer calories than most other digestible carbohydrates. The caloric values of polyols range from 0.2 to 3 kcal/g (Warshaw and Powers, 1999); however, for labeling purposes, the European Union has established a standard value of 2.3 kcal/g for sugar alcohols, whereas the United States assigns values on an individual-case basis (Zumbe et al., 2001). The American Diabetes Association (2000) advises health professionals to use a value of 2 kcal/g for sugar alcohols.

Fate of Absorbed Monosaccharides

Absorbed monosaccharides are transported through the bloodstream to tissues, where they are used as an energy source. Cellular uptake is achieved by GLUT transporters. All three monosaccharides can be taken up in the liver by non-insulin-dependent GLUT2 transporters (Scheepers et al., 2004). In the liver, galactose is phosphorylated and converted to glucose-1-phosphate, the precursor for glycogen synthesis. Fructose is phosphorylated to an intermediate in the glycolytic pathway (fructose-1-phosphate). As it continues through the glycolytic pathway, it will be cleaved to form dihydroxyacetone phosphate and glyceraldehyde. These intermediates can then continue through glycolysis or, under certain conditions, serve as precursors for glycogen and triglyceride synthesis. Glucose is also taken up by most cells in the body to be used for energy. A number of tissue-specific isoforms of GLUT transporters are responsible for glucose uptake, including: GLUT2 in the liver, pancreas, kidney, and small intestine; GLUT3, primarily in the brain; GLUT4, in insulin-sensitive tissues such as adipose and skeletal muscle; and GLUT1, which is ubiquitously expressed but predominates in erythrocytes and the brain. Many other glucose transporters have been identified and are more thoroughly discussed by Scheepers et al. (2004).

Glycolysis

The initial steps in the metabolism of glucose, which occurs in the cytoplasm of all cells, is called glycolysis, and results in the generation of ATP and two three-carbon molecules of pyruvate. If the cell is under anaerobic conditions (or lacks mitochondria in the case of erythrocytes), pyruvate will be reduced to lactate and exported to the liver for gluconeogenesis (the Cori cycle). Under aerobic conditions, pyruvate can enter the mitochondria and be decarboxylated to acetyl coenzyme A, which then enters the citric acid cycle. This cycle completes the catabolism of glucose to carbon dioxide and water, accompanied by the oxidation of coenzymes (NAD$^+$ and FAD), which can then pass off their electrons in the electron transport system to generate large amounts of ATP.

Gluconeogenesis

Because glucose is the primary energy source for the body, it is critical that blood glucose levels be maintained (70–100 mg/dL or 3.9–5.5 mmol/L) to supply tissues with needed fuel. Glucose can be generated from a number of precursors, including pyruvate, lactate, glycerol, and most amino acids. The synthesis of glucose is basically a reversal of glycolysis, with many of the same enzymes utilized; however, gluconeogenesis occurs only in the liver and kidney. The glucose produced is then released into the bloodstream for use by all tissues.

Regulation of Glycolysis and Gluconeogenesis

A number of controls are present in the glycolytic and gluconeogenic pathways to insure that adequate energy is supplied to cells and that blood glucose levels are maintained. These controls include allosteric and/or covalent modification of key enzymes, alterations in the expression of enzymes, and hormonal regulation. The three key regulatory enzymes in the glycolytic pathway are glucokinase/hexokinase, phosphofructokinase-1, and pyruvate kinase. Because these steps in glycolysis are irreversible, the gluconeogenic pathway utilizes four corresponding enzymes (glucose 6-phosphatase, fructose 1,6-bisphosphatase, phosphoenolpyruvate carboxykinase, and pyruvate carboxylase), which are also irreversible in the pathway of glucose generation. These "paired" enzymes are regulated such that the stimulation of one coordinates with the inhibition of the other (Figure 7.2). For example, elevated blood glucose levels will positively affect the glycolytic

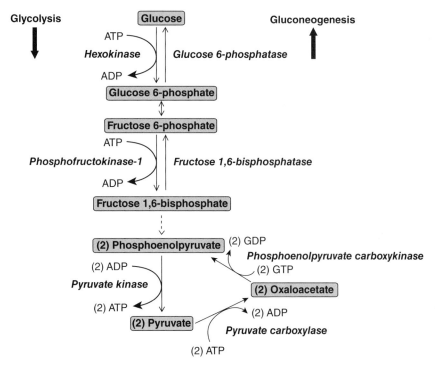

FIG. 7.2 Glycolysis and gluconeogenesis pathways. Left side of the diagram represents glycolysis, and the right side represents gluconeogenesis. Dashed arrow represents steps that were left out of the diagram.

enzyme glucokinase/hexokinase, while simultaneously inhibiting the activity of glucose 6-phosphatase, the corresponding gluconeogenic enzyme.

These enzymes are also subject to hormonal regulation by insulin, glucagon, epinephrine, and glucocorticoids. Insulin, an anabolic hormone, is secreted by the β-cells of the pancreas in response to an increase in blood glucose, such as that which follows a carbohydrate-containing meal. Insulin acts to decrease blood glucose levels by increasing glucose uptake by tissues and by decreasing gluconeogenesis by the liver. To increase tissue uptake, insulin triggers the translocation of GLUT4 receptors to the cell surface in skeletal muscle and adipose tissue. Insulin also stimulates each of the regulatory enzymes in the glycolytic pathway, while also inhibiting the key enzymes of gluconeogenesis. An increase in glucose storage in the form of glycogen is also stimulated by insulin. Glucagon, epinephrine, and glucocorticoids are counter-regulatory hormones to insulin, and are released when blood glucose levels are low, such as during fasting or starvation. Glucagon, produced by the α-cells of the pancreas, and epinephrine and glucocorticoids, produced by the adrenal gland, enhance gluconeogenesis and glycogenolysis (release of glucose from glycogen storage) and inhibit glycolysis. Epinephrine also increases lipolysis during fasting (McGrane, 2000).

Storage of Glucose

The liver and skeletal muscle are able to store excess glucose in the form of glycogen, a branched-chain glucose polymer. The liver is able to store 10% of its weight as glycogen, while skeletal muscle stores approximately 1% (McGrane, 2000). When blood glucose levels fall, the breakdown of liver glycogen is triggered and the glucose released is used to maintain blood glucose levels. During continued fasting, the liver will be depleted of its glycogen stores within 24 hours. Skeletal muscle glycogen can be broken down and used as fuel by the skeletal muscle, which occurs primarily during exercise. Skeletal muscle glycogen is not as effective as liver glycogen at normalizing blood glucose levels during fasting; however, lactate generated in the muscle can be circulated to the liver for gluconeogenesis. Glycogen synthesis and degradation are regulated by hormones, as described in the previous section.

Contribution to Amino Acid and Triglyceride Synthesis

Some metabolites of glucose, such as pyruvate and intermediates in the citric acid cycle, can be used in the synthesis of certain amino acids. Additionally, fatty acids can be formed from oxaloacetic acid and acetyl-coenzyme A (cleavage products of the tricarboxylic acid cycle intermediate citrate). Intermediates in the glycolysis pathway can be modified to serve as the glycerol backbone for triglycerides.

Inborn Errors in Metabolism

A number of disease states associated with deficiencies or genetic defects in certain key enzymes responsible for carbohydrate metabolism have been characterized. Some errors in metabolism, such as those involved in fructose or galactose metabolism, are discovered early and are treated by removal of those monosaccharides from the diet. However, genetic defects in enzymes involved in gluconeogenesis or glycogenolysis are much more life-threatening because individuals with these diseases suffer from frequent hypoglycemia, hepatomegaly, and acidosis. Treatment typically involves small, frequent feedings of carbohydrate to prevent hypoglycemia and acidosis.

Carbohydrate Requirements and Recommendations

In 2002 the US Institute of Medicine established a recommended dietary allowance (RDA) for carbohydrates of 130 g/day for adults and children which is based on the average minimum amount of glucose used by the brain (Institute of Medicine, 2002). This recommendation was based on human studies in which arteriovenous gradients of glucose were measured with estimates of brain blood flow. Although there is not an absolute requirement for glucose, since the brain can switch to using ketone bodies (primarily from fat metabolism), the 130 g/day represents a recommendation that would not require the brain to resort to the use of ketone bodies. This RDA is not the recommendation for overall carbohydrate intake, but rather the recommendation for what is needed by the brain. Most people consume well over the RDA for carbohydrate.

A second recommendation for carbohydrate is the acceptable macronutrient distribution range (AMDR) value of 45% to 65% of total calories in the form of carbohydrate (Institute of Medicine, 2002). The low end of the range was set to allow for sufficient intake of dietary fiber, which would be very difficult to obtain from foods below a level of 45% of calories coming from carbohydrate since all fiber (with the exception of lignin) is carbohydrate. Also, as the intake of one macronutrient gets too low, another macronutrient (either fat or protein in this case) could become too high. There was concern that less than 45% of calories from carbohydrate could result in the intake of excess fat, which in turn could contribute to obesity. At the higher end of the range (65% of calories from carbohydrate), the concern was hypertriglyceridemia and that intakes of fat or protein could be too low.

There is also an adequate intake (AI) value for total fiber of 14 g/1000 calories, which equates to 38 g/day for men under 50 and 25 g/day for women under 50. The fiber recommendation was based on decreased risk of coronary heart disease with higher-fiber diets.

Added Sugars Recommendations

The dietary reference intake (DRI) macronutrient report (Institute of Medicine, 2002) made a recommendation that added sugar intake should not exceed 25% of total calories. This recommendation was based on diminishing intake of micronutrients as the percent of calories from added sugars increased. Although the significant "drop-off" in micronutrient intake was not always at the 25% added sugar intake level for each age and gender group, the overall pattern showed a decline at the 25% intake level. Since the release of the Macronutrient Report in 2002, the 2010 US Dietary Guidelines Advisory Committee (DGAC) completed an evidence-based review of human studies on added sugar intake, particularly from sugar-sweetened beverages, and the relationship to energy intake and body weight (DGAC, 2010). Sugar-sweetened beverages were targeted as numerous studies (Block, 2004; Wang *et al.*, 2008; Bleich *et al.*, 2009; Nelson *et al.*, 2009; Duffey *et al.*, 2010) show them to be the largest contributor of energy in the US and intake has increased significantly since the 1970s. Likewise the prevalence of obesity has also increased since the 1970s. The 2010 DGAC reviewed 14 scientific articles published since 1990 (including systematic reviews, randomized control trials and prospective observational studies) which evaluated intake of sugar-sweetened beverages and energy intake and body weight. The panel concluded the following (DGAC, 2010):

> Limited evidence shows that intake of sugar-sweetened beverages is linked to higher energy intake in adults. A moderate body of epidemiological evidence suggests that greater consumption of sugar-sweetened beverages is associated with increased body weight in adults. A moderate body of evidence suggests that under isocaloric controlled conditions, added sugars, including sugar-sweetened

beverages, are no more likely to cause weight gain than any other sources.

While the 2010 DGAC acknowledged that some studies show an association between added sugars from sugar-sweetened beverages and weight gain, they concluded it was not possible to determine if the relationship was due specifically to added sugars or just a result of increased caloric consumption. Furthermore, additional calories from added sugars are not different from calories from other sources in the diet. The DGAC recommended reducing intake of added sugars from multiple sources as a strategy to reduce caloric intake in the US population (DGAC, 2010).

Whole-Grain Recommendations

In continuation of the 2005 Dietary Guidelines recommendation to increase whole-grain servings to three per day at the expense of refined grains (USDA, 2005), the 2010 DGAC reviewed literature published since June 2004 examining the relationship of whole-grain intake to cardiovascular disease, type 2 diabetes and body weight (DGAC, 2010). What constitutes a whole grain as opposed to a refined grain? Whole grains consist of the entire kernel or seed of the grain, which consists of three components: the bran layer (which contains most of the fiber), the endosperm (which is primarily starch), and the germ (which contains some fat and other nutrients). When whole grains are refined, most of the bran and germ are lost, leaving the endosperm. Refined grains are then enriched with thiamin, riboflavin, iron, and niacin, fortified with folic acid, and are called "enriched grains." Whole grains do not have to be intact in the food product to be called "whole grains" but they do have to have the same ratio of bran to endosperm to germ as they had in the intact kernel. Based on the new data that they reviewed, they concluded (DGAC, 2010):

> A moderate body of evidence from large prospective cohort studies shows that whole-grain intake, which includes cereal fiber, protects against cardiovascular disease. Limited evidence shows that consumption of whole grains is associated with a reduced incidence of type 2 diabetes in large prospective cohort studies. Moderate evidence shows that intake of whole grains and grain fiber is associated with lower body weight.

Considering that most Americans are consuming large amounts of predominantly refined grains (Lin and Yen, 2007), the recommendation was made to replace refined grains with fiber-rich whole grains in the diet. An

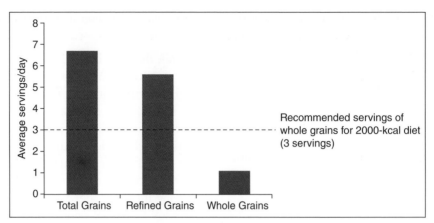

FIG. 7.3 Typical US consumption of total, whole and refined grains based on USDA report on grain consumption (Gibson, 2008). For someone consuming 2000 kcal/day, the 2005 dietary guidelines recommended six total servings of grain per day with at least half of these servings from whole grains. The typical US consumer is eating more grains than recommended, and the majority of those servings are from refined grains.

emphasis was placed on fiber-rich whole grains since not all whole grains or whole-grain foods are high in fiber. For example, brown rice and corn are both whole grains; yet a typical half-cup serving of either contains less than 2 g of fiber. Also foods made from these whole grains, such as rice cakes or corn chips, are also often low in fiber. While there is evidence that whole grains, independent of fiber, have beneficial effects on health, the DGAC acknowledged that when studies on the bran and or/germ components of grain were included with the whole-grain evidence, the scientific support for the health benefit (e.g. CVD) became stronger.

Current Intakes

According to statistics from the FAO/WHO (1998), carbohydrate consumption worldwide ranges from 40% to 80% of energy intake. Most industrialized countries fall at the bottom of this range, whereas underdeveloped countries fall closer to the top of the range. Approximately 50% of carbohydrates consumed are in the form of starch, but this proportion is higher in countries where starches and grains are staple food items. Industrialized nations have shown an increase in sugar intake to 20% to 25% of calories from sugars, and a substantial portion of these calories are from added sugars such as corn syrups and sucrose. In the US, 13% of the population currently consumes more than 25% of their calories from added sugars (Marriott *et al.*, 2010).

Whole-grain consumption varies worldwide. Food consumption data from the USDA indicates that most Americans only consume around one serving of whole grains per day and only 7% of the population meets the recommended three servings per day (Lin and Yen, 2007). Most Americans are consuming more than the recommended amounts of total grains, indicating overconsumption of refined grains (Figure 7.3). Studies in Scandinavian populations show consumption of whole-grain foods to be almost four times the amount consumed in the United States (Lang and Jebb, 2003).

Carbohydrates in Chronic Disease

Energy Balance and Obesity

While the evidence is limited, a number of epidemiological studies have shown an increased intake of added sugars to be associated with an increase in overall energy intake and body weight (DGAC, 2010). Several studies have estimated that consumption of sugar-sweetened beverages in adults adds approximately 200–275 excess calories per day (Reid *et al.*, 2007; Stookey *et al.*, 2007; Duffey *et al.*, 2010). However, when compared with other sources of energy (e.g. fat), calories from added sugars are no more likely to cause weight gain (Vartanian *et al.*, 2007; Gibson, 2008). Since non-diet soft drinks are the largest source of added sugars in the US diet and consumption has increased (Block, 2004), much of the recent research has focused on this area. Vartanian *et al.* (2007) conducted a systematic review and meta-analysis of 88 studies that investigated the effect of sweetened-beverage consumption on energy intake and body weight. While the size of the effect was small, there was a significant relationship between added sugars and energy intake and body weight. Alternatively, a recent review by Ruxton *et al.* (2010) concluded that there is no relationship between added sugar intake and BMI. Many of the discrepancies in these different reports are due to differences in how the reviews were conducted as well as differences in the methods used to measure intake and body weight in the studies. Despite limited evidence, the DGAC recommended that reduction of added sugars from all sources in the diet is advisable to control caloric intake (DGAC, 2010).

Recently, more attention has become focused on different sources of added sugars in the diet (e.g. HFCS, sucrose, fructose, glucose, etc.). A recent workshop reviewed the science in this area and determined key areas that need further investigation. Research was presented and there was scientific agreement that the metabolic effects of HFCS and sucrose are similar. However, it was determined that more science is needed to directly compare the effects of fructose with those of other sweeteners with regard to energy metabolism and chronic disease endpoints. As fructose is metabolized differently from glucose, some research suggests fructose may contribute more than other sweeteners to weight gain or other chronic diseases, such as type 2 diabetes, but more research is needed directly comparing the different monosaccharides (Murphy, 2009).

A few short-term studies have linked low glycemic index diets to weight loss, but longer term controlled studies show no difference in weight loss compared with other calorically restricted diets (e.g. low-fat diets) or high glycemic index diets (DGAC, 2010). Based on these data, the DGAC concluded that there is "strong and consistent evidence that glycemic index and/or glycemic load are not associated with body weight and do not lead to greater weight loss or better weight maintenance" (DGAC, 2010).

The impact of carbohydrates on satiety has also been investigated as a means of controlling energy intake. The glucostatic theory, introduced in the 1950s, suggested that blood glucose levels impacted appetite. When blood glucose levels were high, feelings of satiety were increased and when blood glucose dropped, this triggered feelings of hunger. It has been shown that consuming carbohy-

drates prior to a meal does increase satiety and decrease caloric intake at the next meal. However, this same effect can be seen when protein or fat is given prior to a meal, independent of the glycemic effect. Furthermore, comparisons of high and low glycemic index foods showed no differences in satiety, energy intake, or weight loss (DGAC, 2010).

Diabetes and Insulin Sensitivity

Diabetes is a disorder of carbohydrate metabolism characterized primarily by hyperglycemia resulting from ineffective uptake of glucose by tissues. Type 1 diabetes is an autoimmune disease that typically occurs early in life and results in total loss of insulin production, whereas type 2 diabetes develops over time as tissues develop a resistance to insulin, and insulin release from the pancreas slowly diminishes. As carbohydrates have the greatest effect on blood glucose of all macronutrients, their role in the development of diabetes has been closely examined. Evidence from prospective studies with follow-up periods as long as 16 years have shown no relationship between the amount of carbohydrate in the diet and the development of diabetes. However, recent studies have evaluated the intake of added sugars, particularly from sugar-sweetened beverages, on the incidence of type 2 diabetes and found mixed results. Some studies looking specifically at sugar-sweetened beverages have found a positive relationship to intake and the development of type 2 diabetes (Schulze *et al.*, 2004; Ruxton *et al.*, 2010). However, studies evaluating overall sugar intake as well as intake of overall carbohydrate and refined grains found no association with type 2 diabetes (Meyer *et al.*, 2000; Janket *et al.*, 2003). In most studies the positive association between sugar intake and diabetes is attenuated when overall energy intake is accounted for, suggesting that it is the excess calories provided by the added sugar intake that may be the primary contributor.

Whole grains and dietary fiber, particularly cereal fiber, have been shown in a number of epidemiological studies to be inversely associated with the risk of type 2 diabetes (de Munter *et al.*, 2007). In fact, it appears that the risk reduction due to whole grains may be attributed, in part, to the fiber or bran content of the whole grain (de Munter *et al.*, 2007). One systematic review of six different epidemiological studies, totaling 286 125 people, found that increasing intake of whole grains by two servings per day resulted in a 21% decrease in risk for type 2 diabetes (de Munter *et al.*, 2007).

A number of recent prospective studies have shown mixed results as to an association of glycemic index with type 2 diabetes (DGAC, 2010). Whereas several have shown a positive association of glycemic index and incidence of type 2 diabetes (Schulz *et al.*, 2006; Villegas *et al.*, 2007; Halton *et al.*, 2008), the same number of studies show no association or a negative association (Stevens *et al.*, 2002; Hodge *et al.*, 2004; Barclay *et al.*, 2007; Mosdøl *et al.*, 2007; Sahyoun *et al.*, 2008). Similarly, glycemic load has shown an inconsistent association with the incidence of type 2 diabetes.

Cardiovascular Disease and Blood Lipids

Several epidemiological studies have found a consistent relationship between increased intake of whole grains and reduced risk of cardiovascular disease (CVD) (DGAC, 2010). Additionally, when studies on added bran/germ are included, these inverse relationships are strengthened, suggesting that the fiber content of the whole grain may play an important role in CVD prevention. However, there may be additional bioactive components in whole grain that may act synergistically with the fiber to contribute to the prevention of CVD (Liu *et al.*, 1999; De Moura *et al.*, 2009). The primary mechanisms by which whole grains have been shown to influence CVD is through lowering of blood lipids and decreasing blood pressure. Additional biomarkers of enhanced antioxidant protection and decreases in inflammation have also been suggested as part of the protective mechanism of whole grains against CVD, but have not been confirmed (Brownlee *et al.*, 2010, DGAC, 2010).

There have been no well-established associations between sugar intake and CVD; however, some prospective studies have shown a positive association between sugar-sweetened beverage intake and certain markers for CVD (Malik *et al.*, 2010). Most of these studies report increased incidence of hypertension and hypertriglyceridemia with increasing intakes of sugar-sweetened beverages. Only one study has found a positive association between sugar-sweetened beverage intake and coronary heart disease in women, but adjustment for energy intake attenuated these associations, indicating a contribution of increased energy intake with elevated sugar intake (Fung *et al.*, 2009).

Cancer

Carbohydrate intake has not been shown to be strongly linked to cancer incidence, with the exception of colorectal cancer. Generally, diets high in refined carbohydrates and sugars appear to increase the risk of colon cancer whereas diets high in whole grains appear to be protective (USDA, 2005). Numerous studies in the past 5 years have evaluated the association of glycemic index and cancers of the stomach, ovary, breast, pancreas, and colon. A review of this literature by the 2010 DGAC found that "evidence for an association . . . is overwhelmingly negative" (DGAC, 2010).

Future Directions

A tremendous amount of scientific research and many regulatory changes have occurred in the past decade in the area of carbohydrates' impact on health. Yet there remain areas where research and regulatory clarification are needed. A critical area is establishing a universally accepted definition for whole grains. There is currently inconsistency in how whole-grain foods are defined, which makes it difficult to assess the true effect of whole grains on health when different studies use different inclusion criteria for what constitutes a whole-grain food. Furthermore, an acceptable definition for whole grains would also help consumer understanding and assist them in meeting the dietary recommendations. Future research should also examine the role of other bioactive components (phenolics, etc.) in whole grains beyond just the fiber portion that may be contributing to some of the health benefits seen with whole grains. Additionally, much recent research has focused on liquid calories, such as sugar-sweetened beverages, and the variety of beverages on the market has vastly increased in recent years. The 2010 DGAC recognized that the methods for reporting liquid calories in epidemiological studies should be better developed in order to accurately determine the contribution of carbohydrate sweeteners to energy intake and health endpoints. An important issue to resolve is the substitution of carbohydrates for saturated fats and whether or not that substitution results in an improved blood lipid profile and subsequent decreased risk of coronary heart disease. There has also been a rapid rise in high-throughput technologies, such as metabolomics, that may lead to the discovery of new biomarkers of health and/or disease and a better indication of how carbohydrates may impact disease and metabolic pathways that may lead to disease.

Suggestions for Further Reading

De Moura, F.F., Lewis, K.D., and Falk, M.C. (2009) Applying the FDA definition of whole grains to the evidence for cardiovascular disease health claims. *J Nutr* **139**, 2220S–2226S.

DGAC (2010) Report of the Dietary Guidelines Advisory Committee on the Dietary Guidelines for Americans. http://www.cnpp.usda.gov/DGAs2010-DGACReport.htm

Gibson, S. (2008) Sugar-sweetened soft drinks and obesity: a systematic review of the evidence from observational studies and interventions. *Nutr Res Rev* **21**, 134–147.

Murphy, S.P. (2009) The state of science on dietary sweeteners containing fructose: summary and issues to be resolved. *J Nutr* **139**, 1269S–1270S.

References

American Diabetes Association (2000) Nutrition recommendations and principles for people with diabetes mellitus. *Diabetes Care* **23**, S43–S46.

Atkinson, F.S., Foster-Powell, K., and Brand-Miller, J.C. (2008) International tables of glycemic index and glycemic load values: 2008. *Diabetes Care* **31**, 2281–2283.

Barclay, A.W., Flood, V.M., Rochtchina, E., *et al.* (2007) Glycemic index, dietary fiber, and risk of type 2 diabetes in a cohort of older Australians. *Diabetes Care* **30**, 2811–2813.

Bleich, S.N., Wang, Y.C., Wang, Y., *et al.* (2009) Increasing consumption of sugar-sweetened beverages among US adults: 1988–1994 to 1999–2004. *Am J Clin Nutr* **89**, 372–381.

Block, G. (2004) Foods contributing to energy intake in the US: data from NHANES III and NHANES 1999–2000. *J Food Comp Anal* **17**, 439–447.

Brannon, P.M., Carpenter, T.O., Fernandez, J.R., *et al.* (2010) NIH Consensus Development Conference Statement: Lactose intolerance and health. *NIH Consens State Sci Statements* **27**, 1–27.

Brownlee, I.A., Moore, C., Chatfield, M., *et al.* (2010) Markers of cardiovascular risk are not changed by increased whole-grain intake: the WHOLEheart study, a randomised, controlled dietary intervention. *Br J Nutr* **104**, 125–134.

De Moura, F.F., Lewis, K.D., and Falk, M.C. (2009) Applying the FDA definition of whole grains to the evidence for cardiovascular disease health claims. *J Nutr* **139**, 2220S–2226S.

de Munter, J.S., Hu, F.B., Spiegelman, D., *et al.* (2007) Whole grain, bran, and germ intake and risk of type 2 diabetes: a prospective cohort study and systematic review. *PLoS Med* **4**, e261.

DGAC (2010) Report of the Dietary Guidelines Advisory Committee on the Dietary Guidelines for Americans. http://www.cnpp.usda.gov/dgas2010-dgacreport.htm.

Duffey, K.J., Gordon-Larsen, P., Steffen, L.M., *et al.* (2010) Drinking caloric beverages increases the risk of adverse cardiometabolic outcomes in the Coronary Artery Risk Development in Young Adults (CARDIA) Study. *Am J Clin Nutr* **92**, 954–959.

FAO/WHO (1998) Food and Agriculture Organization/World Health Organization Expert Consultation on Carbohydrates in Human Nutrition. *Carbohydrates in Human Nutrition: A Report of a Joint FAO/WHO Expert Consultation.* FAO Food and Nutrition Paper no. 66. FAO, Rome.

FDA (1997) Food and Drug Administration, HHS. Rules and regulations – food labeling: health claims, dietary sugar alcohols and dental caries. *Federal Register* 63653–63655.

Fung, T.T., Malik, V., Rexrode, K.M., *et al.* (2009) Sweetened beverage consumption and risk of coronary heart disease in women. *Am J Clin Nutr* **89**, 1037–1342.

Gibson, S. (2008) Sugar-sweetened soft drinks and obesity: a systematic review of the evidence from observational studies and interventions. *Nutr Res Rev* **21**, 134–147.

Halton, T. L., Liu, S., Manson, J.E., *et al.* (2008) Low-carbohydrate-diet score and risk of type 2 diabetes in women. *Am J Clin Nutr* **87**, 339–346.

Hanover, L. and White, J. (1993) Manufacturing, composition, and applications of fructose. *Am J Clin Nutr* **58**, 724S–732S.

Hodge, A.M., English, D.R., O'Dea, K., *et al.* (2004) Glycemic index and dietary fiber and the risk of type 2 diabetes. *Diabetes Care* **27**, 2701–2706.

Hu, F.B. and Malik, V.S. (2010) Sugar-sweetened beverages and risk of obesity and type 2 diabetes: epidemiologic evidence. *Physiol Behav* **100**, 47–54.

Institute of Medicine (2002) *Dietary Reference Intakes for Energy, Carbohydrate, Fiber, Fat, Fatty Acids, Cholesterol, Protein, and Amino Acids.* National Academies Press, Washington, DC.

Janket, S.J., Manson, J.E., Sesso, H., *et al.* (2003) A prospective study of sugar intake and risk of type 2 diabetes in women. *Diabetes Care* **26**, 1008–1015.

Jenkins, D.J., Wolever, T.M., Taylor, R.H., *et al.* (1981) Glycemic index of foods: a physiological basis for carbohydrate exchange. *Am J Clin Nutr* **34**, 362–366.

Lang, R. and Jebb, S.A. (2003) Who consumes whole grains, and how much? *Proc Nutr Soc* **62**, 123–127.

Lin, B.H. and Yen, S.T. (2007) The US Grain Consumption Landscape: Who Eats Grain, in What Form, Where, and How Much? ERR-50. US Department of Agriculture, Economic Research Service, Washington, DC.

Liu, S., Stampfer, M.J., Hu, F.B., *et al.* (1999) Whole-grain consumption and risk of coronary heart disease: results from the Nurses' Health Study. *Am J Clin Nutr* **70**, 412–419.

Malik, V.S., Popkin, B.M., Bray, G.A., *et al.* (2010) Sugar-sweetened beverages, obesity, type 2 diabetes mellitus, and cardiovascular disease risk. *Circulation* **121,** 1356–1364.

Marriott, B.P., Olsho, L., Haddon, L., *et al.* (2010) Intake of added sugars and selected nutrients in the United States, National Health and Nutrition Examination Survey (NHANES) 2003–2006. *Crit Rev Food Sci Nutr* **50,** 228–258.

McGrane, M.M. (2000) Carbohydrate metabolism – synthesis and oxidation. In M.H. Stipanuk (ed.), *Biochemical and Physiological Aspects of Human Nutrition.* WB Saunders, Philadelphia, pp. 158–205.

Merrill, A.L. and Watt, B.K. (1973) *Energy Value of Foods: Basis and Derivation. Agriculture Handbook No. 74.* US Government Printing Office; Washington, DC, pp. 2–3.

Meyer, K.A., Kushi, L.H., Jacobs, D.R. Jr, *et al.* (2000) Carbohydrates, dietary fiber, and incident type 2 diabetes in older women. *Am J Clin Nutr* **71,** 921–929.

Meyer, P.D. (2004) Nondigestible oligosaccharides as dietary fiber. *J AOAC Int* **87,** 718–726.

Mosdøl, A., Witte, D.R., Frost, G., *et al.* (2007) Dietary glycemic index and glycemic load are associated with high-density-lipoprotein cholesterol at baseline but not with increased risk of diabetes in the Whitehall II study. *Am J Clin Nutr* **86,** 988–994.

Murphy, S.P. (2009) The state of science on dietary sweeteners containing fructose: summary and issues to be resolved. *J Nutr* **139,** 1269S–1270S.

Nelson, M.C., Neumark-Sztainer, D., Hannan, P.J., *et al.* (2009) Five-year longitudinal and secular shifts in adolescent beverage intake: findings from project EAT (Eating Among Teens) – II. *J Am Diet Assoc* **109,** 308–312.

Reid, M., Hammersley, R., Hill, A.J., *et al.* (2007) Long-term dietary compensation for added sugar: effects of supplementary sucrose drinks over a 4-week period. *Br J Nutr* **97,** 193–203.

Ruxton, C.H., Gardner, E.J., and McNulty, H.M. (2010) Is sugar consumption detrimental to health? A review of the evidence 1995–2006. *Crit Rev Food Sci Nutr* **50,** 1–19.

Sahyoun, N.R., Anderson, A.L., Tylavsky, F.A., *et al.* (2008) Dietary glycemic index and glycemic load and the risk of type 2 diabetes in older adults. *Am J Clin Nutr* **87,** 126–131.

Scheepers, A., Joost, H.G., and Schurmann, A. (2004) The glucose transporter families SGLT and GLUT: molecular basis of normal and aberrant function. *JPEN J Parenter Enteral Nutr* **28,** 364–371.

Schulz, M., Liese, A.D., Fanq, F., *et al.* (2006) Is the association between dietary glycemic index and type 2 diabetes modified by waist circumference? *Diabetes Care* **29,** 1102–1104.

Schulze, M.B., Manson, J.E., and Ludwig, D.S. (2004) Sugar-sweetened beverages, weight gain, and incidence of type 2 diabetes in young and middle-aged women. *JAMA* **292,** 927–934.

Smith, T., Brown, J.C., and Livesey, G. (1998) Energy balance and thermogenesis in rats consuming nonstarch polysaccharides of various fermentabilities. *Am J Clin Nutr* **68,** 802–819.

Stevens, J., Ahn, K., Juhaeri, J., *et al.* (2002) Dietary fiber intake and glycemic index and incidence of diabetes in African-American and white adults: the ARIC study. *Diabetes Care* **25,** 1715–1721.

Stookey, J.D., Constant, F., Gardner, C.D., *et al.* (2007) Replacing sweetened caloric beverages with drinking water is associated with lower energy intake. *Obesity (Silver Spring)* **15,** 3013–3022.

Tungland, B.C. and Meyer, D. (2002) Nondigestible oligo- and polysaccharides (dietary fiber): their physiology and role in human health and food. *Comp Rev Food Sci Food Safety* **1,** 73–92.

USDA (2005) Dietary Guidelines Advisory Committee. *Dietary Guidelines Advisory Committee Report.* Available at: http://www.health.gov/dietaryguidelines/dga2005/report. Accessed February 22, 2006.

Vartanian, L.R., Schwartz, M.B., and Brownell, K.D. (2007) Effects of soft drink consumption on nutrition and health: a systematic review and meta-analysis. *Am J Publ Health* **97,** 667–675.

Villegas, R., Liu, S., Gao, Y.T., *et al.* (2007) Prospective study of dietary carbohydrates, glycemic index, glycemic load, and incidence of type 2 diabetes mellitus in middle-aged Chinese women. *Arch Intern Med* **167,** 2310–2316.

Wang, Y.C., Bleich, S.N., and Gortmaker, S.L. (2008) Increasing caloric contribution from sugar-sweetened beverages and 100% fruit juices among US children and adolescents, 1988–2004. *Pediatrics* **121,** e1604–1614.

Warshaw, H.S. and Powers, M.A. (1999) A search for answers about foods with polyols (sugar alcohols). *Diabetes Educ* **25,** 307–321.

White, J. (1992) Fructose syrup: production, properties and applications. In F. Shenck and R. Hebeda (eds), *Starch Hydrolysis Products – Worldwide Technology, Production, and Applications.* VCH Publishers, New York, pp. 177–200.

Wright, E.M., Martin, M.G., and Turk, E. (2003) Intestinal absorption in health and disease – sugars. *Best Pract Res Clin Gastroenterol* **17,** 943–956.

Zumbe, A., Lee, A., and Storey, D. (2001) Polyols in confectionery: the route to sugar-free, reduced sugar and reduced calorie confectionery. *Br J Nutr* **85,** S31–S45.

8

DIETARY FIBER

IAN T. JOHNSON, PhD

Institute of Food Research, Norwich, UK

Summary

Dietary fiber is a collective term for the many carbohydrate polymers that escape hydrolysis by human digestive enzymes, enter the large bowel and contribute to fecal bulk, either directly or after fermentation by gut bacteria. The presence of dietary fiber within the partially digested intraluminal food matrix modifies gastrointestinal function at every stage of the digestive process, but the physiological effects of the different components of the fiber complex vary, depending upon their physical properties and their chemical interactions within the gut lumen. By modifying the rate and site of nutrient absorption, and by increasing fecal mass and delivering fermentation products to the circulation, the various components of the dietary fiber complex can modify human metabolism to a degree which is of major significance for health. Dietary fiber contributes to the maintenance of normal bowel function, and epidemiological evidence suggests that high intakes are associated with reduced incidences of various dyslipidemias, with type 2 diabetes and coronary heart disease, and with several abnormalities of the metabolic syndrome, which predisposes to these major pathologies. In spite of recommendations by public health bodies to consume higher levels of fiber, average intakes remain low in most industrialized countries. There is a continuing need for research to clarify the mechanisms of action of fiber of most relevance to human alimentary and metabolic health, and to facilitate increased levels of fiber intake at all ages, both by public health initiatives and through the development of novel sources and products.

Introduction

Early physicians were well aware that human bowel movements were influenced by the foods eaten, and knew that some constituents of the diet remained undigested in the alimentary tract. Hippocrates, in the fourth century BC, is said to have recommended the consumption of breads made from unrefined flour. During the nineteenth century in the USA, the brothers J.H. and W.K. Kellogg developed food products based on the perceived benefits of wholegrain cereals, but the formal scientific investigation of the various different sources of carbohydrates in the human diet really began with the work of McCance and Lawrence, who first quantified what they termed the "unavailable carbohydrate" component of plant foods, by which they meant those carbohydrate polymers that, unlike starch,

Present Knowledge in Nutrition, Tenth Edition. Edited by John W. Erdman Jr, Ian A. Macdonald and Steven H. Zeisel.
© 2012 International Life Sciences Institute. Published 2012 by John Wiley & Sons, Inc.

cannot be hydrolyzed by human digestive enzymes (McCance and Lawrence, 1929). The modern concept of "dietary fiber" emerged in the early 1970s, when two colonial medical officers, Denis Burkitt and Hugh Trowell, building on ideas and observations by Cleave (1974), Walker (1949), and others, popularized the hypothesis that many chronic non-infectious diseases of Western society were caused by consumption of diets that lacked adequate quantities of polysaccharides derived from the cell walls of plants used as human foods (Burkitt and Trowell, 1975). This hypothesis was focused initially on the physiology and health of the alimentary tract, but it was soon broadened in scope to include mechanisms related to the prevention of other metabolic and systemic disorders. In the last 35 years much epidemiological research has been carried out to test the fiber hypothesis at the population level, and an immense amount of experimental work has been done to explore the physiological properties and metabolic effects of fiber in humans and animal models. This chapter is concerned with the definition, composition and analysis of dietary fiber, with its physiological effects, both within and beyond the alimentary tract, and with our current understanding of its importance for the maintenance of human health. The use of dietary fiber in the treatment of disease is discussed only where it is relevant to these overall objectives.

The Definition, Composition, and Analysis of Dietary Fiber

"Dietary fiber" is a collective term for various carbohydrates that escape digestion in the human small intestine. This concept seems simple enough, and yet its unexpected complexities have delayed the development of an agreed formal definition of dietary fiber for over 40 years. The term was probably first used by Hipsley, in an early paper on toxaemia of pregnancy (Hipsley, 1953), but both the concept of dietary fiber and its broader implications became more widely recognized with papers by Painter and Burkitt on the causes of diverticular disease (Painter and Burkitt, 1971), and by Trowell, on dietary fiber and ischemic heart disease (Trowell, 1972b). In his paper, Trowell defined dietary fiber simply as "that portion of food which is derived from cellular walls of plants which are digested very poorly by human beings" but a growing awareness of the chemistry of plant cell walls prompted the development of a more precise definition published by

Trowell and colleagues in 1976: "The sum of the lignin and the plant polysaccharides that are not digested by the endogenous secretions of the mammalian digestive tract (Trowell et al., 1976).

Apart from starch, which is the principal storage polysaccharide in plants used as human foods, plant polysaccharides function as the mechanical, supportive elements of tissues and cell walls. They vary considerably in composition and structure, both between plant varieties, and between tissues within the same plant, but they consist mainly of polymers of glucose, galactose, arabinose, xylose, and uronic acids. Cellulose is a linear polymer of beta-linked glucose molecules. Individual polymers, which attain molecular weights of a million Daltons or more, aggregate by means of hydrogen bonding to form cellulose fibrils. A typical, relatively thin, plant cell wall from the undifferentiated parenchyma cells of fruits and vegetables is composed of cellulose fibrils within a matrix of water-soluble polymers of galactose and arabinose and various branching xylose polymers. In supporting tissues, the mechanical strength of the cells is increased by the deposition of additional cellulose and matrix polysaccharides, and in vascular tissues the cell walls are toughened by deposition of a highly complex phenolic compound, lignin. In cereals and other seeds, which provide a very high proportion of the carbohydrates in human diets, the outer polysaccharide layers, forming the bran in cereals, are often thickened and strengthened by lignin and other complex polyphenolic substances. A simplified illustration of the distribution of non-starch polysaccharides and starch granules within the main tissues of a grain of wheat is given in Figure 8.1.

The physical properties of the various polysaccharides differ widely, but they all consist of polymers of beta-linked saccharides, completely resistant to hydrolysis by human digestive enzymes. A summary of the major components of dietary fiber and their sources in the human diet is given in Table 8.1. Lignin, which is a branching polymer of phenyl propane units rather than a polysaccharide, is included in most definitions of dietary fiber, largely because of the difficulty of separating it from cell-wall polysaccharides during analysis. It contributes relatively little to the total mass of fiber in foods, but its presence is very important because of its effects on the physical properties of the polysaccharides with which it is associated.

The development of analytical methods for fiber in foods soon drew attention to the fact that a significant

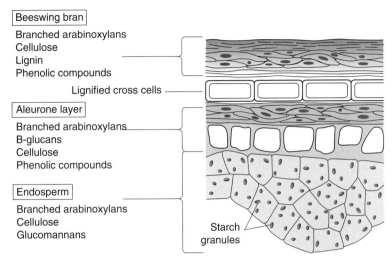

Beeswing bran
Branched arabinoxylans
Cellulose
Lignin
Phenolic compounds

Lignified cross cells

Aleurone layer
Branched arabinoxylans
B-glucans
Cellulose
Phenolic compounds

Endosperm
Branched arabinoxylans
Cellulose
Glucomannans

Starch granules

FIG. 8.1 The distribution of the major non-starch polysaccharides, and starch granules, within the major tissues of a typical wheat grain. Adapted from Waldron and Selvendran (1990).

TABLE 8.1 Major sources and components of dietary fibre in the human diet

Food source	Non-starch polysaccharides	Associated substances
Cereal grains	Cellulose, branched arabinoxylans, xyloglucans, beta-glucans, glucomannans	Lignin, phenolic esters
Leguminous seeds	Cellulose, xyloglucans, mannans, galactomannans, pectic substances	Oligosaccharides
Vegetables and fruits	Cellulose, xyloglucans, pectic polysaccharides	Lignin, suberin, glycoproteins
Manufactured foods	Galactomannan gums (guar, locust bean), beta-glucans, pectins, alginates, carageenans, modified cellulose gums (carboxymethyl cellulose, methyl cellulose)	

proportion of dietary starch resists hydrolysis by pancreatic amylase. Subsequent research has confirmed that some starch escapes digestion in the small intestine and enters the colon together with intact cell-wall polysaccharides. Starch is chemically quite distinct from cell-wall polysaccharides because the two glucose polymers of which it is composed, amylose and amylopectin, both contain only alpha linkages, which are rapidly and completely hydrolysed by human digestive enzymes. In practice, however, the digestion of starch in the human small intestine is often incomplete (Asp *et al.*, 1996). Englyst and Cummings (1988) developed a technique for the complete removal of starch from the cell-wall polysaccharides during analysis, and recommended that dietary fiber should always be defined as *non-starch polysaccharides* (NSP), with *resistant starch* quantified and reported separately. An alternative view is that, since the behavior of resistant starch in the alimentary tract is physiologically similar to that of cell-wall polysaccharides, it should be regarded as dietary fiber and included in the definition (Asp, 1987).

The task of defining dietary fiber became increasingly complex during the 1980s with the widespread use of isolated and purified non-starch polysaccharides, both as research tools and later as food constituents. For example, the galactomannan polymers, guar gum, locust bean gum, and carob bean gum, are storage polysaccharides from leguminous seeds that have long been used in small quantities as thickening agents in foods. Though very different in their physical properties from the structural polysaccharides of plant cell walls, these water-soluble and often viscous polysaccharides also remain undigested in the small intestine, and can exert important effects on digestive physiology. Another group of carbohydrates that have grown in importance as food constituents since the concept of dietary fiber was first proposed are the beta-linked oligosaccharides with chain lengths of three or more saccharide units. These include natural food constituents such as inulin, and purified or synthetic galactose and fructose oligosaccharides used to stimulate the growth of beneficial bacteria in the colonic microflora (prebiotics). Again, since these carbohydrates resist digestion in the small intestine and are readily fermented by the colonic microflora, many argue that they should be included in the general definition of dietary fiber (Flamm *et al.*, 2001), whereas others have maintained that they should be excluded because of their low molecular weight and general lack of similarity to the structural polysaccharides of plant cell walls (Englyst *et al.*, 2007).

Recent definitions of dietary fiber have been designed to take account of the full range of carbohydrates that resist human digestive enzymes and exert beneficial physiological effects. The definition published by the Institute of Medicine of the National Academy of Sciences of the USA makes a distinction between *dietary fiber*, defined as "non-digestible carbohydrates and lignin that are intrinsic and intact in plants" and *functional fiber,* which consists of isolated, non-digestible carbohydrate components that have beneficial physiological effects in humans (Institute of Medicine, 2005). Oligosaccharides, whether from natural or synthetic sources, are excluded from the first category but can be included in the second. Under this scheme, *total dietary fiber* is defined as the sum of dietary and functional fiber. A scientific panel of the European Food Safety Authority published a statement on dietary fiber in 2007, in which it noted that in practice no analytical technique was available to distinguish between dietary fiber and functional fiber when they occur as a mixture in food products, and recommended a simple definition of dietary fiber as "all carbohydrates occurring in foods that are non-digestible in the human small intestine" (European Food Safety Agency, 2007). In 2009 the Commission on Nutrition and Foods for Special Dietary Uses of the Codex Alimentarius Commission, which is the food regulation arm of the World Health Organization, adopted a new definition of dietary fiber for the guidance of national governments when formulating their own legislation. The definition (FAO/WHO Food Standards Programme Codex Committee on Methods of Analysis and Sampling, 2010) is as follows:

Dietary fibre means carbohydrate polymers with ten or more monomeric units, which are not hydrolysed by the endogenous enzymes in the small intestine of humans and belong to the following categories:

- Edible carbohydrate polymers naturally occurring in the food as consumed,
- Carbohydrate polymers, which have been obtained from food raw material by physical, enzymatic or chemical means and which have been shown to have a physiological effect of benefit to health as demonstrated by generally accepted scientific evidence to competent authorities,
- Synthetic carbohydrate polymers which have been shown to have a physiological effect of benefit to health as demonstrated by generally accepted scientific evidence to competent authorities.

This definition does include both resistant starch and purified polysaccharide supplements, but it excludes all oligosaccharides with degrees of polymerization (DP) between 3 and 9. However, a pragmatic footnote to the definition states that a "decision on whether to include carbohydrates from three to nine monomeric units should be left to national authorities."

The Analysis of Dietary Fiber in Foods

Clearly the definition of fiber and the design of analytical methods to quantify it in foods are closely related problems. The earliest methods for fiber analysis were developed to measure the indigestible fraction of animal feeds (Goering and Van Soest, 1970). Among such methods, the neutral detergent fiber technique has been applied most frequently to human foods (Van Soest *et al.*, 1991), but it suffers from the disadvantage that soluble polysaccharides, including pectin, are not included in the analysis. To overcome this and similar problems, Southgate developed a method for the analysis of unavailable carbohydrates in foods (Southgate, 1969), based on enzymatic hydrolysis of polysaccharides and analysis of the liberated sugars by colorimetry, and this was used to determine the values in the fourth edition of the official UK food tables, *The Composition of Foods*, published in 1978 (Paul and Southgate, 1978). This approach was refined by Englyst and colleagues (Englyst *et al.*, 1982), who used carbohydrate analysis by gas liquid chromatography (GLC) to obtain a more definitive analysis of the residual non-starch polysaccharides (NSP) after the removal of starch. This definition of dietary fiber, which is much narrower than the more recent definitions described above, was used in later editions of the UK food tables. Asp *et al.* (1983) and Prosky *et al.* (1984) published methods that relied on gravimetric analysis (i.e. by weight) of residual undigested carbohydrates, after enzymatic hydrolysis and correction for protein and ash. This approach formed the basis for the Association of Official Analytical Chemists (AOAC) method (Prosky *et al.*, 1988) for total dietary fiber (TDF). Standardized versions of the AOAC method are used in the USA, and have now become widely accepted and officially endorsed for routine use elsewhere (FAO, 2010). Variants of both the NSP and TDF methods also support the analysis of *soluble fiber* as a separate component of the total figure. However, the validity of this distinction is problematic because solubility in water is, without other information, a poor predictor of physiological activity, and it is usually not known whether the fraction defined as soluble fiber *in vitro* is actually solubilized in the gut lumen during digestion of foods. A report on carbohydrates published by FAO/WHO in 1998 suggested that the distinction between insoluble and soluble fiber should be phased out (FAO, 1998), but the terminology is still widely used, both in food tables and research papers.

The essential characteristics of the two principal approaches to dietary fiber analysis are summarized in Figure 8.2. In practice, methods based on gravimetric determination of fiber are faster and less expensive than those requiring analysis of sugars, and so are better suited to commercial applications. The TDF method gives higher analytical values than the NSP method, largely because of the inclusion of resistant starch (Tables 8.2, 8.3, and 8.4).

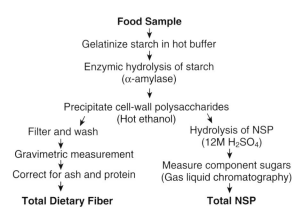

FIG. 8.2 A summary of the essential steps in both the gravimetric (total dietary fiber) and non-starch polysaccharide approaches to dietary fiber analysis.

TABLE 8.2 Values for dietary fiber from some representative foods, measured as NSP and as total dietary fiber

Food source	Non-starch polysaccharide (Englyst method)	Total dietary fiber (AOAC method)
Wholemeal bread	5.0	7.0
Brown bread	3.5	5.0
White bread	2.1	2.9
Green vegetables	2.7	3.3
Fresh fruit	1.4	1.9
Potatoes	1.9	2.4

Data from Food Standards Agency (2002).

TABLE 8.3 Values for dietary fiber from some cereal products, measured as total NSP, insoluble NSP, and soluble NSP

Food source	Non-starch polysaccharides (g/100 g fresh weight)		
	Total NSP	Insoluble NSP	Soluble NSP
Wholemeal bread	4.8	3.2	1.6
Brown bread	3.6	2.5	1.1
White bread	1.5	0.6	0.9
Cornflakes	0.9	0.5	0.4
Crunchy oat cereal	6.0	2.7	3.3

Data from Englyst *et al.* (1989).

TABLE 8.4 Values for dietary fiber from some fruits, vegetables, and nuts, measured as total NSP, insoluble NSP, and soluble NSP

Food source	Non-starch polysaccharides (g/100 g fresh weight)		
	Total NSP	Insoluble NSP	Soluble NSP
Apples	1.7	1.0	0.7
Oranges	2.1	0.7	1.4
Bananas	1.1	0.4	0.7
Tomatoes	1.1	0.7	0.4
Brussels sprouts	4.8	2.3	2.5
Runner beans	2.3	1.4	0.9
Celery	1.3	0.7	0.6
Potatoes	1.1	0.5	0.6
Brazil nuts	4.3	3.0	1.3
Walnuts	3.5	2.0	1.5
Peanuts	6.2	4.3	1.9

Data from Englyst *et al.* (1989).

This is consistent with the broad definitions of dietary fiber now recommended by the Codex Alimentarius Commission and other bodies, but, when reading the physiological or epidemiological literature, it is important to consider how any quoted fiber values have been determined. In any case a single gravimetric measurement of residual carbohydrates of unknown composition cannot predict the physiological effects of any particular food. The NSP method, when combined with a full analysis of carbohydrates by gas liquid chromatography, is more technically demanding and expensive, but gives much more information about the individual polysaccharide components of a food sample, and is therefore more suitable for research on the physiological effects of dietary fiber. Most of the techniques recommended by the Codex Alimentarius Commission for analysis of fiber are AOAC methods for TDF, but the NSP method is also included in recognition of its importance for research purposes (FAO, 2010).

Physiological Effects of Dietary Fiber

During digestion, food is conveyed progressively through the alimentary organs while undergoing a tightly regulated sequence of physical changes and chemical reactions. The presence of intact carbohydrate polymers within the partially digested intraluminal matrix modifies this process at every stage, but the physiological effects of the different constituents of the fiber complex depend upon their physical properties, their chemical interactions with other food components and digestive secretions, and their susceptibility to bacterial fermentation in the large intestine.

Oropharyngeal Effects

The earliest stages of digestion begin with the addition of saliva, which is both a lubricant and a source of salivary amylase, and the mechanical disruption of food during mastication. Raw or lightly processed plant foods usually contain relatively high levels of cell-wall polysaccharides, and often retain much of the three-dimensional cellular structure of the original plant tissue. The presence of intact cell-wall polysaccharides tends to inhibit the physical disruption of food before it reaches the stomach, and thus can inhibit the rate of starch digestion at a very early stage. Hard foods need to be chewed more thoroughly than soft ones, and there is evidence from animal studies that the physical properties of foods consumed during early life influence craniofacial development. It is not clear whether consumption of foods rich in dietary fiber has develop-

mental consequences for human infants, but, at the other end of life, poor dentition among the elderly has been shown to be associated with low intakes of dietary fiber and it has been suggested that this increases the risk of gastrointestinal disease (Moynihan et al., 1994).

Gastric Effects

The transit of food through the digestive tract is delayed in the stomach, where residual food fragments are further degraded by vigorous muscular activity in the presence of hydrochloric acid and proteolytic enzymes. The rate of gastric emptying is partly regulated by particle size, and so the prolonged disruption and dispersion of intractable food particles can delay the digestive process significantly. For example, it has been shown that coarse but not finely dispersed wheat bran slows gastric emptying in humans (Vincent et al., 1995), and the rate at which the starch is digested and absorbed from cubes of cooked potato has been shown to be much slower when they are swallowed whole than when they are chewed normally (Read et al., 1986). Thus simple physical factors can limit the rate at which glucose from carbohydrate foods enters the circulation (Bjorck et al., 1994) but it is important to emphasize that these potentially important effects, though related to the retention of intact cell walls within food, cannot be predicted from single analytical values for dietary fiber.

Small Intestinal Effects

After the physical disruption of food particles and the partial hydrolysis of macromolecules in the stomach, the semi-liquid products of the gastric phase of digestion are released at intervals into the duodenum. Starch, proteins, and triglycerides are further hydrolyzed to oligomers by pancreatic enzymes in the upper jejunal lumen. The final stages of digestion occur at the mucosal surface in the presence of the brush-border hydrolases of the epithelial cells, through which the newly released monosaccharides, fatty acids, peptides, and amino acids, together with water and electrolytes, are absorbed into the circulation. The peristaltic waves of the small intestinal musculature and the rhythmic contractions of the villi ensure that the partially digested chyme is well stirred. In adults, the first residual polysaccharides from a meal containing dietary fiber enter the cecum approximately 4.5 h after ingestion. Soluble polysaccharides, such as guar gum and beta-glucan from oats, have the property of forming extremely viscous solutions in water at low concentrations. Test meals containing such polysaccharides can delay gastric emptying and increase the resistance to peristaltic flow in the small intestine, thereby increasing mouth-to-cecum transit time. On the other hand, coarse insoluble wheat bran, but not finely ground bran, has been reported to accelerate small intestinal transit (Vincent *et al.*, 1995).

The functional significance of dietary fiber in the small intestine lies mainly in its ability to slow the rate of glucose absorption, and thus to modify the metabolic response to a meal. Much of the research to explore the effects of fiber on glucose absorption and metabolism has been done by measuring the glycemic index (GI), either of naturally fiber-rich foods, or of liquid or solid test-meals to which dietary fiber has been added as a supplement. The GI of a food is defined as the incremental area under the blood glucose response curve after consumption of a standardized sample, expressed as a percentage of the response to an equivalent amount of carbohydrate consumed as glucose (Jenkins *et al.*, 1981). Studies on dietary fiber are usually conducted using healthy individuals who have fasted overnight. The technique has undergone a number of methodological refinements in recent years, and it has been shown that, when carefully controlled, the method gives consistent results, which allow foods to be classified according to GI (Wolever *et al.*, 2008). Complex carbohydrates rich in fiber tend to have glycemic indices below 100%, indicating that the rate of glucose absorption is lower than that from pure glucose, but the mechanism of action differs for different types of fiber. In the case of cell walls that remain intact in the small intestine, their presence will impede the access of pancreatic amylase to starch, thus slowing the release of glucose, and often enabling a significant fraction of ingested starch to reach the colon. This is particularly important in the case of certain beans and other leguminous seeds, which have been shown to retain much of their cellular integrity during digestion (Wursch *et al.*, 1986). In general, wheat bran and other insoluble types of fiber have little effect on glucose metabolism when added to test meals of glucose or starch, whereas soluble polysaccharides that form viscous solutions in the stomach and small intestine delay the absorption of glucose (Jenkins and Jenkins, 1985). Their primary mechanism of action appears to be to increase the viscosity of the fluid layer adjacent to the epithelial cells at the mucosal surface. To sustain a high rate of influx, the concentration of glucose and other actively transported substrates must be maintained within the boundary layer, either by convective mixing, or by the much slower process of diffusion. If the physical stirring effects of gut motility are inhibited by a high viscosity, then the effect is to increase the resistance of the boundary layer and slow the overall rate of transport (Johnson and Gee, 1981). A similar mechanism inhibits the uptake of cholesterol (Gee *et al.*, 1983), and probably also the re-absorption of bile salts in the distal ileum.

Apart from the effects of fiber on macronutrient transport and metabolism, there has been much interest in the possibility that both the polysaccharides and complex phenolic components of cell walls interact with and bind ionized substances such as mineral micronutrients in the stomach and small intestinal contents, thereby reducing their availability for absorption (Torre *et al.*, 1991). Intraluminal binding of heavy metals and organic carcinogens might be a valuable protective mechanism against toxicity, but binding of micronutrients could seriously compromise nutritional status. Interactions of this type can be shown to occur *in vitro*, and studies with animals and humans suggest that charged polysaccharides such as pectin can bind inorganic cations in the small intestinal lumen and displace them into the colon under experimental conditions, but there is little objective evidence that dietary fiber *per se* has much of an adverse effect on mineral metabolism in humans. However, phytate (myo-inositol hexaphosphate), which is an organic compound often present in close association with the cell-wall polysaccharides of unprocessed legume seeds, oats, and other cereals, does exert potent binding effects on minerals, and has been shown to significantly reduce the availability of magnesium, zinc, and calcium for absorption in humans (Hurrell *et al.*, 2003). Phytate levels in foods can be reduced by the activity of endogenous phytase enzymes in plant tissue, or by hydrolysis with exogenous phytase enzymes. Such measures may be used to process foods for consumption by populations at risk of mineral deficiency (Troesch *et al.*, 2009).

Metabolic Effects of Dietary Fiber

Long-term supplementation with the viscous polysaccharide guar gum improves control of blood glucose in patients with non-insulin-dependent diabetes mellitus (Groop *et al.*, 1993), and similar effects can be achieved using diets designed to provide a low glycemic index (Jenkins *et al.*, 2008). The glycemic response to carbohydrate ingestion is the major determinant of insulin secretion. Glucose uptake also regulates the release of the incretins, glucagon-like peptide 1 (GLP-1) and gastric inhibitory peptide (GIP), which act to amplify the release of insulin by the pancreatic beta cells, reduce secretion of glucagon by pancreatic alpha cells, and inhibit the motility of the upper gastrointestinal tract. There is evidence that the presence of dietary fiber in foods modulates this system, but neither the mechanisms of action nor the consequences are fully understood. For example, the release of insulin, GLP-1, and GIP has been shown to be lower after ingestion of rye bread than after an equivalent test-meal of white bread, but the effect was apparently attributable to differences in the physical structure of the bread, rather than to the level of dietary fiber (Juntunen *et al.*, 2002). In another study, concerned with soluble dietary fiber, the addition of the viscous polysaccharide beta-glucan from oats to a test-beverage was shown to suppress the absorption of glucose, and to inhibit the release of insulin, cholecystokinin, GLP-1, and peptide YY (PYY). In this example, the importance of the viscosity of the polysaccharide was confirmed by the fact that the effect was abolished by hydrolysis of the beta-glucan, although the total fiber content of the beverage was unchanged (Juvonen *et al.*, 2009).

The distal small intestine is richly endowed with endocrine cells that secrete regulatory peptides including enteroglucagon, GLP-1, and PYY into the circulation in response to intraluminal signals. Soluble, viscous types of dietary fiber can modulate the secretion of these hormones, probably by slowing the absorption of glucose and lipid in the duodenum and thereby increasing their concentrations in the distal intestine, where they can interact with mucosal endocrine cells. In one study, human volunteers consumed varying doses of oat beta-glucan, incorporated into a cereal product. There was evidence of a dose-related increase in plasma PYY levels after meals containing 4–6 g of beta-glucan compared with a control meal (Beck *et al.*, 2009). The significance of such endocrine effects lies in the regulatory role of PYY and other gut peptides in relation to gut motility and appetite. PYY in particular is implicated in the control of food intake in experimental animals but its precise role in humans is unclear (Neary and Batterham, 2009).

Lipid metabolism is also modified by dietary fiber consumption in humans, but again the mechanisms are not well understood. The effects on cholesterol metabolism are of particular interest because of its role in the etiology of coronary heart disease, which is discussed in more detail below. It is well established that soluble polysaccharides, including oat beta-glucan, guar gum, and pectin, exert hypocholesterolemic effects in humans. Brown *et al.*

(1999) undertook a meta-analysis of randomized, controlled intervention trials and concluded that the soluble polysaccharides most commonly used in intervention studies all modified plasma cholesterol levels to a similar though limited extent, amounting in the case of oat beta-glucans to a reduction of about 0.13 mmol/L total cholesterol for every 3 g soluble fiber consumed per day. This is a relatively modest reduction, but one that would be potentially significant for those with total plasma cholesterol levels close to the generally recognized desirable level of 5.2 mmol/L. The most probable mechanism is that the viscosity of these polysaccharides in the distal small intestine inhibits bile-salt reabsorption, thus increasing fecal bile losses. To compensate for this, hepatic bile salt synthesis increases, and draws upon the plasma cholesterol pool. In experimental trials, various types of dietary fiber have been shown also to modify the lipid composition of chylomicrons entering the circulation from the small intestine after fatty test-meals (Cara *et al.*, 1992) but the metabolic significance of these effects in free-living humans consuming mixed diets is not clear.

Colorectal Effects

After their passage through the small intestine, all of the components of dietary fiber enter the proximal colon via the ileocecal valve. In contrast to the upper alimentary tract of healthy human beings, where a number of physiological adaptations ensure that bacterial numbers are kept to a minimum, the colon and rectum are adapted to facilitate colonization by bacteria. Humans do not possess the enlarged cecum typical of herbivores, but the proximal colon does contain around 200 g of bacteria, dietary residues, mucus, and other intestinal secretions, in a semiliquid state that favors fermentation. Estimates differ as to the number of different bacterial species present in the human colon, but it is one of the richest bacterial ecosystems known. The largest single groups present are Gram-negative anaerobes of the genus *Bacteroides*, and Gram-positive organisms including bifidobacteria, eubacteria, lactobacilli, and clostridia. A full understanding of this complexity has been difficult to achieve because a large proportion of the species present cannot be cultured *in vitro* using classical methods, but new genomic techniques are rapidly transforming this situation (Streit and Schmitz, 2004).

The gut microflora and their human host exist in a symbiotic relationship that has evolved over the millennia like any other aspect of human biology. Unlike the endogenous digestive enzymes, which only hydrolyze the alpha linkages of dietary carbohydrates, the gut microflora expresses a diverse array of enzymes capable of degrading most of the components of the plant cell wall. The advantage to the host lies in the ability of the bacteria to break down the residual oligo- and polysaccharides of the dietary fiber complex to the short-chain fatty acids acetate, propionate and butyrate, some of which can be reabsorbed and utilized as a source of metabolic energy. Propionate is metabolized in the liver, whereas acetate enters the circulation and is used as an energy source by various peripheral tissues. The colorectal epithelial cells are adapted to utilize butyrate as their primary source of energy (Roediger, 1980). Although there is no doubt that the human body derives energy from the fermentation of dietary fiber, the precise contribution to total energy needs is difficult to quantify. Dietary energy values are usually calculated using energy conversion factors, applied separately to the protein, fat, and carbohydrate components, and summed to give a total value for the food or diet. The commonly used conversion factor for carbohydrate, based on the empirical work of Atwater (Atwater and Benedict, 1902) is 16.7 kJ/g (4 kcal/g), and assumes that all the carbohydrate is absorbed and metabolized as glucose. If dietary fiber is included in the total carbohydrate content of a food or diet, then the energy content will be overestimated, whereas if it is assumed to contribute zero energy, and is subtracted from total carbohydrates, the energy content will be underestimated (Livesey, 1995). Both non-starch polysaccharides and the various types of resistant starch that occur in foods of plant origin differ significantly in their susceptibility to fermentation, but this is difficult to account for, particularly if only a gravimetric analysis of fiber, with no separate determination of individual polysaccharides, is available. In practice, a figure of 8.4 kJ/g (2.0 kcal/g) is considered a realistic approximation for the energy value of fiber derived from mixed diets (Livesey, 1992) and this figure has been endorsed by the Food and Agriculture Organization of the United Nations (FAO, 2002). It is, however, important to be aware that this is only an approximation, and that the capacity to derive energy from fermentation of carbohydrate differs between individuals, presumably because of differences in the composition of the colonic microflora and the transit time of feces through the colon (Wisker and Feldheim, 1990). A further complication is that high levels of fiber in the diet have been shown to decrease the metabolizable energy available from fat and protein (Baer et al., 1997).

Although most of the bacteria of the human colon exploit carbohydrates, not all can degrade polysaccharides directly, and many are adapted to utilize the initial degradation products of other bacterial species in the community. The amount of fermentable carbohydrates reaching the human colon each day has proven difficult to quantify, but it is clear that it differs considerably between individuals and populations because of the great variation in human diets (Stephen et al., 1995). A minimum quantity of around 20 g can be deduced from estimates of total dietary fiber intake in Western populations consuming mainly refined carbohydrates (Cust et al., 2009). Estimates of resistant-starch intake range up to 30–40 g for the populations of developing countries (Stephen et al., 1995), but these are based largely on the estimation of resistant starch by in vitro techniques. Using an isotope tracer method in human volunteers, Wang et al. (2008) observed that as much as 25% of the starch in some unrefined cereal foods escaped hydrolysis in the small intestine. Thus upper limits in excess of 50 g of fermentable carbohydrate reaching the human colon seem feasible for populations such as those of rural and urban South Africa that consume diets based largely on maize porridge (Ahmed et al., 2000).

Much remains to be discovered about gut bacteria, but, whatever the significance of the gut microflora for the overall metabolic health of human beings turns out to be, there is no doubt of its importance for the proper maintenance of normal bowel function. Nor is there any doubt that the quantity and types of dietary fiber consumed are major determinants of the bulk and the frequency of passage of stool (Stephen et al., 1986). The magnitude of this laxative effect of fiber depends upon the types of polysaccharides consumed. At one extreme are the soluble cell-wall polysaccharides such as pectin, which are readily fermented by bacteria, and at the other are the lignified plant tissues such as wheat bran, which are resistant to bacterial enzymes, and tend to remain at least partially intact in the feces. All components of dietary fiber increase fecal bulk to some extent, but the size of this laxative effect differs markedly between food sources (Table 8.5). The more than five-fold difference in the fecal bulking capacity of wheat bran compared with pectin reflects the fact that, whereas the increment in stool mass caused by wheat bran depends mainly on water retention by the intact bran within the fecal matrix, that caused by fermentable polysaccharides such as pectin is due mainly to increased bacterial cell mass (Stephen and Cummings, 1980). In this as in other physiological effects of fiber, the fecal bulking effect

TABLE 8.5 Mean and range of increased fecal output measured in response to different types of dietary fiber fed to human volunteers

Fiber type or food source	Increase in fecal weight (g/g fiber eaten)
Wheat bran	7.2 (3.0–14.4)
Fruits and vegetables	6.0 (1.4–19.6)
Oats	3.4 (1–5.5)
Legumes	1.5 (0.3–3.1)
Pectin	1.3 (0–3.6)

Data from Elia and Cummings (2007).

of a food cannot, without other information, be predicted from a simple analysis of its total dietary fiber content.

The composition of the residual carbohydrates reaching the colon determines not only the quantity but to some extent also the composition of the bacterial microflora that lives upon it. In health, an individual's gut microflora remains relatively stable over long periods of time. Most types of dietary fiber seem to stimulate a general increase in microbial numbers, with little effect on the relative proportions of different bacterial species present. However, certain oligosaccharides provide a selective stimulus for the growth of species of bifidobacteria, which are thought to be beneficial to health, and this is the basis for the supplementation of diets with galactose or fructose oligosaccharides, or *prebiotics* as they have come to be known (Gibson and Roberfroid, 1995).

Although fermentation tends to reduce the laxative effect of a polysaccharide, the fermentation products do have other very important effects in the colon. Besides providing metabolic energy for the colorectal epithelial cells (Roediger, 1980), butyrate causes differentiation of tumor cells, suppresses cell division, and induces programmed cell death (apoptosis). All of these phenomena have been studied extensively *in vitro*. If the same effects occur in the intact human gut, they may have the beneficial effect of eliminating precancerous cells from the epithelial population (Johnson, 2001), but this remains to be established. The physiological effects of butyrate observed *in vitro* appear to be mediated via the inhibition of the histone deacetylases, a group of enzymes that modify the protein structure of chromosomes and thus regulate gene transcription. These effects are consistent with an anticarcinogenic role for butyrate, but it is not yet clear to what extent they also occur in the intact human intestine.

Although, as mentioned previously, inhibition of nutrient absorption by viscous fiber can initially inhibit the release of GLP-1, butyrate, and acetate derived from fermentation of carbohydrate in the colon can stimulate the release of GLP-1 and PYY by colonic mucosal endocrine cells, and this may provide another mechanism influencing human metabolism. It has been suggested that GLP-1 derived from this source may increase insulin sensitivity in humans, but there is a need for further studies with human subjects to fully evaluate the physiological importance of this mechanism (Freeland and Wolever, 2010). Research continues on the importance of butyrate and other short-chain fatty acids derived from fermentation of dietary fiber for human health.

The other major breakdown products of carbohydrate fermentation are hydrogen, methane, and carbon dioxide, which together comprise flatus gas. Excess gas production may cause distension and pain in some individuals, especially if using supplements such as guar gum (Bianchi and Capurso, 2002), or if they attempt to increase their fiber consumption too abruptly. In many cases, however, extreme flatus is probably caused more by fermentation of oligosaccharides such as stachyose and verbascose, which are found principally in legume seeds, rather than by fermentation of long-chain polysaccharides from the cell wall (Suarez *et al.*, 1999).

Dietary Fiber in the Management and Prevention of Disease

The founders of the dietary fiber hypothesis believed that the populations of Western industrialized societies had become chronically malnourished because of a deficiency of dietary fiber from complex carbohydrate foods, and that the inability of humans to adapt successfully to such a diet accounted for the prevalence of a variety of gastrointestinal and metabolic diseases. As Burkitt put it, "We have so changed our environmental cogs that they no longer engage harmoniously with our genetic constitution which cannot be changed" (Kritchevsky and Bonfield, 1997). This general paradigm of the maladaption of populations in developed societies to many aspects of modern lifestyles continues to evolve and to gain credence among biomedical scientists, but the precise role of dietary fiber in this context remains uncertain. In this section the evidence for the importance of fiber as a determinant of the major types of non-infectious diseases will be briefly reviewed.

Diabetes and the Metabolic Syndrome

Interest in the possibility that a deficiency of fiber might play a role in the etiology of type 2 diabetes began very early in the development of the dietary fiber hypothesis, with the work of Trowell and others (Trowell, 1972a). As we have seen, the rate of delivery of glucose from the gut to the circulation is modified by the presence of intact cell walls, and by certain soluble polysaccharides dispersed in the small intestinal lumen. Epidemiological research published in recent years supports at least some of the early theoretical arguments for the benefits of dietary fiber, and provides strong evidence that the physiological effects revealed under experimental conditions do have important consequences at the population level, even if the mechanisms underlying these effects are unclear. It has become increasingly clear that type 2 diabetes is often preceded by a combination of clinical abnormalities associated with obesity, collectively termed the *metabolic syndrome* (Zimmet *et al.*, 1999), involving impaired glucose tolerance due to insulin resistance, raised plasma LDL cholesterol, raised blood pressure, and signs of increased low-grade systemic inflammation. Remarkably, there is growing evidence that consumption of dietary fiber is associated with protection against all of these abnormalities.

Salmerón and colleagues conducted prospective studies to investigate the relationship between the glycemic index and dietary fiber content of the habitual diets of men (Salmerón *et al.*, 1997a) and women (Salmerón *et al.*, 1997b) and their risk of developing type 2 diabetes during 6 years of follow-up. In both sexes there was an adverse effect of dietary glycemic index and a protective effect of cereal fiber intake. The combined effect of high glycemic index and low intake of cereal fiber more than doubled the risk of disease. More recently, de Munter *et al.* (2007) evaluated the intake of whole grain, bran, and cereal germ in a cohort of 161 737 healthy American women participating in the Nurses' Health Studies I and II, and identified 6486 cases of type 2 diabetes over 12–19 years of follow-up. After adjustment for confounders and for body mass index (BMI), the relative risks for development of type 2 diabetes in the highest consumers of whole grain were 0.75 (95% CI 0.68–0.83) and 0.86 (95% CI 0.72–1.02) in the NHS 1 and 2 cohorts, respectively. The protective effect was similar for cereal bran, but was not significant for cereal germ. Combining these data in a meta-analysis with four other previously published studies, the authors concluded that an increment in whole-grain consumption of two 16 g servings of whole-grain constitu-

ents per day was associated with a 21% (95% CI 13%–28%) decrease in risk of type 2 diabetes. It should be noted of course that "whole grain" contains many constituents other than dietary fiber, and that the correlation with bran intake is consistent with, but does not prove, a direct protective effect of cell-wall polysaccharides.

In a recent prospective study Sluijs and colleagues examined the relationship between carbohydrate consumption and risk of diabetes in 37 846 Dutch members of the European Prospective Investigation of Cancer and Nutrition (EPIC) cohort (Sluijs *et al.*, 2010). The food intake data were used to calculate total carbohydrate, total starch, glycemic index (GI), and glycemic load (the product of carbohydrate intake and average GI). After 10 years of follow-up, 915 cases of type 2 diabetes were identified. Total carbohydrate intake, starch, and glycemic load were all positively correlated with risk of diabetes, but there was an inverse association with total dietary fiber intake (hazard ratio = 0.92; 95% CI: 0.85, 0.99).

Overall, epidemiological data support the concept that diets rich in refined carbohydrate, having a high GI and low content of dietary fiber, carry an increased risk of type 2 diabetes, and conversely that a high intake of fiber is protective. One paradox that remains to be resolved, however, is that whereas it is viscous soluble fiber that attenuates glucose absorption and the insulin response most effectively in acute experimental studies, epidemiological data indicate that habitual consumption of insoluble cereal fiber is most strongly associated with a reduced risk of type 2 diabetes (Schulze *et al.*, 2007). Perhaps, in the context of epidemiological studies, dietary fiber intake merely acts as a surrogate marker for some other protective component or characteristic of the diet. There are, however, experimental data to show that even a short-term intervention with insoluble dietary fiber supplements can improve insulin sensitivity in overweight subjects (Weickert *et al.*, 2006), an effect which, given the nature of the dietary fiber used, seems likely to be independent of any direct effects on glucose absorption in the small intestine.

One interesting possibility is that, at the population level, dietary fiber intake may be acting through a reduction in low-grade systemic inflammation, which is itself a risk factor for type 2 diabetes (Kolb and Mandrup-Poulsen, 2010). Direct evidence for this hypothesis comes from studies on the relationship between fiber consumption and C-reactive protein (CRP) in humans. CRP is a blood-borne protein synthesized in the liver in response to a variety of pathologies ranging from infections to the chronic inflammatory changes associated with abdominal obesity. CRP has a specific functional role in the immune response to infections, and it is widely used as a clinical marker of general inflammatory status. A chronic elevation of CRP is a risk factor for diabetes and cardiovascular disease. Epidemiological studies reveal an inverse relationship between dietary fiber intake and serum CRP levels in the general population. For example, Ajani *et al.* (2004) used data from the National Health and Nutrition Examination Survey 1999–2000 (NHANES) to show that in the USA the odds ratio for having an abnormally high CRP level (>3.0 mg/L) was 0.49 (95% CI 0.37–0.65) for the highest quintile of fiber intake compared with the lowest. In the Finnish Diabetes Prevention Study, Herder *et al.* (2009) showed that of the various aspects of lifestyle investigated, dietary fiber intake and physical activity both independently predicted a reduction in CRP after correction for weight loss. Confidence in a causal relationship between fiber intake and CRP is strengthened by intervention studies with fiber. In a systematic review of the literature, North *et al.* (2009) identified six out of seven intervention trials with fiber, at daily doses of 3.3–7.8 g/MJ energy, in which statistically significantly reductions in CRP concentrations of 25–54% were observed. However, the mechanisms by which dietary fiber modifies systemic inflammation are not known, and at the present time it is difficult to separate them from a relationship between fiber intake and body weight.

Obesity

In general, epidemiological studies tend to support the hypothesis that dietary fiber intake is inversely associated with body-mass index (BMI) in adults, but experimental evidence for a causal relationship remains ambiguous. Population studies have shown that the average daily intake of dietary fiber by individuals with BMI in the normal range is significantly lower than that of overweight and clinically obese subjects (Alfieri *et al.*, 1995; van de Vijver *et al.*, 2009), but this does not necessarily indicate that fiber consumption has any direct influence on body weight gain. The use of prospective studies to explore the issue of causation has been partly successful. Koh-Banerjee *et al.* (2004) studied dietary intake and self-reported weight gain over an 8-year period in 27 082 American men aged 40–75 years. Multivariate analyses indicated a statistically significant inverse association between whole-grain intake and weight gain, such that for every 40-g/day incre-

ment in whole-grain intake, weight gain was 0.49 kg lower. A reduction in weight gain associated independently with the presence of cereal bran in the diet was identified, such that, for every 20 g/day increase in intake, weight gain was reduced by 0.36 kg. The authors therefore concluded that the effects of whole grain on body weight were due both to dietary fiber and to other unidentified constituents of cereal grains. Liu (2003) studied whole-grain and dietary fiber intake in a large cohort of American women enrolled in the Nurses' Health Study and came to similar conclusions. In contrast, a study of a large Danish cohort failed to identify any relationship between weight gain and fiber intake after adjustment for covariates (Iqbal *et al.*, 2006).

Intervention studies designed to test the hypothesis that increased intakes of dietary fiber lead directly to weight loss in humans have produced mixed findings. In a review of published research, Howarth *et al.* (2001) concluded that, in most intervention studies in which energy intakes were maintained constant, an increased intake of either soluble or insoluble fiber led to an increase in postprandial satiety, which would favor weight loss. In studies where energy intake was uncontrolled, an average consumption of an additional 4 g/day fiber was associated with a reduction in energy intake, and a reduction in body weight of 1.9 kg over 3.8 months. Nevertheless, intervention studies with well-defined supplements of soluble dietary fiber, the type which has been shown to exert the most potent effects on gastric emptying and satiety, have not always been successful. Howarth *et al.* (2003) studied the effects of 27-g supplements containing either pectin and beta-glucan, which are soluble, fermentable, non-starch polysaccharides, or methyl cellulose, a soluble but non-fermentable polysaccharide, given to 11 men and women for 3 weeks. They observed no significant effects on energy intake, body weight or body fat. Pittler and Ernst (2001) conducted a meta-analysis of intervention studies with the soluble, viscous, and fermentable polysaccharide guar gum and concluded that, on the basis of the 11 trials identified as suitable for detailed statistical analysis, there was no overall evidence of an effect on weight loss in humans. They noted also that a significant number of unpleasant gastrointestinal side-effects were associated with regular intake of guar gum supplements at the levels used in such studies.

Overall, the epidemiological evidence shows that the consumption of relatively fiber-rich diets in Western countries is associated with lower BMI in adults, but it is unclear whether this can be attributed to any direct effect of dietary fiber on energy intake or metabolism. Dietary fiber, and foods containing high levels of dietary fiber, have a lower energy density and are often bulkier than refined carbohydrate foods. This may tend to promote satiety at relatively low levels of energy intake, so the general concept that a high intake of fiber is associated with greater postprandial satiety seems plausible. However, in view of the complexity of self-selected human diets and the difficulty of correcting for all the variables involved, this general hypothesis is very difficult to test (Elia and Cummings, 2007). At any rate it has proven difficult to consistently demonstrate direct effects of dietary fiber on appetite control in humans under experimental conditions.

Hypertension

Several randomized controlled-intervention trials have explored the hypothesis that supplementation with dietary fiber is an effective means of reducing blood pressure in humans. Two independent meta-analyses have explored this issue and have concluded that dietary fiber supplements are effective as a means of reducing blood pressure in hypertensive and non-hypertensive subjects. Whelton et al. (2005) estimated that, overall, fiber supplementation was associated with a significant reduction of -1.65 mm Hg (95% confidence interval -2.70 to -0.61) in diastolic blood pressure, and a non-significant reduction of -1.15 mm Hg (95% confidence interval -2.68 to 0.39) in systolic blood pressure. Streppel et al. (2005) concluded that an average dose of 11.5 g dietary fiber per day reduced systolic blood pressure by -1.13 mm Hg (95% confidence interval -2.49 to 0.23) and diastolic blood pressure by -1.26 mm Hg (95% confidence interval -2.04 to -0.48). The effects were greater in older hypertensive subjects and in studies with longer duration, but the mechanism of action remains largely unexplored. Although these reductions in blood pressure seem modest, they should be seen in the context of estimates that a reduction of just 2.0 mm Hg in the average systolic blood pressure of the US population would lead to reductions in annual mortality from coronary heart disease and stroke of 4% and 6% respectively (Stamler et al., 1989).

Cardiovascular Disease

The ability of dietary fiber to modify, under experimental conditions, several of the metabolic factors linked to car-

diovascular physiology in humans has encouraged a sustained interest in the possibility that fiber-rich diets may reduce the risk of coronary heart disease (CHD). In most of the large-scale prospective studies that have addressed the issue, good evidence for a protective effect has been obtained. Pereira and colleagues pooled the data from 10 such studies in a systematic analysis (Pereira et al., 2004) that included 91 058 men and 245 186 women, among whom a total of 5249 incident cases of CHD and 2011 deaths occurred during the years of follow-up. In each of the studies analysed, dietary intakes were measured using questionnaires, and intakes of total fiber and fiber from cereals, fruits, and vegetables were estimated. After correction for confounding factors, each 10-g increment in total dietary fiber intake was found to be associated with a 14% reduction in risk of coronary events, and a 27% reduction in risk of death from CHD. Cereal fiber and fruit fiber were protective to similar extents, but there was apparently no protective effect of fiber from vegetables. The findings of this large-scale study of pooled data are generally consistent with those of other smaller studies, including a more recent Japanese cohort (Eshak et al., 2010) in which those in the highest quintiles for consumption of dietary fiber from cereals and fruits were all at lower risk of death from cardiovascular disease compared with those in the lowest quintiles. The protective effects of cereal fiber against death from CHD seem to extend to patients who are already at increased risk of cardiovascular disease because of established type 2 diabetes. In a prospective study of 7822 diabetic women in the USA, identified within the Nurses' Health Study, He et al. (2010) explored the relationship between wholegrain consumption and death from CHD. When participants with the highest versus the lowest quintiles of intakes of whole grain, cereal fiber, bran, and germ were compared, the highest consumers experienced up to 31% lower mortality from all causes. After adjustment for confounders, a statistically significant protective effect of bran intake against both all-cause and CHD mortality was confirmed.

The consistent evidence from cohort studies supporting a protective effect of dietary fiber against CHD is impressive, but when interpreting such data one must remain aware that correlations do not prove causality. Dietary fiber intake is difficult to measure with precision at the population level, intakes may alter over the years of follow-up, and fiber may simply be acting as a marker for other dietary or environmental factors with which it is associated. Statistical corrections for such confounding factors are difficult to achieve, and it is particularly hard to assess whether there are real differences in the effectiveness of fiber from different dietary sources. Ideally a randomized intervention trial should be used to test the hypothesis that dietary fiber protects against CHD, but in practice such experiments are extremely difficult and when attempted they have been inconclusive. One approach to the problem is to measure recurrence of infarction in patients who have already been treated for a cardiac event. An example is the Diet and Reinfarction Trial (DART), in which a group of 2033 men with a history of CHD were randomly allocated to receive either no advice on diet, or advice targeted to dietary intake of fish, dietary lipids or cereal fiber. After 2 years the compliance with advice to consume more cereal fiber was good in that the mean daily intake in those men given advice was 15 g compared with 9 g in those given no advice, but there was no reduction in risk of coronary reinfarction (Burr, 2007). The only conclusion to be drawn is that, assuming that the epidemiology is correct and dietary fiber does indeed protect against CHD, the protective mechanisms probably act over a long period of time and begin well before the pathology has become fully established.

Constipation and Associated Disorders

It is well established that dietary fiber increases fecal frequency and bulk in healthy volunteers, and so it is natural to conclude that it is likely to be of value as a treatment for the symptoms and complications of constipation. According to widely accepted clinical criteria, constipation can be regarded as a pathological condition in patients who regularly experience fewer than three bowel movements per week, where this is coupled with hard stools, a sense of incomplete evacuation or excessive straining (Drossman, 2006). Such patients are usually advised to increase their consumption of dietary fiber, and may be prescribed pharmaceutical preparations based on isphagula husk derived from the seeds of *Plantago psyllium* (Lennard-Jones, 1993), which has been shown to improve symptoms significantly (Fenn *et al.*, 1986). Epidemiological evidence supports the conclusion that a higher intake of dietary fiber from self-selected diets is associated with a reduced incidence of constipation in the general population (Dukas *et al.*, 2003) but the field is in need of further randomized intervention trials to identify the most effective types of fiber and their mechanisms of action.

Diverticular disease is a common condition in which small protrusions called diverticulae bulge through the muscular wall of the colon at sites of penetration by blood vessels. It is much more common in Western populations than in the rural African populations first studied by Burkitt and colleagues, and is strongly associated with increasing age. It was one of the first disorders to be attributed to a chronic deficiency of fiber in the diet (Painter and Burkitt, 1971), and it has long been thought to be caused by the increased intracolonic pressure associated with constipation. There is good epidemiological evidence to support the hypothesis that a high intake of dietary fiber protects against diverticular disease in the male population of the USA (Aldoori *et al.*, 1998), but there appears to be little evidence that increased consumption of dietary fiber is of any value in the management of established disease (Tursi and Papagrigoriadis, 2009).

Irritable Bowel Syndrome

The term "irritable bowel syndrome" (IBS) is applied to a common functional bowel disorder with a variable set of symptoms, the most characteristic of which is abdominal pain in association with changes in bowel habit for which no organic cause can be found. The condition is common in Europe and North America, where the prevalence may be about 10% of the adult population. However, there is some uncertainty about this figure as diagnostic criteria vary between studies and at least half of those who report the recognized symptoms never seek advice from healthcare providers (Hungin *et al.*, 2005). Both the colicky pain of IBS, and the frequent occurrence of constipation, suggest a motility disorder, but there is no convincing evidence that IBS is fiber deficiency disease, and the causes of the condition are unknown. Nevertheless, many general practitioners/family physicians give dietary advice for the management of the condition, and increased consumption of dietary fiber from high-fiber foods or from supplements is frequently prescribed although the clinical basis for this is not well established.

Various types of dietary fiber have been used in the management of IBS but the most common have been wheat bran, which, as we have seen, is insoluble and poorly fermentable, but with good laxative properties, and ispaghula, which is largely soluble, and partially fermentable. Ispaghula, though commonly used as a bulk laxative in hospital settings and as an ingredient of functional foods, is of course not found in traditional diets. In a systematic review Bijkerk *et al.* (2004) analyzed 17 randomized controlled trials and concluded that there was evidence for a statistically significant beneficial effect of dietary fiber on the global symptoms of IBS, particularly in patients with constipation, but no evidence for relief from pain. The beneficial effects were confined to soluble fiber. Wheat bran had no significant beneficial effects, and in some studies was found to worsen symptoms slightly, an effect that has been noted before (Lewis and Whorwell, 1998). In a more recent analysis of placebo-controlled intervention trials, Ford *et al.* (2008) concluded that ispaghula was significantly more effective than placebo, whereas wheat bran was not. These conclusions have now been confirmed in a further randomized placebo-controlled trial (Bijkerk *et al.*, 2009).

Cancers of the Alimentary Tract and Other Sites

The mechanism for the supposedly protective effects of dietary fiber against colorectal cancer proposed by Burkitt was a largely mechanical one, based on the laxative properties of undigested polysaccharides. Burkitt observed that the normal bowel habit of rural Africans consuming traditional diets was very different from that observed in the United Kingdom and other industrialized countries. He proposed that the normal bowel habit for human beings was frequent passage of soft bulky stools, and that Western dietary patterns led to chronic constipation and hence prolonged exposure of the colon to carcinogens in the faecal stream. As we have seen, high intakes of dietary fiber do lead to bulkier stools and more frequent defecation. An influential paper by Cummings and colleagues (Cummings *et al.*, 1992) provided evidence for an inverse relationship between fecal weight and the incidence of colorectal cancer across many population groups, but we cannot be certain that these correlations reflect a causal mechanism.

Much has been learned about the etiology of colorectal cancer in the years since the development of the fiber hypothesis. The disease is now known to result from multiple mutations and long-term modifications of gene expression in developing colorectal epithelial cells, leading to the progressive disruption of normal cellular proliferation and differentiation. These changes occur over decades and are thought to be caused partly by mutagens in the fecal stream, coupled with metabolic risk factors related to obesity, insulin sensitivity, and physical activity (Johnson and Lund, 2007). Thus, apart from the bulking and laxative effects of fiber, it may exert protective effects by reducing the risk of obesity, insulin resistance, and other aspects of the metabolic syndrome. Another possibility is that the supply of butyrate in the fecal stream, which, as mentioned previously, regulates the proliferation, differentiation, and apoptosis of colorectal epithelial cells, may be sub-optimal in Western diets because they lack sufficient fermentable carbohydrate to support the production of butyrate in sufficient quantities to maintain epithelial homeostasis (Scharlau *et al.*, 2009).

It is something of a paradox that although our understanding of the potential mechanisms by which fiber may reduce the risk of colorectal cancer has deepened in the years since the hypothesis was formulated, the epidemiological evidence to support the hypothesis has weakened. For example, in a large prospective study of 88 757 middle-aged North American women, Fuchs *et al.* (1999) observed no protective effects of fiber. Similarly, Pietinen *et al.* (1999) and Terry *et al.* (2001) failed to detect any protective effect of fiber intake in prospective trials with Finnish men and Swedish women, respectively. In contrast, the results of the very large European Prospective Investigation of Cancer and Nutrition (EPIC) project have been much more positive. EPIC was designed to overcome the limitations of prospective studies conducted with relatively small population groups consuming similar diets. The cohort of 519 978 individuals was drawn from several geographically and culturally distinct European countries, and so encompassed a very broad range of fiber intakes from varying sources. Bingham *et al.* (2003) estimated that the relative risk of colorectal cancer for the highest quintile of fiber intake (mean 35 g/day) versus the lowest (mean 15 g/day) was 0.58 (95% CI 0.41–0.85). In a subsequent analysis based on an increased number of cases, these results were confirmed (Bingham, 2006). The authors concluded that in the EPIC cohort there was a significant reduction in colorectal cancer of approximately 9% for each quintile increase in fiber (p < 0.001), and the possibility that the protective effects might have been due to the confounding effects of folate intake from plant foods was tested and eliminated (Bingham, 2006). The EPIC study also provided evidence that the increased risk of colorectal cancer associated with red-meat consumption was substantially reduced in subjects who also consumed relatively large amounts of dietary fiber, though no mechanism for this interactive effect was identified.

Systematic reviews, in which the results of large cohort studies are pooled in order to maximize the numbers of subjects studied, substantially increase the statistical power of the overall analysis. Park *et al.* (2005) pooled 13 cohort studies to give a total of 725 628 participants and 8081 cases, although the analysis did not include the EPIC study. The analysis revealed a statistically significant reduction in risk of 16% when the highest quintile of fiber consumption was compared with the lowest, but this difference was reduced to only 6%, and ceased to be statistically significant, when the data were adjusted for a range of other risk factors. There was no overall evidence of a dose–response relationship, although the 11% of the total population who consumed less than 10 g of fiber per day were found to be at significantly greater risk than the remaining population. The most recent systematic review of dietary fiber and colorectal cancer was that of the World Cancer Research Fund in 2007 (World Cancer Research Fund/American Institute for Cancer Research, 2007) based on a formal meta-analysis of eight studies including EPIC. The results did indicate a dose-dependent protective effect, with a reduction in risk of about 10% for each increment in fiber intake of 10 g per day. The overall judgment of the panel was that foods containing dietary fiber "probably protect against colon cancer," though confounding effects due to other risk factors could not be entirely excluded.

Colorectal cancer develops from adenomatous polyps, which are relatively common precancerous lesions of the colorectal mucosa. Removal of small precancerous polyps at endoscopy is a routine preventative measure, and there have been a number of intervention trials in which supplementation with dietary fiber of various types has been given after polypectomy, with the aim of reducing the risk of polyp recurrence. None of these studies has produced unequivocal evidence for a protective effect of fiber supplementation, although there is some evidence that men may benefit more than women, and that this may have masked a small protective effect in some studies (Jacobs et al., 2006). It is also arguable that, being focused on middle-aged individuals with an already established vulnerability to colorectal cancer, such studies only address a narrow window of time, late in the adenoma–carcinoma sequence, and that they do not rule out a greater protective effect of high dietary fiber consumption extending over a lifetime.

Adverse Effects of Dietary Fiber

There are few well authenticated adverse effects of dietary fiber in humans. Although it is often stated that increased intakes of dietary fiber may lead to abdominal discomfort or flatulence, the effect appears to be mild and short-lived in most individuals. Well-controlled studies with fermentable fructose polysaccharides (Bruhwyler et al., 2008) or resistant maltodextrins (Storey et al., 2007) have suggested that only relatively mild symptoms are reported by healthy volunteers. The possible adverse effects of high-fiber diets on mineral status have been mentioned previously, but are thought to be almost entirely due to phytate, rather than to the polysaccharides with which it is closely associated in some foods. There are occasional reports of intestinal obstruction due to abnormally high intakes of wheat bran; these are usually associated with pre-existing intestinal abnormalities, but occasional reports suggest it is possible to consume enough bran to cause obstruction in an otherwise normal intestine (Harries et al., 1998). Oesophageal obstruction due to consumption of other types of dietary fiber, such as guar gum marketed in the form of "weight-loss pills" is also occasionally reported (Seidner et al., 1990).

One interesting argument against the widening of the definition of dietary fiber to include rapidly fermented polysaccharides and oligosaccharides has been advanced by Goodlad and Englyst, who have suggested that although the supply of butyrate from slowly fermented cell-wall polysaccharides may be beneficial, a very high production of butyrate from rapidly fermented substrates might enhance mucosal cell proliferation in the colon to an extent that could promote rather than inhibit the development of cancer (Goodlad and Englyst, 2001). This argument is supported to some extent by studies with experimental animals, but there is no evidence that fermentable carbohydrate poses such a threat to humans.

Future Directions

Leaving aside the many problems of definition and measurement, the essential idea shared by all the founders of the dietary fiber hypothesis was that the quantity of fiber consumed by the populations of prosperous industrialized societies was much too low. It is a striking fact that, after four decades of research, debate, publicity, and campaigning by public health bodies, much the same can be said today. In 2002, the US National Academy of Sciences Institute of Medicine published Dietary Reference Intakes (Institute of Medicine, 2002) for total dietary fiber in the

USA. The *adequate intake* (AI) for healthy individuals older than 12 months was estimated to be 14 g/1000 kcal/day, which equates to about 38 g/day for an adult man in mid-life and 25 g/day for a woman. In contrast, the actual average intake of dietary fiber was estimated to be 15 g/day for American adults. In the United Kingdom the recommended intake of dietary fiber (defined as NSP) set by the Department of Health is 18 g/day (DoH, 1991), which is equivalent to about 24 g of fiber measured by the AOAC method. In contrast, according to the National Diet and Nutrition Survey, in 2003 the estimated daily intake of fiber by adults was only 15.2 g/day for men and 12.6 g/day for women (Henderson *et al.*, 2003). Higher average intakes of dietary fiber intake do occur in some European countries, but across most of the industrialized world there is a general tendency for fiber intakes to fall significantly below recommended levels (Buttriss and Stokes, 2008). It is probably inevitable that Western diets rich in manufactured foods, dairy products, and meat, will tend to be low in fiber from fruits, vegetables, and lightly processed cereal foods. To achieve the recommended levels of fiber intake, consumers will need to rely on fiber-enriched manufactured foods or on supplements of various kinds. According to the Codex Alimentarius recommendations, a product qualifies as a source of fiber if it contains 3 g/100 g, and it can be described as high in fiber if it contains 6 g/100 g or more (FAO, 2010). The creation of palatable food products that meet or exceed these criteria is something of a challenge, and food technologists will increasingly make use of novel carbohydrate polymers. However, the requirement to go beyond the simple analytical value for fiber, and demonstrate that such novel carbohydrate polymers "have physiological effect of benefit to health", as the Codex Alimentarius definition of dietary fiber requires, poses an even greater challenge. The growing evidence from epidemiological studies showing that a high fiber intake is associated with a reduced risk of several components of the metabolic syndrome is particularly relevant in an industrialized world where obesity and its co-morbidities are of growing concern. There is therefore a continuing need for experimental studies to explore in greater detail the physiological mechanisms whereby dietary fiber interacts with human metabolism beyond the alimentary tract, and to determine which of the many novel components of dietary fiber now available in the human food chain are of most benefit to human health.

Suggestions for Further Reading

Asp, N.G., van Amelsvoort, J.M.M., and Hautvast, J.G.A.J. (1996) Nutritional implications of resistant starch. *Nutr Res Rev* **9**, 1–31.

Elia, M. and Cummings, J.H. (2007) Physiological aspects of energy metabolism and gastrointestinal effects of carbohydrates. *Eur J Clin Nutr* **61** (Suppl 1), S40–S74.

McCleary, B.V. and Prosky, L. (2001) *Advanced Dietary Fiber Technology*. Blackwell Science, Oxford.

Selvendran, R.R. (1984) The plant cell wall as a source of dietary fiber: chemistry and structure. *Am J Clin Nutr* **39**, 320–337.

Spiller, G.A. (2001) (ed.) *CRC Handbook of Dietary Fiber in Human Nutrition*, 3rd edition. CRC Press, Boca Raton, FL.

References

Ahmed, R., Segal, I., and Hassan, H. (2000) Fermentation of dietary starch in humans. *Am J Gastroenterol* **95**, 1017–1020.

Ajani, U.A., Ford, E.S., and Mokdad, A.H. (2004) Dietary fiber and C-reactive protein: findings from national health and nutrition examination survey data. *J Nutr* **134**, 1181–1185.

Aldoori, W.H., Giovannucci, E.L., Rockett, H.R., *et al.* (1998) A prospective study of dietary fiber types and symptomatic diverticular disease in men. *J Nutr* **128**, 714–719.

Alfieri, M.A., Pomerleau, J., Grace, D.M., *et al.* (1995) Fiber intake of normal weight, moderately obese and severely obese subjects. *Obes Res* **3**, 541–547.

Asp, N.G. (1987) Dietary fibre – definition, chemistry and analytical determination. *Mol Aspects Med* **9**, 17–29.

Asp, N.G., Johansson, C.G., Hallmer, H., *et al.* (1983) Rapid enzymatic assay of insoluble and soluble dietary fiber. *J Agric Food Chem* **31**, 476–482.

Asp, N.G., van Amelsvoort, J.M., and Hautvast, J.G. (1996) Nutritional implications of resistant starch. *Nutr Res Rev* **9**, 1–31.

Atwater, W.O. and Benedict, F.G. (1902) Experiments on the metabolism of matter and energy in the human body, 1898–1900. *US Office of Experiment Stations Bulletin* No. 109, Government Printing Office, Washington, DC.

Baer, D.J., Rumpler, W.V., Miles, C.W., *et al.* (1997) Dietary fiber decreases the metabolizable energy content and nutrient digestibility of mixed diets fed to humans. *J Nutr* **127**, 579–586.

Beck, E.J., Tosh, S.M., Batterham, M.J., et al. (2009) Oat beta-glucan increases postprandial cholecystokinin levels, decreases insulin response and extends subjective satiety in overweight subjects. Mol Nutr Food Res 53, 1343–1351.

Bianchi, M. and Capurso, L. (2002) Effects of guar gum, ispaghula and microcrystalline cellulose on abdominal symptoms, gastric emptying, orocaecal transit time and gas production in healthy volunteers. Dig Liver Dis 34 Suppl 2, S129–133.

Bijkerk, C.J., de Wit, N.J., Muris, J.W., et al. (2009) Soluble or insoluble fibre in irritable bowel syndrome in primary care? Randomised placebo controlled trial. BMJ 339, b3154.

Bijkerk, C.J., Muris, J.W., Knottnerus, J.A., et al. (2004) Systematic review: the role of different types of fibre in the treatment of irritable bowel syndrome. Aliment Pharmacol Ther 19, 245–251.

Bingham, S. (2006) The fibre–folate debate in colo-rectal cancer. Proc Nutr Soc 65, 19–23.

Bingham, S.A., Day, N.E., Luben, R., et al. (2003) Dietary fibre in food and protection against colorectal cancer in the European Prospective Investigation into Cancer and Nutrition (EPIC): an observational study. Lancet 361, 1496–1501.

Bjorck, I., Granfeldt, Y., Liljeberg, H., et al. (1994) Food properties affecting the digestion and absorption of carbohydrates. Am J Clin Nutr 59, 699S–705S.

Brown, L., Rosner, B., Willett, W.W., et al. (1999) Cholesterol-lowering effects of dietary fiber: a meta-analysis. Am J Clin Nutr 69, 30–42.

Bruhwyler, J., Carreer, F., Demanet, E., et al. (2008) Digestive tolerance of inulin-type fructans: a double-blind, placebo-controlled, cross-over, dose-ranging, randomized study in healthy volunteers. Int J Food Sci Nutr 1–11. PMID18608562.

Burkitt, D.P. and Trowell, H.C. (1975) Refined Carbohydrate Foods: Some Implications of Dietary Fibre. Academic Press, London.

Burr, M.L. (2007) Secondary prevention of CHD in UK men: the Diet and Reinfarction Trial and its sequel. Proc Nutr Soc 66, 9–15.

Buttriss, J.L. and Stokes, C.S. (2008) Dietary fibre and health: an overview. Nutr Bull 33, 186–200.

Cara, L., Dubois, C., Borel, P., et al. (1992) Effects of oat bran, rice bran, wheat fiber, and wheat germ on postprandial lipemia in healthy adults. Am J Clin Nutr 55, 81–88.

Cleave, T.L. (1974) The saccharine disease. Nurs Times 70, 1274–1275.

Cummings, J.H., Bingham, S.A., Heaton, K.W., et al. (1992) Fecal weight, colon cancer risk, and dietary intake of nonstarch polysaccharides (dietary fiber). Gastroenterology 103, 1783–1789.

Cust, A.E., Skilton, M.R., van Bakel, M.M., et al. (2009) Total dietary carbohydrate, sugar, starch and fibre intakes in the European Prospective Investigation into Cancer and Nutrition. Eur J Clin Nutr 63 Suppl 4, S37–60.

de Munter, J.S., Hu, F.B., Spiegelman, D., et al. (2007) Whole grain, bran, and germ intake and risk of type 2 diabetes: a prospective cohort study and systematic review. PLoS Med 4, e261.

Department of Health (1991) Dietary Reference Values for Food Energy and Nutrients for the United Kingdom. Reports on Public Health and Medical Subjects, No. 41. HMSO, London.

Drossman, D.A. (2006) The functional gastrointestinal disorders and the Rome III process. Gastroenterology 130, 1377–1390.

Dukas, L., Willett, W.C., and Giovannucci, E.L. (2003) Association between physical activity, fiber intake, and other lifestyle variables and constipation in a study of women. Am J Gastroenterol 98, 1790–1796.

Elia, M. and Cummings, J.H. (2007) Physiological aspects of energy metabolism and gastrointestinal effects of carbohydrates. Eur J Clin Nutr 61 Suppl 1, S40–74.

Englyst, H., Wiggins, H.S., and Cummings, J.H. (1982) Determination of the non-starch polysaccharides in plant foods by gas-liquid chromatography of constituent sugars as alditol acetates. Analyst 107, 307–318.

Englyst, H.N. and Cummings, J.H. (1988) Improved method for measurement of dietary fiber as non-starch polysaccharides in plant foods. J Assoc Off Anal Chem 71, 808–814.

Englyst, H.N., Bingham, S.A., Runswick, S.S., et al. (1989) Dietary fiber (non-starch polysaccharides) in cereal products. J Hum Nutr Diet 2, 253–271.

Englyst, K.N., Liu, S., and Englyst, H.N. (2007) Nutritional characterization and measurement of dietary carbohydrates. Eur J Clin Nutr 61 Suppl 1, S19–39.

Eshak, E.S., Iso, H., Date, C., et al. (2010) Dietary fiber intake is associated with reduced risk of mortality from cardiovascular disease among Japanese men and women. J Nutr 140, 1445–1453.

European Food Safety Agency (2007) Statement of the Scientific Panel on Dietetic Products, Nutrition and Allergies on a Request from the Commission Related to Dietary Fibre (Request No. EFSA-Q-2007-121). EFSA, Parma.

Fenn, G.C., Wilkinson, P.D., Lee, C.E., et al. (1986) A general practice study of the efficacy of Regulan in functional constipation. Br J Clin Pract 40, 192–197.

Flamm, G., Glinsmann, W., Kritchevsky, D., et al. (2001) Inulin and oligofructose as dietary fiber: a review of the evidence. Crit Rev Food Sci Nutr 41, 353–362.

Food and Agriculture Organization of the United Nations (1998) Carbohydrates in Human Nutrition. (FAO Food and Nutrition Paper 66). Report of a Joint FAO/WHO Expert Consultation, Rome, April 14–18, 1997. FAO, Rome.

Food and Agriculture Organization of the United Nations (2003) *Food Energy – Methods of Analysis and Conversion Factors* (FAO Food and Nutrition Paper 77). Report of a Technical Workshop, Rome, December 3–6, 2002. FAO, Rome.

Food and Agriculture Organization of the United Nations/World Health Organization Food Standards Programme Codex Committee on Methods of Analysis and Sampling (2010) Thirty-first Session, Budapest, Hungary, March 8–12, 2010. Agenda Item 5. CX/MAS 10/31/5. *Endorsement of Methods of Analysis Provisions in Codex Standards 1.* FAO, Rome.

Food Standards Agency (2002) *McCance and Widdowson's The Composition of Foods*, 6th Edn. Cambridge, Royal Society of Chemistry.

Ford, A.C., Talley, N.J., Spiegel, B.M., et al. (2008) Effect of fibre, antispasmodics, and peppermint oil in the treatment of irritable bowel syndrome: systematic review and meta-analysis. *BMJ* **337**, a2313.

Freeland, K.R. and Wolever, T.M. (2010) Acute effects of intravenous and rectal acetate on glucagon-like peptide-1, peptide YY, ghrelin, adiponectin and tumour necrosis factor-alpha. *Br J Nutr* **103**, 460–466.

Fuchs, C.S., Giovannucci, E.L., Colditz, G.A., et al. (1999) Dietary fiber and the risk of colorectal cancer and adenoma in women. *N Engl J Med* **340**, 169–176.

Gee, J.M., Blackburn, N.A., and Johnson, I.T. (1983) The influence of guar gum on intestinal cholesterol transport in the rat. *Br J Nutr* **50**, 215–224.

Gibson, G.R. and Roberfroid, M.B. (1995) Dietary modulation of the human colonic microbiota: introducing the concept of prebiotics. *J Nutr* **125**, 1401–1412.

Goering, H.K. and Van Soest, P.J. (1970) Forage fiber analyses (apparatus, reagents, procedures, and some applications). ARS/USDA Handbook No. 379, Superintendent of Documents, US Government Printing Office, Washington, DC.

Goodlad, R.A. and Englyst, H.N. (2001) Redefining dietary fibre: potentially a recipe for disaster. *Lancet* **358**, 1833–1834.

Groop, P.H., Aro, A., Stenman, S., et al. (1993) Long-term effects of guar gum in subjects with non-insulin-dependent diabetes mellitus. *Am J Clin Nutr* **58**, 513–518.

Harries, K., Edwards, D., and Shute, K. (1998) Hazards of a "healthy" diet. *Ann R Coll Surg Engl* **80**, 72.

He, M., van Dam, R.M., Rimm, E., et al. (2010) Whole-grain, cereal fiber, bran, and germ intake and the risks of all-cause and cardiovascular disease-specific mortality among women with type 2 diabetes mellitus. *Circulation* **121**, 2162–2168.

Henderson, L., Gregory, J., K., Irving, K., et al. (2003), *The National Diet and Nutrition Survey: Adults Aged 19 to 64 Years: Vol. 2: Energy, Protein, Carbohydrate, Fat and Alcohol Intake.* TSO, London.

Herder, C., Peltonen, M., Koenig, W., et al. (2009) Anti-inflammatory effect of lifestyle changes in the Finnish Diabetes Prevention Study. *Diabetologia* **52**, 433–442.

Hipsley, E.H. (1953) Dietary "fibre" and pregnancy toxaemia. *Br Med J* **2**, 420–422.

Howarth, N.C., Saltzman, E., McCrory, M.A., et al. (2003) Fermentable and nonfermentable fiber supplements did not alter hunger, satiety or body weight in a pilot study of men and women consuming self-selected diets. *J Nutr* **133**, 3141–3144.

Howarth, N.C., Saltzman, E., and Roberts, S.B. (2001) Dietary fiber and weight regulation. *Nutr Rev* **59**, 129–139.

Hungin, A.P., Chang, L., Locke, G.R., et al. (2005) Irritable bowel syndrome in the United States: prevalence, symptom patterns and impact. *Aliment Pharmacol Ther* **21**, 1365–1375.

Hurrell, R.F., Reddy, M.B., Juillerat, M.A., et al. (2003) Degradation of phytic acid in cereal porridges improves iron absorption by human subjects. *Am J Clin Nutr* **77**, 1213–1219.

Institute of Medicine (2002) *Dietary Reference Intakes for Energy, Carbohydrate, Fiber, Fat, Fatty Acids, Cholesterol, Protein, and Amino Acids.* National Academies Press, Washington, DC.

Institute of Medicine (2005) *Dietary Reference Intakes for Energy, Carbohydrate, Fiber, Fat, Fatty Acids, Cholesterol, Protein, and Amino Acids (Macronutrients).* National Academies Press, Washington, DC.

Iqbal, S.I., Helge, J.W., and Heitmann, B.L. (2006) Do energy density and dietary fiber influence subsequent 5-year weight changes in adult men and women? *Obesity (Silver Spring)* **14**, 106–114.

Jacobs, E.T., Lanza, E., Alberts, D.S., et al. (2006) Fiber, sex, and colorectal adenoma: results of a pooled analysis. *Am J Clin Nutr* **83**, 343–349.

Jenkins, D.J. and Jenkins, A.L. (1985) Dietary fiber and the glycemic response. *Proc Soc Exp Biol Med* **180**, 422–431.

Jenkins, D.J., Kendall, C.W., McKeown-Eyssen, G., et al. (2008) Effect of a low-glycemic index or a high-cereal fiber diet on type 2 diabetes: a randomized trial. *JAMA* **300**, 2742–2753.

Jenkins, D.J., Wolever, T.M., Taylor, R.H., et al. (1981) Glycemic index of foods: a physiological basis for carbohydrate exchange. *Am J Clin Nutr* **34**, 362–366.

Johnson, I.T. (2001) Mechanisms and anticarcinogenic effects of diet-related apoptosis in the intestinal mucosa. *Nutr Res Rev* **14**, 229–256.

Johnson, I.T. and Gee, J.M. (1981) Effect of gel-forming gums on the intestinal unstirred layer and sugar transport in vitro. *Gut* **22**, 398–403.

Johnson, I.T. and Lund, E.K. (2007) Review article: nutrition, obesity and colorectal cancer. *Aliment Pharmacol Ther* **26**, 161–181.

Juntunen, K.S., Niskanen, L.K., Liukkonen, K.H., *et al.* (2002) Postprandial glucose, insulin, and incretin responses to grain products in healthy subjects. *Am J Clin Nutr* **75**, 254–262.

Juvonen, K.R., Purhonen, A.K., Salmenkallio-Marttila, M., *et al.* (2009) Viscosity of oat bran-enriched beverages influences gastrointestinal hormonal responses in healthy humans. *J Nutr* **139**, 461–466.

Koh-Banerjee, P., Franz, M., Sampson, L., *et al.* (2004) Changes in whole-grain, bran, and cereal fiber consumption in relation to 8-y weight gain among men. *Am J Clin Nutr* **80**, 1237–1245.

Kolb, H. and Mandrup-Poulsen, T. (2010) The global diabetes epidemic as a consequence of lifestyle-induced low-grade inflammation. *Diabetologia* **53**, 10–20.

Kritchevsky, D. and Bonfield, C. (1997) (eds) *Dietary Fibre in Health and Disease.* Plenum Publishing, New York.

Lennard-Jones, J.E. (1993) Clinical management of constipation. *Pharmacology* **47** Suppl 1, 216–223.

Lewis, M.J. and Whorwell, P.J. (1998) Bran: may irritate irritable bowel. *Nutrition* **14**, 470–471.

Liu, S. (2003) Whole-grain foods, dietary fiber, and type 2 diabetes: searching for a kernel of truth. *Am J Clin Nutr* **77**, 527–529.

Livesey, G. (1992) The energy values of dietary fibre and sugar alcohols for man. *Nutr Res Rev* **5**, 61–84.

Livesey, G. (1995) Metabolizable energy of macronutrients. *Am J Clin Nutr* **62**, 1135S–1142S.

McCance, R.A. and Lawrence, R.D. (1929) The carbohydrate content of foods. Special Report No. 135. Medical Research Council, London.

Moynihan, P.J., Snow, S., Jepson, N.J., *et al.* (1994) Intake of non-starch polysaccharide (dietary fibre) in edentulous and dentate persons: an observational study. *Br Dent J* **177**, 243–247.

Neary, M.T. and Batterham, R.L. (2009) Peptide YY: food for thought. *Physiol Behav* **97**, 616–619.

North, C.J., Venter, C.S., and Jerling, J.C. (2009) The effects of dietary fibre on C-reactive protein, an inflammation marker predicting cardiovascular disease. *Eur J Clin Nutr* **63**, 921–933.

Painter, N.S. and Burkitt, D.P. (1971) Diverticular disease of the colon: a deficiency disease of Western civilization. *Br Med J* **2**, 450–454.

Park, Y., Hunter, D.J., Spiegelman, D., *et al.* (2005) Dietary fiber intake and risk of colorectal cancer: a pooled analysis of prospective cohort studies. *JAMA* **294**, 2849–2857.

Paul, A.A. and Southgate, D.A.T. (1978) (eds) *McCance and Widdowson's The Composition of Foods.* HMSO, London.

Pereira, M.A., O'Reilly, E., Augustsson, K., *et al.* (2004) Dietary fiber and risk of coronary heart disease: a pooled analysis of cohort studies. *Arch Intern Med* **164**, 370–376.

Pietinen, P., Malila, N., Virtanen, M., *et al.* (1999) Diet and risk of colorectal cancer in a cohort of Finnish men. *Cancer Causes Control* **10**, 387–396.

Pittler, M.H. and Ernst, E. (2001) Guar gum for body weight reduction: meta-analysis of randomized trials. *Am J Med* **110**, 724–730.

Prosky, L., Asp, N.G., Furda, I., *et al.* (1984) Determination of total dietary fiber in foods, food products and total diets: interlaboratory study. *J Assoc Off Anal Chem* **67**, 1044–1052.

Prosky, L., Asp, N.G., Schweizer, T.F., *et al.* (1988) Determination of insoluble, soluble, and total dietary fiber in foods and food products: interlaboratory study. *J Assoc Off Anal Chem* **71**, 1017–1023.

Read, N.W., Welch, I.M., Austen, C.J., *et al.* (1986) Swallowing food without chewing; a simple way to reduce postprandial glycaemia. *Br J Nutr* **55**, 43–47.

Roediger, W.E. (1980) Role of anaerobic bacteria in the metabolic welfare of the colonic mucosa in man. *Gut* **21**, 793–798.

Salmerón, J., Ascherio, A., Rimm, E.B., *et al.* (1997a) Dietary fiber, glycemic load, and risk of NIDDM in men. *Diabetes Care* **20**, 545–550.

Salmerón, J., Manson, J.E., Stampfer, M.J., *et al.* (1997b) Dietary fiber, glycemic load, and risk of non-insulin-dependent diabetes mellitus in women. *JAMA* **277**, 472–477.

Scharlau, D., Borowicki, A., Habermann, N., *et al.* (2009) Mechanisms of primary cancer prevention by butyrate and other products formed during gut flora-mediated fermentation of dietary fibre. *Mutat Res* **682**, 39–53.

Schulze, M.B., Schulz, M., Heidemann, C., *et al.* (2007) Fiber and magnesium intake and incidence of type 2 diabetes: a prospective study and meta-analysis. *Arch Intern Med* **167**, 956–965.

Seidner, D.L., Roberts, I.M., and Smith, M.S. (1990) Esophageal obstruction after ingestion of a fiber-containing diet pill. *Gastroenterology* **99**, 1820–1822.

Sluijs, I., van der Schouw, Y.T., van der A, D.L., *et al.* (2010) Carbohydrate quantity and quality and risk of type 2 diabetes in the European Prospective Investigation into Cancer and Nutrition-Netherlands (EPIC-NL) study. *Am J Clin Nutr* **92**, 905–911.

Southgate, D.A. (1969) Determination of carbohydrates in foods. II. Unavailable carbohydrates. *J Sci Food Agric* **20**, 331–335.

Stamler, J., Rose, G., Stamler, R., *et al.* (1989) INTERSALT study findings. Public health and medical care implications. *Hypertension* **14**, 570–577.

Stephen, A.M. and Cummings, J.H. (1980) Mechanism of action of dietary fibre in the human colon. *Nature* **284**, 283–284.

Stephen, A.M., Sieber, G.M., Gerster, Y.A., *et al.* (1995) Intake of carbohydrate and its components – international comparisons, trends over time, and effects of changing to low-fat diets. *Am J Clin Nutr* **62,** 851S–867S.

Stephen, A.M., Wiggins, H.S., Englyst, H.N., *et al.* (1986) The effect of age, sex and level of intake of dietary fibre from wheat on large-bowel function in thirty healthy subjects. *Br J Nutr* **56,** 349–361.

Storey, D., Lee, A., Bornet, F., *et al.* (2007) Gastrointestinal responses following acute and medium term intake of retrograded resistant maltodextrins, classified as type 3 resistant starch. *Eur J Clin Nutr* **61,** 1262–1270.

Streit, W.R. and Schmitz, R.A. (2004) Metagenomics – the key to the uncultured microbes. *Curr Opin Microbiol* **7,** 492–498.

Streppel, M.T., Arends, L.R., van 't Veer, P., *et al.* (2005) Dietary fiber and blood pressure: a meta-analysis of randomized placebo-controlled trials. *Arch Intern Med* **165,** 150–156.

Suarez, F.L., Springfield, J., Furne, J.K., *et al.* (1999) Gas production in human ingesting a soybean flour derived from beans naturally low in oligosaccharides. *Am J Clin Nutr* **69,** 135–139.

Terry, P., Giovannucci, E., Michels, K.B., *et al.* (2001) Fruit, vegetables, dietary fiber, and risk of colorectal cancer. *J Natl Cancer Inst* **93,** 525–533.

Torre, M., Rodriguez, A.R., and Saura-Calixto, F. (1991) Effects of dietary fiber and phytic acid on mineral availability. *Crit Rev Food Sci Nutr* **30,** 1–22.

Troesch, B., Egli, I., Zeder, C., *et al.* (2009) Optimization of a phytase-containing micronutrient powder with low amounts of highly bioavailable iron for in-home fortification of complementary foods. *Am J Clin Nutr* **89,** 539–544.

Trowell, H. (1972a) Fiber: a natural hypocholesteremic agent. *Am J Clin Nutr* **25,** 464–465.

Trowell, H. (1972b) Ischemic heart disease and dietary fiber. *Am J Clin Nutr* **25,** 926–932.

Trowell, H., Southgate, D.A., Wolever, T.M., *et al.* (1976) Letter: Dietary fibre redefined. *Lancet* **1,** 967.

Tursi, A. and Papagrigoriadis, S. (2009) Review article: the current and evolving treatment of colonic diverticular disease. *Aliment Pharmacol Ther* **30,** 532–546.

van de Vijver, L.P., van den Bosch, L.M., van den Brandt, P.A., *et al.* (2009) Whole-grain consumption, dietary fibre intake and body mass index in the Netherlands cohort study. *Eur J Clin Nutr* **63,** 31–38.

Van Soest, P.J., Robertson, J.B., and Lewis, B.A. (1991) Methods for dietary fiber, neutral detergent fiber, and nonstarch polysaccharides in relation to animal nutrition. *J Dairy Sci* **74,** 3583–3597.

Vincent, R., Roberts, A., Frier, M., *et al.* (1995) Effect of bran particle size on gastric emptying and small bowel transit in humans: a scintigraphic study. *Gut* **37,** 216–219.

Waldron, K. and Selvendran, R. (1990) Changes in dietary fibre polymers during storage and cooking In D.A.T. Southgate, K. Waldron, and I.T. Johnson, *et al.* (eds), *Dietary Fiber: Chemical and Biological Aspects.* Royal Society of Chemistry, Cambridge.

Walker, A.R.P. (1949) Effect of low fat intakes of crude fibre on the absorption of fat. *Nature* **164,** 825–827.

Wang, H., Weening, D., Jonkers, E., *et al.* (2008) A curve fitting approach to estimate the extent of fermentation of indigestible carbohydrates. *Eur J Clin Invest* **38,** 863–868.

Weickert, M.O., Mohlig, M., Schofl, C., *et al.* (2006) Cereal fiber improves whole-body insulin sensitivity in overweight and obese women. *Diabetes Care* **29,** 775–780.

Whelton, S.P., Hyre, A.D., Pedersen, B., *et al.* (2005) Effect of dietary fiber intake on blood pressure: a meta-analysis of randomized, controlled clinical trials. *J Hypertens* **23,** 475–481.

Wisker, E. and Feldheim, W. (1990) Metabolizable energy of diets low or high in dietary fiber from fruits and vegetables when consumed by humans. *J Nutr* **120,** 1331–1337.

Wolever, T.M., Brand-Miller, J.C., Abernethy, J., *et al.* (2008) Measuring the glycemic index of foods: interlaboratory study. *Am J Clin Nutr* **87,** 247S–257S.

World Cancer Research Fund/American Institute for Cancer Research (2007) *Food, Nutrition, Physical Activity, and the Prevention of Cancer: A Global Perspective.* AICR, Washington, DC.

Wursch, P., Del Vedovo, S., and Koellreutter, B. (1986) Cell structure and starch nature as key determinants of the digestion rate of starch in legume. *Am J Clin Nutr* **43,** 25–29.

Zimmet, P., Boyko, E.J., Collier, G.R., *et al.* (1999) Etiology of the metabolic syndrome: potential role of insulin resistance, leptin resistance, and other players. *Ann NY Acad Sci* **892,** 25–44.

9

LIPIDS: ABSORPTION AND TRANSPORT

ALICE H. LICHTENSTEIN[1], DSc AND PETER J.H. JONES[2], PhD

[1]*Tufts University, Boston, Massachusetts, USA*
[2]*University of Manitoba, Winnipeg, Manitoba, Canada*

Summary

Because of the hydrophobic nature of lipids, dietary fat is handled differently than protein or carbohydrate with respect to digestion and absorption. Dietary fats are broken down throughout the gastrointestinal system. A unique group of enzymes and cofactors allows this process to proceed in an efficient manner. Elegant systems operate to digest lipid, and to ferry it from the gastrointestinal tract through the unstirred water layer into the enterocyte. Within the enterocyte, complex lipids are resynthesized and packaged into lipoprotein particles for release into the lymph system for subsequent metabolism by peripheral tissue. Once in the body, the apolar nature of lipids necessitates multiple complex transport systems that are unique relative to protein and carbohydrate. Through the coordination of numerous factors, including plasma enzymes and cofactors, cell surface receptors, and intracellular trafficking molecules dietary lipids are ultimately delivered to their targeted sites.

Introduction

Lipid has long been recognized as an important dietary component. Dietary lipid (fat) is a critical source of metabolic energy, a substrate for the synthesis of metabolically active compounds (essential fatty acids) and regulator of gene expression, and serves as a carrier for other nutrients such as the fat-soluble vitamins A, D, E, and K and vitamin precursors in both the gastrointestinal tract and plasma. The bioavailability of dietary lipid-soluble compounds is dependent on fat absorption. With the exception of essential fatty acids, phytosterols, and fat-soluble vitamins, humans have the capacity to synthesize lipids from carbohydrate and protein. In the body, lipid serves as a critical component of cell membranes, as structural moieties of lipoprotein particles, as a precursor for bioactive compounds involved in a wide range of biological functions, and in some cases a regulator of gene expression.

Chemistry

Fatty Acids

Fatty acids are composed of a hydrocarbon (acyl) chain with a methyl and carboxyl group at either end. Most fatty acids have an even number of carbon atoms that are arranged in a straight chain. The majority of dietary fatty acids range in chain length from 4 to 22 carbons (Table 9.1). Although by no means the most metabolically active, fatty acids with 16 and 18 carbons comprise the

Present Knowledge in Nutrition, Tenth Edition. Edited by John W. Erdman Jr, Ian A. Macdonald and Steven H. Zeisel.

TABLE 9.1 Common fatty acids found in foods and in the body

Code	Common name	Formula
Saturated		
4:0	butyric acid	$CH_3(CH_2)_2COOH$
6:0	caproic acid	$CH_3(CH_2)_4COOH$
8:0	caprylic acid	$CH_3(CH_2)_6COOH$
10:0	capric acid	$CH_3(CH_2)_8COOH$
12:0	lauric acid	$CH_3(CH_2)_{10}COOH$
14:0	myristic acid	$CH_3(CH_2)_{12}COOH$
16:0	palmitic acid	$CH_3(CH_2)_{14}COOH$
18:0	stearic acid	$CH_3(CH_2)_{16}COOH$
Monounsaturated		
16:1n-7 *cis*	palmitoleic acid	$CH_3(CH_2)_5CH=(c)CH(CH_2)_7COOH^a$
18:1n-9 *cis*	oleic acid	$CH_3(CH_2)_7CH=(c)CH(CH_2)_7COOH$
18:1n-9 *trans*	elaidic acid	$CH_3(CH_2)_7CH=(t)CH(CH_2)_7COOH$
Polyunsaturated		
18:2n-6,9 all *cis*	linoleic acid	$CH_3(CH_2)_4CH=(c)CHCH_2CH=(c)CH(CH_2)_7COOH$
18:3n-3,6,9 all *cis*	α-linolenic acid	$CH_3CH_2CH=(c)CHCH_2CH=(c)CHCH_2CH$ $=(c)CH(CH_2)_7COOH$
18:3n-6,9,12 all *cis*	γ-linolenic acid	$CH_3(CH_2)_4CH=(c)CHCH_2CH=(c)CHCH_2CH$ $=(c)CH(CH_2)_4COOH$
20:4n-6,9,12,15 all *cis*	arachidonic acid	$CH_3(CH_2)_4CH=(c)CHCH_2CH=(c)CHCH_2CH$ $=(c)CHCH_2CH=(c)CH(CH_2)_3COOH$
20:5n-3,6,9,12,15 all *cis*	eicosapentaenoic acid	$CH_3(CH_2CH=(c)CH)_5(CH_2)_3COOH$
22:6n-3,6,9,12,15,18 all *cis*	docosahexaenoic acid	$CH_3(CH_2CH=(c)CH)_6(CH_2)_2COOH$

^{a}c, *cis*; t, *trans*.

bulk of fatty acids in both the diet and the human body. Individual fatty acids are distinguished from each by chain length, degree of saturation, and double-bond number, conformation, and location. A fatty acid with no double bonds is termed saturated; with a single double bond is termed monounsaturated; and with two or more double bonds is termed polyunsaturated (Figure 9.1A). The double bonds within unsaturated fatty acids can appear in the more common *cis* configuration, with hydrogen atoms on the same side of the carbon atoms, or in the *trans* configuration, with hydrogen atoms on opposite sides of the carbon atoms (Figure 9.1B). Most double bonds occur in a non-conjugated sequence; a carbon atom with single carbon–carbon bonds separates the carbons forming the double bonds. Some occur in the conjugated form: no intervening carbon separates the carbons forming the double bonds (Figure 9.1C). Double-bond number, position, and conformation allow fatty acids to occur as multiple isomers (same number of carbon, hydrogen, and oxygen atoms, yet different structure).

Geometric isomers of fatty acids result from differences in the conformation (spatial orientation) of the double bond(s). The presence of a *cis* relative to a *trans* double bond results in a greater bend or kink in the acyl chain. This kink impedes the fatty acids from aligning or close packing with neighboring lipids, thereby altering the physical properties of the fat. The presence of a *trans* double bond reduces the internal rotational mobility of carbon atoms and makes them less reactive to chemical change than a *cis* double bond.

Positional isomers of fatty acids are defined by differences in the location of double bonds within the acyl chain. These differences result in small alterations to the physical properties of the fatty acid and large changes in the metabolic fate of the fatty acid. The most common distinction among positional isomers is the location of the first double bond from the methyl end of the acyl chain. Fatty acids in which the first double bond occurs three carbons from the methyl end are designated as omega-3 fatty acids, denoted as ω-3 or n-3 fatty acids. Fatty acids in which the first double bond occurs six carbons from the

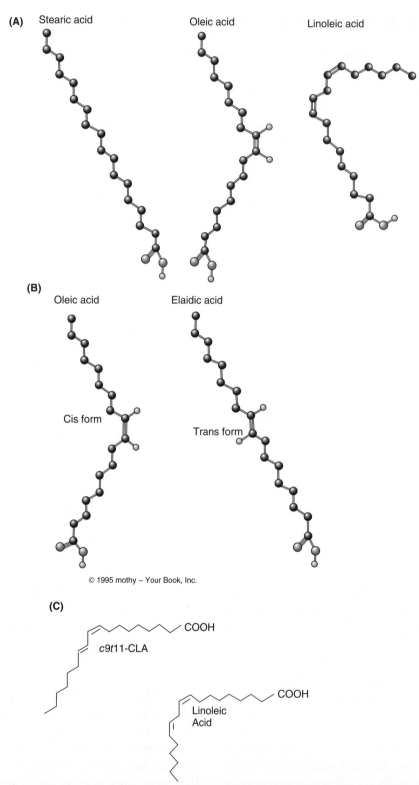

© 1995 mothy – Your Book, Inc.

FIG. 9.1   (A) Examples of fatty acids: a saturated fatty acid (stearic acid), a monounsaturated fatty acid containing a *cis* double bond (oleic acid), and a polyunsaturated fatty acid containing a *trans* double bond (linoleic acid). (B) Conformational difference between *cis* (oleic acid) and *trans* (elaidic acid) double bond containing fatty acids. (C) Structures of *c9t11*-conjugated linoleic acid (CLA) and linoleic acid (18:2[n-6]). Adapted from Belury (2002).

methyl end are termed ω-6 or *n*-6 fatty acids (Leonard *et al.*, 2004; Dupont, 2005).

Fatty acid isomers with conjugated double bonds tend to be more reactive chemically than non-conjugated double bonds (Bretillon *et al.*, 1999). Although there is considerable speculation regarding their role in disease progression, the current state of knowledge is insufficient to make any firm conclusion (Plourde *et al.*, 2008).

Enzymes that metabolize fatty acids distinguish among isomers. The metabolic products are different and can have at times opposing biological effects (Wijendran and Hayes, 2004). For example, omega-3 polyunsaturated fatty acids result in eicosanoids that have vasodilatory properties whereas omega-6 polyunsaturated fatty acids result in eicosanoids that have vasoconstrictor properties.

Triacylglycerols

Triacylglycerols, commonly referred to as triglycerides, are composed of three fatty acids esterified to a glycerol molecule. Each position of the three carbons comprising the glycerol molecule allows for a stereochemically distinct fatty acid bond position; sn-1, sn-2, and sn-3. The fatty acid moieties of the triacylglycerol molecule account for ~90% of its weight, depending on the length of the constituent fatty acids. The physical form of a triacylglycerol is determined by the fatty acids esterified to the glycerol moiety on the basis of chain length; number, position, and conformation of the double bonds; and the stereochemical position of each fatty acid. In vivo, triacylglycerol serves as a storage form of energy and a substrate reservoir for synthesis of bioactive compounds.

Phospholipids

A phospholipid is composed of two fatty acids esterified to a glycerol molecule and one polar head group attached via a phosphate linkage. Phospholipid molecules are amphipathic. The fatty acids confer hydrophobic properties and the polar head group confers hydrophilic properties. Long-chain fatty acids are preferentially esterified to the sn-2 position of glycerol. The most predominant polar head groups include choline, serine, inositol, and ethanolamine.

In vivo, due to their amphipathic nature, phospholipids serve as the structural components of cellular membranes and lipoprotein particles. The fluidity of cell membranes is determined, in part, by the fatty acid profile of the constituent phospholipids. Membrane phospholipid serves as a reservoir of fatty acids necessary

for the synthesis of bioactive compounds. For example, cell-membrane-associated phosphatidylinositol is the predominant source of arachidonic acid. Arachidonic acid is a substrate for cyclooxygenase and 5-lipoxygenase, resulting in the formation of prostaglandins. Additionally, phosphatidylinositol-derived compounds, inositol triphosphate and diacylglycerol, play important roles in cell signal transduction.

Cholesterol and Cholesteryl Ester

Cholesterol is an amphipathic molecule that is composed of a steroid nucleus and a branched hydrocarbon tail. Its presence in the food supply is for the most part restricted to fats of animal origin. It is found in two forms, either unesterified or esterified to a fatty acid at carbon number 3. Unesterified cholesterol is a component of cell membranes, and, along with the phospholipid fatty acid profile, modifies fluidity (Jaureguiberry *et al.*, 2010). Intracellularly, unesterified cholesterol mediates cholesterol homeostasis in three ways (Lillis *et al.*, 2008). Unesterified cholesterol inhibits 3-hydroxy 3-methylglutaryl CoA (HMG CoA) reductase activity, the rate-limiting enzyme in de novo cholesterol biosynthesis. Unesterified cholesterol increases acyl CoA cholesterol acyltransferase (ACAT) activity, the intracellular enzyme that esterifies unesterified cholesterol thereby lowering intracellular concentrations. Lastly, unesterified cholesterol decreases the synthesis of low-density lipoprotein (LDL) cell surface receptors, thereby diminishing the uptake of additional cholesterol from plasma. These three factors protect against excess intracellular cholesterol accumulation, particularly important because a high concentration of intracellular unesterified cholesterol is cytotoxic due the formation of micelles which have detergent properties.

Esterified cholesterol is less polar than free cholesterol. As a consequence, whereas free cholesterol is localized on the surface, cholesteryl ester is sequestered in the core of lipoprotein particles. The majority of cholesterol in plasma, two-thirds, is carried on LDL. In plasma, cholesteryl ester is formed as a result of lecithin cholesterol acyltransferase (LCAT) activity. Intracellularly, cholesteryl ester is formed as a result of ACAT activity and is stored in lipid droplets (Chang *et al.*, 1997; Buhman *et al.*, 2000; Rudel *et al.*, 2001). Cholesteryl ester forms the core of atherosclerotic plaques (Degirolamo *et al.*, 2009). Long-chain saturated fatty acids have been reported to suppress LDL receptor activity (Knopp, 2000).

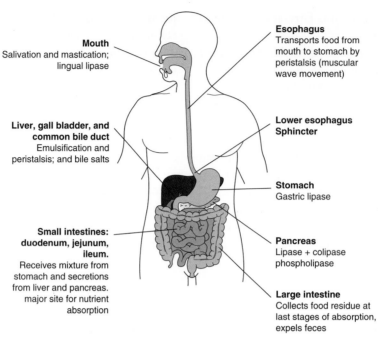

FIG. 9.2   Diagram of absorption.

Plant Sterols

Fats derived from plant materials contain phytosterols, compounds structurally related to cholesterol, commonly referred to as plant sterols. Cholesterol and phytosterols differ chemically with regard to their side-chain configuration and steroid-ring bonding patterns. The most common dietary phytosterols are β-sitosterol, campesterol, and stigmasterol (Abumweis *et al.*, 2008; Demonty *et al.*, 2009). In contrast to cholesterol, phytosterols are poorly absorbed and levels in plasma tend to be low. Because of their ability to displace cholesterol from intestinal micelles, phytosterols can reduce the absorption efficiency of cholesterol, lowering circulating LDL levels.

Digestion

Typical intakes of dietary fat range from 25% to 35% of energy. For a 2000-calorie diet this represents 56 to 78 g of fat and for a 3000-calorie diet 83–117 g of fat. In contrast to dietary carbohydrate and protein, fat does not interface with the aqueous milieu of the gastrointestinal tract, so a different system exists to accommodate the unique challenges posed for the digestion and absorption of dietary fat.

Triacylglycerols
Mouth, Esophagus, and Stomach

Fat digestion begins at the point of entry, the oral cavity where salivation and mastication occur (Figure 9.2). Lingual lipase, released from the von Ebner (serous) glands of the tongue along with saliva, can cause the release of small amounts of fatty acids from triacylglycerol (Lohse *et al.*, 1997; Kawai and Fushiki, 2003). Lingual lipase cleaves the sn-3 position of the triacylglycerol molecule, with higher efficiency towards shorter-chain fatty acids. For this reason the impact is thought to be greater in infants due to their high intake of milk fat, which contains a high proportion of short-chain fatty acids. When active, lingual lipase activity continues as food travels through the esophagus and into the stomach. In the stomach, gastric lipase is released from the gastric mucosa (Canaan *et al.*, 1999a; Pafumi *et al.*, 2002; Mu and Hoy, 2004). This enzyme cleaves triacylglycerol at the sn-3 position. It has been estimated that 10–30% of fat hydrolysis occurs prior to the masticated bolus of food entering the small intestine (Mu and Hoy, 2004). The increased pH of the intestine on entry of the food bolus decreases the activity of the lingual and gastric lipases.

Intestine

The majority of triacylglycerol digestion and absorption occurs in the small intestine (Mu and Hoy, 2004). This process is co-dependent on pancreatic lipase and liver-derived bile salts. Bile is secreted from the gall bladder or directly from the liver in response to the presence of fat in the duodenum. Bile, per se, is composed of bile salts, phospholipid and cholesterol. The major function of bile is to emulsify the intestinal contents, referred to as chyme. Emulsification serves to increase the surface area of the hydrophilic mass. Bile salts have a steroid nucleus and an aliphatic side chain conjugated in an amide bond with taurine or glycine (Canaan *et al.*, 1999b; Chiang, 2004). Bile acids are synthesized from cholesterol in the liver. The rate-limiting enzyme in this process is 7α-hydroxylase (Davis *et al.*, 2002; Hofmann, 2009). The hydroxyl and ionized sulfonate or carboxylate groups of the conjugate make bile salts water soluble. The primary bile salts are cholate and chenodeoxycholate (tri- and dihydroxy bile salts, respectively) which are synthesized directly from cholesterol. The secondary bile salts, deoxycholate and lithocholate, are synthesized from primary bile salts (cholate and chenodeoxycholate, respectively) by bacteria normally present in the intestinal microflora. Secondary bile salts can be further modified by hepatocytes or bacteria. The products are sulfated esters of lithocholate and ursodezylcholate.

The entry of fat into the duodenum, in addition to stimulating the contraction of the gall bladder, causes cholecystokinin secretion and the release of pancreatic lipase and colipase. The amount of fat habitually entering the duodenum regulates gene expression of pancreatic lipase. In the intestine pancreatic lipase is responsible for the majority of the triacylglycerol hydrolysis (Canaan *et al.*, 1999a,b; Whitcomb and Lowe, 2007). Pancreatic lipase hydrolyzes the sn-1 and sn-3 positions of triglyceride. The sn-2 (middle) position of glycerol is resistant to hydrolysis by lipases. Pancreatic lipase is inhibited by bile salts via displacement from the lipid droplet. Colipase, synthesized by the pancreas, binds pancreatic lipase and facilitates the enzyme's adhesion to the lipid droplets (Aloulou *et al.*, 2006; Whitcomb and Lowe, 2007). The hydrolytic products of triacylglycerol (2-monoacylglycerol and free fatty acids), along with bile salts, phospholipids, cholesterol, and other fat-soluble substances, form micelles in the small intestine. Micelles form when the critical micellar concentration of bile, about 2 mM, is reached. The presence of monoacylglycerol increases the capacity of the micelle to accommodate free fatty acids and cholesterol. Deficits in the availability of an adequate amount of pancreatic lipase or bile acids can result in steatorrhea (presence of undigested fat in the stool).

Phospholipid

The majority of the phospholipid in the small intestine is derived from bile with a smaller component coming from the diet. Phospholipase A_2, a pancreatic enzyme secreted in bile, mediates phospholipid digestion. This enzyme hydrolyzes the ester bond at the sn-2 position of the phospholipid, resulting in a free fatty acid and lysophosphoglyceride. These products are incorporated into micelles for subsequent absorption.

Cholesterol and Cholesteryl Ester

Both bile and, to a lesser and more variable extent, diet and sloughed intestinal cells contribute cholesterol to the contents of the small intestine (Nordskog *et al.*, 2001). Cholesterol originating from bile and intestinal cells is present in the free form. Cholesterol originating from the diet occurs as free cholesterol and cholesteryl ester. Prior to absorption, cholesteryl ester hydrolase hydrolyzes cholesteryl ester to free cholesterol and a fatty acid.

Absorption

Triacylglycerol

The efficiency of triacylglycerol absorption is approximately 95% in adults and 85–90% in infants, and is similar over a wide range of the total fat intakes. Fatty acids with 12 or more carbon atoms are absorbed into the lymphatic system as chylomicrons (see later section headed "Intestinal particles"). Fatty acids with 10 or fewer carbon atoms, sometimes referred to as short- and medium-chain fatty acids, are absorbed directly into the portal circulation.

Absorption of micellar components into intestinal mucosal cells is dependent on the penetration of micelles across the unstirred water layer that separates the intestinal contents from the brush border of the small intestine (Nordskog *et al.*, 2001; Iqbal and Hussain, 2009) (Figure 9.3). Under normal circumstances micellar components exist in dynamic equilibrium with the surrounding environment and spontaneously exchange among micellar particles. This process is facilitated by the peristaltic action of the small intestine. Micelles traverse the unstirred water layer because of their relatively small size (30–100 Å) and

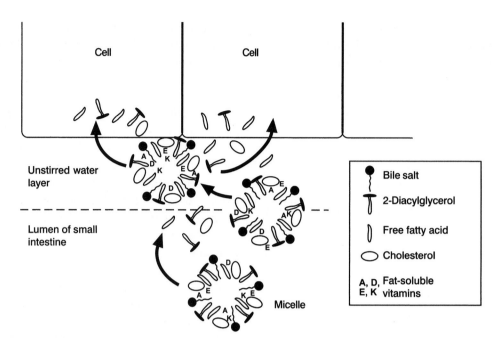

FIG. 9.3 Fat absorption from the smalll intestine. VLDL, very-low-density lipoprotein; IDI, intermediate-density lipoprotein; LDL, low-density lipoprotein; HDL, high-density lipoprotein; LCAT, lecithin cholesterol acyltransferase; ACAT, acyl coenzyme A cholesterol acyltransferase.

hydrophilic nature, due to the presence of bile salts and phospholipid. Since the concentration of the components in the unstirred water layer and intracellularly is lower than in the surrounding environment, the products of hydrolysis flow down the concentration gradient; hence, the mechanism of absorption is passive diffusion. This net loss of micellar constituents results in a shift in the distribution of hydrolytic products from micelles in the intestinal lumen to micelles in the unstirred water layer, and from the unstirred water layer to intestinal cells.

Micellar bile salts are recycled with high efficiency, being reabsorbed in both the small intestine and colon, and resecreted via bile in the duodenum. Bile salts are absorbed independently by both passive and active mechanisms. Passive absorption of unconjugated bile salts occurs along the entire length of the small intestine and colon. Active absorption occurs in the ileum and involves a brush-border membrane receptor, cytosolic bile acid-binding protein, and basolateral anion-exchange proteins. Approximately 97–98% of bile acids are absorbed (Chiang, 2004; Keating and Keely, 2009). Interfering with the reabsorption of bile acids forces the liver to use cholesterol for the synthesis. This cause/effect relationship has been exploited for treatment of hypercholesterolemic patients with bile acid sequestrants and plant sterols, specifically intended to interfere with this process.

Short-chain fatty acids are absorbed directly into the portal circulation and transported bound to albumin via the peripheral circulation rather than undergoing incorporation into chylomicrons as occurs for longer-chain fatty acids. The majority of short-chain fatty acids are either oxidized directly as energy sources or converted to other metabolites within the hepatocyte (White *et al.*, 1999). As such, short-chain fatty acids have been identified as possessing greater thermogenic action than longer-chain fatty acids.

Phospholipid

The products of phospholipid digestion, free fatty acid and lysophosphoglyceride, are incorporated into intestinal micelles and absorbed by a process similar to that described for the hydrolytic products of triacylglycerol.

Cholesterol and Cholesteryl Ester

The efficiency of free and esterified cholesterol absorption is similar, approximately 40–60%. Free cholesterol and the free fatty acids resulting from the hydrolysis of cholesteryl esters are incorporated into intestinal micelles. Absorption efficiency is regulated by the balance between the incorporation of cholesterol into a newly synthesized chylomicron particle and trafficking of cholesterol out of the enterocyte back into the small intestine (Sehayek, 2003; Wilund *et al.*, 2004). These processes are regulated by ATP-binding cassette (ABC) G5 and G8 transporters and Niemann-Pick C1-Like 1 (NPC1L1) (Altmann *et al.*, 2004; Davis *et al.*, 2004; Wang *et al.*, 2004; Rudkowska and Jones, 2008).

Plant Sterols and Sterol Esters

The efficiency of plant sterol absorption is relatively low, approximately 1–10% depending on the specific plant sterol, and somewhat lower for the saturated form of the compounds, stanols (Katan *et al.*, 2003). The poor efficiency of absorption is attributed to multiple factors. These include the activity of the ATP-binding cassette proteins G5 and G8 that transport plant sterols but not cholesterol out of the enterocyte (Sehayek, 2003), the low solubility of the sterols in micelles, and the inability of the intestinal cell to re-esterify the sterols once absorbed (Field and Mathur, 1983). Despite their poor solubility in micelles, plant sterols interfere with cholesterol's incorporation into the intestinal particles, diminishing cholesterol absorption efficiency (Meijer *et al.*, 2003; Sudhop *et al.*, 2003; Talati *et al.*, 2010). Lower rates of cholesterol absorption result in, on average, a 10% reduction in plasma LDL cholesterol concentrations in most individuals (Talati *et al.*, 2010).

Transport and Metabolism

Lipid is transported out of the intestine and in plasma in the form of lipoprotein particles. A common feature of lipoprotein particles is their structure. The core of the spherical particle is composed primarily of apolar components: triacylglycerol and cholesteryl ester. The surface of the particle is composed of the more polar constituents: a phospholipid monolayer, apolipoproteins, and free cholesterol (Babin and Gibbons, 2009). Fat-soluble vitamins are sequestered in the core of the chylomicron particle.

Intestinal Particles

Chylomicrons are intestinally derived lipoprotein particles formed and secreted after the ingestion of fat. Their main function is to provide a mechanism whereby dietary triacylglycerol, cholesterol, and other fat-soluble compounds are carried from the site of absorption (intestine) to other parts of the body for subsequent uptake and metabolism or storage (Redgrave, 2004; Williams *et al.*, 2004).

The first step in the formation of chylomicron particles is the resynthesis of triacylglycerol and phospholipids from fatty acids, and glycerol, sn-2 monoacylglycerides, or lysophospholipids, respectively (Gordon *et al.*, 1994; White *et al.*, 2004). This process occurs on the smooth endoplasmic reticulum. The fatty acid composition of the chylomicron triacylglycerol reflects the fatty acid composition of the diet (Hussain, 2000). A large proportion of the cholesterol that enters the enterocyte is re-esterified, a reaction catalyzed by ACAT, prior to incorporation into the chylomicron particle (Chang *et al.*, 1997; Buhman *et al.*, 2000; Rudel *et al.*, 2001). The re-esterification processes are facilitated by fatty acid-binding protein (Joyce *et al.*, 1999). Chylomicron particles are the largest of all the lipoprotein subclasses (Joyce *et al.*, 1999) (Table 9.2).

In humans, the distinguishing apolipoprotein of intestinally derived lipoprotein particles is apolipoprotein (apo) B-48, in contrast to the distinguishing apolipoprotein of hepatically derived particles, apo B-100. Apo B-48 is a large hydrophobic protein synthesized on the rough endoplasmic reticulum. It results from mRNA editing and is approximately 48% of the molecular weight of apo B-100. Once released into the circulation, additional

TABLE 9.2 Characteristics of lipoproteins

Lipoprotein	Density (g/dL)	Molecular mass (daltons)	Diameter (nm)	Lipid (%)[a]		
				Triacylglyerol	Cholesterol	Phospholipid
Chylomicron	0.95	1400×10^6	75–1200	80–95	2–7	3–9
VLDL	0.95–1.006	$10–80 \times 10^6$	30–80	55–80	5–15	10–20
IDL	1.006–1.019	$5–10 \times 10^6$	25–35	20–50	20–40	15–25
LDL	1.019–1.063	2.3×10^6	18–25	5–15	40–50	20–25
HDL	1.063–1.21	$1.7–3.6 \times 10^5$	5–12	5–10	15–25	20–30

Reproduced with permission from Ginsberg (1994). Copyright Elsevier.
[a]Percentage composition of lipids; apolipoproteins make up the rest.
VLDL, very-low-density lipoprotein; IDL, intermediate-density lipoprotein; LDL, low-density lipoprotein; HDL, high-density lipoprotein.

apolipoproteins are added to the surface of chylomicron particles include apo A-I, apo A-IV, apo A-II, apo C, and apo E (Brown, 2007). It has been suggested that the release of apo A-IV is stimulated by dietary fat and has a role in the regulation of upper gut function and satiety (Tso and Liu, 2004). It has further been suggested that apo A-IV may be involved in the long-term regulation of food intake and that chronic ingestion of a high-fat diet blunts the intestinal apo A-IV response to dietary fat and hence predisposes to obesity (Tso and Liu, 2004).

Chylomicrons are assembled from apo B-48 and triacylglycerol accumulated in the smooth endoplasmic reticulum. Microsomal triacylglycerol transfer protein (MTP) is responsible for transporting and inserting the triacylglycerol into the nascent chylomicron core as the particle is then transferred into the lumen of the endoplasmic reticulum (White et al., 1998). Some data suggest that small apo B-48-containing particles fuse with large, independently formed triacylglycerol apo B-48 free particles prior to secretion (Mu and Hoy, 2004; Kindel et al., 2010). Carbohydrate is added to the nascent chylomicron particle just before release from the Golgi apparatus by exocytosis from the cell.

Chylomicrons are released from enterocytes into the lymph before being channeled from the thoracic duct to the subclavian vein. Some of the apolipoproteins associated with chylomicron particles are acquired by transfer after the lipoprotein is released into the bloodstream. Once in circulation, the triacylglycerol component of chylomicron particles is hydrolyzed by lipoprotein lipase. During this process, apolipoproteins are transferred to other lipoprotein particles. Lipoprotein lipase is synthesized in adipose tissue, heart, and skeletal muscle, and migrates to the capillaries where it functions to hydrolyze triglyceride (Merkel et al., 2002; Stein and Stein, 2003). Apo C-II is a critical cofactor for the reaction whereas apo C-I and apo C-III inhibit the reaction (Shachter, 2001; Merkel et al., 2002; Saito et al., 2004). The hydrolysis of chylomicron triacylglycerol in the circulation accounts for the delivery of fatty acids from the gastrointestinal system to peripheral tissue for oxidation, metabolism, and storage. Chylomicron particles depleted of the triacylglycerol component are taken up by the liver via either the LDL receptor or LDL-receptor-like protein receptor (Cooper, 1997; Havel, 2000). The components of chylomicron particles are either used by the liver directly or are incorporated into newly synthesized hepatically derived lipoprotein particles.

Lipoprotein Particles

Very-low-density (VLDL) and Intermediate-density (IDL) Lipoproteins

VLDL are hepatically derived particles that mediate the transport of fat from the liver to peripheral tissue (Frost and Havel, 1998; Karpe, 1999). The triacylglycerol in VLDL is synthesized from fatty acids derived from de novo lipogenesis (using monosaccharides as substrate), cytoplasmic triacylglycerol, lipoproteins taken up directly by the liver, and exogenous free fatty acids. The major apolipoprotein in VLDL is apo B-100 (Tessari et al., 2009). Apo B-100 is synthesized on the rough endoplasmic reticulum and transferred to the Golgi apparatus where, with the involvement of MTP, it is incorporated into the nascent VLDL particle. Inadequate triacylglycerol or the absence of MTP results in internal degradation of apo B-100 (Olofsson et al., 2007). This degradation is facilitated by the association of nascent apo B with a cytosolic chaperone protein, heat shock protein 70 (Ginsberg, 1997). In plasma, VLDL also contains apo E and apo C, which are either present at the time of secretion or acquired once in the circulation (Frost and Havel, 1998; Karpe, 1999). The lipid components of VLDL particles are similar to those of chylomicrons; however, the relative proportion of triacylglycerol is less (Table 9.2). This results in smaller, denser particles. Once in circulation, the initial stages of VLDL metabolism are similar to that of chylomicron metabolism. Lipoprotein lipase hydrolyzes the core triacylglycerol (Choi et al., 2002; Cilingiroglu and Ballantyne, 2004). The resulting fatty acids are taken up by cells locally and are oxidized for energy, used for the synthesis of structural components (phospholipid) or bioactive compounds (leukotrienes, thromboxanes), or stored (triacylglycerol). Triacylglycerol-depleted particles, VLDL remnants, can either be taken up directly by receptor-mediated mechanisms in the liver or remain in circulation and be progressively depleted of triacylglycerol. The delipidation of VLDL results in the progressive shift in the composition of the lipoprotein particle from one defined as VLDL to IDL and eventually LDL (Choi et al., 2002; Cilingiroglu and Ballantyne, 2004). This process is facilitated not only by lipoprotein lipase, but also by hepatic lipase (Choi et al., 2002; Zambon et al., 2003; Cilingiroglu and Ballantyne, 2004). This second lipase has the capacity to hydrolyze both triacylglycerol and phospholipid, and is localized to the liver. The progressive depletion of triacylglycerol from the lipoprotein particle results in a marked increase in the relative proportion of cholesterol. In circulation, as VLDL is depleted of triacylglycerol, all apolipo-proteins with the exception of apo B-100 are transferred to other lipoprotein particles. The ultimate product is LDL, a cholesterol-rich particle containing only a single copy of apo B-100.

Low-density Lipoprotein

LDL particles can be taken up by an apolipoprotein-mediated (LDL receptor family) or scavenger receptor (Van Berkel et al., 2000; Linton and Fazio, 2001). Several LDL receptor family members exist including the LDL receptor itself, LDL receptor-related protein (LRP), apo E receptor 2 protein, multiple epidermal growth factor-containing protein 7, VLDL receptor, LRP1B, megalin, LRP 5, and LRP 6 (May et al., 2007; Lillis et al., 2008; Goldstein and Brown, 2009). LDL receptors predominate in tissues such as liver, smooth muscle cells, fibroblasts, central nervous system neurons and astrocytes, epithelial cells of the gastrointestinal tract, testis Leydig cells, ovarian granulosa cells, and kidney dendritic interstitial cells (Moestrup et al., 1992). Whereas the LDL receptor mediates the uptake of apo B-100 or apo E-containing lipoproteins, other members of the LDL receptor family recognize multiple apolipoproteins, proteases, and protease/inhibitor complexes, and additional signaling molecules as well as playing other diverse biological roles (Bajari et al., 2005). Once LDL particles are taken up by the cell, they disassociate from the receptor which in turn allows the receptor to be recycled. The LDL particle then fuses with a lysosome and is subsequently degraded. This step is critical for whole-body cholesterol homoeostasis because the cholesterol taken up from circulation and released from the lysosome has three distinct effects as discussed earlier in the "Cholesterol and cholesteryl ester" section. Alternatively, LDL can be taken up by a scavenger receptor on macrophages in various tissues. Scavenger receptors predominate in macrophages. This system predominates after LDL particles are modified or oxidized as they circulate in plasma (Van Berkel et al., 2000; Linton and Fazio, 2001). Whereas the LDL receptor-mediated uptake is rate limited by the ability of unesterified cholesterol to inhibit the synthesis of new receptors, scavenger receptor uptake is proportional to circulating LDL cholesterol concentrations.

Lipoprotein(a) (Lp[a])

Lipoprotein(a) (Lp[a]) contains an LDL-like particle and a single copy of apo(a), covalently bounded to apoB on the LDL-like particle. Blood Lp(a) concentrations are highly heritable and affected by the apo(a) gene (LPA) located on chromosome 6q26-27. Apo(a) proteins comprise a family of proteins differing in size. The size of apo(a) is determined by the number of kringle IV repeats incorporated into the protein as a function of the LPA gene size polymorphism [KIV-2 VNTR]. Although the precise function of Lp(a) remains to be established, high blood Lp(a) concentrations are associated with increased coronary heart disease and stroke risk (Tziomalos et al., 2009; Spence, 2010).

High-density Lipoprotein (HDL)

HDL particles are derived from the liver and intestine. In addition, during delipidation of chylomicrons in the periphery, excess phospholipid and apolipoproteins from the surface of these particles serve as a source of HDL (Merkel et al., 2002). The primary role of HDL particles is to participate in "reverse cholesterol transport" by shuttling cholesterol from the peripheral tissues to the liver for excretion, metabolism, or storage (Meagher, 2004; Morgan et al., 2004). An integral part of this process is scavenger receptor (SR)-B1. This hepatic HDL receptor selectively takes up the cholesteryl ester component of HDL, thus enabling HDL to continually pick up additional cholesterol from peripheral tissue and shuttle it to the liver (Tall, 1998; Marcil et al., 2004).

HDL is a heterogeneous group of particles that differ in both the apolipoprotein composition and size. All HDL particles contain apo A-I. Additional apolipoproteins (apo) associated with HDL can include apo A-II, A-IV, and Cs (Brown, 2007). HDL particles appear to protect other lipoproteins from oxidative modification. This activity appears to be related to the presence of apo A-I, paraoxonase, and platelet-activating factor acetylhydrolase (Ji et al., 1999; Navab et al., 2004, 2007). Plasma HDL levels are inversely related to triglyceride and risk of developing cardiovascular disease (Taskinen, 2003; Szapary and Rader, 2004).

Tangier disease is an autosomal recessive disorder characterized by the virtual absence of HDL cholesterol. HDL-mediated cholesterol efflux, and intracellular lipid trafficking and turnover, are abnormal in fibroblasts from Tangier patients. The genetic defect encoding for a member of the ATP-binding cassette transporter family has been identified in these individuals (Burris et al., 2002; Oram, 2002; Kolovou et al., 2006). The ABC transporter is integral to the process of reverse cholesterol transport. Individuals with a mutation in the ABC transporter have very low levels of HDL cholesterol and develop premature atherosclerosis.

In addition to delipidation, lipoproteins are altered while in circulation (Borggreve *et al.*, 2003; Miller *et al.*, 2003; Wirtz, 2006; Masson *et al.*, 2009). This includes both exchange and modification of lipoprotein constituents. LCAT esterifies free cholesterol on the surface of HDL particles. Apo A-I serves as a co-factor and HDL-associated phosphotidylcholine as the source of fatty acid (Miller *et al.*, 2003; Masson *et al.*, 2009). The formation of cholesteryl ester and its subsequent migration to the core of the HDL particle creates an environment receptive to the addition of more free cholesterol from peripheral tissue and ensures that the cholesterol already on the HDL particle does not transfer back to peripheral tissue. Cholesterol ester transfer protein (CETP) facilitates the exchange of cholesteryl ester from HDL to VLDL or chylomicrons for triacylglycerol (Borggreve *et al.*, 2003; Masson *et al.*, 2009). Phospholipid transfer protein activity results in HDL remodeling through the exchange of phospholipid (Wirtz, 2006). These processes enhance reverse cholesterol transport.

Future Directions

Several areas of lipid nutrition exist at the forefront of research. First, lipid cellular regulators have been identified recently that affect processes including fat synthesis and breakdown. In particular, a group of ethanolamides has been identified as being derived through a series of enzymatic steps from dietary fatty acids in the intestinal cells. Oleoylethanolamide, derived from oleic acid, appears to suppress fat synthesis as well as perhaps to affect appetite (Capasso and Izzo, 2008). Another future area of discovery involves transesterified fats. Repositioning the three fatty acids configured across a glycerol molecule can profoundly alter the manner by which that triacylglycerol is absorbed and metabolized (Berry, 2009). Further research is required to fully define how transesterified triacylglycerol impacts on processes of lipid digestion and utilization.

Another area of current research focus involves the genetic modification of plants to produce vegetable oils with non-traditional fatty acid profiles. For example, plant-based oils enriched in stearidonic or docosahexaenoic acid through genetic enhancement are now available for dietary consumption (Damude and Kinney, 2007). Similarly, fats enriched in oleic acid which function well as substitutes for *trans* fats are available to the food industry. The health effects of such oils need to be more precisely defined.

Suggestions for Further Reading

Betters, J.L. and Yu, L. (2010) NPC1L1 and cholesterol transport. *FEBS Lett* **584**, 2740–2747.

Caesar, R., Fåk, F., and Bäckhed, F. (2010) Effects of gut microbiota on obesity and atherosclerosis via modulation of inflammation and lipid metabolism. *J Intern Med* **268**, 320–328.

Rothblat, G.H. and Phillips, M.C. (2010) High-density lipoprotein heterogeneity and function in reverse cholesterol transport. *Curr Opin Lipidol* **21**, 229–238.

Van der Velde, A.E., Brufau, G., and Groen, A.K. (2010) Transintestinal cholesterol efflux. *Curr Opin Lipidol* **21**, 167–171.

References

Abumweis, S.S., Barake, R., and Jones, P.J. (2008) Plant sterols/stanols as cholesterol lowering agents: a meta-analysis of randomized controlled trials. *Food Nutr Res* **52**, 1811–1820.

Aloulou, A., Rodriguez, J.A., Fernandez, S., *et al.* (2006) Exploring the specific features of interfacial enzymology based on lipase studies. *Biochim Biophys Acta* **1761**, 995–1013.

Altmann, S.W., Davis, H.R., Jr, Zhu, L.J., *et al.* (2004) Niemann-Pick C1 Like 1 protein is critical for intestinal cholesterol absorption. *Science* **303**, 1201–1204.

Babin, P.J. and Gibbons, G.F. (2009) The evolution of plasma cholesterol: direct utility or a "spandrel" of hepatic lipid metabolism? *Progr Lipid Res* **48**, 73–91.

Bajari, T.M., Strasser, V., Nimpf, J., *et al.* (2005) LDL receptor family: isolation, production, and ligand binding analysis. *Methods* **36**, 109–116.

Belury, M.A. (2002) Inhibition of carcinogenesis by conjugated linoleic acid: potential mechanisms of action. *J Nutr* **132**, 2995–2998.

Berry, S.E.E. (2009) Triacylglycerol structure and interesterification of palmitic and stearic acid-rich fats: an overview and implications for cardiovascular disease. *Nutr Res Rev* **22**, 3–17.

Borggreve, S.E., De Vries, R., and Dullaart, R.P. (2003) Alterations in high-density lipoprotein metabolism and reverse cholesterol transport in insulin resistance and type 2 diabetes mellitus: role of lipolytic enzymes, lecithin:cholesterol acyltransferase and lipid transfer proteins. *Eur J Clin Invest* **33**, 1051–1069.

Bretillon, L., Chardigny, J.M., Gregoire, S., *et al.* (1999) Effects of conjugated linoleic acid isomers on the hepatic microsomal desaturation activities in vitro. *Lipids* **34**, 965–969.

Brown, W.V. (2007) High-density lipoprotein and transport of cholesterol and triglyceride in blood. *J Clin Lipidol* **1**, 7–19.

Buhman, K.F., Accad, M., and Farese, R.V. (2000) Mammalian acyl-CoA:cholesterol acyltransferases. *Biochim Biophys Acta* **1529**, 142–154.

Burris, T.P., Eacho, P.I., and Cao, G. (2002) Genetic disorders associated with ATP binding cassette cholesterol transporters. *Mol Genet Metab* **77**, 13–20.

Canaan, S., Riviere, M., Verger, R., *et al.* (1999a) The cysteine residues of recombinant human gastric lipase. *Biochem Biophys Research Commun* **257**, 851–854.

Canaan, S., Roussel, A., Verger, R., *et al.* (1999b) Gastric lipase: crystal structure and activity. *Biochim Biophys Acta* **1441**, 197–204.

Capasso, R. and Izzo, A.A. (2008) Gastrointestinal regulation of food intake: general aspects and focus on anandamide and oleoylethanolamide. *J Neuroendocrinol* **20** Suppl 1, 39–46.

Chang, T.Y., Chang, C.C., and Cheng, D. (1997) Acyl-coenzyme A:cholesterol acyltransferase. *Annu Rev Biochem* **66**, 613–638.

Chiang, J.Y. (2004) Regulation of bile acid synthesis: pathways, nuclear receptors, and mechanisms. *J Hepatol* **40**, 539–551.

Choi, S.Y., Hirata, K., Ishida, T., *et al.* (2002) Endothelial lipase: a new lipase on the block. *J Lipid Res* **43**, 1763–1769.

Cilingiroglu, M. and Ballantyne, C. (2004) Endothelial lipase and cholesterol metabolism. *Curr Atheroscler Rep* **6**, 126–130.

Cooper, A.D. (1997) Hepatic uptake of chylomicron remnants. *J Lipid Res* **38**, 2173–2192.

Damude, H.G. and Kinney, A.J. (2007) Engineering oilseed plants for a sustainable, land-based source of long chain polyunsaturated fatty acids. *Lipids* **42**, 179–185.

Davis, H.R., Jr, Zhu, L.J., Hoos, L.M., *et al.* (2004) Niemann-Pick C1 Like 1 (NPC1L1) is the intestinal phytosterol and cholesterol transporter and a key modulator of whole-body cholesterol homeostasis. *J Biol Chem* **279**, 33586–33592.

Davis, R.A., Miyake, J.H., Hui, T.Y., *et al.* (2002) Regulation of cholesterol-7alpha-hydroxylase: BAREly missing a SHP. *J Lipid Res* **43**, 533–543.

Degirolamo, C., Shelness, G.S., and Rudel, L.L. (2009) LDL cholesteryl oleate as a predictor for atherosclerosis: evidence from human and animal studies on dietary fat. *J Lipid Res* **50** Suppl, S434–439.

Demonty, I., Ras, R.T., Van der Knaap, H.C.M., *et al.* (2009) Continuous dose–response relationship of the LDL-cholesterol-lowering effect of phytosterol intake. *J Nutr* **139**, 271–284.

Dupont, J.L. (2005) Lipids: chemistry and classification. In B. Caballero, L. Allen, and A Prentice (eds), *Encyclopedia of Human Nutrition*. Academic Press, New York, pp. 126–132.

Field, F.J. and Mathur, S.N. (1983) Beta-sitosterol: esterification by intestinal acylcoenzyme A: cholesterol acyltransferase (ACAT) and its effect on cholesterol esterification. *J Lipid Res* **24**, 409–417.

Frost, P.H. and Havel, R.J. (1998) Rationale for use of non-high-density lipoprotein cholesterol rather than low-density lipoprotein cholesterol as a tool for lipoprotein cholesterol screening and assessment of risk and therapy. *Am J Cardiol* **81**, 26B–31B.

Ginsberg, H.N. (1994) Lipoprotein metabolism and its relationship to atherosclerosis. *Med Clin North Am* **78**, 1–20.

Ginsberg, H.N. (1997) Role of lipid synthesis, chaperone proteins and proteasomes in the assembly and secretion of apoprotein B-containing lipoproteins from cultured liver cells. *Clin Exp Pharmacol Physiol* **24**, A29–32.

Goldstein, J.L. and Brown, M.S. (2009) The LDL receptor. *Arterioscler Thromb Vasc Biol* **29**, 431–438.

Gordon, D.A., Jamil, H., Sharp, D., *et al.* (1994) Secretion of apolipoprotein B-containing lipoproteins from HeLa cells is dependent on expression of the microsomal triglyceride transfer protein and is regulated by lipid availability. *Proc Natl Acad Sci USA* **91**, 7628–7632.

Havel, R.J. (2000) Remnant lipoproteins as therapeutic targets. *Curr Opin Lipidol* **11**, 615–620.

Hofmann, A. F. (2009) Bile acids: trying to understand their chemistry and biology with the hope of helping patients. *Hepatology* **49**, 1403–1418.

Hussain, M.M. (2000) A proposed model for the assembly of chylomicrons. *Atherosclerosis* **148**, 1–15.

Iqbal, J. and Hussain, M.M. (2009) Intestinal lipid absorption. *Am J Physiol Endocrinol Metab* **296**, E1183–1194.

Jaureguiberry, M.S., Tricerri, M.A., Sanchez, S.A., *et al.* (2010) Membrane organization and regulation of cellular cholesterol homeostasis. *J Membr Biol* **234**, 183–194.

Ji, Y., Wang, N., Ramakrishnan, R., *et al.* (1999) Hepatic scavenger receptor BI promotes rapid clearance of high density lipoprotein free cholesterol and its transport into bile. *J Biological Chem* **274**, 33398–33402.

Joyce, C., Skinner, K., Anderson, R A., *et al.* (1999) Acyl-coenzyme A:cholesteryl acyltransferase 2. *Curr Opin Lipidol* **10**, 89–95.

Karpe, F. (1999) Postprandial lipoprotein metabolism and atherosclerosis. *J Intern Med* **246**, 341–355.

Katan, M.B., Grundy, S.M., Jones, P., *et al.* (2003) Efficacy and safety of plant stanols and sterols in the management of blood cholesterol levels. *Mayo Clin Proc* **78**, 965–978.

Kawai, T. and Fushiki, T. (2003) Importance of lipolysis in oral cavity for orosensory detection of fat. *Am J Physiol Regul Integr Comp Physiol* **285,** R447–454.

Keating, N. and Keely, S.J. (2009) Bile acids in regulation of intestinal physiology. *Curr Gastroenterol Rep* **11,** 375–382.

Kindel, T., Lee, D.M., and Tso, P. (2010) The mechanism of the formation and secretion of chylomicrons. *Atheroscler Suppl* **11,** 11–16.

Knopp, R.H. (2000) Introduction: low-saturated fat, high-carbohydrate diets: effects on triglyceride and LDL synthesis, the LDL receptor, and cardiovascular disease risk. *Proc Soc Exp Biol Med* **225,** 175–177.

Kolovou, G.D., Mikhailidis, D.P., Anagnostopoulou, K.K., *et al.* (2006) Tangier disease four decades of research: a reflection of the importance of HDL. *Curr Med Chem* **13,** 771–782.

Leonard, A.E., Pereira, S.L., Sprecher, H., *et al.* (2004) Elongation of long-chain fatty acids. *Progr Lipid Res* **43,** 36–54.

Lillis, A.P., Van Duyn, L.B., Murphy-Ullrich, J.E., *et al.* (2008) LDL receptor-related protein 1: unique tissue-specific functions revealed by selective gene knockout studies. *Physiol Rev* **88,** 887–918.

Linton, M.F. and Fazio, S. (2001) Class A scavenger receptors, macrophages, and atherosclerosis. *Curr Opin Lipidol* **12,** 489–495.

Lohse, P., Chahrokh-Zadeh, S., and Seidel, D. (1997) Human lysosomal acid lipase/cholesteryl ester hydrolase and human gastric lipase: site-directed mutagenesis of Cys227 and Cys236 results in substrate-dependent reduction of enzymatic activity. *J Lipid Res* **38,** 1896–1905.

Marcil, M., O'Connell, B., Krimbou, L., *et al.* (2004) High-density lipoproteins: multifunctional vanguards of the cardiovascular system. *Exp Rev Cardiovasc Ther* **2,** 417–430.

Masson, D., Jiang, X.-C., Lagrost, L., *et al.* (2009) The role of plasma lipid transfer proteins in lipoprotein metabolism and atherogenesis. *J Lipid Res* **50** Suppl, S201–206.

May, P., Woldt, E., Matz, R.L., *et al.* (2007) The LDL receptor-related protein (LRP) family: an old family of proteins with new physiological functions. *Ann Med* **39,** 219–228.

Meagher, E.A. (2004) Addressing cardiovascular risk beyond low-density lipoprotein cholesterol: the high-density lipoprotein cholesterol story. *Curr Cardiol Rep* **6,** 457–463.

Meijer, G.W., Bressers, M.A., De Groot, W.A., *et al.* (2003) Effect of structure and form on the ability of plant sterols to inhibit cholesterol absorption in hamsters. *Lipids* **38,** 713–721.

Merkel, M., Eckel, R.H., and Goldberg, I.J. (2002) Lipoprotein lipase: genetics, lipid uptake, and regulation. *J Lipid Res* **43,** 1997–2006.

Miller, M., Rhyne, J., Hamlette, S., *et al.* (2003) Genetics of HDL regulation in humans. *Curr Opin Lipidol* **14,** 273–279.

Moestrup, S.K., Gliemann, J., and Pallesen, G. (1992) Distribution of the alpha 2-macroglobulin receptor/low density lipoprotein receptor-related protein in human tissues. *Cell Tissue Res* **269,** 375–382.

Morgan, J., Carey, C., Lincoff, A., *et al.* (2004) High-density lipoprotein subfractions and risk of coronary artery disease. *Curr Atheroscler Rep* **6,** 359–365.

Mu, H. and Hoy, C.E. (2004) The digestion of dietary triacylglycerols. *Progr Lipid Res* **43,** 105–133.

Navab, M., Ananthramaiah, G.M., Reddy, S.T., *et al.* (2004) The oxidation hypothesis of atherogenesis: the role of oxidized phospholipids and HDL. *J Lipid Res* **45,** 993–1007.

Navab, M., Yu, R., Gharavi, N., *et al.* (2007) High-density lipoprotein: antioxidant and anti-inflammatory properties. *Curr Atheroscler Rep* **9,** 244–248.

Nordskog, B.K., Phan, C.T., Nutting, D.F., *et al.* (2001) An examination of the factors affecting intestinal lymphatic transport of dietary lipids. *Adv Drug Deliv Rev* **50,** 21–44.

Olofsson, S.-O., Wiklund, O., and Boren, J. (2007) Apolipoproteins A-I and B: biosynthesis, role in the development of atherosclerosis and targets for intervention against cardiovascular disease. *Vasc Health Risk Manag* **3,** 491–502.

Oram, J.F. (2002) ATP-binding cassette transporter A1 and cholesterol trafficking. *Curr Opin Lipidol* **13,** 373–381.

Pafumi, Y., Lairon, D., De la Porte, P.L., *et al.* (2002) Mechanisms of inhibition of triacylglycerol hydrolysis by human gastric lipase. *J Biol Chem* **277,** 28070–28079.

Plourde, M., Jew, S., Cunnane, S.C., *et al.* (2008) Conjugated linoleic acids: why the discrepancy between animal and human studies? *Nutr Rev* **66,** 415–421.

Redgrave, T.G. (2004) Chylomicron metabolism. *Biochem Soc Trans* **32,** 79–82.

Rudel, L.L., Lee, R.G., and Cockman, T.L. (2001) Acyl coenzyme A: cholesterol acyltransferase types 1 and 2: structure and function in atherosclerosis. *Curr Opin Lipidol* **12,** 121–127.

Rudkowska, I. and Jones, P.J.H. (2008) Polymorphisms in ABCG5/G8 transporters linked to hypercholesterolemia and gallstone disease. *Nutr Rev* **66,** 343–348.

Saito, H., Lund-Katz, S., and Phillips, M.C. (2004) Contributions of domain structure and lipid interaction to the functionality of exchangeable human apolipoproteins. *Progr Lipid Res* **43,** 350–380.

Sehayek, E. (2003) Genetic regulation of cholesterol absorption and plasma plant sterol levels: commonalities and differences. *J Lipid Res* **44,** 2030–2038.

Shachter, N.S. (2001) Apolipoproteins C-I and C-III as important modulators of lipoprotein metabolism. *Curr Opin Lipidol* **12,** 297–304.

Spence, J.D. (2010) The role of lipoprotein(a) in the formation of arterial plaques, stenoses and occlusions. *Can J Cardiol* **26** Suppl A, 37A–40A.

Stein, Y. and Stein, O. (2003) Lipoprotein lipase and atherosclerosis. *Atherosclerosis* **170**, 1–9.

Sudhop, T., Lutjohann, D., Agna, M., *et al.* (2003) Comparison of the effects of sitostanol, sitostanol acetate, and sitostanol oleate on the inhibition of cholesterol absorption in normolipemic healthy male volunteers. A placebo controlled randomized cross-over study. *Arzneimittel-Forsch* **53**, 708–713.

Szapary, P.O. and Rader, D.J. (2004) The triglyceride-high-density lipoprotein axis: an important target of therapy? *Am Heart J* **148**, 211–221.

Talati, R., Sobieraj, D.M., Makanji, S.S., *et al.* (2010) The comparative efficacy of plant sterols and stanols on serum lipids: a systematic review and meta-analysis. *J Am Diet Assoc* **110**, 719–726.

Tall, A.R. (1998) An overview of reverse cholesterol transport. *Eur Heart J* **19** Suppl A, A31–35.

Taskinen, M.R. (2003) LDL-cholesterol, HDL-cholesterol or triglycerides–which is the culprit? *Diabetes Res Clin Pract* **61** Suppl 1, S19–26.

Tessari, P., Coracina, A., Cosma, A., *et al.* (2009) Hepatic lipid metabolism and non-alcoholic fatty liver disease. *Nutr Metab Cardiovasc Dis* **19**, 291–302.

Tso, P. and Liu, M. (2004) Ingested fat and satiety. *Physiol Behav* **81**, 275–287.

Tziomalos, K., Athyros, V.G., Wierzbicki, A.S., *et al.* (2009) Lipoprotein a: where are we now? *Curr Opin Cardiol* **24**, 351–357.

Van Berkel, T.J., Van Eck, M., Herijgers, N., *et al.* (2000) Scavenger receptor classes A and B. Their roles in atherogenesis and the metabolism of modified LDL and HDL. *Ann NY Acad Sci* **902**, 113–126; discussion 126–127.

Wang, J., Williams, C.M., and Hegele, R.A. (2004) Compound heterozygosity for two non-synonymous polymorphisms in NPC1L1 in a non-responder to ezetimibe. *Clin Genet* **67**, 175–177.

Whitcomb, D.C. and Lowe, M.E. (2007) Human pancreatic digestive enzymes. *Digestive Dis Sci* **52**, 1–17.

White, D.A., Bennett, A.J., Billett, M.A., *et al.* (1998) The assembly of triacylglycerol-rich lipoproteins: an essential role for the microsomal triacylglycerol transfer protein. *Br J Nutr* **80**, 219–229.

White, D.A., Morris, A.J., Burgess, L., *et al.* (2004) Facilitators and barriers to improving the quality of referrals for potential oral cancer. *Br Dental J* **197**, 537–540.

White, M.D., Papamandjaris, A.A., and Jones, P.J. (1999) Enhanced postprandial energy expenditure with medium-chain fatty acid feeding is attenuated after 14 d in premenopausal women. *Am J Clin Nutr* **69**, 883–889.

Wijendran, V. and Hayes, K.C. (2004) Dietary n-6 and n-3 fatty acid balance and cardiovascular health. *Annu Rev Nutr* **24**, 597–615.

Williams, C.M., Bateman, P.A., Jackson, K.G., *et al.* (2004) Dietary fatty acids and chylomicron synthesis and secretion. *Biochem Soc Trans* **32**, 55–58.

Wilund, K.R., Yu, L., Xu, F., *et al.* (2004) High-level expression of ABCG5 and ABCG8 attenuates diet-induced hypercholesterolemia and atherosclerosis in Ldlr-/- mice. *J Lipid Res* **45**, 1429–1436.

Wirtz, K.W.A. (2006) Phospholipid transfer proteins in perspective. *FEBS Lett* **580**, 5436–5441.

Zambon, A., Bertocco, S., Vitturi, N., *et al.* (2003) Relevance of hepatic lipase to the metabolism of triacylglycerol-rich lipoproteins. *Biochem Soc Trans* **31**, 1070–1074.

10

LIPIDS: CELLULAR METABOLISM

PETER J.H. JONES[1], PhD AND ANDREA A. PAPAMANDJARIS[2], PhD

[1]*University of Manitoba, Winnipeg, Manitoba, Canada*
[2]*Nestlé Inc., North York, Ontario, Canada*

Summary

The biology and essentiality of fatty acids and other lipids have been well established. Similarly, structural roles for and cellular pathways of lipids have been clearly defined. Given the diversity of fatty acids across edible oils, the role of dietary fatty acid selection in subsequent cellular structure–function and its downstream implications for disease risk reduction are being increasingly recognized. Recently, focus has shifted to the development of functional foods that incorporate essential fatty acids and other lipids to offer added health benefits to consumers. Overall, research suggests that dietary lipid selection plays a central role in the prevention and development of several important chronic diseases.

Introduction

The objective of this chapter is to provide a general overview of dietary control of lipid metabolism, emphasizing cellular regulatory processes and dietary fatty acid requirements. The discovery of the importance of lipids in healthy nutrition has been a process spanning the twentieth century. Before the 1920s, it was believed that fat did not play an essential dietary role if sufficient vitamins and minerals were in the diet. However, in 1927, Evans and Burr demonstrated that animals fed semi-purified, fat-free diets had impaired growth and reproductive failure (Evans and Burr, 1927). This demonstration that fat was required for health led these authors to postulate that fat contained a new essential substance, which they called vitamin F. Subsequently, Burr and Burr (1929) documented the nutritional essentiality of a specific essential component of fat, linoleic acid (C18:2n-6). In the absence of this nutrient, symptoms developed, including scaliness of the skin, water retention, impaired fertility, and growth retardation (Evans and Burr, 1927; Burr and Burr, 1929, 1930). Thus, the concept of "essential" fatty acids was introduced to represent those dietary fatty acids required by mammals that are not synthesized in vivo.

Fatty acids are classified as essential based on the position of the first double bond from the methyl end of the acyl chain. Mammals do not possess enzymes that are able to synthesize double bonds at the n-6 and n-3 positions of the carbon chain of a fatty acid. Therefore, humans must obtain the essential fatty acids, linoleic acid and α-linolenic acid (C18:3n-3), and their chain-elongated derivatives, from dietary sources. Specific amounts of

Present Knowledge in Nutrition, Tenth Edition. Edited by John W. Erdman Jr, Ian A. Macdonald and Steven H. Zeisel.
© 2012 International Life Sciences Institute. Published 2012 by John Wiley & Sons, Inc.

essential fatty acids required for optimal growth and development are provided later in this chapter.

Identification of the dietary importance of essential fatty acids in humans followed discovery of their importance in animals. Beginning in 1958, studies in infants using skim-milk-based, fat-free diets demonstrated a requirement for essential fatty acids in humans when the introduction of linoleic acid into the diet alleviated skin symptoms (Hansen et al., 1958). In human adults, the use of fat-free parenteral solutions containing only glucose, amino acids, and micronutrients resulted in clinical fatty acid deficiency, which was reversed by the inclusion of linoleic acid in the solution. In the 1970s, dietary deficiency of n-3 fatty acids was linked to abnormal electroretinographic recordings in animals (Futterman et al., 1971; Wheeler et al., 1975). A human n-3 fatty acid requirement was demonstrated in 1982, when deficiency symptoms, including neuropathy, were linked to a parenteral solution deficient in n-3 fatty acids in a young girl (Holman et al., 1982). Symptoms were reversed with the addition of n-3 fatty acids to the solution.

Recent essential fatty acid research has focused on the importance of the dietary ratio of linoleic acid to α-linolenic acid, particularly as it is related to the development of disease (Stanley et al., 2007; Simopoulos, 2009; Harris, 2010). Characterization of dietary needs of individual long-chain polyunsaturated fatty acids, arachidonic acid (ARA) (C20:4n-6), docosahexaenoic acid (DHA) (C22:6n-3), and eicosapentaenoic acid (EPA) (C20:5n-3), is also under investigation, notably in infant populations (Koletzko et al., 2008; Ramakrishnan et al., 2009; Makrides et al., 2010). Additionally, the evolutionary importance of DHA in human brain development has been stressed (Cunnane and Crawford, 2003).

Recent studies show that some polyunsaturated fatty acids play a role in regulating gene expression involved in lipid and energy metabolism. α-Linolenic acid regulates transcription factors such as peroxisome proliferator-activated receptors (PPARs). These transcription factors are important in modulating the expression of genes controlling both systemic and tissue-specific lipid homeostasis and membrane composition (Sampath and Ntambi, 2005).

In addition to their important roles in membrane phospholipids and as energy sources, polyunsaturated fatty acids are required in the formation of metabolic regulators called eicosanoids. Eicosanoids, as a class of diverse components, function in cardiovascular, pulmonary, immune, secretory, and regulatory systems. The discovery of the unique properties of eicosanoids dates back to the 1930s, when the effect of seminal fluid on the relaxation of the uterus was documented. After further research, Von Euler (1967) characterized the active lipid-soluble compound, naming it prostaglandin. In the 1960s, prostaglandin E1 and prostaglandin F1a were isolated from sheep prostate glands (Bergstrom and Sjovall, 1960a,b). Characterization of other prostaglandins followed (Baker, 1990). The biologically active compounds derived from 20-carbon unsaturated fatty acids were classified as eicosanoids in 1979 (Baker, 1990). The effects and mechanisms of eicosanoids in health and disease represent the focus of active, ongoing investigation. These and additional aspects of essential fatty acid research are leading to a better understanding of their role in human nutrition and health.

Dietary Sources of Lipids

Lipids are found in a variety of foods (Table 10.1; see also Table 9.1 in Chapter 9, "Lipids: Absorption and Transport," for fatty acid formulas). Butter is a source of short-chain fatty acids. Medium-chain fatty acids are found in coconut oil. Meat contains longer-chain saturates and monounsaturates, whereas vegetable oils are major dietary sources of essential fatty acids and other unsaturated fatty acids. The fatty acid profile of vegetable oils varies widely, and therefore different oils have different proportions of linoleic acid and α-linolenic acid. Safflower, sunflower, corn, and soybean oils are high in linoleic acid, yet, of these, only soybean oil is a significant source of α-linolenic acid. Flaxseed, linseed, and canola oils are also high in α-linolenic acid but relatively low in linoleic acid. Olive and canola oils have a higher content of monounsaturated oleic acid. Consequently, the consumption of specific vegetable oils as a sole dietary fat source can lead to a deficiency of essential fatty acids. Long-chain polyenoic fatty acids, products of intracellular elongation and desaturation of essential fatty acids, are not present in vegetable oils but are found in some animal products, as well as algae. Particularly, high-fat fish and marine mammals contain larger amounts of long-chain n-3 fatty acids, EPA and DHA. The longer-chain n-6 fatty acids, such as arachidonic acid, are found in foods of animal origin, including organ meats. Smaller quantities of very long chain fatty acids (VLCFAs) and alcohols (more than 24 carbons) are found in plant-derived foods. Cholesterol is found only in

TABLE 10.1 Average triacylglycerol fatty acid composition of various foods and oils

Food	Average fat %	Total[a]	Saturated			Mono- and polyunsaturated		
			16:00	18:00	18:1n-9	18:2n-6	18:3n-3	20:4n-6
Almond oil	100	8	6	1	65	23	Trace	–
Avocado oil	100	11	10	1	67	15	–	–
Beef tallow	100	53	29	20	42	2	Trace	–
Butter	81	53	22	10	20	3	0.3	–
Canola	100	7	4	2	62	19	9	–
Cashew nut	68	24	14	10	30	35	Trace	–
Coconut oil	100	88[a]	10	3	6	2	–	–
Corn oil	100	13	11	2	25	55	Trace	–
Cottonseed oil	100	30	25	3	18	51	Trace	–
Flaxseed oil	100	9	5	4	20	13	53	–
Grapeseed oil	100	11	7	4	20	68	Trace	–
Groundnut oil	100	19[†]	11	3	40–55[b]	20–43[b]	–	–
Hazelnut oil	100	7	5	2	80	11	Trace	–
Hemp oil	100	9	6	3	13	55	16[c]	–
Herring (menhaden)	16–25	30	19	4	13	1	1[d]	–
Mackerel	25	25	17	5	18	1	–	–
Milk (cow's)	3.5	65[a]	25	11	26	1–3	2	Trace
Olive oil	100	17	14	3	71	10	Trace	–
Palm kernel oil	100	80[a]	7	2	14	1	–	–
Palm oil	100	52	45	5	38	10	–	–
Pork fat (lard)	100	42	28	13	46	6–8	2	2
Rapeseed oil	100	7	5	2	53	22	10[e]	–
Safflower seed oil	100	10	7	3	15[f]	75[f]	Trace	–
Salmon	13	3	2	0.5	3	0.2	Trace	Trace
Sesame oil	100	15	9	5	39	40	1	–
Soybean oil	100	15	11	4	23	51	7	–
Sunflower seed oil	100	12	6	4	24	60–70	Trace	–
Tuna	5	1	0.1	0.3	1	Trace	–	Trace
Walnut	63	10	7	2	15	60	10	–
Wheatgerm oil	100	18	17	Trace	17	55	6	–

Note: The percentages given are approximations because climate, species, fodder composition, etc., cause great variations. Trace, 1% detected.

–, Non-detectable amount.

[a]The balance of saturated fatty acids is formed by fatty acids with chain length 12 (butter 14%) and chain lengths of 12 and 14 (butter 16%, coconut and palm kernel 65–70%).

[b]~4% of C20:0 and C22:0; groundnuts from Argentina have relatively low C18:1 and high C18:2 concentrations.

[c]Also contains 18:3n-6.

[d]Menhaden herring oil has 11% C20:5n-3 and 9% C22:6n-3, but Norwegian herring oil has 13% C20:1n-9, 21% C22:1n-11, 7% C20:5n-3, and 7% C22:6n-3. Depending on fishing grounds, mackerel oil is similar to menhaden or to Norwegian/North Sea herring.

[e]Contrary to new rapeseed varieties like canola and low erucic acid rapeseed (LEAR), old varieties of rapeseed oil as well as mustard seed oil have 10% C20:1n-9 and 30–50% C22:1n-9.

[f]Safflower seed oil with the reverse C18:1/18:2 composition is also available.

products of animal origin, while phytosterols (or plant sterols) occur in plant oils.

Recently, focus has shifted to the development of functional foods that incorporate essential fatty acids and other lipids to offer added healthful benefits to consumers. Examples include bakery products made with flaxseed oil, eggs containing marine n-3 fatty acids, and spreads incorporating phytosterols, or their saturated derivatives, phytostanols. Additionally, foods that require oil during preparation are currently made with vegetable-based oils, such as high-oleic vegetable oils, rather than with oils that are animal-based, thereby decreasing the amount of saturated and/or trans fats incorporated in the diet.

Cellular Roles of Lipids

Lipid constituents are required for a diverse array of cellular processes, including structure, function, and energy-related roles. Polyenoic fatty acids provide the hydrophobic moiety of phospholipids, which are critical for membrane structure and serve as precursors for eicosanoids, which regulate cellular activity. Fatty acids also play a pivotal role in providing fuel for adenosine triphosphate (ATP) and reducing equivalents and in generating body heat. Fat contains more than twice the energy per gram (9 kcal/g) as does carbohydrate or protein (4 kcal/g), which explains why humans preferentially store fat as the primary energy reservoir. Dietary lipids are also a source of lipid-soluble vitamins and sterols. Although not essential in the diet, cholesterol is needed as an integral component of membranes to increase their fluidity. Cholesterol is also converted to bile salts through hepatic hydroxylation and conjugation. Bile salts are required for normal digestion and absorption of dietary lipids. Additionally, cholesterol serves as a precursor for steroid-based hormone systems, including sex and adrenocorticoid hormones. Cholesterol, as 7-dehydrocholesterol, exists as the precursor of vitamin D, formed at the skin surface through the action of ultraviolet irradiation. Approximately 50 mg of cholesterol is converted to steroid hormones daily.

To ensure normal cellular function, an elaborate system of control regulates lipid biosynthesis, oxidation, and intracellular trafficking. This homeostatic regulatory system ensures that pathways of lipid anabolism and catabolism mesh with those of other macronutrients. Dominating this regulatory system is the ability of dietary lipid selection to modulate several key metabolic pathways. For example, the fatty acid composition of the diet alters the composition of membrane phospholipids, which in turn changes membrane functions. Similarly, the blend of dietary fatty acids substantially alters adipose tissue fatty acid profiles (Field *et al.*, 1985). Dietary fatty acid selection also modulates cellular synthesis of regulatory eicosanoids, influencing a series of physiological responses. Similarly, alterations in cholesterol or phytosterol intake modulate cholesterol synthesis, absorption, and subsequent metabolism. Consequently, the metabolism of fatty acids, sterols, and their derivatives responds to manipulation in dietary lipid intakes in many important ways. To appreciate the link between dietary lipid consumption and disease risk modification, it is important to individually consider the fundamental processes of cellular lipid metabolism.

Lipid Biosynthesis

Fatty Acid Synthesis

Fatty acids are synthesized *de novo* from acetyl coenzyme A (CoA) in the extramitochondrial space by a group of enzymes classified as fatty acid synthetases. The synthesis of fatty acids is governed by the enzyme acetyl CoA carboxylase, which converts acetyl CoA to malonyl CoA. A series of malonyl CoA units are added to the growing fatty acid chain to culminate in the formation of palmitic acid (C16:0). From this point, more complex fatty acids can be formed through elongation and desaturation; however, humans do not possess the enzymes capable of inserting points of unsaturation at sites below the n-7 carbon, making the n-6 and the n-3 fatty acids essential (see Chapter 9, "Lipids: Absorption and Transport," for a discussion of nomenclature). Desaturase enzymes are membrane bound and occur in the endoplasmic reticulum of several tissues. Desaturases are specific for the position of the double bond in the carbon chain and require electrons supplied by nicotinamide adenine dinucleotide (NADH) or nicotinamide adenine dinucleotide phosphate (NADPH), which are catalyzed by cytochrome b5.

Longer-chain fatty acids are synthesized from C16:0, C18:0, C18:2n-6, and C18:3n-3 by alternating desaturation and elongation. The synthesis of C20:4n-6 from C18:2n-6 and of C20:5n-3 from C18:3n-3 is achieved through D6 desaturation followed by elongation and D5 desaturation (Figure 10.1). The synthesis of C22:6n-3 from C20:5n-3 occurs through elongation, desaturation, and partial α-oxidation (Catalá, 2010). It was recently demonstrated that fatty acid elongation need not

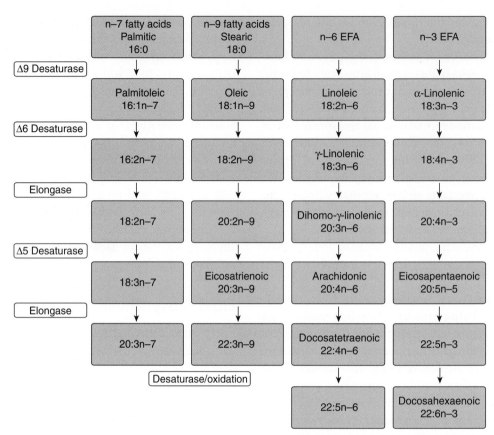

FIG. 10.1   Interconversions of non-essential and essential fatty acids. EFA, essential fatty acid.

commence with 18-carbon precursors. To meet n-6 fatty acid requirements, it is possible to use C16:2n-6, derived from plant materials, in place of linoleic acid, thereby effectively reducing the requirement for the latter fatty acid (Cunnane, 2003). The extent to which this pathway contributes substantially to in vivo linoleic acid levels remains to be assessed.

The synthesis of longer-chain fatty acids has been shown to be regulated by the D6 desaturase enzyme, which in turn is influenced by hormones and dietary constituents. The D6 desaturase preferentially targets the most highly unsaturated fatty acid; the preferential desaturation order is therefore C18:3n-3 > C18:2n-6 > C18:1n-9. As such, the competitive nature of the fatty acid desaturation and elongation among the three classes of fatty acids (Figure 10.1) has nutritional implications. The consumption of diets rich in n-6 fatty acids can result in suppression of the elongation and desaturation of C18:3n-3 to C20:5n-3 and C22:6n-3. An example of this situation is infant formulas, in which high ratios of C18:2n-6 to C18:3n-3 potentially depress the production of important n-3 poly-

enoic fatty acids required for the developing nervous system. Alternatively, changing prostaglandin profiles through elevated intakes of n-3 fatty acids such as EPA and DHA from fish and fish oils can decrease the clotting capacity of blood. Hormonal shifts may also perturb desaturase activity: insulin increases, but glucagon and epinephrine decrease, desaturase enzyme activity (El-Badry et al., 2007).

Reversal of the elongation and desaturation process may also occur intracellularly. Very long chain and long chain n-3 and n-6 fatty acids may undergo shortening and saturation through retroconversion to other, shorter, fatty acids (Mebarek et al., 2009). This process occurs in peroxisomes and is probably necessary for some, if not all, of the endogenous synthesis of DHA in animals (Catalá, 2010).

Cholesterol Biosynthesis

Cholesterol is synthesized in almost all human tissues in a process that possesses more than 20 steps; indeed, the pathway is one of the longest of any lipid produced intracellularly. Humans likely once relied extensively on endogenously produced cholesterol for cellular requirements, as ancestral daily dietary intakes have been estimated at as low as 50 mg. However, today, most people consume diets in which the dietary intake of cholesterol and fat is increased such that cholesterogenesis is less relied on to serve cellular cholesterol needs. Unlike animals, humans appear to synthesize most cholesterol in extrahepatic tissues. The total body pool of cholesterol is estimated to be 75 g. Of the 1200 mg cholesterol turned over daily, 300 to 500 mg is absorbed from the diet, and de novo synthesis accounts for 700 to 900 mg (Dietschy, 1984). How synthesis is coordinated across tissues remains to be defined.

As with fatty acids, the process of cholesterol synthesis begins with acetyl CoA generated through the oxidative decarboxylation of pyruvate or the oxidation of fatty acids. In the initial phase of the pathway, acetyl CoA molecules combine to form mevalonic acid. The final enzyme of this initial phase, hydroxymethylglutaryl (HMG) CoA reductase, is considered to be rate limiting in the overall cascade of cholesterogenesis and has been studied widely in relation to pathway control. In fact, statin drugs, currently the most widespread pharmacological intervention to lower cholesterol levels, work through inhibition of HMG CoA reductase. The later phase of cholesterol biosynthesis involves steps of phosphorylation, isomerization, and conversion to geranyl-B and farnesyl-pyrophosphate, which in turn form squalene (Figure 10.2). From the squalene stage, loss of three methyl groups, side-chain saturation, and bond rearrangement result in the formation of cholesterol.

Diet modulates cholesterol biosynthesis in several ways. Curiously, it is a common misconception that high levels of dietary cholesterol increase circulating levels of cholesterol; however, total and low-density lipoprotein (LDL) cholesterol levels as well as cholesterol biosynthesis are minimally affected by even sizable increases in dietary cholesterol concentration (Jones *et al.*, 1996; Greene *et al.*, 2005). Conversely, qualitative dietary fat intake more substantially perturbs the rate of cholesterol biosynthesis and circulating lipid levels. In particular, dietary polyunsaturated fat intake enhances (Jones, 1997), whereas trans fatty acid intake suppresses (Matthan *et al.*, 2000), cholesterol biosynthesis. Despite this observed effect of trans fatty acids on cholesterol synthesis, overall these fats lower HDL and raise LDL cholesterol levels (Mozaffarian *et al.*, 2006). Increasing the number of meals consumed per day, while holding total caloric intake constant, has also been shown to reduce cholesterol biosynthesis rates (Jones, 1997). Of the dietary factors capable of modifying cholesterol syn-

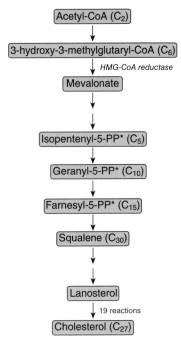

FIG. 10.2 Stages of cholesterol biosynthesis.

thesis, energy restriction has the greatest effect. Humans who fast for 24 hours exhibit complete cessation of cholesterol biosynthesis (Jones, 1997). How synthesis responds to more minor energy imbalances has not been examined; however, substantial suppression of human de novo cholesterogenesis has been demonstrated with even modest levels of energy restriction and weight loss (Di Buono *et al.*, 1999).

Fatty Acid Oxidation

Fatty acid oxidation generates acetyl CoA and occurs through β-oxidation, predominantly in mitochondria. During this process, the fatty acyl chain undergoes cyclical degradation through four stages, including dehydrogenation (removal of hydrogen), hydration (addition of water), dehydrogenation, and cleavage. At points of unsaturation within the acyl chain, the initial dehydration step does not take place. The four-stage oxidation process is repeated until the fatty acid is completely degraded to acetyl CoA, as shown by the absence of chain-shortened n-3 or n-6 fatty acids within cells or in the bloodstream. Fatty acids containing 18 carbons or fewer enter the mitochondria as fatty acyl CoA through transport by carnitine. Short- and medium-chain fatty acids do not require the presence of the carnitine shuttle to enter the mitochondria for oxidation.

Beta-oxidation also occurs in peroxisomes through a similar, but not identical, process that is tailored to the oxidation of long-chain fatty acids with more than 18 carbons. Also, the initial desaturation reaction in peroxisomal oxidation occurs via a fatty acyl CoA oxidase, whereas an acyl CoA dehydrogenase is the first enzyme in the mitochondrial pathway. Last, peroxisomal β-oxidation is not tightly linked to the electron transfer chain. Thus, in peroxisomes, electrons produced during the initial stage of oxidation transfer directly to molecular oxygen. This oxygen generates hydrogen peroxide that is degraded to water by catalase. The energy produced in the second oxidation step is conserved in the form of the high energy level electrons of NADH. Without β-oxidation in peroxisomes, abnormal accumulation of VLCFAs will ensue in plasma and different tissues, leading to peroxisomal disorders such as Zellweger syndrome (ZS) and adrenoleukodystrophy (Fidaleo, 2010).

Evidence is emerging that the rate of fatty acid oxidation is not identical across all chain lengths and degrees of unsaturation, but exhibits structural specificity. For decades it has been suggested that short- and medium-chain saturated fatty acids undergo more rapid combustion for energy compared with long-chain fatty acids, probably because of the preferential transport of the former linked to albumin through the portal circulation and the lack of need for carnitine to enter the mitochondria (Papamandjaris et al., 1998).

In addition, the notion that more highly unsaturated long-chain fatty acids are preferentially oxidized has also received some support (DeLany et al., 2000), although this concept is paradoxical given the essentiality of these highly unsaturated polyunsaturated fatty acids. Intriguingly, carbon from oxidized linoleic and α-linolenic acid is extensively recycled into de novo synthesis of long-chain fatty acids and cholesterol. This pathway is particularly evident in the brain during early development (Cunnane et al., 2003), but is quantitatively important even when intake of these parent polyunsaturates is severely deficient (Cunnane et al., 2006).

In addition to the effect exerted by the type of fatty acid consumed, variations in the metabolic state also influence the rate of fat oxidation. Conditions such as fasting and exercise at moderate intensity result in increased lipolysis and oxidation (Achten and Jeukendrup, 2004; Solomon et al., 2008). With respect to substrates and hormones, raised glucose and insulin levels suppress fatty acid oxidation (Wolfe, 1998).

Eicosanoid Production and Regulation

Structurally, as oxygenated 20-carbon derivatives from the n-3 and n-6 family of fatty acids, eicosanoid members include prostaglandins, thromboxanes, leukotrienes, hydroxy acids, and lipoxins. The production of specific categories of eicosanoids is governed by fast-acting and rapidly inactivated enzyme systems. Whereas prostaglandins and thromboxanes are generated via cyclooxygenase (COX) enzymes, leukotrienes, hydroxy acids, and lipoxins are produced through the action of lipoxygenase (LOX) enzymes. Major pathways for eicosanoid synthesis are depicted in Figure 10.3. The process begins with the action of phospholipase A2 on cell-membrane phospholipids, splitting off fatty acids from the sn-2 position of the molecule. All membrane phospholipid species serve as substrates in the cleavage process; the resultant cleaved fatty acids serve directly as substrates for eicosanoid production via the cyclooxygenase and lipoxygenase enzyme cascades. With respect to the n-6 series, cleaved arachidonic acid is transformed to prostaglandins by prostaglandin H synthase-1 (PGHSB1) and prostaglandin H synthase-2 (PGHSB2). These enzymes catalyze the conversion of arachidonic acid to prostaglandin G2 (PGG2) via a cyclooxygenase reaction, and then the reduction of PGG2 to PGH2 via a peroxidase reaction. This latter intermediate then undergoes rapid conversion to other active forms of prostaglandins, thromboxanes, or prostacyclins. As an alternative pathway, arachidonic acid undergoes oxidation via a series of LOX enzymes to form a series of active eicosanoids. The 5-LOX pathway generates leukotrienes B4, C4, and D4 (LTB4, LTC4, and LTD4), which are believed to serve as mediators in the immune response. The 12-LOX pathway generates 12-L-hydroxyeicosatetranoic acid (12-HETE) and 12-hydroperoxyeicosatetranoic acid (12-HPETE), which are also involved in the inflammatory response. The action of a third LOX reaction pathway, 15-LOX, results in the formation of 15-hydroeicosatetranoic acid (15-HETE), which possesses anti-inflammatory actions and may inhibit the activities of both 5-LOX and 12-LOX. Thus, several eicosanoid subtypes may be generated from arachidonic acid intracellularly.

Eicosanoids are also derived from the n-3 series of fatty acids cleaved from membrane phospholipids. Eicosanoids derived from n-3 fatty acids evoke less-active responses than do those of the corresponding n-6 eicosanoids. Thus, PGE3 formed from EPA possesses less inflammatory action than does PGE2 formed from arachidonic acid.

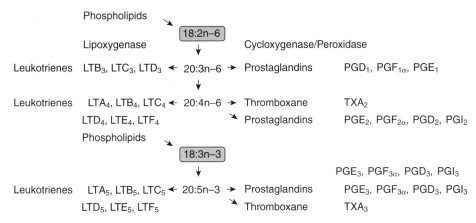

FIG. 10.3 Synthesis of major eicosanoids from n-6 and n-3 fatty acids.

Similarly, LTB5 derived from EPA is less active in the proinflammatory response than is LTB4, which is produced from arachidonic acid. On these bases, the two classes of eicosanoids compete, evoking opposing biological actions.

Dietary fatty acid composition has been shown to play an important role in eicosanoid-mediated function. The consumption of diets high in n-3-rich fats produces higher levels of n-3 fatty acids in phospholipids. These fatty acids, when cleaved from phospholipids, compete with arachidonic acid for incorporation into eicosanoids. The enhanced bleeding times observed in Inuit populations who consume higher levels of n-3 fatty-acid-containing fish reflect the shift from n-6- to n-3-based eicosanoid formation. PGI3, produced from EPA, has anti-aggregatory action. The prolonged bleeding times in individuals consuming high amounts of n-3 fatty-acid-containing marine-based foods are believed to be mediated through such anti-aggregatory action of n-3-based eicosanoids. Conversely, eicosanoid overproduction from arachidonic acid, a result of diets poor in n-3 fatty acids, may result in a number of disorders associated with the inflammatory and immune systems, including thrombosis, arthritis, lupus, and cancer (see section on dietary fatty acids and disease risk). For instance, arthritic patients appear to benefit from increasing their intake of fish oil (Calder, 2009a), likely to be due to the inhibition by n-3 fatty acids of the production of the proinflammatory eicosanoids LTB4 and PGE2. The demonstration that dietary fatty acid selection may modulate physiological function through eicosanoid generation underscores the impor-

tance of food selection in the prevention and treatment of disease.

Dietary Requirements for Fatty Acids

The USDA recommends 20–35% of the daily food intake should come from fat. Currently, dietary recommendations for omega-3 fatty acids are 1.6 g/day for men and 1.1 g/day for women, whereas omega-6 fatty acids recommendations are 17 g/day for men and 12 g/day for women (Institute of Medicine 2002/2005). These values were established based on the levels of fatty acids required to prevent or alleviate essential fatty acid deficiency. Deficiency symptoms were documented when patients were fed total parenteral nutrition solutions devoid of essential fatty acids in the 1960s. Skin irritations that developed during fat-free diets were alleviated when patients were fed solutions containing linoleic acid (Hansen *et al.*, 1958). Recent evidence indicates that pure linoleate deficiency, in contrast to general unsaturated fatty acid deficiency categorized previously, can be reversed with as little as 2% of dietary energy fed as linoleic acid in the rat (Cunnane, 2003). For α-linolenic acid, classification of deficiency symptoms has been difficult, since related deficiencies are more subtle than those found with linoleic acid. Also, pure deficiencies are hard to induce because symptoms may remain absent in the presence of DHA.

Based on essential fatty acid metabolism, an indicator for essential fatty acid deficiency is the triene-to-tetraene ratio, which assesses the ratio of C20:3n-9 to C20:4n-6. The triene, C20:3n-9, is the product of the desaturation of C18:1n-9 to C20:3n-9 (Figure 10.1). Because of the affinity of the D6 desaturase for essential fatty acids more than 16 carbons in length, triene concentrations increase only during essential fatty acid deficiency, when C16:0 and C18:1n-9 are the major substrates available. A triene-to-tetraene ratio above 0.4 indicates essential fatty acid deficiency. However, the ratio is not specific to deficiency of linoleic or α-linolenic acid. To assess for α–linolenic deficiency, the ratio of DPA (n-6) to DHA can be a valuable index, because the absence of n-3 fatty acids results in the increased formation of n-6 elongation and desaturation products.

As the roles of essential fatty acids and their products in the achievement and maintenance of optimal health are further elucidated through research, dietary recommendations may be set on the basis of health promotion rather than on the avoidance of deficiency. An example is the recognition of the contribution of the ratio of linoleic acid to α-linolenic acid in the diet to a healthy essential fatty acid profile. The competitive desaturation of n-3, n-6, and n-9 fatty acids by D6 desaturase is of major significance consistent with this rationale. If α-linolenic acid is lacking in the diet or if there is a large amount of linoleic acid present, EPA production will become elevated and little or no DHA will be produced. If both essential fatty acids are lacking, C20:3n-9 will accumulate. Inhibition of arachidonic acid and DHA production achieved through high levels of linoleic acid or essential fatty acid deficiency may be undesirable, based on the metabolic functions of these compounds and their roles in disease onset and progression (see below).

Beginning in the 1920s, the levels of linoleic acid in the Western diet have been increasing and the levels of α-linolenic acid have been decreasing (Uauy et al., 1999; Simopoulos, 2009). Estimates of the current ratio of linoleic to α-linolenic acid in North America range from 9.8:1 to 15:1 to 30:1 (Kris-Etherton et al., 2000; Simopoulos, 2008). A ratio of 2:1 to 5:1 is currently recommended (Holman, 1998; Kris-Etherton et al., 2000; Simopoulos, 2008), with the World Health Organization (WHO, 1994) recommended level at 5:1 to 10:1. Achieving this recommended ratio would require a reversal in the trend of fatty acid consumption, with the inclusion of greater amounts of n-3 fatty acids from plant and marine oils in tandem with the consumption of lower amounts of n-6 fatty acids from seed oil in the diet. The consequences of the long-term consumption of a high ratio of n-6 to n-3 fatty acids are being studied and will

provide further insight into healthy dietary essential fatty acid levels. At present, arachidonic acid and DHA are not considered essential to a healthy adult diet, unless the capacity for desaturation and elongation of essential fatty acids is compromised.

Dietary essential fatty acid requirements in infants are being widely investigated, because there might be a need to provide not only essential fatty acids, but arachidonic acid and DHA as well. Preterm infants, depending on age at birth, may not receive an intrauterine supply of arachidonic acid and DHA (Lapillonne and Jensen, 2009) and, if formula fed, may not receive arachidonic acid and DHA, but only 18-carbon essential fatty acids. Recently, conventional infant formulas have been produced that contain added DHA and ARA. DHA and ARA are often added at levels concurrent with the WHO (1994) guidelines, which are based on international levels of DHA and ARA in breast milk (Innis, 2007). Because both brain and retina have high levels of DHA, it has been hypothesized that DHA in breast milk may confer a developmental advantage to both term and preterm infants, as has been reported with breast feeding (Lucas et al., 1994; Michaelsen et al., 2009). These findings have been somewhat supported by the results of clinical intervention studies, in which direct supplementation of formula with n-3 fatty acids resulted in improvements in development-associated parameters (Neuringer et al., 2000; Uauy et al., 2003; Fleith and Clandinin, 2005). Without the inclusion of arachidonic acid and DHA, there may not be sufficient capacity to convert essential fatty acids into arachidonic acid and, more specifically, into DHA to meet requirements for brain and visual function (Cunnane, et al., 2000). Results in preterm infants have demonstrated evidence that DHA supplementation may affect visual acuity and development (Lapillonne et al., 2000; Uauy et al., 2000; Agostoni, 2008; Henriksen et al., 2008), but not all studies show positive benefits (Simmer and Patole, 2004). A recent review of the clinical trials published to date in preterm infants has concluded that the long-term benefits of DHA and ARA formula supplementation have yet to be demonstrated (Simmer et al., 2008b). For infants born at term, research has demonstrated that formula supplementation with DHA may (Larque et al., 2002; Hoffman et al., 2003, 2009; Birch et al., 2005, 2010; Eilander et al., 2007) or may not (Simmer et al., 2008a; Beyerlein et al., 2010) affect development, and that any effect may disappear over time (Agostoni et al., 1995, 1997). No differences were reported in age-appropriate tests of receptive and expressive language, IQ, visual or motor function, or visual acuity in infants at 39 months who had either been breast-fed or formula-fed with formula that either did or did not contain DHA and ARA (Uauy *et al.*, 2003). Continued research in this area in both term and preterm infants using well-controlled studies with large sample sizes will address the long-term and short-term effects of DHA and arachidonic acid supplementation on visual and cognitive development.

Dietary Fatty Acids and Disease Risk

Scientists and the general public alike are interested in the importance of comparative fatty acid selection in relation to health and longevity. Consensus is beginning to emerge concerning the role of qualitative fat intake in the management of disease risk. For certain diseases common to Western civilization, the evidence for reducing risk by adopting certain fat intake profiles is compelling; for other diseases, the link remains speculative. This rapidly progressing field will undoubtedly see further development as research advances our knowledge. Quantitative fat intake is undergoing renewed scrutiny as scientists debate the percentage of daily energy from fat that is necessary for optimal health.

Current recommendations relating to quantitative fat intake call for a reduction in total fat and saturated fat intakes (National Cholesterol Education Program, 2002; Lichtenstein *et al.*, 2006; Hall, 2009). The basis for such recommendations comes from epidemiological evidence indicating that body weight is positively correlated with quantitative fat and not carbohydrate intake (Astrup, 2005; Acheson, 2010). Additionally, research has shown that increasing the fat content of a diet promotes fat storage in adipose tissue rather than fat oxidation (Jequier, 1993; Fernández-Quintela *et al.*, 2007) (see Chapters 45, 61, 62, and 68). However, not all evidence establishes a link between quantitative fat intake and obesity. Willett (1998) demonstrated that a decrease in dietary fat as a percentage of energy has not resulted in a decrease in overweight and obesity. Indeed, there is insufficient evidence to link percentage energy from dietary fat with obesity (Astrup, 2005). It may be more effective to focus on qualitative fat consumption – notably, decreased saturated fat and increased unsaturated fat – combined with recommendations to restrict energy intakes (Lichtenstein, 2003; Purnell, 2009). Such an approach would acknowledge the overall importance of the metabolic actions of all

> ## BOX 10.1 Diseases influenced by qualitative polyunsaturated fatty acid intake in humans
>
> Coronary heart disease and stroke
> Essential fatty acid deficiency during development
> Autoimmune disorders, including lupus and nephropathy
> Type 2 diabetes
> Inflammatory bowel disease
> Breast, colon, and prostate cancers
> Rheumatoid arthritis

fatty acids in the diet, which is an increasing area of focus in fatty acid research. This approach would also recognize the link between percent fat and energy density, and the influence on total caloric intake (French and Robinson, 2003; Prentice and Jebb, 2003).

Box 10.1 lists diseases linked to the relationship between polyunsaturated and other fatty acids in the diet. Of these disorders, coronary heart disease is the most strongly linked to qualitative fat intake. Although it has been well established that consumption of n-9 and n-6 fatty acids favorably reduces circulating levels of total cholesterol and LDL cholesterol, n-3 fatty acids recently have been the focus of much attention (Lichtenstein, 2003; McCowen and Bistrian, 2005; Erkkilä *et al.*, 2008; Harris *et al.*, 2008; Wall *et al.*, 2010). The surprisingly low cardiovascular mortality rate in Native Alaskans consuming traditional diets high in EPA and DHA alerted researchers to the fact that, in the presence of elevated total fat intakes, n-3 fatty acids are effective in reducing disease risk. The influence of fish oils on cardiovascular disease risk is multifactorial. Fish oils reduce very-low-density-lipoprotein (VLDL) secretion, lower triacylglycerol transport, and may enhance VLDL clearance (McEwen *et al.*, 2010). The net effect often is a reduction of circulating triacylglycerol levels. For LDL cholesterol, the data are clearer for n-9 and n-6 fatty acids, as the consumption of these fats results in unequivocal depression of circulating levels. However, for n-3 fatty acids, the data are more controversial; evidence indicates that LDL cholesterol may increase marginally in humans fed fish oil. Similarly, in vitro plasma lipid oxidizability is enhanced in animals fed fish oil. The consumption of diets high in n-6 fatty acids generally results in the suppression of HDL cholesterol levels, whereas n-9 fatty acid intake does not affect values. Studies of the effects on blood lipids of n-3-containing fish oils suggest that HDL cholesterol levels are maintained or elevated with fish-oil consumption.

The action of n-3 fatty acids in reducing coronary heart disease risk is not related solely to effects on circulating lipids. Fish-oil-derived fatty acids may also increase endothelium-dependent dilatation of arteries, which is thought to be beneficial in risk reduction for atherosclerosis. Moreover, polyenoic n-3 fatty acids are receiving considerable attention as potential anti-inflammatory agents (Calder, 2004; Flickinger and Huth, 2004; Singer *et al.*, 2008). In vitro studies comparing the action of various long-chain polyunsaturated fatty acids on endothelial tissue activation as assessed by surface enzyme immunoassay or flow cytometry found no effect. However, a progressive increase in the inhibition of cytokine-induced expression of adhesion molecules was observed with increasing degrees of fatty acid unsaturation from monounsaturated fatty acids to polyenoic n-3 fatty acids. Endothelial activation was most highly inhibited with n-3 versus n-6 or n-9 fatty acids.

In addition, the beneficial effects of dietary n-3 fatty acids on coronary heart disease risk are thought to be mediated via the prevention of arrhythmias, particularly ventricular tachycardia and fibrillation, as well as by favorable modulation of prostaglandin and leukotriene production to reduce thrombogenesis (Gerber *et al.*, 2000; Renaud, 2001). It can be surmised that dietary fat selection consistent with maximal reduction in cardiovascular disease risk would result in lower levels of saturated fats and higher intakes of EPA and DHA from fish oil. Based on current knowledge, this approach would be appropriate for both primary and secondary disease prevention.

A second critical health issue regarding the selection of dietary fatty acids is the need for adequate intakes of essential fatty acids during fetal development and shortly following birth. As noted above, polyenoic unsaturated fatty acids are important components of neural structure membrane phospholipids. Major phospholipid classes in brain and retina contain high levels of DHA. DHA is considered a conditionally essential nutrient for adequate growth in humans (Saldanha *et al.*, 2009). Prolonged absence of dietary n-6 or n-3 fatty acids results in depressed levels of phospholipid polyenoic fatty acids. Of particular interest is the definition of what constitutes adequate dietary n-3 fatty acid levels; neural tissue DHA levels fall to one-fifth the normal amount in animals deprived of n-3

fats (Neuringer *et al.*, 1986). In addition to structural changes, n-3 fatty acid deficiency also results in pronounced behavioral changes. In rhesus monkeys, perinatal n-3 deficiency resulted in functional changes in offspring including reduced vision, electroretinogram irregularities, polydipsia, and possibly cognition disturbances (Reisbick *et al.*, 1996). Although the behavioral changes in animals deprived of n-3 fatty acids may be due directly to impaired neural cell function, secondary neurotransmitter-related effects arise from n-3 fatty acid deficiency. In rats deficient in n-3 fatty acids, behavioral disturbances were shown to be associated with changes in dopaminergic neurotransmission in the nucleus accumbens region of the brain (Zimmer *et al.*, 2000).

By extension, a critical issue relating to human health is the quantity and composition of n-3 fatty acids in infant formulas. Probably because of reduced levels of polyenoic long-chain fatty acids in infant formulas compared with human breast milk, formula-fed infants have lower levels of DHA in the brain (Makrides *et al.*, 1994). Although earlier formulas had notoriously imbalanced ratios of n-3 to n-6 fatty acids, the use of soybean oil has markedly improved this ratio in modern formulas. However, the n-3 fatty acids are provided largely as α-linolenic acid, which may not be fully converted to DHA by developing infants. Current debate focuses on whether infant formula would benefit from direct supplementation with highly polyunsaturated fatty acids of both the n-6 and the n-3 classes. Manufacturing processes presently add specific antioxidants to reduce the possibility of oxidative damage, which allows the routine addition of long-chain polyunsaturated fatty acids. Results at this time remain equivocal, but continued study with reliable sources of DHA and ARA, such as single-cell oils and standardized developmental tests, should permit the establishment of consensus in the near future.

The relationship between dietary fat composition and inflammatory bowel disease is increasingly recognized (Calder, 2009b; Uchiyama *et al.*, 2010). Although it has been proposed that olive oil and oils containing n-6 fatty acids are potentially beneficial, most interest is centered on the use of dietary fish oil to improve remission rates of Crohn's disease and to suppress the symptoms and histological appearance of ulcerative colitis. Results from recent studies are not unequivocal; however, evidence suggests that the consumption of n-3 fatty acids, particularly as fish oil, improves the clinical management of inflammatory bowel disease (Turner *et al.*, 2007). The likely reason is that n-3 fatty acids suppress LTB4 and thromboxane A2, both of which are derived from arachidonic acid and are associated with mucosal inflammation.

The role of dietary fat composition in cancer risk remains controversial. It has been demonstrated that the effects of specific fatty acids on mammary carcinogenesis vary in both in vitro and in vivo animal models, with stimulatory effects observed for linoleic acid compared with saturated fatty acids (Rose et al., 1995; Rose, 1997). Mechanistically, cyclooxygenase and lipoxygenase products derived from n-6 fatty acids may stimulate the growth factors and oncogenes that are responsible for the increased carcinogenesis. Alternatively, the inhibition of calcium mobilization, which is linked to cell signaling and cell proliferation, may be affected by the presence of higher cellular concentrations of EPA and DHA (Calviello et al., 2000). The link with n-6 fatty acid consumption and prostate cancer remains weak. Mounting evidence does, however, suggest a beneficial role of n-3 fatty acids compared with other fats in the suppression of breast and prostate cancers (Rose et al., 1995; Judé et al., 2006; Berquin et al., 2008; Giacosa and Rondanelli, 2008; Hurst et al., 2010; Shaikh et al., 2010).

Evidence linking the consumption of n-3 fatty acids with reduced severity of arthritic symptoms remains controversial despite reported improvements in the incidence of tender joints and joint stiffness in a meta-analysis of studies reporting n-3 fatty acid supplement use (Hurst et al., 2010). The effect probably involves altered eicosanoid metabolism and interleukin-1 levels. In general, patients are advised to consume 3–6 g/day of n-3 fatty acids to achieve benefits against arthritis, although further confirmation of this association is needed.

Several studies raise the possibility that certain dietary fatty acids can lower the risks of developing type 2 diabetes mellitus (T2DM). Research has shown that increasing the amounts of dietary n-3 long-chain polyunsaturated fatty acids may reduce T2DM as these fatty acids are linked to cell membrane function, enzyme activity, and gene expression, all of which influence glucose metabolism (Risérus et al., 2009). Also, increased intake of omega-3 fatty acids has been shown to increase insulin sensitivity, reduce circulatory TG levels, and increase HDL concentrations. In addition, fatty acids are now linked to reducing adiposity and lipid accumulation in the visceral area (Fruchart, 2009). These actions not only reduce the progression in T2DM but also decrease the risks of obesity and cardiovascular disease.

A model demonstrating the possible effects of different levels of essential fatty acids and long-chain polyunsaturated fatty acids on the disease states discussed above is illustrated in Figure 10.4 (Okuyama et al., 1996; Uauy et al., 1999; Steinberg, 2007; Simopoulos, 2008). The model demonstrates the interrelated manner in which various dietary lipid components interact to influence disease outcome, and highlights the heterogeneity of dietary lipid constituents. It also points out potential beneficial actions of increasing the ratio of n-3 to n-6 fatty acid intake; however, the possible risk of increasing peroxidative status with the elevation in degree of unsaturation of the fat consumed must also be considered.

Overall, research suggests that dietary lipid selection plays a central role in the prevention and development of several important chronic diseases (McCowen and Bistrian, 2005). An emerging conclusion is that the ratio of linoleic acid to α-linolenic acid may be of importance in the etiology of several of these conditions. Evidence suggests that a lower ratio may be protective. Given the present high ratio of 18:2n-6 to 18:3n-3 in the Western-style diet (Simopoulos, 2008), dietary recommendations to include greater amounts of n-3 fatty acids may be valuable in preventing disease (Holman, 1998; Uauy et al., 1999; Harris, 2006; Simopoulos, 2008; Calder, 2009a). However, safety issues related to increased n-3 fatty acid intakes also need to be fully explored, because it cannot be ruled out that peroxidative status increases along with the degree of unsaturation of dietary fat (Catalá, 2010). Future well-controlled clinical trials are necessary to clearly elucidate the effects of qualitative fatty acid intake in relation to disease risk.

Future Directions

Resolvins and Protectins: Novel Lipid Mediators

Eicosanoids derived from 20-carbon PUFAs provide a pivotal link between the dietary balance of n-6 and n-3 PUFAs and their association with the progression of inflammatory diseases. Recently, novel lipid mediators have been identified that actively induce the resolution of acute inflammation, termed resolvins (resolution phase interaction products) and protectins (Serhan et al., 2008). These proresolution products are synthesized from the oxygenation of EPA and DHA. A series of reactions via the 5-LOX pathway produces the EPA E-series resolvins (RvE1, RvE2) and DHA D-series resolvins (RvD1 through

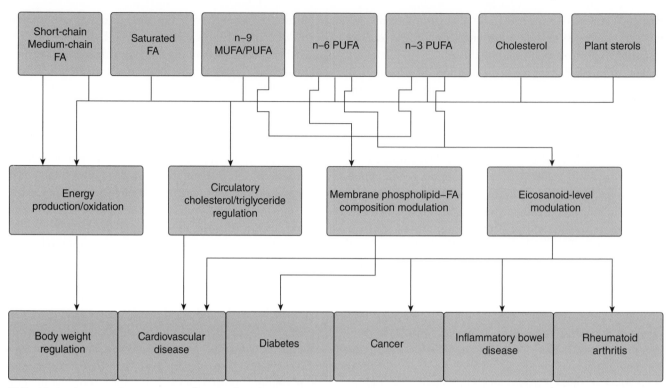

FIG. 10.4 Interaction among dietary lipid components, metabolic systems, and disease/health outcomes.

RvD6), as well as neuroprotectin D1 (Serhan *et al.*, 2008). Since DHA is highly concentrated in neurological tissue, protectins comprise the DHA metabolites docosatrienes and the D-series resolvins and are specifically associated with neuroprotective and anti-inflammatory effects (Serhan, 2005). Resolvins and protectins act locally to reduce PMN infiltration and proinflammatory gene expression, block inflammatory cytokines such as TNF-α and IL-1, and induce macrophage uptake of apoptotic cells. Although preliminary in vitro studies have been conducted with isolated human cells, future studies are needed to investigate the in vivo functions of resolvins and protectins and their role in amelioration of chronic disease.

PPARs

Peroxisome proliferator-activated receptors (PPARs), which include the isoforms PPARα, PPARγ, and PPARδ, are a group of ligand-regulated nuclear transcription factors regulating the expression of genes involved in lipid and lipoprotein metabolism, inflammation, and vascular function (Fruchart, 2009). EPA and DHA have a high affinity for PPARs, therefore current research is focusing on the metabolic effects associated with regulation of

transcription factors by PUFAs and implications in chronic disease.

Acknowledgments

We thank Stephanie Jew, Meriam Mohammed, and Leah Gillingham for their assistance in preparing this chapter.

Suggestions for Further Reading

Adkins, Y. and Kelley, D.S. (2010) Mechanisms underlying the cardioprotective effects of omega-3 polyunsaturated fatty acids. *J Nutr Biochem* **21**, 781–792.

Burdge, G.C. and Calder, P.C. (2007) Conversion of α-linolenic acid to longer-chain polyunsaturated fatty acids in human adults. *Reprod Nutr Devel* **45**, 581–597.

Calder, P.C. (2006) Long-chain polyunsaturated fatty acids and inflammation. *Scand J Food Nutr* **50** (Suppl 2), 54–61.

Plourde, M. and Cunnane, S.C. (2007) Extremely limited synthesis of long chain polyunsaturates in adults: implications for their dietary essentiality and use as supplements. *Appl Physiol Nutr Metab* **32**, 619–634.

References

Acheson, K.J. (2010) Carbohydrate for weight and metabolic control: where do we stand? *Nutrition* **26,** 141–145.

Achten, J. and Jeukendrup, A.E. (2004) Optimizing fat oxidation through exercise and diet. *Nutrition* **20,** 716–727.

Agostoni, C. (2008) Role of long-chain polyunsaturated fatty acids in the first year of life. *J Pediatr Gastroenterol Nutr* **47** (Suppl 2), S41–44.

Agostoni, C., Trojan, S., Bellù, R., *et al.* (1995) Neurodevelopmental quotient of healthy term infants at 4 months and feeding practice: the role of long-chain polyunsaturated fatty acids. *Pediatr Res* **38,** 262–266

Agostoni, C., Trojan, S., Bellù, R., *et al.* (1997) Developmental quotient at 24 months and fatty acid composition of diet in early infancy: a follow up study. *Arch Dis Child* **76,** 421–424.

Astrup, A. (2005) The role of dietary fat in obesity. *Semin Vasc Med* **5,** 40–47.

Baker, R.R. (1990) The eicosanoids: a historical overview. *Clin Biochem* **23,** 455–458.

Bergstrom, S. and Sjovall, J.(1960a) The isolation of prostaglandin F from sheep prostate glands. *Acta Chem Scand* **14,** 1693–1700.

Bergstrom, S. and Sjovall, J. (1960b) The isolation of prostaglandin E from sheep prostate glands. *Acta Chem Scand* **14,** 1701–1705.

Berquin, I.M., Edwards, I.J., and Chen, Y.Q. (2008) Multi-targeted therapy of cancer by omega-3 fatty acids. *Cancer Lett* **269,** 363–377.

Beyerlein, A., Hadders-Algra, M., Kennedy, K., *et al.* (2010) Infant formula supplementation with long-chain polyunsaturated fatty acids has no effect on Bayley developmental scores at 18 months of age – IPD meta-analysis of four large clinical trials. *J Pediatr Gastroenterol Nutr* **50,** 79–84.

Birch, E.E., Carlson, S.E., Hoffman, D.R., *et al.* (2010) The DIAMOND (DHA Intake And Measurement Of Neural Development) Study: a double-masked, randomized controlled clinical trial of the maturation of infant visual acuity as a function of the dietary level of docosahexaenoic acid. *Am J Clin Nutr* **91,** 848–859.

Birch, E.E., Castañeda,Y.S., Wheaton, H.D., *et al.* (2005) Visual maturation of term infants fed long-chain polyunsaturated fatty acid–supplemented or control formula for 12 months. *Am J Clin Nutr* **81,** 871–879.

Burr, G.O. and Burr, M.M. (1929) A new deficiency disease produced by the rigid exclusion of fat from the diet. *J Biol Chem* **82,** 345–367.

Burr, G.O. and Burr, M.M. (1930) On the nature and the role of fatty acids essential in nutrition. *J Biol Chem* **86,** 587–621.

Calder, P.C. (2004) n-3 Fatty acids and cardiovascular disease: evidence explained and mechanisms explored. *Clin Sci* **107,** 1–11.

Calder, P.C. (2009a) Polyunsaturated fatty acids and inflammation: therapeutic potential in rheumatoid arthritis. *Curr Rheumatol Rev* **5,** 214–225.

Calder, P.C. (2009b) Fatty acids and immune function: relevance to inflammatory bowel diseases. *Int Rev Immunol* **28,** 506–534.

Calviello, G., Palozza, P., Di Nicuolo, F., *et al.* (2000) n-3 PUFA dietary supplementation inhibits proliferation and store-operated calcium influx in thymoma cells growing in Balb/c mice. *J Lipid Res* **41,** 182–188.

Catalá, A. (2010) A synopsis of the process of lipid peroxidation since the discovery of the essential fatty acids. *Biochem Biophys Res Commun* **399,** 318–323.

Cunnane, S.C. (2003) Problems with essential fatty acids: time for a new paradigm? *Prog Lipid Res* **42,** 544–568.

Cunnane, S.C. and Crawford, M.A. (2003) Survival of the fattest: fat babies were the key to evolution of the large human brain. *Comp Biochem Physiol A Mol Integr Physiol* **136,** 17–26.

Cunnane, S.C., Francescutti, V., Brenna, J.T., *et al.* (2000) Breast-fed infants achieve a higher rate of brain and whole body docosahexaenoate accumulation than formula-fed infants not consuming dietary docosahexaenoate. *Lipids* **35,** 105–111.

Cunnane, S.C., Ryan, M.A., Nadeau, C.R., *et al.* (2003) Why is lipid synthesis an integral target of β-oxidized and recycled carbon from polyunsaturates in neonates? *Lipids* **38,** 477–484.

Cunnane, S.C., Ryan, M.A., Yu, H.L., *et al.* (2006) Suckling rats actively recycle carbon from α-linolenate into newly synthe-sized lipids even during extreme dietary deficiency of n-3 poly-unsaturates. *Pediatr Res* **59,** 107–110.

DeLany, J.P., Windhauser, M.M., Champagne, C.M., *et al.* (2000) Differential oxidation of individual dietary fatty acids in humans. *Am J Clin Nutr* **72,** 905–911.

Di Buono, M., Hannah, J.S., Katzel, L.I., *et al.* (1999) Weight loss due to energy restriction suppresses cholesterol biosynthesis in overweight, mildly hypercholesterolemic men. *J Nutr* **129,** 1545–1548.

Dietschy, J.M. (1984) Regulation of cholesterol metabolism in man and in other species. *Klin Wochenschr* **62,** 338–345.

Eilander, A., Hundscheid, D.C., Osendarp, S.J., *et al.* (2007) Effects of n-3 long chain polyunsaturated fatty acid supple-mentation on visual and cognitive development throughout childhood: a review of human studies. *Prostaglandins Leukot Essent Fatty Acids* **76,** 189–203.

El-Badry, A.M., Graf, R., and Clavien, P. (2007) Omega 3–omega 6: what is right for the liver? *J Hepatol* **47,** 718–725.

Erkkilä, A., de Mello, V.D.F., Risérus, U., *et al.* (2008) Dietary fatty acids and cardiovascular disease: an epidemiological approach. *Prog Lipid Res* **47,** 172–187.

Evans, H.M. and Burr, G.O. (1927) New dietary deficiency with highly purified diets. *Proc Soc Exp Biol Med* **24**, 740–743.

Fernández-Quintela, A., Churruca, I., and Portillo, M.P. (2007) The role of dietary fat in adipose tissue metabolism. *Public Health Nutr* **10**, 1126–1131.

Fidaleo, M (2010) Peroxisomes and peroxisomal disorders: the main facts. *Exp Toxicol Pathol* **62**, 615–625.

Field, C.J., Angel, A., and Clandinin, M.T. (1985) Relationship of diet to the fatty acid composition of human adipose tissue structural and stored lipids. *Am J Clin Nutr* **42**, 1206–1220.

Fleith, M. and Clandinin, M.T. (2005) Dietary PUFA for preterm and term infants: review of clinical studies. *Crit Rev Food Sci Nutr* **45**, 205–229.

Flickinger, B.D. and Huth, P.J. (2004) Dietary fats and oils: technologies for improving cardiovascular health. *Curr Atheroscleros Rep* **6**, 468–476.

French, S. and Robinson, T. (2003) Fats and food intake. *Curr Opin Clin Nutr Metab Care* **6**, 629–634.

Fruchart, J. (2009) Peroxisome proliferator-activated receptor-alpha (PPARα): at the crossroads of obesity, diabetes and cardiovascular disease. *Atherosclerosis* **205**, 1–8.

Futterman, S., Downer, J.L., and Hendrickson, A. (1971) Effect of essential fatty acid deficiency on the fatty acid composition, morphology, and electroretinographic response of the retina. *Invest Ophthalmol* **10**, 151–156.

Gerber, M.J., Scali, J.D., Michaud, A., et al. (2000) Profiles of a healthful diet and its relationship to biomarkers in a population sample from Mediterranean southern France. *J Am Diet Assoc* **100**, 1164–1171.

Giacosa, A. and Rondanelli, M. (2008) Fish oil and treatment of cancer cachexia. *Genes Nutr* **3**, 25–28.

Greene, C.M., Zern, T.L., Wood, R.J., et al. (2005) Maintenance of the LDL cholesterol:HDL cholesterol ratio in an elderly population given a dietary cholesterol challenge. *J Nutr* **135**, 2793–2798.

Hall, W.L. (2009) Dietary saturated and unsaturated fats as determinants of blood pressure and vascular function. *Nutr Res Rev* **22**, 18–38.

Hansen, A.E., Haggard, M.E., Boelsche, A.N., et al. (1958). Essential fatty acids in infant nutrition. III. Clinical manifestations of linoleic acid deficiency. *J Nutr* **66**, 565–576.

Harris, W.S. (2006) The omega-6/omega-3 ratio and cardiovascular disease risk: uses and abuses. *Curr Atheroscler Rep* **8**, 453–459.

Harris, W.S. (2010) Omega-6 and omega-3 fatty acids: partners in prevention. *Curr Opin Clin Nutr Metab Care* **13**, 125–129.

Harris, W.S., Miller, M., Tighe, A.P., et al. (2008) Omega-3 fatty acids and coronary heart disease risk: clinical and mechanistic perspectives. *Atherosclerosis* **197**, 12–24.

Henriksen, C., Haugholt, K., Lindgren, M., et al. (2008) Improved cognitive development among preterm infants attributable to early supplementation of human milk with docosahexaenoic acid and arachidonic acid. *Pediatrics* **121**, 1137–1145.

Hoffman, D.R., Birch, E.E., Castañeda, Y.S., et al. (2003) Visual function in breast-fed term infants weaned to formula with or without long-chain polyunsaturates at 4 to 6 months: a randomized clinical trial. *J Pediatr* **142**, 669–677.

Hoffman, D.R., Boettcher, J.A., and Diersen-Schade, D.A. (2009) Toward optimizing vision and cognition in term infants by dietary docosahexaenoic and arachidonic acid supplementation: a review of randomized controlled trials. *Prostaglandins Leukot Essent Fatty Acids* **81**, 151–158.

Holman, R.T. (1998) The slow discovery of the importance of ω3 essential fatty acids in human health. *J Nutr* **128** (2 Suppl), 427S–433S.

Holman, R.T., Johnson, S.B., and Hatch, T.F. (1982) A case of human linolenic acid deficiency involving neurological abnormalities. *Am J Clin Nutr* **35**, 617–623.

Hurst, S., Zainal, Z., Caterson, B., et al. (2010) Dietary fatty acids and arthritis. *Prostaglandins Leukot Essent Fatty Acids* **82**, 315–318.

Innis, S.M. (2007) Human milk: maternal dietary lipids and infant development. *Proc Nutr Soc* **66**, 397–404.

Institute of Medicine (2002/2005) *Dietary Reference Intakes for Energy, Carbohydrate, Fiber, Fat, Fatty Acids, Cholesterol, Protein, and Amino Acids (Macronutrients*. National Academies Press, Washington, DC. Available online at: http://www.nap.edu/openbook.php?isbn=0309085373; record_id=10490. Accessed July 15, 2010.

Jequier, E. (1993) Body weight regulation in humans: the importance of nutrient balance. *News Physiol Sci* **8**, 273–276.

Jones, P.J. (1997) Regulation of cholesterol biosynthesis by diet in humans. *Am J Clin Nutr* **66**, 438–446.

Jones, P.J., Pappu, A.S., Hatcher, L., et al. (1996). Dietary cholesterol feeding suppresses human cholesterol synthesis measured by deuterium incorporation and urinary mevalonic acid levels. *Arterioscler Thromb Vasc Biol* **16**, 1222–1228.

Judé, S., Roger, S., Martel, E., et al. (2006) Dietary long-chain omega-3 fatty acids of marine origin: a comparison of their protective effects on coronary heart disease and breast cancers. *Prog Biophys Mol Biol* **90**, 299–325.

Koletzko, B., Lien, E., Agostoni, C., et al. (2008) The roles of long-chain polyunsaturated fatty acids in pregnancy, lactation and infancy: review of current knowledge and consensus recommendations. *J Perinat Med* **36**, 5–14.

Kris-Etherton, P.M., Taylor, D.S., Yu-Poth, S., et al. (2000) Polyunsaturated fatty acids in the food chain in the United States. *Am J Clin Nutr* **71** (1 Suppl.), 179S–188S.

Lapillonne, A. and Jensen, C.L. (2009) Reevaluation of the DHA requirement for the premature infant. *Prostaglandins Leukot Essent Fatty Acids* **81**, 143–150.

Lapillonne, A., Picaud, J., Chirouze, V., *et al.* (2000) The use of low-EPA fish oil for long-chain polyunsaturated fatty acid supplementation of preterm infants. *Pediatr Res* **48**, 835–841.

Larque, E., Demmelmair, H., and Koletzko, B. (2002) Perinatal supply and metabolism of long-chain polyunsaturated fatty acids: importance for the early development of the nervous system. *Ann NY Acad Sci* **967**, 299–310.

Lichtenstein, A.H. (2003) Dietary fat and cardiovascular disease risk: quantity or quality? *J Womens Health (Larchmt)* **12**, 109–114.

Lichtenstein, A.H., Appel, L.J., Brands, M., *et al.* (2006) Diet and lifestyle recommendations revision 2006: a scientific statement from the American Heart Association Nutrition Committee. *Circulation* **114**, 82–96.

Lucas, A., Morley, R., Cole, T.J., *et al.* (1994) A randomised multicentre study of human milk versus formula and later development in preterm infants. *Arch Dis Child* **70** (2 Suppl.), F141–F146.

Makrides, M., Neumann, M.A., Byard, R.W., *et al.* (1994) Fatty acid composition of brain, retina, and erythrocytes in breast- and formula-fed infants. *Am J Clin Nutr* **60**, 189–194.

Makrides, M., Smithers, L.G., and Gibson, R.A. (2010) Role of long-chain polyunsaturated fatty acids in neurodevelopment and growth. *Nestlé Nutr Workshop Ser Pediatr Program* **65**, 123–136.

Matthan, N.R., Ausman, L.M., Lichtenstein, A.H., *et al.* (2000) Hydrogenated fat consumption affects cholesterol synthesis in moderately hypercholesterolemic women. *J Lipid Res* **41**, 834–839.

McCowen, K.C. and Bistrian, B.R. (2005) Essential fatty acids and their derivatives. *Curr Opin Gastroenterol* **21**, 207–215.

McEwen, B., Morel-Kopp, M.C., Tofler, G., *et al.* (2010). Effect of omega-3 fish oil on cardiovascular risk in diabetes. *Diabetes Educ* **36**, 565–584.

Mebarek, S., Ermak, N., Benzaria, A., *et al.* (2009) Effects of increasing docosahexaenoic acid intake in human healthy volunteers on lymphocyte activation and monocyte apoptosis. *Br J Nutr* **101**, 852–858.

Michaelsen K.F., Lauritzen, L., and Mortensen, E.L. (2009) Effects of breast-feeding on cognitive function. *Adv Exp Med Biol* **639**, 199–215.

Mozaffarian, D., Katan M.B., Ascherio A., *et al.* (2006) Trans fatty acids and cardiovascular disease. *New Engl J Med* **354**, 1601–1613.

National Cholesterol Education Program (2002) Third Report of the National Cholesterol Education Program (NCEP) Expert Panel on Detection, Evaluation, and Treatment of High Blood Cholesterol in Adults (Adult Treatment Panel III) final report. *Circulation* **106**, 3143–3421.

Neuringer, M., Adamkin, D., Auestad, N., *et al.* (2000) Efficacy of dietary long-chain polyunsaturated fatty acids (LCP) for preterm (PT) infants. *FASEB J* **14**, LB179.

Neuringer, M., Connor, W.E., Lin, D.S., *et al.* (1986) Biochemical and functional effects of prenatal and postnatal omega-3 fatty acid deficiency on retina and brain in rhesus monkeys. *Proc Natl Acad Sci USA* **83**, 40021–40025.

Okuyama, H., Kobayashi, T., and Watanabe, S. (1996) Dietary fatty acids – the N-6/N-3 balance and chronic elderly diseases. Excess linoleic acid and relative N-3 deficiency syndrome seen in Japan. *Prog Lipid Res* **35**, 409–457.

Papamandjaris, A.A., Macdougall, D.E., and Jones, P.J.H. (1998) Medium chain fatty acid metabolism and energy expenditure: obesity treatment implications. *Life Sci* **62**, 1203–1215.

Prentice, A.M. and Jebb, S.A. (2003) Fast foods, energy density and obesity: a possible mechanistic link. *Obesity Rev* **4**, 187–194.

Purnell, J.Q. (2009) Obesity: calories or content: what is the best weight-loss diet? *Nat Rev Endocrinol* **5**, 419–420.

Ramakrishnan, U., Imhoff-Kunsch, B., and Digirolamo, A.M. (2009) Role of docosahexaenoic acid in maternal and child mental health. *Am J Clin Nutr* **89**, 958S–962S.

Reisbick, S., Neuringer, M., and Connor, W.E. (1996) Effects of n-3 fatty acid deficiency in non-human primates. In J.G. Bindels, A.C. Goedhardt, and H.K.A. Visser (eds), *Nutrica Symposium*. Kluwer Academic, Lancaster, pp. 157–172.

Renaud, S.C. (2001) Diet and stroke. *J Nutr Health Aging* **5**, 167–172.

Risérus, U., Willett, W., and Hu, F. (2009) Dietary fats and prevention of type 2 diabetes. *Prog Lipid Res* **48**, 44–51.

Rose, D.P., Connolly, J.M., Rayburn, J., *et al.* (1995) Influence of diets containing eicosapentaenoic or docosahexaenoic acid on growth and metastasis of breast cancer cells in nude mice. *J Natl Cancer Inst* **87**, 587–592.

Saldanha, L.G., Salem, N., Jr, and Brenna, J.T. (2009) Workshop on DHA as a required nutrient: overview. *Prostaglandins Leukot Essent Fatty Acids* **81**, 233–236.

Sampath, H. and Ntambi, J.M. (2005) Polyunsaturated fatty acid regulation of genes of lipid metabolism. *Annu Rev Nutr* **25**, 317–340.

Serhan, C.N. (2005) Novel eicosanoid and docosanoid mediators: resolvins, docosatrienes, and neuroprotectins. *Curr Opin Clin Nutr Metab Care* **8**, 115–121.

Serhan, C.N., Yacoubian, S., and Yang, R. (2008) Anti-inflammatory and proresolving lipid mediators. *Annu Rev Pathol Mech Dis* **3**, 279–312.

Shaikh, I.A., Brown, I., Wahle, K.W.J., *et al.* (2010) Enhancing cytotoxic therapies for breast and prostate cancers with polyunsaturated fatty acids. *Nutr Cancer* **62**, 284–296.

Simmer, K. and Patole, S. (2004) Long chain polyunsaturated fatty acid supplementation in preterm infants. *Cochrane Database Syst Rev* CD000375.

Simmer, K., Patole, S.K., and Rao, S.C. (2008a) Longchain polyunsaturated fatty acid supplementation in infants born at term. *Cochrane Database Syst Rev* CD000376.

Simmer, K., Schulzke, S.M., and Patole, S. (2008b). Longchain polyunsaturated fatty acid supplementation in preterm infants. *Cochrane Database Syst Rev* CD000375.

Simopoulos, A.P. (2008) The importance of the omega-6/omega-3 fatty acid ratio in cardiovascular disease and other chronic diseases. *Exp Biol Med* **233**, 674–688.

Simopoulos, A.P. (2009) Evolutionary aspects of the dietary omega-6:omega-3 fatty acid ratio: medical implications. *World Rev Nutr Diet* **100**, 1–21.

Singer, P., Shapiro, H., Theilla, M., *et al.* (2008) Anti-inflammatory properties of omega-3 fatty acids in critical illness: novel mechanisms and an integrative perspective. *Intensive Care Med* **34**, 1580–1592.

Solomon, T.P.J., Sistrun, S.N., Krishnan, R.K., *et al.* (2008) Exercise and diet enhance fat oxidation and reduce insulin resistance in older obese adults. *J Appl Physiol* **104**, 1313–1319.

Stanley, J.C., Elsom, R.L., Calder, P.C., *et al.* (2007) UK Food Standards Agency Workshop Report: The effects of the dietary. *Br J Nutr* **98**, 1305–1310.

Steinberg, G.R. (2007) Inflammation in obesity is the common link between defects in fatty acid metabolism and insulin resistance. *Cell Cycle* **6**, 888–894.

Turner, D., Zlotkin, S.H., Shah, P.S., *et al.* (2007) Omega 3 fatty acids (fish oil) for maintenance of remission in Crohn's disease. *Cochrane Database Syst Rev* CD006320.

Uauy, R., Hoffman, D.R., Mena, P., *et al.* (2003) Term infant studies of DHA and ARA supplementation on neurodevelopment: results of randomized controlled trials. *J Pediatr* **143** (4 Suppl), S17–S25.

Uauy, R., Mena, P., and Rojas, C. (2000) Essential fatty acids in early life: structural and functional role. *Proc Nutr Soc* **59**, 3–15.

Uauy, R., Mena, P., and Valenzuela, A. (1999) Essential fatty acids as determinants of lipid requirements in infants, children and adults. *Eur J Clin Nutr* **53** (Suppl 1), S66–S77.

Uchiyama, K., Nakamura, M., Odahara, S., *et al.* (2010) N-3 polyunsaturated fatty acid diet therapy for patients with inflammatory bowel disease. *Inflamm Bowel Diseases* **16**, 1696–1707.

Von Euler, U.S. (1967) Welcoming address. In S. Bergstrom and B. Samuelsson (eds), *Prostaglandins: Proceedings of the Second Nobel Symposium*. Interscience Publishers, New York, pp. 17–21.

Wall, R., Ross, R.P., Fitzgerald, G.F., *et al.* (2010) Fatty acids from fish: the anti-inflammatory potential of long-chain omega-3 fatty acids. *Nutr Rev* **68**, 280–289.

Wheeler, T.G., Benolken, R.M., and Anderson, R.E. (1975) Visual membranes: specificity of fatty acid precursors for the electrical response to illumination. *Science* **188**, 1312–1314.

Willett, W.C. (1998) Is dietary fat a major determinant of body fat? *Am J Clin Nutr* **67** (3 Suppl.), 556S–562S.

Wolfe, R.R. (1998) Metabolic interactions between glucose and fatty acids in human subjects. *Am J Clin Nutr* **67**, 519S–526S.

World Health Organization (1994) Fats and oils in human nutrition. Report of a Joint Expert Consultation. Food and Agriculture Organization of the United Nations and the World Health Organization. FAO Food and Nutrition Paper 57, pp. i–xix, 1–147.

Zimmer, L., Delion-Vancassel, S., Durand, G., *et al.* (2000) Modification of dopamine neurotransmission in the nucleus accumbens of rats deficient in n-3 polyunsaturated fatty acids. *J Lipid Res* **41**, 32–40.

11

VITAMIN A

NOEL W. SOLOMONS, MD

Center for Studies of Sensory Impairment, Guatemala City, Guatemala

Summary

Vitamin A is a fat-soluble compound essential for functions of the retinal pigments for vision, intercellular communication via the connexin mechanisms, and regulation of nuclear transcription via nuclear receptor coupling related to cellular growth and differentiation. Its actions include retinoid analogs' anti-proliferative action against proliferative disorders, and a putative enhancement of the biological availability of dietary iron. The vitamin can be obtained from foods of animal origin, such as organ meats, fish oil, dairy products, in the preformed vitamin (retinoid) form, and from plant-origin foods, such as orange, yellow, and green vegetables and fruits, as provitamin A (carotene). The latter is enzymatically oxidized to yield the active vitamin, although a number of intestinal, dietary, and genetic factors influence the efficiency of bioconversion of provitamin A to the active form. The limited intake of vitamin A sources, absorptive disorders of the intestines, and inflammatory diseases are common predisposing conditions for deficiency. The manifestations of vitamin A deficiency include functional and anatomic ocular degeneration, diverse changes in epithelial tissues, immune deficits, and excessive mortality from childhood diseases. The hepatic concentration of vitamin A is a true reflection of nutritional status. The ideal diagnostic biomarker for assessing vitamin A status of individuals has yet to be devised. Circulating retinol concentration has severe limitations for reflecting vitamin A status of an individual and cannot be easily interpreted in a survey context to assess the vitamin A status of a population. When adequate vitamin A cannot be provided from the diet, periodic vitamin supplementation and food fortification constitute common public health intervention strategies. Home fortification of complementary foods and enriching provitamin A content in plants (biofortification) are recently developed approaches in the area of fortification. Vitamin A supplementation has diverse applications in clinical medicine from treating severe clinical deficiency to supporting recovery from measles and protein energy malnutrition. Excess intakes of preformed vitamin A can produce congenital malformations and possibly thinning of the bones. Severe overdoses of preformed vitamin A damage the liver and nervous system, with potentially lethal consequences.

Present Knowledge in Nutrition, Tenth Edition. Edited by John W. Erdman Jr, Ian A. Macdonald and Steven H. Zeisel.
© 2012 International Life Sciences Institute. Published 2012 by John Wiley & Sons, Inc.

Introduction

McCollum and his co-workers recognized vitamin A as the first of the vitamins in 1913. By 1929, Moore had shown that oxidation of the carotenoid family (provitamin A compounds) could be oxidized to yield the retinoid forms of the vitamin. Vitamin A deficiency is a public health problem. The highest specific prevalence rates of hypovitaminosis A are seen in southern Asia and sub-Saharan Africa among pregnant women and young children (Ramakrishnan, 2002). Specifically, it has been estimated that approximately 127 million preschool children have vitamin A deficiency at any time, and 4.4 million have some stage of xerophthalmia (West, 2002) . Annually, over 6 million women in developing countries develop night blindness during pregnancy. Vitamin A and other retinoids have important health-related actions beyond a nutritional role.

Nomenclature and Chemical Properties

The term "vitamin A" refers to a subgroup of retinoids that possess the biological activity of all-*trans*-retinol. Retinol has a molecular weight of 286.5 kDa. Retinoids typically have four isoprenoid units joined head to tail, and contain five conjugated carbon–carbon double bonds. Figure 11.1 provides the molecular structures for selected retinoid and carotenoid compounds. The numbering system for the carbons of retinol is illustrated in Figure 11.1A (American Institute of Nutrition, 1990). Retinol can be reversibly oxidized to retinal (Figure 11.1B), which exhibits all of the biological activities of retinol, or further oxidized to retinoic acid (Figure 11.1C). Exogenous retinoic acid is insufficient for vision and reproduction. The form of vitamin A involved in vision is 11-*cis*-retinal (Figure 11.1D), whereas the primary storage form is retinyl palmitate (Figure 11.1E) (Blomhoff *et al.*, 1994). Beyond

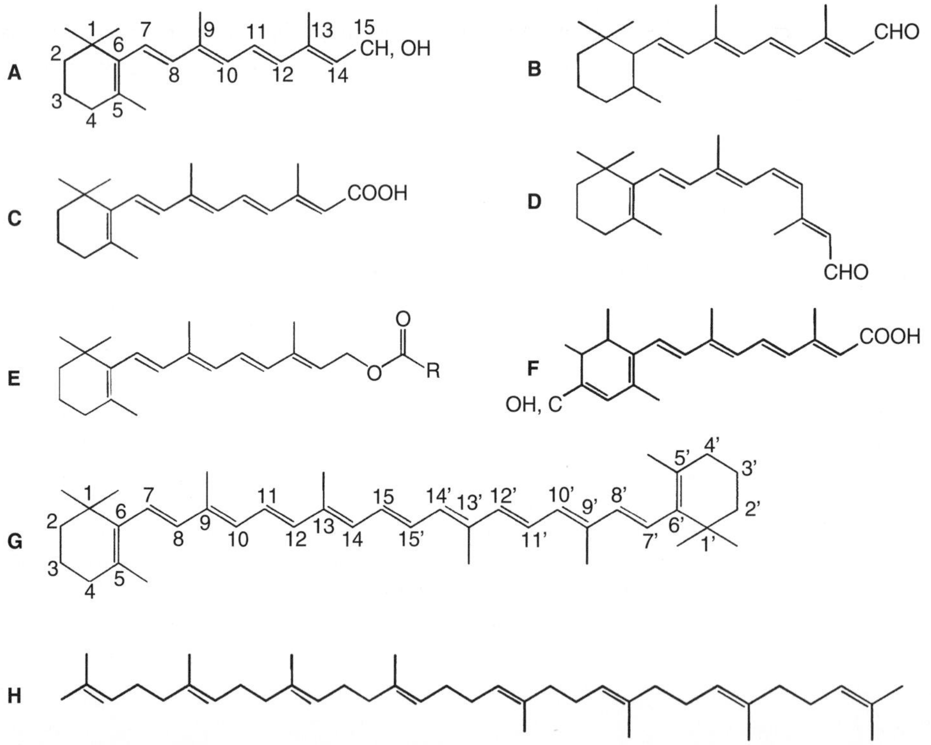

FIG. 11.1 Vitamin A. (A) All-*trans*-retinol; (B) all-*trans*-retinal; (C) all-*trans*-retinoic acid; (D) 11-*cis*-retinal; (E) retinyl esters, mainly retinyl palmitate; (F) all-*trans* β-carotene; (G) trimethyl methoxyphenol retinoic acid (etrin, acitretin); (H) lycopene.

their nutritional function, skin disorders, and some cancers are therapeutic targets of retinoids (Dawson and Okamura, 1990). Acitretin (Figure 11.1F) is one example of a less toxic, highly active, synthetic retinoid. The term "provitamin A" is given to several carotenoids, the archetype of which, B-carotene (Figure 11.1G), has a molecular weight of 536.9 kDa and can be cleaved to yield active retinoids. An unsubstituted β-ionone ring is necessary for this function. Lycopene, by contrast (Figure 11.1H), is an example of a carotene that lacks the properties to be a provitamin A compound. Although more than 700 carotenoids have been isolated from natural sources, only about 50 possess vitamin A activity.

Retinoids and carotenoids are susceptible to oxidation and isomerization when exposed to light, oxygen, reactive metals, and thermal effects. Both are insoluble in water but soluble to varying degrees in most organic solvents. Under ideal storage conditions, both retinoids and carotenoids will remain stable for long periods in serum, tissue, or crystalline forms (Comstock *et al.*, 1993).

Analytical Methods

The conjugated polyene structures of these compounds give them unique light absorption spectra and high molar absorptivities, producing characteristic ultraviolet or visible absorption spectra, constituting physical properties useful for its analysis (Furr, 2004). The absorption maxima and molar extinction coefficients in ethanol are 325 nm (~52 480) for all-*trans*-retinol, 381 nm (~43 400) for all-*trans*-retinal, and 350 nm (~45 200) for all-*trans*-retinoic acid. Retinol fluoresces at 470 nm when excited with UV light at 325 nm. Its ability to form a blue color with Lewis acids in anhydrous chloroform has been used as the basis of quantitation for decades. β-Carotene, with nine conjugated double bonds, absorbs maximally in petroleum ether at 450 nm (~138 900).

The historical approach to quantifying retinoids and carotenoids using their absorption or fluorescence properties has given way in recent years to reverse-phase high-performance liquid chromatography (HPLC) (Furr, 2004). Reverse-phase HPLC (C18 column) followed by visible detection for carotenoids (approximately 450 nm) or UV detection for retinoids is the most common method of analysis. In many cases, *cis–trans* isomers can be better separated using normal-phase HPLC (silica or alumina columns). During sample preparation and analysis, samples should be protected from heat, light, and oxidizing sub-

stances. Other techniques, such as gas chromatography (GC) and mass spectroscopy (coupled with GC and HPLC), immunoassays, supercritical fluid chromatography, and capillary electrophoresis, have proven useful in certain applications (Furr, 2004). To analyze serum retinol, the retinol binding protein (RBP) is denatured with alcohol or acetonitrile to release the retinol for organic-solvent extraction prior to analysis.

Relevant in pathology and in food composition analysis is the fact that vitamin A in tissues is stored as retinyl esters, predominantly retinyl palmitate. Although retinyl esters can be extracted directly into organic solvents, cellular proteins are usually precipitated prior to hydrolysis of the esters to release free retinol. Guidance for the analysis of provitamin A compounds in foods by both traditional open-column and advanced HPLC techniques has been published (Rodriguez-Amaya, 1999; Blake, 2007).

Intestinal Absorption of Preformed Vitamin A and Provitamin A

The first requirement for a nutrient to nourish is for it to be absorbed. Host vitamin nutriture depends on the sequence of digestion of vitamin A source foods, uptake of preformed vitamin A or carotenoids into intestinal cells, and its handling within the enterocyte.

Mechanisms of Absorption

Accessing vitamin A may begin with food matrix factors, dissociated by chewing and gastric action. In green leafy vegetables, carotenes are embedded in chloroplasts, whereas they form part of chromoplasts in orange fruits, vegetables, and tubers of hue (West *et al.*, 2002). Thereafter, as dietary lipids, digestion is fundamental for access of carotenes and vitamin A. This includes the constellation of actions by bile salts and pancreatic lipases within an appropriate pH milieu, in conjunction with forming mixed micelles within the intestinal lumen. In foods such as dairy items, and especially some fatty fruits, the carotenoids are dispersed and emulsified in an oily milieu within the foods. Not unlike other nutrients in their absorption, provitamin A carotenes are more efficiently converted to the active vitamin at lower oral intakes (Novotny *et al.*, 2010).

Once taken up into enterocytes, an intracellular transport system for vitamin A, not dissimilar to that in peripheral tissue cells (see below), is mediated by a complement of cellular transport proteins. Cellular mechanisms of vitamin A absorption have been reviewed by Harrison

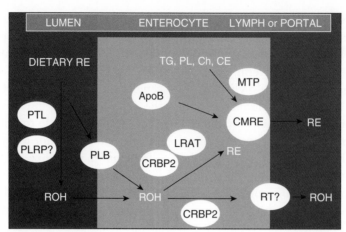

FIG. 11.2 Overview of digestion and absorption of vitamin A. Dietary retinyl esters (REs) are hydrolyzed in the lumen by the pancreatic enzyme pancreatic triglyceride lipase (PTL) and intestinal brush-border enzyme phospholipase B (PLB). Studies of the carboxylester lipase (CEL) knockout mouse suggested that CEL is not involved in dietary RE digestion. The possible roles of the pancreatic lipase-related proteins (PLRPs) 1 and 2 and other enzymes require further investigation. Unesterified retinol (ROH) is taken up by the enterocyte, perhaps facilitated by an as-yet-unidentified retinol transporter. Once in the cell, retinol is complexed with cellular RBP type 2 (CRBP2), and the complex serves as substrate for re-esterification of the retinol by the enzyme lecithin retinol acyltransferase (LRAT). The REs are then incorporated into chylomicrons, intestinal lipoproteins containing other dietary lipids such as triglycerides (TGs), phospholipids (PLs), cholesterol (Ch), cholesteryl esters (CEs), and apolipoprotein B (ApoB). The incorporation of some of the lipids is dependent on the activity of microsomal triglyceride-transfer protein (MTP). Chylomicrons containing newly absorbed retinyl esters (CMREs) are then secreted into the lymph. Unesterified retinol is also absorbed into the portal circulation and its efflux from the basolateral cell membrane may also be facilitated by retinol transporter (RT) proteins. Reproduced with permission from Harrison (2005).

et al. (2005). The particular routes of transport and roles and functions of transporters are illustrated diagrammatically in Figure 11.2 (Harrison, 2005).

As to provitamin A carotenes, options include being passed intact into the lymphatic circulation, cleaved and converted into a retinoid, metabolized to an inactive species, or retained intact until the cell is desquamated. The history of discovery and the mechanisms of bioconversion of provitamin A to the active (retinoid) form of the vitamin have been reviewed (Krinsky *et al.*, 1993; Yuem and Russell, 2002; Lietz *et al.*, 2010). The conventional mechanism for conversion of β-carotene to retinaldehyde involves oxygen-mediated oxidative cleavage in the center of the molecule by the intestinal enzyme, carotene monooxygenase 1 (CMO1, EC 1.13.11.21, formerly the 15,15′ monooxygenase enzyme); this central cleavage leads to the formation of up to two retinal molecules from each carotenoid moiety. The enzyme has been

cloned (Lindqvist and Andersson, 2002). Early on, peroxisome proliferator-activated receptor-alpha (PPAR-α) was thought to be a transcriptional regulator in the expression of this monooxygenase (Boulanger *et al.*, 2003), but later a role for PPAR-γ in the expression of CMO1 was confirmed (Gong *et al.*, 2006). Understanding of a more complex and elaborated scenario for the regulation of the intestinal handling of provitamin A β-carotene has advanced importantly over the past 5 years, as recently reviewed by von Lintig (2010). In addition to CMO1, a membrane protein, scavenger receptor class B type 1 (SR-B1), is involved as part of a negative feedback homeostatic regulation mechanism. More than through retinoid receptor or PPAR transcription factors, the intestine-specific transcription factor, ISX, suppresses both SR-B1 and CMO1 in an independent fashion. When sufficient dietary vitamin A is available, it exerts a suppressive effect on the further oxidative cleavage of β-carotene to avoid vitamin A production in excess of nutritional needs (von Lintig, 2010).

Eccentric cleavage of β-carotene also occurs, with the conversion of β-carotene into β-apo-carotenals and eventually retinoids. This is not exclusively related to spontaneous oxidation, and it has been found to be present in at least four mammalian species by enzymatic action (carotene monooxygenase 2 or CMO2) (Biesalski *et al.*, 2007).

Considerations of Bioavailability and Bioconversion of Provitamin A

It is the consensus of experts in the field that provitamin A carotenoids are an important contributor to the vitamin A nutrition of the world's population (Grune *et al.*, 2010). A series of factors influence the yield of vitamin A derived from provitamin A carotenoids, both those extrinsic to the body (i.e diets that provide vitamin A) and those intrinsic to the host (i.e. the consequence of one's digestive and absorptive capacities). These factors can enhance or inhibit the uptake of vitamin A or provitamin A and the conversion of the latter into the active vitamin. This topic has been comprehensively reviewed (Grune *et al.*, 2010).

Extrinsic Factors

Our understanding of the dietary factors influencing the efficacy of conversion of provitamin A in foods has been aided by rapid advances in isotope tracer techniques and mathematical modeling (van Lieshout *et al.*, 2003; Furr *et al.*, 2005). It is known that the yield of vitamin A from carrots, for example, is generally low, and highly variable depending on the preparation: juiced, puréed, grated, or cooked (Edwards *et al.*, 2002; Thurmann *et al.*, 2002). When the provitamin A is in leaves or pulp of plants, the bioefficacy is well below 6:1 in relation to active vitamin A (Haskell *et al.*, 2004; Tang *et al.*, 2005) in both marginal and replete subjects. Pectin also interferes with dietary carotene utilization, but not non-starch polysaccharides. Weight-control drugs, which induce fat malabsorption, do not affect vitamin A status, but plant sterols consumed for cholesterol lowering can interfere with β-carotene uptake.

As carotenes dispersed and emulsified in fat or oil approach the biological efficacy of preformed vitamin A itself (West *et al.*, 2002), the amount of dietary fat accompanying vitamin A and provitamin A in meals is an enhancing factor. The presence of fat ensures the absorption of preformed vitamin A, but a minimum of 3–5 g is required to enhance the uptake of provitamin A for bio-

conversion (Ribaya-Mercado, 2002). In two situations in Asia in which fat intake is habitually low, addition of fat to the diet resulted in improvement in circulating levels of retinol (Alam *et al.*, 2010) or increased body stores of the vitamin (Maramag *et al.*, 2010). Nagao (2004) also suggests that lipids modulate the action of CMO1.

Intrinsic Factors

The intrinsic factors for intestinal uptake begin with the nutritional demand of the organism for vitamin A, by which the intestine homeostatically regulates the conversion of provitamin A carotenoids to vitamin A. That is, in the healthy individual, it depends upon the underlying adequacy of vitamin A status. Individuals who are replete have a low bioconversion drive (Hickenbottom *et al.*, 2002), and aging may reduce the efficiency of the conversion further (Wang *et al.*, 2004). The physical health of the alimentary tract is an additional factor for both preformed and provitamin A, insofar as fat maldigestion or injury or malfunction of the intestinal cells impairs the release of the constituents from the food and their transport out of the intestinal lumen.

Genetic Factors

Suspicion regarding heterogeneity and an adaptation of the efficiency of bioconversion has existed for decades (Solomons and Bulux, 1994). Evidence to that effect has appeared more recently. Two variant allelic polymorphisms exist for the CMO1 carotene-splitting enzyme: A379V and R267S (Leung *et al.*, 2009). With respect to the non-mutant genotypes, the A379V variant reduces carotene bioconversion efficiency by 32% and the combination of both variant alleles produces a 69% reduction. Comparisons across populations show Europeans to have higher frequencies of the variant alleles, and hence less efficiency of provitamin A conversion than Asian and African groups, suggesting a selection for greater production of vitamin A in areas historically more dependent on plant sources in the diet.

Post-intestinal (Systemic) Bioconversion of Provitamin A Carotenes

Enzymes capable of oxidative cleavage of carotenes, both in a central and eccentric manner, have long been identified in extra-intestinal peripheral tissues including liver, lungs, and kidney (Wyss *et al.*, 2001; Leung *et al.*, 2009). Wyss *et al.* (2001) noted that "beta-carotene 15,15′-dioxygenase is also expressed in epithelial structures, where it serves to provide the tissue-specific vitamin A supply," and Lindqvist and Andersson (2004) stated that "the finding that the enzyme is expressed in all epithelia examined thus far leads us to suggest that BCMO1 may be important for local synthesis of vitamin A, constituting a back-up pathway of vitamin A synthesis during times of insufficient dietary intake of vitamin A." To date, however, no firm quantitative estimate of extra-intestinal enzymatic bioconversion of provitamin A of nutritional importance has been made.

Metabolism of Preformed Vitamin A and Provitamin A

The appropriate fate of an absorbed nutrient is to become inserted into the sites of its essential physiological or structural roles or to be maintained in a storage reserve until needed.

Storage and Transport

At any given time, the majority of the body's vitamin A, up to 90%, is in storage, with the remainder in active sites in peripheral tissues and undertaking vitamin A-dependent functions.

Cellular Uptake and Intracellular Metabolism

As shown in the entero- and hepatocyte metabolic schemes in Figure 11.3 (Napoli, 2000), the chemical actors are RBP from the circulation, cellular RBPs (CRBP I and CRBP II), cellular retinoic acid binding proteins (CRABP I and CRABP II), the retinaldehyde dehydrogenase type 2 (RALDH-2) and other enzymes, the retinoic acid receptors (RARs), and the retinoid X receptors (RXRs). Since the composition of those schemata, cytochrome P450 must be added to the scene. The RARs are primed for activation by retinoic acid and its analogs, whereas the RXRs are receptors for the vitamin A metabolite 9-*cis* retinoic acid (Glass *et al.*, 1997; Rowe, 1997; Troen *et al.*, 1999). It has also been noted by Biesalski and Nohr (2004) that under certain circumstances and in selected tissues, such as buccal mucosa and vaginal epithelium, retinyl ester forms can be taken up directly by cells for nutritional purposes.

The transport of retinoids intracellularly is the purview of the cellular retinol-binding proteins. Retinol first encounters the CRBP class of transport proteins to carry retinol to either esterifying or oxidizing enzymes (Troen *et al.*, 1999). Metabolic transformation of the step of all-

trans RA to 4-hydroxylated RA appears to be primarily catalyzed by the cytochrome P450 (Gidlof *et al.*, 2006; Heise *et al.*, 2006). After oxidation to the aldehyde, and further on to an acid, the CRABP class assumes a relevant regulatory role as well (Rowe, 1997; Napoli, 2000). These intracellular binding proteins show high specificity and affinity for specific retinoids, and seem to control retinoid metabolism both qualitatively and quantitatively. On the former side, they protect retinoids from non-specific interactions, and, on the quantitative side, they have been stated to "chaperone" access of metabolic enzymes to retinoids (Napoli, 1999).

Hepatic Storage

The storage organ for vitamin A is the liver, with 80% of the body's vitamin in the liver, and 50–80% of that located in the fat-storing stellate cells (Senoo *et al.*, 2010). Newly absorbed retinyl esters are packaged in chylomicra, circulated through the mesenteric lymph to the systemic circulation and eventually taken up by the liver (hepatocyte) cells (Napoli, 2000), as shown in Figure 11.3. Its uptake by the liver follows the normal metabolism and degradation of chylomicra to their remnants. Aging greatly retards the clearance rate of retinyl esters from the circulation.

Circulatory Transport

Transport of vitamin A to peripheral tissues occurs primarily by way of a shuttle of recently absorbed vitamin from the liver to the tissues as part of the retinol–RBP–transthyretin (TTR) complex. Within the hepatocyte, retinol forms a complex with RBP, a 183-amino acid residue, 21-23-kDa peptide, and accumulates in the endoplasmic reticulum until retinol for transport becomes available (Gaetani *et al.*, 2002); this in turn joins a binding site on TTR after secretion into the circulation. Stability of RBP's binding to retinol is enhanced by complexing with TTR, increasing the binding affinity of RBP for retinol (Zanotti and Berni, 2004). This undergoes further complexing with the 55-kDa homotetramer TTR to prevent glomerular filtration and urinary excretion of the smaller RBP (Raghu and Sivakumar, 2004).

In states of vitamin A sufficiency, RBP synthesis and accumulation are modest, and little if any newly absorbed vitamin moves out of the liver. In states of vitamin A deficiency, hepatic RBP builds up in the hepatocyte. Consumption of a vitamin A-rich meal translates into a major release of RBP-bound retinol to feed deprived

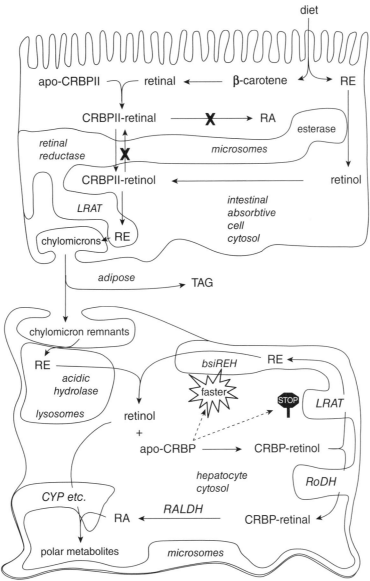

FIG. 11.3 A model of retinol metabolism and retinoic acid (RA) biosynthesis that integrates cumulative data of interactions between cellular retinol-binding protein (CRBP) and CRBP (II) and enzymes that catalyze retinol metabolism. Top panel: Dietary carotenoids undergo central cleavage into retinal, which binds to CRBP (II). A microsomal retinal reductase recognizes retinal bound with CRBP (II) and converts it into retinol. Dietary retinol esters (RE) undergo hydrolysis into retinol, which bind to CRBP (II). Lecithin retinol acyltransferase (LRAT) recognizes the complex CRBP (II)-retinol and synthesizes RE. CRBP(II) prevents oxidation of retinal and retinol, optimizing RE formation. Chylomicrons incorporate and deliver RE to the liver as chylomicron remnants formed after hydrolysis of triacylglycerol (TAG). Bottom panel: Chylomicron remnants deliver RE to the liver, where lysosomes engulf them and an acidic hydrolase releases retinol to bind with CRBP. The holo-CRBP formed serves as substrate for retinol esterification catalyzed by LRAT. A neutral bile salt-independent RE hydrolase (bsiREH) catalyzes RE mobilization. Apo-CRBP controls retinol metabolism by inhibiting LRAT and increasing the rate of hydrolysis via the bsiREH. Holo-CRBP also serves as substrate for retinal formation, catalyzed by retinol dehydrogenase (RoDH). Retinal dehydrogenase (RALDH) isozymes catalyse the irreversible and possibly rate-determining conversion of retinal into RA. Absence of CRBP potentially would allow numerous enzymes access to retinol, in addition to LRAT and RoDH, including perhaps medium-chain alcohol dehydrogenases, cytochromes P-450 (CY), oxidoreductases, etc. Reactive oxygen species, nucleophiles and other intracellular reactive molecules also would have access to retinol in the absence of CRBP. The enhanced access of enzymes and reactive smaller molecular species would accelerate retinol metabolism and RE depletion. Reproduced with permission from Napoli (2000).

peripheral tissues. This is the biological basis for the relative dose–response test (Loerch *et al.*, 1979).

Transplacental Transport

Given the essential role of retinoids in cell proliferation and differentiation and the teratogenic role of retinol and its analogs, the width of the gaps in knowledge concerning the transplacental transport of vitamin A and the dearth of research interest are astounding. What appears to be most likely is that RBP-free retinol diffuses across the intravillous spaces to be captured by RBP of fetal amnio-chorionic membrane origin (Artacho *et al.*, 1993). Two scenarios have been proposed for the enigma of vitamin A nutriture of the fetus: (1) that the vitamin A is derived from the 15 mL of amniotic fluid swallowed daily in utero; or (2) that it derives from the placenta as an extra-intestinal site of bioconversion of β-carotene to the active vitamin (Dimenstein *et al.*, 1996).

Secretory Transport in Lactation

The vitamin A supplied by lactation is adequate to supply all of the needs of the growing infant through the first 6 months of life (Dewey *et al.*, 2004). In a multinational collaborative study involving developed and transitional nations (Australia, Canada, China, Chile, Japan, Mexico, the Philippines, and the United Kingdom), milk retinol levels were generally adequate, but varied two-fold across countries (Canfield *et al.*, 2003). Nevertheless, experience from dairy sciences and laboratory animals provides an inference for the mechanisms by which vitamin A is mobilized to the mammary glands for milk secretion. Rodent (Valentine and Tanumihardjo, 2005) and piglet (Akohoue *et al.*, 2006) studies suggest that recently absorbed vitamin A is preferentially delivered to the milk, as compared with that stored in the liver. The human literature is inconsistent, however, as to the determinance of the specific intake of vitamin A from meals on milk content of the vitamin (Olafsdottir *et al.*, 2001; Menses *et al.*, 2004; Menses and Trugo, 2005). Even more inconsistency about diet's determinance comes from reports on the degree to which high-dose oral supplements of retinyl palmitate to lactating mothers improve vitamin A concentrations or augment circulating retinol in the offspring (Oliveira-Menegozzo and Bergamaschi, 2010).

Findings related to carotenoids as a source of infant vitamin A were even more interesting. Overall, provitamin A species constituted 50% of total milk carotenoids. In the aforementioned multinational study (Canfield *et al.*, 2003), total carotenoids were highest in Japanese milk samples and lowest in the Philippines, whereas β-carotene content was highest in Chile and lowest in the Philippines. In Brazilian mothers, the plasma-to-milk ratio for β-carotene was 17:1, with modest mutual association (Menses and Trugo, 2005). Observations comparing carotenoid patterns in colostrum and mature milk may provide some inferential insights into the distribution of provitamin A to human milk. In colostrum, the carotenoid pattern resembled that in LDL lipoproteins, whereas at 19 days (mature milk) it reflected that in HDL, suggesting that the transfer of carotenoids to milk involves different lipoproteins at different specific times of lactation (Schweigert *et al.*, 2004).

Excretion

The primary excretion route for vitamin A metabolites from the body is in the bile. In rodent models (Skare and DeLuca, 1983; Hicks *et al.*, 1984), vitamin A is excreted with a fixed concentration in bile, with net losses depending on biliary volume. With increased hepatic stores, output increases in a responsive manner (Skare and DeLuca, 1983). The fractional loss of vitamin A in the urine is minuscule under usual circumstances. Eclampsia, acute renal failure, multiple myeloma, and febrile infections, however, are pathological situations producing excessive urinary losses. An estimated 20–40% of a child's liver reserve can be lost in the urine during a severe diarrheal episode (Mitra *et al.*, 2002).

Physiology of Vitamin A: Functions and Actions

The late Professor James A. Olson defined the "function" of a food constituent as "an essential role played by the nutrient in growth, development, and maturation"; by contrast, he defined "actions" as "demonstrable effects in various biologic systems that may or may not have general physiologic significance" (Olson, 1998).

Physiological Functions of Vitamin A

Some form of retinoid is involved in the functions of every cell in the body. Vision, intercellular communication, mucin production, embryogenesis, cell growth, and cell differentiation are prominent among the gamut of functions related to vitamin A.

Retinal Isomer and Visual Pigments in the Visual Cycle

The classical function for which vitamin A is known is in the visual cycle. The vitamin A metabolite retinaldehyde (retinal) is an active component of the visual pigments in the rods and cones of the retina. For dim-light (scotopic) vision with the dark-adapted eye, the cycle involves the regeneration of the rhodopsin pigment, with the insertion of 11-*cis*-retinal. Low-intensity photons produce the cleavage of the pigment–retinoid complex, liberating dissociated all-*trans*-retinal, and exciting neural transmission, as originally described by George Wald (1968). The regeneration of the retinol from the aldehyde form was the primary feature, and the molecular biology of this visual pathway has subsequently been elucidated. For high-resolution, color (photopic) vision in daylight, the retinal cones of the retinal epithelium are involved in a similar, although less well understood, photon-activated excitation and neural signal transmission. The regeneration of 11-*cis*-retinal via all-*trans*-retinol to 11-*cis*-retinal has been shown to be distinct in the photopic vision cycle (Wolf, 2004).

Retinoids and Intercellular Communication

One of the macro-level functions for the integrity and function of tissues is the communication among adjacent cells. This can occur by various signaling mechanisms, the best understood of which is the connexin 36 mechanism at so-called "gap junctions" across the intercellular space. All-*trans*-retinal and retinoic acid have been shown to be potent inhibitors of connexin-36-mediated gap junctional communication (Pulukuri and Sitaramayya, 2004). On the other hand, within the cell nucleus, retinoic acid induces adhesion proteins and membrane complexes necessary for cell-to-cell adhesion and communication among hepatocytes (Ara *et al.*, 2004).

Mechanism of Action as a Nuclear Hormone

The functions, metabolism, and relationship to their nuclear receptors of natural retinoids have been reviewed (Ziouzenkova and Plutzky, 2008; Rochette-Egly and Germain, 2009; Lefebvre *et al.*, 2010; Amman *et al.*, 2011). Much of the wide variety of functions of vitamin A enumerated earlier are derived from a complex retinoid signaling pathway system in which various isometric forms of retinoic acid act as nuclear hormones (Evans, 2005). These include all-*trans*-retinoic acid and 9-*cis*-retinoic acid as the principal players, with additional participation by 13-*cis*-retinoic acid. As alluded to below, a wide array of synthetic retinoid analogs can also participate in the signaling system in pharmacological situations.

The retinoids act as transcription factors, modulating and regulating either the activation or repression of messenger RNA formation in cell nuclei (Lefebvre *et al.*, 2010). This is effected by their serving as binding ligands in nuclear receptor complexes. The basic elements of the genetic signaling system are the nuclear receptors. The receptors for retinoic acid (RAR) and its 9-*cis* isomer (RXR) each have three subtypes (alpha, beta, and gamma). RARs can bind and respond to both retinoic acid and its isomer, whereas RXRs are specific for an isometric form (9-*cis*-retinoic acid). The receptors act through either dimerization to form homodimers (RAR–RAR, RXR–RXR) or heterodimers (RAR–RXR) with the various permutations of the Greek-letter subtypes. Cooperative binding to hormone response elements coordinates the regulation of target genes by RXR ligands. The transcription regulation, moreover, can involve further heterodimer formation between the RXR receptor and either thyroid hormone receptor or the peroxisome proliferator-activated receptor-gamma (PPAR-γ) (Higgins and Depaoli, 2010).

The best-known roles of the retinoid receptor system involve the regulation of the division and differentiation of cells. Signals involving the RXR reduce cellular proliferation and enhance programmed cell death (apoptosis) (Nohara *et al.*, 2009). The pivotal action of intracellular retinoid regulatory roles via RAR in cellular differentiation involves influencing the cell cycle proteins (Chen and Ross, 2004).

An alternative mechanism for influencing genetic expression involves epigenetic regulation at the level of conformation of the chromatin backbone of the helical nucleic acid strands of DNA. Mammalian reflections of the uncoupling of histone acetylation in the HIV1 virus are postulated (Kiefer *et al.*, 2004). Interestingly, the alcohol form, retinol, has been shown possibly to have epigenetic potential in modifying the chromatin conformation of a zinc-finger domain of the gene for serine/threonine kinase expression (Hoyos *et al.*, 2005).

Up-regulated expression of mRNA for mucin proteins of the conjunctiva and the respiratory tract by retinoic acid is a classical example of signaling related to intracellular protein synthesis (Hori *et al.*, 2004). The retinoid signaling system is central to embryogenesis such as of the brachial arches (Mark *et al.*, 2004) and the alveolar membrane of the lungs (Maden and Hind, 2004).

Retinoic acid, circulating in nanomolar concentrations in blood, accounts for the majority of the supply for the brain and liver, but is also locally produced in other tissues (Ross, 2004). Beyond the serial oxidation of retinol is the intracorporeal bioconversion of carotenoids as a potential source of retinoids at the tissue and cellular level (Tang *et al.*, 2003).

Actions of Vitamin A

Outside of the evolutionary functions of vitamin A for the metabolism in normal health, vitamin A exhibits a series of actions that assist in the correction of various pathological conditions.

Antiproliferative Action

The ability of vitamin A and its isomeric forms to promote terminal differentiation, inhibit proliferation, and promote apoptosis comes into play in neoplasia. High-dose retinoids have shown anti-neoplastic activity in vitro in a diverse array of cancer cell lines as discussed below (Dawson and Zhang, 2002; Abu *et al.*, 2005; Evans, 2005).

Improved Iron Uptake from Meals

Iron is a vitally essential but generally poorly bioavailable dietary trace element. There are a series of conflicting observations related to enhancement of the biological availability of iron. Vitamin A, including provitamin A forms, improved iron absorption, presumably by nullifying the interference of phytates (Layrisse *et al.*, 1997, 1998; Garcia-Casal *et al.*, 1998). Swiss investigators examined iron absorption efficiency from iron-fortified maize porridge in vitamin A-deficient African children in the presence or absence of retinyl palmitate, and found no enhancement (Davidsson *et al.*, 2003). Since the settings and systems used in Venezuela and Africa are so different, the final word on this potential dietary action of vitamin A is not yet established.

Manifestations and Consequences of Vitamin A Deficiency and Variation in Vitamin A Nutriture

Deficiency of vitamin A is associated with clinical and functional manifestations. However, apparent variations of vitamin A status within the range that would be considered adequate also can influence human health and modulate physiological function.

Ocular Manifestations

Xerophthalmia (literally, dryness of the eye) is the hallmark clinical feature of clinical vitamin A deficiency. It has been classified by stages according to specific ocular manifestations. Stage XN, the earliest stage, involves night blindness due to impaired dark adaptation. Stage X1A is conjunctival xerosis due to reduction in goblet cell mucus, followed by stage X1B, which is manifested by Bitot's spots, foamy excrescences on the temporal surface of the conjunctiva. Corneal xerosis constitutes the advancing stages, with X2 being simple drying of the cornea, with involvement of less than (X3A) or more than (X3B) one-third of the corneal surface with ulceration or corneal liquefaction, respectively. Past involvement leaves a corneal scar (XS), and a globe destroyed by advanced keratomalacia is xerophthalmic fundus.

Other Epithelial Dysfunction Syndromes

Other epithelial tissues are affected by vitamin A deficiency. Thickening of the hair follicles (follicular hyperkeratosis) is a cutaneous manifestation of vitamin A deficiency. The reduction in mucin production in mucous membranes from the adenopharyngeal passages, bronchial and pulmonary tissue to the digestive tract, produces symptomatic distress and susceptibility to microbial invasion. Overt esophagitis is a recently recognized consequence of the mucosal alterations of impaired vitamin A status (Herring *et al.*, 2010).

Excessive Mortality Rates

The pioneering epidemiological observations of Sommer *et al.* (1983) in the Ache region of Indonesia in the 1980s first informed us that marginal vitamin A status was associated with excessive mortality from childhood infections. This was confirmed first by a vitamin A intervention study in the same population (Sommer *et al.*, 1986) and then by meta-analyses across six sites (Beaton *et al.*, 1993). Additional confirmatory intervention studies continue to emerge, including a 22% mortality reduction in newborn infants in southern India (Rahmathullah *et al.*, 2003) and a 46% reduction in HIV-infected children in Uganda (Semba *et al.*, 2005).

In developed countries, sudden infant death syndrome (SIDS) may bear some relationship to differential vitamin A status. Observations from Sweden suggested a high association between SIDS and infants not being given vitamin A supplements during the first year of life (Alm *et al.*, 2003).

Excess Infectious Morbidity

Although deaths from childhood infectious diseases are more common in low-income societies, and immune defense deficiencies result from marginal vitamin A deficiency, little evidence for reduced *incidence* (new occurrences) of infectious episodes has been gleaned from community intervention trials. The odds ratio was 1.08 for the effect of prophylactic vitamin A supplementation on acute respiratory infections in a meta-analysis (Grotto *et al.*, 2003), whereas a comparable analysis for efficacy also showed no efficacy (Brown and Roberts, 2004). Supplementation was effective to prevent cough among HIV-infected children in Uganda (Semba *et al.*, 2005). The prevention of diarrhea is another domain in which meta-analyses revealed no efficacy (Grotto *et al.*, 2003). In the situation of HIV, however, reductions in the incidence of acute and chronic diarrhea (Semba *et al.*, 2005) have been noted. As tentative resolution of this apparent mortality–morbidity paradox, it is postulated that the specific intensity and lethality of infections is aggravated in the child with marginal vitamin A status.

Hematological Support

Observational studies have documented an independent association of vitamin A status with hematological adequacy (Kafwembe, 2001; Gamble *et al.*, 2004; Osório *et al.*, 2004) beyond any direct action of meal vitamin A to enhance iron absorption. Historically, vitamin A interventions were shown to improve hemoglobin or hematocrits in a multiply deficient, anemic population. Semba and Bloem (2002) propose several metabolic mechanisms whereby modulation of vitamin A exposure and status could influence red cell biology: stimulating progenitor cells, promoting resistance to infection, and mobilization of iron to the erythron. Basic research provides evidence for retinoids regulating hematopoiesis from the yolk sac stage in the embryo to the fetal liver production in utero to the bone marrow (Oren *et al.*, 2003).

Not only is the erythropoietic line of bone marrow proliferation related to vitamin A, but platelet production is also influenced by retinoid biology. Japanese oncologists observed increased thrombocytosis and thrombopoietin levels in patients treated with all-*trans*-retinoic acid for acute promyelocytic leukemia. In subsequent in vitro studies in bone marrow stromal cell culture, all-*trans*-retinoic acid triples thrombopoietin mRNA expression (Kinjo *et al.*, 2004).

Miscellaneous Considerations

Endemic vitamin A deficiency and controlled observations of responses to vitamin A supplementation interventions have received so much interest in observational and intervention studies that commentary on consequences that do not appear to be part of the hypovitaminosis A context may not receive specific attention. Two situations of benefits from vitamin A unrelated to initial deficiency are of interest. For instance, in the situation of HIV-infected preschoolers, vitamin A supplementation to non-deficient women improved postnatal growth of children in Tanzania (Villamor *et al.*, 2005), while direct child supplementation improved growth in the same milieu (Villamor *et al.*, 2002). A curious, but potentially important, recent observation in hemodialysis patients is that a lower circulating retinol level is an independent predictor of overall cardiovascular mortality in this population (Kalousová *et al.*, 2010).

Causes of Variation in Vitamin A Status and the Epidemiology of Vitamin A Deficiency

Secondary vitamin A deficiency can arise in any situation or clinical condition or illness in which there is reduced absorption, increased excretion, enhanced destruction, impaired utilization, or exaggerated requirement for the nutrient.

Conditions Predisposing to Impaired Vitamin A Status

A standard list of predisposing causes of vitamin A deficiency has been recognized for decades. These include a myriad of situations of low intake and reduced bioconvertibility of dietary vitamin A, along with poor intestinal absorption, impaired utilization of the vitamin, and its increased destruction or wastage. Recent concerns focus on impairment in vitamin A nutriture in novel conditions or emergent or re-emergent diseases. These include: bariatric surgical procedures for weight loss (Slater *et al.*, 2004; Mason *et al.*, 2005), pancreaticoduodenostomy ablation surgery for malignancies (Armstrong *et al.*, 2005), peritoneal dialysis (Aguilera *et al.*, 2002), hematopoietic stem cell transplant (High *et al.*, 2002), acute respiratory syndromes (Schmidt *et al.*, 2004), pulmonary tuberculosis (van Lettow *et al.*, 2004), cigarette smoking (Tiboni *et al.*, 2004), HIV/AIDS (Visser *et al.*, 2003; Vorster *et al.*, 2004), and asthma (Arora *et al.*, 2002).

Population Epidemiology of Hypovitaminosis A

The current estimates of hypovitaminosis A on a worldwide basis suggest that it is the second most common micronutrient deficiency. Singh and West (2004) estimate that 23% of children between the ages of 5 and 15 years in Southeast Asian nations have deficient vitamin A status. In a nationally representative sample of Mexico (Villalpando *et al.*, 2003), low retinol levels were found in a quarter of the sample, with highest rates in indigenous communities in the southern part of the country. Diverse, contemporary surveys have identified a prevalence of impaired vitamin A status in Inuit and First Nation newborns (Dallaire *et al.*, 2003), Israeli Bedouin toddlers (Coles *et al.*, 2004), black toddlers in the Western Cape of South Africa (Oelofse *et al.*, 2002), nomadic herder women in Chad (Zinsstag *et al.*, 2002), and pregnant urban women in Nigeria (Ajose *et al.*, 2004). Risk factors found variously across sites of hypovitaminosis A endemicity were male gender (Semba *et al.*, 2004), young age of children (Villalpando *et al.*, 2003; Semba *et al.*, 2004), low body-mass index (BMI) (Villalpando *et al.*, 2003), stunting (Semba *et al.*, 2004), familial xerophthalmia history (Semba *et al.*, 2004), history of maternal diarrhea (Semba *et al.*, 2004), the nutritional quality of pastoralists' milk (Zinsstag *et al.*, 2002), and warm seasons (Semba *et al.*, 2004).

Nutrient Requirements and Recommended Intakes for Dietary Vitamin A

Quantitative Expression of Dietary Vitamin A Activity

Units of expression of vitamin A in foods and pharmaceutical preparations have a tortuous history, and present confusion to consumers and professionals alike. Historically, we have international units (IU) from early food science literature, retinol equivalents (RE), adopted by a Food and Agriculture Organization of the United Nations/World Health Organization (FAO/WHO) panel in 1967 (FAO/WHO, 1967), and retinol *activity* equivalents (RAE), created by the US Institute of Medicine for the 2001 *Dietary Reference Intakes* (Institute of Medicine, 2001). Certain measures can be taken to promote harmonization and reduce inconsistencies.

The IU expression can be found in food composition tables, and is still widely used in medicinal contexts. The conversion relationship is 1 IU = 3.3 RE (1 RE = 0.3 IU), which is valid only for preformed vitamin A. Where *preformed* vitamin A in foods or supplements are concerned, RE and RAE are completely interchangeable. Interconversions involving the IU and provitamin A are universally invalid, and expression of dietary vitamin A in mixed diets in RE or RAE will grossly overestimate true vitamin content.

The RE is related to vitamin A compounds in gravimetric units in the following manner:

1 RE = 1 μg of retinol
1 RE = 6 μg of all-*trans* β-carotene
1 RE = 12 μg of other provitamin A carotenes

The equivalency definitions for RAEs provided in the DRI (Institute of Medicine, 2001) were:

1 RAE = 1 μg of retinol
1 RAE = 2 μg of all-*trans* β-carotene as supplement
1 RAE = 12 μg of all-*trans* β-carotene in food matrix
1 RAE = 24 μg of other provitamin A carotenes in food matrix

The aforementioned considerations regarding the inferior conversion for carotenes in the plant matrices and the superior bioconversion of isolated carotenes in an oily matrix, reviewed above, guided the creation of the RAE. For clarification, the "other" provitamin A carotenes include the stereoisomers of β-carotene, as well as compounds such as α-carotene and β-cryptoxanthin. Moreover, it must be clarified that, implicitly, 4 μg of other provitamin A carotenoids alone or in oil could also be equivalent to 1 RAE. What still may be unresolved within the RAE convention is an appropriate value for carotenes that are free of plant matrices but in a relatively modest fatty milieu. This would apply to provitamin A in milk and most cheeses, as well as in eggs.

Estimated Human Requirements and Recommended Dietary Intakes

For planning and evaluation, it is important to have estimates of the daily requirements of vitamin A. The recommendable intakes for vitamin A from both the 2001 DRIs for the United States and Canada (Institute of Medicine, 2001) and the 2004 WHO and Food and Nutrition Organization *Human Vitamin and Mineral Requirements* (FAO/WHO, 2004) are outlined in Table 11.1. The former are based, when possible, around estimated average requirements (EAR) for relevant age

TABLE 11.1 Recommendations for Daily Intake of vitamin A from the US Institute of Medicine and the World Health Organization

Population	United Nations System (WHO/FAO)		United States and Canada dietary reference intakes	
	Recalculated estimated average requirements[a]	Recommended nutrient intake	Estimated average requirement	Recommended dietary allowance
	RE/day		RAE/day	
0–6 months	–	375	–	400 AI
7–12 months	–	400	–	500 AI
0–1 years	290	400	–	–
1–3 years	320	450	210	300
4–6 years	320	450	–	–
4–8 years	–	–	275	400
7–9 years	360	500	–	–
9–13 years	–	–	445[b]; 420[c]	600
10–18 years	430	600	–	–
14–18 years males	–	–	630	900
14–18 years females	–	–	485	700
Adult males	430	600	625	900
Adult females	360	500	500	750
Pregnant	570	800	550	770
Lactating	610	850	900	1300

AI, adequate intake; RE, retinol equivalents; RAE, retinol activity equivalents.
[a]Using modeling provided on p. 292 of Allen et al. (2006) and rounded off to the nearest zero. They can only be applied after 1 year of age.
[b]Males.
[c]Females.

groups, sexes, and physiological status. When individual recommended nutrient intakes are considered, for an intake level of reference to assure upwards of a 90% probability of covering the requirement of vitamin A for a healthy individual, the DRI calculates a recommended dietary allowance (RDA) and the United Nations (UN) agencies provide a recommended nutrient intake (RNI). Returning to the EARs, their primary purpose is to allow for probabilistic estimates for the prevalence of individuals at risk in a *population* (Murphy and Poos, 2002). EARs were not originally part of the UN system at the time of its publication in 2004 (FAO/WHO, 2004), but a WHO document on food fortification (Allen *et al.*, 2006) provides for a back-calculated modeling of these population means.

The discrepancy between the units of dietary vitamin A activity, RAE for the DRI (Institute of Medicine, 2001) and RE for the UN system (FAO/WHO, 2004), compli-

cates the discussion of recommended intakes of vitamin A for an international forum. Nevertheless, there is a certain degree of correspondence in the estimates for protective intakes, RNI, and RDA for vitamin A between the two options in Table 11.1. The recommended intakes of the UN system agencies are slightly lower for infancy, higher for childhood, and lower again for adolescence and adulthood. The major discrepancy between the two panels of recommendations relates to the disproportion in estimated requirements for lactation.

Food Sources and Dietary Intakes of Vitamin A

The richest animal sources of vitamin A in the human diet are fish liver oils, liver, other organ meats, cream, butter, and fortified milks. Certain tropical fatty fruits are the richest sources of provitamin A.

Estimates of Average Dietary Intake and Adequacy of Vitamin Consumption

There is a large dietetic and nutritional literature on vitamin A intakes by different populations. Nevertheless, differences in dietary methodology, use of different food compositions and different units of measurement, and variation in expression (median vs. mean), with different ways of adjusting and modeling are among the challenges to its synthesis and comparison. For instance, the RAE unit is not fully accepted or used outside of the US and Canada, and little if any survey results using the RAE have been published in the decade since its creation. One survey, denominated in RAE, was published for *pregnant* Mexican-American women in 2005 by Harley *et al.* For the US-born subjects in the survey (Harley *et al.*, 2005), the vitamin A intake from foods and beverages was 1035 RAE, but this rose to 2156 RAE when prenatal vitamin supplement content was included in the summation. Surprisingly these totals were about 300 RAE lower than corresponding Mexican-born subjects in the same study, whose higher intakes related exclusively to additional consumption of the vitamin on the dietary side.

Erwin *et al.* (2004) disaggregated the mean contribution of preformed vitamin A to the sex-combined representative samples of United States adults from the era of 1999–2000. Still estimated in RE, the average preformed vitamin A was 1484 RE, and with an estimated contribution from provitamin A in plants of 450 RE, and a total of 1934 RE; insofar as the use of the RE expression tends to overvalue the contribution of carotene sources, equivalency in RAE would be somewhat lower, at 225 RE, for a revised combination in the Erwin *et al.* (2004) data of 1610 RE. This is far greater than estimates for European populations, with the RE-based average intake of the vitamin from foods in surveys estimated at 900 RE (Goldbohm *et al.*, 1998) for Dutch women and 549 RE for British women (Henderson *et al.*, 2003). Across a broad selection of the data in surveys and convenience samples in low-income societies of the tropical regions, women's estimated intakes, expressed in RE, are on the order of that for the British sample or lower.

Children are theoretically the most vulnerable segment of society for ill effects from hypovitaminosis A. Clearly, central tendencies of juveniles' intake of the vitamin from the era in which the contribution of provitamin A was overvalued by two-fold, were much higher in Europe (Serra-Majem *et al.*, 2001; Sichert-Hellert *et al.*, 2001a;

Watt *et al.*, 2001) than on the Indian subcontinent (Venkaiah *et al.*, 2002).

With respect to adequacy of intakes, preformed vitamin A levels were above the EAR in adult women of all ethnic groups in small towns of the contemporary rural south of the United States (Lewis *et al.*, 2003) and generally among pregnant Mexican-American women (Harley *et al.*, 2005). From studies in selected European adult samples, over 10% of the Spanish population was shown to be consuming less than two-thirds of the referent standard for vitamin A intake (Aranceta *et al.*, 2001); among Portuguese elderly, 78% of men and 73% of women had intakes below the lowest European recommended dietary intake levels (Martins *et al.*, 2002).

Dietary Sources of Vitamin A

The comparative aspects for the contribution of different foods and beverages to vitamin A intake is relatively less susceptible to the vagaries that confound quantitative estimates. Dietary sources from two representative national survey samples, for the United States and The Netherlands, are available. Sixty-seven percent of cumulative intake of vitamin A in the US diet, as calculated in RE, comprised, in descending order: carrots, organ meats, ready-to-eat cereals, cheese, margarine, tomatoes, and eggs (Cotton *et al.*, 2004). Carrots constitute 27% of all estimated intake. Comparable data for The Netherlands, also in RE but organized by food groups, found 91% of all vitamin A consumed came from meats (35%), fats and oils (24%), vegetables (16%), and dairy foods (16%) (Goldbohm *et al.*, 1998).

Among Inuits of Canada, the livers of seals, caribou, and fish provide half of the vitamin A, and market foods provide the other half (Egeland *et al.*, 2004). It has been estimated that fortified dairy products can contribute 39% of the RDA in three standard portions in Spain (Herrero *et al.*, 2002). In central Java, where 83% of pregnant women consumed less than 700 RE in the first trimester of pregnancy, plant sources contributed 64% to 79% of total vitamin A (Persson *et al.*, 2002). As noted above, dietary supplements make an important contribution to vitamin A intake. Through interval nationally representative surveys in the United States from 1987 to 1992 to 2000, the use of dietary supplements has increased steadily from 23.2% to 23.7% to 33.9% across the successive time points (Millen *et al.*, 2004). Supplement use is credited with reducing the number of adults consuming substandard amounts of vitamin A by Irish adults from 20% to 5% (Kiely *et al.*, 2001).

With respect to juvenile populations, German children and adolescents received 50–65% of reference intake needs of vitamin A from non-fortified foods in their diets, and an additional 10–20% from fortified foods (Sichert-Hellert *et al.*, 2001a, b). This cohort had shown a 5–15% increase in the amount of the vitamin obtained from fortified beverages during the previous 15-year period (Sichert-Hellert *et al.*, 2001b). On the island of Guam in the South Pacific, fruit drinks, milk, and fortified cereals contributed most of the vitamin A in Guamanian children, the median vitamin A intake was 76% of the age-appropriate RDA (Pobocic and Richer, 2002). For the children living on the mainland of the United States, however, concern has been expressed that excessive sweetened drink consumption is associated with displacement of milk from children's diets, higher daily energy intake, and greater weight gain (Mrdjenovic and Levitsky, 2003).

Human milk can be a relatively important source of vitamin A, even beyond the first year of life. According to a study in Kenya, breast milk supplies more vitamin A than the complementary foods that replace it, making it an "irreplaceable source of fat and vitamin A" (Onyango *et al.*, 2002). The role of supplements as the source of vitamin A for juvenile populations is now beginning to emerge, even in the first two years of life. Among a cohort followed from infants to toddlers in the US state of Iowa, 32% were consuming vitamin A-containing supplements 40–60% of days by the age of 24 months (Eichenberger-Gilmore *et al.*, 2005).

Factors Affecting Vitamin A Consumption

The influence of cultural, behavioral, and physical factors on vitamin A intake has been studied in various adult populations. In a study among pregnant women in the United States, Mexican-born women consumed more vitamin A than US-born Mexican-American women during pregnancy (Cotton *et al.*, 2004). Edentulous US white elderly consumed less vitamin A and carotene than peers with adequate dentition, although no gradient was seen in African-American contemporaries compared in an analogous manner related to mastication capacity. Smoking behavior – smokers, ex-smokers, or never smokers – had no effect on vitamin A intake in Greater Chicago residents (Dyer *et al.*, 2003). In an analysis of US Department of Agriculture (USDA) survey data, estimated vitamin A

intakes were highest in those who derived the greatest portion of energy from carbohydrates (Bowman and Spence, 2002). Meals containing traditional native foods provide more vitamin A than non-traditional commodities among indigenous populations of the Arctic of Canada (Kuhnlein *et al.*, 2004).

In children, adequacy of vitamin A intakes decreases with age (Serra-Majem *et al.*, 2001; Lytle *et al.*, 2002). Moreover, a gender gap emerges and widens over time, with boys' relative intakes better maintained than those of girls (Lytle *et al.*, 2002). Ethnicity joins sex as a factor among US children, with the Continuing Survey of Food Intakes showing that being black or being a female child of any race conferred the highest risk of consuming less than two-thirds of the RDA for vitamin A (Ganji *et al.*, 2003).

A predictor of a preschool child's not meeting the RNI in the northern regions of the United Kingdom was being the son or daughter of a manual laborer (Thane *et al.*, 2004). In the metro Manila area, schoolchildren of higher socioeconomic status consumed more vitamin A than those of low socioeconomic status (Florentino *et al.*, 2002). In British youth, low intake was inverse to dairy food consumption (Thane *et al.*, 2004). Finally, consuming a more "Mediterranean" diet did not influence the relative adequacy of vitamin A intake (Serra-Majem *et al.*, 2003).

Diagnostic Assessment of Vitamin A Nutriture

The Biomarkers of Nutrition for Development (BOND) project is giving impetus to the re-examination of diagnostic assessment of nutritional status by pointing out some obvious discrepancies and weaknesses in the current application and interpretation of nutritional biomarkers (Raiten *et al.*, 2011). After a period of dormancy and reliance on established conventions, renewed emphasis on evidence-based decision making and expanding technological and logistic capacity to measure nutrients and metabolites in the clinic and in populations have provided incentives for more objective, transparent, and robust documentation and analysis.

The BOND biomarker paradigm is divided into three levels of interest for any nutrient: (1) magnitude of exposure to the nutrient; (2) nutrient (nutritional) status; and (3) functional consequences of exposure. It seeks primarily material (chemical) markers, with less tangible (behavioral) indicators as a second level of marker. It recognizes for a nutrient such as vitamin A that health and policy issues revolve around how much of the nutrient is actually offered and consumed. Since there is no stoichiometric relationship between consumption with uptake, retention, and utilization, the first level of quantifying exposure is somewhat discrete from nutrient status; the latter refers to the amount of the nutrient within stores and functional pathways. Finally, insofar as nutrients have functions and actions, as discussed earlier, the third element of the paradigm looks for concrete measures of functional consequence attributable to a given degree of nutrient exposure. In general terms, all three of the aforementioned elements can refer to individuals (a specific diagnosis), or to groups of individuals (as prevalence and rates).

A virtual plethora of diagnostic options are displayed in Table 11.2. The key to rational selection depends, in part, on whether the application is for individuals in a clinical context or for a population for epidemiological and public health purposes. In the former, it is our interest to get an accurate measurement for the individual patient to diagnose the underlying disease or take a decision for supplement therapy. When it comes to a population, the issue is the risk of a substantial number of individuals having suboptimal vitamin A status to merit a collective or targeted intervention program. In general, the limits on diagnostic methods for clinical practice derive from the day-to-day variation or distortion by clinical conditions, which combine to create imprecision in reflecting the underlying status of an individual, or both. The limits on assessment testing at the public health and population level derive from constraints of cost, convenience, acceptability, and ethical application in otherwise healthy persons.

Evolution of Vitamin A Assessment

It was the emergence of interest in vitamin A and childhood mortality (Sommer et al., 1983), in which preclinical ("marginal") vitamin A deficiency was a risk factor, that stimulated creation of assessment tools. In 1993, in a guideline book from the International Vitamin A Consultative Group, Underwood and Olson (1993) set forth its mission: to provide tools for "assessing the regional distribution and magnitude of vitamin A deficiency." It covered 13 assessment areas, 10 of which would be firmly considered biomarkers. This was followed, in 1996, by a largely derivative official WHO publication (WHO, 1996) which claimed to provide "principles governing the use of biological indicators for vitamin A deficiency (VAD) surveillance [providing] the rationale behind each indicator and its limitations and cut-off points for interpretation in terms of public health significance." Almost a decade later, Tanumihardjo (2004) comments, in published proceedings: "having many choices of vitamin A assessment methods, laboratory sophistication and resources available will usually dictate which methods are chosen." As part of the BOND, she has updated her consideration: "biomarkers of vitamin A status are still needed for the near future in order to more specifically identify populations at risk for vitamin A deficiency and to evaluate the effectiveness of different interventions or programs" (Tanumihardjo, 2011).

TABLE 11.2 Clinical assessment of vitamin A status and estimation of population risk of vitamin A deficiency

Dietary intake assessment	Test type
Biological fluid markers	Circulating retinol
	Retinol binding protein (RBP)
	RBP/transthyretin (TTR) ratio
	Breast-milk retinol
Isotope dilution tests	Deuterated retinol dilution test (DRD)
Tissue biopsy markers	Invasive:
	-Hepatic biopsy assay
	Non-invasive:
	-Buccal cell vitamin A
Functional tests	Invasive:
	-Relative dose–response (RDR)
	-Modified RDR
	-30-day RDR
	Mildly invasive:
	-Conjunctival impression
	-Cytology
	Non-invasive:
	-Dark adaptation tests
	-Self-reported night blindness

Gold Standards of Vitamin A Status for Reference to Biomarkers

A chemical rendering of a cadaver postmortem is the most definitive gold standard, but of little clinical relevance. Since 80% of vitamin stores are in the liver, chemical analysis of a percutaneous liver biopsy is the second best approximation (Figures 11.4 and 11.5), and reflection of

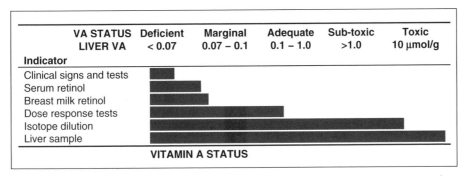

VA STATUS LIVER VA	Deficient < 0.07	Marginal 0.07 – 0.1	Adequate 0.1 – 1.0	Sub-toxic >1.0	Toxic 10 μmol/g
Indicator					
Clinical signs and tests					
Serum retinol					
Breast milk retinol					
Dose response tests					
Isotope dilution					
Liver sample					

VITAMIN A STATUS

FIG. 11.4 The horizontal axis represents a continuum of hepatic vitamin A concentrations in μmol/g, with corresponding division into range bands categorizing specific states of vitamin A status. For each of the six approaches (one clinical method and five biomarkers), the range of liver concentration in which an abnormal result can provide diagnostic validity is represented by the horizontal solid bars in each row. Reproduced with permission from Tanumihardjo (2011).

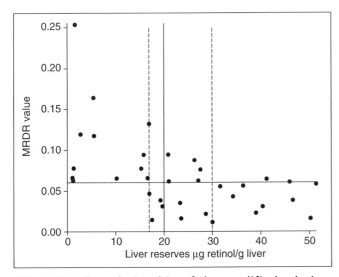

FIG. 11.5 The relationship of the modified relative-dose–response value to liver retinol concentration in piglets. Below 17 μg/g liver, the MRDR value is invariably positive, i.e. >0.060; between 17 and 29 μg/g, the response is split; and above 29 μg/g liver, the MRDR value is usually <0.060. Reproduced with permission from Tanumihardjo (2011).

hepatic stores is the metric of other biomarkers (WHO, 1996; Tanumihardjo, 2004, 2011). Underwood and Olson (1993) consider 1.05 μmol of vitamin A per gram of liver tissue (equivalent to 30 μg/g in gravimetric units) the lower threshold for normal vitamin A status. The safest surrogate "gold standard" method for assessment of total body vitamin A is deuterated-retinol, stable-isotopic dilution technique (Tang *et al.*, 2002; Ribaya-Mercado *et al.*, 2003, 2004a,b); it reflects hepatic vitamin A levels across the entire spectrum from depletion to intoxication (Figure 11.4).

Biomarkers for Patient Management in Clinical Practice

If vitamin A status is severely deficient, clinical acumen in the physical examination may provide suspicion of hypovitaminosis A. In general, the majority of the screening tests listed in Table 11.2 are not relevant to hospital or clinic practice. Only the circulating retinol for routine application and the tissue biopsy for extraordinary use are of major interest. With respect to the former, however, for clinical assessment retinol has a series of recognized limitations. It is often low in situations of deficiency. It can be falsely normal in the situation of recent ingestion of preformed vitamin, dehydration, or hyperproteinemia, or falsely low with hypoproteinemia, infection, inflammatory states, obesity, hormonal replacement, or oral contraception. It has been suggested that only circulating concentrations <10 μg/dL (0.35 μmol) have any robust diagnostic significance for vitamin A inadequacy (Underwood and Olson, 1993), but it is probably more prudent to be guided by the established limits of normality for circulating retinol in the clinical laboratory of record. A lower-than (or higher-than) limit result should guide the practitioner to pursue the implications for differential diagnosis in an individual case.

Biomarkers for Population Assessment in Surveys and Epidemiology

In the era of concern surrounding "marginal" vitamin A deficiency and the populations in which it is endemic, the relevance of biomarkers relates to action for public health (Underwood and Olson, 1993; WHO, 1996; Tanumihardjo, 2004, 2011). Among the selected biomarkers listed in Table 11.2, those with the lowest degree of invasiveness, complexity, and cost are the initial candidates for application in the field survey setting. According to the recent review by Tanumihardjo (2011), only four biomarkers (serum retinol, breast-milk retinol, dose–response tests, isotope dilution) have been cross-calibrated with grades of liver vitamin A concentration, and only the first three are appropriate for the field assessment for marginal vitamin A status of a population. Serum retinol and breast-milk retinol would both be susceptible to distortion by inflammation and infection, which are prevalent in low-income populations; they would be limited as monitoring indices for improvement in response to interventions by not bridging from the marginal to the adequate band of hepatic vitamin stores.

The family of dose–response tests, the relative dose response (RDR) (Stephensen et al., 2002; Verhoef and West, 2005) and the modified RDR (Tanumihardjo and Olson, 1988; Tanumihardjo et al., 1990a,b) merit special attention because of their putative ability to respond across a wider range of vitamin A status and through the range of the spectrum most relevant to public health (Figure 11.4). Both are based on the same physiological principle, namely that apo-RBP builds up in the liver during vitamin A deprivation; hence, an acute dosing with oral retinol leads to an exaggerated export of vitamin A. This response can be tracked as a quantitative post-dose elevation in retinol concentrations in the standard RDR, which requires two serial blood samples at a 5-hour interval (Verhoef and West, 2005), or an increment in a variant vitamin A isomer (3,4-didehydroretinol) in the modified RDR, which requires only a single (4-hour post-dose) blood sampling (Tanumihardjo et al., 1990b; Tanumihardjo, 2011). The sensitivity and specificity of the modified RDR (MRDR) in relation to the $30\,\mu g/g$ ($1.05\,\mu mol/g$) hepatic vitamin A concentration, posited as the cutoff for marginal versus adequate vitamin A status (Underwood and Olson, 1993) are illustrated by original work by Tanumihardjo (2011) in Figure 11.5. A normal MRDR ratio value of <0.06 was seen in all but one instance of liver vitamin A in the adequate range, for a virtually 100% diagnostic specificity to detect vitamin A-adequate individuals. Abnormal ratios begin to appear below the critical liver value, but the test is only 100% sensitive for a deficient classification at liver vitamin A concentrations less than $18\,\mu g/g$ ($0.63\,\mu mol/g$). For applications, such as to exclude populations from interventions and to monitor improvement (correction) of vitamin A status to adequate, the MRDR is a minimally invasive biomarker of exceptional promise.

We should not neglect or discard, however, the other creative – and even less invasive and certainly less expensive – assessment tools that came out of the test-generating brainstorming of the 1980s and 1990s. Among these are ocular-response tests (Wondmikun, 2002; Taren et al., 2004), conjunctival histology (Courtright et al., 2002), buccal sampling (Sobeck et al., 2002), and others, which are yet to be calibrated with hepatic stores. However, by cross-calibrating the rates of test-result abnormalities in a population known to meet the objective threshold for intervention, one might develop population-based criteria for the diagnosis of hypovitaminosis A endemicity. The caveats are two-fold: (1) selecting appropriate criteria for normal and abnormal rating of the tests, and (2) making any feasible adjustments for ethnic, environmental or other confounders of test response. As it is the population itself that is the target of policy action and programmatic intervention, the status of the collective – rather than the individuals within it – would seem to be a viable viewpoint for the interpretation of screening biomarkers for vitamin A. The BOND process (Raiten et al., 2011) must grapple with a subtle conceptual issue of whether population assessment inherently needs to be based on measurement of the *prevalence* of individuals with truly marginal vitamin A stores in a population of interest or merely on an index of the *rate* of abnormal screening test occurrences.

Assessment for Vitamin A Excess

The concern for exposure and status assessment does not only reside at the lower end and the center of the vitamin A continuum. The upper end of individual status or collective exposure can produce adverse consequences on unborn fetuses and on overly exposed individuals. Early in the course of toxic exposure, circulating levels of retinol may rise above $300\,\mu g/dL$ ($10.5\,\mu mol$), in association with elevations of fasting retinyl esters (Underwood and Olson,

1993). When severe hypervitaminosis A is suspected on clinical grounds, a liver biopsy is medically justified.

The risk of damage to the developing fetus is based on dietary intake criteria (Institute of Medicine, 2001). In the absence of any imminent prospects for a salivary, urinary or fecal metabolite as a biomarker for individuals' chronic exposure, mathematical modeling, using data on food selection, food preformed vitamin A content, and extent of fortification (Dary, 2006), is likely to offer the best promise for identifying community risk and taking remedial action at the public education or food regulation levels or both.

Vitamin A Interventions in Preventive Medicine and Public Health

As part of the global call to action, the UN Special Session on Children in 2002 set as one of its goals the elimination of vitamin A deficiency and its consequences by the year 2010. The strategy to achieve this goal is to ensure that young children living in areas where the intake of vitamin A is inadequate receive the vitamin through a combination of breastfeeding, dietary improvement, food fortification, and supplementation.

General Health Interventions

A healthy individual is better able to absorb, retain, and utilize vitamin A than an impaired host. Sanitation and hygienic measures that reduce diarrhea and control intestinal parasites optimize the intestinal health and the capacity to take up the vitamin from the diet. As inflammation and fevers provoke urinary wastage of the vitamin, prevention of febrile episodes would limit the loss of vitamin A. Routine immunizations and control of systemic parasites can act to limit catabolic losses of micronutrients including vitamin A.

Food-Choice Approaches

Dietary diversification is the most fundamental and sustainable format to prevent hypovitaminosis A and has recently been acclaimed as the ideal approach (Latham, 2010). It is based on increasing the selection and consumption of foods rich in dietary vitamin A activity to bring the habitual consumption into the range of recommended intakes. Constraints in culture, cuisine, and household economics, however, often interfere with achieving adequate intakes in low-income societies. To succeed with dietary approaches, strategies appropriate to the endogenous possibilities and limitations of the settings must be devised.

Preformed vitamin A is the more utilizable form. In Bangladesh, the consumption of small indigenous fish is widespread and promotes adequacy of intake (Roos et al., 2003a,b). In Kenya, the addition of milk or meat to the school snack (a vegetable stew) improved overall vitamin A intake (Murphy et al., 2003). When animal source foods can be made affordable and directed to vulnerable segments of the population, they constitute the most potent underpinning for a food-based strategy.

Plant sources of vitamin A are considerably more problematic as strategies for ensuring adequacy given the bioconversion issues of plant matrices. Nevertheless, home-gardening interventions in South Africa (Faber et al., 2002a) and Thailand (Schipani et al., 2002) were shown to support better vitamin A status. Varieties of bananas, extraordinarily rich in provitamin A carotenes, are cultivated throughout the Micronesian islands of the Pacific and have been recommended as a complement for that region (Englberger et al., 2003). To enhance the bioefficacy of mango's provitamin A, its consumption with fat has been advanced in Gambia (Drammeh et al., 2002).

A number of oil-bearing fruits with high contents of vitamin A are available but underutilized. Gac fruit (*Momordica cochinchinensis*) from Vietnam (Vuong and King, 2003) and aguage or buriti fruit (*Mauritia vinifera* Mart) from the Amazon valley (Mariath et al., 1989) are the two tropical fatty fruits with the highest specific concentrations of provitamin A. Derivatives of the palm fruit (*Elaeis* spp.), such as red palm oil, are in third place, containing in excess of 50 mg of mixed provitamin A per 100 g of oil (Nagendran et al., 2000). Intervention trials in India (Sivan et al., 2002; Radhika et al., 2003) and Burkina Faso (Zagre et al., 2003) demonstrate the efficacy of cooking with red palm oil to improve vitamin A status. Tailored shortenings (Benade, 2003) or dishes of local cuisine (Solomons and Orozco, 2003) prepared with red palm oil represent the most highly developed approaches to dietary fortification with derivatives of oil-bearing fruits. With the caveat of potential health risks from certain saturated fatty acid patterns, the provitamin A in oil matrices optimizes the nutritional potential for the carotenes. (Institute of Medicine, 2001).

Food Fortification with Vitamin A and Provitamin A

The addition of vitamin A to foods began in the 1930s with the enrichment of margarine so that it supported vitamin nutrition in a manner similar to natural butter. Homogenized milk, with its lower butterfat content, is also enriched with vitamin A, as is skim and low-fat milk and their powdered forms. Beginning in the 1970s, the idea of fortifying foods that were never natural sources of vitamin A emerged into public-health thinking (Dary and Mora, 2002; Mora, 2003). This has been expanded and developed, and an overview and guideline for food fortification with micronutrients serve as a contemporary guide to understanding and effecting this strategy (Allen et al., 2006).

For the selection of the vehicle for mass fortification, it is important that the item reach those segments most at risk, which would include those with the lowest incomes and the young and the pregnant and lactating within that class (Allen et al., 2002). Two food items, sugar and cooking oil, are currently leading in the context of public-health fortification of staple foods. Sugar is fortified with retinyl palmitate in four of the five republics of Central America, as well as in Zambia. A survey showed that 89% of Ugandan households consumed sugar during any given week, making this sweetener a feasible vehicle in that African country as well (Kawuma, 2002). Oil is the other potentially useful vehicle. A pilot fortification of coconut oil in the Philippines made it the leading single source of the vitamin, providing one-third of dietary vitamin A and improved retinol status in the population (Candelária et al., 2005). Salt may soon become a third staple food vehicle because a triple-fortification strategy involving microencapsulation, which adds vitamin A to table salt without displacing iodine and iron, has been developed (Zimmermann et al., 2004).

A variation on the theme of fortification is that of specific products. At the public health level, vitamin A fortification can also be targeted to a specific segment of the population, as shown in a low-cost complementary food for infants and toddlers that was pilot tested in South Africa (Oelofse et al., 2003). Outside of public health programs, industrial fortification of commercial foods has growing prominence; this has been termed "market-driven" fortification (Allen et al., 2006; Dary, 2006). Breakfast cereals and fruit-flavored drinks are among the commercial items offered with additional vitamin A. Although this approach adds more vitamin A to national food supplies, critics suggest that vitamin A in commercial foods does not reach the vulnerable sectors due to cost, but may expose the more affluent consumers to additional and unneeded preformed vitamin (Dary, 2006).

Home Fortification and Its Variants

The accompanying with or mixing of micronutrient preparations with the non-breast-milk component of the weanling's diet, termed home fortification, is a promising modality for combating deficiencies in later infancy and in the toddler years (Nestel et al., 2003). Home fortification of complementary diets originally arose as a response to anemia, but multiple micronutrients, including vitamin A, are added to each of the common formats: micronutrient lipid spreads (Briend, 2001; Adu-Afarwuah et al., 2008), nutrient mix in sachets (Sprinkles™, MixMe™) (Lundeen et al., 2010), and crushable food-based tablets (foodLETs) (Smuts et al., 2003, 2005). Although each of the options for home fortification has been demonstrated as effective to decrease anemia, only the foodLETs have been explicitly analyzed for their effects on hypovitaminosis A. In a randomized, four-regimen, multi-center study in Peru, South Africa, Indonesia, and Vietnam (Smuts et al., 2005), 6 months of daily or weekly supplementation with a multinutrient foodLET preparation significantly reduced the prevalence of retinol values of <0.7 μmol/L (<20 μg/dL), without any effects with the placebo or iron-only regimens. An analogous approach, but for schoolchildren, has been adopted in India; fortifying a school meal for Himalayan children over an 8-month school year with 75% of RDA for vitamin A improved circulating vitamin A concentration (Osei et al., 2010).

Biofortification of the Food Supply

Biofortification is an example of a food-based approach to improving vitamin A status in which food sources are modified to include greater than usual contents of dietary vitamin A. It has generally been applied to foods of vegetable origin, in which the provitamin A content is enhanced by genetic means, either cross-breeding hybridization or genetic modification (Welch, 2005). Vegetables such as carrots (Mills et al., 2008), roots and tubers such as potatoes (Diretto et al., 2010), sweet potatoes (Low et al., 2007; Failla et al., 2009), cassava (Thakkar et al., 2007; Welsch et al., 2010), and staple grains such as maize (Naqvi et al., 2009; Vallabhaneni et al., 2009; Yan et al., 2010) and rice (Beyer, 2010) are among the examples of foods biofortified with provitamin A. Some are enriched spontaneously or through traditional hybridization cross-breeding (Low *et al.*, 2007; Thakkar *et al.*, 2007; Mills *et al.*, 2008; Failla *et al.*, 2009; Diretto *et al.*, 2010; Yan *et al.*, 2010), whereas others are genetically modified by gene insertion (Naqvi *et al.*, 2009; Vallabhaneni *et al.*, 2009; Beyer, 2010; Diretto *et al.*, 2010; Welsch *et al.*, 2010). Another genetically modified plant identified for potential contribution of provitamin A is golden mustard (*Brassica juncea*) (Chow *et al.*, 2010); oil extracted from mustard seed has wide distribution and has had a profound impact against hypovitaminosis A in India.

One might first consider enhancing the carotene content of fruits and vegetables. We have hybrid carrots as a beginning (Mills *et al.*, 2008). Carrot provitamin A is not of high bioavailability, the consumption frequency is occasional, and the amount consumed is limited. It is really in the main staple crops relied upon by low-income populations, such as maize and rice, in which hopes for biofortification's public-health role have been invested (Nestel *et al.*, 2006; Hotz and McClafferty, 2007). These two grains, along with cassava, potatoes, and sweet potatoes, cover much of the caloric needs of developing countries.

It was widely speculated that provitamin A would be poorly available to provide active vitamin from the matrices of staple crops. In stark contrast to predictions, at least with newer varieties of golden rice, ingenious studies with cultivars isotopically labelled hydroponically revealed a carotene-to-retinol conversion factor in healthy adults of ~4:1 (Tang *et al.*, 2009). Similarly, with carotene-rich natural hybrids of orange-flesh sweet potatoes, field trials in East Africa showed significant increases in serum retinol with the supplemented diets (Low *et al.*, 2007).

In the final analysis, the acceptability by the public of a yellow or orange hue in normally white-fleshed foods, such as rice, cassava, potatoes or cauliflower, or even of pigmented plants of a deeper hue, such as maize and sweet potato, remains to be assessed in large-scale consumer trials. The other acceptability (and safety) issue emerges as with any edible genetically modified organism, especially in developing countries. There is greater skepticism in governments and civil society in tropical societies, and the concerns for human health and environmental safety of consuming and cultivating these plants have yet to be entirely allayed.

Vitamin A Supplementation Interventions

Since the pioneering field trial by Sommer *et al.* (1986), a myriad of vitamin A supplementation trials for prophy-laxis against adverse health outcomes have been conducted. With their ongoing evaluation and meta-analyses, the recommendations for target populations and schedules of public-health vitamin A supplementation for prophylaxis against endemic hypovitaminosis A continue in flux.

Current Prophylactic Vitamin A Supplementation Recommendations

Over the years, recommendations have been based on one or a number of studies, transient evidence for routine, prophylactic administration to all of the groups listed in Table 11.3, and programs sanctioned by the WHO, Centers for Disease Control and Prevention, or the International Vitamin A Consultative Group, alone or in conjunction. On August 11, 2011, however, a revised and updated, target-group-specific set of guidelines from the WHO were disseminated: http://www.who.int/nutrition/publications/micronutrients/guidelines; these were the product of Cochrane-style systematic reviews, assessed by a panel of experts specific to the population groups. These contemporary guidelines are summarized in the second column of Table 11.3. Prophylactic "high-dose" oral supplementation of vitamin A is routinely recommended only for 6- to 59-month-old children, with the caveat that supplementation of pregnant women can be recommended where evidence of maternal night blindness is found. Delivery of these periodic doses is linked to the immunization schedules for infants and children.

Caution in supplementation is warranted in areas of high endemicity of HIV, as vitamin A supplementation to seropositive mothers has demonstrated adverse effects on the health and viral progression of mothers and offspring (Mehta *et al.*, 2007). As noted, earlier recommendations for neonatal dosing have been largely abandoned. In fact, in the setting of Guinea Bissau in West Africa, adverse health effects and excess mortality occur in female low- and normal-birth-weight neonates, but it is safe for newborn boys (Benn *et al.*, 2010). In the specific instance of HIV-infected infants, however, the delivery of an age-appropriate supplement dosage (~50 000 IU) of vitamin A to infants of HIV-positive mothers within 2 days of birth improved survival (Sommer, 2005; Humphreys *et al.*, 2010).

Programmatic and Pragmatic Challenges to the Delivery of Vitamin A Supplements

After a brisk take-off in the early 1990s, the worldwide effort to maintain dosing every 6 months with age-appropriate, high-dose vitamin A has subsequently run

TABLE 11.3 World Health Organization Guidelines on Vitamin A supplementation (2011)

Population category	Guideline for vitamin A supplementation
Neonates	The WHO does not recommend vitamin A supplementation for neonates as a public health intervention.
Infants 1–5 months of age	The WHO does not recommend vitamin A supplementation for infants 1–5 months of age as a public health intervention. Mothers should continue to be encouraged to exclusively breastfeed infants for the first 6 months to achieve optimal growth, health, and development.
Infants and children 6–59 months of age	The WHO recommends high-dose vitamin A supplementation every 4–6 months for infants and children 6–59 months of age, as a public health intervention to reduce child morbidity and mortality.
Pregnant women	The WHO does not recommend vitamin A supplementation during pregnancy as part of routine antenatal care. However, in areas where there is a severe public health problem of vitamin A deficiency, the WHO recommends giving vitamin A supplementation during pregnancy for the prevention of night blindness.
Postpartum women	The WHO does not recommend vitamin A supplementation for postpartum women as a public health intervention for the prevention of maternal and infant morbidity and mortality.
During pregnancy for reducing the risk of mother-to-child transmission of HIV	Currently the WHO does not recommend vitamin A supplementation in HIV-positive women as a public health intervention for the prevention of mother-to-child transmission of HIV.

The WHO standard for "high-dose" vitamin A supplementation refers to an oral dose of 100 000 IU (30 303 RE) for 6- to 12-month-old infants and 200 000 IU (60 606 RE) from 1 year onward, including in adults. These are also the age-specific dosages for specific therapeutic indications for oral vitamin A supplementation. Modified from guidelines on routine immunization from the World Health Organization. (Available at: http://www.who.int/nutrition/publications/micronutrients/guidelines/en/index.html.)

into obstacles. It was forced to move from campaign-style vaccination campaigns, associated with polio eradication, to the more routine, health-post-based schedules, which are far less universal across populations. It has also been shown in Indonesia (Pangaribuan *et al.*, 2004), the Philippines (Choi *et al.*, 2005), and Bangladesh (Semba *et al.*, 2010) that poorer (and theoretically more vulnerable) target families were less likely to have access to the vitamin A distribution system.

The safety reputation of the measure came under assault as the result of a highly publicized incident in Assam State, India, in 2002, in which excessive doses of a vitamin A syrup allegedly produced inadvertent lethal overdose during a regional campaign (Kapil, 2002). However, the emergent concern has shifted to the dependency issues of a medically controlled and health-sector-linked measure. Latham (2010) has argued that the only sustainable approach to coverage of the vitamin A needs of infants and young children will be a food-based strategy; the insistence

on maintaining high-dose prophylaxis in policy circles is seen as deferring a serious and concerted effort to transfer the burden of protection to an improved vitamin A content of complementary food and home diets of the children (and mothers) at risk of hypovitaminosis A in the world's low-income societies.

Vitamin A in Clinical Medicine and Therapeutics

Uses for Vitamin A and Provitamin A

Vitamin A supplements of both high and lower doses have been studied, and therapeutic supplementation is potentially indicated in a number of conditions and explicitly recommended in others.

Xerophthalmia

Xerophthalmia is a medical emergency. An immediate administration of 200 000 IU (60 606 RE) of vitamin A is indicated, followed by a second dose on the following day, to respond to the danger of rapid deterioration of the ocular tissues.

Measles

Vaccination has dramatically reduced the worldwide incidence of this viral exanthem. Complications from measles are more common in vitamin A-deficient populations (Perry and Halsey, 2004). First indicated as efficacious intervention trials in hospitalized children with measles complications in Africa, systematic reviews confirmed that intra-infection supplementation with vitamin A is effective in reducing measles mortality (D'Souza and D'Souza, 2004; Sudfeld *et al.*, 2010). Two consecutive day's worth of age-appropriate "high doses", as established for prophylactic administration by the WHO (Table 11.3, footnotes), is indicated.

Clinical Protein-Energy Malnutrition

The severe, endemic protein-energy malnutrition had been in decline in recent decades, resulting in a loss of the clinical acumen to manage sporadic cases. Recent famines, natural disasters, civil conflicts, and refugee situations, however, have produced a recrudescence in clinical protein-energy malnutrition. It has long been appreciated that multiple micronutrient deficiencies, including that of vitamin A, are common in these patients. The WHO initiative to improve care for protein-energy malnutrition (Ashworth *et al.*, 2004) includes a provision to administer high-dose vitamin A, with the same "high-dose" dosage as shown in the footnotes of Table 11.3.

Vitamin A Supplementation Indications in Other Diseases and Conditions

Aside from the three major public-health situations discussed above, evidence for efficacy of vitamin A supplementation has been reported in at least six areas of note (Box 11.1). Multiple therapeutic trials have shown that daily administration of retinyl palmitate slows the progression of the ocular defect in patients with retinitis pigmentosa (Hartong *et al.*, 2006). Vitamin A cycles from retinal pigment epithelia to photoreceptors of the neural retina with the conversion of all-*trans*-retinol to 11-*cis*-retinal. Gene mutations in these pathways explain a series of retinal dystrophies (Thompson and Gal, 2003).

Complications associated with premature birth are another vitamin A-responsive condition. Because hepatic vitamin A stores are laid down in late gestation, babies

> ### BOX 11.1   Additional situations in which evidence for efficacy of vitamin A supplementation has been reported
>
> Retinitis pigmentosa
> Complications associated with premature birth
> Malaria
> Tuberculosis
> Radiation proctitis
> Prevention of malignant transformation of hydatidiform moles

born before term are notably deficient in vitamin A (Mactier and Weaver, 2005). Moreover, lung prematurity or bronchopulmonary dysplasia, a common affliction of the small preterm infant, is more frequent the lower the circulating retinol concentration (Spears *et al.*, 2004). Vitamin A has been found to up-regulate genes necessary for fetal lung growth and increase surfactant production in animal models. A major multicenter collaborative randomized clinical trial of thrice-weekly doses of 5000 IU (1515 RAE) of intramuscular retinyl palmitate over the first 4 weeks of life in extremely low-birth-weight infants (under 1000 g), was conducted in US neonatal intensive care units in the 1990s (Tyson *et al.*, 1999); it demonstrated a slight, but significant, 11% reduction in the combined outcomes of death or chronic lung disease at 36 weeks. Darlow and Graham (2007), in their systematic review, comment:

> Supplementing very low birthweight infants with vitamin A is associated with a reduction in death or oxygen requirement at one month of age and oxygen requirement among survivors at 36 weeks postmenstrual age, with this latter outcome being confined to infants with birthweight less than 1000 g.

With respect to infections, vitamin A supplementation has shown beneficial effects in malaria and tuberculosis. Vitamin A administration has had a positive effect on malaria by reducing the severity of attacks. Shankar *et al.* (1999) demonstrated reduced morbidity from this parasitosis in an area of hyperendemicity of *Plasmodium falciparum* malaria in Papua New Guinea, with periodic high-dose vitamin A supplementation. Serghides and Kain (2002) speculate that the mechanism could lie in enhancing protozoal clearance by phagocytic cells and in suppressing the tumor necrosis factor-alpha response. It also decreases C-reactive protein (Cusick *et al.*, 2005). Moreover, vitamin A supplementation ameliorated the adverse effect on growth of malaria-infected children in Tanzania (Sazawal *et al.*, 2006). With respect to tuberculosis, a double-blind, placebo-controlled study of vitamin A and zinc supplementation in persons with tuberculosis was conducted in central Java in Indonesia (Karyadi *et al.*, 2002). A daily regimen of 5000 IU (1515 RAE) and 15 mg zinc in patients with tuberculosis under treatment produced earlier sputum clearance and radiographic resolution. The authors recommended this micronutrient combination as an adjunctive therapy for tuberculosis.

In several applications in oncology, vitamin A supplementation has a role. In proctitis due to pelvic field radiotherapy, preliminary encouraging findings in a randomized clinical trial using 10 000 IU (3030 RAE) of retinyl palmitate for 90 days in oncology patients reduced rectal symptoms 6 months post-radiation (Ehrenpreis *et al.*, 2005). A preliminary observation in Indonesia of a five-fold reduction in the malignant transformation of hydatidiform moles (non-viable conceptuses giving rise to vesicular placenta, occurring in one in 100 pregnancies) with short-term daily supplementation with 200 000 IU of vitamin A has been reported (Andrijono and Muhilal, 2010).

Well conducted studies have also tested supplementation and found it to be ineffective. Clinical trials with vitamin A supplementation during episodes of acute diarrhea have shown mixed and selective results, generally with no greater efficacy for reducing disease severity than placebo (Biswas *et al.*, 1994; Bhandari *et al.*, 1997; Andreozzi *et al.*, 2006). Such is also the case for reducing the vaginal shedding of herpes simplex virus in HIV infection (Baeten *et al.*, 2004).

Uses for Retinoids

Retinoic acid and various isomers and synthetic analogs are being used in pharmacological dosages for an increasing number of therapeutic purposes.

Severe Acne Vulgaris

Both topical and systematic administration of retinoids have been successfully applied to the treatment of severe cases of acne vulgaris. Retinoids act to lyse the microcomedo before they develop into full-blown comedones (Chivot, 2003). Both all-*trans*-retinoic acid (tretinoin) and 13-*cis*-retinoic acid (isotretinoin) have successful track records in acne therapy.

Malignancies

Retinoids have also found application in therapy of both solid tumors and hematological malignancies. They are used to treat cancer, in part because of their ability to induce differentiation and arrest proliferation (Bushue and Wan, 2010; Tang and Gudas, 2011). It also inhibits angiogenesis, depriving tissues of new vasculature (Siddikuzzaman *et al.*, 2010).

It was first observed that long-term remissions of chronic myelogenous leukemia could be induced by systemic application of all-*trans*-retinoic acid (ATRA), and later its efficacy in chronic promyelocytic leukemia was also shown. In both dyscrasias, the retinoid induces terminal differentiation of the myeloid cells (Oren *et al.*, 2003). It is also effective in the treatment of Wilms' tumors (Johanning and Piyathilake, 2003). Also among the human tumors for which ATRA has shown therapeutic value are: Kaposi's sarcoma, head and neck squamous cell carcinoma, ovarian carcinoma, bladder cancer, and neuroblastoma (Siddikuzzaman *et al.*, 2010). Rapid metabolism and resistance are problems such that combination therapy with drugs such as DNA methyltransferase and histone deacetylase inhibitors, which regulate the epigenome, are required (Tang and Gudas, 2011).

Adjunctive Therapy in Hepatitis C Treatment

Insight into a potential advance in adjunctive interferon-1 therapy for hepatitis C virus comes from in vitro studies with 9-*cis*-retinoic acid on hepatic cells. The retinoid increases expression of the IFN-1 receptors, enhancing the antiviral effect of the drug (Hamamoto *et al.*, 2003).

Adverse and Toxic Consequences of Exposures to Vitamin A and Retinoids

By virtue of their chemical nature and persistence in the body, exposure to retinoids has recognized adverse consequences, and even toxic effects, which can prove lethal under certain conditions (Fenaux *et al.*, 2001, 2007). In conjunction with the considerations of nutritional adequacy, at least two organizations have offered systematic advice regarding tolerable upper intake levels (ULs) for habitual daily dietary intakes of preformed vitamin A: (1) the Food and Nutrition Board of the US Institute of

TABLE 11.4 Summary of estimated tolerable upper intake levels for average daily consumption of preformed vitamin A supplementation with vitamin A

Population group	Estimated tolerable upper level (micrograms[a])
EU Commission Scientific Committee on Food[b]	
1–3 years	800
4–6 years	1100
7–10 years	1500
11–14 years	2000
15–17 years	2600
Adults	3000
Older adults	No finding
Dietary reference intakes[c]	
0–1 years	600
1–3 years	600
4–8 years	900
9–13 years	1700
14–18 years	2800
Adults	3000
Pregnant women	3000
Lactating women	3000

[a]Assumes micrograms of preformed vitamin A.
[b]Data from European Union Commission, Scientific Committee on Food, Task-Force on Upper Levels for Vitamins and Minerals (2002).
[c]Data from Institute of Medicine (2001).

Medicine (Institute of Medicine, 2001); and (2) a panel of the European Union on Food (European Union Commission, 2002). The respective estimates of tolerable levels are shown in Table 11.4. They are largely homologous, indicating that habitual intake of 3000 μg of preformed vitamin A is the consensus UL.

Systemic Toxicity of Vitamin A

A hepatic concentration of over 300 mg/g of vitamin A is considered excessive, and could be associated with clinical toxicity manifestations. In fulminant overdoses of vitamin A, signs include severe skin rash, headache, double vision, and coma due to pseudotumor cerebri, resulting in rapid demise (Khasru *et al.*, 2007). In more chronic, but massive overdoses, hepatic fibrosis and ascites and skin lesions share the syndrome with central nervous system disturbances. More recently recognized toxic manifestations include bone-marrow suppression in an infant with hypervitaminosis A (Perrotta *et al.*, 2002) and hypercalcemia in

an adult consuming commercial enteral formula for a prolonged period (Bhalia *et al.*, 2005).

In an interesting observation at the interface of pharmacology and toxicology, Myhre *et al.* (2003) reported that oil-based vitamin A and liver have one-tenth the toxic potential as water-miscible, emulsified, and solid forms of retinol supplements. In recent years, two prospective studies in healthy adult volunteers have compared daily consumption of oil-based retinyl ester supplements at dosages of 25000 IU (7575 RAE), 50000 IU (15152 RAE), and 75000 IU (23727 RAE) for periods of 12 months (Alberts *et al.*, 2004) and 16 months (Sedjo *et al.*, 2004) with this latter dose representing 7.5 times the UL. No evidence of toxicity or adverse consequences was detected over the respective intervals.

With a public health perspective, Allen and Haskell (2002) have examined the supplementation regimens current in 2002, and conclude that, on a single-dose or periodic basis, the schedules for high-dose supplements were safe for infants, children, and postpartum women. Although some exceeded the daily UL on a prorated basis, none would surpass the no-observed-adverse-effect level.

Systemic Toxicity of Retinoic Acid and Isomers

Since the advent of high-dose treatment with systemic retinoic acid for leukemia and other malignant conditions, a condition known as "retinoic acid syndrome" has been recognized. It is characterized by weight gain, episodes of hypotension, acute renal failure, unexplained fever, and respiratory distress associated with interstitial pulmonary infiltrates and pleural and pericardial effusions seen on chest X-rays (Larson and Tallman, 2003). High doses of retinoid analogs can increase intracranial pressure as well (Friedman, 2005).

Teratogenesis

Congenital birth defects can be induced by vitamin A deficiency and excess. The UL of vitamin A (Institute of Medicine, 2001) is based on increased risk of teratogenesis, which is estimated to begin with habitual intakes of preformed vitamin A in excess of 10000 IU (3030 RAE). The damage occurs in the embryogenic phase within days of conception. The manifestations of excess vitamin A include a spectrum of malformations including ocular, pulmonary, cardiovascular, and urogenital defects (Lefebvre *et al.*, 2010). These same birth defects can arise when systemic doses of the retinoid analogs are administered in dermatological practice to treat acne (Miller *et al.*, 1998). Provisional evidence suggests, however, that the topical use of these analogs in early pregnancy presents minimal to no risk of teratogenesis (Loureiro *et al.*, 2005).

Other Adverse Consequences

Interest has arisen regarding adverse consequences of vitamin A interaction with HIV infections, bone mineralization, cardiovascular risk, and repletion of iodine-deficient populations.

Interaction with HIV infection

A series of adverse effects of vitamin A in the maternal–infant dyad with maternal HIV infection have been identified (Mehta *et al.*, 2007). Subclinical mastitis, common among HIV-infected women, was exacerbated in its incidence when vitamin A supplements were given to seropositive Tanzanian lactating women (Arsenault *et al.*, 2010).

Bone Demineralization and Osteoporotic Fracture Risk

One of the areas of most recent toxicological concern is that of an adverse effect of vitamin A on bone mineralization and structural integrity. Spontaneous bone fractures are a common manifestation from vitamin A overfeeding in animals (Genaro and Martini, 2004), and it is well established that vitamin A stimulates bone resorption and inhibits bone formation (Kawahara *et al.*, 2006). A concern for humans arose from a study in Swedish women (Melhus *et al.*, 1998), in which an inverse association was reported between consumption of preformed vitamin A intake and bone mineral density in a cross-sectional analysis, with adverse effect arising for habitual daily vitamin A intakes above 1500 μg equivalents, one-half the UL level (Institute of Medicine, 2001). Subsequently, numerous publications based on estimated preformed vitamin A intake or circulating retinol showed inconsistent results (Crandall, 2004; Ribaya-Mercado and Blumberg, 2007; Morgan *et al.*, 2009). Of important note is that intakes of provitamin A carotenes are in no way suspected of adverse effects on bone mineralization. Also, with respect to vitamin A analog retinoids and bone loss, a survey from the nation-wide registry of Denmark failed to show any association between fractures at any site and retinoid therapy histories (Vestergaard *et al.*, 2010).

The public-health importance of this constellation of observations has yet to be defined. A prudent interim conclusion comes from Crandall (2004), however: "It is not yet possible to set a specific level of retinol intake above which bone health is compromised. Pending further investigation, Vit A supplements should not be used with the express goal of improving bone health."

Future Directions

The future of vitamin A may involve a return to basics and to revisiting issues addressed in previous decades. An emerging notion is that the conventional application of biomarkers to assessment of vitamin A status has not been providing guidance for policy decisions. The BOND effort along with a forthcoming World Health Organization reissuing of guidance needs to rationalize the way in which biomarkers are used in assessment, while preserving the features of low-cost, non-invasive nature and subject-friendliness. The recent re-evaluation of interpretation of biomarkers calls for the setting aside of conventional approaches to assessment of vitamin A status and points out the need to become more circumscriptive and attentive to the BOND process and the WHO reassessment.

Another legacy of the 1980s, the population-wide supplementation with high-dose retinyl palimate, has come under scrutiny as permanent programs. Detractors feel that reliance on supplementation focuses on only one of many micronutrients that may be problematic, and deters a serious mobilization in developing food-based approaches (Allen *et al.*, 2006). To replace supplementation, any food-based approaches must cover the foods consumed by the most vulnerable sub-segment of the population, children under 5 years. Addition of vitamin A to the diet through voluntary fortification of commercial foods is expanding (Allen *et al.*, 2006); however, contribution of such foods to the diets of young children in the poorest of communities is questionable. For the more affluent consumers of such products, however, the ability to add retinyl palmitate to commercial processed foods, as well as public health programs, raises safety issues about excess vitamin A exposure as a prominent health concern. For vulnerable populations, biofortification and carotene fortification present potential intervention opportunities. Plant sources of provitamin A and added carotenes have absolute safety, but variable efficacy, depending on food-matrix factors and accompanying fat. Moreover, newly acquired insights into polymorphisms in the enzymes governing bioconversion of provitamin A sources (Allen *et al.*, 2006) may guide public health authorities in selection of populations in which plant-source intervention might hold greater or lesser promise.

Suggestions for Further Reading

Allen, L.H., de Benoist, B., Dary, O., *et al.* (2006) *Guidelines on Food Fortification with Micronutrients.* WHO, Geneva.

Grune, T., Lietz, G., Palou, A., *et al.* (2010) β-Carotene is an important vitamin A source for humans. *J Nutr* **140**, 2268S–2285S.

Harrison, E.H. (2005) Mechanisms of digestion and absorption of dietary vitamin A. *Annu Rev Nutr* **25**, 87–103.

Raiten, D.J., Namasté, S., Brabin, B., *et al.* (2011) Executive summary: Biomarkers of Nutrition for Development (BOND): Building a consensus. *Am J Clin Nutr* (Suppl) **94**, 633S–650S.

Vitamin A supplementation: http://www.who.int/vaccines/en/vitamina.shtml [accessed on October 29, 2010].

References

Abu, J., Batuwangala, M., Herbert, K., *et al.* (2005) Retinoic acid and retinoid receptors: potential chemopreventive and therapeutic role in cervical cancer. *Lancet Oncol* **6**, 712–720.

Adu-Afarwuah, S., Lartey, A., Brown,K.H., *et al.* (2008) Home fortification of complementary foods with micronutrient supplements is well accepted and has positive effects on infant iron status in Ghana. *Am J Clin Nutr* **87**, 929–938.

Aguilera, A., Bajo, M.A., del Peso, G., *et al.* (2002) True deficiency of antioxidant vitamins E and A in dialysis patients. Relationship with clinical patterns of atherosclerosis. *Adv Perit Dial* **18**, 206–211.

Ajose, O.A., Adelekan, D.A., and Ajewole, E.O. (2004) Vitamin A status of pregnant Nigerian women: relationship to dietary habits and morbidity. *Nutr Health* **17**, 325–333.

Akohoue, S.A., Green, J.B., and Green, M.H. (2006) Dietary vitamin A has both chronic and acute effects on vitamin A indices in lactating rats and their offspring. *J Nutr* **136**, 128–132.

Alam, D.S., van Raaij, J.M., Hautvast, J.G., *et al.* (2010) Effect of dietary fat supplementation during late pregnancy and first six months of lactation on maternal and infant vitamin A status in rural Bangladesh. *J Health Popul Nutr* **28**, 333–342.

Alberts, D., Ranger-Moore, J., Einspahr, J., *et al.* (2004) Safety and efficacy of dose-intensive oral vitamin A in subjects with sun-damaged skin. *Clin Cancer Res* **10**, 1875–1880.

Allen, L.H. and Haskell, M. (2002) Estimating the potential for vitamin A toxicity in women and young children. *J Nutr* **132** (9 Suppl), 2907S–2919S.

Allen, L.H., de Benoist, B., Dary, O., *et al.* (2006) *Guidelines on Food Fortification with Micronutrients.* WHO, Geneva.

Alm, B., Wennergren, G., Norvenius, S.G., *et al.* (2003) Nordic Epidemiological SIDS Study. Vitamin A and sudden infant death syndrome in Scandinavia 1992–1995. *Acta Pediatr* **92**, 162–164.

Amann, P.M., Eichmüller, S.B., Schmidt. J., *et al.* (2011) Regulation of gene expression by retinoids. *Curr Med Chem* **18**, 1405–1412.

American Institute of Nutrition (1990) Nomenclature policy: generic descriptions and trivial names for vitamins and related compounds. *J Nutr* **120**, 12–19.

Andreozzi, V.L., Bailey, T.C., Nobre, F.F., *et al.* (2006) Random-effects models in investigating the effect of vitamin A in childhood diarrhea. *Ann Epidemiol* **16**, 241–247.

Andrijono, A. and Muhilal, M. (2010) Prevention of post-mole malignant trophoblastic disease with vitamin A. *Asian Pac J Cancer Prev* **11**, 567–570.

Ara, C., Devirgiliis, L.C., and Massimi, M. (2004) Influences of retinoic acid on adhesion complexes in human hepatoma cells: a clue to its antiproliferative effects. *Cell Commun Adhes* **11**, 13–23.

Aranceta, J., Serra-Majem, L., Perez-Rodrigo, C., *et al.* (2001) Vitamins in Spanish food patterns: the eVe Study. *Public Health Nutr* **4**, 1317–1323.

Armstrong, T., Walters, E., Varshney, S., *et al.* (2002) Deficiencies of micronutrients, altered bowel function, and quality of life during late follow-up after pancreaticoduodenectomy for malignancy. *Pancreatology* **2**, 528–534.

Arora, P., Kumar, V., and Batra, S. (2002) Vitamin A status in children with asthma. *Pediatr Allergy Immunol* **13**, 223–226.

Arsenault, J.E., Aboud, S., Manji, K.P., *et al.* (2010) Vitamin supplementation increases risk of subclinical mastitis in HIV-infected women. *J Nutr* **140**, 1788–1792.

Artacho, C.A., Piantedosi, R., and Blaner, W.S. (1993) Placental transfer of vitamin A. *Sight and Life Newsletter* **3**, 23–28.

Ashworth, A., Chopra, M., McCoy, D., *et al.* (2004) WHO guidelines for management of severe malnutrition in rural South African hospitals: effect on case fatality and the influence of operational factors. *Lancet* **363**, 1110–1115.

Baeten, J.M., McClelland, R.S., Corey, L., *et al.* (2004) Vitamin A supplementation and genital shedding of herpes simplex virus among HIV-1-infected women: a randomized clinical trial. *J Infect Dis* **189**, 1466–1471.

Beaton, G.H., Martorell, R., Aronson, K.J., *et al.* (1993) Effectiveness of vitamin A supplementation in the control of young child morbidity and mortality in developing countries.

ACC/SCN State-of-the-art Series Nutrition Policy Discussion Paper No.13. SubCommittee on Nutrition, Geneva.

Benade, A.J. (2003) A place for palm fruit oil to eliminate vitamin A deficiency. *Asia Pacific J Clin Nutr* **12**, 369–372.

Benn, C.S., Fisker, A.B., Napirna, B.M., *et al.* (2010) Vitamin A supplementation and BCG vaccination at birth in low birth-weight neonates: two by two factorial randomised controlled trial. *Br Med J* **340**, c1101.

Beyer, P. (2010) Golden rice and "Golden" crops for human nutrition. *Biotechnology* **27**, 478–481.

Bhalia, K., Ennis. D.M., and Ennis, E.D. (2005) Hypercalcemia caused by iatrogenic hypervitaminosis A. *J Am Diet Assoc* **105**, 119–121.

Bhandari, N., Bahl, R., Sazawal, S., *et al.* (1997) Breast-feeding status alters the effect of vitamin A treatment during acute diarrhea in children. *J Nutr* **127**, 59–63.

Biesalski, H.K. and Nohr, D. (2004) New aspects in vitamin A metabolism: the role of retinyl esters as systemic and local sources for retinol in mucous epithelia. *J Nutr* **134** (12 Suppl), 3453S–3457S.

Biesalski, H.K., Chichili, G.R., Frank, J., *et al.* (2007) Conversion of beta-carotene to retinal pigment. *Vitam Horm* **75**, 117–130.

Biswas, R., Biswas, A.B., Manna, B., *et al.* (1994) Effect of vitamin A supplementation on diarrhea and acute respiratory tract infection in children. A double blind placebo controlled trial in a Calcutta slum community. *Eur J Epidemiol* **10**, 57–61.

Blake, C.J. (2007) Status of methodology for the determination of fat-soluble vitamins in foods, dietary supplements, and vitamin premixes. *J AOAC Int* **90**, 897–910.

Blomhoff, R., Green, M.H., Berg, T., *et al.* (1994) Transport and storage of vitamin A. *Science* **250**, 399–404.

Boulanger, A., McLemore, P., Copeland, N.G., *et al.* (2003) Identification of beta-carotene 15,15'-monooxygenase as a peroxisome proliferator-activated receptor target gene. *FASEB J* **17**, 1304–1306.

Bowman, S.A. and Spence, J.T. (2002) A comparison of low-carbohydrate vs. high-carbohydrate diets: energy restriction, nutrient quality and correlation to body mass index. *J Am Coll Nutr* **21**, 268–274.

Briend, A. (2001) Highly nutrient-dense spreads: a new approach to delivering multiple micronutrients to high-risk groups. *Br J Nutr* **85** (Suppl 2), S175–S179.

Brown, N. and Roberts, C. (2004) Vitamin A for acute respiratory infection in developing countries: a meta-analysis. *Acta Pediatrica* **93**, 437–442.

Bushue, N. and Wan, Y.J. (2010) Retinoid pathway and cancer therapeutics. *Adv Drug Deliv Res* **62**, 1285–1298.

Candelária, L.V., Magsadia, C.R., Velasco, R.E., *et al.* (2005) The effect of vitamin A-fortified coconut cooking oil on the serum retinol concentration of Filipino children 4–7 years old. *Asia Pac J Clin Nutr* **14**, 43–53.

Canfield, L.M., Clandinin, M.T., Davies, D.P., *et al.* (2003) Multinational study of major breast milk carotenoids of healthy mothers. *Eur J Nutr* **42**, 133–141.

Chen, Q. and Ross, A.C. (2004) Retinoic acid regulates cell cycle progression and cell differentiation in human monocytic THP-1 cells. *Exp Cell Res* **297**, 68–81.

Chivot, M. (2005) Retinoid therapy for acne. A comparative review. *Am J Clin Dermatol* **6**, 13–19.

Choi, Y., Bishai, D., and Hill, K. (2005) Socioeconomic differentials in supplementation of vitamin A: evidence from the Philippines. *J Health Popul Nutr* **23**, 156–164.

Chow, J., Klein, E.Y., and Laxminarayan, R. (2010) Cost-effectiveness of "golden mustard" for treating vitamin A deficiency in India. *PLoS One* **5**, e12046.

Coles, C.L., Levy, A., Gorodischer, R., *et al.* (2004) Subclinical vitamin A deficiency in Israeli-Bedouin toddlers. *Eur J Clin Nutr* **58**, 796–802.

Comstock, G.W., Alberg, A.J., and Helzlsouer, K.J. (1993) Reported effects of long-term freezer storage on concentrations of retinol, beta-carotene, and alpha-tocopherol in serum or plasma summarized. *Clin Chem* **39**, 1075–1078.

Cotton, P.A., Subar, A.F., Friday, J.E., *et al.* (2004) Dietary sources of nutrients among US adults. 1994 to 1996. *J Am Diet Assoc* **104**, 921–930.

Courtright, P., Fine, D., Broadhead, R.L., *et al.* (2002) Abnormal vitamin A cytology and mortality in infants aged 9 months and less with measles. *Ann Trop Pediatr* **22**, 239–243.

Crandall, C. (2004) Vitamin A intake and osteoporosis: a clinical review. *J Women's Health (Larchmont)* **13**, 939–953.

Cusick, S.E., Tielsch, J.M., Ramsan, M., *et al.* (2005) Short-term effects of vitamin A and antimalarial treatment on erythropoiesis in severely anemic Zanzibari preschool children. *Am J Clin Nutr* **82**, 406–412.

Dallaire, F., Dewailly, E., Shademani, R., *et al.* (2003) Vitamin A concentration in umbilical cord blood of infants from three separate regions of the province of Quebec (Canada). *Can J Public Health* **94**, 386–390.

Darlow, B.A. and Graham, P.J. (2007) Vitamin A supplementation to prevent mortality and short- and long-term morbidity in very low birthweight infants. *Cochrane Database Syst Rev* CD000501.

Dary, O. (2006) The importance and limitations of food fortification for the management of nutritional deficiencies. In K. Kraemer (ed.), *Nutritional Anemia*. Sight and Life Press, Basel, pp. 315–336.

Dary, O. and Mora, J.O., International Vitamin A Consultative Group (2002) Food fortification to reduce vitamin A deficiency: International Vitamin A Consultative Group recommendations. *J Nutr* **132** (9 Suppl), 2927S–2933S.

Davidsson, L., Adou, P., Zeder, C., *et al.* (2003) The effect of retinyl palmitate added to iron-fortified maize porridge on erythrocyte incorporation of iron in African children with vitamin A deficiency. *Br J Nutr* **90**, 337–343.

Dawson, M.I. and Okamura, W.H. (1990) *Chemistry and Biology of Synthetic Retinoids*. CRC Press, Boca Raton, FL.

Dawson, M.I. and Zhang, X.K. (2002) Discovery and design of retinoic acid receptor and retinoid X receptor class- and subtype-selective synthetic analogs of all-*trans*-retinoic acid and 9-*cis*-retinoic acid. *Curr Med Chem* **9**, 623–637.

Dewey, K.G., Cohen, R.J., and Brown, K.H. (2004) Exclusive breast-feeding for 6 months, with iron supplementation, maintains adequate micronutrient status among term, low-birthweight, breast-fed infants in Honduras. *J Nutr* **134**, 1091–1098.

Dimenstein, R., Trugo, N.M.F., Donangelo, C.M., *et al.* (1996) Effect of subadequate maternal vitamin A status on placental transfer of retinol and β-carotene to the human fetus. *Biol Neonate* **69**, 230–234.

Diretto, G., Al-Babili, S., Tavazza, R., *et al.* (2010) Transcriptional-metabolic networks in beta-carotene-enriched potato tubers: the long and winding road to the Golden phenotype. *Plant Physiol* **54**, 899–912.

Drammeh, B.S., Marquis, G.S., Funkhouser, E., *et al.* (2002) A randomized, 4-month mango and fat supplementation trial improved vitamin A status among young Gambian children. *J Nutr* **132**, 3693–3699.

D'Souza, R.M. and D'Souza, R. (2002) Vitamin A for treating measles in children. *Cochrane Database Syst Rev* CD001479.

Dyer, A.R., Elliot, P., Stamler, J., *et al.* (2003) Dietary intake in male and female smokers, ex-smokers, and never smokers: the INTERMAP study. *J Hum Hypertens* **17**, 641–654.

Edwards, A.J., Nguyen, C.H., You, C.S., *et al.* (2002) Alpha- and beta-carotene from a commercial purée are more bioavailable to humans than from boiled-mashed carrots, as determined using an extrinsic stable isotope reference method. *J Nutr* **132**, 159–167.

Egeland, G.M., Berti, P., Soueida, R., *et al.* (2004) Age differences in vitamin A intake among Canadian Inuit. *Can J Public Health* **95**, 465–469.

Ehrenpreis, E.D., Jani, A., Levitsky, J., *et al.* (2005) A prospective, randomized, double-blind, placebo-controlled trial of retinol palmitate (vitamin A) for symptomatic chronic radiation proctopathy. *Dis Colon Rectum* **48**, 1–8.

Eichenberger-Gilmore, J.M., Hong, L., Broffit, B., *et al.* (2005) Longitudinal patterns of vitamin and mineral supplement use in young white children. *J Am Diet Assoc* **105**, 763–772.

Englberger, L., Darnton-Hill, I., Coyne, T., *et al.* (2003) Carotenoid-rich bananas: a potential food source for alleviating vitamin A deficiency. *Food Nutr Bull* **24**, 303–318.

European Union Commission, Scientific Committee on Food, Task-Force on Upper Levels for Vitamins and Minerals (2002) *Draft Opinion of the Scientific Committee on Food on the Tolerable Upper Intake Level of Preformed Vitamin A (Retinol and Retinyl Esters)*. European Commission, Brussels.

Evans, T. (2005) Regulation of hematopoiesis by retinoid signaling. *Exp Hematol* **33**, 1055–1561.

Faber, M., Phungula, M.A., Venter, S.L., *et al.* (2002a) Home gardens focusing on the production of yellow and dark green leafy vegetables increase the serum retinol concentrations of 2-5-y-old children in South Africa. *Am J Clin Nutr* **76**, 1048–1054.

Failla, M.L., Thakkar, S.K., and Kim, J.Y. (2009) In vitro bioaccessibility of beta-carotene in orange fleshed sweet potato (*Ipomoea batatas*, Lam.). *J Agric Food Chem* **57**, 10922–10927.

Fenaux, P., Chomienne, C., and Degos, L. (2001) Treatment of acute promyelocytic leukaemia. *Best Pract Res Clin Haematol* **14**, 153–174.

Fenaux, P., Wang, Z.Z., and Degos, L. (2007) Treatment of acute promyelocytic leukemia by retinoids. *Current Topics Microbiol Immunol* **313**, 101–128.

FAO/WHO (Food and Agricultural Organization/World Health Organization) (1967) *Requirement of Vitamin A, Thiamine, Riboflavin and Niacin*. FAO Food and Nutrition Series B. FAO, Rome.

FAO/WHO (Food and Agricultural Organization/World Health Organization) (2004) *Vitamin and Mineral Requirements in Human Nutrition*. WHO, Geneva.

Florentino, R.F., Villavieja, G.M., and Lana, R.D. (2002) Dietary and physical activity patterns of 8- to 10-years-old urban school children in Metro Manila, Philippines. *Food Nutr Bull* **23**, 267–273.

Friedman, D.I. (2005) Medication-induced intracranial hypertension in dermatology. *Am J Clin Dermatol* **6**, 29–37.

Furr, H.C. (2004) Analysis of retinoids and carotenoids: problems resolved and unsolved. *J Nutr* **134**, 281S–285S.

Furr, H.C., Green, M.H., Haskell, M., *et al.* (2005) Stable isotope dilution techniques for assessing vitamin A status and bioefficacy of provitamin A carotenoids in humans. *Public Health Nutr* **8**, 596–607.

Gaetani, S., Bellovino, D., Apreda, M., *et al.* (2002) Hepatic synthesis, maturation and complex formation between retinol-binding protein and transthyretin. *Clin Chem Lab Med* **40**, 1211–1220.

Gamble, M.V., Palafox, N.A., Dancheck, B., *et al.* (2004) Relationship of vitamin A deficiency, iron deficiency, and inflammation to anemia among preschool children in the

Republic of the Marshall Islands. *EurJ ClinNutr* **58**, 1396–1401.

Ganji, V., Hampl, J.S., and Betts, N.M. (2003) Race-, gender- and age-specific differences in dietary micronutrient intakes of US children. *Int J Food Sci Nutr* **54**, 485–490.

Garcia-Casal, M.N., Layrisse, M., Solano, L., *et al.* (1998) A new property of vitamin A and β-carotene on human non-heme iron absorption in rice, wheat and corn. *J Nutr* **128**, 646–650.

Genaro, P. de S. and Martini, L.A. (2004) Vitamin A supplementation and risk of skeletal fracture. *Nutr Rev* **62**, 65–67.

Gidlof, A.C., Ocaya, P., Olofsson, P.S., *et al.* (2006) Differences in retinol metabolism and proliferative response between neointimal and medial smooth muscle cells. *J Vasc Res* **43**, 392–398.

Glass, C.K., Rosenfeld, M.G., Rose, D.W., *et al.* (1997) Mechanisms of transcriptional activation by retinoic acid receptors. *Biochem Soc Trans* **25**, 602–605.

Goldbohm, R.A., Brants, H.A., Hulshof, K.F., *et al.* (1998) The contribution of various foods to intake of vitamin A and carotenes in the Netherlands. *Int J Vitam Nutr Res* **68**, 378–383.

Gong, X., Tsai, S.W., Yan, B., *et al.* (2006) Cooperation between MEF2 and PPARgamma in human intestinal beta,beta-carotene 15,15′-monooxygenase gene expression. *BMC Mol Biol* **7**, 7.

Grotto, I., Mimouni, M., Gdalevich, M., *et al.* (2003) Vitamin A supplementation and childhood morbidity from diarrhea and respiratory infections: a meta-analysis. *J Pediatrics* **142**, 297–304.

Grune, T., Lietz, G., Palou, A., *et al.* (2010) Beta-carotene is an important vitamin A source for humans. *J Nutr* **140**, 2268S–2285S.

Hamamoto, S., Fukuda, R., Ishimura, N., *et al.* (2003) 9-*cis* retinoic acid enhances the antiviral effect of interferon on hepatitis C virus replication through increased expression of type I interferon receptor. *J Lab Clin Med* **141**, 58–66.

Harley, K., Eskenazi, B., and Block, G. (2005) The association of time in the US and diet during pregnancy in low income women of Mexican descent. *Pediatr Perinat Epidemiol* **19**, 125–134.

Harrison, E.H. (2005) Mechanisms of digestion and absorption of dietary vitamin A. *Annu Rev Nutr* **25**, 87–103.

Hartong, D.T., Berson, E.L., and Dryja, T.P. (2006) Retinitis pigmentosa. *Lancet* **368**, 1795–1809.

Haskell, M.J., Jamil, K.M., Hassan. F., *et al.* (2004) Daily consumption of Indian spinach (*Basella alba*) or sweet potatoes has a positive effect on total-body vitamin A stores in Bangladeshi men. *Am J Clin Nutr* **80**, 705–714.

Heise, R., Mey, J., Neis, M.M., *et al.* (2006) Skin retinoid concentrations are modulated by CYP26AI expression restricted to basal keratinocytes in normal human skin and differentiated 3D skin models. *J Invest Dermatol* **126**, 2473–2480.

Henderson, L., Irving, K., Bates, C., *et al.* (2003) Vitamin and mineral intake and urinary analytes. In *The National Diet and Nutrition Survey, Adults Aged 19 to 64 Years*, Vol. 3. Office for National Statistics, Food.

Herrero, C., Granado, F., Blanco, I., *et al.* (2002) Vitamin A and E content in dairy products: their contribution to the recommended dietary allowances (RDA) for elderly people. *J Nutr Health Aging* **6**, 57–59.

Herring, W., Nowicki, M.J., and Jones, J.K. (2010) An uncommon cause of esophagitis. *Gastroenterology* **139**, e6–7.

Hickenbottom, S.J., Follet, J.R., Lin, Y., *et al.* (2002) Variability in conversion of beta-carotene to vitamin A in men as measured by using a double-tracer study design. *Am J Clinical Nutr* **75**, 900–907.

Hicks, V.A., Gunning, D.B., and Olson, J.A. (1984) Metabolism, plasma transport and biliary excretion of radioactive vitamin A and its metabolites as a function of liver reserves of vitamin A in the rat. *J Nutr* **114**, 1327–1333.

Higgins, L.S. and Depaoli, A.M. (2010) Selective peroxisome proliferator-activated receptor gamma (PPARgamma) modulation as a strategy for safer therapeutic PPARgamma activation. *Am J Clin Nutr* **91**, 267S–272S.

High, K.P., Legault, C., Sinclair, J.A., *et al.* (2002) Low plasma concentrations of retinol and alpha-tocopherol in hematopoietic stem cell transplant recipients: the effect of mucositis and the risk of infection *Am J Clin Nutr* **76**, 1358–1366.

Hori, Y., Spurr-Michaud, S., Russo, C.L., *et al.* (2004) Differential regulation of membrane-associated mucins in the human ocular surface epithelium. *Invest Ophthalmol Vis Sci* **45**, 114–122.

Hotz, C. and McClafferty, B. (2007) From harvest to health: challenges for developing biofortified staple foods and determining their impact on micronutrient status. *Food Nutr Bull* **28** (2 Suppl), S271–S279.

Hoyos, B., Jiang, S., and Hammerling, U. (2005) Location and functional significance of retinol-binding sites on the serine/theorine kinase, c-Raf. *J Biol Chem* **280**, 6872–6878.

Humphreys, E.H., Smith, N.A., Azman, H., *et al.* (2010) Prevention of diarrhoea in children with HIV infection or exposure to maternal HIV infection. *Cochrane Database Syst Rev* CD008563.

Institute of Medicine (2001) Food and Nutrition Board. *Dietary Reference Intakes for Vitamin A, Vitamin K, Arsenic, Boron, Chromium, Copper, Iodine, Iron, Manganese, Molybdenum, Nickel, Silicon, Vanadium and Zinc*. National Academy Press, Washington, DC.

Johanning, G.L. and Piyathilake, C.J. (2003) Retinoids and epigenetic silencing in cancer. *Nutr Rev* **61**, 284–289.

Kafwembe, E.M. (2001) Iron and vitamin A status of breastfeeding mothers in Zambia. *East Afr Med J* **78**, 454–457.

Kalousová, M., Kubena, A.A., Kostírová, M., *et al.* (2010) Lower retinol levels as an independent predictor of mortality in long-term hemodialysis patients: a prospective observational cohort study. *Am J Kidney Dis* **56**, 513–521.

Kapil, U. (2002) Deaths in Assam during vitamin A pulse distribution: the needle of suspicion is on the new measuring cup. *Indian Pediatr* **39**, 114–115.

Karyadi, E., West, C.E., Schultink, W., *et al.* (2002) A double-blind, placebo-controlled study of vitamin A and zinc supplementation in persons with tuberculosis in Indonesia: effects on clinical response and nutritional status. *Am J Clin Nutr* **75**, 720–727.

Kawahara, T.N., Krueger, D.C., Engelke, J.A., *et al.* (2002) Short-term vitamin A supplementation does not affect bone turnover in men. *J Nutr* **132**, 1169–1172.

Kawuma, M. (2002) Sugar as a potential vehicle for vitamin A fortification: experience from Kamuli district in Uganda. *Afr Health Sci* **2**, 11–15.

Khasru, M.R., Yasmin, R., Salek, A.K., *et al.* (2010) Acute hypervitaminosis A in a young lady. *Mymensingh Med J* **19**, 294–298.

Kiefer, H.L., Hanley, T.M., Marcello, J.E., *et al.* (2004) Retinoic acid inhibition of chromatin remodeling at the human immunodeficiency virus type 1 promoter. Uncoupling of histone acetylation and chromatin remodeling. *J Biol Chem* **279**, 43604–43613.

Kiely, M., Flynn, A., Harrington, K.E., *et al.* (2001) The efficacy and safety of nutritional supplement use in a representative sample of adults in the North/South Ireland Food Consumption Survey. *Public Health Nutr* **4**, 1089–1097.

Kinjo, K., Miyakawa, Y., Uchida, H., *et al.* (2004) All-*trans* retinoic acid directly upregulates thrombopoietin transcription in human bone marrow stromal cells. *Exp Hematol* **32**, 45–51.

Krinsky, N.I., Wang, X.-D., Tang, G., *et al.* (1993) Mechanism of carotenoid cleavage to retinoids. *Ann NY Acad Sci* **681**, 167–176.

Kuhnlein, H.V., Receveur, O., Soueida, R., *et al.* (2004) Arctic indigenous peoples experience the nutrition transition with changing dietary patterns and obesity. *J Nutr* **134**, 1447–1453.

Larson, R.S. and Tallman, M.S. (2003) Retinoic acid syndrome: manifestations, pathogenesis, and treatment. *Best Pract Rest Clin Haematol* **16**, 453–461.

Latham, M. (2010) The great vitamin A fiasco. *World Nutr* **1**, 12–15.

Layrisse, M., Garcia-Casal, M.N., Solano, L., *et al.* (1997) The role of vitamin A on the inhibition of nonheme iron absorption: preliminary results. *J Nutr Biochem* **8**, 61–67.

Layrisse, M., Garcia-Casal, M.N., Solano, L., *et al.* (1998) Vitamin A reduces the inhibition of iron absorption by phytates and polyphenols. *Food Nutr Bull* **19**, 3–5.

Lefebvre, P., Benomar, Y., and Staels, B. (2010) Retinoid X receptors: common heterodimerization partners with distinct functions. *Trends Endocrinol Metab* **21**, 676–683.

Leung, W.C., Hessel, S., Méplan, C., *et al.* (2009) Two common single nucleotide polymorphisms in the gene encoding beta-carotene 15,15′-monooxygenase alter beta-carotene metabolism in female volunteers. *FASEB J* **23**, 1041–1053.

Lewis, S.M., Mayhugh, M.A., Freni, S.C., *et al.* (2003) Assessment of antioxidant nutrient intake of a population of southern US African-American and Caucasian women of various ages when compared to dietary reference intakes. *J Nutr Health Aging* **7**, 121–128.

Lietz, G., Lange, J., and Rimbach, G. (2010) Molecular and dietary regulation of beta-carotene 15,15′-monooxygenase 1 (BCMO1). *Arch Biochem Biophys* **502**, 8–16.

Lindqvist, A. and Andersson, S. (2002) Biochemical properties of purified recombinant human beta-carotene 15,15′-monooxygenase. *J Biol Chem* **277**, 23942–23948.

Lindqvist, A. and Andersson, S. (2004) Cell type-specific expression of beta-carotene 15,15′-mono-oxygenase in human tissues. *J Histochem Cytochem* **52**, 491–499.

Loerch, J.D., Underwood, B.A., and Lewis, K.C. (1979) Response of plasma levels of vitamin A to a dose of vitamin A as an indicator of hepatic vitamin A reserves in rats. *J Nutr* **109**, 778–788.

Loureiro, K.D., Kao, K.K., Jones, K.L., *et al.* (2005) Minor malformations characteristic of the retinoic acid embryopathy and other birth outcomes in children of women exposed to topical tretinoin during early pregnancy. *Am J Med Genet* **136**, 117–121.

Low, J.W., Arimond, M., Osman, N., *et al.* (2007) A food-based approach introducing orange-fleshed sweet potatoes increased vitamin A intake and serum retinol concentrations in young children in rural Mozambique. *J Nutr* **137**, 1320–1327.

Lundeen, E., Schueth, T., Toktobaev, N., *et al.* (2010) Daily use of Sprinkles micronutrient powder for 2 months reduces anemia among children 6 to 36 months of age in the Kyrgyz Republic: a cluster-randomized trial. *Food Nutr Bull* **31**, 446–460.

Lytle, L.A., Himes, J.H., Feldman, H., *et al.* (2002) Nutrient intake over time in a multi-ethnic sample of youth. *Public Health Nutr* **5**, 319–328.

Mactier, H. and Weaver, L.T. (2005) Vitamin A and preterm infants: what we know, what we don't know, and what we need to know. *Arch Dis Child Fetal Neonatal Ed* **90**, F103–F108.

Maden, M. and Hind, M. (2004) Retinoic acid in alveolar development, maintenance and regeneration. *Philos Trans R Soc Lond B Biol Sci* **359**, 799–780.

Maramag, C.C., Ribaya-Mercado, J.D., Rayco-Solon, P., *et al.* (2010) Influence of carotene-rich vegetable meals on the prevalence of anaemia and iron deficiency in Filipino schoolchildren. *Eur J Clin Nutr* **64**, 468–474.

Mariath, J.G.R., Lima, M.C.C., and Santos, L.M.P. (1989) Vitamin A activity of buriti (*Maurita vinifera* Mart) and its effectiveness in the treatment and prevention of xerophthalmia. *Am J Clin Nutr* **49**, 849–853.

Mark, M., Ghyselinck, N.B., and Chambon, P. (2004) Retinoic acid signaling in the development of branchial arches. *Curr Opin Genet Devel* **14**, 591–598.

Martins, I., Dantas, A., Guiomar, S., *et al.* (2002) Vitamin and mineral intakes in elderly. *J Nutr Health Aging* **6**, 63–65.

Mason, M.E., Jalagani, H., and Vinik, A.I. (2005) Metabolic complications of bariatric surgery: diagnosis and management issues. *Gastroenterol Clin North Am* **34**, 25–33.

Mehta, S., Finkelstein, J.L., and Fawzi, W.W. (2007) Nutritional interventions in HIV-infected breastfeeding women. *Annales Nestlé* [English version] **65**, 39–48.

Melhus, H., Michaelsson, K., Kindmark, A., *et al.* (1998) Excessive dietary intake of vitamin A is associated with reduced bone mineral density and increased risk for hip fracture. *Ann Intern Med* **129**, 770–778.

Menses, F. and Trugo, N.M.F. (2005) Retinol, β-carotene, and lutein + zeaxanthin in the milk of Brazilian nursing women: associations with plasma concentrations and influences of maternal characteristics. *Nutr Res* **25**, 443–451.

Menses, F., Torres, A.C., and Trugo, N.M.F. (2004) Influence of recent dietary intake on plasma and human milk levels of carotenoids and retinol in Brazilian nursing women. *Adv Exp Med Biol* **554**, 351–354.

Millen, A.E., Dodd, K.W., and Subar, A.F. (2004) Use of vitamin, mineral, nonvitamin and nonmineral supplements in the United States: The 1987, 1992, and 2000 National Health Interview Survey results. *J Am Diet Assoc* **104**, 942–950.

Miller, R.K., Hendrickx, A.G., Mills, J.L., *et al.* (1998) Periconceptional vitamin A use: how much is teratogenic? *Reprod Toxicol* **8**, 75–88.

Mills, J.P., Simon, P.W., and Tanumihardjo, S.A. (2008) Biofortified carrot intake enhances liver antioxidant capacity and vitamin A status in Mongolian gerbils. *J Nutr* **138**, 1692–1698.

Mitra, A.K., Wahed, M.A., Chowdhury, A.K., *et al.* (2002) Urinary retinol excretion in children with acute watery diarrhea. *J Health Popul Nutr* **20**, 12–17.

Mora, J.O. (2003) Proposed vitamin A fortification levels. *J Nutr* **133**, 2990S–2993S.

Morgan, S.L. (2009) Nutrition and bone: it is more than calcium and vitamin D. *Women's Health (Lond Engl)* **5**, 727–737.

Mrdjenovic, G. and Levitsky, D.A. (2003) Nutritional and energetic consequences of sweetened drink consumption in 6- to 13-year-old children. *J Pediatrics* **142**, 604–610.

Murphy, S.P. and Poos, M.I. (2002) Dietary Reference Intakes: summary of applications in dietary assessment. *Public Health Nutr* **5**, 843–849.

Murphy, S.P., Gewa, C., Liang, L.J., *et al.* (2003) School snacks containing animal source foods improve dietary quality for children in rural Kenya. *J Nutr* **133** (11 Suppl 2), 3950S–3956S.

Myhre, A.M., Carlsen, M.H., Bohn, S.K., *et al.* (2003) Water-miscible, emulsified, and solid forms of retinol supplements are more than oil-based preparations. *Am J Clin Nutr* **78**, 1152–1159.

Nagao, A. (2004) Oxidative conversion of carotenoids to retinoids and other products. *J Nutr* **134**, 237S–240S.

Nagendran, B., Unnithan, U.R., Choo, Y.M., *et al.* (2000) Characteristics of red palm oil, a carotene- and vitamin E-rich refined oil for food uses. *Food Nutr Bull* **21**, 189–194.

Napoli, J.L. (1999) Interactions of retinoid binding proteins and enzymes in retinoid metabolism. *Biochim Biophys Acta* **1440**, 139–162.

Napoli, J.L. (2000) A gene knockout corroborates the integral function of cellular retinol-binding protein in retinoid metabolism. *Nutr Rev* **58**, 230–235.

Naqvi, S., Zhu, C., Farre, G., *et al.* (2009) Transgenic multivitamin corn through biofortification of endosperm with three vitamins representing three distinct metabolic pathways. *Proc Natl Acad Sci USA* **106**, 7762–7767.

Nestel, P., Bouis, H.E., Meenakshi, J.V., *et al.* (2006) Biofortification of staple food crops. *J Nutr* **136**, 1064–1067.

Nestel, P., Briend, A., de Benoist, B., *et al.* (2003) Complementary food supplements to achieve micronutrient adequacy for infants and young children. *J Pediatr Gastroenterol Nutr* **36**, 316–328.

Nohara, A., Kobayashi, J., and Mabuchi, H. (2009) Retinoid X receptor heterodimer variants and cardiovascular risk factors. *J Atheroscler Thromb* **16**, 303–318.

Novotny, J.A., Harrison, D.J., Pawlosky, R., *et al.* (2010) Beta-carotene conversion to vitamin A decreases as the dietary dose increases in humans. *J Nutr* **140**, 915–918.

Oelofse, A., Van Raaij, J.M., Benade, A.J., *et al.* (2002) Disadvantaged black and coloured infants in two urban communities in the Western Cape, South Africa differ in micronutrient status. *Public Health Nutr* **5**, 289–294.

Oelofse, A., Van Raaij, J.M., Benade, A.J., *et al.* (2003) The effect of a micronutrient-fortified complementary food on micronutrient status, growth and development of 6- to12-month-old disadvantaged urban South African infants. *Int J Food Sci Nutr* **54**, 399–407.

Olafsdottir, A.S., Wagner, K.H., Thorsdottir, I., *et al.* (2001) Fat-soluble vitamins in the maternal diet, influence of cod liver oil supplementation and impact of the maternal diet on human milk composition. *Ann Nutr Metab* **45**, 265–272.

Oliveira-Menegozzo, J.M. and Bergamaschi, D.P. (2010) Vitamin A supplementation for postpartum women. *Cochrane Database Syst Rev* CD005944.

Olson, J.A. (1998) Carotenoids. In M.E. Shils, J.A. Olson, A.C. Ross, *et al.* (eds), *Modern Nutrition in Health and Disease*, 9th Edn. W.B. Saunders, Philadelphia, pp. 525–541.

Onyango, A.W., Receveur, O., and Esrey, S.A. (2002) The contribution of breast milk to toddler diets in western Kenya. *Bull World Health Organ* **80**, 292–299.

Oren, T., Sher, J.A., and Evans, T. (2003) Hematopoiesis and retinoids: development and disease. *Leuk Lymphoma* **44**, 1881–1891.

Osei, A.K., Rosenberg, I.H., Houser, R.F., *et al.* (2010) Community-level micronutrient fortification of school lunch meals improved vitamin A, folate, and iron status of schoolchildren in Himalayan villages in India. *J Nutr* **140**, 1146–1154.

Osório, M.M., Lira, P.I., and Ashworth, A. (2004) Factors associated with Hb concentration in children aged 6–59 months in the state of Pernambuco, Brazil. *Br J Nutr* **91**, 307–315.

Pangaribuan, R., Scherbaum, V., Erhardt, J.G., *et al.* (2004) Socioeconomic and familial characteristics influence caretakers' adherence to the periodic vitamin A capsule supplementation program in Central Java, Indonesia. *J Trop Pediatr* **50**, 143–148.

Perrotta, S., Nobili, B., Rossi, F., *et al.* (2002) Infant hypervitaminosis A causes severe anemia and thrombocytopenia evidence of a retinol-dependent bone marrow cell growth inhibition. *Blood* **99**, 2017–2022.

Perry, R.T. and Halsey, N.A. (2004) The clinical significance of measles: a review. *J Infect Dis* **189** (Suppl 1), S4–S16.

Persson, V., Hartini, T.N., Greiner. T., *et al.* (2002) Vitamin A intake is low among pregnant women in central Java, Indonesia. *Int J Vit Nutr Res* **72**, 124–132.

Pobocic, R.S. and Richer, J.J. (2002) Estimated intake and food sources of vitamin A, folate, vitamin C, vitamin E, calcium, iron, and zinc for Guamanian children aged 9 to 12. *Pac Health Dialog* **9**, 193–202.

Pulukuri, S. and Sitaramayya, A. (2004) Retinaldehyde, a potent inhibitor of gap junctional intercellular communication. *Cell Commun Adhes* **11**, 25–33.

Radhika, M.S., Bhaskaram, P., Balakrishna, N., *et al.* (2003). Red palm oil supplementation: a feasible diet-based approach to improve the vitamin A status of pregnant women and their infants. *Food Nutr Bull* **24**, 208–217.

Raghu, P. and Sivakumar, B. (2004) Interactions amongst plasma retinol-binding protein, transthyretin and their ligands: implications in vitamin A homeostasis and transthyretin amyloidosis. *Biochim Biophys Acta* **1703**, 1–9.

Rahmathullah, L., Tielsch, J.M., Thulasiraj, R.D., *et al.* (2003) Impact of supplementing newborn infants with vitamin A on early infant mortality: community based randomized trial in southern India. *Br Med J* **327**, 254.

Raiten, D.J., Namasté, S., Brabin, B., *et al.* (2011) Executive summary: Biomarkers of Nutrition for Development (BOND): building a consensus. *Am J Clin Nutr* (Suppl) **94**, 633S–650S.

Ramakrishnan, U. (2002) Prevalence of micronutrient malnutrition worldwide. *Nutr Rev* **60**, S46–S52.

Ribaya-Mercado, J.D. (2002) Influence of dietary fat on beta-carotene absorption and bioconversion into vitamin A. *Nutr Rev* **60**, 104–110.

Ribaya-Mercado, J.D. and Blumberg, J.B. (2007) Vitamin A: is it a risk factor for osteoporosis and bone fracture? *Nutr Rev* **65**, 425–438.

Ribaya-Mercado, J.D., Solomons, N.W., Medrano, Y., *et al.* (2004a) Use of the deuterated-retinol-dilution technique to monitor the vitamin A status of Nicaraguan schoolchildren 1 y after initiation of the Nicaraguan national program of sugar fortification with vitamin A. *Am J Clin Nutr* **80**, 1291–1298.

Ribaya-Mercado, J.D., Solon, F.S., Dallal, G.E., *et al.* (2003) Quantitative assessment of total body stores of vitamin A in adults with the use of a 3-d deuterated-retinol-dilution procedure. *Am J Clin Nutr* **77**, 694–699.

Ribaya-Mercado, J.D., Solon, F.S., Fermin, L.S., *et al.* (2004b) Dietary vitamin A intakes of Filipino elders with adequate or low liver vitamin A concentrations as assessed by the deuterated-retinol-dilution method: implications for dietary requirements. *Am J Clin Nutr* **79**, 633–641.

Rochette-Egly, C. and Germain, P. (2009) Dynamic and combinatorial control of gene expression by nuclear retinoic acid receptors (RARs). *Nucl Recept Signal* **6**, e005.

Rodriguez-Amaya, D.B. (1999) *A Guide to Carotenoid Analysis in Foods*. ILSI Press, Washington, DC.

Roos, N., Islam, M.M., and Thilsted, S.H. (2003a) Small indigenous fish species in Bangladesh: contribution to vitamin A, calcium and iron intakes. *J Nutr* **133** (11 Suppl 2), 4021S–4026S.

Roos, N., Islam, M., and Thilsted, S.H. (2003b) Small fish is an important dietary source of vitamin A and calcium in rural Bangladesh. *Int J Food Sci Nutr* **54**, 329–339.

Ross, A.C. (2004) On the sources of retinoic acid in the lung: understanding the local conversion of retinol to retinoic acid. *Am J Physiol Lung Cell Mol Physiol* **286**, L247–L248.

Rowe, A. (1997) Retinoid X receptors. *Biochem Cell Biol* **29**, 275–278.

Sazawal, S., Black, R.E., Ramsan, M., *et al.* (2006) Effects of routine prophylactic supplementation with iron and folic acid on admission to hospital and mortality in preschool children in a high malaria transmission setting: community-based, randomised, placebo-controlled trial. *Lancet* **367,** 133–143.

Schipani, S., van der Haar, F., Sinawar, S., *et al.* (2002) Dietary intake and nutritional status of young children in families practicing mixed home gardening in northeast Thailand. *Food Nutr Bull* **23,** 175–180.

Schmidt, R., Luboeinski, T., Markart, P., *et al.* (2004) Alveolar antioxidant status in patients with acute respiratory distress syndrome. *Eur Resp J* **24,** 994–999.

Schweigert, F.J., Bathe, K., Chen, F., *et al.* (2004) Effect of the stage of lactation in humans on carotenoid levels in milk, blood plasma and plasma lipoprotein fractions. *Eur J Nutr* **43,** 39–44.

Sedjo, R.L., Ranger-Moore, J., Foote, J., *et al.* (2004) Circulating endogenous retinoic acid concentrations among participants enrolled in a randomized placebo-controlled clinical trial of retinyl palmitate. *Cancer Epidemiol Biomarkers Prev* **13,** 1687–1692.

Semba, R.D. and Bloem, M.W. (2002) The anemia of vitamin A deficiency: epidemiology and pathogenesis. *Eur J Clin Nutr* **56,** 271–281.

Semba, R.D., de Pee, S., Panagides, D., *et al.* (2004) Risk factors for xerophthalmia among mothers and their children and for mother–child pairs with xerophthalmia in Cambodia. *Arch Ophthalmol* **122,** 517–523.

Semba, R.D, de Pee, S., Sun, K., *et al.* (2010) Coverage of vitamin A capsule programme in Bangladesh and risk factors associated with non-receipt of vitamin A. *J Health Popul Nutr* **28,** 143–148.

Semba, R.D., Ndugwa, C., Perry, R.T., *et al.* (2005) Effect of periodic vitamin A supplementation on mortality and morbidity of human immunodeficiency virus-infected children in Uganda: a controlled clinical trial. *Nutrition* **21,** 25–31.

Senoo, H., Yoshikawa, K., Morii, M., *et al.* (2010) Hepatic stellate cell (vitamin A-storing cell) and its relative – past, present and future. *Cell Biol Int* **34,** 1247–1272.

Serghides, L. and Kain, K.C. (2002) Mechanism of protection induced by vitamin A in falciparum malaria. *Lancet* **359,** 1404–1406.

Serra-Majem, L., Ribas, L., Garcia, A., *et al.* (2003) Nutrient adequacy and Mediterranean diet in Spanish school children and adolescents. *Eur J Clin Nutr* **57**(Suppl 1), S35–S39.

Serra-Majem, L., Ribas, L., Ngo, J., *et al.* (2001) Risk of inadequate intakes of vitamin A, B1, B6, C, E, folate, iron and calcium in the Spanish population aged 4 to 18. *Int J Vitam Nutr Res* **71,** 325–331.

Shankar, A.H., Genton, B., Semba, R.D., *et al.* (1999) Effect of vitamin A supplementation on morbidity due to *Plasmodium falciparum* in young children in Papua New Guinea: a randomized trial. *Lancet* **354,** 203–209.

Sichert-Hellert, W., Kersting, M., Dortmund Nutritional and Anthropometric Longitudinally Designed Study (2001a) Significance of fortified beverages in the long-term diet of German children and adolescents: 15-year results of the DONALD Study. *Int J Vitam Nutr Res* **71,** 356–363.

Sichert-Hellert, W., Kersting, M., and Manz, F. (2001b) Changes in time-trends of nutrient intake from fortified and non-fortified food in German children and adolescents – 15 year results of the DONALD study. Dortmund Nutritional and Anthropometric Longitudinally Designed Study. *Eur J Nutr* **40,** 49–55.

Siddikuzzaman, Guruvayoorappan, C. and Berlin Grace, V.M. (2011) All-*trans* retinoic acid and cancer. *Immunopharmacol Immunotoxicol* **33,** 241–249.

Singh, V. and West, K.P., Jr (2004) Vitamin A deficiency and xerophthalmia among school-aged children in southeastern Asia. *Eur J Clin Nutr* **58,** 1342–1349.

Sivan, Y.S., Alwin Jayakumar, Y., Arumughan, C., *et al.* (2002) Impact of vitamin A supplementation through different dosages of red palm oil and retinol palmitate on preschool children. *J Trop Pediatr* **48,** 24–28.

Skare, K.L. and DeLuca, H.F. (1983) Biliary metabolites of all-*trans*-retinoic acid in the rat. *Arch Biochem Biophys* **224,** 13–18.

Slater, G.H., Ren, C.J., Siegel, N., *et al.* (2004) Serum fat-soluble vitamin deficiency and abnormal calcium metabolism after malabsorptive bariatric surgery. *J Gastrointest Surg* **8,** 48–55.

Smuts, C.M., Benadé, A.J., Berger, J., *et al.* (2003) IRIS I: a FOODlet-based multiple-micronutrient intervention in 6- to 12-month-old infants at high risk of micronutrient malnutrition in four contrasting populations: description of a multicenter field trial. *Food Nutr Bull* **24** (3 Suppl), S27–S33.

Smuts, C.M., Lombard, C.J., Benadé, A.J., *et al.* (2005) Efficacy of a foodlet-based multiple micronutrient supplement for preventing growth faltering, anemia, and micronutrient deficiency of infants: the four country IRIS trial pooled data analysis. *J Nutr* **135,** 631S–638S.

Sobeck, U., Fischer, A., and Bieslaski, H.K. (2002) Determination of vitamin A palmitate in buccal mucosal cells: a pilot study. *Eur J Med Res* **7,** 287–289.

Solomons, N.W. and Bulux, J. (1994) Plant sources of vitamin A and human nutrition revisited: recent evidence from developing countries. *Nutr Rev* **52,** 62–64.

Solomons, N.W. and Orozco, M. (2003) Alleviation of vitamin A deficiency with palm fruit and its products. *Asia Pac J Clin Nutr* **12,** 373–384.

Sommer, A. (2005) Innocenti Micronutrient Report No.1. *Sight and Life Newsletter* **3**, 13–18.

Sommer, A., Tarwotjo, I., Djunaedi, E., *et al.* (1986) The impact of vitamin A supplementation on childhood mortality. A randomized controlled community trial. *Lancet* **1**, 1169–1173.

Sommer, A., Tarwojto, I., and Hussaini, G. (1983) Increased mortality in children with mild vitamin A deficiency. *Lancet* **2**, 585–588.

Spears, K., Cheney, C., and Zerzan, J. (2004) Low plasma retinol concentrations increase the risk of developing bronchopulmonary dysplasia and long-term respiratory disability in very-low-birth-weight infants. *Am J Clin Nutr* **80**, 1589–1594.

Stephensen, C.B., Franchi, L.M., Hernandez, H., *et al.* (2002) Assessment of vitamin A status with the relative-dose-response test in Peruvian children recovering from pneumonia. *Am J Clin Nutr* **76**, 1351–1357.

Sudfeld, C.R., Navar, A.M., and Halsey, N.A. (2010) Effectiveness of measles vaccination and vitamin A treatment. *Int J Epidemiol* **39** (Suppl 1), 1148–1155.

Tang, H.S. and Gudas, L.J. (2011) Retinoids, retinoic acid receptors, and cancer. *Annu Rev Pathol* **6**, 345–364.

Tang, G., Qin, J., Dolnikowski, G.G., *et al.* (2003) Short-term (intestinal) and long-term (postintestinal) conversion of beta-carotene to retinol in adults as assessed by a stable-isotope reference method. *Am J Clin Nutr* **78**, 259–266.

Tang, G., Qin, J, Dolnikowski, G.G., *et al.* (2005) Spinach or carrots can supply significant amounts of vitamin A as assessed by feeding with intrinsically deuterated vegetables. *Am J Clin Nutr* **82**, 821–828.

Tang, G., Qin, J., Dolnikowski, G.G., *et al.* (2009) Golden Rice is an effective source of vitamin A. *Am J Clin Nutr* **89**, 1776–1783.

Tang. G., Qin, J., Hao, L.Y., *et al.* (2002) Use of a short-term isotope-dilution method for determining the vitamin A status of children. *Am J Clin Nutr* **76**, 413–418.

Tanumihardjo, S.A. (2004) Assessing vitamin A status: past, present and future. *J Nutr* **134**, 290S–293S.

Tanumihardjo, S.A. (2011) Vitamin A: biomarkers of nutrition for development. *Am J Clin Nutr* **94**, 658S–665S.

Tanumihardjo, S.A. and Olson, J.A. (1988) A modified relative dose–response assay employing 3,4-didehydroretinol (vitamin A2) in rats. *J Nutr* **118**, 598–603.

Tanumihardjo, S.A., Furr, H.C., Erdman, J.W., Jr, *et al.* (1990a) Use of the modified relative dose response (MRDR) assay in rats and its application to humans for the measurement of vitamin A status. *Eur J Clin Nutr* **44**, 219–224.

Tanumihardjo, S.A., Koellner, P.G., and Olson, J.A. (1990b) The modified relative-dose-response assay as an indicator of vitamin A status in a population of well-nourished American children. *Am J Clin Nutr* **52**, 1064–1067.

Taren, D.L., Duncan, B., Shrestha, K., *et al.* (2004) The night vision threshold test is a better predictor of low serum vitamin A concentration than self-reported night blindness in pregnant urban Nepalese women. *J Nutr* **134**, 2573–2578.

Thakkar, S.K., Huo, T., Maziya-Dixon, B., *et al.* (2009) Impact of style of processing on retention and bioaccessibility of beta-carotene in cassava (*Manihot esculenta* Crantz). *J Agric Food Chem* **57**, 1344–1348.

Thane, C.W., Bates, C.W., and Prentice, A. (2002) Zinc and vitamin A intake and status in a national sample of British young people aged 4–18 y. *Eur J Clin Nutr* **58**, 363–375.

Thompson, D.A. and Gal, A. (2003) Vitamin A metabolism in the retinal pigment epithelium: genes, mutations, and diseases. *Prog Retin Eye Res* **22**, 683–703.

Thurmann, P.A., Steffen, J., Zwernemann, C., *et al.* (2002) Plasma concentration response to drinks containing beta-carotene as carrot juice or formulated as a water dispersible powder. *Eur J Nutr* **41**, 228–235.

Tiboni, G.M., Bucciarelli, T., Giampietro. F., *et al.* (2004) Influence of cigarette smoking on vitamin E, vitamin A, beta-carotene and lycopene concentrations in human pre-ovulatory folicular fluid. *Int J Immunopathol Pharmacol* **17**, 389–393.

Troen, G., Eskild, W., Fromm, S.H., *et al.* (1999) Vitamin A-sensitive tissues in transgenic mice expressing high levels of human cellular retinol-binding protein type I are not altered phenotypically. *J Nutr* **129**, 1621–1627.

Tyson, J.E., Wright, L.L., Oh, W., *et al.* (1999) Vitamin A supplementation for extremely-low-birth-weight infants. National Institute of Child Health and Human Development Neonatal Research Network. *N Engl J Med* **340**, 1962–1968.

Underwood, B.A. and Olson, J.A. (1993) *A Brief Guide to Current Methods of Assessing Vitamin A Status*. The Nutrition Foundation, Washington, DC.

Valentine, A.R. and Tanumihardjo, S.A. (2005) One-time vitamin A supplementation of lactating sows enhances hepatic retinol in their offspring independent of dose size. *Am J Clin Nutr* **81**, 427–433.

Vallabhaneni, R., Gallagher, C.E., Licciardello, N., *et al.* (2009) Metabolite sorting of a germplasm collection reveals the hydroxylase3 locus as a new target for maize provitamin A biofortification. *Plant Physiol* **151**, 1635–1645.

van Lettow, M., Harries, A.D., Kumwenda, J.J., *et al.* (2004) Micronutrient malnutrition and wasting in adults with pulmonary tuberculosis with and without HIV co-infection in Malawi. *BMC Infect Dis* **4**, 61.

van Lieshout, M., West, C.E., and van Breemen, R.B. (2003) Isotopic tracer techniques for studying the bioavailability and bioefficacy of dietary carotenoids, particularly beta-carotene, in humans: a review. *Am J Clin Nutr* **77**, 12–28.

Venkaiah, K., Damayanti, K., Nayak, M.U., *et al.* (2002) Diet and nutritional status of rural adolescents in India. *Eur J Clin Nutr* **56**, 1119–1125.

Verhoef, H. and West, C.E. (2005) Validity of the relative-dose–response test and the modified-relative-dose–response test as indicators of vitamin A stores in liver. *Am J Clin Nutr* **81**, 835–839.

Vestergaard, P., Rejnmark, L., and Mosekilde, L. (2010) High-dose treatment with vitamin A analogues and risk of fractures. *Arch Dermatol* **146**, 478–482.

Villalpando, S., Montalvo-Velarde, I., Zambrano, N., *et al.* (2003) Vitamins A and C and folate status in Mexican children under 12 years and women 12–49 years: a probabilistic national survey. *Salud Publica (Mexico)* **45** (Suppl 4), S508–S519.

Villamor, E., Mbise, R., Spiegelman, D., *et al.* (2002) Vitamin A supplements ameliorate the adverse effect of HIV-1, malaria, and diarrheal infections on child growth. *Pediatrics* **109**, E6.

Villamor, E., Saathoff, E., Bosch, R.J., *et al.* (2005) Vitamin supplementation of HIV-infected women improves postnatal child growth. *Am J Clin Nutr* **81**, 880–888.

Visser, M.E., Maartens, G., Kossew, G., *et al.* (2003) Plasma vitamin A and zinc levels in HIV-infected adults in Cape Town, South Africa. *Br J Nutr* **89**, 475–482.

Von Lintig, J. (2010) Colors with functions: elucidating the biochemical and molecular basis of carotenoid metabolism. *Annu Rev Nutr* **30**, 35–56.

Vorster, H.H., Kruger, A., Margetts, B.M., *et al.* (2004) The nutritional status of asymptomatic HIV-infected Africans: directions for dietary intervention. *Public Health Nutr* **7**, 1055–1064.

Vuong, L.T. and King, J. C. (2003) A method of preserving and testing the acceptibility of gac fruit oil, a good source of β-carotene and essential fatty acids. *Food Nutr Bull* **24**, 224–230.

Wald, G. (1968) Molecular basis of visual excitation. *Science* **162**, 230–239.

Wang, Z., Yin, S., Zhao, X., *et al.* (2004) Beta-carotene–vitamin A equivalence in Chinese adults assessed by an isotope dilution technique. *Br J Nutr* **91**, 121–131.

Watt, R.G., Dykes, J., and Shelham, A. (2001) Socio-economic determinants of selected dietary indicators in British preschool children. *Public Health Nutr* **4**, 1229–1233.

Welch, R.M. (2005) Biotechnology, biofortification, and global health. *Food Nutr Bull* **26**, 419–421.

Welsch, R., Arango, J., Bär, C., *et al.* (2010) Provitamin A accumulation in cassava (*Manihot esculenta*) roots driven by a single nucleotide polymorphism in a phytoene synthase gene. *Plant Cell* **22**, 3348–3356.

West, C.E., Eilander, A., and van Lieshout, M. (2002) Consequences of revised estimates of carotenoid bioefficacy for dietary control of vitamin A deficiency in developing countries. *J Nutr* **132** (9 Suppl), 2920S–2926S.

West, K.P., Jr (2002) Extent of vitamin A deficiency among preschool children and women of reproductive age. *J Nutr* **132** (9 Suppl), 2857S–2866S.

Wolf, G. (2004) The visual cycle of the cone photoreceptors of the retina. *Nutr Rev* **62**, 283–286.

Wondmikun, Y. (2002) Dark adaptation pattern of pregnant women as an indicator of functional disturbance at acceptable serum vitamin A levels. *Eur J Clin Nutr* **56**, 462–466.

World Health Organization (1996) *Indicators for Assessing Vitamin A Deficiency and their Application in Monitoring and Evaluating Intervention Programmes.* WHO/NUT/96.10. WHO, Geneva.

Wyss, A., Wirtz, G.M., Woggon, W.D., *et al.* (2001) Expression pattern and localization of beta-carotene 15,15′-dioxygenase in different tissues. *Biochem J* **354**, 521–529.

Yan, J., Kandianis, C.B., Harjes, C.E., *et al.* (2010) Rare genetic variation at *Zea mays* crtRB1 increases beta-carotene in maize grain. *Nature Genet* **42**, 322–327.

Yeum, K.J. and Russell, R.M. (2002) Carotenoid bioavailability and bioconversion. *Annu Rev Nutr* **22**, 483–504.

Zagre, N.M., Delpeuch, F., Traissac, P., *et al.* (2003) Red palm oil as a source of vitamin A for mothers and children: impact of a pilot project in Burkina Faso. *Public Health Nutr* **6**, 733–742.

Zanotti, G. and Berni, R. (2004) Plasma retinol-binding protein: structure and interactions with retinol, retinoids, and transthyretin. *Vitam Horm* **69**, 271–295.

Zimmermann, M.B., Wegmueller, R., Zeder, C., *et al.* (2004) Triple fortification of salt with microcapsules of iodine, iron, and vitamin A. *Am J Clin Nutr* **80**, 1283–1290.

Zinsstag, J., Schelling, E., Daoud, S., *et al.* (2002) Serum retinol of Chadian nomadic pastoralist women in relation to their livestocks' milk retinol and beta-carotene content. *Int J Vitam Nutr Res* **72**, 221–228.

Ziouzenkova, O. and Plutzky, J. (2008) Retinoid metabolism and nuclear receptor responses: new insights into coordinated regulation of the PPAR–RXR complex. *FEBS Lett* **582**, 32–38.

Zulet, M.A., Puchau, B., Hermsdorff, H.H., *et al.* (2008) Vitamin A intake is inversely related with adiposity in healthy young adults. *J Nutr Sci Vitaminol (Tokyo)* **54**, 347–352.

12

CAROTENOIDS

BRIAN L. LINDSHIELD, PhD

Kansas State University, Manhattan, Kansas, USA

Summary

Carotenoids are 40-carbon fat-soluble compounds. Many carotenoids are pigmented; the six main carotenoids consumed and found in the body are: β-carotene, α-carotene, β-cryptoxanthin, lutein, zeaxanthin, and lycopene. β-Carotene, α-carotene, and β-cryptoxanthin are provitamin A carotenoids, meaning they can be cleaved to form retinal primarily by the carotenoid cleavage enzyme carotenoid monooxygenase 1 (CMO1). Retinol activity equivalents (RAEs) were established by the Dietary Reference Intakes Committee to estimate the vitamin A contribution of provitamin A carotenoids. Evidence suggests that the second carotenoid cleavage enzyme carotenoid monooxygenase 2 (CMO2) cleaves non-provitamin A carotenoids. A number of factors influence carotenoid bioavailability and bioconversion, which are summarized by the mnemonic "SLAMENGHI" (Species, Linkage, Amount, Matrix, Effectors, Nutrient status, Genetic factors, Host-related factors, and Interactions). The relationship between carotenoids and chronic diseases has been and remains an active area of investigation. Three of the most researched areas are β-carotene and lung cancer, lycopene and prostate cancer, and lutein/zeaxanthin and macular degeneration. Golden rice, genetically modified to produce β-carotene, was designed to combat vitamin A deficiency in countries that consume rice as a staple food. Despite being developed over a decade ago it continues to face regulatory hurdles in making it to market.

Introduction

Carotenoids are non-polar, 40-carbon poly-isoprenoid compounds found throughout nature. Of the approximately 600 known carotenoids, only 40 are typically ingested by humans and of these only 20 are commonly found in human tissues (Young *et al.*, 2004). The six main carotenoids found in the diet, blood, and tissues are: β-carotene, α-carotene, β-cryptoxanthin, lutein, zeaxanthin, and lycopene. The latter carotenoid, lycopene, is the predominant carotenoid found in the diet and blood in the United States (Holden *et al.*, 1999) (Table 12.1 and Figure 12.1). Carotenoids are classified in two ways: first, based on whether or not the carotenoid is capable of being converted to vitamin A (provitamin A activity), and secondly on structural differences and polarity. Oxygenated carotenoids are known as xanthophylls, while hydrocarbon carotenoids are known as carotenes.

Present Knowledge in Nutrition, Tenth Edition. Edited by John W. Erdman Jr, Ian A. Macdonald and Steven H. Zeisel.
© 2012 International Life Sciences Institute. Published 2012 by John Wiley & Sons, Inc.

Table 12.1 Color, xanthophyll/carotene classification, retinol conversion factors, US mean serum and intake levels, and good food sources of selected carotenoids.

Carotenoid	Color	Xanthophyll or Carotene	RE	RAE	US mean serum levels[a]		US mean intake from foods[a]		Good food sources[b]
					M	F	M	F	
					μg/dL		mg/d		
Lycopene	Red	Carotene	–	–	26.4	23.9	11.27	6.71	Tomatoes, watermelon, guava, pink grapefruit
β-Carotene	Yellow-orange	Carotene	6	12	14.6	18.4	2.22	1.87	Carrots, sweet potatoes, pumpkin, spinach, apricots
α-Carotene	Light yellow	Carotene	12	24	3.8	4.4	0.44	0.36	Carrots, pumpkin
β-Cryptoxanthin	Orange	Xanthophyll	12	24	8.6	8.1	0.13	0.10	Sweet red peppers, tangerines, papaya, persimmons
Lutein	Yellow	Xanthophyll	–	–	20.1[c]	18.2[c]	2.11	1.86	Kale, spinach, corn, collard greens, broccoli, eggs
Zeaxanthin	Yellow	Xanthophyll	–	–					
Canthaxanthin	Red-orange	Xanthophyll	–	–	–	–	–	–	Not consumed in significant quantities
Astaxanthin	Red	Xanthophyll	–	–	–	–	–	–	Not consumed in significant quantities

RE, retinol equivalent; RAE, retinol activity equivalent; M, male; F, female.
[a]US mean serum levels and food intakes were calculated using the values for the 19–30 and 30–51 age groups (DRI 2000, DRI 2001).
[b]Foods from: Holden et al. (1999).
[c]Serum and intake levels are the sum of lutein and zeaxanthin.

Carotenoid structures contain multiple conjugated double bonds that are responsible for their ability to efficiently scavenge free radicals (and thus serve as antioxidants) and to absorb light in the visible region. This absorption causes them to reflect their respective colors. Differences in the number of double bonds result in carotenoids ranging from colorless (owing to an insufficient number of conjugated double bonds) to bright red (Deming et al., 2001) (Figure 12.1 and Table 12.1). This unsaturated structure also causes carotenoids to be labile to oxygen, light, and heat.

In plants, carotenoids are part of the light-harvesting complex that captures light for photosynthesis. Carotenoids are also found in bacteria, yeasts, molds, bird feathers, and crustaceans; however, mammals do not synthesize carotenoids and must obtain them from their diet. The carotenoids astaxanthin, lutein, and zeaxanthin are commonly used as animal feed supplements. Astaxanthin is responsible for the pink color of salmon, while lutein and zeaxanthin are used in poultry to increase the yellow pigmentation of egg yolks (Table 12.1 and Figure 12.1).

In this chapter, the factors that influence carotenoid bioavailability (how much carotenoid is actually absorbed) and bioconversion (how much carotenoid is converted to vitamin A) will be initially addressed, followed by a discussion of the conversion of provitamin A carotenoids. The transport and accumulation of carotenoids, factors affecting circulating serum levels, deficiency, and toxicity will

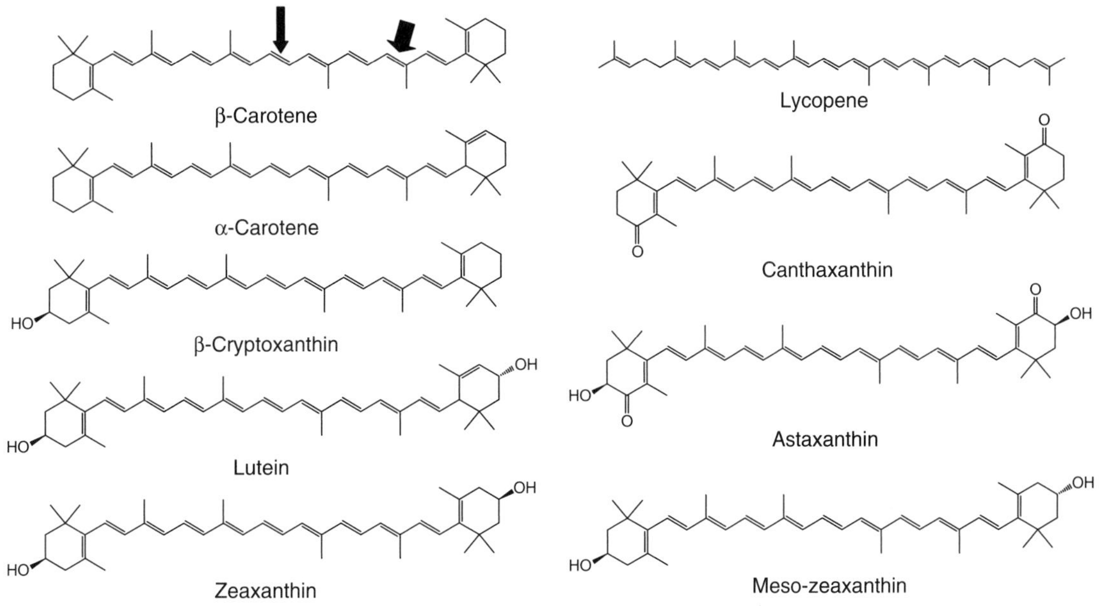

FIG. 12.1 All-*trans* structures of common carotenoids.
Note: Narrow arrow on β-carotene indicates 15,15′ CMO1 central cleavage site; wide arrow on β-carotene indicates 9′,10′ CMO2 eccentric cleavage site.

next be reviewed. The carotenoid cleavage enzymes will then be discussed, followed by sections on β-carotene and lung cancer, lycopene and prostate cancer, lutein/zeaxanthin and macular degeneration and cataract formation, carotenoids and skin, and carotenoids and cardiovascular disease. Finally, future directions of carotenoid research will be suggested.

Bioavailability and Bioconversion

A number of factors influence the absorption of carotenoids and conversion of provitamin A carotenoids to vitamin A. To help remember these factors, the mnemonic "SLAMENGHI" (for Species, Linkage, Amount, Matrix, Effectors, Nutrient status, Genetic factors, Host-related factors, and Interactions) was coined by Clive West and colleagues (Castenmiller and West, 1998). The major SLAMENGHI factors impacting carotenoid bioavailability and bioconversion to vitamin A are addressed below.

Species
Among carotenoids, xanthophylls are generally more readily absorbed than carotenes. This is believed to be

because the more hydrophilic nature of xanthophylls allows them to be incorporated into the outer portion of lipid micelles in the gastrointestinal tract (Yeum and Russell, 2002). Carotenoids are normally found in nature in the all-*trans* form; however, they are easily isomerized to form *cis* isomers following exposure to heat and/or light. The relative absorption of *cis* isomers apparently differs between carotenoids. For example, absorption is decreased for β-carotene *cis* isomers, whereas uptake is increased for lycopene *cis* isomers compared with their respective all-*trans* forms (Castenmiller and West, 1998).

Molecular Linkage
In many fruits and vegetables, the hydroxyl groups of xanthophylls are esterified to fatty acids. Before esterified xanthophylls can be absorbed, the fatty acids must be cleaved to form free xanthophylls in the gastrointestinal tract. Xanthophyll ester hydrolysis appears to be an efficient process because the absorption of lutein and β-cryptoxanthin esters is similar to that of the free carotenoid forms (Breithaupt *et al.*, 2003; Chung *et al.*, 2004), while the uptake of zeaxanthin esters may actually be greater than that of free forms of this carotenoid (Breithaupt *et al.*, 2004).

Matrix

The context, or matrix, in which carotenoids are provided appears to be the greatest factor affecting their bioavailability. For example, orange fruits such as papaya, mango, squash, and pumpkin yield twice as much vitamin A activity and four-fold higher serum β-carotene levels than green leafy vegetables and carrots (Boileau and Erdman, 2004). The difference between these fruits and vegetables is that in these fruits the carotenoids are found dissolved in oil droplets, whereas in vegetables they are sequestered as crystals, bound in chloroplasts, or associated with macromolecules such as fiber or protein. It is difficult for crystalline or bound carotenoids to become solubilized in micelles in the gastrointestinal tract, thus hindering their absorption. Mild heating and food processing increase the bioavailability of carotenoids by disrupting plant cell walls, binding proteins, and organelles, thus freeing carotenoids for uptake. In addition, because there is no matrix inhibiting their release, carotenoids provided in oil (e.g. red palm oil), or commercially available water-soluble beadlets, have superior bioavailability compared with fruits or vegetables (Boileau and Erdman, 2004). In rats, however, lycopene from tomato powder was more bioavailable than water-soluble beadlets (Canene-Adams et al., 2007).

Effectors

There are many effectors of carotenoid absorption. Fat intake, like a modest amount of salad dressing on a salad, increases carotenoid uptake by facilitating the formation of mixed micelles. Mixed micelles are needed for lipid-soluble carotenoids to cross the unstirred water layer for uptake into enterocytes. Fiber, olestra, plant sterol, and stanol esters are dietary compounds that decrease the absorption of carotenoids. When provided at high levels, the consumption of one carotenoid can decrease carotenoid absorption. This most likely occurs because carotenoids share similar uptake and transport pathways (Yeum and Russell, 2002). In contrast, cosupplementation with other antioxidants may actually increase the bioavailability of carotenoids. Antioxidants, such as vitamins C and E, may increase the stability of the carotenoids in the gastrointestinal tract and thereby facilitate their absorption (Tanumihardjo et al., 2005).

Nutrient Status of Host

Higher vitamin A status is believed to decrease carotenoid bioconversion (Yeum and Russell, 2002), whereas low vitamin A status increases the conversion to vitamin A to help meet the body's needs. In addition, protein deficiency decreases the level of the carotenoid central cleavage enzyme in rats (Barua, 2004; Tang and Russell, 2004). Furthermore, because the central cleavage enzyme requires ferrous iron as a cofactor, iron status also is likely important to its activity (von Lintig et al., 2005).

Host-Related Factors

Atrophic gastritis, a common condition of aging that results in insufficient gastric acid secretion, decreases carotenoid uptake by disturbing the formation and absorption of mixed micelles (Yeum and Russell, 2002). Parasitic infections, which are prevalent in vitamin A deficient populations, can also have a dramatic negative effect on carotenoid absorption (Barua, 2004).

Carotenoid Retinol Equivalents and Retinol Activity Equivalents

In 1989, the Food and Nutrition Board of the National Academies of Science established the conversion value of $2 \mu g$ of purified all-trans-β-carotene from supplements to be one retinol equivalent (RE = $1 \mu g$ all-trans-retinol). Because of decreased bioavailability, $3 \mu g$ of dietary all-trans-β-carotene from food was considered to be equivalent to $1 \mu g$ of purified all-trans-β-carotene in oil. Thus, $6 \mu g$ of dietary all-trans-β-carotene was equivalent to 1 RE. Other dietary provitamin A carotenoids (mainly α-carotene and β-cryptoxanthin) were believed to have half the vitamin A activity of dietary all-trans-β-carotene and set at $12 \mu g$ = 1 RE (Table 12.1). However, in 2001 the Food and Nutrition Board revised these conversion values based on human trials revealing that the bioavailability of all-trans-β-carotene from foods was half of what was originally believed. To help alleviate the confusion in making the changes, a new term was coined: "retinol activity equivalent" (RAE = $1 \mu g$ all-trans-retinol). The RAE ratios of conversion for purified all-trans-β-carotene in oil, dietary all-trans-β-carotene, and other dietary provitamin A carotenoids were set at 2:1, 12:1, and 24:1, respectively (Table 12.1) (Institute of Medicine, 2001). However, recent work in Mongolian gerbils suggests that the bioconversion of dietary provitamin A carotenoids may be more efficient than the RAE ratios (Howe and Tanumihardjo, 2006; Davis et al., 2008; Howe et al., 2009; Arscott et al., 2010; Ejoh et al., 2010). A recent study found evidence suggesting that the relative bioavailability of β-cryptoxanthin and α-carotene is greater than that of β-carotene, a fact that would partly explain the more efficient bioconversion (Burri et al., 2010).

Transport and Accumulation

In the lumen of the small intestine, carotenoids are first incorporated into mixed micelles, which facilitate their absorption through an unresolved mechanism(s). Evidence suggests that carotenoids are absorbed by simple diffusion and transporters such as scavenger receptor class B type I (SR-BI) (Nagao, 2009). Following absorption, carotenoids are incorporated primarily into chylomicrons and released into the lymph before entering general circulation. Carotenoids may be partially taken up by peripheral tissues before chylomicron remnants are taken up by the liver (Deming *et al.*, 2001). In the liver, carotenoids are repackaged into very-low-density lipoproteins (VLDL) and secreted back into the blood.

Carotenoids are not equally distributed among lipoproteins; the hydrophobic carotenes are found predominantly in low-density lipoproteins (LDL), while the more hydrophilic xanthophylls tend to be found in higher amounts in high-density lipoproteins (HDL) (Furr and Clark, 2004). The uptake of carotenoids also varies between tissues. Table 12.2 gives the concentrations of the six major carotenoids in selected human tissues. Quantitatively, carotenoids are highest in the liver and adipose; however, carotenoid concentrations are highest in the liver, adrenal, and reproductive tissues (such as the prostate). The reason for this differential accumulation is not known, but it has been hypothesized that the differential uptake is a result of either high levels of LDL receptors in these tissues or specific carotenoid-binding proteins and/or transporters that have not yet been identified (Deming *et al.*, 2001). Recently lutein keto-carotenoid metabolites were found to accumulate at higher levels than lutein in the liver and fat, suggesting they are actively metabolized in the body

(Yonekura *et al.*, 2011). Similar metabolites of lutein and zeaxanthin accumulated at high levels in CMO2 knockout mice (Amengual *et al.*, 2011). It remains to be seen what the functions of these metabolites are and whether β-cryptoxanthin forms similar metabolite(s).

Factors Affecting Circulating Levels

Body composition is a major factor that affects the circulating levels of carotenoids. A number of studies have reported an inverse association between body mass index (BMI) and plasma carotenoid concentrations. Further dissection of this association suggests that carotenoid plasma concentrations are inversely related not only to fat mass, but also to lean body mass. This indicates that non-fat tissues, such as muscle, may also serve as a reservoir for carotenoids (Furr and Clark, 2004). Accordingly, people with anorexia nervosa have very high levels of plasma carotenoids, most likely due to high levels of mobilization in this catabolic condition (Curran-Celentano and Erdman, 1993).

In general, circulating carotenoid levels are correlated with serum triglyceride and cholesterol levels. There are reported increases in serum levels as people age, which could be related to the upward shift in the serum lipid profile of older adults. In females, the concentrations of different carotenoids peak at different points of the menstrual cycle. The reason or significance is not known, but in men there also appears to be an inverse interaction between androgens and lycopene (Furr and Clark, 2004). Smoking is associated with lower carotenoid levels, presumably owing to an increase in oxidative stress, and alcohol intake has been shown to be inversely related to β-carotene levels. However, both smoking and alcohol

TABLE 12.2   Carotenoid concentrations in selected human tissues

Tissue	Lycopene	β-Carotene	α-Carotene	β-Cryptoxanthin	Lutein	Zeaxanthin
	ng/g tissue					
Colon	534	256	128	35	452	32
Liver	352	470	67	363	1701	591
Lung	300	226	47	121	212	90
Prostate	374	163	50	–	128	35
Skin	69	26	8	–	26	6
Retinal pigment epithelium[a]	8.64	10.80	2.97	–	18.27	4.85

[a]Concentrations in approximately 0.2 g of pooled retinal pigment epithelium/choroid.
Data from Furr and Clark (2004) and Khachik *et al.* (2002).

intake are also associated with reduced dietary intakes of carotenoids. It is not clear whether diet or metabolic differences are responsible for these decreased serum carotenoid levels (Institute of Medicine, 2000).

Toxicity and Deficiency

Unlike vitamin A, there are no deficiencies or toxicities for carotenoids *per se*. Low levels of carotenoids may increase people's risk for developing certain chronic diseases, but no classical deficiencies have been described. High intakes of β-carotene and lycopene can lead to carotenodermia and lycopenodermia, respectively. Carotenodermia is a condition that results in a yellowing of the skin due to accumulation of high levels of β-carotene. This disorder has been reported in subjects consuming large amounts of foods such as carrots or supplementing with 30 mg β-carotene per day or more for long periods of time. Carotenodermia does not result in discoloring of the ocular sclera as occurs in jaundice, thus allowing carotenodermia to be distinguished from this malady. Similarly, lycopenodermia results from high intakes of tomatoes or lycopene and causes the skin to become orange (Institute of Medicine, 2000). Both of these conditions reverse days or weeks after reducing carotenoid intake. Two examples of adverse effects of high-dose carotenoid supplementation that are discussed below are β-carotene and lung cancer risk in smokers, and canthaxanthin-induced retinopathy in the eye.

Carotenoid-Cleavage Enzymes

The small intestine and selected other tissues contain high levels of the two main carotenoid-cleavage enzymes, carotenoid monooxygenase 1 (CMO1) and carotenoid monooxygenase 2 (CMO2). Both of these enzymes are capable of cleaving provitamin A carotenoids to form different retinoids. CMO1 primarily catalyzes the central cleavage of the 15,15′ β-carotene bond to form two retinal molecules (Figure 12.1), along with cleavage of the other provitamin A carotenoids. Characterization of a human mutation and studies with CMO1 knockout mice have found increased β-carotene levels and decreased vitamin A levels, as expected given its function (Hessel *et al.*, 2007; Lindqvist *et al.*, 2007). In addition, dyslipidemia, increased risk of obesity, and steatosis have been reported in CMO1 knockout mice, suggesting alterations in lipid metabolism (Hessel *et al.*, 2007). However, another study in CMO1

knockout mice failed to find these lipid alterations (Lindshield *et al.*, 2008). Two common CMO1 single nucleotide polymorphisms (SNPs) have been identified that decrease β-carotene cleavage in women (Leung *et al.*, 2009), meaning they are less efficient at converting β-carotene to retinal. It does not appear that CMO1 cleaves non-provitamin A carotenoids to any great extent.

CMO2 catalyzes the eccentric cleavage of the 9′,10′ β-carotene bond that subsequently can be shortened to one retinoic acid molecule by a mechanism similar to β-oxidation of fatty acids (Figure 12.1). Unlike CMO1, evidence suggests that CMO2 cleaves non-provitamin A carotenoids. For lycopene this evidence includes the following:

- *E. coli* engineered to express CMO2 and produce lycopene experience a color shift compared with *E. coli* producing lycopene alone (Kiefer *et al.*, 2001);
- ferret CMO2 in insect cells cleave lycopene *cis* isomers, but not all-*trans* lycopene (Hu *et al.*, 2006);
- CMO1 knockout mice that have increased expression of CMO2 exhibit altered tissue lycopene biodistribution (Lindshield *et al.*, 2008);
- CMO2 knockout mice have increased serum and tissue lycopene levels (Ford *et al.*, 2010).

In addition, ferret CMO2 *in vitro* has been shown to preferentially cleave zeaxanthin and lutein (Mein *et al.*, 2011), and CMO2 knockout mice have been shown to accumulate 3,3′-didehydrozeaxanthin and 3-dihydrolutein, derivatives of zeaxanthin and lutein, respectively. In addition to cleavage alterations in accumulation of xanthophylls, mitochondrial dysfunction and increased oxidative stress were reported in CMO2 knockout mice fed lutein or zeaxanthin (Amengual *et al.*, 2011).

Table 12.3 shows the relative tissue levels of CMO1 in mice and humans and CMO2 expression in mice. The expression varies between tissues, and the two different carotenoid cleavage enzymes are not always expressed in the same tissue. The significance of this differential tissue expression is under investigation.

Health and Disease States Related to Carotenoids

β-Carotene and Lung Cancer
Lung cancer is the leading fatal cancer in both men and women in the United States, with the main risk factor being smoking (American Cancer Society, 2010). In the

TABLE 12.3 Relative carotenoid monooxygenase 1 (CMO1) and carotenoid monooxygenase (CMO2) tissue mRNA expression levels in mice (CMO1 and CMO2 mRNA levels) and CMO1 humans mRNA and protein levels

Tissue	Mouse mRNA		Human CMO1	
	CMO1[a]	CMO2[b]	mRNA[c]	Protein[d]
Colon	−	−	+	+++
Liver	++	+++	++	+++
Lung	−	+	−	nm
Prostate	nm	nm	++	+
Retinal pigment epithelium	nm	nm	+++	nm
Skin	nm	nm	nm	+++
Adrenal	nm	nm	nm	++
Brain	−	++	nm	nm
Endometrium	nm	nm	nm	+++
Heart	−	+	−	nm
Kidney	+++	+++	+++	++
Ovary	nm	nm	++	+
Pancreas	+	nm	nm	+++
Retina	+	nm	−	nm
Skeletal muscle	nm	nm	+	+
Small intestine	+++	+++	+++	+++
Spleen	−	+	−	nm
Stomach	−	−	+	+++
Testis	++	++	++	++
Thymus	+	nm	nm	nm

−, Not detected; +, low; ++, medium; +++, high; nm, not measured.
[a]Data from Kiefer *et al.* (2001) and Wyss (2004);
[b]Kiefer *et al.* (2001);
[c]Lindqvist and Andersson (2002) and Yan *et al.* (2001);
[d]Lindqvist and Andersson (2004).

early 1990s, there was strong epidemiological evidence indicating an inverse association between consumption of β-carotene-rich fruits and vegetables and lung cancer risk. Thus two large randomized placebo-controlled trials were undertaken to determine whether high-dose β-carotene supplementation could decrease lung cancer incidence in high-risk populations. These two studies infamously found that β-carotene supplementation increased lung cancer risk (Lindshield and Erdman, 2010). A recent systematic review and meta-analysis found that high-dose β-carotene supplementation (20–30 mg/day) is associated with an increased risk of lung cancer in smokers and asbestos workers (Druesne-Pecollo *et al.*, 2010). However, lower-dose β-carotene supplementation and dietary β-carotene are more protective than detrimental to lung cancer development (Gallicchio *et al.*, 2008; Druesne-Pecollo *et al.*, 2010).

These dose-dependent effects of β-carotene have also been found in smoking ferrets, an appropriate animal model used because they metabolize and accumulate β-carotene in a manner similar to humans (Lee *et al.*, 1999). The mechanism through which high-dose β-carotene has these deleterious effects in smokers has not been elucidated, but a number of mechanisms have been suggested such as an increased oxidative stress, altered retinoic acid signaling, and cytochrome P450 induction (Goralczyk, 2009). These mechanisms have been found *in vitro* and in some animal models, but not in human samples from those who developed lung cancer in the β-carotene clinical trials (Liu *et al.*, 2009; Wright *et al.*, 2010).

Accordingly, with the evidence discussed above, after reviewing the evidence the American Institute for Cancer Research (AICR) panel determined "that foods containing carotenoids probably protect against lung cancer" and that the evidence was convincing "that β-carotene supplements cause lung cancer in current smokers" (AICR, 2007).

Lycopene and Prostate Cancer

The prostate is the most frequent site of cancer in males in the United States, estimated to account for nearly one-third of all diagnosed cases in 2010 (American Cancer Society, 2010). In 1995, the Health Professional Follow-up Study, a prospective male cohort in the United States, found that lycopene intake, as well as the consumption of raw tomatoes, tomato sauce, and pizza, were all significantly associated with a decreased risk of prostate cancer (Giovannucci et al., 1995). As reviewed recently (Lindshield and Erdman, 2010), along with publications since that review (Karppi et al., 2009; Beilby et al., 2010; Kristal et al., 2010), epidemiological evidence when considered as a whole suggests a moderate decrease in prostate cancer risk with increased dietary tomato/lycopene consumption and/or serum levels. A number of small clinical trials/intervention studies have been reviewed recently (Lindshield and Erdman, 2010). When considered with those published since or not included in that review (Barber et al., 2006; Schwenke et al., 2009), these suggest that there may be some benefit of tomato/lycopene consumption for men with prostate cancer. However, larger, longer, better-designed studies are needed to determine whether tomato/lycopene conclusively improves outcomes for men with prostate cancer (Haseen et al., 2009). No intervention study has looked at whether lycopene or tomato consumption can prevent the development of prostate cancer.

Why the association between lycopene and prostate cancer? For reasons that are still not understood, lycopene preferentially accumulates in the prostate. In this tissue, the androgens testosterone and dihydrotestosterone play an important role in stimulating proliferation and the development of prostate cancer. There appears to be an interaction between androgens and lycopene levels, such that castration of male rats leads to a two-fold increase in hepatic lycopene, an effect that is normalized by testosterone replacement (Boileau et al., 2001). In addition, some animal studies have found that lycopene reduces the expression of androgen-signaling genes (Wertz, 2009); however, other animal studies have failed to find evidence of these alterations (Lindshield et al., 2010). There are a variety of other proposed mechanisms (Wertz, 2009); evidence however suggests that antioxidant action is unlikely to be the primary mechanism of action (Erdman et al., 2009).

A common question is whether lycopene is responsible for the inverse association between tomato consumption and prostate cancer, or if there are other compounds in tomatoes that may also have anti-cancer action. This is a question that is hard to address in human studies or epidemiology, but animal studies recently reviewed (Lindshield and Erdman, 2010), and one published since (Lindshield et al., 2010), suggest that lycopene is not as efficacious as the whole tomato. It should, however, be noted that a recent animal study found lycopene to be superior to the tomato-paste diet in decreasing the incidence of prostate cancer (Konijeti et al., 2010).

In 2004 the FDA was petitioned to create a health claim for tomatoes, lycopene, and prostate cancer. After reviewing the evidence the FDA issued the following qualified health claim (Kavanaugh et al., 2007) for tomatoes and prostate cancer: "very limited and preliminary scientific research suggests that eating one-half to one cup of tomatoes and/or tomato sauce a week may reduce the risk of prostate cancer." For lycopene and prostate cancer, the FDA concluded "that there was no credible evidence to support lycopene consumption, either as a food ingredient, a component of food, or as a dietary supplement, and any of the cancers evaluated in the studies" (Kavanaugh et al., 2007). In contrast, the American Institute for Cancer Research (AICR) panel, which considered more studies than the FDA, concluded that "foods containing lycopene (particularly tomato products) probably protect against prostate cancer," while not assigning an evidence ranking to consumption of lycopene alone (AICR, 2007).

Lutein/Zeaxanthin and Macular Degeneration

In the United States and Europe, age-related macular degeneration (AMD) is the leading cause of blindness in people aged 60 or older (Barker, 2010). AMD is characterized by the formation of druzen, oxidized lipids and proteins that can lead to the separation of photoreceptor cells from their nutrient and oxygen source (Bernstein, 2009). Photoreceptor cell death follows, leading to permanent vision loss.

The retina, which is located at the back of the human eye, contains a depression known as the fovea, on which light is focused after entering the lens (Figure 12.2). This region contains a high concentration of color-sensitive cones that afford humans our clearest, sharpest vision. The fovea is in the center of the macula lutea, which is Latin

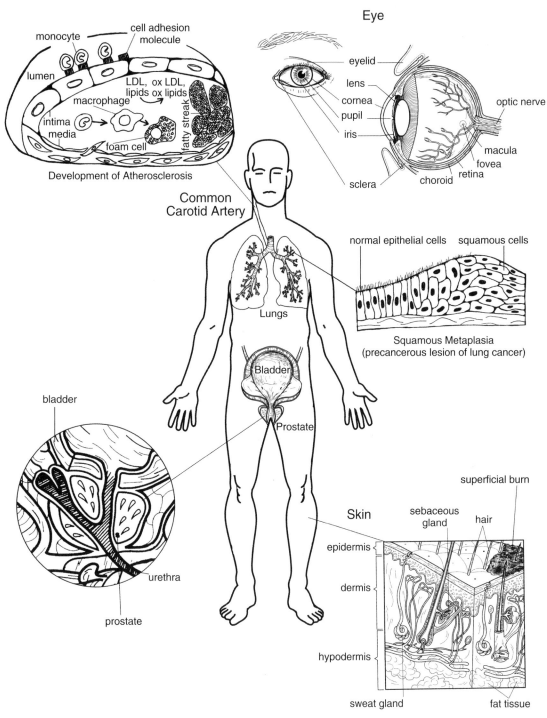

FIG. 12.2 Health and disease states related to carotenoids. ox, oxidized.

for "yellow spot." This yellow color is the result of large amounts of lutein and zeaxanthin in this area, collectively referred to as the macular pigment. The levels of carotenoids in this macula lutea are by far the highest found in the body. Lutein and zeaxanthin concentrations vary throughout the retina. In the central fovea, zeaxanthin and its isomer meso-zeaxanthin are each found in equal concentrations to lutein; however, with increasing distance from the fovea the concentration of lutein increases, making lutein the predominant carotenoid in the peripheral regions of the retina (Bhosale *et al.*, 2009).

Meso-zeaxanthin is not found in the diet to any great extent. Instead it is believed to be formed from a double-bond shift of lutein in the central fovea (Figure 12.1) (Johnson *et al.*, 2005). How this occurs is unknown, but glutathione S-transferase Pi isoform is a zeaxanthin-binding protein found in high levels in the macula near the fovea, and at lower levels elsewhere in the retina. Glutathione S-transferases have been shown to catalyze reactions similar to the double-bond shift from lutein to meso-zeaxanthin, so it is possible that this protein may be enzymatically involved in this transformation (Bhosale *et al.*, 2004). A lutein-binding protein has been identified from the human peripheral retina that is believed to be a member of the steroidogenic acute regulatory (StAR) family of proteins. The location of these binding proteins in the retina corresponds to the distribution of the carotenoids (Bhosale *et al.*, 2009).

The connection between lutein, zeaxanthin, and AMD is that autopsied retinas from individuals with AMD have decreased macular pigment levels in comparison with non-diseased retinas. The macular pigment is believed to be protective in two ways: by absorbing blue light, and by acting as an antioxidant (Bernstein, 2009). Monkeys raised on a carotenoid-free diet lack macular pigment and form druzen, mimicking the early stages of AMD (Landrum and Bone, 2004). Epidemiologic studies, as well as feeding and supplementation studies, suggest that macular pigment levels can be increased by lutein and zeaxanthin intake (Barker, 2010).

Some, but not all, epidemiologic studies have found that both intake and serum lutein and zeaxanthin levels are associated with reduced risk of AMD (Barker, 2010). To determine whether supplementation with lutein and zeaxanthin, along with omega-3 fatty acids, can prevent the development of advanced AMD, the Age-Related Eye Disease Study 2 (AREDS2) is currently underway. AREDS2 is a randomized clinical trial that completed enrollment in June 2008. The subjects will be followed for 5–6 years, so results are expected in 2013–2014 (AREDS2, 2010).

In addition to AMD, lutein and zeaxanthin intake/blood levels have been associated with decreased cataract incidence. Lutein and zeaxanthin are the only detectable carotenoids present in the lens, albeit at much lower levels than in the retina. Cataracts are believed to be caused by photo-induced oxidation and precipitation of lens proteins. It is believed that lutein and zeaxanthin lower the risk of cataract formation by preventing the oxidation of proteins, which ultimately leads to the development of this condition (Barker, 2010). AREDS2 is looking at cataract formation as an outcome; its results should give the strongest evidence to date on whether lutein and zeaxanthin are efficacious in preventing this condition (AREDS2, 2010).

Skin

Excess sunlight can lead to ultraviolet (UV)-induced erythema, a reddening of the skin more commonly referred to as sunburn. There is evidence to suggest that carotenoids can provide modest skin protection. Studies suggest that at least 10 weeks of supplementation is needed before benefits can be expected; for example, a recent meta-analysis found that β-carotene supplementation for at least 10 weeks is associated with a significant decrease in sunburn (Kopcke and Krutmann, 2008). It is also important to note that beneficial interactions occur between carotenoids, and probably other dietary components such as flavonoids, meaning diets rich in these compounds will likely provide better protection against UV-induced skin damage than the individual compounds alone (Stahl and Sies, 2007; Shapira, 2010).

The red-orange carotenoid canthaxanthin is marketed at high doses as a natural tanning pill because it accumulates in the fat pads below the skin, giving skin a bronze color. However, the high-dose long-term supplementation needed to sustain skin's tanned color may lead to the development of canthaxanthin-induced retinopathy, a condition in which canthaxanthin crystals form in the retina. Luckily this condition is reversible and does not result in vision loss (Goralczyk *et al.*, 2000; Sujak, 2009).

Cardiovascular Disease

Epidemiological studies have supported the relationship between carotenoid-rich foods and decreased risk of developing cardiovascular disease. There are a number of potential mechanisms through which carotenoid consumption may maintain endothelial function and prevent atherosclerosis. The most commonly cited is through the antioxidant action of carotenoids, which would then decrease lipid and LDL oxidation. The oxidation of lipids and LDL increases their uptake by macrophages. After macrophages accumulate high levels of these lipids, they become what are known as foam cells. Foam cells aggregate to form the fibrous plaque that leads to the development of fatty streaks and ultimately atherosclerosis (Figure 12.2). Research indicating that carotenoids act as antioxidants in this manner to prevent cardiovascular disease is, however, limited (Erdman *et al.*, 2009; Riccioni, 2009).

Future Directions

To date, β-carotene has been the primary carotenoid studied, but far less is known about other carotenoids commonly found in human diets and tissues. This includes potential cleavage of non-provitamin A carotenoids by CMO2. If carotenoids are cleaved, products that are produced and whether they are bioactive are questions of great interest. We coined the term "lycopenoids" to refer to potential lycopene metabolites produced by CMO2 that we hypothesize are metabolically active like retinoids (Lindshield *et al.*, 2007). Similar hypotheses can be made for other non-provitamin A carotenoids; however, very little is known in this area. The role of the carotenoid cleavage enzymes CMO1 and CMO2 in lipid metabolism still remains to be elucidated. The results thus far suggest that the enzymes have other metabolic functions besides cleaving carotenoids. The role of CMO1 and CMO2 SNPs in carotenoid and potentially lipid metabolism also remains to be investigated.

Reasons for varying carotenoid concentrations in different tissues are not clear, with the exception of the accumulation of lutein and zeaxanthin in the eye. For example, it is not known why lycopene preferentially accumulates in the prostate compared to its precursor carotenoids, phytoene, phytofluene, and ζ-carotene, which are remarkably similar in structure (Campbell *et al.*, 2007). Factors that regulate carotenoid storage in tissues and/or degradation still need to be elucidated. Identifying factors that influence the levels of carotenoids in tissues is likely to help us to begin to understand the role of individual carotenoids in tissues, and potentially, roles in health and disease prevention.

The genetic modification of plants to increase their carotenoid level is also an active area in research. Golden rice, which is genetically engineered to accumulate β-carotene, was produced to help combat vitamin A deficiency in developing countries. However, the levels of β-carotene in the rice were believed to be too low to realistically ameliorate this condition. In response to this concern, a corn-derived enzyme was inserted that increased the production of β-carotene 20-fold in golden rice 2. This new β-carotene concentration is closer to a range that may be relevant to preventing vitamin A deficiency (Grusak, 2005; Paine *et al.*, 2005). Recently it was shown that the β-carotene in golden rice 2 is bioavailable and it will probably reach the market in 2012 after more than a decade clearing regulatory hurdles (Tang *et al.*, 2009; Potrykus, 2010). It remains to be seen whether golden rice 2 will finally make it to intended populations and be accepted for growing and consumption.

Suggestions for Further Reading

Castenmiller, J.J. and West, C.E. (1998) Bioavailability and bioconversion of carotenoids. *Annu Rev Nutr* **18**, 19–38.

Institute of Medicine (2000) Beta-carotene and other carotenoids. In *Dietary Reference Intakes for Vitamin C, Vitamin E, Selenium, and Carotenoids*. National Academies Press, Washington, DC, pp. 325–382.

Kiefer, C., Hessel, S., Lampert, J.M., *et al.* (2001) Identification and characterization of a mammalian enzyme catalyzing the asymmetric oxidative cleavage of provitamin A. *J Biol Chem* **276**, 14110–14116.

Lindshield, B.L. and Erdman, J.W., Jr (2010) Carotenoids. In J.A. Milner and D.F. Romagnolo (eds), *Bioactive Compounds and Cancer*. Humana Press, New York, pp. 311–333.

References

AICR (2007) *Food, Nutrition, Physical Activity, and the Prevention of Cancer: a Global Perspective*. World Cancer Research Fund/American Institute for Cancer Research, Washington, DC.

Amengual, J., Lobo, G., Golczak, M., *et al.* (2011) A mitochondrial enzyme degrades carotenoids and protects against oxidative stress. *FASEB J* **25**, 948–959.

American Cancer Society (2010) *Cancer Facts and Figures 2010*. American Cancer Society, Atlanta, GA.

AREDS2 (2010) *Age-Related Eye Disease Study 2 (AREDS2)* Homepage of National Eye Institute: https://web.emmes.com/study/areds2/index.htm.

Arscott, S., Howe, J., Davis, C., *et al.* (2010) Carotenoid profiles in provitamin A-containing fruits and vegetables affect the bioefficacy in Mongolian gerbils. *Exp Biol Med* **235,** 839–848.

Barber, N.J., Zhang, X., Zhu, G., *et al.* (2006) Lycopene inhibits DNA synthesis in primary prostate epithelial cells in vitro and its administration is associated with a reduced prostate-specific antigen velocity in a phase II clinical study. *Prostate Cancer Prostatic Dis* **9,** 407–413.

Barker, F. (2010) Dietary supplementation: effects on visual performance and occurrence of AMD and cataracts. *Curr Med Res Opin* **26,** 2011–2023.

Barua, A.B. (2004) Bioconversion of provitamin A carotenoids. In N.I. Krinsky, S.T. Mayne, and H. Sies (eds), *Carotenoids in Health and Disease*. Marcel Dekker, New York, pp. 295–312.

Beilby, J., Ambrosini, G.L., Rossi, E., *et al.* (2010) Serum levels of folate, lycopene, β-carotene, retinol and vitamin E and prostate cancer risk. *Eur J Clin Nutr* **64,** 1235–1238.

Bernstein, P.S. (2009) Nutritional interventions against age-related macular degeneration. *Acta Hort* **841,** 103–112.

Bhosale, P., Larson, A.J., Frederick, J.M., *et al.* (2004) Identification and characterization of a Pi isoform of glutathione S-transferase (GSTP1) as a zeaxanthin-binding protein in the macula of the human eye. *J Biol Chem* **279,** 49447–49454.

Bhosale, P., Li, B., Sharifzadeh, M., *et al.* (2009) Purification and partial characterization of a lutein-binding protein from human retina. *Biochemistry* **48,** 4798–4807.

Boileau, A.C. and Erdman, J.W., Jr (2004) Impact of food processing on content and bioavailability of carotenoids. In N.I. Krinsky, S.T. Mayne, and H. Sies (eds), *Carotenoids in Health and Disease*. Marcel Dekker, New York, pp. 209–228.

Boileau, T.W., Clinton, S.K., Zaripheh, S., *et al.* (2001) Testosterone and food restriction modulate hepatic lycopene isomer concentrations in male F344 rats. *J Nutr* **131,** 1746–1752.

Breithaupt, D.E., Weller, P., Wolters, M., *et al.* (2003) Plasma response to a single dose of dietary beta-cryptoxanthin esters from papaya (*Carica papaya* L.) or non-esterified beta-cryptoxanthin in adult human subjects: a comparative study. *Br J Nutr* **90,** 795–801.

Breithaupt, D.E., Weller, P., Wolters, M., *et al.* (2004) Comparison of plasma responses in human subjects after the ingestion of 3R,3R′-zeaxanthin dipalmitate from wolfberry (*Lycium barbarum*) and non-esterified 3R,3R′-zeaxanthin using chiral high-performance liquid chromatography. *Br J Nutr* **91,** 707–713.

Burri, B.J., Chang, J.S.T., and Neidlinger, T.R. (2011) β-Cryptoxanthin- and α-carotene-rich foods have greater apparent bioavailability than β-carotene-rich foods in Western diets. *Br J Nutr* **105,** 212–219.

Campbell, J.K., Engelmann, N.J., Lila, M.A., *et al.* (2007) Phytoene, phytofluene, and lycopene from tomato powder differentially accumulate in tissues of male Fisher 344 rats. *Nutr Res* **27,** 794–801.

Canene-Adams, K., Lindshield, B.L., Wang, S., *et al.* (2007) Combinations of tomato and broccoli enhance antitumor activity in dunning R3327-H prostate adenocarcinomas. *Cancer Res* **67,** 836–843.

Castenmiller, J.J. and West, C.E. (1998) Bioavailability and bioconversion of carotenoids. *Annu Rev Nutr* **18,** 19–38.

Chung, H.Y., Rasmussen, H.M., and Johnson, E.J. (2004) Lutein bioavailability is higher from lutein-enriched eggs than from supplements and spinach in men. *J Nutr* **134,** 1887–1893.

Curran-Celentano, J. and Erdman, J.W., Jr (1993) A case study of carotenemia in anorexia nervosa may support the interrelationship of vitamin A and thyroid hormone. *Nutr Res* **13,** 379.

Davis, C., Jing, H., Howe, J., *et al.* (2008) Beta-cryptoxanthin from supplements or carotenoid-enhanced maize maintains liver vitamin A in Mongolian gerbils (*Meriones unguiculatus*) better than or equal to beta-carotene supplements. *Br J Nutr* **100,** 786–793.

Deming, D.M., Boileau, T.W., Heintz, K.H., *et al.* (2001) Carotenoids: linking chemistry, absorption, and metabolism to potential roles in human health and disease. In E. Cadenas and L. Packer (eds), *Handbook of Antioxidants*, 2nd Edn. Marcel Dekker, New York, pp. 189–221.

Druesne-Pecollo, N., Latino-Martel, P., Norat, T., *et al.* (2010) Beta-carotene supplementation and cancer risk: a systematic review and metaanalysis of randomized controlled trials. *Int J Cancer* **127,** 172–184.

Ejoh, R., Dever, J., Mills, J., *et al.* (2010) Small quantities of carotenoid-rich tropical green leafy vegetables indigenous to Africa maintain vitamin A status in Mongolian gerbils (*Meriones unguiculatus*). *Br J Nutr* **103,** 1594–1601.

Erdman, J., Ford, N., and Lindshield, B. (2009) Are the health attributes of lycopene related to its antioxidant function? *Arch Biochem Biophys* **483,** 229–235.

Ford, N., Clinton, S., von Lintig, J., *et al.* (2010) Loss of carotene-9′,10′-monooxygenase expression increases serum and tissue lycopene concentrations in lycopene-fed mice. *J Nutr* **140,** 2134–2138.

Furr, H.C. and Clark, R.M. (2004) Transport, uptake, and target tissue storage of carotenoids. In N.I. Krinsky, S.T. Mayne, and H. Sies (eds), *Carotenoids in Health and Disease*. Marcel Dekker, New York, pp. 229–278.

Gallicchio, L., Boyd, K., Matanoski, G., *et al.* (2008) Carotenoids and the risk of developing lung cancer: a systematic review. *Am J Clin Nutr* **88,** 372–383.

Giovannucci, E., Ascherio, A., Rimm, E.B., *et al.* (1995) Intake of carotenoids and retinol in relation to risk of prostate cancer. *J Natl Cancer Inst* **87**, 1767–1776.

Goralczyk, R. (2009) Beta-carotene and lung cancer in smokers: review of hypotheses and status of research. *Nutr Cancer* **61**, 767–774.

Goralczyk, R., Barker, F.M., Buser, S., *et al.* (2000) Dose dependency of canthaxanthin crystals in monkey retina and spatial distribution of its metabolites. *Invest Ophthalmol Vis Sci* **41**, 1513–1522.

Grusak, M.A. (2005) Golden rice gets a boost from maize. *Nature Biotechnol* **23**, 429–430.

Haseen, F., Cantwell, M.M., O'Sullivan, J.M., *et al.* (2009) Is there a benefit from lycopene supplementation in men with prostate cancer? A systematic review. *Prostate Cancer Prostatic Dis* **12**, 325–332.

Hessel, S., Eichinger, A., Isken, A., *et al.* (2007) CMO1 deficiency abolishes vitamin A production from beta-carotene and alters lipid metabolism in mice. *J Biol Chem* **282**, 33553–33561.

Holden, J.M., Eldridge, A.L., Beecher, G.R., *et al.* (1999) Carotenoid content of food: an update of the database. *J Food Comp Anal* **12**, 169–196.

Howe, J. and Tanumihardjo, S. (2006) Carotenoid-biofortified maize maintains adequate vitamin A status in Mongolian gerbils. *J Nutr* **136**, 2562–2567.

Howe, J., Maziya-Dixon, B., and Tanumihardjo, S. (2009) Cassava with enhanced beta-carotene maintains adequate vitamin A status in Mongolian gerbils (*Meriones unguiculatus*) despite substantial cis-isomer content. *Br J Nutr* **102**, 342–349.

Hu, K.Q., Liu, C., Ernst, H., *et al.* (2006) The biochemical characterization of ferret carotene-9′,10′-monooxygenase catalyzing cleavage of carotenoids in vitro and in vivo. *J Biol Chem* **281**, 19327–19338.

Institute of Medicine (2000) Beta-carotene and other carotenoids. In *Dietary Reference Intakes for Vitamin C, Vitamin E, Selenium, and Carotenoids*. National Academies Press, Washington, DC, pp. 325–382.

Institute of Medicine (2001) *Dietary Reference Intakes for Vitamin A, Vitamin K, Arsenic, Boron, Chromium, Copper, Iodine, Iron, Manganese, Molybdenum, Nickel, Silicon, Vanadium, and Zinc*. National Academies Press, Washington, DC.

Johnson, E.J., Neuringer, M., Russell, R.M., *et al.* (2005) Nutritional manipulation of primate retinas, III: Effects of lutein or zeaxanthin supplementation on adipose tissue and retina of xanthophyll-free monkeys. *Invest Ophthalmol Vis Sci* **46**, 692–702.

Karppi, J., Kurl, S., Nurmi, T., *et al.* (2009) Serum lycopene and the risk of cancer: the Kuopio Ischaemic Heart Disease Risk Factor (KIHD) study. *Ann Epidemiol* **19**, 512–518.

Kavanaugh, C.J., Trumbo, P.R., and Ellwood, K.C. (2007) The US Food and Drug Administration's evidence-based review for qualified health claims: tomatoes, lycopene, and cancer. *J Natl Cancer Inst* **99**, 1074–1085.

Khachik, F., Carvalho, L., Bernstein, P.S., *et al.* (2002) Chemistry, distribution, and metabolism of tomato carotenoids and their impact on human health. *Exp Biol Med (Maywood)* **227**, 845–851.

Kiefer, C., Hessel, S., Lampert, J.M., *et al.* (2001) Identification and characterization of a mammalian enzyme catalyzing the asymmetric oxidative cleavage of provitamin A. *J Biol Chem* **276**, 14110–14116.

Konijeti, R., Henning, S., Moro, A., *et al.* (2010) Chemoprevention of prostate cancer with lycopene in the TRAMP model. *Prostate* **70**, 1547–1554.

Kopcke, W. and Krutmann, J. (2008) Protection from sunburn with beta-carotene – a meta-analysis. *Photochem Photobiol* **84**, 284–288.

Kristal, A., Arnold, K., Neuhouser, M.L., *et al.* (2010) Diet, supplement use, and prostate cancer risk: results from the prostate cancer prevention trial. *Am J Epidemiol* **172**, 566–577.

Landrum, J.T. and Bone, R.A. (2004) Mechanistic evidence for eye disease and carotenoids. In N.I. Krinsky, S.T. Mayne, and H. Sies (eds), *Carotenoids in Health and Disease*. Marcel Dekker, New York, pp. 445–472.

Lee, C.M., Boileau, A.C., Boileau, T.W., *et al.* (1999) Review of animal models in carotenoid research. *J Nutr* **129**, 2271–2277.

Leung, W.C., Hessel, S., Meplan, C., *et al.* (2009) Two common single nucleotide polymorphisms in the gene encoding beta-carotene 15,15′-monooxygenase alter beta-carotene metabolism in female volunteers. *FASEB J* **23**, 1041–1053.

Lindqvist, A. and Andersson, S. (2002) Biochemical properties of purified recombinant human beta-carotene 15,15′-monooxygenase. *J Biol Chem* **277**, 23942–23948.

Lindqvist, A. and Andersson, S. (2004) Cell type-specific expression of beta-carotene 15,15′-mono-oxygenase in human tissues.. *J Histochem Cytochem* **52**, 491–499.

Lindqvist, A., Sharvill, J., Sharvill, D.E., *et al.* (2007) Loss-of-function mutation in carotenoid 15,15′-monooxygenase identified in a patient with hypercarotenemia and hypovitaminosis A. *J Nutr* **137**, 2346–2350.

Lindshield, B.L. and Erdman, J.W., Jr (2010) Carotenoids. In J.A. Milner and D.F. Romagnolo (eds), *Bioactive Compounds and Cancer*. Humana Press, New York, pp. 311–333.

Lindshield, B.L., Canene-Adams, K., and Erdman, J.W., Jr (2007) Lycopenoids: are lycopene metabolites bioactive? *Arch Biochem Biophys* **458**, 136–140.

Lindshield, B.L., Ford, N.A., Canene-Adams, K., *et al.* (2010) Selenium, but not lycopene or vitamin E, decreases growth of transplantable dunning R3327-H rat prostate tumors. *PLoS One* **5**, e10423–e10423.

Lindshield, B.L., King, J.L., Wyss, A., *et al.* (2008) Lycopene biodistribution is altered in 15,15′-carotenoid monooxygenase knockout mice. *J Nutr* **138**, 2367–2371.

Liu, C., Wang, X., Mucci, L., *et al.* (2009) Modulation of lung molecular biomarkers by beta-carotene in the Physicians' Health Study. *Cancer* **115**, 1049–1058.

Mein, J., Dolnikowski, G., Ernst, H., *et al.* (2011) Enzymatic formation of apo-carotenoids from the xanthophyll carotenoids lutein, zeaxanthin and β-cryptoxanthin by ferret carotene-9′,10′-monooxygenase. *Arch Biochem Biophys* **506**, 109–121.

Nagao, A. (2009) Absorption and function of dietary carotenoids. *Forum Nutr* **61**, 55–63.

Paine, J.A., Shipton, C.A., Chaggar, S., *et al.* (2005) Improving the nutritional value of golden rice through increased pro-vitamin A content. *Nature Biotechnol* **23**, 482–487.

Potrykus, I. (2010) Regulation must be revolutionized. *Nature* **466**, 561–561.

Riccioni, G. (2009) Carotenoids and cardiovascular disease. *Curr Atheroscler Rep* **11**, 434–439.

Schwenke, C., Ubrig, B., Thürmann, P., *et al.* (2009) Lycopene for advanced hormone refractory prostate cancer: a prospective, open phase II pilot study. *J Urology* **181**, 1098–1103.

Shapira, N. (2010) Nutritional approach to sun protection: a suggested complement to external strategies. *Nutr Rev* **68**, 75–86.

Stahl, W. and Sies, H. (2007) Carotenoids and flavonoids contribute to nutritional protection against skin damage from sunlight. *Molec Biotechnol* **37**, 26–30.

Sujak, A. (2009) Interactions between canthaxanthin and lipid membranes – possible mechanisms of canthaxanthin toxicity. *Cell Mol Biol Lett* **14**, 395–410.

Tang, G. and Russell, R.M. (2004) Bioequivalence of provitamin A carotenoids. In N.I. Krinsky, S.T. Mayne, and H. Sies (eds), *Carotenoids in Health and Disease*, Marcel Dekker, New York, pp. 279–294.

Tang, G., Qin, J., Dolnikowski, G., *et al.* (2009) Golden rice is an effective source of vitamin A. *Am J Clin Nutr* **89**, 1776–1783.

Tanumihardjo, S.A., Li, J., and Dosti, M.P. (2005) Lutein absorption is facilitated with cosupplementation of ascorbic acid in young adults. *J Am Diet Assoc* **105**, 114–118.

von Lintig, J., Hessel, S., Isken, A., *et al.* (2005) Towards a better understanding of carotenoid metabolism in animals. *Biochim Biophys Acta* **1740**, 122–131.

Wertz, K. (2009) Lycopene effects contributing to prostate health. *Nutr Cancer* **61**, 775–783.

Wright, M., Groshong, S., Husgafvel-Pursiainen, K., *et al.* (2010) Effects of beta-carotene supplementation on molecular markers of lung carcinogenesis in male smokers. *Cancer Prev Res (Phila)* **3**, 745–752.

Wyss, A. (2004) Carotene oxygenases: a new family of double bond cleavage enzymes. *J Nutr* **134**, 246S–250S.

Yan, W., Jang, G.F., Haeseleer, F., *et al.* (2001) Cloning and characterization of a human beta,beta-carotene-15,15′-dioxygenase that is highly expressed in the retinal pigment epithelium. *Genomics* **72**, 193–202.

Yeum, K.J. and Russell, R.M. (2002) Carotenoid bioavailability and bioconversion. *Annu Rev Nutr* **22**, 483–504.

Yonekura, L., Kobayashi, M., Terasaki, M., *et al.* (2011) Keto-carotenoids are the major metabolites of dietary lutein and fucoxanthin in mouse tissues. *J Nutr* **140**, 1824–1831.

Young, A.J., Phillip, D.M., and Lowe, G.M. (2004) Carotenoid antioxidant activity. In N.I. Krinsky, S.T. Mayne, and H. Sies (eds), *Carotenoids in Health and Disease*. Marcel Dekker, New York, pp. 105–126.

13

VITAMIN D

ANTHONY W. NORMAN, PhD AND HELEN L. HENRY, PhD

University of California, Riverside, California, USA

Summary

It is established that the classical biological actions of the nutritionally important vitamin D in mediating calcium homeostasis are supported by a complex vitamin D endocrine system which coordinates the metabolism of vitamin D_3 into $1\alpha,25(OH)_2D_3$ and $24R,25(OH)_2D_3$. The biologically inert vitamin D_3 must be converted to its daughter steroid hormone, $1\alpha,25(OH)_2D_3$, which acts in partnership with the vitamin D receptor (VDR) to mediate both genomic and rapid responses. Our updated understanding of the vitamin D endocrine system includes many more target tissues than simply the calcium-homeostasis-related intestine, bone, kidney, and parathyroid gland. It is now accepted that five previously unrecognized physiological systems respond to $1\alpha,25(OH)_2D_3$ working with VDR. These include the heart and cardiovascular system, the immune system (both innate and adaptive), muscle, pancreas, and metabolic homeostasis, and the brain. Vitamin D nutritionists and scientists in many countries agree that about half of elderly Western Europeans and North Americans and probably two-thirds of the rest of the world are not receiving enough vitamin D to maintain healthy bone. It is also agreed that the best marker of an individual's vitamin D nutritional status is the level of the serum 25(OH)D. A level of 25(OH)D of <20 ng/mL (50 nmol/L) reflects a state of vitamin D insufficiency or worse. A circulating level of 25(OH)D >30 ng/mL or 75 nmol/L is reflective of a vitamin D sufficient state. Given its recently recognized importance in important physiological systems, the fact that so many people throughout the world have much lower 25(OH)D levels is a public health challenge of major proportions.

Introduction

Background

Vitamin D is essential for life in higher animals. Classically it has been shown to be one of the most important biological regulators of calcium homeostasis. It has been established that these biological effects are only achieved as a consequence of the metabolism of vitamin D into a family of daughter metabolites, including the two key kidney-produced metabolites, $1\alpha,25(OH)_2$-vitamin D_3 [$1\alpha,25(OH)_2D_3$] and $24R,25(OH)_2$-vitamin D_3 [$24R,25(OH)_2D_3$] (see Figure 13.2). $1\alpha,25(OH)_2D_3$ is considered to be a steroid hormone and there is evidence that $24R,25(OH)_2D_3$ may also act as a steroid hormone (Feldman *et al.*, 2005).

Since the 1980s it has become increasingly apparent that $1\alpha,25(OH)_2D_3$, in addition to its role in calcium homeostasis, plays an important role in differentiation and

Present Knowledge in Nutrition, Tenth Edition. Edited by John W. Erdman Jr, Ian A. Macdonald and Steven H. Zeisel.
© 2012 International Life Sciences Institute. Published 2012 by John Wiley & Sons, Inc.

proliferation of a wide variety of cells and tissues not primarily related to mineral metabolism; these include cells of the hematopoietic system, keratinocytes, and cells secreting parathyroid hormone and insulin. In addition, many types of cancer cells, including breast and prostate cancer cells, possess the vitamin D receptor (VDR) and therefore are targets of $1\alpha,25(OH)_2D_3$ action. And in the last decade, it has become clear that five new physiological roles for $1\alpha,25(OH)_2D_3$ have been added to its list of responsibilities.

The purpose of this chapter is to provide a succinct overview of our current understanding of the important nutritional substance vitamin D, the mechanisms by which its biologically active metabolite, the steroid hormone $1\alpha,25(OH)_2D_3$, mediates biological responses, and its role in several important human diseases In addition, the nutritional aspects of vitamin D are presented from the perspective that there is widespread vitamin D deficiency in all countries of the world.

Historical Review

The first scientific description of rickets, the hallmark of vitamin D deficiency, was provided by Dr Daniel Whistler in 1645 and Professor Francis Glisson in 1650 (Norman, 1979). The major breakthrough in understanding the causative factors of rickets was the development of nutrition as an experimental science, followed by the appreciation of the existence of vitamins more than two centuries later. Although vitamin D, through a historical accident, was originally classified as a vitamin, it is now known that the "D-vitamin" is produced in the skin and it is widely accepted that its biologically active form is a steroid hormone. In 1919–1920 Sir Edward Mellanby, working with dogs raised exclusively in the absence of sunlight or ultraviolet light, devised a diet which allowed him to unequivocally establish that rickets was caused by a deficiency of a trace component in the diet. In 1921 he wrote, "The action of fats in rickets is due to a vitamin or accessory food factor which they contain, probably identical with the fat-soluble vitamin." Furthermore he established that cod-liver oil was an excellent antirachitic agent, leading to the classification of the antirachitic factor as a vitamin (Norman, 1979).

The chemical structures of the D vitamins were determined in the 1930s in the laboratory of Professor A. Windaus at the University of Göttingen. Vitamin D_2, produced by ultraviolet irradiation of the plant/yeast steroid ergosterol, was chemically characterized in 1932

(Norman, 1979). Vitamin D_3, the form that is produced in the skin of vertebrate animals, was not chemically characterized until 1936 when it was shown to result from the ultraviolet irradiation of 7-dehydrocholesterol (Norman, 1979). Virtually simultaneously, the elusive antirachitic component of cod-liver oil was shown to be identical to the newly characterized vitamin D_3 (Norman, 1979). These results clearly established that the antirachitic substance vitamin D was chemically a steroid, more specifically a seco-steroid (see below).

The modern era of vitamin D began in the interval of 1965–1970 with the discovery (Haussler et al., 1968) and chemical characterization of $1\alpha,25(OH)_2D_3$ (Norman et al., 1971) and its nuclear receptor, the VDR (Haussler and Norman, 1969).

Chemistry of Vitamin D

The structures of vitamin D_3 (cholecalciferol) and its provitamin, 7-dehydrocholesterol, are presented in Figure 13.1. Vitamin D is a generic term and indicates a molecule of the general structure shown for rings A, B, C, and D with differing side-chain structures. The ring structure is derived from the cyclopentanoperhydrophenanthrene ring structure for steroids but with the 9,10 carbon–carbon bond of ring B broken, as indicated by the inclusion of "9,10-seco" in the official nomenclature. A discussion of the conformational shapes attainable by vitamin D is given in the legend to Figure 13.1.

Vitamin D (synonym calciferol) is named according to the revised rules of IUPAC (the International Union of Pure and Applied Chemists: IUPAC, 1960). Because it is derived from a steroid, vitamin D retains its numbering from the parent compound cholesterol (see Figure 13.1). Asymmetric centers are designated by using the R,S notation (Norman and Litwack, 1987); the configurations of the double bonds are indicated as E (trans) and Z (cis). Thus the official name of vitamin D_3 is 9,10-seco(5Z,7E)-5,7,10(19)cholestatriene-3β-ol. Vitamin D_2 differs from D_3 by virtue of the presence of a 22,23 double bond and a 24-methyl group in the side chain. The official name of vitamin D_2 is 9,10-seco(5Z,7E)-5,7,10(19),22-ergostatetraene-3β-ol. From 1940 until about 1960, vitamin D_2 was used as the food supplement to supply vitamin D activity, but since the 1970s, in the United States, vitamin D_3 has been the form of calciferol that is routinely used for food supplementation (Norman, 1979).

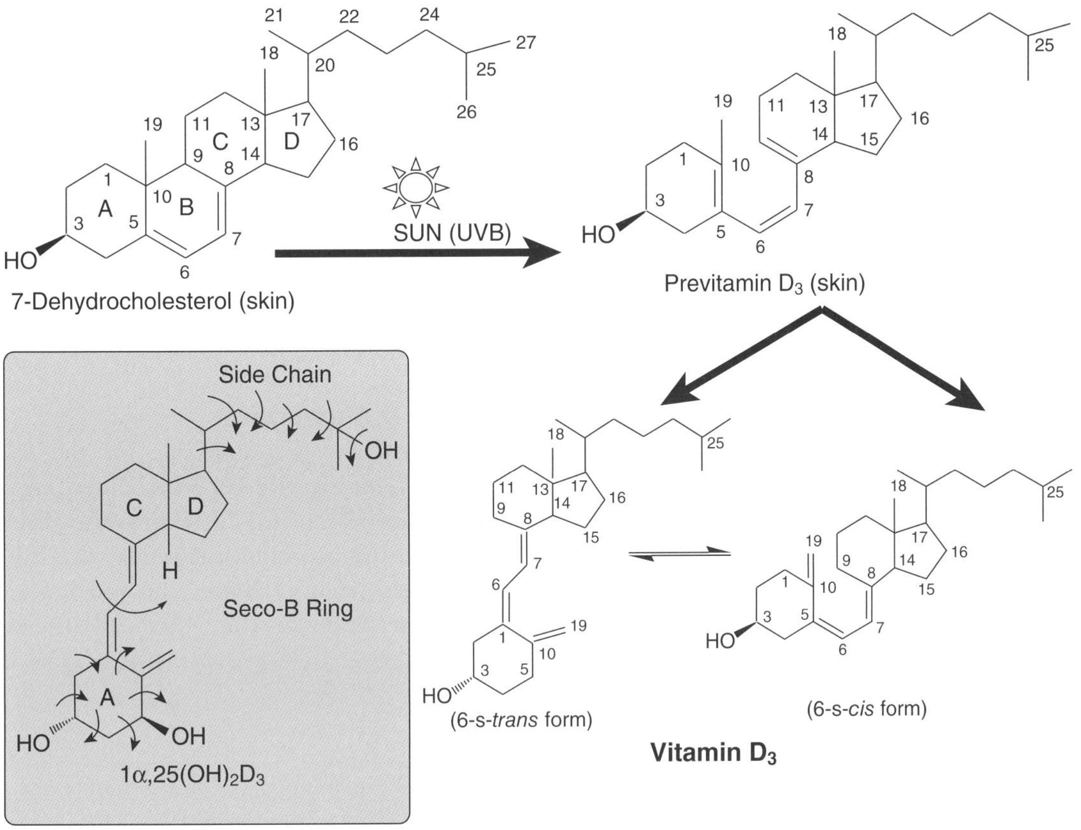

FIG. 13.1 Chemistry and irradiation pathway for production of vitamin D₃. The provitamin 7-dehydrocholesterol (in the skin), which is characterized by the presence in the B ring of a Δ5, Δ7 conjugated double-bond system, when exposed to ultraviolet light is converted to the seco B previtamin D₃ steroid when the 9,10 carbon–carbon bond has been broken. Then the previtamin D₃, in a process independent of ultraviolet light, thermally isomerizes to the "vitamin" form, which is characterized by a Δ5,6, Δ7,8, Δ10,19 conjugated triple bond system.

The extreme conformational flexibility potential of all vitamin D metabolites is illustrated in the inset box for the principal metabolite, 1α,25(OH)₂D₃. Each of the arrows indicates carbon–carbon single bonds present (in the side chain, the seco B ring, and the A ring) that have complete 360° rotational freedom. This results, for the various vitamin D molecules, in the generation in solution and in biological systems of a multitude of different shapes (Bouillon *et al.*, 1995). The main portion of the figure also illustrates the two principal conformations of the molecule that result as a consequence of rotation about the 6,7 carbon single bond of the seco B ring. These are the 6-s-*cis* conformer (the steroid-like shape) and the 6-s-*trans* conformer (the extended shape).

Vitamin D₃ is produced photochemically in the epidermis of most higher animals from the provitamin D, 7-dehydrocholesterol, by the action of sunlight or artificial ultraviolet light. The conjugated double bond system in ring B (see Figure 13.1) allows the absorption of light quanta in the UV range 280–310 nm to initiate a complex series of transformations of the provitamin into vitamin D₃ (Figure 13.1). Thus it is important to appreciate that, as long as the animal (or human) has access to adequate sunlight on a regular basis, vitamin D₃ can be endog-

enously produced and there may be no need for a dietary requirement for this "vitamin".

Physiology and Biochemistry of Vitamin D

Vitamin D Endocrine System

Vitamin D₃ itself is not known to have any intrinsic biological activity but must be metabolized, first to 25(OH) D₃ in the liver and then to 1α,25(OH)₂D₃ and/or

24R,25(OH)₂D₃ by the kidney. Altogether, some 37 vitamin D_3 metabolites have been isolated and chemically characterized (Bouillon *et al.*, 1995).

The elements of the vitamin D endocrine system (Bouillon *et al.*, 1995) include the following:

(a) the photoconversion of 7-dehydrocholesterol to vitamin D_3 in the skin or dietary intake of vitamin D_3 (Figure 13.1);
(b) metabolism of vitamin D_3 by the liver to 25(OH)D_3 which is the major form of vitamin D circulating in the blood (Figure 13.2);
(c) conversion of 25(OH)D_3 by the kidney (functioning as an endocrine gland) to produce the two principal dihydroxylated metabolites, 1α,25(OH)₂D_3 and 24R,25(OH)₂D_3;
(d) systemic transport of the dihydroxylated metabolites 24R,25(OH)₂D_3 and 1α,25(OH)₂D_3 to distal target organs (Figure 13.2);

(e) binding of the dihydroxylated metabolites, particularly 1,25(OH)₂D_3, to the vitamin D receptor (VDR) in the target organs followed by the subsequent generation of appropriate biological responses (Figure 13.3).

An additional key component in the operation of the vitamin D endocrine system is the plasma vitamin D binding protein (DBP) which carries vitamin D_3 and all its metabolites to their sites of metabolism and various target organs (Laing and Cooke, 2005).

Vitamin D Metabolism

The three enzymes responsible for the conversion of vitamin D_3 into its two key metabolites (Figure 13.2) are the hepatic vitamin D_3-25-hydroxylase (Feldman *et al.*, 2005) and the two kidney enzymes, the 25(OH)D_3-1α-hydroxylase (Henry, 2005) and the 25(OH)D_3-24R-hydroxylase (Feldman *et al.*, 2005). All three enzymes have

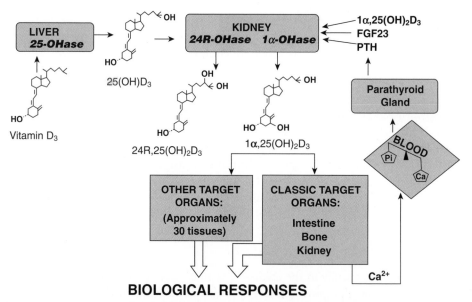

FIG. 13.2 Elements of the vitamin D endocrine system. The biologically inactive vitamin D is first hydroxylated at C-25 on the side chain in the liver to form 25(OH)D_3, the principal circulating member of vitamin D steroids. 25(OH)D_3 serves as the substrate for one of two hydroxylases in the kidney to result in either 24R,25(OH)₂D_3 or 1α,25(OH)₂D_3, the predominant biologically active steroid-hormone form of the parent vitamin. The regulation of these two hydroxylases is exerted by parathyroid hormone, which reflects serum calcium levels; the steroid hormone 1α,25(OH)₂D_3 itself; and FGF23 as a feedback regulator representing blood phosphate levels. The biological actions of the two dihydroxylated metabolites of vitamin D are represented in general form here and described in the text.

PROPOSED MECHANISM

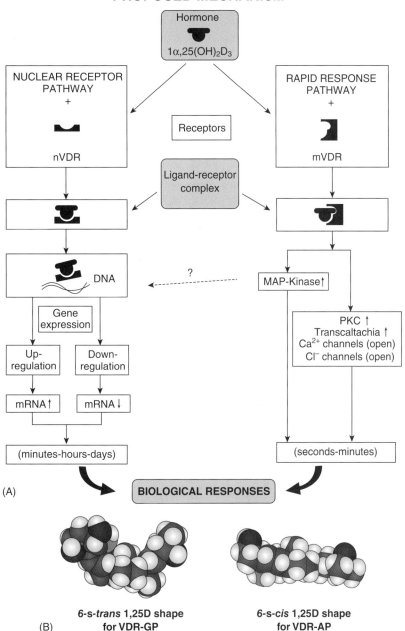

**6-s-*trans* 1,25D shape
for VDR-GP**

**6-s-*cis* 1,25D shape
for VDR-AP**

(B)

FIG. 13.3 Model to describe how $1\alpha,25(OH)_2D_3$ generates biological responses. (A) Biological responses to $1\alpha,25(OH)_2D_3$ occur as a consequence of different shapes of the conformationally flexible $1\alpha,25(OH)_2D_3$ interacting with two ligand binding domains (a VDR–GP, genomic pocket, and a VDR-AP, alternative pocket) on the classic vitamin D receptor (VDR). In the genomic pathway, occupancy of the VDR-GP by a 6-s-*trans*-shaped $1\alpha,25(OH)_2D_3$ that is localized to the nucleus of the cell (top of the hat icon) leads to up- or down-regulation of genes subject to hormone regulation. In the rapid response pathway, occupancy of the VDR-AP, which is localized to the cell membrane/caveolae by a (6-s-*cis*) shape (half-hat icon) of $1\alpha,25(OH)_2D_3$, can produce a variety of rapid responses which depend upon the cell type. These can include activation of protein kinase C (PKC), opening of voltage-gated Ca^{2+} or Cl^- channels, or activation of MAP-kinase which are linked to the generation of biological response(s). (B) The 6-s-*trans* and 6-s-*cis* space-filling molecular shapes of $1\alpha,25(OH)_2D_3$ are shown.

been demonstrated to be cytochrome P-450 mixed-function oxidases (Henry, 2000). Both renal enzymes are localized in mitochondria of the proximal tubules of the kidney. The genes for all three cytochrome P-450 molecules have been cloned (Feldman *et al.*, 2005). The specific sites of mutations of the 25(OH)D$_3$-1α-hydroxylase which result in vitamin D-resistant rickets type I (VDRR-I) have been identified (Kitanaka *et al.*, 1998).

A crucial point of regulation of the vitamin D endocrine system occurs through the stringent control of the activity of the renal 25(OH)D$_3$-1α-hydroxylase (1α-hydroxylase) so that the production of the hormone 1α,25(OH)$_2$D$_3$ can be modulated according to the calcium and other endocrine needs of the organism (Henry, 2005). It is well known that the chief determinant of kidney 1α-hydroxylase activity is the vitamin D status of the animal whereby the activity is elevated in vitamin D deficiency and muted by vitamin D repletion. This is accomplished by 1α,25(OH)$_2$D$_3$ itself, which down-regulates its own production in a tight negative feedback loop. Parathyroid hormone (PTH), secreted in response to low serum-calcium levels, stimulates the renal production of 1α,25(OH)$_2$D$_3$ so that it can contribute to normalizing blood calcium (Henry *et al.*, 1992). The other endocrine factor that contributes to maintaining the balance between calcium and phosphate in the blood through modulation of vitamin D metabolism is fibroblast growth factor 23 (FGF23) which is secreted by bone cells in response to elevated serum phosphate levels and down-regulates 1α-hydroxylase activity in the kidney.

The 25(OH)D$_3$-24R-hydroxylase in the kidney produces circulating 24R,25(OH)$_2$D$_3$, whose biological significance is discussed below (Norman and Henry, 2003). In the kidney the 24R-hydroxylase is sensitive to vitamin D status (i.e. circulating 1α,25[OH]$_2$D$_3$ levels) and is also subject to regulation by parathyroid hormone. An equally important function of the 24R-hydroxylase, which occurs in the vast majority if not all target cells of 1α,25(OH)$_2$D$_3$, is the inactivation and degradation of this steroid hormone. In target cells exposed to 1α,25(OH)$_2$D$_3$, the 24R-hydroxylase is rapidly increased from virtually undetectable levels to those several orders of magnitude higher. The enzyme not only catalyzes the formation of 1α,24R,25(OH)$_3$D$_3$ but also subsequent oxidation steps on the side chain, resulting in the inactive catabolite, 1α(OH)-23-OH-24,25,26,27-tetranor-vitamin D$_3$. Thus, the 24-hydroxylase can be considered to have two functions depending on its location: production of circulating 24R,25(OH)$_2$D$_3$ in the kidney and inactivating 1α,25(OH)$_2$D$_3$ in target cells throughout the body (Henry, 2001).

Mechanisms of Action of 1α,25(OH)$_2$D$_3$

The steroid hormone 1α,25(OH)$_2$D$_3$, as well as many other steroid hormones (e.g. estradiol, progesterone, testosterone, cortisol, aldosterone), generates biological responses both by regulation of gene transcription (the classic genomic responses) and through the rapid activation of signal transduction pathways at or near the plasma membrane. These are referred to as either rapid or non-genotropic responses (Mizwicki *et al.*, 2004; Norman *et al.*, 2004).

The genomic responses to 1α,25(OH)$_2$D$_3$ result from its stereospecific interaction with its nuclear receptor, VDR (see Figure 13.3). VDR is a protein of 50 kDa which binds 1α,25(OH)$_2$D$_3$ with high affinity ($K_d \approx 0.5$ nM). 25(OH)D$_3$ and 1α(OH)D$_3$ only bind 0.1–0.3% as well as 1α,25(OH)$_2$D$_3$ and the parent vitamin D does not bind to the VDR at all. As is the case for all nuclear steroid hormone receptors, the primary amino acid sequence of the VDR consists of five functional domains: nuclear localization (A/B), DNA binding (the C domain), heterodimerization, ligand binding (the E domain) and transcriptional activation (F) (Pike and Shevde, 2005). A detailed discussion of the VDR and its participation in the regulation of gene transcription is available (Whitfield *et al.*, 2005).

The receptors for all classic steroid hormones and the nuclear receptors for 1α,25(OH)$_2$D$_3$, retinoic acid, and thyroid hormone are members of the same superfamily (Mangelsdorf *et al.*, 1995); accordingly there is substantial conservation of their amino acid sequences, particularly in the DNA binding domains. Although there is considerably less conservation of amino acid sequence in the ligand binding domains (LBDs) of the nuclear receptors, X-ray crystallographic studies of many of these LBDs show the same overall secondary and tertiary structures (Weatherman *et al.*, 1999). These LBD structures, including that of the VDR, consist of 12 α-helices arranged to create a three-layer sandwich that completely encompasses the ligand 1α,25(OH)$_2$D$_3$ in a hydrophobic core.

Nuclear-receptor-mediated regulation of gene transcription is exquisitely dependent upon the structural relationship between the unoccupied receptor, which is, in general, transcriptionally inactive, and its cognate ligand. Formation of the ligand–receptor complex results in conformational

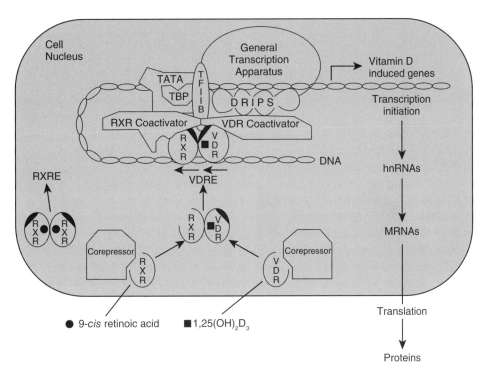

FIG. 13.4 Model of 1α,25(OH)$_2$D$_3$ and VDR activation of transcription. The VDR after binding its cognate ligand 1α,25(OH)$_2$D$_3$ forms a heterodimer with RXR. This heterodimer complex then interacts with the appropriate VDRE on the promoter of genes (in specific target cells) which are destined to be up- or down-regulated. The heterodimer–DNA complex then recruits necessary coactivator proteins, TATA, TBP, TFIIB and other proteins to generate a competent transcriptional complex capable of modulating mRNA production. A detailed discussion is given by Whitfield *et al.* (2005).

changes in the receptor protein, allowing it to interact with the transcriptional machinery. A detailed understanding of the complementarity of the ligand shape with that of the interior surface of the nuclear VDR receptor ligand binding domain is the key to understanding the structural basis of its formation of heterodimers and interactions with coactivators (see Figure 13.4). Such an understanding is also fundamental to designing new drug forms of the steroid hormones, including 1α,25(OH)$_2$D$_3$.

Mice in which the gene for the VDR has been deleted or rendered non-functional (VDR-KO) by targeted disruption of the DNA encoding the first or second zinc finger of the DNA-binding domain of the VDR (Bula *et al.*, 2005) display the phenotype of vitamin D-dependent rickets type II (VDDR-II). Except for the alopecia that appears at about 7 weeks, most of the features of this phenotype can be "rescued" by feeding the mice a diet high in calcium and lactose. Additionally, in spite of the widespread tissue distribution of the VDR,

these animals are phenotypically normal at birth. These results suggest that there is biological redundancy with respect to many of the functions of the VDR. Interestingly, VDR knockout (KO) mice have an impaired insulin secretory capacity (Zeitz *et al.*, 2003) which may presage involvement of vitamin D nutritional status with glucose homeostasis.

The "rapid" or non-genomic responses to 1α,25(OH)$_2$D$_3$ are mediated through its interaction with the classic VDR that is associated with caveolae present in the plasma membrane of a variety of cells (Huhtakangas *et al.*, 2004). For example, studies with VDR KO mice demonstrated that rapid modulation of osteoblast ion channel responses by 1α,25(OH)$_2$D$_3$ requires the presence of a functional vitamin D nuclear/caveolae receptor (Zanello and Norman, 2004).

Rapid responses stimulated by 1α,25(OH)$_2$D$_3$ or 6-s-*cis* locked analogs of 1α,25(OH)$_2$D$_3$ (see below) acting through the VDR include the following: rapid stimulation by $1\alpha,25(OH)_2D_3$ of intestinal Ca^{2+} absorption (trans-caltachia) (Norman *et al.*, 1993); opening of voltage-gated Ca^{2+} and Cl^- (Zanello and Norman, 2007) RM channels; store-operated Ca^{2+} influx in skeletal muscle cells as modulated by phospholipase C, protein kinase C, and tyrosine kinases (Vazquez *et al.*, 1998); activation of protein kinase C (PKC) (Schwartz *et al.*, 2002); and inhibition of activation of apoptosis in osteoblasts mediated by rapid activation of Src, phosphatidyl inositol 3′-kinase and JNK kinases (Vertino *et al.*, 2005).

Careful study using structural analogs of $1,25(OH)_2D_3$ has shown that the genomic and non-genomic responses to this conformationally flexible steroid hormone have different requirements for ligand structure (Mizwicki *et al.*, 2004, 2010). The results indicate that the classic nuclear VDR can orchestrate both genomic and nongenomic responses (see Figure 13.3A). A plausible mechanism by which it could carry out these two disparate functions is that specific structural features of the VDR permit differently shaped ligands (see Figure 13.3B) to activate different classes of biological responses via either the VDR-GP (genomic pocket) or the VDR-AP (alternative pocket).

For example, a key consideration is the position of rotation about the 6,7 single carbon–carbon bond which can either be in the 6-s-*cis* or 6-s-*trans* orientation (see Figure 13.1). The preferred shape of the ligand for VDR, determined from the X-ray crystal structure of the VDR-GP receptor occupied with ligand, is a 6-s-*trans*-shaped bowl with the A-ring 30° above the plane of the C/D rings. In contrast, structure–function studies of rapid non-genomic actions of $1,25(OH)_2D_3$ and its analogs show that the VDR-AP prefers its ligand to have a 6-s-*cis* shape (Mizwicki and Norman, 2009).

Biological Properties of 24R,25(OH)₂D₃

In comparison with $1\alpha,25(OH)_2D_3$, the biological actions of $24R,25(OH)_2D_3$ have been relatively less studied. One key question that has attracted attention is whether $1\alpha,25(OH)_2D_3$ acting alone can generate *all* the biological responses that are attributed to the parent vitamin D_3 or whether, for some responses, a second vitamin D_3 metabolite may be required. Evidence has been presented to support the view that the combined presence of $1\alpha,25(OH)_2D_3$ and $24R,25(OH)_2D_3$ is required to generate the complete spectrum of biological responses attributable to the parent vitamin D_3 (Norman *et al.*, 1980). The key experiments demonstrated that, when hens were raised

from hatching to sexual maturity with $1\alpha,25(OH)_2D_3$ as their sole source of vitamin D, fertile eggs appear to develop normally but failed to hatch. However, when the hens received a combination of $1\alpha,25(OH)_2D_3$ and $24R,25(OH)D_3$, hatchability equivalent to that with hens given vitamin D_3 was obtained (Henry and Norman, 1978; Norman *et al.*, 1983).

Evidence of a biological role for $24R,25(OH)_2D_3$ in the fracture-healing process has also been obtained using a chicken model system (Seo *et al.*, 1997). Recent studies in mice deficient in the 24R-hydroxylase have extended the evidence for a role for $24R,25(OH)_2D_3$ in fracture healing to a mammalian system by demonstrating delayed callus mineralization in these mice relative to wild-type control animals (St-Arnaud, 2010).

Disease States in Man Related to Vitamin D

Newly Recognized Vitamin D Target Organs and Their Associated Diseases

Over the past several decades it has emerged that the vitamin D endocrine system is not restricted to calcium homeostasis and that at least 38 tissues express the VDR (Norman and Bouillon, 2010). In just the last 10 years, several lines of investigation have resulted in striking new insights into the new responsibilities of vitamin D. The following approaches were employed:

(a) studies of the cellular and molecular effects of $1\alpha,25(OH)_2D_3$ in a wide range of cell types (Norman, 2006);
(b) experimental studies in VDR KO mouse models (Bouillon *et al.*, 2006);
(c) several large observational epidemiological studies in subjects with variable degrees of vitamin D status (Thacher and Clarke, 2011).

Figure 13.5 summarizes the newly expanded vitamin D endocrine systems. The five new physiological systems known to be influenced by vitamin D are the immune system (both innate and adaptive), the pancreas and glucose and fat metabolism, and the heart–cardiovascular, muscle, and brain systems. Examples of documented biological responses are provided for each new system, except for the brain, as well as disease states that have been found to be associated with vitamin D deficiency (see Figure 13.5 legend). A more detailed presentation and discussion are provided by Norman and Bouillon (2010).

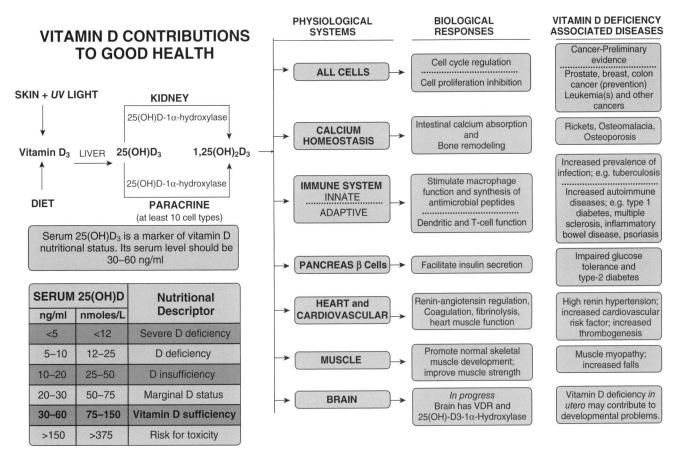

FIG. 13.5 Vitamin D contributions to good health. The three columns on the right-hand side summarize (a) the six physiological systems that are dependent upon a proper vitamin D nutritional status; (b) biological responses mediated by $1\alpha,25(OH)_2D_3$, in collaboration with its VDR; and (c) disease states associated with vitamin D deficiency. These six systems are dependent upon the availability of the essential vitamin D_3, and its subsequent metabolism to $25(OH)D_3$ and then to the steroid hormone, $1\alpha,25(OH)_2D_3$. The inset table (lower left) summarizes the serum 25(OH)D concentrations that define the spectrum of vitamin D nutritional states. These range from severe D deficiency to vitamin D sufficiency and then to levels of 25(OH)D that are associated with a risk of toxicity. Selected literature citations for disease states that have been found to have some association with vitamin D deficiency for each new system (except for the brain) are as follows: innate immune system, Williams *et al.* (2008) and Talat *et al.* (2010); adaptive immune system – inflammation, Munger *et al.* (2006); pancreas – metabolic syndrome, adiposity, Pittas *et al.* (2007) and Ochs-Balcom *et al.* (2011); heart – cardiovascular, Shea *et al.* (2008) and Bouillon (2009); and muscle, Bischoff-Ferrari (2009). There are also associations between low levels of serum 25(OH)D (20 ng/mL or 50 nmol/mL) and a higher incidence of digestive system cancers (Giovannucci *et al.*, 2006; Garland *et al.*, 2007).

Traditional Vitamin D Deficiency Diseases (Rickets, Osteomalacia, Osteoporosis)

The classic deficiency state of vitamin D, due to either its absence from the diet or inadequate exposure to sunlight, is the bone disease termed rickets in children or osteomalacia in adults; the clinical features depend upon the age of onset. Rickets includes deformity of the bones, especially in the knees, wrists, and ankles, as well as changes in the costochondral joint functions, sometimes referred to as the rachitic rosary. If rickets develops in the first 6 months, infants may suffer from convulsions or develop tetany due to a low blood calcium level (usually <7 mg/100 mL), but may have only minor skeletal changes. After 6 months, bone pain as well as tetany are likely to be present. Since osteomalacia occurs in adulthood after growth and development of the skeleton are complete, its main symptoms are muscular weakness and bone pain with little bone deformity (Norman and Litwack, 1987).

The differences between osteomalacia and osteoporosis are subtle but important. Osteomalacia arises from a problem in the bone-building process, whereas osteoporosis arises from a weakening of mature bone via a general loss of bone calcium from the ongoing daily process of bone remodeling.

Osteoporosis is the most common generalized disorder of bone; it is estimated that in the US over 30 million people, 80% of whom are female, have some form of osteoporosis. Chronic vitamin D deficiency in the elderly (>70 years) can result in an imbalance in the remodeling rate of bone and exacerbate the bone loss.

Nutritional Aspects of Vitamin D

Vitamin D Deficiency

Vitamin D nutritionists and scientists in many countries agree that about half of elderly Western Europeans and North Americans and probably two-thirds of the rest of the world are not receiving enough vitamin D to maintain healthy bone and that this is a major public health issue (Norman et al., 2007; Henry et al., 2010). It is possible that there are as many as 1 billion people in the world who are vitamin D deficient. Given the emerging data supporting a worldwide pandemic of vitamin D deficiency (Norman et al., 2007), this represents an enormous challenge to the nutrition and health agencies of the world's nations.

Substantial proportions of the population of the US and of Canada are exposed to suboptimal levels of sunlight, particularly during winter months (Webb and Holick, 1988). Under these conditions vitamin D becomes a true vitamin, which dictates that it must be supplied in the diet on a regular basis. One report (Vieth et al., 2001) suggests that winter-time vitamin D insufficiency is common in young Canadian women, and makes the observation that the levels of vitamin D in food did not prevent the deficiency. Other reports document the widespread deficiency of vitamin D in all regions and on all continents of the world (Lips, 2007). These observations have led to the question as to whether the optimal requirement of vitamin

D should be much higher than what is officially recommended (Vieth, 2004).

The nutritional availability of vitamin D is particularly important in both the newborn and young child and in the elderly. Deprivation of sunlight through seasonal variation (winter) (Harris and Dawson-Hughes, 1998), skin pigmentation in Africans (Thacher et al., 1999) or African-Americans (Kreiter et al., 2000), or certain cultural groups or clothing habits such as those of Muslims (Mawer et al., 1986), all can lead to the onset of clinical rickets or osteomalacia, characterized by low serum $25(OH)D_3$ levels. If the clothing covers the nursing infant as well, she or he will be at risk for rickets if the mother is vitamin D deficient.

When vitamin D deficiency is encountered in the clinical setting (e.g. older or sick individuals; newborn infants), the physician naturally will want to provide replacement or supplemental vitamin D; this could be in the form of either vitamin D_3 or vitamin D_2. It has been taught for the last seven decades that in humans vitamin D_3 and vitamin D_2 are equally biologically efficacious. However, with the realization that the serum $25(OH)D$ clinical assay provides the best assessment of vitamin D status (see Figure 13.5, inset table), it became appropriate to determine whether vitamin D_2 is as effective in elevating serum $25(OH)D$ levels in humans as vitamin D_3. Four studies in humans have compared the relative abilities of vitamin D_2 and vitamin D_3 to elevate serum $25(OH)D$. Three studies (Trang et al., 1998; Armas et al., 2004; Heaney et al., 2011) reported that vitamin D_3 is significantly more effective than vitamin D_2, but there was one report (Holick et al., 2008) that, for a dose of 1000 IU/day, vitamin D_3 and vitamin D_2 were equivalent.

Unfortunately, for patients who have a poor vitamin D status, there are currently no high-dose vitamin D_3 formulations approved by the USA FDA for clinical use. Similarly no drug formulations of $25(OH)D_3$ are approved in the USA.

Recommended Dietary Reference Intake (DRI) of Vitamin D

The former dietary reference intake (DRI: average daily requirements) allowance of vitamin D recommended in 1997 by an Institute of Medicine (IOM) special committee was 200 IU/day (5 μg/day) for infants, children, and adult males and females (including during pregnancy and lactation) up to age 51. The adequate intake level was set at 400 IU/day (10 μg) for males and females aged 51–70 and at 600 IU/day (15 μg) for ages > 70 (Institute of Medicine, 1997).

These 1997 DRI guidelines were updated on November 30, 2010, by a newly convened IOM Expert Committee of 13 members (Institute of Medicine, 2011). The US and Canadian governments asked the IOM committee to assess the current data on health outcomes associated with vitamin D and calcium. For vitamin D the recommended dietary allowance is now 600 IU/day for ages 1–70 years, regardless of pregnancy or lactation, and 800 IU/day for ages > 70. For infants (0–12 months), the RDA is 800 IU/day.

Vitamin D: Safety, Serum 25(OH)D Levels, and Toxicity

Safety

The 1997 IOM committee set the tolerable upper level intake (TULI) at 1000 IU/day for infants and 2000 IU/day for all other age groups. The 2010 IOM committee raised the TULI to 4000 IU/day for individuals of 9 years or older. The TULI dose for infants 0–6 months is 1000 IU/day, 1500 IU/day for infants 6–12 months, 2500 IU/day for ages 1–3 years, and 3000 IU/day for ages 4–8 years. Others have argued, based on the absence of toxicity in a number of human clinical trials, that the TULI should be 10 000 IU/day (Hathcock, 2007).

25(OH)D Levels

The Institute of Medicine (IOM) committee has emphasized that, although a serum 25(OH)D level of 20 ng/mL is adequate to ensure good bone health, there is not enough evidence to make any recommendations with respect to non-skeletal benefits. Both of the authors of this chapter as well as many other scientists in the vitamin D field (Norman *et al.*, 2007; Henry *et al.*, 2010) believe that there are at least four new physiological systems (the immune system, the pancreas and metabolic homeostasis, heart and cardiovascular system, and muscle) in which there is a clear and strong positive association between serum 25(OH)D levels (dependent on vitamin D intake) and optimal function that is contributory to good health (Figure 13.5, right-hand column). Support for the fifth biological system, the brain, is just now emerging.

The inset table in Figure 13.5 provides alternative guidelines concerning serum 25(OH)D levels as a measure of relative vitamin D nutritional status. It lists six categories: severe D deficiency; vitamin D deficiency; vitamin D insufficiency; marginal vitamin D status; vitamin D sufficiency; and risk for toxicity. The serum 25(OH)D levels that define the first three categories, severe D deficiency, vitamin D deficiency, and vitamin D insufficiency, are also endorsed by the IOM committee. In deviation from the IOM committee, we and many other scientists in the field believe that the range of 20–30 μg/mL is a state of marginal vitamin D status and that, to insure an adequate response by the calcium homeostatic system as well as the four new biological systems, it is essential to have achieved a state of "*vitamin D sufficiency*"; that is, a serum 25(OH)D concentration in the range of 30–60 ng/mL (75–150 nmol/L). Heaney and Holick (2011) have enunciated a "rule of thumb" that states that, for vitamin D intake, each additional increment of 100 IU/day will raise serum 25(OH)D by about 1 ng/mL (2.5 nmol/L). Thus a daily dose of vitamin D of 3000 IU should elevate the serum 25(OH)D to 30 ng/day.

In support of safety concerns for 25(OH)D levels in the 50–70 ng/mL (125–175 nmol/L) interval, it is known that outdoor construction workers and lifeguards routinely have serum 25(OH)D levels in the summer in the range of 50–65 ng/mL (125–160 nmol/L) without adverse consequences (Barger-Lux and Heaney, 2002).

Toxicity

Excessive amounts of vitamin D are not normally available from the usual dietary sources and thus reports of vitamin D intoxication are rare. However, there is always the possibility that vitamin D intoxication may occur in individuals who are taking excessive amounts of supplemental vitamins. One report describes vitamin D intoxication occurring from drinking milk that had been fortified with inappropriately high amounts of vitamin D_3 (5.1 mg or 230 000 IU/L levels per liter) (Jacobus *et al.*, 1992). This resulted in an average serum 25(OH)D level of 300 ng/mL or 750 nmol/L in eight subjects, seven of whom had hypercalcemia levels that are associated with vitamin D intoxication.

Symptoms of vitamin D intoxication include hypercalcemia, hypercalciuria, anorexia, nausea, vomiting, thirst, polyuria, muscular weakness, joint pains, diffuse demineralization of bones, and general disorientation. If the condition is allowed to go unchecked, it will likely be fatal. The extent of vitamin D toxicity has been shown in some instances to be related to the level of dietary intake of calcium (Beckman *et al.*, 1995).

Future Directions

New Ideas about Vitamin D Intake Levels

There is emerging evidence that a state of vitamin D sufficiency can contribute to longevity of life. One example was reported in hemodialysis patients (Wolf *et al.*, 2008). A second example reported that low serum 25(OH)D levels (<17 ng/mL or 42 nmol/L) were associated with a higher rate of mortality (Melamed *et al.*, 2008). Finally, 25(OH)D deficiency has been found to be associated with hypertension, obesity, glucose intolerance, and the metabolic syndrome, which may be responsible, at least in part, for its association with increased cardiovascular mortality rate (Michos and Blumenthal, 2007).

Will the D-responsive physiological systems data be derived from evidence-based medicine (randomized clinical trials in the appropriate target populations) or via observational approaches? An important concern is what are the frequency and severity of vitamin D toxicity when vitamin D supplementation is implemented in a very large population of many millions of people over a lifetime?

Policy: Food Supplementation versus Daily Intake

Under the right circumstances, sunlight UVB exposure can generate significant amounts of vitamin D. But since sunlight exposure can also result in skin cancer as well as non-lethal skin damage, the use of UVB as source of vitamin D is not encouraged. Given that the 2009 world population was 6.8 billion (Wright, 2010), then approximately one-third of the world's citizens (2.3 billion) live between 40°N and 90°N, where, for a significant portion of the year, levels of UVB are limited and there is a risk of vitamin D deficiency.

Given the worldwide pandemic of vitamin D insufficiency, a major goal for the health and nutritional agencies of each of the world's countries is to elucidate the severity of the vitamin D deficiency for each ethnic group and document their dietary practices. This may facilitate the decision as to whether food fortification or individual supplementation is the best approach. This is a complex public health and policy matter that is beyond the scope of this presentation.

In the US, the FDA has approved fortification of milk and milk products, breakfast cereal, orange juice, pastas, infant formulas, and margarines. In developing-world countries there are no reliable sources of vitamin D-enriched food.

Suggestions for Further Reading

The interested reader is referred to five articles in the recent scientific literature which provide differing perspectives and more detailed elaboration. These include the following:

VDR and 1α,25(OH)$_2$D$_3$ mediated genomic and rapid responses (Mizwicki *et al.*, 2010);

Vitamin D nutritional policy (Norman and Bouillon, 2010);

Use of vitamin D deficient mice to make new observations (Bouillon *et al.*, 2006);

25(OH)D levels and the risk of mortality in the general population (Melamed *et al.*, 2008);

Vitamin D and human health – lessons from vitamin D receptor null mice (Bouillon *et al.*, 2008).

References

Armas, L.A.G., Hollis, B.W., and Heaney, R.P. (2004) Vitamin D$_2$ is much less effective than vitamin D$_3$ in humans. *J Clin Endocrinol Metab* **89**, 5387–5391.

Barger-Lux, M.J. and Heaney, R.P. (2002) Effects of above average summer sun exposure on serum 25-hydroxyvitamin D and calcium absorption. *J Clin Endocrinol Metab* **87**, 4952–4956.

Beckman, M.J., Johnson, J.A., Goff, J.P., *et al.* (1995) The role of dietary calcium in the physiology of vitamin D toxicity: excess dietary vitamin D$_3$ blunts parathyroid hormone induction of kidney 1-hydroxylase. *Arch Biochem Biophys* **319**, 535–539.

Bischoff-Ferrari, H.A., Dawson-Hughes, B., Staehelin, H.B., *et al.* (2009) Fall prevention with supplemental and active forms of vitamin D: a meta-analysis of randomised controlled trials. *Br Med J* **339**, b3692.

Bouillon, R. (2009) Vitamin D as potential baseline therapy for blood pressure control. *Am J Hypertens* **22**, 867–870.

Bouillon, R., Carmeliet, G., Verlinden, L., *et al.* (2008) Vitamin D and human health: lessons from vitamin D receptor null mice. *Endocrinol Rev* **29**, 726–776.

Bouillon, R., Okamura, W.H., and Norman, A.W. (1995) Structure–function relationships in the vitamin D endocrine system. *Endocrinol Rev* **16**, 200–257.

Bouillon, R., Verstuyf, A., Mathieu, C., *et al.* (2006) Vitamin D resistance. *Best Pract Res Clin Endocrinol Metab* **20**, 627–645.

Bula, C.M., Huhtakangas, J., Olivera, C.J., *et al.* (2005) Presence of a truncated form of the vitamin D receptor (VDR) in a strain of VDR-knockout mice. *Endocrinology* **146**, 5581–5586.

Feldman, D., Pike, J.W., and Glorieux, F.H. (2005) (eds) *Vitamin D*, 2nd Edn. Elsevier Academic Press, San Diego.

Garland, C.F., Gorham, E.D., Mohr, S.B., *et al.* (2007) Vitamin D and prevention of breast cancer: pooled analysis. *J Steroid Biochem Mol Biol* **103**, 708–711.

Giovannucci, E., Liu, Y., Rimm, E.B., *et al.* (2006) Prospective study of predictors of vitamin D status and cancer incidence and mortality in men. *J Natl Cancer Inst* **98**, 451–459.

Harris, S.S. and Dawson-Hughes, B. (1998) Seasonal changes in plasma 25-hydroxyvitamin D concentrations of young American black and white women. *Am J Clin Nutr* **67**, 1232–1236.

Hathcock, J.N., Shao, A., Vieth, R., *et al.* (2007) Risk assessment for vitamin D. *Am J Clin Nutr* **85**, 6–18.

Haussler, M.R. and Norman, A.W. (1969) Chromosomal receptor for a vitamin D metabolite. *Proc Natl Acad Sci USA* **62**, 155–162.

Haussler, M.R., Myrtle, J.F., and Norman, A.W. (1968) The association of a metabolite of vitamin D_3 with intestinal mucosa chromatin, *in vivo*. *J Biol Chem* **243**, 4055–4064.

Heaney, R.P. and Holick, M.F. (2011) Why the IOM recommendations for vitamin D are deficient. *J Bone Miner Res* PMID 21207378.

Heaney, R.P., Recker, R.R., Grote, J., *et al.* (2011) Vitamin D_3 is more potent than vitamin D_2 in humans. *J Clin Endocrinol Metab* **96**, E447–452. PMID 21177785.

Henry, H.L. (2000) Vitamin D. In H.M. Goodman (ed.), *Handbook of Physiology, Section 7: The Endocrine System*. Oxford University Press, New York, pp. 699–718.

Henry, H.L. (2001) The $25(OH)D_3/1\alpha,25(OH)_2D_3$-24R-hydroxylase: a catabolic or biosynthetic enzyme? *Steroids* **66**, 391–398.

Henry, H.L. (2005) The 25-hydroxyvitamin D3 -1a-hydroxylase in vitamin D. In D. Feldman, F.H. Glorieux, and J.W. Pike (eds), *Vitamin D*, 2nd Edn. Academic Press, San Diego, pp. 69–83.

Henry, H.L. and Norman, A.W. (1978) Vitamin D: two dihydroxylated metabolites are required for normal chicken egg hatchability. *Science* **201**, 835–837.

Henry, H.L., Bouillon, R., Norman, A.W., *et al.* (2010) 14th Vitamin D Workshop consensus on vitamin D nutritional guidelines. *J Steroid Biochem Mol Biol* **121**, 4–6.

Henry, H.L., Dutta, C., Cunningham, N., *et al.* (1992) The cellular and molecular regulation of $1,25(OH)_2D_3$ production. *J Steroid Biochem Mol Biol* **41**, 401–407.

Holick, M.F., Biancuzzo, R.M., Chen, T.C., *et al.* (2008) Vitamin D_2 is as effective as vitamin D_3 in maintaining circulating concentrations of 25-hydroxyvitamin D. *J Clin Endocrinol Metab* **93**, 677–681.

Huhtakangas, J.A., Olivera, C.J., Bishop, J.E., *et al.* (2004) The vitamin D receptor is present in caveolae-enriched plasma membranes and binds $1\alpha,25(OH)_2$-vitamin D_3 *in vivo* and *in vitro*. *Mol Endocrinol* **18**, 2660–2671.

Institute of Medicine (1997) *Dietary Reference Intakes for Calcium, Magnesium, Phosphorus, Vitamin D, and Fluoride*. National Academies Press, pp. 250–287.

Institute of Medicine (2011) *Dietary Reference Intakes for Calcium and Vitamin D*. National Academies Press, Washington, DC. http://books.nap.edu/openbook.php?record_id=13050.

IUPAC (1960) Definitive rules for the nomenclature of amino acids, steroids, vitamins, and carotenoids. *J Am Chem Soc* **82**, 5575–5586.

Jacobus, C.H., Holick, M.F., Shao, Q., *et al.* (1992) Hypervitaminosis D associated with drinking milk. *New Engl J Med* **326**, 1173–1177.

Kitanaka, S., Takeyama, K., Murayama, A., *et al.* (1998) Inactivating mutations in the 25-hydroxyvitamin D_3 1α-hydroxylase gene in patients with pseudovitamin D-deficiency rickets. *N Engl J Med* **338**, 653–661.

Kreiter, S.R., Schwartz, R.P., Kirkman, H.N., Jr, *et al.* (2000) Nutritional rickets in African American breast-fed infants. *J Pediatr* **137**, 153–157.

Laing, C.J. and Cooke, N.E. (2005) Vitamin D binding protein. In D. Feldman, F.H. Glorieux, and J.W. Pike (eds), *Vitamin D*, 2nd Edn. Elsevier Academic Press, San Diego, pp. 117–134.

Lips, P. (2007) Vitamin D status and nutrition in Europe and Asia. *J Steroid Biochem Mol Biol* **103**, 620–625.

Mangelsdorf, D.J., Thummel, C., Beato, M., *et al.* (1995) The nuclear receptor superfamily: the second decade. *Cell* **83**, 835–839.

Mawer, E.B., Stanbury, S.W., Robinson, M.J., *et al.* (1986) Vitamin D nutrition and vitamin D metabolism in the premature human neonate. *Clin Endocrinol (Oxf)* **25**, 641–649.

Melamed, M.L., Michos, E.D., Post, W., *et al.* (2008) 25-hydroxyvitamin D levels and the risk of mortality in the general population. *Arch Intern Med* **168**, 1629–1637.

Michos, E.D. and Blumenthal, R.S. (2007) Vitamin D supplementation and cardiovascular disease risk. *Circulation* **115**, 827–828.

Mizwicki, M. and Norman, A.W. (2009) The vitamin D sterol–vitamin D receptor ensemble model offers unique insights into both genomic and rapid-response signaling. *Sci Signal* **2**, re4. PMID 19531804.

Mizwicki, M.T., Keidel, D., Bula, C.M., *et al.* (2004) Identification of an alternative ligand-binding pocket in the nuclear vitamin D receptor and its functional importance in $1\alpha,25(OH)_2$-vitamin D_3 signaling. *Proc Natl Acad Sci USA* **101**, 12876–12881.

Mizwicki, M.T., Menegaz, D., Yaghmaei, S., *et al.* (2010) A molecular description of ligand binding to the two overlapping binding pockets of the nuclear vitamin D receptor (VDR): structure–function implications. *J Steroid Biochem Mol Biol* **121**, 98–105.

Munger, K.L., Levin, L.I., Hollis, B.W., *et al.* (2006) Serum 25-hydroxyvitamin D levels and risk of multiple sclerosis. *JAMA* **296**, 2832–2838.

Norman, A.W. (1979) *Vitamin D: The Calcium Homeostatic Steroid Hormone*, 1st Edn. Academic Press, New York.

Norman, A.W. (2006) Minireview: vitamin D receptor: new assignments for an already busy receptor. *Endocrinology* **147**, 5542–5548.

Norman, A.W.and Bouillon, R. (2010) Vitamin D nutritional policy needs a vision for the future. *Exp Biol Med* **235**, 1034–1045.

Norman, A.W. and Henry, H.L. (2003) Vitamin D: 24,25-dihydroxy vitamin D. In H.L. Henry and A.W. Norman (eds), *Encyclopedia of Hormones*. Academic Press, San Diego, pp. 635–638.

Norman, A.W. and Litwack, G. (1987) *Hormones*. Academic Press, Orlando, FL.

Norman, A.W., Bouillon, R., Whiting, S.J., *et al.* (2007) 13th Workshop consensus for vitamin D nutritional guidelines. *J Steroid Biochem Mol Biol* **103**, 204–205.

Norman, A.W., Henry, H.L., and Malluche, H.H. (1980) 24R,25-dihydroxyvitamin D_3 and 1α,25-dihydroxyvitamin D_3 are both indispensable for calcium and phosphorus homeostasis. *Life Sci* **27**, 229–237.

Norman, A.W., Leathers, V.L., and Bishop, J.E. (1983) Studies on the mode of action of calciferol. XLVIII. Normal egg hatchability requires the simultaneous administration to the hen of 1α,25-dihydroxyvitamin D_3 and 24R,25-dihydroxyvitamin D_3. *J Nutr* **113**, 2505–2515.

Norman, A.W., Mizwicki, M.T., and Norman, D.P.G. (2004) Steroid hormone rapid actions, membrane receptors and a conformational ensemble model. *Nat Rev Drug Discov* **3**, 27–41.

Norman, A.W., Myrtle, J.F., Midgett, R.J., *et al.* (1971) 1,25-Dihydr oxycholecalciferol: identification of the proposed active form of vitamin D_3 in the intestine. *Science* **173**, 51–54

Norman, A.W., Okamura, W.H., Farach-Carson, M.C., *et al.* (1993) Structure–function studies of 1,25-dihydroxyvitamin D_3 and the vitamin D endocrine system. 1,25-dihydroxy-pentadeuterio-previtamin D_3 (as a 6-s-*cis* analog) stimulates nongenomic but not genomic biological responses. *J Biol Chem* **268**, 13811–13819.

Ochs-Balcom, H.M., Chennamaneni, R., Millen, A.E., *et al.* (2011) Vitamin D receptor gene polymorphisms are associated with adiposity phenotypes. *Am J Clin Nutr* **93**, 5–10.

Pike, J.W. and Shevde, N.K. (2005) The vitamin D receptor. In D. Feldman, F.H. Glorieux, and J.W. Pike (eds), *Vitamin D*, 2nd Edn. Academic Press, San Diego, pp. 167–191.

Pittas, A.G., Lau, J., Hu, F.B., *et al.* (2007) The role of vitamin D and calcium in type 2 diabetes. A systematic review and meta-analysis. *J Clin Endocrinol Metab* **92**, 2017–2029.

Schwartz, Z., Sylvia, V.L., Larsson, D., *et al.* (2002) 1α,25(OH)$_2$D$_3$ regulates chondrocyte matrix vesicle protein kinase D (PKC) directly via G protein-dependent mechanisms and indirectly via incorporation of PKC during matrix vexicle biogenesis. *J Biol Chem* **277**, 11828–11837.

Seo, E-G., Einhorn, T.A., and Norman, A.W. (1997) 24R,25-Dihydroxyvitamin D_3: an essential vitamin D_3 metabolite for both normal bone integrity and healing of tibial fracture in chicks. *Endocrinology* **138**, 3864–3872.

Shea, M.K., Booth, S.L., Massaro, J.M., *et al.* (2008) Vitamin K and vitamin D status: associations with inflammatory markers in the Framingham Offspring Study. *Am J Epidemiol* **167**, 313–320.

St-Arnaud, R. (2010) CYP24A1-deficient mice as a tool to uncover a biological activity for vitamin D metabolites hydroxylated at position 24. *J Steroid Biochem Mol Biol* **121**, 254–256.

Talat, N., Perry, S., Parsonnet, J., *et al.* (2010) Vitamin D deficiency and tuberculosis progression. *Emerg Infect Dis* **16**, 853–855.

Thacher, T.D. and Clarke, B.L. (2011) Vitamin D insufficiency. *Mayo Clin Proc* **86**, 50–60.

Thacher, T.D., Fischer, P.R., Petitfor, J.M., *et al.* (1999) A comparison of calcium, vitamin D, or both for nutritional rickets in Nigerian children. *N Engl J Med* **341**, 563–568.

Trang, H., Cole, D.E., Rubin, L.A., *et al.* (1998) Evidence that vitamin D_3 increases serum 25-hydroxyvitamin D more efficiently than does vitamin D_3. *Am J Clin Nutr* **68**, 854–858.

Vazquez, G., De Boland, A.R., and Boland, R.L. (1998) 1α,25-Dihydroxy-vitamin-D_3-induced store-operated Ca^{2+} influx in skeletal muscle cells – modulation by phospholipase C, protein kinase C, and tyrosine kinases. *J Biol Chem* **273**, 33954–33960.

Vertino, A.M., Bula, C.M., Chen, J-R., *et al.* (2005) Nongenotropic, and anti-apoptotic signaling of vitamin D analogs through the ligand binding domain (LBD) of the vitamin D receptor (VDR) in osteoblasts and osteocytes: mediation by Src, P13 and JNK kinases. *J Biol Chem* **280**, 14130–14137.

Vieth, R. (2004) Why the optimal requirement for vitamin D_3 is probably much higher than what is officially recommended for adults. *J Steroid Biochem Mol Biol* **89–90**, 575–579.

Vieth, R., Cole, D.E., Hawker, G.A., *et al.* (2001) Wintertime vitamin D insufficiency is common in young Canadian women, and their vitamin D intake does not prevent it. *Eur J Clin Nutr* **55**, 1091–1097.

Weatherman, R.V., Fletterick, R.J., and Scanlon, T.S. (1999) Nuclear receptor ligands and ligand-binding domains. *Annu Rev Biochem* **68,** 559–582.

Webb, A.R. and Holick, M.F. (1988) The role of sunlight in the cutaneous production of vitamin D_3. *Annu Rev Nutr* **8,** 375–399.

Whitfield, G.K., Jurutka, P.W., Haussler, C.A., *et al.* (2005) Nuclear vitamin D receptor: structure–function, molecular control of gene transcription and novel bioactions. In D. Feldman, F.H. Glorieux, and J.W. Pike (eds), *Vitamin D*, 2nd Edn. Academic Press, San Diego, pp. 219–328.

Williams, B., Williams, A.J., and Anderson, S.T. (2008) Vitamin D deficiency and insufficiency in children with tuberculosis. *Pediatr Infect Dis J* **27,** 941–942.

Wolf, M., Betancourt, J., Chang, Y., *et al.* (2008) Impact of activated vitamin D and race on survival among hemodialysis patients. *J Am Soc Nephrol* **19,** 1379–1388.

Wright, J.W. (ed.) (2010) World population. *New York Times 2010 Almanac*. Penguin Books, London, pp. 484–486.

Zanello, L.P. and Norman, A.W. (1997) Stimulation by $1\alpha,25(OH)_2$-vitamin D_3 of whole cell chloride currents in osteoblastic ROS 17/2.8 cells: a structure–function study. *J Biol Chem* **272,** 22617–22622.

Zanello, L.P. and Norman, A.W. (2004) Rapid modulation of osteoblast ion channel responses by $1\alpha,25(OH)_2$-vitamin D_3 requires the presence of a functional vitamin D nuclear receptor. *Proc Natl Acad Sci USA* **101,** 1589–1594.

Zeitz, U., Weber, K., Soegiarto, D.W., *et al.* (2003) Impaired insulin secretory capacity in mice lacking a functional vitamin D receptor. *FASEB J* **17,** 509–511.

14

VITAMIN E

MARET G. TRABER, PhD

Oregon State University, Corvallis, Oregon, USA

Summary

α-Tocopherol acts as a peroxyl and alkoxyl radical scavenger in lipid environments, and thus halts lipid peroxidation in lipoproteins and membranes. Nervous tissues in humans are particularly susceptible to vitamin E deficiency, resulting in a progressive peripheral sensory neuropathy. A growing body of evidence suggests that it is not only free-radical-mediated reactions, but also inflammatory responses, that play major roles in chronic diseases such as heart disease, diabetes, and neurodegenerative diseases. Epidemiologic studies suggest that chronic disease risk can be reduced by a lifetime of consuming higher dietary vitamin E intakes. However, more than 90% of Americans consume less than 40% of the 15 mg (22 IU) α-tocopherol recommended daily by the Food and Nutrition Board. Is the usual 6 mg consumed sufficient? The evidence-based data necessary to answer this question are currently unavailable. The Women's Health Study, a 10-year prevention trial in normal, healthy women, found that 600 IU vitamin E every other day decreased overall cardiovascular mortality by 24%, and in women over 65 by 49%. In contrast, randomized clinical trials of vitamin E therapeutic benefit in the treatment of heart disease were overly optimistic in their expectation that a vitamin could reverse poor dietary habits and a sedentary lifestyle, as well as provide benefits beyond those of pharmaceutical agents in treating heart disease. Thus, nearly 100 years after the discovery of vitamin E, we are still searching for the answer to the question, why is α-tocopherol required by humans?

Introduction

Vitamin E is unique in human nutrition because its major, if not sole, function is that of an antioxidant and it is thus unlike most vitamins that are co-factors or have specific metabolic functions (Traber and Atkinson, 2007). Consequently, vitamin E deficiency symptoms in target tissues are dependent not only upon vitamin E concentrations, but also on the degree of oxidative stress and the level of other antioxidants and antioxidant enzymes (Macevilly and Muller, 1996). Potentially, nerve degeneration caused by lipid peroxidation could be reversed by adequate vitamin E (Butterfield *et al.*, 2010). This chapter will describe vitamin E structures and antioxidant proper-

Present Knowledge in Nutrition, Tenth Edition. Edited by John W. Erdman Jr, Ian A. Macdonald and Steven H. Zeisel.
© 2012 International Life Sciences Institute. Published 2012 by John Wiley & Sons, Inc.

ties; distribution in food; lipoprotein transport, delivery to tissues, and metabolism; and safety and its role in chronic disease prevention.

Definitions, Structures, Antioxidant Activity

Vitamin E is the collective name for molecules synthesized by plants that exhibit the antioxidant activity of α–tocopherol. Vitamin E was discovered in 1922 when it was found that α–tocopherol was required by pregnant rats to prevent the resorption of fetuses (Evans and Bishop, 1922). At least eight different molecules (tocopherols and tocotrienols) have α–tocopherol antioxidant activity (Institute of Medicine, 2000). These forms vary in the number of methyl groups on the chromanol ring: trimethyl (α–), dimethyl (β– or γ–), and monomethyl (δ–). The tocopherols have a chromanol ring with a phytyl side chain, while the tocotrienols have an unsaturated side chain.

Vitamin E Form Required by Humans: α-Tocopherol

α-Tocopherol, as synthesized by plants, is *RRR-α-*tocopherol (Institute of Medicine, 2000). This nomenclature means that the chiral carbons are in the *R*-conformation at positions 2, 4′ and 8′. Unlike most other vitamins, commercially, chemically synthesized α–tocopherol is not identical to the naturally occurring form. Synthetic α–tocopherol is called *all-rac-*α-tocopherol (*all racemic*, or *dl*) and contains an equal mixture of eight different stereoisomers (*RRR, RSR, RRS, RSS, SRR, SSR, SRS, SSS*), which differ in the stereochemistry of the side chain. Thus, all of the stereoisomers have equal in vitro antioxidant but differing biologic activities. Recent efforts have been published describing the purification using chiral columns that allow separation of 2*R*- and 2*S*-α-tocopherol from the racemic product (Netscher, 2007). Enzymatic methods for *RRR-*α-tocopherol synthesis have been described (Nozawa *et al.*, 2000), but these are not in commercial production.

The 2 position of α-tocopherol (the junction of the ring and side chain) is critical for α-tocopherol biologic activity. Only 2*R*-α-tocopherol forms meet human vitamin E requirements (Institute of Medicine, 2000). *SRR-*α-tocopherol is prototypic of the 2*S*-forms and has been used to study synthetic vitamin E kinetics.

Vitamin E supplements often contain esters of α–tocopherol, such as α–tocopheryl acetate, succinate, or nicotinate. The ester form prevents the oxidation of vitamin E and prolongs its shelf life. Following oral administration, these esters are readily hydrolyzed and α-tocopherol (unesterified form) is absorbed (Cheeseman *et al.*, 1995).

Antioxidant Activity

Vitamin E, a potent peroxyl radical scavenger, is a chain-breaking antioxidant that prevents the propagation of free radicals in membranes and in plasma lipoproteins (Traber and Atkinson, 2007). When peroxyl radicals (ROO•) are formed, these react 1000 times faster with vitamin E (Vit E-OH) than with polyunsaturated fatty acids (PUFA, or RH in Figure 14.1) (Buettner, 1993). The hydroxyl group of tocopherol reacts with the peroxyl radical to form the corresponding hydroperoxide and the tocopheroxyl radical (Vit E–O•):

In the presence of vitamin E:

$$ROO\bullet + \text{Vit E–OH} \rightarrow ROOH + \text{Vit E–O}\bullet$$

In the absence of vitamin E:

$$ROO + RH \rightarrow ROOH + R\bullet$$
$$R\bullet + O_2 \rightarrow ROO$$

The tocopheroxyl radical (Vit E–O•) reacts with vitamin C (or other hydrogen donors, AH), thereby oxidizing the latter and returning vitamin E to its reduced state.

$$\text{Vit E–O}\bullet + AH \rightarrow \text{Vit E–OH} + A$$

This phenomenon has led to the idea of "vitamin E recycling", where the antioxidant function of oxidized vitamin E is continuously restored by other antioxidants. This "antioxidant network" depends upon the supply of aqueous antioxidants and the metabolic activity of cells. It should be noted that free metals, such as iron or copper, can reinitiate lipid peroxidation by reaction with ROOH to form an alkoxyl radical. Additionally, if other antioxidants are not present, Vit E–O• can reinitiate lipid peroxidation (Thomas and Stocker, 2000).

The interaction of vitamins E and C has been demonstrated in humans under oxidative stress. Specifically, cigarette smokers with the lowest plasma ascorbic acid concentrations had the fastest vitamin E disappearance rates (Bruno *et al.*, 2005). Furthermore, when cigarette smokers were supplemented with vitamin C, their vitamin

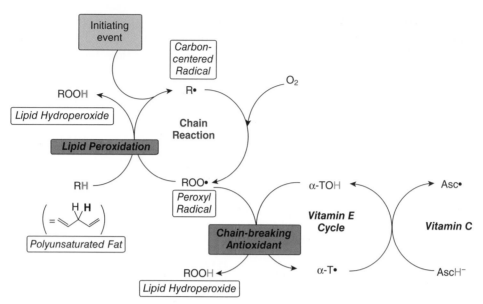

FIG. 14.1 Vitamin E antioxidant activity. When peroxyl radicals (ROO•) are formed, these react 1000 times faster with vitamin E (Vit E-OH) than with PUFA (RH); thus, membranes and lipoproteins are protected from the chain reaction of lipid peroxidation by vitamin E. The hydroxyl group of tocopherol reacts with the peroxyl radical to form the corresponding hydroperoxide (ROOH) and the tocopheroxyl radical (Vit E-O). The tocopheroxyl radical reacts with vitamin C (or other hydrogen donors, AH), thereby oxidizing the latter and returning vitamin E to its reduced state. It should be noted that free metals, such as iron or copper, can reinitiate lipid peroxidation by reaction with ROOH to form an alkoxyl radical. Additionally, if other antioxidants are not present, Vit E-O• can reinitiate lipid peroxidation (Thomas and Stocker, 2000).

E disappearance rates returned to levels seen in normal subjects (Bruno *et al.*, 2006a). Additionally, studies in rodents have shown that a combined vitamin E and C deficiency causes devastating neurologic damage in guinea pigs (Burk *et al.*, 2006) and increases the severity of atherosclerosis in susceptible mice unable to synthesize vitamin C (Babaev *et al.*, 2010).

Since the tocopheroxyl radical can be reduced back to tocopherol by ascorbate or other reducing agents, oxidized tocopherols are usually not found in vivo. Biologically relevant oxidation products formed from α−tocopherol include 4a,5-epoxy- and 7,8-epoxy-8a(hydroperoxy)-tocopherones and their respective hydrolysis products, 2,3-epoxy-tocopherol quinone and 5,6-epoxy-α−tocopherol quinone (Liebler *et al.*, 1996). However, these products are formed during in vitro oxidation; their importance in vivo is unknown (Brigelius-Flohé and Traber, 1999).

The search for a specific vitamin E function has continued since its discovery. Various authors have claimed "non-antioxidant" functions, or various signaling functions. It is likely, however, that all of the observations concerning the in vivo mechanism of action of α-tocopherol, as a vitamin, result from its role as a lipid-soluble antioxidant (Traber and Atkinson, 2007). The importance of this function is to maintain the integrity of long-chain polyunsaturated fatty acids in the membranes of cells and thus maintain their bioactivity. Thus, these bioactive lipids are important signaling molecules, and changes in their amounts, or in their loss due to oxidation, are the key cellular events to which cells respond, not the amount or oxidation state of α-tocopherol (Traber and Atkinson, 2007). This premise was elegantly tested using the comparison of α-tocopherol and α-tocotrienol in the protection against glutamate-induced neurotoxicity in vitro. Saito *et al.* (2010) demonstrated that, when both tocols were delivered to cells in similar concentrations, α-tocopherol was a better antioxidant and protected against the oxidative stress induced by glutamate.

Various authors have also used esters of α-tocopherol to deliver vitamin E to cells in culture and study gene regulation. This approach has shown that α-tocopheryl

TABLE 14.1   2R-α-tocopherol contents of foods

Food item	Weight (g)	Measure	mg per measure
Cereals, ready-to-eat, fortified	30	¾ cup	13.50
Tomato paste, canned	262	1 cup	11.27
Sunflower seeds, dry roasted	32	¼ cup	8.35
Almonds	28	1 oz (24 nuts)	7.43
Spinach, cooked	190	1 cup	6.73
Tomato pasta sauce, ready-to-serve	250	1 cup	6.00
Oil, sunflower	14	1 tbsp	5.59
Tomato purée	250	1 cup	4.93
Oil, safflower	14	1 tbsp	4.63
Turnip greens, cooked	164	1 cup	4.36
Hazelnuts	28	1 oz	4.26
Tomato sauce	245	1 cup	3.48
Potato chips	28	1 oz	3.23
Carrot juice	236	1 cup	2.74
Beet greens, cooked	144	1 cup	2.61
Fish, swordfish, cooked	106	piece	2.56
Sweet potato, canned	255	1 cup	2.55
Blue crab, canned	135	1 cup	2.48
Oil, canola	14	1 tbsp	2.44
Broccoli, cooked	184	1 cup	2.43
Red peppers, cooked	136	1 cup	2.24
Peanuts, dry-roasted	28	1 oz (approx 28)	2.21
Margarine, regular	14	1 tbsp	2.19
Asparagus, cooked	180	1 cup	2.16

Adapted from USDA National Nutrient Database for Standard Reference, Release 23, http://www.nal.usda.gov/fnic/foodcomp/search/.

succinate (Neuzil *et al.*, 2001; Yu *et al.*, 2003; Li *et al.*, 2010; Saito *et al.*, 2010; Wang *et al.*, 2010), or other non-hydrolyzable analogues such as α-tocopherol ether-linked acetic acid (Tiwary *et al.*, 2010), may be potent anti-cancer agents. However, these are not vitamin E functions, but functions of α-tocopheryl esters. Careful reading of protocols to ascertain that α-tocopheryl succinate, not tocopherol, was used, and ensuring that the concentrations used are high relative to those achieved in vivo are necessary to avoid misleading conclusions.

Content of Foods

γ-Tocopherol is the most abundant tocopherol found in the US diet (Eitenmiller and Lee, 2004). However, α–tocopherol, not γ–tocopherol, and specifically only the 2R-forms of α-tocopherol, were defined by the Food and Nutrition Board to meet human vitamin E requirements (Institute of Medicine, 2000). Only 8% of men and 2% of women in the United States had dietary vitamin E intakes (Maras *et al.*, 2004) that met the 2000 estimated average requirement (EAR, 12 mg α-tocopherol/day) (Institute of Medicine, 2000). Moreover, most individuals obtain dietary vitamin E from high-energy, high-fat foods that are not particularly α-tocopherol-rich (Maras *et al.*, 2004). Some examples of vitamin E food sources are shown in Table 14.1. It is therefore not surprising that the USDA's Dietary Guidance 2010, in an effort to limit fat intakes, does not try to optimize vitamin E intakes (http://www.cnpp.usda.gov/DGAs2010-DGACReport.htm, August 27, 2010).

Dietary Reference Intakes

Recommended Dietary Allowance for α–Tocopherol

In 2000, the Food and Nutrition Board published the Dietary Reference Intakes for Vitamin C, Vitamin E, Selenium and the Carotenoids (Institute of Medicine, 2000). The recommended dietary allowances (RDAs) represent the daily α–tocopherol intakes required to ensure adequate nutrition in 95–97.5% of the population and are

TABLE 14.2 Criteria and dietary reference intake values for vitamin E by life-stage group[a]

Life-stage group	Criterion	EAR[b] (mg/day)	RDA[c] (mg/day)	AI[d] (mg/day)	UL[e] (mg/day)
Premature infants					21
0–6 months	Average vitamin E intake from human milk			4	
7–12 months	Extrapolation from 0 to 6 months AI			5	
1–3 years	Extrapolation from adult EAR	5	6		200
4–8 years	Extrapolation from adult EAR	6	7		300
9–13 years	Extrapolation from adult EAR	9	11		600
14–18 years	Extrapolation from adult EAR	12	15		800
>18 years	Intakes sufficient to prevent hydrogen peroxide-induced erythrocyte hemolysis in vitro	12	15		1000
Pregnancy					
≤18 years	Adolescent EAR	12	15		800
19–50 years	Adult EAR	12	15		1000
Lactation					
≤18 years	Adolescent EAR plus average amount of vitamin E secreted in human milk	16	19		800
19–50 years	Adolescent EAR plus average amount of vitamin E secreted in human milk	16	19		1000

[a]Adapted from Institute of Medicine (2000).
[b]EAR, estimated average requirement. The intake that meets the estimated nutrient needs of half the individuals in a group.
[c]RDA, recommended dietary allowance. The intake that meets the nutrient needs of almost all (97–98%) individuals in a group.
[d]AI, adequate intake. The observed average or experimentally determined intake by a defined population or subgroup that appears to sustain a defined nutritional status. For healthy infants receiving human milk, the AI is the mean intake.
[e]UL, tolerable upper intake level. The highest level of daily nutrient intake that is likely to pose no risk of adverse health effects in almost all individuals.

an overestimation of the level needed for most people in any given age or gender group (Institute of Medicine, 2000): see Table 14.2.

The vitamin E requirement is based on the observation that only supplements containing α–tocopherol have been shown to reverse vitamin E deficiency symptoms in humans. The α–tocopherol amounts were based primarily on the amounts necessary to correct abnormal erythrocyte hemolysis in physically healthy subjects who had consumed experimental vitamin E-deficient diets for 5 to 7 years (Institute of Medicine, 2000). Serum concentrations (in response to known supplemental vitamin E intakes) that prevented in vitro peroxide-induced erythrocyte hemolysis were used to determine the EAR. Supplements containing either *RRR*- or *all rac*-α-tocopherol were used to reverse vitamin E abnormal erythrocyte hemolysis; therefore, correction factors were developed to convert IU to milligrams of 2R-α-tocopherol.

The factors to convert IU to milligrams are 0.45 times the IU for *all rac*- and 0.67 times the IU for *RRR*-α-tocopherol (see Table 6.1 in Institute of Medicine, 2000). For example, if a vitamin E supplement is labeled 400 IU *dl*-α-tocopheryl acetate, then 400 times 0.45 equals 180 mg 2R-α–tocopherol, but if it is labeled 400 IU *d*-α-tocopheryl acetate, then 400 times 0.67 equals 268 mg 2R-α–tocopherol. These conversions are used only to estimate intakes relative to the RDA; different conversion factors are used to assess intakes relative to the upper limit

(UL). For labeling, the vitamin E daily value (DV) is 30 IU, which is based on a Daily Reference Value established in FDA regulations 21 CFR 101.9(c)(9) (Food and Drug Administration, 2009).

The amount of vitamin E to be recommended for daily consumption is controversial, and various organizations have proposed different values. For example, the FAO (Food and Agriculture Organization of the United Nations, 2004) found as follows:

> At present, data are not sufficient to formulate recommendations for vitamin E intake for different age groups except for infancy…Thus a human-milk-fed infant consuming 850 ml would have an intake of 2.7 mg α-TE (α-tocopherol equivalents). It seems reasonable that formula milk should not contain less than 0.3 mg α-TE/100 ml of reconstituted feed and not less than 0.4 mg α-TE/g PUFA.

Note that this unit of α-TE takes into account that the various forms of vitamin E in the diet have different biologic activities that are based on the rat fetal resorption assay. This assay has been called into question because the placenta and uterus express the α-tocopherol transfer protein and therefore suggest that α-tocopherol is required by the feto-placental unit (Kaempf-Rotzoll et al., 2002, 2003; Muller-Schmehl et al., 2004; Rotzoll et al., 2008).

Safety and Upper Limits

The recommendation by the Food and Nutrition Board is that the UL for any supplements containing α-tocopherol is 1000 mg for adults (Institute of Medicine, 2000). Reports of adverse effects of vitamin E supplements in humans are sufficiently rare that data from multi-year studies in rats fed high dietary vitamin E levels were used to set the ULs (Institute of Medicine, 2000). No UL was set for infants as food was recommended as the only vitamin E source for infants. However, a UL of 21 mg/day was suggested for premature infants with birth weights of 1.5 kg, based on the adult UL. The ULs are also shown in Table 14.2.

The UL was set only for vitamin E supplements, not for food, because it is almost impossible to consume 1000 mg α–tocopherol from foods daily for prolonged periods of time. The UL was defined for both 2R- and 2S-α–tocopherols because all of the stereoisomeric forms in all rac-α-tocopherol are absorbed and delivered to the liver. The appropriate conversion factors are different from those above for all rac-α-tocopherol. The factors to convert IU to milligrams are 0.9 times the IU for all rac- and 0.67 times the IU for RRR-α-tocopherol. The UL amounts

given in IU are 1100 IU for all rac- and 1500 IU for RRR-α-tocopherol. The UL for RRR-α–tocopherol is apparently higher because each capsule of RRR-α–tocopherol contains fewer milligrams of α–tocopherol than does one containing all rac-α–tocopherol.

The UK established an Expert Group on Vitamins and Minerals which in 2003 reported their evaluation of the toxicity data for vitamin E (Expert Group on Vitamins and Minerals, 2003). They recommended that the Safe Upper Level supplemental for daily consumption over a lifetime should be 800 IU (540 mg d-α-tocopherol equivalents per day), which they estimated is equivalent to 9.0 mg/kg body weight per day in a 60-kg adult. Note that, as of October 1, 2010, the responsibility for nutrition policy transferred from the Food Standards Agency to the Department of Health in England and to the Assembly Government in Wales (web accessed Jan 6, 2011, http://www.food.gov.uk/healthiereating/).

A review of the literature on vitamin E safety has been published (Hathcock et al., 2005). However, reports from three clinical trials have suggested adverse vitamin E effects in humans under special circumstances (Biesalski et al., 2010). One study was a 3-year double-blind trial of antioxidants (vitamins E and C, β-carotene, and selenium) in 160 subjects on simvastatin–niacin therapy (Brown et al., 2001). In subjects taking antioxidants, there was less benefit of the drugs in raising HDL cholesterol than was expected and there was an increase in clinical endpoints (arteriographic evidence of coronary stenosis, or the occurrence of a first cardiovascular event [death, myocardial infarction, stroke, or revascularization]) (Brown et al., 2001). The Women's Angiographic Vitamin and Estrogen (WAVE) trial was a randomized, double-blind trial of 423 postmenopausal women with at least one coronary stenosis at baseline coronary angiography. In the postmenopausal women on hormone replacement therapy, all-cause mortality was increased in women assigned to antioxidant vitamins compared with placebo (HR, 2.8; 95% CI, 1.1–7.2; $p = 0.047$) (Waters et al., 2002). Finally, the HopeToo trial suggested that patients at high risk for coronary heart disease taking vitamin E were at increased risk of left-ventricular dysfunction (Lonn et al., 2005). Interestingly, none of these trials had the same adverse effect of vitamin E. Moreover, a meta-analysis evaluating the relationship of vitamin E supplements with all-cause mortality did not associate any adverse effects with a vitamin E-specific mechanism (Miller et al., 2005). Studies using the meta-analysis approach to evaluating clinical trials have reached very dramatically different conclusions ranging from increased risk of mortality to virtually no risk from anti-oxidant supplements (Miller *et al.*, 2005; Bjelakovic *et al.*, 2007; Berry *et al.*, 2009; Biesalski *et al.*, 2010). In fact, the use of randomized clinical trials to assess nutrient benefits has been called into question given the fact that the known adverse effect of a nutrient in humans results from its deficiency and that subjects in the placebo group do not consume inadequate intakes (Blumberg *et al.*, 2010). Biesalski *et al.* (2010) evaluated benefit as well as harm, and suggested that a risk/benefit ratio be used to evaluate vitamin E effects.

Another potential source of the adverse effects seen in clinical trials is that the patients who are studied are likely consuming a variety of pharmaceutical agents. In general, interactions between nutrients and xenobiotic metabolism has not been taken into account, and there is the possibil-ity that the nutrients are consumed with drugs (Traber, 2004). Potentially, an increase in vitamin E metabolism in response to supplements could alter xenobiotic metabo-lism and disposition, thereby decreasing the efficacy of pharmaceutical agents. However, when vitamin E supple-ments were given to patients taking statin drugs that are metabolized by cytochrome P450 3A (CYP3A), no effect on cholesterol levels was observed (Leonard *et al.*, 2007). In contrast, γ-tocopherol levels increased when a statin drug was administered (Werba *et al.*, 2007), suggesting that tocopherol levels may be influenced by xenobiotic metabolism in humans.

High vitamin E intakes are associated with an increased tendency to bleed (Institute of Medicine, 2000). It is not known if increased bleeding is a result of decreased platelet aggregation caused by an inhibition of protein kinase C by α-tocopherol (Freedman *et al.*, 2000), some other platelet-related mechanism (Steiner and Anastasi, 1976; Steiner, 1981), or decreased clotting due to vitamin K and E interactions (Glynn *et al.*, 2007) causing abnormal blood clotting (Institute of Medicine, 2000). Importantly, in the Women's Health Study, vitamin E supplements (600 IU every other day for 10 years) decreased incidence of thromboembolism (Glynn *et al.*, 2007). Thus, there may be a benefit from vitamin E supplements, as well as harm, by altering blood clotting.

Biological Activities of the Tocopherols

Intestinal Absorption

All vitamin E forms are absorbed along with fats into intestinal cells and incorporated in chylomicrons for secre-tion into lymph (Traber, 1999). The major steps from micellar uptake, to enterocyte trafficking and incorpora-tion into chylomicrons, are largely unknown. Along with other transporters, Niemann-Pick C1-like 1 (NPC1L1) facilitates cholesterol absorption into the enterocyte (Hui *et al.*, 2008). Similarly, vitamin E absorption is facilitated by NPC1L1 (Narushima *et al.*, 2008), but the exact mech-anisms for its transfer across the intestinal mucosa remain undiscovered.

Fat malabsorption syndromes (e.g. cholestatic liver disease) and genetic abnormalities in either lipoprotein synthesis (e.g. abetalipoproteinemia) or the α–tocopherol transfer protein (e.g. ataxia with vitamin E deficiency, AVED) result in vitamin E malabsorption or abnormally low plasma α–tocopherol transport, respectively (Traber, 1999).

Vitamin E absorption from supplements is poor when the supplement is consumed without fat, as was observed when vitamin E pills were consumed without food (Leonard *et al.*, 2004). Moreover vitamin E bioavailability is highly influenced by prandial status (Iuliano *et al.*, 2001). Indeed, studies using apples fortified with deuterium-labeled vitamin E demonstrated that vitamin E absorption increased as the fat in the meal increased (Bruno *et al.*, 2006b). Depending on the fat content of the meal, the bioavailability of vitamin E that occurs natu-rally in foods, that is present as a food fortificant, or is consumed as a supplement may be different.

Lipoprotein Transport

Unlike other fat-soluble vitamins that have specific plasma transport proteins, vitamin E is transported non-specifically in all of the plasma lipoproteins (Figure 14.2). Once chy-lomicron remnants containing dietary vitamin E reach the liver, only one form of vitamin E, α–tocopherol, is prefer-entially secreted by the liver into the plasma in-very-low density lipoproteins (VLDL) (Traber, 1999). In the circulation, VLDL are delipidated to form LDL. During this process, vitamin E is transferred to HDL, which can transfer vitamin E to all of the circulating lipoproteins (Traber, 1999). Thus, the liver, not the intestine, discriminates between tocophe-rols. All lipoproteins transport vitamin E, and all mecha-nisms for delivery of lipids from lipoproteins to tissues (e.g. receptors) deliver vitamin E along with the lipoprotein contents. This phenomenon was demonstrated in a porcine blood–brain barrier model where both the SR-B1 receptor and lipoprotein lipase were demonstrated to deliver α–tocopherol to cells (Goti *et al.*, 2002).

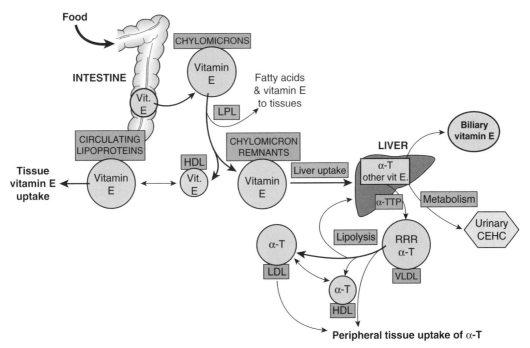

FIG. 14.2 Determinants of vitamin E biologic activity. The various dietary forms of vitamin E are absorbed by the intestine and secreted in chylomicrons. During chylomicron catabolism some vitamin E is transferred to circulating lipoproteins; the remainder is delivered to the liver. The liver α-TTP selects α-tocopherol for re-secretion into the plasma, while "excess" α-tocopherol and other dietary vitamin E forms are metabolized and excreted as CEHCs. Thus, metabolism is a major determinant of plasma vitamin E concentrations.

All forms of vitamin E are absorbed and transported by chylomicrons and are delivered to the tissues. Thus, forms in addition to α-tocopherol can be detected in tissues (Burton *et al.*, 1998). However, it should be noted that metabolism and excretion of non-α-tocopherol forms result in their relatively rapid removal from the body. This rapid excretion was demonstrated in α-tocotrienol-fed rats (Patel *et al.*, 2006) and in increased metabolism of deuterium-labeled γ-tocopherol in humans (Leonard *et al.*, 2005b). Moreover, sesame oil, which interferes with the metabolism of γ-tocopherol, slowed plasma γ-tocopherol disappearance (Frank *et al.*, 2008). These findings emphasize that the body prefers α-tocopherol despite the presence of other non-α-tocopherol forms in the diet.

α–Tocopherol Transfer Protein

The liver preferentially secretes α–tocopherol into plasma under the control of the hepatic α–tocopherol transfer protein (α–TTP), as shown in patients with genetic α–TTP defects (Traber *et al.*, 1990b, 1993) and in α–TTP null mice (Terasawa *et al.*, 2000).

Liver α–TTP has been isolated, its cDNA sequences have been reported and α–TTP crystallized, and the α–tocopherol binding pocket has been identified (Meier *et al.*, 2003; Min *et al.*, 2003). Interestingly, the pocket causes α–tocopherol to fold such that the 2-position is critical for the fit into the pocket. This preference of α–TTP for the 2R-α-tocopherol stereoisomers is the basis for the statement that only 2R-α-tocopherols (*RRR, RSR, RSS, RRS*) meet the human requirement for vitamin E (Institute of Medicine, 2000).

α-TTP belongs to a family of hydrophobic ligand-binding proteins that have a *cis*-retinal binding motif sequence (CRAL_TRIO). All of these can bind α-tocopherol, but only α-TTP appears to have sufficient affinity to be a physiological mediator of its transport (Panagabko *et al.*, 2003). The selective transfer of α–tocopherol is hypothetically responsible for the in vivo α–TTP action enriching nascent VLDL secreted with

RRR-α–tocopherol (Traber et al., 1990a). However, when tested directly, α-TTP-mediated α-tocopherol secretion was not coupled with VLDL secretion (Arita et al., 1997). Studies to elucidate the mechanism by which α-TTP facilitates α-tocopherol secretion into plasma have used fluorescent α-tocopherol analogs to follow trafficking (West et al., 2010) and assessment of ligand binding by native and naturally occurring human mutations in α-TTP (Morley et al., 2008). Thus far the mechanisms by which α-TTP delivers α-tocopherol to the plasma remain unclear and are under investigation.

Plasma Vitamin E Kinetics

A kinetic model of vitamin E transport in plasma has been described (Traber et al., 1994). In normal subjects, the fractional disappearance rates of RRR-α–tocopherol (0.4 ± 0.1 pools per day) were significantly (p < 0.01) slower than for SRR-α–tocopherol (1.2 ± 0.6). The apparent half-life of RRR-α–tocopherol was about 48 hours, whereas SRR-α–tocopherol had a half-life of approximately 13 hours (Traber et al., 1994).

Vitamin E kinetics of α- and γ-tocopherols have also been studied (Leonard et al., 2005b). Plasma γ–tocopherol exponential disappearance rates (1.39 ± 0.44 pools per day) were triple those of α-tocopherol (0.33 ± 0.11, p < 0.001). The γ–tocopherol half-lives were 13 ± 4 hours compared with 57 ± 19 hours for α-tocopherol. Thus, RRR-α-tocopherol remains in the plasma around four times longer than does SRR-α–tocopherol or γ-tocopherol. The similarity in the disappearance rates for γ–tocopherol and SRR-α–tocopherol strongly support the idea that forms of vitamin E that are not actively re-secreted by α–TTP into the plasma are excreted or metabolized.

Biliary Excretion

Vitamin E is not accumulated in the liver to "toxic" levels, suggesting that excretion and metabolism are important in preventing adverse effects of vitamin E excess. However, the regulation of hepatic vitamin E concentrations has not been extensively studied. α–Tocopherol is excreted into bile via multi-drug resistance gene 2 (MDR2, ABC B4, or p-glycoprotein) (Mustacich et al., 1998), an ATP-binding cassette transporter that also facilitates biliary phospholipid excretion.

The ATP-binding cassette transporter (ABCAI) mediates the α-tocopherol efflux from cells to HDL, similarly to "cholesterol reverse transport" (Oram et al., 2001).

HDL has been shown to deliver α-tocopherol to the liver via scavenger receptor-BI (SR-BI) (Mardones et al., 2001). In SR-BI-null compared with wild-type mice, plasma α–tocopherol concentrations increased, biliary α–tocopherol decreased but liver α–tocopherol was unchanged (Mardones et al., 2002); therefore, it appears that SR-BI-mediated hepatic α–tocopherol uptake is coupled to its biliary excretion (Mardones et al., 2002). Importantly, SR-BI protein is increased in vitamin E-deficient rats, suggesting that the liver can increase SR-BI to increase hepatic α–tocopherol delivery (Witt et al., 2000). Under normal conditions, α-tocopherol transport via HDL to the liver would allow uptake of α-tocopherol into a liver pool destined for excretion in bile or perhaps metabolism.

Vitamin E Metabolism

Vitamin E metabolites (α–CEHC and γ-CEHC [carboxyethyl hydroxychromans]) are derived from α- and γ-tocopherol (as well as from α- and γ-tocotrienols), respectively, and have been detected in urine, bile, and plasma (Brigelius-Flohé and Traber, 1999), and from liver homogenates (Leonard et al., 2005a). When equimolar amounts of labeled tocopherols (~50 mg each d_6-α- and d_2-γ–tocopheryl acetates) were administered to normal humans (Leonard et al., 2005b), plasma d_6-α-CEHC concentrations were below levels of detection for all subjects at all time points. Rates of plasma γ–CEHC and γ–tocopherol disappearance were not different from each other and were much faster than α–tocopherol disappearance (Leonard et al., 2005b). These studies confirm that vitamin E metabolism is important in discriminating between various tocopherols and tocotrienols and is thus a key regulator of vitamin E bioavailability.

Vitamin E metabolism is mediated by cytochrome P450s (CYPs), in that the tocopherols or tocotrienols are initially ω-oxidized by CYPs, then following β-oxidation are conjugated with sulfate or glucuronide and excreted in urine or bile (Brigelius-Flohé and Traber, 1999). CYP4F2 has been demonstrated to be the major P450 enzyme involved in the ω-oxidation of vitamin E (Sontag and Parker, 2002, 2007). However, there is cross-talk between the P450 enzymes, and CYP3A may also play a role when liver vitamin E concentrations are particularly high (Traber, 2010). The subsequent β-oxidation of the metabolite has been localized to the mitochondria (Mustacich et al., 2010). Sulfation may be an important early step in intracellular trafficking to guide vitamin E metabolism, or at least γ-tocopherol metabolism. Sulfated-γ-CEHC is the major CEHC conjugate both in rats and in human cells in culture, and sulfated intermediates were found between 13′-OH-γ-tocopherol and γ-CEHC (Jiang et al., 2007; Freiser and Jiang, 2009a,b). Intermediates of γ-tocopherol metabolism, including 9-COOH, 11-COOH, 13-COOH, and 13-OH-γ-tocopherol, have been identified using a novel mass spectrometric approach (Yang et al., 2010).

Because of their rapid metabolism, orally administered γ-tocopherol or tocotrienols are not very effective at raising their own plasma and tissue concentrations (Khanna et al., 2005; Patel et al., 2006). In humans, Wiser et al. (2008) used a γ-tocopherol-rich preparation (containing 623 mg γ-tocopherol, 61.1 mg α-tocopherol, 11.1 mg β-tocopherol, and 231 mg of d-δ-tocopherol per capsule). Taken daily for 2 weeks this preparation raised plasma γ-tocopherol concentrations to nearly those of α-tocopherol, but, within 1 week of stopping the dosing, γ-tocopherol concentrations returned to baseline. Therefore, to take advantage of the possibility that γ-tocopherol could scavenge reactive nitrogen species, nebulized tocopherols have been used in lung studies (Hamahata et al., 2008).

Deficiency

Although rare, overt vitamin E deficiency occurs in humans as a result of genetic abnormalities in α–TTP or lipoprotein synthesis and as a result of various fat malabsorption syndromes (Traber, 1999). Vitamin E deficiency occurs secondary to fat malabsorption because vitamin E absorption requires biliary and pancreatic secretions (Traber, 1999).

The large-caliber myelinated axons in peripheral sensory nerves are the predominant target tissue in vitamin E deficiency in humans. A progressive peripheral neuropathy is observed with a dying back of the large-caliber axons in the sensory neurons (Sokol, 1993). In deficient humans, axonal degeneration rather than demyelination is the primary sensory nerve abnormality (Traber et al., 1987; Sokol et al., 1988). Thus, the axons degenerate first, then demyelination occurs.

Genetic defects in α–TTP are associated with a characteristic syndrome, ataxia with vitamin E deficiency, AVED (Ben Hamida, C. et al., 1993; Ben Hamida, M. et al., 1993; Doerflinger et al., 1995; Ouahchi et al., 1995). The

ataxia observed in these patients has also been mimicked in α–TTP-null mice (Yokota et al., 2001).

AVED patients have extraordinarily low plasma vitamin E concentrations (as low as 1/100 of normal), but if they are given vitamin E supplements, plasma concentrations reach normal within hours (Sokol et al., 1988). A dose of 800–1200 mg/day is usually sufficient to prevent further deterioration of neurologic function, and in some cases improvements have been noted (Sokol, 1993; Gabsi et al., 2001). Post-mortem analysis of an AVED patient demonstrated that vitamin E supplementation did allow brain vitamin E accumulation and prevention of Purkinje cell loss (Yokota et al., 2000). If supplementation is halted, plasma vitamin E concentrations fall within days to deficient levels. The biochemical defect in AVED patients, shown using deuterated tocopherols, demonstrated that hepatic α–TTP is required to maintain plasma RRR-α–tocopherol concentrations (Traber et al., 1990b, 1993) via secretion in VLDL. Over 20 mutations have been identified in patients with AVED (Di Donato et al., 2010).

Chronic Disease Protection and Public Health Implications

Given that vitamin E deficiency is very rare and that the vitamin E intakes of most Americans are very much less than their estimated requirements, the question arises as to whether the dietary α-tocopherol recommendations are too high. Conversely, given the potential for adverse effects, is there benefit to vitamin E supplements? The questions would be easier to answer if there were specific metabolic pathways that required vitamin E such that a marginal deficiency could be defined. Certainly, signaling pathways and specific genes have been identified that are altered by low or high α-tocopherol concentrations (Azzi et al., 2004), but there is no consensus concerning such "molecular" effects and they are difficult to separate from changes in oxidative stress-dependent mechanisms (Saito et al., 2010). One area of particular importance is that of impaired immune function in the elderly, which can be improved with vitamin E supplementation (Meydani et al., 2004). Again, it is not clear if the elderly are an example of long-term sub-optimal intakes of vitamin E that allow increased oxidative stress to alter T-cell function. Similarly, aged patients with eye disease (macular degeneration) were benefited by a supplement cocktail that included vitamin E (Age-Related Eye Disease Study Research Group, 2001). Eyes are an extension of the nervous system, and vitamin E is particularly necessary for the maintenance of normal nerve function. It is therefore interesting that vitamin E supplements were associated with a decreased risk of amyotrophic lateral sclerosis (Ascherio *et al.*, 2005) and that supplements have been reported to delay progression of Alzheimer disease (Sano *et al.*, 1997). However, meta-analysis of vitamin E intervention trials in Alzheimer disease have not found a benefit of vitamin E supplements in prevention of the onset of the disease (Isaac *et al.*, 2008).

Oxidative stress increases plasma vitamin E disappearance in endurance exercise (Mastaloudis *et al.*, 2001) and in cigarette smokers (Bruno *et al.*, 2005). Thus, increased oxidative stress might increase chronic disease risk; however, measures of oxidative stress are frequently not obtained. Vitamin E supplements have decreased heart-attack risk in subjects with demonstrably inadequate antioxidant protection. For example, haptoglobin 2-2 genotype results in a dysfunctional protein and causes increased oxidation by free heme (Levy *et al.*, 2010). In a placebo-controlled study carried out in diabetics who have the haptoglobin 2-2 genotype, daily vitamin E supplementation (400 IU) reduced cardiovascular events (Milman *et al.*, 2008). Additionally, haptoglobin 2-2 genotype subjects are more susceptible to vitamin C deficiency as a result of impaired haptoglobin antioxidant function (Cahill and El-Sohemy, 2010). The lower vitamin C status may also increase vitamin E depletion (Bruno *et al.*, 2005, 2006a).

Taken together these findings suggest that long-term sub-optimal vitamin E intakes will indeed allow the accumulation of oxidative damage. Certainly, it is generally agreed that chronic diseases are associated with increased, accumulated, oxidative damage (Institute of Medicine, 2000). What remains an open question is whether vitamin E supplements in excess of daily requirements will decrease the risk of chronic disease. Although many vitamin E supplementation studies carried out in patients with various kinds of chronic diseases have failed to show benefit, these studies have largely attempted to reverse existing disease. The question as to whether increased oxidative stress as a result of suboptimal vitamin E intakes increases the risk of chronic disease has not yet been answered. However, a follow-up study of the Alpha-Tocopherol Beta-Carotene Cancer Prevention trial showed (Wright *et al.*, 2006) that men in the

higher quintiles of serum α-tocopherol had significantly lower risks of total and cause-specific mortality than did those in the lowest quintile (relative risk [RR] = 0.82 [95% CI: 0.78, 0.86] for total mortality and 0.79 [0.72, 0.86], 0.81 [0.75, 0.88], and 0.70 [0.63, 0.79] for deaths due to cancer, cardiovascular disease, and other causes, respectively; P for trend for all <0.0001).

Importantly, these benefits were found for those subjects consuming 12 mg α-tocopherol daily, a level equivalent to the vitamin E EAR (Institute of Medicine, 2000).

Future Directions

Oxidative stress in humans more rapidly depletes plasma vitamin E (Bruno *et al.*, 2005, 2006a) and sufficient vitamin C intake counters the accelerated vitamin E depletion (Bruno *et al.*, 2006a). In response to oxidative stressors, vitamin E can decrease biomarkers of lipid peroxidation, is itself sacrificed, and requires optimal vitamin C status to function most effectively. Thus, adequate vitamin E intakes are clearly needed, but what is adequate, and for what function, have yet to be defined. Studies are needed to define why humans require vitamin E and how much they need. Vitamin E kinetic studies will allow determination of key measures of vitamin E status including fractional absorption, rates of delivery to tissues, and whole-body efflux. Hypothetically, the delivery of α-tocopherol to the target tissues will be increased if ascorbic acid is limiting, or if oxidative stress is high in those tissues.

Additionally, we are learning that there are certain genetic abnormalities that lead to increased vitamin E requirements. It is becoming increasingly apparent that each individual's "nutrigenomic biome" may have important consequences for nutrient requirements. Personalized nutrition will require the recognition of factors that alter needs. A biomarker for vitamin E status has yet to be defined; moreover, we do not have any specific indicators of vitamin E function that might be altered in health or disease.

Acknowledgment

This work was supported in part by a grant to MGT (NIH DK081761).

Suggestions for Further Reading

Biesalski, H.K., Grune, T., Tinz, J., *et al.* (2010) Reexamination of a meta-analysis of the effect of antioxidant supplementation on mortality and health in randomized trials. *Nutrients* **2**, 929–949.

Di Donato, I., Bianchi, S., and Federico, A. (2010) Ataxia with vitamin E deficiency: update of molecular diagnosis. *Neurol Sci* **31**, 511–515.

Morley, S., Cecchini, M., Zhang, W., *et al.* (2008) Mechanisms of ligand transfer by the hepatic tocopherol transfer protein. *J Biol Chem* **283**, 17797–17804.

Traber, M.G. (2010) Regulation of xenobiotic metabolism, the only signaling function of alpha-tocopherol? *Mol Nutr Food Res* **54**, 661–668.

References

Age-Related Eye Disease Study Research Group (2001) A randomized, placebo-controlled, clinical trial of high-dose supplementation with vitamins C and E, beta carotene, and zinc for age-related macular degeneration and vision loss: AREDS Report No. 8. *Arch Ophthalmol* **119**, 1417–1436.

Arita, M., Nomura, K., Arai, H., *et al.* (1997) Alpha-tocopherol transfer protein stimulates the secretion of alpha-tocopherol from a cultured liver cell line through a brefeldin A-insensitive pathway. *Proc Natl Acad Sci USA* **94**, 12437–12441.

Ascherio, A., Weisskopf, M.G., O'Reilly E, J., *et al.* (2005) Vitamin E intake and risk of amyotrophic lateral sclerosis. *Ann Neurol* **57**, 104–110.

Azzi, A., Gysin, R., Kempna, P., *et al.* (2004) Regulation of gene expression by alpha-tocopherol. *Biol Chem* **385**, 585–591.

Babaev, V.R., Li, L., Shah, S., *et al.* (2010) Combined vitamin C and vitamin E deficiency worsens early atherosclerosis in apolipoprotein E-deficient mice. *Arterioscler Thromb Vasc Biol* **30**, 1751–1757.

Ben Hamida, C., Doerflinger, N., Belal, S., *et al.* (1993) Localization of Friedreich ataxia phenotype with selective vitamin E deficiency to chromosome 8q by homozygosity mapping. *Nature Genet* **5**, 195–200.

Ben Hamida, M., Bilal, S., Sirugo, G., *et al.* (1993) Friedreich's ataxia phenotype not linked to chromosome 9 and associated with selective autosomal recessive vitamin E deficiency in two inbred Tunisian families. *Neurology* **43**, 2179–2183.

Berry, D., Wathen, J.K., and Newell, M. (2009) Bayesian model averaging in meta-analysis: vitamin E supplementation and mortality. *Clin Trials* **6**, 28–41.

Biesalski, H.K., Grune, T., Tinz, J., *et al.* (2010) Reexamination of a meta-analysis of the effect of antioxidant supplementation

on mortality and health in randomized trials. *Nutrients* **2**, 929–949.

Bjelakovic, G., Nikolova, D., Gluud, L.L., *et al.* (2007) Mortality in randomized trials of antioxidant supplements for primary and secondary prevention: systematic review and meta-analysis. *JAMA* **297**, 842–857.

Blumberg, J., Heaney, R.P., Huncharek, M., *et al.* (2010) Evidence-based criteria in the nutritional context. *Nutr Rev* **68**, 478–484.

Brigelius-Flohé, R. and Traber, M.G. (1999) Vitamin E: function and metabolism. *FASEB J* **13**, 1145–1155.

Brown, B.G., Zhao, X.Q., Chait, A., *et al.* (2001) Simvastatin and niacin, antioxidant vitamins, or the combination for the prevention of coronary disease. *N Engl J Med* **345**, 1583–1592.

Bruno, R.S., Leonard, S.W., Atkinson, J.K., *et al.* (2006a) Faster vitamin E disappearance in smokers is normalized by vitamin C supplementation. *Free Radic Biol Med* **40**, 689–697.

Bruno, R.S., Leonard, S.W., Park, S.-I., *et al.* (2006b) Human vitamin E requirements assessed with the use of apples fortified with deuterium-labeled α-tocopheryl acetate. *Am J Clin Nutr* **83**, 299–304.

Bruno, R.S., Ramakrishnan, R., Montine, T.J., *et al.* (2005) α-Tocopherol disappearance is faster in cigarette smokers and is inversely related to their ascorbic acid status. *Am J Clin Nutr* **81**, 95–103.

Buettner, G.R. (1993) The pecking order of free radicals and antioxidants: lipid peroxidation, alpha-tocopherol, and ascorbate. *Arch Biochem Biophys* **300**, 535–543.

Burk, R.F., Christensen, J.M., Maguire, M.J., *et al.* (2006) A combined deficiency of vitamins E and C causes severe central nervous system damage in guinea pigs. *J Nutr* **136**, 1576–1581.

Burton, G.W., Traber, M.G., Acuff, R.V., *et al.* (1998) Human plasma and tissue alpha-tocopherol concentrations in response to supplementation with deuterated natural and synthetic vitamin E. *Am J Clin Nutr* **67**, 669–684.

Butterfield, D.A., Bader Lange, M.L., and Sultana, R. (2010) Involvements of the lipid peroxidation product, HNE, in the pathogenesis and progression of Alzheimer's disease. *Biochim Biophys Acta* **1801**, 924–929.

Cahill, L.E. and El-Sohemy, A. (2010) Haptoglobin genotype modifies the association between dietary vitamin C and serum ascorbic acid deficiency. *Am J Clin Nutr* **92**, 1494–1500.

Cheeseman, K.H., Holley, A.E., Kelly, F.J., *et al.* (1995) Biokinetics in humans of RRR-alpha-tocopherol: the free phenol, acetate ester, and succinate ester forms of vitamin E. *Free Radic Biol Med* **19**, 591–598.

Di Donato, I., Bianchi, S., and Federico, A. (2010) Ataxia with vitamin E deficiency: update of molecular diagnosis. *Neurol Sci* **31**, 511–515.

Doerflinger, N., Linder, C., Ouahchi, K., *et al.* (1995) Ataxia with vitamin E deficiency: refinement of genetic localization and analysis of linkage disequilibrium by using new markers in 14 families. *Am J Hum Genet* **56**, 1116–1124.

Eitenmiller, R. and Lee, J. (2004) *Vitamin E: Food Chemistry, Composition, and Analysis*. Marcel Dekker, New York.

Evans, H.M. and Bishop, K.S. (1922) On the existence of a hitherto unrecognized dietary factor essential for reproduction. *Science* **56**, 650–651.

Expert Group on Vitamins and Minerals (2003) Risk assessment: vitamin E. In M.J.S. Langman (ed.), *Safe Upper Levels for Vitamins and Minerals*. Food Standards Agency, London. www.food.gov.uk/multimedia/pdfs/vitmin2003.pdf

FAO (2004) Vitamin E. In K. Tontisirin and G. Clugston (eds), *Vitamin and Mineral Requirements in Human Nutrition*, 2nd Edn. World Health Organization, Geneva, pp. 94–107.

Food and Drug Administration (2009) 14, Appendix F: Calculate the Percent Daily Value for the Appropriate Nutrients. Guidance for Industry; A Food Labeling Guide. http://www.fda.gov/Food/GuidanceComplianceRegulatoryInformation/GuidanceDocuments/FoodLabelingNutrition/FoodLabelingGuide/ucm064928.htm. Jan 2, 2011.

Frank, J., Lee, S., Leonard, S.W., *et al.* (2008) Sex differences in the inhibition of γ-tocopherol metabolism by a single dose of dietary sesame oil in healthy subjects *Am J Clin Nutr* **87**, 1723–1729.

Freedman, J.E., Li, L., Sauter, R., *et al.* (2000) Alpha-tocopherol and protein kinase C inhibition enhance platelet-derived nitric oxide release. *FASEB J* **14**, 2377–2379.

Freiser, H. and Jiang, Q. (2009a) Gamma-tocotrienol and gamma-tocopherol are primarily metabolized to conjugated 2-(beta-carboxyethyl)-6-hydroxy-2,7,8-trimethylchroman and sulfated long-chain carboxychromanols in rats. *J Nutr*, **139**, 884–889.

Freiser, H. and Jiang, Q. (2009b) Optimization of the enzymatic hydrolysis and analysis of plasma conjugated gamma-CEHC and sulfated long-chain carboxychromanols, metabolites of vitamin E. *Anal Biochem* **388**, 260–265.

Gabsi, S., Gouider-Khouja, N., Belal, S., *et al.* (2001) Effect of vitamin E supplementation in patients with ataxia with vitamin E deficiency. *Eur J Neurol* **8**, 477–481.

Glynn, R.J., Ridker, P.M., Goldhaber, S.Z., *et al.* (2007) Effects of random allocation to vitamin E supplementation on the occurrence of venous thromboembolism: report from the Women's Health Study. *Circulation* **116**, 1497–1503.

Goti, D., Balazs, Z., Panzenboeck, U., *et al.* (2002) Effects of lipoprotein lipase on uptake and transcytosis of low density lipoprotein (LDL) and LDL-associated alpha-tocopherol in a porcine in vitro blood–brain barrier model. *J Biol Chem* **277**, 28537–28544.

Hamahata, A., Enkhbaatar, P., Kraft, E.R., *et al.* (2008) gamma-Tocopherol nebulization by a lipid aerosolization device improves pulmonary function in sheep with burn and smoke inhalation injury. *Free Radic Biol Med* **45**, 425–433.

Hathcock, J.N., Azzi, A., Blumberg, J., *et al.* (2005) Vitamins E and C are safe across a broad range of intakes. *Am J Clin Nutr* **81**, 736–745.

Hui, D.Y., Labonte, E.D., and Howles, P.N. (2008) Development and physiological regulation of intestinal lipid absorption. III. Intestinal transporters and cholesterol absorption. *Am J Physiol Gastrointest Liver Physiol* **294**, G839–843.

Institute of Medicine (2000) *Dietary Reference Intakes for Vitamin C, Vitamin E, Selenium, and Carotenoids*. Food and Nutrition Board and Institute of Medicine. National Academy Press, Washington, DC.

Isaac, M.G., Quinn, R., and Tabet, N. (2008) Vitamin E for Alzheimer's disease and mild cognitive impairment. *Cochrane Database Syst Rev* CD002854.

Iuliano, L., Micheletta, F., Maranghi, M., *et al.* (2001) Bioavailability of vitamin E as function of food intake in healthy subjects: effects on plasma peroxide-scavenging activity and cholesterol-oxidation products. *Arterioscler Thromb Vasc Biol* **21**, E34–37.

Jiang, Q., Freiser, H., Wood, K.V., *et al.* (2007) Identification and quantitation of novel vitamin E metabolites, sulfated long-chain carboxychromanols, in human A549 cells and in rats. *J Lipid Res* **48**, 1221–1230.

Kaempf-Rotzoll, D.E., Horiguchi, M., Hashiguchi, K., *et al.* (2003) Human placental trophoblast cells express alpha-tocopherol transfer protein. *Placenta* **24**, 439–444.

Kaempf-Rotzoll, D.E., Igarashi, K., Aoki, J., *et al.* (2002) Alpha-tocopherol transfer protein is specifically localized at the implantation site of pregnant mouse uterus. *Biol Reprod* **67**, 599–604.

Khanna, S., Patel, V., Rink, C., *et al.* (2005) Delivery of orally supplemented alpha-tocotrienol to vital organs of rats and tocopherol-transport protein deficient mice. *Free Radic Biol Med* **39**, 1310–1319.

Leonard, S.W., Good, C.K., Gugger, E.T., *et al.* (2004) Vitamin E bioavailability from fortified breakfast cereal is greater than that from encapsulated supplements. *Am J Clin Nutr* **79**, 86–92.

Leonard, S.W., Gumpricht, E., Devereaux, M.W., *et al.* (2005a) Quantitation of rat liver vitamin E metabolites by LC-MS during high-dose vitamin E administration. *J Lipid Res* **46**, 1068–1075.

Leonard, S.W., Joss, J.D., Mustacich, D.J., et al. (2007) Effects of vitamin E on cholesterol levels of hypercholesterolemic patients receiving statins. Am J Health-System Pharm **64**, 2257–2266.

Leonard, S.W., Paterson, E., Atkinson, J.K., et al. (2005b) Studies in humans using deuterium-labeled alpha- and gamma-tocopherol demonstrate faster plasma gamma-tocopherol disappearance and greater gamma-metabolite production. Free Radic Biol Med **38**, 857–866.

Levy, A.P., Asleh, R., Blum, S., et al. (2010) Haptoglobin: basic and clinical aspects. Antioxid Redox Signal **12**, 293–304.

Li, C.J., Li, R.W., and Elsasser, T.H. (2010) Alpha-tocopherol modulates transcriptional activities that affect essential biological processes in bovine cells. Gene Regul Syst Biol **4**, 109–124.

Liebler, D.C., Burr, J.A., Philips, L., et al. (1996) Gas chromatography–mass spectrometry analysis of vitamin E and its oxidation products. Anal Biochem **236**, 27–34.

Lonn, E., Bosch, J., Yusuf, S., et al. (2005) Effects of long-term vitamin E supplementation on cardiovascular events and cancer: a randomized controlled trial. JAMA **293**, 1338–1347.

Macevilly, C.J. and Muller, D.P. (1996) Lipid peroxidation in neural tissues and fractions from vitamin E-deficient rats. Free Radic Biol Med **20**, 639–648.

Maras, J.E., Bermudez, O.I., Qiao, N., et al. (2004) Intake of alpha-tocopherol is limited among US adults. J Am Diet Assoc **104**, 567–575.

Mardones, P., Quinones, V., Amigo, L., et al. (2001) Hepatic cholesterol and bile acid metabolism and intestinal cholesterol absorption in scavenger receptor class B type I-deficient mice. J Lipid Res **42**, 170–180.

Mardones, P., Strobel, P., Miranda, S., et al. (2002) Alpha-tocopherol metabolism is abnormal in scavenger receptor class B type I (SR-BI)-deficient mice. J Nutr **132**, 443–449.

Mastaloudis, A., Leonard, S.W., and Traber, M.G. (2001) Oxidative stress in athletes during extreme endurance exercise. Free Radic Biol Med **31**, 911–922.

Meier, R., Tomizaki, T., Schulze-Briese, C., et al. (2003) The molecular basis of vitamin E retention: structure of human alpha-tocopherol transfer protein. J Mol Biol **331**, 725–734.

Meydani, S.N., Leka, L.S., Fine, B.C., et al. (2004) Vitamin E and respiratory tract infections in elderly nursing home residents: a randomized controlled trial. JAMA **292**, 828–836.

Miller, E.R., 3rd, Paston-Barriuso, R., Dalal, D., et al. (2005) Meta-analysis: high-dosage vitamin E supplementation may increase all-cause mortality. Ann Intern Med **142**, 37–46.

Milman, U., Blum, S., Shapira, C., et al. (2008) Vitamin E supplementation reduces cardiovascular events in a subgroup of middle-aged individuals with both Type 2 diabetes mellitus and the haptoglobin 2-2 genotype. A prospective double-blinded clinical trial. Arterioscler Thromb Vasc Biol **28**, 1–7.

Min, K.C., Kovall, R.A., and Hendrickson, W.A. (2003) Crystal structure of human alpha-tocopherol transfer protein bound to its ligand: implications for ataxia with vitamin E deficiency. Proc Natl Acad Sci USA **100**, 14713–14718.

Morley, S., Cecchini, M., Zhang, W., et al. (2008) Mechanisms of ligand transfer by the hepatic tocopherol transfer protein. J Biol Chem **283**, 17797–17804.

Muller-Schmehl, K., Beninde, J., Finckh, B., et al. (2004) Localization of alpha-tocopherol transfer protein in trophoblast, fetal capillaries' endothelium and amnion epithelium of human term placenta. Free Radic Res **38**, 413–420.

Mustacich, D.J., Shields, J., Horton, R.A., et al. (1998) Biliary secretion of alpha-tocopherol and the role of the mdr2 P-glycoprotein in rats and mice. Arch Biochem Biophys **350**, 183–192.

Mustacich, D.J., Leonard, S.W., Patel, N.K., et al. (2010) Alpha-tocopherol beta-oxidation localized to rat liver mitochondria. Free Radic Biol Med **48**, 73–81.

Narushima, K., Takada, T., Yamanashi, Y., et al. (2008) Niemann-Pick C1-like 1 mediates alpha-tocopherol transport. Mol Pharmacol **74**, 42–49.

Netscher, T. (2007) Synthesis of vitamin E. Vitam Horm **76**, 155–202.

Neuzil, J., Weber, T., Schroder, A., et al. (2001) Induction of cancer cell apoptosis by alpha-tocopheryl succinate: molecular pathways and structural requirements. FASEB J **15**, 403–415.

Nozawa, M., Takahashi, K., Kato, K., et al. (2000) Enantioselective synthesis of (2R,4′R,8′R)-alpha-tocopherol (vitamin E) based on enzymatic function. Chem Pharm Bull (Tokyo) **48**, 272–277.

Oram, J.F., Vaughan, A.M., and Stocker, R. (2001) ATP-binding cassette transporter A1 mediates cellular secretion of alpha-tocopherol. J Biol Chem **276**, 39898–39902.

Ouahchi, K., Arita, M., Kayden, H., et al. (1995) Ataxia with isolated vitamin E deficiency is caused by mutations in the alpha-tocopherol transfer protein. Nature Genet **9**, 141–145.

Panagabko, C., Morley, S., Hernandez, M., et al. (2003) Ligand specificity in the CRAL-TRIO protein family. Biochemistry **42**, 6467–6474.

Patel, V., Khanna, S., Roy, S., et al. (2006) Natural vitamin E alpha-tocotrienol: retention in vital organs in response to long-term oral supplementation and withdrawal. Free Radic Res **40**, 763–771.

Rotzoll, D.E., Scherling, R., Etzl, R., et al. (2008) Immunohistochemical localization of alpha-tocopherol transfer protein and lipoperoxidation products in human first-trimester and term placenta. Eur J Obstet Gynecol Reprod Biol **140**, 183–191.

Saito, Y., Nishio, K., Akazawa, Y.O., *et al.* (2010) Cytoprotective effect of vitamin E homologues against glutamate-induced cell death in immature primary cortical neuron cultures: tocopherols and tocotrienols exert similar effects by antioxidant function. *Free Radic Biol Med* **49**, 1542–1549.

Sano, M., Ernesto, C., Thomas, R.G., *et al.* (1997) A controlled trial of selegiline, alpha-tocopherol, or both as treatment for Alzheimer's disease. The Alzheimer's Disease Cooperative Study. *N Engl J Med* **336**, 1216–1222.

Sokol, R.J. (1993) Vitamin E deficiency and neurological disorders. In L. Packer and J. Fuchs (eds), *Vitamin E in Health and Disease*. Marcel Dekker, New York, pp. 815–849.

Sokol, R.J., Kayden, H.J., Bettis, D.B., *et al.* (1988) Isolated vitamin E deficiency in the absence of fat malabsorption – familial and sporadic cases: characterization and investigation of causes. *J Lab Clin Med* **111**, 548–559.

Sontag, T.J. and Parker, R.S. (2002) Cytochrome P450 omega-hydroxylase pathway of tocopherol catabolism: Novel mechanism of regulation of vitamin E status. *J Biol Chem* **277**, 25290–25296.

Sontag, T.J. and Parker, R.S. (2007) Influence of major structural features of tocopherols and tocotrienols on their omega-oxidation by tocopherol-omega-hydroxylase. *J Lipid Res* **48**, 1090–1098.

Steiner, M. (1981) Vitamin E changes the membrane fluidity of human platelets. *Biochim Biophys Acta* **640**, 100–105.

Steiner, M. and Anastasi, J. (1976) Vitamin E. An inhibitor of the platelet release reaction. *J Clin Invest* **57**, 732–737.

Terasawa, Y., Ladha, Z., Leonard, S.W., *et al.* (2000) Increased atherosclerosis in hyperlipidemic mice deficient in alpha-tocopherol transfer protein and vitamin E. *Proc Natl Acad Sci USA* **97**, 13830–13834.

Thomas, S.R. and Stocker, R. (2000) Molecular action of vitamin E in lipoprotein oxidation: implications for atherosclerosis. *Free Radic Biol Med* **28**, 1795–1805.

Tiwary, R., Yu, W., Sanders, B.G., *et al.* (2010) Alpha-TEA cooperates with MEK or mTOR inhibitors to induce apoptosis via targeting IRS/PI3K pathways. *Br J Cancer* **104**, 101–109.

Traber, M.G. (1999) Vitamin E. In M.E. Shils, J.A. Olson, M. Shike *et al.* (eds), *Modern Nutrition in Health and Disease*. Williams and Wilkins, Baltimore, pp. 347–362.

Traber, M.G. (2004) Vitamin E, nuclear receptors and xenobiotic metabolism. *Arch Biochem Biophys* **423**, 6–11.

Traber, M.G. (2010) Regulation of xenobiotic metabolism, the only signaling function of alpha-tocopherol? *Mol Nutr Food Res* **54**, 661–668.

Traber, M.G. and Atkinson, J. (2007) Vitamin E, antioxidant and nothing more. *Free Radic Biol Med*, **43**, 4–15.

Traber, M.G., Ramakrishnan, R., and Kayden, H.J. (1994) Human plasma vitamin E kinetics demonstrate rapid recycling of plasma *RRR*-α-tocopherol. *Proc Natl Acad Sci USA* **91**, 10005–10008.

Traber, M.G., Rudel, L.L., Burton, G.W., *et al.* (1990a) Nascent VLDL from liver perfusions of cynomolgus monkeys are preferentially enriched in *RRR*- compared with *SRR*-α tocopherol: studies using deuterated tocopherols. *J Lipid Res* **31**, 687–694.

Traber, M.G., Sokol, R.J., Burton, G.W., *et al.* (1990b) Impaired ability of patients with familial isolated vitamin E deficiency to incorporate alpha-tocopherol into lipoproteins secreted by the liver. *J Clin Invest* **85**, 397–407.

Traber, M.G., Sokol, R.J., Kohlschütter, A., *et al.* (1993) Impaired discrimination between stereoisomers of α-tocopherol in patients with familial isolated vitamin E deficiency. *J Lipid Res* **34**, 201–210.

Traber, M.G., Sokol, R.J., Ringel, S.P., *et al.* (1987) Lack of tocopherol in peripheral nerves of vitamin E-deficient patients with peripheral neuropathy. *N Engl J Med* **317**, 262–265.

Wang, X.F., Xie, Y., Wang, H.G., *et al.* (2010) Alpha-tocopheryl succinate induces apoptosis in erbB2-expressing breast cancer cell via NF-kappaB pathway. *Acta Pharmacol Sin* **31**, 1604–1610.

Waters, D.D., Alderman, E.L., Hsia, J., *et al.* (2002) Effects of hormone replacement therapy and antioxidant vitamin supplements on coronary atherosclerosis in postmenopausal women: a randomized controlled trial. *JAMA* **288**, 2432–2440.

Werba, J.P., Cavalca, V., Veglia, F., *et al.* (2007) A new compound-specific pleiotropic effect of statins: modification of plasma gamma-tocopherol levels. *Atherosclerosis* **193**, 229–233.

West, R., Panagabko, C., and Atkinson, J. (2010) Synthesis and characterization of BODIPY-alpha-tocopherol: a fluorescent form of vitamin E. *J Org Chem* **75**, 2883–2892.

Wiser, J., Alexis, N.E., Jiang, Q., *et al.* (2008) In vivo gamma-tocopherol supplementation decreases systemic oxidative stress and cytokine responses of human monocytes in normal and asthmatic subjects. *Free Radic Biol Med* **45**, 40–49.

Witt, W., Kolleck, I., Fechner, H., *et al.* (2000) Regulation by vitamin E of the scavenger receptor BI in rat liver and HepG2 cells. *J Lipid Res* **41**, 2009–2016.

Wright, M.E., Lawson, K.A., Weinstein, S.J., *et al.* (2006) Higher baseline serum concentrations of vitamin E are associated with lower total and cause-specific mortality in the Alpha-Tocopherol, Beta-Carotene Cancer Prevention Study. *Am J Clin Nutr* **84**, 1200–1207.

Yang, W.C., Regnier, F.E., Jiang, Q., *et al.* (2010) In vitro stable isotope labeling for discovery of novel metabolites by liquid chromatography-mass spectrometry: confirmation of gamma-tocopherol metabolism in human A549 cell. *J Chromatogr A*, **1217**, 667–675.

Yokota, T., Uchihara, T., Kumagai, J., *et al.* (2000) Postmortem study of ataxia with retinitis pigmentosa by mutation of the alpha-tocopherol transfer protein gene. *J Neurol Neurosurg Psychiatry* **68**, 521–525.

Yokota, T., Igarashi, K., Uchihara, T., *et al.* (2001) Delayed-onset ataxia in mice lacking alpha-tocopherol transfer protein: model for neuronal degeneration caused by chronic oxidative stress. *Proc Natl Acad Sci USA* **98**, 15185–15190.

Yu, W., Sanders, B.G., and Kline, K. (2003) RRR-alpha-tocopheryl succinate-induced apoptosis of human breast cancer cells involves Bax translocation to mitochondria. *Cancer Res* **63**, 2483–2491.

15

VITAMIN K

GUYLAINE FERLAND, PhD

Université de Montréal, Montréal, Québec, Canada

Summary

Historically discovered for its role in blood coagulation, vitamin K is emerging as a vitamin of wide-ranging physiological implications. Whether through the vitamin K-dependent protein family or specific K vitamers, vitamin K is now known to be involved in bone and cardiovascular metabolism, cell proliferation, brain function, and energy metabolism. In this chapter we will go over the most recent scientific literature relating to vitamin K and point to ongoing and future research efforts.

Introduction

The history of vitamin K dates back to 1929 when, as part of his work on sterol metabolism, Henrik Dam observed that chicks fed fat-free diets developed subcutaneous hemorrhages and anemia. Further work by Dam determined that the antihemorrhagic substance was fat soluble and occurred in extracts of liver and various plant tissues. In 1935 Dam named this new substance vitamin K. By 1939 the two naturally occurring forms of the vitamin – vitamin K_1 and vitamin K_2 – had been isolated from alfalfa and putrefied fish meal, respectively (Suttie, 2009). In 1941 the first vitamin K antagonist was discovered when a new substance identified in spoiled sweet clover hay had been reported to cause hemorrhagic disease in cattle in the US and western Canada in the 1920s. This substance, 3,3'-methyl-bis-(4-hydroxycoumarin), later became known as dicoumarol. In the period after the discovery

of dicoumarol, several derivatives of coumarin were synthesized for use as clinical agents in anticoagulant therapy. One of these, warfarin (3-[a-acetonyl-benzyl]-4-hydroxycoumarin), has been used successfully as a clinical agent since 1941. Access to vitamin K antagonists eventually helped specify the role of vitamin K in blood coagulation and proved to be invaluable to vitamin K research in general.

Although the bleeding condition reported by Dam was originally associated with decreased prothrombin (Factor II) activity, it was later established that three other coagulation proteins (factors VII, IX, and X) were also depressed in vitamin K deficiency states. For many years this participation in blood coagulation was assumed to be the sole physiological role for vitamin K. However, the discovery in the early 1970s of γ-carboxyglutamic acid (Gla), a new amino acid common to all vitamin K proteins, later led to the discovery of additional vitamin K-dependent proteins

Present Knowledge in Nutrition, Tenth Edition. Edited by John W. Erdman Jr, Ian A. Macdonald and Steven H. Zeisel.
© 2012 International Life Sciences Institute. Published 2012 by John Wiley & Sons, Inc.

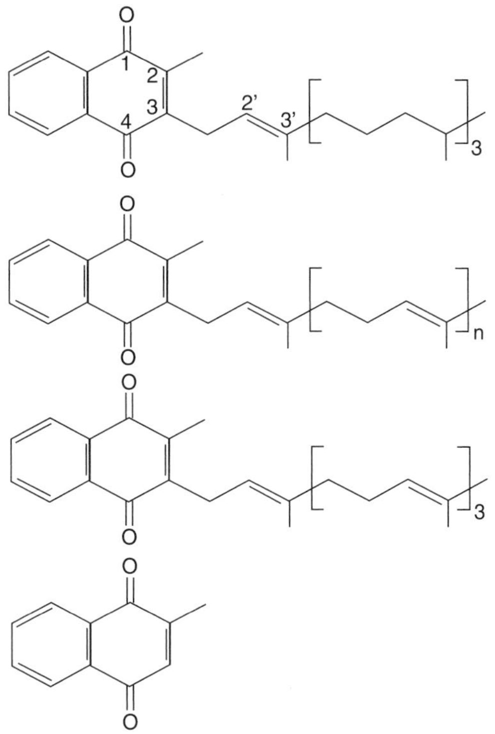

FIG. 15.1 Chemical structures of phylloquinone, the menaquinones, MK-4, and menadione.

not involved in hemostasis, and greatly contributed to our present understanding of the action of vitamin K at the molecular level. To this day, the participation of vitamin K in Gla synthesis remains the only well defined function of this vitamin (Berkner and Runge, 2004).

Chemistry and Nomenclature

Compounds with vitamin K activity have a common 2-methyl-1,4-naphthoquinone ring but differ in the structure at the 3-position. Vitamin K occurs naturally in two forms. Phylloquinone (2-methyl-3-phytyl-1,4-naphthoquinone; also referred to as vitamin K_1), is synthesized in plants and represents the main source of dietary vitamin K in Western countries (Institute of Medicine, 2001). Menaquinones (2-methyl-1,4-naphthoquinones; also referred to as vitamin K_2), are produced by bacteria and form a family of compounds with unsaturated isoprenyl side chains of varying length at the 3 position. The predominant forms of the menaquinone series contain 6–10 isoprenoid units, but menaquinones containing up to 13 units have been isolated (Suttie, 1995). One of the

menaquinones, MK-4, is not a common product of bacterial synthesis but is synthesized from phylloquinone with menadione as an intermediate (see later in this chapter). The parent structure of all K vitamins, 2-methyl-1,4 naphthoquinone, also called menadione or vitamin K_3, does not occur in nature but can be alkylated to MK-4 in avian and mammalian tissues. This synthetic form has been used as a source of vitamin K in a wide range of animal feeds (Suttie, 2009). The different K vitamers are illustrated in Figure 15.1.

Current methods to assess vitamin K in plasma, biological tissues, and foods are based on high performance liquid chromatography (HPLC). Vitamin K is first extracted from matrices with organic solvents, then by solid phase chromatography, before being selectively isolated by HPLC. Quantitation is usually achieved using fluorescence detection, and procedures enabling simultaneous determination of phylloquinone and the menaquinones have been developed and applied reliably (Davidson and Sadowski, 1997; Wang et al., 2004). Methods combining chromatographic and mass spectrometry techniques have also been developed and used in studies involving labeled phylloquinone (Ducros *et al.*, 2010). A vitamin K external quality assurance scheme (KEQAS) was recently established to assist in the harmonization of phylloquinone analysis among laboratories worldwide and to improve the comparability of clinical and nutritional studies (Card *et al.*, 2009). Finally, a method using HPLC was recently published for the measurement of menadione in urine (Al Rajabi *et al.*, 2010).

Absorption, Transport, Turnover, and Storage

Absorption/Bioavailability

Vitamin K is absorbed from the proximal intestine into the lymphatic system by a process that requires the presence of bile and pancreatic juices (Shearer *et al.*, 1974). Consequently, conditions interfering with these functions or associated with fat malabsorption will impair vitamin K absorption (Savage and Lindenbaum, 1983). In healthy adults, absorption of phylloquinone has been estimated to be ~80% when administered in its free form, but decreases significantly when it is absorbed from foods (Shearer *et al.*, 1974). When investigated using the area under an absorption curve, absorption of phylloquinone from spinach was found to be 4–17% that of phylloquinone from a suspension or a tablet (Gijsbers *et al.*, 1996; Garber *et al.*, 1999). A similar estimate was recently reported for phylloquinone from kale using compartmental modelling (Novotny *et al.*, 2010). Phylloquinone absorption from vegetables can be improved when consumed with fat (Gijsbers *et al.*, 1996) but absorption efficiency remains lower than when phylloquinone is being consumed in an oil form (Booth *et al.*, 2002). Moreover, a recent study that used stable isotope methodology suggests that absorption of phylloquinone is influenced by meal components (Jones *et al.*, 2009). Data for the menaquinones are more limited but when MK-4 was administered with butter (Gijsbers *et al.*, 1996) and MK-7 as part of the Japanese food natto (Schurgers and Vermeer, 2000), the bioavailability of these two vitamers was higher than that of phylloquinone from spinach.

Transport and Cellular Uptake

Absorbed phylloquinone is incorporated into chylomicrons and transported to the liver, where it is cleared from chylomicron remnants through an apolipoprotein E (apoE) receptor. Unlike other fat-soluble vitamins, vitamin K has no known carrier protein. In the circulation, phylloquinone is principally carried in triacylglycerol-rich lipo-

proteins (TGRLP; >50%) with each of the LDL and HDL fractions accounting for ~15% of the circulating vitamer (Lamon-Fava *et al.*, 1998; Erkkila *et al.*, 2004). This likely explains the strong positive correlation observed between circulating phylloquinone and triacylglycerols in various studies (Sadowski *et al.*, 1989; Azharuddin *et al.*, 2007). Data on the lipoprotein distribution of ingested menaquinones is more limited. In a comparative study that involved the administration of equimolar amounts of phylloquinone, MK-4 and MK-9, the menaquinones were associated with both the TGRLP and LDL fractions while MK-4 was also observed in the HDL fraction (Schurgers and Vermeer, 2002). This study also highlighted a much longer half-life time in the circulation for MK-9 compared with phylloquinone, a finding also observed for MK-7 (Schurgers *et al.*, 2007). Compared to the other fat-soluble vitamins, phylloquinone circulates in blood in very small concentrations, and a normal range of 0.25–2.7 nmol/L has been published by Sadowski *et al.* (1989). Fasting plasma phylloquinone has been linked to the genetic polymorphism of apolipoprotein E (apoE); however, results have been inconsistent, differing in healthy subjects and certain groups of patients (Kohlmeier *et al.*, 1995; Yan *et al.*, 2005). Normal ranges for menaquinones are not yet available. Uptake of phylloquinone into tissues including bone is deemed to be via clearance of chylomicron remnants by apoE. Furthermore, internalization of phylloquinone in osteoblasts appears to vary according to apoE genotype (Newman *et al.*, 2002). Cellular uptake of menaquinones has not been investigated specifically, but it was recently suggested that long-chain menaquinones could enter osteoblasts via the LDL receptor in light of their close association with this lipoprotein fraction (Shearer and Newman, 2008).

Catabolism and Turnover

Older studies that used pharmacological dosage protocols showed phylloquinone to be rapidly metabolized with about 20% being excreted in the urine and 40–50% excreted in the feces via the bile. Urinary vitamin K metabolites consist mainly of glucuronide conjugates of derivatives in which the phytyl side chain has been oxidized and cleaved. Biliary metabolites have not been clearly identified. A method for measuring two major urinary metabolites of phylloquinone, 5C- and 7C-aglycones, by HPLC with electrochemical detection in the redox mode, has been published (Harrington *et al.*, 2005) and used successfully in metabolic studies (Harrington *et al.*, 2010).

When consumed in physiological amounts, postprandial plasma phylloquinone concentration peaks after about 6 hours, returning to baseline by 24 hours (Erkkila *et al.*, 2004). This is in contrast to the long-chain menaquinones which remain in the circulation for much longer periods when ingested in similar quantities (up to 72 hours in the case of MK-7: Schurgers and Vermeer, 2000). Studies on the clearance kinetics of phylloquinone following an intravenous dose have been conducted using various approaches and point to a biphasic disappearance profile comprised of a rapid phase with a half-life of ~0.3 hour and a slower phase with a half-life of ~2.5 hours (Shearer *et al.*, 1974; Jones *et al.*, 2008). Other studies have reported slower clearance rates (Olson *et al.*, 2002; Novotny *et al.*, 2010) suggesting that other body pools of vitamin K, e.g. adipose tissue or bone, could turn over much more slowly. A detailed review of vitamin K metabolism has been published (Shearer and Newman, 2008).

Tissue Stores and Biosynthesis of MK-4

As the site of synthesis of the coagulation proteins, liver has traditionally been considered the main storage organ and consists of around 90% menaquinones, with MK-10 and MK-11 being particularly abundant, and 10% phylloquinone (Suttie, 2009). However, phylloquinone and the menaquinones are also present in extrahepatic tissues. In post-mortem specimens, phylloquinone concentrations in heart and pancreas were found to be comparable to that in liver while those in lung, kidney, and brain were much lower. Menaquinone-4 is also widely distributed and is present in tissues in variable amounts. In brain and kidney, for instance, MK-4 concentrations largely exceed those of phylloquinone whereas, in the pancreas, MK-4 and phylloquinone are present in comparable amounts (Thijssen and Drittij-Reijnders, 1996). Vitamin K is also present in bone, phylloquinone predominating over the menaquinones (MK-4 through MK-8) (Shearer and Newman, 2008).

The presence of MK-4 in tissues has been the object of investigation for over 50 years. It is only recently, however, that the origin of this menaquinone has been elucidated. It is now well established that MK-4, which is not a common product of bacterial synthesis, is synthesized from phylloquinone with menadione as an intermediate (Thijssen *et al.*, 2006). In a series of studies conducted in mice, data suggest that MK-4 in cerebra could originate from two sources: (1) phylloquinone following the release of menadione in the intestine and subsequent prenylation of mena-

dione in the cerebra, and (2) cleavage of phylloquinone and generation of menadione within the target cells followed by prenylation (Okano *et al.*, 2008). Very recently, this team established that the human UbiA prenyltransferase domain-containing protein 1 (UBIAD1) enzyme is responsible for MK-4 biosynthesis. This enzyme, which is located in the endoplasmic reticulum, was found to be expressed in several tissues in mice (Nakagawa *et al.*, 2010).

Biochemical and Physiological Function

Vitamin K-dependent Carboxylation

Over 40 years after its discovery, vitamin K was shown to act as a cofactor in the post-translational synthesis of Gla from glutamic acid (Glu) residues contained in precursor proteins. γ-Carboxyglutamic acid is common to all vitamin K-dependent proteins (VKDP) and increases the affinity of these proteins for calcium (Berkner and Runge, 2004). As illustrated in Figure 15.2, the γ-carboxylation of glutamate residues is catalyzed by a microsomal enzyme called γ-glutamyl carboxylase (GGCX) located at the luminal surface of the endoplasmic reticulum in a reaction that requires the reduced form of vitamin K, hydroquinone, as well as carbon dioxide and oxygen. It is currently believed that the vitamin K hydroquinone and oxygen react to form a strong base capable of abstracting a proton from the γ-carbon of the Glu residue to form a carbanion intermediate, which then undergoes carboxylation to yield a Gla residue (Dowd *et al.*, 1995). The carboxylase hence uses the energy of vitamin K hydroquinone oxygenation to convert Glu residues to Gla residues in the VKDPs. Carboxylation of the Glu residues is accomplished by a processive mechanism and is facilitated by a carboxylase recognition signal propeptide that tethers the Glu residues to the enzyme (reviewed in Berkner, 2008).

Once formed, vitamin K 2,3-epoxide is recycled to its quinone and hydroquinone forms in successive reactions catalyzed by a vitamin K oxidoreductase (VKOR). Activity of VKOR is dependent on dithiol cofactors and is inhibited by 4-hydroxycoumarin derivatives such as warfarin. The blocking action of coumarin-type drugs towards this enzyme forms the basis of their pharmacological action as anticoagulants. However, at least in the liver, reduction of the vitamin K quinone to hydroquinone is also possible by a NAD(P)H-dependent quinone reductase that is insensitive to coumarin drugs, but cannot reduce vitamin K epoxide to the quinone form. This enzyme operates at high tissue concentrations of vitamin K and can therefore

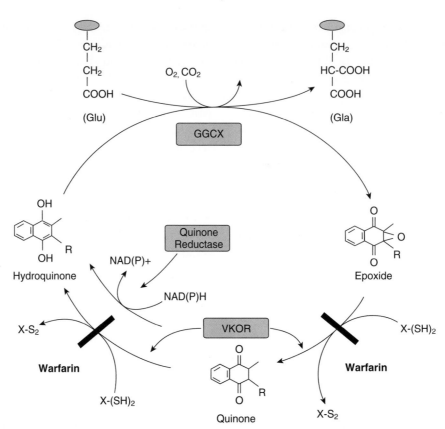

FIG. 15.2 The vitamin K cycle. GGCX refers to the γ-glutamyl carboxylase and VKOR to the vitamin K oxi-doreductase enzymes, respectively. X-$(SH)_2$ and X-S_2 denote reduced and oxidized dithiols, respectively. The dithiol-dependent reductases are inhibited by coumarin-type drugs such as warfarin whereas the NAD(P)H-dependent reductase is not.

support carboxylation of the hepatic VKDP in the presence of coumarins (reviewed in Berkner and Runge, 2004; Suttie, 2009). Collectively, these reactions make up the vitamin K cycle (Figure 15.2).

In the absence of vitamin K or in the presence of vitamin K antagonists, carboxylation of precursor proteins is incomplete and proteins are secreted in plasma in various undercarboxylated forms. These proteins, referred to as PIVKAs (protein induced by vitamin K absence or antagonism), lack biological activity and have been used to assess vitamin K nutritional status. Specific antibodies for the undercarboxylated forms of prothrombin, osteocalcin, and matrix Gla protein have been developed and their presence in blood and tissues is usually interpreted as reflecting a suboptimal VK status (see below).

Vitamin K-dependent Proteins

Although gamma-carboxyglutamic acid residues have been detected in both vertebrate and invertebrate species, only proteins of mammalian origin will be discussed here.

Blood Coagulation Proteins

There are seven vitamin K-dependent proteins involved in blood coagulation, namely prothrombin (factor II), factors VII, IX and X, protein C, protein S, and protein Z. All the vitamin K-dependent coagulation proteins (46 000–80 000 Da) are synthesized in the liver and contain between 10 and 12 Gla residues. The Gla residues enable Ca^{2+}-mediated binding of the proteins to the negatively charged phospholipid surfaces provided by blood platelets and endothelial cells at the site of injury. With the exception of proteins S and Z, Gla-containing blood proteins are zymogen forms of serine proteases and have considerable structural homology. Prothrombin was among the proteins associated with the coagulation cascade as described in the middle of the 19th century. The identification of factors VII, IX, and X came much later (1950s) through the study of patients with hereditary bleeding tendencies, and proteins C, S, and Z were discovered in the mid-1970s (Davie, 2003; Suttie, 2009). Prothrombin and factors VII, IX, and X represent the classical vitamin K-dependent plasma clotting factors and participate in the cascade resulting in the formation of a fibrin clot. A key element in the formation of fibrin is the generation of thrombin from prothrombin by activated factor X. Vitamin K-dependent factors VII and IX activate factor X by the extrinsic and intrinsic pathways, respectively. In contrast, proteins C, S, and Z are inhibitors of the procoagulant system. Protein C exerts its inhibitory activity by inactivating factors Va and VIIIa and enhances fibrinolysis with protein S as a cofactor, and protein Z serves as a cofactor for the inhibition of factor Xa by protein Z-dependent protease inhibitor (Berkner and Runge, 2004). An abbreviated diagram of the coagulation cascade is presented in Figure 15.3.

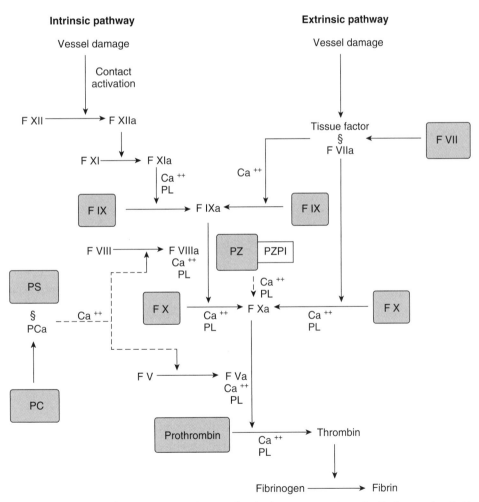

FIG. 15.3 The coagulation cascade. Factors and proteins in boxes are vitamin K-dependent. Numbered factors are abbreviated as F VII, F IX, etc. PC and PS denote protein C and protein S, respectively. Active proteins are represented as "a". PZPI, protein Z–dependent protease inhibitor; PL, phospholipid. Procoagulant reactions are shown as solid lines whereas inhibition reactions are shown as dotted lines.

In addition to their hemostatic action at the cell surface, many of the coagulation proteins are now known to also possess cell signaling activity and influence a wide range of cellular events. Hence, through its interaction with protease-activated receptors (PARs), thrombin has been shown to promote platelet aggregation and to be involved in such phenomena as tumor growth and metastasis, angiogenesis, atherosclerosis and inflammation, survival of glial cells, neurons and myoblasts, and chemotaxis of neutrophils and monocytes (Sokolova and Reiser, 2008; Chen and Dorling, 2009). When complexed to tissue factor, factors VII and Xa activate PAR-1 and PAR-2 receptors and participate in pro-inflammatory cell signaling (Levi and Van der Poll, 2010). In contrast, protein C (PC) and its activated form (APC) have been shown to possess anti-inflammatory and anti-apoptotic properties through mechanisms that appear to involve interactions with the endothelial PC receptor (EPCR) and PAR-1 in the membrane. Clinically, alterations in the PC system have been linked to conditions such as sepsis, asthma, inflammatory bowel disease, atherosclerosis, and lung and heart inflammation (Danese et al., 2010). In contrast to the other VK-dependent blood factors, which are principally associated with the liver, protein S (PS) is synthesized by different cell types (e.g. megakaryocytes, endothelial and vascular smooth muscle cells [VSMCs], and osteoblasts) and has been found in many extrahepatic tissues including brain, testes, spleen, heart, endothelium, and bone. Like the parent vitamin K-dependent protein, Gas6 (cf. later in this chapter), protein S is a ligand for the receptor tyrosine kinases Axl, Sky, and Mer, and is involved in important cell functions. Specifically, protein S has been shown to possess anti-inflammatory activity, to mediate phagocytosis of apoptotic cells, to be a potent mitogen for VSMCs, and to confer neuronal protection (Hafizi and Dahlback, 2006).

Bone Proteins

There are three Gla proteins in bone, namely osteocalcin, matrix Gla protein, and protein S, although two recently discovered VKDP (Gla-rich protein and periostin, cf. below) could probably also be included in this category. Osteocalcin, also known as bone Gla protein, is synthesized in osteoblasts and odontoblasts, and accounts for 15–20% of the non-collagenous bone protein in most vertebrate species. Osteocalcin (OC) has a molecular weight of ~5.7 kDa and three Gla residues, which allow binding to hydroxyapatite crystals in bone. Synthesis of OC by osteoblasts is stimulated by the active metabolite of vitamin D, $1,25(OH)2D_3$. About 20% of the newly synthesized protein is released into the circulation and is used as a measure of bone formation. In states of dietary restriction or following treatment with vitamin K antagonists, partially carboxylated osteocalcin (ucOC) appears in the circulation. Despite the interest osteocalcin has raised since its discovery, its physiological function remains elusive. Reports have shown that rats rendered OC deficient following treatment with warfarin exhibit excessive bone mineralization and premature closure of the growth plate (Price, 1988) and that mice lacking the osteocalcin gene exhibit a phenotype characterized by increased bone mass and improved functional qualities (Ducy et al., 1996). Collectively, these data suggest a role for OC as a negative regulator of bone formation. The second vitamin K-dependent bone protein to be discovered, matrix Gla protein (MGP), has a molecular weight of ~9.6 kDa and contains five Gla residues. In contrast to osteocalcin, which is exclusively associated with mineralized tissues, MGP is expressed in many soft tissues and cell types including vascular smooth muscle cells, although the protein itself only accumulates in calcified tissues. The physiological function of MGP as an inhibitor of calcification was established when mice lacking the gene coding for MGP showed calcification of their arteries that led to hemorrhagic death due to vessel rupture within 2 months (Luo et al., 1997). A similar phenotype, i.e. calcification of the arteries and of the aortic valves, was subsequently observed, although to a lesser degree of severity, in MGP-depleted rats treated with warfarin (Price et al., 1998). Although the mechanism of action for MGP remains to be fully elucidated (Proudfoot and Shanahan, 2006), the protein has been shown to bind calcium ions and inhibit crystal growth (Roy and Nishimoto, 2002), and to modulate the action of bone morphometric protein type 2 (Zebboudj et al., 2003) and type 4 (Yao et al., 2006). Finally, protein S is also present in bone. The protein has been shown to be synthesized and secreted by osteoblasts (Maillard et al., 1992) and to enhance the bone-resorbing activity of mature osteoclasts, an action that appears to be related to its ability to bind tyrosine kinase receptors (Nakamura et al., 1998).

Other VKDPs

Gas6

Discovered in 1993, Gas6, thus named after it was found to be the product of the growth-arrest-specific gene 6, is a high molecular weight protein (75 kDa) that contains

11–12 Gla residues. It has a structure similar to that of protein S (44% amino acid homology) and is expressed in numerous tissues (Manfioletti *et al.*, 1993). Gas6 binds and activates the receptor tyrosine kinases of the TAM family (Tyro3, Axl, and Mer), a property that is dependent on Gla residues. Since its discovery, Gas6 has been involved in a wide range of cellular processes that include cell differentiation, proliferation and activation, cell adhesion and chemotaxis, phagocytosis, and protection against apoptosis. Physiologically, Gas6 has been involved in the nervous system and the retina, in platelet metabolism and hemostasis, in vascular calcification, and in osteogenic differentiation and osteoclast function. In light of these actions, Gas6 has been linked to conditions such as inflammation, thrombotic events, atherosclerosis, glomerular kidney disease, and cancer. The multiple actions of Gas6 have recently been reviewed (Bellido-Martín and de Frutos, 2008; Benzacour, 2008; Tjwa *et al.*, 2009).

Transmembrane Gla Proteins

Among the other VKDPs that have been identified are those of the transmembrane Gla family (TMG), which comprises four proteins: proline-rich Gla proteins 1 and 2 (PRPG1, PRPG2; Kulman *et al.*, 1997) and transmembrane Gla proteins 3 and 4 (TMG3 and TMGP4; Kulman *et al.*, 2001). In contrast to the previously discussed VKDPs, these are not secreted but rather are single-pass integral membrane proteins. Like Gas6, however, the TGMs have a wide tissue distribution. Their functions *in vivo* are presently unclear but their chemical conformations suggest that they could be involved in cell transduction and have broad physiological activities.

Gla-rich Protein

In 2008, a new Gla-rich protein (GRP) was isolated from calcified cartilage. This 10.2-kDa protein contains 16 Gla residues, which is the highest proportion of Glas reported among the VKDPs (Viegas *et al.*, 2008). It is widely distributed but its expression is highest in cartilage with chondrocytes, chondroblasts, osteoblasts, and osteocytes expressing the protein. In a recent report, GRP was found to accumulate in pathological calcification (Viegas *et al.*, 2009). Although the exact function of GRP is presently unknown, it could regulate extracellular calcium.

Periostin

Associated with the extracellular matrix known to promote cell migration and angiogenesis, periostin was recently identified as a VKDP (Coutu *et al.*, 2008). Specifically, it was shown to be secreted by mesenchymal stromal cells and to be present in mineralized bone nodules. In addition to its known functions, periostin could have a role in extracellular matrix mineralization.

Transthyretin

A protein known for its association with thyroid hormones and retinol-binding protein, transthyretin was recently found to contain a Gla residue (Ruggeberg *et al.*, 2008). The role of this vitamin K-dependent modification is presently unknown. A summary of the VKDPs and their functions is given in Table 15.1.

Vitamin K and Health

Bone Health

The discovery of osteocalcin and the evidence that the glutamic acid residues it contained needed to be carboxylated for its function in bone soon fostered interest in the role of vitamin K nutriture in bone health. Numerous observational studies have been conducted over the years, opening the way to randomized control trials of vitamin K supplementation which have just recently become available. In observational studies, high phylloquinone intakes have been associated with lower risk of hip fracture in most studies in contrast to the relationship between phylloquinone intake and bone mineral density (BMD) which has been more variable. Reports from Japan have pointed to higher BMD and lower risk of hip fracture in individuals with a high consumption of the MK-7-rich food, natto. When investigated with respect to vitamin K nutritional status, increased levels of the ucOC, reflective of a low status, have been associated with increased risk of hip fracture in the elderly and lower BMD in both adults and children. However, and as reviewed in detail by Gundberg *et al.* (1998), the methodology for the estimation of ucOC is subject to numerous sources of variation, and, without proper standardization of the assay, ucOC values may not be reliable.

Associations between plasma phylloquinone, the menaquinones, and bone health have been more variable. These studies have recently been reviewed (Shea and Booth, 2008; Booth, 2009). One caveat of dietary associations is that they make it difficult to discern the specific role of vitamin K from those of other nutrients in the diet. Diets rich in vitamin K also tend to be rich in fruits and vegetables which in themselves are beneficial to

TABLE 15.1 Summary of the vitamin K-dependent proteins and their functions

Protein category	Physiological functions	
Blood coagulation	Hemostasis	Cell Signaling-Related Actions
Prothrombin	Procoagulant	*Thrombin*
Factor VII	Procoagulant	Platelet aggregation
		Tumor growth and metastasis
		Angiogenesis
		Atherosclerosis and inflammation
		Cell survival
		Chemotaxis
Factor IX	Procoagulant	*FVII-FIX-tissue factor complex*
Factor X	Procoagulant	Pro-inflammatory action
Protein C	Anticoagulant	*Protein C*
Protein S	Anticoagulant	Anti-inflammatory action
		Anti-apoptotic actions
Protein Z	Anticoagulant	*Protein S*
		Anti-inflammatory and anti-apoptotic actions
		Phagocytosis of apoptotic cells
		Mitogenesis (VSMC)
		Neuronal protection
Bone		
Osteocalcin	Negative regulator of bone formation	
	Endocrine function	
Matrix Gla protein	Inhibitor of calcification*	
Protein S	Undetermined	
Others		
Gas6	Cell differentiation, proliferation, adhesion, and chemotaxis	
	Phagocytosis and protection from apoptosis	
TMGs	Undetermined	
Gla rich protein	Undertermied	
Periostin	Cell migration and angiogenesis	
Transthyretin	Ligand for thyroid hormones and retinol-binding protein	

TMG, transmembrane Gla; VSMC, vascular smooth muscle cells.
*This role as calcification inhibitor applies to soft tissues as well as bone.

bone health (Tucker, 2009). Our recent access to large randomized control trials of vitamin K supplementation have been helpful in this regard. Data from five trials of phylloquinone (Braam *et al.*, 2003; Bolton-Smith *et al.*, 2007; Booth *et al.*, 2008; Cheung *et al.*, 2008; Binkley *et al.*, 2009) and four trials (one open label) of MK-4 (Shiraki *et al.*, 2000; Knapen *et al.*, 2007; Binkley *et al.*, 2009; Inoue *et al.*, 2009) of 1–3 years' duration are now available. Studies were mostly conducted in postmenopausal women (with or without osteoporosis) and included dosages ranging from 200 μg/day to 5 mg/day for phylloquinone and 45 mg/day for MK-4. In most studies calcium and vitamin D were also provided with the K vitamer. As

summarized in recent reviews (Booth, 2009; Iwamoto *et al.*, 2009), supplementation protocols led to increased circulating vitamers, decreased levels of ucOC and little or no change in bone resorption markers. With respect to bone outcomes, supplementation had little impact on BMD when assessed at the hip or other anatomical sites, with only one trial reporting increased BMD at the ultra-distal radius following 2-year supplementation with 200 μg/day phylloquinone (no effects were observed at the femoral neck and mid-radius) (Bolton-Smith *et al.*, 2007). In another trial, women who had been supplemented with 5 mg phylloquinone for 2 years presented fewer clinical fractures. As pointed out by the authors, however, this result should be viewed with caution as the study had not been powered to examine fractures and their numbers were small (Cheung *et al.*, 2008). Results from a recent large MK-4 trial are also at odds with previous smaller studies. In the two trials that included their assessment, MK-4 supplementation had no effect on bone resorption markers. Furthermore, impact on bone was in general limited with one trial reporting improved bone mineral content and femoral neck width, but no effect on BMD (Knapen *et al.*, 2007), and another trial reporting, in post-hoc analysis, a lower incidence of vertebral fractures in patients with at least five vertebral fractures, but not in the whole group (*n* ≈ 2000) (Inoue *et al.*, 2009). None of the other trials reported any benefit from high phylloquinone or MK-4 intakes on bone. Clearly, results from these well-designed trials do not support the conclusions of previous observational studies and those of the smaller phylloquinone and MK-4 supplementation trials (Cockayne *et al.*, 2006). However, the role of vitamin K in bone is complex, and research needs to be pursued. In vitro studies have shown MK-4 to be a potent agonist of the steroid and xenobiotic nuclear receptor and to regulate the transcription of various bone-related genes including those of the extracellular matrix involved in collagen accumulation (reviewed in Horie-Inoue and Inoue, 2008). Finally, because individuals on warfarin therapy are by definition in states of chronic vitamin K deficiency, bone status in these patients has been investigated. A meta-analysis conducted some years ago associated warfarin treatment with a modest reduction in BMD at the radius but not at other sites (Caraballo *et al.*, 1999a). Studies of warfarin treatment and risk of fractures have also been discordant, some reporting negative impact (Caraballo *et al.*, 1999b) or no impact (Woo *et al.*, 2008) on bone fractures. Warfarin is used for a wide range of clinical entities and this may explain the inconsistencies of the current literature.

Cardiovascular Health

In addition to the animal work described earlier, evidence for a role of vitamin K in calcification came with reports from genetic diseases. Individuals suffering from Keutel syndrome, a disorder characterized by abnormal cartilage calcification, have been shown to possess mutations of the MGP gene that result in non-functional MGP (Munroe *et al.*, 1999). Similarly, patients presenting with pseudoxanthoma elasticum, a multi-system disorder characterized by dystrophic mineralization of soft connective tissues, had a lower concentration of total MGP

compared with healthy controls (Hendig *et al.*, 2008). Immunohistochemical studies comparing normal and atherosclerotic human tissues showed MGP to be constitutively expressed in the vessel wall during calcification and in atherosclerotic plaque (Erkkila and Booth, 2008). However, the association between circulating MGP and calcification has been inconsistent. In one study, total MGP was inversely correlated with the severity of coronary artery calcification (Jono *et al.*, 2004) whereas it was positively associated with risk factors for atherosclerosis but not with coronary artery disease in another study (O'Donnell *et al.*, 2006). Assays targeting the inactive uncarboxylated form of MGP (ucMGP) have recently been developed (Schurgers *et al.*, 2005, 2010); however, reports using these assays have been difficult to interpret due to the different specificity of the antibodies. Whether circulating level of ucMGP is a useful surrogate marker of the calcification process requires further investigation. Furthermore, although the role of vitamin K in cardiovascular health has thus far been assumed to be through MGP, it must be kept in mind that other VKDPs, i.e. Gas6, GRP, and periostin, have been associated with the calcification process. Future studies should include these proteins as well.

The influence of dietary vitamin K in cardiovascular health has also been investigated through epidemiological studies. In the majority of cases, phylloquinone intakes have not been associated with cardiovascular disease (CVD) after adjustments for other risk factors. In contrast, high menaquinone intakes have been linked to reduced incidence of CVD and coronary calcification in three studies (reviewed in Erkkila and Booth, 2008; Booth, 2009; Rees *et al.*, 2010). The lack of association between phylloquinone intake and CVD is not surprising given that a high phylloquinone intake has been associated with a heart-healthy dietary pattern (Braam *et al.*, 2004a). The reported association between menaquinone intake and CVD is certainly interesting but will need to be replicated in future studies as issues have been raised regarding the relative validity of the food frequency questionnaires (FFQ) used in these studies. In contrast to phylloquinone (Presse *et al.*, 2009), no FFQ have been specifically validated for the menaquinones. Furthermore, because menaquinones are found in the diet in low amounts except for MK-7 in the Japanese diet, circulating MKs are usually at the limit of detection of current assessment methods. In light of this and as we aspire to better understand the impact of dietary MKs in cardiovascular health, future studies should include state-of-the-art diet assessment tools. Two randomized control trials aimed at assessing the effect of phylloquinone on vascular health have been conducted to date. Supplementation with 1 mg of phylloquinone plus vitamin D and a mineral cocktail for 3 years improved the elastic and compliance properties of the common carotid artery in a group of postmenopausal women (Braam *et al.*, 2004b). More recently, supplementing older men and women with 500 µg of phylloquinone along with a multivitamin for 3 years slowed the progression of coronary artery calcification (CAC). In this study, the beneficial effect of phylloquinone on CAC was independent of changes in serum MGP (Shea *et al.*, 2009a). Additional intervention studies, notably trials of menaquinone supplementation, are warranted before it can be determined whether dietary vitamin K influences cardiovascular health in a clinically significant manner. Finally, there has been limited investigation of the impact of warfarin treatment on vascular calcification. Available cross-sectional studies have reported warfarin treatment to be associated with aortic valve (Koos *et al.*, 2009) and extra-coronary arterial (Rennenberg *et al.*, 2010) calcification. In contrast, warfarin exposure has not been associated with extent of coronary calcification in patients without apparent coronary heart disease participating in the Warfarin and Coronary Calcification Study (Villines *et al.*, 2009). Here also, large prospective studies are needed to determine whether warfarin treatment has a significant clinical impact on vascular health (Danziger, 2008).

Emerging Functions for Vitamin K

Sphingolipid Synthesis

Vitamin K is involved in the synthesis of sphingolipids, a group of complex lipids present in brain cell membranes and which possess important cell signaling properties. Administration of the vitamin K antagonist warfarin to growing rats has been shown to reduce brain sphingolipids and perturb key synthetic enzymes (reviewed in Denisova and Booth, 2005). MK-4, which represents >98% of total vitamin K in rat brain, is present in significantly higher concentrations in myelinated regions of the brain and is strongly correlated to the sphingolipids, sulfatides, sphingomyelin, and gangliosides (Carrié *et al.*, 2004). In a recent report, changes in sphingolipid profile were associated with cognitive deficits in old rats (Carrié *et al.*, 2011). Whether vitamin K through its action in sphingolipid metabolism has a role in neurodegenerative diseases such

as Alzheimer's disease (Presse *et al.*, 2008) remains to be determined.

Inflammation

Menaquinone-4 has been shown to limit the production of interleukin-6 (IL-6) and of prostaglandins *in vitro*, and to limit inflammation in models of encephalomyelitis. Similarly, phylloquinone has been reported to suppress lipopolysaccharide-induced inflammation in the rat (reviewed in Shearer and Newman, 2008). Furthermore, recent epidemiological cohort studies have reported that a high vitamin K nutritional status is associated with lower levels of the proinflammatory markers IL-6, intracellular adhesion molecule-1, tumor necrosis factor receptor 2, and C-reactive protein (reviewed in Booth, 2009). The role of vitamin K in the inflammation process is a topic of much research interest.

Endocrine Function

Menaquinone-4 is present in pancreatic juices (Thomas *et al.*, 2004), and studies conducted over 20 years ago have suggested that both phylloquinone and MK-4 could have a protective role against insulin resistance (reviewed in Booth, 2009). More recently, high phylloquinone intakes were reported to have beneficial effects on insulin resistance in healthy men and women, as determined by the homeostasis model assessment of insulin resistance (HOMA-IR) (Yoshida *et al.*, 2008a,b). It has been suggested that the VKDP osteocalcin could act as a hormone. In a series of reports, osteocalcin, notably its undercarboxylated form (ucOC), was shown to regulate glucose metabolism and fat mass in a transgenic mouse model (Lee *et al.*, 2007; Ferron *et al.*, 2008). The fact that only ucOC was associated with the endocrine effect of osteocalcin in these studies was not confirmed in recent epidemiologic cohort studies where the protective effect of a high phylloquinone intake on insulin resistance was associated with the carboxylated form of osteocalcin (Shea *et al.*, 2009b). Research aimed at elucidating the mechanisms of action of vitamin K in energy metabolism is ongoing.

Anti-cancer Effect

Numerous in vitro and a few in vivo studies have suggested anti-carcinogenic effects for vitamin K, notably for MK-4. This protective role of vitamin K has been linked to its ability to influence cell differentiation and induce apoptosis (reviewed in Shearer and Newman, 2008). Recently, intakes of menaquinones, but not of phylloquinone, were associated with reduced risk of cancer and mortality in the large EPIC-Heidelberg study (Nimptsch *et al.*, 2008, 2010). As for the other actions of vitamin K, its anti-cancer potential will have to be investigated in rigorous intervention trials.

Deficiency

Clinically significant vitamin K deficiency is associated with an increase in prothrombin time and, in severe cases, bleeding. However, overt vitamin K deficiency is uncommon in adults and has mainly been associated with gastrointestinal disorders associated with fat malabsorption (e.g. bile-duct obstruction, inflammatory bowel disease, chronic pancreatitis, cystic fibrosis) and liver disease (Savage and Lindenbaum, 1983). Hospitalized patients with low food intake or poor nutritional status may also be at increased risk of vitamin K deficiency, especially if treated with antibiotics or other drugs interfering with vitamin K metabolism. Although bleeding episodes in antibiotic-treated patients have often been attributed to an acquired vitamin K deficiency resulting from a suppression of menaquinone-synthesizing organisms in the gut, data to substantiate this hypothesis are lacking. Furthermore, interpretation of these reports has generally been complicated by the possibility of general malnutrition in the patients under investigation (Institute of Medicine, 2001). However, newborn infants are a clinical population with a well established risk for vitamin K deficiency. Factors contributing to the condition are poor placental transfer, low concentrations of plasma clotting factors due to hepatic immaturity, and low vitamin K content of breast milk. Individually or in concert, these factors increase the risk of bleeding in infants in the first weeks of life, a condition known as vitamin K deficiency bleeding (VKDB) (Shearer, 2009). Because VKDB can be effectively prevented by administration of vitamin K, the American Academy of Pediatrics recommends that phylloquinone be given to all newborns as a single, intramuscular dose of 0.5–1 mg within 6 hours of birth (American Academy of Pediatrics Committee on Fetus and Newborn, 2003). Similarly, the WHO/FAO recommends that all breast-fed babies receive vitamin K supplementation at birth according to nationally approved guidelines, vitamin K formulations and prophylactic regimes differing from country to country (WHO/FAO, 2004). In preterm infants, a bolus of 0.2 mg (or 0.3 mg/kg) appears to be sufficient to protect during the neonatal period (Clarke,

2010). Reports in the early 1990s of an increased risk of leukemia and other forms of cancer in children who had received vitamin K intramuscularly at birth were not corroborated in subsequent studies, confirming the innocuousness of this prophylactic measure.

High doses of vitamin E have been shown to interfere with vitamin K and precipitate deficiency states, especially in subjects with low vitamin K status. In a study, 12 weeks' supplementation with 1000 IU *RRR*-α-tocopherol per day increased PIVKA-prothrombin (PIVKA-II) levels in adults not receiving oral anticoagulant therapy. In contrast, neither plasma phylloquinone nor ucOC was significantly affected by the supplementation regimen (Booth *et al.*, 2004). Although the clinical significance of the PIVKA-II changes observed in this study warrants further investigation, this study shows that high-dose vitamin E supplementation has the potential to interfere with vitamin K status. The interaction between vitamin K and E has recently been reviewed (Traber, 2008).

Patients treated with coumarin drugs undergo a particular drug–nutrient interaction as warfarin blocks the vitamin K cycle by inhibiting vitamin K epoxide reductase activity. In light of this tight coupling, alteration in vitamin K intake will influence warfarin efficacy, as has been reported on numerous occasions. The Institute of Medicine recommends that once the dose of warfarin has been established, individuals can avoid any complications resulting from variations in vitamin K intake by continuing to follow their normal dietary patterns (Institute of Medicine, 2001). However, recent studies have shown that anticoagulated patients who have low dietary intake of vitamin K are more likely to present unstable anticoagulation (Rombouts *et al.*, 2010). In fact a growing number of reports indicate beneficial effects of high intakes of vitamin K with respect to anticoagulation control (Kim *et al.*, 2010), and supplementing patients with small amounts of phylloquinone has also been shown to be beneficial (Sconce *et al.*, 2007). In a recent report, high usual dietary vitamin K intake was found to be associated with low relative variability in vitamin K intake, a finding that could partly explain the beneficial effect of high dietary vitamin K intake on anticoagulant therapy (Presse *et al.*, 2011).

Requirements

The Food and Nutrition Board of the National Academy of Sciences updated the recommendations for vitamin K in 2001 (Institute of Medicine, 2001). The recommended adequate intake (AI) for vitamin K is 120 µg/day for men and 90 µg/day for females. The AI for children during the first 6 months of life is 2 µg/day and from 7 to 12 months is 2.5 µg/day. AIs for children are 30 µg/day for ages 1–3 years, 55 µg/day for ages 4–8 years, 60 µg/day for ages 9–13 years, and 75 µg/day for ages 14–18 years. The recommendations for pregnancy and lactation are the same as for non-pregnant females of similar age (90 µg/day). No Tolerable Intake Level for vitamin K has been established.

In the United Kingdom, an amount of 1 µg of phylloquinone per kilogram body weight per day is being used as the official guideline for vitamin K and is based on the estimated average daily requirement for its role in blood clotting (Department of Health, 1991). This amount is also used by the WHO/FAO as part of their recommended nutrient intakes (RNI). Values for respective categories are: infants 0–6 months 5 µg/day, an intake that cannot be met by infants who are exclusively breast-fed; infants 7–12 months 10 µg/day; children 1–3 years 15 µg/day; children 4–6 years 20 µg/day; children 7–9 years 25 µg/day; adolescents 10–18 years 35–55 µg/day; adult females >19 years 55 µg/day; adult males >19 years 65 µg/day. The recommendations for pregnancy and lactation are the same as for non-pregnant females of similar age (55 µg/day) (WHO/FAO, 2004).

Sources and Dietary Intakes of Vitamin K

The application of high performance liquid chromatography analysis to vitamin K and the development of relatively straightforward assay procedures have enabled analysis of a large number of foods in the last decade in both the US and in Europe. Vitamin K is found in a limited number of foods, with the green leafy vegetables contributing 40–50% of total intake, followed by certain oils. Mixed dishes were reported to contribute 15% of total intake by virtue of the oils added to the foods. Vegetables such as Swiss chard, spinach, and kale contain in excess of 300 µg phylloquinone/100 g, while broccoli, brussels sprouts, and cabbage contain between 100 and 200 µg phylloquinone/100 g (Booth and Suttie, 1998). The phylloquinone content of oils is variable, soybean and canola oils being the richest sources (100 and 200 µg/100 g), followed by olive oil whose content is slightly lower (50–100 µg/100 g). Oils derived from corn and sunflower seeds are not good sources of phylloquinone, with a content of

<10 µg/100 g. Hydrogenation of plant oils to form solid shortenings results in some conversion of phylloquinone to 2′,3′-dihydrophylloquinone. This form of the vitamin is most prevalent in margarines and prepared foods and has been reported to contribute 15–30% of total phylloquinone intakes in the United States. The bioavailability and the relative biological activity of dihydrophylloquinone were shown to be lower than those of phylloquinone (Booth et al., 2001). The menaquinones are not widely distributed in commonly consumed foods but can be found in animal-based foods (chicken, meats, etc.) and some cheeses (Schurgers and Vermeer, 2000; Elder et al., 2006). Natto, a traditional Japanese dish made of fermented soybeans, is an excellent source of MK-7 (Kamao et al., 2007).

The availability of reliable data on the vitamin K content of foods has now made it possible to obtain reasonable estimates of the dietary phylloquinone intake of the North American, European, and Asian populations. The results of a number of studies on phylloquinone intake have been summarized by Booth and Suttie (1998). These data are somewhat variable but indicate a mean phylloquinone intake of about 150 µg/day for older (>55 years) and 80 µg/day for younger men and women. Reported phylloquinone intakes in the UK and Ireland are comparable to these, albeit slightly lower, while those in The Netherlands and in China are higher (reviewed in Shearer and Newman, 2008). Intake and sources of phylloquinone from British children have also been published (Prynne et al., 2005). Dietary intake data for the menaquinones are more limited but available data suggest that their contribution to total vitamin K intake does not exceed 10% (Shurgers and Vermeer, 2000).

Toxicity

No toxicity for the natural form of vitamins K_1 and K_2 has been documented even when large amounts are administered (Institute of Medicine, 2001). However, synthetic menadione has been shown to produce hemolytic anemia, hyperbilirubinemia, and kernicterus when administered in amounts of more than 5 mg/day to infants. Consequently, menadione is no longer used as a therapeutic agent.

Future Directions

Significant ground has been covered since the discovery of vitamin K. From a nutrient assumed to be strictly involved in blood coagulation, this vitamin has become a nutrient of many physiological systems. The family of the vitamin K-dependent proteins now comprises proteins involved in bone remodeling, calcification processes, endocrine function, and cell-signaling events. Still, many aspects of vitamin K metabolism remain to be specified. For instance, although recent clinical trials do not appear to support a role for dietary vitamin K in bone health, research into the underlying action of vitamin K in bone should be pursued. Similarly, the role of vitamin K in cardiovascular health needs to be further investigated using randomized clinical trials to determine whether vitamin K nutriture has the potential to significantly influence cardiovascular risks. Finally, research efforts should focus on the emerging actions of the various K vitamers, i.e. sphingolipid metabolism, inflammation, endocrine function and anti-cancer effects, as they could have important public health impact. In light of this research agenda, the vitamin K field will continue to be an exciting one in the years to come.

Suggestions for Further Reading

Booth, S.L. (2009) Roles for vitamin K beyond coagulation. *Annu Rev Nutr* **29**, 89–110.

Shearer, M.J. and Newman, P. (2008) Metabolism and cell biology of vitamin K. *Thromb Haemost* **100**, 530–547.

Suttie, J.W. (2009) *Vitamin K in Health and Disease*. CRC Press, Boca Raton, FL.

References

Al Rajabi, A., Peterson, J., Choi, S.W., *et al.* (2010) Measurement of menadione in urine by HPLC. *J Chromatogr B* **878**, 2457–2460.

American Academy of Pediatrics Committee on Fetus and Newborn (2003) Controversies concerning vitamin K and the newborn. *Pediatrics* **112**, 191–192.

Azharuddin, M.K., O'Reilly, D.S., Gray, A., *et al.* (2007) HPLC method for plasma vitamin K1: effect of plasma triglyceride and acute-phase response on circulating concentrations. *Clin Chem* **53**, 1706–1713.

Bellido-Martín, L. and de Frutos, P.G. (2008) Vitamin K-dependent actions of Gas6. *Vitam Horm* **78**, 185–209.

Benzakour, O. (2008) Vitamin K-dependent proteins: functions in blood coagulation and beyond. *Thromb Haemost* **100**, 527–529.

Berkner, K.L. (2008) Vitamin K-dependent carboxylation. *Vitam Horm* **78**, 131–156.

Berkner, K.L. and Runge, K.W. (2004) The physiology of vitamin K nutriture and vitamin K-dependent protein function in atherosclerosis. *J Thromb Haemost* **2**, 2118–2132.

Binkley, N., Harke, J., Krueger, D., *et al.* (2009) Vitamin K treatment reduces undercarboxylated osteocalcin but does not alter bone turnover, density, or geometry in healthy postmenopausal North American women. *J Bone Min Res* **24**, 983–991.

Bolton-Smith, C., McMurdo, M.E., Paterson, C.R., *et al.* (2007) Two-year randomized controlled trial of vitamin K1 (phylloquinone) and vitamin D3 plus calcium on the bone health of older women. *J Bone Min Res* **22**, 509–519.

Booth, S.L. (2009) Roles for vitamin K beyond coagulation. *Annu Rev Nutr* **29**, 89–110.

Booth, S.L. and Suttie, J.W. (1998) Dietary intake and adequacy of vitamin K. *J Nutr* **128**, 785–788.

Booth, S.L., Dallal, G., Shea, M.K., *et al.* (2008) Effect of vitamin K supplementation on bone loss in elderly men and women. *J Clin Endocrinol Metab* **93**, 1217–1223.

Booth, S.L., Golly, I., Sacheck, J.M., *et al.* (2004) Effect of vitamin E supplementation on vitamin K status in adults with normal coagulation status. *Am J Clin Nutr* **80**, 143–148.

Booth, S.L., Lichtenstein, A.H., and Dallal, G.E. (2002) Phylloquinone absorption from phylloquinone-fortified oil is greater than from a vegetable in younger and older men and women. *J Nutr* **132**, 2609–2612.

Booth, S.L., Lichtenstein, A.H., O'Brien-Morse, M., *et al.* (2001) Effects of a hydrogenated form of vitamin K on bone formation and resorption. *Am J Clin Nutr* **74**, 783–790.

Braam, L.A., Knapen, M.H., Geusens, P., *et al.* (2003) Vitamin K1 supplementation retards bone loss in postmenopausal women between 50 and 60 years of age. *Calcif Tissue Int* **73**, 21–26.

Braam, L., McKeown, N., Jacques, P., *et al.* (2004a) Dietary phylloquinone intake as a potential marker for a heart-healthy dietary pattern in the Framingham Offspring cohort. *J Am Diet Assoc* **104**, 1410–1414.

Braam, L.A., Hoeks, A.P., Brouns, F., *et al.* (2004b) Beneficial effects of vitamins D and K on the elastic properties of the vessel wall in postmenopausal women: a follow-up study. *Thromb Haemost* **91**, 373–380.

Caraballo, P.J., Gabriel, S.E., Castro, M.R., *et al.* (1999a) Changes in bone density after exposure to oral anticoagulants: a meta-analysis. *Osteoporos Int* **9**, 441–448.

Caraballo, P.J., Heit, J.A., Atkinson, E.J., *et al.* (1999b) Long-term use of oral anticoagulants and the risk of fracture. *Arch Int Med* **159**, 1750–1756.

Card, D.J., Shearer, M.J., Schurgers, L.J., *et al.* (2009) The external quality assurance of phylloquinone (vitamin K(1)) analysis in human serum. *Biomed Chromatogr* **23**, 1276–1282.

Carrié, I., Bélanger, E., Portoukalian, J., *et al.* (2011) Life-long low phylloquinone intake is associated with cognitive impairments in old rats. *J Nutr* **141**, 1495–1501.

Carrié, I., Portoukalian, J., Vicaretti, R., *et al.* (2004) Menaquinone-4 concentration is correlated with sphingolipid concentrations in rat brain. *J Nutr* **134**, 167–172.

Chen, D. and Dorling, A. (2009) Critical roles for thrombin in acute and chronic inflammation. *J Thromb Haemost* **7** (Suppl 1), 122–126.

Cheung, A.M., Tile, L., Lee, Y., *et al.* (2008) Vitamin K supplementation in postmenopausal women with osteopenia (ECKO trial): a randomized controlled trial. *PLoS Med* **5**, e196.

Clarke, P. (2010) Vitamin K prophylaxis for preterm infants. *Early Hum Dev* **86** (Suppl 1), 17–20.

Cockayne, S., Adamson, J., Lanham-New, S., *et al.* (2006) Vitamin K and the prevention of fractures: systematic review and meta-analysis of randomized controlled trials. *Arch Int Med* **166**, 1256–1261.

Coutu, D.L., Wu, J.H., Monette, A., *et al.* (2008) Periostin, a member of a novel family of vitamin K-dependent proteins, is expressed by mesenchymal stromal cells. *J Biol Chem* **283**, 17991–18001.

Danese, S., Vetrano, S., Zhang, L., *et al.* (2010) The protein C pathway in tissue inflammation and injury: pathogenic role and therapeutic implications. *Blood* **115**, 1121–1130.

Danziger, J. (2008) Vitamin K-dependent proteins, warfarin, and vascular calcification. *Clin J Am Soc Nephrol* **3**, 1504–1510.

Davidson, K.W. and Sadowski, J.A. (1997) Determination of vitamin K compounds in plasma or serum by high-performance liquid chromatography using postcolumn chemical reduction and fluorimetric detection. *Methods Enzymol* **282**, 408–421.

Davie, E.W. (2003) A brief historical review of the waterfall/cascade of blood coagulation. *J Biol Chem* **278**, 50819–50832.

Denisova, N.A. and Booth, S.L. (2005) Vitamin K and sphingolipid metabolism: evidence to date. *Nutr Rev* **63**, 111–121.

Department of Health (1991) *Dietary Reference Values for Food Energy and Nutrients for the United Kingdom*. Report on Health and Social Subjects No. 41. HMSO, London.

Dowd, P., Hershline, R., Ham, S.W., *et al.* (1995) Vitamin K and energy transduction: a base strength amplification mechanism. *Science* **269**, 1684–1691.

Ducros, V., Pollicand, M., Laporte, F., *et al.* (2010) Quantitative determination of plasma vitamin K1 by high-performance liquid chromatography coupled to isotope dilution tandem mass spectrometry. *Anal Biochem* **401**, 7–14.

Ducy, P., Desbois, C., Boyce, B., *et al.* (1996) Increased bone formation in osteocalcin-deficient mice. *Nature* **382**, 448–452.

Elder, S.J., Haytowitz, D.B., Howe, J., *et al.* (2006) Vitamin K contents of meat, dairy, and fast food in the US diet. *J Agric Food Chem* **54**, 463–467.

Erkkila, A.T. and Booth, S.L. (2008) Vitamin K intake and atherosclerosis. *Curr Opin Lipidol* **19**, 39–42.

Erkkila, A.T., Lichtenstein, A.H., Dolnikowski, G.G., *et al.* (2004) Plasma transport of vitamin K in men using deuterium-labeled collard greens. *Metabolism* **53**, 215–221.

Ferron, M., Hinoi, E., Karsenty, G., *et al.* (2008) Osteocalcin differentially regulates beta cell and adipocyte gene expression and affects the development of metabolic diseases in wild-type mice. *Proc Natl Acad Sci USA* **105**, 5266–5270.

Garber, A.K., Binkley, N.C., Krueger, D.C., *et al.* (1999) Comparison of phylloquinone bioavailability from food sources or a supplement in human subjects. *J Nutr* **129**, 1201–1203.

Gijsbers, B.L., Jie, K.S., and Vermeer, C. (1996) Effect of food composition on vitamin K absorption in human volunteers. *Br J Nutr* **76**, 223–229.

Gundberg, C.M., Nieman, S.D., Abrams, S., *et al.* (1998) Vitamin K status and bone health: an analysis of methods for determination of undercarboxylated osteocalcin. *J Clin Endocrinol Metab* **83**, 3258–3266.

Hafizi, S. and Dahlback, B. (2006) Gas6 and protein S. Vitamin K-dependent ligands for the Axl receptor tyrosine kinase subfamily. *FEBS J* **273**, 5231–5244.

Harrington, D.J., Clarke, P., Card, D.J., *et al.* (2010) Urinary excretion of vitamin K metabolites in term and preterm infants: relationship to vitamin K status and prophylaxis. *Pediatr Res* **68**, 508–512.

Harrington, D.J., Soper, R., Edwards, C., *et al.* (2005) Determination of the urinary aglycone metabolites of vitamin K by HPLC with redox-mode electrochemical detection. *J Lipid Res* **46**, 1053–1060.

Hendig, D., Zarbock, R., Szliska, C., *et al.* (2008) The local calcification inhibitor matrix Gla protein in pseudoxanthoma elasticum. *Clin Biochem* **41**, 407–412.

Horie-Inoue, K. and Inoue, S. (2008) Steroid and xenobiotic receptor mediates a novel vitamin K2 signaling pathway in osteoblastic cells. *J Bone Min Metab* **26**, 9–12.

Inoue, T., Fujita, T., Kishimoto, H., *et al.* (2009) Randomized controlled study on the prevention of osteoporotic fractures (OF study): a phase IV clinical study of 15-mg menatetrenone capsules. *J Bone Min Metab* **27**, 66–75.

Institute of Medicine (2001) *Dietary Reference Intakes for Vitamin A, Vitamin K, Arsenic, Boron, Chromium, Copper, Iodine, Iron, Manganese, Molybdenum, Nickel, Silicon, Vanadium, and Zinc*. National Academy Press, Washington, DC.

Iwamoto, J., Sato, Y., Takeda, T., *et al.* (2009) High-dose vitamin K supplementation reduces fracture incidence in postmenopausal women: a review of the literature. *Nutr Res* **29**, 221–228.

Jones, K.S., Bluck, L.J., Wang, L.Y., *et al.* (2008) A stable isotope method for the simultaneous measurement of vitamin K1 (phylloquinone) kinetics and absorption. *Eur J Clin Nutr* **62**, 1273–1281.

Jones, K.S., Bluck, L.J., Wang, L.Y., *et al.* (2009) The effect of different meals on the absorption of stable isotope-labelled phylloquinone. *Br J Nutr* **102**, 1195–1202.

Jono, S., Ikari, Y., Vermeer, C., *et al.* (2004) Matrix Gla protein is associated with coronary artery calcification as assessed by electron-beam computed tomography. *Thromb Haemost* **91**, 790–794.

Kamao, M., Suhara, Y., Tsugawa, N., *et al.* (2007) Vitamin K content of foods and dietary vitamin K intake in Japanese young women. *J Nutr Sci Vitaminol* **53**, 464–470.

Kim, K.H., Choi, W.S., Lee, J.H., *et al.* (2010) Relationship between dietary vitamin K intake and the stability of antico-agulation effect in patients taking long-term warfarin. *Thromb Haemost* **104**, 755–759.

Knapen, M.H., Schurgers, L.J., and Vermeer, C. (2007) Vitamin K2 supplementation improves hip bone geometry and bone strength indices in postmenopausal women. *Osteoporos Int* **18**, 963–972.

Kohlmeier, M., Saupe, J., Drossel, H.J., *et al.* (1995) Variation of phylloquinone (vitamin K1) concentrations in hemodialysis patients. *Thromb Haemost* **74**, 1252–1254.

Koos, R., Krueger, T., Westenfeld, R., *et al.* (2009) Relation of circulating matrix Gla-protein and anticoagulation status in patients with aortic valve calcification. *J Thromb Haemost* **101**, 706–713.

Kulman, J.D., Harris, J.E., Haldeman, B.A., *et al.* (1997) Primary structure and tissue distribution of two novel proline-rich gamma-carboxyglutamic acid proteins. *Proc Natl Acad Sci USA* **94**, 9058–9062.

Kulman, J.D., Harris, J.E., Xie, L., *et al.* (2001) Identification of two novel transmembrane gamma-carboxyglutamic acid pro-teins expressed broadly in fetal and adult tissues. *Proc Natl Acad Sci USA* **98**, 1370–1375.

Lamon-Fava, S., Sadowski, J.A., Davidson, K.W., *et al.* (1998) Plasma lipoproteins as carriers of phylloquinone (vitamin K1) in humans. *Am J Clin Nutr* **67**, 1226–1231.

Lee, N.K., Sowa, H., Hinoi, E., *et al.* (2007) Endocrine regula-tion of energy metabolism by the skeleton. *Cell* **130**, 456–469.

Levi, M. and Van Der Poll, T. (2010) Inflammation and coagula-tion. *Crit Care Med* **38**, (2 suppl) S26–34.

Luo, G., Ducy, P., McKee, M.D., *et al.* (1997) Spontaneous calci-fication of arteries and cartilage in mice lacking matrix GLA protein. *Nature* **386**, 78–81.

Maillard, C., Berruyer, M., Serre, C.M., *et al.* (1992) Protein-S, a vitamin K-dependent protein, is a bone matrix component synthesized and secreted by osteoblasts. *Endocrinology* **130**, 1599–1604.

Manfioletti, G., Brancolini, C., Avanzi, G., *et al.* (1993) The protein encoded by a growth arrest-specific gene (gas6) is a new member of the vitamin K-dependent proteins related to protein S, a negative coregulator in the blood coagulation cascade. *Mol Cell Biol* **13**, 4976–4985.

Munroe, P.B., Olgunturk, R.O., Fryns, J.P., *et al.* (1999) Mutations in the gene encoding the human matrix Gla protein cause Keutel syndrome. *Nature Genet* **21**, 142–144.

Nakagawa, K., Hirota, Y., Sawada, N., *et al.* (2010) Identification of UBIAD1 as a novel human menaquinone-4 biosynthetic enzyme. *Nature* **468**, 117–121.

Nakamura, Y.S., Hakeda, Y., Takakura, N., *et al.* (1998) Tyro 3 receptor tyrosine kinase and its ligand, Gas6, stimulate the function of osteoclasts. *Stem Cells* **16**, 229–238.

Newman, P., Bonello, F., Wierzbicki, A.S., *et al.* (2002) The uptake of lipoprotein-borne phylloquinone (vitamin K1) by osteob-lasts and osteoblast-like cells: role of heparan sulfate proteogly-cans and apolipoprotein E. *J Bone Min Res* **17**, 426–433.

Nimptsch, K., Rohrmann, S., Kaaks, R., *et al.* (2010) Dietary vitamin K intake in relation to cancer incidence and mortality: results from the Heidelberg cohort of the European Prospective Investigation into Cancer and Nutrition (EPIC-Heidelberg). *Am J Clin Nutr* **91**, 1348–1358.

Nimptsch, K., Rohrmann, S., and Linseisen, J. (2008) Dietary intake of vitamin K and risk of prostate cancer in the Heidelberg cohort of the European Prospective Investigation into Cancer and Nutrition (EPIC-Heidelberg). *Am J Clin Nutr* **87**, 985–992.

Novotny, J.A., Kurilich, A.C., Britz, S.J., *et al.* (2010) Vitamin K absorption and kinetics in human subjects after consumption of 13C-labelled phylloquinone from kale. *Br J Nutr* **104**, 858–862.

O'Donnell, C.J., Shea, M.K., Price, P.A., *et al.* (2006) Matrix Gla protein is associated with risk factors for atherosclerosis but not with coronary artery calcification. *Arterioscler Thromb Vasc Biol* **26** (12), 2769–2774.

Okano, T., Shimomura, Y., Yamane, M., *et al.* (2008) Conversion of phylloquinone (vitamin K1) into menaquinone-4 (vitamin K2) in mice: two possible routes for menaquinone-4 accumulation in cerebra of mice. *J Biol Chem* **283**, 11270–11279.

Olson, R.E., Chao, J., Graham, D., *et al.* (2002) Total body phyl-loquinone and its turnover in human subjects at two levels of vitamin K intake. *Br J Nutr* **87**, 543–553.

Presse, N., Kergoat, M.J., and Ferland, G. (2011) High usual dietary vitamin K intake is associated with low relative variabil-ity in vitamin K intake: implications for anticoagulant therapy. *Br J Haematol* **153**, 129–130.

Presse, N., Shatenstein, B., Kergoat, M.J., *et al.* (2008) Low vitamin K intakes in community-dwelling elders at an early stage of Alzheimer's disease. *J Am Diet Assoc* **108,** 2095–2099.

Presse, N., Shatenstein, B., Kergoat, M.J., *et al.* (2009) Validation of a semiquantitative food-frequency questionnaire measuring dietary vitamin K intake in elderly people. *J Am Diet Assoc* **109,** 1251–1255.

Price, P.A. (1988) Role of vitamin-K-dependent proteins in bone metabolism. *Annu Rev Nutr* **8,** 565–583.

Price, P.A., Faus, S.A., and Williamson, M.K. (1998) Warfarin causes rapid calcification of the elastic lamellae in rat arteries and heart valves. *Arterioscler Thromb Vasc Biol* **18,** 1400–1407.

Proudfoot, D. and Shanahan, C.M. (2006) Molecular mechanisms mediating vascular calcification: role of matrix Gla protein. *Nephrology* **11,** 455–461.

Prynne, C.J., Thane, C.W., Prentice, A., *et al.* (2005) Intake and sources of phylloquinone (vitamin K(1)) in 4-year-old British children: comparison between 1950 and the 1990s. *Public Health Nutr* **8,** 171–180.

Rees, K., Guraewal, S., Wong, Y.L., *et al.* (2010) Is vitamin K consumption associated with cardio-metabolic disorders? A systematic review. *Maturitas* **67,** 121–128.

Rennenberg, R.J., Van Varik, B.J., Schurgers, L.J., *et al.* (2010) Chronic coumarin treatment is associated with increased extracoronary arterial calcification in humans. *Blood* **115,** 5121–5123.

Rombouts, E.K., Rosendaal, F.R., and Van Der Meer, F.J. (2010) Influence of dietary vitamin K intake on subtherapeutic oral anticoagulant therapy. *Br J Haematol* **149,** 598–605.

Roy, M.E. and Nishimoto, S.K. (2002) Matrix Gla protein binding to hydroxyapatite is dependent on the ionic environment: calcium enhances binding affinity but phosphate and magnesium decrease affinity. *Bone* **31,** 296–302.

Ruggeberg, S., Horn, P., Li, X., *et al.* (2008) Detection of a gamma-carboxy-glutamate as novel post-translational modification of human transthyretin. *Protein Pept Lett* **15,** 43–46.

Sadowski, J.A., Hood, S.J., Dallal, G.E., *et al.* (1989) Phylloquinone in plasma from elderly and young adults: factors influencing its concentration. *Am J Clin Nutr* **50,** 100–108.

Savage, D. and Lindenbaum, J. (1983) Clinical and experimental human vitamin K deficiency. In J Lindenbaum (ed.), *Nutrition in Hematology*. Churchill Livingstone, New York, pp. 271–320.

Schurgers, L.J. and Vermeer, C. (2000) Determination of phylloquinone and menaquinones in food. Effect of food matrix on circulating vitamin K concentrations. *Haemostasis* **30,** 298–307.

Schurgers, L.J. and Vermeer, C. (2002) Differential lipoprotein transport pathways of K-vitamins in healthy subjects. *Biochim Biophys Acta* **1570,** 27–32.

Schurgers, L.J., Barreto, D.V., Barreto, F.C., *et al.* (2010) The circulating inactive form of matrix gla protein is a surrogate marker for vascular calcification in chronic kidney disease: a preliminary report. *Clin J Am Soc Nephrol* **5,** 568–575.

Schurgers, L.J., Teunissen, K.J., Hamulyak, K., *et al.* (2007) Vitamin K-containing dietary supplements: comparison of synthetic vitamin K1 and natto-derived menaquinone-7. *Blood* **109,** 3279–3283.

Schurgers, L.J., Teunissen, K.J., Knapen, M.H., *et al.* (2005) Novel conformation-specific antibodies against matrix gamma-carboxyglutamic acid (Gla) protein: undercarboxylated matrix Gla protein as marker for vascular calcification. *Arterioscler Thromb Vasc Biol* **25,** 1629–1633.

Sconce, E., Avery, P., Wynne, H., *et al.* (2007) Vitamin K supplementation can improve stability of anticoagulation for patients with unexplained variability in response to warfarin. *Blood* **109,** 2419–2423.

Shea, M.K. and Booth, S.L. (2008) Update on the role of vitamin K in skeletal health. *Nutr Rev* **66,** 549–557.

Shea, M.K., Gundberg, C.M., Meigs, J.B., *et al.* (2009b) Gamma-carboxylation of osteocalcin and insulin resistance in older men and women. *Am J Clin Nutr* **90,** 1230–1235.

Shea, M.K., O'Donnell, C.J., Hoffmann, U., *et al.* (2009a) Vitamin K supplementation and progression of coronary artery calcium in older men and women. *Am J Clin Nutr* **89,** 1799–1807.

Shearer, M.J. (2009) Vitamin K deficiency bleeding (VKDB) in early infancy. *Blood Rev* **23,** 49–59.

Shearer, M.J. and Newman, P. (2008) Metabolism and cell biology of vitamin K. *Thromb Haemost* **100,** 530–547.

Shearer, M.J., McBurney, A., and Barkhan, P. (1974) Studies on the absorption and metabolism of phylloquinone (vitamin K1) in man. *Vitam Horm* **32,** 513–542.

Shiraki, M., Shiraki, Y., Aoki, C., *et al.* (2000) Vitamin K2 (menatetrenone) effectively prevents fractures and sustains lumbar bone mineral density in osteoporosis. *J Bone Min Res* **15,** 515–521.

Sokolova, E. and Reiser, G. (2008) Prothrombin/thrombin and the thrombin receptors PAR-1 and PAR-4 in the brain: localization, expression and participation in neurodegenerative diseases. *Thromb Haemost* **100,** 576–581.

Suttie, J.W. (1995) The importance of menaquinones in human nutrition. *Annu Rev Nutr* **15,** 399–417.

Suttie, J.W. (2009) *Vitamin K in Health and Disease*. CRC Press, Boca Raton, FL.

Thijssen, H.H. and Drittij-Reijnders, M.J. (1996) Vitamin K status in human tissues: tissue-specific accumulation of phylloquinone and menaquinone-4. *Br J Nutr* **75,** 121–127.

Thijssen, H.H., Vervoort, L.M., Schurgers, L.J., *et al.* (2006) Menadione is a metabolite of oral vitamin K. *Br J Nutr* **95,** 260–266.

Thomas, D.D., Krzykowski, K.J., Engelke, J.A., *et al.* (2004) Exocrine pancreatic secretion of phospholipid, menaquinone-4, and calveolin-1 in vivo. *Biochem Biophys Res Commun* **319,** 974–979.

Tjwa, M., Moons, L., and Lutgens, E. (2009) Pleiotropic role of growth arrest-specific gene 6 in atherosclerosis. *Curr Opin Lipidol* **20,** 386–392.

Traber, M.G. (2008) Vitamin E and K interactions – a 50-year-old problem. *Nutr Rev* **66,** 624–629.

Tucker, K.L. (2009) Osteoporosis prevention and nutrition. *Curr Osteopor Rep* **7,** 111–117.

Viegas, C.S., Cavaco, S., Neves, P.L., *et al.* (2009) Gla-rich protein is a novel vitamin K-dependent protein present in serum that accumulates at sites of pathological calcifications. *Am J Pathol* **175,** 2288–2298.

Viegas, C.S., Simes, D.C., Laize, V., *et al.* (2008) Gla-rich protein (GRP), a new vitamin K-dependent protein identified from sturgeon cartilage and highly conserved in vertebrates. *J Biol Chem* **283,** 36655–36664.

Villines, T.C., O'Malley, P.G., Feuerstein, I.M., *et al.* (2009) Does prolonged warfarin exposure potentiate coronary calcification in humans? Results of the warfarin and coronary calcification study. *Calcif Tissue Int* **85,** 494–500.

Wang, L., Bates, C.J., Yan, L., *et al.* (2004) Determination of phylloquinone (vitamin K1) in plasma and serum by HPLC with fluorescence detection. *Clin Chim Acta* **347,** 199–207.

WHO/FAO (World Health Organization, Food and Agricultural Organization of the United Nations) (2004) *Vitamin and Mineral Requirements in Human Nutrition*, 2nd Edn. WHO, Geneva, Chapter 10

Woo, C., Chang, L.L., Ewing, S.K., *et al.* (2008) Single-point assessment of warfarin use and risk of osteoporosis in elderly men. *J Am Geriatr Soc* **56,** 1171–1176.

Yan, L., Zhou, B., Nigdikar, S., *et al.* (2005) Effect of apolipoprotein E genotype on vitamin K status in healthy older adults from China and the UK. *Br J Nutr* **94,** 956–961.

Yao, Y., Zebboudj, A.F., Shao, E., *et al.* (2006) Regulation of bone morphogenetic protein-4 by matrix GLA protein in vascular endothelial cells involves activin-like kinase receptor 1. *J Biol Chem* **281,** 33921–33930.

Yoshida, M., Booth, S.L., Meigs, J.B., *et al.* (2008a) Phylloquinone intake, insulin sensitivity, and glycemic status in men and women. *Am J Clin Nutr* **88,** 210–215.

Yoshida, M., Jacques, P.F., Meigs, J.B., *et al.* (2008b) Effect of vitamin K supplementation on insulin resistance in older men and women. *Diabetes Care* **31,** 2092–2096.

Zebboudj, A.F., Shin, V., and Bostrom, K. (2003) Matrix GLA protein and BMP-2 regulate osteoinduction in calcifying vascular cells. *J Cell Biochem* **90,** 756–765.

16

VITAMIN C

CAROL S. JOHNSTON, PhD, RD

Arizona State University, Phoenix, Arizona, USA

Summary

Vitamin C is a potent reducing agent/antioxidant in animal species and land plants. Humans rely on vitamin C for the activity of enzymes involved in collagen, carnitine, and norepinephrine synthesis, and vitamin C status may impact physiological health, including risk for infections, cardiovascular disease, and cancer. The recommended daily intake for vitamin C is 90 mg/day for adult men and 75 mg/day for adult women, and the tolerable upper limit is 2000 mg/day. Supplemental vitamin C should not replace high intakes of fruits and vegetables, but may offer health benefits under certain circumstances for some individuals. Low intakes of fresh fruits and vegetables, either by choice or due to scarcity, increase the risk for scurvy, a concern for isolated populations, refugees, cancer patients, the critically ill, and the elderly. Smokers, individuals with diabetes, and adult men living alone are also at risk for suboptimal vitamin C status; in developed countries, current vitamin C deficiency rates range from 8% to 19%. Individuals with a history of renal stone formation or conditions associated with iron overload should use caution when supplementing vitamin C.

Introduction

Long before vitamin C was utilized as a cofactor for enzymes in mammalian systems, it was a ubiquitous constituent of plants. The presence of duplicative biosynthetic pathways for vitamin C in algae and land plants suggests an important role for vitamin C in the evolutionary success of higher plants (Wolucka and Van Montagu, 2007). In the animal kingdom, invertebrates and teleost fish, the dominant fishes in oceans and fresh water, cannot manufacture vitamin C; however, primitive fish, amphibians, and reptiles produce vitamin C as do most mammals.

The extremely stressful conditions associated with terrestrial life, including high oxygen tension, desiccation by dry air, and hot sun, may have necessitated selection pressure for species capable of vitamin C synthesis (Chatterjee, 1973). However, several divergent lines of mammals (bats, guinea pigs, non-human primates, and man) lost the ability to synthesize vitamin C due to the absence of the terminal enzyme of the ascorbic acid synthetic pathway. Yet, vitamin C-dependent species possess a marked increase in both copper and zinc superoxide dismutases compared with the vitamin C-synthesizing amphibians, reptiles, and mammals, thereby maintaining

Present Knowledge in Nutrition, Tenth Edition. Edited by John W. Erdman Jr, Ian A. Macdonald and Steven H. Zeisel.
© 2012 International Life Sciences Institute. Published 2012 by John Wiley & Sons, Inc.

a strong defense system against oxygen toxicity (Nandi et al., 1997).

Chatterjee (1973) calculated that the rate of vitamin C synthesis in small mammals ranged from 150 mg/kg body weight/day in rats to nearly 275 mg/kg body weight/day in rabbits and mice. In these species, the body pool of vitamin C ranged from 30 to 100 mg/kg and blood vitamin C concentrations varied from 0.5 to 1.0 mg/dL (28–57 μmol/L) (Dash et al., 1984). In contrast, vitamin C-dependent humans consume only about 1 mg of vitamin C/kg body weight/day and maintain a body pool of vitamin C near 20 mg/kg and a plasma vitamin C concentration near 0.5–0.7 mg/dL (28–40 μmol/L)(Bluck et al., 1996). Also, the half-life for vitamin C in humans (range: 14–40 days) appears to be orders of magnitude above that for rats or guinea pigs (3–6 days) (Blanchard, 1991). However, direct interspecies comparisons for ascorbate body-pool size and turnover are probably invalid owing to confounding related to variability in dosage level, baseline vitamin C status, stress level of subject, and/or analytical methods (Levine, 1986). Although incapable of manufacturing vitamin C, humans are particularly adept at conserving the vitamin since adequate plasma concentrations are maintained at lower intakes of vitamin C (~1 mg/kg per day) as compared with other vitamin C-dependent species (3–6 mg/kg per day) (Tillotson and O'Connor, 1980).

In guinea pigs and rats, as well as in primates, there is considerable conversion of vitamin C to carbon dioxide. Over 65% of an injected dose was excreted as carbon dioxide within 10 days in guinea pigs, with 20% of the dose catabolized to carbon dioxide within the first 24 hours (Burns et al., 1951). In humans, this respiratory pathway seems insignificant since less than 5% of an injected dose appeared as carbon dioxide after a 10-day period. The principal route of excretion of vitamin C and its metabolites in humans is through the urine, mainly as oxalate and unmetabolized ascorbic acid. In 10 days, about 40% of an injected dose of ascorbic acid is excreted in the urine in humans compared with only 10% in guinea pigs (Hellman and Burns, 1958).

Chemistry and Metabolism

Vitamin C was first isolated from the adrenal glands of cows in 1928 and termed "hexuronic acid" by the Hungarian scientist, Albert Szent-Györgyi. By 1932 the antiscorbutic property of hexuronic acid was established

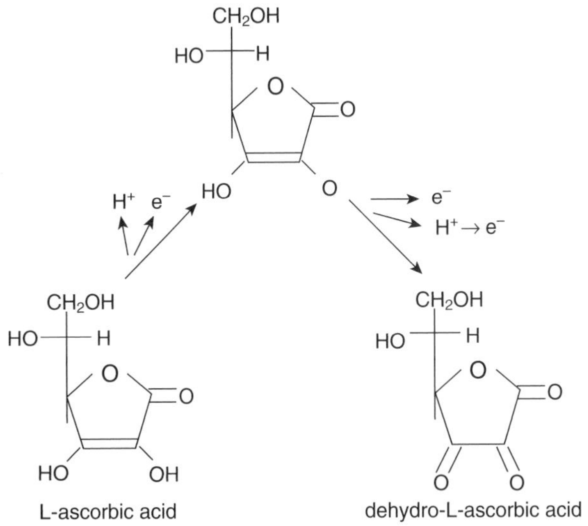

FIG. 16.1 Oxidation of ascorbic acid.

independently by Szent-Györgyi and C.G. King of the University of Pittsburgh, and the compound was renamed "ascorbic acid." Chemist Norman Haworth, in Birmingham, England, working in collaboration with Szent-Györgyi, elucidated the structure of ascorbic acid in 1933. Both men received a Nobel Prize in 1937 for their work leading to the discovery and structure of vitamin C.

Vitamin C is a redox-active system comprising L-ascorbic acid, the free radical monodehydro-L-ascorbic acid (AFR), and oxidized ascorbate or dehydro-L-ascorbic acid (DHA) (Figure 16.1). The ascorbate radical/ascorbate thermodynamic couple, the one-electron reduction potential, is below that of most physiological redox systems. Hence, ascorbic acid is a primary nonenzymatic antioxidant for many reactive compounds in vivo, including the α-tocopherol free radical, the glutathione radical, peroxyl radicals, the hydroxyl free radical, the superoxide radical, and the urate free radical (Buettner and Jurkiewicz, 1993). AFR can be detected directly by electron spin resonance spectroscopy and is a useful measure of radical formation in biological systems and plasma (Stefansson et al., 2008).

Ascorbic acid is a six-carbon, water-soluble (33 g/100 cm^3 at 20°C) γ-lactone (MW 176.14). Its acidic nature results from the ionization of the enolic OH on C-3 (pK_a 4.25) at neutral pH. Liquid chromatography–electrochemical detection methods are considered the most sensitive and precise systems for measuring ascorbic acid in biological samples. Currently, DHA cannot be detected directly in these systems and is measured indirectly by subtraction after its pre- or post-column reduction to ascorbic acid (Li and Franke, 2009). Ascorbic acid degrades rapidly in extracted plasma; hence, samples must be carefully handled and rapidly preserved and frozen. Procedures vary dependent on preservatives used. Plasma samples preserved with trichloroacetic acid should be collected in EDTA tubes and supernatants frozen at -70°C within 1.5 hours of collection (Salminen and Alfthan, 2008). This preparation and storage preserves the ascorbic acid for up to 10 years. If meta-phosphoric acid is the precipitant, heparin vacutainers should be used, and the samples should be analyzed within 80 days (Karlsen et al., 2007).

A simple and rapid enzymatic procedure using ascorbate oxidase and o-phenylenediamine was automated for use in clinical settings and correlated well with standard chromatographic analyses (Ihara et al., 2000). A colorimetric procedure utilizing the reducing properties of ascorbic acid was also shown to provide plasma ascorbic acid results comparable to those from HPLC analyses (Chung et al., 2001). Schaus et al. (1986) demonstrated that total ascorbic acid (ascorbate + DHA) analyses of isolated leukocytes using the 2,4-dinitrophenylhydrazine colorimetric method yielded results comparable to those from HPLC methodology.

In all plant species tested, ascorbic acid is synthesized from GDP-D-mannose in the L–galactose pathway; in mammals the vitamin is synthesized from L-gulonate in the hexuronic acid pathway of the liver or kidney. In the vitamin C-dependent mammals, a genetic lesion inhibits the synthesis of L-gulonolactone oxidase, the terminal enzyme for ascorbic acid synthesis, and L-gulonate is processed via the pentose pathway to re-enter carbohydrate metabolism (Linster and Van Schaftingen, 2006).

Ascorbic acid is transported into cells via the sodium-dependent transporter SVCT1, located on epithelial cells; the sodium and Ca^{2+}/Mg^{2+}-dependent transporter SVCT2, widely distributed in metabolically active and specialized tissues, including brain, eye, placenta, osteoblast cells, adrenals, and endothelial tissues, transports ascorbic acid into metabolically active tissue cells (Godoy et al., 2007). Hence, SVCT2 likely regulates ascorbic acid metabolism in tissues while SVCT1 regulates whole-body homeostasis. Oxidative stressors increase SVCT2 mRNA expression, whereas aging decreases SVCT1 mRNA expression (Rivas et al., 2008).

Genetic variation in the gene that codes for the ascorbic acid transporter SVCT1, SLC23A1, has been associated with variations in circulating ascorbic acid concentrations in large population studies (Cahill and El-Sohemy, 2009; Timpson et al., 2010). Also, glutathione S-transferase genotypes have been associated with risk for serum vitamin C deficiency, but only for individuals whose diets were marginal in vitamin C (Cahill et al., 2009). These results demonstrate the important roles that this transport system plays in vitamin C homeostasis. Genetic variations in the SVCT2 transporter are associated with risk for cancer (Wright et al., 2009) and preterm delivery (Erichsen et al., 2006) indicating an important role for this transporter in vitamin C functionality.

In its metabolic roles, ascorbic acid is converted to AFR in blood and tissues. This radical does not contribute to free radical chain reactions in vivo since it is rapidly recycled to ascorbic acid via NADPH-dependent reduction by thioredoxin reductases or by microsomal or mitochondrial oxidoreductases which are present in all cell types (Kennett and Kuchel, 2006). At sites of marked oxidant stress, the dismutation of two molecules of AFR to DHA and ascorbic acid likely occurs. Although DHA undergoes irreversible hydrolysis with a half-life of less than 2 minutes, nearby cells can bind DHA via specific facilitative glucose transporter isoforms: GLUT1 (ubiquitous distribution), GLUT3 (largely confined to neuronal tissues), and GLUT4 (largely confined to muscle and adipose tissues) (Corti et al., 2010). This uptake of DHA via glucose transporters by many cell types, followed by the immediate two-electron reduction of DHA to ascorbic acid by several mechanisms (glutathione-dependent systems or NADPH-dependent systems mediated by thioredoxin reductase or by 3α-hydroxysteroid dehydrogenase), suggests an efficient system for the recycling and salvaging of vitamin C at sites of high oxidative stress (Nualart et al., 2003).

Possibly this "bystander effect" would increase the intracellular antioxidant defense capacity of targeted tissues when the need is greatest. Yet, under normal physiologic conditions, DHA concentrations would be low and the circulating glucose would successfully compete with DHA for the GLUT transporters minimizing this recycling pathway (Corti et al., 2010). Moreover, research in SVCT2 knockout mice clearly demonstrates that this recycling pathway is not sufficient in the absence of direct ascorbic acid transfer into cells. In mutant mice lacking SVCT2 as a result of allele deletion, respiratory failure and severe

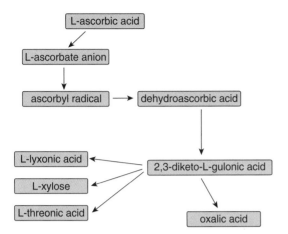

FIG. 16.2 Catabolism of ascorbic acid.

cerebral hemorrhaging occurred immediately after birth, indicating the vital role of ascorbic acid transport via SVCT2 (Sotiriou *et al.*, 2002).

If not recycled to ascorbate, DHA is irreversibly delactonized to 2,3-diketogulonic acid, and its further degradation to oxalic acid likely represents the major catabolic pathway of vitamin C in nonsupplementing individuals. Other possible catabolic products of vitamin C include L-threonic acid, L-xylonic acid, L-lyxonic acid, and L-xylose (Figure 16.2). In a carefully conducted vitamin C depletion–repletion pharmacokinetic study in seven healthy in-patient volunteers, the bioavailability of an orally administered dose of ascorbic acid ranged from 100% at 200 mg, 73% at 500 mg, and 49% at 1250 mg (Levine *et al.*, 1996). At these same doses, the fraction of ascorbic acid excreted unmetabolized after 24 hours was approximately 50%, and at steady state (once plasma ascorbic acid reached a plateau) the 24-hour oxalate excretion was approximately 30, 35, and 40 mg.

In subjects administered intravenous ascorbic acid (1.5 g/kg or approximately 100 g), within 6 hours, about 80% of the administered dose was excreted unmetabolized and <0.5% of the administered dose was excreted as oxalic acid (80 mg oxalic acid) (Robitaille *et al.*, 2009). In healthy adults, oxalate excretion averages about 25 mg/day, and normal oxalate excretion is considered to be less than 40 mg/day. Thus, practitioners utilizing high-dose intravenous vitamin C therapy need to recognize the possibility of hyperoxaluria.

Biochemical Functions

As a cofactor for mixed function oxidases, vitamin C participates in the synthesis of various macromolecules including collagen, carnitine, and norepinephrine. In these reactions, vitamin C promotes enzyme activity by maintaining metal ions in the reduced form. In collagen and carnitine syntheses, α-ketoglutarate-dependent dioxygenases incorporate one atom of oxygen into succinate and one into the oxidized product of the substrate in the presence of ferrous iron. Three ascorbate-dependent dioxygenases are required for the synthesis of collagen (prolyl 4-hydroxylase, prolyl 3-hydroxylase, and lysylhydroxylase), and two are involved in carnitine biosynthesis (6-N-trimethyl-L-lysine hydroxylase and γ-butyrobetaine hydroxylase). Many of the symptoms of the vitamin C deficiency disease scurvy are attributed to weakened collagenous structures and insufficient tissue carnitine: fatigue and lassitude, bleeding and gum deterioration, impaired wound healing, and epiphyseal and metaphyseal plate lesions in bone. Oral vitamin C repletion (10–15 mg/kg/day) results in rapid resolution of the hemorrhagic and bone abnormalities in scurvy (Karthiga *et al.*, 2008; Vitale *et al.*, 2009).

Hughes *et al.* (1980) first postulated that reduced muscle carnitine was responsible for the marked fatigue characteristic of vitamin C depletion and early scurvy. Carnitine is necessary for the transport of long-chain fatty acids into the mitochondrial matrix for oxidation, and plays an important role in energy metabolism. Individuals with myopathies associated with primary carnitine deficiency report muscle weakness and fatigability (Vielhaber *et al.*, 2004); however, to date, muscle carnitine analyses in human scurvy have not been conducted. In cultured guinea-pig hepatocytes, supplemental vitamin C resulted in enhanced carnitine synthesis and the stimulation of beta-oxidation (Ha *et al.*, 1994).

Vitamin C is also considered to be the predominant reductant for two copper-dependent enzymes: dopamine β-hydroxylase (used in the synthesis of norepinephrine from dopamine in the adrenal medulla) and peptidylglycine α-amidating monooxygenase (used in the amidation, and therefore activation, of various hormones and neurotransmitters)(Bornstein *et al.*, 2003; Bousquet-Moore *et al.*, 2010). A role for vitamin C in these reactions may explain the high concentrations of vitamin C in the adrenal and pituitary glands, 30–40 mg/100 g versus 10–15 mg/100 g in most other tissues. Given the roles of norepinephrine in the regulation of arousal and adaptation to stressors, and the fact that peptidylglycine α-amidating monooxygenase controls the production of more than one half of all neuropeptides, the involvement of vitamin C in these synthetic pathways suggests an important yet largely unexplored role of this nutrient in neuroendocrine biology.

Although the impact of ascorbic acid in cell culture media is difficult to interpret (Osiecki *et al.*, 2010), recent investigations utilizing cDNA microarray analysis showed that vitamin C affects gene expression in human skin fibroblasts (increasing expression of DNA replication and repair genes) and in rat CNS precursor cells (increasing expression of pro-collagen type 1 alpha 2, transferrin, tyrosine hydroxylase, and interferon alpha-inducible protein) (Yu *et al.*, 2004; Duarte *et al.*, 2009). Vitamin C-induced cell differentiation is a novel molecular mechanism of vitamin C and suggests an important role for vitamin C in intracellular signaling cascades. Other work demonstrates a facilitator role for vitamin C in the reprogramming of somatic cells to pluripotent stem cells, possibly by increasing the activity of epigenetic regulating factors such as histone demethylases (Esteban *et al.*, 2010).

Physiological Functions

Supplemental vitamin C has been demonstrated to enhance immune parameters in certain patient populations, including neutrophil activation in sepsis and Chediak-Higashi syndrome, natural killer cell activity in thalassemia, and improved neutrophil motility in furunculosis (Weening *et al.*, 1981; Vohra *et al.*, 1990; Levy *et al.*, 1996; Atasever *et al.*, 2006). However, these are isolated reports amid many that show no benefit, and a definitive role for vitamin C in immunoresponsiveness has not been established. As an effective scavenger of reactive oxygen species, vitamin C may minimize the oxidative stress associated with the respiratory burst of activated phagocytic leukocytes, thereby functioning to control the inflammation and tissue damage associated with immune responses (Wintergerst *et al.*, 2006). *In vitro*, vitamin C directly inhibited NF-κB activation and selectively inhibited inflammatory cytokine production in monocytes, suggesting a possible antioxidant-independent effect of vitamin C in controlling inflammatory responses (Bowie and O'Neill, 2000; Härtel *et al.*, 2004).

The addition of ascorbic acid to virally infected cultured cells reduced virus multiplication, but this antiviral activity was related specifically to ascorbic acid-derived oxidation products including dehydroascorbic acid and hydroxyl radicals (Furuya *et al.*, 2008). Topical application of ascorbic acid in patients with herpes simplex virus infections decreased the duration of the lesions and viral shedding (Hamuy and Berman, 1998), and intravenous ascorbic acid in the treatment of herpetic neuralgia resulted in immediate remission of the neuropathic pain and remission of the cutaneous lesions within 10 days in two patients (Schencking *et al.*, 2010). In a randomized clinical trial, intravenous administration of ascorbic acid for 1 week reduced spontaneous pain in postherpetic neuralgia patients as compared with the saline control, but ascorbate therapy did not improve brush-evoked mechanical pain in these patients (Chen *et al.*, 2009). In patients recovering from wrist fractures, oral vitamin C dosing (200–1500 mg/day) reduced the occurrence of complex regional pain syndrome for up to 350 days (Zollinger *et al.*, 2007). These reports suggest a possible role for vitamin C therapy in pain management.

Serum vitamin C was inversely related to seroprevalence of *Helicobacter pylori* in a large, population-based US sample (Simon *et al.*, 2003). In a randomized, controlled trial (*n* = 312 patients with *H. pylori* infection), the addition of vitamin C (500 mg/day) to the standard *H. pylori* treatment regimen significantly improved the *H. pylori* eradication rate by nearly 60% (from 49% to 78%) (Zojaji *et al.*, 2009). Others have also noted beneficial effects of supplemental vitamin C in combination with *H. pylori* eradication regimens in randomized clinical trials (Kaboli *et al.*, 2009; Sezikli *et al.*, 2009). However, these improvements in eradication rates may be related to reductions in antibiotic resistance, differences in genetic composition, and/or geographical localization, and not to a direct antiviral effect of vitamin C (Filik, 2010).

The role of supplemental vitamin C in combating the common cold has long been debated, and although the majority of randomized clinical trials show no effect of vitamin C for reducing the incidence or duration of colds in the general population, there are some notable exceptions. A meta-analysis of 30 controlled trials concluded that vitamin C supplementation reduced the incidence of colds in people under stressful conditions such as severe physical activity or cold environments but not in normal, unstressed people (Douglas *et al.*, 2007). A 5-year randomized, double-blinded, placebo-controlled trial demonstrated that vitamin C supplementation (500 mg/day) reduced the frequency of colds by 20%, and reduced the risk of suffering more than two cold episodes over a 3-year period by 66% compared with the placebo treatment (50 mg vitamin C/day) (Sasazuki *et al.*, 2006).

In a randomized controlled trial, vitamin C (1500 mg/day for 2 weeks) protected against exercise-induced airway narrowing in patients with asthma, possibly due to reductions in the proinflammatory eicosanoids related to bronchoconstriction (Tecklenburg *et al.*, 2007). Also, supplementation with 250 mg of vitamin C/day for 6 weeks significantly reduced (by 50%) monocyte ICAM-1 mRNA expression in healthy male subjects (Rayment *et al.*, 2003); ICAM-1 is an adhesion molecule associated with the airway hyperresponsiveness that is characteristic of the common cold, allergic asthma, and seasonal allergic rhinitis. Low vitamin C status has also been associated with risk of lung infections, particularly pneumonia (Hemilä and Louhiala, 2007).

Current evidence suggests possible roles of vitamin C in the promotion of vascular health beyond its role as a general antioxidant (Frikke-Schmidt and Lykkesfeldt, 2009). In coronary heart disease (CHD) oxidative stress reduces intracellular concentrations of the vasodilator nitric oxide (NO) and elevates vascular cell adhesion molecules and proinflammatory substances. Vitamin C stimulates endothelial NO synthesis by attenuating the oxidative degradation of tetrahydrobiopterin, an essential cofactor for endothelial NO synthase (Kim *et al.*, 2006). Additionally, vitamin C reduced plasma concentrations of the cell adhesion molecule P selectin and the inflammatory cytokine, IL-6, a mediator of local inflammation and vascular dysfunction (Tahir *et al.*, 2005; Böhm *et al.*, 2007). Vitamin C administration has been shown to reverse endothelial dysfunction in patients with hypertension, diabetes, and stable angina (Anderson *et al.*, 2006; Holowatz and Kenney, 2007) and to reverse ischemia-reperfusion-induced endothelial dysfunction in healthy subjects, subjects with peripheral arterial disease, and smokers (de Sousa *et al.*, 2005; Pleiner *et al.*, 2008).

Although several large randomized clinical trials did not show clear benefits of supplemental vitamin C for reducing risk of CHD or for improving clinical symptoms in patient populations (Hasnain and Mooradian, 2004; Willcox *et al.*, 2008), other evidence suggests that vitamin C regimens may have clinical value. In a randomized controlled trial, vitamin C (500 mg/day) reduced restenosis 26% and increased the minimal lumen diameter 30% in patients recovering from coronary angioplasty (Tomoda *et al.*, 1996). Pooled analyses from several clinical trials (*n* = 156 949) revealed that subjects who took >700 mg

vitamin C daily had a significant 25% lower risk for CHD compared with subjects who did not take supplemental vitamin C, a finding that remained significant after adjustment for healthy lifestyles (Knekt *et al.*, 2004). However, in the subjects that did not supplement vitamin C, dietary vitamin C was not related to CHD risk. In a 5-year prospective study of 1605 randomly selected men (42–60 years), those with vitamin C deficiency at baseline (plasma vitamin C <0.2 mg/dL) were at significantly increased risk of myocardial infarction after controlling for confounding variables (Nyyssonen *et al.*, 1997). For patients receiving cardiac catheterization treatment, a low plasma vitamin C concentration predicted the presence of an unstable coronary syndrome as indicated by atherosclerotic lesion activity (Vita *et al.*, 1998).

Many large prospective trials show modest, inverse relationships between vitamin C status and cancer incidence and/or mortality, particularly in men; and, recent meta-analyses suggest that vitamin C may possibly protect against lung, breast, and esophageal cancers (Cho *et al.*, 2006; Kubo and Corley, 2007). Yet, short-term prospective intervention trials did not demonstrate an anti-cancer role for supplemental vitamin C (120 mg/day for 5 years on the incidence of esophageal, stomach, or colon cancers or 500 mg/day for 8 years on the incidence of prostate or total cancer in men) (Blot *et al.*, 1993; Gaziano *et al.*, 2009). However, the progression of *H. pylori* infection to gastric dysplasia or gastric cancer was reduced by 80% in individuals with adequate serum vitamin C status (>0.55 mg/dL) compared with those who had below-adequate status (You *et al.*, 2000).

Although investigations show that vitamin C reduces DNA and protein oxidative damage *in vivo*, providing plausible mechanisms for an anti-cancer effect of vitamin C, current interest is focused on the efficacy of high-dose vitamin C injection therapy as a cancer treatment (Frei and Lawson, 2008). At pharmaceutical concentrations in biological systems, vitamin C acts as a pro-oxidant generating H_2O_2 that directly destroys cancer cells but not normal cells. Although case studies report success with high-dose intravenous vitamin C therapy (Padayatty *et al.*, 2006), a phase I clinical trial in 24 patients with advanced cancers did not demonstrate an objective anti-cancer response with intravenous vitamin C (0.4 to 1.5 g/kg fixed dosages three times weekly) in any patient (Hoffer *et al.*, 2008). Vitamin C may also promote anti-cancer effects by inhibiting cancer metastases although the mechanism of this effect is not known (Pollard *et al.*, 2010).

For the many pathological conditions associated with oxidative stress and reactive radicals, including cataract, macular degeneration, Alzheimer's disease, and rheumatoid arthritis, the total antioxidant capacity of tissues is an important preventive measure. Vitamin C regenerates vitamin E as well as antioxidant polyphenols and acts in synergy with these antioxidants, and with glutathione and selenium, to promote maximal antioxidant protection (Cuddihy *et al.*, 2008; Iglesias *et al.*, 2009).

High intakes of vitamin C have been related to higher bone mineral density in older adults (Sahni *et al.*, 2008). Recent research suggested that vitamin C has cofactor roles in several transcription and enzymatic reactions that regulate osteoblast differentiation (Gabbay *et al.*, 2010). Vitamin C status is also inversely related to adiposity in adults (Johnston *et al.*, 2007). Plausibly, obesity-induced inflammation may accelerate the metabolism of vitamin C *in vivo*, reducing plasma concentrations of the vitamin; however, some evidence has shown that vitamin C promotes locomotive behaviors and lipolytic responses in cafeteria-diet-fed rats (García-Díaz *et al.*, 2009) and inhibited gene expression linked to obesity onset (García-Díaz *et al.*, 2007).

Non-heme iron absorption from test meals is enhanced two- to threefold in the presence of 25 to 70 mg of vitamin C, a consequence of the ascorbate-induced reduction of ferric iron to ferrous iron, the form less likely to bind phytates. Recent evidence suggests that vitamin C also promotes duodenal ferric reductase activity in iron-deficient subjects but not in iron-replete subjects (Atanasova *et al.*, 2005). In animal models, vitamin C deficiency reduces the activity of hepatic cholesterol 7 alpha-hydroxylase, affecting the catabolism of cholesterol to bile acids and the risk for gall-bladder disease, and reduces serum uric acid via a uricosuric effect. Prospective trials in adult populations have demonstrated protective effects of vitamin C for reducing risk for gallstones and for gout (Choi *et al.*, 2009; Walcher *et al.*, 2009).

Deficient and Marginal Status

Functional measures of vitamin C status are not currently available, and vitamin C concentrations in plasma or leukocytes are used to determine vitamin C status. Leukocyte concentrations are difficult to measure and interpret; hence, the measurement of plasma vitamin C is the most widely applied test for vitamin C status. Plasma concentrations <0.2 mg/dL (11 μmol/L) indicate vitamin C defi-

ciency, and concentrations between 0.2 and 0.5 mg/dL (11 and 28 μmol/L) represent marginal vitamin C status, defined as moderate risk for developing vitamin C deficiency due to inadequate tissue stores. Intakes at the recommended level, 75–90 mg/day, are associated with plasma vitamin C concentrations near 0.8 mg/dL (45 μmol/L), and tissue saturation is achieved at intakes from 100 to 200 mg/day, corresponding to plasma concentrations near 1.0 mg/dL (about 60 μmol/L) (Levine *et al.*, 1996).

Subcutaneous and intramuscular hemorrhages, leg edema, neuropathy, and cerebral hemorrhage characterize scurvy, the vitamin C deficiency disease, and these symptoms are generally attributed to weakened collagenous structures. If untreated, the condition is ultimately fatal. Throughout the course of civilization, scurvy has plagued whole populations without access to fresh fruits and vegetables. Scurvy continues to be observed in developed nations, particularly among alcoholics, institutionalized elderly, men who live alone, and individuals who consume restrictive diets. Patients complain of lassitude, weakness, and general malaise, and seek medical advice following the appearance of a skin rash, lower extremity edema, and bone pain.

Data from the second National Health and Nutrition Examination Survey (NHANES II) conducted in the US from 1976 to 1980 indicated that the prevalence of vitamin C deficiency ranged from 0.1% in children (3–5 years) to 3% in females (25–44 years) and 7% in males (45–64 years) (Fulwood *et al.*, 1982). The prevalence of marginal vitamin C status ranged from 17% in adult females to 24% in adult males. In the most recent NHANES data analyses (2003–2004), vitamin C deficiency rates ranged from 8 to 11% for women and men (20–39 years and 20–59 years, respectively) (Schleicher *et al.*, 2009). Marginal vitamin C prevalence rates for adults have remained fairly stable over the past 25 years (20–23%) (Hampl *et al.*, 2004). Vitamin C deficiency rates for Canadian and low-income European citizens have also been reported recently (14% and 19% respectively) (Mosdøl *et al.*, 2008; Cahill *et al.*, 2009).

Dietary Requirements

In 2000 the Panel on Dietary Antioxidants and Related Compounds of the Institute of Medicine, a part of the United States National Academies, released the Dietary Reference Intakes (DRI) for vitamin C (Table 16.1)

TABLE 16.1 Daily vitamin C recommendations for age and gender groups by various health agencies

Age (gender) group	Vitamin C/day (mg)			
	RDA IOM	RNI WHO/FAO	RNI UK	RDA NIHN
0–6 months	40[a]	25	25	40[b]
7–12 months	50[a]	30	25	40[b]
1–3 years	15	30	30	40–45
4–8 years	25	30–35	30	45–70
9–13 years (boys)	45	35–40	30–35	70–100
14–17 years (boys)	75	40	35–40	100
9–13 years (girls)	45	35–40	30–35	70–100
14–17 years (girls)	65	40	35–40	100
19+ years (men)	90	45	40	100
19+ years (women)	75	45	40	100
14–18 years (pregnant)	80	55	50	110
19–50 years (pregnant)	85	55	50	110
14–18 years (lactating)	115	70	70	150
19–50 years (lactating)	120	70	70	150

RDA, recommended dietary allowance; RNI, reference nutrient intake; IOM, Institute of Medicine of the United States National Academies; WHO/FAO, World Health Organization/Food and Agricultural Organization of the United Nations; UK, United Kingdom; NIHN, National Institute of Health and Nutrition, Japan.
[a]Estimated average requirement.
[b]Adequate intake.

(Institute of Medicine, 2000). For adult men, the estimated average requirement (EAR) for vitamin C, the level of intake that is estimated to meet the requirements of half the healthy individuals in a life stage and gender group, was set at 75 mg/day to maintain near-maximal tissue concentrations of vitamin C and provide antioxidant protection. The estimated requirement for adult women, 60 mg/day, was extrapolated based on body weight differences from the EAR for men.

The RDAs were calculated as 120% of the EAR, and are believed to cover the needs of 97–98% of individuals in a group (90 and 75 mg/day for adult men and women, respectively). Older age groups (>50 years) have decreased lean body mass compared with their younger counterparts; however, the DRIs for older men and women were not decreased from that for younger adults because oxidative stress, which causes higher vitamin C needs, increases with age. Smokers should consume an additional 35 mg of vitamin C daily, totaling 125 mg/day for adult men and 110 mg/day for adult women, due to increased oxidative stress.

Higher vitamin C intakes were recommended for pregnant and lactating women to offset losses from maternal body pools (Table 16.1). RDAs for children ranged from 15 to 25 mg/day for younger children and from 45 to 75 mg/day for preadolescents and adolescents. Since there were no functional criteria for vitamin C status in infants, the recommended intakes of vitamin C at this age level were based on adequate intakes (AI), reflecting the vitamin C ingestion of mainly breast-fed infants (Table 16.1).

The World Health Organization and Food and Agriculture Organization of the United Nations (WHO/FAO, 2002) set the recommended nutrient intake for vitamin C at 45 mg/day for all adults and elderly individuals including smokers, a value estimated to achieve 50% tissue saturation in 97.5% of this population. Pregnant and lactating women require an additional 10 and 20 mg daily; recommended intakes were arbitrarily set at 25 mg/day for infants, gradually rising to 40 mg/day for adolescents (Table 16.1). The United Kingdom's Food Standards Agency recommended vitamin C intakes of 40 mg/day for adults and 50 and 70 mg/day for pregnant and lactating women respectively (COMA, 1991). The Ministry of Health, Labour and Welfare of Japan set the dietary reference intakes for vitamin C at 40 mg/day for infants and children up to 2 years of age; the recommendation gradually rises to 80 mg/day for children 10–11 years of age and to 100 mg daily for all age categories 12 years and older (Sasaki, 2008). For pregnant and lactating women, the recommendations are 110 and 150 mg daily (Table 16.1).

High doses of vitamin C (as high as 2 g/day) are well tolerated by healthy individuals. Based strictly on reports of gastrointestinal disturbances, a tolerable upper intake level for vitamin C was set at 2000 mg/day for adults by the Institute of Medicine (2000). The upper intake level represents a dosage level that with high probability is tolerated biologically and provides guidance to individuals using dietary supplements. Claims that high-dose vitamin C regimens may lead to rebound scurvy, the iron-catalyzed oxidation of ascorbic acid, red blood cell hemolysis, and vitamin B_{12} deficiency do not withstand scientific scrutiny.

Because dietary vitamin C may enhance mealtime iron absorption, high-dose vitamin C regimens may aggravate conditions associated with increased iron absorption and storage, notably hemochromatosis. About 0.5% and 10% of the US population are homozygous and heterozygous, respectively, for the hemochromatosis *HFE* gene mutation. The addition of vitamin C fortified orange juice to a test meal did increase non-heme iron absorption in homozygous patients compared with controls (Lynch *et al.*, 1989), but increased iron absorption was not observed in patients heterozygous for the *HFE* gene mutation (Hunt and Zeng, 2004). Analyses of NHANES data from 1976 to 1980 showed that women with the highest serum vitamin C concentrations (>2.1 mg/dL or 116 μmol/L) had a twofold increased prevalence of elevated serum ferritin levels (Simon and Hudes, 1999).

Vitamin C supplementation may also have adverse effects on thalassemia major, an iron-overload disease characterized by impaired globin chain synthesis. Cases are usually diagnosed in the first year of life, and blood transfusions are often required for survival. In the absence of chelation therapy, iron accumulation in parenchymal tissues is associated with progressive dysfunction of the heart, liver, and endocrine glands. Vitamin C supplementation by patients may mobilize iron stores, creating iron-overloaded plasma and risk for increased oxidative stress (Diav-Citrin *et al.*, 1999). Vitamin C supplementation in these patients should be coordinated with chelation therapy.

High-dose vitamin C regimens increase urinary excretion of oxalic acid and uric acid, constituents of renal calculi, and, theoretically, may promote the formation of kidney stones. Epidemiologic investigations have reported mixed results regarding a direct association between vitamin C supplementation and stone incidence. In one large prospective trial (51 529 men), the annual number of additional incidental kidney stones was 0.84 per 1000 for those consuming >90 mg vitamin C daily (Taylor *et al.*, 2004).

Future Directions

Research into the contribution of vitamin C deficiency to morbidity and mortality is needed since 8–19% of North American and European citizens fall into this category. Diet–gene interactions are important considerations for trials examining associations between vitamin C intake and disease risk. Also, because it is inexpensive and relatively non-toxic, continued investigation of the potential benefits of supplemental vitamin C should be pursued.

Suggestions for Further Reading

Li, Y. and Schellhorn, H.E. (2007) New developments and novel therapeutic perspectives for vitamin C. *J Nutr* **137**, 2171–2184.

Mandl, J., Szarka, A., and Banhegyi, G. (2009) Vitamin C: update on physiology and pharmacology. *Br J Pharmacol* **157**, 1097–1110.

References

Anderson, R.A., Evans, L.M., Ellis, G.R., *et al.* (2006) Prolonged deterioration of endothelial dysfunction in response to postprandial lipaemia is attenuated by vitamin C in Type 2 diabetes. *Diabet Med* **23**, 258–264.

Atanasova, B.D., Li, A.C., Bjarnason, I., *et al.* (2005) Duodenal ascorbate and ferric reductase in human iron deficiency. *Am J Clin Nutr* **81**, 130–133.

Atasever, B., Ertan, N.Z., Erdem-Kuruca, S., *et al.* (2006) In vitro effects of vitamin C and selenium on NK activity of patients with beta-thalassemia major. *Pediatr Hematol Oncol* **23**, 187–197.

Blanchard, J. (1991) Depletion and repletion kinetics of vitamin C in humans. *J Nutr* **121**, 170–176.

Blot, W.J., Li, J.Y., Taylor, P.R., *et al.* (1993) Nutrition intervention trials in Linxian, China: supplementation with specific vitamin/mineral combinations, cancer incidence, and disease-specific mortality in the general population. *J Natl Cancer Inst* **85**, 1483–1492.

Bluck, L.J., Izzard, A.P., and Bates, C.J. (1996) Measurement of ascorbic acid kinetics in man using stable isotopes and gas chromatography/mass spectrometry. *J Mass Spectrom* **31**, 741–748.

Böhm, F., Settergren, M., and Pernow, J. (2007) Vitamin C blocks vascular dysfunction and release of interleukin-6 induced by endothelin-1 in humans in vivo. *Atherosclerosis* **190**, 408–415.

Bornstein, S.R., Yoshida-Hiroi, M., Sotiriou, S., *et al.* (2003) Impaired adrenal catecholamine system function in mice with deficiency of the ascorbic acid transporter (SVCT2). *FASEB J* **17**, 1928–1930.

Bousquet-Moore, D., Mains, R.E., and Eipper, B.A. (2010) Peptidylglycine alpha-amidating monooxygenase and copper: a gene–nutrient interaction critical to nervous system function. *J Neurosci Res* **88**, 2535–2545.

Bowie, A.G. and O'Neill, L.A. (2000) Vitamin C inhibits NF-κB activation by TNF via the activation of p38 mitogen-activated protein kinase. *J Immunol* **165**, 7180–7188.

Buettner, G.R. and Jurkiewicz, B.A. (1993) Ascorbate free radical as a marker of oxidative stress: an EPR study. *Free Radic Biol Med* **14**, 49–55.

Burns, J.J., Burch, H.B., and King, C.G. (1951) The metabolism of 1-C14-L-ascorbic acid in guinea pigs. *J Biol Chem* **191**, 501–514.

Cahill, L., Corey, P.N., and El-Sohemy, A. (2009) Vitamin C deficiency in a population of young Canadian adults. *Am J Epidemiol* **170**, 464–471.

Cahill, L.E. and El-Sohemy, A. (2009) Vitamin C transporter gene polymorphisms, dietary vitamin C and serum ascorbic acid. *J Nutrigenet Nutrigenomics* **2**, 292–301.

Cahill, L.E., Fontaine-Bisson, B., and El-Sohemy, A. (2009) Functional genetic variants of glutathione S-transferase protect against serum ascorbic acid deficiency. *Am J Clin Nutr* **90**, 1411–1417.

Chatterjee, I.B. (1973) Evolution and the biosynthesis of ascorbic acid. *Nature* **182**, 1271–1272.

Chen, J.Y., Chang, C.Y., Feng, P.H., *et al.* (2009) Plasma vitamin C is lower in postherpetic neuralgia patients and administration of vitamin C reduces spontaneous pain but not brush-evoked pain. *Clin J Pain* **25**, 562–569.

Cho, E., Hunter, D.J., Spiegelman, D., *et al.* (2006) Intakes of vitamins A, C and E and folate and multivitamins and lung cancer: a pooled analysis of 8 prospective studies. *Int J Cancer* **118**, 970–978.

Choi, H.K., Gao, X., and Curhan, G. (2009) Vitamin C intake and the risk of gout in men: a prospective study. *Arch Intern Med* **169**, 502–507.

Chung, W.Y., Chung, J.K., Szeto, Y.T., *et al.* (2001) Plasma ascorbic acid: measurement, stability and clinical utility revisited. *Clin Biochem* **34**, 623–627.

COMA (1991) Dietary Reference Values for Food Energy and Nutrients for the United Kingdom. Report of the Panel on Dietary Reference Values of the Committee on the Medical Aspects of Food Policy (COMA). Department of Health RHSS 41. HMSO, London.

Corti, A., Casini, A.F., and Pompell, A. (2010) Cellular pathways for transport and efflux of ascorbate and dehydroascorbate. *Arch Biochem Biophys* **500**, 107–115.

Cuddihy, S.L., Parker, A., Harwood, D.T., *et al.* (2008) Ascorbate interacts with reduced glutathione to scavenge phenoxyl radicals in HL60 cells. *Free Radic Biol Med* **44**, 1637–1644.

Dash, J.A., Jenness, R., and Hume, I.D. (1984) Ascorbic acid turnover and excretion in two arboreal marsupials and in laboratory rabbits. *Comp Biochem Physiol B* **77**, 391–397.

de Sousa, M.G., Yugar-Toledo, J.C., Rubira, M., *et al.* (2005) Ascorbic acid improves impaired venous and arterial endothelium-dependent dilation in smokers. *Acta Pharmacol Sin* **26**, 447–452.

Diav-Citrin, O., Atanackovic, G., and Koren, G. (1999) An investigation into variability in the therapeutic response to deferiprone in patients with thalassemia major. *Ther Drug Monit* **21**, 74–81.

Douglas, R.M., Hemilä, H., Chalker, E., *et al.* (2007) Vitamin C for preventing and treating the common cold. *Cochrane Database Syst Rev* CD000980.

Duarte, T.L., Cooke, M.S., and Jones, G.D. (2009) Gene expression profiling reveals new protective roles for vitamin C in human skin cells. *Free Radic Biol Med* **46**, 78–87.

Erichsen, H.C., Engel, S.A., Eck, P.K., *et al.* (2006) Genetic variation in the sodium-dependent vitamin C transporters, SLC23A1, and SLC23A2 and risk for preterm delivery. *Am J Epidemiol* **163**, 245–254.

Esteban, M.A., Wang, T., Qin, B., *et al.* (2010) Vitamin C enhances the generation of mouse and human induced pluripotent stem cells. *Cell Stem Cell* **6**, 71–79.

Filik, L. (2010) Comment to "The efficacy of *Helicobacter pylori* eradication regimen with and without vitamin C supplementation". *Dig Liver Dis* **42**, 596.

Frei, B. and Lawson, S. (2008) Vitamin C and cancer revisited. *Proc Natl Acad Sci USA* **105**, 11037–11038.

Frikke-Schmidt, H. and Lykkesfeldt, J. (2009) Role of marginal vitamin C deficiency in atherogenesis: in vivo models and clinical studies. *Basic Clin Pharmacol Toxicol* **104**, 419–433.

Fulwood, R., Johnson, C.L., Bryner, J.D., *et al.* (1982) Hematological and nutritional biochemistry reference data for persons 6 months–74 years of age: United States, 1976–1980. DHHS Publication No. (PHS) 83-1682. US Department of Health and Human Services, Public Health Service, National Center for Health Statistics, Hyattsville, MD.

Furuya, A., Uozaki, M., Yamasaki, H., *et al.* (2008) Antiviral effects of ascorbic and dehydroascorbic acids in vitro. *Int J Mol Med* **22**, 541–545.

Gabbay, K.H., Bohren, K.M., Morello, R., *et al.* (2010) Ascorbate synthesis pathway: dual role of ascorbate in bone homeostasis. *J Biol Chem* **285**, 19510–19520.

García-Díaz, D.F., Campión, J., Milagro, F.I., *et al.* (2007) Adiposity dependent apelin gene expression: relationships with oxidative and inflammation markers. *Mol Cell Biochem* **305**, 87–94.

García-Díaz, D.F., Campion, J., Milagro, F.I., *et al.* (2009) Ascorbic acid oral treatment modifies lipolytic response and behavioural activity but not glucocorticoid metabolism in cafeteria diet-fed rats. *Acta Physiol* **195**, 449–457.

Gaziano, J.M., Glynn, R.J., Christen, W.G., *et al.* (2009) Vitamins E and C in the prevention of prostate and total cancer in men: the Physicians' Health Study II randomized controlled trial. *J Am Med Assoc* **301**, 52–62.

Godoy, A., Ormazabal, V., Moraga-Cid, G., *et al.* (2007) Mechanistic insights and functional determinants of the transport cycle of the ascorbic acid transporter SVCT2. Activation by sodium and absolute dependence on bivalent cations. *J Biol Chem* **282**, 615–624.

Ha, T.Y., Otsuka, M., and Arakawa, N. (1994) Ascorbate indirectly stimulates fatty acid utilization in primary cultured guinea pig hepatocytes by enhancing carnitine synthesis. *J Nutr* **124**, 732–737.

Hampl, J.S., Taylor, C.A., and Johnston, C.S. (2004) Vitamin C deficiency and depletion in the United States: the Third National Health and Nutrition Examination Survey, 1988 to 1994. *Am J Public Health* **94**, 870–875.

Hamuy, R. and Berman, B. (1998) Treatment of herpes simplex virus infections with topical antiviral agents. *Eur J Dermatol* **8**, 310–319.

Härtel, C., Strunk, T., Bucsky, P., *et al.* (2004) Effects of vitamin C on intracytoplasmic cytokine production in human whole blood monocytes and lymphocytes. *Cytokine* **27**, 101–106.

Hasnain, B.I. and Mooradian, A.D. (2004) Recent trials of antioxidant therapy: what should we be telling our patients? *Cleve Clin J Med* **71**, 327–334.

Hellman, L. and Burns, J.J. (1958) Metabolism of L-ascorbic acid-1-C14 in man. *J Biol Chem* **230**, 923–930.

Hemilä, H. and Louhiala, P. (2007) Vitamin C for preventing and treating pneumonia. *Cochrane Database Syst Rev* CD005532.

Hoffer, L.J., Levine, M., Assouline, S., *et al.* (2008) Phase I clinical trial of i.v. ascorbic acid in advanced malignancy. *Ann Oncol* **19**, 1969–1974.

Holowatz, L.A. and Kenney, W.L. (2007) Local ascorbate administration augments NO- and non-NO-dependent reflex cutaneous vasodilation in hypertensive humans. *Am J Physiol Heart Circ Physiol* **293**, H1090–1096.

Hughes, R.E., Hurley, R.J., and Jones, E. (1980) Dietary ascorbic acid and muscle carnitine (β-OH-γ-(trimethyl amino) butyric acid) in guinea pigs. *Br J Nutr* **43**, 385–387.

Hunt, J.R. and Zeng, H. (2004) Iron absorption by heterozygous carriers of the HFE C282Y mutation associated with hemochromatosis. *Am J Clin Nutr* **80**, 924–931.

Iglesias, J., Pazos, M., Andersen, M.L., *et al.* (2009) Caffeic acid as antioxidant in fish muscle: mechanism of synergism with endogenous ascorbic acid and alpha-tocopherol. *J Agric Food Chem* **57**, 675–681.

Ihara, H., Shino, Y., Aoki, Y., *et al.* (2000) A simple and rapid method for the routine assay of total ascorbic acid in serum and plasma using ascorbate oxidase and o-phenylenediamine. *J Nutr Sci Vitaminol* **46**, 321–324.

Institute of Medicine (2000) *Dietary Reference Intakes for Vitamin C, Vitamin E, Selenium, and Carotenoids*. National Academies Press, Washington, DC. Available online at: http://www.nap.edu/openbook/0309069351/html/index.html. Accessed August 27, 2010.

Johnston, C.S., Beezhold, B.L., Mostow, B., *et al.* (2007) Plasma vitamin C is inversely related to body mass index and waist circumference but not to plasma adiponectin in nonsmoking adults. *J Nutr* **137**, 1757–1762.

Kaboli, S.A., Zojaji, H., Mirsattari, D., *et al.* (2009) Effect of addition of vitamin C to clarithromycin–amoxicillin–omeprazol triple regimen on *Helicobacter pylori* eradication. *Acta Gastroenterol Belg* **72**, 222–224.

Karlsen, A., Blomhoff, R., and Gundersen, T.E. (2007) Stability of whole blood and plasma ascorbic acid. *Eur J Clin Nutr* **61**, 1233–1236.

Karthiga, S., Dubey, S., Garber, S., *et al.* (2008) Scurvy: MRI appearances. *Rheumatology* **47**, 1109.

Kennett, E.C. and Kuchel, P.W. (2006) Plasma membrane oxidoreductases: effects on erythrocyte metabolism and redox homeostasis. *Antioxid Redox Signal* **8**, 1241–1247.

Kim, H.J., Lee, S.I., Lee, D.H., *et al.* (2006) Ascorbic acid synthesis due to L-gulono-1,4-lactone oxidase expression enhances NO production in endothelial cells. *Biochem Biophys Res Commun* **345**, 1657–1662.

Knekt, P., Ritz, J., Pereira, M.A., *et al.* (2004) Antioxidant vitamins and coronary heart disease risk: a pooled analysis of nine cohorts. *Am J Clin Nutr* **80**, 1508–1520.

Kubo, A. and Corley, D.A. (2007) Meta-analysis of antioxidant intake and the risk of esophageal and gastric cardia adenocarcinoma. *Am J Gastroenterol* **102**, 2323–2330.

Levine, M. (1986) New concepts in the biology and biochemistry of ascorbic acid. *N Engl J Med* **314**, 892–902.

Levine, M., Conry-Cantilena, C., Wang, Y., *et al.* (1996) Vitamin C pharmacokinetics in healthy volunteers: evidence for a recommended dietary allowance. *Proc Natl Acad Sci USA* **93**, 3704–3709.

Levy, R., Shriker, O., Porath, A., *et al.* (1996) Vitamin C for the treatment of recurrent furunculosis in patients with impaired neutrophil functions. *J Infect Dis* **173**, 1502–1505.

Li, X. and Franke, A.A. (2009) Fast HPLC–ECD analysis of ascorbic acid, dehydroascorbic acid and uric acid. *J Chromatogr B Analyt Technol Biomed Life Sci* **877**, 853–856.

Linster, C.L. and Van Schaftingen, E. (2006) Vitamin C. Biosynthesis, recycling and degradation in mammals. *FEBS J* **274**, 1–22.

Lynch, S.R., Skikne, B.S., and Cook, J.D. (1989) Food iron absorption in idiopathic hemochromatosis. *Blood* **74**, 2187–2193.

Mosdøl, A., Erens, B., and Brunner, E.J. (2008) Estimated prevalence and predictors of vitamin C deficiency within UK's low-income population. *J Public Health* **30**, 456–460.

Nandi, A., Mukhopadhyay, C.K., Ghosh, M.K., *et al.* (1997) Evolutionary significance of vitamin C biosynthesis in terrestrial vertebrates. *Free Radic Biol Med* **22**, 1047–1054.

Nualart, F.J., Rivas, C.I., Montecinos, V.P., *et al.* (2003) Recycling of vitamin C by a bystander effect. *J Biol Chem* **278**, 10128–10133.

Nyyssonen, K., Parviainen, M.T., Salonen, R., *et al.* (1997) Vitamin C deficiency and risk of myocardial infarction: prospective population study of men from Eastern Finland. *Br Med J* **314**, 634–638.

Osiecki, M., Ghanavi, P., Atkinson, K., *et al.* (2010) The ascorbic acid paradox. *Biochem Biophys Res Commun* **400**, 466–470.

Padayatty, S.J., Riordan, H.D., Hewitt, S.M., *et al.* (2006) Intravenously administered vitamin C as cancer therapy: three cases. *CMAJ* **174**, 937–942.

Pleiner, J., Schaller, G., Mittermayer, F., *et al.* (2008) Intra-arterial vitamin C prevents endothelial dysfunction caused by ischemia-reperfusion. *Atherosclerosis* **197**, 383–391.

Pollard, H.B., Levine, M.A., Eidelman, O., *et al.* (2010) Pharmacological ascorbic acid suppresses syngeneic tumor growth and metastases in hormone-refractory prostate cancer. *In Vivo* **24**, 249–255.

Rayment, S.J., Shaw, J., Woollard, K.J., *et al.* (2003) Vitamin C supplementation in normal subjects reduces constitutive ICAM-1 expression. *Biochem Biophys Res Commun* **308**, 339–345.

Rivas, C.I., Zuniga, F.A., Salas-Burgos, A., *et al.* (2008) Vitamin C transporters. *J Physiol Biochem* **64**, 357–376.

Robitaille, L., Mamer, O.A., Miller, W.H., *et al.* (2009) Oxalic acid excretion after intravenous ascorbic acid administration. *Metabolism* **58**, 263–269.

Sahni, S., Hannan, M.T., Gagnon, D., *et al.* (2008) High vitamin C intake is associated with lower 4-year bone loss in elderly men. *J Nutr* **138**, 1931–1938.

Salminen, I. and Alfthan, G. (2008) Plasma ascorbic acid preparation and storage for epidemiological studies using TCA precipitation. *Clin Biochem* **41**, 723–727.

Sasaki, S. (2008) Dietary Reference Intakes (DRIs) in Japan. *Asia Pac J Clin Nutr* **17**(Suppl 2), 420–444.

Sasazuki, S., Sasaki, S., Tsubono, Y., *et al.* (2006) Effect of vitamin C on common cold: randomized controlled trial. *Eur J Clin Nutr* **60**, 9–17.

Schaus, E.E., Kutnink, M.A., O'Conner, D.K., *et al.* (1986) A comparison of leukocyte ascorbate levels measured by the 2,4-dinitrophenylhydrazine method with high-performance liquid chromatography using electrochemical detection. *Biochem Med Metab Biol* **36**, 369–376.

Schencking, M., Sandholzer, H., and Frese, T. (2010) Intravenous administration of vitamin C in the treatment of herpetic neuralgia: two case reports. *Med Sci Monit* **28**, CS58–61.

Schleicher, R.L., Carroll, M.D., Ford, E.S., *et al.* (2009) Serum vitamin C and the prevalence of vitamin C deficiency in the United States: 2003–2004 National Health and Nutrition Examination Survey (NHANES). *Am J Clin Nutr* **90**, 1252–1263.

Sezikli, M., Cetinkaya, Z.A., Sezikli, H., *et al.* (2009) Oxidative stress in *Helicobacter pylori* infection: does supplementation with vitamins C and E increase the eradication rate? *Helicobacter* **14**, 280–285.

Simon, J.A. and Hudes, E.S. (1999) Relation of serum ascorbic acid to serum vitamin B12, serum ferritin, and kidney stones in US adults. *Arch Intern Med* **159**, 619–624.

Simon, J.A., Hudes, E.S., and Perez-Perez, G.I. (2003) Relation of serum ascorbic acid to *Helicobacter pylori* serology in US adults: the Third National Health and Nutrition Examination Survey. *J Am Coll Nutr* **22**, 283–289.

Sotiriou, S., Gispert, S., Cheng, J., *et al.* (2002) Ascorbic-acid transporter Slc23a1 is essential for vitamin C transport into the brain and for perinatal survival. *Nat Med* **8**, 514–517.

Stefansson, B.V., Haraldsson, B., and Nilsson, U. (2008) Ascorbyl free radical reflects catalytically active iron after intravenous iron saccharate injection. *Free Rad Biol Med* **45**, 1302–1307.

Tahir, M., Foley, B., Pate, G., *et al.* (2005) Impact of vitamin E and C supplementation on serum adhesion molecules in chronic degenerative aortic stenosis: a randomized controlled trial. *Am Heart J* **150**, 302–306.

Taylor, E.N., Stampfer, M.J., and Curhan, G.C. (2004) Dietary factors and the risk of incident kidney stones in men: new insights after 14 years of follow-up. *J Am Soc Nephrol* **15**, 3225–3232.

Tecklenburg, S.L., Mickleborough, T.D., Fly, A.D., *et al.* (2007) Ascorbic acid supplementation attenuates exercise-induced bronchoconstriction in patients with asthma. *Respir Med* **101,** 1770–1778.

Tillotson, J.A. and O'Connor, R. (1980) Ascorbic acid requirements of the trained monkey as determined by blood ascorbate levels. *Int J Vitam Nutr Res* **50,** 171–178.

Timpson, N.J., Forouhi, N.G., Brion, M.J., *et al.* (2010) Genetic variation at the SLC23A1 locus is associated with circulating concentrations of L-ascorbic acid (vitamin C): evidence from five independent studies with >15,000 participants. *Am J Clin Nutr* **92,** 375–382.

Tomoda, H., Yoshitake, M., Morimoto, K., *et al.* (1996) Possible prevention of postangioplasty restenosis by ascorbic acid. *Am J Cardiol* **78,** 1284–1286.

Vielhaber, S., Feistner, H., Weis, J., *et al.* (2004) Primary carnitine deficiency: adult onset lipid storage myopathy with a mild clinical course. *J Clin Neurosci* **11,** 919–924.

Vita, J.A., Keaney, J.F., Raby, K.E., *et al.* (1998) Low plasma ascorbic acid independently predicts the presence of an unstable coronary syndrome. *J Am Coll Cardiol* **31,** 980–986.

Vitale, A., La Torre, F., Martini, G., *et al.* (2009) Arthritis and gum bleeding in two children. *J Paediatr Child Health* **45,** 158–160.

Vohra, K., Khan, A.J., Telang, V., *et al.* (1990) Improvement of neutrophil migration by systemic vitamin C in neonates. *J Perinatol* **10,** 134–136.

Walcher, T., Haenle, M.M., Kron, M., *et al.* (2009) Vitamin supplement use may protect against gallstones: an observational study on a randomly selected population. *BMC Gastroenterol* **9,** 74.

Weening, R.S., Schoorel, E.P., Roos, D., *et al.* (1981) Effect of ascorbate on abnormal neutrophil, platelet and lymphocytic function in a patient with the Chediak-Higashi syndrome. *Blood* **57,** 856–865.

Willcox, B.J., Curb, J.D., and Rodriguez, B.L. (2008) Antioxidants in cardiovascular health and disease: key lessons from epidemiologic studies. *Am J Cardiol* **101,** 75D–86D.

WHO/FAO (World Health Organization and Food and Agriculture Organization of the United Nations) (2002) Human Vitamin and Mineral Requirements. Rome. Available online at: http://www.fao.org/docrep/004/y2809e/y2809e0c.htm#bm12. Accessed January 22, 2011.

Wintergerst, E.S., Maggini, S., and Hornig, D.H. (2006) Immune-enhancing role of vitamin C and zinc and effect on clinical conditions. *Ann Nutr Metab* **50,** 85–94.

Wolucka, B.A. and Van Montagu, M. (2007) The VTC2 cycle and the de novo biosynthesis pathways for vitamin C in plants: an opinion. *Phytochemistry* **68,** 2602–2613.

Wright, M.E., Andreotti, G., Lissowska, J., *et al.* (2009) Genetic variation in sodium-dependent ascorbic acid transporters and risk of gastric cancer in Poland. *Eur J Cancer* **45,** 1824–1830.

You, W.C., Zhang, L., Gail, M.H., *et al.* (2000) Gastric dysplasia and gastric cancer: *Helicobacter pylori*, serum vitamin C, and other risk factors. *J Natl Cancer Inst* **92,** 1607–1612.

Yu, D.H., Lee, K.H., Lee, J.Y., *et al.* (2004) Changes of gene expression profiles during neuronal differentiation of central nervous system precursors treated with ascorbic acid. *J Neurosci Res* **78,** 29–37.

Zojaji, H., Talaie, R., and Mirsattari, D. (2009) The efficacy of *Helicobacter pylori* eradication regimen with and without vitamin C supplementation. *Dig Liver Dis* **41,** 644–647.

Zollinger, P.E., Tuinebreijer, W.E., Breederveld, R.S., *et al.* (2007) Can vitamin C prevent complex regional pain syndrome in patients with wrist fractures? A randomized, controlled, multicenter dose–response study. *J Bone Joint Surg Am* **89,** 1424–1431.

17

THIAMIN

LUCIEN BETTENDORFF, PhD

University of Liège – GIGA-Neurosciences, Liège, Belgium

Summary

Thiamin (vitamin B_1) was the first vitamin to be characterized and from its discovery originated the vitamin concept. Thiamin deficiency mainly affects the nervous system and causes two classical diseases, beriberi (a polyneuritic syndrome) and Wernicke–Korsakoff syndrome (anterograde amnesia resulting from brain lesions in alcoholics). Thiamin transport across cell membranes requires specific carriers. As this process is slow, various lipid-soluble thiamin precursors with better bioavailability have been developed. In the cytosol, thiamin is pyrophosphorylated to thiamin diphosphate (ThDP), an indispensable cofactor in cell energy metabolism. Therefore, thiamin deficiency causes decreased cofactor function, leading to neuronal death. In addition, the non-cofactor roles of the triphosphorylated derivatives thiamin triphosphate and adenosine thiamin triphosphate may play a part in metabolic regulation and may contribute to the pathology of thiamin-deficiency-induced brain lesions. Current research interest is focused on the metabolism and role of thiamin derivatives (especially in catalysis by ThDP-dependent enzymes) and the biochemical and pathophysiological mechanisms by which thiamin deficiency induces specific brain lesions and may be implicated in other disorders such as Alzheimer's disease and diabetes.

Introduction

Thiamin (thiamine, Figure 17.1A) is a water-soluble vitamin of the B group (vitamin B_1, aneurin). Most bacteria, fungi, and plants are able to synthesize thiamin *de novo*, whereas animals solely rely on exogenous sources. Nutritional thiamin deficiency leads to beriberi, a polyneuritic syndrome. Beriberi used to be a major public health problem in East Asia, especially in the nineteenth century, because the population in these countries relied heavily on polished rice (poor in thiamin) as staple food. A rare cardiovascular form of beriberi (wet beriberi, shoshin beriberi) leading to congestive heart failure is also sometimes observed. Another, relatively common form of thiamin deficiency, Wernicke–Korsakoff syndrome, affects the central nervous system and is generally associated with chronic alcoholism.

Free thiamin has no known physiological role, but thiamin diphosphate (ThDP, Figure 17.1A), formerly called thiamin pyrophosphate or cocarboxylase, is an

Present Knowledge in Nutrition, Tenth Edition. Edited by John W. Erdman Jr, Ian A. Macdonald and Steven H. Zeisel.
© 2012 International Life Sciences Institute. Published 2012 by John Wiley & Sons, Inc.

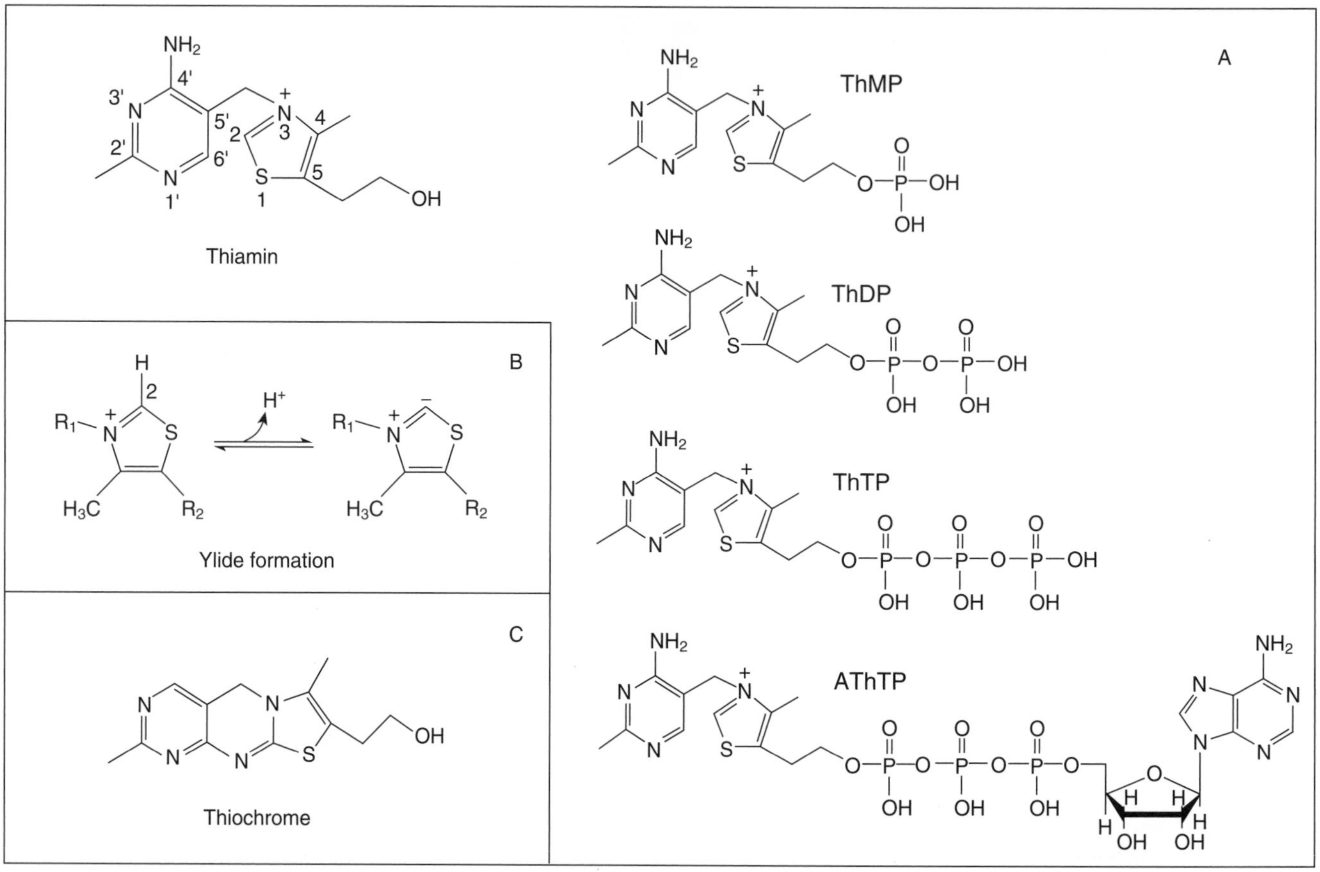

FIG. 17.1 Structure of thiamin derivatives. A, Natural derivatives; B, formation of the catalytic ylide intermediate; C, tricyclic fluorescent thiochromes.

essential cofactor in cell energy metabolism. As is the case for thiamin, several other B vitamins such as riboflavin (B_2), niacin (B_3), and pantothenic acid (B_5) are also precursors of cofactors required for mitochondrial energy production (Depeint et al., 2006). In addition to ThDP, two other phosphorylated derivatives, thiamin monophosphate (ThMP) and thiamin triphosphate (ThTP), have been known for many years (Makarchikov et al., 2003). More recently, adenylated thiamin derivatives, adenosine thiamin triphosphate (AThTP) and adenosine thiamin diphosphate have been described (Bettendorff et al., 2007; Frédérich et al., 2009). The biological roles of derivatives other than ThDP are still unclear, especially in eukaryotic organisms.

The Discovery of Vitamins: Thiamin and the Biochemical Lesion

The discovery of thiamin is a well-known story (Carpenter, 2000) from which originated the concept of vitamins and other food accessory factors. Beriberi was described in Chinese medical texts as early as 4000 years ago. The first description of beriberi in Japan appeared in the ninth century, but its relationship with diet was not suspected until the end of the nineteenth century. In 1884, a Japanese navy surgeon, Kanehiro Takaki, noticed that sailors were protected from beriberi when their diet was supplemented with condensed milk, bread, and meat in addition to the basic food consisting of polished rice (Takaki, 1885). In

1890, the Dutch physician, Christiaan Eijkman, working at the Laboratory of Bacteriology and Pathology in Batavia (now Djakarta), made the significant observation that fowl, when fed on polished rice, soon died from paralysis. Their peripheral nerves revealed histological signs of degeneration analogous to those described in human beri-beri (Eijkman, 1990). In chickens, the early symptoms could be reversed by switching to whole rice.

Gerrit Grijns, Eijkman's successor in Batavia, correctly recognized that polyneuritis was caused by the lack of an essential substance virtually absent in the endosperm but present in the husk of the rice (Grijns, 1901). At the same time, the vitamin concept started to be developed by the English biochemist Frederick Hopkins, who first postulated that food must contain, in addition to the well-known fundamental components, i.e. proteins, sugars, and fats, "accessory factors" that, although present in only low amounts, are none the less indispensable for the normal functioning of the organism. The anti-beriberi factor had been called "vitamine" because it contained an amino group, but the final e was dropped when it was recognized that not all accessory factors were amines. It took many years to isolate the anti-beriberi factor, which was finally obtained in pure crystals by B.C.P. Jansen and W.F. Donath in 1926, also in Batavia (Jansen and Donath, 1926). The American chemist R.R. Williams determined its structure in 1934 and synthesized the vitamin for the first time (Williams and Cline, 1936). It was first called "aneurin" for *anti-neur*itic vita*min* but later it was internationally agreed that it should be named "thiamin" for "sulfur-containing vitamin"; however, its exact properties and role remained unknown.

The first clues concerning the fundamental role of thiamin in carbohydrate metabolism were provided by the classical studies carried out from 1929 to 1940 by Peters and associates, using the thiamin-deficient pigeon as a model. The deficient birds (fed on polished rice) show a typical head retraction behavior called opisthotonos. Remarkably, thiamin administration at an early stage of the deficiency allows a complete recovery within 30 minutes. As no morphological brain lesions were observed before or after thiamin treatment, these observations led to the concept of "biochemical lesion."

What is the nature of this biochemical lesion? In 1937, Lohman and Schuster demonstrated that ThDP was an indispensable cofactor for the oxidative decarboxylation of pyruvate, an end product of glycolysis. It was subsequently demonstrated that ThDP is also a cofactor for the oxidative decarboxylation of 2-oxoglutarate, another 2-oxo acid. Between 1950 and 1960, Breslow and coworkers investigated the mechanism by which the thiamin moiety of ThDP catalyzes the decarboxylation of pyruvate in the reaction catalyzed by yeast pyruvate decarboxylase (Breslow, 1958). The same mechanism is involved in the first step of oxidative decarboxylation of 2-oxo acids by mitochondrial pyruvate and oxoglutarate dehydrogenase complexes. These studies revealed that ThDP exerts its function by proton substitution on the carbon in position 2 of the thiazolinium ring (Figure 17.1B).

Chemical Properties of Thiamin and Thiamin Phosphate Derivatives

Thiamin (3-[(4-amino-2-methyl-5-pyrimidinyl)methyl]-5-(2-hydroxyethyl)-4-methylthiazole) contains a pyrimidine and a thiazole moiety linked through a methylene bridge. Whereas the pyrimidine ring is found in many natural compounds, such as the pyrimidine nucleotides, thiamin is the only coenzyme of the primary metabolism containing a thiazole ring. Thiamin, generally available as the double chloride salt ($C_{12}H_{17}N_4OSCl.HCl$, molecular weight 337.28), is highly soluble in water, but poorly soluble in alcohol and other organic solvents. Thiamin is therefore unable to diffuse through lipid membranes and its uptake by living cells requires specific transporters. As this carrier-mediated transport is relatively slow, lipid-soluble thiamin precursors with higher bioavailability have been synthesized. The properties of these compounds will be discussed later in this chapter.

Thiamin is highly reactive and may undergo various transformations in the presence of OH^- and other nucleophilic agents (thiazolium ring opening, Figure 17.1B) or oxidizers (thiochrome formation, Figure 17.1C). Thiamin is stable at acid pH (2–4) and unstable at alkaline pH and high temperatures. While the $N_{1'}$ and $N_{3'}$ have a basic character and can be protonated, the primary amine $C_{4'}$-NH_2 is never protonated. Phosphorylated derivatives with phosphoanhydride bonds (in particular ThDP and ThTP) are spontaneously hydrolyzed to ThMP in aqueous solutions, especially at high or low pH. At physiological temperatures and pH, ThDP is stable for several hours.

The biosynthesis of thiamin occurs in most prokaryotes, plants, and fungi. During this complex process, phosphorylated thiazolium and pyrimidinium moieties are synthesized separately and then assembled to yield ThMP (Jurgenson *et al.*, 2009). In enterobacteria, ThMP is phosphorylated to ThDP by a ThMP kinase, whereas in eukaryotic organisms ThMP is dephosphorylated and thiamin is pyrophosphorylated to ThDP by the enzyme thiamin pyrophosphokinase (EC 2.7.6.2). In most cell types, the cofactor ThDP is the major thiamin compound (≥ 80% of total thiamin). Free thiamin and other phosphorylated derivatives are found in variable amounts (Makarchikov *et al.*, 2003; Frédérich *et al.*, 2009; Gangolf *et al.*, 2010a).

Determination of Thiamin in Biological Samples and Food Preparations

Many different methods have been described for the determination of thiamin derivatives (Kawasaki, 1992). In most cases, detection involves transformation of thiamin derivatives to the corresponding tricyclic thiochrome derivative (Figure 17.1C). Quantitative derivatization is obtained after oxidation (e.g. with potassium ferricyanide or bromocyanogen) in highly alkaline medium. Thiochrome derivatives are highly fluorescent at pH >8 with an excitation maximum around 370 nm and an emission maximum at 433 nm.

Thin-layer chromatography, electrophoresis, and low pressure liquid chromatography were used until the 1970s for the separation of thiamin derivatives, but since then HPLC has become the method of choice for the separation and quantification of thiamin derivatives in tissue samples, food or pharmaceutical preparations. Most methods rely on reversed-phase columns with or without ion-pairing agents (Kawasaki, 1992; Fayol, 1997). They are based on either a precolumn or a postcolumn derivatization procedure. According to our experience, precolumn procedures are preferable for several reasons. First, thiochromes, because of their lack of a positive charge on the thiazole ring and their tricyclic structure, have a more hydrophobic character (resulting in better chromatographic parameters) than the corresponding thiamin compounds. Second, postcolumn derivatization implies the presence of a reaction coil introducing additional void volumes responsible for decreased resolution. However, thiochromes are only fluorescent at alkaline pH, conditions under which silica-based columns are unstable. This drawback can be avoided by the use of postcolumn derivatization. Alternatively, stationary phases resistant to alkaline pH, such as polystyrene-divinylbenzene resins, can be used (Bettendorff

et al., 1991). Most of these methods are highly sensitive, and amounts as low as several femtomoles can be detected, allowing the detection of thiamin or its derivatives at nanomolar concentrations.

Nutritional Requirements and Toxicity

Thiamin is found in most foods, but whole grains, meat, fish, and yeast are particularly rich sources for this vitamin, containing approximately 3 mg/kg of wet weight (Davis and Icke, 1983). Vegetables contain two to three times less thiamin than meat per unit weight. Thiamin is stable on storage, but it should be emphasized that food processing may have an impact on the final thiamin content. Thiamin is heat-labile, and procedures such as overcooking, pasteurization of milk or heating of canned food may result in considerable loss of the vitamin.

For that reason, many processed foodstuffs such as cereals, bread, dairy products, and infant formulas are enriched with thiamin along with other vitamins such as niacin, riboflavin or folic acid. The recommended dietary allowance (RDA) is 1.2 mg/day for adult males and 1.1 mg/day for adult females. The RDA is increased to 1.4 mg/day during pregnancy and even 1.5 mg/day for lactating women. In children, the RDA increases with age and is 0.5, 0.6, and 0.9 mg/day respectively for 1–3, 4–8, and 9–13 years of age.

Thiamin supplementation is advisable for alcohol abusers and is sometimes suggested for elderly people as both might have decreased intestinal thiamin absorption. High thiamin intake (100 mg/day orally or intravenously) is needed in some rare conditions such as Wernicke's encephalopathy and in some rare genetic diseases, e.g. thiamin-responsive megaloblastic anemia or thiamin-responsive maple syrup urine disease. In these cases, thiamin derivatives with higher bioavailability than thiamin may be of advantage (benfotiamine, sulbutiamine or fursultiamine, see below).

Therapeutic doses generally range between 10 and 100 mg/day. For instance, cardiovascular beriberi is treated with 100 mg thiamin intravenously for several days. Note that intravenous thiamin administration should precede intravenous glucose administration as glucose may worsen thiamin deficiency. Indeed, it has been consistently observed that thiamin requirement, in contrast to that of other vitamins, increases when carbohydrate intake is high. This might be linked to the role of the cofactor ThDP in glucose catabolism. A recent study suggested an instability of enzyme-bound ThDP during the catalytic reactions (McCourt *et al.*, 2006). Therefore, increased glucose uptake would result in increased flux through ThDP-dependent enzymes and in increased breakdown of ThDP, worsening the thiamin status.

Oral intake of large doses generally has no adverse effects. However, intravenous administration of large doses (125 mg/kg in mice) can lead to respiratory depression and neuromuscular blockade. In dogs, blood thiamin levels of 10 μg/100 ml (300 μmol/L) are invariably fatal (Davis and Icke, 1983). In humans, allergic reactions (anaphylactic shock) are a rare complication of intravenous thiamin administration.

Thiamin Transport and Homeostasis

Intestinal Absorption

Thiamin homeostasis is maintained by balancing intestinal uptake and renal loss. Thiamin phosphate esters taken up from the food are hydrolyzed to thiamin or ThMP by intestinal alkaline phosphatase and transported across the brush-border membrane to the portal system. At low concentration (<1 μM), thiamin is absorbed through an active process, while at high intraluminal concentration a passive process seems to prevail. As a result, a larger proportion of small doses of thiamin is absorbed when its concentration is low.

The high-affinity transport process ($K_m = 0.1–1 \, \mu M$) across the brush-border membrane of the enterocyte involves an electroneutral thiamin/H^+ antiport and is thus facilitated by an outwardly directed H^+ gradient (Casirola *et al.*, 1988).

Therefore, the pH gradient (more alkaline in the intestinal lumen) is probably the driving force for intestinal thiamin transport. Chronic ethanol consumption was shown to decrease intestinal thiamin transport (Balaghi and Neal, 1977; Gastaldi *et al.*, 1989; Subramanya *et al.*, 2010). Furthermore, enterocyte thiamin transport seems to be affected by age. Aging is associated with decreased affinity and increased rate of high-affinity thiamin transport, while low-affinity transport is decreased (Gastaldi *et al.*, 1992).

Transport and Distribution of Thiamin Derivatives in Other Tissues

In most cell types, as in enterocytes, there is a dual, active high-affinity and passive low-affinity thiamin uptake mechanism. For active transport, different mechanisms have been shown to exist: a pH dependence similar to that observed in enterocytes has been demonstrated in human-derived liver cells (Said *et al.*, 2002), rat renal brush-border membrane (Gastaldi *et al.*, 2000), and human-derived renal epithelial cells (Ashokkumar *et al.*, 2006). However, a Na^+–thiamin cotransport mechanism has been suggested in hepatocytes (Lumeng *et al.*, 1979; Yoshioka, 1984). Intracellular thiamin pyrophosphorylation, subsequent uptake of ThDP by mitochondria and binding to apoenzymes are additional factors favoring the intracellular accumulation of thiamin derivatives.

In rats, only 1.5% of total thiamin is found in the brain, while 22% is found in the liver (Balaghi and Pearson, 1966; Ishii *et al.*, 1979; Sanemori *et al.*, 1980). However, during thiamin deficiency, thiamin levels decrease less steeply in the brain than in the liver (De Caro *et al.*, 1961; Balaghi and Pearson, 1966). Administration of high doses of thiamin (or thiamin precursors with a higher bioavailability) leads to a marked increase in total thiamin in the blood and in the liver, but not in the brain (see below). These results can be explained if the rate of thiamin transport across the blood–brain barrier is low compared with the rate of uptake by hepatocytes. As many studies use different units, it is difficult to compare the relative rates of transport in various preparations. There is no doubt, however, that the administration of radioactively labeled thiamin in rats leads to a much more rapid and higher accumulation of radioactivity in the blood and the liver than in the brain (Rindi *et al.*, 1980). This is in agreement with the observation that thiamin is not actively transported across the blood–brain barrier (Greenwood *et al.*, 1982, 1986), except maybe in the choroid plexus (Spector and Johanson, 2007). In brain cells, thiamin is probably not exchanged for H^+ nor cotransported with Na^+. Rather, the driving force for thiamin uptake appears to be its pyrophosphorylation to ThDP and subsequent strong binding to apoenzymes such as transketolase and oxoglutarate dehydrogenase complex (Bettendorff and Wins, 1994). Active accumulation of ThDP by mitochondria is another possibility (see below).

Net thiamin accumulation by the brain is also influenced by efflux of thiamin through the blood–brain barrier (Lockman *et al.*, 2003), an efflux considerably increased by trans-stimulation. Thiamin efflux was also stimulated by extracellular thiamin in cultured rat neuroblastoma cells, possibly by a self-exchange mechanism (Bettendorff, 1995). Such a trans-stimulation of thiamin efflux would limit excess thiamin uptake by the brain. It has been shown by different groups that, even in the presence of blood thiamin levels several orders of magnitude above control, brain thiamin content hardly changed whereas levels in liver and erythrocytes greatly increased (Sanemori and Kawasaki, 1982; Bettendorff *et al.*, 1990; Volvert *et al.*, 2008).

In conclusion, the emerging picture is that thiamin entering the bloodstream is mostly captured and phosphorylated by the liver (which is the main organ storing the vitamin) and, to a lesser extent, by erythrocytes which act as a thiamin buffer. In contrast, thiamin levels in the brain are highly regulated to minimize variations in thiamin and thiamin phosphate levels: regulatory mechanisms control both the influx and efflux of thiamin. Similar considerations hold for other vitamins (Spector and Johanson, 2007). Thus, vitamins B_3 (niacin) and B_6 (pyridoxine/pyridoxal) enter the brain through high-affinity transporters, whereas pantothenic acid and biotin enter through active transport. Homeostatic mechanisms tend to keep plasma levels and, even more, brain levels constant.

Thiamin Excretion

Excess thiamin and some of its metabolites (2-methyl-4-amino-5-pyrimidine carboxylic acid and 4-methyl-thiazole-5-acetic acid) are excreted in the urine. Urinary thiamin excretion is decreased during fasting (Fukuwatari *et al.*, 2010). Human urine thiamin concentrations are ~0.5 µg/ml or 1.5 µM (Roser *et al.*, 1978). In the rat, after intraperitoneal administration of ^{14}C-pyrimidine-labeled thiamin, ~30% of the vitamin taken up is eliminated by urinary excretion and 13% in the feces (Pearson *et al.*, 1966). However, only ~6% of the excreted radioactivity was genuine thiamin, the rest being found in at least 22 degradation products (Neal and Pearson, 1964). Probably most of these are products of detoxification enzymes present in liver and kidney. None of these enzymes is known to be specific for thiamin.

Thiamin Transport Proteins

Thiamin-responsive megaloblastic anemia is accompanied by diabetes mellitus and sensorineural deafness. Patients affected by this genetic disease lack the high-affinity thiamin transporter in erythrocytes (Poggi *et al.*, 1984; Rindi *et al.*, 1992, 1994; Stagg *et al.*, 1999). As the low-affinity thiamin transporter is still present, the patients respond, at least partly, to high doses of thiamin. The gene location was restricted to the chromosomal 1q23.3 region, and the identification of the genes in this region led to the

identification of a new gene (*SLC19A2* for solute carrier family 19 member 2) homologous to *SLC19A1* encoding the reduced folate carrier protein (RFC-1) (Fleming *et al.*, 1999). In humans it is highly expressed in skeletal muscle, heart, and placenta, but in mice the highest expression is observed in liver, kidney, and brain, with practically no expression in skeletal muscle (Fleming *et al.*, 2001; Oishi *et al.*, 2001). As these tissues are not affected in the patients and they have normal plasma thiamin levels (Oishi *et al.*, 2002), it is plausible that alternative routes for transporting thiamin are present in many cells except in tissues affected in thiamin-responsive megaloblastic anemia, i.e. bone marrow (where blood cells are formed), beta cells of the islets of Langerhans and inner-ear cells. The identity of alternative transporters is still unclear but it has been shown that RFC-1 is able to transport ThMP and ThDP but not thiamin (Zhao *et al.*, 2001, 2002). While ThDP is not physiologically encountered in extracellular media, ThMP is present in plasma and cerebrospinal fluid and therefore RFC-1 may be an alternative route for cells to capture thiamin. The choroid plexus, which plays an important role in brain thiamin homeostasis, accumulates the vitamin by an active process and releases thiamin and ThMP on the apical (CSF) side (Spector and Johanson, 2007). RFC-1 is highly expressed on the apical side of the choroid plexus (Wang *et al.*, 2001) and may thus be responsible for the release of ThMP into the CSF.

A third member of the same gene family, *SLC19A3*, located on chromosome 2q37, encodes a 55.6-kDa protein with 56% similarity to RFC-1 and 64% identity to ThTR1 (Eudy *et al.*, 2000). ThTR2, the *SLC19A3* gene product, was shown to transport thiamin (Rajgopal *et al.*, 2001), with a very high apparent affinity for thiamin ($K_m = 27 \pm 8$ nM) (Said *et al.*, 2004). In contrast, ThTR1 has a K_m of 2.5 ± 0.6 µM (Dutta *et al.*, 1999).

ThTR2 is rather ubiquitously expressed, with the highest levels in placenta, liver, kidney, and heart, which might explain why these tissues are spared in thiamin-responsive megaloblastic anemia. Furthermore, its expression is low in bone marrow. ThTR2 is expressed along the whole length of the human digestive tract, with the highest expression in the proximal part (duodenal and jejunal areas), which has the highest capacity of the intestine to absorb thiamin (Rindi and Ferrari, 1977; Laforenza *et al.*, 1997). Nevertheless the transporter is also present on colonocytes where it might play a role in the absorption of thiamin produced by the microflora of the large intestine (Said *et al.*, 2001). Differentiation of intestinal epithelial cells is associated with an up-regulation of thiamin transport, in a process involving transcriptional regulation of both the *SLC19A2* and *SLC19A3* genes (Nabokina *et al.*, 2005; Reidling and Said, 2005).

That mutations in *SLC19A2* are indeed responsible for thiamin-responsive megaloblastic anemia was shown by targeted disruption of the gene in mice (Oishi *et al.*, 2002). These mice exhibited the hallmarks of the disease: mega-loblastosis, diabetes, and sensorineural deafness when put on a thiamin-deficient diet (Oishi *et al.*, 2002). The fact that gene disruption alone does not cause these symptoms suggests that differences in thiamin metabolism and in tissue distribution of thiamin transporters exist between humans and mice, as was indeed shown for *SLC19A3* (Eudy *et al.*, 2000). An intriguing point is that recent results suggest that mutations in *SLC19A3* are responsible for biotin-responsive basal ganglia disease (Zeng *et al.*, 2005), a rare recessive disorder with onset in childhood and with brain-specific pathology involving bilateral lesions of the caudate nucleus and the putamen. At an early stage the disease is associated with subacute encepha-lopathy, progressing to acute encephalopathy. These symp-toms are reversed by high doses of biotin (vitamin B_7). Many transporters have overlapping substrate specificity, as illustrated by the case of RFC-1, able, for instance, to transport reduced folate, ThMP, and ThDP. Therefore, the hypothesis that ThTR2 might transport biotin was very appealing. However, it was shown (Subramanian *et al.*, 2006) that the mutations identified in *SLC19A3* in patients with biotin-responsive basal ganglia disease inhibit the thiamin transport capacity of ThTR2 but that the normal as well as the mutated proteins were all unable to transport biotin.

Thiamin Diphosphate Synthesis and Transport into Mitochondria

In animal cells, thiamin transported into the cells is rapidly phosphorylated to ThDP according to the reaction: thiamin + ATP ⇌ ThDP + AMP, catalyzed by thiamin pyrophosphokinase. The equilibrium of this reaction is far towards the reactants (Peterson *et al.*, 1975). However, inside the cells the equilibrium is shifted to the right because of the binding of ThDP to cytosolic transketolase and transport into mitochondria.

A mitochondrial ThDP transporter (*SLC25A19*) was recently characterized in yeast (Marobbio *et al.*, 2002) and in animals (Lindhurst *et al.*, 2006). Mutations in *SLC25A19* cause Amish lethal microcephaly, an autosomal

recessive disease characterized by extreme microcephaly, severe 2-oxoglutarate aciduria, and fatal outcome within the first year. *SLC25A19* seems to act as an antiporter, exchanging extramitochondrial ThDP against intramito-chondrial nucleotides. The concentration of free ThDP is probably higher in the mitochondrial matrix than in the cytosol, but the exact mechanism of active ThDP transport – if any – in mitochondria remains unclear.

Tissue Content and Metabolism of Thiamin Phosphate Derivatives

Thiamin phosphate derivatives are found in all organisms. In most cases the cofactor ThDP is the major thiamin compound. In most animal cells, ThDP represents 70 to 90% of total thiamin, and in the brain most of it is bound to apoenzymes. However, free ThDP is more concentrated in hepatocytes, enterocytes, and skeletal muscle fibers. ThDP is synthesized from thiamin and ATP in the cytosol (see above) and is hydrolyzed by thiamin diphosphatases yielding ThMP, which can be hydrolyzed to thiamin. Several enzymes have been reported to hydrolyze ThDP, but all thiamin diphosphatases studied so far also hydro-lyze nucleoside diphosphates. Likewise, no hydrolase has been found to be specific for ThMP, which may be hydro-lyzed by alkaline phosphatases, acid phosphatases or an ecto-5′-nucleotidase. ThMP and free thiamin generally amount to less than 15% of total thiamin in animal cells. The triphosphorylated derivative, ThTP, is generally a minor compound (less than 1% of total thiamin), but it is found in most organisms, including humans (Makarchikov *et al.*, 2003; Gangolf *et al.*, 2010a). In *E. coli*, ThTP is transiently synthesized when the bacteria are switched from an amino acid rich medium to one that is amino acid poor, suggesting that it might be a signal involved in the adaptation to amino acid starvation (Lakaye *et al.*, 2004). In animal tissues, ThTP is consistently found in nervous tissue and skeletal muscle. At least two kinds of enzymes have been shown to hydrolyze ThTP. A soluble 25-kDa thiamin triphosphatase (EC 3.6.1.28) has been characterized at the molecular level (Lakaye *et al.*, 2002; Song *et al.*, 2008). It is very specific for ThTP and rela-tively ubiquitously expressed in mammalian tissues, and in the brain it seems mainly localized in neurons (Czerniecki *et al.*, 2004). A membrane-bound thiamin triphosphatase has been described in animal tissues, but this enzyme has never been purified and its specificity remains to be dem-onstrated (Barchi and Braun, 1972; Bettendorff *et al.*,

1987, 1988). The mechanism of ThTP synthesis is controversial. Adenylate kinase 1 (EC 2.7.4.3) may synthesize ThTP according to the reaction ThDP + ADP ⇆ ThTP + AMP (Shikata *et al.*, 1989a,b; Gigliobianco *et al.*, 2008), but the rate of this reaction is six to seven orders of magnitude lower than the natural reaction 2 ADP ⇆ ATP + AMP. Nevertheless, this enzyme may be responsible for the accumulation of cytosolic ThTP in tissues, such as skeletal muscle, where AK1 activity is particularly high. In brain, ThTP is localized in mitochondria and might be synthesized by a chemiosmotic mechanism resembling that of ATP synthesis (Gangolf *et al.*, 2010b).

AThTP was only recently discovered in *E. coli*, where it accumulates during acute energy stress (Bettendorff *et al.*,

2007; Gigliobianco *et al.*, 2010). It might be synthesized by a ThDP adenylyl transferase (Makarchikov *et al.*, 2007). It is found in the roots of plants and in animal cells, but we have no indication as to its potential roles. The diphosphate analog, adenosine thiamin diphosphate, was found in low amounts in bacteria and rodent liver (Frédérich *et al.*, 2009).

Cofactor Role of Thiamin Diphosphate

Vitamins of the B group or their derivatives are essential cofactors in many basic enzyme-catalyzed reactions. In the case of thiamin, ThDP is the cofactor of several enzymes involved in key metabolic pathways (Figure 17.2). ThDP

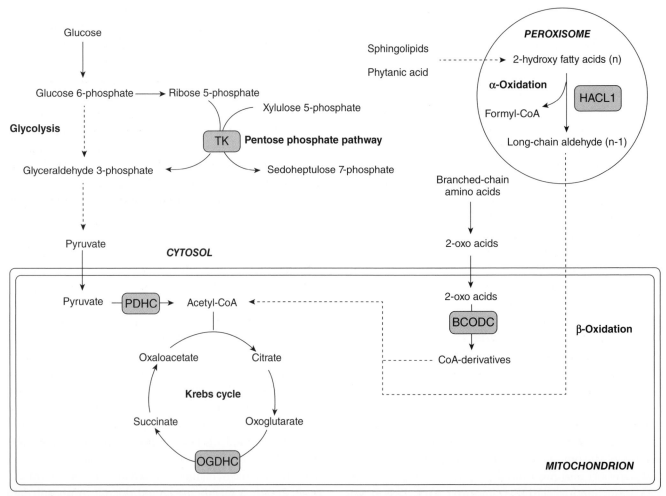

FIG. 17.2 Thiamin diphosphate-dependent enzymes in mammalian cells. TK, transketolase; PDHC, pyruvate dehydrogenase complex; OGDHC, oxoglutarate dehydrogenase complex; BCODC; branched-chain 2-oxo acid dehydrogenase; HACL1, 2-hydroxyacyl-CoA lyase.

bound to apoenzymes is considered the "slow turnover ThDP pool" (Bettendorff, 1994a; Bettendorff *et al.*, 1994), although the stability of the different coenzyme–apoenzyme complexes varies: ThDP dissociates faster from pyruvate dehydrogenase than from oxoglutarate dehydrogenase complex and transketolase. It can be estimated that, in brain cells or neuroblastoma cells, the slow ThDP pool represents 90–95% of the total cellular ThDP and has a turnover of 6–20 hours. For the smaller pool, the turnover is of the order of 1–3 hours. In other cell types such as hepatocytes or red blood cells, the free cytosolic ThDP pool may be much more important, particularly after administration of thiamin.

ThDP-Dependent Enzymes and Their Roles

In mammalian cells, ThDP is a cofactor for the cytosolic transketolase (EC 2.2.1.1), and in mitochondria ThDP is the cofactor of E1 subunits of pyruvate dehydrogenase complex (EC 1.2.4.1), oxoglutarate dehydrogenase complex (EC 1.2.4.2), and branched-chain 2-oxo acid (EC 1.2.4.4) dehydrogenase. More recently, 2-hydroxyacyl-CoA lyase (EC 4.1.-.-) has been described in peroxisomes where it is involved in the degradation of 3-methyl-branched-chain and 2-hydroxy long-chain fatty acids (Foulon *et al.*, 1999).

In yeast, pyruvate decarboxylase (EC 4.1.1.1), catalyzing the non-oxidative decarboxylation of pyruvate to acetaldehyde, is the committed step in alcoholic fermentation. It is a key reaction involved in the production of beer, wine, and other alcoholic beverages.

Pyruvate and oxoglutarate dehydrogenase complexes are essential for mitochondrial oxidative metabolism, which, especially in neurons, is crucial for survival. Mutations in pyruvate dehydrogenase (among other enzymes involved in mitochondrial energy metabolism) have been associated with subacute necrotizing encephalomyelopathy (Leigh's disease) (Barnerias *et al.*, 2010), a rare heterogeneous neurodegenerative disorder of early childhood characterized by focal, symmetric necrotic brain lesions, leading to death generally before the age of 5. Administration of thiamin in these patients may at best delay but will not prevent the fatal outcome. Oxoglutarate dehydrogenase complex is the rate-limiting enzyme of the Krebs cycle in the brain. Its activity is decreased in the brains of patients with Alzheimer's disease (Mastrogiacomo *et al.*, 1996b).

Transketolase is cytosolic and is a key enzyme in the pentose phosphate pathway, a major source of NADPH for reductive biosynthesis (of fatty acids, for instance) and of ribose (nucleic acid synthesis). It has been suggested that carriers of variants with decreased affinity for ThDP might have a predisposition for Wernicke–Korsakoff's syndrome, but no mutations were found in the coding sequence in Wernicke–Korsakoff compared with non Wernicke–Korsakoff individuals (Mukherjee *et al.*, 1987; McCool *et al.*, 1993; Alexander-Kaufman and Harper, 2009). In humans, three isoforms of the enzyme have been described: transketolase, transketolase-like 1, and transketolase-like 2 (Coy *et al.*, 1996, 2005; Xu *et al.*, 2009). Transketolase-like 1 expression is up-regulated in various forms of cancer, and specific inhibitors of transketolase-like 1 (antithiamins) might have antitumor effects (Cascante *et al.*, 2000).

Branched-chain 2-oxo acid dehydrogenase complex plays a central role in the degradation of the branched-chain amino acids leucine, isoleucine, and valine. Deficiency of this activity due to mutations leads to the accumulation of toxic 2-oxo acid products leading to maple syrup urine disease, also called branched-chain ketoaciduria. This autosomal recessive metabolic disorder is characterized by a maple-syrup-like odor of the urine of affected children. If untreated, severe brain damage will rapidly lead to coma and death. The patients must observe a strict diet, poor in the three incriminated amino acids. As they are essential amino acids, they must be present in minimal amounts in the daily ration so their levels have to be carefully adjusted on an individual basis. The patients may respond to administration of high-dose thiamin when the E1 component of the branched chain 2-oxo acid dehydrogenase complex is affected.

2-Hydroxyacyl-CoA lyase was the first ThDP-dependent enzyme to be discovered in peroxisomes (Foulon *et al.*, 1999). In liver it is involved in the degradation of 3-methyl-branched fatty acids, essentially phytanic acid (3,7,11,15-tetramethyl hexadecanoic acid) present in human diet as a degradation product of chlorophyll. Accumulation of phytanic acid in blood and tissues leads to Refsum's disease, an autosomal, recessive, and progressive metabolic disorder presenting neurologic damage, cerebellar degeneration, and peripheral neuropathy.

Several other ThDP-dependent enzymes have been described in prokaryotes, but they will not be discussed here.

Mechanism of ThDP-Dependent Catalysis

In all ThDP-catalyzed enzymatic reactions, ThDP catalyzes the cleavage or the formation of a C–C bond immediately adjacent to a carbonyl group (α-cleavage or α-condensation) such as in the decarboxylation of 2-oxo acids (Eq. 1, 2-oxo acid dehydrogenases, pyruvate decarboxylase and 2-hydroxyacyl-CoA lyase) or the cleavage of α-hydroxyketones (Eq. 2, transketolase):

$$R-\overset{\overset{\displaystyle O}{\|}}{C}-COO^- + H^+ \longrightarrow R-\overset{\overset{\displaystyle O}{\|}}{C}H + CO_2 \qquad (1)$$

$$R-\overset{\overset{\displaystyle HO}{|}}{\underset{\underset{\displaystyle H}{|}}{C}}-\overset{\overset{\displaystyle O}{\|}}{C}-R' \longrightarrow R-\overset{\overset{\displaystyle O}{\|}}{C}H + H\overset{\overset{\displaystyle O}{\|}}{C}-R' \qquad (2)$$

As there is no simple acid–base-catalyzed mechanism for such reactions, a special catalyst is required. The catalytic action of ThDP is linked to the ability of its thiazolium ring to form an ylide (carbanion) intermediate (Figure 17.1B) by deprotonation of the thiazolium C-2 and attack of the resulting carbanion on a substrate carbonyl. The diphosphate group plays no role in catalysis itself and is only required for tight binding of ThDP to the apoenzymes. The anionic carbon of the thiazolium ring readily reacts with substrates by addition to the carbonyl group, forming a covalent adduct undergoing cleavage that ultimately leads to the formation of acetyl-CoA in the case of oxidative decarboxylation of pyruvate.

Non-Cofactor Roles of Thiamin Phosphate Derivatives in Animals

Non-cofactor roles of thiamin or its phosphorylated derivatives have been postulated since the 1940s (Bettendorff, 1994b). Such hypotheses take root in the well-known particular sensitivity of the nervous system to thiamin deficiency and to more specific observations, e.g. that electrical stimulation of isolated nerves leads to a release of thiamin, probably as a consequence of the dephosphorylation of ThDP and ThTP. This result has sometimes been interpreted as consumption of ThTP during nerve activity, for instance for protein phosphorylation. ThTP has indeed been shown to be able to phosphorylate proteins in the electric organ of *Torpedo marmorata* or rodent brain (Nghiêm *et al.*, 2000). Furthermore, ThTP activated a high-conductance chloride channel, possibly by a phosphorylation-dependent mechanism (Bettendorff *et al.*, 1993). However, the physiological significance of these events remains to be established. The recent observation that ThTP is synthesized in brain but not in liver mitochondria suggests that this compound might play a role in neuronal energy metabolism (Gangolf *et al.*,

2010b). Several studies showed complex effects of free thiamin on the neuromuscular junction (Eder *et al.*, 1976; Romanenko, 1990), but in all cases relatively high concentrations (>0.1 mM) were required, casting doubt on the physiological significance of these data. Adenylated thiamin derivatives also exist in animals in small quantities (Bettendorff *et al.*, 2007; Frédérich *et al.*, 2009). Therefore, it appears that thiamin biochemistry is more complex than that of other B vitamins. The existence of mono-, di-, and triphosphates is more reminiscent of nucleotides than of vitamins.

Diseases Specifically Related to Thiamin Deficiency

Assessment of Thiamin Status in Humans

As discussed above, HPLC is the method of choice for the determination of thiamin in body fluids. The most direct measure is the determination of ThDP in blood samples (Korner *et al.*, 2009). This method is direct, rapid, suitable for pediatric diagnostics, highly sensitive, and easy to standardize. However, such methods are generally not routinely available in most medical laboratories. The erythrocyte transketolase activity assay is a widely used method to assess thiamin status in humans. It is based on the increased activity of erythrocyte transketolase after addition of ThDP. An abnormally large ThDP effect can be interpreted as a low saturation of transketolase by the cofactor, as a consequence of thiamin deficiency. A good correlation is obtained between direct erythrocyte ThDP determination and the ThDP effect. The latter is, however, an indirect determination of the thiamin status that can be influenced by factors other than thiamin deficiency and it is less sensitive.

Dry and Wet Beriberi

Beriberi is the typical manifestation of alimentary thiamin deficiency. It was a major health problem in Eastern and Southern Asia during the nineteenth century as polished rice had become the staple food in these countries. Such chronic deficiency (unrelated to alcohol abuse) most often results in dry beriberi, characterized by symmetrical peripheral neuritis. The condition, which mainly affects the lower limbs, results in weakness in the legs and cramps, followed at later stages by hyperesthesia and deep muscle pain. If not treated it may lead to death, but administration of thiamin results in a rapid cure. Wet (shoshin) beriberi is a rarer form of the disease with a difficult diagnostic, ultimately leading to fatal congestive heart failure. It is characterized by edema, pulmonary hypertension, and lactic acidosis. The improvement can be rapid and spectacular after treatment with thiamin. Just like the nervous system, the heart muscle relies heavily on oxidative metabolism, which explains its high sensitivity to thiamin deficiency.

Wernicke–Korsakoff Syndrome

In developed countries, beriberi is now virtually non-existent, but thiamin deficiency related to chronic alcohol abuse leads to a severe impairment of brain function known as Wernicke–Korsakoff syndrome. This remains the third most common cause of dementia after Alzheimer's disease and vascular dementia, contributing to between 10 and 24% of all cases of dementia (Victor *et al.*, 1989; Butterworth, 2003; Harper, 2009; Kopelman *et al.*, 2009). It seems that alcohol interferes with intestinal thiamin absorption, in particular by reducing the expression of ThTR1 in the intestine (Subramanya *et al.*, 2010). An impairment of phosphorylation of thiamin to ThDP has also been suggested (Rindi *et al.*, 1986; Laforenza *et al.*, 1990).

The clinical features of Wernicke's encephalopathy (which is the first acute stage of the syndrome) include ophthalmoplegia, global confusional state, and ataxia. Korsakoff's psychosis appears as a consequence of chronic thiamin deficiency in the alcoholic patient, often after several episodes of Wernicke's encephalopathy. Clinical features are anterograde amnesia, disorientation, confabulation, and learning defects, probably arising from irreversible diencephalic lesions. Administration of thiamin at an early stage of Wernicke's encephalopathy leads to rapid improvement, but if high doses of thiamin are not administered early enough, there are irreversible sequelae such as residual ataxia and horizontal nystagmus, deficits in learning, memory loss, and personality changes, which are hallmarks of Korsakoff's psychosis. This is linked to irreversible brain lesions that are rather specific, affecting the thalamus, the mammillary bodies, and sometimes the cerebellum, the cerebral cortex being largely spared. The lesions probably arise from decreased 2-oxoglutarate dehydrogenase activity impairing energy metabolism in endothelial cells and neurons (Heroux and Butterworth, 1995). Neuronal loss actually results from a combination of several factors, including excitotoxicity, inflammation and oxidative stress (Hazell and Butterworth, 2009). The reason for the selective vulnerability of certain brain regions remains largely unknown and is a subject of active investigation. A recent hypothesis links the origin of the lesions to an impairment of the blood cerebrospinal fluid barrier at the level of the choroid plexus (Nixon *et al.*, 2008).

Not all alcoholics develop Wernicke–Korsakoff syndrome, and environmental and genetic factors may also play a role. Some variants of transketolase (Alexander-Kaufman and Harper, 2009) and ThTR1 (Guerrini *et al.*, 2005) have been associated with Wernicke–Korsakoff syndrome, but it remains to be proven that there is a causal relationship. Furthermore, while Wernicke–Korsakoff syndrome is most often associated with alcoholism, it can also occur as a result of general malnutrition after gastrectomy (Shimomura *et al.*, 1998), in patients with fast-growing hematologic malignant tumors (van Zaanen and van der Lelie, 1992), in drug abusers, and in AIDS patients (Butterworth *et al.*, 1991). Rare cases of accidental thiamin deficiency may also occur, such as an episode of encephalopathy in infants in Israel in 2003, caused by a defective soy-based formula (Fattal-Valevski *et al.*, 2005).

Subclinical Thiamin Deficiency

Subclinical thiamin deficiency in humans is probably more widespread in developed countries than initially thought, especially in elderly people (Smidt *et al.*, 1991; Chen *et al.*, 1996; Thurman and Mooradian, 1997; Wilkinson *et al.*, 1997; Vognar and Stoukides, 2009), as well as in some risk groups such as infants, and pregnant and lactating women (Butterworth, 1987). Maternal thiamin deficiency may be a problem in displaced populations, as a result either of insufficient thiamin intake or of the consumption of thiaminase-containing food (McGready *et al.*, 2001). Low circulating thiamin levels were also observed in patients with Alzheimer's disease (Gold *et al.*, 1995; Molina *et al.*, 2002) and ThDP levels are decreased in postmortem brains of patients with Alzheimer's disease (Heroux *et al.*, 1996; Mastrogiacomo *et al.*, 1996a) and frontal lobe degeneration of the non-Alzheimer's type (Bettendorff *et al.*, 1997). It is important to emphasize that circulating and brain thiamin levels are much lower in humans than in rodents (Bettendorff *et al.*, 1996; Gangolf *et al.*, 2010a). This might be one reason why humans are more prone to thiamin deficiency than rodents and most other animals. It has also been reported that loop diuretic therapy in patients with heart failure results in increased renal thiamin loss and these patients are therefore at a higher risk of developing thiamin deficiency (Sica, 2007).

Nutritional, Alcohol-Related, and Genetically Induced Thiamin Deficiencies Are Symptomatically Distinct

It is worth commenting on the various forms of thiamin-deficiency-related diseases. While purely nutritional thiamin deficiency mainly leads to peripheral symptoms such as polyneuritis (dry beriberi) or congestive heart failure (wet beriberi), alcohol-induced thiamin deficiency mainly affects the central nervous system (Wernicke–Korsakoff syndrome) although polyneuritis is also present in many cases. This may suggest that alcohol toxicity may contribute to the symptoms observed, as discussed by some authors (Harper, 1998). On the other hand, deficiency in thiamin transport due to mutations in ThTR1 (*SLC19A2*) leads to the peripheral symptoms (though unrelated to beriberi) in thiamin-responsive megaloblastic anemia: anemia, diabetes, and deafness. This suggests that the main transporter in the brain is ThTR2. Indeed, patients with known loss-of-function mutations in ThTR2 suffer from brain lesions and respond to thiamin administration (Kono *et al.*, 2009). However, some mutations in ThTR2 lead to a lethal familial form of encephalopathy as a result of necrosis of the basal ganglia (Vlasova *et al.*, 2005; Zeng *et al.*, 2005; Debs *et al.*, 2010). Strangely, this disease responds to biotin administration, or sometimes to a combination of biotin and thiamin, though biotin is not transported by ThTR2. ThTR2-knockout mice have reduced intestinal thiamin uptake and are relatively normal, but die at age of 1 year of unknown causes (but not from brain lesions) (Reidling *et al.*, 2010). This does not seem to be due to compensation by ThTR1 but could be the result of a different expression pattern of thiamin transporters in humans compared with mice. Finally, the fact that ThDP deficiency in mitochondria plays a key role in thiamin deficiency-induced brain lesions is illustrated by the extremely severe phenotype observed in mutation of the mitochondrial ThDP transporter *SLC25A19* (Amish lethal microcephaly, see above) (Lindhurst *et al.*, 2006).

Thiamin Precursors and Lipid-Soluble Thiamin Compounds

Unlike other B-vitamins, oral administration of thiamin does not lead to significantly increased plasma vitamin levels (Davis and Icke, 1983), probably because intestinal thiamin absorption is a relatively slow process, especially in humans. This probably contributes to the fact that

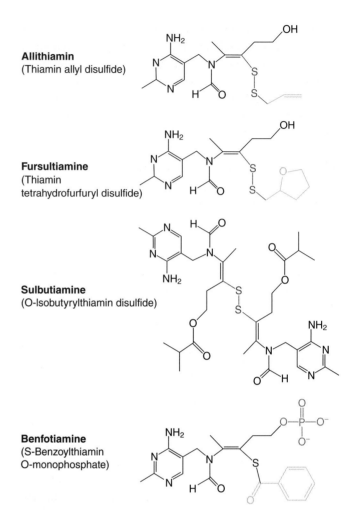

FIG. 17.3 Thiamin precursors with high bioavailability. Note the thioester bond in benfotiamine as compared with the disulfide bridge in the other compounds, as well as the phosphate group making this molecule lipid insoluble. Note that in contrast to the other three molecules, sulbutiamine is a symmetric dimer. Modified from Volvert *et al.* (2008).

marginal thiamin deficiency in humans is more common than initially thought. In order to overcome this problem, several thiamin precursors with higher bioavailability were developed (Figure 17.3).

In the 1950s, M. Fujiwara and colleagues in Tokyo discovered that a thiamin derivative with high bioavailability was formed in crushed garlic (*Allium sativum*) bulbs through the action of a plant enzyme on thiamin and allicin (diallyl thiosulphinate) (Fujiwara *et al.*, 1954). They named this compound allithiamin, which they later identified as thiamin allyl disulfide. Other synthetic thiamin disulfides such as sulbutiamine (O-isobutyrylthiamin disulfide) and fursultiamine (thiamin tetrahydrofurfuryl disulfide) were developed. All have a higher bioavailability than thiamin, probably because their hydrophobic character means that they easily cross intestinal membranes and no transporter is required. In the bloodstream, these disulfide compounds are easily reduced to thiamin in the presence of cysteine or glutathione. Intraperitoneal administration of sulbutiamine in rats leads to a significant increase in the levels of thiamin phosphate esters in the brain and it has a documented effect on the central nervous system as a psychotropic drug (Bizot *et al.*, 2005). Fursultiamine improves energy metabolism and physical performance during physical fatigue loading in rats (Nozaki *et al.*, 2009). Central nervous effects of fursultiamine are less well documented but it was suggested to have beneficial effects on speech, behavior and sleep in autistic children (Lonsdale *et al.*, 2002).

Benfotiamine (S-benzoylthiamin O-monophosphate), another synthetic thiamin precursor, is being extensively studied. In contrast to the lipophilic thiamin disulfides, benfotiamine, a thioester, because of its hydrophilic phosphoryl group is not lipid-soluble. In contrast, it dissolves in aqueous solvents at slightly alkaline pH. To be absorbed, benfotiamine must be dephosphorylated to S-benzoylthiamin by ecto-alkaline phosphatases present in the intestinal mucosa (Volvert *et al.*, 2008). The more lipophilic S-benzoylthiamin may then cross the brush-border membrane. It can be hydrolyzed to thiamin by thioesterases present in the liver. The different modes of transport and degradation of these three compounds probably explain their different effects, though all raise blood thiamin levels well above those obtained by administration of an equivalent dose of thiamin. Benfotiamine mainly acts on peripheral tissues through increase in transketolase activity and thus is effective in preventing diabetic complications such as retinopathy (Hammes *et al.*, 2003). However, benfotiamine is unable to significantly raise thiamin phosphate levels in the rodent brain, which probably explains why, until recently, it had no documented central nervous system effects. However, very recently, benfotiamine was shown to improve cognitive functions and to dramatically decrease amyloid plaques and neurofibrillary tangles in a mouse model of Alzheimer's disease (Pan *et al.*, 2010).

Antithiamins

Several synthetic thiamin antagonists have been developed. The most potent is pyrithiamin, a highly competitive inhibitor of thiamin transport and thiamin pyrophosphokinase. Other analogs such as oxythiamin, amprolium, and the chemically unrelated diuretic amiloride also inhibit thiamin transport (Bettendorff and Wins, 1994). While pyrithiamin has an affinity comparable to that of thiamin ($K_{m,app}$ <1 μM) for thiamin pyrophosphokinase, oxythiamin has a 1000 times lower affinity. Both compounds may be pyrophosphorylated by thiamin pyrophosphokinase. Oxythiamin diphosphate is a potent inhibitor of thiamin-dependent enzymes, whereas pyrithiamin diphosphate is not. Pyrithiamin, in combination with a thiamin-deficient diet, is used in rodents as a model of Wernicke–Korsakoff syndrome (Desjardins and Butterworth, 2005). Indeed, nutritional deprivation of thiamin alone takes at least 4 weeks in rats before thiamin deficiency symptoms develop. Administration of pyrithiamin in addition to thiamin deprivation reduces the delay to about 10 days. Pyrithiamin, in contrast to oxythiamin, crosses the blood–brain barrier, and the lesions observed closely resemble those in human Wernicke–Korsakoff syndrome. In contrast, oxythiamin-treated animals have no neurological symptoms, but suffer weight loss, anorexia, and cardiac enlargement, probably as a result of inhibition of ThDP-dependent enzymes by oxythiamin diphosphate.

Sulfites, added as preservatives to food, cleave the vitamin at the level of the methylene bridge yielding separate pyrimidine and thiazole moieties, and cases of thiamin deficiency in dogs due to feeding on sulfite-preserved meat have been described (Singh *et al.*, 2005). Earlier studies had suggested that 3,4-dihydroxycinnamic acid (caffeic acid) and similar substances had an antithiamin activity, but this was later disproved (Horman and Brambilla, 1982).

Some foodstuffs may contain thiaminases (thiamin-destroying) enzymes. Some fish (carp, eel, Baltic herring or catfish, for instance) and shellfish may contain thermolabile thiaminase I, a pyrimidine transferase (EC 2.5.1.2). This is also the case for some ferns (*Pteris aquilina*), which, when consumed by grazing cattle or horses, may result in severe thiamin deficiency. Thiaminase is destroyed by cooking, but consumption of raw food containing thiaminase may cause beriberi in humans. Another thiaminase found in microorganisms, thiaminase II (EC 3.5.99.2), catalyzes the hydrolysis of thiamin in separate pyrimidine and thiazole moieties. Recent results suggest that this enzyme may be involved in thiamin salvage, rather than a thiamin degradation pathway (Jenkins *et al.*, 2007). Indeed, thiamin degradation in the soil leads to the formation of aminopyrimidine, and thiaminase II catalyzes the conversion of aminopyrimidine to hydroxypyrimidine, a building block for the biosynthesis of thiamin by some bacteria.

Future Directions

Thiamin was the first vitamin characterized and from its discovery the concept of vitamins originated. Nearly a century later, many questions remain. Several phosphorylated thiamin derivatives exist in practically all cell types, but only the cofactor role of ThDP has been clearly demonstrated and extensively studied. Future work should be devoted to the study of the biological roles of all phosphorylated derivatives, as compounds other than ThDP, in particular the triphosphates, might also participate in the symptoms observed during thiamin deficiency. Though we have learned a lot concerning the effects of thiamin deficiency on cell survival, many questions remain open. In particular, we must clarify the mechanism leading to selective vulnerability of certain brain regions to thiamin deficiency, but also the possible beneficial effects of benfotiamine in diabetes and Alzheimer's disease open exciting new fields in thiamin research.

Acknowledgments

LB is Research Director at the Funds for Scientific Research (FRS-FNRS, Belgium). The author is grateful to Dr Pierre Wins for reading the manuscript.

Suggestions for Further Reading

Bettendorff, L. (1994) Thiamine in excitable tissues: reflections on a non-cofactor role. *Metab Brain Dis* **9**, 183–209.

Bettendorff, L. and Wins, P. (2009) Thiamin diphosphate in biological chemistry: new aspects of thiamin metabolism, especially triphosphate derivatives acting other than as cofactors. *FEBS J* **276**, 2917–2925.

Bettendorff, L., Wirtzfeld, B., Makarchikov, A.F., *et al.* (2007) Discovery of a natural thiamine adenine nucleotide. *Nature Chem Biol* **3**, 211–212.

Carpenter, K.J. (2000) *Beriberi, White Rice, and Vitamin B: a Disease, a Cause, and a Cure*. University of California Press, Berkeley, CA.

Harper, C. (2009) The neuropathology of alcohol-related brain damage. *Alcohol Alcohol* **44**, 136–140.

Jordan, J. and Patel, M.S. (2004) *Thiamine. Catalytic Mechanisms in Normal and Disease States*. Marcel Dekker, New York.

Jurgenson, C.T., Begley, T.P., and Ealick, S.E. (2009) The structural and biochemical foundations of thiamin biosynthesis. *Annu Rev Biochem* **78**, 569–603.

Kawasaki, T. (1992) Vitamin B1: thiamine. In A.P. De Leenheer, W.E. Lambert, and H.J. Nelis (eds), *Modern Chromatographic Analysis of Vitamins*, Vol. 60. Marcel Dekker, New York, pp. 319–354.

Kluger, R. and Tittmann, K. (2008) Thiamin diphosphate catalysis: enzymic and nonenzymic covalent intermediates. *Chem Rev* **108**, 1797–1833.

McCandless, D.W. (2010) *Thiamine Deficiency and Associated Clinical Disorders*. Humana Press, New York.

References

Alexander-Kaufman, K. and Harper, C. (2009) Transketolase: observations in alcohol-related brain damage research. *Int J Biochem Cell Biol* **41**, 717–720.

Ashokkumar, B., Vaziri, N.D., and Said, H.M. (2006) Thiamin uptake by the human-derived renal epithelial (HEK-293) cells: cellular and molecular mechanisms. *Am J Physiol Renal Physiol* **291**, F796–805.

Balaghi, M. and Neal, R.A. (1977) Effect of chronic ethanol administration on thiamin metabolism in the rat. *J Nutr* **107**, 2144–2152.

Balaghi, M. and Pearson, W.N. (1966) Tissue and intracellular distribution of radioactive thiamine in normal and thiamine-deficient rats. *J Nutr* **89**, 127–132.

Barchi, R.L. and Braun, P.E. (1972) A membrane-associated thiamine triphosphatase from rat brain. Properties of the enzyme. *J Biol Chem* **247**, 7668–7673.

Barnerias, C., Saudubray, J.M., Touati, G., *et al.* (2010) Pyruvate dehydrogenase complex deficiency: four neurological phenotypes with differing pathogenesis. *Dev Med Child Neurol* **52**, e1–9.

Bettendorff, L. (1994a) Thiamine in excitable tissues: reflections on a non-cofactor role. *Metab Brain Dis* **9**, 183–209.

Bettendorff, L. (1994b) The compartmentation of phosphorylated thiamine derivatives in cultured neuroblastoma cells. *Biochim Biophys Acta* **1222**, 7–14.

Bettendorff, L. (1995) Thiamine homeostasis in neuroblastoma cells. *Neurochem Int* **26**, 295–302.

Bettendorff, L. and Wins, P. (1994) Mechanism of thiamine transport in neuroblastoma cells. Inhibition of a high affinity carrier by sodium channel activators and dependence of thiamine uptake on membrane potential and intracellular ATP. *J Biol Chem* **269**, 14379–14385.

Bettendorff, L., Kolb, H.A., and Schoffeniels, E. (1993) Thiamine triphosphate activates an anion channel of large unit conductance in neuroblastoma cells. *J Mem Biol* **136**, 281–288.

Bettendorff, L., Mastrogiacomo, F., Kish, S.J., et al. (1996) Thiamine, thiamine phosphates, and their metabolizing enzymes in human brain. *J Neurochem* **66**, 250–258.

Bettendorff, L., Mastrogiacomo, F., Wins, P., et al. (1997) Low thiamine diphosphate levels in brains of patients with frontal lobe degeneration of the non-Alzheimer's type. *J Neurochem* **69**, 2005–2010.

Bettendorff, L., Michel-Cahay, C., Grandfils, C., et al. (1987) Thiamine triphosphate and membrane-associated thiamine phosphatases in the electric organ of *Electrophorus electricus*. *J Neurochem* **49**, 495–502.

Bettendorff, L., Peeters, M., Jouan, C., et al. (1991) Determination of thiamin and its phosphate esters in cultured neurons and astrocytes using an ion-pair reversed-phase high-performance liquid chromatographic method. *Anal Biochem* **198**, 52–59.

Bettendorff, L., Weekers, L., Wins, P., et al. (1990) Injection of sulbutiamine induces an increase in thiamine triphosphate in rat tissues. *Biochem Pharmacol* **40**, 2557–2560.

Bettendorff, L., Wins, P., and Lesourd, M. (1994) Subcellular localization and compartmentation of thiamine derivatives in rat brain. *Biochim Biophys Acta* **1222**, 1–6.

Bettendorff, L., Wins, P., and Schoffeniels, E. (1988) Thiamine triphosphatase from *Electrophorus* electric organ is anion-dependent and irreversibly inhibited by 4,4′-diisothiocyanostilbene-2,2'disulfonic acid. *Biochem Biophys Res Commun* **154**, 942–947.

Bettendorff, L., Wirtzfeld, B., Makarchikov, A.F., et al. (2007) Discovery of a natural thiamine adenine nucleotide. *Nature Chem Biol* **3**, 211–212.

Bizot, J.C., Herpin, A., Pothion, S., et al. (2005) Chronic treatment with sulbutiamine improves memory in an object recognition task and reduces some amnesic effects of dizocilpine in a spatial delayed-non-match-to-sample task. *Prog Neuro-Psychopharmacol Biol Psychiatr* **29**, 928–935.

Breslow, R. (1958) On the mechanism of thiamine action. IV.1 Evidence from studies on model systems. *J Am Chem Soc* **80**, 3719–3726.

Butterworth, R.F. (1987) Thiamin malnutrition and brain development. In Rassin, D.K., Haber, B., and Drujan, B. (eds)., *Basic and Clinical Aspects of Nutrition and Brain Development*, Vol. 16. Alan R Liss, New York, pp. 287–304.

Butterworth, R.F. (2003) Thiamin deficiency and brain disorders. *Nutr Res Rev* **16**, 277–284.

Butterworth, R.F., Gaudreau, C., Vincelette, J., et al. (1991) Thiamine deficiency and Wernicke's encephalopathy in AIDS. *Metab Brain Dis* **6**, 207–212.

Carpenter, K.J. (2000) *Beriberi, White Rice, and Vitamin B: a Disease, a Cause, and a Cure*. University of California Press, Berkeley, CA.

Cascante, M., Centelles, J.J., Veech, R.L., et al. (2000) Role of thiamin (vitamin B-1) and transketolase in tumor cell proliferation. *Nutr Cancer* **36**, 150–154.

Casirola, D., Ferrari, G., Gastaldi, G., et al. (1988) Transport of thiamine by brush-border membrane vesicles from rat small intestine. *J Physiol* **398**, 329–339.

Chen, M.F., Chen, L.T., Gold, M., et al. (1996) Plasma and erythrocyte thiamin concentrations in geriatric outpatients. *J Am Coll Nutr* **15**, 231–236.

Coy, J.F., Dressler, D., Wilde, J., et al. (2005) Mutations in the transketolase-like gene TKTL1: clinical implications for neurodegenerative diseases, diabetes and cancer. *Clin Lab* **51**, 257–273.

Coy, J.F., Dubel, S., Kioschis, P., et al. (1996) Molecular cloning of tissue-specific transcripts of a transketolase-related gene: implications for the evolution of new vertebrate genes. *Genomics* **32**, 309–316.

Czerniecki, J., Chanas, G., Verlaet, M., et al. (2004) Neuronal localization of the 25-kDa specific thiamine triphosphatase in rodent brain. *Neuroscience* **125**, 833–840.

Davis, R.E. and Icke, G.C. (1983) Clinical chemistry of thiamin. *Adv Clin Chem* **23**, 93–140.

Debs, R., Depienne, C., Rastetter, A., et al. (2010) Biotin-responsive basal ganglia disease in ethnic Europeans with novel SLC19A3 mutations. *Arch Neurol* **67**, 126–130.

De Caro, L., Rindi, G., and De Giuseppe, L. (1961) Contents in rat tissue of thiamine and its phosphates during dietary thiamine deficiency. *Int Z Vitaminforsch* **31**, 333–340.

Depeint, F., Bruce, W.R., Shangari, N., et al. (2006) Mitochondrial function and toxicity: role of the B vitamin family on mitochondrial energy metabolism. *Chem Biol Interact* **163**, 94–112.

Desjardins, P. and Butterworth, R.F. (2005) Role of mitochondrial dysfunction and oxidative stress in the pathogenesis of selective neuronal loss in Wernicke's encephalopathy. *Mol Neurobiol* **31**, 17–26.

Dutta, B., Huang, W., Molero, M., *et al.* (1999) Cloning of the human thiamine transporter, a member of the folate transporter family. *J Biol Chem* **274,** 31925–31929.

Eder, L., Hirt, L., and Dunant, Y. (1976) Possible involvement of thiamine in acetylcholine release. *Nature* **264,** 186–188.

Eijkman, C. (1990) Report of the investigations carried out in the laboratory of pathology and bacteriology, Weltevreden, during the year 1895. VI. Polyneuritis in chickens. New contributions to the etiology of the disease. 1896. *Nutr Rev* **48,** 243–246.

Eudy, J.D., Spiegelstein, O., Barber, R.C., *et al.* (2000) Identification and characterization of the human and mouse SLC19A3 gene: a novel member of the reduced folate family of micronutrient transporter genes. *Mol Genet Metab* **71,** 581–590.

Fattal-Valevski, A., Kesler, A., Sela, B.A., *et al.* (2005) Outbreak of life-threatening thiamine deficiency in infants in Israel caused by a defective soy-based formula. *Pediatrics* **115,** e233–e238.

Fayol, V. (1997) High-performance liquid chromatography determination of total thiamin in biological and food products. *Methods Enzymol* **279,** 57–66.

Fleming, J.C., Steinkamp, M.P., Kawatsuji, R., *et al.* (2001) Characterization of a murine high-affinity thiamine transporter, Slc19a2. *Mol Genet Metab* **74,** 273–280.

Fleming, J.C., Tartaglini, E., Steinkamp, M.P., *et al.* (1999) The gene mutated in thiamine-responsive anaemia with diabetes and deafness (TRMA) encodes a functional thiamine transporter. *Nature Genet* **22,** 305–308.

Foulon, V., Antonenkov, V.D., Croes, K., *et al.* (1999) Purification, molecular cloning, and expression of 2-hydroxyphytanoyl-CoA lyase, a peroxisomal thiamine pyrophosphate-dependent enzyme that catalyzes the carbon–carbon bond cleavage during alpha-oxidation of 3-methyl-branched fatty acids. *Proc Natl Acad Sci* **96,** 10039–10044.

Frédérich, M., Delvaux, D., Gigliobianco, T., *et al.* (2009) Thiaminylated adenine nucleotides. Chemical synthesis, structural characterization and natural occurrence *FEBS J* **276,** 3256–3268.

Fujiwara, M., Watanabe, H., and Katsui, K. (1954) Allithiamine, a newly found derivative of vitamin B1. *J Biochem* **41,** 29–39.

Fukuwatari, T., Yoshida, E., Takahashi, K., *et al.* (2010) Effect of fasting on the urinary excretion of water-soluble vitamins in humans and rats. *J Nutr Sci Vitaminol (Tokyo)* **56,** 19–26.

Gangolf, M., Czerniecki, J., Radermecker, M., *et al.* (2010a) Thiamine status in humans and content of phosphorylated thiamine derivatives in biopsies and cultured cells. *PLoS One* **5,** e13616.

Gangolf, M., Wins, P., Thiry, M., *et al.* (2010b) Thiamine triphosphate synthesis in rat brain occurs in mitochondria and is coupled to the respiratory chain. *J Biol Chem* **285,** 583–594.

Gastaldi, G., Casirola, D., Ferrari, G., *et al.* (1989) Effect of chronic ethanol administration on thiamine transport in microvillous vesicles of rat small intestine. *Alcohol Alcohol* **24,** 83–89.

Gastaldi, G., Cova, E., Verri, A., *et al.* (2000) Transport of thiamin in rat renal brush border membrane vesicles. *Kidney Int* **57,** 2043–2054.

Gastaldi, G., Laforenza, U., Ferrari, G., *et al.* (1992) Age-related thiamin transport by small intestinal microvillous vesicles of rat. *Biochim Biophys Acta* **1105,** 271–277.

Gigliobianco, T., Lakaye, B., Makarchikov, A.F., *et al.* (2008) Adenylate kinase-independent thiamine triphosphate accumulation under severe energy stress in *Escherichia coli.* *BMC Microbiol* **8,** 16.

Gigliobianco, T., Lakaye, B., Wins, P., *et al.* (2010) Adenosine thiamine triphosphate accumulates in *Escherichia coli* cells in response to specific conditions of metabolic stress. *BMC Microbiol* **10,** 148.

Gold, M., Chen, M.F., and Johnson, K. (1995) Plasma and red blood cell thiamine deficiency in patients with dementia of the Alzheimer's type. *Arch Neurol* **52,** 1081–1086.

Greenwood, J., Love, E.R., and Pratt, O.E. (1982) Kinetics of thiamine transport across the blood–brain barrier in the rat. *J Physiol* **327,** 95–103.

Greenwood, J., Luthert, P.J., Pratt, O.E., *et al.* (1986) Transport of thiamin across the blood–brain barrier of the rat in the absence of aerobic metabolism. *Brain Res* **399,** 148–151.

Grijns, G. (1901) Over polyneuritis gallinarum. I. *Geneeskundig Tijdschr Nederlandsch Indië* **41,** 3–110.

Guerrini, I., Thomson, A.D., Cook, C.C., *et al.* (2005) Direct genomic PCR sequencing of the high affinity thiamine transporter (SLC19A2) gene identifies three genetic variants in Wernicke Korsakoff syndrome (WKS). *Am J Med Genet B Neuropsychiatr Genet* **137B,** 17–19.

Hammes, H.P., Du, X., Edelstein, D., *et al.* (2003) Benfotiamine blocks three major pathways of hyperglycemic damage and prevents experimental diabetic retinopathy. *Nature Med* **9,** 294–299.

Harper, C. (1998) The neuropathology of alcohol-specific brain damage, or does alcohol damage the brain? *J Neuropathol Exp Neurol* **57,** 101–110.

Harper, C. (2009) The neuropathology of alcohol-related brain damage. *Alcohol Alcohol* **44,** 136–140.

Hazell, A.S. and Butterworth, R.F. (2009) Update of cell damage mechanisms in thiamine deficiency: focus on oxidative stress, excitotoxicity and inflammation. *Alcohol Alcohol* **44,** 141–147.

Heroux, M. and Butterworth, R.F. (1995) Regional alterations of thiamine phosphate esters and of thiamine diphosphate-dependent enzymes in relation to function in experimental Wernicke's encephalopathy. *Neurochem Res* **20,** 87–93.

Heroux, M., Raghavendra Rao, V.L., Lavoie, J., *et al.* (1996) Alterations of thiamine phosphorylation and of thiamine-dependent enzymes in Alzheimer's disease. *Metab Brain Dis* **11**, 81–88.

Horman, I. and Brambilla, E. (1982) The alleged antithiamine activity of o-diphenols: an artefact of oxygen in the thiochrome method? *Int J Vitaminol Nutr Res* **52**, 134–142.

Ishii, K., Sarai, K., Sanemori, H., *et al.* (1979) Concentrations of thiamine and its phosphate esters in rat tissues determined by high-performance liquid chromatography. *J Nutr Sci Vitaminol (Tokyo)* **25**, 517–523.

Jansen, B.C.P. and Donath, W.F. (1926) On the isolation of anti-beriberi vitamin. *Proc Koninklijke Ned Akad Wetensch* **29**, 1390–1400.

Jenkins, A.H., Schyns, G., Potot, S., *et al.* (2007) A new thiamin salvage pathway. *Nat Chem Biol* **3**, 492–497.

Jurgenson, C.T., Begley, T.P., and Ealick, S.E. (2009) The structural and biochemical foundations of thiamin biosynthesis. *Annu Rev Biochem* **78**, 569–603.

Kawasaki, T. (1992) Vitamin B1: Thiamine. In A.P. De Leenheer, W.E. Lambert, and H.J. Nelis (eds), *Modern Chromatographic Analysis of Vitamins*, Vol. 60. Marcel Dekker, New York, pp. 319–354.

Kono, S., Miyajima, H., Yoshida, K., *et al.* (2009) Mutations in a thiamine-transporter gene and Wernicke's-like encephalopathy. *New Engl J Med* **360**, 1792–1794.

Kopelman, M.D., Thomson, A.D., Guerrini, I., *et al.* (2009) The Korsakoff syndrome: clinical aspects, psychology and treatment. *Alcohol Alcohol* **44**, 148–154.

Korner, R.W., Vierzig, A., Roth, B., *et al.* (2009) Determination of thiamin diphosphate in whole blood samples by high-performance liquid chromatography – a method suitable for pediatric diagnostics. *J Chromatogr B* **877**, 1882–1886.

Laforenza, U., Patrini, C., Alvisi, C., *et al.* (1997) Thiamine uptake in human intestinal biopsy specimens, including observations from a patient with acute thiamine deficiency. *Am J Clin Nutr* **66**, 320–326.

Laforenza, U., Patrini, C., Gastaldi, G., *et al.* (1990) Effects of acute and chronic ethanol administration on thiamine metabolizing enzymes in some brain areas and in other organs of the rat. *Alcohol Alcohol* **25**, 591–603.

Lakaye, B., Makarchikov, A.F., Antunes, A.F., *et al.* (2002) Molecular characterization of a specific thiamine triphosphatase widely expressed in mammalian tissues. *J Biol Chem* **277**, 13771–13777.

Lakaye, B., Wirtzfeld, B., Wins, P., *et al.* (2004) Thiamine triphosphate, a new signal required for optimal growth of *Escherichia coli* during amino acid starvation. *J Biol Chem* **279**, 17142–17147.

Lindhurst, M.J., Fiermonte, G., Song, S., *et al.* (2006) Knockout of Slc25a19 causes mitochondrial thiamine pyrophosphate depletion, embryonic lethality, CNS malformations, and anemia. *Proc Natl Acad Sci USA* **103**, 15927–15932.

Lockman, P.R., Mumper, R.J., and Allen, D.D. (2003) Evaluation of blood–brain barrier thiamine efflux using the in situ rat brain perfusion method. *J Neurochem* **86**, 627–634.

Lonsdale, D., Shamberger, R.J., and Audhya, T. (2002) Treatment of autism spectrum children with thiamine tetrahydrofurfuryl disulfide: a pilot study. *Neuroendocrinol Lett* **23**, 303–308.

Lumeng, L., Edmondson, J.W., Schenker, S., *et al.* (1979) Transport and metabolism of thiamin in isolated rat hepatocytes. *J Biol Chem* **254**, 7265–7268.

Makarchikov, A.F., Brans, A., and Bettendorff, L. (2007) Thiamine diphosphate adenylyl transferase from *E. coli*: functional characterization of the enzyme synthesizing adenosine thiamine triphosphate *BMC Biochemistry* **8**, 17.

Makarchikov, A.F., Lakaye, B., Gulyai, I.E., *et al.* (2003) Thiamine triphosphate and thiamine triphosphatase activities: from bacteria to mammals. *Cell Mol Life Sci* **60**, 1477–1488.

Marobbio, C.M., Vozza, A., Harding, M., *et al.* (2002) Identification and reconstitution of the yeast mitochondrial transporter for thiamine pyrophosphate. *EMBO J* **21**, 5653–5661.

Mastrogiacomo, F., Bettendorff, L., Grisar, T., *et al.* (1996a) Brain thiamine, its phosphate esters, and its metabolizing enzymes in Alzheimer's disease. *Ann Neurol* **39**, 585–591.

Mastrogiacomo, F., Lindsay, J.G., Bettendorff, L., *et al.* (1996b) Brain protein and alpha-ketoglutarate dehydrogenase complex activity in Alzheimer's disease. *Ann Neurol* **39**, 592–598.

McCool, B.A., Plonk, S.G., Martin, P.R., *et al.* (1993) Cloning of human transketolase cDNAs and comparison of the nucleotide sequence of the coding region in Wernicke–Korsakoff and non-Wernicke–Korsakoff individuals. *J Biol Chem* **268**, 1397–1404.

McCourt, J.A., Nixon, P.F., and Duggleby, R.G. (2006) Thiamin nutrition and catalysis-induced instability of thiamin diphosphate. *Br J Nutr* **96**, 636–638.

McGready, R., Simpson, J.A., Cho, T., *et al.* (2001) Postpartum thiamine deficiency in a Karen displaced population. *Am J Clin Nutr*, **74**, 808–813.

Molina, J.A., Jimenez-Jimenez, F.J., Hernanz, A., *et al.* (2002) Cerebrospinal fluid levels of thiamine in patients with Alzheimer's disease. *J Neural Transm* **109**, 1035–1044.

Mukherjee, A.B., Svoronos, S., Ghazanfari, A., *et al.* (1987) Transketolase abnormality in cultured fibroblasts from familial chronic alcoholic men and their male offspring. *J Clin Invest* **79**, 1039–1043.

Nabokina, S.M., Reidling, J.C., and Said, H.M. (2005) Differentiation-dependent up-regulation of intestinal thiamin uptake: cellular and molecular mechanisms. *J Biol Chem* **280**, 32676–32682.

Neal, R.A. and Pearson, W.N. (1964) Studies of thiamine metabolism in the rat. I. Metabolic products found in urine. *J Nutr* **83**, 343–350.

Nghiêm, H.O., Bettendorff, L., and Changeux, J.P. (2000) Specific phosphorylation of *Torpedo* 43K rapsyn by endogenous kinase(s) with thiamine triphosphate as the phosphate donor. *FASEB J* **14**, 543–554.

Nixon, P.F., Jordan, L., Zimitat, C., *et al.* (2008) Choroid plexus dysfunction: the initial event in the pathogenesis of Wernicke's encephalopathy and ethanol intoxication. *Alcohol Clin Exp Res* **32**, 1513–1523.

Nozaki, S., Mizuma, H., Tanaka, M., *et al.* (2009) Thiamine tetrahydrofurfuryl disulfide improves energy metabolism and physical performance during physical-fatigue loading in rats. *Nutr Res*, **29**, 867–872.

Oishi, K., Hirai, T., Gelb, B.D., *et al.* (2001) Slc19a2: cloning and characterization of the murine thiamin transporter cDNA and genomic sequence, the orthologue of the human TRMA gene. *Mol Genet Metab* **73**, 149–159.

Oishi, K., Hofmann, S., Diaz, G.A., *et al.* (2002) Targeted disruption of Slc19a2, the gene encoding the high-affinity thiamin transporter Thtr-1, causes diabetes mellitus, sensorineural deafness and megaloblastosis in mice. *Hum Mol Genet* **11**, 2951–2960.

Pan, X., Gong, N., Zhao, J., *et al.* (2010) Powerful beneficial effects of benfotiamine on cognitive impairment and beta-amyloid deposition in amyloid precursor protein/presenilin-1 transgenic mice. *Brain* **133**, 1342–1351.

Pearson, W.N., Hung, E., Darby, W.J.J., *et al.* (1966) Excretion of metabolites of 14C-pyrimidine-labeled thimine by the rat at different levels of thiamine intake. *J Nutr* **89**, 133–142.

Peterson, J.W., Gubler, C.J., and Kuby, S.A. (1975) Partial purification and properties of thiamine pyrophosphokinase from pig brain. *Biochim Biophys Acta* **397**, 377–394.

Poggi, V., Longo, G., DeVizia, B., *et al.* (1984) Thiamin-responsive megaloblastic anaemia: a disorder of thiamin transport? *J Inher Metab Dis* **7**(Suppl 2), 153–154.

Rajgopal, A., Edmondson, A., Goldman, I.D., *et al.* (2001) SLC19A3 encodes a second thiamine transporter ThTr2. *Biochim Biophys Acta* **1537**, 175–178.

Reidling, J.C. and Said, H.M. (2005) Adaptive regulation of intestinal thiamin uptake: molecular mechanism using wild-type and transgenic mice carrying hTHTR-1 and -2 promoters. *Am J Physiol Gastrointest Liver Physiol* **288**, G1127–1134.

Reidling, J.C., Lambrecht, N., Kassir, M., *et al.* (2010) Impaired intestinal vitamin B1 (thiamin) uptake in thiamin transporter-2-deficient mice. *Gastroenterology* **138**, 1802–1809.

Rindi, G. and Ferrari, G. (1977) Thiamine transport by human intestine in vitro. *Experientia* **33**, 211–213.

Rindi, G., Casirola, D., Poggi, V., *et al.* (1992) Thiamine transport by erythrocytes and ghosts in thiamine-responsive megaloblastic anaemia. *J Inherit Metab Dis* **15**, 231–242.

Rindi, G., Imarisio, L., and Patrini, C. (1986) Effects of acute and chronic ethanol administration on regional thiamin pyrophosphokinase activity of the rat brain. *Biochem Pharmacol* **35**, 3903–3908.

Rindi, G., Patrini, C., Comincioli, V., *et al.* (1980) Thiamine content and turnover rates of some rat nervous regions, using labeled thiamine as a tracer. *Brain Res* **181**, 369–380.

Rindi, G., Patrini, C., Laforenza, U., *et al.* (1994) Further studies on erythrocyte thiamin transport and phosphorylation in seven patients with thiamin-responsive megaloblastic anaemia. *J Inherit Metab Dis* **17**, 667–677.

Romanenko, A.V. (1990) A new way of muscle activity regulation: thiamine participation in neuromuscular transmission. *Muscle Motil* **2**, 151–153.

Roser, R.L., Andrist, A.H., Harrington, W.H., *et al.* (1978) Determination of urinary thiamine by high-pressure liquid chromatography utilizing the thiochrome fluorescent method. *J Chromatogr* **146**, 43–53.

Said, H.M., Balamurugan, K., Subramanian, V.S., *et al.* (2004) Expression and functional contribution of hTHTR-2 in thiamin absorption in human intestine. *Am J Physiol Gastrointest Liver Physiol* **286**, G491–498.

Said, H.M., Ortiz, A., Subramanian, V.S., *et al.* (2001) Mechanism of thiamine uptake by human colonocytes: studies with cultured colonic epithelial cell line NCM460. *Am J Physiol Gastrointest Liver Physiol* **281**, G144–150.

Said, H.M., Reidling, J.C., and Ortiz, A. (2002) Cellular and molecular aspects of thiamin uptake by human liver cells: studies with cultured HepG2 cells. *Biochim Biophys Acta* **1567**, 106–112.

Sanemori, H. and Kawasaki, T. (1982) Thiamine triphosphate metabolism and its turnover in the rat liver. *Experientia* **38**, 1044–1045.

Sanemori, H., Ueki, H., and Kawasaki, T. (1980) Reversed-phase high-performance liquid chromatographic analysis of thiamine phosphate esters at subpicomole levels. *Anal Biochem* **107**, 451–455.

Shikata, H., Egi, Y., Koyama, S., *et al.* (1989a) Properties of the thiamin triphosphate-synthesizing activity catalyzed by adenylate kinase (isoenzyme 1). *Biochem Int* **18**, 943–949.

Shikata, H., Koyama, S., Egi, Y., *et al.* (1989b) Cytosolic adenylate kinase catalyzes the synthesis of thiamin triphosphate from thiamin diphosphate. *Biochem Int* **18**, 933–941.

Shimomura, T., Mori, E., Hirono, N., *et al.* (1998) Development of Wernicke–Korsakoff syndrome after long intervals following gastrectomy. *Arch Neurol* **55**, 1242–1245.

Sica, D.A. (2007) Loop diuretic therapy, thiamine balance, and heart failure. *Congestive Heart Failure* **13**, 244–247.

Singh, M., Thompson, M., Sullivan, N., *et al.* (2005) Thiamine deficiency in dogs due to the feeding of sulphite preserved meat. *Aust Vet J* **83**, 412–417.

Smidt, L.J., Cremin, F.M., Grivetti, L.E., *et al.* (1991) Influence of thiamin supplementation on the health and general well-being of an elderly Irish population with marginal thiamin deficiency. *J Gerontol* **46**, M16–22.

Song, J., Bettendorff, L., Tonelli, M., *et al.* (2008) Structural basis for the catalytic mechanism of mammalian 25-kDa thiamine triphosphatase. *J Biol Chem* **283**, 10939–10948.

Spector, R. and Johanson, C.E. (2007) Vitamin transport and homeostasis in mammalian brain: focus on vitamins B and E. *J Neurochem* **103**, 425–438.

Stagg, A.R., Fleming, J.C., Baker, M.A., *et al.* (1999) Defective high-affinity thiamine transporter leads to cell death in thiamine-responsive megaloblastic anemia syndrome fibroblasts. *J Clin Invest* **103**, 723–729.

Subramanian, V.S., Marchant, J.S., and Said, H.M. (2006) Biotin-responsive basal ganglia disease-linked mutations inhibit thiamine transport via the human thiamine transporter-2 (hTHTR2): biotin is not a substrate for hTHTR2. *Am J Physiol Cell Physiol* **291**, C851–C859.

Subramanya, S.B., Subramanian, V.S., and Said, H.M. (2010) Chronic alcohol consumption and intestinal thiamin absorption: effects on physiological and molecular parameters of the uptake process. *Am J Physiol Gastrointest Liver Physiol* **299**, G23–31.

Takaki, K. (1885) On the cause and prevention of Kak'ke. *Sei-i-kai Medical J* **4** (Suppl 4), 29–37.

Thurman, J.E. and Mooradian, A.D. (1997) Vitamin supplementation therapy in the elderly. *Drugs Aging* **11**, 433–449.

van Zaanen, H.C. and van der Lelie, J. (1992) Thiamine deficiency in hematologic malignant tumors. *Cancer* **69**, 1710–1713.

Victor, M., Adams, R.D., and Collins, G.H. (1989) *The Wernicke-Korsakoff Syndrome and Related Neurological Disorders due to Alcoholism and Malnutrition.* F.A. Davies, Philadelphia.

Vlasova, T.I., Stratton, S.L., Wells, A.M., *et al.* (2005) Biotin deficiency reduces expression of SLC19A3, a potential biotin transporter, in leukocytes from human blood. *J Nutr* **135**, 42–47.

Vognar, L. and Stoukides, J. (2009) The role of low plasma thiamin levels in cognitively impaired elderly patients presenting with acute behavioral disturbances. *J Am Geriatr Soc* **57**, 2166–2168.

Volvert, M.L., Seyen, S., Piette, M., *et al.* (2008) Benfotiamine, a synthetic S-acyl thiamine derivative, has different mechanisms of action and a different pharmacological profile than lipid-soluble thiamine disulfide derivatives. *BMC Pharmacol* **8**, 10.

Wang, Y., Zhao, R., Russell, R.G., *et al.* (2001) Localization of the murine reduced folate carrier as assessed by immunohistochemical analysis. *Biochim Biophys Acta* **1513**, 49–54.

Wilkinson, T.J., Hanger, H.C., Elmslie, J., *et al.* (1997) The response to treatment of subclinical thiamine deficiency in the elderly. *Am J Clin Nutr* **66**, 925–928.

Williams, R.R. and Cline, J.K. (1936) Synthesis of vitamin B1. *J Am Chem Soc* **58**, 1504–1505.

Xu, X., Zur Hausen, A., Coy, J.F., *et al.* (2009) Transketolase-like protein 1 (TKTL1) is required for rapid cell growth and full viability of human tumor cells. *Int J Cancer* **124**, 1330–1337.

Yoshioka, K. (1984) Some properties of the thiamine uptake system in isolated rat hepatocytes. *Biochim Biophys Acta* **778**, 201–209.

Zeng, W.Q., Al-Yamani, E., Acierno, J.S., Jr, *et al.* (2005) Biotin-responsive basal ganglia disease maps to 2q36.3 and is due to mutations in SLC19A3. *Am J Human Genet* **77**, 16–26.

Zhao, R., Gao, F., and Goldman, I.D. (2002) Reduced folate carrier transports thiamine monophosphate: an alternative route for thiamine delivery into mammalian cells. *Am J Physiol Cell Physiol* **282**, C1512–C1517.

Zhao, R., Gao, F., Wang, Y., *et al.* (2001) Impact of the reduced folate carrier on the accumulation of active thiamin metabolites in murine leukemia cells. *J Biol Chem* **276**, 1114–1118.

18

RIBOFLAVIN

DONALD B. MCCORMICK, PhD
Emory University, Atlanta, Georgia, USA

Summary

Riboflavin (vitamin B_2) is the principal flavin among a larger group of natural substituted iso-alloxazines that can be biosynthesized by many bacteria, yeasts, and higher plants. However, most animals cannot make riboflavin and it must be supplied by dietary intake either as the free vitamin or as flavocoenzymes that are hydrolyzed in the gut to release the vitamin. After both specific and facilitated uptake, as well as passive diffusion into cells, the vitamin is largely converted by kinase- and synthetase-catalyzed reactions to the coenzymes, flavin mononucleotide (FMN) and flavin adenine dinucleotide (FAD), which operate in numerous enzymatic oxidation–reduction catalyses. Two among many such enzyme systems are FAD-dependent glutathione reductase and FMN-dependent pyridoxine (pyridoxamine) phosphate oxidase, both useful as erythrocyte biochemical indicators of riboflavin nutritional status in humans. Less frequently encountered are enzymes that have flavocoenzymes covalently attached to the polypeptide backbone, such as the mammalian mitochondrial 8α-S-cysteinyl-FAD of monoamine oxidase and the 8α-N^3-histidyl-FAD of dehydrogenases for succinate and sarcosine.

Riboflavin has a wide distribution in foodstuffs, and is present at especially high levels in kidney, liver, cheese, eggs, and milk, where it is largely bound in coenzymes that can be hydrolyzed in the gut to release the free vitamin. Limited solubility of riboflavin precludes tissue overload and potential toxicity. Specific and saturable absorption mechanisms for the vitamin occur at cellular level, and the transport by albumin and more tightly bound immunoglobulins follows in the blood plasma of mammals. A significant fraction of the vitamin and derived flavin products are excreted in urine and secreted in milk by humans and other mammals. The diverse degradative products from flavin that are excreted in the urine reflect hydrolytic and oxidative processes including tissue mixed-function oxidation of methyl groups of the free flavin and ribityl side-chain cleavage that is largely the result of microfloral activity in the gut and exposure of skin to light.

Causes for nutritional deficiency are ascribed not only to inadequate intake but also, less frequently, to impairment in metabolic disposition. There is an expansion of our knowledge of genetic defects in the formation of functional flavoproteins such as reflect mitochondrial electron transfer and β-oxidation of fatty acyl-CoAs. Some of these relatively rare diseases benefit from supplementation, but normal individuals receive ample vitamin by eating a variety of foods, some already fortified with riboflavin.

Present Knowledge in Nutrition, Tenth Edition. Edited by John W. Erdman Jr, Ian A. Macdonald and Steven H. Zeisel.
© 2012 International Life Sciences Institute. Published 2012 by John Wiley & Sons, Inc.

Introduction

Riboflavin is so named because it has a ribose-like part of its structure and is yellow (Latin, *flavus*); it was historically designated as the second vitamin in the B-complex of water-soluble vitamins so it is also called vitamin B_2. Much of the early history of this vitamin has been detailed in volume series such as that edited by Sebrell and Harris during the 1940s, and has been summarized in more recent book chapters (McCormick, 1988; Combs, 1998). Most of the methods for isolation or syntheses, characterization, and quantitation of flavin systems have been collated in the series on *Vitamins and Coenzymes* that was edited by McCormick *et al.* (1970–1997). The ongoing discovery of new flavins, the proteins they associate with, and the diverse oxidation–reduction (redox) reactions in which they participate have been periodically enlarged upon in volumes resulting from symposia held every three years since 1960; a recent (sixteenth) volume of such proceedings was published in 2008 (Frago *et al.*, 2008a). Augmentation of this largely biochemical information can be found in recent papers on flavoprotein systems (see Gadda, 2010). Relatively current reviews that include brief coverage of the history of riboflavin and coenzymes, including chemistry and properties, are to be found in books dealing with all the vitamins required by humans (McCormick, 2006; Rivlin, 2007). The present chapter provides an update on this vitamin since the preceding editions of *Present Knowledge in Nutrition* (McCormick, 1990; Rivlin, 2006).

Natural Flavins

All known natural flavins but one (5-deazaflavin) are isoalloxazines, which are 10-substituted derivatives of alloxazine, the parent tricyclic ring system, with nitrogens in positions 1, 3, and 5. The variations in structures of naturally occurring flavins, with a dashed line between atoms in positions 1 and 5 to allow for oxidized (quinoid), half-reduced (semiquinoid or radical), and fully reduced (hydroquinoid) forms, are summarized in Figure 18.1. Approximately 35 different flavoquinones have been isolated from natural sources.

Riboflavin (7,8-dimethyl-10-[1′-D-ribityl]isoalloxazine) is a yellow fluorescent compound that is widely distributed throughout the plant and animal kingdoms. Studies with bacteria and fungi, particularly *Ashbya gossypii* and *Eremothecium ashbyii*, which can biosynthesize

rather large quantities of riboflavin, have revealed a pathway from guanosine triphosphate (GTP). Most of the intermediates and enzymes involved were characterized over the past half-century; however, continuing work has provided more molecular details (Bacher *et al.*, 2000, 2001). Recent examination of the crystal structure of a bifunctional enzyme from *Bacillus subtilis* revealed an N-terminal deaminase domain belonging to the cytidine deaminase superfamily and a C-terminal reductase domain similar to that found in dihydrofolate reductase (Chen *et al.*, 2006). The two reductases involved in riboflavin and folate biosyntheses probably evolved from an ancestral gene and remind us of the similar initial steps in the pathways that result in isoalloxazine and pterin systems, both of which originate from GTP and require cyclohydrolases. Dismutation of 6,7-dimethyl-8-ribityllumazine yields diastereomeric pentacyclic intermediates in archaeal (*Methanococcus jannaschii*) and non-archaeal (*Escherichia coli*) riboflavin synthases that yield 5-amino-6-ribitylamino-2,4(1H,3H)-pyrimidinedione and riboflavin (Illarionov *et al.*, 2005). Though most flavins derive from further actions upon riboflavin, at least two, namely roseoflavin with an 8-dimethylamino function produced by *Streptomyces davawensis* and coenzyme F_{420} with a 5-carba-5-deaza nucleus formed in *Methanobacterium* sp., must arise in variations of the usual biosynthetic pathway. Structures of these native flavins, with substituents noted in respect to Figure 18.1, are summarized in Table 18.1. Higher organisms, notably the human and other mammals, cannot biosynthesize the isoalloxazine system; therefore, riboflavin is a water-soluble vitamin (i.e. a required nutrient) for such species.

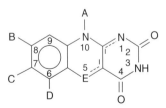

FIG. 18.1 Generalized structure for flavins and derivatives that occur naturally. Particular substituents are given in the text and tables that refer to diverse types.

Flavocoenzyme Types and Functions

The major coenzyme forms of riboflavin function as prosthetic groups of numerous holoenzymes that catalyze diverse and often essential one- and two-electron redox reactions. The five physiologically relevant redox forms have been structurally detailed in an earlier review (McCormick, 1988). Flavin mononucleotide (FMN, also named riboflavin 5'-phosphate) may account for as much as 10% of the total flavin in diverse cells, and the more frequently encountered flavin adenine dinucleotide (FAD) comprises nearly 90%. Moreover, a small but significant fraction of both coenzymes (5–10% of FAD) occurs in some organelles and organisms as forms altered at positions 6, 8, or 8α. Structures of the coenzyme-level flavins with substituents noted in respect to Figure 18.1 are summarized in Table 18.2.

Sources for the coenzyme-level flavins were summarized in a previous review (Merrill *et al.*, 1981a). Briefly, however, it can be noted that the 6-hydroxy derivatives of both FMN and FAD may arise from oxidative turnover of the predominant natural coenzymes during function. The

6-S-cysteinyl-FMN, 8-hydroxy flavins, and 8α-O-tyrosyl-FAD have been found in certain bacterial systems, but the 8α-S-cysteinyl- and both 8α-N^1- and N^3-histidyl-FAD forms are found in several lower and higher organisms. Berberine bridge enzyme, a plant enzyme involved in alkaloid biosynthesis, was isolated from the California poppy (*Eschscholzia californica*), expressed at a higher level in the methylotropic yeast (*Pischia pastoris*), and found to contain an FAD linked in the 8α-position to a histidyl residue and in the 6-position to a cysteinyl thiol function (Winkler *et al.*, 2006). The bi-covalently attached FAD has the highest redox potential so far known for any flavoprotein and may predispose the enzyme for a hydride ion transfer from substrate (Winkler *et al.*, 2007). Examination of the crystal structure of berberine bridge enzyme and such mutants as lack one of the linkages to FAD revealed that both linkages are involved in increasing redox potential and fine-tuning the active-site geometry for optimal substrate binding (Winkler *et al.*, 2009). The covalent attachment of FAD via an 8α-linkage to a cysteinyl residue in mitochondrial monoamine oxidase (both A and B types) and such linkage to the N^3 of an imidazole of histidyl residues in mitochondrial succinate and sarcosine dehydrogenases are important examples in our bodies. The N^1-histidyl linkage occurs, among other places, in L-gulonolactone oxidase, which allows certain animals, e.g. rats, to biosynthesize L-ascorbic acid.

Absorption, Transport, and Uptake

Methods to assess the bioavailability of riboflavin from foods continue to be improved. As determined by

TABLE 18.1 Native flavins formed by microorganisms

Name	Substituent				
	A	B	C	D	E
Riboflavin	1'-D-ribityl	CH$_3$	CH$_3$	H	N
Roseoflavin	1'-D-ribityl	(CH$_3$)$_2$N	CH$_3$	H	N
5-Deazaflavin	1'-D-ribityl	HO	H	H	CH

TABLE 18.2 Flavocoenzymes found with flavoenzymes

Name	Substituent				
	A	B	C	D	E
FMN	1'-D-ribityl-5'-phosphate	CH$_3$	CH$_3$	H	N
6-Hydroxy-FMN	1'-D-ribityl-5'-phosphate	CH$_3$	CH$_3$	HO	N
6-S-Cysteinyl-FMN	1'-D-ribityl-5'-phosphate	CH$_3$	CH$_3$	S-Cys	N
Coenzyme F$_{420}$	1'-D-ribityl-5'-phospholactyldiglutamate	HO	H	H	CH
FAD	1'-D-ribityl-5'-ADP	CH$_3$	CH$_3$	H	N
6-Hydroxy-FAD	1'-D-ribityl-5'-ADP	CH$_3$	CH$_3$	HO	N
8-Hydroxy-FAD	1'-D-ribityl-5'-ADP	HO	CH$_3$	H	N
8α-O-Tyrosyl-FAD	1'-D-ribityl-5'-ADP	CH$_2$-O-Tyr	CH$_3$	H	N
8α-S-Cysteinyl-FAD	1'-D-ribityl-5'-ADP	CH$_2$-S-Cys	CH$_3$	H	N
8α-N^1-Histidyl-FAD	1'-D-ribityl-5'-ADP	CH$_2$-N^1-His	CH$_3$	H	N
8α-N^3-Histidyl-FAD	1'-D-ribityl-5'-ADP	CH$_2$-N^3-His	CH$_3$	H	N
6-S-Cysteinyl-8α-N^3-HistidylFAD	1'-D-ribityl-5'-ADP	CH$_2$-N^3-His	CH$_3$	S-Cys	N

stable-isotope labels and kinetic modeling (Dainty et al., 2007), a large fraction of newly absorbed riboflavin in the human is removed by the liver on "first pass" so that appearance in plasma underestimates bioavailability from foodstuffs. Urinary monitoring suggests that riboflavin from spinach is as bioavailable as it is from milk. After ingestion of diverse natural flavins, most of which occur as coenzymes and traces of flavinyl peptides, release occurs by non-specific hydrolytic activities in the gastrointestinal tract. Earlier investigations on general aspects of absorption in humans were updated by studies with sections of gut (Daniel et al., 1983) and isolated cells (Hegazy and Schwenk, 1983) from other mammals. The vitamin is primarily absorbed in the human in the proximal small intestine by a saturable uptake that is rapid and proportional to dose before leveling off in adults at about 25 mg of riboflavin (Zempleni et al., 1996a). Bile salts appear to facilitate uptake, and a modest amount of the vitamin circulates via the enterohepatic system. Active transport at lower concentrations may be Na^+ dependent and involve phosphorylation. However, a recently studied Na^+-independent transport protein that is pH sensitive may also contribute in jejunal and ileal regions (Yamamoto et al., 2009). Most recently human riboflavin transporters (hRFTs) have been identified and found to be expressed differentially in various tissues (Fujimura et al., 2010; Yao et al., 2010). The mRNAs for both hRFT 1 and 2 are strongly expressed in the small intestine, whereas hRFT 3 is expressed in the brain. As reported earlier, intestinal absorption seems to be affected by aging, fiber intake, antacids, and uremic conditions (McCormick, 1990). Metabolic trapping by conversion to coenzymes generally occurs before release of the vitamin to circulation by pyrophosphatase and phosphatase activities.

Transport of flavin by blood plasma is known to involve both loose association with albumin and tight associations with some globulins. Among the latter, immunoglobulins were identified as the major binding proteins for riboflavin in serum from normal humans (Merrill et al., 1981b; Innis et al., 1985) and from patients with certain types of cancer (Innis et al., 1986; Zhu et al., 2006). By use of flavinyl-affinity chromatography, different immunoglobulin subclasses, namely IgG, IgM, and IgA, were isolated and shown to have both κ and λ light chains (Merrill et al., 1987). Papain cleavage of the immunoglobulins yielded Fab fragments that still bound riboflavin. Hence, at least a portion of the antigenic binding site may be involved. In this connection it is interesting to note that riboflavin

antibodies were elicited in response to haptenic challenges (Barber et al., 1987).

Some riboflavin-binding proteins are pregnancy specific, including the classic case of the estrogen-induced egg white protein. This subject has been reviewed both in particular (Kozik, 1985; White and Merrill, 1988) and as part of past general reviews of riboflavin (McCormick, 1990, 2006). Examples include binding proteins from pregnant cows, rats, bonnet monkeys, and humans. These proteins appear similar to the avian riboflavin-binding protein because their epitopes are recognized by monoclonal antibodies to the chicken riboflavin-binding protein. They are essential for fetal development because immunization of animals with the avian protein or injection of antibodies against the avian protein terminates pregnancy in rats, mice, and the bonnet monkey. Fetal degeneration accompanies lowering of FAD levels in the fetus. The exact cause of the effect on level of flavocoenzyme is not known, but an interaction between chick liver flavokinase and riboflavin-binding protein has been demonstrated (Kozik, 1985; White and Merrill, 1988; McCormick, 1990, 2006). Placental transfer of riboflavin seems to involve binding proteins that help vector the vitamin and enhance supply to the fetus. In perfused human placenta, differential rates of uptake were noted at maternal and fetal surfaces (McCormick, 2006). There are differences in riboflavin concentrations in maternal and cord blood in the human, carrier proteins were isolated from both, and a flavin-containing placental protein was isolated (McCormick, 2006).

Uptake processes for flavins by mammalian cells have some characteristics in common, but there are both qualitative and quantitative differences among different cell types (Bowman et al., 1989; McCormick, 1990, 2006). Hepatocytes exhibit an initial rapid and specific intake followed by slower passive diffusion of the vitamin, which becomes metabolically trapped by flavokinase-catalyzed phosphorylation (Aw et al., 1983). The uptake process is relatively insensitive to both Na^+ and ouabain and probably reflects a facilitated, carrier-mediated system. A riboflavin-binding protein has been reported to occur in the plasma membrane of rat liver cells (Nokubo et al., 1989). With proximal tubular epithelial cells from rat kidney, the faster facilitated phase of flavin uptake exhibits Na^+ dependence (like small intestine but unlike liver) but is insensitive to oubain (like liver but unlike small intestine) (Bowers-Komro and McCormick, 1987). An ATP requirement reflects, as for other cells, the trapping of

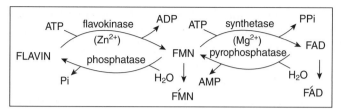

FIG. 18.2 Interconversions of flavin and flavocoenzymes.

riboflavin by phosphorylation, a process that can be impeded by other flavin substrates or inhibitors of flavokinase.

Coenzyme Formations and Interconversions

Knowledge on the way in which flavins are interconverted to coenzymatic forms is summarized in Figure 18.2.

As noted in a summary on this subject (McCormick et al., 1987), relatively homogeneous preparations of flavokinase (now also called riboflavin kinase) were obtained first from rat liver (Merrill and McCormick, 1980), then from mung beans (Sobhanaditya and Appaji Rao, 1981) and more recently from a bacterium (Manstein and Pai, 1986). Though not identical in molecular properties, the mammalian (28 000 MW) and plant (30 000–35 000 MW) kinases cannot further catalyze formation of FAD from FMN, whereas the bacterial enzyme (38 000 MW) is both a flavokinase and an FAD synthetase. This type of dual-functional enzyme is found in many prokaryotes wherein the N-terminal and C-terminal domains are related to nucleotidyl transferase and riboflavin kinases, respectively (Frago et al., 2008b). The FAD synthetase from liver is a larger enzyme (100 000 MW dimer) but cannot function as a flavokinase (Oka and McCormick, 1987). Seemingly in all cases, Zn^{2+} is preferred for kinase activity and Mg^{2+} for synthetase activity. The phylogenetic differences among flavokinases and FAD synthetases located in the cytosol are interesting and may have a bearing on the controls that can modulate levels of flavocoenzyme formed in higher organisms with separate but probably interactive enzymes. The kinetics of substrate and product interactions with the kinase/synthetase system of rat liver has been discerned (Yamada et al., 1990). FAD as an inhibitory end-product may regulate its own formation. There is significant endocrine control of mammalian flavocoenzyme level, most especially as involves thyroid-hormone induced increase in biosynthesis (Rivlin, 2001). Increase in triiodothyronine in rats leads to an increase in a more active form of liver flavokinase and a concomitant decrease in a less active form (Lee and McCormick, 1985). Recent work suggests that tumor necrosis factor, through activation of flavokinase, enhances the incorporation of FAD in NADPH oxidases (Yazdanpanah et al., 2009).

The non-specific hydrolytic enzymes that break down FMN and FAD have been observed in extracts from numerous sources (McCormick, 1975). Mammalian phosphatases that can hydrolyze FMN to riboflavin and inorganic phosphate not only include those with somewhat acidic pH optima (McCormick and Russell, 1962), such as those located in lysosomes, but also include those with alkaline optima (Akiyama et al., 1982), such as in the intestinal brush border. FAD pyrophosphatases from both liver and intestine are optimal at alkaline pH. There are age-related decreases in the hydrolytic activities for both FMN and FAD in liver (Lee and McCormick, 1983). It has been found recently that a C-terminal flavokinase homolog in plants (*Arabidopsis thaliana*) is fused with an FMN hydrolase (Sandoval and Roje, 2005). Subcellular localization of these and the FAD synthetase activities within plastids has also been delineated (Sandoval et al., 2008).

The means by which subsequent modifications of flavo-coenzymes occur is not yet completely understood. However, it is certain that FMN and more commonly FAD are preformed before fractions of these coenzymes are covalently attached to specific apoenzymes. Studies on incorporation of ^{14}C-riboflavin into covalently bound FAD of enzymes from rat liver mitochondria indicate that formation of FAD preceded attachment (Yagi et al., 1976; Addison and McCormick, 1978; Sato et al., 1984). The fact that certain synthetic 8α-substituted riboflavins (e.g. S-cysteinyl or N[3]-histidyl derivatives) were not converted by flavokinase to the corresponding FMN analog (Merrill and McCormick, 1979, 1980) and that synthetic 8α-imidazole-FMN is not a substrate for the FAD synthetase (Bowers-Komro et al., 1989) would also argue against covalent linkage of FAD to the peptide in such systems as are in monoamine oxidase or succinate dehydrogenase until after FAD is formed.

Work with cell-free synthesis of 6-hydroxy-D-nicotine oxidase from *Arthrobacter oxidans*, an enzyme with an 8α-N[3]-histidyl-FAD, has established that intact FAD is incorporated into nascent polypeptide chains during ribosomal translation (Hamm and Decker, 1978, 1980). This has been extended to the similarly linked FAD within bacterial succinate and fumarate dehydrogenases (Brandsch and Bichler, 1985, 1986). The apoenzyme of the hydroxy-nicotine oxidase could be transformed into holoenzyme in the presence of FAD, ATP, phosphoenolpyruvate, and pyruvate kinase (Brandsch and Bichler, 1987). This indicates that flavinylation is enzyme catalyzed and may proceed through a phospho-intermediate. A protein fraction in the mitochondrial matrix has been reported to stimulate flavination of dimethylglycine dehydrogenase (Brizio et al., 2000).

Catabolism, Excretion, and Secretion

Certain bacteria of the genus *Pseudomonas* can extensively degrade both the ring system (Tsai and Stadtman, 1971) and side chains (Yanagita and Forster, 1956; Yang and McCormick, 1967) of flavins, but mammals are more limited in their abilities to catabolize the vitamin (McCormick, 1975; McCormick et al., 1984, 1987). The diversity of flavin-derived products in mammalian urine, however, reflects metabolic events that occur in gastrointestinal microbes as well as in the somatic cells and additionally is augmented by photochemical events that occur at the dermal level. These diverse compounds and their interconnections are summarized in Figure 18.3.

Cleavage of the side chain at position 10 seems mainly if not entirely attributable to intestinal microflora and light. Action of the former on riboflavin was shown to lead to partial fragmentation to form the 10-formylmethylflavin found in urine from ruminants (Owen and West, 1971a) which can interconvert this product with the 10-hydroxyethylflavin formed as a result of pyridine-nucleotide-dependent dehydrogenase in tissues (Owen and West, 1971b). The 10-hydroxymethylflavin is also found in urine from rats (Chastain and McCormick, 1987a) and humans (Chastain and McCormick, 1987b). Lumichrome-level compounds not only may result from complete removal of the side chain by microflora, which can be decreased by antibiotic administration (Yang and McCormick, 1978; Chastain and McCormick, 1987a), but may also accompany lumiflavin as a photoproduct from action of light on flavin within the dermal tissue (Yang and McCormick, 1978; Chastain and McCormick, 1987a,b). A significant fraction of fecal radioactivity obtained from rats administered [2-^{14}C]riboflavin was also found to be chloroform soluble and at the level of lumi-

chrome (Yang and McCormick, 1978). A portion of the formylmethylflavin can also be oxidized by alimentary bacteria of the ruminant and human to form the 10-carboxymethylflavin (West and Owen, 1973).

No enzymatic activity able to lead to such chain-shortened products has been identified within tissues (Oka and McCormick, 1985). Rather, those catabolites of riboflavin that primarily derive from oxidations within tissue are the 7- and 8-hydroxymethylriboflavins (7α- and 8α-hydroxyriboflavins) found especially in human urine (Ohkawa et al., 1983a; Chastain and McCormick, 1987b). The 7α-compound is also the main catabolite to appear in plasma of humans administered the vitamin orally (Zempleni et al., 1996b). The 7- and 8-carboxyllumichromes occur in considerable amounts in rat urine (Ohkawa et al., 1983b; Chastain and McCormick, 1987a). These methyl oxidized products reflect microsomal mixed-function oxidase activity (Ohkawa et al., 1983c). Other flavin catabolites include those from 8α-(amino acid)riboflavins released from covalently bonded FAD (Chia et al., 1978). An 8α-sulfonylriboflavin found in human urine may derive from the 8α-cysteinyl-FAD of monoamine oxidase (Chastain and McCormick, 1987b). A peptide ester of riboflavin has also been found in human urine (Chastain and McCormick, 1988). We can account for > 95% of flavins excreted in human urine. For normal adults eating varied diets, riboflavin comprises about two-thirds; 7-hydroxymethylriboflavin, 10–15%; a few to several percent of the 8-hydroxymethyl- and 8α-sulfonyl-riboflavins occur; there are lesser amounts of riboflavinyl peptide ester and such side-chain-altered flavins as the 10-hydroxyethyl and 10-formylmethyl compounds; and only traces of carboxymethylflavins and lumiflavin. It has been reported that such compounds as boric acid and chlorpromazine increase urinary excretion of riboflavin (Rivlin, 2006).

Secretion of flavins into milk has been reviewed (McCormick, 2006). As with urinary flavins, output reflects dietary status of the mother. In milk from cows (Roughead and McCormick, 1990a) and from humans (Roughead and McCormick, 1990b), the flavin in highest concentration other than the free vitamin is FAD, which can account for more than one-third of total flavin. Much of this is hydrolyzed during pasteurization. Fairly significant quantities of the 10-(2′-hydroxyethyl)flavin are notable, because this catabolite has antivitaminic activities as reflected in competitive inhibition of both cellular uptake (Aw et al., 1983) and subsequent flavokinase-catalyzed phosphorylation of

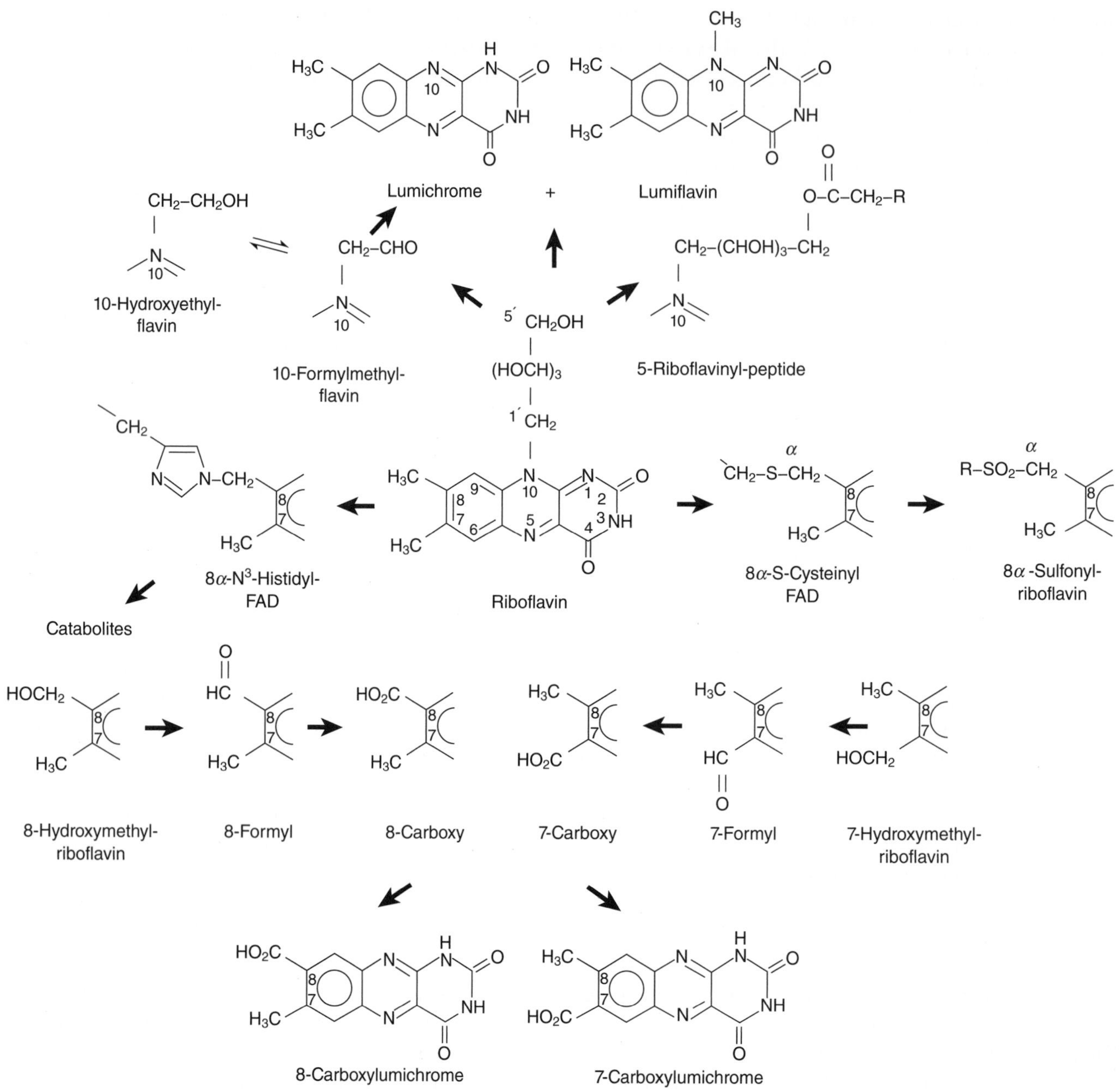

FIG. 18.3 Catabolism and photodegradation of riboflavin reflected by urinary products from mammals.

riboflavin (McCormick, 1962). Hence, this catabolite subtracts modestly from the biologic activity of the milk. Several percent of both 7- and 8-hydroxymethylriboflavins are also present, with more of the former. Smaller amounts of other catabolites, including the 10-formylmethylflavin and lumichrome, account for most of the rest (Roughead and McCormick 1990a,b).

There are other metabolic derivatives of flavin known to occur naturally. Among these are glycosides (Whitby, 1971) and a cyclic phosphodiester (Tachibana, 1967) of the ribityl side chain, and even schizoflavins (Tachibana and Murakami, 1980) that derive from oxidations at the 5'-hydroxymethyl terminus (Kekelidze et al., 1994; Chen and McCormick, 1997a,b). A riboflavinyl 5'-malonate has been obtained from *Avena* coleoptiles (Ghisla *et al.*, 1984). However, these compounds are generally associated with bacterial, fungal, or plant organisms and are not normally of consequence to the human. The riboflavinyl α-D-glucoside was reported in rat urine (Ohkawa *et al.*, 1983d) and its uptake and metabolism have been studied in rat liver cells (Joseph and McCormick, 1995).

Status and Deficiency

Human riboflavin requirements, biochemical indicators for these, and factors affecting the requirements have been covered in earlier reviews (Sauberlich, 1984; Bates, 1987) and were summarized in a report by the Institute of Medicine (1998). The current RDAs for adults are 1.1 mg for women and 1.3 mg for men. The median intake from foods in the US, especially including supplements, is considerably higher than requirements. As previously listed (Ensminger *et al.*, 1994; Rivlin, 2007), foods especially rich in bioavailable riboflavin are yeast, kidney, liver, cheese, eggs, and milk. Green vegetables are reasonably good sources. Natural grains and cereals are relatively poor sources, but fortification and enrichment have led to a considerable increase in intake of riboflavin from these food items. The mean intake of the vitamin by the US population is well above the estimated requirements. There are many who take over-the-counter supplements of micronutrients, which are commonly pills and drinks that contain riboflavin as well as other vitamins and trace essential elements; however, few gain from such misguided practice, especially as concerns riboflavin which has limited absorption (McCormick, 2010). Among factors affecting the requirement are bioavailability (~ 95% of food flavin), nutrient–nutrient interactions, and perhaps energy intake and physical activity. There is also some increase in urinary flavin loss with the use of such drugs as chlorpromazine and in the accidental drinking of boric acid solutions (Rivlin, 2006).

Biochemical indicators for estimating riboflavin requirements and determining status include assays of red cell and urinary flavin (both enhanced by HPLC and fluorometry) and the erythrocyte assays of glutathione reductase (± FAD) and pyridoxine (pyridoxamine) phosphate (± FMN). Although widely used, the erythrocyte glutathione reductase assay using freshly lysed red cells (Sauberlich *et al.*, 1972; McCormick and Green, 1999) has known limitations. The test cannot be used in persons with glucose-6-phosphate dehydrogenase deficiency, which

occurs in about 10% of African-Americans, because of an increased avidity in the glutathione reductase for FAD in this disease (Nicholads, 1981). A study of mutations in the glutathione reductase gene among Saudi Arabians showed that both genetic causes and deficiency can lead to a decrease in the reductase (Warsy and El-Hazmi, 1999). Moreover, in vitro treatment of blood with inosine and adenine elevates activity coefficients (Trout, 1989). In a study of piglets, the erythrocyte glutathione reductase activity coefficient was not significantly correlated with either total vitamin B_2 metabolites in the circulation or liver, which may suggest that it is not useful as a status determinant in this species (Giguère *et al.*, 2002). However, the erythrocyte reductase activity coefficient increased and liver flavins concomitantly decreased during induction of riboflavin deficiency in the rat (Yates *et al.*, 2001). More recently used is the FMN-dependent pyridoxine (pyridoxamine) phosphate oxidase assay which is unaffected by differences in glucose-6-phosphate status. The oxidase is an interface between riboflavin and vitamin B_6 (McCormick, 1989). The oxidase was shown to require FMN as coenzyme with the pure liver apoenzyme (Kazarinoff and McCormick, 1975). Its sensitivity to riboflavin status was then demonstrated with rats (Rasmussen *et al.*, 1979, 1980). Extension of this oxidase assay as an indicator for flavin status in the human was forthcoming (Mushtaq *et al.*, 2009). A low oxidase activity due to a red cell deficiency of FMN, confirmed by response to oral riboflavin, was reported in the majority of subjects with glucose-6-phosphate dehydrogenase deficiency (Powers and Bates, 1985; Anderson *et al.*, 1987). Such cases seem to have an accelerated conversion of FMN to FAD so that glutathione reductase is saturated. This contrasts with heterozygous β-thalassemia, where there is an inherited slow red-cell conversion of riboflavin to FMN, a decrease in subsequent FAD, and a high stimulation of the glutathione reductase by extraneous FAD (Anderson *et al.*, 1984, 1987).

Clinical signs of deficiency (ariboflavinosis) have been reviewed (Wilson, 1983; Institute of Medicine, 1998; Rivlin, 2006). In all animals there is retardation of growth. Additional effects include loss of hair, disturbances of the skin, etc. In humans, symptoms include sore throat; hyperemia and edema of the pharyngeal and oral mucous membranes; cheilosis; angular stomatitis; glossitis (magenta tongue); seborrheic dermatitis; and normochromic, normocytic anemia associated with pure red cell cytoplasia of the bone marrow. Because riboflavin deficiency is most often accompanied by deficiency of other B-complex vita-mins, some of the symptoms described may reflect such complications. In general where there are populations that receive too little food, such as in parts of Africa, one still finds deficiency of riboflavin and other vitamins. However, there have also been reports of poor riboflavin status in European groups that do not show overt clinical signs of riboflavin deficiency, but reflect a possible biochemically detected subclinical deficiency. One recent example is the high activity coefficient of erythrocyte glutathione reduct-ase measured in a group of young Irish women (Powers *et al.*, 2011).

There has been an expansion in our knowledge of those inborn errors of metabolism that are the result of genetic defects in formation of functional flavoproteins (Bartlett, 1983; Gregersen, 1985; Vianey-Liaud *et al.*, 1987). Some involve enzymes of mitochondrial general electron trans-fer, as in amyotrophic lateral sclerosis (Lin *et al.*, 2009) and a myopathic form of coenzyme Q10 deficiency (Gempel *et al.*, 2007), whereas others are associated with β-oxidation of fatty acyl-CoA (Chioang *et al.*, 2007; Henriques *et al.*, 2009). In most cases, therapeutic levels of riboflavin have a beneficial effect.

Other diseases also affect riboflavin status, as previously noted (McCormick, 1990). Some effects arise as a result of treatment, e.g. dialysis required with chronic renal failure or phototherapy in the potentially kernicteric infant. In these cases supplements are warranted. Supplementation also may be reasonable with the use of certain drugs, including antimalarials, some of which are flavin analogs (Cowden *et al.*, 1988). In this latter connec-tion, it is interesting that a relative riboflavin deficiency confers some protection against plasmodial infection in humans (Thumham *et al.*, 1983).

Future Directions

Some points that still require further investigation were raised in the last edition of *Present Knowledge in Nutrition* (Rivlin, 2006). However, it seems clear that studies at the molecular to cellular levels can reveal more. The relative sensitivity of the numerous flavin-dependent enzymes needs to be better defined and the criticality of their for-mation understood. Ultimately clinical symptoms are a reflection of these parameters. Ideally one should know which systems are most affected by limitation of flavoen-zyme availability, whether due to impaired intake of vitamin, formation of coenzymes, or improper holoen-zyme formation and function. Clearly both biochemical and genetic approaches will continue to be useful for a more complete nutritional understanding. Certain too is the need to expand our knowledge on how age, gender, and disease interplay with the need for riboflavin.

Suggestions for Further Reading

As has been pointed out in the Introduction, several earlier volumes contain more information concerning the history of discovery of riboflavin and its natural forms, and details of the isolation and chemistry of these, and there is an ever-expanding literature on the biological actions of the myriad related flavins. In par-ticular, there are three volume series that can be perused by any who are looking for a fuller account of how we accrued our present level of understanding in this area:

Present Knowledge in Nutrition, editions from the first to the current (10th) published by the International Life Sciences Institute.
Modern Nutrition in Health and Disease, editions from first to current (10th) published by Lippincott Williams & Wilkins.
Vitamins and Coenzymes, 12 volumes intermittent from Vol. 18 to Vol. 282 spanning 1970–1997 in the *Methods in Enzymology* series published by Academic Press.

References

Addison, R. and McCormick, D.B. (1978) Biogenesis of flavopro-tein and cytochrome components in hepatic mitochondria from riboflavin-deficient rats. *Biochem Biophys Commun* **81**, 133–138.

Akiyama, T., Selhub, J., Rosenberg, I.H., *et al.* (1982) FMN phos-phatase and FAD pyrophosphatase in rat intestinal brush borders: role in intestinal absorption of dietary riboflavin. *J Nutr* **112**, 263–268.

Anderson, B.B., Clements, J.E., Perry, G.M., *et al.* (1987) Glutathione reductase activity in GPDH deficiency. *Eur J Haematol* **38**, 12–20.

Anderson, B.B., Perry, G.M., and Clements, J.E. (1984) Red cell enzyme activities in thalassaemia. *Br J Haematol* **57**, 711–714.

Aw, T.Y., Jones, D.W., and McCormick, D.B. (1983) Uptake of riboflavin by isolated rat liver cells. *J Nutr* **113**, 1249–1254.

Bacher, A., Eberhardt, S., Eisenreich, W., *et al.* (2001) Biosynthesis of riboflavin. *Vitam Horm* **61**, 1–49.

Bacher, A., Eberhardt, S., Fischer, M., *et al.* (2000) Biosynthesis of vitamin B$_2$ (riboflavin). *Annu Rev Nutr* **20**, 153–167.

Barber, M.J., Eichler, D.C., Solomonson, L.P., *et al.* (1987) Anti-flavin antibodies. *Biochem J* **242**, 89–95.

Bartlett, K. (1983) Vitamin-responsive inborn errors of metabolism. *Adv Clin Chem* **23**, 141–198.

Bates, C.J. (1987) Human riboflavin requirements, and metabolic consequences of deficiency in man and animals. *World Rev Nutr Diet* **50**, 215–265.

Bowers-Komro, D.M. and McCormick, D.B. (1987) Riboflavin uptake by isolated rat kidney cells. In D.E. Edmondson and D.B. McCormick (eds) *Flavins and Flavoproteins.* de Gruyter, Berlin, pp. 449–453.

Bowers-Komro, D.M., Yamada, Y., and McCormick, D.B. (1989) Substrate specificity and variables affecting efficiency of mammalian flavin adenine dinucleotide synthetase. *Biochemistry* **28**, 8439–8446.

Bowman, B.B., McCormick, D.B., and Rosenberg, I.H. (1989) Epithelial transport of water-soluble vitamins. *Annu Rev Nutr* **9**, 187–199.

Brandsch, R. and Bichler, V. (1985) In vivo and in vitro expression of the 6-hydroxy-D-nicotine oxidase gene of *Arthrobacter oxidans*, cloned into *Escherichia coli*, as an enzymatically active, covalently flavinylated polypeptide. *FEBS Lett* **192**, 204–208.

Brandsch, R. and Bichler, V. (1986) Studies in vivo on the flavinylation of 6-hydroxy-D-nicotine oxidase. *Eur J Biochem* **160**, 285–289.

Brandsch, R. and Bichler, V. (1987) Covalent flavinylation of 6-hydroxy-D-nicotine oxidase involves an energy-requiring process. *FEBS Lett* **224**, 121–124.

Brizio, C., Otto, A., Brandsch, R., *et al.* (2000) A protein factor of rat liver mitochondrial matrix involved in flavinylation of dimethylglycine dehydrogenase. *Eur J Biochem* **267**, 4346–4354.

Chastain, J.L. and McCormick, D.B. (1987a) Clarification and quantitation of primary (tissue) and secondary (microbial) catabolites of riboflavin that are excreted in mammalian (rat) urine. *J Nutr* **117**, 468–475.

Chastain, J.L. and McCormick, D.B. (1987b) Flavin catabolites: identification and quantitation in human urine. *Am J Clin Nutr* **46**, 830–834.

Chastain, J.L. and McCormick, D.B. (1988) Characterization of a new flavin metabolite from human urine. *Biochim Biophys Acta* **967**, 131–134.

Chen, H. and McCormick, D.B. (1997a) Riboflavin 5′-hydroxymethyl oxidation: molecular cloning, expression, and glycoprotein nature of the 5′-aldehyde-forming enzyme from *Schizophyllum commune*. *J Biol Chem* **272**, 20077–20081.

Chen, H. and McCormick, D.B. (1997b) Fungal riboflavin 5′-hydroxymethyl dehydrogenase catalyzes formation of both the aldehyde (riboflavinal) and the acid (riboflavoic acid). *Biochim Biophys Acta* **1342**, 116–118.

Chen, S-C., Chang, Y-C., Lin, C-H., *et al.* (2006) Crystal structure of a bifunctional deaminase and reductase from *Bacillus subtilis* involved in riboflavin biosynthesis. *J Biol Chem* **281**, 7605–7613.

Chia, C.P., Addison, R., and McCormick, D.B. (1978) Absorption, metabolism, and excretion of 8α-(amino acid)riboflavins in the rat. *J Nutr* **108**, 373–381.

Chiong, M.A., Sim, K.G., Carpenter, K., *et al.* (2007) Transient multiple acyl-CoA dehydrogenation deficiency in a newborn female caused by maternal riboflavin deficiency. *Mol Genet Metab* **92**, 109–114.

Combs, G.F., Jr (1998) Riboflavin. In *The Vitamins. Fundamental Aspects in Nutrition and Health* 2nd Edn. Academic Press, San Diego, pp. 295–510..

Cowden, W.B., Clark, I.A., and Hunt, N.H. (1988) Flavins as potential antimalarials. 1. 10-(Halophenyl)-3-methylflavins. *J Med Chem* **31**, 799–801.

Dainty, J.R., Bullock, N.R., Hart, D.J., *et al.* (2007) Quantification of the bioavailability of riboflavin from foods by use of stable-isotope labels and kinetic modeling. *Am J Clin* **85**, 1557–1564.

Daniel, H., Wille, U., and Rehner, G. (1983) In vitro kinetics of the intestinal transport of riboflavin in rats. *J Nutr* **113**, 636–643.

Ensminger, A.M., Ensminger, M.E., Konlande, J.E., *et al.* (1994) *Food and Nutrition Encyclopedia*, CRC Press, Boca Raton, FL, p. 1927

Frago, S., Gomez-Moreno, C., and Medina, M. (2008a) (eds) *Flavins and Flavoproteins*, 16th Edn. International Symposium of Flavins and Flavoproteins. Prensas Universitarias de Zaragoza, Spain.

Frago, S., Martinez-Julvez, M., Serrano, A., *et al.* (2008b) Structural analysis of FAD synthetase from *Corynebacterium ammoniagenes*. *MBC Microbiol* **8**, 160.

Fujimura, M., Yamamoto, S., Murata, T., *et al.* (2010) Functional characteristics of the human ortholog of riboflavin transporter 2 and riboflavin-responsive expression of its rat ortholog in the small intestine indicate its involvement in riboflavin absorption. *J Nutr* **140**, 1722–1727.

Gadda, G. (2010) (ed.) Oxidative enzymes. *Arch Biochem Biophys* **493**, 1–124.

Gempel, K., Topaloglu, H., Talim, B., *et al.* (2007) The myopathic form of coenzyme Q10 deficiency is caused by mutations in the electron-transferring-flavoprotein dehydrogenase (ETFDH) gene. *Brain* **130**, 2037–2044.

Ghisla, S., Mack, R., Blankenhorn, G., et al. (1984) Structure of a novel flavin chromophore from avena coleoptiles, the possible "blue light" photoreceptor. Eur J. Biochem 138, 339–344.

Giguère, A., Girard, C.L., and Matte, J.G. (2002) Erythrocyte glutathione reductase activity and riboflavin status in early-weaned piglets. Int J Vitam Nutr Res 72, 383–387.

Gregersen, N. (1985) Riboflavin-responsive defects of beta-oxidation. J. Inherit Metab Dis 1(Suppl 8), 65–69.

Hamm, H.H. and Decker, K. (1978) FAD is covalently attached to peptidyl-tRNA during cell-free synthesis of 6-hydroxy-D-nicotine oxidase. Eur J Biochem 92, 449–454.

Hamm, H.H. and Decker, K. (1980) Cell-free synthesis of a flavoprotein containing the 8α-(N^3-histidyl)-riboflavin linkage. Eur J Biochem 104, 391–395.

Hegazy, E. and Schwenk, M. (1983) Riboflavin uptake by isolated enterocytes of guinea pigs. J Nutr 113, 1702–1707.

Henriques, B.J., Rodrigues, J.V., Olsen, R.K., et al. (2009) Role of flavinylation in a mild variant of multiple acyl-CoA dehydrogenation deficiency: a molecular rationale for the effects of riboflavin supplementation. J Biol Chem 284, 4222–4229.

Illarionov, B., Eisenreich, W., Schramek, N., et al. (2005) Biosynthesis of vitamin B$_2$. Diasteromeric reaction intermediates of archaeal and non-archaeal riboflavin synthases. J Biol Chem 280, 28541–28546.

Innis, W.S.A., McCormick, D.B., and Merrill, A.H., Jr (1985) Variations in riboflavin binding by human plasma: identification of immunoglobulins as the major proteins responsible. Biochem Med 34, 151–165.

Innis, W.S.A., Nixson, D.W., Murray, D.R., et al. (1986) Immunoglobulins associated with elevated riboflavin binding by plasma from cancer patients. Proc Soc Exp Biol Med 181, 237–231.

Institute of Medicine (1998) Dietary Reference Intakes.. Thiamin, Riboflavin, Niacin, Vitamin B$_6$, Folate, Vitamin B$_{12}$, Pantothenic Acid, .Biotin, and Choline. National Academy Press, Washington, DC.

Joseph, T. and McCormick, D.B. (1995) Uptake and metabolism of riboflavin-5′-α-D-glucoside by rat and isolated liver cells. J Nutr 125, 2194–2198.

Kazarinoff, M.N. and McCormick, D.B. (1975) Rabbit liver pyridoxamine (pyridoxine) 5′-phosphate oxidase: purification and properties. J Biol Chem 250, 3436–3442.

Kekelidze, T.N., Edmondson, D.E., and McCormick, D.B. (1994) Flavin substrate specificity of the vitamin B$_2$-aldehyde-forming enzyme from Schizophyllum commune. Arch Biochem Biophys 315, 100–103.

Kozik, A. (1985) Riboflavin binding proteins. Postepy Biochem 31, 263–281.

Lee, S.S. and McCormick, D.B. (1983) Effect of riboflavin status on hepatic activities of flavin-metabolizing enzymes in rats. J Nutr 113, 2274–2279.

Lee, S.S. and McCormick, D.B. (1985) Thyroid hormone regulation of flavocoenzyme biosynthesis. Arch Biochem Biophys 237, 197–201.

Lin, J., Diamanduos, A., Chowdhury, S.A., et al. (2009) Specific electron transport chain abnormalities in amyotropic lateral sclerosis. J Neurol 256, 774–782.

Manstein, D.J. and Pai, E.F. (1986) Purification and characterization of FAD synthetase from Brevebacterium ammoniagenes. J Biol Chem 261, 16169–16173.

McCormick, D.B. (1962) The intracellular localization, partial purification, and properties of flavokinase from rat liver. J Biol Chem 237, 959–962.

McCormick, D.B. (1975) Metabolism of riboflavin. In R.S. Rivlin (ed.), Riboflavin. Plenum Press, New York, pp. 153–198.

McCormick, D.B. (1988) Riboflavin. In M.E. Shils and V.R. Young (eds), Modern Nutrition in Health and Disease, 7th Edn. Lea and Febiger, Philadelphia, pp. 362–382.

McCormick, D.B. (1989) Two interconnected B vitamins: riboflavin and pyridoxine. Physiol Rev 69, 1170–1198.

McCormick, D.B. (1990) Riboflavin. In M.L. Brown (ed.), Present Knowledge in Nutrition, 6th Edn, ILSI Press, Washington, DC, pp. 146–154.

McCormick, D.B. (2006) Riboflavin. In M.E. Shils, M. Shike, A.C. Ross, et al. (eds), Modern Nutrition in Health and Disease, 10th Edn. Lippincott Williams and Wilkins, Philadelphia, pp. 434–441.

McCormick, D.B. (2010) Vitamin/mineral supplements: of questionable benefit for the general population. Nutr Rev 68, 207–213.

McCormick, D.B. and Green, H.L. (1999) Vitamins. In C.A. Burtis and E.R. Ashwood (eds), Tietz Textbook on Clinical Chemistry. WB Saunders, Philadelphia, pp. 999–1028.

McCormick, D.B. and Russell, M. (1962) Hydrolysis of flavin mononucleotide by acid phosphatases from animal tissues. Comp Biochem Physiol 5, 113–121.

McCormick, D.B. et al. (1970–1997) (eds) Vitamins and Coenzymes, Methods in Enzymology series, intermittent volumes from 18 to 282. Academic Press, New York, and Orlando, FL.

McCormick, D.B., Innis, W.S.A., Merrill, A.H., Jr, et al. (1984) Mammalian metabolism of flavins. In R.C. Bray, P.C. Engel, and S.G. Mayhew (eds), Flavins and Flavoproteins. de Gruyter, Berlin, pp. 833–846:

McCormick, D.B., Innis, W.S.A., Merrill, A.H., Jr, et al. (1987) An update on flavin metabolism in rats and humans. In E. Edmondson and D.B. McCormick (eds), Flavins and Flavoproteins. de Gruyter, Berlin, pp. 459–471.

Merrill, A.H., Jr, and McCormick, D.B. (1979) Preparation and properties of immobilized flavokinase. *Biotechnol Bioeng* **21**, 1629–1638.

Merrill, A.H., Jr, and McCormick, D.B. (1980) Affinity chromatographic purification and properties of flavokinase (ATP: riboflavin 5′-phosphotransferase) from rat liver. *J Biol Chem* **255**, 1335–1338.

Merrill, A.H., Jr, Froelich, J.A., and McCormick, D.B.(1981b) Isolation and identification of alternative riboflavin-binding proteins from human plasma. *Biochem Med* **25**, 198–206.

Merrill, A.H., Jr, Innis-Whitehouse, W.S.A., and McCormick, D.B. (1987) Characterization of human riboflavin-binding immunoglobulins. In D.E. Edmondson and D.B. McCormick (eds), *Flavins and Flavoproteins*. de Gruyter, Berlin, pp. 445–448.

Merrill, A.H., Jr, Lambeth, J.D., Edmondson, D.E., *et al.* (1981a) Formation and mode of action of flavoproteins. *Annu Rev Nutr* **1**, 281–317.

Mushtaq, S., Su, H., Marilyn, M.H.E., *et al.* (2009) Erythrocyte pyridoxamine phosphate oxidase activity: a potential biomarker of riboflavin status. *Am J Clin Nutr* **90**, 1151–1159.

Nichoalds, G.E. (1981) Riboflavin. Symposium in Laboratory Medicine. In R.F. Labbae (ed.), *Symposium on Laboratory Assessment of Nutritional Status*, Clinics in Laboratory Medicine Series, Vol. 1, WB Saunders, Philadelphia, pp. 685–698.

Nokubo, M., Ohta, M., and Kitani, K. (1989) Identification of protein bound riboflavin in rat hepatocyte plasma membrane as a source of autofluorescence. *Biochim Biophys Acta* **981**, 303–308.

Ohkawa, H., Ohishi, N., and Yagi, K. (1983a) New metabolites of riboflavin appear in human urine. *J Biol Chem* **258**, 5623–5628.

Ohkawa, H., Ohishi, N., and Yagi, K. (1983b) New metabolites of riboflavin appeared in rat urine. *Biochem Int* **6**, 239–247.

Ohkawa, H., Ohishi, N., and Yagi, K. (1983c) Hydroxylation of the 7- and 8-methyl groups of riboflavin by the microsomal electron transfer system of rat liver. *J Biol Chem* **258**, 5629–5633.

Ohkawa, H., Ohishi, N., and Yagi, K. (1983d) Occurrence of riboflavinyl glucoside in rat urine. *J Nutr Sci Vitaminol (Tokyo)* **29**, 515–522.

Oka, M. and McCormick, D.B. (1985) Urinary lumichrome-level catabolites of riboflavin are due to microbial and photochemical events and not tissue enzymic cleavage of the ribityl chain. *J Nutr* **115**, 496–499.

Oka, M. and McCormick, D.B. (1987) Complete purification and general characterization of FAD synthetase from rat liver. *J Biol Chem* **262**, 7418–7422.

Owen, E.C. and West, D.W. (1971a) Isolation and identification of 7,8-dimethyl-10–formylmethylisoalloxazine as a product of the bacterial degradation of riboflavin. In D.B. McCormick and L.D. Wright (eds), *Vitamins and Coenzymes, Methods in Enzymology*, Vol. 18B. Academic Press, New York, pp. 579–581.

Owen, E.C. and West, D.W. (1971b) Isolation and identification of 7,8-dimethyl-10-(2-′-hydroxyethyl)isoalloxazine from natural sources. In D.B. McCormick and L.D. Wright (eds), *Vitamins and Coenzymes*, Methods in Enzymology series, Vol. 18B. Academic Press, New York, pp. 574–579.

Powers, H.J. and Bates, C.J. (1985) A simple fluorimetric assay for pyridoxamine phosphate oxidase in erythrocyte haemolysates: effects of riboflavin supplementation and of glucose 6-phosphate dehydrogenase deficiency. *Hum Nutr Clin Nutr* **39**, 107–115.

Powers, H.J., Hill, M.H., Mushtaq, S., *et al.* (2011) Correcting a marginal riboflavin deficiency improves hematologic status in young women in the United Kingdom (RIBOFEM). *Am J Clin Nutr* **93**, 1274–1284.

Rasmussen, K.M., Barsa, P.M., and McCormick, D.B. (1979) Pyridoxamine (pyridoxine)-5′- phosphate oxidase activity in rat tissues during development of riboflavin or pyridoxine deficiency. *Proc Soc Exp Biol Med* **161**, 527–530.

Rasmussen, K.M, Barsa, P.M., McCormick, D.B., *et al.* (1980) Effect of strain, sex, and dietary riboflavin on pyridoxamine (pyridoxine)-5′-phosphate oxidase activity in rat tissues. *J Nutr* **110**, 1940–1946.

Rivlin, R.S. (2001) Riboflavin. In B.A. Bowman and R.M. Russell (eds), *Present Knowledge in Nutrition*, 8th Edn. ILSI Press, Washington, DC, pp. 191–198.

Rivlin, R.S. (2006) Riboflavin. In R. Russell and B.B. Bowman (eds), *Present Knowledge in Nutrition*, 9th Edn. ILSI Press, Washington, DC, pp. 250–259.

Rivlin, R.S. (2007) Riboflavin. In J. Zempleni, R.B. Rucker, D.B. McCormick, *et al.* (eds), *Handbook of Vitamins*, 4th Edn. CRC Press, Boca Raton, FL, pp. 233–251.

Roughead, Z.K. and McCormick, D.B. (1990a) A qualitative and quantitative assessment of flavins in cow's milk. *J Nutr* **120**, 382–388.

Roughead, Z.K. and McCormick, D.B. (1990b) Flavin composition of human milk. *Am. J. Clin. Nutr* **52**, 854–857.

Sandoval, F.J. and Roje, S. (2005) An FMN hydrolase is fused to ribokinase homolog in plants. *J Biol Chem* **280**, 38337–38345.

Sandoval, F.J., Zhang, Y., and Roje, S. (2008) Flavin nucleotide metabolism in plants: monofunctional enzymes synthesize FAD in plastids. *J Biol Chem* **283**, 30890–30900.

Sato, M., Ohishi, O., and Yagi, K. (1984) Localization and identification of covalently bound flavoproteins in rat liver mitochondria by prelabeling of their flavin moiety. *J Biochem* **96**, 553–562.

Sauberlich, H.E. (1984) Implications of nutritional status on human biochemistry, physiology, and health. *Clin Chem* **17**, 132–142.

Sauberlich, H.E., Judd, J.H., Jr, Nichoalds, G.E., *et al.* (1972) Application of the erythrocyte glutathione reductase assay in evaluating riboflavin nutritional status in a high school student population. *Am J Clin Nutr* **25**, 756–762.

Sobhanaditya, J. and Appaji Rao, N. (1981) Plant flavokinase. Affinity-chromatographic procedure for the purification of the enzyme from mung-bean (*Phaseolus aureus*) seeds and conformational changes in its interaction with orthophosphate. *Biochem J* **197**, 227–232.

Tachibana, S. (1967) The formation of new flavin phosphates by molds. *J Vitaminol (Kyoto)* **13**, 70–79.

Tachibana, S. and Murakami, T. (1980) Isolation and identification of schizoflavins. In D.B. McCormick and L.D. Wright (eds), *Vitamins and Coenzymes*, Methods in Enzymology Series, Vol. 66. Academic Press, New York,. pp. 333–338.

Thumham, D.I., Oppenheimer, S.J., and Bull, R. (1983) Riboflavin status and malaria in infants in Papua, New Guinea. *Trans R Soc Trop Med Hyg* **77**, 423–424.

Trout, G.E. (1989) Elevated glutathione reductase activity coefficients in erythrocytes after treatment in vitro with inosine and adenine. *Proc Soc Exp Biol Med* **191**, 12–17.

Tsai, L. and Stadtman, E.R. (1971) Riboflavin degradation. In D.B. McCormick and L.D. Wright (eds), *Vitamins and Coenzymes, Vol. 18B*, Methods in Enzymology series. Academic Press, New York, pp. 557–571.

Vianey-Liaud, C., Divry, P., Gregersen, N., *et al.* (1987) The inborn errors of mitochondrial fatty acid oxidation. *J. Inher Metab Dis* **1**(Suppl. 10), 159–200.

Warsy, A.S. and El-Hazmi, M.A. (1999) Glutathione reductase deficiency in Saudi Arabia. *East Mediterr Health J* **5**, 1208–1212.

West, D.W. and Owen, E.C. (1973) Degradation of riboflavin by alimentary bacteria of the .ruminant and man: production of 7,8-dimethyl-10-carboxymethylisoalloxazine. *Br J Nutr* **29**, 33–41.

Whitby, L.G. (1971) Glycosides of riboflavin. In D.B. McCormick and L.D. Wright (eds), *Vitamins and Coenzymes*, Methods in Enzymology Series, Vol. 18B. Academic Press, New York, pp. 404–413.

White, H.B., III, and Merrill, A.H. Jr (1988) Riboflavin-binding proteins. *Annu Rev Nutr* **8**, 279–299.

Wilson, J.A. (1983) Disorders of vitamins. In R.G. Petersdorf and T.R. Harrison (eds), *Harrison's Principles of Internal Medicine*, 10th Edn. McGraw-Hill, New York, pp. 461–470.

Winkler, A., Hartner, F., Kutchan, T.M., *et al.* (2006) Biochemical evidence that berberine bridge enzyme belongs to a novel family of flavoproteins containing a bi-covalently attached FAD cofactor. *J Biol Chem* **281**, 21276–21285.

Winkler, A., Kutchan, T.M., and Macheroux, P. (2007) 6-S-Cysteinylation of bi-valently attached FAD in berberine bridge enzyme tunes the redox potential for optimal activity. *J Biol Chem* **282**, 24437–24443.

Winkler, A., Motz, K., Riedl, S., *et al.* (2009) Hold on to that flavin. *J Biol Chem* **284**, 19993–20001.

Yagi, K., Nakagawa, Y., Suzuki, O., *et al.* (1976) Incorporation of riboflavin into covalently-bound flavins in rat liver. *J. Biochem* **79**, 841–843.

Yamada, Y., Merrill, A.H., Jr, and McCormick, D.B. (1990) Probable reaction mechanisms of flavokinase and FAD synthetase from rat liver. *Arch Biochem Biophys* **278**, 125–130.

Yamamoto, S., Katsuhisa, I., Ohta, K-Y., *et al.* (2009) Identification and functional characterization of rat riboflavin transporter 2. *J Biochem* **145**, 437–443.

Yanagita, T. and Forster, J.W. (1956) A bacterial riboflavin hydrolase. *J Biol Chem* **221**, 593–607.

Yang, C.S. and McCormick, D.B. (1967) Substrate specificity of a riboflavin hydrolase from *Pseudomonas riboflavina*. *Biochim Biophys Acta* **132**, 511–513.

Yang, C.S. and McCormick, D.B. (1978) Degradation and excretion of riboflavin in the rat. *J Nutr* **93**, 445–453.

Yao, Y., Yonezawa, A., Yoshimatsu, H., *et al.* (2010) Identification and comparative functional characterization of a new human riboflavin transporter hRFT3 expressed in the brain. *J Nutr* **140**, 1220–1226.

Yates, C.A., Evans, G.S., and Powers, H.J. (2001) Riboflavin deficiency: early effects on post-weaning development of the duodenum in rats. *Br J Nutr* **86**, 593–599.

Yazdanpanah, B., Wiegmann, K., Tchikov, V., *et al.* (2009) Riboflavin kinase couples TNF receptor 1 to NADPH oxidase. *Nature* **460**, 1159–1163.

Zempleni, J., Galloway, J.R., and McCormick, D.B. (1996a) Pharmacokinetics of orally and intravenously administered riboflavin in healthy humans. *Am J Clin Nutr* **63**, 54–66.

Zempleni, J., Galloway, J.R., and McCormick, D.B. (1996b) The identification and kinetics of 7α-hydroxyriboflavin (7-hydroxymethylriboflavin) in blood plasma from humans following oral administration of riboflavin supplements. *Int J Vit Nutr Res* **66**, 151–157.

Zhu, X., Wentworth, P., Jr, Kyle, R.A., *et al.* (2006) Cofactor-containing antibodies: crystal structure of the original yellow antibody. *Proc Natl Acad Sci* **103**, 3581–3585.

19

NIACIN

W. TODD PENBERTHY[1], PhD AND JAMES B. KIRKLAND[2], PhD

[1]*University of Central Florida College of Medicine, Orlando, Florida, USA*
[2]*University of Guelph, Guelph, Ontario, Canada*

Summary

The niacin deficiency disease pellagra was the most devastating nutritional disease in modern American history. Even today, after enrichment of refined foods, niacin deficiencies may occur through poor food habits. Niacin is transformed to the essential pyridine nucleotides nicotinamide adenine dinucleotide (NAD[P]). Used by at least 470 proteins, these are involved in more reactions than any other vitamin-derived molecule. Nicotinic acid may also activate the GPR109 receptors, which mediate many of the dyslipidemia-correcting activities. An active area of therapeutic research involves increased nicotinamide adenine dinucleotide (NAD) working through sirtuin activation to provide benefit in many disease settings. The development of poly(ADP)-ribose polymerase inhibitors to simultaneously preserve NAD levels while decreasing genomic stability is also an area of great interest, particularly in cancer research. Nicotinic acid, nicotinamide, nicotinamide riboside, tryptophan, and the more recently considered nicotinamide mononucleotide all possess distinguishable characteristics as NAD precursors that continue to be examined. Other nutrients affecting NAD metabolism have potential as combinatorial modifiers of niacin status. These include glutamine, thiamin, and others required for completion of the de novo pathway from tryptophan: ascorbate, riboflavin, and pyridoxal phosphate. Further study of NAD metabolism will excite scientists and clinicians, and will lead to improved health.

Introduction

Niacin deficiency was first described by Casal in 1762 in Europe as a condition characterized by extreme weakness and crusty skin (Carpenter, 1981). Accordingly, Casal coined the disease "pellagra," meaning angry skin. Just over 100 years later, pellagra would reach epidemic proportions in the southern United States due to the invention and distribution of industrial-scale milling devices in the 1870s. Suddenly the first refined foods, white flour and rice, became available to the American masses. Thereafter pellagra and beriberi became pervasive depending on the variety of individual diets. Pellagra exerted many effects on psychiatric health and was the leading cause of death in mental hospitals in 1907. By the 1920s, pellagra had become the most severe deficiency disease in the history of the United States. Over 120 000 people died from pellagra epidemics in the US during the first two decades of the twentieth century (Etheridge, 1972; Carpenter, 1981).

Present Knowledge in Nutrition, Tenth Edition. Edited by John W. Erdman Jr, Ian A. Macdonald and Steven H. Zeisel.
© 2012 International Life Sciences Institute. Published 2012 by John Wiley & Sons, Inc.

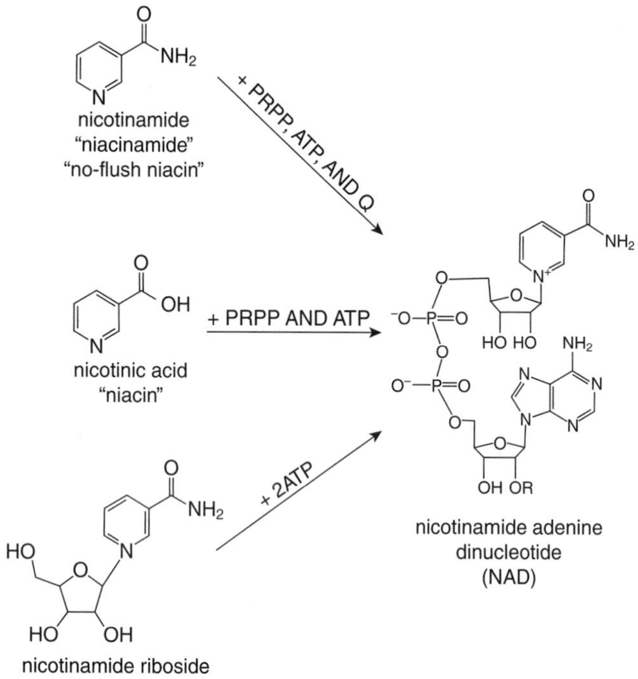

FIG. 19.1 Forms of vitamin B$_3$. Various dietary precursors can support the formation of the essential molecule, nicotinamide adenine dinucleotide (NAD). The cofactors required to convert each vitamin B$_3$ precursor to NAD are shown. PRPP, 5-phosphoryl-ribose-1-pyrophosphate; Q, glutamine.

Pellagra was finally understood in the 1930s thanks in large part to the work of the epidemiologist Dr Joseph Goldberger. Initially Dr Goldberger's hypothesis that pellagra was a dietary deficiency disease was rejected in favor of corn toxins or poor sanitation. Elvjeham identified the pellagra-preventing factor in 1937 as the molecule nicotinic acid. First a dietary-deficiency dog model that caused tongue discoloration was created. Then, a rice-polishing component that prevented tongue discoloration was isolated and named the pellagra-preventing factor. The government established legally mandated standards of niacin enrichment of flour in 1942. Niacin refers to the chemical nicotinic acid, while niacinamide refers to the chemical nicotinamide. However, niacin is commonly used to refer to either form. This is unfortunate because there are significant physiological differences between niacin and niacinamide.

Doctors who witnessed pellagrous dementia noticed many similarities to schizophrenia and theorized that schizophrenics might have a genetic disorder that required far greater levels of niacin. Experiments performed in the 1950s revealed that administration of gram quantities of niacin to schizophrenic patients frequently exerted therapeutic benefits with no adverse reaction (Hoffer *et al.*, 1957). However, this approach remains controversial today. This may be due, in part, to the fact that schizophrenia could enter a stage of irreversible change that is no longer responsive to chemical approaches. These same researchers discovered that high-dose nicotinic acid, but not nicotinamide, effectively lowered blood cholesterol (Altschul *et al.*, 1955). Today, high-dose niacin is a more effective elevator of the high-density lipoprotein ("good" cholesterol) than any pharmaceutical. This approach also lowers triglycerides, and very-low-density lipoprotein ("bad" cholesterol). Amazingly, high-dose niacin will also raise cholesterol for individuals with abnormally low cholesterol. Administration of high doses of the various alternative nicotinamide adenine dinucleotide (NAD) precursors nicotinic acid/niacin, nicotinamide/niacinamide, and/or nicotinamide riboside remains an ongoing area of clinical research.

Niacin Structure and Nomenclature

Niacin, which commonly refers to nicotinic acid or nicotinamide, is vitamin B$_3$. Nicotinic acid has many effects that differ from nicotinamide due to the presence of a ketone body receptor, which also recognizes nicotinic acid and mediates the flush response. Niacin is also known as nicotinic acid or pyridine-3-carboxylic acid, while niacinamide is also known as nicotinamide or pyridine-3-carboxamide. Together nicotinic acid and nicotinamide are vitamin B$_3$. Vitamin B$_3$ is defined as the dietary precursors to nicotinamide adenine dinucleotide, other than the amino acid tryptophan. Most recently, a third form of vitamin B$_3$, nicotinamide riboside, was discovered (Bieganowski and Brenner, 2004). Structures for the three molecules are shown in Figure 19.1.

Assessment and Maintenance of Niacin Nutriture

Biochemical Determination of Niacin Status

Biochemical assessment of niacin status is ideally determined by measuring tissue NAD levels (Jacobson et al., 1999; Shah et al., 2005). Alternatively, measures of the urinary metabolites N′-methylnicotinamide and 2-pyridone are frequently used as indirect indicators of niacin status (McCormick and Greene, 1999). Measures of 41 nM/mL human blood are increased by approximately fourfold after supplementation, while consumption of a low-niacin diet causes a decrease of about 50% in whole blood NAD (Jacobson et al., 1999). Another frequently used measure is the niacin number, which is a ratio of NAD to NADP in whole blood (Fu et al., 1989; Jacobson and Jacobson, 1997). As NADP levels are relatively stable during niacin deficiency whereas NAD declines (Tang et al., 2008), this ratio is a convenient measure of niacin status. Analysis of over 1000 women in 1980s Sweden using this technique surprisingly revealed that 15–20% of modern-day populations in developed countries may have significant niacin deficiency (Jacobson, 1993).

"Niacin" is a term that refers to direct vitamin precursors for NAD formation whereas "niacin equivalents" takes into consideration the non-vitamin NAD precursor, tryptophan. The conversion factor for the endogenous transformation of tryptophan to NAD is approximately 60 mg of tryptophan per 1 mg of NAD. Thus ingestion of 60 mg of trytophan counts as 1 niacin equivalent (NE). The tryptophan content of protein is approximately 1%. Thus, a diet of approximately 100 g of protein would presumably result in approximately 16 mg of niacin, thus meeting the recommended daily allowance for NAD without inclusion of the vitamin forms of niacin.

Daily Recommended Intake and Food Sources

Recommended dietary allowances (RDA) originated during World War II as minimal standards for food relief, and have continued to evolve. The RDA represents the amount of vitamin necessary to meet the needs of 97.5% of the population. Restricting niacin intake to 50% of RDA decreases NAD by 70% within 5 weeks, while nicotinamide adenine dinucleotide phosphate (NADP) levels remain constant (Fu et al., 1989). These decreased NAD levels precede pellagra symptoms and are frequently seen in carcinoid syndrome patients (Shah et al., 2005). Most significantly, more niacin is needed during pregnancy and lactation (Table 19.1) (Otten et al., 2006). Since tryptophan can also be converted to nicotinic acid mononucleotide (Figure 19.2), but with 1/60th the efficiency of nicotinic acid, 60 mg of tryptophan is considered 1 niacin equivalent.

Table 19.1 Recommended dietary allowance (RDA) values for niacin across the lifespan

Population group	NE/day[a]
Infants	
0–0.5 years	2
0.5–1.0 years	4
Children	
1–3 years	6
4–8 years	8
9–13 years	12
Males	
≥14	16
Females	
≥14	14
Pregnant	18
Lactating	17

[a]NE (niacin equivalents) = mg niacin + 1/60 mg tryptophan.
Reproduced with permission from Otten et al. (2006).

TABLE 19.2 Food sources of preformed niacin

Food source	Amount of niacin
Dairy	0.2 mg per 1 cup whole milk
	0.05 mg per 1 egg
Meats (per 3oz, 85 g)	14 mg beef liver
	10–11 mg tuna, halibut, swordfish
	7 mg rainbow trout
	2–6 mg beef, lamb, pork, poultry, other fish
Cereals and grain products	2–10 mg per 1 cup ready-to-eat cereal
	3 mg per cup barley or rice, cooked
	3–4 mg per 4-in (3-oz/85-g) bagel
	2 mg per 2-oz/56-g hard roll
	2 mg per cup noodles or pasta
Vegetables (per cup)	4 mg canned tomato product
	3 mg mushrooms
	2 mg corn
	2 mg potatoes
	0.5 mg of mustard greens
Other	4 mg per oz (28 g) peanuts

Data from USDA/ARS (2005) USDA National Nutrient Standard Database, Release 18. USDA/ARS, Washington, DC. Retrieved December 23, 2005, from www.ars.usda.gov/ba/bhnrc/ndl.

The simple but essential niacin pyridine molecules are first made in plants and thereafter distributed in the food chain (Table 19.2) (USDA/ARS, 2005). For example, niacin can be synthesized in grasses, which are ingested by cows. Then bacteria can synthesize more niacin. Ultimately

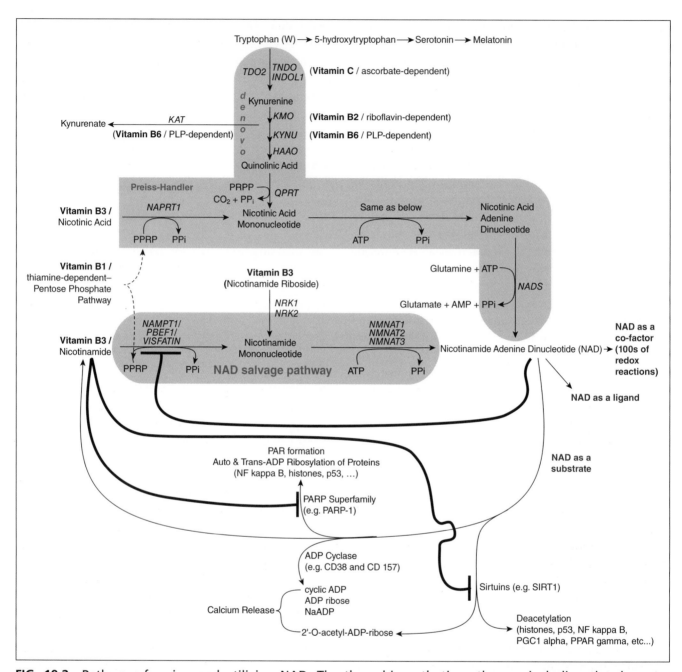

FIG. 19.2 Pathways forming and utilizing NAD. The three biosynthetic pathways, including the de novo, Preiss-Handler, and salvage pathways, are followed with grey shading. Vitamin B_2 (riboflavin), vitamin B_6 (pyridoxyl phosphate), and vitamin C (ascorbate) are all required for completion of the NAD de novo pathway starting from tryptophan. Otherwise, vitamin B_1 (thiamin) is required for synthesis of phosphoribosyl pyrophosphate (PRPP) in the pentose phosphate pathway. The uses of NAD as a co-factor, ligand, or substrate are shown to the right. Gene names are in italics.

the vitamin can be transmitted through milk or meat consumption to people.

Physiological Functions of NAD

Molecular biologists use gene deletion to determine gene function. We can consider similar loss of function analysis for determining nutrient function. More significantly, however, we are able to readily perform pharmacological complementary rescue of loss of function symptoms by administering the vitamin molecule. Experiments involving vitamin deficiencies can only be performed on humans for brief periods (Fu *et al.*, 1989); however, we can still learn from the history of pellagra and through experimentally controllable animal models of niacin deficiency.

Dietary Deficiency Disease

The three classic "Ds" of pellagra include diarrhea, dermatitis, and dementia, which occur in unpredictable orders and combinations, depending perhaps on genetics, lifestyle or infectious conditions. These are followed ultimately by death of the patient if the diet is not improved. Pellagrous dermatitis has a characteristic appearance on parts of the body that is triggered by exposure to sunlight, heat, or mild trauma, such as the face, neck, hands, feet, and elbows. These lesions are typically bilaterally symmetric about the head. Accordingly they were first termed "Casal's necklace." Mental symptoms include irritability, headaches, sleeplessness, loss of memory, and emotional instability. Women were more suicidal, while men were more violent during the pellagra epidemics. Pellagra-like symptoms are also caused by chronic alcoholism, carcinoid syndrome (Shah *et al.*, 2005), and some drugs such as the anti-tuberculosis medicine isoniazid or chemotherapeutics (Dreizen *et al.*, 1990).

Niacin-Responsive Genetic Disorders

Ultimately niacin is converted to NAD, which is used in more reactions than any other vitamin-derived cofactor. Over 400 proteins use NAD for chemical reactions. Ultimately amino acid polymorphisms residing within cofactor binding domains result in decreased binding affinity with associated decreased enzyme kinetics (increased K_m). There are known examples where administration of vitamin co-factor supplements can rescue the symptoms arising from decreased enzyme efficiency due to these mutations (Ames *et al.*, 2002). Known niacin-responsive genetic diseases include mutations in either the

neutral amino acid transporter encoded by the SLC6A19 gene, the aldehyde dehydrogenase encoded by ALDH2, or the glucose-6-phosphate-1-dehydrogenase gene. Mutations causing a loss of SLC6A19 function result in Hartnup disease, which resembles pellagra and leads to death unless treated early. This occurs due to an inability to transport tryptophan into cells. Symptoms are rescued via the administration of niacin, thus supporting the vital importance of tryptophan as a NAD precursor (Nozaki *et al.*, 2001). Up to one-third of all known enzyme-encoding gene mutations may result in decreased enzyme efficiency due to altered binding affinity for the cofactor (Ames *et al.*, 2002). Given that there are more NAD-binding proteins than any other cofactor and most have never been examined, it is expected that many more undiscovered mutations are in fact responsive to administration of high doses of NAD precursors.

NAD Metabolism

Humans cannot specifically synthesize nicotinic acid or nicotinamide endogenously. Rather we depend on plants and microorganisms to introduce these chemicals into the food chain. NAD is essential to all forms of life, and humans convert various sources of niacin to NAD by distinct metabolic pathways.

Pathways to and from NAD

The NAD precursors (nicotinic acid/niacin, nicotinamide/niacinamide, nicotinamide riboside, or tryptophan) follow separate pathways to generate NAD within the cell, but all of these pathways ultimately require the one enzyme, nicotinamide mononucleotide phosphoribosyltransferase (NMNAT). There are three different NMNAT isoforms (encoded by *NMNAT1*, *NMNAT2*, and *NMNAT3*) expressed in distinguishable subcellular locations. Overexpression of any of these enzymes dramatically increases cell viability when challenged by otherwise lethal stress in general through maintaining vital NAD concentrations (Sasaki *et al.*, 2006; Feng *et al.*, 2010; Gilley and Coleman, 2010; Mayer *et al.*, 2010; Yan *et al.*, 2010). In this section we review the NAD-producing pathways as shown in Figure 19.2.

Nicotinamide produced by NAD glycohydrolases is recycled back to NAD via the *NAD salvage pathway* (Figure 19.2). The first enzyme, nicotinamide phosphoribosyltransferase, is rate-limiting in controlling NAD synthesis (Revollo *et al.*, 2004). Changes in NMNAT levels become more important in controlling NAD production during times of stress, which are known to highly induce expression of NAMPT. Increases in the efficiency of the NAD salvage pathway have been repeatedly shown to provide greater protection against otherwise lethal shocks in a wide variety of cell types.

Nicotinic acid is converted to NAD via the *Preiss-Handler pathway* starting with nicotinic acid phosphoribosyltransferase (encoded by the *NPT1* gene). This enzyme is not inhibited by nicotinamide, whereas the equivalent mononucleotide-generating enzyme for nicotinamide (encoded by the *NAMPT* gene) is inhibited. Accordingly, high doses of nicotinic acid are known to increase the amount of NAD within cells to a greater level than does nicotinamide. Whether this greater increase in intracellular NAD is part of the reason for nicotinic acid's superior performance in preventing atherosclerosis is not very clear. Next, nicotinic acid mononucleotide is converted to nicotinic acid adenine dinucleotide via NMNAT, which requires ATP. Lastly glutamine is used by NAD synthase to replace the acid with the amide to produce NAD.

Lastly, nicotinamide riboside was discovered in 2004 to be a third form of vitamin B_3 (Bieganowski and Brenner, 2004). By contrast, nicotinic acid and nicotinamide were discovered and have been studied for over 60 years to date. Nicotinamide riboside is converted to NAD by a simple two-step pathway starting with a reaction catalyzed by nicotinamide riboside kinase (Figure 19.2). Less is known about nicotinamide riboside, but it is present in milk. None the less, experiments to date indicate that nicotinamide riboside boosts NAD levels, activates Sir2, and extends replicative lifespan in yeast, thus supporting the high likelihood that there will be positive therapeutic benefits in humans (Belenky *et al.*, 2007). Nicotinamide riboside is distinguished in vertebrate development for serving essential pathways in muscular development (Goody *et al.*, 2010).

The de novo pathway of NAD synthesis starts with tryptophan. Requiring over seven chemical reactions, this is the longest NAD biosynthetic pathway. One intermediate, 2-amino-3-carboxymuconate-6-semialdehyde (ACMS), has to accumulate and degrade nonenzymatically to allow the pathway to be completed. The enzyme that degrades ACMS towards acetyl CoA lowers the efficiency of tryptophan to niacin conversion (Fukuwatari *et al.*, 2002), likely explaining the individual and interspecies variation that is observed. Tryptophan has two distinctly essential characteristics. It is required for the biosynthesis of NAD starting from endogenous sources, and tryptophan is found at the lowest concentrations of any amino acid under basal conditions. The importance of tryptophan as a precursor to NAD is particularly evident with Hartnup disease, which arises from a mutation in a transporter that is required to assist delivery of tryptophan into the cell. Hartnup disease presents with many symptoms that resemble pellagra, most of which are rescuable by administration of preformed niacin or niacinamide (Oakley and Wallace, 1994; Symula *et al.*, 1997; Patel and Prabhu, 2008). The NAD de novo pathway also requires riboflavin (vitamin B_2), pyridoxyl phosphate (vitamin B_6), ascorbate (vitamin C), and glutamine in order to go to completion to NAD (Figure 19.2). Much of the tryptophan to NAD conversion occurs via the hepatic tryptophan dioxygenase (TDO) catalyzed pathway. However, the de novo pathway is highly regulated by the immune system in specific cell types as well. Interferon gamma activates the rate-limiting enzyme indoleamine-2,3-dioxygenase (IDO) which is required for interferon's biological activities. The intermediates in this NAD synthetic pathway such as kynurenine and kynurenate have significant physiological roles. IDO is also expressed in endothelial cells, which are vulnerable to excessive immune-cell depletion of plasma tryptophan (Niinisalo *et al.*, 2010). Persistent activation of IDO is seen in many autoimmune diseases and cancer, where decreased serum tryptophan is a common diagnostic indicator of poor prognosis. Complementary administration of high doses of NAD precursors have been repeatedly shown to rescue these pathogenic processes in animal models as well as in examined clinical cases (Penberthy, 2007).

NAD-utilizing Proteins

NAD participates in more reactions than any other vitamin-derived molecule. At least 470 proteins use NAD(P(H)), see supplementary Table, NAD-Utilizing Proteins (http://web.me.com/wtpenber/NAD-Utilizing_Enzymes/1.html). NAD functions in hundreds of redox reactions as a *cofactor*; tens of reactions as a *substrate*, and single-digit numbers of proteins use NAD as a *ligand*. More and more proteins are being discovered by biochemists to be directly involved in NAD(P(H))-connected activities at the biochemical level. The importance of NAD concentrations in regulating these various processes is a perennial area of vibrant clinical research interest.

NAD as a Cofactor in Redox Reactions

In general, redox enzymes use NAD(H) for catabolic reactions and NADP(H) more commonly for anabolic (biosynthetic) reactions. For example, NADPH serves as an important reducing agent for the synthesis of lipids and steroids, while NAD^+ is required to oxidize substrates in the Krebs cycle.

Both NAD and NADP serve essential bioenergetic functions in the intracellular respiratory chain of all cells. NAD assists in the stepwise transfer of electrons from various energy substrates to the cytochromes. NADH usually donates its electrons to a flavin coenzyme in the mitochondrial electron transport chain responsible for ATP production. Reducing equivalents are carried to the mitochondria by the malate–aspartate or the glycerol phosphate–dihydroxyacetone shuttles. The approximately 57 different cytochrome P450 monooxygenase proteins are used by humans for a wide variety of metabolic processes including synthesis and degradation of: drugs, xenobiotics, prostaglandins, leukotrienes, retinoic acid, vitamin D, cholesterol, bile, and steroids (Nebert and Russell, 2002). Pyridine nucleotides and flavocoenzymes funnel reducing equivalents to the mitochondrial respiratory chain.

NAD as a Substrate and NAD Depletion

Four categorical enzymes play conditionally dominant roles in controlling NAD levels. These enzymes respond to DNA damage, immune activation, and other stimuli. This section covers aspects of these NAD concentration-controlling enzymes: poly(ADP-ribose) polymerase (PARPs 1–18), NAD-dependent deacetylases (sirtuins 1–7), ADP cyclases (CD38 and CD157), and indoleamine 2,3-dioxygenases (IDO). The first three categorical enzymes produce nicotinamide as a side product that is recycled back to NAD via the salvage pathway as shown in Figure 19.2.

PARP1 and PARP2 NAD-consuming activities are highly activated by any kind of DNA damage (Schraufstatter et al., 1986). These enzymes use NAD to produce the anionic polymer poly(ADP)ribose. Also they transfer ADP-ribose directly to histones and other proteins including p53, NF kappa B, and other important proteins. There are up to 18 different ADP-ribose transferring enzymes identified, based on genome sequencing. The degree of PARP activation is directly proportional to the degree of DNA damage. This response serves a critical function in stopping cell division after the DNA is damaged, thus minimizing rogue cancer cell expansion and enabling DNA repair. However, hyperactivation of PARP1 leads to severe depletion of intracellular NAD and ATP. This results in uncontrolled necrotic cell death. In fact PARP inhibition prevents a wide variety of otherwise lethal shocks in mammals, but it does come with a slightly increased likelihood for tumor formation (Shall and de Murcia, 2000).

We cannot change our genetic makeup significantly during our lifetime, but epigenetics are very responsive to nutritional status. Increased NAD levels can activate SIRT1, which alters chromatin structure through histone deacetylation. SIRT1 activation has been attracting interest as it is thought to be the mechanism underlying the lifespan extension associated with caloric restriction. While other histone deacetylates only possess constitutive activity, the sirtuins are activated by increases in NAD concentrations. This NAD-dependent activation of sirtuin HDAC activity is thus quite unique because we can alter our NAD levels to ultimately alter chromatin structure. However, NAD-dependent PARP1 activity also tends to relax chromatin structure, and the combination of these two influences of niacin status on chromatin structure has not been properly investigated (Kirkland, 2009a).

Activated NAD-dependent sirtuins deacetylate histones, p53, NF kappa B, and many other important proteins. Sirtuins can negatively regulate PARP activity by deacetylation (Gupta et al., 2008). A tremendous amount of investment has been devoted to sirtuin research owing in large part to the excitement surrounding SIRT1-dependent caloric restriction-mediated lifespan extension (Howitz et al., 2003). Animal models have revealed that sirtuin activation is beneficial for treatment of diabetes (Ramsey et al., 2008) and neurodegeneration (Araki et al., 2004; Qin et al., 2006).

The ADP cyclase enzyme CD38 uses NAD as a substrate to generate known mediators of intracellular calcium release (De Flora et al., 2004). This mechanism is required for chemotaxis of many types of immune cells. The CD38-deficient mouse has persistent elevated NAD levels and increased energy, and does not become obese even when fed a high-fat diet (Barbosa et al., 2007). However, CD38-deficient mice are more susceptible to infections (Partida-Sanchez et al., 2007). CD38 levels and activity are chiefly regulated at the transcriptional level. Tumor necrosis factor-alpha (TNF-alpha) especially increases CD38 expression. CD157 is another NAD-dependent ADP cyclase that has important but less studied functions.

CD38 is highly expressed in the brain, where its potential neurological role is an active area of research (Young and Kirkland, 2008).

Indoleamine 2,3-dioxygenase (IDO) is highly regulated by the immune responses (Mellor and Munn, 2004). IDO plays significant roles by decreasing available plasma tryptophan concentrations and potentially controlling NAD concentrations, similar to Hartnup disease. Tryptophan is present at the lowest concentrations of all amino acids under basal conditions, and it is used for the NAD biosynthesis de novo pathway. During pregnancy IDO is highly expressed in the trophoblasts surrounding the developing fetus. This starves local immune cells, thus conferring fetal immunotolerance and preventing rejection of the foreign fetus by the immune system. During infections and in autoimmune disease, IDO is highly activated by interferons in specific professional antigen-presenting immune cells (dendritic cells, macrophages, and B cells). Activation of IDO also exerts antibacterial and antiviral activities, particularly intracellularly. IDO is frequently persistently activated in autoimmune disease and cancer (Uyttenhove et al., 2003). Persistent or acute excessive activation of IDO during autoimmune disease or cancer weakens neighboring cells due to exceedingly low serum tryptophan levels. Accordingly high doses of vitamin B$_3$ have been shown to complement many effects of this deficiency of de novo NAD precursor tryptophan, thus relieving many of the pellagra-like symptoms similar to the effects seen in Hartnup disease (Penberthy, 2007).

NAD as a Ligand

NAD binds to the receptors P2Y1 (colonic cells) or P2Y11 (in monocytes and granulocytes) to function as a neurotransmitter (Mutafova-Yambolieva et al., 2007; Klein et al., 2009). NAD functions as an inhibitory neurotransmitter inhibiting colonic muscle contraction. This causes an increase in intracellular calcium. Some of these NAD effects are ultimately due to associations between the P2Y receptors and other G-protein coupled receptors.

Physiological Concentrations of NAD Precursors

Baseline sera concentrations of nicotinic acid are in the low nanomolar range, while nicotinamide concentrations are somewhat higher and more responsive to normal dietary intakes. Treatment of dyslipidemia, pharmacological administration of 3–5 g/day of nicotinic acid, elevates serum levels of nicotinic acid above 10 μM. Peak concentrations vary up to 240 μM depending on whether immediate-release niacin or timed-release niacin is used (Kirkland, 2009b). This high concentration exerts many therapeutically desirable effects for preventing cardiovascular disease, including raising HDL while lowering triglycerides, LDL, and VLDL. By contrast, high doses of nicotinamide do not exert these effects on blood lipids.

Nicotinic acid mediates some of these beneficial effects on the lipid profile via the nicotinic acid high affinity (100 nM equilibrium binding) G-protein coupled receptors, GPR109a and GPR109b (Gille et al., 2008). Nicotinamide does not bind to these receptors, and the binding by nicotinic acid appears to represent an unphysiological binding to receptors meant to respond to high circulating ketone bodies. Nicotinic acid–GPR109 signaling causes a flush response: vasodilation, reddening of the skin, alterations in temperature, and sometimes itching. The flush response occurs with as little as 35 mg of nicotinic acid and is considered unpleasant by most individuals, but it is not associated with any known tissue injury. The nicotinic acid-mediated flush is linked to beneficial effects in the correction of dyslipidemia, whereas nicotinamide does not exert these beneficial effects on lipid profiles.

Niacin and Disease

The questions as to which is the most effective NAD precursor in pharmacological use and which diseases are most responsive to these treatments are among the most exciting in molecular therapeutic clinical research today. We therefore briefly review here what happens to concentrations of NAD, tryptophan, poly(ADP)ribose, and other relevant molecules over the course of pathogenesis for several diseases.

Pharmacological Niacin

Gram-level quantities of standard/immediate release or prescription sustained release niacin have been used with large populations of hyperlipidemic patients with only rare adverse events. Sustained release niacin, however, has resulted in chemical hepatitis (Carlson, 2005; Guyton and Bays, 2007). Other rare side-effects include cystoid macular edema. Inositol hexanicotinate has also been prescribed as a form of niacin ("flush free"); however, there is evidence that the nicotinic acid is poorly released from the inositol and that correction of dyslipidemia is less effective.

Cardiovascular Disease

More people ultimately die due to cardiovascular events than as a result of any other disease. High-dose niacin is well known as one of the most effective agents preventing atherosclerosis-related strokes and heart attacks (Carlson, 2005). Niacin increases HDL (the good cholesterol) levels more than any other pharmaceutical, while simultaneously decreasing cholesterol, VLDL, and triglycerides in otherwise dyslipidemic individuals. A 15-year follow-up to a cohort receiving 3 g niacin per day showed a 15% reduction in mortality (Canner *et al.*, 1986). Similar reductions in mortality were seen in patients with previous myocardial infarctions (Carlson and Rosenhamer, 1988). The book *The Eight-Week Cure for Cholesterol* written by a medical journalist described his struggle to treat severe dyslipidemia using niacin (Kowalski, 2001).

The mechanism of action of niacin in correcting dyslipidemia is a perennial cardiovascular research question. The high-affinity nicotinic acid G-protein-coupled receptors GPR109a and GPR109b serve primary roles in the niacin dyslipidemia-correcting mechanism of action. These are highly expressed in adipose tissue, but also in neutrophils, professional antigen presenting cells (dendritic cells, macrophages, and B cells), intestine, retina, and other areas within the central nervous system. In adipocytes nicotinic acid signaling through GPR109 causes a decrease in cyclic AMP levels, which decreases hormone-sensitive lipase (Karpe and Frayn, 2004). In other cells a wide variety of prostaglandins are produced at high levels, mediating potentially beneficial effects including increased peripheral circulation. The endogenously produced prostaglandin PGJ_2 most potently activates PPAR gamma and other PPARs similar to the diabetes and dyslipidemia drugs, thiazolidinediones and clofibrate, respectively. NAD working through sirtuin–PPAR pathways is also potentially involved in positive lipid-correcting activities. Still other nicotinic acid associated pathways, including regulation of membrane-bound ATP synthases and diacylglycerol acyltransferase, are potentially involved in the myriad of high-dose niacin/nicotinic acid benefits (Kamanna and Kashyap, 2008).

Cancer

While the death rate for cardiovascular disease has dropped by over 60% over the past 50 years, that for cancer has been disappointingly unchanged by comparison, having decreased by merely 5% adjusted for age and population (Kolata, 2009). Cancer is initiated by unrepaired DNA damage. Under healthy conditions, cells with too much DNA damage commit apoptosis. NAD plays significant roles in controlling both genomic stability and the cell death process. Moreover, later in the progression of cancer disease, NAD can become a dominant theme in metabolic chemotherapy.

The rate of NAD turnover in cancerous transformed cells is much higher than that of normal cells. This is due to an increased demand for NAD in glycolysis and also the increased PARP1/2 activity associated with genomic instability. Cancer cells have a far greater essential requirement for glycolysis than for oxidative phosphorylation as a means of generating ATP. Tumor cells typically perform glycolysis at a 30 times greater rate than that of normal cells (Ganapathy *et al.*, 2009). Moreover the rate of entry of glucose into cancer cells is also 20 to 30 times greater than into untransformed cells in order to supply essential levels of glucose. Oxygen-independent glycolytic ATP production requires regeneration of NAD by lactate dehydrogenase. Interestingly, clinical pellagra may be observed during chemotherapy (Dreizen *et al.*, 1990).

Today, chemotherapeutics are being developed to decrease NAD via inhibition of NAMPT and/or IDO (Yang *et al.*, 2010). Other interesting areas of niacin cancer research include the observation that GPR109a can function as a tumor suppressor in the colon (Thangaraju *et al.*, 2009). Whether administration of niacin can help in colon cancer is unknown. However, niacin is well known to provide therapeutic benefit in the related ectodermal skin cancer models (Gensler *et al.*, 1999; Jacobson *et al.*, 1999; Benavente *et al.*, 2009).

Neurodegenerative Disease

As excitable energy-demanding tissues, neural cells (neurons and glia) have distinct metabolic NAD-dependent requirements. Similar to tumor cells, neurons are very dependent on glycolysis as a source of ATP generation. Oxidizing glucose in glycolysis and the pentose phosphate pathway, with low mitochondrial activity, decreases oxidant stress in these sensitive tissues. Glial cells function as support cells to neurons, synthesizing cholesterol and lactate, which are both delivered to neurons. Increases in baseline NAD or NAD salvage pathway efficiency are well known to prevent otherwise lethal stress-induced neurodegeneration in cells and animal models. Thus, we must understand what happens to NAD levels in the diseases of neurodegeneration: dementia/Alzheimer's disease (AD), Parkinson's disease (PD), Huntington's disease (HD), amyotrophic lateral sclerosis, multiple sclerosis, and even schizophrenia. Alzheimer's disease is the most common form of dementia recognized today. This is followed by vascular dementia. The NAD-deficiency disease pellagra is characterized by dementia, where niacin is one of the rare molecules known to prevent a form of dementia while also providing many therapeutic vascular benefits.

Diseases defined by the formation of insoluble protein plaques include AD (amyloid protein; tauopathies), HD (huntingtin protein), and PD (α-synuclein; Lewy bodies). While surgery and stem cells may hold promise for the future, currently these latter diseases are irreversible after a certain point in disease progression. Primary emphasis is placed on prevention or stay of progression. An increase in dietary niacin from 15 mg to 40 mg/day has been correlated with a 70% decrease in the likelihood of Alzheimer's disease, in a study examining 6158 patients over 65 years of age (Morris et al., 2004). NAD, potentially through activation of SIRT1, can reduce amyloid precursor protein processing to plaques in transgenic mouse models of AD (Qin et al., 2006). Studies show that high apolipoprotein A-1 (apoA-1) decreases AD risk (Scarmeas, 2007), and high-dose niacin is effective in raising apoA-1 containing HDL, suggesting that this might be effective in delaying the progression of brain injury. Meanwhile, high ApoE is associated with increased risk of AD (Corder et al., 1993, 1994) and is found in the chylomicrons, VLDL and LDL particles. ApoE mutations can cause familial AD and dyslipidemia. ApoE-deficient mice are used as a model of dyslipidemia, where administration of niacin is able to correct the elevations in cholesterol and triglycerides but not the decrease in HDL unless cholesteryl ester transfer protein is over-expressed (van der Hoorn et al., 2008). More research is needed to understand how niacin nutrition and pharmacological use relate to the frequency of AD, ApoE, and vascular dementia as well as how best to incorporate niacin into treatments. Parkinson's disease occurs due to a deficiency of dopamine-producing neurons in the substantia nigra part of the midbrain. The mechanisms of Parkinson's disease are poorly understood; however, excessive methyl-nicotinamide (MN) has been proposed to be part of the cause of PD pathogenesis (Ying, 2007). Urinary MN is elevated in Parkinson's disease. Since this is the metabolic byproduct of niacin metabolism, this suggests that NAD metabolism is somehow involved. By contrast, administration of NADH has been tested on PD patients and found to stimulate increased dopamine production. Future work will be required to understand the role in brain metabolism of various NAD precursors and metabolites.

Multiple sclerosis (MS) is the most commonly diagnosed disease of the central nervous system. Animal models of MS have revealed that NAD precursors can prevent the onset and damage of MS pathogenesis. Poly (ADP-ribose) (PAR) formation increases at sites of pathogenesis, where preservation of NAD levels is key to maintaining health (reviewed by Penberthy and Tsunoda, 2009).

Other ongoing areas of neurobiology research involve the slow Wallerian degeneration (Wld^s) mouse, which is remarkably resilient to stress-induced neuronal cell death. Razor excision of wild-type neurons leads to degeneration in less than 24 hours. Remarkably, Wld^s mouse neurons survive for up to 2 weeks and are still capable of depolarization (Adalbert et al., 2005). The gene mediating this effect includes the NAD biosynthetic enzyme, nicotinamide adenine mononucleotide adenylyl transferase-1 (Ube4b/NMNAT1) (Mack et al., 2001). Follow-up research has determined that increased expression of NMNAT1, NMNAT2, or NMNAT3 is extremely neuroprotective and that NAD itself can exert a similar survival effect (Araki et al., 2004; Sasaki et al., 2009; Gilley and Coleman, 2010; Yan et al., 2010). NAD-mediated neuroprotection may be mediated by increased sirtuin activity (Araki et al., 2004), but NAD-chaperone survival activities have also been observed for NMNAT (Zhai et al., 2008).

Autoimmune Disease

Some autoimmune diseases, listed from more to less common include hypothyroiditis, rheumatoid arthritis, hyperthyroiditis, type 1 diabetes, systemic lupus erythematosus, myocarditis, multiple sclerosis, and inflammatory bowel disease. Autoimmune diseases commonly arise from an undesirable clonal expansion of autoreactive T cells. One of the best-understood mechanisms for controlling this expansion involves starving the T cells of tryptophan by interaction with tryptophan-hoarding professional antigen-presenting cells (dendritic cells, macrophages, B cells, and microglia [Mellor and Munn, 2004]). IDO is frequently activated in autoimmune diseases as the immune system works to control this undesirable expansion. This ultimately contributes to depletion of extracellular tryptophan where low tryptophan levels are characteristic and correlate highly with a poor prognosis (Schrocksnadel et al., 2006). This activated immune system may also activate PARP-1, which additively contributes to NAD depletion. Ultimately, the complementary administration of NAD precursors to this situation makes sense and has been repeatedly shown to prevent onset of pathogenesis or even to cure the disease in many animal models of disease as well as in some clinical examples (Penberthy, 2007).

Future Directions

There is much that remains to be determined in niacin research. The impact of low and high niacin status on basic energy metabolism is poorly appreciated and is a logical area in which to apply cutting-edge techniques in metabolomics. The use of NAD as a substrate in the formation of poly, mono, and cyclic ADP-ribose, as well as in support of sirtuin activities, suggests that there are complex interactions between intermediary metabolism and control through ADP-ribosylation reactions. It is clear that ADP-ribosyltransferases, sirtuins, and metabolic families of enzymes all play important roles in cancer and in autoimmune and neurodegenerative diseases, with much still to be learned. With the benefits of inhibiting ADP-ribose metabolism under certain conditions (ischemia-reperfusion, treatment of certain cancers), and the risks of doing so at other times, clinical management of ADP-ribose metabolism is in its infancy. Given the extremely large number of niacin-dependent proteins in metabolism, cataloging polymorphisms and individual variation in niacin requirements is another long-term goal.

Suggestions for Further Reading

Expanded coverage of basic niacin and ADP-ribose metabolism: Kirkland, J.B. (2009) Niacin status, NAD distribution and ADP-ribose metabolism. *Curr Pharm Des* **15**, 3–11.

Health benefits versus risks of PARP activation in various disease states: Kirkland, J.B. (2010) Poly ADP-ribose polymerase-1 and health. *Exp Biol Med* **235**, 561–568.

Historical perspective on niacin in the treatment of dyslipidemia: Carlson, L.A. (2005) Nicotinic acid: the broad-spectrum lipid drug. A 50th anniversary review. *J Intern Med* **258**, 94–114.

Further readings on the sirtuins: Imai, S. and Guarente, L. (2010) Ten years of NAD-dependent SIR2 family deacetylases: implications for metabolic diseases. *Trends Pharmacol Sci* **31**, 212–220.

A review of the exciting area of niacin and skin health: Benavente, C.A., Jacobson, M.K., and Jacobson, E.L. (2009) NAD in skin: therapeutic approaches for niacin. *Curr Pharm Des* **15**, 29–38.

A review of known polymorphisms that cause altered vitamin requirements: Ames, B.N., Elson-Schwab, I., and Silver, E.A. (2002) High-dose vitamin therapy stimulates variant enzymes with decreased coenzyme binding affinity (increased K(m)): relevance to genetic disease and polymorphisms. *Am J Clin Nutr* **75**, 616–658.

References

Adalbert, R., Gillingwater, T.H., Haley, J.E., *et al.* (2005) A rat model of slow Wallerian degeneration (WldS) with improved preservation of neuromuscular synapses. *Eur J Neurosci* **21**, 271–277.

Altschul, R., Hoffer, A., and Stephen, J.D. (1955) Influence of nicotinic acid on serum cholesterol in man. *Arch Biochem* **54**, 558–559.

Ames, B.N., Elson-Schwab, I., and Silver, E.A. (2002) High-dose vitamin therapy stimulates variant enzymes with decreased coenzyme binding affinity (increased K(m)): relevance to genetic disease and polymorphisms. *Am J Clin Nutr* **75**, 616–658.

Araki, T., Sasaki, Y., and Milbrandt, J. (2004) Increased nuclear NAD biosynthesis and SIRT1 activation prevent axonal degeneration. *Science* **305**, 1010–1013.

Barbosa, M.T., Soares, S.M., Novak, C.M., *et al.* (2007) The enzyme CD38 (a NAD glycohydrolase, EC 3.2.2.5) is necessary for the development of diet-induced obesity. *FASEB J* **21**, 3629–3639.

Belenky, P., Racette, F.G., Bogan, K.L., *et al.* (2007) Nicotinamide riboside promotes Sir2 silencing and extends lifespan via Nrk and Urh1/Pnp1/Meu1 pathways to NAD+. *Cell* **129**, 473–484.

Benavente, C.A., Jacobson, M.K., and Jacobson, E.L. (2009) NAD in skin: therapeutic approaches for niacin. *Curr Pharm Des* **15**, 29–38.

Bieganowski, P. and Brenner, C. (2004) Discoveries of nicotinamide riboside as a nutrient and conserved NRK genes establish a Preiss-Handler independent route to NAD+ in fungi and humans. *Cell* **117**, 495–502.

Canner, P.L., Berge, K.G., Wenger, N.K., *et al.* (1986) Fifteen year mortality in Coronary Drug Project patients: long-term benefit with niacin. *J Am Coll Cardiol* **8**, 1245–1255.

Carlson, L.A. (2005) Nicotinic acid: the broad-spectrum lipid drug. A 50th anniversary review. *J Intern Med* **258**, 94–114.

Carlson, L.A. and Rosenhamer, G. (1988) Reduction of mortality in the Stockholm Ischaemic Heart Disease Secondary Prevention Study by combined treatment with clofibrate and nicotinic acid. *Acta Med Scand* **223**, 405–418.

Carpenter, K.J. (1981) Effects of different methods of processing maize on its pellagragenic activity. *Fed Proc* **40**, 1531–1535.

Corder, E.H., Saunders, A.M., Risch, N.J., *et al.* (1994) Protective effect of apolipoprotein E type 2 allele for late onset Alzheimer disease. *Nat Genet* **7**, 180–184.

Corder, E.H., Saunders, A.M., Strittmatter, W.J., *et al.* (1993) Gene dose of apolipoprotein E type 4 allele and the risk of Alzheimer's disease in late onset families. *Science* **261**, 921–923.

De Flora, A., Zocchi, E., Guida, L., *et al.* (2004) Autocrine and paracrine calcium signaling by the CD38/NAD+/cyclic ADP-ribose system. *Ann N Y Acad Sci* **1028**, 176–191.

Dreizen, S., McCredie, K.B., Keating, M.J., *et al.* (1990) Nutritional deficiencies in patients receiving cancer chemotherapy. *Postgrad Med* **87**, 163–167, 170.

Etheridge, E.W. (1972) *The Butterfly Caste: A Social History of Pellagra in the South*. Greenwood Publishing, Westport, Conn.

Feng, Y., Yan, T., Zheng, J., *et al.* (2010) Overexpression of Wld(S) or Nmnat2 in mauthner cells by single-cell electroporation delays axon degeneration in live zebrafish. *J Neurosci Res* **88**, 3319–3327.

Fu, C.S., Swendseid, M.E., Jacob, R.A., *et al.* (1989) Biochemical markers for assessment of niacin status in young men: levels of erythrocyte niacin coenzymes and plasma tryptophan. *J Nutr* **119**, 1949–1955.

Fukuwatari, T., Sugimoto, E., and Shibata, K. (2002) Growth-promoting activity of pyrazinoic acid, a putative active compound of antituberculosis drug pyrazinamide, in niacin-deficient rats through the inhibition of ACMSD activity. *Biosci Biotechnol Biochem* **66**, 1435–1441.

Ganapathy, V., Thangaraju, M., and Prasad, P.D. (2009) Nutrient transporters in cancer: relevance to Warburg hypothesis and beyond. *Pharmacol Ther* **121**, 29–40.

Gensler, H.L., Williams, T., Huang, A.C., *et al.* (1999) Oral niacin prevents photocarcinogenesis and photoimmunosuppression in mice. *Nutr Cancer* **34**, 36–41.

Gille, A., Bodor, E.T., Ahmed, K., *et al.* (2008) Nicotinic acid: pharmacological effects and mechanisms of action. *Annu Rev Pharmacol Toxicol* **48**, 79–106.

Gilley, J. and Coleman, M.P. (2010) Endogenous Nmnat2 is an essential survival factor for maintenance of healthy axons. *PLoS Biol* **8**, e1000300.

Goody, M.F., Kelly, M.W., Lessard, K.N., *et al.* (2010) Nrk2b-mediated NAD+ production regulates cell adhesion and is required for muscle morphogenesis in vivo: Nrk2b and NAD+ in muscle morphogenesis. *Dev Biol* **344**, 809–826.

Gupta, M.P., Rajamohan, S.B., Sundarasean, N.R., *et al.* (2008) SIRT1 prevents cell death by deacetylating PARP1 and suppressing its enzymatic activity. Paper presented at: PARP 2008 (Tucson, Arizona).

Guyton, J.R. and Bays, H.E. (2007) Safety considerations with niacin therapy. *Am J Cardiol* **99**, 22C–31C.

Hoffer, A., Osmond, H., Callbeck, M.J., *et al.* (1957) Treatment of schizophrenia with nicotinic acid and nicotinamide. *J Clin Exp Psychopathol* **18**, 131–158.

Howitz, K.T., Bitterman, K.J., Cohen, H.Y., *et al.* (2003) Small molecule activators of sirtuins extend *Saccharomyces cerevisiae* lifespan. *Nature* **425**, 191–196.

Jacobson, E.L. (1993) Niacin deficiency and cancer in women. *J Am Coll Nutr* **12**, 412–416.

Jacobson, E.L. and Jacobson, M.K. (1997) Tissue NAD as a biochemical measure of niacin status in humans. *Methods Enzymol* **280**, 221–230.

Jacobson, E.L., Shieh, W.M., and Huang, A.C. (1999) Mapping the role of NAD metabolism in prevention and treatment of carcinogenesis. *Mol Cell Biochem* **193**, 69–74.

Kamanna, V.S. and Kashyap, M.L. (2008) Mechanism of action of niacin. *Am J Cardiol* **101**, 20B–26B.

Karpe, F. and Frayn, K.N. (2004) The nicotinic acid receptor – a new mechanism for an old drug. *Lancet* **363**, 1892–1894.

Kirkland, J.B. (2009a) Niacin status impacts chromatin structure. *J Nutr* **139**, 2397–2401.

Kirkland, J.B. (2009b) Niacin status, NAD distribution and ADP-ribose metabolism. *Curr Pharm Des* **15**, 3–11.

Klein, C., Grahnert, A., Abdelrahman, A., *et al.* (2009) Extracellular NAD(+) induces a rise in [Ca(2+)](i) in activated human monocytes via engagement of P2Y(1) and P2Y(11) receptors. *Cell Calcium* **46**, 263–272.

Kolata, G. (2009) Advances elusive in the drive to cure cancer. *New York Times*. http://www.nytimes.com/2009/04/24/health/policy/24cancer.html?pagewanted=all

Kowalski, R.E. (2001) *The New 8-Week Cholesterol Cure: The Ultimate Program for Preventing Heart Disease*. Harper Collins, New York.

Mack, T.G., Reiner, M., Beirowski, B., *et al.* (2001) Wallerian degeneration of injured axons and synapses is delayed by a Ube4b/Nmnat chimeric gene. *Nat Neurosci* **4**, 1199–1206.

Mayer, P.R., Huang, N., Dewey, C.M., *et al.* (2010) Expression, localization and biochemical characterization of NMN adenylyltransferase 2. *J Biol Chem* **285**, 40387–40396.

McCormick, D.B. and Greene, H.L. (1999) Vitamins. In C.A. Burtis and E.R. Ashwood (eds), *Textbook of Clinical Chemistry*. WH Saunders, Philadelphia, pp. 999–1029.

Mellor, A.L. and Munn, D.H. (2004) IDO expression by dendritic cells: tolerance and tryptophan catabolism. *Nat Rev Immunol* **4**, 762–774.

Morris, M.C., Evans, D.A., Bienias, J.L., *et al.* (2004) Dietary niacin and the risk of incident Alzheimer's disease and of cognitive decline. *J Neurol Neurosurg Psychiatr* **75**, 1093–1099.

Mutafova-Yambolieva, V.N., Hwang, S.J., Hao, X., *et al.* (2007) Beta-nicotinamide adenine dinucleotide is an inhibitory neurotransmitter in visceral smooth muscle. *Proc Natl Acad Sci USA* **104**, 16359–16364.

Nebert, D.W. and Russell, D.W. (2002) Clinical importance of the cytochromes P450. *Lancet* **360**, 1155–1162.

Niinisalo, P., Oksala, N., Levula, M., *et al.* (2010). Activation of indoleamine 2,3-dioxygenase-induced tryptophan degradation in advanced atherosclerotic plaques: Tampere vascular study. *Ann Med* **42**, 55–63.

Nozaki, J., Dakeishi, M., Ohura, T., *et al.* (2001) Homozygosity mapping to chromosome 5p15 of a gene responsible for Hartnup disorder. *Biochem Biophys Res Commun* **284**, 255–260.

Oakley, A. and Wallace, J. (1994) Hartnup disease presenting in an adult. *Clin Exp Dermatol* **19**, 407–408.

Otten, J.J., Hellwig, J.P., and Meyers, L.D. (eds) (2006) *Dietary Reference Intakes: The Essential Guide to Nutrient Requirements.* National Academies Press, Washington, DC.

Partida-Sanchez, S., Rivero-Nava, L., Shi, G., *et al.* (2007) CD38: an ecto-enzyme at the crossroads of innate and adaptive immune responses. *Adv Exp Med Biol* **590**, 171–183.

Patel, A.B. and Prabhu, A.S. (2008) Hartnup disease. *Indian J Dermatol* **53**, 31–32.

Penberthy, W.T. (2007) Pharmacological targeting of IDO-mediated tolerance for treating autoimmune disease. *Curr Drug Metab* **8**, 245–266.

Penberthy, W.T. and Tsunoda, I. (2009) The importance of NAD in multiple sclerosis. *Curr Pharm Des* **15**, 64–99.

Qin, W., Yang, T., Ho, L., *et al.* (2006) Neuronal SIRT1 activation as a novel mechanism underlying the prevention of Alzheimer disease amyloid neuropathology by calorie restriction. *J Biol Chem* **281**, 21745–21754.

Ramsey, K.M., Mills, K.F., Satoh, A., *et al.* (2008) Age-associated loss of Sirt1-mediated enhancement of glucose-stimulated insulin secretion in beta cell-specific Sirt1-overexpressing (BESTO) mice. *Aging Cell* **7**, 78–88.

Revollo, J.R., Grimm, A.A., and Imai, S. (2004). The NAD biosynthesis pathway mediated by nicotinamide phosphoribosyltransferase regulates Sir2 activity in mammalian cells. *J Biol Chem* **279**, 50754–50763.

Sasaki, Y., Araki, T., and Milbrandt, J. (2006) Stimulation of nicotinamide adenine dinucleotide biosynthetic pathways delays axonal degeneration after axotomy. *J Neurosci* **26**, 8484–8491.

Sasaki, Y., Vohra, B.P., Baloh, R.H., *et al.* (2009) Transgenic mice expressing the Nmnat1 protein manifest robust delay in axonal degeneration in vivo. *J Neurosci* **29**, 6526–6534.

Scarmeas, N. (2007) Invited commentary: lipoproteins and dementia – is it the apolipoprotein A-I? *Am J Epidemiol* **165**, 993–997.

Schraufstatter, I.U., Hinshaw, D.B., Hyslop, P.A., *et al.* (1986) Oxidant injury of cells. DNA strand-breaks activate polyadenosine diphosphate-ribose polymerase and lead to depletion of nicotinamide adenine dinucleotide. *J Clin Invest* **77**, 1312–1320.

Schrocksnadel, K., Wirleitner, B., Winkler, C., *et al.* (2006) Monitoring tryptophan metabolism in chronic immune activation. *Clin Chim Acta* **364**, 82–90.

Shah, G.M., Shah, R.G., Veillette, H., *et al.* (2005) Biochemical assessment of niacin deficiency among carcinoid cancer patients. *Am J Gastroenterol* **100**, 2307–2314.

Shall, S. and de Murcia, G. (2000) Poly(ADP-ribose) polymerase-1: what have we learned from the deficient mouse model? *Mutat Res* **460**, 1–15.

Symula, D.J., Shedlovsky, A., Guillery, E.N., *et al.* (1997) A candidate mouse model for Hartnup disorder deficient in neutral amino acid transport. *Mamm Genome* **8**, 102–107.

Tang, K., Sham, H., Hui, E., *et al.* (2008) Niacin deficiency causes oxidative stress in rat bone marrow cells but not through decreased NADPH or glutathione status. *J Nutr Biochem* **19**, 746–753.

Thangaraju, M., Cresci, G.A., Liu, K., *et al.* (2009) GPR109A is a G-protein-coupled receptor for the bacterial fermentation product butyrate and functions as a tumor suppressor in colon. *Cancer Res* **69**, 2826–2832.

USDA/ARS (2005) USDA National Nutrient Standard Database, Release 18. US Department of Agriculture/Agricultural Research Service, Washington, DC. Retrieved December 23, 2005, from www.ars.usda.gov/ba/bhnrc/ndl.

Uyttenhove, C., Pilotte, L., Theate, I., *et al.* (2003) Evidence for a tumoral immune resistance mechanism based on tryptophan degradation by indoleamine 2,3-dioxygenase. *Nat Med* **9**, 1269–1274.

van der Hoorn, J.W., de Haan, W., Berbee, J.F., *et al.* (2008) Niacin increases HDL by reducing hepatic expression and plasma levels of cholesteryl ester transfer protein in APOE*3Leiden. CETP mice. *Arterioscler Thromb Vasc Biol* **28**, 2016–2022.

Yan, T., Feng, Y., Zheng, J., *et al.* (2010) Nmnat2 delays axon degeneration in superior cervical ganglia dependent on its NAD synthesis activity. *Neurochem Int* **56**, 101–106.

Yang, H.J., Yen, M.C., Lin, C.C., *et al.* (2010) A combination of the metabolic enzyme inhibitor APO866 and the immune adjuvant L-1-methyl tryptophan induces additive antitumor activity. *Exp Biol Med (Maywood)* **235**, 869–876.

Ying, W. (2007) NAD+ and NADH in brain functions, brain diseases and brain aging. *Front Biosci* **12,** 1863–1888.

Young, G.S. and Kirkland, J.B. (2008) The role of dietary niacin intake and the adenosine-5′-diphosphate-ribosyl cyclase enzyme CD38 in spatial learning ability: is cyclic adenosine diphosphate ribose the link between diet and behaviour? *Nutr Res Rev* **21,** 42–55.

Zhai, R.G., Zhang, F., Hiesinger, P.R., *et al.* (2008) NAD synthase NMNAT acts as a chaperone to protect against neurodegeneration. *Nature* **452,** 887–891.

20

VITAMIN B$_6$

VANESSA R. DA SILVA[1], PhD, KATELYN A. RUSSELL[2], BS, AND
JESSE F. GREGORY III[2], PhD

[1]*University of Georgia, Athens, Georgia, USA*
[2]*University of Florida, Gainesville, Florida, USA*

Summary

Vitamin B$_6$ is a family of related compounds comprised of pyridoxine (PN), pyridoxal (PL), and pyridoxamine (PM), along with their phosphate esters and glucosides. The primary vitamin B$_6$ coenzymic form, pyridoxal 5′-phosphate, is an obligatory cofactor in over 140 enzymatic reactions primarily in the metabolism of amino acids but also in reactions of carbohydrates and lipids. Vitamin B$_6$ also plays a vital role in one-carbon metabolism, facilitating cellular methylation processes, methionine recycling, regulation of homocysteine, and synthesis of cysteine. Recent findings indicate that marginal vitamin B$_6$ status remains a concern in human nutrition, at least in segments of the population. The consequence of marginal vitamin B$_6$ status is unclear but serves as cause for concern in view of associations between low vitamin B$_6$ status, risk of cardiovascular disease and stroke, and certain cancers. This chapter provides an overview of vitamin B$_6$ bioavailability, metabolism and metabolic function, nutritional status and assessment, and roles in human health and disease.

Introduction

Background, Chemistry, Sources, and Bioavailability

Evidence of the existence of an unknown water-soluble factor later termed vitamin B$_6$ first emerged in the late 1920s, and its purification, identification, and synthesis followed quickly thereafter in the 1930s (for historical review, see Gyorgy, 1956). Identification of pyridoxal (PL) and pyridoxamine (PM) as natural forms of the vitamin, and the recognition of a phosphorylated form of PL, eventually identified as pyridoxal 5′-phosphate, followed in the 1940s (for review, see Snell, 1990). Much of this work

evolved from bioassays involving the growth of rats and the prevention of a characteristic skin condition termed acrodynia (Beaton *et al.*, 1952; Gyorgy, 1956) and the use of vitamin B$_6$-dependent bacteria (Snell, 1990). We are indebted to these early researchers for their biochemical ingenuity, insight, and experimental skills in an era when modern analytical tools were lacking.

Vitamin B$_6$ is the term for the family of water-soluble vitamin species with the basic structure of 2-methyl,3-hydroxy,5-hydroxymethyl-pyridines (Figure 20.1). Through its coenzymatic function in processes including amino acid metabolism, one-carbon metabolism and nucleotide synthesis, neurotransmitter metabolism,

Present Knowledge in Nutrition, Tenth Edition. Edited by John W. Erdman Jr, Ian A. Macdonald and Steven H. Zeisel.
© 2012 International Life Sciences Institute. Published 2012 by John Wiley & Sons, Inc.

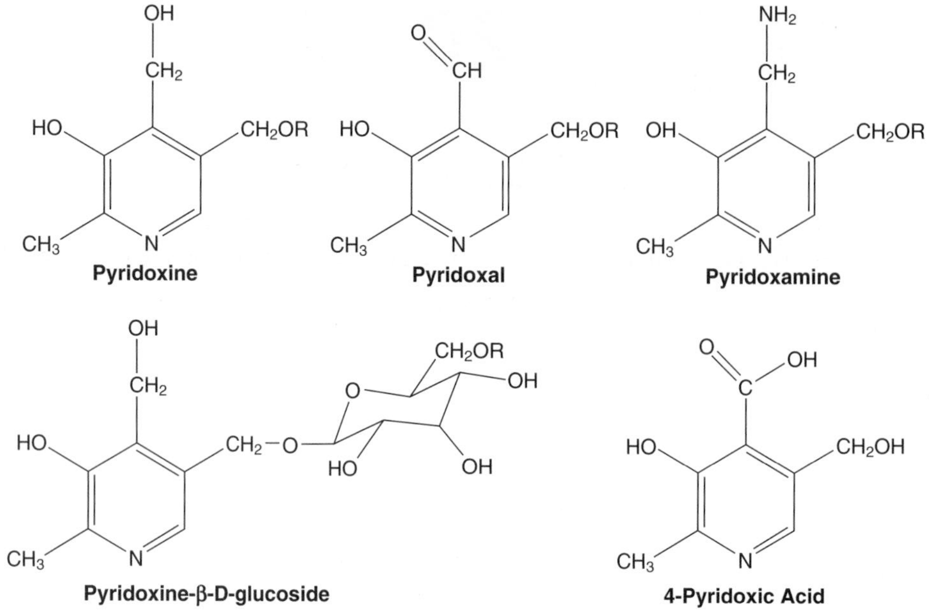

FIG. 20.1 Chemical forms of vitamin B₆. R = -H for non-phosphorylated pyridoxine, pyridoxal, and pyridox-amine, and R = -PO₃H for their 5′-phosphates.

heme synthesis, gluconeogenesis, and glycogenolysis, vitamin B₆ affects nearly all aspects of metabolic function and cellular homeostasis. The various forms differ with respect to the nature of the C-4 substituent which defines pyridoxal (PL, aldehyde, -CHO), pyridoxine (PN, alcohol, -CH₂OH), and pyridoxamine (PM, amine, -CH₂NH₂). Further variation among the constituents of this family exists through the ability of PN, PM, and PL to exist as a phosphate ester (designated PLP, PNP, and PMP for pyridoxal 5′-phosphate, pyridoxine 5′-phosphate, and pyridoxamine 5′-phosphate, respectively) or with pyridoxine as a glucoside derivative (PNG). 4-Pyridoxic acid (4-PA) is the primary catabolic product. Pyridoxine (PN), as the HCl salt, is the synthetic form used in food fortification and dietary supplements, mainly for reasons of its superior stability.

The ability of PLP (and PL to a lesser extent) to condense with the uncharged amino group of amines and amino acids to form Schiff base (aldimine) and related complexes is well known and, indeed, serves as the basis for the coenzyme function of vitamin B₆. This reactivity with amines and aldehydes also accounts for the observed non-enzymatic interconversions between PLP and/or PL with PMP and/or PM during food processing (Gregory, 2007). In addition, PLP is very sensitive to photochemical oxidation, forming 4-pyridoxic acid phosphate, and other vitamin B₆ species also exhibit some photochemical insta-

bility. Consequently, care must be taken to minimize light exposure in vitamin B₆ analysis and other research procedures. The greater reactivity of PLP toward amines is due to the presence of the phosphate group which prevents the formation of an internal hemiacetal bridge between the C-5 hydroxymethyl group and the C-4 aldehyde, as occurs readily in PL. PL and PLP also can undergo reductive binding to the €-amino groups of protein lysyl side chains to form €-pyridoxyllysine during the thermal processing of food. This complexed form of the vitamin is enigmatic as it is not detected in common vitamin B₆ assays, and it exhibits partial vitamin B₆ activity but also competes with other vitamin B₆ species for cellular uptake (Gregory, 1997).

Vitamin B₆ is widely distributed in foods of plant and animal origin. Muscle-derived foods including beef, pork, chicken, and fish are good sources, and organ meats are particularly rich in vitamin B₆. The distribution of vitamin B₆ in plants is rather enigmatic, although certain generalizations can be made as follows. Whole grains are good sources of vitamin B₆, as are bananas and, to a lesser extent, potatoes. Whereas whole-wheat flour is a good source of the vitamin, white flour is low (which reflects the relative lack of vitamin B₆ in the endosperm). The presence of glycosylated forms of PN in plants, particularly as PNG, complicates their nutritional evaluation. This is because dietary PNG exhibits only about 50% bioavailability in humans and it also exerts weak antagonistic effects on the utilization of non-glycosylated PN (Nakano *et al.*, 1997; Gregory, 1998). The content of PNG in plant foods varies widely, ranging, for example, from 5% in bananas to 75% in carrots as a fraction of total vitamin B₆. The overall bioavailability of vitamin B₆ in a mixed diet has been reported to be approximately 75% (Tarr *et al.*, 1981). In spite of the potential for lower bioavailability of vitamin B₆ in certain plant foods due to the presence of PNG and potential effects of fiber and cellular structure, there is little evidence that vegetarians with sufficiently varied diet and good total intake of the vitamin would be particularly at risk of insufficient vitamin B₆ status (Shultz and Leklem, 1987). However, individuals with marginal intake of total vitamin B₆ would be more prone to reduced nutritional status due to this incomplete bioavailability.

Whereas sources of vitamin B₆ in the US diet are distributed over a wide range of foods, breakfast cereals fortified with PN constitute an important source. Various fortified sports bars, meal-replacement products, and beverages also constitute major sources of vitamin B₆ intake in many individuals. Unlike thiamin, niacin, riboflavin, and folic acid, PN is not added to enriched flour and other enriched grain products.

Vitamin B₆ Disposition and Metabolic Function

The in vivo disposition of vitamin B₆ is summarized in Figure 20.2, which was adapted from McCormick (2006).

Uptake

Intestinal absorption of vitamin B₆ from dietary sources occurs both in the small intestine and from bacterial production in the large intestine. Uptake of dietary vitamin B₆ occurs primarily in the jejunum, with rate of absorption varying according to the B₆ species present (Hamm *et al.*, 1979; Mehansho *et al.*, 1979; Buss *et al.*, 1980). Glycosylated forms of vitamin B₆ found in plant foods are hydrolyzed partially by brush-border lactase-phlorizin hydrolase (Mackey *et al.*, 2004) prior to absorption. Some absorption of intact PNG also occurs, after which it may be partially hydrolyzed by β-glucosidase apparently in the kidney or excreted in the urine (Ink *et al.*, 1986; Gregory

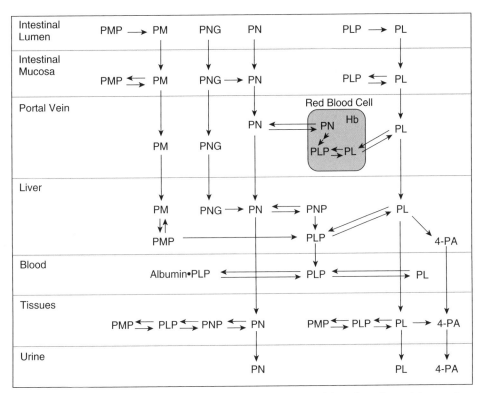

FIG. 20.2 In vivo disposition of ingested forms of vitamin B₆. PL, pyridoxal; PM, pyridoxamine; PN, pyridoxine; PLP, PMP, PNP, their respective phosphorylated forms; PNG, pyridoxine β-D-glucoside; 4-PA, 4-pyridoxic acid. Hb, hemoglobin.

et al., 1991; Nakano *et al.*, 1997). PMP and PLP usually are major vitamin B$_6$ species in animal products and also exist in lesser proportions in plant-derived foods. All such phosphorylated vitamers require dephosphorylation by alkaline phosphatase and other phosphatases prior to absorption. Kinetics reported in many studies are consistent with intestinal absorption of PL, PM, and PN by simple, non-saturable diffusion. However, evidence exists for carrier-mediated intestinal absorption of the vitamin, with rate of transport both pH dependent and saturable (Kozik and McCormick, 1984; Said *et al.*, 2008). Vitamin B$_6$ synthesized by the microflora in the human colon may be a secondary exogenous source available for absorption. Studies with mouse and human colonic cells have provided evidence of colonic absorption of vitamin B$_6$ (Said *et al.*, 2008). While the contribution of bacterially produced vitamin B$_6$ to overall nutritional status warrants further investigation, dietary intake certainly constitutes the major source of vitamin B$_6$ nutrition.

Phosphorylation catalyzed by pyridoxal kinase in the enterocytes provides metabolic trapping of the newly absorbed PL, PM, and PN (Mehansho *et al.*, 1979). The negative charge provided by the phosphate moiety hinders diffusion of the vitamin across the cell membrane and promotes protein binding. PNP, PMP, and PLP are dephosphorylated before crossing the basolateral membrane and entering portal circulation (Mehansho *et al.*, 1979). Uptake by the liver is facilitated by metabolic trapping.

The liver is at the core of vitamin B$_6$ metabolism. Whereas most tissues can phosphorylate PL, PN, and PM, the liver is the site where the various species of vitamin B$_6$ undergo interconversion to form PLP. The latter serves as the primary coenzymatic form of vitamin B$_6$ and is the major form of the vitamin in the body (Johansson *et al.*, 1974; Merrill *et al.*, 1984; Coburn *et al.*, 1988a). Upon absorption to the liver, the non-phosphorylated forms of vitamin B$_6$ are first phosphorylated by pyridoxal kinase, which uses zinc and ATP as cofactor and phosphoryl donor (Merrill *et al.*, 1984). Hepatic activity of pyridoxal kinase is ten-fold that of the phosphatase, therefore phosphorylated species of vitamin B$_6$ predominate (Merrill *et al.*, 1984). Binding of PLP to high-abundance PLP-dependent enzymes such as serine-hydroxymethyltransferase, aminotransferases and glycogen phosphorylase also renders PLP less accessible to phosphatases for dephosphorylation. The formation of PLP by oxidation of PNP and PMP occurs by the action of the flavin mononucleotide-dependent pyridoxine (pyridoxamine) phosphate oxidase (PNP–PMP oxidase) (Kazarinoff and McCormick, 1975; McCormick and Chen, 1999).

Transport

Vitamin B$_6$ is carried to organs and tissues primarily in plasma. There the main form is PLP and to a lesser extent PL, which are bound to albumin (Lumeng *et al.*, 1974a). In erythrocytes, PLP and PL are bound to hemoglobin (Mehansho and Henderson, 1980; Coburn *et al.*, 1988b). Tissue uptake of circulating plasma PLP requires prior removal of the 5′-phosphate group, whereas plasma PL is immediately available. The importance of alkaline phosphatase in vitamin B$_6$ metabolism is evident in the transport as well as in the initial absorption of the vitamin. Prior to uptake by tissue or transfer between cell compartments, membrane phosphatase converts PLP to PL (Van Hoof and de Broe, 1994). Metabolic trapping by phosphorylation, as seen in the enterocyte, is repeated in tissues in order to retain the vitamin.

Vitamin B$_6$ Metabolism and Role as a Coenzyme

The largest body pool of vitamin B$_6$ is in skeletal muscle, which constitutes 70–80% of the whole-body vitamin B$_6$ mainly as PLP associated with glycogen phosphorylase (Krebs and Fischer, 1964; Coburn, 1990). An analysis of the vitamin B$_6$ content of human muscle via biopsy estimated the total body pool in adult humans to be ~1000 µmol (~170 mg) (Coburn *et al.*, 1988a). Muscle concentration of vitamin B$_6$ has been found to be quite resilient to effects of dietary restriction and even supplementation, whereas plasma vitamin B$_6$ showed marked changes under the same conditions (Coburn *et al.*, 1991). Studies in rats have shown that muscle PLP concentration and glycogen phosphorylase activity decreased in response to a caloric deficit but not to dietary depletion of vitamin B$_6$ (Black *et al.*, 1978), but functional consequences of these findings are unclear.

The PLP molecule readily condenses with free amino groups of proteins and small molecules to form a Schiff base. As the coenzyme for aminotransferases and most other PLP-dependent enzymes, the pyridine ring and the C-4 carbonyl group enable PLP to facilitate many reactions involving amino acid substrates. In the absence of substrate, PLP is bound to an €-amino group of a specific lysine residue. In the case of aminotransferases, the binding of the incoming substrate amino acid to the enzyme-PLP complex allows migration of the PLP to yield a new Schiff base with the amino acid. Subsequent shifting of charge in this complex allows bond labilization at the α-carbon, with hydrolysis of the complex to release the keto acid product and concurrent generation of PMP. Schiff base formation of an alternate keto acid leads to an analogous process of charge transfer, bond labilization, and transfer of the NH$_2$ group from PMP (i.e. originally from the first substrate amino acid) to the keto acid to generate a new amino acid. See Figure 20.3 for a depiction of the mechanism by which the Schiff base formation labilizes the α-carbon bond of an amino acid.

Whereas this reactivity of PLP with lysyl residues of PLP-dependent enzymes and the α-amino groups of their substrates accounts for the primary coenzymatic mechanism of PLP, its ability to form such Schiff bases indiscriminately when present at higher concentrations probably explains why an over-accumulation of cellular PLP would have adverse effects. The body minimizes the risk of detrimental levels of PLP when vitamin B$_6$ intake is high by the combined action of phosphatases and oxidases. The strong inhibition of PNP–PMP oxidase by its product, PLP, retards accumulation of the latter (Merrill *et al.*, 1978). Dephosphorylation of the phosphorylated forms also contributes to cellular homeostasis of PLP by promoting vitamin B$_6$ turnover, through enhanced conversion of PL to a biologically inactive form, 4-pyridoxic acid (4-PA), with a carboxyl group at the 4′-carbon (Huff and Perlzweig, 1944). This irreversible conversion is known to occur in the liver, and has not been well examined in other tissues. Perfusion studies with isolated rat kidney have suggested that the kidney may also be a site of 4-PA production (Hamm *et al.*, 1980). 4-PA, the major vitamin B$_6$ catabolite, is then excreted in the urine.

PLP-dependent processes are involved either directly or indirectly in almost all phases of metabolism. Many processes in amino acid interconversion and catabolism involve PLP-dependent enzymes. Aside from playing important roles in amino acid metabolism, the formation of α-keto

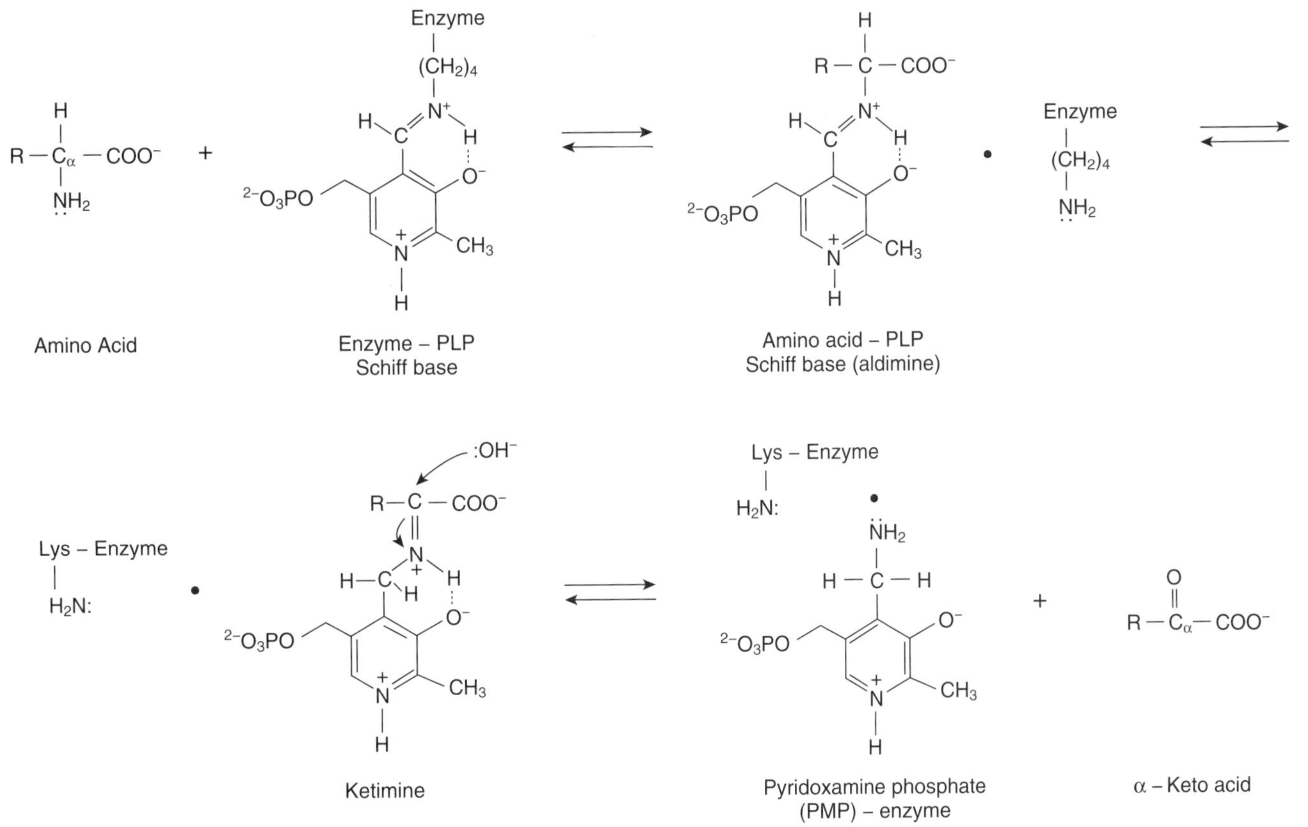

FIG. 20.3 Mechanism of bond labilization via Schiff-base formation in PLP-dependent transamination reactions.

acids constitutes an important anapleurotic process generating and interconverting metabolic intermediates. An indirect role of PLP in the metabolism of n-3 and n-6 fatty acids can be inferred from reported changes in fatty acid profiles during vitamin B$_6$ deficiency (Tsuge *et al.*, 2000); however, the biochemical mechanism is unknown.

Another important role of PLP-dependent enzymes is in the area of one-carbon metabolism which constitutes a collection of reactions in the folate cycle and methionine cycle that generate methyl groups (as S-adenosylmethionine), facilitate methionine recycling, and regulate homocysteine concentration, incorporate one-carbon units in thymidylate and purine synthesis, and provide synthesis of cysteine. Figure 20.4 illustrates the PLP-dependent reactions in the one-carbon pathway. Serine hydroxymethyltransferase (SHMT) isoforms exist

One-Carbon Metabolism

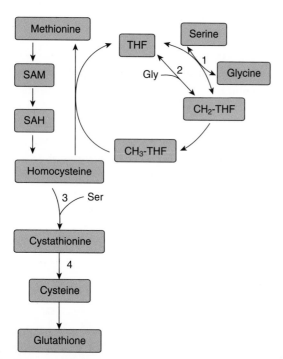

FIG. 20.4 PLP-dependent reactions in the one-carbon pathway. 1, Serine hydroxymethyltransferase; 2, glycine decarboxylase; 3, cystathionine β-synthase; 4, cystathionine γ-lyase. SAH, S-adenosylhomocysteine; SAM, adenosylmethionine; THF, tetrahydrofolate. PLP-dependent metabolism of serine, glycine, and cysteine not shown.

in both cytoplasm and mitochondria and catalyze the reversible reaction: glycine + 5,10-methylenetetrahydrofolate ⇔ serine + tetrahydrofolate. These reactions mediate vital components of cellular one-carbon metabolism by allowing the interconversion of serine and glycine as well as providing a means of supplying the folate one-carbon pool by generating 5,10-methylenetetrahydrofolate. The mitochondrial glycine cleavage system is a four-enzyme complex containing a PLP-dependent glycine decarboxylase. This glycine cleavage process has been shown to yield at least 20 times as much 5,10-methylenetetrahydrofolate as needed for methylation demands and to maintain glycine cleavage flux that far exceeds the rate of SHMT-catalyzed processes (Lamers *et al.*, 2009b). Stable isotopic tracer studies conducted before and after vitamin B$_6$ restriction in humans showed the resiliency of these critical processes in maintaining one-carbon metabolism (Davis *et al.*, 2005, 2006; Lamers *et al.*, 2009b).

PLP also serves as the coenzyme for both components of the transsulfuration pathway, which is responsible for the catabolism of homocysteine and the synthesis of cysteine. The first step, cystathionine β-synthase (CBS), exhibits allosteric stimulation by S-adenosylmethionine (SAM), and exhibits little change in activity as a result of moderate vitamin B$_6$ deficiency. The second enzyme, cystathionine γ-lyase (CGL), catalyzes the cleavage of cystathionine to form cysteine and α-aminobutyrate. CGL exhibits much greater susceptibility to loss of its PLP coenzyme during vitamin B$_6$ deficiency. Unexpectedly, cysteine production and cysteine concentration in tissue and plasma are maintained over a wide range of suboptimal levels of vitamin B$_6$ nutriture (Davis *et al.*, 2006; Lima *et al.*, 2006; Nijhout *et al.*, 2009) apparently because the greatly elevated cystathionine concentration tends to maintain CGL flux (Davis *et al.*, 2006).

Assessment of Vitamin B$_6$ Nutritional Status

Methods

Vitamin B$_6$ nutritional status can be measured by either direct or indirect methods. The most commonly used direct criterion is plasma PLP concentration, which is typically measured by the tyrosine decarboxylase assay or by HPLC. Plasma PLP has been shown to correlate well with tissue stores in rats (Lui *et al.*, 1985) and serves as a reasonable indicator of long-term vitamin B$_6$ nutritional status.

In spite of its widespread utility, plasma PLP may be influenced by factors other than vitamin B$_6$ intake that complicate its interpretation as a status indicator. These factors include pregnancy (Lumeng *et al.*, 1974b), age (Lee and Leklem, 1985), exercise (Manore *et al.*, 1987), sex (Manore *et al.*, 1989; Morris *et al.*, 2008), inflammation (Morris *et al.*, 2010), smoking (Ulvik *et al.*, 2010), and alcohol intake (Lumeng and Li, 1974). Whereas rigorous assessment of vitamin B$_6$ status is best accomplished when using an alternative indicator to accompany plasma PLP measurement, in practice such efforts are duplicative and rarely performed. Regardless, the complexity of plasma PLP data should be recognized.

Other direct measures of vitamin B$_6$ status include total plasma vitamin B$_6$, erythrocyte PLP, urinary 4-pyridoxic acid (4-PA), and total urinary vitamin B$_6$ excretion, all of which have been used widely in previous nutritional evaluations. Approximately 50% of total vitamin B$_6$ intake is excreted as urinary 4-PA. The measurement of urinary 4-PA as a nutritional status indicator is limited because it is influenced by both vitamin B$_6$ tissue stores and short-term dietary intake. Whereas assessments using urinary 4-PA generally involve burdensome complete 24-h urine collections, the validity of assays based on a 4-PA/creatinine ratio in untimed urine collections has been reported and may alleviate this issue (Schuster *et al.*, 1984). The value of plasma 4-PA measurements in vitamin B$_6$ status assessment requires further evaluation.

Indirect methods of vitamin B$_6$ status evaluate concentrations of metabolites or the activity of PLP-dependent enzymes. Before plasma PLP became the preferred method of vitamin B$_6$ status assessment, the tryptophan load test was widely used as a functional indicator of vitamin B$_6$ status (Leklem, 1990). The activity of kynureninase, a PLP-dependent enzyme involved in the catabolism of tryptophan, is decreased in vitamin B$_6$ deficiency, altering the flux of the pathway (Yess *et al.*, 1964). Following a 2-g oral bolus of tryptophan, metabolites can be measured in the urine. In vitamin B$_6$ deficiency, the urinary excretion of xanthurenic acid and other tryptophan metabolites is increased (Yess *et al.*, 1964). However, the tryptophan load test is not a highly specific measure of vitamin B$_6$ status as tryptophan metabolism can be affected by various factors including certain drugs.

The methionine load test, which involves a 3-g oral methionine load (Ubbink *et al.*, 1996), is similar to the tryptophan load test in that it measures the functioning of a vitamin B$_6$-dependent pathway. In effect, the methionine load test evaluates the balance of homocysteine production from the bolus of methionine versus the capacity for its metabolic clearance (Selhub, 1999). Under the conditions of this procedure, homocysteine remethylation is suppressed while homocysteine production is extensive. Thus, the methionine load test as applied to vitamin B$_6$ status assessment is a functional evaluation of the transsulfuration pathway of homocysteine catabolism. As stated above, both cystathionine β-synthase and cystathionine γ-lyase are PLP-dependent, with the latter highly subject to effects of inadequate vitamin B$_6$ status (Davis *et al.*, 2006; Lima *et al.*, 2006). In contrast to the utility of post-methionine-load plasma homocysteine as a diagnostic criterion of vitamin B$_6$ status, fasting plasma homocysteine is only weakly related to vitamin B$_6$ status (Selhub, 1999). Fasting plasma cystathionine also can be used as a functional biomarker of vitamin B$_6$ nutritional insufficiency. In vitamin B$_6$ deficiency, rat liver cystathionine and human plasma cystathionine exhibit elevation over a wide range of vitamin B$_6$ deficiency states ranging from marginal to severe (e.g. Stabler *et al.*, 1997; Davis *et al.*, 2006; Lima *et al.*, 2006). Further investigation and standardization of the use of cystathionine as a nutritional index is required. Elevation of plasma glycine also commonly occurs in vitamin B$_6$ deficiency but to a lesser extent than that of cystathionine.

Erythrocyte alanine aminotransferase (EALT) and aspartic aminotransferase (EAST) activity and stimulation can also be used to measure vitamin B$_6$ status indirectly. Coenzyme stimulation is the increase in enzyme activity following the addition of PLP in vitro, as vitamin B$_6$ deficiency increases the proportion of apoenzyme to holoenzyme in the erythrocyte. EALT and EAST are viewed as indicators of long-term vitamin B$_6$ status (Leklem, 1990). In principle one would expect that these coenzyme stimulation assays would correlate closely with erythrocyte PLP concentration.

Deficiency

Vitamin B$_6$ deficiency can contribute to adverse health effects because of the many metabolic roles played by PLP. Overt vitamin B$_6$ deficiency is rare in developed countries, but includes clinical manifestations such as microcytic anemia, convulsions, and dermatitis. PLP is a cofactor for δ-aminolevulinate synthase, the rate-limiting enzyme in heme biosynthesis. In vitamin B$_6$ deficiency, heme synthesis is depressed, which limits hemoglobin synthesis and leads to the production of smaller than normal red blood cells and a condition known as microcytic anemia (Verloop and Rademaker, 1960). PLP also is involved in the synthesis of neurotransmitters, such as δ-aminobutyric acid and serotonin. Depressed neurotransmitter levels have been observed in vitamin B$_6$-deficient animals (Paulose et al., 1988). PLP's role in neurotransmitter production may explain the seizures observed in infants fed vitamin B$_6$-deficient formula; administration of PN alleviated the problem (Nelson, 1956). The risk of all such disorders associated with vitamin B$_6$ deficiency would undoubtedly be affected by the vitamin B$_6$ intake relative to the requirement, the rate of depletion if associated with an abrupt change in intake, and the duration and extent of a chronic deficiency.

Vitamin B$_6$ deficiency can be caused by inadequate intake, impaired absorption, and inefficient conversion of absorbed forms of the vitamin to PLP (Merrill et al., 1984). Certain drugs, such as isoniazid (Cilliers et al., 2010), phenelzine (Stewart et al., 1984), dopamine (Weir et al., 1991), and gentamicin (Weir et al., 1990), bind to the carbonyl group of PLP or PL and can induce functional vitamin B$_6$ deficiency. Theophylline, an asthma drug, inhibits PL kinase, which interferes with PLP synthesis (Ubbink et al., 1990). The effect of oral contraceptives on vitamin B$_6$ status has been debated (Miller et al., 1975; Leklem, 1986; Miller, 1986), but several studies report significantly lower plasma PLP concentration in oral contraceptive users compared with non-users (Lumeng et al., 1974b; Lussana et al., 2003; Morris et al., 2008).

More relevant in developed countries is the issue of marginal vitamin B$_6$ status, which often is viewed as that associated with the range of plasma PLP concentration of 20–30 nmol/L. Though not accompanied by clinical symptoms of deficiency, marginal status may increase risk for chronic diseases such as cancer and cardiovascular disease. Studies involving controlled depletion of healthy adults frequently show changes in plasma amino acids, specifically mild elevation of glycine and a doubling of cystathionine concentration (Davis et al., 2006; Lamers et al., 2009b), and alterations in glutathione synthesis in certain individuals (Lamers et al., 2009a). Whereas this level of deficiency yields little or no elevation in fasting plasma homocysteine, a transient postprandial rise in homocysteine could occur. The relationship between these metabolic changes and disease processes remains unclear.

Abnormal electroencephalographic patterns were observed in women consuming a controlled diet providing less than 0.05 mg of vitamin B$_6$ per day having mean plasma PLP of 9.8 nmol/L (Kretsch et al., 1991). Therefore, plasma PLP concentrations of at least 10 nmol/L are suggested as a lower limit of nutritional adequacy based on this physiological criterion.

Toxicity

Pyridoxine supplements of over 500 mg/day have been reported to cause sensory neuropathy (Berger et al., 1992). In order to minimize this risk, the tolerable upper limit for vitamin B$_6$ has been set at 100 mg/day for adults (Institute of Medicine, 1998). This range far exceeds the formulation of typical multivitamin supplements that provide 2 mg/daily dose.

Several types of genetic disorders are vitamin B$_6$-responsive, and therapeutic vitamin B$_6$ supplementation is used in their management. These conditions include inborn errors that affect enzymes involved in the interconversion of vitamin B$_6$ isoforms, reduce absorption of vitamin B$_6$, or affect PLP-dependent enzymes; for example, pyridoxine-responsive anemia, cystathioniuria, and homocysteinuria (Clayton, 2006). Furthermore, certain inborn errors result in the generation of metabolites that inactivate PLP. Similar high doses of pyridoxine have been used therapeutically in pyridoxine-responsive disorders with few reports of toxic effects, although health-care professionals should be cognizant of risks of toxicity (Clayton, 2006).

Requirements

Many controlled dietary studies and observational investigations have concluded that vitamin B$_6$ intake and dietary protein intake (Miller et al., 1985; Hansen et al., 1996) are the most significant determinants of plasma PLP concentration. Plasma PLP concentrations appear to increase 12 nmol/L for every 1 mg/day increase in vitamin B$_6$ intake (Morris et al., 2008), whereas high protein intake lowers plasma PLP concentrations (Pannemans et al., 1994; Hansen et al., 1996). Extensive literature exists regarding the relationship between vitamin B$_6$ intake and various other indices of vitamin B$_6$ status such as urinary total vitamin B$_6$, urinary 4-PA, EALT and EAST activity and PLP stimulation, plasma total vitamin B$_6$, plasma 4-PA, plasma PLP, and the methionine and tryptophan load tests. However, none of these provides the truly functional information from a biochemical or physiological basis on which to base the absolute requirement. As mentioned earlier, the observation of altered electroencephalographic patterns in a vitamin B$_6$ depletion study that induced plasma PLP ~10 nmol/L provides evidence of a functional inadequacy in this very low and undoubtedly inadequate range.

As reviewed previously (Institute of Medicine, 1998), many studies have shown that plasma PLP values in the range of 20–30 nmol/L are common and have not been associated with obvious health effects. Leklem (1990) recommended that 30 nmol/L plasma PLP be viewed as indicative of the lower end of the normal range of vitamin B$_6$ status, and the range of 20–30 nmol/L has been considered as marginal deficiency (Leklem, 1999; Gregory, 2001). The Institute of Medicine used a cutoff of 20 nmol/L on which to base the estimated average requirement (EAR) and commented that even this conservative criterion may overestimate the actual requirement for half of the population on the basis of health maintenance (Institute of Medicine, 1998). In spite of this conservative view on which the current RDA is based, the dilemma remains how to define the requirement in the absence of obvious causal relationships between vitamin B$_6$ and health. The revision of an RDA based on a 30 nmol/L plasma PLP cutoff would provide greater assurance of adequacy as indicated by the biochemical effects of marginal status and growing associations between marginal vitamin B$_6$ status and chronic disease. The current recommended dietary allowances (RDA) for vitamin B$_6$ across the lifespan are given in Table 20.1.

Recent NHANES data estimate average vitamin B$_6$ intake in the US to be 1.86 mg/day for non-users of dietary supplements and 1.94 mg/day for supplement users (Morris et al., 2008). Relative to the vitamin B$_6$ RDA of 1.3 mg/day for adults, this suggests adequate intake by most of the population, with the exception of lower percentiles. However, measurement of plasma PLP revealed concentrations <20 nmol/L in all subgroups examined, which suggests that the current RDA may be insufficient. These data also showed at-risk populations, such as the elderly, blacks, and oral contraceptive users, that may require above 3–4.9 mg/day to maintain adequate plasma PLP concentrations (Morris et al., 2008). The reason for the large discrepancy between these observations and those based on controlled dietary studies has not been determined.

Vitamin B$_6$ in Health and Disease

The lower ranges of vitamin B$_6$ intake, especially among women, are well below recommended levels, and this marginal range is associated with increased risk of cardiovascular disease, stroke, and venous thrombosis. These lower ranges also have been associated recently with incidence of certain cancers. At present the key word is association: the mechanistic connections (if any) between low vitamin B$_6$ status and chronic disease remain to be determined.

Chronically inadequate vitamin B$_6$ nutritional status has been associated with aberrant one-carbon metabolism and health. Suboptimal vitamin B$_6$ nutriture was first associated with vascular disease in monkeys (Rinehart and Greenberg, 1949), a relationship confirmed in human epidemiological studies. Verhoef et al. (1996) reported that the frequency of myocardial infarction was negatively associated with both folate and vitamin B$_6$ nutriture. Rimm et al. (1998) confirmed these findings in the Nurses' Health Study. Women in the highest quintile of B$_6$, folate, or folate plus B$_6$ intake had less coronary heart disease than those in the lowest quintile of each intake category. An Italian study (Friso et al., 2004) also reported an independent association of low plasma PLP concentration with coronary artery disease risk. Dalery et al. (1995) described the results of large trials examining plasma PLP concentration and risk of vascular disease. Even in healthy control subjects, low folate or B$_6$ status increased the risk of vascular disease, and risk of vascular disease in low vitamin B$_6$ status was independent of plasma homocysteine concentration. Kelly et al. observed that low vitamin B$_6$ status (plasma PLP <30 nmol/L) was associated with more than a two-fold increase in risk of stroke or transient ischemic attack (Kelly et al., 2003, 2004) independent of folate

TABLE 20.1 Current recommended dietary allowances for vitamin B$_6$

Life stage and age		Amount (mg/day)	
		Female	Male
Infants	0–5 months	0.1	0.1
	6–11 months	0.3	0.3
Children	1–3 years	0.5	0.5
	4–6 years	0.6	0.6
	7–9 years	1.0	1.0
	10–18 years	1.2	1.3
Adults	19–50 years	1.3	1.3
	>50 years	1.5	1.7
Pregnancy		1.9	
Lactation		2.0	

status or plasma total homocysteine (tHcy). Further, a prospective study has shown that people with plasma PLP <23.3 nmol/L had 1.8-fold higher recurrent risk of venous thromboembolism than those with PLP >23.3 nmol/L (Hron *et al.*, 2007). In spite of the strength of these associations, acute supplementation trials with mixed folic acid, vitamin B$_{12}$ and vitamin B$_6$ (e.g. Albert *et al.*, 2008; Hankey *et al.*, 2010) or pyridoxine alone compared with mixed vitamins (e.g. Ebbing *et al.*, 2008, 2010) for *secondary* prevention (i.e. preventing *recurrence* of cardiovascular disease) have yielded largely negative results.

The mechanism by which low vitamin B$_6$ intake is associated with risk of vascular disease is not known. Since vitamin B$_6$ deficiency has little tendency to raise fasting plasma total homocysteine and primarily yields an elevation following a methionine load, low B$_6$ nutriture may lead to repeated transient mild hyperhomocysteinemia following meal consumption.

Several reports of associations between elevated plasma C-reactive protein (CRP) and low vitamin B$_6$ status have raised the hypothesis that systemic inflammation is prone to occur during vitamin B$_6$ deficiency or contributes to low B$_6$ status (Friso *et al.*, 2001; Morris *et al.*, 2010). The mechanism behind this association is unclear because controlled dietary restriction of vitamin B$_6$ in healthy adults does not cause a change in CRP (Davis *et al.*, 2006). In light of the reports of a relationship between CRP, vascular disease, and low vitamin B$_6$ status in observational studies such as NHANES (Morris *et al.*, 2010), it appears that vitamin B$_6$ deficiency alone is not an inflammatory condition, but the deficiency may predispose an individual to the effects of other inflammatory processes. Alternatively, inflammation may lead to tissue-specific deficiency (Chiang *et al.*, 2005) by altering vitamin B$_6$ cellular metabolism, turnover or transport. Altered glutathione metabolism (Lima *et al.*, 2006; Lamers *et al.*, 2009a) may be one such metabolic connection between impaired vitamin B$_6$ status and inflammatory response. These questions indicate the need for a more thorough understanding of the metabolic changes occurring in low vitamin B$_6$ status, inflammatory conditions, and disease risk.

A linkage between vitamin B$_6$ status and certain aspects of cancer risk has also been reported. For example, a meta-analysis evaluated prospective studies and found a significant inverse relationship between plasma PLP concentration and colorectal cancer risk (Larsson *et al.*, 2010). In this study, the evidence was less conclusive regarding vitamin B$_6$ intake and risk, possibly as a result of greater uncer-

tainty in assessing vitamin B$_6$ consumption patterns. Risk of lung cancer also has been shown to be inversely associated with plasma PLP concentration (Johansson *et al.*, 2010). Little consistent evidence of other connections between vitamin B$_6$ and cancer has been reported, and further investigation is needed.

Future Directions

Vitamin B$_6$ is a family of related compounds consisting of pyridoxine, pyridoxal, pyridoxamine, and their 5'-phosphates. Fruits and vegetables also contain pyridoxine β-D-glucoside in variable and often substantial amounts. The development of more complete food composition tables would improve dietary assessment by accounting for differences in bioavailability among various dietary forms of the vitamin.

The development of a better understanding of the linkage between vitamin B$_6$ nutritional status and disease susceptibility is an important need. Smaller scale controlled mechanistic studies examining connections of metabolomic patterns, dietary intake, genetics, and in vivo kinetics may help in the development of diagnostic tools and biomarkers for use in larger population studies.

Understanding vitamin B$_6$ nutrition on a personalized level will be important in assessing optimal intakes and consequences of deficiency. For example, how do genetic and nutritional factors interact to define an individual's health and susceptibility to chronic disease?

Further characterization of the interaction of inflammatory processes and vitamin B$_6$ status may be an important key in understanding optimal nutrition and in interpreting biomarkers such as plasma PLP and CRP.

It is also important to determine the role of vitamin supplementation and food fortification in human health, specifically with respect to primary prevention of cardiovascular and other forms of chronic disease.

Suggestions for Further Reading
Clarke, R., Halsey, J., Bennett, D., *et al.* (2011) Homocysteine and vascular disease: review of published results of the homocysteine-lowering trials. *J Inher Metab Dis* **34**, 83–91.
Coburn, S.P. (1996) Modeling vitamin B6 metabolism. *Adv Food Nutr Res* **40**, 107–132.

Ebbing, M., Bønaa, K.H., and Arnesen, E. (2010) Combined analyses and extended follow-up of two randomized controlled homocysteine-lowering B-vitamin trials. *J Int Med* **268**, 367–382.

Gregory, J.F. (1997) Bioavailability of vitamin B-6. *Eur J Clin Nutr* **51**, S43–S48.

Gregory, J.F. (1998) Nutritional properties and significance of vitamin glycosides. *Annu Rev Nutr* **18**, 277–296.

Gyorgy, P. (1956) The history of vitamin B6. *Am J Clin Nutr* **4**, 313–317.

Institute of Medicine (1998) *DRI Reference Intakes for Thiamin, Riboflavin, Niacin, Vitamin B$_6$, Folate, Vitamin B$_{12}$, Pantothenic Acid, Biotin, and Choline.* National Academy Press, Washington, DC.

Morris, M.S., Picciano, M.F., Jacques, P.F., et al. (2008) Plasma pyridoxal 5′-phosphate in the US population: the National Health and Nutrition Examination Survey, 2003–2004. *Am J Clin Nutr* **87**, 1446–1454.

Nijhout, H.F., Reed, M.C., and Ulrich, C.M. (2008) Mathematical models of folate-mediated one-carbon metabolism. *Vitam Horm* **79**, 45–82.

Snell, E.E. (1990). Vitamin-B6 and decarboxylation of histidine. *Ann NY Acad Sci* **585**, 1–12.

References

Albert, C.M., Cook, N.R., Gaziano, J.M., et al. (2008) Effect of folic acid and B vitamins on risk of cardiovascular events and total mortality among women at high risk for cardiovascular disease – a randomized trial. *JAMA* **299**, 2027–2036.

Beaton, J.R., Beare, J.L., and McHenry, E.W. (1952) Factors affecting the development of acrodynia in pyridoxine-deficient rats. *J Nutr* **48**, 325–334.

Berger, A.R., Schaumburg, H.H., Schroeder, C., et al. (1992) Dose response, coasting, and differential fiber vulnerability in human toxic neuropathy: a prospective study of pyridoxine neurotoxicity. *Neurology* **42**, 1367–1370.

Black, A.L., Guirard, B.M., and Snell, E.E. (1978) Behavior of muscle phosphorylase as a reservoir for vitamin-B6 in rat. *J Nutr* **108**, 670–677.

Buss, D.D., Hamm, M.W., Mehansho, H., et al. (1980) Transport and metabolism of pyridoxine in the perfused small-intestine and the hindlimb of the rat. *J Nutr* **110**, 1665–1663.

Chiang, E.P., Smith, D.E., Selhub, J., et al. (2005) Inflammation causes tissue-specific depletion of vitamin B6. *Arthritis Res Ther* **7**, R1254–1262.

Cilliers, K., Labadarios, D., Schaaf, H.S., et al. (2010) Pyridoxal-5-phosphate plasma concentrations in children receiving tuberculosis chemotherapy including isoniazid. *Acta Paediatr* **99**, 705–710.

Clayton, P.T. (2006) B6-responsive disorders: a model of vitamin dependency. *J Inher Metab Dis* **29**, 317–326.

Coburn, S.P. (1990) Location and turnover of vitamin B6 pools and vitamin B6 requirements of humans. *Ann NY Acad Sci* **585**, 76–85.

Coburn, S.P., Lewis, D.L.N., Fink, W.J., et al. (1988a) Human vitamin-B-6 pools estimated through muscle biopsies. *Am J Clin Nutr* **48**, 291–294.

Coburn, S.P., Mahuren, J.D., Kennedy, M.S., et al. (1988b) B6 vitamer content of rat tissues measured by isotope tracer and chromatographic methods. *Biofactors* **1**, 307–312.

Coburn, S.P., Ziegler, P.J., Costill, D.L., et al. (1991) Response of vitamin-B6 content of muscle to changes in vitamin-B6 intake in men. *Am J Clin Nutr* **53**, 1436–1442.

Dalery, K., Lussiercacan, S., Selhub, J., et al. (1995) Homocysteine and coronary-artery disease in French-Canadian subjects – relation with vitamins B-12, B-6, pyridoxal-phosphate, and folate. *Am J Cardiol* **75**, 1107–1111.

Davis, S.R., Quinlivan, E.P., Stacpoole, P.W., et al. (2006) Plasma glutathione and cystathionine concentrations are elevated but cysteine flux is unchanged by dietary vitamin B-6 restriction in young men and women. *J Nutr* **136**, 373–378.

Davis, S.R., Scheer, J.B., Quinlivan, E.P., et al. (2005) Dietary vitamin B-6 restriction does not alter rates of homocysteine remethylation or synthesis in healthy young women and men. *Am J Clin Nutr* **81**, 648–655.

Ebbing, M., Bleie, O., Ueland, P.M., et al. (2008) Mortality and cardiovascular events in patients treated with homocysteine-lowering B vitamins after coronary angiography – a randomized controlled trial. *JAMA* **300**, 795–804.

Ebbing, M., Bonaa, K.H., Arnesen, E., et al. (2010) Combined analyses and extended follow-up of two randomized controlled homocysteine-lowering B-vitamin trials. *J Intern Med* **268**, 367–382.

Friso, S., Girelli, D., Martinelli, N., et al. (2004) Low plasma vitamin B-6 concentrations and modulation of coronary artery disease risk. *Am J Clin Nutr* **79**, 992–998.

Friso, S., Jacques, P.F., Wilson, P.W.F., et al. (2001) Low circulating vitamin B-6 is associated with elevation of the inflammation marker C-reactive protein independently of plasma homocysteine levels. *Circulation* **103**, 2788–2791.

Gregory, J.F. (1997) Bioavailability of vitamin B-6. *Eur J Clin Nutr* **51**, S43–S48.

Gregory, J.F. (1998) Nutritional properties and significance of vitamin glycosides. *Annu Rev Nutr* **18**, 277–296.

Gregory, J.F. (2001) Vitamin B6 deficiency. In R. Carmel and D.W. Jacobsen (eds), *Homocysteine in Health and Disease.* Cambridge University Press, Cambridge, pp. 307–320.

Gregory, J.F. (2007) Vitamins. In S.P.K. Damodaran, K.L. Parkin, and O.R. Fennema (eds), *Fennema's Food Chemistry*, 4th Edn. CRC Press, Boca Raton, FL.

Gregory, J.F., Trumbo, P.R., Bailey, L.B., *et al.* (1991) Bioavailability of pyridoxine-5'-beta-d-glucoside determined in humans by stable-isotopic methods. *J Nutr* **121**, 177–186.

Gyorgy, P. (1956) The history of vitamin B6. *Am J Clin Nutr* **4**, 313–317.

Hamm, M.W., Mehansho, H., and Henderson, L.M. (1979) Transport and metabolism of pyridoxamine and pyridoxamine phosphate in the small-intestine of the rat. *J Nutr* **109**, 1552–1559.

Hamm, M.W., Mehansho, H., and Henderson, L.M. (1980) Management of pyridoxine and pyridoxal in the isolated kidney of the rat. *J Nutr* **110**, 1597–1609.

Hankey, G.J., Eikelboom, J.W., Baker, R.I., *et al.* (2010) B vitamins in patients with recent transient ischaemic attack or stroke in the VITAmins TO Prevent Stroke (VITATOPS) trial: a randomised, double-blind, parallel, placebo-controlled trial. *Lancet Neurol* **9**, 855–865.

Hansen, C.M., Leklem, J.E., and Miller, L.T. (1996) Vitamin B-6 status of women with a constant intake of vitamin B-6 changes with three levels of dietary protein. *J Nutr* **126**, 1891–1901.

Hron, G., Lombardi, R., Eichinger, S., *et al.* (2007) Low vitamin B6 levels and the risk of recurrent venous thromboembolism. *Haematologica* **92**, 1250–1253.

Huff, J.W. and Perlzweig, W.A. (1944) A product of oxidative metabolism of pyridoxine, 2-methyl-3-hydroxy-4-carboxy-5-hydroxymethylpyridine (4-pyridoxic acid) I. Isolation from urine, structure, and synthesis. *J Biol Chem* **155**, 345–355.

Ink, S.L., Gregory, J.F., and Sartain, D.B. (1986) Determination of vitamin-B6 bioavailability in animal-tissues using intrinsic and extrinsic labeling in the rat. *J Agric Food Chem* **34**, 998–1004.

Institute of Medicine (1998) Vitamin B6. *Dietary Reference Intakes for Thiamin, Riboflavin, Niacin, Vitamin B$_6$, Folate, Vitamin B$_{12}$, Pantothenic Acid, Biotin, and Choline.* National Academy Press, Washington, DC.

Johansson, M., Relton, C., Ueland, P.M., *et al.* (2010) Serum B vitamin levels and risk of lung cancer. *JAMA* **303**, 2377–2385.

Johansson, S., Lindsted, S., and Tiselius, H.G. (1974) Metabolic interconversions of different forms of vitamin-B6. *J Biol Chem* **249**, 6040–6046.

Kazarinoff, M.N. and McCormick, D.B. (1975) Rabbit liver pyridoxamine (pyridoxine) 5'-phosphate oxidase – purification and properties. *J Biol Chem* **250**, 3436–3442.

Kelly, P.J., Kistler, J.P., Shih, V.E., *et al.* (2004) Inflammation, homocysteine, and vitamin B6 status after ischemic stroke. *Stroke* **35**, 12–15.

Kelly, P.J., Shih, V.E., Kistler, J.P., *et al.* (2003) Low vitamin B6 but not homocyst(e)ine is associated with increased risk of stroke and transient ischemic attack in the era of folic acid grain fortification. *Stroke* **34**, E51–E54.

Kozik, A. and McCormick, D.B. (1984) Mechanism of pyridoxine uptake by isolated rat-liver cells. *Arch Biochem Biophys* **229**, 187–193.

Krebs, E.G. and Fischer, E.H. (1964) Phosphorylase and related enzymes of glycogen metabolism. *Vitam Horm* **22**, 399–410.

Kretsch, M.J., Sauberlich, H.E., and Newbrun, E. (1991) Electroencephalographic changes and periodontal status during short-term vitamin B-6 depletion of young, nonpregnant women. *Am J Clin Nutr* **53**, 1266–1274.

Lamers, Y., O'Rourke, B., Gilbert, L.R., *et al.* (2009a) Vitamin B-6 restriction tends to reduce the red blood cell glutathione synthesis rate without affecting red blood cell or plasma glutathione concentrations in healthy men and women. *Am J Clin Nutr* **90**, 336–343.

Lamers, Y., Williamson, J., Ralat, M., *et al.* (2009b) Moderate dietary vitamin B-6 restriction raises plasma glycine and cystathionine concentrations while minimally affecting the rates of glycine turnover and glycine cleavage in healthy men and women. *J Nutr* **139**, 452–460.

Larsson, S.C., Orsini, N., and Wolk, A. (2010) Vitamin B-6 and risk of colorectal cancer a meta-analysis of prospective studies. *JAMA* **303**, 1077–1083.

Lee, C.M. and Leklem, J.E. (1985) Differences in vitamin B6 status indicator responses between young and middle-aged women fed constant diets with two levels of vitamin B6. *Am J Clin Nutr* **42**, 226–234.

Leklem, J.E. (1986) Vitamin B-6 requirement and oral contraceptive use – a concern? *J Nutr* **116**, 475–477.

Leklem, J.E. (1990) Vitamin-B6 – a status report. *J Nutr* **120**, 1503–1507.

Leklem, J.E. (1999) Vitamin B6. In M. Shils, J. Olson, and M. Shike (eds), *Modern Nutrition in Health and Disease*, 9th Edn. Lea and Febinger, Philadelphia.

Lima, C.P., Davis, S.R., Mackey, A.D., *et al.* (2006) Vitamin B-6 deficiency suppresses the hepatic transsulfuration pathway but increases glutathione concentration in rats fed AIN-76a or AIN-93g diets. *J Nutr* **136**, 2141–2147.

Lui, A., Lumeng, L., Aronoff, G.R., *et al.* (1985) Relationship between body store of vitamin-B6 and plasma pyridoxal-p clearance – metabolic balance studies in humans. *J Lab Clin Med* **106**, 491–497.

Lumeng, L. and Li, T.K. (1974) Vitamin B6 metabolism in chronic alcohol abuse. Pyridoxal phosphate levels in plasma and the effects of acetaldehyde on pyridoxal phosphate synthesis and degradation in human erythrocytes. *J Clin Invest* **53**, 693–704.

Lumeng, L., Brashear, R.E., and Li, T.K. (1974a) Pyridoxal 5′-phosphate in plasma – source, protein-binding, and cellular transport. *J Lab Clin Med* **84**, 334–343.

Lumeng, L., Cleary, R.E., and Li, T.K. (1974b) Effect of oral contraceptives on the plasma concentration of pyridoxal phosphate. *Am J Clin Nutr* **27**, 326–333.

Lussana, F., Zighetti, M.L., Bucciarelli, P., *et al.* (2003) Blood levels of homocysteine, folate, vitamin B-6 and B-12 in women using oral contraceptives compared to non-users. *Thromb Res* **112**, 37–41.

Mackey, A.D., McMahon, R.J., Townsend, J.H., *et al.* (2004) Uptake, hydrolysis, and metabolism of pyridoxine-5′-beta-D-glucoside in Caco-2 cells. *J Nutr* **134**, 842–846.

Manore, M., Leklem, J., and Walter, M. (1987) Vitamin B-6 metabolism as affected by exercise in trained and untrained women fed diets differing in carbohydrate and vitamin B-6 content. *Am J Clin Nutr* **46**, 995–1004.

Manore, M.M., Vaughan, L.A., Carroll, S.S., *et al.* (1989) Plasma pyridoxal 5′-phosphate concentration and dietary vitamin B-6 intake in free-living, low-income elderly people. *Am J Clin Nutr* **50**, 339–345.

McCormick, D.B. (2006) Vitamin B6. In B.A. Bowman and R.M. Russell (eds), *Present Knowledge in Nutrition*, 7th Edn. ILSI Press, International Life Sciences Institute, Washington, DC.

McCormick, D.B. and Chen, H.Y. (1999) Update on interconversions of vitamin B-6 with its coenzyme. *J Nutr* **129**, 325–327.

Mehansho, H. and Henderson, L.M. (1980) Transport and accumulation of pyridoxine and pyridoxal by erythrocytes. *J Biol Chem* **255**, 1901–1907.

Mehansho, H., Hamm, M.W., and Henderson, L.V.M. (1979) Transport and metabolism of pyridoxal and pyridoxal-phosphate in the small-intestine of the rat. *J Nutr* **109**, 1542–1551.

Merrill, A.H., Henderson, J.M., Wang, E., *et al.* (1984) Metabolism of vitamin-B6 by human liver. *J Nutr* **114**, 1664–1674.

Merrill, A.H., Horiike, K., and McCormick, D.B. (1978) Evidence for regulation of pyridoxal 5′-phosphate formation in liver by pyridoxamine (pyridoxine) 5′-phosphate oxidase. *Biochem Biophys Res Commun* **83**, 984–990.

Miller, L.T. (1986) Do oral contraceptive agents affect nutrient requirements – vitamin B-6? *J Nutr* **116**, 1344–1345.

Miller, L.T., Johnson, A., Benson, E.M., *et al.* (1975) Effect of oral contraceptives and pyridoxine on the metabolism of vitamin B6 and on plasma tryptophan and alpha-amino nitrogen. *Am J Clin Nutr* **28**, 846–853.

Miller, L.T., Leklem, J.E., and Shultz, E.D. (1985) The effect of dietary protein on the metabolism of vitamin B-6 in humans. *J Nutr* **83**, 1663–1672.

Morris, M.S., Picciano, M.F., Jacques, P.F., *et al.* (2008) Plasma pyridoxal 5′-phosphate in the US population: the National Health and Nutrition Examination Survey, 2003–2004. *Am J Clin Nutr* **87**, 1446–1454.

Morris, M.S., Sakakeeny, L., Jacques, P.F., *et al.* (2010) Vitamin B-6 intake is inversely related to, and the requirement is affected by, inflammation status. *J Nutr* **140**, 103–110.

Nakano, H., McMahon, L.G., and Gregory, J.F. (1997) Pyridoxine-5′-beta-D-glucoside exhibits incomplete bioavailability as a source of vitamin B-6 and partially inhibits the utilization of co-ingested pyridoxine in humans. *J Nutr* **127**, 1508–1513.

Nelson, E.M. (1956) Association of vitamin B6 deficiency with convulsions in infants. *Public Health Rep* **71**, 445–448.

Nijhout, H.F., Gregory, J.F., Fitzpatrick, C., *et al.* (2009) A mathematical model gives insights into the effects of vitamin B-6 deficiency on 1-carbon and glutathione metabolism. *J Nutr* **139**, 784–791.

Pannemans, D.L., Van Den Berg, H., and Westerterp, K.R. (1994) The influence of protein intake on vitamin B-6 metabolism differs in young and elderly humans. *J Nutr* **124**, 1207–1214.

Paulose, C., Dakshinamurti, K., Packer, S., *et al.* (1988) Sympathetic stimulation and hypertension in the pyridoxine-deficient adult rat. *Hypertension* **11**, 387–391.

Rimm, E.B., Willett, W.C., Hu, F.B., *et al.* (1998) Folate and vitamin B-6 from diet and supplements in relation to risk of coronary heart disease among women. *JAMA* **279**, 359–364.

Rinehart, J.F. and Greenberg, L.D. (1949) Arteriosclerotic lesions in pyridoxine-deficient monkeys. *Am J Pathol* **25**, 481–491.

Said, Z.M., Subramanian, V.S., Vaziri, N.D., *et al.* (2008) Pyridoxine uptake by colonocytes: a specific and regulated carrier-mediated process. *Am J Physiol Cell Physiol* **294**, C1192–C1197.

Schuster, K., Bailey, L., Cerda, J., *et al.* (1984) Urinary 4-pyridoxic acid excretion in 24-hour versus random urine samples as a measurement of vitamin B6 status in humans. *Am J Clin Nutr* **39**, 466–470.

Selhub, J. (1999) Homocysteine metabolism. *Annu Rev Nutr* **19**, 217–246.

Shultz, T.D. and Leklem, J.E. (1987) Vitamin-B6 status and bioavailability in vegetarian women *Am J Clin Nutr* **46**, 647–651.

Snell, E.E. (1990) Vitamin-B6 and decarboxylation of histidine. *Ann NY Acad Sci* **585**, 1–12.

Stabler, S.P., Sampson, D.A., Wang, L.P., *et al.* (1997) Elevations of serum cystathionine and total homocysteine in pyridoxine-, folate-, and cobalamin-deficient rats. *J Nutr Biochem* **8**, 279–289.

Stewart, J.W., Harrison, W., Quitkin, F., *et al.* (1984) Phenelzine-induced pyridoxine deficiency. *J Clin Psychopharmacol* **4,** 225–226.

Tarr, J.B., Tamura, T., and Stokstad, E.L.R. (1981) Availability of vitamin-B6 and pantothenate in an average American diet in man. *Am J Clin Nutr* **34,** 1328–1337.

Tsuge, H., Hotta, N., and Hayakawa, T. (2000) Effects of vitamin B-6 on (n-3) polyunsaturated fatty acid metabolism. *J Nutr* **130,** 333S–334S.

Ubbink, J.B., Delport, R., Bissbort, S., *et al.* (1990) Relationship between vitamin B-6 status and elevated pyridoxal kinase levels induced by theophylline therapy in humans. *J Nutr* **120,** 1352–1359.

Ubbink, J.B., Van Der Merwe, A., Delport, R., *et al.* (1996) The effect of a subnormal vitamin B-6 status on homocysteine metabolism. *J Clin Invest* **98,** 177–184.

Ulvik, A., Ebbing, M., Hustad, S., *et al.* (2010) Long- and short-term effects of tobacco smoking on circulating concentrations of B vitamins. *Clin Chem* **56,** 755–763.

Van Hoof, V.O. and De Broe, M.E. (1994) Interpretation and clinical significance of alkaline-phosphatase isoenzyme patterns. *Crit Rev Clin Lab Sci* **31,** 197–293.

Verhoef, P., Stampfer, M.J., Buring, J.F., *et al.* (1996) Homocysteine metabolism and risk of myocardial infarction: relation with vitamins B6, B12, and folate. *Am J Epidemiol* **143,** 845–859.

Verloop, M.C. and Rademaker, W. (1960) Anaemia due to pyridoxine deficiency in man. *Br J Haematol* **6,** 66–80.

Weir, M.R., Keniston, R.C., Enriquez, J.I., Sr, *et al.* (1990) Depression of vitamin B6 levels due to gentamicin. *Vet Hum Toxicol* **32,** 235–238.

Weir, M.R., Keniston, R.C., Enriquez, J.I., Sr, *et al.* (1991) Depression of vitamin B6 levels due to dopamine. *Vet Hum Toxicol* **33,** 118–121.

Yess, N., Price, J.M., Brown, R.R., *et al.* (1964) Vitamin B6 depletion in man: urinary excretion of tryptophan metabolites. *J Nutr* **84,** 229–236.

21

FOLATE

LYNN B. BAILEY[1], PhD AND MARIE A. CAUDILL[2], PhD, RD

[1]*University of Georgia, Athens, Georgia, USA*
[2]*Cornell University, Ithaca, New York, USA*

Summary

Key metabolic reactions involving the transfer and acceptance of one-carbon entities are dependent on folate consumed as polyglutamyl food folate or as monoglutamyl synthetic folic acid in fortified foods or supplements. Intestinal absorption of folate vitamers involves deconjugation, if in the polyglutamyl form, followed by absorption of the monoglutamate form primarily by the proton-coupled folate transporter (PCFT). Circulating folate is free or bound to proteins prior to cellular uptake by specific transporters. Intracellular folate is converted to a series of coenzymes whose functions include the acceptance and donation of one-carbon (1-C) entities critical to nucleotide and amino acid synthesis as well as numerous regulatory and structural compounds. Genetic variants of the genes involved in the synthesis and regulation of folate metabolism may lead to metabolic abnormalities which have been linked in some cases with disease and birth-defect risk, particularly under conditions of sub-optimal folate status. Alcohol and specific drugs are recognized to impair folate metabolism, increasing the risk for folate deficiency. Folate intake recommendations consider differences in the bioavailability of folate which vary depending on the source (naturally occurring food folate or folic acid in fortified foods). A special folic acid intake recommendation coupled with folic acid fortification in the US (and numerous other countries globally) are specifically designed to reduce the risk of neural tube defects (NTDs). Evolving research studies have linked folate status/metabolism to key congenital and chronic diseases and have defined a challenging research agenda to address unanswered questions.

Introduction

Folate is a generic term for this water-soluble vitamin and includes naturally occurring food folate and synthetic folic acid in supplements and fortified foods. Folate coenzymes function in the acceptance and transfer of 1-C moieties involved in the synthesis, interconversion, and modification of nucleotides, amino acids, and other cellular components. This chapter provides a review of current knowledge related to folate mediated 1-C metabolism. Factors that may cause metabolic abnormalities in folate mediated 1-C metabolism including inadequate folate intake, incomplete bioavailability of folate, and folate-related genetic polymorphisms are discussed. The chapter

Present Knowledge in Nutrition, Tenth Edition. Edited by John W. Erdman Jr, Ian A. Macdonald and Steven H. Zeisel.
© 2012 International Life Sciences Institute. Published 2012 by John Wiley & Sons, Inc.

also provides an overview of current knowledge regarding the interactions between the physiological, biochemical, and genetic aspects of folate metabolism coupled with an extrapolation to human health including developmental abnormalities and chronic disease. In addition, folate–alcohol/drug interactions, dietary folate intake recommendations, folate status assessment, current estimates of intake and blood concentrations, and issues related to folic acid safety are highlighted.

Chemistry and Sources

Common structural features of the folate family include a pteridine bicyclic ring system, p-aminobenzoic acid, and one or more glutamic acid residues (Figure 21.1). Naturally occurring food folates are present in the reduced, tetrahydrofolate (THF) form and typically have side chains com-

posed of five to eight glutamate residues joined in γ-peptide linkages. Folic acid, the fully oxidized monoglutamate synthetic form of the vitamin, is found in fortified foods and supplements but rarely occurs in nature. Reduction of the pteridine moiety to dihydrofolate (DHF) and THF, elongation of the glutamate chain, and acquisition of single carbons on the N-5, N-10, or both positions are required for folate to participate in cellular 1-C metabolism (Shane, 2009). The 1-C substituted folates exist with methyl (CH₃), methylene (–CH₂–), methenyl (–CH=), formyl (–CH=O), or formimino (–CH=NH) groups mainly in the polyglutamyl form of the THF molecule.

Naturally occurring dietary folate is concentrated in foods such as orange juice, dark green leafy vegetables, asparagus, strawberries, peanuts, and certain legumes (e.g., black beans and kidney beans) (Kauwell, 2009). As of January 1, 1998, all US cereal grain products labeled as

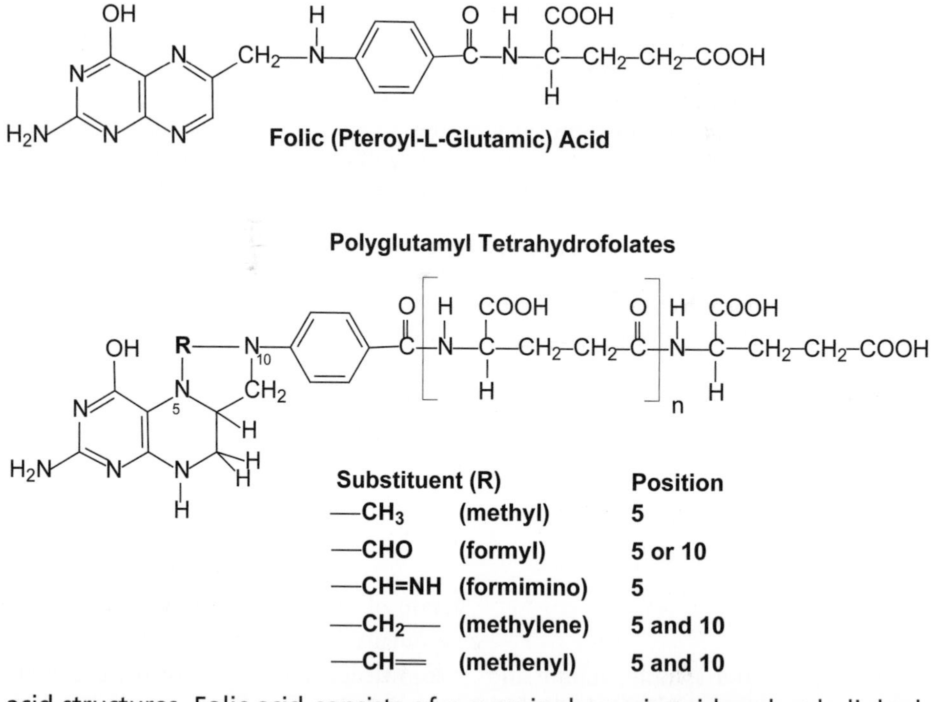

FIG. 21.1 Folic acid structures. Folic acid consists of a p-aminobenzoic acid molecule linked at one end to a pteridine ring and at the other end to a molecule of glutamic acid. Food folates exist in various forms, containing from two to ten additional glutamate residues joined to the first glutamate. The folate/folic acid structure can vary by reduction of the pteridine moiety to form dihydrofolic acid and tetrahydrofolic acid (THF), elongation of the glutamate chain, and substitution of 1-C units at the N5, N10, or both positions. Folate coenzymes are formed by the attachment of 1-C units including methyl (CH₃), methylene (–CH₂–), methenyl (–CH=), formyl (–CH=O), or formimino (–CH=NH) groups to the polyglutamyl form of the THF molecule.

"enriched" (i.e., bread, pasta, flour, breakfast cereal, and rice) and mixed food items containing these grains were required by the Food and Drug Administration (FDA) to be fortified with folic acid (Department of Health and Human Services Food and Drug Administration, 1996). In addition to the US, more than 50 countries are now implementing mandatory folic acid fortification programs (Berry et al., 2009).

Physiology and Metabolism

Absorption

Naturally occurring food folate occurs predominantly in the polyglutamate form which must be converted to the monoglutamate form prior to absorption. The hydrolysis of polyglutamyl folates occurs primarily in the proximal part of the jejunum with the involvement of the brush-border enzyme glutamate carboxypeptidase II (GCPII; EC 3.4.17.21), previously also known as folate hydrolase, folylpolyglutamate hydrolase, pteroylpolyglutamate hydrolase or pteroylpoly-γ-glutamate carboxypeptidase. The enzyme acts as an exopeptidase, cleaving terminal γ-linked glutamate residues from polyglutamyl folates (Chandler et al., 1986; Gregory et al., 1987). The optimal pH for GCPII is 6.5 (Chandler et al., 1986) and studies have shown that the maintenance of this optimal pH is critical for the complete deconjugation of polyglutamyl folates in the jejunum (Tamura et al., 1976; Chandler et al., 1986).

Membrane transport of folates into intestinal cells is mediated mainly by the facilitative carrier, protein-coupled folate transporter (PCFT), as described in the next section. When pharmacological doses (>10 μM) of folate are consumed, absorption takes place by a nonsaturable diffusion-like process and most of the diffused vitamin appears unchanged in portal circulation (Shane, 2009).

In the large intestine another potential source of folate is that produced by microorganisms. Evidence for the absorption of folate across the large intestine was provided by a study in which participants were infused with a physiological dose of stable-isotopically labeled folate during colonoscopy (Aufreiter et al., 2009).

Transport

Folate transport systems are classified as either transmembrane carriers or systems mediated by folate binding proteins (i.e. folate receptors) (Shane, 2009). The reduced folate carrier (RFC) is a bi-directional transmembrane protein that is saturable and has a fairly high affinity for reduced folates with K_m values in the low micromolar range (~1–3 μM) (Zhao et al., 2002; Matherly and Goldman, 2003) but a greatly reduced affinity for folic acid (K_m ~200 μM). PCFT is a more recently identified transmembrane unidirectional transport protein whose proton coupling allows the concentrative transport of folates at acidic pH (Qiu et al., 2006; Zhao et al., 2009). Unlike RFC, this carrier has similar affinity for reduced folates and folic acid (K_m values 0.5 to 0.8 μM at pH 5.5). PCFT appears to play a primary role in intestinal folate absorption since it is expressed in the apical brush border of the duodenum and the jejunum (as is RFC) and, in addition, has characteristics consistent with the requirements for folate transport in the small intestine (acidic pH optimum, high affinity for both folic acid and reduced folates) (Subramanian et al., 2008; Zhao et al., 2009). Intestinal basolateral transport occurs via the multidrug resistance-associated proteins (Mutch et al., 2004).

When synthetic folic acid is consumed, it shares both a common transport mechanism and metabolic fate with most naturally occurring dietary folates since the different chemical forms are metabolized to 5-methylTHF during passage across the intestinal mucosa into portal circulation (Pietrzik et al., 2010). Folic acid is first reduced to DHF and then to THF by DHF reductase in the mucosal cells with some of this metabolism occurring in the liver prior to the release of 5-methylTHF into peripheral circulation (Whitehead and Cooper, 1967; Melikian et al., 1971). Unmetabolized folic acid may appear in the circulation when the metabolic capacity of DHF reductase is exceeded (Kelly et al., 1997; Sweeney et al., 2006).

Once folate enters portal circulation, it is transported into the liver by one of several transporters (Matherly and Goldman, 2003) where it is metabolized to the polyglutamate form which can be used intracellularly, stored, or released into blood or bile (following its conversion back to the monoglutamate form). The predominant form of folate in circulation is the monoglutamyl form of 5-methylTHF. Low- and high-affinity proteins bind folate in circulation with the largest percentage (~50%) bound loosely to albumin (Ratnam and Freisheim, 1990).

Cellular uptake by peripheral tissues utilizes mainly RFC (Herbert and Das, 1994), although PCFT is widely expressed and prominent in kidney, liver, and brain (Yuasa et al., 2009; Zhao et al., 2009). Folate receptors (FRα), high-affinity binding proteins, mediate folate uptake (via an endocytotic process) in the central nervous system

(Matherly and Goldman, 2003) and are also involved in folate reabsorption from the kidney proximal tubules (Matherly and Goldman, 2003; Matherly and Hou, 2008). In addition to internalization of folate, PCFT plays a role in FRα-mediated endocytosis by serving as a route of export of folates from acidified endosomes (Zhao *et al.*, 2009).

Cellular Storage

Once within cells, 5-methylTHF is demethylated through the action of methionine synthase (EC 1.16.1.8) and converted to a polyglutamyl form by folylpolyglutamate synthetase (EC 6.3.2.17) (Shane, 1989). Since folate polyglutamates do not cross cell membranes due to their charge and binding to folate enzymes, polyglutamylation serves as a mechanism to help sequester folate inside the cell (Shane, 1989). Prior to release from tissues, folate polyglutamates are reconverted to the monoglutamate form by γ-glutamyl hydrolase (EC 3.4.19.9) (Shane, 2009). Tissues are limited in their ability to store folate beyond that required for metabolic function. The total body content of humans is estimated to be approximately 15–30 mg based on measurements of liver tissue concentration (Whitehead, 1973; Hoppner and Lampi, 1980), assumptions of liver mass (~1400 g) and relative folate content (i.e. ~50% of total body folate) (Herbert and Zalusky, 1962). Calculations based on in vivo kinetic studies yield similar estimates of body folate pools (Gregory *et al.*, 1998, 2001), but conflicting data have been reported (Lin *et al.*, 2004).

Excretion

The fraction of plasma folate that is not associated with protein is freely filtered at the glomerulus and most folate is reabsorbed in the proximal renal tubules (Shane, 2009). Folate is effectively reabsorbed in the kidney proximal tubules and little or no folate is lost in the urine at normal folate intakes. Urinary excretion occurs mainly as the products of folate cleavage, and the urinary excretion of intact folates represents only a small percentage of dietary folate except in populations exposed to folic acid fortification and/or consuming multivitamins with folic acid (Caudill *et al.*, 1998; Shane, 2009). Biliary secretion of folate has been estimated to be as high as 100 μg/day providing for enterohepatic circulation of folate (Shane, 2009). Fecal folate losses are difficult to assess due to the contribution of colonic microbial synthesis of folate.

Excretion of fecal folate has been estimated to be similar to that of total urinary excretion of intact folate and cleavage products based on data from a study involving radiolabeled folate (Krumdieck *et al.*, 1978).

In Vivo Kinetics

Knowledge of in vivo kinetics (study of rates) aids in understanding the requirements of a nutrient and provides an insight into experimental design in interventions to alter nutritional status (Gregory *et al.*, 2009). Most kinetic studies of folate metabolism in humans utilizing either stable or radiolabeled folate have shown one or more fast-turnover pools and larger slow-turnover pools (Krumdieck *et al.*, 1978; Stites *et al.*, 1997; Clifford *et al.*, 1998; Gregory *et al.*, 1998). The folate pools that exhibit fastest turnover in whole-body kinetic studies typically have half-lives of a few hours or less and appear to be comprised mostly of monoglutamyl species primarily in plasma. In contrast, the far slower-turnover folate pools often exhibit half-lives of the order of months and are comprised primarily of polyglutamatyl folates in tissues (Gregory *et al.*, 2009).

Bioavailability

The concept of folate bioavailability as reviewed refers to the overall efficiency of utilization, including the physiological and biochemical processes involved in intestinal absorption, transport, metabolism, and excretion (McNulty and Pentieva, 2009; Caudill, 2010). In contrast to supplemental folic acid, folate from naturally occurring food sources exhibits variable and often incomplete bioavailability. Many dietary variables, physiological conditions, and pharmaceuticals may affect the bioavailability of food folate. These include: (a) entrapment of naturally occurring folates in the cellular structure or insoluble matrix of certain foods; (b) instability of labile tetrahydrofolates during passage through the stomach; (c) inhibition of the intestinal deconjugation of polyglutamyl folates by food constituents; and (d) indirect impairment of folate deconjugation and absorption by alteration of jejunal pH. Because of variation among individuals in folate digestion, absorption, and metabolism, variability in the bioavailability of food folate is a common finding, and conflicts exist among published studies (Tamura and Stokstad, 1973; Babu and Srikantia, 1976; Prinz-Langenohl *et al.*, 1999). The higher bioavailability of folic acid consumed as fortified food relative to food folate provided the rationale for the derived term dietary folate equivalents (DFEs) cur-

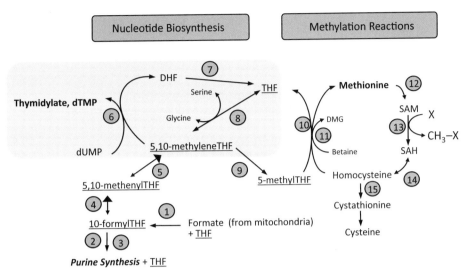

FIG. 21.2 Cytosolic folate-mediated biosynthetic reactions and interconversions of folates (polyglutamates) emphasizing the mostly unidirectional flow of 1-C units through reactions 4 and 5. The thymidylate cycle denoted by the gray background also occurs in the nucleus. Each reaction shows the product plus THF, which is recycled to accept another formate from the mitochondria. The enzymes and reactions are described in Table 21.1. DHF, dihydrofolate; DMG, dimethylglycine; SAM, S-adenosylmethionine; SAH, S-adenosylhomocysteine; THF, tetrahydrofolate; X, methyl group acceptor.

rently used for dietary folate intake recommendations as described in more detail later in this chapter.

Biochemical Functions

Folate coenzymes function in the acquisition and donation of 1-C units and are localized to three cellular compartments: cytosol, nucleus, and mitochondrion. Cytosolic 1-C metabolism is involved in phases of amino acid metabolism, purine and thymidylate biosynthesis, and the formation of the primary methylating agent, S-adenosylmethionine (SAM). The pyrimidine, thymidylate, is also generated in the nucleus during DNA replication and repair. The 1-Cs used in cytosolic folate-mediated 1-C metabolism are derived primarily from the mitochondria in the form of formate through mitochondrial catabolism of serine, glycine, and choline (Stover, 2009).

Cytosolic Folate Metabolism

Cytosolic folate-mediated 1-C metabolism includes three interconnected biosynthetic pathways that catalyze the de novo biosynthesis of purines and thymidylate, and remethylation of homocysteine to methionine (Figure 21.2 and Table 21.1). The trifunctional cytosolic enzyme C_1-THF synthase, encoded by *MTHFD1*, (Figure 21.2, reactions

1, 4, and 5) (Christensen and MacKenzie, 2008), enables entry of mitochondrial 1-Cs into the cytosol with its 10-formylTHF synthetase activity (reaction 1) and facilitates the interconversions of 10-formylTHF, 5,10-methenylTHF and 5,10-methyleneTHF in reactions catalyzed by the activities of 5,10-methenylTHF cyclohydrolase (MTHFC) and 5,10-methyleneTHF dehydrogenase (MTHFD), respectively (Figure 21.2, reactions 4 and 5). Although mitochondria are a primary source of single carbons for these biosynthetic reactions, 1-Cs can be also be generated in the cytosol from serine via the action of cytosolic serine hydroxymethyltransferase (cSHMT) (Figure 21.2, reaction 8), as well as from histidine and purines, which enter the cytosolic pool as 5,10-methenylTHF (Stover, 2009).

Purine Biosynthesis

10-FormylTHF is the required folate coenzyme for the de novo synthesis of the purines, adenine and guanine. The formyl group of 10-formylTHF is incorporated at the C-2 and C-8 positions of the purine ring during de novo purine biosynthesis by reactions catalyzed by glycinamide ribonucleotide formyltransferase (GARFT) and aminoimidazole carboxamide ribonucleotide (AICARFT) (Figure 21.2, reactions 2 and 3). 10-Formyl is generated

TABLE 21.1   Major cytosolic metabolic reactions for folate (as shown in Figure 21.2)

Reaction[a]	Enzyme (abbreviation)	EC number
1	10-FormylTHF synthetase	6.3.4.3
2	Glycinamide ribonucleotide formyltransferase (GARFT)	2.1.2.2
3	Aminoimidazole carboxamide ribonucleotide formyltransferase (AICARFT)	2.1.2.3
4	5,10-MethenylTHF cyclohydrolase (MTHFC)	3.5.4.9
5	5,10-MethyleneTHF dehydrogenase (MTHFD)	1.5.1.5
6	Thymidylate synthase (TS)	2.1.1.45
7	Dihydrofolate reductase (DHFR)	1.5.1.3
8	Serine hydroxymethyltransferase (SHMT)	2.1.2.1
9	5,10-MethyleneTHF reductase (MTHFR)	1.5.1.20
10	Methionine synthase	2.1.1.13
11	Betaine: homocysteine methyltransferase (BHMT)	2.1.1.5
12	S-Adenosylmethionine synthase	2.5.1.6
13	Cellular methyltransferases	Various
14	S-Adenosylhomocysteine hydrolase	3.3.1.1
15	Cystathionine β-synthase (CBS)	4.2.1.22

[a]Enzymes 1, 4, and 5 represent the three activities associated with the trifunctional C1-THF synthase.

by the coupling of formate to THF catalyzed by the activity of 10-formylTHF synthetase of the C_1-THF synthase trifunctional enzyme (Figure 21.2, reaction 1). 5,10-MethyleneTHF is not believed to be a significant contributor to 10-formylTHF production because the reductive environment in the cytosol favors the conversion of 10-formylTHF to 5,10-methyleneTHF (Christensen and MacKenzie, 2008) in reactions catalyzed by the activities of MTHFC and MTHFD of the C_1-THF synthase trifunctional enzyme (Figure 21.2, reactions 4 and 5, respectively)

Thymidylate Biosynthesis

The synthesis of the pyrimidine, thymidylate, is dependent on the availability of 5,10-methyleneTHF, a required coenzyme of thymidylate synthase (TS) which catalyzes the rate-limiting step during the cell cycle thereby enabling DNA replication to proceed. 5,10-MethyleneTHF can be generated from THF in conjunction with the conversion of serine to glycine by cSHMT (Figure 21.2, reaction 8) or from 10-formylTHF by the trifunctional C_1-THF synthase (Figure 21.2, reactions 4 and 5). In the biosynthesis of thymidylate, 5,10-methyleneTHF donates the 1-C group to deoxyuridine monophosphate (dUMP), forming deoxythymidine monophosphate (dTMP) (Figure 21.2, reaction 6). This reaction is unique in folate 1-C transfers in that the THF carrier is oxidized to DHF, with the electrons being used to reduce the 1-C unit to the methyl level. THF is subsequently regenerated in a reaction cata-

lyzed by dihydrofolate reductase (DHFR) (Figure 21.2, reaction 7).

De novo thymidylate biosynthesis also occurs in the nucleus. During cell division, the cytosolic enzymes, constituting the thymidylate cycle (SHMT, TS, and DHFR), are translocated to the nucleus by small ubiquitin-like modification (Anderson *et al.*, 2007; Woeller *et al.*, 2007).

Methylation Reactions

5,10-MethyleneTHF can also be reduced to the methyl donor, 5-methylTHF, in a unidirectional reaction catalyzed by methylenetetrahydrofolate reductase (MTHFR) (Figure 21.2, reaction 9). The production of 5-methylTHF by MTHFR is an important functional and regulatory step in the regeneration of methionine from homocysteine. The folate-dependent remethylation process is catalyzed by methionine synthase, and requires cobalamin and 5-methylTHF (Figure 21.2, reaction 10). Homocysteine remethylation is the only known reaction involving 5-methylTHF. In the methionine synthase reaction, a methyl group is sequentially transferred from 5-methylTHF to cobalamin, and then to homocysteine, thus forming methionine. The dependence of methionine synthase on both folate and cobalamin provides a biochemical explanation of why a single deficiency of either vitamin leads to the same megaloblastic changes in the bone marrow and other tissues with rapidly dividing cells. In a cobalamin deficiency, folate is "trapped" in the 5-methylTHF form and THF is not regenerated for the formation of

5,10-methyleneTHF, required for thymidylate and thus DNA synthesis.

Methionine, either from dietary protein or produced from homocysteine, can be activated to SAM, the principal methylating agent in all cells (Figure 21.2, reaction 12). SAM is the methyl donor in over 100 transmethylation reactions, including methylation of DNA, RNA, histones, neurotransmitters, and phospholipids. The main consumers of SAM include phosphatidylethanolamine *N*-methyltransferase, guanidinoacetate methyltransferase, and glycine *N*-methyltransferase (GNMT) which synthesize phosphatidylcholine, creatine, and sarcosine, respectively. Sarcosine is a source of 1-C units following its degradation in the mitochondria as discussed in subsequent text. As a result of methyl-group transfer by a variety of methyltransferases, SAM is converted to S-adenosylhomocysteine (SAH) (Figure 21.2, reaction 13), which is subsequently hydrolyzed to homocysteine and adenosine by SAH hydrolase (Figure 21.2, reaction 14). This reaction is reversible and, although the equilibrium favors SAH synthesis (Melnyk *et al.*, 2000), utilization of adenosine and the remethylation of homocysteine provide the kinetic impetus that drives this reaction in the direction of homocysteine formation.

Homocysteine can be removed permanently from the methionine cycle via the transsulfuration pathway leading ultimately to cysteine. Cystathionine β-synthase (CBS) (Figure 21.2, reaction 15) catalyzes the committing step in transsulfuration in which homocysteine and serine are coupled to form cystathionine in a pyridoxal phosphate-dependent reaction that is activated by SAM. This promotes CBS activation and favors the transsulfuration pathway under conditions of ample methionine.

Mitochondrial Folate Metabolism

Mitochondria generate 1-C units in the form of formate for cytosolic folate-mediated 1-C metabolism (Figure 21.3 and Table 21.2). The C3 of serine, derived from the diet, glycolytic intermediates and serine produced by cSHMT, is a primary source of 1-C units from which 5,10-methyleneTHF is formed through the action of mitochondrial SHMT (Figure 21.3, reaction 1). 5,10-MethyleneTHF is converted to 10-formylTHF by a bifunctional enzyme encoded by *MTHFD2* (embryos) or the putative *MTHFD2L* (adults) with MTHFD and MTHFC activities (Christensen and MacKenzie, 2006; Tibbetts and Appling, 2010) (Figure 21.3, reactions 2 and 3 respectively). In the final step, 10-formylTHF is hydrolyzed to formate and THF by mitochondrial 10-formylTHF

synthetase (Figure 21.3, reaction 4), a monofunctional enzyme encoded by *MTHFD1L* (Christensen *et al.*, 2005). The formate is then delivered to the cytosol where it is converted to 10-formylTHF for purine synthesis (Figure 21.2, reaction 1) or is reduced to 5,10-methyleneTHF which can be diverted to cellular methylation reactions (Figure 21.2, reaction 9) or thymidylate biosynthesis (Figure 21.2, reaction 6). Alternatively, the 1-C unit in the form of 10-formylTHF may be oxidized to CO_2 by the enzyme, 10-formylTHF dehydrogenase, which removes excess 1-C groups (Figure 21.3, reaction 8).

Additional sources of 1-C units in select tissues (e.g., liver) include the mitochondrial glycine cleavage system and the oxidative catabolism of choline. The glycine cleavage system is a multienzyme complex that cleaves glycine to produce CO_2, ammonia and 5,10-methyleneTHF (Figure 21.3, reaction 7), the latter of which can be oxidized to 10-formylTHF to recover 1-C units. Choline catabolism involves its oxidation to betaine which, like 5-methylTHF, is used in the remethylation of homocysteine to methionine in a reaction catalyzed by cytosolic betaine-homocysteine methyltransferase (BHMT) (Figure 21.2, reaction 11) (also, see Chapter 26). The other product of this reaction, dimethylglycine, undergoes two sequential mitochondrial oxidations catalyzed by dimethylglycine dehydrogenase and sarcosine dehydrogenase to form glycine and two molecules of 5,10-methyleneTHF (Figure 21.3, reactions 5 and 6 respectively).

Only a limited exchange of free folate occurs between the cytosolic and mitochondrial compartments. However, these compartments are metabolically connected by transport of 1C donors (serine, glycine, and formate) across the mitochondrial membranes, supporting a mostly unidirectional flow from serine to formate (mitochondria) and on to methionine (cytosol) (Tibbetts and Appling, 2010).

Regulation of Cytosolic One-Carbon Metabolism

Methylation Reactions

SAM and SAH are major regulators of the use of methyl groups and exert control at several regulatory points.

SAM Regulation

Surplus SAM binds to the regulatory domain of MTHFR and inhibits enzyme activity thereby reducing the production of 5-methylTHF which is required for the recycling of homocysteine through the methionine synthase reaction. Diminished production of 5-methylTHF by MTHFR

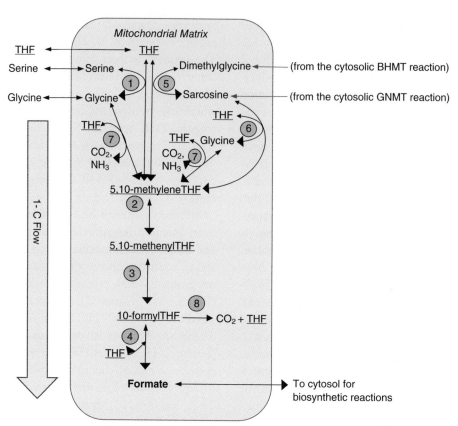

FIG. 21.3   Mitochondrial folate-mediated 1-C metabolism emphasizing the generation of formate from the catabolism of serine, choline, and glycine. Serine, glycine, and dimethylglycine (from oxidative choline catabolism) can traverse the mitochondrial inner membrane enabling their entry from the cytosolic compartment and their conversion to formate. The enzymes and reactions in this diagram are described in Table 21.2.

TABLE 21.2   Major mitochondrial enzymes and reactions (as shown in Figure 21.3)

Reaction[a]	Enzyme (abbreviation)	EC number
1	Serine hydroxymethyltransferase (SHMT)	2.1.2.1
2	5,10-MethyleneTHF dehydrogenase (MTHFD)	1.5.1.5
3	5,10-MethenylTHF cyclohydrolase (MTHFC)	3.5.4.9
4	10-FormylTHF synthetase	6.3.4.3
5	Dimethylglycine dehydrogenase	1.5.99.2
6	Sarcosine dehydrogenase	1.5.99.1
7	Glycine cleavage system (GCS)	2.1.2.10
8	10-FormylTHF dehydrogenase	1.5.1.6

[a]Enzymes 2 and 3 represent the two activities associated with the bifunctional C-1 THF synthase.

also yields an active GNMT which is normally inhibited by 5-methylTHF. GNMT catalyzes the SAM-dependent methylation of glycine to sarcosine (Ogawa *et al.*, 1998) thereby metabolizing excess SAM. Sarcosine is converted back to glycine and 5,10-methyleneTHF via sarcosine dehydrogenase following its transport into the mitochondria (Figure 21.3, reaction 6), which allows for the conservation of 1-C units. SAM also activates CBS (Figure 21.2, reaction 15), the first step in the transsulfuration pathway that initiates homocysteine catabolism and its permanent removal from the methionine cycle.

Under conditions of inadequate SAM concentration, methionine conservation is preserved by recycling homocysteine to methionine through activation of MTHFR and inhibition of CBS. Further, as a result of enhanced MTHFR activity and greater production of 5-methylTHF, GNMT is inhibited, sparing SAM for essential methylation reactions.

SAH Regulation

SAH is a potent product inhibitor of most methyltransferases (Melnyk *et al.*, 1999, 2000). Accumulation of SAH and the associated inhibition of cellular methyltransferases will occur under metabolic conditions that interfere with product removal of homocysteine or adenosine (Melnyk *et al.*, 2000). Increased cytosolic SAH concentrations have also been reported to up-regulate CBS activity, decrease BHMT activity, and decrease MTHFR activity in certain tissues (Melnyk *et al.*, 2000).

Purine and Thymidylate Biosynthesis

10-FormylTHF is essential for purine biosynthesis and is also the primary source of 5,10-methyleneTHF which is required for thymidylate biosynthesis. The availability of 10-formylTHF for de novo nucleotide synthesis is regulated at multiple points (Stover, 2009). *MTHFD1* encodes the trifunctional enzyme, C_1-THF synthase, which harbors 10-formylTHF synthethase, MTHFD and MTHFC activities and thus influences the availability of 10-formylTHF and 5,10-methyleneTHF which exist in equilibrium (Pelletier and MacKenzie, 1995). Although the transcriptional levels of *MTHFD1* are not modified by growth factors in cultured fibroblasts, mRNA is stabilized post-transcriptionally by growth factors, which in turn decreases the loss of message due to mRNA turnover (Peri and MacKenzie, 1991). Additional enzymes with regulatory functions include: 10-formylTHF dehydrogenase, which regulates the availability of folate coenzymes

for nucleotide biosynthesis by depleting 10-formylTHF pools (Anguera *et al.*, 2006); MTHFR, which mediates the flow of 1-C units between thymidylate biosynthesis and methylation reactions; and cSHMT, which preferentially partitions cSHMT-derived 5,10-methyleneTHF towards thymidylate biosynthesis at the expense of methylation reactions (Herbig *et al.*, 2002).

Mitochondrial 1-Carbon Metabolism

Redox and equilibrium conditions support the flow of 1-C units through the mitochondria in the oxidative direction of 5,10-methyleneTHF to 10-formylTHF to formate (Tibbetts and Appling, 2010) as shown in Figure 21.3. In adult hepatic cells, however, the mitochondria may transiently favor serine production for use in gluconeogenesis (Christensen and MacKenzie, 2008). Although *MTHFD1L*, which encodes mitochondrial 10-formyl synthetase, is up-regulated under conditions requiring increased DNA synthesis (Christensen and MacKenzie, 2006), many questions remain regarding the control of 1-C flux through the mitochondria.

Genetic Polymorphisms

Normal folate metabolism is dependent on genes encoding the ~150 proteins directly or indirectly involved in folate metabolism and transport. Hundreds of single nucleotide polymorphisms (SNPs) have been identified in these genes. These genetic variants or polymorphisms can alter enzyme activity or regulation, or influence gene expression, resulting in changes in the concentrations of critical metabolites, or they could have no effect (Christensen and Rozen, 2009). Examples of select SNPs which do result in metabolic alterations and have been associated with increased disease or birth-defect risk are discussed below. More in-depth descriptions of these and other folate-related genetic variants and their relevance to birth defects and chronic diseases are available elsewhere (Christensen and Rozen, 2009; Molloy *et al.*, 2009; Shaw *et al.*, 2009).

The most extensively studied of the folate-related polymorphisms is a C to T substitution at base pair 677 in the gene encoding the enzyme MTHFR that catalyzes the reduction of 5,10-methyleneTHF to 5-methylTHF, the methyl donor for homocysteine remethylation to methionine (Frosst *et al.*, 1995). Individuals who are homozygous for the *MTHFR* C677T (rs1801133) variant (i.e. TT genotype) exhibit lower specific activity of

MTHFR, and reduced stability of the enzyme in vitro (Frosst *et al.*, 1995).

The prevalence of the 677TT genotype varies widely between regions and ethnic groups (Christensen and Rozen, 2009). In North American Caucasians the frequency has been reported as 8–14%. In European populations, the frequency appears to increase from north to south: 6–14% in Northern Europe and 15–24% in Southern Europe. The genotype is particularly common in Mexican and other Hispanic populations at 15–35%, whereas less than 2% of African and African-American populations are homozygous for the variant. In Asia, the reported frequencies may also be quite high, ranging from ~15% to 39% (Christensen and Rozen, 2009; Crider *et al.*, 2011).

The C677→T variant leading to reduced MTHFR activity increases homocysteine concentrations by decreasing the 5-methylTHF available for homocysteine methylation. Elevations in homocysteine in individuals with the 677TT genotype compared with 677CC individuals have been reported in numerous studies, however, the evidence indicates that homocysteine may only be elevated in individuals with the TT genotype when folate status is low (Jacques *et al.*, 1996; Hustad *et al.*, 2007).

The distribution of folate derivatives is altered when MTHFR activity is reduced, resulting in an increase in 5,10-methyleneTHF which can then be used for dTMP synthesis or converted to other folate forms, such as 10-formylTHF. As 5-methylTHF is the major transport form of folate, reduced MTHFR activity is expected to decrease the amount of circulating folate, possibly exacerbating its metabolic impact (Christensen and Rozen, 2009). Altered distribution of folate forms appears to confound the measurement of total RBC folate by certain assay methods (Molloy *et al.*, 1998b), leading to conflicting results regarding the association between *MTHFR* variants and RBC folate. However, the measurement of folate in plasma/serum is unaffected by these technical difficulties; the variant TT genotype is usually associated with a 10 to 35% reduction in circulating folate (Gueant-Rodriguez *et al.*, 2006; Yang *et al.*, 2008).

The methionine synthase reductase (MTRR) enzyme reactivates the cobalamin cofactor of MTR when it is oxidized to cobalt(II) (Olteanu *et al.*, 2002). The *MTRR* A66G (rs1801394) polymorphism has a relatively high frequency in Caucasians (20–38%) but a much lower frequency in other ethnic groups (Christensen and Rozen, 2009). The *MTRR* A66G (rs1801394) variant may modu-

late homocysteine concentrations when coupled with other genetic variants and/or low vitamin B_{12} concentrations (Christensen and Rozen, 2009).

RFC has a higher affinity for circulating 5-methylTHF relative to folic acid, therefore the common gene variant *RFC* A80G (rs1051266) theoretically may disturb folate metabolism by reducing the cellular pool of 1-C donors, although there is limited evidence to support this (Christensen and Rozen, 2009). It is possible that other folate transporters may compensate for reduced RFC activity and therefore the variant may affect folate metabolism only under specific circumstances (Christensen and Rozen, 2009).

Severe Clinical Deficiency, Pregnancy Complications, Fetal Growth

Severe Clinical Deficiency

Chronic severe folate deficiency is associated with decreased DNA synthesis which leads to impaired maturation of erythropoietic precursors resulting in a gradual increase in red blood cell mean cell volume. The resulting megaloblastic anemia is characterized by large abnormal nucleated erythrocytes that accumulate in the bone marrow (Lindenbaum and Allen, 1995; Stabler, 2009). There are also decreased numbers of white cells and platelets, as a result of general impairment of cell division related to folate's role in nucleic acid synthesis (Lindenbaum and Allen, 1995; Stabler, 2009). Since the intestinal mucosa undergoes continuous regeneration, with replacement of epithelial cells every 3 days, its folate requirements are greater than other tissues (Lindenbaum and Allen, 1995; Stabler, 2009). Gastrointestinal symptoms frequently result from severe folate deficiency and are often associated with impaired absorption (Lindenbaum and Allen, 1995; Stabler, 2009). Overconsumption of alcohol is the most likely cause of folate deficiency anemia due to alcohol's well documented negative effects on folate metabolism that result in a depletion of folate body stores (Halsted *et al.*, 2009).

Pregnancy Complications and Fetal Growth

Pregnant women are at increased risk of developing a folate deficiency due to the accelerated demands placed on the supply of folate for the synthesis of DNA and other 1-C transfer reactions (Tamura and Picciano, 2006). A number of pregnancy complications including placental abruption, preeclampsia, spontaneous abortion, stillbirths, and fetal growth restriction have been inversely associated with impaired folate status and linked to hyperhomocysteinemia; however, data are inconclusive, and definitive conclusions cannot be drawn (as recently reviewed: Tamura *et al.*, 2009).

Infant birth-weight has been reported to positively respond to folic acid supplementation in some studies but not others (Tamura *et al.*, 2009). Improved birth-weight in response to folic acid supplementation is likely associated with impaired maternal folate status (Tamura *et al.*, 2009). Analysis of data from over 5 million birth records in California indicated significant reductions in rates of low- and very-low-birth-weight incidence as well as preterm delivery after initiation of the folic acid fortification program (Shaw *et al.*, 2004).

Neural Tube Defects

Embryological malformations of the central nervous system, commonly referred to as NTDs, result from a failure of fusion of the neural folds in the developing embryo (Botto *et al.*, 1999). Folic acid taken periconceptionally significantly reduces the risk of NTDs, a conclusion based on definitive evidence from randomized controlled intervention trials (RCT) and supported by observational studies (Hobbs *et al.*, 2009). The implementation of mandatory folic acid fortification programs has resulted in convincing reductions in NTDs during the post-fortification era, providing further evidence of the efficacy of this nutrient for NTD risk reduction (Berry *et al.*, 2009).

The mechanism(s) by which folic acid facilitates the reduction in NTD risk is unknown and is the focus of on-going research endeavors by numerous research groups around the globe. It is hypothesized that folic acid intake reduces the risk of NTDs by overcoming metabolic inefficiencies linked to genetic abnormalities (Wallis *et al.*, 2009). The research evidence to date suggests that maternal/fetal folate metabolism is disordered in some cases and this metabolic error may affect uptake and/or metabolism of folate which can in turn adversely affect gene expression critical to normal embryogenesis.

The *MTHFR 677T* variant, either in the mother or in the child, has been associated with an increased risk for NTD (Botto and Yang, 2000; Amorim *et al.*, 2007; Molloy *et al.*, 2009; Shaw *et al.*, 2009). The association between the *MTHFR C677T* variant and NTDs is not always observed, possibly due to various modifiers including vitamin use/folate status (Molloy *et al.*, 1998a, 2009; Shaw *et al.*, 1998). The impact of the *MTRR* A66G variant in the mother has been found to significantly increase NTD risk in some but not all studies (O'Leary *et al.*, 2005) with low vitamin B_{12} and high MMA magnifying the risk significantly (Wilson *et al.*, 1999; van der Linden *et al.*, 2006).

Homozygosity for the variant RFC 80G allele has been associated with a significant increase in NTD risk by some investigators (De Marco *et al.*, 2003; Pei *et al.*, 2005) but not others (O'Leary *et al.*, 2006). The inconsistency may be due to potential interaction between maternal genotype and folate intake since it has been reported by multiple investigators that the combination of low folate intake and maternal GG genotype is associated with an increased risk for NTD (Shaw *et al.*, 2002; Pei *et al.*, 2005).

Congenital Heart Defects

Congenital heart defects are the most common birth defect with the highest prevalence among stillbirths and miscarriages (Tennstedt *et al.*, 1999; Botto *et al.*, 2003). A considerable body of evidence does support the conclusion that maternal use of folic-acid-containing supplements in early pregnancy significantly reduces the risk for some heart defects (Botto *et al.*, 2003; Hobbs *et al.*, 2009). Finnell and coworkers (Wallis *et al.*, 2009) have provided an in-depth description of how folate may be involved in overcoming select metabolic/genetic abnormalities that may increase the risk for congenital heart defects. Of interest is the fact that the development of both the neural tube and cardiac tissue depends on neural crest cells which have a high demand for folate to support cellular differentiation, growth, and migration (Wallis *et al.*, 2009).

The risk for congenital heart defects has also been mildly associated with the *MTHFR* C677T variant (van Beynum, *et al.*, 2007; Verkleij-Hagoort *et al.*, 2007). Shaw *et al.* (2009) reported that the risk for conotruncal heart defects was not strongly associated with any of the 118 folate-related SNPs evaluated by this research group. The folate status of the mother as well as the heterogeneity of the type of defect should be considered when examining the potential impact of gene variants on risk.

Vascular Disease

A large number of epidemiological and mechanistic studies have provided evidence for the "homocysteine hypothesis" linking elevated homocysteine to increased risk for vascular disease thus providing the impetus for folic acid intervention strategies and controlled trials to lower homocysteine and related vascular disease risk (Hannibal *et al.*, 2009; Kalin and Rimm, 2009). Recently, results from numerous major randomized controlled trials of high-dose folic acid, vitamin B_6, and vitamin B_{12} supplementation for secondary prevention of cardiovascular disease (CVD) have been reported (Baker *et al.*, 2002; Toole *et al.*, 2004; Bonaa *et al.*, 2006; Lonn *et al.*, 2006; Jamison *et al.*, 2007; Albert *et al.*, 2008; Ebbing *et al.*, 2008). This large body of evidence from these controlled intervention trials support the conclusion that folic acid alone or in combination with other B vitamins is not efficacious in the secondary prevention of CVD.

While these secondary intervention trials have largely failed to find any benefit for folic acid supplementation, the interpretation of some of these studies has been complicated by the advent of mandatory folic acid fortification in the US and Canada in 1998. The most recent data suggest that post-fortification, average homocysteine concentrations in the US dropped by about 10% (Pfeiffer *et al.*, 2008), enough to potentially obscure any benefit of additional folic acid supplementation. In addition, since the intervention trials were secondary in nature, they may not reflect a protective effect of ensuring adequate folate status and normal homocysteine concentrations on risk reduction for vascular disease in healthy individuals.

Cancer

Epidemiological studies have provided convincing evidence that inadequate folate status enhances the risk of colorectal cancer as reviewed (Giovannucci, 2002; Sanjoaquin *et al.*, 2005; Chen *et al.*, 2009). There is also more limited support for an inverse relationship between folate status and cancer risk at other sites including the breast (Beilby *et al.*, 2004; Ericson *et al.*, 2007), lung (Voorrips *et al.*, 2000), pancreas (Larsson *et al.*, 2006), esophagus (Larsson *et al.*, 2006), and others. In addition to this ever increasing body of evidence demonstrating that enhancing folate status reduces the risk of cancer initiation, it is also recognized that once foci of pre-cancerous cells are established, increasing folate intake may increase cancer risk (Stolzenberg-Solomon *et al.*, 2006; Cole *et al.*, 2007; Ciappio and Mason, 2009).

There are a number of proposed mechanisms by which inadequate folate status may initiate or promote carcinogenesis (Ciappio and Mason, 2009). One of the prevailing hypotheses is that, under the conditions of low folate, enhanced uracil "misincorporation" increases the risk of

mutagenic DNA strand breaks (Dianov *et al.*, 1991; Elliott and Jasin, 2002; Ciappio and Mason, 2009). A second proposed mechanism by which folate status modulates carcinogenesis relates to observed abnormalities in DNA methylation (hypo and hyper) that are common in cancer (Gronbaek *et al.*, 2007). In contrast, it is widely accepted that excess folate intake may accelerate the growth of premalignant cells and established cancerous cells because the rapidly proliferating cells have an elevated requirement for folate to meet the demands for increased DNA synthesis (Voeller *et al.*, 2004; Ciappio and Mason, 2009).

Evidence suggests that the risk for colorectal cancer is lower in individuals with the MTHFR 677TT genotype who have high folate status but that protection is lost, or the TT genotype may become a risk factor, if folate concentrations are low (Sharp and Little, 2004). The protective effect of this variant may be due to an increase in 5,10-methyleneTHF for conversion of dUMP to dTMP, reducing DNA damage resulting from uracil misincorporation into DNA (Chen *et al.*, 1996; Blount *et al.*, 1997).

Cognitive Function

Morris and Jacques (2009) have thoroughly reviewed epidemiological evidence linking folate status and a wide array of neurological functions. In patients with Alzheimer's disease with associated brain infarcts, low folate status has been linked to neuropathological indicators and to cognitive impairment (Morris and Jacques, 2009). Proposed mechanisms by which folate status could be involved in the etiology of cognitive dysfunction include direct neurotoxic effects of elevated homocysteine associated with low folate status as well as homocysteine-independent mechanisms such as biogenic amine metabolism and/or folate's role in the synthesis of SAM as previously reviewed (Bottiglieri and Reynolds, 2009). There is a great deal of inconsistency in the literature related to the potential association between folate status and cognition. The heterogeneity in findings is likely due to the complexity of assessing neurological function including consideration and control for a wide array of potentially confounding factors (Morris and Jacques, 2009).

Drug and Alcohol Impairment of Folate Metabolism

Antifolate Drugs

The enzymes involved in folate metabolism have been therapeutic targets for the treatment of neoplastic diseases since the 1940s. Antifolates disrupt purine and thymidylate biosynthesis, thereby resulting in impaired DNA replication and cell death (Assaraf, 2007). Methotrexate (MTX), a derivative of aminopterin, is a primary antifolate and structural analogue of folic acid differing only by an amino group replacing the 4-hydroxyl group on the pteridine ring and a methyl group at the N-10 position. These modifications give MTX more affinity for its target, DHFR, than the natural folate substrate (Priest and Bunni, 1995). MTX and/or MTX-polyglutamates bind tightly to DHFR and inhibit it, causing accumulation of DHF and a lack of substrate for TS. A newer antifolate drug, pemetrexed, targets and inhibits various enzymes of folate metabolism including TS, DHFR, C1-THF synthase, and enzymes that catalyze the final folate-dependent steps of purine biosynthesis, GARFT and AICARFT (Exinger et al., 2003).

Methotrexate, at low doses, is also a standard treatment for several inflammatory disorders, particularly rheumatoid arthritis and psoriasis. Although the precise mechanism by which MTX exerts its anti-inflammatory effects is unclear, a variety of pharmacological actions are likely to contribute including inhibition of cellular proliferation of lymphocytes involved in the inflammation process, as well as the enhanced release of adenosine, an anti-inflammatory molecule, into the intracellular space (Whittle and Hughes, 2004; Wessels et al., 2008).

Folate status declines in patients on high- and low-dose methotrexate (Hellman et al., 1964) and folate deficiency increases the risk of MTX toxicity (Hellman et al., 1964). Folinic acid, under the drug name leucovorin, is a form of folate (5-formyl-THF) that can help "rescue" or reverse the toxic effects of methotrexate. Folic acid and folinic acid are equally effective in patients with rheumatoid arthritis, and in the US folic acid is routinely prescribed along with the MTX to prevent toxicity and prolong the use of the medication (Whittle and Hughes, 2004). However, a careful balance must be maintained between drug therapy and adjunct folic acid supplementation to ensure both drug efficacy and prevention of severe folate deficiency (van Ede et al., 2001).

Anticonvulsants

There are numerous reports of impaired folate status associated with chronic use of the anticonvulsants, diphenylhydantoin (phenytoin, Dilantin®) and phenobarbital; however, the mechanism of the drug–nutrient interaction has not been determined.

Sulfonamides

Salicylazosulfapyridine (Aztilfidine®, sulfasalazine) is an anti-inflammatory drug with antifolate properties (Selhub et al., 1978) and is commonly used for the treatment of ulcerative colitis. Sulfasalazine is a potent inhibitor of PCFT (Yuasa et al., 2009) and supplementation with folic acid is often advised (Jansen et al., 2004).

Alcohol

Alcohol consumed chronically in large amounts has been shown to contribute to folate deficiency by interfering with folate absorption, decreasing hepatic folate uptake, and increasing urinary folate excretion as reviewed by Halsted et al. (2009). The combination of a folate-deficient diet and chronic alcohol consumption accentuates abnormal hepatic methionine metabolism and accelerates the development of alcoholic liver injury (Halsted et al., 2009).

Recommended and Estimated Folate/Folic Acid Intakes in the US and the Impact of Fortification

Dietary Reference Intakes

The Institute of Medicine (IOM) established the dietary reference intakes (DRIs), which include a series of reference values for folate intake including the estimated average requirement (EAR), recommended dietary allowance (RDA), adequate intake (AI), and the tolerable upper intake level (UL) (Table 21.3) (IOM, 1998). The EAR is defined as the median usual intake of folate needed to meet the requirements of 50% of the population. The RDA is estimated from the EAR by correcting for population variance and represents the average daily dietary intake level sufficient to meet the nutrient requirement of approximately 98% of the population (Table 21.3). The AI was estimated when there were insufficient data on which to derive an EAR and is defined as the quantity of folate consumed by a group with no evidence of folate inadequacy (Table 21.3). The UL pertains specifically to folic acid (rather than food folate) and is characterized as the maximum daily usual intake at which consumption would pose no risk of adverse health effects (IOM, 1998).

The IOM considered differences in bioavailability between synthetic folic acid in fortified foods and naturally occurring dietary folate when expressing the DRIs as DFEs (IOM, 1998). The conversion of dietary folate

TABLE 21.3 Folate dietary reference intakes (μg of DFE/day)

Group	Adequate intake	Recommended dietary allowance
Infants		
0–6 months	65	
6–11 months	80	
Children and adolescents		
1–3 years		150
4–8 years		200
9–13 years		300
14–18 years		400
Adults		
≥19 years		400
Pregnant women		
All ages		600
Lactating women		
All ages		500

intake to DFE is a method to convert all forms of dietary folate, including folic acid in fortified food, to an amount that is equivalent to naturally occurring food folate. DFEs are defined as micrograms of naturally occurring food folate plus 1.7 times the micrograms of synthetic folate. The use of the 1.7 multiplier for converting folic acid to DFE was based on the assumption that added folic acid (consumed with a meal as a supplement or fortificant) is ~85% available (Pfeiffer *et al.*, 1997) and food folate is ~50% available (Sauberlich *et al.*, 1987); thus the ratio 85/50 yielded the multiplier of 1.7 in the DFE calculation.

A UL was estimated (IOM, 1998) for folic acid (1000 μg/day); however, no UL was established for naturally occurring food folate. The UL for folic acid is primarily based on case reports describing vitamin B_{12}-deficient patients whose anemia responded to folic acid alone, which is referred to as "masking" (IOM, 1998). In addition, the IOM committee considered evidence that excessive folic acid may precipitate or exacerbate neuropathy in vitamin B_{12}-deficient patients (IOM, 1998). Unlike the case for other nutrients for which there is a UL; there are no substantiated toxic side-effects and no dose response associated with the reported masking on which the UL is based (IOM, 1998).

Folic Acid Intake Recommendation for Neural Tube Defect Risk Reduction

The IOM recommendation for NTD risk reduction is not the same as the RDA, a common misconception, since the recommendation specifies that the supplemental form of the vitamin, folic acid (400 μg/day), be taken (or consumed as a fortified food) in addition to folate in a varied diet (IOM, 1998). This recommendation is consistent with that of the US Public Health Service (CDC, 1992).

Effect of Folic Acid Fortification on Folate Intake and Status in the United States and NTDs

In the United States, total dietary folate intake includes food folate plus folic acid from enriched cereal grain products (140 μg/100 g flour) and fortified RTE cereals, including those with up to 400 μg/serving (FDA, 1996). Estimates of dietary folate intake (μg/day) can be determined and categorized as (1) naturally occurring food folate; (2) folic acid; (3) total folate as μg/day; and (4) total folate as μg/day DFEs using the USDA Food and Nutrient Database for Dietary Studies (USDA, 2009). Total folate intake (μg/day DFEs) in the US has been estimated to be 813 for men and 724 for women (Bailey *et al.*, 2010).

Yang *et al.* (2010) estimated that usual median intake of folic acid differed across folic acid consumption groups for the non-pregnant adult US population aged ≥19 years from the National Health and Nutrition Examination Surveys (NHANES) 2003–2004 and 2005–2006 using the US Department of Agriculture (USDA) Food and Nutrient Databases for Dietary Studies (USDA, 2009). The usual median intakes (μg/day) of folic acid for enriched cereal grain products (ECGP) only, ECGP plus ready-to-eat cereals (RTE), ECGP plus supplements (SUPP), and ECGP + RTE + SUPP were 138, 274, 479, and 635, respectively (Yang *et al.*, 2010).

During the first post-fortification survey period (1999–2000) median serum folate concentrations for the population increased by approximately three times compared with the pre-fortification period (1988–1994) (Pfeiffer *et al.*, 2007). A comprehensive evaluation of blood folate concentrations from 1988 to 2006 demonstrates that the median serum and RBC folate concentrations of the US population 4 years of age and older have increased significantly over the time period from 1988 to 2006 (McDowell *et al.*, 2008). The large increases that occurred between 1988–1994 and 1999–2000 were followed by small fluctuations from 1999 to 2006 (McDowell *et al.*, 2008).

Mandatory fortification of flour with folic acid has proven to be one of the most successful public-health interventions in preventing morbidity and mortality from NTDs. The reduction in birth prevalence rates of NTDs has been substantial in every country that has implemented mandatory fortification, with overall declines ranging from 19% to 55% (Berry *et al.*, 2009).

Analytical Methods

Essentially all aspects of research related to folate nutrition are predicated on reliable measurement of the vitamin in biological specimens and diet components. The major approaches to the measurement of folate in biological specimens and foods or diet samples include microbiological growth procedures, protein–ligand binding methods, and chromatographic and mass-spectrometry methods as extensively reviewed by Pfeiffer *et al.* (2009).

The selection of the best method for folate analysis is dependent on the setting in which the assay will be used and the type of data needed. When one is monitoring trends in folate concentrations in a population over time, either the microbiological assay (low-resource settings) or ID-LC-MS/MS (specialized laboratories) are suitable tools; commercial assays are less suited because they will likely change over time (Pfeiffer *et al.*, 2009). In contrast, in the clinical setting, where assay accuracy and continuity are trumped by the need for throughput and low cost, commercial assays may be the answer. Finally, in the research setting, the various types of chromatographic assays would be best suited for the analysis of specific folate species (Pfeiffer *et al.*, 2009).

Status Assessment

Folate status assessment in the research setting and in population surveys routinely includes blood folate concentrations and some indicators of metabolic function, as previously reviewed (IOM, 1998). Since hematological findings such as macrocytic anemia occur late in the development of a folate deficiency, the emphasis in status assessment studies is on changes that precede clinical indicators (IOM, 1998).

Static Indicators

Serum folate concentrations are generally determined when folate status is assessed; however, changes may indicate a transient reduction in folate intake and not represent body stores (IOM, 1998). Serum folate is considered to be a sensitive indicator of recent dietary folate intake and may require repeated measurements over time in the same individual to reflect long-term status (IOM, 1998). The criterion for serum folate concentration routinely used to define inadequate folate status is <7 nmol/L (<3 ng/mL) (IOM, 1998).

In contrast to serum folate concentration, red blood cell (RBC) folate concentration is considered an indicator of long-term status. Since folate is not taken up by the mature erythrocytes in circulation, RBC folate concentration represents folate taken up in the developing reticulocytes early in the ~120-day erythrocyte lifespan. RBC folate concentration is considered representative of tissue folate stores based on associations with liver folate concentration determined by biopsy (IOM, 1998). A cut-off value of <305 nmol/L (<140 ng/mL) is the criterion commonly used to define inadequate folate status (IOM, 1998).

Functional Indices

In addition to blood folate concentrations, it is also considered important to evaluate folate status indices that may indicate changes in metabolic function. One such "functional" indicator is plasma total homocysteine concentration, which increases when there is a deficiency of 5-methylTHF, the folate form necessary to convert homocysteine to methionine. The inverse association between blood folate concentrations and plasma total homocysteine concentration is well established (IOM, 1998). Although plasma homocysteine concentration is considered a sensitive functional indicator, it is not specific for folate status since it may be influenced by a number of other nutrient deficiencies, genetic abnormalities, and renal insufficiency (IOM, 1998). Various cutoff values for elevated homocysteine have been reported to define normal folate status and most frequently have ranged from >10 to >16 μmol/L (IOM, 1998).

Human studies in postmenopausal women have shown that global DNA methylation decreases as a function of dietary folate depletion (Jacob *et al.*, 1998; Rampersaud *et al.*, 2000). DNA methylation is dependent on an adequate supply of 5-methylTHF for the synthesis of SAM. However, like homocysteine, global DNA methylation is not specific to folate and can be modified by other nutritional and environmental factors.

Estimation of uracil misincorporation into DNA may also serve as a functional index of folate status (Blount *et al.*, 1997; Jacob *et al.*, 1998). Folate in the form of

5,10-methyleneTHF is required for the conversion of dUMP to dTMP, by thymidylate synthase (Figure 21.2, reaction 6). When this reaction is impaired due to poor folate status, deoxyuridylate may accumulate leading to deoxynucleotide pool imbalances and an increase in the dUMP:dTTP ratio. As a result, uracil, which is normally only present in RNA, may be incorporated into DNA in place of thymine, initiating an excision–repair cycle that may cause DNA strand breaks and chromosome damage (Blount *et al.*, 1997).

Safety of Folic Acid

Safety concerns include the detection of folic acid versus the metabolically reduced form in circulation; the reported association between high folic acid intake and impaired cognitive function; and the potential for folic acid intake to promote the growth of established tumors. Unmetabolized folic acid will be found circulating in the blood if the capacity of dihydrofolate reductase is exceeded. The amount of folic acid as a bolus dose that may result in the appearance of folic acid in circulation has been reported to be >200 μg (Sweeney *et al.*, 2007). Intakes exceeding this threshold are common in the United States since the average dose of folic acid in supplements is 400 μg which is taken in addition to folic acid consumed in enriched grain products and fortified breakfast cereals (Rock, 2007). The presence of unmetabolized folic acid has been detected in many groups evaluated, including older adults in the US (Bailey *et al.*, 2010) and newborn infants (Obeid *et al.*, 2010). High intakes of folic acid have been hypothesized to be associated with cognitive impairment among seniors (Morris *et al.*, 2010), although the findings might have been confounded by the presence of vitamin B_{12} deficiency pernicious anemia and related neurological decline. As reviewed by Ciappio and Mason (2009), folate deficiency has been associated with an increased risk of cancer. Of concern, however, is the potential for folic acid to promote the growth of tumors that may already exist, and this is the focus of on-going research investigations (Ciappio and Mason, 2009). The potential for supplemental folic acid to increase cancer risk was evaluated in a recent meta-analysis involving >37,000 individuals who participated in vitamin D intervention trials designed to assess cardiovascular disease endpoints (Clarke *et al.*, 2010). No increase in cancer risk was associated with supplemental folic acid intake in these large-scale intervention trials.

Future Directions

There are still fundamental gaps in our knowledge of 1-C metabolism and its regulation. Much can still be learned about the interactions among mitochondrial, cytosolic, and nuclear 1-C metabolism and their role in gene expression and genome stability. In addition, the entire metabolic pathway for the folate-dependent conversion of serine to formate and glycine has yet to be established and is the focus of on-going and future research investigations. One-carbon metabolism can be disrupted by folate-related genetic polymorphisms with outcomes modulated by nutrient (e.g. folate, choline, betaine) status. Future studies in genetically engineered mice will be required to model and elucidate the gene–nutrient interactions and associated mechanisms that can alter 1-C metabolism and increase risk for folate-related pathologies.

It is well established that NTD risk is significantly reduced in response to increased folate intake. The biological mechanism by which the vitamin is protective is not, however, fully understood. It is recognized that folate is only one component of a complex metabolic pathway consisting of multiple metabolites, enzymes, and other micronutrients, thus presenting a major challenge to research scientists. New technologies and strategies for investigating biomarkers, genetic variants, and epigenetic phenomena will be essential to further understand the complex relationship between folate and NTDs as well as other birth defects that may be folate responsive.

Reports of the presence of circulating "oxidized unreduced" folic acid will likely increase as the amount and number of sources of this synthetic form of the vitamin increase. Future research studies are warranted to investigate potential physiological consequences of "unmetabolized" folic acid.

The complexity of the relationship between folate intake, cancer, and vascular diseases presents future research challenges. Definitive data from controlled intervention trials are often difficult to interpret for healthy population groups since the studies have been conducted in patients with established histories of disease. Since primary prevention trials are unlikely to be conducted, other means to address this question would need to be considered. With the advent of network analyses from genome-wide association studies, the most important biological pathways in the etiology of cardiovascular disease and cancer can be investigated to determine whether these pathways are folate responsive.

Many additional polymorphisms in genes associated with folate metabolism are yet to be identified. Genome-wide technologies will facilitate conduction of numerous association studies to evaluate the impact of genetic variation on human health in a variety of populations across the globe.

Suggestions for Further Reading

Folate's role in health and disease with accompanying metabolic background is the highlight of a recently published book with more than 50 experts in the folate field as contributing authors (Bailey, 2009). Present knowledge of compartmentalization of folate-mediated 1-C metabolic pathways has been detailed in a comprehensive review (Tibbetts and Appling, 2010).

The basis of our current DRIs for folate was written by scientific experts in the folate field, and their report (IOM, 1998) provides a fundamental overview of the derivation of intake recommendations including the folic acid intake recommendation for NTD risk reduction (IOM, 1998).

References

Albert, C.M., Cook, N.R., Gaziano, J.M., *et al.* (2008) Effect of folic acid and B vitamins on risk of cardiovascular events and total mortality among women at high risk for cardiovascular disease: a randomized trial. *JAMA* **299**, 2027–2036.

Amorim, M.R., Lima, M.A., Castilla, E.E., *et al.* (2007) Non-Latin European descent could be a requirement for association of NTDs and MTHFR variant 677C > T: a meta-analysis. *Am J Med Genet A* **143A**, 1726–1732.

Anderson, D.D., Woeller, C.F., and Stover, P.J. (2007) Small ubiquitin-like modifier-1 (SUMO-1) modification of thymidylate synthase and dihydrofolate reductase. *Clin Chem Lab Med* **45**, 1760–1763.

Anguera, M.C., Field, M.S., Perry, C., *et al.* (2006) Regulation of folate-mediated one-carbon metabolism by 10-formyltetrahydrofolate dehydrogenase. *J Biol Chem* **281**, 18335–18342.

Assaraf, Y.G. (2007) Molecular basis of antifolate resistance. *Cancer Metastasis Rev* **26**, 153–181.

Aufreiter, S., Gregory, J.F., 3rd, Pfeiffer, C.M., *et al.* (2009) Folate is absorbed across the colon of adults: evidence from cecal infusion of (13)C-labeled [6S]-5-formyltetrahydrofolic acid. *Am J Clin Nutr* **90**, 116–123.

Babu, S. and Srikantia, S.G. (1976) Availability of folates from some foods. *Am J Clin Nutr* **29**, 376–379.

Bailey, L.B. (ed.) (2009) *Folate in Health and Disease*, 2nd Edn. CRC Press, Boca Raton, FL.

Bailey, R.L., Dodd, K.W., Gahche, J.J., *et al.* (2010) Total folate and folic acid intake from foods and dietary supplements in the United States: 2003–2006. *Am J Clin Nutr* **91**, 231–237.

Baker, F., Picton, D., Blackwood, S., *et al.* (2002) Blinded comparison of folic acid and placebo in patients with ischemic heart disease: an outcome trial. *Circulation* **106**, 3642 (abstract).

Beilby, J., Ingram, D., Hahnel, R., *et al.* (2004) Reduced breast cancer risk with increasing serum folate in a case-control study of the C677T genotype of the methylenetetrahydrofolate reductase gene. *Eur J Cancer* **40**, 1250–1254.

Berry, R., Mullinare, J., and Hamner HC. (2009) Folic acid fortification: Neural tube defect risk reduction – global perspective. In L. Bailey (ed.), *Folate in Health and Disease*, 2nd Edn, CRC Press, Boca Raton, FL, pp. 179–204.

Blount, B.C., Mack, M.M., Wehr, C.M., *et al.* (1997) Folate deficiency causes uracil misincorporation into human DNA and chromosome breakage: implications for cancer and neuronal damage. *Proc Natl Acad Sci USA* **94**, 3290–3295.

Bønaa, K.H., Njølstad, I., Ueland, P.M., *et al.* (2006). Homocysteine lowering and cardiovascular events after acute myocardial infarction. *N Engl J Med* **354**, 1578–1588.

Bottiglieri, T. and Reynolds, E. (2009) Folate and neurological disease. Basic mechanisms. In L.B. Bailey (ed.), *Folate in Health and Disease*, 2nd Edn. CRC Press, Boca Raton, FL, pp. 355–380.

Botto, L. and Yang, Q. (2000) 5,10-Methylenetetrahydrofolate reductase gene variants and congenital anomalies: a HuGE review. *Am J Epidemiol* **151**, 862–877.

Botto, L.D., Moore, C.A., Khoury, M.J., *et al.* (1999) Neural-tube defects. *N Engl J Med* **341**, 1509–1519.

Botto, L.D., Mulinare, J., and Erickson, J.D. (2003) Do multivitamin or folic acid supplements reduce the risk for congenital heart defects? Evidence and gaps. *Am J Med Genet* **121A**, 95–101.

Caudill, M.A. (2010) Folate bioavailability: implications for establishing dietary recommendations and optimizing status. *Am J Clin Nutr* **91**, 1455S–1460S.

Caudill, M.A., Gregory, J.F., Hutson, A.D., *et al.* (1998) Folate catabolism in pregnant and nonpregnant women with controlled folate intakes. *J Nutr* **128**, 204–208.

CDC (1992) Recommendations for the use of folic acid to reduce the number of cases of spina bifida and other neural tube defects. *MMWR Recomm Rep* **41**, 1–7.

Chandler, C.J., Wang, T.T., and Halsted, C.H. (1986) Pteroylpolyglutamate hydrolase from human jejunal brush borders. Purification and characterization. *J Biol Chem* **261**, 928–933.

Chen, J., Giovannucci, E., Kelsey, K., *et al.* (1996) A methylenetetrahydrofolate reductase polymorphism and the risk of colorectal cancer. *Cancer Res* **56**, 4862–4864.

Chen, J., Xu, X., Liu, A., *et al.* (2009) Folate and cancer: epidemiological perspective. In L.B. Bailey (ed.), *Folate in Health and Disease*, 2nd Edn. CRC Press, Boca Raton, FL, pp. 205–233.

Christensen, K.E. and MacKenzie, R.E. (2006) Mitochondrial one-carbon metabolism is adapted to the specific needs of yeast, plants and mammals. *Bioessays* **28**, 595–605.

Christensen, K.E. and MacKenzie, R.E. (2008) Mitochondrial methylenetetrahydrofolate dehydrogenase, methenyltetrahydrofolate cyclohydrolase, and formyltetrahydrofolate synthetases. *Vitam Horm* **79**, 393–410.

Christensen, K.E. and Rozen, R. (2009) Genetic variation: effect on folate metabolism and health. In L.B. Bailey (ed.), *Folate in Health and Disease*, 2nd Edn. CRC Press, Boca Raton, pp. 75–110.

Christensen, K.E., Patel, H., Kuzmanov, U., *et al.* (2005) Disruption of the mthfd1 gene reveals a monofunctional 10-formyltetrahydrofolate synthetase in mammalian mitochondria. *J Biol Chem* **280**, 7597–7602.

Ciappio, E. and Mason, J.B. (2009) Folate and carcinogenesis: basic mechanisms. In L.B. Bailey (ed.), *Folate in Health and Disease*, 2nd Edn. CRC Press, Boca Raton, FL, pp. 205–233.

Clarke, R., Halsey, J., Lewington, S., *et al.* (2010) Effects of lowering homocysteine levels with B vitamins on cardiovascular disease, cancer, and cause-specific mortality: meta-analysis of 8 randomized trials involving 37,485 individuals. *Arch Intern Med* **170**, 1622–1631.

Clifford, A.J., Arjomand, A., Dueker, S.R., *et al.* (1998). The dynamics of folic acid metabolism in an adult given a small tracer dose of 14C-folic acid. *Adv Exp Med Biol* **445**, 239–251.

Cole, B.F., Baron, J.A., Sandler, R.S., *et al.* (2007). Folic acid for the prevention of colorectal adenomas: a randomized clinical trial. *JAMA* **297**, 2351–2359.

Crider, K.S., Zhu, J., Hao, L., *et al.* (2011) MTHFR 677C→T genotype is associated with folate and homocysteine concentrations in a large, population-based, double-blind trial of folic acid supplementation. *Am J Clin Nutr* **93**, 1365–1372.

De Marco, P., Calevo, M.G., Moroni, A., *et al.* (2003). Reduced folate carrier polymorphism (80A→G) and neural tube defects. *Eur J Hum Genet* **11**, 245–252.

Department of Health and Human Services, Food and Drug Administration (1996) Food standards: amendment of standards of identity for enriched grain products to require addition of folic acid. *Fed Reg* **61**, 8781–8797.

Dianov, G.L., Timchenko, T.V., Sinitsina, O.I., *et al.* (1991) Repair of uracil residues closely spaced on the opposite strands of plasmid DNA results in double-strand break and deletion formation. *Mol Gen Genet* **225**, 448–452.

Ebbing, M., Bleie, O., Ueland, P.M., *et al.* (2008). Mortality and cardiovascular events in patients treated with homocysteine-lowering B vitamins after coronary angiography: a randomized controlled trial. *JAMA* **300**, 795–804.

Elliott, B. and Jasin, M. (2002) Double-strand breaks and translocations in cancer. *Cell Mol Life Sci* **59**, 373–385.

Ericson, U., Sonestedt, E., Gullberg, B., *et al.* (2007). High folate intake is associated with lower breast cancer incidence in postmenopausal women in the Malmo Diet and Cancer cohort. *Am J Clin Nutr* **86**, 434–443.

Exinger, D., Exinger, F., Mennecier, B., *et al.* (2003) Multitargeted antifolate (pemetrexed): a comprehensive review of its mechanisms of action, recent results and future prospects. *Cancer Therapy* **1**, 315–322.

FDA (1996) Food standards: amendment of standards of identity for enriched grain products to require addition of folic acid, Final Rule, 21. CFR Parts 136, 137, and 139. *Fed Reg* **64**, 8781–8789).

Frosst, P., Blom, H. J., Milos, R., *et al.* (1995) A candidate genetic risk factor for vascular disease: a common mutation in methylenetetrahydrofolate reductase. *Nat Genet* **10**, 111–113.

Giovannucci, E. (2002) Epidemiologic studies of folate and colorectal neoplasia: a review. *J Nutr* **132** (8 Suppl), 2350S–2355S.

Gregory, I.J., DaSilva, V., and Lamers, Y. (2009) Kinetics of folate and one-carbon metabolism. In L.B. Bailey (ed.), *Folate in Health and Disease*, 2nd Edn. CRC Press, Boca Raton, FL, pp. 491–519

Gregory, J.F., 3rd, Caudill, M.A., Opalko, F.J., *et al.* (2001) Kinetics of folate turnover in pregnant women (second trimester) and nonpregnant controls during folic acid supplementation: stable-isotopic labeling of plasma folate, urinary folate and folate catabolites shows subtle effects of pregnancy on turnover of folate pools. *J Nutr* **131**, 1928–1937.

Gregory, J.F., 3rd, Ink, S.L., and Cerda, J.J. (1987) Comparison of pteroylpolyglutamate hydrolase (folate conjugase) from porcine and human intestinal brush border membrane. *Comp Biochem Physiol B* **88**, 1135–1141.

Gregory, J.F., 3rd, Williamson, J., Liao, J.F., *et al.* (1998) Kinetic model of folate metabolism in nonpregnant women consuming [^{2}H$_2$]folic acid: isotopic labeling of urinary folate and the catabolite para-acetamidobenzoylglutamate indicates slow, intake-dependent, turnover of folate pools. *J Nutr* **128**, 1896–1906.

Gronbaek, K., Hother, C., and Jones, P.A. (2007) Epigenetic changes in cancer. *APMIS* **115**, 1039–1059.

Gueant-Rodriguez, R.-M., Gueant, J.-L., Debard, R., *et al.* (2006) Prevalence of methylenetetrahydrofolate reductase 677T and 1298C alleles and folate status: a comparative study in Mexican, West African, and European populations. *Am J Clin Nutr* **83**, 701–707.

Halsted, C.H., Medici, V., and Esfandiari, F. (2009) Influence of alcohol on folate status and methionine metabolism in relation to alcoholic liver disease. In L.B. Bailey (ed.), *Folate in Health and Disease*, 2nd Edn. CRC Press, Boca Raton, FL, pp. 429–448.

Hannibal, L., Glushchenko, A.V., and Jacobsen, D.W. (2009) (ed.), *Folate in Health and Disease*, 2nd Edn. CRC Press, Boca Raton, FL, pp. 291–323.

Hellman, S., Iannotti, A.T., and Bertino, J.R. (1964) Determinations of the levels of serum folate in patients with carcinoma of the head and neck treated with methotrexate. *Cancer Res* **24**, 105–113.

Herbert, V. and Das, K.C. (1994) Folic acid and vitamin B12. In M. Shils, J.A. Olson, and M. Shike (eds), *Modern Nutrition in Health and Disease*, 8th Edn. Lea and Fabiger, Philadelphia, pp. 402–425

Herbert, V. and Zalusky, R. (1962) Interrelations of vitamin B12 and folic acid metabolism: folic acid clearance studies. *J Clin Invest* **41**, 1263–1276.

Herbig, K., Chiang, E.-P., Lee, L.-R., *et al.* (2002) Cytoplasmic serine hydroxymethyltransferase mediates competition between folate-dependent deoxyribonucleotide and S-adenosylmethionine biosyntheses. *J Biol Chem* **277**, 38381–38389.

Hobbs, C.A., Shaw, G.M., Werler, M.M., *et al.* (2009) Folate status and birth defect risk. In L.B. Bailey (ed.), *Folate in Health and Disease*, 2nd Edn. CRC Press, Boca Raton, FL, pp. 133–153.

Hoppner, K. and Lampi, B. (1980) Folate levels in human liver from autopsies in Canada. *Am J Clin Nutr* **33**, 862–864.

Hustad, S., Midttun, O., Schneede, J., *et al.* (2007) The methylenetetrahydrofolate reductase 677C→T polymorphism as a modulator of a B vitamin network with major effects on homocysteine metabolism. *Am J Hum Genet* **80**, 846–855.

Institute of Medicine (1998) Folate. In *Dietary Reference Intakes for Thiamin, Riboflavin, Niacin, Vitamin B6, Folate, Vitamin B12, Pantothenic Acid, Biotin, and Choline*. National Academies Press, Washington, DC, pp. 196–305.

Jacob, R.A., Gretz, D.M., Taylor, P.C., *et al.* (1998) Moderate folate depletion increases plasma homocysteine and decreases lymphocyte DNA methylation in postmenopausal women. *J Nutr* **128**, 1204–1212.

Jacques, P.F., Bostom, A.G., Williams, R.R., *et al.* (1996) Relation between folate status, a common mutation in methylenetetrahydrofolate reductase, and plasma homocysteine concentrations. *Circulation* **93**, 7–9.

Jamison, R.L., Hartigan, P., Kaufman, J.S., *et al.* (2007) Effect of homocysteine lowering on mortality and vascular disease in advanced chronic kidney disease and end-stage renal disease: a randomized controlled trial. *JAMA* **298**, 1163–1170.

Jansen, G., van der Heijden, J., Oerlemans, R., *et al.* (2004) Sulfasalazine is a potent inhibitor of the reduced folate carrier: implications for combination therapies with methotrexate in rheumatoid arthritis. *Arthritis Rheum* **50**, 2130–2139.

Kalin, S.R. and Rimm, E.B. (2009) Folate and vascular disease: epidemiological perspective. In L.B. Bailey (ed.), *Folate in Health and Disease*, 2nd Edn. CRC Press, Boca Raton, FL, pp. 263–290.

Kauwell, P., Diaz, M.L., Yang, Q., *et al.* (2009). Folate: recommended intakes, consumption, and status. In L.B. Bailey (ed.), *Folate in Health and Disease*, 2nd Edn. CRC Press, Boca Raton, FL, pp. 467–490

Kelly, P., McPartlin, J., Goggins, M., *et al.* (1997). Unmetabolized folic acid in serum: Acute studies in subjects consuming fortified food supplements. *Am J Clin Nutr* **65**, 1790–1795.

Krumdieck, C.L., Fukushima, K., Fukushima, T., *et al.* (1978) A long-term study of the excretion of folate and pterins in a human subject after ingestion of 14C folic acid, with observations on the effect of diphenylhydantoin administration. *Am J Clin Nutr* **31**, 88–93.

Larsson, S.C., Giovannucci, E., and Wolk, A. (2006) Folate intake, MTHFR polymorphisms, and risk of esophageal, gastric, and pancreatic cancer: a meta-analysis. *Gastroenterology* **131**, 1271–1283.

Lin, Y., Dueker, S.R., Follett, J.R., *et al.* (2004) Quantitation of in vivo human folate metabolism. *Am J Clin Nutr* **80**, 680–691.

Lindenbaum, J. and Allen, R. (1995) Clinical spectrum and diagnosis of folate deficiency. In L.B. Bailey (ed.), *Folate in Health and Disease*. Marcel Decker, New York, pp. 43–73.

Lonn, E., Yusuf, S., Arnold, M.J., *et al.* (2006) Homocysteine lowering with folic acid and B vitamins in vascular disease. *N Engl J Med* **354**, 1567–1577.

Matherly, L.H. and Goldman, D.I. (2003) Membrane transport of folates. *Vitam Horm* **66**, 403–456.

Matherly, L.H. and Hou, Z. (2008) Structure and function of the reduced folate carrier a paradigm of a major facilitator superfamily mammalian nutrient transporter. *Vitam Horm* **79**, 145–184.

McDowell, M.A., Lacher, D.A., Pfeiffer, C.M., *et al.* (2008) Blood folate levels: the latest NHANES results. *NCHS Data Brief* (6), 1–8.

McNulty, H. and Pentieva, K. (2009) Folate bioavailability. In L.B. Bailey (ed.), *Folate in Health and Disease*, 2nd Edn. CRC Press, Boca Raton, FL, pp. 25–47.

Melikian, V., Paton, A., and Leeming, R.J., *et al.* (1971). Site of reduction and methylation of folic acid in man. *Lancet* **2**, 955–957.

Melnyk, S., Pogribna, M., Pogribny, I., *et al.* (1999) A new HPLC method for the simultaneous determination of oxidized and reduced plasma aminothiols using coulometric electrochemical detection. *J Nutr Biochem* **10**, 490–497.

Melnyk, S., Pogribna, M., Pogribny, I.P., *et al.* (2000) Measurement of plasma and intracellular S-adenosylmethionine and S-adenosylhomocysteine utilizing coulometric electrochemical detection: alterations with plasma homocysteine and pyridoxal 5′-phosphate concentrations. *Clin Chem* **46**, 265–272.

Molloy, A.M., Mills, J.L., Kirke, P.N., *et al.* (1998a) Low blood folates in NTD pregnancies are only partly explained by thermolabile 5,10-methylenetetrahydrofolate reductase: low folate status alone may be the critical factor. *Am J Med Genet* **78**, 155–159.

Molloy, A.M., Mills, J.L., Kirke, P.N., *et al.* (1998b) Whole-blood folate values in subjects with different methylenetetrahydrofolate reductase genotypes: differences between the radioassay and microbiological assays. *Clin Chem* **44**, 186–188.

Molloy, A.M., Brody, L.C., Mills, J.L., *et al.* (2009) The search for genetic polymorphisms in the homocysteine/folate pathway that contribute to the etiology of human neural tube defects. *Birth Defects Res A Clin Mol Teratol* **85**, 285–294.

Morris, M.S. and Jacques, P.F.E. (2009) Folate and neurological disease. Epidemiological perspective. In L.B. Bailey (ed.), *Folate in Health and Disease*, 2nd Edn. CRC Press, Boca Raton, FL, pp. 325–353.

Morris, M.S., Jacques, P.F., Rosenberg, I.H., *et al.* (2010) Circulating unmetabolized folic acid and 5-methyltetrahydrofolate in relation to anemia, macrocytosis, and cognitive test performance in American seniors. *Am J Clin Nutr* **91**, 1733–1744.

Mutch, D.M., Anderle, P., Fiaux, M., *et al.* (2004) Regional variations in ABC transporter expression along the mouse intestinal tract. *Physiol Genomics* **17**, 11–20.

Obeid, R., Kasoha, M., Kirsch, S.H., *et al.* (2010) Concentrations of unmetabolized folic acid and primary folate forms in pregnant women at delivery and in umbilical cord blood. *Am J Clin Nutr* **92**, 1416–1422.

Ogawa, H., Gomi, T., Takusagawa, F., *et al.* (1998) Structure, function and physiological role of glycine N-methyltransferase. *Int J Biochem Cell Biol* **30**, 13–26.

O'Leary, V.B., Mills, J.L., Pangilinan, F., *et al.* (2005) Analysis of methionine synthase reductase polymorphisms of neural tube defects risk association. *Mol Genet Metab* **85**, 220–227.

O'Leary, V.B., Pangilinan, F., Cox, C., *et al.* (2006) Reduced folate carrier polymorphisms and neural tube defect risk. *Mol Genet Metab* **87**, 364–369.

Olteanu, H., Munson, T., and Banerjee, R. (2002) Differences in the efficiency of reductive activation of methionine synthase and exogenous electron acceptors between the common polymorphic variants of human methionine synthase reductase. *Biochemistry* **41**, 13378–13385.

Pei, L., Zhu, H., Ren, A., *et al.* (2005) Reduced folate carrier gene is a risk factor for neural tube defects in a Chinese population. *Birth Defects Res A Clin Mol Teratol* **73**, 430–433.

Pelletier, J.N. and MacKenzie, R.E. (1995) Binding and interconversion of tetrahydrofolates at a single site in the bifunctional methylenetetrahydrofolate dehydrogenase/cyclohydrolase. *Biochemistry* **34**, 12673–12680.

Peri, K.G. and MacKenzie, R.E. (1991) Transcriptional regulation of murine NADP(+)-dependent methylenetetrahydrofolate dehydrogenase-cyclohydrolase-synthetase. *FEBS Lett* **294**, 113–115.

Pfeiffer, C.M., Fazili, Z., and Zhang, M. (2009) Folate analytical methodology. In L.B. Bailey (ed.), *Folate in Health and Disease*, 2nd Edn. CRC Press, Boca Raton, FL, pp. 517–574.

Pfeiffer, C.M., Johnson, C.L., Jain, R.B., *et al.* (2007) Trends in blood folate and vitamin B-12 concentrations in the United States, 1988–2004. *Am J Clin Nutr* **86**, 718–727.

Pfeiffer, C.M., Osterloh, J.D., Kennedy-Stephenson, J., *et al.* (2008) Trends in circulating concentrations of total homocysteine among US adolescents and adults: findings from the 1991–1994 and 1999–2004 National Health and Nutrition Examination Surveys. *Clin Chem* **54**, 801–813.

Pfeiffer, C.M., Rogers, L.M., Bailey, L.B., *et al.* (1997) Absorption of folate from fortified cereal-grain products and of supplemental folate consumed with or without food determined by using a dual-label stable-isotope protocol. *Am J Clin Nutr* **66**, 1388–1397.

Pietrzik, K., Bailey, L., and Shane, B. (2010) Folic acid and L-5-methyltetrahydrofolate. *Clin Pharmacokinet* **49**, 535–548.

Priest, D.G. and Bunni, M.A. (1995) Folates and folate antagonists in cancer chemotherapy. In L.B. Bailey (ed.), *Folate in Health and Disease*. Marcel Dekker, New York, pp. 379–404.

Prinz-Langenohl, R., Bronstrup, A., Thorand, B., *et al.* (1999) Availability of food folate in humans. *J Nutr* **129**, 913–916.

Qiu, A., Jansen, M., Sakaris, A., *et al.* (2006). Identification of an intestinal folate transporter and the molecular basis for hereditary folate malabsorption. *Cell* **127**, 917–928.

Rampersaud, G.C., Kauwell, G.P., Hutson, A.D., *et al.* (2000) Genomic DNA methylation decreases in response to moderate folate depletion in elderly women. *Am J Clin Nutr* **72**, 998–1003.

Ratnam, M. and Freisheim, J.H. (1990). Proteins involved in the transport of folates and antifolates by normal and neoplastic cells. In M.F. Picciano, E.L.R. Stokstad, and J.F. Gregory (eds), *Contemporary Issues in Clinical Nutrition*, Vol. 13. Wiley-Liss, New York, pp. 91–120.

Rock, C.L. (2007) Multivitamin–multimineral supplements: who uses them? *Am J Clin Nutr* **85**, 277S–279S.

Sanjoaquin, M.A., Allen, N., Couto, E., *et al.* (2005) Folate intake and colorectal cancer risk: a meta-analytical approach. *Int J Cancer* **113**, 825–828.

Sauberlich, H.E., Kretsch, M.J., Skala, J.H., *et al.* (1987) Folate requirement and metabolism in nonpregnant women. *Am J Clin Nutr* **46**, 1016–1028.

Selhub, J., Dhar, G.J., and Rosenberg, I.H. (1978) Inhibition of folate enzymes by sulfasalazine. *J Clin Invest* **61**, 221–224.

Shane, B. (1989) Folylpolyglutamate synthesis and role in the regulation of one-carbon metabolism. *Vitam Horm* **45**, 263–335.

Shane, B. (2009) Folate chemistry and metabolism. In L.B. Bailey (ed.), *Folate in Health and Disease*, 2nd Edn. CRC Press, Boca Raton, FL, pp. 1–24.

Sharp, L. and Little, J. (2004) Polymorphisms in genes involved in folate metabolism and colorectal neoplasia: A HuGE Review. *Am J Epidemiol* **159**, 423–443.

Shaw, G.M., Carmichael, S.L., Nelson, V., *et al.* (2004) Occurrence of low birthweight and preterm delivery among California infants before and after compulsory food fortification with folic acid. *Public Health Rep* **119**, 170–173.

Shaw, G.M., Lammer, E.J., Zhu, H., *et al.* (2002) Maternal periconceptional vitamin use, genetic variation of infant reduced folate carrier (A80G), and risk of spina bifida. *Am J Med Genet* **108**, 1–6.

Shaw, G.M., Lu, W., Zhu, H., *et al.* (2009) 118 SNPs of folate-related genes and risk of spina bifida and conotruncal heart defects. *BMC Med Genet* **10**, 49.

Shaw, G.M., Rozen, R., Finnell, R.H., *et al.* (1998) Maternal vitamin use, genetic variation of infant methylenetetrahydrofolate reductase, and risk for spina bifida. *Am J Epidemiol* **148**, 30–37.

Stabler, S.S. (2009) Clinical folate deficiency. In L.B. Bailey (ed.) *Folate in Health and Disease*, 2nd Edn. CRC Press, Boca Raton, FL, pp. 409–448.

Stites, T.E., Bailey, L.B., Scott, K.C., *et al.* (1997) Kinetic modeling of folate metabolism through use of chronic administration of deuterium-labeled folic acid in men. *Am J Clin Nutr* **65**, 53–60.

Stolzenberg-Solomon, R.Z., Chang, S.C., Leitzmann, M.F., *et al.* (2006) Folate intake, alcohol use, and postmenopausal breast cancer risk in the Prostate, Lung, Colorectal, and Ovarian Cancer Screening Trial. *Am J Clin Nutr* **83**, 895–904.

Stover, P. (2009) Folate biochemical pathways and their regulation. In L.B. Bailey (ed.), *Folate in Health and Disease*, 2nd Edn. CRC Press, Boca Raton, FL, pp. 49–74

Subramanian, V.S., Marchant, J.S., and Said, H.M. (2008) Apical membrane targeting and trafficking of the human proton-coupled transporter in polarized epithelia. *Am J Physiol Cell Physiol* **294**, C233–240.

Sweeney, M., McPartlin, J., and Scott, J. (2007) Folic acid fortification and public health: Report on threshold doses above which unmetabolised folic acid appears in serum. *BMC Public Health* **7**, 41.

Sweeney, M.R., McPartlin, J., Weir, D.G., *et al.* (2006) Postprandial serum folic acid response to multiple doses of folic acid in fortified bread. *Br J Nutr* **95**, 5–51.

Tamura, T. and Picciano, M.F. (2006) Folate and human reproduction. *Am J Clin Nutr* **83**, 993–1016.

Tamura, T. and Stokstad, E.L. (1973) The availability of food folate in man. *Br J Haematol* **25**, 513–532.

Tamura, T., Picciano, M.F., and McGuire, M.K. (2009) Folate in pregnancy and lactation. In L.B. Bailey (ed.), *Folate in Health and Disease*, 2nd Edn. CRC Press, Boca Raton, FL, pp. 111–131.

Tamura, T., Shin, Y.S., Buehring, K.U., *et al.* (1976) The availability of folates in man: effect of orange juice supplement on intestinal conjugase. *Br J Haematol* **32**, 123–133.

Tennstedt, C., Chaoui, R., Korner, H., *et al.* (1999) Spectrum of congenital heart defects and extracardiac malformations associated with chromosomal abnormalities: results of a seven year necropsy study. *Heart* **82**, 34–39.

Tibbetts, A.S. and Appling, D.R. (2010) Compartmentalization of mammalian folate-mediated one-carbon metabolism. *Annu Rev Nutr* **30**, 57–81.

Toole, J.F., Malinow, M.R., Chambless, L.E., *et al.* (2004) Lowering homocysteine in patients with ischemic stroke to prevent recurrent stroke, myocardial infarction, and death: the Vitamin Intervention for Stroke Prevention (VISP) randomized controlled trial. *JAMA* **291**, 565–575.

USDA (2009) Food and Nutrient Database for Dietary Studies Version 1.0. [internet database].: US Department of Agriculture and Agricultural Research Service, Food Surveys Research Group;. c 2004. Beltsville, MD Available from: http://www.ars.usda.gov/services/docs.htm?docid=7673.

van Beynum, I.M., den Heijer, M., Blom, H.J., *et al.* (2007) The MTHFR 677C→T polymorphism and the risk of congenital heart defects: a literature review and meta-analysis. *QJM* **100**, 743–753.

van der Linden, I.J., den Heijer, M., Afman, L.A., *et al.* (2006) The methionine synthase reductase 66A>G polymorphism is a maternal risk factor for spina bifida. *J Mol Med* **84**, 1047–1054.

van Ede, A.E., Laan, R.F., Rood, M.J., *et al.* (2001) Effect of folic or folinic acid supplementation on the toxicity and efficacy of methotrexate in rheumatoid arthritis: a forty-eight week, multicenter, randomized, double-blind, placebo-controlled study. *Arthritis Rheum* **44,** 1515–1524.

Verkleij-Hagoort, A., Bliek, J., Sayed-Tabatabaei, F., *et al.* (2007) Hyperhomocysteinemia and MTHFR polymorphisms in association with orofacial clefts and congenital heart defects: a meta-analysis. *Am J Med Genet A* **143A,** 952–960.

Voeller, D., Rahman, L., and Zajac-Kaye, M. (2004) Elevated levels of thymidylate synthase linked to neoplastic transformation of mammalian cells. *Cell Cycle* **3,** 1005–1007.

Voorrips, L.E., Goldbohm, R.A., Brants, H.A., *et al.* (2000) A prospective cohort study on antioxidant and folate intake and male lung cancer risk. *Cancer Epidemiol Biomarkers Prev* **9,** 357–365.

Wallis, D., Ballard, J.L., Shaw, G.M., *et al.* (2009) Folate-related birth defects: embryonic consequences of abnormal folate transport and metabolism. In L.B. Bailey (ed.), *Folate in Health and Disease*, 2nd Edn. CRC Press, Boca Raton, FL, pp. 155–178.

Wessels, J.A., Huizinga, T.W., and Guchelaar, H.J. (2008) Recent insights in the pharmacological actions of methotrexate in the treatment of rheumatoid arthritis. *Rheumatology (Oxford)* **47,** 249–255.

Whitehead, V.M. (1973) Polygammaglutamyl metabolites of folic acid in human liver. *Lancet* **1,** 743–745.

Whitehead, V.M. and Cooper, B.A. (1967) Absorption of unaltered folic acid from the gastrointestinal tract in man. *Br J Haematol* **13,** 679–686.

Whittle, S.L. and Hughes, R.A. (2004) Folate supplementation and methotrexate treatment in rheumatoid arthritis: a review. *Rheumatology (Oxford)* **43,** 267–271.

Wilson, A., Platt, R., Wu, Q., *et al.* (1999) A common variant in methionine synthase reductase combined with low cobalamin (vitamin B12) increases risk for spina bifida. *Mol Genet Metab* **67,** 317–323.

Woeller, C.F., Anderson, D.D., Szebenyi, D.M., and Stover, P.J. (2007) Evidence for small ubiquitin-like modifier-dependent nuclear import of the thymidylate biosynthesis pathway. *J Biol Chem* **282,** 17623–17631.

Yang, Q., Cogswell, M.E., Hamner, H.C., *et al.* (2010) Folic acid source, usual intake, and folate and vitamin B-12 status in US adults: National Health and Nutrition Examination Survey (NHANES) 2003–2006. *Am J Clin Nutr* **91,** 64–72.

Yang, Q.H., Botto, L.D., Gallagher, M., *et al.* (2008) Prevalence and effects of gene–gene and gene–nutrient interactions on serum folate and serum total homocysteine concentrations in the United States: findings from the third National Health and Nutrition Examination Survey DNA Bank. *Am J Clin Nutr* **88,** 232–246.

Yuasa, H., Inoue, K., and Hayashi, Y. (2009) Molecular and functional characteristics of proton-coupled folate transporter. *J Pharm Sci* **98,** 1608–1616.

Zhao, R., Gao, F., and Goldman, I.D. (2002) Reduced folate carrier transports thiamine monophosphate: an alternative route for thiamine delivery into mammalian cells. *Am J Physiol Cell Physiol* **282,** C1512–1517.

Zhao, R., Matherly, L.H., and Goldman, I.D. (2009) Membrane transporters and folate homeostasis: intestinal absorption and transport into systemic compartments and tissues. *Expert Rev Mol Med* **11,** e4.

Zhao, R., Min, S.H., Wang, Y., *et al.* (2009) A role for the proton-coupled folate transporter (PCFT-SLC46A1) in folate receptor-mediated endocytosis. *J Biol Chem* **284,** 4267–4274.

22

VITAMIN B$_{12}$

SALLY P. STABLER, MD

University of Colorado School of Medicine, Denver, Colorado, USA

Summary

Vitamin B$_{12}$ (cobalamin) is a cobalt-containing corrin ring cofactor required for two enzymes in higher animals, methionine synthase and L-methylmalonyl-CoA mutase. It is a product of microbial synthesis, and therefore elaborate mechanisms of uptake and transport have evolved to insure availability of this rare nutrient in higher animals. Vitamin B$_{12}$ ingested in the diet binds to intrinsic factor and is internalized in the distal small intestine by the cubam receptor. It is delivered to all the cells in the body by transcobalamin, a binding protein. Human B$_{12}$ deficiency is caused by lack of animal source food, or lack of intrinsic factor due to the autoimmune disease, pernicious anemia, and other malabsorption syndromes. Human deficiency causes megaloblastic anemia and/or demyelinating neurologic syndromes. A deficiency of vitamin B$_{12}$ causes a build-up of methylmalonic acid and homocysteine which can be assayed for diagnostic purposes. Treatment with parenteral or high-dose oral vitamin B$_{12}$ is effective in malabsorption syndromes and will completely correct megaloblastic anemia. Neurologic abnormalities due to B$_{12}$ deficiency may only partially correct, especially in infants. The development of inexpensive B$_{12}$-containing foods acceptable to populations unwilling to eat or unable to afford animal source foods would be of benefit because of the high prevalence of B$_{12}$ deficiency worldwide.

Introduction

Vitamin B$_{12}$ (cobalamin, Cbl) holds a unique position in the science of human nutrition since there is a specific disease (pernicious anemia) which results in the isolated malabsorption of vitamin B$_{12}$, and was ultimately fatal prior to the development of vitamin therapy. This unique syndrome of megaloblastic anemia and demyelinating lesions of the central nervous system was recognized and described by Thomas Addison as early as 1855 (Castle, 1975). Pernicious anemia has such specific manifestations and such a dramatic response to the replacement of vitamin B$_{12}$ that a patient response could actually be used as a bioassay. In 1926 Minot and Murphy showed that a diet containing large amounts of liver would stimulate red blood cell production in patients with pernicious anemia (Minot and Murphy, 1926). Their early work eventually culminated in the purification of vitamin B$_{12}$ from liver by Folkers at Merck, Sharp & Dohme in 1948, and Smith and Parker at Glaxo in the same year (Folkers, 1982).

Present Knowledge in Nutrition, Tenth Edition. Edited by John W. Erdman Jr, Ian A. Macdonald and Steven H. Zeisel.
© 2012 International Life Sciences Institute. Published 2012 by John Wiley & Sons, Inc.

During the next 50 years the structure, X-ray crystallography, synthesis of coenzyme forms, and chemistry and biochemistry of the cobamides have been elucidated (Hogenkamp, 1999). Much of what we know about the role of vitamin B$_{12}$ in metabolism and the pathophysiology of the deficient state has been determined by studying patients with pernicious anemia since this accident of nature results in a very selective model of a deficiency disease not complicated by protein-calorie malnutrition or multiple vitamin and mineral deficiencies.

Structure of Vitamin B$_{12}$

The structure of vitamin B$_{12}$ (OH-Cbl) is shown in Figure 22.1. It is a very complex molecule containing a corrin ring (which coordinates a cobalt molecule), 5,6-dimethylbenzimidazole, a sugar, and an aminopropanol group. An upper axial ligand is coordinated to the cobalt and can be hydroxy, cyano, glutathione or the coenzyme forms, methyl (CH$_3$) and adenosyl (Banerjee and Ragsdale, 2003). The chemistry of the carbon–cobalt bond found in the coenzyme forms is unique and has been studied extensively (Ludwig and Matthews, 1997; Randaccio et al., 2010). Only microorganisms retain the ability to synthesize cobalamins, and microbial synthesis

FIG. 22.1   The structure of OH-cobalamin.

pathways have been elucidated in a series of elegant studies (Martens et al., 2002). Plants do not use Cbl, therefore the source of Cbl in all higher animals is the product of microbial synthesis. Analogues of Cbl with bases other than 5,6-dimethylbenzimidazole are widely found in nature including in the human intestinal tract (Allen and Stabler, 2008), but do not support coenzyme activity in higher animals, though they are utilized by various microorganisms.

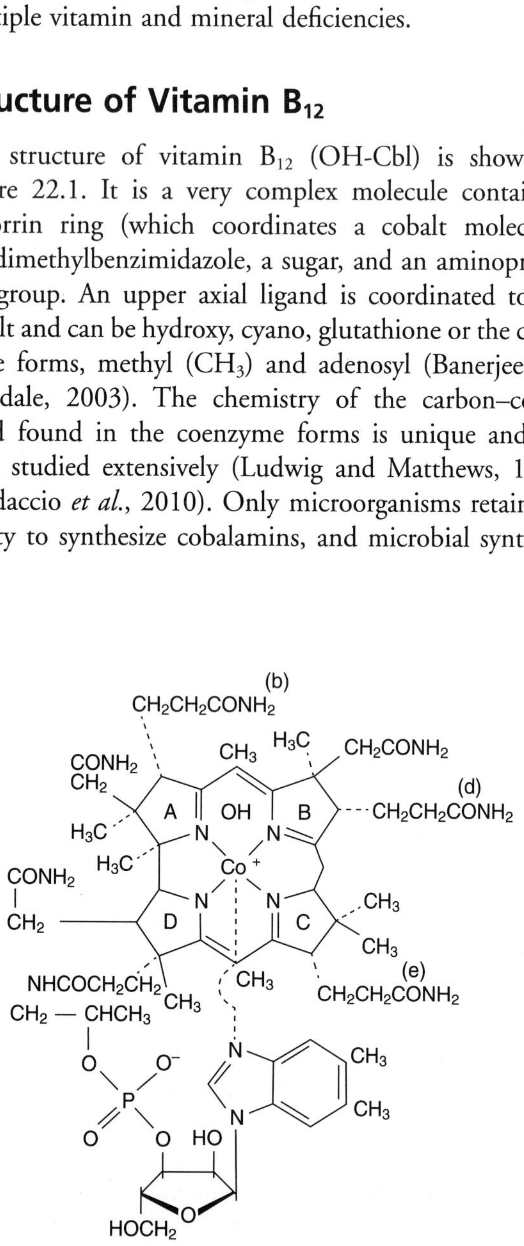

Vitamin B$_{12}$-Dependent Enzyme Reactions

Microorganisms use different forms of Cbl in many reactions, including methionine synthesis, carbon skeleton mutation, elimination reactions, aminomutations, and acetate and methane synthesis (Randaccio et al., 2010). Higher animals require Cbl as a cofactor for only two enzymes, L-methylmalonyl-CoA mutase and methionine synthase (Banerjee and Ragsdale, 2003). The binding of the coenzyme forms to these two enzymes has been studied by X-ray crystallography (Drennan et al., 1994; Mancia et al., 1996; Randaccio et al., 2010). It appears that the dimethylbenzimidazole is displaced from the cobalt and a histidine residue from the enzyme coordinates at that position. Although both of these enzymes use vitamin B$_{12}$, they perform very different types of chemical reaction. During methionine synthesis and other methyltransfer reactions, the methyl–cobalt bond undergoes heterolytic cleavage, whereas the mutase performs a homolytic cleavage of adenosyl-Cbl which results in the formation of a radical. Methionine synthase must be reactivated since the cobalamin cofactor is occasionally oxidized (every 2000 cycles) (Koutmos et al., 2009). A recent review describes structural–functional relationships of the cobalt–carbon bonds in the coenzymes and the role that bond cleavage plays in the specific reactions (Randaccio et al., 2010).

L-Methylmalonyl CoA Mutase

The pathway of propionyl-CoA metabolism is shown in Figure 22.2. The metabolism of various amino acids such as valine, isoleucine, and odd-chain fatty acids results in the formation of propionyl-CoA which is carboxylated to form D-methylmalonyl-CoA. A racemase interconverts the two isomers, and L-methylmalonyl-CoA is a substrate for the adenosyl-Cbl-dependent enzyme L-methylmalonyl-CoA mutase (Fenton et al., 2001). D-Methylmalonyl-CoA

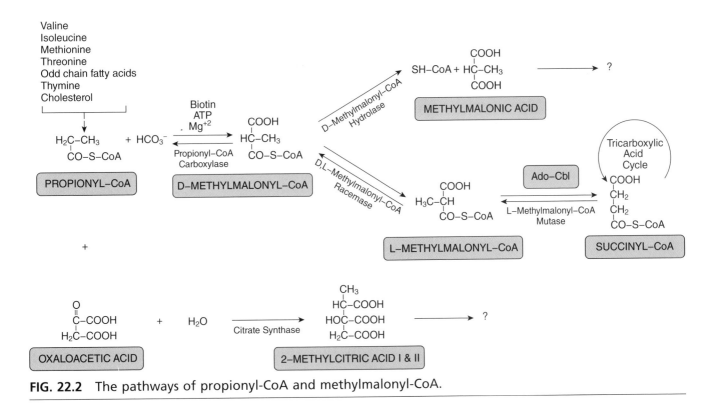

FIG. 22.2 The pathways of propionyl-CoA and methylmalonyl-CoA.

can be hydrolyzed to methylmalonic acid (MMA). The mutase is a mitochondrial matrix enzyme. It has been purified from humans (Kolhouse et al., 1980) and other sources and the genes have been cloned and sequenced also from human (Jansen et al., 1989) and bacterial sources. The enzyme is a homodimer which binds 2 mol of adenosyl-Cbl per dimer. During the last decade the reaction mechanisms have been intensively studied (Randaccio et al., 2010).

The mutase is not completely saturated with adenosyl-Cbl in vivo (Kondo et al., 1981). OH-Cbl infusions in rats over 14 days increased holo-L-methylmalonyl-CoA mutase activity and decreased the serum MMA (Stabler et al., 1991c). High-dose oral vitamin B$_{12}$ lowered mean MMA concentrations in normal subjects who had baseline concentrations > 240 nmol/L (Rasmussen et al., 1996).

This pathway is an important source of energy in ruminants since the bacterial fermentation in the rumen produces large quantities of propionic acid. However, this pathway is also important in humans since congenital defects of the mutase or of the ability to synthesize adenosyl-Cbl result in life-threatening methylmalonicaciduria which is complicated by severe metabolic ketoacidosis (Fenton et al., 2001). Serum, urine or CSF MMA concen-

trations are always increased in conditions of B$_{12}$ deficiency (Cox and White, 1962; Lindenbaum et al., 1990; Savage et al., 1994b), human or animal nitrous-oxide-induced cobalamin inactivation (Stabler et al., 1991b,c), experimental animal deficiency (Stabler et al., 1991c), ruminants with cobalt deficiency (Rice et al., 1989), and tissue culture cells (Kolhouse et al., 1993).

Methionine Synthase

The pathway of methionine metabolism is shown in Figure 22.3 (Allen et al., 1993a). Methionine is an essential amino acid which is necessary for protein synthesis but also is a crucial methyl donor after activation to S-adenosylmethionine (SAM). SAM is a source of methyl groups for the synthesis of creatine and phospholipids (quantitatively the most important together) and also for synthesis of neurotransmitters, DNA, RNA, and protein methylation (Mudd et al., 2007). After donating the methyl group, S-adenosylhomocysteine (SAH) is formed which is cleaved to homocysteine and adenosine by SAH-hydrolase. The homocysteine that is generated can either be remethylated to form methionine or condensed with serine to form cystathionine by a vitamin B$_6$-dependent

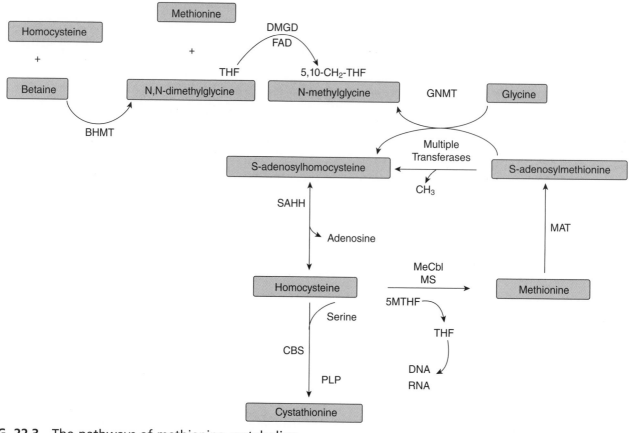

FIG. 22.3 The pathways of methionine metabolism.

enzyme, cystathionine beta-synthase. Cystathionine is further metabolized to cysteine and alpha-ketobutyrate by another vitamin B₆-dependent enzyme, gamma-cystathionase (Mudd *et al.*, 2007).

Methionine can be synthesized by two different enzymes, Cbl-dependent methionine synthase and betaine-homocysteine methyltransferase (Erickson, 1960; Matthews *et al.*, 2008). Methionine synthase transfers a methyl group from 5-methyltetrahydrofolate to homocysteine. The methyl-Cbl bound to the methionine synthase is demethylated in the reaction with the homocysteine and then remethylated by the reaction with 5-methyltetrahydrofolate. SAM is also required because occasionally the active Cbl form, cob(1)alamin is oxidized and must be reduced by obtaining a methyl group from SAM (Koutmos *et al.*, 2009). Recent investigations show that there is also a human methionine synthase reductase which is a flavoprotein (Leclerc *et al.*, 1998). Methionine synthase is a cytoplasmic enzyme. It contains 1 mol of Cbl

per mol of protein. Mechanisms of methionine synthase have been studied extensively (Matthews *et al.*, 2008).

It is readily appreciated from Figure 22.3 that the balance of methionine metabolism is dependent on three vitamins, vitamin B₁₂, folate, and vitamin B₆. Congenital defects of the methionine synthase, methionine synthase reductase or the synthesis of methyl-Cbl have been described and they cause severe hyperhomocysteinemia (Rosenblatt and Fenton, 2001). Deficiencies of either vitamin B₁₂ or folic acid also result in hyperhomocysteinemia (Stabler *et al.*, 1988; Savage *et al.*, 1994a). Elevations of serum total homocysteine (tHcy) are associated with accelerated vascular disease and thrombosis. The field of congenital and acquired defects has therefore generated much interest (Fowler, 2005).

Homocysteine is at a branch point between the remethylation to methionine or the reaction to form cystathionine which is termed transsulfuration. Transsulfuration is not reversible and eventually results in removal of the sulfhydral group. Cystathionine beta-synthase is activated by SAM; thus, in conditions of high methionine intake, transsulfuration is stimulated and homocysteine is removed (Finkelstein, 1990). The concentrations of SAM are regulated by the methylation of glycine by glycine N-methyltransferase, an enzyme that is found in a high concentration in the liver (Cook and Wagner, 1984). This reaction is inhibited by 5-methyltetrahydrofolate, a form of folate which may build up in B$_{12}$ deficiency because methionine synthase activity is impaired.

Another area of interest is in the regulation of the concentrations of cystathionine since both vitamin B$_{12}$ and folate deficiency cause marked rises in serum cystathionine, despite the fact that there is experimental evidence and theoretical reasons to believe that the deficiency of SAM in these conditions should result in a decrease in transsulfuration and the formation of cystathionine (Stabler *et al.*, 1993).

Metabolic Abnormalities in Vitamin B$_{12}$ Deficiency

Box 22.1 shows the metabolites, MMA, homocysteine, S-adenosylhomocysteine, cystathionine, 2-methylcitric acid, and N,N-dimethylglycine, that are found in elevated concentrations in body fluids (serum, urine, cerebrospinal fluid) and tissues in both humans with pernicious anemia and in other forms of vitamin B$_{12}$ deficiency as well as in experimental models of vitamin B$_{12}$ deficiency. Cox and White in 1962 demonstrated that 95% of symptomatic vitamin B$_{12}$-deficient humans had elevated concentrations of urine MMA which responded to therapy. Their work has been repeatedly confirmed and it is now well accepted that virtually every patient who has clinical abnormalities that will respond to vitamin B$_{12}$ replacement has elevated MMA (Stabler *et al.*, 1986, 1990; Moelby *et al.*, 1990; Savage *et al.*, 1994a). Elevations of MMA are highly specific to Cbl metabolism with the exception of modest elevations seen in chronic renal insufficiency (Rasmussen *et al.*, 1990; Allen *et al.*, 1993b). Thus, monitoring MMA is extremely useful in diagnosis, for studying responses to treatment, and in documenting vitamin B$_{12}$ deficiency in animal or cellular models.

Figure 22.2 showed that propionyl-CoA can be condensed with oxaloacetic acid to form 2-methylcitric acid. Elevated concentrations of 2-methylcitric acid are found in patients with inborn errors of mutase and in severely affected vitamin B$_{12}$-deficient subjects (Allen *et al.*, 1993a).

BOX 22.1 Laboratory abnormalities in vitamin B$_{12}$ deficiency

Metabolites
High methylmalonic acid
High total homocysteine
High cystathionine
High 2-methylcitric acid
High N,N-dimethylglycine
High S-adenosylhomocysteine

Megaloblastic anemia
Peripheral blood
  Low red blood cell count
  Low hemoglobin and hematocrit
  Low white blood cell count
  Low platelet count
  High mean cell volume
  High red cell distribution width
  Hypersegmented granulocytes
Bone marrow
  Hypercellularity
  Nuclear-cytoplasmic dys-synchrony
  Open immature nuclear chromatin pattern
  Giant metamyelocytes and bands
  Intramedullary cell death

Blood chemistry
  Increased unconjugated bilirubin
  Increased lactate dehydrogenase
  Decreased haptoglobin

Total homocysteine is frequently elevated in the serum in humans with pernicious anemia (Stabler *et al.*, 1988; Savage, 1994a) and other forms of vitamin B$_{12}$ deficiency as well as animal models of vitamin B$_{12}$ deficiency (Stabler *et al.*, 1991a). Elevated homocysteine is not specific to vitamin B$_{12}$ deficiency, in contrast to MMA, but is found in folate deficiency, and in defects of cystathionine beta-synthase, methionine adenosyltransferase, 5,10-methylenetetrahydrofolate reductase, and methionine synthase, and in the methyl-Cbl reductive pathway (Fowler, 2005). Homocysteine concentration is highly correlated with the serum creatinine, at least partly because of the role of SAM in the formation of creatine, the precursor of creatinine (Soria *et al.*, 1990). The mean homocysteine value of a population is highly dependent on the dietary and supplement intake of folate and vitamin B$_{12}$. These additional influences make elevated tHcy less specific as a diagnostic tool for vitamin B$_{12}$ deficiency. However, it has been shown

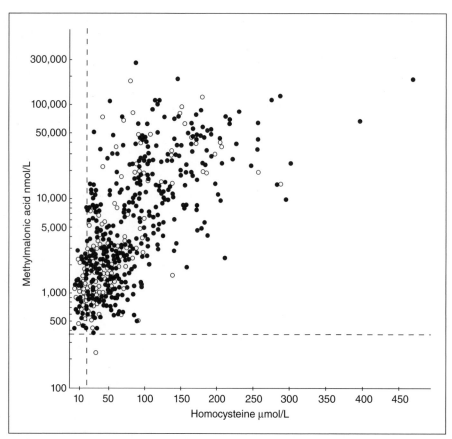

FIG. 22.4 Serum methylmalonic acid and total homocysteine concentrations in 491 episodes of B₁₂ deficiency. Closed circles represent patients with hematocrit <38% and open circles ≥38%. Patient values are collated from the following references: Lindenbaum *et al.*, 1988, 1990, 1994; Stabler *et al.*, 1988, 1990, 1997, 1999; Pennypacker *et al.*, 1992; Savage *et al.*, 1994a,b; Kuzminski *et al.*, 1998; Sekhar and Stabler, 2007; Guerra-Shinohara *et al.*, 2007. The hatched lines represent three standard deviations above the mean for normal controls, MMA, 376 nmol/L and total homocysteine, 21.3 µmol/L.

that elevated homocysteine due to vitamin B₁₂ deficiency will not correct with folic acid treatment (Allen *et al.*, 1990).

The serum cystathionine concentration is elevated in most subjects with severe vitamin B₁₂ deficiency (Stabler *et al.*, 1993). Like the total homocysteine, it is not specific to vitamin B₁₂ deficiency since folate deficiency and especially vitamin B₆ deficiency also cause elevated concentrations.

Both the serum MMA and homocysteine concentrations can reach extremely high levels in symptomatic vitamin B₁₂ deficiency, as shown in Figure 22.4. Only three out of 313 episodes of well documented vitamin B₁₂-deficient megaloblastic anemia had normal concentrations of both metabolites (Savage *et al.*, 1994a). The MMA and

homocysteine were elevated in 121 subjects who had neurologic syndromes without anemia in the same report, and, as can be seen in Figure 22.4, patients with normal hematocrit are found at all levels of metabolites.

There are alterations in the total coenzyme-A pools and in carnitine metabolism as a result of the build-up of methylmalonyl-CoA in animal models of vitamin B₁₂ deficiency (Brass *et al.*, 1990a,b). The increase in propionyl-CoA appears to lead to increased formation of branched-chain and odd-chain fatty acids in both inborn errors of the mutase and severe vitamin B₁₂ deficiency (Frenkel, 1973; Coker *et al.*, 1996).

Figure 22.3 demonstrates that there are interactions between vitamin B₁₂ and folate metabolism. The irreversible reaction forming 5-methyltetrahydrofolate results in a metabolically inactive form of folate unless it is demethylated by methionine synthase. 5-Methyltetrahydrofolate is a poor substrate for folyl polyglutamate synthase and thus is not retained intracellularly and can be lost in the urine (Cichowicz and Shane, 1987). Thus there is "trapping" of folate as 5-methyltetrahydrofolate in severe vitamin B$_{12}$ deficiency and this may result in secondary folate deficiency (Savage and Lindenbaum, 1995; Smulders et al., 2006). N-Methylglycine is elevated in folate-deficient but not B$_{12}$-deficient patients, suggesting that "trapped" methylfolate may be bound to and inhibiting glycine N-methyltransferase (Allen et al., 1993a) further sparing SAM but not SAH concentrations in B$_{12}$ deficiency (Guerra-Shinohara et al., 2007). Since other forms of folate are necessary for thymidine and purine synthesis, there are resulting impairments in DNA synthesis likely causing megaloblastosis (see the section of megaloblastic anemia). There are also abnormalities in one-carbon metabolism in vitamin B$_{12}$ deficiency, probably due to the secondary folate deficiency (Deacon et al., 1990).

Clinical Manifestations

The clinical manifestations of vitamin B$_{12}$ deficiency have been best studied in the human with pernicious anemia. Although there are spontaneously occurring animal models of vitamin B$_{12}$ deficiency such as ruminants pastured on cobalt-deficient soil (Rice et al., 1989) and dogs (Fyfe et al., 1989) with selective malabsorption of vitamin B$_{12}$, these animals do not display similar syndromes. In one investigation, Cbl analogue treatment of mini-pigs caused spinal lesions and mild anemia and leucopenia, although the rise in mean red cell volume and morphologic changes in the bone marrow were very subtle as compared with what would be expected in a human (Stabler et al., 1991c). The lack of convenient animal models has certainly been a detriment to the study of the pathophysiology of vitamin B$_{12}$.

Megaloblastic Anemia

In humans, vitamin B$_{12}$ and folate deficiency cause identical forms of megaloblastic anemia (Koury and Ponka, 2004; Wickramasinghe, 2006). Thus, the secondary block in folate metabolism in vitamin B$_{12}$ deficiency must be the underlying cause. This constellation of morphologic changes and clinical and laboratory abnormalities is due to an imbalance of decreased DNA synthesis with adequate RNA synthesis. Impaired methylation due to an increase in SAH, which inhibits methyltransferases, may also be important (Guerra-Shinohara et al., 2007). The nuclei of the developing hematopoietic precursor cells in the bone marrow remain immature as compared with the cytoplasm. The morphologic result is a macrocytic red blood cell precursor (high mean cell volume), with an open chromatin pattern. The white blood cells are enlarged with hypersegmentation of granulocyte nuclei. Many cells die in the bone marrow (ineffective erythropoiesis), possibly by apoptosis which leads to the cellular release of bilirubin and lactate dehydrogenase. The megaloblastic nuclei demonstrate decreased DNA synthesis, increased precursors in S phase, misincorporation of uracil into DNA, little evidence for decreased DNA methylation, chromosomal breakage and rescue by both purines and thymidine (Koury and Ponka, 2004). The cellular bone marrow packed with very immature-appearing erythroblasts has led to the mistaken diagnosis of acute leukemia. The fragmentation of the red blood cells may also lead to erroneous diagnoses such as hemolysis, or thrombotic microangiopathies (Sekhar and Stabler, 2007). Megaloblastic anemia can be completely cured with vitamin B$_{12}$ treatment, and can be partially corrected with folate treatment which leads to diagnostic errors, as has been thoroughly reviewed by Savage and Lindenbaum (1995). Ultimately, many of such incorrectly treated patients succumbed to relapse of anemia and/or neurologic disease.

The megaloblastic anemia outlined above is the classic picture of severe vitamin B$_{12}$-deficient anemia. More recently it has been noted that there are many patients who have only mild abnormalities of blood cells and bone marrow but who may have severe abnormalities of the nervous system (Lindenbaum et al., 1988). Figure 22.4 demonstrates that many of the patients with normal or near-normal hematocrit (open circles) had profound elevation of MMA and/or homocysteine. The reason an individual is susceptible to megaloblastic anemia vs. neurologic abnormalities is unknown. The use of MMA and homocysteine as screening tests has also led to the realization that there is a significant fraction of individuals with biochemically severe vitamin B$_{12}$ deficiency who appear to have no signs of megaloblastic anemia, or neurologic abnormalities.

Neurologic Abnormalities

Vitamin B$_{12}$ deficiency, whether naturally occuring or induced by nitrous oxide (which inactivates methionine synthase), leads to a demyelinating disorder of the central nervous system in humans (Healton *et al.*, 1991; Stabler *et al.*, 1991a; Singer *et al.*, 2008), non-human primates (Scott *et al.*, 1981), fruit bats (Metz, 1992), and swine (Weir *et al.*, 1988; Stabler *et al.*, 1991c), but no other animal species. This lesion was described long before the underlying vitamin B$_{12}$ dependence was recognized. It has been termed "subacute combined degeneration" or "combined systems disease." The pathology includes swelling of myelin sheaths and patchy vacuolation of myelin with spongy degeneration of the spinal cord, starting in the thoracic and cervical dorsal columns and progressing to the lateral columns. Lesions are also seen in the brain and optic nerves and possibly peripheral nerves (Stabler, 2006). Signs and symptoms vary considerably. The most common symptom seen in a large review of well-documented cases was painful paresthesia of the extremities (Healton *et al.*, 1991). The most common sign was loss of proprioception and vibration sense in the toes or ankles. One of the most intriguing discoveries has been the strong inverse relationship between the severity of the hematologic and neurologic abnormalities (Healton *et al.*, 1991; Savage *et al.*, 1994a). Only about one-third of patients with pernicious anemia will develop the neurologic abnormalities, and 25% of these will have almost completely normal hematologic parameters, which has caused great difficulty in diagnosis in the past (Lindenbaum *et al.*, 1988). Serum MMA and homocysteine and all of the other metabolic changes are similar in the subjects with involvement of the nervous system as compared with those with just hematologic involvement (Allen *et al.*, 1993c). Vitamin B$_{12}$ treatment will partially or completely correct the lesions if begun promptly (Healton *et al.*, 1991).

The underlying biochemical abnormalities leading to demyelination of the central nervous system are not understood. There is intriguing negative data from observation of individuals with methylmalonicaciduria due to mutase defects who do not develop the demyelinating disease of the spinal cord seen in vitamin B$_{12}$ deficiency (Fenton *et al.*, 2001). Likewise patients with severe folate deficiency and elevations of homocysteine similar to the levels seen in vitamin B$_{12}$ deficiency do not develop myelopathy (Savage and Lindenbaum, 1995). However, the combined defects (cbl-C, D, F) do cause central nervous system disease very similar to that seen with B$_{12}$ deficiency. It appears that the activity of both cobalamin-dependent enzymes need to be impaired in order to cause the demyelinating disease, although defects of methionine synthase

might be an exception (Rosenblatt and Fenton, 2001). There is also no explanation for why most animal species are resistant to the development of spinal cord defects. A gastrectomized rat model has shown abnormalities of cytokines and growth factors (Scalabrino and Peracchi, 2006), in the nervous system. Similar changes were found in humans with B$_{12}$ deficiency (Scalabrino *et al.*, 2004). Magnetic resonance imaging techniques of the brain and spinal column demonstrate the areas of demyelination and surprisingly often show improvement long before signs and symptoms abate (Singer *et al.*, 2008). Functional studies have shown brain choline depletion, especially in infants (Horstmann *et al.*, 2003; Dror and Allen, 2008).

Clinical Spectrum of Vitamin B$_{12}$ Deficiency

Vitamin B$_{12}$ deficiency has a very wide spectrum of severity and manifestations (Stabler, 2006). In addition to anemia and/or neurologic disease, some subjects may have additional symptoms such as glossitis of the tongue, megaloblastic gut, weight loss, mental changes, and even infertility. The clinical spectrum in infants is also markedly different from that in adults (Whitehead, 2006; Dror and Allen, 2008), with failure to thrive, irritability, movement disorders, and poor brain growth leading to permanent developmental delay in some cases (Graham *et al.*, 1992).

Causes of Vitamin B$_{12}$ Deficiency

All animals require vitamin B$_{12}$ and obtain it ultimately from the products of microbial synthesis. Ruminant animals actually carry bacteria that synthesize cobalamins in their rumen (Girard *et al.*, 2009). Humans obtain vitamin B$_{12}$ from products of animal origin including meats, fish, shellfish, dairy products, and eggs (Watanabe, 2007). Improved methods of corrinoid analysis have shown that fermented vegetable foods, some algae and other plant products may contain B$_{12}$ (Watanabe, 2007). Synthetic vitamin B$_{12}$ has been added to cereal and other supplemented foods in the western world.

Absorption and Intracellular Metabolism of Vitamin B$_{12}$

Vitamin B$_{12}$ is generally bound to one of the two enzymes or other carrier proteins in food. It must therefore be released prior to absorption. This process starts when food is chewed and mixed with saliva, which contains a Cbl binding protein, haptocorrin (R-protein). The bound Cbl is further released in the acid environment of the stomach where peptic digestion of proteins begins. The released vitamin B$_{12}$ is bound to haptocorrin and carried to the duodenum. The specific Cbl binding protein intrinsic factor (IF) is released by the gastric parietal cells, but does not bind Cbl until stomach acid is neutralized in the duodenum, and digestive enzymes remove the haptocorrin from the vitamin (reviewed by Quadros, 2010). The binding of IF is very specific for Cbl and thus may prevent the binding and absorption of Cbl analogues also found in foods. The IF-Cbl is carried to the ileum where it is taken up by the cubam receptor (formed from cubulin and amnionless, a transmembrane protein [Fyfe *et al.*, 2004; Andersen *et al.*, 2010]). The IF-Cbl then goes to the lysosomes and is eventually released bound to transcobalamin. Inborn errors of IF, cubulin or amnionless cause juvenile megaloblastic anemia and Imerslund–Grasbeck syndrome (Tanner *et al.*, 2004, 2005). The Cbl F defect has now been shown to be a defective lysosomal membrane transporter (Rutsch *et al.*, 2011).

It is not known exactly how the absorbed Cbl is then processed so that a complex of transcobalamin-Cbl (TC-Cbl) is secreted into the portal blood and thus delivered to the liver and ultimately all tissues. TC is the primary serum transport protein for vitamin B$_{12}$. The TC-Cbl is taken up by receptor-mediated endocytosis by the recently purified TCblR (Quadros, 2010) and fused to lysosomes in which the Cbl is released. Recent evidence suggests that Cbl export from cells may be mediated by the ATP-binding cassette drug transporter, ABCC1 (Beedholm-Ebssen *et al.*, 2010). Cobalamin in the circulation is bound to haptocorrin (R-binder, TCI and III), 70–90%, and transcobalamin, 10–30%. The function of haptocorrin is unclear but could be protective since it also binds corrinoids other than cobalamin and can deliver them to the liver (Alpers, 2005). Defects of TC cause a severe megaloblastic anemia, elevations of MMA and homocysteine, neurologic disease, and immune deficiency in the first few months of life (Whitehead, 2006). Deficient haptocorrin appears to be relatively common and a cause of the "false positive" low serum B$_{12}$ level.

After the Cbl is released from the lysosomes, the coenzyme forms must be synthesized. A number of defects of intracellular Cbl metabolism have been described which form eight complementation groups with three generally similar clinical syndromes (Whitehead, 2006). If there is a defect in methionine synthase or in regenerating CH$_3$-Cbl (MS, cblE, cblG), the patients have only hyperhomocysteinemia. Other complementation groups have defects in L-methylmalonal-CoA mutase or in the formation of adenosyl-Cbl (mut°, mut⁻, cblA, cblB) and these patients have only methylmalonicacidemia. However, there are also patients who have difficulty with the lysosomol release of Cbl (cblF), described above, or with a reduction step common to the synthesis of both coenzymes (cblC, cblD) who have combined hyperhomocysteinemia and methylmalonicaciduria (Lerner-Ellis *et al.*, 2009). Recently cblD has been shown to be associated also with isolated hyperhomocysteinemia or methylmalonicacidemia (Miousse *et al.*, 2009).

Acquired Vitamin B$_{12}$ Deficiency

The major causes of acquired vitamin B$_{12}$ deficiency are shown in Box 22.2. By far the most common causes of vitamin B$_{12}$ deficiency relate to acquired malabsorption.

Dietary deficiency of vitamin B$_{12}$ develops if foods of animal origin are not consumed (Stabler and Allen, 2004;

BOX 22.2 Causes of vitamin B$_{12}$ deficiency

Animals
Cobalt-deficient soil – ruminants only
Congenital ileal malabsorption – dogs and cats

Human
Dietary
  Lack of foods of animal origin
  Vitamin B$_{12}$-deficient breast milk
Malabsorption
  Pernicious anemia
  Protein-bound B$_{12}$ malabsorption
  Pancreatic insufficiency
  Jejunal bacterial overgrowth
  Fish tapeworm
  Tropical sprue
  Total or partial gastric resection or bypass
  Ileal disease or resection
  Ileal–urinary conduit
Drugs
  Nitrous oxide
  Metformin
  Stomach acid blockers
Congenital
  Intrinsic factor defect
  Transcobalamin defect
  Immerslund–Gräsbeck syndrome
  CblA–CblG defects

Gilsing *et al.*, 2010). The bioavailability of vitamin B$_{12}$ may vary between foods. Many meat-substitute foods in the United States are supplemented with vitamin B$_{12,}$ thus deficiency is rare if such products are consumed. Exclusively breast-fed infants of mothers with untreated pernicious anemia or a vegetarian diet are at risk for deficiency since the breast milk may be deficient in vitamin B$_{12}$ at a time when a mother is asymptomatic (Dror and Allen, 2008).

The autoimmune disease pernicious anemia is the most common cause of severe malabsorption of vitamin B$_{12}$ (Stabler, 2006). Chronic autoimmune atrophic gastritis (Type A atrophic gastritis) develops with antibodies to gastric parietal cells and in 50% of the individuals also to IF (Toh *et al.*, 1997; Lahner and Annibale, 2009). The gastric parietal cell H$^+$/K$^+$-ATPase has been shown to be the antigen against which parietal-cell antibodies are directed. There is a complete loss of IF so vitamin B$_{12}$ malabsorption ensues. The disease is found in all races and ethnic groups throughout the world (Savage *et al.*, 1994a,b; Chui *et al.*, 2001; Stabler and Allen, 2004) and the prevalence increases with age and female sex (Stabler, 2006). Though rare, pernicious anemia occurs even in young people, and those of African origin may be at higher risk for young onset (Carmel, 1992). One study found that the prevalence in persons over age 65 years was 1.9% (Carmel, 1996). In pernicious anemia there is impaired enterohepatic circulation of Cbl since the Cbl secreted in the bile cannot be bound to IF and is lost in the stool leading to more rapid depletion of Cbl when treatment is discontinued (Lindenbaum *et al.*, 1990).

Surgical manipulations of the gastrointestinal tract including total and partial gastrectomy, gastric bypass operations, ileal resections or ileal urinary conduit constructions frequently lead to vitamin B$_{12}$ malabsorption (Sumner *et al.*, 1996; Lahner and Annibale, 2009). Parasitic infection with the fish tapeworm and jejunal bacterial overgrowth, chronic inflammatory diseases of the ileum such as Crohn's disease and tropical sprue or resection have been shown to cause vitamin B$_{12}$ deficiency. *Helicobactor pylori* may be a cause of atrophic gastritis also (Lahner and Annibale, 2009).

Up to 15% of elderly subjects are found to have mild to moderate vitamin B$_{12}$ deficiency documented by elevated MMA and homocysteine concentrations and decreased serum Cbl levels (Pennypacker *et al.*, 1992; Lindenbaum *et al.*, 1994; Johnson *et al.*, 2010). Only a minority of the subjects discovered in screening studies have true pernicious anemia; the others may have abnor-malities in the release of vitamin B$_{12}$ from food and varying degrees of atrophic gastritis and achlorhydria (Carmel, 1997).

Recent reports suggest that, if borderline vitamin B$_{12}$-deficient patients are treated with nitrous oxide anesthesia, they can develop a rapid onset of the demyelinating syndrome in the weeks to months postoperatively (Singer *et al.*, 2008). The widespread use of stomach acid blockers such as the histamine blockers or the proton pump inhibitors may lead to a syndrome similar to the malabsorption of protein-bound B$_{12}$. Metformin (widely used in treatment of diabetes) may induce vitamin B$_{12}$ deficiency (de Jager *et al.*, 2010).

Diagnosis

The mainstay of diagnosis of vitamin B$_{12}$ deficiency has been the demonstration of a low serum-Cbl level (Hvas and Nexo, 2006; Stabler, 2006), although the specificity and sensitivity vary according to the lab cut-off values. Many methods can be used to assay total Cbl in serum, including microbiologic assays with *Lactobacillus leichmanii*, intrinsic factor competitive binding assays, utilizing radioisotope, chemiluminescence or enzyme-linked detection methods and chromatographic methods (Kumar *et al.*, 2010). Standardization between assays is problematic (Carmel *et al.*, 2000; Thorpe *et al.*, 2007). The use of serum assays for diagnosis is complicated by the fact that only about 20% of total serum Cbl is carried by TC (the cellular delivery protein) and the known roles for Cbl are all intracellular so tissue levels may not necessarily reflect those found in the plasma. In general, there is a rough correlation with the serum Cbl values such that extremely low concentrations often do indicate clinical deficiency, and values above the mean for a population generally can be interpreted as adequate (Lindenbaum *et al.*, 1990, 1994). There is a theoretical advantage to measuring Cbl on TC, known as holo-TC; however, diagnostic accuracy for elevated MMA is about equal between total Cbl and holo-TC (Hvas and Nexo, 2005; Miller *et al.*, 2006).

A comparison of the serum Cbl concentration versus serum or red-cell folate concentration has been frequently used to distinguish between the megaloblastic anemia resulting from deficiencies of either Cbl or folate. This is problematic because red-cell folate can be low in both vitamin B$_{12}$- and folate-deficient subjects and serum folate can occasionally be low in vitamin B$_{12}$ deficiency (Savage and Lindenbaum, 1995). However, since MMA concentrations are elevated only due to vitamin B$_{12}$ deficiency, it is possible to determine that a patient with megaloblastic anemia has at least vitamin B$_{12}$ deficiency, although in some cases there may also be coexisting folate deficiency (Savage *et al.*, 1994a). The lack of hematologic abnormalities should never prevent assessment of Cbl status in a patient with compatible neurologic disease because of the strong inverse correlation between the two.

In some cases there will be clinical utility in determining the cause of deficiency since there may be gastrointestinal pathology that needs to be treated. The presence of blocking anti-IF antibodies is diagnostic of pernicious anemia but the test is not very sensitive (Carmel, 1992; Khan *et al.*, 2009). The Schilling test determines the quantity of radioactive Cbl that is excreted in the urine after an oral dose of crystalline Cbl, with or without added IF; however, it is not routinely available (Carmel, 2007). A new absorptive test has been proposed based on the appearance of an increase in holo-TC after oral Cbl loading (Hvas *et al.*, 2007). Children who are found to have metabolic Cbl deficiency should obviously be evaluated for inborn errors of metabolism or the congenital defects of malabsorption, and such individuals will need lifelong surveillance and treatment as well as case finding among siblings.

Treatment of Vitamin B$_{12}$ Deficiency

The minimum quantity of B$_{12}$ required to sustain life is not known, but is likely less than 0.5 μg/day, and would not maintain normal biochemical values. Although the United States has set an RDA of 2.4 μg (Institute of Medicine, 1998), MMA is higher in those with an intake less than 6 μg; dietary supplements should therefore reflect this (Bor *et al.*, 2010). Vegetarians can be treated with small doses of oral vitamin B$_{12}$ supplements. Parenteral vitamin B$_{12}$ has been primarily used in the United States for the treatment of vitamin B$_{12}$ deficiency due to pernicious anemia and other forms of malabsorption. A standard regimen would be to start with weekly intramuscular injections of 1000 μg of CN-Cbl for 4–8 weeks until the clinical response is clearly evident, followed by monthly injections for life. An occasional patient will have serum MMA levels above the normal range on monthly injections and will require more frequent treatment (Kuzminski *et al.*, 1998). Hydroxy-Cbl is used in Europe and is claimed to need less frequent dosing; however, that has not been proven (Hvas and Nexo, 2006). High-dose daily oral therapy may be a good alternative to intermittent parenteral

treatment. Whereas IF-mediated Cbl uptake is limited, investigations from 40 years ago showed that subjects with or without pernicious anemia will absorb about 1% of a radioactively labeled oral dose (Berlin *et al.*, 1978). It has been shown that subjects with pernicious anemia can be maintained on daily oral doses of greater than 500 μg/day (Waife *et al.*, 1963), also 2000 μg oral daily resulted in much higher serum Cbl concentrations and lower MMA concentrations than monthly injections of Cbl (Kuzminski *et al.*, 1998). Patients should be offered a choice of high oral dose vs. parenteral therapy (Andrès *et al.*, 2010). The commonly available multivitamin preparations in the United States contain much lower quantities of vitamin B$_{12}$, usually 6–9 μg although some marketed to seniors contain up to 100 μg. Although serum Cbl concentrations are higher in seniors who take multivitamins, the serum MMA concentrations are not corrected in many individuals (Stabler *et al.*, 1999). Also, subjects with pernicious anemia and other malabsorption syndromes cannot be treated with standard multivitamin preparations containing low quantities of vitamin B$_{12}$. In most cases, vitamin B$_{12}$ therapy must be continued for life, thus it is imperative to have fully documented the deficiency prior to treatment and to convince the patient that this treatment is an ongoing necessity.

Future Directions

Folic acid has been added to fortified grain products in the United States since January 1998 (and in many other countries). Since then, low serum-folate concentrations have virtually been eliminated in the United States (Pfeiffer *et al.*, 2007), whereas Cbl status has been largely unchanged. Patients with pernicious anemia or other forms of severe Cbl deficiency may have been put at risk by masking of megaloblastic anemia. New concerns that B$_{12}$-deficient seniors with cognitive disorders may have been harmed by high folate intake have surfaced, although this is controversial. Vitamin B$_{12}$-deficient seniors may have impairments in cognition and abnormalities on neurophysiologic testing despite having no evidence of megaloblastic anemia (Carmel *et al.*, 1995). Because it has been difficult to prove clinical benefit with mild deficiency in seniors, there is controversy about the benefits of screening and treating (Stanger *et al.*, 2009; Werder, 2010). Another approach would be to fortify the food supply with B$_{12}$ as well as folic acid. Questions about adequate dose, stability of B$_{12}$ after cooking and storage (since B$_{12}$ analogs could be harmful) and the intended target population all remain (Allen *et al.*, 2010; Carmel, 2010). The recognition that B$_{12}$ deficiency may be related to birth defects and poor pregnancy outcomes is part of the impetus driving these recommendations (Li *et al.*, 2009). Evaluating inexpensive microbial or fermented vegetarian food sources of B$_{12}$ may have a large impact for the world populations who either cannot afford or choose not to consume animal source foods (Stabler and Allen, 2004; Watanabe, 2007). Newer methods of analysis which distinguish B$_{12}$ analogs from true B$_{12}$ will be necessary for this endeavor. Finally, the actual biochemical lesion in demyelination of the vitamin B$_{12}$-deficient nervous system continues to elude us. Further research should be directed to the role of vitamin B$_{12}$ in these processes since the basic mechanisms learned may be important in other demyelinating syndromes.

Suggestions for Further Reading

Savage, D.G., Lindenbaum, J., Stabler, S.P., *et al.* (1994) Sensitivity of serum methylmalonic acid and total homocysteine determinations for diagnosing cobalamin deficiency and folate deficiencies. *Am J Med* **96**, 239–246.

Stabler, S.P. and Allen, R.H. (2004) Vitamin B12 deficiency as a worldwide problem. *Ann Rev Nutr* **24**, 299–326.

Watanabe, F. (2007) Vitamin B12 sources and bioavailability. *Exp Biol Med* **232**, 1266–1274.

Whitehead, V.M. (2006) Acquired and inherited disorders of cobalamin and folate in children. *Br J Haematol* **134**, 125–136.

References

Allen, R.H. and Stabler, S.P. (2008) Identification and quantitation of cobalamin and cobalamin analogues in human feces. *Am J Clin Nutr* **87**, 1324–1335.

Allen, L.H., Rosenberg, I.H., Oakley, G.P., *et al.* (2010) Considering the case for vitamin B12 fortification of flour. *Food Nutr Bull* **31**, S36–S46.

Allen, R.H., Stabler, S.P., and Lindenbaum, J. (1993a) Serum betaine, *N-N*-dimethylglycine and *N*-methylglycine levels in patients with cobalamin and folate deficiency and related inborn errors of metabolism. *Metabolism* **42**, 1448–1460.

Allen, R.H., Stabler, S.P., Savage, D.G., *et al.* (1990) Diagnosis of cobalamin deficiency I: usefulness of serum methylmalonic acid and total homocysteine concentrations. *Am J Hematol* **34**, 90–98.

Allen, R.H., Stabler, S.P., Savage, D.G., *et al.* (1993b) Elevation of 2-methylcitric acid I and II levels in serum, urine and cerebrospinal fluid of patients with cobalamin deficiency. *Metabolism* **42**, 978–988.

Allen, R.H., Stabler, S.P., Savage, D.G., *et al.* (1993c) Metabolic abnormalities in cobalamin (vitamin B12) and folate deficiency. *FASEB J* **7**, 1344–1353.

Alpers, D.H. (2005) What is new in vitamin B(12)? *Curr Opin Gastroenterol* **21**, 183–186.

Andersen, C.B., Madsen, M., Storm, T., *et al.* (2010) Structural basis for receptor recognition of vitamin B(12)-intrinsic factor complexes. *Nature* **464**, 445–448.

Andrès, E., Fothergill, H., and Mecili, M. (2010) Efficacy of oral cobalamin (vitamin B12) therapy. *Expert Opin Pharmacother* **11**, 249–256.

Banerjee, R. and Ragsdale, S.W. (2003) The many faces of vitamin B12: catalysis by cobalamin-dependent enzymes. *Annu Rev Biochem* **72**, 209–247.

Beedholm-Ebsen, R., van de Wetering, K., Hardlei, T., *et al.* (2010) Identification of multidrug resistance protein 1 (MRP1/ABCC1) as a molecular gate for cellular export of cobalamin. *Blood* **115**, 1632–1639.

Berlin, R., Berlin, H., Bronte, G., *et al.* (1978) Vitamin B$_{12}$ body stores during oral and parenteral treatment of pernicious anemia. *Acta Med Scand* **204**, 81–84.

Bor, M.V., von Castel-Roberts, K.M., Kauwell, G.P., *et al.* (2010) Daily intake of 4 to 7 microg dietary vitamin B12 is associated with steady concentrations of vitamin B12-related biomarkers in a healthy young population. *Am J Clin Nutr* **91**, 571–577.

Brass, E.P., Allen, R.H., Arung, T., *et al.* (1990a) Coenzyme-A metabolism in vitamin B$_{12}$ deficient rats. *J Nutr* **120**, 290–297.

Brass, E.P., Allen, R.H., Ruff, L.J., *et al.* (1990b) Effect of hydroxycobalamin [c-lactam] on propionate and carnitine metabolism in the rat. *Biochem J* **266**, 809–815.

Carmel, R. (1992) Reassessment of the relative prevalences of antibodies to gastric parietal cell and to intrinsic factor in patients with pernicious anaemia: influence of patient age and race. *Clin Exp Immunol* **89**, 74–77.

Carmel, R. (1996) Prevalence of undiagnosed pernicious anemia in the elderly. *Arch Intern Med* **156**, 1097–1100.

Carmel, R. (1997) Cobalamin, the stomach and aging. *Am J Clin Nutr* **66**, 750–759.

Carmel, R. (2007) The disappearance of cobalamin absorption testing: a critical diagnostic loss. *J Nutr* **137**, 2481–2484.

Carmel, R. (2011) Mandatory fortification of the food supply with cobalamin: an idea whose time has not yet come. *J Inherit Metab Dis* **34**, 67–73.

Carmel, R., Brar, S., Agrawal. A., *et al.* (2000) Failure of assay to identify low cobalamin concentrations. *Clin Chem* **46**, 2017–2018.

Carmel, R., Gott, P.S., Waters, C.H., *et al.* (1995) The frequently low cobalamin levels in dementia usually signify treatable metabolic, neurologic and electrophysiologic abnormalities. *Eur J Haematol* **54**, 245–253.

Castle, W.B. (1975) The history of corrinoids. In B.M. Babior (ed.), *Cobalamin Biochemistry and Pathophysiology*, 20th Edn. Wiley-Interscience, New York, pp. 1–17.

Chui, C.H., Lau, F.Y., Wong, R., *et al.* (2001) Vitamin B12 deficiency – need for a new guideline. *Nutrition* **17**, 917–920.

Cichowicz, D.J. and Shane, B. (1987) Mammalian folylpoly-γ-glutamate synthase 2. Substrate specificity and kinetic properties. *Biochemistry* **26**, 513–521.

Coker, M., de Klerk, J.B., Poll-The, B.T., *et al.* (1996) Plasma total odd-chain fatty acids in the monitoring of disorders of propionate, methylmalonate and biotin metabolism. *J Inherit Metab Dis* **19**, 743–751.

Cook, R.J. and Wagner, C. (1984) Glycine N-methyltransferase is a folate binding protein of rat liver cytosol. *Proc Natl Acad Sci USA* **81**, 3631–3634.

Cox, E.M. and White, A.M. (1962) Methylmalonic acid excretion: an index of vitamin B$_{12}$ deficiency. *Lancet* **ii**, 853–856.

Deacon, R., Perry, J., Lumb, M., *et al.* (1990) Formate metabolism in the cobalamin-inactivated rat. *Br J Haematol* **74**, 354–359.

de Jager, J., Kooy, A., Lehert, P., *et al.* (2010) Long term treatment with metformin in patients with type 2 diabetes and risk of vitamin B-12 deficiency: randomised placebo controlled trial. *Br Med J* **340**, c2181.

Drennan, C.L., Haang, S., Drummond, J.T., *et al.* (1994) How a protein binds B$_{12}$: A 3.0 x-ray structure of B$_{12}$-binding domains of methionine synthase. *Science* **266**, 1669–1674.

Dror, D.K. and Allen, L.H. (2008) Effect of vitamin B12 deficiency on neurodevelopment in infants: current knowledge and possible mechanisms. *Nutr Rev* **66**, 250–255.

Erickson, L.E. (1960) Betaine-homocysteine-methyl-transferases. *Acta Chem Scand* **14**, 2102–2112.

Fenton, W.A., Gravel, R.A., and Rosenblatt, D.S. (2001) Disorders of propionate and methylmalonate metabolism. In C.R. Scriver, A.L. Beaudet, W.S. Sly, *et al.* (eds), *The Metabolic and Molecular Bases of Inherited Disease*, Vol. 2, 8th Edn. McGraw-Hill, New York, pp. 2165–2193.

Finkelstein, J.D. (1990) Methionine metabolism in mammals. *J Nutr Biochem* **1**, 228–237.

Folkers, K. (1982) History of B$_{12}$: pernicious anemia to crystalline cyanocobalamin. In D. Dolphin (ed.), *B$_{12}$*, Vol. 1. Wiley-Interscience, New York, pp. 1–5.

Fowler, B. (2005) Homocysteine: overview of biochemistry, molecular biology, and role in disease processes. *Semin Vasc Med* **5**, 77–86.

Frenkel, E.P. (1973) Abnormal fatty acid metabolism in peripheral nerves of patients with pernicious anemia. *J Clin Invest* **52**, 1237–1245.

Fyfe, J.C., Jezyk, P.F., Giger, U., *et al.* (1989) Inherited selective malabsorption of vitamin B$_{12}$ in giant schnauzers. *J Am Animal Hosp Assoc* **25**, 533–539.

Fyfe, J.C., Madsen, M., Højrup, P., *et al.* (2004) The functional cobalamin (vitamin B12)-intrinsic factor receptor is a novel complex of cubilin and amnionless. *Blood* **103**, 1573–1579.

Gilsing, A.M., Crowe, F.L., Lloyd-Wright, Z., *et al.* (2010) Serum concentrations of vitamin B12 and folate in British male omnivores, vegetarians and vegans: results from a cross-sectional analysis of the EPIC-Oxford cohort study. *Eur J Clin Nutr* **64**, 933–939

Girard, C.L., Berthiaume, R., Stabler, S.P., *et al.* (2009) Identification of cobalamin and cobalamin analogues along the gastrointestinal tract of dairy cows. *Arch Anim Nutr* **63**, 379–388.

Graham, S.H., Arvela, O.M., and Wise, G.A. (1992) Long term neurologic consequences of nutritional vitamin B$_{12}$ deficiency in infants. *J Pediatr* **121**, 710–714.

Guerra-Shinohara, E.M., Morita, O.E., Pagliusi, R.A., *et al.* (2007) Elevated serum S-adenosylhomocysteine in cobalamin-deficient megaloblastic anemia. *Metabolism* **56**, 339–347.

Healton, E.B., Savage, D.G., Brust, J.C.M., *et al.* (1991) Neurological aspects of cobalamin deficiency. *Medicine* **70**, 229–245.

Hogenkamp, H.P.C. (1999) B$_{12}$: 1948–1998. In R. Banerjee (ed.), *Chemistry and Biochemistry of B$_{12}$*, Vol. 1. Wiley-Interscience, New York, pp. 3–8. .

Horstmann, M., Neumaier-Probst, E., Lukacs, Z., *et al.* (2003) Infantile cobalamin deficiency with cerebral lactate accumulation and sustained choline depletion. *Neuropediatrics* **34**, 261–264.

Hvas, A.M. and Nexo, E. (2005) Holotranscobalamin–a first choice assay for diagnosing early vitamin B deficiency? *J Intern Med* **257**, 289–298.

Hvas, A.M. and Nexo, E. (2006) Diagnosis and treatment of vitamin B12 deficiency–an update. *Haematologica* **91**, 1506–1512.

Hvas, A.M., Morkbak, A.L., and Nexo, E. (2007) Plasma holotranscobalamin compared with plasma cobalamins for assessment of vitamin B12 absorption; optimisation of a non-radioactive vitamin B12 absorption test (CobaSorb). *Clin Chim Acta* **376**, 150–154.

Institute of Medicine (1998) *Dietary Reference Intakes: Thiamin, Riboflavin, Niacin, Vitamin B6, Folate, Vitamin B12,*

Pantothenic Acid, Biotin, and Choline. National Academy Press, Washington, DC.

Jansen, R., Kalousek, F., Fenton, W.A., *et al.* (1989) Cloning of full-length methylmalonyl-CoA mutase from a cDNA library using the polymerase chain reaction. *Genomics* **4**, 198–205.

Johnson, M.A., Hausman, D.B., Davey, A., *et al.* (2010) Vitamin B12 deficiency in African-American and white octogenarians and centenarians in Georgia. *J Nutr Health Aging* **14**, 339–345.

Khan, S., Del-Duca, C., Fenton, E., *et al.* (2009) Limited value of testing for intrinsic factor antibodies with negative gastric parietal cell antibodies in pernicious anaemia. *J Clin Pathol* **62**, 439–441.

Kolhouse, J.F., Stabler, S.P., and Allen, R.H. (1993) Identification and perturbation of mutant human fibroblasts based on measurements of methylmalonic acid and total homocysteine in the culture media. *Arch Biochem Biophys* **303**, 355–360.

Kolhouse, J.F., Utley, C., and Allen, R.H. (1980) Isolation and characterization of methylmalonyl-CoA mutase from human placenta. *J Biol Chem* **255**, 2708–2712.

Kondo, H., Osborne, M.L., Kolhouse, J.F., *et al.* (1981) Nitrous oxide has multiple deleterious effects on cobalamin metabolism and causes decreases in activities of both mammalian cobalamin-dependent enzymes in rats. *J Clin Invest* **67**, 1270–1283.

Koury, M.J. and Ponka, P. (2004) New insights into erythropoiesis: the roles of folate, vitamin B12, and iron. *Ann Rev Nutr* **24**, 105–131.

Koutmos, M., Datta, S., Pattridge, K.A., *et al.* (2009) Insights of cobalamin-dependent methionine synthase. *Proc Natl Acad Sci USA* **44**, 18527–18532.

Kumar, S.S., Chouhan R.S., and Thakur, M.S. (2010) Trends in analysis of vitamin B12. *Anal Biochem* **398**, 139–149.

Kuzminski, A.M., Del Giacco, E.J., Allen, R.H., *et al.* (1998) Effective treatment of cobalamin deficiency with oral cobalamin. *Blood* **92**, 1191–1198.

Lahner, E. and Annibale, B. (2009) Pernicious anemia: new insights from a gastroenterological point of view. *World J Gastroenterol* **15**, 5121–5128.

Leclerc, D., Wilson, A., Dumas, R., *et al.* (1998) Cloning and mapping of a cDNA for methionine synthase reductase, a flavoprotein defective in patients with homocystinuria. *Proc Natl Acad Sci USA* **95**, 3059–3064.

Lerner-Ellis, J.P., Anastasio, N., Liu, J., *et al.* (2009) Spectrum of mutations in MMACHC, allelic expression, and evidence for genotype–phenotype correlations. *Hum Mutat* **30**, 1072–1081.

Li, F., Watkins, D., and Rosenblatt, D.S. (2009) Vitamin B(12) and birth defects. *Mol Genet Metab* **98**, 166–172.

Lindenbaum, J., Healton, E.B., Savage, D.G., *et al.* (1988) Neuropsychiatric disorders caused by cobalamin deficiency in the absence of anemia or macrocytosis. *New Engl J Med* **318**, 1720–1728.

Lindenbaum, J., Rosenberg, I., Wilson, P., *et al.* (1994) Prevalence of cobalamin deficiency in the Framingham elderly population. *Am J Clin Nutr* **60**, 2–11.

Lindenbaum, J., Stabler, S.P., and Allen, R.H. (1990) Diagnosis of cobalamin deficiency. II Relative sensitivities of serum cobalamin, methylmalonic acid and total homocysteine concentrations. *Am J Hematol* **34**, 99–107.

Ludwig, M.L. and Matthews, R.G. (1997) Structure-based perspectives on B₁₂-dependent enzymes. *Annu Rev Biochem* **66**, 269–313.

Mancia, F., Keep, N.H., Nakagawa, A., *et al.* (1996) How coenzyme B₁₂ radicals are generated: the crystal structure of methylmalonyl-coenzyme A mutase at 2 A resolution. *Structure* **4**, 339–350.

Martens, J.H., Barg, H., Warren, M.J., *et al.* (2002) Microbial production of vitamin B12. *Appl Microbiol Biotechnol* **58**, 275–285.

Matthews, R.G., Koutmos, M., and Datta, S. (2008) Cobalamin-dependent and cobamide-dependent methyltransferases. *Curr Opin Struct Biol* **18**, 658–666.

Metz, J. (1992) Cobalamin deficiency and the pathogenesis of nervous system disease. *Ann Rev Nutr* **12**, 59–79.

Miller, J.W., Garrod, M.G., Rockwood, A.L., *et al.* (2006) Measurement of total vitamin B12 and holotranscobalamin, singly and in combination, in screening for metabolic vitamin B12 deficiency. *Clin Chem* **52**, 278–285.

Minot, G.R. and Murphy, W.P. (1926) Treatment of pernicious anemia by a special diet. *J Am Med Assoc* **87**, 470–476.

Miousse, I.R., Watkins, D., Coelho, D., *et al.* (2009) Clinical and molecular heterogeneity in patients with the *CblD* inborn error of cobalamin metabolism. *J Pediatr* **154**, 551–556.

Moelby, L., Rasmussen, K., Jensen, M.K., *et al.* (1990) The relationship between clinically confirmed cobalamin deficiency and serum methylmalonic acid. *J Intern Med* **228**, 373–378.

Mudd, S.H., Brosnan, J.T., Brosnan, M.E., *et al.* (2007) Methyl balance and transmethylation fluxes in humans. *Am J Clin Nutr* **85**, 19–25.

Pennypacker, L.C., Allen, R.H., Kelly, J.P., *et al.* (1992) High prevalence of cobalamin deficiency in elderly outpatients. *J Am Geriatr Soc* **40**, 1197–1204.

Pfeiffer, C.M., Johnson, C.L., Jain, R.B., *et al.* (2007) Trends in blood folate and vitamin B-12 concentrations in the United States, 1988 2004. *Am J Clin Nutr* **86**, 718–727.

Quadros, E.V. (2010) Advances in the understanding of cobalamin assimilation and metabolism. *Br J Haematol* **148**, 195–204.

Randaccio, L., Geremia, S., Demitri, N., *et al.* (2010) Vitamin B12: unique metalorganic compounds and the most complex vitamins. *Molecules* **15**, 3228–3259.

Rasmussen, K., Moller, J., Lyngbak, M., *et al.* (1996) Age-and-gender-specific reference intervals for total homocysteine and methylmalonic acid in plasma before and after vitamin supplementation. *Clin Chem* **42**, 630–636.

Rasmussen, K., Vyberg, B., Pedersen, K.O., *et al.* (1990) Methylmalonic acid in renal insufficiency: evidence of accumulation and implications for diagnosis of cobalamin deficiency. *Clin Chem* **36**, 1523–1524.

Rice, D.A., McLoughlin, M., Blanchflower, W.J., *et al.* (1989) Sequential changes in plasma methylmalonic acid and vitamin B12 in sheep eating cobalt-deficient grass. *Biol Trace Elem Res* **22**, 153–163.

Rosenblatt, D.A. and Fenton, W.A. (2001) Inherited disorders of cobalamin transport and metabolism. In C.R. Scriver, A.L. Beaudet, W.S. Sly, *et al.* (eds), *The Metabolic and Molecular Bases of Inherited Disease*, Vol. 3, 8th Edn. pp. 3897–3933. McGraw-Hill, New York.

Rutsch, F., Gailus, S., Suormala, T., *et al.* (2011) LMBRD1: the gene for the cblF defect of vitamin B(12) metabolism. *J Inherit Metab Dis* **34**, 121–126.

Savage, D.G. and Lindenbaum, J. (1995) Folate–cobalamin interactions. In L.B. Bailey (ed.), *Folate in Health and Disease*, Vol. 1. Marcel-Dekker, New York, pp. 237–285.

Savage, D., Gangaidzo, I., Lindenbaum, J, *et al.* (1994a) Vitamin B12 deficiency is the primary cause of megaloblastic anaemia in Zimbabwe. *Br J Haematol* **86**, 844–850.

Savage, D.G., Lindenbaum, J., Stabler, S.P., *et al.* (1994b) Sensitivity of serum methylmalonic acid and total homocysteine determinations for diagnosing cobalamin deficiency and folate deficiencies. *Am J Med* **96**, 239–246.

Scalabrino, G. and Peracchi, M. (2006) New insights into the pathophysiology of cobalamin deficiency. *Trends Molec Med* **12**, 247–254.

Scalabrino, G., Carpo, M., Bamonti, F., *et al.* (2004) High tumor necrosis factor-alpha [corrected] levels in cerebrospinal fluid of cobalamin-deficient patients. *Ann Neurol* **56**, 886–890.

Scott, J.M., Wilson, P., Dinn, J.J., *et al.* (1981) Pathogenesis of subacute combined degeneration: a result of methyl group deficiency. *Lancet* **2**, 334–337.

Sekhar, J. and Stabler, S.P. (2007) Life-threatening megaloblastic pancytopenia with normal mean cell volume: case series. *Eur J Int Med* **18**, 548–550.

Singer, M.A., Lazaridis, C., Nations, S.P., *et al.* (2008) Reversible nitrous oxide-induced myeloneuropathy with pernicious anemia: case report and literature review. *Muscle Nerve* **37**, 125–129.

Smulders, Y.M., Smith, D.E., Kok, R.M., *et al.* (2006) Cellular folate vitamer distribution during and after correction of vitamin B12 deficiency: a case for the methylfolate trap. *Br J Haematol* **132**, 623–629.

Soria, C., Chadefaux, B., Coude, M., *et al.* (1990) Concentrations of total homocysteine in plasma in chronic renal failure. *Clin Chem* **36**, 2137–2138.

Stabler, S.P. (2006) Megaloblastic anemias: pernicious anemia and folate deficiency. In N.S. Young, S.L. Gerson, and K.A. High (eds), *Clinical Hematology*, Vol. 1. Mosby, Philadelphia, pp. 242–251

Stabler, S.P. and Allen, R.H. (2004) Vitamin B12 deficiency as a worldwide problem. *Annu Rev Nutr* **24**, 299–326.

Stabler, S.P., Allen, R.H., Barrett, R.E., *et al.* (1991a) Cerebrospinal fluid methylmalonic acid levels in normal subjects and patients with cobalamin deficiency. *Neurology* **41**, 1627–1632.

Stabler, S.P., Allen, R.H., Fried, L.P., *et al.* (1999) Racial differences in prevalence of cobalamin and folate deficiencies in disabled elderly women. *Am J Clin Nutr* **70**, 911–919.

Stabler, S.P., Allen, R.H., Savage, D.G., *et al.* (1990) Clinical spectrum and diagnosis of cobalamin deficiency. *Blood* **76**, 871–881.

Stabler, S.P., Brass, E.P., Allen, R.H., *et al.* (1991b) Inhibition of cobalamin-dependent enzymes by cobalamin analogues in rats. *J Clin Invest* **87**, 1422–1430.

Stabler, S.P., DeMasters, B.K., and Allen, R.H. (1991c) Cobalamin (Cbl) analogue-induced Cbl deficiency in pigs – a new model for human disease. *Blood* **78**, 253a.

Stabler, S.P., Lindenbaum, J., and Allen, R.H. (1997) Vitamin B12 deficiency in the elderly: current dilemmas. *Am J Clin Nutr* **66**, 741–749.

Stabler, S.P., Lindenbaum, J., Savage, D.G., *et al.* (1993) Elevation of serum cystathionine levels in patients with cobalamin and folate deficiency. *Blood* **81**, 3104–3113.

Stabler, S.P., Marcell, P.D., Podell, E.R., *et al.* (1986) Assay of methylmalonic acid in the serum of patients with cobalamin deficiency using capillary gas chromatography–mass spectrometry. *J Clin Invest* **77**, 1606–1612.

Stabler, S.P., Marcell, P.D., Podell, E.R., *et al.* (1988) Elevation of total homocysteine in the serum of patients with cobalamin or folate deficiency detected by capillary gas chromatography–mass spectrometry. *J Clin Invest* **81**, 466–474.

Stanger, O., Fowler, B., Piertzik, K., *et al.* (2009) Homocysteine, folate and vitamin B12 in neuropsychiatric diseases: review and treatment recommendations. *Exp Rev Neurother* **9**, 1393–1412.

Sumner, A.E., Chin, M.M., Abrahm, J.L., *et al.* (1996) Elevated methylmalonic acid and total homocysteine levels show high prevalence of vitamin B$_{12}$ deficiency after gastric surgery. *Ann Int Med* **124**, 469–476.

Tanner, S.M., Li, Z., Bisson, R., *et al.* (2004) Genetically heterogeneous selective intestinal malabsorption of vitamin B12: founder effects, consanguinity, and high clinical awareness explain aggregations in Scandinavia and the Middle East. *Hum Mutat* **23,** 327–333.

Tanner, S.M., Li, Z., Perko, J.D., *et al.* (2005) Hereditary juvenile cobalamin deficiency caused by mutations in the intrinsic factor gene. *Proc Natl Acad Sci USA* **102,** 4130–4133.

Thorpe, S.J., Heath, A., Blackmore, S., *et al.* (2007) International Standard for serum vitamin B(12) and serum folate: international collaborative study to evaluate a batch of lyophilised serum for B(12) and folate content. *Clin Chem Lab Med* **45,** 380–386.

Toh, B.H., van Driel, I.R., and Gleeson, P.A. (1997) Pernicious anemia. *New Engl J Med* **337,** 1441–1448.

Waife, S.O., Jansen, C.J., Crabtree, R.E., *et al.* (1963) Oral vitamin B$_{12}$ without intrinsic factor in the treatment of pernicious anemia. *Ann Intern Med* **58,** 810–817.

Watanabe, F. (2007) Vitamin B12 sources and bioavailability. *Exp Biol Med* **232,** 1266–1274.

Weir, D.G., Keating, S., Molloy, A., *et al.* (1988) Methylation deficiency causes vitamin B$_{12}$ associated neuropathy in the pig. *J Neurochem* **51,** 1949–1952.

Werder, S.F. (2010) Cobalamin deficiency, hyperhomocysteinemia, and dementia. *Neuropsychiatr Dis Treat* **6,** 159–195.

Whitehead, V.M. (2006) Acquired and inherited disorders of cobalamin and folate in children. *Br J Haematol* **134,** 125–136.

Wickramasinghe, S.N. (2006) Diagnosis of megaloblastic anaemias. *Blood Rev* **20,** 299–318.

23

BIOTIN

JANOS ZEMPLENI, PhD, SUBHASHINEE S.K. WIJERATNE, PhD
AND TOSHINOBU KUROISHI, PhD

University of Nebraska–Lincoln, Lincoln, Nebraska, USA

Summary

Biotin is a water-soluble vitamin and serves as a coenzyme for five carboxylases, which catalyze key steps in the metabolism of fatty acids, glucose, and amino acids in humans. Biotin also regulates gene expression, mediated by biotinylation of lysine residues in histones H2A, H3, and H4, and by various transcription factors. Holocarboxylase synthetase, biotinidase, sodium-dependent multivitamin transporter, and the biotin transporters SMVT and MCT1 play crucial roles in biotin homeostasis in mammals. Human biotin requirements are unknown, and recommendations for dietary intake are based on estimates of biotin intake in apparently healthy populations ("adequate intake"). Individuals carrying mutations in genes coding for holocarboxylase synthetase and biotinidase require lifelong supplementation with pharmacological doses of biotin. Reliable markers for biotin status include the activity of propionyl-CoA carboxylase in lymphocytes, and the urinary excretion of biotin and the metabolite 3-hydroxyisovaleric acid. Anticonvulsants and lipoic acid may interfere with biotin metabolism, thereby increasing biotin requirements. Severe biotin deficiency has been linked to birth defects and impaired immune function in animal studies. Whether these effects of marginal biotin deficiency occur spontaneously in humans remains unclear.

Introduction

Humans and other metazoans cannot synthesize the water-soluble vitamin biotin and depend on dietary biotin that originated in plants and microorganisms (Zempleni *et al.*, 2009). Major advances have been made over the past 10 years, leading to a more complete understanding of the roles of biotin as a key regulator at various crossroads of intermediary metabolism and gene regulation. Biotin is now known to play key roles in the metabolism of macronutrients, in histone modification, and in various signal transduction pathways. Importantly, clinical evidence now exists that life stages (e.g. pregnancy) and lifestyle factors (e.g. smoking) affect biotin requirements. This chapter reviews the current state of knowledge in biotin nutrition in humans and, occasionally, other organisms.

History

Boas demonstrated a requirement for the water-soluble vitamin biotin in mammals over 80 years ago (Boas, 1927).

Present Knowledge in Nutrition, Tenth Edition. Edited by John W. Erdman Jr, Ian A. Macdonald and Steven H. Zeisel.
© 2012 International Life Sciences Institute. Published 2012 by John Wiley & Sons, Inc.

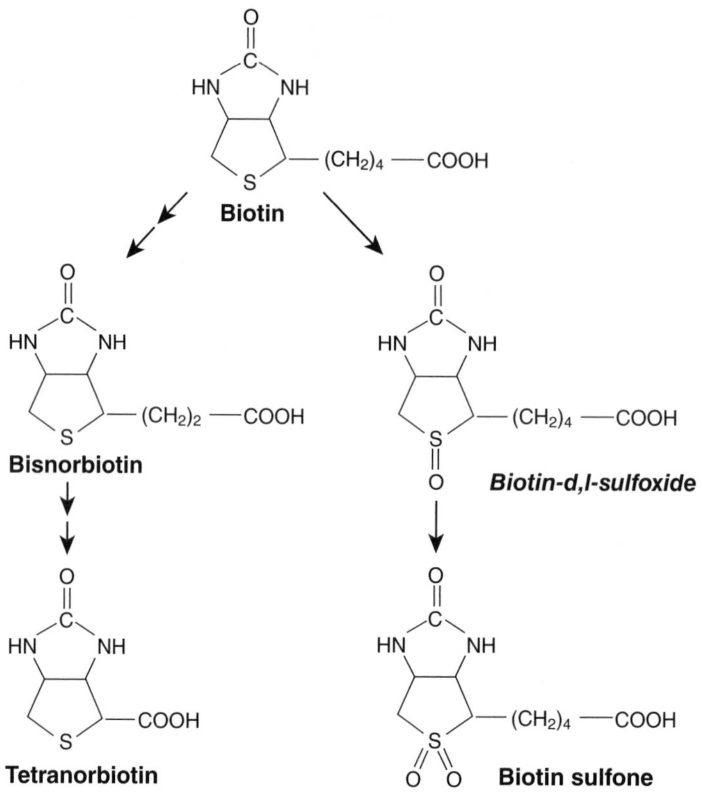

FIG. 23.1   Pathways of biotin catabolism (data from McCormick and Wright, 1971).

Biotin was first isolated by Kögl and Tönnis (1932) and its chemical structure was determined by du Vigneaud *et al.* (1942). Biotin was first chemically synthesized by Harris *et al.* (1943).

Biosynthesis

Mammals and other metazoans cannot synthesize biotin and depend on dietary biotin originating in microbial and plant biosynthetic pathways. The route of biosynthesis of biotin was largely elaborated by Eisenberg *et al.* working with *Escherichia coli* (Rolfe and Eisenberg, 1968; Eisenberg *et al.*, 1975). In this pathway, dethiobiotin is formed from pimelyl-CoA (which can be synthesized from oleic acid) and carbamyl phosphate (Hatakeyama *et al.*, 1997). Sulfur is incorporated into dethiobiotin in a synthase-dependent step, generating biotin (Flint and Allen, 1997).

Catabolism of Biotin

McCormick and co-workers identified two pathways of biotin catabolism in microorganisms and mammals (Figure

23.1). In one pathway, biotin is catabolized by β-oxidation of the valeric acid side chain (McCormick and Wright, 1971). The repeated cleavage of two-carbon units leads to the formation of bisnorbiotin, tetranorbiotin, and related catabolites that are known to result from β-oxidation of fatty acids (i.e. α,β-dehydro-, β-hydroxy, and β-keto-intermediates). β-Ketobiotin and β-ketobisnorbiotin are unstable and may decarboxylate spontaneously to form bisnorbiotin methyl ketone and tetranorbiotin methyl ketone (McCormick and Wright, 1971). After degradation of the valeric acid side chain to one carbon (tetranorbiotin), microorganisms cleave and degrade the heterocyclic ring (McCormick and Wright, 1971); degradation of the heterocyclic ring is quantitatively minor in mammals (Lee *et al.*, 1972). In a second pathway of biotin catabolism, the sulfur in the heterocyclic ring is oxidized to produce biotin-*l*-sulfoxide, biotin-*d*-sulfoxide, and biotin sulfone (McCormick and Wright, 1971). It is likely that sulfur oxidation in the biotin molecule occurs in the smooth endoplasmic reticulum in a reaction that depends on nicotinamide adenine dinucleotide phosphate (Lee *et al.*, 1970). Finally, biotin is also catabolized by a combination of both β-oxidation and sulfur oxidation, producing compounds such as bisnorbiotin sulfone.

Biological Functions of Biotin

Biotin serves as a covalently bound coenzyme for five human carboxylases (Zempleni *et al.*, 2009). In addition, biotin also plays unique roles in gene regulation, mediated by both biotinylation of histones and "classical" pathways of cell signaling (Zempleni *et al.*, 2009).

Biotin-Dependent Carboxylases

In mammals, biotin serves as a covalently bound coenzyme for acetyl-CoA carboxylases (ACC) 1 and 2, pyruvate carboxylase (PC), propionyl-CoA carboxylase (PCC), and 3-methylcrotonyl-CoA carboxylase (MCC) (Zempleni *et al.*, 2009). The attachment of biotin to the ε-amino group of a specific lysine residue in holocarboxylases is catalyzed by holocarboxylase synthetase (HCS); biotinylation of carboxylases requires ATP and proceeds in the following two steps.

1. $ATP + biotin + HCS \rightarrow Biotinyl-5'-AMP-HCS$
$+ pyrophosphate$

2. $Biotinyl-5'-AMP-HCS + apocarboxylase$
$\rightarrow holocarboxylase + AMP + HCS$

$$\overline{}$$

(*Net*) $ATP + biotin + apocarboxylase$
$\rightarrow holocarboxylase + AMP + pyrophosphate$

Both the N- and C-termini in HCS are important for recognition of carboxylases (Hassan *et al.*, 2009). Holocarboxylases mediate the covalent binding of bicarbonate (not carbon dioxide), using 1'-N-carboxybiotinyl as an HCS-bound carboxyl donor (Knowles, 1989).

Both the cytoplasmic ACC1 and the mitochondrial ACC2 catalyze the binding of bicarbonate to acetyl-CoA to generate malonyl-CoA, but the two isoforms play distinct roles in intermediary metabolism (Kim *et al.*, 1997). ACC1 produces malonyl-CoA for the synthesis of fatty acid synthesis in the cytoplasm; ACC2 is an important regulator of fatty acid oxidation in mitochondria. The malonyl-CoA produced by ACC2 inhibits mitochondrial uptake of fatty acids for β-oxidation.

PC, PCC, and MCC localize in mitochondria. PC is a key enzyme in gluconeogenesis. PCC catalyzes an essential step in the metabolism of propionyl-CoA, which is pro-

duced in the metabolism of some amino acids, the cholesterol side chain, and odd-chain fatty acids. MCC catalyzes an essential step in leucine metabolism (Figure 23.2). Both PCC and MCC are composed of non-identical subunits, i.e. biotinylated α subunits and non-biotinylated β subunits, which are encoded by distinct genes.

Proteolytic degradation of holocarboxylases leads to the formation of biotinyl peptides and biocytin (biotin-ε-lysine). These compounds are further degraded by biotinidase to release biotin, which is then recycled in holocarboxylase synthesis (Wolf *et al.*, 1985).

Biotinylation of Histones

Histones are quantitatively the most important proteins in chromatin and play essential roles in processes such as DNA packaging and repair, replication, and gene regulation (Wolffe, 1998). Mammals express five major classes of histones: linker histone H1, and core histones H2A, H2B, H3, and H4. Histones consist of a globular domain and a flexible N-terminal tail. Chromatin is made of repetitive nucleoprotein complexes, the nucleosomes. Each nucleosome ("nucleosomal core particle") consists of 146 base pairs of DNA, wrapped around an octamer of core histones (one H3/H3/H4/H4 tetramer, two H2A/H2B dimers). The N-terminal tails of core histones protrude from the nucleosomal surface; covalent modifications of these tails affect the structure of chromatin and play critical roles in gene regulation. Some modifications also exist in the globular domain and C-terminal regions (Kouzarides and Berger, 2007; Zempleni *et al.*, 2009) (Figure 23.3).

Biotinylation of distinct lysine (K) residues is among the recognized modification marks in histones (Hymes *et al.*, 1995; Stanley *et al.*, 2001). As of today, 11–13 biotinylation sites have been identified in histones H2A, H3, and H4 (Zempleni *et al.*, 2009). Initially, it was believed that biotinylation of histones is catalyzed by biotinidase (Hymes *et al.*, 1995). However, subsequent studies revealed that HCS is much more important than biotinidase for biotinylation of histones *in vivo* (Camporeale *et al.*, 2006; Bao *et al.*, 2011), while acknowledging that biotinidase has histone biotinyl transferase activity *in vitro* (Camporeale *et al.*, 2004). HCS can be detected in both nuclear and extranuclear compartments (Narang *et al.*, 2004; Chew *et al.*, 2006); nuclear HCS is a chromatin protein (Camporeale *et al.*, 2006) and its binding to chromatin might be mediated by physical interactions with histones H3 and H4 (Bao

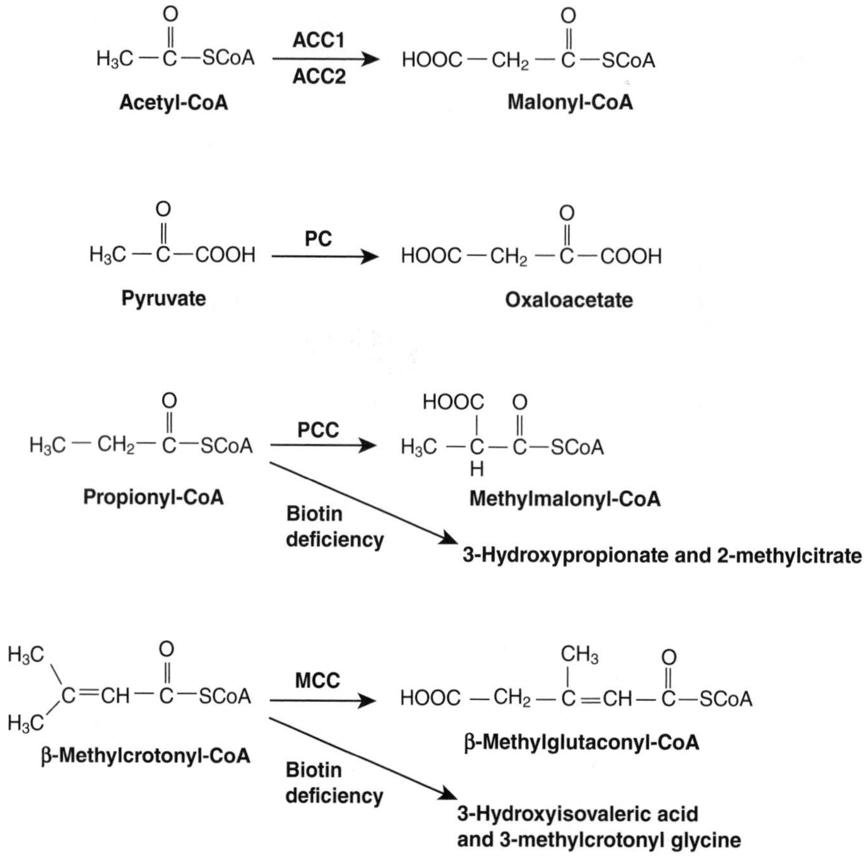

FIG. 23.2   Biotin-dependent carboxylases (data from Zempleni et al., 2009). ACC, acetyl-CoA carboxylase; MCC, 3-methylcrotonyl-CoA carboxylase; PC, pyruvate carboxylase; PCC, propionyl-CoA carboxylase.

et al., 2011). Phenotypes of HCS knockdown include decreased lifespan and heat survival in *Drosophila melanogaster* (Camporeale et al., 2006).

Evidence is emerging for the biological functions of K12-biotinylated histone H4 (H4K12bio), while information regarding other biotinylation marks is scarce. The H4K12bio mark is enriched in heterochromatin repeats (telomeres, long-terminal repeats, and pericentromeric alpha satellite repeats) and transcriptionally repressed genes (Zempleni et al., 2009). H4K12bio plays a role in the regulation of biotin transporter expression and the repression of long-terminal repeats (Chew et al., 2008; Gralla et al., 2008). Importantly, the abundance of histone biotinylation marks depends on biotin supply (Chew et al., 2008). Low levels of histone biotinylation in biotin-deficient cells and model organisms has been linked to increased frequency of retrotransposition events, suggest-

ing a role for histone biotinylation in chromosomal stability (Chew et al., 2008). Biotinylation of lysines other than K12 in histone H4 appears to have biological functions similar to that described for H4K12bio (Pestinger et al., 2010).

Gene Expression

Pioneering studies by Dakshinamurti and co-workers suggested a role for biotin in the regulation of the *glucokinase* gene (Dakshinamurti and Cheah-Tan, 1968). Subsequently, it was shown that biotin affects gene regulation by "classical" signaling pathways such as cGMP, NF-κB, Sp1 and Sp3, nitric oxide, and receptor tyrosine kinases, and by the intermediate biotinyl-5'-AMP (Solorzano-Vargas et al., 2002; Zempleni et al., 2009). Biotin also affects gene expression at the post-transcriptional level (Collins et al., 1988).

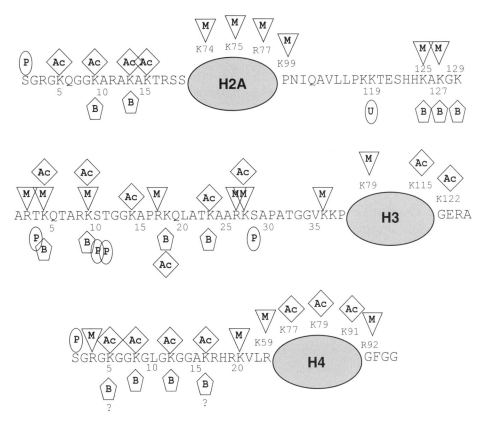

FIG. 23.3 Modification sites in histones H2A, H3, and H4 (data from Kouzarides and Berger (2007) and Zempleni et al. (2009). Ac, acetate; B, biotin; M, methyl; P, phosphate; U, ubiquitin.

Methods of Biotin Analysis

Microbial Growth Assays

Biotin auxotroph microorganisms have been used for biotin analysis, but these microbes lack chemical specificity and show variable growth responses to biotin and the various biotin precursors, catabolites, and analogs (Zempleni and Mock, 2000a). In addition, binding of biotin to proteins can be a meaningful confounder in microbial growth assays.

(Strept)Avidin-Binding Assays

The proteins avidin and streptavidin are widely used in biotin analysis because they bind biotin with extraordinary strength and specificity; the dissociation constant of the avidin–biotin complex is 1.3×10^{-15} M (Green, 1975). Avidin and streptavidin are purified from egg white and *Streptomyces* sp., respectively. Streptavidin has greater spe-

cificity for biotin compared with avidin, and is the probe of choice in avidin-binding assays. In our laboratory, we are currently relying on an assay developed by Kuroishi et al. (2008).

Biotin catabolites and compounds that are structurally similar to biotin also bind to avidin, causing the following potential pitfalls in biotin analysis. First, avidin binds biotin catabolites less tightly compared with biotin (Zempleni and Mock, 2000a). Hence, avidin-binding assays may underestimate the true concentration of biotin plus catabolites if calibrated by using biotin. Second, compounds other than biotin or catabolites may bind to avidin and cause artificially large readings for "apparent biotin." Therefore, avidin-binding compounds in biological samples need to be resolved by chromatography prior to analysis of individual chromatographic fractions against authentic standards, as reviewed elsewhere (Zempleni and Mock, 2000a).

4′-Hydroxyazobenzene-2-Carboxylic Acid

4′-Hydroxyazobenzene-2-carboxylic acid is a robust probe to quantify chemically pure biotin at concentrations that exceed those typically found in biological samples, e.g. in pharmaceutical preparations (Zempleni and Mock, 2000a).

Biotin Analogs

Synthetic biotin analogs (e.g. iminobiotin) and some naturally occurring biotin metabolites (e.g. biocytin) are available commercially. Likewise, a large number of reagents are available for chemical biotinylation of amines, sulfhydryl groups, carboxyl groups, nucleic acids, and others.

Absorption, Transport Proteins, Storage, and Excretion

Digestion

Biotin in foods is largely protein bound (Wolf *et al.*, 1985). Several gastrointestinal proteases may hydrolyze biotin-containing proteins to generate biotinyl peptides. Biotinyl peptides are further hydrolyzed by intestinal biotinidase to release biotin. Intestinal biotinidase is found in pancreatic juice, secretions of the intestinal glands, bacterial flora, and the brush-border membranes. Biotinidase activities are similar in mucosa from duodenum, jejunum, and ileum. The primary site or sites for hydrolysis of biotinyl peptides are unknown. Small quantities of biotinyl peptides may be absorbed without prior hydrolysis (Said *et al.*, 1993).

Intestinal Transport and Bioavailability

Early investigations of biotin transport in rat jejunum suggested that intestinal biotin uptake is mediated by both saturable and non-saturable components (Bowman *et al.*, 1986). At biotin concentrations less than 5 µmol/L, biotin absorption proceeds largely by the saturable process, whereas, at concentrations above 25 µmol/L, non-saturable uptake predominates (Bowman *et al.*, 1986). The saturable mechanism of biotin transport is sodium dependent (Said and Redha, 1987). Transport of biotin is faster in the jejunum than in the ileum, and is minimal in the colon (85 vs. 36 vs. 2.8 pmol/g tissue wet weight/25 min, respectively); the apparent Km (Michaelis–Menten constant) of the transporter for biotin in rat jejunum is 3.7 µmol/L. The biotin transporter was cloned and has comparable affinities for biotin, pantothenic acid, and lipoic acid, if overexpressed in mammalian cells (Prasad *et al.*, 1998). Consequently, this transporter was named the sodium-

dependent multivitamin transporter (SMVT) (Prasad *et al.*, 1998). Four splicing variants of SMVT transcripts have been identified in rats (Said, 2004). The expression of SMVT is regulated by protein kinase C and histone biotinylation (Said, 2004; Gralla *et al.*, 2008).

The 5′-regulatory regions of *SMVT* genes in rats and humans have been cloned and characterized (Dey *et al.*, 2002). The rat and human *SMVT* genes contain three and two distinct promoters, respectively. Both promoter sequences in the human gene are TATA-less, CAAT-less, contain highly GC-rich sites, and have multiple putative regulatory *cis*-elements, e.g. AP-1, AP-2, C/EBP, SP1, NF1, and GATA (Dey *et al.*, 2002). The minimal region required for basal activity of the human SMVT promoter is encoded by a sequence between −5846 to −5313 for promoter 1 and between −4417 to −4244 for promoter 2 relative to the translation initiation codon. The three promoters in the rat SMVT gene contain *cis*-elements similar to the elements observed in the human promoters, but the rat 5′-regulatory region also contains two TATA-like elements (Chatterjee *et al.*, 2001).

Chemically pure biotin is about 100% bioavailable, even if the dose administered is 600 times the normal dietary intake (Zempleni and Mock, 1999a). Biotin exits enterocytes at the basolateral membrane by a carrier-mediated, sodium-independent process that does not accumulate biotin against a concentration gradient (Said *et al.*, 1988).

Protein-Binding in Plasma

Human albumin, α-globulin, and β-globulin bind biotin rather unspecifically (Dakshinamurti and Chauhan, 1994). Biotinidase has one high-affinity (dissociation constant $K_d = 0.5$ nmol/L) and one low-affinity ($K_d = 50$ nmol/L) binding site for biotin and might serve as a biotin-carrier protein in the plasma of normal adults (Chauhan and Dakshinamurti, 1988). A biotin-binding glycoprotein (mol. wt. 66000) is present in serum of pregnant and estrogenized female rats and appears to be essential for embryonic survival (Seshagiri and Adiga, 1987). The protein binding of biotin in plasma is somewhat controversial; evidence has been provided for the importance of a low-affinity, high-capacity system such as albumin (Mock and Malik, 1992).

Biotin Uptake into Liver and Peripheral Tissues

The SMVT is the most important transporter for mediating biotin uptake into liver and most peripheral tissues

(Said, 2004). In contrast, monocarboxylate transporter 1 contributes importantly towards biotin uptake into lymphoid cells and perhaps keratinocytes (Daberkow *et al.*, 2003).

Cell Compartments

Biotin is distributed unequally across cellular compartments (Petrelli *et al.*, 1979). For example, the vast majority of biotin in rat liver localizes in mitochondria and cytoplasm, whereas only a small fraction localizes in microsomes. The relative enrichment of biotin in mitochondria and cytoplasm is consistent with the role of biotin as a coenzyme for carboxylases in these compartments. A quantitatively small but qualitatively important fraction of biotin localizes in the cell nucleus, i.e. about 0.7% of total biotin in human lymphoid cells can be recovered from the nuclear fraction (Stanley *et al.*, 2001). The relative abundance of nuclear biotin increases to about 1% of total biotin in response to proliferation, consistent with a possible role for biotinylated histones in cell proliferation.

Storage

A relatively large fraction of intravenously administered biotin accumulates in rat liver, consistent with a role for this organ in biotin storage (Petrelli *et al.*, 1979). Depletion and repletion experiments of biotin-dependent carboxylases in rat liver suggest that ACC2 serves as a reservoir for biotin (Shriver *et al.*, 1993), but our own studies are not consistent with a role of any holocarboxylase as a biotin reservoir (Kaur Mall *et al.*, 2010).

Urinary Excretion

Healthy adults excrete approximately 100 nmol/day of biotin and catabolites into urine (Zempleni *et al.*, 1997b). Biotin accounts for approximately half of the total; bisnorbiotin, biotin-*d,l*-sulfoxides, bisnorbiotin methyl ketone, biotin sulfone, and tetranorbiotin-*l*-sulfoxide account for most of the balance. If physiological or pharmacological doses of biotin are administered parenterally to humans, rats, or pigs, 43% to 75% of the dose is excreted into urine (Lee *et al.*, 1972; Zempleni and Mock, 1999a); the remainder is unaccounted for and might be due to excretion of metabolites not detectable by avidin assays; incorporation into biotin sinks such as histones or carboxylases; or excretion via non-renal routes. Renal epithelia reclaim biotin that is filtered in the glomeruli in an SMVT-mediated process (Nabokina *et al.*, 2003).

Biliary Excretion

The biliary excretion of biotin and catabolites is quantitatively minor, i.e. <2% of an intravenous dose of [14C] biotin (Zempleni *et al.*, 1997a). The concentration ratios of biotin, bisnorbiotin, and biotin-*d,l*-sulfoxide (bile versus serum) in pigs are at least one order of magnitude smaller than the ratio measured for the cholephil compound, bilirubin.

Pharmacokinetics

[3H]Biotin efflux from human lymphocytes is best described by using a three-compartment model; the half-lives of the three elimination phases are approximately 0.2 hours, 1.2 hours, and 22 hours (Zempleni and Mock, 1999c). Likely, the half-life of [3H]biotin during the terminal, slow phase of efflux is determined by the breakdown of biotin-dependent carboxylases to release free [3H]biotin, followed by efflux of [3H]biotin from lymphocytes. The half-life of [3H]biotin during the terminal phase of efflux (22 hours) resembles the half-lives of pyruvate carboxylase (28 hours) and acetyl-CoA carboxylase (4.6 days). Studies in pigs also generated valuable insights into biotin pharmacokinetics (Mock *et al.*, 1997c).

Biotin Status

Direct Measures

The serum concentrations and the urinary excretions of biotin and catabolites are potential markers of biotin status. Biotin accounts for about half of the total of all biotinyl compounds in human urine and serum (Zempleni *et al.*, 2009) (Table 23.1). Tetranorbiotin-*l*-sulfoxide was detected in human urine but its avidin affinity is too low to allow meaningful quantitation.

The urinary excretion of biotin and biotin catabolites decreases rapidly and substantially in biotin-deficient individuals (Mock *et al.*, 1997d), suggesting that the urinary excretion is an early and sensitive indicator of biotin deficiency. In contrast, serum concentrations of biotin, bisnorbiotin, and biotin-*d,l*-sulfoxide do not decrease in biotin-depleted individuals and in patients on biotin-free total parenteral nutrition (Velazquez *et al.*, 1990) during reasonable periods of observation. Hence, serum concentrations are not good indicators of marginal biotin deficiency.

TABLE 23.1 Serum concentrations and urinary excretions of biotin and catabolites

Compound	Serum (pmol/L)	Urine (nmol/24 hours)
Biotin	244 ± 61	35 ± 14
Bisnorbiotin	189 ± 135	68 ± 48
BSO[a]	15 ± 33	5 ± 6
BNBMK[a]	ND[a]	9 ± 9
Biotin sulfone	ND[a]	5 ± 5
Total biotin	464 ± 178[b]	122 ± 66

Means ± SD are reported (n = 15 for serum; n = 6 for urine).
[a]BSO, Biotin-d,l-sulfoxides; BNBMK, bisnorbiotin methyl ketone; ND, not determined (BNBMK and biotin sulfone had not been identified at the time when this study of serum was conducted and, hence, quantification of these "unknowns" was based on using biotin as a standard).
[b]Including three unidentified biotin catabolites.
Data from Zempleni et al., 2009.

Indirect Measures

Lymphocyte PCC and its activation by biotin *ex vivo* are reliable markers for human biotin status (Stratton et al., 2006). The carboxylase activation index equals the ratio of PCC activities in lymphocytes incubated with and without excess biotin (Velazquez et al., 1990). High values for the activation index suggest that a substantial fraction of total PCC is apo-PCC, indicating biotin deficiency.

Reduced carboxylase activities in biotin deficiency cause metabolic blocks in intermediary metabolism (Figure 23.2). Reduced activity of MCC impairs leucine catabolism. As a consequence, 3-methylcrotonyl-CoA is shunted to alternative pathways, leading to an increased formation of 3-hydroxyisovaleric acid and 3-methylcrotonyl glycine. The urinary excretion of 3-hydroxyisovaleric acid is an early and sensitive indicator of biotin status (Mock et al., 2002a). The derivative, carnityl-3-hydroxyisovaleric acid, also appears to be a robust indicator of biotin status (Stratton et al., 2010).

Reduced activity of PCC causes a metabolic block in propionic acid metabolism. Consequently, propionic acid is shunted to alternative metabolic pathways. In these pathways, 3-hydroxypropionic acid and 2-methylcitric acid are formed. The urinary excretion of 3-hydroxypropionic acid and 2-methylcitric acid is not a good indicator of marginal biotin deficiency (Mock et al., 2004). The accumulation of propionyl-CoA likely leads to occasional incorporation of a three-carbon fragment

(instead of the usual acetyl group) in fatty acid elongation and consequently to significant accumulation of odd-chain fatty acids in plasma phospholipids, plasma triglycerides and RBC membrane phospholipids (Mock et al., 1988).

ACC and PC activities might also be reduced in biotin deficiency, but the responses of these pathways to biotin depletion have not yet been thoroughly investigated. Apparently, lactate levels increase in biotin-depleted *Drosophila melanogaster* compared with biotin-sufficient controls, presumably due to decreased PC activity (Smith et al., 2007). This observation is consistent with the biotin responsiveness of lactate and pyruvate levels observed in an individual with inborn biotin transporter deficiency (Mardach et al., 2002).

Biotin Deficiency

Clinical Findings of Frank Biotin Deficiency

Signs of frank biotin deficiency have been described in patients receiving parenteral nutrition without biotin supplementation (Zempleni and Mock, 1999b) and in patients with biotinidase deficiency (Wolf and Heard, 1991). Frank biotin deficiency may also be observed in individuals consuming large amounts of raw egg white, which contains non-denatured avidin. Binding of biotin to avidin in the gastrointestinal tract prevents absorption of biotin (Spencer and Brody, 1964).

Clinical findings of frank biotin deficiency include periorificial dermatitis, conjunctivitis, alopecia, ataxia, hypotonia, ketolactic acidosis/organic aciduria, seizures, skin infection, and developmental delay in infants and children (Wolf and Heard, 1991). In addition, the following symptoms were observed in adults and adolescents on egg white diet:

- thinning hair, often with loss of hair color;
- skin rash described as scaly (seborrheic) and red (eczematous); in several cases the rash was distributed around the eyes, nose, and mouth;
- depression, lethargy, hallucinations, and paresthesias of the extremities.

Immune System

Biotin deficiency has adverse effects on cellular and humoral immune functions. For example, children with hereditary abnormalities of biotin metabolism developed candida dermatitis; these children had absent delayed-hypersensitivity skin-test responses, IgA deficiency, and subnormal percentages of T lymphocytes in peripheral blood (Cowan *et al.*, 1979). In biotin-deficient rats, the synthesis of antibodies is reduced (Kumar and Axelrod, 1978). Biotin deficiency in mice decreases the number of spleen cells and the percentage of B lymphocytes in spleen (Báez-Saldaña *et al.*, 1998); inhibits thymocyte maturation (Baez-Saldaña and Ortega, 2004); and increases the production of pro-inflammatory cytokines (Kuroishi *et al.*, 2009).

Cell Proliferation

Biotin deficiency causes decreased rates of cell proliferation and cell cycle arrest in HeLa cells and choriocarcinoma cells (Zempleni *et al.*, 2009). Human lymphoid cells respond to mitogen-induced proliferation with a 200% to 600% increase in biotin uptake compared with quiescent controls. This effect is mediated by an increased expression of biotin transporters rather than by an increased affinity of transporters for biotin (Zempleni and Mock, 1999d; Stanley *et al.*, 2002). The increased biotin uptake in proliferating cells is paralleled by increased activities of MCC (180% increase compared with quiescent controls) and PCC (50% increase), and by increased biotinylation of histones (400% increase) (Stanley *et al.*, 2001, 2002). These observations suggest that cell proliferation generates an increased demand for biotin.

Cell Stress and Survival

HCS deficiency mimics biotin deficiency. HCS knockdown flies exhibited a decreased survival in response to heat stress in comparison with wild-type controls (Camporeale *et al.*, 2006). In contrast, biotin deficiency increased survival of human lymphoid cell cultures treated with cell death signals and anti-neoplastic agents, possibly due to increased nuclear translocation of the transcription factor NF-κB (Rodriguez-Melendez *et al.*, 2004). *Drosophila melanogaster* exhibits greater survival rates in response to stress compared with biotin-sufficient controls, if fed biotin-defined diets for 11 days (Landenberger *et al.*, 2004). The reason for the differences in HCS- and biotin-deficient organisms is unknown.

Lipid Metabolism

Three biotin-dependent carboxylases are directly linked to lipid metabolism: ACC 1 and 2 (fatty acid synthesis and β-oxidation) and PCC (metabolism of odd-chain fatty acids). Biotin deficiency causes alterations of the fatty acid

profile in liver, skin, and serum of several animal species, which was paralleled by a >80% decrease in carboxylase activities (Zempleni and Mock, 2000b). The observed increase in the abundance of odd-chain fatty acids suggests that odd-chain fatty acid accumulation might be a marker for reduced PCC activity in biotin-deficient individuals. In patients who developed biotin deficiency during parenteral alimentation, the percentage of odd-chain fatty acids (15:0, 17:0) in serum increased for each of the four major lipid classes, i.e. cholesterol esters, phospholipids, triglycerides, and free fatty acids, but the relative changes have not always been consistent among studies (Zempleni and Mock, 2000b). Some tissues might be more susceptible than others, e.g. biotin deficiency affected the fatty acid composition in liver to a much greater extent than in brain tissue (Zempleni and Mock, 2000b).

Teratogenic Effects of Biotin Deficiency

Severe biotin deficiency is teratogenic in several animal species, including cleft palate, micrognathia, and micromelia in rats and mice (Mock, 2005). About half of the pregnant women in the US are marginally biotin deficient despite a normal dietary biotin intake (Mock *et al.*, 2002b), judged by increased urinary 3-hydroxyisovaleric acid, and decreased urinary biotin and PCC activity in lymphocytes. Marginal biotin deficiency in pregnant women might be caused by accelerated biotin catabolism and fetal accumulation of biotin (Mock and Stadler, 1997; Mock *et al.*, 1997a). The fetal-to-maternal concentration ratio of biotin plus metabolites is about 6:1, suggesting that fetal biotin accumulation might contribute to maternal biotin depletion (Mantagos *et al.*, 1998). Yet, the activity of PCC is reduced by approximately 90% in the fetus at term in response to feeding an egg-white diet that causes only a 50% reduction in maternal hepatic PCC activity in mice, suggesting that the fetus may not really be an efficient biotin parasite (Sealey *et al.*, 2005). If conclusive evidence was provided that marginal biotin deficiency causes birth defects in a quantitatively important fraction of pregnant women, this line of research would have major implications for health-care professionals and policy makers.

Biotin Homeostasis in the Central Nervous System (CNS)

Disturbances in biotin homeostasis in the CNS cause encephalopathies (Ozand *et al.*, 1998). Factors leading to biotin imbalances in CNS include deficiencies of biotinidase, HCS, and perhaps biotin transporters as described below. Afflicted patients typically respond to the administration of large doses of biotin by maintaining normal neurologic function. The reader should note that the biotin-responsive defect observed by Ozand *et al.* (1998) turned out to be a thiamin transporter defect (Subramanian *et al.*, 2006); the link between biotin and thiamin transport remains to be elucidated.

Moderate dietary biotin deficiency is typically not associated with neurologic symptoms, because the CNS maintains normal concentrations of biotin at the expense of other tissues. Evidence has been provided that biotin deficiency causes a >90% decrease in holocarboxylases in rat liver, whereas brain carboxylases remain unchanged (Pacheco-Alvarez *et al.*, 2005). Apparently, biotin deficiency decreases expression of SMVT in rat liver while maintaining normal expression of SMVT in brain.

Disorders of Biotin Metabolism

Biotinidase Deficiency

Low activities of the enzyme biotinidase cause a failure to recycle biotin from degraded carboxylases, i.e. to release biotin from biocytin (Wolf and Heard, 1991). Substantial amounts of biocytin are excreted into urine (Suormala *et al.*, 1988), eventually leading to biotin deficiency. Thus, clinical and biochemical features in children with biotinidase deficiency are similar to those described for biotin deficiency (Wolf and Heard, 1991).

Typically, symptoms of biotinidase deficiency appear at age 1 week to >1 year (Wolf and Heard, 1991). Wolf proposed to distinguish between patients with profound biotinidase deficiency (<10% of normal serum biotinidase activity), and patients with partial deficiency (10–30% of normal biotinidase activity). The estimated incidence of profound biotinidase deficiency is 1 in 112 000 and the incidence of partial biotinidase deficiency is 1 in 129 000. The combined incidence of profound and partial deficiency is 1 in 60 000 live births; an estimated 1 in 123 individuals is heterozygous for the disorder. Most of the children in whom biotinidase deficiency has been diagnosed are Caucasian. Mutations of the *biotinidase* gene have been well characterized at the molecular level (Neto *et al.*, 2004). Children with profound biotinidase deficiency are treated with 5–20 mg of biotin per day to compensate for urinary loss of biotin (Wolf and Heard, 1991). If identified early, symptomatic patients improve rapidly after lifelong biotin supplementation is initiated.

Procedures for prenatal diagnosis of biotinidase activity in cultured amniotic fluid cells and for neonatal screening using blood samples have been proposed (Wolf and Heard, 1991). Biotinidase activity is measured by quantifying the release of *p*-aminobenzoic acid from *N*-biotinyl-*p*-aminobenzoate (Wolf *et al.*, 1983). The mean (± SD) normal activity of biotinidase is 5.8 ± 0.9 nmol *p*-aminobenzoate liberated/min/mL serum (Wolf *et al.*, 1983). Synthetic inhibitors are available for studies of biotinidase *in vitro* (Kobza *et al.*, 2008).

Carboxylase Deficiencies

Afflicted individuals present with either isolated deficiencies of individual carboxylases or multiple deficiencies of multiple biotin-dependent carboxylases, i.e. multiple carboxylase deficiency (MCD) (Wolf and Feldman, 1982). MCD is caused by mutations in the *HCS* gene (reducing binding of biotin to carboxylases) or mutations in biotin transporter genes (reducing intracellular concentrations of biotin). MCD patients characteristically exhibit low activities of all five biotin-dependent carboxylases. Mutations of the *HCS* gene (Suzuki *et al.*, 1994) have been well characterized at the molecular level (Suzuki *et al.*, 2005). The incidence of HCS deficiency is less than 1 in 100 000 live births in Japan (Suzuki *et al.*, 2005). Afflicted individuals typically respond well to administration of pharmacological doses of biotin, in particular if the mutation of the gene resides in the biotin-binding region of the protein. In addition to the ~30 mutations in the human *HCS* gene that have been described, 2200 SNPs have been mapped in the *HCS* locus (National Center for Biotechnology Information, 2008) but their importance for HCS activity and human health is unknown.

Isolated PCC deficiency is a rare disorder with an estimated incidence of one in 350 000 individuals (Wolf and Feldman, 1982). Afflicted individuals become symptomatic during early infancy with vomiting, lethargy, and hypotonia (Wolf and Feldman, 1982). Treatment by administration of oral biotin may be successful. PCC deficiency can be diagnosed prenatally either by demonstrating deficient enzyme activity in cultured amniotic fluid cells or by detecting the presence of elevated concentrations of methylcitrate in amniotic fluid. Mutations of genes coding for both α and β subunits of PCC have been identified (Perez *et al.*, 2003).

A small number of patients (21 patients as of 1982) with isolated PC deficiency have been reported (Wolf and Feldman, 1982). Symptoms appear in early infancy.

Biotin administration was not a successful treatment. PC deficiency presents either as the North American phenotype (lacticacidemia, hyperalaninemia, hyperprolinemia) or the French phenotype (elevated blood levels of ammonia, citrulline, proline, and lysine) (Robinson *et al.*, 1987). Very little information is available in regard to mutations in genes coding for MCC and ACC (Wolf and Feldman, 1982; Desviat *et al.*, 2003, Baumgartner *et al.*, 2004).

Biotin Transporter Deficiency

Recently, a case of inborn biotin transporter deficiency has been identified (Mardach *et al.*, 2002). Of note, the patient with biotin transporter deficiency did not have any of the cutaneous symptoms of biotin deficiency. Rather, central nervous system signs and profound metabolic disturbances consistent with deficiencies of multiple carboxylases dominated that patient's clinical picture. All resolved with biotin supplementation. Evidence was provided that biotin transporter deficiency was not caused by abnormal SMVT, but the identity of the afflicted transporter remained unknown.

Biotin–Drug Interactions

Anticonvulsants

Biotin requirements may be increased during anticonvulsant therapy. The anticonvulsants primidone and carbamazepine inhibit biotin uptake into brush-border membrane vesicles from human intestine (Zempleni and Mock, 1999b). Long-term therapy with anticonvulsants increases both biotin catabolism and urinary excretion of 3-hydroxyisovaleric acid. Phenobarbital, phenytoin, and carbamazepine displace biotin from biotinidase, conceivably affecting plasma transport, renal handling, or cellular uptake of biotin. This is associated with decreased plasma concentrations of biotin.

Lipoic Acid (Thioctic Acid)

Lipoic acid may be administered to treat heavy-metal intoxication, to reduce signs of diabetic neuropathy, and to enhance glucose disposal in patients with non-insulin-dependent diabetes mellitus (Zempleni *et al.*, 1997c). Lipoic acid competes with biotin for binding to SMVT (Prasad *et al.*, 1998), potentially decreasing the cellular uptake of biotin. Indeed, chronic administration of pharmacological doses of lipoic acid decreased the activities of

TABLE 23.2   Adequate intakes of biotin

Life-stage group	Adequate intake (µg/day)
Infants	
0–6 months	5
7–12 months	6
Children	
1–3 years	8
4–8 years	12
Adults	
9–13 years	20
14–18 years	25
19 years and older	30
Pregnant women	30
Lactating women	35

Data from Institute of Medicine, 1998.

PC and MCC in rat liver to 64–72% of controls (Zempleni *et al.*, 1997c).

Requirements and Recommended Intakes

Adequate Intakes

The Food and Nutrition Board of the National Research Council has released recommendations for adequate intake of biotin (Table 23.2) (Institute of Medicine, 1998). These data are based on estimated biotin intakes (not to be confused with requirements) in a group of healthy people. Adequate intakes may serve as goals for the nutrient intake of individuals. Biotin supplements may contribute substantially to biotin intake. For example, 15–20% of individuals in the United States report consuming biotin-containing dietary supplements (Institute of Medicine, 1998).

Life Stages and Lifestyle Factors that Affect Biotin Requirements

Pregnancy and use of drugs may be associated with an increased requirement for biotin as described above. Smoking might further accelerate biotin catabolism in women (Sealey *et al.*, 2004) and alcohol impairs human placental biotin transport (Schenker *et al.*, 1993).

Lactation may generate an increased demand for biotin. At 8 days postpartum, biotin in human milk is approximately 8 nmol/L and accounts for 44% of biotin plus catabolites; bisnorbiotin and biotin-*d,l*-sulfoxide account for 48% and 8%, respectively (Mock *et al.*, 1997b). By 6 weeks postpartum, the biotin concentration increases to approximately 30 nmol/L and accounts for about 70% of biotin plus catabolites; bisnorbiotin and biotin-*d,l*-sulfoxides account for about 20% and less than 10%, respectively.

Intake and Food Sources

The majority of biotin in meats and cereals appears to be protein bound (Zempleni and Mock, 1999b). Most studies of biotin content in foods have depended on using bioassays. Despite potential analytical limitations due to interfering endogenous compounds, protein binding, and lack of chemical specificity for biotin, there is reasonably good agreement among published reports. Biotin is widely distributed in natural foodstuffs. Foods relatively rich in biotin include egg yolk, liver, and some vegetables. The dietary biotin intake in Western populations is about 35–70 µg/day (143–287 nmol/day). Infants consuming 800 mL of mature breast milk per day ingest approximately 6 µg (24 nmol) of biotin (Mock *et al.*, 1997b). It remains unclear whether biotin synthesis by gut microorganisms contributes importantly to the total biotin absorbed (Zempleni and Mock, 1999b).

Excess and Toxicity

Empirically, ingestion of pharmacological doses of biotin has been considered safe. For example, lifelong treatment of biotinidase deficiency patients with biotin doses that exceed the normal dietary intake by 300 times does not produce frank signs of toxicity (Wolf and Heard, 1991). Likewise, no signs of biotin overdose were reported after acute oral and intravenous administration of doses that exceeded the dietary biotin intake by up to 600 times (Zempleni and Mock, 1999a). Note, however, that biotin supplementation is associated with alterations of gene expression in healthy adults and human cell culture models as described above (Rodriguez-Melendez and Zempleni, 2003). Some of these changes might have undesired effects in cell biology. For example, biotin supplementation decreases expression of the gene coding for sarco/endoplasmic reticulum ATPase 3 in human lymphoid cells; decreased expression of this calcium transporter is associated with impaired protein folding in the endoplasmic reticulum, causing cell stress (Griffin *et al.*, 2006).

Future Directions

In the foreseeable future, biotin research likely will focus on the following priority areas:

1. Decipher the complex role of histone biotinylation in gene regulation and genome stability.
2. Use transgenic animal models to characterize the roles of HCS, biotinidase, and biotin transporters in biotin homeostasis and histone biotinylation.
3. Determine whether marginal biotin deficiency causes birth defects in humans.
4. Quantify human biotin requirements and determine the true prevalence of biotin deficiency in vulnerable subgroups of the population.
5. Determine whether polymorphisms in genes coding for HCS, biotinidase, and biotin transporters affect biotin requirements.
6. Characterize the biological effects of marginal biotin deficiency.

Acknowledgments

A contribution of the University of Nebraska Agricultural Research Division, supported in part by funds provided through the Hatch Act. Additional support was provided by NIH grants DK063945, DK077816, DK082476, and ES015206, USDA CSREES grant 2006-35200-17138, and NSF grants MCB 0615831 and EPS 0701892.

Suggestions for Further Reading

Camporeale, G., Shubert, E.E., Sarath, G., *et al.* (2004) K8 and K12 are biotinylated in human histone H4. *Eur J Biochem* **271**, 2257–2263.

McCormick, D.B. and Wright, L.D. (1971) The metabolism of biotin and analogues. In Florkin, M. and Stotz, E.H. (eds), *Metabolism of Vitamins and Trace Elements*. Elsevier, Amsterdam, pp. 81–110.

Said, H.M. (2004) Recent advances in carrier-mediated intestinal absorption of water-soluble vitamins. *Annu. Rev Physiol* **66**, 419–446.

Suzuki, Y., Yang, X., Aoki, Y., *et al.* (2005) Mutations in the holocarboxylase synthetase gene HLCS. *Hum Mutat* **26**, 285–290.

References

Baez-Saldaña, A. and Ortega, E. (2004) Biotin deficiency blocks thymocyte maturation, accelerates thymus involution, and decreases nose–rump length in mice. *J Nutr* **134,** 1970–1977.

Báez-Saldaña, A., Díaz, G., Espinoza, B., *et al.* (1998) Biotin deficiency induces changes in subpopulations of spleen lymphocytes in mice. *Am J Clin Nutr* **67,** 431–437.

Bao, B., Pestinger, V., Hassan, Y.I., *et al.* (2010) Holocarboxylase synthetase is a chromatin protein and interacts directly with histone H3 to mediate biotinylation of K9 and K18. *J Nutr Biochem* **22,** 470–475.

Baumgartner, M.R., Dantas, M.F., Suormala, T., *et al.* (2004) Isolated 3-methylcrotonyl-CoA carboxylase deficiency: evidence for an allele-specific dominant negative effect and responsiveness to biotin therapy. *Am J Hum Genet* **75,** 790–800.

Boas, M.A. (1927) The effect of desiccation upon the nutritive properties of egg-white. *Biochem J* **21,** 712–724.

Bowman, B.B., Selhub, J., and Rosenberg, I.H. (1986) Intestinal absorption of biotin in the rat. *J Nutr* **116,** 1266–1271.

Camporeale, G., Giordano, E., Rendina, R., *et al.* (2006) *Drosophila* holocarboxylase synthetase is a chromosomal protein required for normal histone biotinylation, gene transcription patterns, lifespan and heat tolerance. *J Nutr* **136,** 2735–2742.

Camporeale, G., Shubert, E.E., Sarath, G., *et al.* (2004) K8 and K12 are biotinylated in human histone H4. *Eur J Biochem* **271,** 2257–2263.

Chatterjee, N.S., Rubin, S.A., and Said, H.M. (2001) Molecular characterization of the 5′ regulatory region of rat sodium-dependent multivitamin transporter gene. *Am J Physiol Cell Physiol* **280,** C548–C555.

Chauhan, J. and Dakshinamurti, K. (1988) Role of human serum biotinidase as biotin-binding protein. *Biochem J* **256,** 265–270.

Chew, Y.C., Camporeale, G., Kothapalli, N., *et al.* (2006) Lysine residues in N- and C-terminal regions of human histone H2A are targets for biotinylation by biotinidase. *J Nutr Biochem* **17,** 225–233.

Chew, Y.C., West, J.T., Kratzer, S.J., *et al.* (2008) Biotinylation of histones represses transposable elements in human and mouse cells and cell lines, and in *Drosophila melanogaster*. *J Nutr* **138,** 2316–2322.

Collins, J.C., Paietta, E., Green, R., *et al.* (1988) Biotin-dependent expression of the asialoglycoprotein receptor in HepG2. *J Biol Chem* **263,** 11280–11283.

Cowan, M.J., Wara, D.W., Packman, S., *et al.* (1979) Multiple biotin-dependent carboxylase deficiencies associated with defects in T-cell and B-cell immunity. *Lancet* **2,** 115–118.

Daberkow, R.L., White, B.R., Cederberg, R.A., *et al.* (2003) Monocarboxylate transporter 1 mediates biotin uptake in human peripheral blood mononuclear cells. *J Nutr* **133,** 2703–2706.

Dakshinamurti, K. and Chauhan, J. (1994) Biotin-binding proteins. In K. Dakshinamurti (ed.), *Vitamin Receptors: Vitamins as Ligands in Cell Communication.* Cambridge University Press, Cambridge, pp. 200–249.

Dakshinamurti, K. and Cheah-Tan, C. (1968) Liver glucokinase of the biotin deficient rat. *Can J Biochem* **46,** 75–80.

Desviat, L.R., Perez-Cerda, C., Perez, B., *et al.* (2003) Functional analysis of MCCA and MCCB mutations causing methylcrotonylglycinuria. *Mol Genet Metab* **80,** 315–320.

Dey, S., Subramanian, V.S., Chatterjee, N.S., *et al.* (2002) Characterization of the 5′ regulatory region of the human sodium-dependent multivitamin transporter, hSMVT. *Biochim Biophys Acta* **1574,** 187–192.

Du Vigneaud, V., Melville, D.B., Folkers, K., *et al.* (1942) The structure of biotin: a study of desthiobiotin. *J Biol Chem* **146,** 475–485.

Eisenberg, M.A., Mee, M., Prakash, O., *et al.* (1975) Properties of alpha-dehydrobiotin-resistant mutants of Escherichia coli K-12. *J Bacteriol* **122,** 66–72.

Flint, D.H. and Allen, R.M. (1997) Purification and characterization of biotin synthases. In D.M. McCormick, J.W. Suttie, and C. Wagner, (eds), *Vitamins and Coenzymes, Part 1.* Academic Press, San Diego, pp. 349–356.

Gralla, M., Camporeale, G., and Zempleni, J. (2008) Holocarboxylase synthetase regulates expression of biotin transporters by chromatin remodeling events at the SMVT locus. *J Nutr Biochem* **19,** 400–408.

Green, N.M. (1975) Avidin. *Adv Protein Chem* **29,** 85–133.

Griffin, J.B., Rodriguez-Melendez, R., Dode, L., *et al.* (2006) Biotin supplementation decreases the expression of the *SERCA3* gene (*ATP2A3*) in Jurkat cells, thus, triggering unfolded protein response. *J Nutr Biochem* **17,** 272–281.

Harris, S.A., Wolf, D.E., Mozingo, R., *et al.* (1943) Synthetic biotin. *Science* **97,** 447–448.

Hassan, Y.I., Moriyama, H., Olsen, L.J., *et al.* (2009) N- and C-terminal domains in human holocarboxylase synthetase participate in substrate recognition. *Mol Genet Metab* **96,** 183–188.

Hatakeyama, K., Kobayashi, M., and Yukawa, H. (1997) Analysis of biotin biosynthesis pathway in coryneform bacteria: *Brevibacterium flavum*. In D.B. McCormick, J.W. Suttie, and C. Wagner (eds), *Vitamins and Coenzymes, Part I.* Academic Press, San Diego, pp. 349–356 .

Hymes, J., Fleischhauer, K., and Wolf, B. (1995) Biotinylation of histones by human serum biotinidase: assessment of biotinyltransferase activity in sera from normal individuals and children with biotinidase deficiency. *Biochem Mol Med* **56**, 76–83.

Institute of Medicine (1998) *Dietary Reference Intakes for Thiamin, Riboflavin, Niacin, Vitamin B6, Folate, Vitamin B12, Pantothenic Acid, Biotin, and Choline*. National Academies Press, Washington, DC.

Kaur Mall, G., Chew, Y.C., and Zempleni, J. (2010) Biotin requirements are lower in human Jurkat lymphoid cells but homeostatic mechanisms are similar to those of HepG2 liver cells. *J Nutr* **140**, 1086–1092.

Kim, K.-H., McCormick, D.B., Bier, D.M., *et al.* (1997) Regulation of mammalian acetyl-coenzyme A carboxylase. *Ann Rev Nutr* **17**, 77–99.

Knowles, J.R. (1989) The mechanism of biotin-dependent enzymes. *Ann Rev Biochem* **58**, 195–221.

Kobza, K.A., Chaiseeda, K., Sarath, G., *et al.* (2008) Biotinylmethyl 4-(amidomethyl) benzoate is a competitive inhibitor of human biotinidase. *J Nutr Biochem* **19**, 826–832.

Kögl, F. and Tönnis, B. (1932) Über das Bios-Problem. Darstellung von krystallisiertem Biotin aus Eigelb. *Z Physiol Chem* **242**, 43–73.

Kouzarides, T. and Berger, S.L. (2007) Chromatin modifications and their mechanism of action. In C.D. Allis, T. Jenuwein, and D. Reinberg (eds), *Epigenetics*. Cold Spring Harbor Press, Cold Spring Harbor, pp. 191–209.

Kumar, M. and Axelrod, A.E. (1978) Cellular antibody synthesis in thiamin, riboflavin, biotin and folic acid-deficient rats. *Proc Soc Exp Biol Med* **157**, 421–423.

Kuroishi, T., Endo, Y., Muramoto, K., *et al.* (2008) Biotin deficiency up-regulates TNF-alpha production in murine macrophages. *J Leukoc Biol* **83**, 912–920.

Kuroishi, T., Kinbara, M., Sato, N., *et al.* (2009) Biotin status affects nickel allergy via regulation of interleukin-1beta production in mice. *J Nutr* **139**, 1031–1036.

Landenberger, A., Kabil, H., Harshman, L.G., *et al.* (2004) Biotin deficiency decreases life span and fertility but increases stress resistance in *Drosophila melanogaster*. *J Nutr Biochem* **15**, 591–600.

Lee, H.M., Wright, L.D., and McCormick, D.B. (1972) Metabolism of carbonyl-labeled [^{14}C] biotin in the rat. *J Nutr* **102**, 1453–1464.

Lee, Y.C., Joiner-Hayes, M.G., and McCormick, D.B. (1970) Microsomal oxidation of α-thiocarboxylic acids to sulfoxides. *Biochem Pharmacol* **19**, 2825–2832.

Mantagos, S., Malamitsi-Puchner, A., Antsaklis, A., *et al.* (1998) Biotin plasma levels of the human fetus. *Biol Neonate* **74**, 72–74.

Mardach, R., Zempleni, J., Wolf, B., *et al.* (2002) Biotin dependency due to a defect in biotin transport. *J Clin Invest* **109**, 1617–1623.

McCormick, D.B. and Wright, L.D. (1971) The metabolism of biotin and analogues. In M. Florkin and E.H. Stotz (eds), *Metabolism of Vitamins and Trace Elements*. Elsevier, Amsterdam, pp. 81–110.

Mock, D.M. (2005) Marginal biotin deficiency is teratogenic in mice and perhaps humans: a review of biotin deficiency during human pregnancy and effects of biotin deficiency on gene expression and enzyme activities in mouse dam and fetus. *J Nutr Biochem* **16**, 435–437.

Mock, D.M. and Malik, M.I. (1992) Distribution of biotin in human plasma: most of the biotin is not bound to protein. *Am J Clin Nutr* **56**, 427–432.

Mock, D.M. and Stadler, D.D. (1997) Conflicting indicators of biotin status from a cross-sectional study of normal pregnancy. *J Am Coll Nutr* **16**, 252–257.

Mock, D.M., Henrich, C.L., Carnell, N. *et al.* (2002a) Indicators of marginal biotin deficiency and repletion in humans: validation of 3-hydroxyisovaleric acid excretion and a leucine challenge. *Am J Clin Nutr* **76**, 1061–1068.

Mock, D.M., Henrich-Shell, C.L., Carnell, N., *et al.* (2004) 3-Hydroxypropionic acid and methylcitric acid are not reliable indicators of marginal biotin deficiency in humans. *J Nutr* **134**, 317–320.

Mock, D.M., Johnson, S.B. and Holman, R.T. (1988) Effects of biotin deficiency on serum fatty acid composition: evidence for abnormalities in humans. *J Nutr* **118**, 342–348.

Mock, N., Malik, M., Stumbo, P., *et al.* (1997d) Increased urinary excretion of 3-hydroxyisovaleric acid and decreased urinary excretion of biotin are sensitive early indicators of decreased status in experimental biotin deficiency. *Am J Clin Nutr* **65**, 951–958.

Mock, D.M., Quirk, J.G., and Mock, N.I. (2002b) Marginal biotin deficiency during normal pregnancy. *Am J Clin Nutr* **75**, 295–259.

Mock, D.M., Stadler, D., Stratton, S., *et al.* (1997a) Biotin status assessed longitudinally in pregnant women. *J Nutr* **127**, 710–716.

Mock, D.M., Stratton, S.L., and Mock, N.I. (1997b) Concentrations of biotin metabolites in human milk. *J Pediatr* **131**, 456–458.

Mock, D.M., Wang, K.-S., and Kearns, G.L. (1997c) The pig is an appropriate model for human biotin catabolism as judged by the urinary metabolite profile of radioisotope-labeled biotin. *J Nutr* **127**, 365–369.

Nabokina, S.M., Subramanian, V.S., and Said, H.M. (2003) Comparative analysis of ontogenic changes in renal and intestinal biotin transport in the rat. *Am J Physiol Renal Physiol* **284**, F737–742.

Narang, M.A., Dumas, R., Ayer, L.M., *et al.* (2004) Reduced histone biotinylation in multiple carboxylase deficiency patients: a nuclear role for holocarboxylase synthetase. *Hum Mol Genet* **13**, 15–23.

National Center for Biotechnology Information (2008) Entrez SNP. National Institutes for Health. http://www.ncbi.nlm.nih.gov (accessed November 23, 2008).

Neto, E.C., Schulte, J., Rubim, R., *et al.* (2004) Newborn screening for biotinidase deficiency in Brazil: biochemical and molecular characterizations. *Braz J Med Biol Res* **37**, 295–299.

Ozand, P.T., Gascon, G.G., Essa, M.A., *et al.* (1998) Biotin-responsive basal ganglia disease: a novel entity. *Brain* **121**, 1267–1279.

Pacheco-Alvarez, D., Solorzano-Vargas, R.S., Gravel, R.A., *et al.* (2005) Paradoxical regulation of biotin utilization in brain and liver and implications for inherited multiple carboxylase deficiencies. *J Biol Chem* **279**, 52312–52318.

Perez, B., Desviat, L.R., Rodriguez-Pombo, P., *et al.* (2003) Propionic acidemia: identification of twenty-four novel mutations in Europe and North America. *Mol Genet Metab* **78**, 59–67.

Pestinger, V., Wijeratne, S.S.K., Rodriguez-Melendez, R., *et al.* (2010) Novel histone biotinylation marks are enriched in repeat regions and participate in repression of transcriptionally competent genes. *J Nutr Biochem* **22**, 328–333.

Petrelli, F., Moretti, P., and Paparelli, M. (1979) Intracellular distribution of biotin-14C COOH in rat liver. *Mol Biol Rep* **4**, 247–252.

Prasad, P.D., Wang, H., Kekuda, R., *et al.* (1998) Cloning and functional expression of a cDNA encoding a mammalian sodium-dependent vitamin transporter mediating the uptake of pantothenate, biotin, and lipoate. *J Biol Chem* **273**, 7501–7506.

Robinson, B.H., Oei, J., Saudubray, J.M., *et al.* (1987) The French and North American phenotypes of pyruvate carboxylase deficiency, correlation with biotin-containing protein by ³H-biotin incorporation, ³⁵S-streptavidin labeling, and northern blotting with a cloned cDNA probe. *Am J Hum Genet* **40**, 50–59.

Rodriguez-Melendez, R. and Zempleni, J. (2003) Regulation of gene expression by biotin. *J Nutr Biochem* **14**, 680–690.

Rodriguez-Melendez, R., Schwab, L.D., and Zempleni, J. (2004) Jurkat cells respond to biotin deficiency with increased nuclear translocation of NF-?B, mediating cell survival. *Int J Vitam Nutr Res* **74**, 209–216.

Rolfe, B. and Eisenberg, M.A. (1968) Genetic and biochemical analysis of the biotin loci of Escherichia coli K-12. *J Bacteriol* **96**, 515–524.

Said, H.M. (2004) Recent advances in carrier-mediated intestinal absorption of water-soluble vitamins. *Annu. Rev Physiol* **66**, 419–446.

Said, H.M. and Redha, R. (1987) A carrier-mediated system for transport of biotin in rat intestine in vitro. *Am J Physiol* **252**, G52–G55.

Said, H.M., Redha, R., and Nylander, W. (1988) Biotin transport in basolateral membrane vesicles of human intestine. *Gastroenterology* **94**, 1157–1163.

Said, H.M., Thuy, L.P., Sweetman, L., *et al.* (1993) Transport of the biotin dietary derivative biocytin (N-Biotinyl-L-lysine) in rat small intestine. *Gastroenterology* **104**, 75–80.

Schenker, S., Hu, Z., Johnson, R.F., *et al.* (1993) Human placental biotin transport: normal characteristics and effect of ethanol. *Alcohol Clin Exp Res* **17**, 566–575.

Sealey, W.M., Stratton, S.L., Mock, D.M., *et al.* (2005) Marginal maternal biotin deficiency in CD-1 mice reduces fetal mass of biotin-dependent carboxylases. *J Nutr* **135**, 973–977.

Sealey, W.M., Teague, A.M., Stratton, S.L., *et al.* (2004) Smoking accelerates biotin catabolism in women. *Am J Clin Nutr* **80**, 932–935.

Seshagiri, P.B. and Adiga, P.R. (1987) Isolation and characterisation of a biotin-binding protein from the pregnant-rat serum and comparison with that from the chicken egg-yolk. *Biochim Biophys Acta* **916**, 474–481.

Shriver, B.J., Roman-Shriver, C., and Allred, J.B. (1993) Depletion and repletion of biotinyl enzymes in liver of biotin-deficient rats: evidence of a biotin storage system. *J Nutr* **123**, 1140–1149.

Smith, E.M., Hoi, J.T., Eissenberg, J.C., *et al.* (2007) Feeding *Drosophila* a biotin-deficient diet for multiple generations increases stress resistance and lifespan and alters gene expression and histone biotinylation patterns. *J Nutr* **137**, 2006–2012.

Solorzano-Vargas, R.S., Pacheco-Alvarez, D., and Leon-Del Rio, A. (2002) Holocarboxylase synthetase is an obligate participant in biotin-mediated regulation of its own expression and of biotin-dependent carboxylases mRNA levels in human cells. *Proc Natl Acad Sci USA* **99**, 5325–5330.

Spencer, R.P. and Brody, K.R. (1964) Biotin transport by small intestine of rat, hamster, and other species. *Am J Physiol* **206**, 653–657.

Stanley, J.S., Griffin, J.B., Mock, D.M., *et al.* (2002) Biotin uptake into human peripheral blood mononuclear cells increases early in the cell cycle, increasing carboxylase activities. *J Nutr* **132**, 1854–1859.

Stanley, J.S., Griffin, J.B., and Zempleni, J. (2001) Biotinylation of histones in human cells: effects of cell proliferation. *Eur J Biochem* **268**, 5424–5429.

Stratton, S.L., Bogusiewicz, A., Mock, M.M., *et al.* (2006) Lymphocyte propionyl-CoA carboxylase and its activation by biotin are sensitive indicators of marginal biotin deficiency in humans. *Am J Clin Nutr* **84**, 384–388.

Stratton, S.L., Horvath, T.D., and Bogusiewicz, A. (2010) Plasma concentration of 3-hydroxyisovaleryl carnitine is an early and sensitive indicator of marginal biotin deficiency in humans. *Am J Clin Nutr* **92**, 1399–1405.

Subramanian, V.S., Marchant, J.S., and Said, H.M. (2006) Biotin-responsive basal ganglia disease-linked mutations inhibit thiamine transport via hTHTR2: biotin is not a substrate for hTHTR2. *Am J Physiol Cell Physiol* **291**, C851–C859.

Suormala, T., Baumgartner, E.R., Bausch, J., *et al.* (1988) Quantitative determination of biocytin in urine of patients with biotinidase deficiency using high-performance liquid chromatography (HPLC). *Clin Chim Acta* **177**, 253–270.

Suzuki, Y., Aoki, Y., Ishida, Y., *et al.* (1994) Isolation and characterization of mutations in the human holocarboxylase synthetase cDNA. *Nat Genet* **8**, 122–128.

Suzuki, Y., Yang, X., Aoki, Y., *et al.* (2005) Mutations in the holocarboxylase synthetase gene HLCS. *Hum Mutat* **26**, 285–290.

Velazquez, A., Zamudio, S., Baez, A., *et al.* (1990) Indicators of biotin status: a study of patients on prolonged total parenteral nutrition. *Eur J Clin Nutr* **44**, 11–16.

Wolf, B. and Feldman, G.L. (1982) The biotin-dependent carboxylase deficiencies. *Am J Hum Genet* **34**, 699–716.

Wolf, B. and Heard, G.S. (1991) Biotinidase deficiency. In L. Barness and F. Oski (eds), *Advances in Pediatrics*. Medical Book Publishers, Chicago, pp. 1–21.

Wolf, B., Grier, R.E., Allen, R.J., *et al.* (1983) Biotinidase deficiency: an enzymatic defect in late-onset multiple carboxylase deficiency. *Clin Chim Acta* **131**, 273–281.

Wolf, B., Heard, G.S., McVoy, J.R.S., *et al.* (1985) Biotinidase deficiency. *Ann NY Acad Sci* **447**, 252–262.

Wolffe, A. (1998) *Chromatin*. Academic Press, San Diego.

Zempleni, J. and Mock, D.M. (1999a) Bioavailability of biotin given orally to humans in pharmacologic doses. *Am J Clin Nutr* **69**, 504–508.

Zempleni, J. and Mock, D.M. (1999b) Biotin biochemistry and human requirements. *J Nutr Biochem* **10**, 128–138.

Zempleni, J. and Mock, D.M. (1999c) The efflux of biotin from human peripheral blood mononuclear cells. *J Nutr Biochem* **10**, 105–109.

Zempleni, J. and Mock, D.M. (1999d) Mitogen-induced proliferation increases biotin uptake into human peripheral blood mononuclear cells. *Am J Physiol Cell Physiol* **276**, C1079–1084.

Zempleni, J. and Mock, D.M. (2000a) Biotin. In W.O. Song and G.R. Beecher (eds), *Modern Analytical Methodologies on Fat and Water-Soluble Vitamins*. Wiley, New York, pp. 389–409.

Zempleni, J. and Mock, D.M. (2000b) Marginal biotin deficiency is teratogenic. *Proc Soc Exp Biol Med* **223**, 14–21.

Zempleni, J., Green, G.M., Spannagel, A.U., *et al.* (1997a) Biliary excretion of biotin and biotin metabolites is quantitatively minor in rats and pigs. *J Nutr* **127**, 1496–1500.

Zempleni, J., McCormick, D.B., and Mock, D.M. (1997b) Identification of biotin sulfone, bisnorbiotin methyl ketone, and tetranorbiotin-*l*-sulfoxide in human urine. *Am J Clin Nutr* **65**, 508–511.

Zempleni, J., Trusty, T.A., and Mock, D.M. (1997c) Lipoic acid reduces the activities of biotin-dependent carboxylases in rat liver. *J Nutr* **127**, 1776–1781.

Zempleni, J., Wijeratne, S.S., and Hassan, Y.I. (2009) Biotin. *Biofactors* **35**, 36–46.

24

PANTOTHENIC ACID

JOSHUA W. MILLER[1], PhD AND ROBERT B. RUCKER[2], PhD

[1]University of California Davis Medical Center, Sacramento, California, USA
[2]University of California, Davis, California, USA

Summary

Identified almost 60 years ago, pantothenic acid is an essential vitamin, which serves as the metabolic precursor for coenzyme A. In the form of coenzyme A and as a component of acyl carrier protein, pantothenic acid is a participant in a myriad of metabolic reactions involving lipids, proteins, and carbohydrates. Though essential, pantothenic acid deficiency in humans is rare owing to its ubiquitous distribution in foods of both animal and plant origin. Pantothenic acid supplementation may have some efficacy, but further investigation into various health claims is necessary before any specific recommendations can be given.

Introduction

The discovery of pantothenic acid followed the same path that led to the discovery of other water-soluble vitamins, i.e. studies utilizing bacteria and single-cell eukaryotic organisms (e.g. yeast), animal models, and thoughtful chemical analysis. It was largely the efforts of research groups associated with R.J. Williams, C.A. Elvehjem, and T.H. Jukes that resulted in the identification of pantothenic acid as an essential dietary factor. Williams *et al.* (1933) established that pantothenic acid was required for the growth of certain bacteria and yeast. Next, Elvehjem and associates (Wooley *et al.*, 1939) and Jukes and associates (Jukes *et al.*, 1939; Spies *et al.*, 1940) demonstrated that

pantothenic acid was a growth and "anti-dermatitis" factor for chickens. Williams coined the name pantothenic acid from the Greek meaning "from everywhere" to indicate its widespread occurrence in foodstuffs (Williams *et al.*, 1933; Williams and Majors, 1940). The eventual characterization of pantothenic acid by Williams took advantage of observations that the anti-dermatitis factor present in acid extracts of various food sources, i.e. pantothenic acid, did not bind to fuller's earth under acidic conditions. Using chromatographic and fractionation procedures that were typical of the 1930s (solvent-dependent chemical partitioning), Williams isolated several grams of pantothenic acid for structural determination from 250 kg of liver as starting material (Williams and Majors, 1940). With this

Present Knowledge in Nutrition, Tenth Edition. Edited by John W. Erdman Jr, Ian A. Macdonald and Steven H. Zeisel.

information, a number of research groups contributed to the chemical synthesis and commercial preparation of pantothenic acid.

In the 1950s, one of the functional forms of pantothenic acid, coenzyme A, was discovered as the cofactor essential for the acetylation of sulfonamides and choline (Plesofsky-Vig and Brambi, 1988). In the mid-1960s, pantothenic acid was next identified as a component of acyl carrier protein (ACP) in the fatty acid synthesis complex (Wakil, 1989). These developments, in addition to a steady series of observations throughout this period on the effects of pantothenic acid deficiency in humans and other animals, provide the foundation for our current understanding of this vitamin.

Chemistry and Nomenclature

The chemical structure of pantothenic acid consists of pantoic acid and β-alanine bound in amide linkage (Figure 24.1A). Metabolic processing of pantothenic acid, described in detail below, produces the important intermediate, 4'-phosphopantetheine (Figure 24.1B), which includes β-mercaptoethylamine (cysteamine) bound in amide linkage to the terminal carboxyl group of the molecule. 4'-Phosphopantetheine serves as a covalently linked prosthetic group for ACP (Figure 24.1C). Further metabolic processing with the addition of adenine and ribose 3'-phosphate produces the essential cofactor, coenzyme A (CoA) (Figure 24.1D).

Pure pantothenic acid is a water-soluble, viscous, yellow oil. It is stable at neutral pH, but is readily destroyed by acid, alkali, and heat. Calcium pantothenate, a white, odorless, crystalline substance, is the form of pantothenic acid usually found in commercial vitamin supplements because it has greater stability than the pure acid (Bird and Thompson, 1967). Early literature referred to pantothenic acid as chick anti-dermatitis factor, filtrate factor, and vitamin B3. Today, it is often referred to as vitamin B5, though the origin of this designation is obscure.

Intestinal Absorption, Cellular Uptake and Efflux, Plasma Transport, and Excretion

The vast majority of pantothenic acid in food is present as a component of CoA or 4'-phosphopantetheine. In order to be absorbed, these substances must first be hydrolyzed (Shibata et al., 1983). This occurs in the intestinal lumen by the sequential activity of two hydrolases, pyrophosphatase and phosphatase, with pantetheine as the product. Pantetheine is either absorbed as is, or further metabolized to pantothenic acid by a third intestinal hydrolase, pantetheinase. In rats, pantothenic acid absorption was initially found to occur in all sections of the small intestine by simple diffusion (Shibata et al., 1983). However, subsequent work in rats and chicks indicated that at low concentrations the vitamin is absorbed by a saturable, sodium-dependent transport mechanism (Fenstermacher and Rose, 1986), sometimes referred to as the sodium-dependent multivitamin transporter (SMVT), which is shared with biotin (Said, 1999). In vitro experiments utilizing Caco-2 cell monolayers as a model of intestinal absorption established that pantothenic acid uptake is inhibited competitively by biotin, and vice versa (Said, 1999).

After absorption, pantothenic acid enters the circulation from which it is taken up by cells in a manner similar to that of intestinal absorption (Spector and Mock, 1987; Beinlich et al., 1990; Grassl, 1992). The process for pantothenic acid cellular uptake appears saturable with an apparent K_m of 15–20 μM. Transport across cell membranes occurs by carrier-mediated, sodium gradient-dependent and electroneutral mechanisms (Smith and Milner, 1985; Lopaschukf et al., 1987; Beinlich et al., 1989, 1990; Said et al., 1998). Pantothenic acid cellular uptake has also been linked to protein kinase C (PKC) and calmodulin-dependent regulatory and signaling pathways (Lopaschukf et al., 1987). The dependence on PKC is based on observations that pretreatment of cells with a PKC activator, such as phorbol 12-myristate 13-acetate (PMA) or 1,2-dioctanoyl-glycerol, significantly inhibits pantothenic acid uptake. If an inward sodium gradient is imposed, a rapid uptake of pantothenic acid is observed. Uptake of pantothenic acid is reduced when sodium is replaced by potassium or if external sodium is reduced below 40 mM. Ouabain, gramicidin D, cyanide, azide, and 2,4-dinitrophenol also act as inhibitors.

With regard to cellular efflux, unlike uptake, the export of pantothenic acid is unaffected by the addition of pantothenic acid, sodium, ouabain, gramicidin D, or 2,4-dinitrophenol to the external medium. Moreover, the metabolic state also has an impact on uptake. For example, in the perfused heart, pantothenic acid transport is significantly increased when hearts are perfused and are acting as "working" hearts because of addition of a fuel source (Lopaschukf et al., 1987). That active uptake of pan-

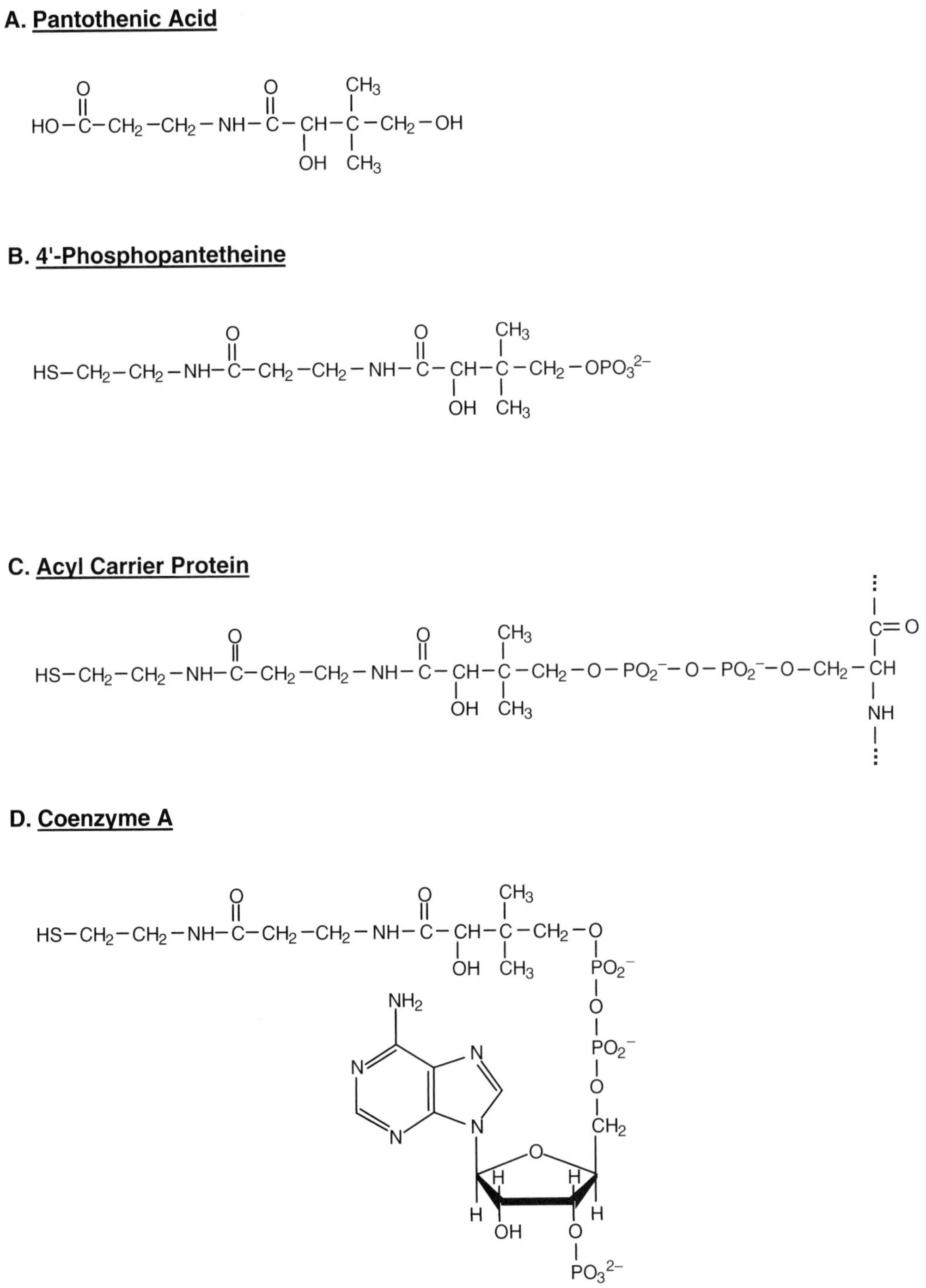

A. Pantothenic Acid

B. 4'-Phosphopantetheine

C. Acyl Carrier Protein

D. Coenzyme A

FIG. 24.1 Chemical structures of pantothenic acid, 4'-phosphopantetheine, acyl carrier protein, and coenzyme A.

tothenic acid is important is underscored by the differences in cellular versus plasma concentrations of free pantothenic acid. The cellular concentration of free pantothenic acid in the liver is 10–15 μM and in the heart ~100 μM compared with 1–5 μM observed in plasma. Similarly, the unidirectional influx of pantothenic acid across cerebral capillaries (the blood–brain barrier) occurs by a low-capacity, saturable transport system with a half-saturation concentration approximately 10 times the plasma pantothenic acid concentration (Spector, 1986, 1987). For comparison, the concentrations of CoA and ACP are 50–100 μM and 10 μM, respectively, in the cytosol of typical cells. In mitochondria, the CoA concentration can be as much as 10- to 20-fold higher, i.e. 70–90% of the total cellular CoA content.

The vitamin is excreted in the urine primarily as pantothenic acid. This occurs after its release from CoA by a series of hydrolysis reactions that cleave off the phosphate and β-mercaptoethylamine moieties.

Cellular Regulation and Functions

CoA and ACP Synthesis

Pantothenic acid is nutritionally essential due to the inability of animal cells to synthesize the pantoic acid moiety of the vitamin. The primary function of pantothenic acid is to serve as substrate for the synthesis of CoA and ACP (Figure 24.2). The first step is phosphorylation of pantothenic acid to 4'-phosphopantothenic acid by pantothenic acid kinase (Fisher *et al.*, 1985; Rock *et al.*, 2000). Three distinct types of pantothenic acid kinase (PanK) have been identified. PanK-I and III are found in bacteria. PanK-II is mainly found in eukaryotes and occurs in four different isoforms (PanK1, PanK2, PanK3, and PanK4) (Leonardi *et al.*, 2005). Pantothenic acid kinase possesses a broad pH optimum (between pH 6 and 9) with a K_m for pantothenic acid of ~20 μM. Mg-ATP is used as the nucleotide substrate for this phosphorylation reaction with a K_m of ~0.6 mM.

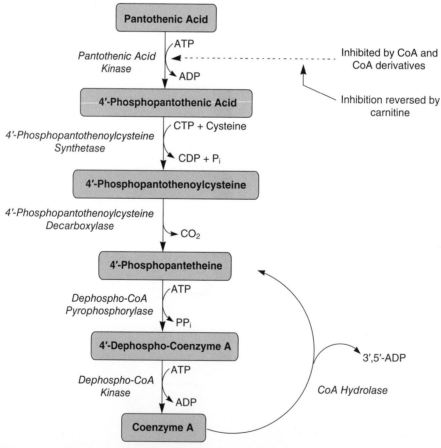

FIG. 24.2 Metabolic conversion of pantothenic acid to coenzyme A.

The pantothenic acid kinase reaction also serves as the primary control point in the synthesis of CoA and ACP. The reaction is activated and inhibited non-specifically by various anions (e.g. thiazolidinediones, sulfonylureas, and steroids are inhibitors and fatty acyl-amides and tamoxifen are activators) (Leonardi *et al.*, 2010). In cells, feedback inhibition of the kinase by CoA or CoA derivatives governs flux through the subsequent steps in the CoA synthesis pathway and defines the upper threshold for intracellular CoA cofactor levels. Inhibition by acetyl-CoA is greater than that of free CoA. The inhibition by free CoA is uncompetitive with respect to pantothenate concentration, with a K_i for inhibition of 0.2 μM. Substrates are added to pantothenic acid kinase sequentially with ATP as the leading substrate. The allosteric regulatory domain responsible for acetyl-CoA inhibition also binds the substrates, pantothenate and pantetheine, and the various small molecule inhibitors and activators that can influence pantothenic acid kinase activity. Thus, descriptive features of mechanisms involving pantothenic acid kinase at the substrate level are often complex.

Of interest, L-carnitine, important for the transport of fatty acids into mitochondria, is a non-essential activator of pantothenic acid kinase. Carnitine has no effect by itself, but specifically reverses the inhibition by CoA. In heart, the free carnitine content varies directly with the phosphorylation of pantothenic acid. Thus, these properties of the kinase provide a potential mechanism for the control of CoA synthesis and regulation of cellular pantothenic acid content, i.e. feedback inhibition by CoA and its acyl esters that is reversed by changes in the concentration of free carnitine. However, it is important to underscore that the free concentration of acyl CoA in cells is low and variable because the bulk of acyl derivatives are protein bound. Moreover, similar to CoA, carnitine exists in both free and acylated forms, and reversal of kinase inhibition by CoA does not occur when carnitine is acylated (Fisher *et al.*, 1985). The ratio of free to acylated carnitine varies considerably depending on feeding and hormonal influences, with insulin particularly important. Fasting and type 1 diabetes (states of low insulin) increase pantothenic acid kinase activity and the total content of CoA (Reibel *et al.*, 1981; Robishaw *et al.*, 1982; Kirschbaum *et al.*, 1990). In addition, perfusion of heart preparations or incubation of liver cells with glucose, pyruvate or palmitate markedly inhibits pantothenic acid phosphorylation, due to reduction in free carnitine and increases in the free and acylated forms of CoA.

Following 4′-phosphopantothenic acid formation, the subsequent steps in CoA synthesis are carried out on a protein complex (~400 000 Da) with multifunctional catalytic sites. Important enzymatic features of this complex include dephospho-CoA-pyrophosphorylase activity, which catalyzes the reaction between 4′-phosphopantetheine and ATP to form 4′-dephospho-CoA; dephospho-CoA-kinase activity, which catalyzes the ATP-dependent final step in CoA synthesis; and coenzyme A hydrolase activity, which catalyzes the hydrolysis of CoA to 3′,5′-ADP and 4′-phosphopantetheine. This sequence of reactions is referred to as the CoA/4′-phosphopantetheine cycle and provides a mechanism by which the 4′-phosphopantetheine can be recycled to form CoA. Each turn of the cycle utilizes two molecules of ATP and produces one molecule of ADP, one molecule of pyrophosphate, and one molecule of 3′,5′-ADP (Figure 24.2) (Bucovaz *et al.*, 1998).

ACP is sometimes referred to as a "macro-cofactor," because, in bacteria, yeast and plants, it is composed of a polypeptide chain (MW ~8500–8700 Da) to which 4′-phosphopantetheine is attached. However, in higher animals, ACP is most often associated with a fatty acid synthase complex that is composed of two very large protein subunits (MW ~250 000 Da each). The carrier segment or domain of the fatty acid synthetic complex is also called acyl carrier protein, i.e. one of seven functional or catalytic domains on each of the two subunits that comprise fatty acid synthase. The inactive ACP apopolypeptide (or domain) is converted to an active holoform (or domain) by the post-translational transfer of a 4′-phosphopantetheinyl moiety to the side-chain hydroxyl of a serine residue at the active center of ACP. The reaction is catalyzed by 4′-phosphopantetheinyl transferase, which uses CoA as the 4′-phosphopantetheine substrate. Although there are few data related to the regulation of holoACP peptide or domain formation, the 4′-phosphopantetheine transferase gene has been cloned from a human source (Praphanphoj *et al.*, 2001). Although data are limited on phosphopantetheine transferase and ACP regulation in animals, in plants the addition of exogenous CoA to intact chloroplasts stimulates the conversion of apoACP to holoACP. It should also be appreciated that, in addition to fatty acid synthesis, phosphopantetheine transferase catalyzes the transfer of 4′-phosphopantetheine from CoA to other proteins. For example, it has been shown that in human cell lines one of the enzymes of folate metabolism, 10-formyltetrahydrofolate dehydrogenase (FDH), requires

TABLE 24.1   Selected functions of CoA and ACP

Function	Importance
Carbohydrate-related	
Citric acid cycle transfer reactions	Oxidative metabolism
Acetylation of sugars (e.g. N-acetylglucosamine)	Production of carbohydrates important to cell structure
Lipid-related	
Phospholipid biosynthesis	Cell membrane formation and structure
Isoprenoid biosynthesis	Cholesterol and bile salt production
Steroid biosynthesis	Steroid hormone production
Fatty acid elongation	Ability to modify cell membrane fluidity
Acyl (fatty acid) and triacyl glyceride synthesis	Energy storage
Protein-related	
Protein acetylation	Altered protein conformation; activation of certain hormones and enzymes, e.g. adrenocorticotropin; transcription, e.g. acetylation of histone
Protein acylation (myristic and palmitic acid additions) and prenylation	Compartmentalization and activation of hormones and transcription factors

a 4′-phosphopantetheine prosthetic group to aid the conversion of 10-formyltetrahydrofolate to tetrahydrofolate and CO_2 (Strickland *et al.*, 2010).

As an additional point, various agonists of fatty acid catabolism can affect CoASH-related metabolism. Peroxisome proliferator-activated receptors, such as PPARα, when activated are often related to an increase in fatty acid β-oxidation. Targets of PPARα also influence PanK and genes encoding proteins involved in the transport and synthesis of acylcarnitines. Using state-of-the-art metabolomic approaches (e.g. high-resolution NMR and mass spectrometry technology), it has been shown in humans that significant depletion of both pantothenic acid (as much as five-fold) and acetylcarnitine (as much as 20-fold) occurs in response to PPAR agonists, such as fenofibrate, based on analysis of urinary metabolites (Patterson *et al.*, 2009). As a transcriptional regulator, PPARα includes pantothenate kinase and genes encoding proteins involved in the transport and synthesis of acylcarnitines.

Selected Functions of CoA and ACP

Important functions of CoA and ACP are listed in Table 24.1. Principally, CoA is involved in acetyl and acyl transfer reactions and processes related to oxidative metabolism and catabolism, whereas ACP is involved primarily in synthetic reactions. The adenosyl moiety of CoA provides a site for tight binding to CoA-requiring enzymes, while allowing the phosphopantetheine portion to serve as a flexible arm to move substrates from one catalytic center to another. Similarly, when pantothenic acid (as 4′-phosphopantetheine) in ACP is used in the transfer reactions associated with the fatty acid synthase process, 4′-phosphopantetheine also functions as a flexible arm that allows for an orderly and systematic presentation of acyl derivatives to each of the active centers of the fatty acid synthase complex. A summary of catalytic sites and their functions in the fatty acid synthase complex is presented in Table 24.2. In addition to fatty acid synthesis, hints that ACP-like factors may perform other functions in humans and animals come from observations that an oligosaccharide-linked acyl carrier protein acts as a transmethylation inhibitor in porcine liver (Seo *et al.*, 2002). ACP is also structurally homologous to acidic ribosomal structural proteins, e.g. ribosomal protein P2 (Raychaudhuri and Rajasekharan, 2003). Moreover, in bacteria and plants, ACP is important in a number of pathways, such as amino acid synthesis and formation of polyketides, a remarkably diverse group of secondary metabolites that include antibiotics, such as erythromycin, cholesterol-lowering drugs, such as lovastatin, and putative anti-aging compounds, such as resveratrol (Khosla and Tang, 2005).

It is also important to appreciate that intermediates arising from the transfer reactions catalyzed by CoA and 4′-phosphopantetheine in ACP may be viewed as "high energy" compounds. CoA or ACP reacts with acetyl or acyl

TABLE 24.2 Catalytic sites associated with the fatty acid synthase complex

Enzyme	Catalytic function
1. Acetyl transferase	Catalyzes the transfer of an activated acetyl group on CoA to the sulfhydryl group of 4′-phosphopantetheine (ACP domain). In a subsequent step, the acetyl group is transferred to a second cysteine-derived sulfhydryl group near the active site of 3-oxoacyl synthase (see step 3) leaving the 4′-phosphopantetheine sulfhydryl group free for step 2
2. Malonyl transferase	Catalyzes the transfer of successive incoming malonyl groups to 4′-phosphopantetheine
3. 3-Oxoacyl synthetase	The first condensation reaction in the process, catalyzed by 3-oxoacyl synthase, in which attack on malonyl-ACP by the acetyl moiety (transferred in step 1) occurs with decarboxylation and condensation to yield a 3-oxobutyryl (acetoacetyl) derivative. In the second through the seventh cycles, it is the newly formed acyl moieties that attack the malonyl group added at each cycle (see step 6)
4. Oxoacyl reductase	Reductions of acetoacetyl or 3-oxoacyl intermediates involve NADPH. The first cycle of this reaction generates D-hydroxybutyrate, and in subsequent cycles, hydroxy fatty acids
5. 3-Hydroxyacyl dehydratase	Catalyzes the removal of a molecule of water from the 3-hydroxyacyl derivatives produced in step 4 to form enoyl derivatives
6. Enoyl reductase	Reduction of the enoyl derivatives (step 5) by a second molecule of NADPH generates a fatty acid. This acyl group is also transferred to the sulfhydryl group adjacent to 3-oxoacyl synthase, as described in step 1, until a 16-carbon palmitoyl group is formed. This group, still attached to the 4′-phosphopantetheine arm, is the highly specific substrate for the remaining enzyme of the complex, thioester hydrolase
7. Thioester hydrolase	Liberates palmitic acid (step 6) from the 4′-phosphopantetheine arm

groups to form thioesters. Thioesters (–S–CO–R) are thermodynamically less stable than typical esters (–O–CO–R) or amides (–N–CO–R). The double-bond character of the C–O bond in –S–CO–R does not extend significantly into the C–S bond. This causes thioesters to have relatively high energy potential, and for most reactions involving CoA or ACP no additional energy, e.g. from ATP hydrolysis, is required for transfer of the acetyl or acyl group. For example, consider that, at pH 7.0, the -ΔG of hydrolysis is ~7.5 kcal for acetyl-CoA and 10.5 kcal for acetoacetyl-CoA compared with 7–8 kcal for the hydrolysis of ATP to AMP and pyrophosphate or ADP and phosphate. The terminal thiol group of CoA and ACP is also ideally suited for nucleophilic substitution reactions involving activated carboxylic acids and α- and β-carbonyl functions (Nicholis and Ferguson, 2002).

Dietary Sources and Requirements

Pantothenic acid is found in a wide variety of foods of both plant and animal origin at levels in the range 20–50 μg/g. Particularly rich sources of pantothenic acid

include chicken, beef, liver and other organ meats, whole grains, potatoes, and tomato products (Walsh *et al.*, 1981). Royal bee jelly and ovaries of tuna and cod also have high levels of the vitamin (Robinson, 1966). Because of its thermal lability and susceptibility to oxidation, significant amounts of pantothenic acid are lost from highly processed foods, including refined grains and cooked or canned meats and vegetables. Processing and refining whole grains results in a 37–47% loss of pantothenic acid, while canning of meats, fish, and dairy products leads to losses of 20–35% (Schroeder, 1971). Greater losses of the vitamin occur during canning (46–78%) and freezing (37–57%) of vegetables. Pantothenic acid is also synthesized by intestinal microorganisms (Stein and Diamond, 1989), though the amount produced and the availability of the vitamin from this source is unknown.

The primary source of pantothenic acid in food is CoA. Intestinal phosphatases and nucleosidases are capable of very efficient hydrolysis of CoA so that near quantitative release of pantothenic acid occurs as a normal part of digestion. Further, the overall K_m for pantothenic acid intestinal uptake is 10–20 μM. At an intake of ~10–15 mg

TABLE 24.3   Adequate intakes (AIs) for pantothenic acid

Age group	AI (mg/day)
Infants	
0–5 months	1.7
6–12 months	1.8
Children	
1–3 years	2.0
4–8 years	3.0
9–13 years	4.0
Adolescents	
14–18 years	5.0
Adults	
19–50 years	5.0
>50 years	5.0
Pregnancy	6.0
Lactation	7.0

Data from Institute of Medicine, 1988.

of CoA, the amount of CoA in a typical meal, the pantothenic acid concentration in luminal fluid would be $\sim$1–2μM. At this concentration, pantothenic acid would not saturate the transport system, and as a consequence should be efficiently and actively absorbed (Said, 1999).

A dietary reference intake has yet to be established for pantothenic acid. Adequate intakes (AI) for men and women throughout the life-cycle have been suggested based on observed mean intakes and estimates of basal excretion in urine (Table 24.3) (Institute of Medicine, 1988). Urinary excretion of pantothenic acid only exceeds basal levels when intakes are greater than 4 mg/day in young adult males. Thus, an intake of 4 mg/day likely reflects the level at which saturation of the body pool occurs (Tarr *et al.*, 1981). Estimates of dietary intake in healthy adults have ranged from 4 to 7 mg/day (Srinivasan *et al.*, 1981; Tarr *et al.*, 1981; Bull and Buss, 1982; Kathman and Kies, 1984). There is no evidence to suggest that this range of intake is inadequate, and 5 mg/day has been set as the AI for adults. For adults older than 51 years, the AI remains the same (5 mg/day) as there is currently no basis for expecting an increased requirement in elderly individuals. During pregnancy, the AI is increased to 6 mg/day based on usual intakes of 5.3 mg/day (Song *et al.*, 1985) with rounding up. During lactation, the AI is increased further to 7 mg/day, accounting for additional secretion of the vitamin in human milk (1.7 mg/day) and the lower maternal blood concentrations reported when intakes are about 5–6 mg/day (Deodhar and Ramakrishnan, 1961; Cohenour and Calloway, 1972; Song *et al.*, 1985). This is likely the result of efficient sequestering of the vitamin in human milk, estimated to be 0.4 mg for every 1 mg pantothenic acid consumed during active lactation (Song *et al.*, 1984).

The AI for infants reflects the mean intake of infants fed principally with human milk. Human milk contains about 5–6 mg of pantothenic acid per 1000 kcal. Values for children and adolescents have largely been extrapolated from adult values. These values are supported by studies comparing intake and urinary excretion of the vitamin in preschool children (Kerrey *et al.*, 1968). Dietary intake of pantothenic acid was 3.8 and 5 mg/day in children of high and low socioeconomic status, respectively, and urinary excretion was 3.36 and 1.74 mg/day, respectively. In a separate study, 35 healthy girls, 7–9 years of age, were fed defined diets, and urinary excretion was measured (Pace *et al.*, 1961). The average daily excretion was 1.3 mg/day when intake was 2.79 mg/day, and 2.7 mg/day when intake was 4.45 mg/day. Therefore, intakes of 2.8–4.5 mg/day exceed urinary excretion of the vitamin. In healthy adolescents (13–19 years of age), 4-day diet records indicated that the average pantothenic acid intake was 6.3 mg/day for males and 4.1 mg/day for females (Eissenstat *et al.*, 1986). Average urinary excretion in this latter study was 3.3 and 4.5 mg/day for males and females, respectively, while whole blood pantothenic acid concentrations averaged 1.86 μmol/L and 1.57 μmol/L respectively. Normal blood concentrations of the vitamin in healthy individuals have been reported to range from 1.6 to 2.7 μmol/L (Wittwer *et al.*, 1989). Taken together, these data indicate that intake of 4 mg/day is sufficient to maintain normal blood concentrations in adolescents.

Using the estimate of 20–50 μg pantothenic acid per gram typically found in edible animal and plant tissues, it is possible to meet the AI for adults with a mixed diet containing as little as 100–200 g of solid food, i.e. the equivalent of a mixed diet corresponding to 600–1200 kcal or 2.4–4.8 MJ. The typical western diet contains 6 mg or more of available pantothenic acid (Tarr *et al.*, 1981). For a more detailed review of the AI for pantothenic acid, see Institute of Medicine (1988).

Deficiency and Toxicity

The essentiality of pantothenic acid has been documented in a wide variety of animal species. The classical signs

TABLE 24.4 Effects of pantothenic acid deficiency in selected species

Species	Symptoms
Chicken	Dermatitis around beak, feet, and eyes; poor feathering; spinal cord myelin degeneration; involution of the thymus; fatty degeneration of the liver (Jukes, 1939; Wooley *et al.*, 1939; Spies *et al.*, 1940; Kratzer and Williams, 1948; Milligan and Briggs, 1949; Gries and Scott, 1972)
Rat	Dermatitis; loss of hair color; loss of hair around the eyes; hemorrhagic necrosis of the adrenals; duodenal ulcer; spastic gait; anemia; leukopenia; impaired antibody production; gonadal atrophy with infertility (Subba Row and Hitchings, 1939; Sullivan and Nicholls, 1942; Axelrod, 1971; Eida *et al.*, 1975; Pietrzik *et al.*, 1975)
Dog	Anorexia; diarrhea; acute encephalopathy; coma; hypoglycemia; leukocytosis; hyperammonemia; hyperlactemia; hepatic steatosis; mitochondrial enlargement (Schaefer *et al.*, 1942; Noda *et al.*, 1991)
Pig	Dermatitis; hair loss; diarrhea with impaired sodium, potassium, and glucose absorption; lachrymation; ulcerative colitis; spinal cord and peripheral nerve lesions with spastic gait (Wintrobe *et al.*, 1943; Nelson, 1968)
Human	Numbness and burning of feet and hands; headache; fatigue; insomnia; anorexia with gastric disturbances; increased sensitivity to insulin; decreased eosinopenic response to adrenocorticotropic hormone (ACTH); impaired antibody production (Glusman, 1947; Hodges *et al.*, 1958, 1959)

of deficiency, first recognized by Elvehjem, Jukes and colleagues in chickens, include growth retardation and dermatitis (Jukes, 1939; Wooley *et al.*, 1939; Spies *et al.*, 1940). Many other physiological systems are affected by pantothenic acid deficiency, owing to the diversity of metabolic functions in which CoA and ACP participate. Neurological, immunological, hematological, reproductive, and gastrointestinal pathologies have been reported. The effects of pantothenic acid deficiency in different species are summarized in Table 24.4 (Subba Row and Hitchings, 1939; Schaefer *et al.*, 1942; Sullivan and Nicholls, 1942; Wintrobe *et al.*, 1943; Glusman, 1947; Kratzer and Williams, 1948; Milligan and Briggs, 1949; Hodges *et al.*, 1958, 1959; Nelson, 1968; Axelrod, 1971; Gries and Scott, 1972; Eida *et al.*, 1975; Pietrzik *et al.*, 1975; Noda *et al.*, 1991).

Assuming that the human adult requirement for pantothenic acid is ~5 mg/day, it may be predicted that, with a severe dietary deficiency, 5–6 weeks would be required before clear signs of deficiency are observed. This is based on the estimate that daily excretion of 5 mg represents a 1–2% loss of the total body pool of pantothenic acid. Consistent with this estimate, limited studies in humans indicate that about 6 weeks of severe depletion are required before urinary pantothenic acid decreases to a basal level of excretion (Fox and Linkswiler, 1961; Fry *et al.*, 1976; Annous and Song, 1985).

Because pantothenic acid is such a ubiquitous component of foods, both animal and vegetable, deficiency of this vitamin in humans is very rare. If present, pantothenic acid deficiency is usually associated with multiple nutrient deficiencies, thus making it difficult to discern effects specific to a lack of pantothenic acid. What is known about pantothenic acid deficiency in humans comes primarily from two sources of information. During World War II, malnourished prisoners of war in Japan, Burma, and the Philippines experienced numbness and burning sensations in their feet. While these individuals suffered multiple deficiencies, this specific syndrome was only reversed upon pantothenic acid supplementation (Glusman, 1947). Experimental pantothenic acid deficiency has also been induced in both animals and humans by administration of the pantothenic acid kinase inhibitor, ω-methylpantothenate, in combination with a diet low in pantothenic acid (Drell and Dunn, 1951; Hodges *et al.*, 1958, 1959). Observed symptoms in humans included numbness and burning of the hands and feet similar to that experienced by the World War II prisoners of war, as well as a myriad of other symptoms listed in Table 24.4. Some of the same symptoms are produced when individuals are fed a semi-synthetic diet from which pantothenic acid has been essentially eliminated, but without addition of ω-methylpantothenate (Fry *et al.*, 1976). Another pantothenic acid antagonist, calcium hopantenate, has been shown to induce encephalopathy with hepatic steatosis and a Reye-like syndrome in both dogs and humans (Noda et al., 1988, 1991).

Further evidence of the essentiality of pantothenic acid metabolism is revealed by an autosomal recessive disorder, initially called Hallervorden-Spatz syndrome and subsequently referred to as pantothenate kinase-associated neurodegenerative disease or neurodegeneration with brain-iron accumulation-1 (Zhou et al., 2001; Hayflick et al., 2003; Johnson et al., 2004; Gregory et al., 2009). Mutations in the gene encoding PANK2 (gene map locus: 20p13-p12.3) underlie this disorder, which is characterized by iron accumulation in the brain, progressive neurodegeneration, and early death. The pathogenesis of the disorder is believed to be related to mitochondrial CoA deficiency, inhibition of fatty acid β-oxidation, and oxidative stress. In addition, lack of phosphopantothenic acid synthesis may lead to accumulation of cysteine, the substrate required for step 2 of pantothenic acid metabolism, i.e. synthesis of phosphopantothenoylcysteine (Figure 24.2). It has been proposed that accumulated cysteine rapidly auto-oxidizes in the presence of free iron, leading to the generation of free radicals and additional oxidative stress (Zhou et al., 2001; Johnson et al., 2004).

Oral pantothenic acid, even in doses as high as 10–20 g/day, is well tolerated (Ralli and Dumm, 1953; Tahiliani and Beinlich, 1991). Occasional mild diarrhea may occur.

Status Determination

Pantothenic acid status is reflected by both whole blood concentration and urinary excretion. As cited above, whole blood concentrations typically range from 1.6 to 2.7 μmol/L (Wittwer et al., 1989), and a value <1 μmol/L is considered low. Urinary excretion is considered a more reliable indicator of status because it is more closely related to dietary intake (Hodges et al., 1958, 1959; Fry et al., 1976; Tarr et al., 1981; Eissenstat et al., 1986). Excretion of <1 mg pantothenic acid per day in urine is considered low. Plasma level of the vitamin is a poor indicator of status because it is not highly correlated with changes in intake or status (Cohenour and Calloway, 1972; Sauberlich, 1999).

Pantothenic acid concentrations in whole blood, plasma, and urine are measured by microbiological assay employing Lactobacillus plantarum. For whole blood, enzyme pre-treatment is required to convert CoA

to free pantothenic acid since L. plantarum does not respond to CoA. Other methods that have been employed to assess pantothenic acid status include radioimmunoassay, ELISA, and gas chromatography. The topic of pantothenic acid status assessment has been reviewed (Sauberlich, 1999).

Health Claims

With the rapid development of the internet, information about nutritional supplements and their putative health benefits is disseminated to the general public with an ease and pace never before possible. However, many health claims for nutritional supplements have little or no scientific basis. Although overt deficiency of pantothenic acid is extremely rare in humans, an internet search for "pantothenic acid" reveals numerous websites providing background information, health claims, and of course an opportunity to buy the vitamin for oral consumption. Many of the claims made on these websites are completely unwarranted. For example, the use of pantothenic acid to prevent and treat graying hair was based on the observation that pantothenic acid deficiency in rodents causes their fur to turn gray (Sullivan and Nicholls, 1942). No association between graying of hair in humans and pantothenic acid status has ever been demonstrated. Moreover, although other claims for pantothenic acid have a more credible scientific basis and are summarized below, it should be noted that many such claims are based on studies that were conducted in the 1940s, 1950s, and 1960s, and still await validation.

Cholesterol Lowering

Pantothenic acid is not particularly effective in lowering serum cholesterol levels. Rather, oral doses of its metabolite, pantetheine, or more specifically the dimer, pantethine, induce favorable effects on serum cholesterol concentrations. Several studies indicated that pantethine, in doses typically ranging from 500 to 1200 mg/day, can lower total serum cholesterol, low-density lipoprotein cholesterol, and triacylglycerols, and raise high-density lipoprotein cholesterol in individuals with dyslipidemia, hypercholesterolemia, and hyperlipoproteinemia associated with diabetes (Avogaro et al., 1983; Gaddi et al., 1984; Miccoli et al., 1984; Arsenio et al., 1986; Bertolini et al., 1986; Binaghi et al., 1990). The effects are favorable when compared with those of the more conventional lipid-lowering drugs, such as lovastatin, which may be associated with side-effects and liver toxicity. There appear to be no adverse side-effects associated with high-dose pantethine therapy. Furthermore, evidence exists that pantethine therapy is more effective than dietary modification in reducing serum cholesterol and lipid concentrations (Avogaro *et al.*, 1983). The mechanism by which pantethine exerts its hypolipemic effects is unclear. A hypothesized site of action is in the regulation of liver sterol biosynthesis. Because pantethine is a coenzyme precursor, it may shunt active acetate from sterol synthesis to mitochondrial oxidative and respiratory pathways (Kameda and Abiko, 1980). Additionally, pantethine may promote improved triacylglycerol and low-density lipoprotein cholesterol catabolism, as well as reduced cholesterol synthesis via inhibition of the enzyme hydroxymethyl glutaryl-CoA-reductase (Cighetti *et al.*, 1986, 1987, 1988).

Enhancement of Athletic Performance

Scientific support for an effect of pantothenic acid supplements on athletic performance is also limited. Until recently, most of the potential benefit has been inferred from animal studies. More than 60 years ago, frog muscles soaked in pantothenic acid solution were shown to do twice as much work as control muscles before exhaustion (Shock and Sebrell, 1944), and more than 30 years ago rats supplemented with high doses of pantothenic acid were shown to withstand exposure to cold water longer than unsupplemented mice (Ralli, 1968). Moreover, rats deficient in pantothenic acid became exhausted more rapidly during exercise than did pantothenic acid replete controls (Smith *et al.*, 1987). In this latter study, deficiency was associated with lower tissue CoA concentrations and greater depletion of glycogen reserves during exercise.

Studies assessing the influence of pantothenic acid on human performance are mixed. In one study, well-trained distance runners were supplemented with 2 g/day of pantothenic acid for 2 weeks (Litoff *et al.*, 1985). These athletes outperformed other equally well-trained distance runners who received placebo. Those who received the supplements also used 8% less oxygen to perform equivalent work and had ~17% less lactic acid accumulation. However, in a separate study, no effect on performance was observed in highly conditioned distance runners after receiving 1 g/day of pantothenic acid for 2 weeks (Nice *et al.*, 1984). Additionally, no difference in performance was observed among highly trained cyclists given either a combination of thiamin (1 g) and pantethine/pantothenic acid (1.9 g) or placebo. The supplement or placebo was given for 7 days before each exercise test. The investigators found no effect on any physiological or performance parameters during steady-state or high-intensity exercise (Webster, 1998).

Rheumatoid Arthritis

Over 50 years ago researchers noted that young rats made acutely deficient in pantothenic acid suffered defects in growth and development of bone and cartilage that were reversed by repletion of the vitamin (Nelson *et al.*, 1950). Subsequently, blood levels of pantothenic acid in humans with rheumatoid arthritis were found to be lower than in healthy controls. On the basis of this finding, a clinical trial was conducted in which 20 patients with rheumatoid arthritis were injected daily with 50 mg calcium pantothenate (Barton-Wright and Elliot, 1963). Blood levels of pantothenic acid increased to normal, and relief from rheumatoid symptoms was achieved in most cases. Symptoms recurred when supplementation was discontinued. Similar results were obtained in arthritic vegetarians (Barton-Wright and Elliot, 1963). More recently, it was found in a double-blind, placebo trial that oral doses of calcium pantothenate (≤2 g/day) reduced the duration of morning stiffness, degree of disability, and severity of pain in patients with rheumatoid arthritis (US General Practitioner Research Group, 1980). Individuals with other forms of arthritis were not helped by the supplements, indicating that the therapeutic effect of pantothenic acid is specific for rheumatoid arthritis.

Wound Healing

Oral administration of pantothenic acid and application of pantothenol ointment to the skin have been shown to accelerate the closure of skin wounds and increase the strength of scar tissue in animals. Adding calcium D-pantothenate to cultured human skin cells given an artificial wound increased the number of skin cells and the distance that they migrated across the edge of the wound (Weimann and Hermann, 1999). These effects are likely to accelerate wound healing. Little in vivo data, however, exist for humans to support the findings of accelerated wound healing in cell culture and animal studies. A randomized, double-blind study examining the effect of supplementing patients undergoing surgery for tattoo removal with 1000 mg of vitamin C and 200 mg of pantothenic acid did not demonstrate any significant improvement in the wound healing process in those that received the supplements (Vaxman *et al.*, 1995). Furthermore, no benefits were observed when the doses were increased to

3000 mg of ascorbic acid and 900 mg of pantothenic acid (Vaxman *et al.*, 1996). A topical form of pantothenic acid, panthenol or dexapanthenol, appears to play some role in the management of minor skin disorders. Dexpanthenol may help maintain skin hydration in cases of radiation dermatitis (Schmuth *et al.*, 2002), and may reduce skin irritation caused by experimental sodium lauryl sulfate exposure (Biro *et al.*, 2003). Dexpanthenol has also been recommended to treat cheilitis and dry nasal mucosa associated with treatment with the acne drug, isotretinoin (Romiti and Romiti, 2002).

Lupus Erythematosus

It has been hypothesized that lupus erythematosus, a systemic autoimmune disorder that affects the skin, joints, and various internal organ systems, may be the result of pantothenic acid deficiency (Leung, 2004). The hypothesis is based on the supposition that pantothenic acid deficiency may be induced by three drugs – procainamide, hydralazine, and isoniazid – that are also known to cause drug-induced lupus erythematosus. These drugs are metabolized via CoA-dependent acetylation, and the increased demand for CoA may cause pantothenic acid deficiency. It must be noted, however, that no data have been generated on the effect of these drugs on cellular CoA or pantothenic acid concentrations. It is further postulated that non-drug-induced systemic lupus erythematosus may be the consequence of an increased need for pantothenic acid in susceptible individuals with genetic polymorphisms in CoA-dependent enzymes. Such polymorphisms remain to be identified. None the less, it is recommended that lupus erythematosus be treated with a combination of vitamins and minerals, including 10 g/day of pantothenic acid (Leung, 2004). Support for such pharmacological doses comes from studies carried out in the 1950s. Some symptoms of lupus erythematosus, but not all, were alleviated with high doses (8–15 g/day) of pantothenic acid derivatives (calcium pantothenate, panthenol, or sodium pantothenate) alone (Goldman, 1950) or in combination with vitamin E supplements (Welsh, 1952, 1954). No improvements in disease symptoms were observed with lower doses (400–600 mg) of calcium pantothenate (Cochrane and Leslie, 1952). With modern technology available to probe genes for polymorphic variability, supplementation trials in lupus erythematosus patients should be repeated to test the hypothesis that a genetic-based increased requirement of pantothenic acid underlies the pathogenesis of this disease.

Antimalarial Drugs

More recently, *inhibitors* of the pantothenic acid pathway have been investigated for use as antimalarial drugs, most specifically related to the malaria parasite *Plasmodium falciparum*, which is the most virulent of the *Plasmodium* species in humans. *Plasmodium falciparum* requires an external supply of pantothenic acid to support its intracellular growth (Saliba *et al.*, 2005). Erythrocytes infected with *P. falciparum* rapidly take up pantothenate via the "new permeability pathways" (NPP) induced in the erythrocyte membrane by the maturing parasite (Saliba *et al.*, 1998). This increased permeability of the membrane via the NPP is not present in uninfected erythrocytes. The *P. falciparum* parasite relies on the endogenous synthesis of CoA from pantothenate and does not require exogenous CoA (Bozdech *et al.*, 2003). Thus, the CoA biosynthesis pathway has been a target for antimicrobial drug discovery. The antiplasmodial activity of the many pantothenic acid analogs already available now needs to be determined for *P. falciparum* in vitro in continuous culture. The compounds that are found to be effective at inhibiting the in vitro growth of the parasite should then be tested in a mammalian model. As the spread of the resistance to antimalarial agents widens, the development of new therapies for the treatment and prevention of malaria is essential.

Future Directions

Although CoA and ACP have been the focus of numerous investigations, far less attention has been paid to pantothenic acid. In part this is due to the rarity of naturally occurring pantothenic acid deficiency, and to the fact that descriptions of pantothenic acid deficiency and functions in humans have largely evolved indirectly from the administration of pantothenic acid antagonists; in particular, inhibitors of pantothenic acid kinase. Though these studies were informative, better information is needed regarding pantothenic acid requirements. The Food and Nutrition Board of the Institute of Medicine has yet to consider an RDA, because scientific evidence is currently insufficient for such estimations, although an AI has been set (Table 24.3) (Institute of Medicine, 1988). An RDA has been difficult to establish because CoA and ACP are involved in so many aspects of metabolism that biochemical markers or clinical deficiency criteria *specific* for pantothenic acid deficiency in humans have been difficult to define. In this regard, more information is needed related to the extent to which dietary pantothenic acid supplementation can stimulate or influence CoA or ACP synthesis.

Another area for future investigation is the potential for pantothenic acid–drug interactions. This could be important given that pantothenic acid and cofactors such as biotin share common receptors (Said *et al.*, 1998). For example, oral contraceptives containing estrogen and progestin may increase the requirement for pantothenic acid (Lewis and King, 1980). Also, though pantetheine has lipid lowering effects (Avogaro *et al.*, 1983; Gaddi *et al.*, 1984; Miccoli *et al.*, 1984; Arsenio *et al.*, 1986; Bertolini *et al.*, 1986; Binaghi *et al.*, 1990), little is known as to whether combining pantetheine with 3-hydroxy-3-methyl-glutaryl-CoA (HMG-CoA) reductase inhibitors (statins) or nicotinic acid will produce additive effects on blood lipid profiles. In this regard, clinical studies are warranted, as well as basic investigations into the mechanisms of these interactions. The potential for pantothenic acid inhibitors to serve as antimalarial agents is also of great interest for future investigation.

Acknowledgment

The authors wish to acknowledge the contribution of Lisa M. Rogers, PhD, in the preparation and writing of this chapter.

Suggestions for Further Reading

Coxon, K.M., Chakauya, E., and Ottenhof, H.H. (2005) Pantothenate biosynthesis in higher plants. *Biochem SocTrans* **33**, 743–746.

Leonardi, R., Zhang, Y.M., Rock, C.O., *et al.* (2005) Coenzyme A: back in action. *Prog Lipid Res* **44**, 125–153.

Rucker, R.B. and Bauerly, K. (2007) Pantothenic acid. In J. Zempleni, R.B. Rucker, D.B. McCormick, *et al.* (eds), *Handbook of Vitamins*, 4th Edn. CRC Press, Boca Raton, FL, pp. 289–313.

Spry, C., van Schalkwyk, D.A., Strauss, E., *et al.* (2010) Pantothenate utilization by *Plasmodium* as a target for antimalarial chemotherapy. *Infect Disord Drug Targets* **10**, 200–216.

Webb, M.E., Alison, G., Smith, A.G., *et al.* (2004) Biosynthesis of pantothenate. *Nat Prod Rep* **21**, 695–721.

References

Annous, K.F. and Song, W.O. (1985) Pantothenic acid uptake and metabolism by red blood cells of rats. *J Nutr* **125**, 2586–2593.

Arsenio, L., Bodria, P., Magnati, G., *et al.* (1986) Effectiveness of long-term treatment with pantethine in patients with dyslipidemia. *Clin Ther* **8**, 537–545.

Avogaro, P., Bittolo Bon, G., and Fusello, M. (1983) Effects of pantethine on lipids, lipoproteins and apolipoproteins in man. *Curr Ther Res* **33**, 488–493.

Axelrod, A.E. (1971) Immune processes in vitamin deficiency states. *Am J Clin Nutr* **24**, 265–271.

Barton-Wright, E.C. and Elliot, W.A. (1963) The pantothenic acid metabolism of rheumatoid arthritis. *Lancet* **2**, 862–863.

Beinlich, C.J., Naumovitz, R.D., Song, W.O., *et al.* (1990) Myocardial metabolism of pantothenic acid in chronically diabetic rats. *J Mol Cell Cardiol* **22**, 323–332.

Beinlich, C.J., Robishaw, J.D., and Neely, J.R. (1989) Metabolism of pantothenic acid in hearts of diabetic rats. *J Mol Cell Cardiol* **21**, 641–650.

Bertolini, S., Donati, C., Elicio, N., *et al.* (1986) Lipoprotein changes induced by pantethine in hyperlipoproteinemic patients: adults and children. *Int J Clin Pharmacol Ther Toxicol* **24**, 630–637.

Binaghi, P., Cellina, G., Lo Cicero, G., *et al.* (1990) Evaluation of the cholesterol-lowering effectiveness of pantethine in women in perimenopausal age. *Minerva Med* **81**, 475–479.

Bird, O.D. and Thompson, R.Q. (1967) Pantothenic acid. In P. Gyorgy and W.N. Pearson (eds), *The Vitamins*, Vol. 7, 2nd Edn. Academic Press, New York, pp. 209–241.

Biro, K., Thaci, D., Ochsendorf, F.R., *et al.* (2003) Efficacy of dexpanthenol in skin protection against irritation: a double-blind, placebo-controlled study. *Contact Dermatitis* **49**, 80–84.

Bozdech, Z., Llinas, M., Pulliam, B.L., *et al.* (2003) The transcriptome of the intraerythrocytic developmental cycle of *Plasmodium falciparum*. *PLoS Biol* **1**, E5.

Bucovaz, E.T., MacLeod, R.M., Morrison, J.C., *et al.* (1998) The coenzyme A–synthesizing protein complex and its proposed role in CoA biosynthesis in bakers' yeast. *Biochimie* **79**, 787–798.

Bull, N.L. and Buss, D.H. (1982) Biotin, pantothenic acid and vitamin E in the British household food supply. *Hum Nutr Appl Nutr* **36**, 190–196.

Cighetti, G., Del Puppo, M., Paroni, R., *et al.* (1986) Effects of pantethine on cholesterol synthesis from mevalonate in isolated rat hepatocytes. *Atherosclerosis* **60**, 67–77.

Cighetti, G., Del Puppo, M., Paroni, R., *et al.* (1987) Pantethine inhibits cholesterol and fatty acid syntheses and stimulates carbon dioxide formation in isolated rat hepatocytes. *J Lipid Res* **28**, 152–161.

Cighetti, G., Del Puppo, M., Paroni, R., *et al.* (1988) Modulation of HMG-CoA reductase activity by pantetheine/pantethine. *Biochim Biophys Acta* **963**, 389–393.

Cochrane, T. and Leslie, G. (1952) The treatment of lupus erythematosus with calcium pantothenate and panthenol. *J Invest Dermatol* **18**, 365–367.

Cohenour, S.H. and Calloway, D.H. (1972) Blood, urine, and dietary pantothenic acid levels of pregnant teenagers. *Am J Clin Nutr* **25**, 512–517.

Deodhar, A.D. and Ramakrishnan, C.V. (1961) Studies on human lactation: relation between the dietary intake of lactating women and the chemical composition of milk with regard to vitamin content. *J Trop Pediatr* **6**, 44–70.

Drell, W. and Dunn, M.S. (1951) Production of pantothenic acid deficiency syndrome in mice with methylpantothenic acid. *Arch Biochem* **33**, 110–119.

Eida, K., Kubato, N., Nishigaki, T., *et al.* (1975) Harderian gland: V. Effect of dietary pantothenic acid deficiency on porphyrin biosynthesis in Harderian gland of rats. *Chem Pharm Bull* **23**, 1–4.

Eissenstat, B.R., Wyse, B.W., and Hansen, R.G. (1986) Pantothenic acid status of adolescents. *Am J Clin Nutr* **44**, 931–937

Fenstermacher, D.K. and Rose, R.C. (1986) Absorption of pantothenic acid in rat and chick intestine. *Am J Physiol* **250**, G155–G160.

Fisher, M.N., Robishaw, J.D., and Neely, J.R. (1985) The properties of and regulation of pantothenate kinase from rat heart. *J Biol Chem* **256**, 15745–15751.

Fox, H.M. and Linkswiler, H. (1961) Pantothenic acid excretion on three levels of intake. *J Nutr* **75**, 451–454.

Fry, P.C., Fox, H.M., and Tao, H.G. (1976) Metabolic response to a pantothenic acid deficient diet in humans. *J Nutr Sci Vitaminol* **22**, 339–346.

Gaddi, A., Descovich, G.C., Noseda, G., *et al.* (1984) Controlled evaluation of pantethine, a natural hypolipidemic compound, in patients with different forms of hyperlipoproteinemia. *Atherosclerosis* **50**, 73–83.

Glusman, M. (1947) The syndrome of "burning feet" (nutritional melagia) as a manifestation of nutritional deficiency. *Am J Med* **3**, 211–223.

Goldman, L. (1950) Intensive panthenol therapy of lupus erythematosus. *J Invest Dermatol* **15**, 291–293.

Grassl, S.M. (1992) Human placental brush-border membrane Na$^+$-pantothenate cotransport. *J Biol Chem* **267**, 22902–22906.

Gregory, A., Polster, B.J., and Hayflick, S.J. (2009) Clinical and genetic delineation of neurodegeneration with brain iron accumulation. *J Med Genet* **46**, 73–80.

Gries, C.L. and Scott, M.L. (1972) The pathology of thiamin, riboflavin, pantothenic acid and niacin deficiencies in the chick. *J Nutr* **102**, 1269–1285.

Hayflick, S.J., Westaway, S.K., Levinson, B., *et al.* (2003) Genetic, clinical, and radiographic delineation of Hallervorden-Spatz syndrome. *New Engl J Med* **348**, 33–40.

Hodges, R.E., Ohlson, M.A., and Bean, W.B. (1958) Pantothenic acid deficiency in man. *J Clin Invest* **37**, 1642–1657.

Hodges, R.E., Bean, W.B., Ohlson, M.A., *et al.* (1959) Human pantothenic acid deficiency produced by omega-methyl pantothenic acid. *J Clin Invest* **38**, 1421–1425.

Institute of Medicine (1988) *Dietary Reference Intakes for Thiamin, Riboflavin, Niacin, Vitamin B6, Folate, Vitamin B12, Pantothenic Acid, Biotin, and Choline.* National Academy Press, Washington, DC.

Johnson, M.A., Kuo, Y.M., Westaway, S.K., *et al.* (2004) Mitochondrial localization of human PANK2 and hypotheses of secondary iron accumulation in pantothenate kinase-associated neurodegeneration. *Ann NY Acad Sci* **1012**, 282–298.

Jukes, T.H. (1939) The pantothenic acid requirements of the chick. *J Biol Chem* **129**, 225–231.

Kameda, K. and Abiko, Y. (1980) Stimulation of fatty acid metabolism by pantethine. In D. Cavallini, G.E. Gaull, and V. Zappia (eds), *Natural Sulfur Compounds*. Plenum Press, New York, pp. 443–452.

Kathman, J.V. and Kies, C. (1984) Pantothenic acid status of free-living adolescent and young adults. *Nutr Res* **4**, 245–250.

Kerrey, E., Crispin, S., Fox, H.M., *et al.* (1968) Nutritional status of preschool children. I. Dietary and biochemical findings. *Am J Clin Nutr* **21**, 1274–1279.

Khosla, C. and Tang, Y. (2005) Chemistry: a new route to designer antibiotics. *Science* **308**, 367–368.

Kirschbaum, N., Climons, R., Marino, K.A., *et al.* (1990) Pantothenate kinase activity in livers of genetically diabetic mice (db/db) and hormonally treated cultured rat hepatocytes. *J Nutr* **120**, 1376–1386.

Kratzer, F.H. and Williams, D.E. (1948) The pantothenic acid requirement for poults for early growth. *Poultry Sci* **27**, 518–523.

Leonardi, R., Zhang, Y.M., Rock, C.O., *et al.* (2005) Coenzyme A: back in action. *Prog Lipid Res* **44**, 125–153.

Leonardi, R., Zhang, Y.M., Yun, M.K., *et al.* (2010) Modulation of pantothenate kinase 3 activity by small molecules that interact with the substrate/allosteric regulatory domain. *Chem Biol* **17**, 892–902.

Leung, L.H. (2004) Systemic lupus erythematosus: a combined deficiency disease. *Med Hypoth* **62**, 922–924.

Lewis, C.M. and King, J.C. (1980) Effect of oral contraceptives agents on thiamin, riboflavin, and pantothenic acid status in young women. *Am J Clin Nutr* **33**, 832–838.

Litoff, D., Scherzer, H., and Harrison, J. (1985) Effects of pantothenic acid supplementation on human exercise. *Med Sci Sports Exercise* **17**(Suppl), 287.

Lopaschukf, G.D., Michalak, M., and Tsang, H. (1987) Regulation of pantothenic acid transport in the heart: involvement of a Na$^+$-cotransport system. *J Biol Chem* **262**, 3615–3619.

Miccoli, R., Marchetti, P., Sampietro, T., *et al.* (1984) Effects of pantethine on lipids and apolipoproteins in hypercholesterolemic diabetic and nondiabetic patients. *Curr Ther Res* **36**, 545–549.

Milligan, J.L. and Briggs, G.M. (1949) Replacement of pantothenic acid by panthenol in chick diets. *Poultry Sci* **28**, 202–205.

Nelson, M.M, Sulon, E., Becks, H., *et al.* (1950) Changes in endochondral ossification of the tibia accompanying acute pantothenic acid deficiency in young rats. *Proc Soc Exp Biol Med* **73**, 31–36.

Nelson, R.A. (1968) Intestinal transport, coenzyme A, and colitis in pantothenic acid deficiency. *Am J Clin Nutr* **21**, 495–501.

Nice, C., Reeves, A., Brinck-Johnson, T., *et al.* (1984) The effects of pantothenic acid on human exercise capacity. *J Sports Med Phys Fitness* **24**, 26–29.

Nicholis, D.G. and Ferguson, S.J. (2002) *Bioenergetics–3*. Academic Press, Boston, pp. 1–207.

Noda, S., Haratake, J., Sasaki, A., *et al.* (1991) Acute encephalopathy with hepatic steatosis induced by pantothenic acid antagonist, calcium hopantenate, in dogs. *Liver* **11**, 134–142.

Noda, S., Umezaki, H., Yamamoto, K., *et al.* (1988) Reye-like syndrome following treatment with the pantothenic acid antagonist, calcium hopantenate. *J Neurol Neurosurg Psychiatr* **51**, 582–585.

Pace, J.K., Stier, L.B., Taylor, D.D., *et al.* (1961) Metabolic patterns in preadolescent children. 5. Intake and urinary excretion of pantothenic acid and folic acid. *J Nutr* **74**, 345–351.

Patterson, A.D., Slanar, O., Krausz, K.W., *et al.* (2009) Human urinary metabolomic profile of PPARalpha induced fatty acid β-oxidation. *J Proteome Res* **8**, 4293–4300.

Pietrzik, K., Hesse, C.H., Zur Wiesch, E.S., *et al.* (1975) Urinary excretion of pantothenic acid as a measurement of nutritional requirements. *Int J Vit NutrRes* **45**, 153–162.

Plesofsky-Vig, N. and Brambi, R. (1988) Pantothenic acid and coenzyme A in cellular modification of proteins. *Annu Rev Nutr* **8**, 461–482.

Praphanphoj, V., Sacksteder, K.A., Gould, S.J., *et al.* (2001) Identification of the alpha-aminoadipic semialdehyde dehydrogenase phosphopantetheinyl transferase gene, the human ortholog of the yeast LYS5 gene. *Mol Genet Metab* **72**, 336–342.

Ralli, E.P. (1968) Effects of dietary supplementation on the ability of rats to withstand exposure to cold. *Nutr Rev* **26**, 124.

Ralli, E.P. and Dumm, M.E. (1953) Relation of pantothenic acid to adrenal cortical function. *Vitam Horm* **11**, 133–158.

Raychaudhuri, S. and Rajasekharan, R. (2003) Nonorganellar acyl carrier protein from oleaginous yeast is a homologue of ribosomal protein P2. *J Biol Chem* **278**, 37648–37657.

Reibel, D.K., Wyse, B.W., Berkich, D.A., *et al.* (1981) Regulation of coenzyme A synthesis in heart muscle: effects of diabetes and fasting. *Am J Physiol* **240**, H606–H611.

Robinson, F.A. (1966) *The Vitamin Co-factors of Enzyme Systems.* Pergamon Press, Oxford.

Robishaw, J.D., Berkich, D., and Neely, J.R. (1982) Rate-limiting step and control of coenzyme A synthesis in cardiac muscle. *J Biol Chem* **257**, 10967–10972.

Rock, C.O., Calder, R.B., Karim, M.A., *et al.* (2000) Pantothenate kinase regulation of the intracellular concentration of coenzyme A. *J Biol Chem* **275**, 1377–1383.

Romiti, R. and Romiti, N. (2002) Dexpanthenol cream significantly improves mucocutaneous side effects associated with isotretinoin therapy. *Pediatr Dermatol* **1**, 368–371.

Said, H.M. (1999) Cellular uptake of biotin: mechanisms and regulation. *J Nutr* **129**, 490S–493S.

Said, H.M., Ortiz, A., McCloud, E., *et al.* (1998) Biotin uptake by human colonic epithelial NCM460 cells: a carrier-mediated process shared with pantothenic acid. *Am J Physiol* **275**, C1365–C1371.

Saliba, K.J., Ferru, I., and Kirk, K. (2005) Provitamin B$_5$ (pantothenol) inhibits growth of the interaerythrocytic malaria parasite. *Antimicrob Agents Chemother* **49**, 632–637.

Saliba, K.J., Horner, H.A., and Kirk, K. (1998) Transport and metabolism of the essential vitamin pantothenic acid in human erythrocytes infected with the malaria parasite *Plasmodium falciparum*. *J Biol Chem* **273**, 10190–10195.

Sauberlich, H.E. (1999) Pantothenic acid. In *Laboratory Tests for the Assessment of Nutritional Status*, 2nd Edn. CRC Press, Boca Raton, FL, pp. 175–183.

Schaefer, A.E., McKibbin, J.M., and Elvehjem, C.A. (1942) Pantothenic acid deficiency in dogs. *J Biol Chem* **143**, 321–330.

Schmuth, M., Wimmer, M.A., Hofer, S., *et al.* (2002) Topical corticosteroid therapy for acute radiation dermatitis: a prospective, randomized, double-blind study. *Br J Dermatol* **146**, 983–991.

Schroeder, H.A. (1971) Losses of vitamins and trace minerals resulting from processing and preservation of foods. *Am J Clin Nutr* **24**, 562–573.

Seo, D.W., Kim, Y.K., Cho, E.J., *et al.* (2002) Oligosaccharide-linked acyl carrier protein, a novel transmethylase inhibitor from porcine liver inhibits cell growth. *Arch Pharmacol Res* **25**, 463–468.

Shibata, K., Gross, C.J., and Henderson, L.M. (1983) Hydrolysis and absorption of pantothenate and its coenzymes in the rat small intestine. *J Nutr* **113**, 2207–2215.

Shock, N.W. and Sebrell, W.H. (1944) The effect of changes in concentration of pantothenate on the work output of perfused frog muscles. *Am J Physiol* **142**, 274–278.

Smith, C.M. and Milner, R.E. (1985) The mechanism of pantothenate transport by rat liver parenchymal cells in primary culture. *J Biol Chem* **260**, 4823–4931.

Smith, C.M., Narrow, C.M., Kendrick, Z.V., *et al.* (1987) The effect of pantothenate deficiency in mice on their metabolic response to fast and exercise. *Metabolism* **36**, 115–121.

Song, W.O., Chan, G.M., Wyse, B.W., *et al.* (1984) Effect of PA status on the content of the vitamin in human milk. *Am J Clin Nutr* **40**, 317–324.

Song, W.O., Wyse, B.W., and Hansen, R.G. (1985) Pantothenic acid status of pregnant and lactating women. *J Am Diet Assoc* **85**, 192–198.

Spector, R. (1986) Pantothenic acid transport and metabolism in the central nervous system. *Am J Physiol* **250**, R292–R297.

Spector, R. (1987) Development and characterization of pantothenic acid transport in brain. *J Neurochem* **47**, 563–568.

Spector, R. and Mock, D.M. (1987) Biotin transport through the blood–brain barrier. *J Neurochem* **48**, 400–404.

Spies, T.D., Stanberry, S.R., Williams, R.J., *et al.* (1940) Pantothenic acid in human nutrition. *J Am Med Assoc* **115**, 523–524.

Srinivasan, V., Christensen, N., Wyse, B.W., *et al.* (1981) Pantothenic acid nutritional status in the elderly – institutionalized and non-institutionalized. *Am J Clin Nutr* **34**, 1736–1742.

Stein, E.D. and Diamond, J.M. (1989) Do dietary levels of pantothenic acid regulate its intestinal uptake in mice? *J Nutr* **119**, 1973–1983.

Strickland, K.C., Hoeferlin, L.A., Oleinik, N.V., *et al.* (2010) Acyl carrier protein-specific 4′-phosphopantetheinyl transferase activates 10-formyltetrahydrofolate dehydrogenase. *J Biol Chem* **285**, 1627–1633.

Subba Row, Y. and Hitchings, G.H. (1939) Pantothenic acid as a factor in rat nutrition. *J Am Chem Soc* **61**, 1615–1618.

Sullivan, M. and Nicholls, J. (1942) Nutritional dermatoses in the rat: VI. The effect of pantothenic acid deficiency. *Arch Dermatol Syphilol* **45**, 917–932.

Tahiliani, A.G. and Beinlich, C.J. (1991) Pantothenic acid in health and disease. *Vitam Horm* **46**, 165–228.

Tarr, J.B., Tamura, T., and Stokstad, E.L. (1981) Availability of vitamin B6 and pantothenate in an average American diet in man. *Am J Clin Nutr* **34**, 1328–1337.

US General Practitioner Research Group (1980) Calcium pantothenate in arthritic conditions. a report from the general practitioner research group. *Practitioner* **224**, 208–211.

Vaxman, F., Olender, S., Lambert, A., *et al.* (1995) Effect of pantothenic acid and ascorbic acid supplementation on human skin wound healing process. A double-blind, prospective and randomized trial. *Eur Surg Res* **27**, 158–166.

Vaxman, F., Olender, S., Lambert, A., *et al.* (1996) Can the wound healing process be improved by vitamin supplementation? Experimental study on humans. *Eur Surg Res* **28**, 306–314.

Wakil, S.J. (1989) Fatty acid synthetase, a proficient multifunctional enzyme. *Biochemistry* **28**, 4523–4530.

Walsh, J.H., Wyse, B.W., and Hansen, R.G. (1981) Pantothenic acid content of 75 processed and cooked foods. *J Am Diet Assoc* **78**, 140–144.

Webster, M.J. (1998) Physiological and performance responses to supplementation with thiamin and pantothenic acid derivatives. *Eur J Appl Physiol Occup Physiol* **77**, 486–491.

Weimann, B.I. and Hermann, D. (1999) Studies on wound healing: effects of calcium D-pantothenate on the migration, proliferation and protein synthesis of human dermal fibroblasts in culture. *Int J Vit Nutr Res* **69**, 113–119

Welsh, A.L. (1952) Lupus erythematosus: treatment by combined use of massive amounts of calcium pantothenate or panthenol with synthetic vitamin E. *AMA Arch Dermatol Syphilol* **65**, 137–148.

Welsh, A.L. (1954) Lupus erythematosus: treatment by combined use of massive amounts of pantothenic acid and vitamin E. *AMA Arch Dermatol Syphilol* **70**, 181–198.

Williams, R.J. and Majors, R.T. (1940) The structure of pantothenic acid. *Science* **91**, 246–248.

Williams, R.J., Lyman, C.M., Goodyear, G.H., *et al.* (1933) Pantothenic acid, a growth determinant of universal biological occurrence. *J Am Chem Soc* **55**, 2912–2927.

Wintrobe, M.M., Follis, R.H., Alcayaga, R., *et al.* (1943) Pantothenic acid deficiency in swine with particular reference to the effects on growth and on the alimentary tract. *Bull Johns Hopkins Hosp* **73**, 313–319.

Wittwer, C.T., Schweitzer, C., Pearson, J., *et al.* (1989) Enzymes for liberation of pantothenic acid in blood: use of plasma pantetheinase. *Am J Clin Nutr* **50**, 1072–1078.

Wooley, D.A., Waisman, H.A., and Elvehjem, C.A. (1939) Nature and partial synthesis of the chick antidermatitic factor. *J Am Chem Soc* **61**, 977–978.

Zhou, B., Westaway, S.K., Levinson, B., *et al.* (2001) A novel pantothenate kinase gene (*PANK2*) is defective in Hallervorden-Spatz syndrome. *Nat Genet* **28**, 345–349.

25

L-CARNITINE

CHARLES J. REBOUCHE, PhD

University of Iowa, Iowa City, Iowa, USA

Summary

L-Carnitine has essential roles in intermediary metabolism. For normal humans, endogenous synthesis of carnitine is adequate and therefore there is no dietary requirement. L-Carnitine has been proven to be useful in treatment in several diseases of genetic and acquired origin. For a number of other conditions L-carnitine and/or its acetyl or propionyl esters may prove useful in alleviation or moderation of symptoms. Use of L-carnitine and/or its esters may be valuable as dietary supplements to maintain or improve physical and mental function and slow decline during the aging process.

Introduction

L-Carnitine (Figure 25.1) is a low-molecular-weight (161.5 g/mol) biologically active amino acid derived from the essential amino acids L-lysine and L-methionine. The optical isomer D-carnitine has no biological activity and is not produced in eukaryotic organisms. At physiological pH carnitine[1] exists as a zwitterion, containing a positively charged quaternary amine and a negatively charged carboxyl group separated by a three-carbon chain. A hydroxyl group is attached to the middle carbon. This hydroxyl group is utilized biologically to form short-, medium-, and long-chain esters of organic and fatty acids with carnitine (e.g. acetyl-L-carnitine, palmitoyl-L-carnitine; Figure 25.1). Transfer of activated acyl moieties between carnitine and coenzyme A, catalyzed by several chain-length-specific carnitine acyltransferases, forms the core of the biological activity of carnitine. Esterification to carnitine permits transfer of activated acyl moieties, most notably acetyl and long-chain fatty acyl units, across membranes of cellular organelles, particularly the inner membrane of mitochondria and the peroxisomal membrane.

Carnitine in the Diet, Bioavailability, and Absorption

For human adults typical omnivorous diets provide 0.1 to 1.0 mmol of L-carnitine per day (2–12 μmol/kg body weight/day) (Rebouche, 1992). Diets rich in animal

---

[1]The term "carnitine" in this text refers specifically to the L stereoisomer.

Present Knowledge in Nutrition, Tenth Edition. Edited by John W. Erdman Jr, Ian A. Macdonald and Steven H. Zeisel.

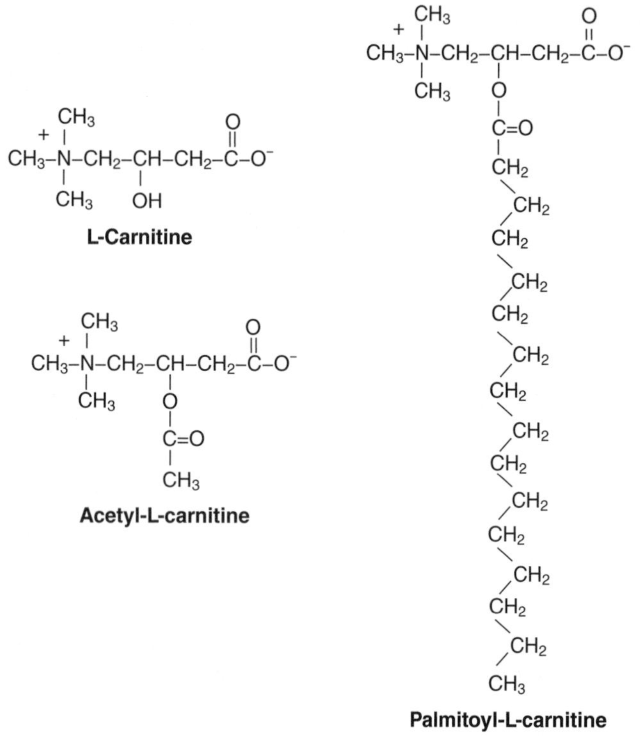

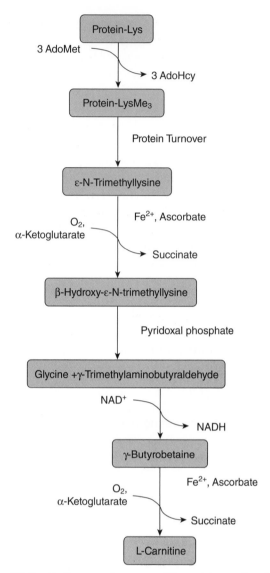

FIG. 25.1 Structures of carnitine and representative acylcarnitine esters.

products (meat, poultry, fish, and dairy products) provide almost all of the carnitine obtained from mixed diets (Rebouche and Engel, 1984; Demarquoy *et al.*, 2004). Fruits and vegetables contain very little carnitine. Vegan diets provide less than 1 μmol of carnitine/kg body weight/day. Fractional absorption of dietary carnitine is variable, generally in the range of 54–86% (Rebouche, 2004). Fractional absorption of dietary supplements (0.6–7 g/day) is 5–25% (Rebouche, 2004). At low carnitine intakes at least part of the absorption process may be facilitated or active. However, carnitine in the form of oral supplements is probably almost entirely absorbed by passive process(es).

Biosynthesis and Metabolism

Carnitine is synthesized from ε-*N*-trimethyllysine, an amino acid derived from post-translational modification of lysine in a variety of proteins (Figure 25.2). Probably the great majority of ε-*N*-trimethyllysine arises from turnover of muscle proteins. Many proteins are known to contain one or a few methylated lysine residues, including

FIG. 25.2 Pathway for carnitine biosynthesis in mammals.

actin, myosin, ATP synthase, histones, cytochrome *c*, and calmodulin. No single protein has been identified that contains a large number of these residues and/or that turns over rapidly such that it could provide a primary source of ε-*N*-trimethyllysine for carnitine synthesis. Rather, from an evolutionary perspective, accrual of this derivative from normal protein synthesis and degradation has been adequate for mammalian requirements for carnitine. It is noted that the fungus *Neurospora crassa* is able to methylate unbound lysine (Rebouche and Broquist, 1976; Borum and Broquist, 1977), but no other organism has been shown to possess this capability.

ε-*N*-Trimethyllysine is converted to carnitine via a series of four enzymatic reactions, catalyzed by two dioxygenases (ε-*N*-trimethyllysine hydroxylase and γ-butyrobetaine hydroxylase), an aldolase (serine hydroxymethyltransferase), and a dehydrogenase (aldehyde dehydrogenase) (Vaz and Wanders, 2002). Thus the process also requires the cofactors Fe^{2+}, ascorbic acid and pyridoxal phosphate, and co-substrates α-ketoglutarate, O_2, and NAD^+. Conversion of ε-*N*-trimethyllysine to carnitine is not quantitative in mammals. Significant amounts of this amino acid and the penultimate precursor of carnitine, γ-butyrobetaine, are normally excreted in urine. The normal rate of carnitine synthesis in humans is estimated to be about 1.2 μmol/kg body weight/day (Rebouche, 1992). This estimate was obtained indirectly from rates of carnitine excretion at steady state in the absence of significant dietary intake of carnitine. The variability among individuals or populations is not known.

Carnitine is not degraded by enzymes of animal origin. However, degradation products of carnitine have been identified in urine and feces of rats and humans. These arise from catabolism of carnitine by bacterial enzymes in the gastrointestinal tract. Enterobacteria metabolize carnitine to γ-butyrobetaine anaerobically via a two-step process (not a reverse of the single-step hydroxylation of γ-butyrobetaine in carnitine biosynthesis) (Figure 25.3). In these organisms carnitine may serve as a growth-promoting electron acceptor in the absence of preferred substrates (Rebouche and Seim, 1998). Carnitine is degraded aerobically by some organisms, by carbon–nitrogen cleavage resulting in trimethylamine and malic semialdehyde (Figure 25.3). Trimethylamine is absorbed from the lumen of the large intestine, and is oxidized in the liver to trimethylamine oxide (Higgins *et al.*, 1972). Following oral administration of carnitine radiolabeled in the methyl groups, radiolabeled trimethylamine oxide and γ-butyrobetaine were the major degradation products observed in urine and feces, respectively, in both rats and humans (Rebouche *et al.*, 1984; Rebouche and Chenard, 1991).

Carnitine and its esters are distributed into three kinetically defined pools in the body (Rebouche and Engel, 1984). The largest corresponds to muscle tissues, and contains 92–97% of total body carnitine. A pool corresponding to other tissues including liver and kidneys contains 2–6% of total body carnitine. The extracellular fluid pool of carnitine accounts for the remaining 0.7–1.5%. Turnover of the muscle carnitine pool is relatively slow (191 hours), but, because of its size, the flux (movement into and out of a compartment) of carnitine is relatively rapid (427 μmol/hour in adult humans). Collective turnover time and flux of carnitine for other tissues are 11.6 hours and 277 μmol/hour, respectively. Turnover time for the extracellular carnitine pool is 1.13 hours, and

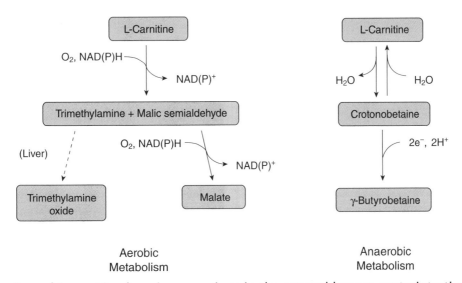

FIG. 25.3 Catabolism of L-carnitine by microorganisms in the rat and human gastrointestinal tract.

whole-body turnover of carnitine is 66 days. The total carnitine pools in tissues and extracellular fluid consist of approximately 10–20% esterified carnitine and 80–90% non-esterified carnitine. The esterified carnitine fraction consists primarily of acetyl-L-carnitine, with smaller amounts of propionyl-L-carnitine and long-chain fatty acyl carnitine esters. The concentration of carnitine is generally greater in tissues than in extracellular fluid. In skeletal muscle and liver, respectively, the total carnitine concentrations are 76 and 50 times that in extracellular fluid. The highest concentrations of carnitine and acetyl-L-carnitine (1–80 mmol/L) are found in seminal plasma and within epididymal tissue and spermatozoa (Jeulin and Lewin, 1996).

Entry of carnitine and its short-chain acyl esters acetyl-L-carnitine and propionyl-L-carnitine into most tissues is facilitated by the organic cation transporter OCTN2. This protein has a high affinity for carnitine and its short-chain acyl esters (K_t = 3–5 μmol/L). Transport is dependent on an inwardly directed sodium-ion gradient, and sodium ions are co-transported with carnitine. This protein is highly expressed in kidney, skeletal muscle, heart, placenta, pancreas, testis and epididymis, and modestly expressed in liver, lung, and brain (Wu *et al.*, 1998). OCTN2 also is expressed in the colon, where it may facilitate salvage of dietary carnitine and γ-butyrobetaine formed from dietary carnitine by action of colonic microbes (Fujiya *et al.*, 2007; D'Argenio *et al.*, 2010). In addition, it has been implicated in transport of a bacterial quorum-sensing peptide that activates cell survival pathways in colonic epithelia (Fujiya *et al.*, 2007). Other proteins that are capable of transporting carnitine across cell membranes include the organic cation transporters OCTN1, OCTN3, Oat9S and the amino acid transporter $ATB^{0,+}$ (Lamhonwah *et al.*, 2003; Rebouche, 2006; Tsuchida *et al.*, 2010). OCTN3 is involved in peroxisomal transport of carnitine and acylcarnitine esters (Lamhonwah *et al.*, 2005). The physiological role(s) of OCTN1, Oat9s, and $ATB^{0,+}$ in carnitine transport and carnitine homeostasis are unknown or are poorly characterized.

A unique carnitine transporter, designated CT-2, is specifically expressed in testes (Enomoto *et al.*, 2002). The transporter is highly specific and has high affinity (K_t = 20 μmol/L) for carnitine. It is located phylogenically between the OAT and OCT/OCTN families of organic ion transporters. CT2 protein is localized to the luminal membrane of the epididymal endothelium and within Sertoli cells.

The major route for excretion of carnitine is via the kidney. Carnitine is filtered across the glomerulus. Normally 90–98% of filtered carnitine is reabsorbed by humans. OCTN2 in the renal brush-border membrane is primarily or totally responsible for reabsorption of carnitine and its short-chain acyl esters, and probably also the immediate precursor of carnitine, γ-butyrobetaine. Renal reabsorption of carnitine is thought to be a primary regulator of carnitine homeostasis in humans (Rebouche, 2004). Carnitine reabsorption is highly efficient when plasma carnitine concentrations are at or below about 60 μmol/L (normal plasma total carnitine concentration is 30–65 μmol/L). When the plasma carnitine concentration is increased above 60 μmol/L, by, for example, intravenous infusion of carnitine or oral consumption of a carnitine supplement, the efficiency of carnitine reabsorption rapidly decreases and a greater proportion of filtered carnitine is lost to urinary excretion.

Renal tubular cells secrete carnitine, short-chain acyl esters of carnitine, and γ-butyrobetaine into the tubular lumen (Rebouche and Engel, 1980; Hokland and Bremer, 1986; Mancinelli *et al.*, 1995). Some of these are reabsorbed and some are lost in the urine. Urine total carnitine typically contains a higher percentage of acylcarnitine esters than does the circulating carnitine pool (Lombard *et al.*, 1989). Under normal conditions the acylcarnitine ester fraction in urine is mostly comprised of acetyl-L-carnitine. Because the affinity of the renal brush-border membrane transporter OCTN2 for carnitine and acetyl-L-carnitine is similar, one should not be selectively reabsorbed from the glomerular filtrate over the other. Thus renal tubular cells may produce and secrete acylcarnitine esters selectively as a means to remove excess acyl burden from the body.

Requirements and Consequences of Deficiency

Carnitine is not required by normal humans. It is often described as a conditionally essential nutrient (Borum, 1995), but this designation applies to abnormal or special circumstances such as prematurity at birth, genetic or acquired diseases, and chronic use of some drugs. Vegan adults and children, who acquire only minimal amounts of carnitine from their diets, have plasma carnitine concentrations approximately 10% and 25%, respectively, lower than their omnivorous counterparts (Lombard *et al.*, 1989). There is no dietary reference intake for L-carnitine.

Primary systemic carnitine deficiency in humans occurs as a result of defects in the gene coding for OCTN2. Clinical features include hypoketotic hypoglycemia, seizures, vomiting, lethargy progressive to coma, cardiomyopathy, and chronic muscle weakness (Nyhan and Ozand, 1998; Laforêt and Vianey-Saban, 2010). Therapeutic treatment with carnitine is highly successful. Plasma and liver carnitine concentrations are restored, attacks of hypoketotic hypoglycemia are prevented, and heart size is reduced to normal within months of treatment initiation. Skeletal muscle weakness improves, despite only slight increases in muscle carnitine concentration. A murine model (the *jvs* mouse) of spontaneous origin has been described (Hashimoto *et al.*, 1998).

Carnitine deficiency or depletion occurs secondary to many genetic inborn errors and acquired medical conditions, and with use of some medications. These have been reviewed extensively elsewhere (Pons and De Vivo, 1995). In numerous case reports of low circulating carnitine concentrations "a defect in carnitine biosynthesis" has been suggested. However, there is no documented case of car-

nitine deficiency in humans caused by absent or defective proteins associated with carnitine biosynthesis.

Mechanisms of Action/ Biological Activity

A primary function of carnitine in cellular metabolism is to facilitate transport of activated long-chain fatty acids into mitochondria (Figure 25.4). Activated long-chain fatty acids (as coenzyme A esters) are transesterified to carnitine on the outer membrane of mitochondria. This reaction is catalyzed by carnitine palmitoyltransferase I (CPT I). Long-chain fatty acylcarnitine is transported across the mitochondrial inner membrane by carnitine-acylcarnitine translocase (CACT) (Iacobazzi *et al.*, 1998), a member of the mitochondrial metabolite carrier protein family (Palmieri *et al.*, 1995). Carnitine palmitoyltransferase II (CPT II) associated with the matrix side of the mitochondrial inner membrane then catalyzes transesterification of the activated fatty acid to intramitochondrial coenzyme A. The activated fatty

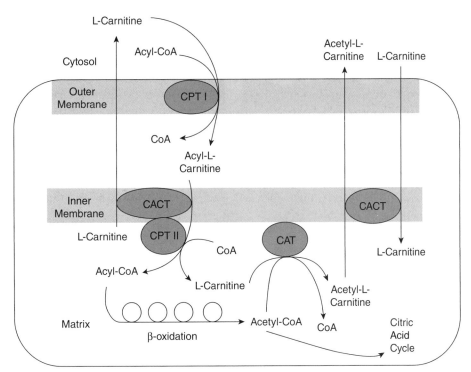

FIG. 25.4 Facilitation of entry of long-chain fatty acids into mitochondria by carnitine. CPT I, carnitine palmitoyltransferase I; CPT II, carnitine palmitoyltransferase II; CACT, carnitine-acylcarnitine translocase; CAT, carnitine acetyltransferase; CoA, coenzyme A.

acids are oxidized through multiple cycles of the β-oxidation pathway.

CPT I is rate-controlling, although not necessarily rate-limiting, for β-oxidation of fatty acids (Eaton, 2002). CPT I is inhibited by malonyl-CoA and stimulated by AMP-activated protein kinase (Bartlett and Eaton, 2004). Two major forms of CPT I have been identified and are products of different genes (*CPT1A* and *CPT1B*) (Ramsay *et al.*, 2001). M-CPT I is found in skeletal muscle and heart, and L-CPT I is found in liver and many other non-muscle tissues. The two forms differ in their affinity for both the inhibitor, malonyl-CoA, and the substrate, carnitine. The carnitine concentration in tissues is not limiting for CPT I activity, unless it is abnormally low. Michaelis constants for carnitine binding to L-CPT I and M-CPT I are 30 and 500 μmol/L, respectively (Ramsay *et al.*, 2001).

Carnitine participates in maintenance of intramitochondrial non-esterified coenzyme A availability. Carnitine is released in the mitochondrial matrix after import of long-chain fatty acylcarnitine and transesterification of the acyl group to coenzyme A. It can exit mitochondria via CACT, or it may be used as a reservoir for excess acetyl groups formed during β-oxidation and/or pyruvate oxidation. This process allows for maintenance of sufficient non-esterified coenzyme A concentration in the mitochondrial matrix to supply the β-oxidation cycle, pyruvate dehydrogenase, and the citric acid cycle. Transesterification of acetyl groups to carnitine from coenzyme A is catalyzed by carnitine acetyltransferase. Acetyl-L-carnitine may exit the mitochondrial matrix via CACT for use in other compartments of the cell, for use by other cells or tissues, or for excretion. The ability of carnitine to act as a reservoir for activated acyl residues is also important in abnormal cellular metabolism, particularly in genetic diseases associated with defects in organic and fatty acid metabolism (Rebouche, 2006). Experimental studies in mice, monkeys, and humans (Yamaguti *et al.*, 1996) show that, during starvation, acetyl-L-carnitine concentration in the circulation increases, perhaps due to higher rates of β-oxidation of fatty acids in some tissues, with consequent export of excess acetyl units. This phenomenon may also provide a means to transfer readily oxidizable carbon to tissues such as kidney and brain in times of metabolic stress. Following glucose re-feeding, the circulating acetyl-L-carnitine concentration decreases as this metabolite is transported into the liver.

Carnitine participates in shuttling of chain-shortened fatty acids from peroxisomes to mitochondria. Very-long-chain fatty acids are partially oxidized in peroxisomes. Activated medium-chain-length organic acid products are transesterified to carnitine in peroxisomes, the acylcarnitine esters are exported from peroxisomes and the acyl moieties are subsequently oxidized in mitochondria. In peroxisomes transesterification of medium-chain acyl groups from coenzyme A to carnitine is catalyzed by carnitine octanoyltransferase (Ramsay, 1999).

In addition to the functions described above, carnitine and its esters have a number of physiological and pharmacological interactions and effects that have been demonstrated in animal, cell culture, and in vitro experimentation. These interactions and effects may be physiological in nature, but may also be magnified by pharmacological use of these compounds.

Carnitine and extra-mitochondrial carnitine palmitoyltransferase function in utilization of long-chain fatty acids for phospholipid biosynthesis and remodeling. Fatty acids bound to carnitine are incorporated into erythrocyte membrane phospholipids during repair after oxidative insult (Arduini *et al.*, 1990a), and into dipalmitoylphosphatidylcholine, a major component of surfactant, in lung alveolar cells (Arduini *et al.*, 2001). Carnitine and acetyl-L-carnitine may increase membrane stability in mature erythrocytes, presumably by a specific interaction with cytoskeletal proteins (Arduini *et al.*, 1990b).

Carnitine at millimolar concentrations reduces binding of dexamethasone to the glucocorticoid receptor α, while itself triggering nuclear translocation of the receptor and stimulating transcription of glucocorticoid receptor α-responsive promoters (Manoli *et al.*, 2004). L-Carnitine mimics several immunomodulatory effects of glucocorticoids, including suppressing lipopolysaccharide-induced cytokine production in rats, promoting fetal lung development in pregnant rats, and decreasing serum levels of tumor necrosis factor α in surgical and HIV-infected patients (Manoli *et al.*, 2004). Carnitine may share some of the therapeutic properties of glucocorticoids, but without their deleterious side-effects.

Carnitine supplementation attenuates hyperammonemia and its toxic effects in a number of clinical and experimentally induced conditions, including primary systemic carnitine deficiency, medium-chain acyl-CoA dehydrogenase deficiency, valproic acid administration and ammonium chloride intoxication. This effect may derive from stabilization of mitochondrial function and/or by maintaining urea cycle activity. In the *jvs* mouse, a model for human primary systemic carnitine deficiency, carnitine administration attenuated hyperammonemia and normalized hepatic expression of urea cycle enzymes suppressed by accumulation of long-chain fatty acids (Horiuchi et al., 1992; Tomomura et al., 1996). These effects may be mediated by the interaction of carnitine with the glucocorticoid receptor (Tomomura et al., 1996; Manoli et al., 2004).

Carnitine and its short-chain acyl esters may block formation or mitigate toxic effects of intracellular reactive oxygen species. Direct antioxidant effects of carnitine have been demonstrated in vitro. Model reactions revealed concentration-dependent reducing power (potassium ferricyanide reduction method) and hydrogen peroxide and radical scavenging (1,1-diphenyl-2-picryl-hydrazyl free radical (DPPH) assay) activities of carnitine similar in magnitude to α-tocopherol (Gülçin, 2006). Ferrous iron chelating ability of carnitine was also demonstrated. Gülçin (2006) speculated that, in the reaction with DPPH, a radical centered on carbon 2 of carnitine is generated with reduction of DPPH· to 1,1-diphenyl-2-picryl hydrazine (DPPH). This reaction is purportedly energetically favorable: ΔH for the reaction was calculated to be -181 kcal/mol.

Carnitine may indirectly attenuate oxidative stress. It has been shown to inhibit arachidonic acid incorporation into platelet lipids, agonist-induced arachidonic acid release, and arachidonic acid-induced NADPH oxidase activation (Pignatelli et al., 2003). Carnitine may also up-regulate expression of redox-sensitive transcription factors, sirtuins, and heat-shock proteins that protect against oxidative damage (Calabrese et al., 2009).

Supplements: Infant Nutrition, Health Maintenance, Performance Enhancement, and Prevention or Retardation of Aging and Chronic Disease

Carnitine and acetyl-L-carnitine are available commercially as diet supplements in the US. Propionyl-L-carnitine is available in Europe. Typical recommendations for use are 0.5 to 4 g/day for children and adults. Little or no toxicity is associated with consumption of these amounts of supplement. Occasional occurrences of diarrhea or body odor ("fish odor syndrome") have been reported.

Carnitine has been described as a conditionally essential nutrient for infants. An Expert Panel commissioned by the

US Food and Drug Administration's Center for Food Safety and Applied Nutrition has recommended a minimum carnitine content in infant formulas of 7.5 μmol/100 kcal, a level similar to that found in human milk, and a maximum level of 12.4 μmol/100 kcal, a value similar to the upper limit reported for human milk (Raitan et al., 1998). These recommendations were made on the basis of reported biochemical differences when infants were fed carnitine-free diets compared with similar diets with carnitine, and despite the lack of evidence that carnitine is essential for the term infant.

Carnitine is not added to premature infant formulas, enteral or parenteral, at the time of manufacture, but these formulas may be supplemented with carnitine at the time of use. The rationale for supplementation is twofold: infants utilize lipids as a primary source for energy and growth after birth, requiring a high rate of mitochondrial oxidation, and the concentration of carnitine in infant circulation and tissues typically is lower without supplementation than in infants fed human milk or formulas containing carnitine. Studies in premature infants have focused on the effect of carnitine supplements on growth rate and lipid metabolism, with mixed results. In one study, no differences in 2-week weight gain over 8 weeks were observed between supplemented and non-supplemented infants (Shortland et al., 1998). In another study, supplemented neonates regained their birth-weight more rapidly than placebo-group neonates, indicating that L-carnitine supplementation may promote more rapid catch-up growth (Crill et al., 2006). An extensive review of these and other relevant studies has been published (Crill and Helms, 2007). For infants expected to be on parenteral nutrition for 7 days or longer, supplementation with carnitine 10–20 mg/kg body weight/day, given intravenously or orally, is recommended (Crill and Helms, 2007).

Carnitine has been investigated for its potential for performance enhancement and recovery from physical exertion. Several commercial entities market carnitine as an ergogenic aid. This strategy is based on the notion that supplemental carnitine will increase oxidative metabolism of fatty acids and perhaps spare muscle glycogen. It presumes that an increase of available carnitine will increase the flux of long-chain fatty acids into mitochondria. Clinical data suggest that muscle function is sensitive to changes in carnitine content when carnitine concentration is less than 25 to 50% of normal, but is insensitive to changes when the carnitine concentration is normal (Brass,

2004). If an increase in carnitine concentration alone is the sole factor in performance enhancement, it is unlikely that improvements would occur with carnitine supplementation, both because normal carnitine concentration is saturating for muscle CPT I kinetics, and only a very modest increase in carnitine concentration would be expected with even the most rigorous supplementation regimen. Even though carnitine supplements are not likely to substantially increase muscle carnitine concentration, they may improve the efficiency of muscle metabolism by exchange of non-esterified carnitine (provided by the supplement) into muscle for excess activated acetate (as acetyl-L-carnitine) formed from β-oxidation, when the citric acid cycle and/or oxidative phosphorylation pathways are operating at maximum capacity. In addition, the antioxidant and radical scavenging activity may assist in preventing damage from reactive oxygen species generated during prolonged physical exertion. Most studies of carnitine use to improve athletic performance have not shown any benefit. However, due to limitations in study design, the lack of evidence should not necessarily be taken to conclude that carnitine supplements are not beneficial (Brass, 2004). Particularly for elite athletes, very small increments in performance enhancement that are not quantifiable or statistically significant by standard experimental paradigms may have substantial impact on competitive outcome.

Propionyl-L-carnitine administered as a dietary supplement may provide some modest enhancement in physical performance. In a double-blind, placebo-controlled, crossover-design clinical trial, propionyl-L-carnitine (as glycine propionyl-L-carnitine), 4.5 g, administered orally to trained athletes significantly enhanced peak power production in resistance-trained males with significantly lower lactate accumulation (Jacobs et al., 2009). The incremental differences in power production were modest and were observed only after repeated short–duration Wingate cycle sprints. Propionyl-L-carnitine may be more effective in enhancement of exercise performance than carnitine, because of its ability to increase nitric oxide production and vasodilation. Moreover, propionyl-L-carnitine may enhance citric acid cycle activity by providing propionyl units that can be converted to succinate.

Carnitine may reduce chemical damage to tissues after exercise and optimize the processes of muscle repair and remodeling (Kraemer et al., 2008). In double-blind, placebo-controlled, crossover studies, 3 weeks of carnitine supplementation 2 g/day, followed by an acute resistance

exercise challenge, biochemical markers of purine metabolism, free radical formation, muscle tissue disruption, and muscle soreness were attenuated in non-trained young men (Spiering et al., 2007) and middle-aged men and women (Ho et al., 2010). The authors of these studies speculate that supplemental carnitine acts to protect vascular endothelial cells, improving regulation of blood flow to deliver oxygen to tissues and reducing hypoxia and oxidative stress generated by physical activity (Ho et al., 2010). Whereas the results of these studies are impressive, the benefit-to-cost of this supplement regimen may only be attractive to competitive athletes and individuals pursuing very active lifestyles.

Some vendors have marketed carnitine as a dietary supplement to promote weight loss. The term "fat burner" has been used to describe carnitine. The rationale for this claim is based mostly on animal studies carried out in very highly controlled settings. In commercial animal husbandry the impetus for use of carnitine is to partition nutrients away from fat accretion and toward muscle deposition. In growing pigs fed energy-limited, fat-containing diets with or without supplemental carnitine, those receiving the supplement for 10 days had improved nitrogen retention and reduced carcass fat (Heo et al., 2000), thus supporting a role for supplemental carnitine to improve body composition. Obesity affects a significant proportion of domestic pets, particularly dogs and cats. Carnitine added to a weight reduction diet for dogs resulted in a substantially greater loss of weight (7% vs. 2%) and fat mass (4% vs. 2%) in dogs receiving the supplement compared with diet alone, over a period of 7 weeks (Anonymous, 2009).

The success observed in animal studies has not been achieved in humans. For example, in a double-blind investigation to test the weight-loss efficacy of L-carnitine, 36 moderately overweight premenopausal women were pair-matched on body mass index and randomly assigned to two groups (Villani et al., 2000). For 8 weeks one group ingested 2 g of carnitine twice daily, and the placebo group ingested the same amount of lactose. All subjects walked for 30 minutes (60–70% maximum heart rate) 4 days per week. No significant changes in mean total body mass, fat mass, and resting lipid utilization occurred over time. The success in animals suggests that it may be possible to achieve weight reduction and more desirable body composition with use of carnitine supplements in humans, but the regimens necessary to achieve these goals may be too rigid to be widely effective.

Carnitine and acetyl-L-carnitine have been investigated for use in maintenance of mental and physical function and reversal of decline with aging. In rats mitochondrial function declines with aging. Mitochondria of old rats have higher levels of products of oxidation of lipids, proteins and nucleic acids than do mitochondria of young rats. In old rats, cellular oxygen uptake and mitochondrial membrane potential, cardiolipin concentration, and respiratory control ratio are lower than in young rats (Ames and Liu, 2004). In heart mitochondria of old rats, DNA transcription and activity of cytochrome oxidase, adenine nucleotide translocase, and CACT are reduced compared with mitochondria of young rats (Gadeleta et al., 1994; Paradies et al., 1994, 1995). Administration of acetyl-L-carnitine to old rats restores cardiolipin concentration and mitochondrial function to near those in young rats (Paradies et al., 1994, 1995; Ames and Liu, 2004). One mechanism proposed to explain these effects is protection afforded by acetyl-L-carnitine against oxidative decline in activity of carnitine acetyltransferase observed *in vivo* and *in vitro* (Liu et al., 2002). Although this effect may contribute to overall restoration of mitochondrial function, the more general effects on membrane-associated enzyme activities and transporters probably are related to the restoration of cardiolipin concentration in the mitochondrial inner membrane.

Administration of acetyl-L-carnitine to old rats improves ambulatory activity and restores some memory loss by improving mitochondrial function and reducing accumulation of oxidation products (Liu et al., 2002; Ames and Liu, 2004). Administration of carnitine to old rats restores activities of citric acid cycle and electron-transferring enzymes to near those of young rats (Kumaran et al., 2005). In one study, acetyl-L-carnitine but not L-carnitine attenuated appearance of malondialdehyde, a lipid oxidation product (Liu et al., 2004), but in another study carnitine supplementation increased the activities of the antioxidant enzymes superoxide dismutase and glutathione peroxidase (Juliet et al., 2005).

In elderly humans, patients with depressive syndrome scored significantly lower on the Hamilton Rating Scale for Depression following supplementation with acetyl-L-carnitine (Tempesta et al., 1987). Elderly subjects with mild mental impairment had better scores on cognitive performance tests following supplementation with acetyl-L-carnitine (Salvioli and Neri, 1994). A meta-analysis of the efficacy of acetyl-L-carnitine for cognitive impairment in mild Alzheimer's disease showed a significant advantage for the supplement over placebo on both clinical scales and psychometric tests (Montgomery et al., 2003). Ames (2003) has advocated a "metabolic tune-up" that includes micronutrients with acetyl-L-carnitine to maintain mitochondrial function during the life cycle and prevent age-related cognitive dysfunction and other degenerative diseases associated with aging.

Therapeutic Use and Health Claims

L-Carnitine is approved by the US Food and Drug Administration for treatment of primary and secondary carnitine deficiency diseases (e.g. OCTN2 deficiency, glutaric aciduria type II, methylmalonic aciduria, propionic acidemia, and medium-chain acyl-CoA dehydrogenase deficiency), and in end-stage renal-disease patients undergoing hemodialysis. It has been suggested that carnitine is beneficial for relief of symptoms in a number of other diseases and medical conditions (see Table 25.1). In most cases these claims are supported by experimental and/or clinical evidence, but additional clinical trials may be required to establish efficacy.

Future Directions

More basic studies are needed to elucidate the chemical basis for antioxidant and anti-apoptotic effects of carnitine and acetyl-L-carnitine. These should include examination of intracellular direct antioxidant effects (neutralizing reactive oxygen species), facilitation of acetylation of proteins that affords protection from oxidative damage from reactive oxygen species, improvement of mitochondrial function by facilitating a more orderly flow of substrates through the tricarboxylic cycle and electrons through the electron transport chain, or direct effects on transcription of genes whose products are important in intracellular antioxidant defense. Any or all of these effects could be operational *in vivo* either physiologically or pharmacologically. Novel experimental approaches may be necessary to sort out the relative importance of one over others. Examples of the obvious importance of the role of carnitine lie in the observations in experimental animals that carnitine supplements can attenuate the nephrotoxicity of cisplatin (Chang et al., 2002) and the cardiotoxicity of doxorubicin (Alberts et al., 1978), two important but perhaps under-utilized chemotherapeutic agents, due to their inherent toxicity toward normal cells.

TABLE 25.1   Potential therapeutic uses for carnitine and/or its esters in humans

Disease or condition	Comment	References
HIV infection and antiretroviral therapy	Increase CD4 cell count, reduce lymphocyte apoptosis; improve symptoms of neuropathy; prevent cardiovascular damage; decrease serum triacylglycerols; treat antiretroviral therapy-associated lipodystrophy	Ilias et al., 2004; Youle et al., 2007
Cancer chemotherapy	Alleviation of chemotherapy-induced fatigue, nephrotoxicity, cardiomyopathy	Graziano et al., 2002; Cruciani et al., 2009
Type 2 diabetes	Improves non-oxidative glucose disposal; enhances effects of treatment with sibutramine or orlistat on lipid profile, insulin resistance parameters, glycemic control and inflammation indices	Mingrone, 2004; Arduini et al., 2008; Derosa, et al., 2010a,b
Chronic diabetic neuropathy	Alleviates pain, improves nerve-fiber regeneration and vibration perception	Sima et al., 2005
Endothelial dysfunction associated with type 2 diabetes mellitus and/or obesity	Attenuates free-fatty-acid-induced endothelial dysfunction	Shankar et al., 2004
Peripheral vascular disease	Improves initial and maximal treadmill walking distance	Hiatt, 2004; Andreozzi, 2009
Congestive heart failure	Increases exercise capacity and reduces ventricular size	Anand et al., 1998
Angina pectoris	Increases exercise workload tolerated prior to onset of angina, and decreases ST segment depression (electrocardiographic evidence of ischemia) during exercise	Higdon and Drake, 2007
Long-term therapy following acute myocardial infarction	Reduction of left ventricular dilation; lowered incidence of death, congestive heart failure, and ischemic events	Iliceto et al., 1995
Seizure disorders treated with valproic acid	Attenuates hyperammonemia; may be particularly effective with anticonvulsant polytherapy that includes valproic acid	Coulter, 1995; Gidal et al., 1997
Treatment of conditions with pivoxil-containing prodrugs	Pivalate is transesterified to carnitine and is quantitatively excreted as pivaloyl-L-carnitine, which may lead to carnitine depletion if exogenous carnitine is not provided	Brass, 2002
Male reproductive dysfunction	Improve sperm concentration, total sperm counts and forward motility, and viability of sperm in patients with astheno- and oligoasthenozoospermia	Agarwal and Said, 2004
Hyperthyroidism	Inhibits thyroid action by inhibiting thyroid hormone entry into the nucleus	Benvenga et al., 2003

Note: Some "therapeutic" uses may also be considered "dietary supplement" use. For example, L-carnitine is included in a formula marketed as a diet supplement to enhance fertility and improve reproductive health.

Controlled clinical trials should be designed and implemented to establish efficacy in the many clinical conditions in which carnitine and/or its esters are presumed to be of benefit. Some health claims for nutritional supplements have little or no scientific or medical basis. For carnitine and its esters, claims have been made based on studies in experimental animals, testimony, anecdotal evidence, and research studies in humans that do not meet accepted standards for proof of efficacy. For some claims the standard placebo-controlled, double-blind paradigm would be very difficult or impossible to implement, due to lack of accessibility of definitive, quantitative endpoint(s), and/or the requirement for large sample sizes to detect small but meaningful physiological or pathological differences in a heterogeneous population. Nevertheless, there is great promise for the use of these supplements to restore and/or maintain healthy metabolic function.

Suggestions for Further Reading

Flanagan, J.L., Simmons, P.A., Vehige, J., et al. (2010) Role of carnitine in disease. Nutr Metab 7, 30 (doi:10.1186/1743-7075-7-30). PMID 20398344.

Jones, L.L., McDonald, D.A., and Borum, P.R. (2010) Acylcarnitines: role in brain. Prog Lipid Res 49, 61–75.

Rebouche, C.J. (2010) L-Carnitine, acetyl-L-carnitine, and propionyl-L-carnitine. In P.M. Coates, J.M. Betz, M.R. Blackman, et al. (eds), Encyclopedia of Dietary Supplements, 2nd Edn. Informa Healthcare, New York, pp. 107–114.

Zammit, V.A., Ramsay, R.R., Bonomini, M., et al. (2009) Carnitine, mitochondrial function and therapy. Adv Drug Deliv Rev 61, 1353–1362.

References

Agarwal, A. and Said, T.M. (2004) Carnitines and male infertility. Reprod Biomed Online 8, 376–384.

Alberts, D.S., Peng, Y.M., Moon, T.E., et al. (1978) Carnitine prevention of adriamycin toxicity in mice. Biomedicine 29, 265–268.

Ames, B.N. (2003) Delaying the mitochondrial decay of aging – a metabolic tune-up. Alzheimer Dis Assoc Dis 17(Suppl 2), S54–S57.

Ames, B.N. and Liu, J. (2004) Delaying the mitochondrial decay of aging with acetylcarnitine. Ann NY Acad Sci 1033, 108–116.

Anand, I., Chandrashekhan, Y., De Giuli, F., et al. (1998) Acute and chronic effects of propionyl-L-carnitine on the hemodynamics, exercise capacity, and hormones in patients with congestive heart failure. Cardiovasc Drugs Ther 12, 291–299.

Andreozzi, G.M. (2009) Propionyl-L-carnitine: intermittent claudication and peripheral arterial disease. Expert Opin Pharmacother 10, 2697–2707.

Anonymous (2009) L-Carnitine effects in overweight dogs. Food for Thought™ Technical Bulletin No. 126R. The P and G Company. http://www.iams.com/pet-health/dog-article/l-carnitine-effects-in-overweight-dogs (accessed 23rd January, 2012).

Arduini, A., Bonomini, M., Savica, V., et al. (2008) Carnitine in metabolic disease: Potential for pharmacological intervention. Pharmacol Ther 120, 149–156.

Arduini, A., Mancinelli, G., and Ramsay, R.R. (1990a) Palmitoyl-L-carnitine, a metabolic intermediate of the fatty acid incorporation pathway in erythrocyte membrane phospholipids. Biochem Biophys Res Commun 173, 212–217.

Arduini, A., Rossi, M., Mancinelli, G., et al. (1990b) Effect of L-carnitine and acetyl-L-carnitine on the human erythrocyte membrane stability and deformability. Life Sci 47, 2395–2400.

Arduini, A., Zibellini, G., Ferrari, L., et al. (2001) Participation of carnitine palmitoyltransferase in the synthesis of dipalmitoylphosphatidylcholine in rat alveolar type II cells. Mol Cell Biochem 218, 81–86.

Bartlett, K. and Eaton, S. (2004) Mitochondrial β-oxidation. Europ J Biochem 271, 462–469.

Benvenga, S., Lapa, D., Cannavò, S., et al. (2003) Successive thyroid storms treated with L-carnitine and low doses of methimazole. Am J Med 115, 417–418.

Borum, P.R. (1995) Carnitine in neonatal nutrition. J Child Neurol 10(Suppl), 2S25–2S31.

Borum, P.R. and Broquist, H.P. (1977) Purification of S-adenosylmethionine:ε-N-L-lysine methyl-transferase. The first enzyme in carnitine biosynthesis. J Biol Chem 252, 5651–5655.

Brass, E.P. (2002) Pivalate-generating prodrugs and carnitine homeostasis in man. Pharmacol Rev 54, 589–598.

Brass, E.P. (2004) Carnitine and sports medicine. Use or abuse? Ann NY Acad Sci 1033, 67–78.

Calabrese, V., Cornelius, C., Dinkova-Kostova, A.T., et al. (2009) Vitagenes, cellular stress response, and acetylcarnitine: relevance to hormesis. BioFactors 35, 146–160.

Chang, B., Nishikawa, M., Sato, E., et al. (2002) L-Carnitine inhibits cisplatin-induced injury of the kidney and small intestine. Arch Biochem Biophys 405, 55–64.

Coulter, D.L. (1995) Carnitine deficiency in epilepsy: risk factors and treatment. J Child Neurol 10(Suppl), 2A32–2A39.

Crill, C.M. and Helms, R.A. (2007) The use of carnitine in pediatric nutrition. *Nutr Clin Pract* **22**, 204–213.

Crill, C.M., Storm, M.C., Christensen, M.L., *et al.* (2006) Carnitine supplementation in premature neonates: effect on plasma and red blood cell concentrations, nutrition parameters and morbidity. *Clin Nutr* **26**, 886–896.

Cruciani, R.A., Dvorkin, E., Homel, P., *et al.* (2009) L-Carnitine supplementation in patients with advanced cancer and carnitine deficiency: a double-blind, placebo-controlled study. *J Pain Symptom Manage* **37**, 622–631.

D'Argenio, G., Petillo, O., Margarucci, S., *et al.* (2010) Colon *OCTN2* gene expression is up-regulated by peroxisome proliferator-activated receptor γ in humans and mice and contributes to local and systemic carnitine homeostasis. *J Biol Chem* **285**, 27078–27087.

Demarquoy, J., Georges, W., Rigault, C., *et al.* (2004) Radioisotopic determination of L-carnitine content in foods commonly eaten in Western countries. *Food Chem* **86**, 137–142.

Derosa, G., Maffioli, P., Ferrari, I., *et al.* (2010a) Orlistat and L-carnitine compared to orlistat alone on insulin resistance in obese diabetic patients. *Endocr J* **57**, 777–786.

Derosa, G., Maffioli, P., Salvadeo, S.A.T., *et al.* (2010b) Effects of combination of silbutramine and L-carnitine compared with silbutramine monotherapy on inflammatory parameters in diabetic patients. *Metabolism* **60**, 421–429.

Eaton, S. (2002) Control of mitochondrial β-oxidation flux. *Prog Lipid Res* **41**, 197–239.

Enomoto, A., Wempe, M.F., Tsuchida, H., *et al.* (2002) Molecular identification of a novel carnitine transporter specific to human testis. Insights into the mechanism of carnitine recognition. *J Biol Chem* **277**, 36262–36271.

Fujiya, M., Musch, M.W., Nakagawa, Y., *et al.* (2007) The *Bacillus subtilis* quorum-sensing molecule CSF contributes to intestinal homeostasis via OCTN2, a host cell membrane transporter. *Cell Host Microbe* **1**, 299–308.

Gadaleta, M.N., Petruzzella, V., Daddabbo, L., *et al.* (1994) Mitochondrial DNA transcription and translation in aged rat. Effect of acetyl-L-carnitine. *Ann NY Acad Sci* **717**, 150–160.

Gidal, B.E., Inglese, C.M., Meyer, J.F., *et al.* (1997) Diet- and valproate-induced transient hyperammonemia: effect of L-carnitine. *Pediatr Neurol* **16**, 301–305.

Graziano, F., Bisonni, R., Catalano, V., *et al.* (2002) Potential role of levocarnitine supplementation for the treatment of chemotherapy-induced fatigue in non-anaemic cancer patients. *Br J Cancer* **86**, 1854–1857.

Gülçin, I. (2006) Antioxidant and antiradical activities of L-carnitine. *Life Sci* **78**, 803–811.

Hashimoto, N., Suzuki, F., Tamai, I., *et al.* (1998) Gene-dose effect on carnitine transport activity in embryonic fibroblasts of JVS mice as a model of human carnitine transporter deficiency. *Biochem Pharmacol* **55**, 1729–1732.

Heo, K., Odle, J., Han, I.K., *et al.* (2000) Dietary carnitine improves nitrogen utilization in growing pigs fed low energy, fat-containing diets. *J Nutr* **130**, 1809–1814.

Hiatt, W.R. (2004) Carnitine and peripheral arterial disease. *Ann NY Acad Sci* **1033**, 92–98.

Higdon, J. and Drake, V.J. (2007) L-Carnitine. The Linus Pauling Institute Micronutrient Information Center. http://lpi.oregonstate.edu/infocenter/othernuts/carnitine/ (accessed 23rd January, 2012).

Higgins, T., Chaykin, S., Hammond, K.B., *et al.* (1972) Trimethylamine N-oxide synthesis: a human variant. *Biochem Med* **6**, 392–396.

Ho, J.Y., Kraemer, W.J., Volek, J.S., *et al.* (2010) L-Carnitine L-tartrate supplementation favorably affects biochemical markers of recovery from physical exertion in middle-aged men and women. *Metabolism* **59**, 1190–1199.

Hokland, B.M. and Bremer, J. (1986) Metabolism and excretion of carnitine and acylcarnitine in the perfused rat kidney. *Biochim Biophys Acta* **886**, 223–230.

Horiuchi, M., Kobayashi, K., Tomomura, M., *et al.* (1992) Carnitine administration to juvenile visceral steatosis mice corrects the suppressed expression of urea cycle enzymes by normalizing their transcription. *J Biol Chem* **267**, 5032–5035.

Iacobazzi, V., Naglieri, M.A., Stanley, C.A., *et al.* (1998) The structure and organization of the human carnitine/acylcarnitine translocase (CACT) gene. *Biochem Biophys Res Commun* **252**, 770–774.

Ilias, I., Manoli, I., Blackman, M.R., *et al.* (2004) L-Carnitine and acetyl-L-carnitine in the treatment of complications associated with HIV infection and antiretroviral therapy. *Mitochondrion* **4**, 163–168.

Iliceto, S., Scrutinio, D., Bruzzi, P., *et al.* (1995) Effects of L-carnitine administration on left ventricular remodeling after acute anterior myocardial infarction: the L-Carnitine Ecocardiografia Digitalizzata Infarto Miocardico (CEDIM) trial. *J Am Coll Cardiol* **26**, 380–387.

Jacobs, P.L., Goldstein, E.R., Blackburn, W., *et al.* (2009) Glycine propionyl-L-carnitine produces enhanced anaerobic work capacity with reduced lactate accumulation in resistance trained males. *J Int Soc Sports Nutr* **6**, 9.

Jeulin, C. and Lewin, L.M. (1996) Role of free L-carnitine and acetyl-L-carnitine in post-gonadal maturation of mammalian spermatozoa. *Human Reprod Update* **2**, 87–102.

Juliet, P.A.R., Joyee, A.G., Jayaraman, G., *et al.* (2005) Effect of L-carnitine on nucleic acid status of aged rat brain. *Exp Neurol* **191**, 33–40.

Kraemer, W.J., Volek, J.S., and Dunn-Lewis, C. (2008) L-Carnitine supplementation: influence upon physiological function. *Curr Sports Med Rep* **7**, 218–223.

Kumaran, S., Subathra, M., Balu, M., *et al.* (2005) Supplementation of L-carnitine improves mitochondrial enzymes in heart and skeletal muscle of aged rats. *Exp Aging Res* **31**, 55–67.

Laforêt, P. and Vianey-Saban, C. (2010) Disorders of muscle lipid metabolism: diagnostic and therapeutic challenges. *Neuromusc Dis* **20**, 693–700.

Lamhonwah, A.M., Ackerley, C.A., Tilups, A., *et al.* (2005) OCTN3 is a mammalian peroxisomal membrane carnitine transporter. *Biochem Biophys Res Commun* **338**, 1966–1972.

Lamhonwah, A.M., Skaug, J., Scherer, S.W., *et al.* (2003) A third human carnitine/organic cation transporter (OCTN3) as a candidate for the 5q31 Crohn's disease locus (IBD5). *Biochem Biophys Res Commun* **301**, 98–101.

Liu, J., Head, E., Kuratsune, H., *et al.* (2004) Comparison of the effects of L-carnitine and acetyl-L-carnitine on carnitine levels, ambulatory activity, and oxidative stress biomarkers in the brain of old rats. *Ann NY Acad Sci* **1033**, 117–131.

Liu, J., Killilea, D.W., and Ames, B.N. (2002) Age-associated mitochondrial oxidative decay: improvement of carnitine acetyltransferase substrate-binding affinity and activity in brain by feeding old rats acetyl-L-carnitine and/or R-α-lipoic acid. *Proc Natl Acad Sci USA* **99**, 1876–1881.

Lombard, K.A., Olson, A.L., Nelson, S.E., *et al.* (1989) Carnitine status of lactoovovegetarians and strict vegetarian adults and children. *Am J Clin Nutr* **50**, 301–306.

Mancinelli, A., Longo, A., Shanahan, K., *et al.* (1995) Disposition of L-carnitine and acetyl-L-carnitine in the isolated perfused rat kidney. *J Pharmacol Exp Ther* **274**, 1122–1128.

Manoli, I., De Martino, M.U., Kino, T., *et al.* (2004) Modulatory effects of L-carnitine on glucocorticoid receptor activity. *Ann NY Acad Sci* **1033**, 147–157.

Mingrone, G. (2004) Carnitine in type 2 diabetes. *Ann NY Acad Sci* **1033**, 99–107.

Montgomery, S.A., Thal, L.J., and Amrein, R. (2003) Meta-analysis of double blind randomized controlled clinical trials of acetyl-L-carnitine versus placebo in the treatment of mild cognitive impairment and mild Alzheimer's disease. *Int Clin Psychopharmacol* **18**, 61–71.

Nyhan, W.L. and Ozand, P.T. (1998) *Atlas of Metabolic Diseases*. Chapman & Hall Medical, London, pp. 212–216.

Palmieri, F., Indiveri, C., Bisaccia, F., *et al.* (1995) Mitochondrial metabolite carrier proteins: purification, reconstitution, and transport studies. In G. Attardi and A. Chomyn (eds), *Methods in Enzymology, vol. 260: Mitochondrial Biogenesis and Genetics, Part A*. Academic Press, San Diego, pp. 349–369.

Paradies, G., Ruggiero, F.M., Petrosillo, G., *et al.* (1994) Effect of aging and acetyl-L-carnitine on the activity of cytochrome oxidase and adenine nucleotide translocase in rat heart mitochondria. *FEBS Lett* **350**, 213–215.

Paradies, G., Ruggiero, F.M., Petrosillo, G., *et al.* (1995) Carnitine-acylcarnitine translocase activity in cardiac mitochondria from aged rats: the effect of acetyl-L-carnitine. *Mech Ageing Dev* **84**, 103–112.

Pignatelli, P., Lenti, L., Sanguigni, V., *et al.* (2003) Carnitine inhibits arachidonic acid turnover, platelet function, and oxidative stress. *Am J Physiol* **284**, H41–H48.

Pons, R. and De Vivo, D.C. (1995) Primary and secondary carnitine deficiency syndromes. *J Child Neurol* **10**(Suppl), 2S8–2S24.

Raiten, D.J., Talbot, J.M., and Waters, J.H. (eds) (1998) Assessment of nutrient requirements for infant formulas. *J Nutr* **128**(Suppl), 2120S–2121S.

Ramsay, R.R. (1999) The role of the carnitine system in peroxisomal fatty acid oxidation. *Am J Med Sci* **318**, 28–35.

Ramsay, R.R., Gandour, R.D., and van der Leij, F.R. (2001) Molecular enzymology of carnitine transfer and transport. *Biochim Biophys Acta* **1546**, 21–43.

Rebouche, C.J. (1992) Carnitine function and requirements during the life cycle. *FASEB J* **6**, 3379–3386.

Rebouche, C.J. (2004) Kinetics, pharmacokinetics, and regulation of L-carnitine and acetyl-L-carnitine metabolism. *Ann NY Acad Sci* **1033**, 30–41.

Rebouche, C.J. (2006) Carnitine. In M.E. Shils, M. Shike, A.C. Ross, *et al.* (eds), *Modern Nutrition in Health and Disease*, 10th Edn. Williams and Wilkins, Baltimore, pp. 537–544.

Rebouche, C.J. and Broquist, H.P. (1976) Carnitine biosynthesis in *Neurospora crassa*: Enzymatic conversion of lysine to ε-*N*-trimethyllysine. *J Bacteriol* **126**, 1207–1214.

Rebouche, C.J. and Chenard, C.A. (1991) Metabolic fate of dietary carnitine in human adults: identification and quantification of urinary and fecal metabolites. *J Nutr* **121**, 539–546.

Rebouche, C.J. and Engel, A.G. (1980) Significance of renal γ-butyrobetaine hydroxylase for carnitine biosynthesis in man. *J Biol Chem* **255**, 8700–8705.

Rebouche, C.J. and Engel, A.G. (1984) Kinetic compartmental analysis of carnitine metabolism in the human carnitine deficiency syndromes. Evidence for alterations in tissue carnitine transport. *J Clin Invest* **73**, 857–867.

Rebouche, C.J. and Seim, H. (1998) Carnitine metabolism and its regulation in microorganisms and mammals. *Annu Rev Nutr* **18**, 39–61.

Rebouche, C.J., Mack, D.L., and Edmonson, P.F. (1984) L-Carnitine dissimilation in the gastrointestinal tract of the rat. *Biochemistry* **23**, 6422–6426.

Salvioli, G. and Neri, M. (1994) L-Acetylcarnitine treatment of mental decline in the elderly. *Drugs Exp Clin Res* **20**, 169–176.

Shankar, S.S., Mirzamohammadi, B., Walsh, J.P., *et al.* (2004) L-Carnitine may attenuate free fatty acid-induced endothelial dysfunction. *Ann NY Acad Sci* **1033**, 189–197.

Shortland, G.J., Walter, J.H., Stroud, C., *et al.* (1998) Randomized controlled trial of L-carnitine as a nutritional supplement in preterm infants. *Arch Dis Child Fetal Neonatal Ed* **78**, F185–F188.

Sima, A.A.F., Calvani, M., Mehra, M., *et al.* (2005) Acetyl-L-carnitine improves pain, nerve regeneration, and vibratory perception in patients with chronic diabetic neuropathy. *Diabetes Care* **28**, 89–94.

Spiering, B.A., Kraemer, W.J., Vingren, J.L., *et al.* (2007) Responses of criterion variables to different supplemental doses of L-carnitine L-tartrate. *J Strength Cond Res* **21**, 259–264.

Tempesta, E., Casella, L., Pirrongelli, C., *et al.* (1987) L-Acetylcarnitine in depressed elderly subjects. A cross-over study vs. placebo. *Drugs Exp Clin Res* **12**, 417–423.

Tomomura, M., Tomomura, A., Abu Musa, D.M.A., *et al.* (1996) Long-chain fatty acids suppress the induction of urea cycle enzyme genes by glucocorticoid action. *FEBS Lett* **399**, 310–312.

Tsuchida, H., Anzai, N., Shin, H.J., *et al.* (2010) Identification of a novel organic anion transporter mediating carnitine transport in mouse liver and kidney. *Cell Physiol Biochem* **25**, 511–522.

Vaz, F.M. and Wanders, R.J.A. (2002) Carnitine biosynthesis in mammals. *Biochem J* **361**, 417–429.

Villani, R.G., Gannon, J., Self, M., *et al.* (2000) L-Carnitine supplementation combined with aerobic training does not promote weight loss in moderately obese women. *Int J Sport Nutr* **10**, 199–207.

Wu, X., Prasad, P.D., Leibach, F.H., *et al.* (1998) cDNA sequence, transport function, and genomic organization of human OCTN2, a new member of the organic cation transporter family. *Biochem Biophys Res Commun* **246**, 589–595.

Yamaguti, K., Kuratsune, H., Watanabe, Y., *et al.* (1996) Acylcarnitine metabolism during fasting and after refeeding. *Biochem Biophys Res Commun* **225**, 740–746.

Youle, M., Osio, M., on behalf of the ALCAR Study Group (2007) A double-blind, parallel-group, placebo-controlled, multicentre study of acetyl L-carnitine in the symptomatic treatment of antiretroviral toxic neuropathy in patients with HIV-1 infection. *HIV Medicine* **8**, 241–250.

26

CHOLINE

STEVEN H. ZEISEL, MD, PhD AND KAREN D. CORBIN, PhD, RD

University of North Carolina at Chapel Hill, Kannapolis, North Carolina, USA

Summary

Choline is an essential nutrient for numerous biological functions. Experience derived from research on choline has pioneered a new way of thinking about nutrition requirements for optimal health. This body of knowledge has demonstrated that the dietary need for choline is highly individual, and is based on several factors including genetics and gender. In addition, measurable biological consequences related to inadequate choline intake can be improved with dietary interventions at various life stages, from the embryo to adulthood. In this chapter, we describe key aspects of choline function and metabolism in health and disease.

Introduction

Function of Choline and Its Metabolites

Choline is needed for the normal function of all cells since its derivatives contribute to the structural integrity and signaling functions of cell membranes. It is a major source of methyl-groups in the diet, directly affects cholinergic neurotransmission, and is required for hepatic lipid homeostasis (Zeisel, 2006a). Growing experimental evidence has identified important roles for choline in multiple metabolic processes such as gene expression (Niculescu *et al.*, 2004), carcinogenesis (Zeisel *et al.*, 1997), apoptosis (Albright *et al.*, 1996), lipid metabolism (Noga *et al.*, 2002; Watkins *et al.*, 2003), and early brain development (Albright *et al.*, 1999b, 2003; Cermak *et al.*, 1999; Craciunescu *et al.*, 2003; Meck and Williams, 2003).

Choline-containing compounds of physiologic importance include betaine, acetylcholine (ACh), phosphatidylcholine (PtdCho), platelet-activating factor, sphingomyelin (SM), lysosphingomyelin, glycerophosphocholine, and phosphocholine (some of these compounds are depicted in Figure 26.1). Choline (via its metabolite betaine), is a methyl group donor that can influence gene expression (discussed later in this chapter) (Zeisel, 2009). Also, betaine is an osmolyte used in the glomerulus of the kidney to help reabsorb water. PtdCho (lecithin) is the predominant phospholipid (>50%) in most mammalian membranes and is also important for regulating hepatic lipid packaging and export (Li and Vance, 2008). SM is another choline-containing phospholipid important for membrane and myelin formation (Diringer and Koch, 1973). Transmembrane signaling processes can involve hydrolysis of both of these choline-phospholipids, thereby generating

Present Knowledge in Nutrition, Tenth Edition. Edited by John W. Erdman Jr, Ian A. Macdonald and Steven H. Zeisel.
© 2012 International Life Sciences Institute. Published 2012 by John Wiley & Sons, Inc.

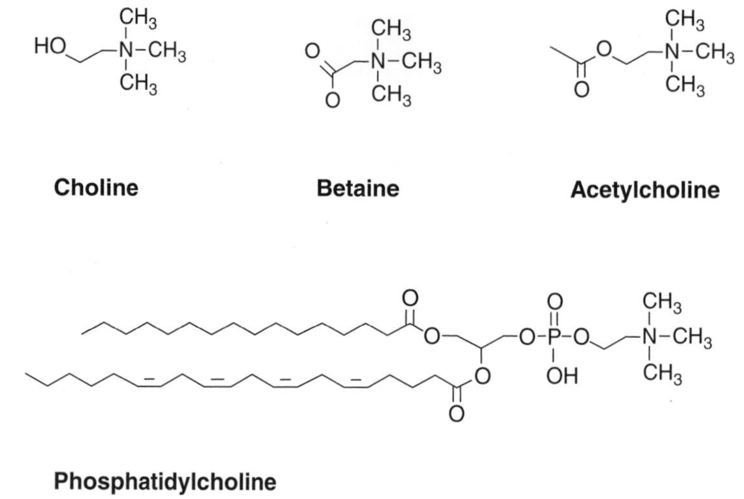

FIG. 26.1 Structures of several important choline-containing molecules.

second messengers (including diacylglycerol, arachidonic acid, and ceramide) that alter cell function (Exton, 1994; Merrill *et al.*, 1995). ACh is a neurotransmitter important in brain functions such as memory and mood (Blusztajn and Wurtman, 1983).

Choline Metabolism

Choline Synthesis and Metabolic Fate
Aside from diet, new choline molecules can only be derived from de novo synthesis of PtdCho that is catalyzed by phosphatidylethanolamine-N-methyltransferase (PEMT) (Vance *et al.*, 1997). This pathway is primarily active in the liver. PEMT catalyzes the methylation of phosphatidylethanolamine (PtdEtn) to PtdCho. During this process, S-adenosylmethionine (SAM) is used as a methyl donor for the formation of a new choline moiety. Free choline can be generated by the catabolism of PtdCho (it can also be formed by the catabolism of SM and ACh). It is important to note that two pathways that use choline molecules to catalyze PtdCho biosynthesis are ubiquitously active in the body: the cytidine diphosphocholine and base-exchange pathways. Neither of these pathways leads to a net synthesis of choline moiety; rather, they allow for redistribution of existing choline molecules (Zeisel, 2006a).

Although the main metabolic fate of choline is the formulation of PtdCho, this fate is, in part, tissue specific. All tissues form PtdCho via the cytidine diphosphocholine pathway, and the first enzyme in this pathway has high affinity for choline. Once this pathway is saturated, the available choline can be oxidized to form betaine (in selected tissues such as kidney and liver) or it can be acetylated to form ACh (in selected tissues such as placenta and neurons). These pathways are highly regulated and interrelated to maintain choline homeostasis (Li and Vance, 2008).

Methyl Group Metabolism
The metabolism of choline, folate, vitamin B$_{12}$, vitamin B$_6$, and methionine are interrelated (Figure 26.2) and disturbances in one of these metabolic pathways are associated with compensatory changes in the others. This means the methyl groups from methyltetrahydrofolate (MTHF), methionine, and choline can be interchangeable. For example, methionine can be formed via two pathways: from homocysteine using methyl groups donated by MTHF (Finkelstein, 2000), or from methyl groups donated by betaine (derived from choline) (Park and Garrow, 1999). MTHF synthesis also has two pathways: via one-carbon units derived from serine or from the methyl groups of choline through dimethylglycine (Gregory *et al.*, 2000). Finally, choline can be formed from methyl groups derived from SAM (Vance *et al.*, 1997). When animals and humans are fed a diet deficient in choline, dietary folate requirements increase because more MTHF is used to remethylate homocysteine in the liver (Selhub *et al.*, 1991; Varela-Moreiras *et al.*, 1992). If instead they are fed a diet deficient in folate, dietary

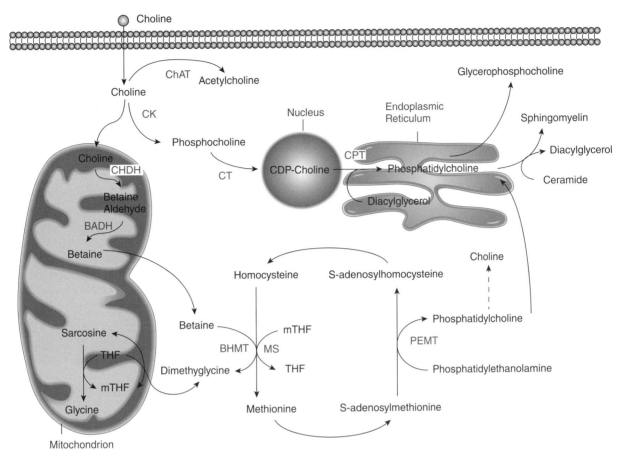

FIG. 26.2 Choline, folate, and homocysteine metabolism are closely interrelated. The pathways for the metabolism of these three nutrients intersect at the formation of methionine from homocysteine. BADH, betaine aldehyde dehydrogenase; BHMT, betaine homocysteine methyltransferase; ChAT, choline acetyl-transferase; CHDH, choline dehydrogenase; CK, choline kinase; CPT, choline phosphotransferase; CT, CTP:phosphocholine cytidylyltransferase; MS, methionine synthase; mTHF, methyl tetrahydrofolate; PEMT, phosphatidylethanolamine-N-methyltransferase; THF, tetrahydrofolate.

choline requirements increase as choline becomes the primary methyl donor (Kim *et al.*, 1995; Jacob *et al.*, 1998, 1999). That several parallel pathways have evolved to help ensure adequate supply of methyl donors demonstrates the physiologic importance of these compounds.

Digestion, Absorption, and Transport

Choline in foods is mostly in the form of phospholipids, phosphocholine, glycerophosphocholine, and choline. After ingestion and subsequent digestion by pancreatic and mucosal enzymes, the water-soluble compounds, choline, phosphocholine, and glycerophosphocholine, enter the portal circulation and are taken up by the liver. They rapidly accumulate in the liver where most are phos-

phorylated and used to make membranes and lipoproteins (Zeisel *et al.*, 1980c). Approximately half of the lipid-soluble choline compounds in foods, PtdCho and SM, persist intact after digestion. They enter via the lymphatic system in chylomicrons, miss first-pass metabolism by the liver, and can reach other organs (Garner *et al.*, 1995). Choline enters tissues by diffusion and mediated transport. Several genes have been identified in the control of choline transport across plasma and mitochondrial membranes (Brandon *et al.*, 2004; Ferguson *et al.*, 2004; Yuan *et al.*, 2004; Michel and Bakovic, 2009). In brain, a specific carrier mechanism transports free choline across the blood–brain barrier at a rate proportional to the serum choline concentration (Cornford *et al.*, 1978; Pardridge,

1986). Cholinergic neurons have a special high-affinity choline transporter that helps them accumulate choline (Vickroy *et al.*, 1984).

Dietary Requirements for Choline

Choline Is an Essential Nutrient

The human requirement for the nutrient choline was officially recognized with the establishment of adequate intake (AI) recommendations by the US Institute of Medicine in 1998 (Institute of Medicine, 1998). Previously, choline was not considered an essential nutrient for humans because there is an endogenous pathway for de novo biosynthesis of the choline moiety as part of PtdCho (Bremer and Greenberg, 1961). Despite this capacity to synthesize some choline in liver, healthy humans with normal folate and vitamin B_{12} status that are fed a choline-deficient diet develop fatty liver, liver damage (elevated plasma alanine [or aspartate] transaminase), or muscle damage (elevated creatine phosphokinase-CPK) that resolves when choline is restored to the diet (da Costa *et al.*, 2004; Fischer *et al.*, 2007). Metabolic abnormalities (decreased clearance of homocysteine) (da Costa *et al.*, 2005), elevations in markers of DNA damage (da Costa *et al.*, 2006b) and alterations in lymphocyte gene expression (Niculescu *et al.*, 2007) are also observed in choline deficiency. In addition, humans fed intravenously with solutions low in choline develop liver dysfunction that resolves when choline is added back to their diets (Buchman *et al.*, 1995). Clearly, endogenous synthesis is not sufficient to prevent signs of choline deficiency, and thus choline is not a dispensable nutrient for some humans. The same is true for most non-ruminant species of animals (Zeisel and Blusztajn, 1994).

The Institute of Medicine suggests an AI for choline for adult men of 550 mg/day and for adult women 425 mg/day (Institute of Medicine, 1998). Pregnancy creates increased demands for dietary choline, and pregnant female rats are susceptible to choline deficiency (Zeisel *et al.*, 1995). In rats, maternal liver choline concentration over the course of pregnancy declines from 130 μmol/L in non-pregnant adult rats to 38 μmol/L in late pregnancy (Gwee and Sim, 1978). The AI for choline during pregnancy is 450 mg/day (Institute of Medicine, 1998). Because lactation further consumes maternal choline stores, sensitivity to choline deficiency is higher in lactating rats than non-lactating rats (Zeisel *et al.*, 1995). Thus, the AI for lactating women is estimated to be 550 mg/day of choline

(Institute of Medicine, 1998). Though no experimental data exists, AIs for infants have been extrapolated from amounts that would be consumed in breast milk, and AIs for children have been extrapolated based on adult requirements per kilogram of body mass, resulting in estimates of the AI that vary between 125 and 375 mg/day, depending on age (Institute of Medicine, 1998). Currently, studies are underway to refine these estimates of human choline requirements; some report that a subset of adult humans become depleted of choline at intakes of 750 mg/day (Fischer *et al.*, 2007), suggesting that the estimates for the AI may be too low for adults.

Dietary Sources of Choline

Many foods contain significant amounts of choline or choline-containing compounds (Zeisel *et al.*, 2003a,b). Eggs, beef, chicken, fish, and milk as well as select plant foods like cruciferous vegetables and certain beans are particularly good sources of choline, providing at least 10% of the daily requirement per serving (Caudill, 2010). (See also http://www.nal.usda.gov/fnic/foodcomp/Data/Choline/Choline.html [last accessed July 5 2010] and Zeisel *et al.*, 2003a,b). Humans on an *ad libitum* diet ingest between 150 mg and 600 mg choline/day (as free choline and choline esters) (Shaw *et al.*, 2004; Fischer *et al.*, 2005; Cho *et al.*, 2006; Bidulescu *et al.*, 2007; Konstantinova *et al.*, 2008; Xu *et al.*, 2009). In the 2005 NHANES study, only a small portion of Americans in all age groups ate diets achieving the recommended intake for choline (Jensen *et al.*, 2007).

Foods also contain the choline metabolite betaine (Zeisel *et al.*, 2003a,b). It cannot be converted to choline, but can be used as a methyl donor, thereby sparing some choline requirements (Craig, 2004; Dilger *et al.*, 2007). Plant-derived foods can be a rich source of betaine (named after beets), with grain products being particularly good sources. Lecithin, a phosphatidylcholine-rich fraction prepared during commercial purification of phospholipids, is often added to foods as an emulsifying agent, or may be taken as a dietary supplement (Zeisel *et al.*, 2003a,b).

Supply of Choline to the Fetus and Infant

In mammals, the placenta delivers choline to the fetus by pumping it against a concentration gradient (Sweiry *et al.*, 1986). The placenta may serve as a special reserve storage pool (in the form of ACh) to ensure adequate delivery of choline to the fetus. Choline concentration in amniotic fluid is several-fold higher than in maternal blood (Ozarda Ilcol *et al.*, 2002). The mammary gland extracts choline from maternal blood, synthesizes important choline metabolites, and secretes all of these into milk (Zeisel *et al.*, 1986; Chao *et al.*, 1988; Yang *et al.*, 1988; Holmes-McNary *et al.*, 1996).

The total choline content of human milk is approximately 1.3–1.5 mmol/L (Holmes-McNary *et al.*, 1996) and is likely important for sustaining tissue choline in the infant. Many commercially available infant formulas were reformulated to deliver amounts of choline similar to that in mature human breast milk; before 2007 many formulas had less than is present in human breast milk (Holmes-McNary *et al.*, 1996). Choline concentrations in the plasma or serum of human infants are elevated during the perinatal period (compared with adults) and slowly decrease after birth until they reach adult levels some time after the first year of life (Zeisel *et al.*, 1980a; Zeisel and Wurtman, 1981; Ozarda Ilcol *et al.*, 2002; Ilcol *et al.*, 2005). Presumably these very high levels ensure enhanced availability of choline to the developing tissues.

Deficiency and Assessment of Choline Nutrition Status

Given that many people consume less than the AI level of choline, it is plausible that some are choline deficient. Animal studies have given us important clues as to the biological consequences of choline deficiency. Choline deficiency in the rat reduces concentrations of choline and choline-containing compounds in the liver (Zeisel *et al.*, 1989). Low intake of dietary choline in rodents is associated with liver dysfunction, compromised renal function, infertility, growth impairment, and hypertension (Zeisel, 2006a). In adults, particularly those with genotypes that increase susceptibility to choline deficiency, low choline intake leads to fatty liver, elevated liver enzymes, and muscle abnormalities (Buchman *et al.*, 2001; Kohlmeier *et al.*, 2005). Low choline intake by women during pregnancy and lactation affects brain development and other important health parameters in offspring (Albright *et al.*, 2001; Zeisel, 2006a,b; Fischer *et al.*, 2007). Further discussions on the role of choline for critical biological functions and health outcomes are found later in this chapter.

Choline nutrition status can be assessed in several ways. Hepatic phosphocholine levels are highly correlated with dietary choline intake, are quite sensitive to even moderate choline deficiency, and can be measured via magnetic reso-

nance spectroscopy in humans (Pomfret *et al.*, 1990; Cohen *et al.*, 1995; da Costa *et al.*, 2005). Plasma concentrations of choline are also responsive to dietary intake; concentrations increase accordingly with intake of choline and decrease with a choline-inadequate diet (Burt *et al.*, 1980; Sheard *et al.*, 1986; Chawla *et al.*, 1989; Zeisel *et al.*, 1991; Buchman *et al.*, 1993). Studies in humans suggest plasma choline concentrations normally exhibit a two-fold variation in response to consumption of common foods (Zeisel *et al.*, 1980b). There appears to be an internal mechanism to keep choline concentrations above a certain minimal level: approximately 50–75% of normal, even after a week-long fast (Savendahl *et al.*, 1997). Plasma PtdCho concentrations also decrease with choline deficiency and have been looked at as another possible marker of choline status, however, this measure may not accurately reflect choline status if lipoprotein metabolism is perturbed. An individual with an elevation in homocysteine concentrations after a methionine load, who has adequate status for folate and vitamins B_6 and B_{12}, should be suspected to be choline deficient (da Costa *et al.*, 2005).

In a recent study, metabolomic profiling of individuals was an effective measure that could predict which individuals would develop organ dysfunction when fed a choline-deficient diet. Metabolites in several pathways, including choline, lipid, carnitine, and amino acid metabolism, predicted which individuals would develop choline deficiency-related fatty liver (Sha *et al.*, 2010). Apparently, there is a complex and interrelated profile of metabolites that can define those at increased risk for the consequences of choline deficiency.

Individual Variation in Choline Requirements

As discussed earlier, choline deficiency in humans leads to liver dysfunction and muscle damage. Susceptibility to organ damage due to choline deficiency is linked to genetics (da Costa *et al.*, 2006a). Dietary choline requirements are governed by an individual's ability to make choline *de novo*, and genes in choline and folate metabolism are intertwined in this process. Several very common single nucleotide polymorphisms (SNPs) in these genes have a profound impact on choline needs (Kohlmeier *et al.*, 2005; da Costa *et al.*, 2006a). For example, the PEMT rs12325817 SNP has an obvious effect in postmenopausal women where one allele is sufficient to increase the risk of developing choline deficiency-induced organ dysfunction by 25-fold (Kohlmeier *et al.*, 2005; da Costa *et al.*, 2006a; Fischer *et al.*, 2007). Another SNP in the PEMT gene (rs7946) is present more often in people with fatty liver (Song *et al.*, 2005).

Premenopausal women who are carriers of the very common 5,10-methylenetetrahydrofolate dehydrogenase SNP (MTHFD1; rs2236225) are more than 15 times as likely as non-carriers to develop choline deficiency-induced organ dysfunction (Kohlmeier *et al.*, 2005). A choline intake exceeding current dietary recommendations also preserves markers of cellular methylation and attenuates DNA damage in a genetic subgroup of folate-compromised men with an SNP in the methylenetetrahydrofolate reductase *MTHFR* gene (Shin *et al.*, 2010). Based on these diet–gene interactions, the polymorphisms in choline-related genes seem to become important when humans eat diets low in choline content.

When deprived of dietary choline, 77% of men and 80% of postmenopausal women, develop fatty liver, liver damage or muscle damage, while only 44% of premenopausal women develop such signs of organ dysfunction (Kohlmeier *et al.*, 2005; da Costa *et al.*, 2006a; Fischer *et al.*, 2007). The promoter for the PEMT gene is estrogen responsive (da Costa *et al.*, 2006a; Resseguie *et al.*, 2007), and this likely explains why premenopausal women are more resistant to developing organ dysfunction when fed a choline-deficient diet (Resseguie *et al.*, 2007). Indeed, an SNP in the promoter region of *PEMT* (rs12325817) marks a haplotype with decreased estrogen-responsive induction of PEMT activity; likely there is a defect in the estrogen-responsive sites in the promoter of *PEMT*. These findings suggest that gender and estrogen status also influence individual requirements for choline.

We now have a much better set of parameters to define an individual's requirement for choline. These parameters include a combination of genetics, gender, and metabolomics, and there are likely additional mechanisms such as epigenetics and proteomics. Research to fine-tune our understanding of these signatures is ongoing.

Role of Choline in Normal Cell and Organ Function

Cell and Mitochondrial Membranes

Choline is an important component of membranes. Choline deficiency significantly decreases the PtdCho concentrations in plasma membranes (da Costa *et al.*, 1995; Yen *et al.*, 1999). Mitochondrial membranes are similarly affected, with resulting loss of mitochondrial membrane potential and leakage of reactive oxygen species (Vrablic

et al., 2001; Albright *et al.*, 2003a). Several species of lipids are components of cell membranes. Docosahexaenoic acid (DHA) is an omega-3 polyunsaturated fatty acid important for cell membranes. It is an essential nutrient, and its metabolism is linked to choline metabolism. DHA and choline work together to promote healthy brain development by affecting gene expression and membrane signaling. The aberrant effects of choline deficiency on brain cell differentiation and apoptosis can be corrected by DHA supplementation via the normalization of membrane lipid composition (da Costa *et al.*, 2010).

Aside from the important role of choline in mitochondrial membrane integrity, several effects of choline on mitochondrial function are known. In choline-deficient rodents, mitochondria have abnormal morphology and bioenergetics (Teodoro *et al.*, 2008). Choline dehydrogenase (CHDH), one of the enzymes catalyzing the formation of betaine from choline, is located on the inner mitochondrial membrane. Deletion of the *Chdh* gene in mice impairs mitochondrial function, especially in sperm (Burg, 1995). These effects of choline on plasma and mitochondrial membranes are vital for normal cellular and organelle function.

Gene Regulation

Through its function as a methyl donor, choline has important roles in regulation of gene expression via epigenetic mechanisms. Epigenetics refers to alterations in gene expression that do not involve changes to the DNA sequence. These modifications include methylation of DNA, several modifications to histones (proteins around which DNA is wrapped), imprinting, and small interfering RNA. Methylation is an important modification on proteins (histones) or DNA (typically on cytosines in regions where cytosines are followed by guanines) that regulates gene expression by altering chromatin structure or promoter activity, respectively (Dolinoy *et al.*, 2007).

Epigenetic patterns are heritable, but can change over an individual's lifetime. Since the inherited DNA code is generally not changeable, with the exception of rare mutations, epigenetics represents a mechanism by which gene expression can be altered differentially throughout one's lifetime. Epigenetics is responsive to many environmental cues including diet, exercise, smoking, and pollution, allowing for integration of environmental signals with genetics (Zeisel, 2009). Even though methylation patterns are inherited, a mother's diet during pregnancy can lead to changes that manifest in altered, permanent health outcomes for offspring. Choline-deficiency during pregnancy induces changes in DNA methylation and gene expression in multiple tissues including brain and liver (Meck and Williams, 1999, 2003; Niculescu *et al.*, 2005; Mehedint *et al.*, 2010b). The functional consequences of choline-mediated epigenetic changes in gene expression are discussed in subsequent sections of this chapter.

Brain

Perhaps the most comprehensive knowledge related to the role of choline in organ function concerns the brain. The perinatal period is a critical time for cholinergic organization of brain function (Meck *et al.*, 1988; Pyapali *et al.*, 1998; Albright *et al.*, 1999a; Jones *et al.*, 1999; Montoya *et al.*, 2000). In rats and mice, choline availability is very important for development of the hippocampus and septum (Meck *et al.*, 1988; Albright *et al.*, 1999b; Craciunescu *et al.*, 2003; Meck and Williams, 2003). In humans, hippocampal development occurs from day 56 of pregnancy through 4 years after birth (Dani *et al.*, 1997; Seress *et al.*, 2001); no experiments have yet been completed to determine if human hippocampal development can be influenced by dietary choline, though there is no reason to believe that it would not be. It should be noted that the hippocampus is one of the few areas of the brain in which nerve cells continue to multiply slowly in adults (Markakis and Gage, 1999; van Praag *et al.*, 1999).

During brain development, neural progenitor cells must proliferate, migrate, differentiate, and survive to form the structures that we recognize in adult brain. Choline regulates neural precursor cell proliferation, migration, differentiation, and apoptosis (Albright *et al.*, 1998, 1999a,b, 2001, 2003b; Craciunescu *et al.*, 2003). The development of the nervous system (neurogenesis) is coordinated with blood-vessel formation (angiogenesis) so that there is adequate delivery of nutrients and oxygen to developing neurons. In mice, choline deficiency during pregnancy prevents normal angiogenesis, and this is presumably tightly associated with the effects of choline deficiency on neurogenesis (Mehedint *et al.*, 2010a).

The effects of dietary choline during embryonic brain development are detectable later in life. Neurons of the hippocampus have larger soma and an increased number of primary and secondary basal dendritic branches in rodents exposed to extra choline during the perinatal period (Loy *et al.*, 1991; Williams *et al.*, 1998; Li *et al.*, 2004). In rodents, choline supplementation during critical periods of neonatal development can have long-term ben-

eficial effects on memory (Wong-Goodrich *et al.*, 2008). The likely mechanisms for these effects of choline involve DNA methylation, altered gene expression, and associated changes in stem-cell proliferation and differentiation (Zeisel, 2006b). In mice, choline deficiency during critical periods of brain development leads to impaired differentiation and function of brain cells due to global and gene-specific alterations in methylation (Niculescu *et al.*, 2006). These types of changes lead to irreversible changes in hippocampal function manifesting in impaired nerve cell potentiation, memory, and behavior that persist into adulthood (Meck and Williams, 1999, 2003; Niculescu *et al.*, 2005; Zeisel, 2009). Overall, substantial evidence exists to support the enduring nature of the changes in brain function induced by choline availability.

Liver

Two key roles for choline in the normal function of the liver have been studied extensively. The first relates to gene expression. A diet devoid of methyl-group donors, including choline, leads to altered expression of proteins that are necessary for the DNA methylation process to function properly. These genetic alterations increase the risk of cancer and fat accumulation in the liver (Ghoshal *et al.*, 2006; Pogribny *et al.*, 2009). A second key role of choline in liver function involves lipid metabolism. The packaging and transport of lipids in the liver are dependent on the formation of very-low-density lipoprotein (VLDL). PtdCho, produced by PEMT in the liver, is indispensable for the export of triglycerides from the liver so they can be delivered to other tissues. Without this function of PEMT, due to either choline deficiency (Varela-Moreiras *et al.*, 1992; Buchman *et al.*, 2001; Kohlmeier *et al.*, 2005; da Costa *et al.*, 2006a) or gene deletion (Noga *et al.*, 2002; Zhu *et al.*, 2003), fat accumulates in the liver and this can lead to significant dysfunction. In addition to its function in the formation of PtdCho, PEMT is involved in regulating the flux of lipids between liver and plasma and the delivery of essential fatty acids (such as DHA) to tissues (Watkins *et al.*, 2003).

Choline in Human Health

Birth Defects

Inhibition of choline uptake and metabolism is associated with the development of NTDs in mice (Fisher *et al.*, 2001, 2002). Recent evidence suggests this may also be the case in humans: A retrospective case-control study

(400 cases and 400 controls) of periconceptional dietary intakes of choline in women in California found that women in the lowest quartile for daily dietary choline intake had four times the risk of having a baby with an NTD than did women in the highest quartile for intake (Shaw *et al.*, 2004). Elevated NTD risk was also associated with lower concentrations of serum total choline in a folate-fortified population (Shaw *et al.*, 2009). Additional birth defects have been associated with choline deficiency including cleft lip (Shaw *et al.*, 2006), hypospadias (defect in male urethra) (Carmichael *et al.*, 2009), heart defects (Chan *et al.*, 2010), and congenital diaphragmatic hernia (Yang *et al.*, 2008).

Cancer

Choline is the only nutrient for which dietary deficiency causes development of hepatocarcinomas without any known carcinogen. Interestingly, choline-deficient rats not only have a higher incidence of spontaneous hepatocarcinoma, but they are markedly sensitized to the effects of administered carcinogens. Choline deficiency is therefore considered to stimulate both cancer-initiating and cancer-promoting activities (Newberne and Rogers, 1986). Breast cancer also has been associated with choline deficiency. In the first study to examine the association between choline and breast cancer, Xu *et al.* (2008) found that breast cancer risk was reduced by 24% among women with high dietary intakes of choline and was increased in women with the PEMT rs12325817 SNP (previously discussed; reduces estrogen-induced PEMT activity). Importantly, a subsequent analysis determined that breast cancer mortality was reduced by high intakes of choline and betaine and by an SNP in the betaine homocysteine methyltransferase gene (BHMT; rs3733890; catalyzes the synthesis of methionine from betaine and homocysteine) (Xu *et al.*, 2009).

Neurological Disorders

In addition to the role of choline in brain development, behavior, and memory (Zeisel, 2006b), there are suggestions that choline supplementation may be a useful treatment in several neurological disorders. Choline and DHA promote neuronal membrane and synapse formation, and diminish the accumulation of amyloid plaque in brain, especially when used in combination (Kamphuis and Wurtman, 2009). These mechanisms are of particular importance in ameliorating the cognitive derangements associated with Alzheimer's disease (Kamphuis and Wurtman, 2009). In addition, Citicoline (cytidine 5′-

diphosphocholine), a choline-containing molecule, is being used to treat stroke and traumatic brain injury (Conant and Schauss, 2004). A recent study in a mouse model of Down syndrome reported improvements in cognitive function and emotion regulation in mice born to mothers supplemented with choline during the perinatal period (Moon *et al.*, 2010). Other studies in mice suggest that perinatal choline supplementation may reduce the neurological consequences of fetal alcohol syndrome (Thomas *et al.*, 2007).

Fatty Liver

As discussed earlier, one important function of the liver is the maintenance of whole-body lipid homeostasis. Choline, especially via its metabolite, PtdCho, is essential for the export of lipids from the liver (Noga *et al.*, 2002; Noga and Vance, 2003). In animal models and humans, choline deficiency is associated with fat accumulation in the liver (steatosis). Such non-alcoholic fatty liver disease (NAFLD) is the most common chronic liver disorder, occurring in 30% of the general population and 65–90% of overweight or obese individuals (Ong and Younossi, 2007). Although choline deficiency in humans is associated with hepatic steatosis, not all individuals are affected equally. Thus far, genetics and gender have been implicated as factors that mediate risk (Kohlmeier *et al.*, 2005; Song *et al.*, 2005; da Costa *et al.*, 2006a; Fischer *et al.*, 2007). However, the mechanisms by which these factors lead to NAFLD, additional factors that are involved, and how these factors are associated with the progression of benign NAFLD to more severe liver disease, are still unknown. It is important to note that fatty liver is tightly associated with metabolic syndrome, obesity, insulin resistance and cardiovascular disease (Moore, 2010), providing further evidence that choline-mediated pathways could have far reaching effects on chronic disease.

Heart Disease

Little is known about the health consequences of choline overnutrition, but emerging evidence suggests this is a cause of concern. Dietary intake of choline results in bacteria-mediated formation of trimethylamine (TMA) which is then absorbed and oxidized by flavin monooxygenases in the liver to form TMAO. These metabolites of choline impart a fishy body odor after very large doses of choline (grams) (Institute of Medicine and National Academy of Sciences USA, 1998; Zeisel *et al.*, 1983). Of greater concern, small molecules formed from dietary choline are associated with increased risk for cardiovascular disease (Wang *et al.*, 2011). Three metabolites present in the blood of humans (choline, betaine and trimethylamine N-oxide (TMAO)) predicted risk for atherosclerotic cardiovascular disease (CVD) in an independent large clinical cohort (Wang *et al.*, 2011). In addition, dietary supplementation of apoliproprotein E knockout mice with choline or TMAO increased the development of atherosclerotic lesions. TMAO, formed by gut bacteria from the choline metabolite trimethylamine (TMA) was the critical intermediate responsible for the atherosclerotic effects of dietary choline as the atherosclerotic effect of choline did not occur in germ-free mice or in mice where there was antibiotic-suppression of intestinal microbiome, while TMAO retained its atherogeneic effect in these mice (Wang *et al.*, 2011). Additional side effects observed due to excess dietary choline include vomiting, sweating, gastrointestinal side effects, and hypotension. A tolerable upper limit of choline for adults has been set at 3.5 g/day (Institute of Medicine and National Academy of Sciences USA, 1998), but at that time, link between dietary choline and CVD was not known. It is evident that research is needed to delineate the individual upper limit for dietary choline.

Future Directions

The decades of research invested in understanding the biological functions of choline in humans have resulted in an impressive body of knowledge about the health implications of choline insufficiency and supplementation. There are several areas of research that warrant further attention to enhance our understanding of the choline needs of individuals and the potential to use this nutrient, and its derivatives, as therapeutic agents. For example, little is known about the role of choline in inflammation, and epidemiological studies have linked low dietary choline intake to higher concentrations of proinflammatory markers (Detopoulou *et al.*, 2008; Fargnoli *et al.*, 2008). Another area where additional research is needed is assessment of the prevalence of choline variants in large populations. Thus far, most of our knowledge about choline variants, particularly as they relate to the role of choline deficiency and organ function, stems from populations in North Carolina. As we broaden our knowledge, it will be important for groups of researchers around the world to assess the impact of ethnicity and environment on the prevalence and consequences of choline-related SNPs. This will greatly enhance our ability to evaluate the role of choline in disease. We are only beginning to understand the wide-reaching effects of choline in systems biology as a direct result of its role as a methyl donor. The implications of epigenetics in health and disease are becoming increasingly evident, and the specific mechanisms by which choline is involved remain to be elucidated. The interesting links between genetics and metabolomics in determining risk for diseases associated with choline deficiency are initial examples of the complexities of the signatures that we will need to define to distinguish those who are at risk of disease from those who are not. This is true not just for choline, but for all nutrients. Finally, the observations that dietary choline influences brain development and can perhaps moderate the severity of several neurological diseases is mostly based on data obtained in rodents. Human studies confirming these effects are needed. The future of choline and nutrition research in general is exciting and complex. The hope is to ultimately understand how all nutrients act in concert with systems biology to determine the health outcomes of individuals.

Acknowledgments

Funded by a grant from the National Institutes of Health (DK55865). Support for this work was also provided by grants from the National Institutes of Health to the University of North Carolina Nutrition and Obesity Research Center (DK56350) and Clinical and Translational Research Center (M01RR00046 and UL1RR025747).

Suggestions for Further Reading
Fischer, L.M., daCosta, K., Kwock, L., *et al.* (2007) Sex and menopausal status influence human dietary requirements for the nutrient choline. *Am J Clin Nutr* **85**, 1275–1285.

References

Albright, C.D., Friedrich, C.B., Brown, E.C., *et al.* (1999) Maternal dietary choline availability alters mitosis, apoptosis and the localization of TOAD-64 protein in the developing fetal rat septum. *Brain Res* **115**, 123–129.

Albright, C.D., Lui, R., Bethea, T.C., *et al.* (1996) Choline deficiency induces apoptosis in SV40-immortalized CWSV-1 rat hepatocytes in culture. *FASEB J* **10**, 510–516.

Albright, C.D., Mar, M.H., Friedrich, C.B., *et al.* (2001) Maternal choline availability alters the localization of p15Ink4B and p27Kip1 cyclin-dependent kinase inhibitors in the developing fetal rat brain hippocampus. *Dev Neurosci* **23**, 100–106.

Albright, C.D., Salganik, R.I., Craciunescu, C.N., *et al.* (2003a) Mitochondrial and microsomal derived reactive oxygen species mediate apoptosis induced by transforming growth factor-beta1 in immortalized rat hepatocytes. *J Cell Biochem* **89**, 254–261.

Albright, C.D., Siwek, D.F., Craciunescu, C.N., *et al.* (2003b) Choline availability during embryonic development alters the localization of calretinin in developing and aging mouse hippocampus. *Nutr Neurosci* **6**, 129–134.

Albright, C.D., Tsai, A.Y., Friedrich, C.B., *et al.* (1999) Choline availability alters embryonic development of the hippocampus and septum in the rat. *Brain Res* **113**, 13–20.

Albright, C.D., Tsai, A.Y., Mar, M.-H., *et al.* (1998) Choline availability modulates the expression of TGFß1 and cytoskeletal proteins in the hippocampus of developing rat brain. *Neurochem Res* **23**, 751–758.

Bidulescu, A., Chambless, L.E., Siega-Riz, A.M., *et al.* (2007) Usual choline and betaine dietary intake and incident coronary heart disease: the Atherosclerosis Risk in Communities (ARIC) study. *BMC Cardiovasc Disord* **7**, 20.

Blusztajn, J.K. and Wurtman, R.J. (1983) Choline and cholinergic neurons. *Science* **221**, 614–620.

Brandon, E.P., Mellott, T., Pizzo, D.P., *et al.* (2004) Choline transporter 1 maintains cholinergic function in choline acetyltransferase haploinsufficiency. *J Neurosci* **24**, 5459–5466.

Bremer, J. and Greenberg, D. (1961) Methyl transferring enzyme system of microsomes in the biosynthesis of lecithin (phosphatidylcholine). *Biochim Biophys Acta* **46**, 205–216.

Buchman, A., Dubin, M., Moukarzel, A., *et al.* (1995) Choline deficiency: a cause of hepatic steatosis during parenteral nutrition that can be reversed with intravenous choline supplementation. *Hepatology* **22**, 1399–1403.

Buchman, A.L., Ament, M.E., Sohel, M., *et al.* (2001) Choline deficiency causes reversible hepatic abnormalities in patients receiving parenteral nutrition: proof of a human choline requirement: a placebo-controlled trial. *JPEN J Parenter Enteral Nutr* **25**, 260–268.

Buchman, A.L., Moukarzel, A., Jenden, D.J., *et al.* (1993) Low plasma free choline is prevalent in patients receiving long term parenteral nutrition and is associated with hepatic aminotransferase abnormalities. *Clin Nutr* **12**, 33–37.

Burg, M. (1995) Molecular basis of osmotic regulation. *Am J Physiol* **268**, F983–996.

Burt, M.E., Hanin, I., and Brennan, M.F. (1980) Choline deficiency associated with total parenteral nutrition. *Lancet* **2**, 638–639.

Carmichael, S.L., Yang, W., Correa, A., *et al.* (2009) Hypospadias and intake of nutrients related to one-carbon metabolism. *J Urol* **181**, 315–321; discussion 321.

Caudill, M.A. (2010) Pre- and postnatal health: evidence of increased choline needs. *J Am Diet Assoc* **110**, 1198–1206.

Cermak, J.M., Blusztajn, J.K., Meck, W.H., *et al.* (1999) Prenatal availability of choline alters the development of acetylcholinesterase in the rat hippocampus. *Dev Neurosci* **21**, 94–104.

Chan, J., Deng, L., Mikael, L.G., *et al.* (2010) Low dietary choline and low dietary riboflavin during pregnancy influence reproductive outcomes and heart development in mice. *Am J Clin Nutr* **91**, 1035–1043.

Chao, C.K., Pomfret, E.A., and Zeisel, S.H. (1988) Uptake of choline by rat mammary-gland epithelial cells. *Biochem J* **254**, 33–38.

Chawla, R.K., Wolf, D.C., Kutner, M.H., *et al.* (1989) Choline may be an essential nutrient in malnourished patients with cirrhosis. *Gastroenterology* **97**, 1514–1520.

Cho, E., Zeisel, S.H., Jacques, P., *et al.* (2006) Dietary choline and betaine assessed by food-frequency questionnaire in relation to plasma total homocysteine concentration in the Framingham Offspring Study. *Am J Clin Nutr* **83**, 905–911.

Cohen, B.M., Renshaw, P.F., Stoll, A.L., *et al.* (1995) Decreased brain choline uptake in older adults. An in vivo proton magnetic resonance spectroscopy study. *JAMA* **274**, 902–907.

Conant, R. and Schauss, A.G. (2004) Therapeutic applications of citicoline for stroke and cognitive dysfunction in the elderly: a review of the literature. *Altern Med Rev* **9**, 17–31.

Cornford, E.M., Braun, L.D., and Oldendorf, W.H. (1978) Carrier mediated blood–brain barrier transport of choline and certain choline analogs. *J Neurochem* **30**, 299–308.

Craciunescu, C.N., Albright, C.D., Mar, M.H., *et al.* (2003) Choline availability during embryonic development alters progenitor cell mitosis in developing mouse hippocampus. *J Nutr* **133**, 3614–3618.

Craig, S.A. (2004) Betaine in human nutrition. *Am J Clin Nutr* **80**, 539–549.

da Costa, K.A., Badea, M., Fischer, L.M., *et al.* (2004) Elevated serum creatine phosphokinase in choline-deficient humans: mechanistic studies in C2C12 mouse myoblasts. *Am J Clin Nutr* **80**, 163–170.

da Costa, K.A., Gaffney, C.E., Fischer, L.M., *et al.* (2005) Choline deficiency in mice and humans is associated with increased plasma homocysteine concentration after a methionine load. *Am J Clin Nutr* **81**, 440–444.

da Costa, K.A., Garner, S.C., Chang, J., *et al.* (1995) Effects of prolonged (1 year) choline deficiency and subsequent refeeding of choline on 1,2,-sn-diradylglycerol, fatty acids and protein kinase C in rat liver. *Carcinogenesis* **16**, 327–334.

da Costa, K.A., Kozyreva, O.G., Song, J., *et al.* (2006a) Common genetic polymorphisms affect the human requirement for the nutrient choline. *FASEB J* **20**, 1336–1344.

da Costa, K.A., Niculescu, M.D., Craciunescu, C.N., *et al.* (2006b) Choline deficiency increases lymphocyte apoptosis and DNA damage in humans. *Am J Clin Nutr* **84**, 88–94.

da Costa, K.A., Rai, K.S., Craciunescu, C.N., *et al.* (2010) Dietary docosahexaenoic acid supplementation modulates hippocampal development in the Pemt-/- mouse. *J Biol Chem* **285**, 1008–1015.

Dani, S., Hori, A., and Walter, G. (eds) (1997) *Principles of Neural Aging*. Elsevier, Amsterdam.

Detopoulou, P., Panagiotakos, D.B., Antonopoulou, S., *et al.* (2008) Dietary choline and betaine intakes in relation to concentrations of inflammatory markers in healthy adults: the ATTICA study. *Am J Clin Nutr* **87**, 424–430.

Dilger, R.N., Garrow, T.A., and Baker, D.H. (2007) Betaine can partially spare choline in chicks but only when added to diets containing a minimal level of choline. *J Nutr* **137**, 2224–2228.

Diringer, H. and Koch, M.A. (1973) Biosynthesis of sphingomyelin. Transfer of phosphorylcholine from phosphatidylcholine to erythro-ceramide in a cell-free system. *Hoppe Seylers Z Physiol Chem* **354**, 1661–1665.

Dolinoy, D.C., Weidman, J.R., and Jirtle, R.L. (2007) Epigenetic gene regulation: linking early developmental environment to adult disease. *Reprod Toxicol* **23**, 297–307.

Exton, J.H. (1994) Phosphatidylcholine breakdown and signal transduction. *Biochim Biophys Acta* **1212**, 26–42.

Fargnoli, J.L., Fung, T.T., Olenczuk, D.M., *et al.* (2008) Adherence to healthy eating patterns is associated with higher circulating total and high-molecular-weight adiponectin and lower resistin concentrations in women from the Nurses' Health Study. *Am J Clin Nutr* **88**, 1213–1224.

Ferguson, S.M., Bazalakova, M., Savchenko, V., *et al.* (2004) Lethal impairment of cholinergic neurotransmission in hemicholinium-3-sensitive choline transporter knockout mice. *Proc Natl Acad Sci USA* **101**, 8762–8767.

Finkelstein, J.D. (2000) Pathways and regulation of homocysteine metabolism in mammals. *Semin Thromb Hemost* **26**, 219–225.

Fischer, L.M., da Costa, K., Kwock, L., *et al.* (2007) Sex and menopausal status influence human dietary requirements for the nutrient choline. *Am J Clin Nutr* **85**, 1275–1285.

Fischer, L.M., Scearce, J.A., Mar, M.H., *et al.* (2005) Ad libitum choline intake in healthy individuals meets or exceeds the proposed adequate intake level. *J Nutr* **135**, 826–829.

Fisher, M.C., Zeisel, S.H., Mar, M.H., *et al.* (2001) Inhibitors of choline uptake and metabolism cause developmental abnormalities in neurulating mouse embryos. *Teratology* **64**, 114–122.

Fisher, M.C., Zeisel, S.H., Mar, M.H., *et al.* (2002) Perturbations in choline metabolism cause neural tube defects in mouse embryos in vitro. *FASEB J* **16**, 619–621.

Garner, S.C., Mar, M.-H., and Zeisel, S.H. (1995) Choline distribution and metabolism in pregnant rats and fetuses are influenced by the choline content of the maternal diet. *J Nutr* **125**, 2851–2858.

Ghoshal, K., Li, X., Datta, J., *et al.* (2006) A folate- and methyl-deficient diet alters the expression of DNA methyltransferases and methyl CpG binding proteins involved in epigenetic gene silencing in livers of F344 rats. *J Nutr* **136**, 1522–1527.

Gregory, J.F., 3rd, Cuskelly, G.J., Shane, B., *et al.* (2000) Primed, constant infusion with [2H3]serine allows in vivo kinetic measurement of serine turnover, homocysteine remethylation, and transsulfuration processes in human one-carbon metabolism. *Am J Clin Nutr* **72**, 1535–1541.

Gwee, M.C. and Sim, M.K. (1978) Free choline concentration and cephalin-N-methyltransferase activity in the maternal and foetal liver and placenta of pregnant rats. *Clin Exp Pharmacol. Physiol* **5**, 649–653.

Holmes-McNary, M., Cheng, W.L., Mar., M.H., *et al.* (1996) Choline and choline esters in human and rat milk and infant formulas. *Am J Clin Nutr* **64**, 572–576.

Ilcol, Y.O., Ozbek, R., Hamurtekin, E., *et al.* (2005) Choline status in newborns, infants, children, breast-feeding women, breast-fed infants and human breast milk. *J Nutr Biochem* **16**, 489–499.

Institute of Medicine (1998) Choline. In *Dietary Reference Intakes for Folate, Thiamin, Riboflavin, Niacin, Vitamin B12, Pantothenic Acid, Biotin, and Choline*, 1. National Academy Press, Washington, DC, pp. 390–422

Jacob, R., Jenden, D., Okoji, R., *et al.* (1998) Choline status of men and women is decreased by low dietary folate. *FASEB J* **12**, A512.

Jacob, R.A., Jenden, D.J., Allman-Farinelli, M.A., *et al.* (1999) Folate nutriture alters choline status of women and men fed low choline diets. *J Nutr* **129**, 712–717.

Jensen, H.H., Batres-Marquez, S.P., Carriquiry, A., *et al.* (2007) Choline in the diets of the U.S. population: NHANES, 2003–2004. *FASEB J* **21**, lb219.

Jones, J.P., Meck, W., Williams, C.L., *et al.* (1999) Choline availability to the developing rat fetus alters adult hippocampal long-term potentiation. *Brain Res* **118**, 159–167.

Kamphuis, P.J. and Wurtman, R.J. (2009) Nutrition and Alzheimer's disease: pre-clinical concepts. *Eur J Neurol* **16**(Suppl 1), 12–18.

Kim, Y.-I., Miller, J.W., da Costa, K.-A., *et al.* (1995) Folate deficiency causes secondary depletion of choline and phosphocholine in liver. *J Nutr* **124**, 2197–2203.

Kohlmeier, M., da Costa, K.A., Fischer, L.M., *et al.* (2005) Genetic variation of folate-mediated one-carbon transfer pathway predicts susceptibility to choline deficiency in humans. *Proc Natl Acad Sci USA* **102**, 16025–16030.

Konstantinova, S.V., Tell, G.S., Vollset, S.E., *et al.* (2008) Dietary patterns, food groups, and nutrients as predictors of plasma choline and betaine in middle-aged and elderly men and women. *Am J Clin Nutr* **88**, 1663–1669.

Li, Q., Guo-Ross, S., Lewis, D.V., *et al.* (2004) Dietary prenatal choline supplementation alters postnatal hippocampal structure and function. *J Neurophysiol* **91**, 1545–1555.

Li, Z. and Vance, D.E. (2008) Phosphatidylcholine and choline homeostasis. *J Lipid Res* **49**, 1187–1194.

Loy, R., Heyer, D., Williams, C.L., *et al.* (1991) Choline-induced spatial memory facilitation correlates with altered distribution and morphology of septal neurons. *Adv Exp Med Biol* **295**, 373–382.

Markakis, E.A. and Gage, F.H. (1999) Adult-generated neurons in the dentate gyrus send axonal projections to field CA3 and are surrounded by synaptic vesicles. *J Comp Neurol* **406**, 449–460.

Meck, W.H. and Williams, C.L. (1999) Choline supplementation during prenatal development reduces proactive interference in spatial memory. *Brain Res* **118**, 51–59.

Meck, W.H. and Williams, C.L. (2003) Metabolic imprinting of choline by its availability during gestation: implications for memory and attentional processing across the lifespan. *Neurosci Biobehav Rev* **27**, 385–399.

Meck, W.H., Smith, R.A., and Williams, C.L. (1988) Pre- and postnatal choline supplementation produces long-term facilitation of spatial memory. *Dev Psychobiol* **21**, 339–353.

Mehedint, M.G., Craciunescu, C.N., and Zeisel, S.H. (2010a) Maternal dietary choline deficiency alters angiogenesis in fetal mouse hippocampus. *Proc Natl Acad Sci USA* **107**, 12834–12839.

Mehedint, M.G., Niculescu, M.D., Craciunescu, C.N., *et al.* (2010b) Choline deficiency alters global histone methylation and epigenetic marking at the Re1 site of the calbindin 1 gene. *FASEB J* **24**, 184–195.

Merrill, A.H., Jr, Liotta, D.C., and Riley, R.E. (1995) Bioactive properties of sphingosine and structurally related compounds. *Handbook Lipid Res* **8**, 205–237.

Michel, V. and Bakovic, M. (2009) The solute carrier 44A1 is a mitochondrial protein and mediates choline transport. *FASEB J* **23**, 2749–2758.

Montoya, D.A., White, A.M., Williams, C.L., *et al.* (2000) Prenatal choline exposure alters hippocampal responsiveness to cholinergic stimulation in adulthood. *Brain Res Dev Brain Res* **123**, 25–32.

Moon, J., Chen, M., Gandhy, S.U., *et al.* (2010) Perinatal choline supplementation improves cognitive functioning and emotion regulation in the Ts65Dn mouse model of Down syndrome. *Behav Neurosci* **124**, 346–361.

Moore, J.B. (2010) Non-alcoholic fatty liver disease: the hepatic consequence of obesity and the metabolic syndrome. *Proc Nutr Soc* **69**(2), 211–220.

Newberne, P.M. and Rogers, A.E. (1986) Labile methyl groups and the promotion of cancer. *Annu Rev Nutr* **6**, 407–432.

Niculescu, M.D., Craciunescu, C.N., and Zeisel, S.H. (2005) Gene expression profiling of choline-deprived neural precursor cells isolated from mouse brain. *Brain Res* **134**, 309–322.

Niculescu, M.D., Craciunescu, C.N., and Zeisel, S.H. (2006) Dietary choline deficiency alters global and gene-specific DNA methylation in the developing hippocampus of mouse fetal brains. *FASEB J* **20**, 43–49.

Niculescu, M.D., da Costa, K.A., Fischer, L.M., *et al.* (2007) Lymphocyte gene expression in subjects fed a low-choline diet differs between those who develop organ dysfunction and those who do not. *Am J Clin Nutr* **86**, 230–239.

Niculescu, M.D., Yamamuro, Y., and Zeisel, S.H. (2004) Choline availability modulates human neuroblastoma cell proliferation and alters the methylation of the promoter region of the cyclin-dependent kinase inhibitor 3 gene. *J Neurochem* **89**, 1252–1259.

Noga, A.A. and Vance, D.E. (2003) A gender-specific role for phosphatidylethanolamine N-methyltransferase-derived phosphatidylcholine in the regulation of plasma high density and very low density lipoproteins in mice. *J Biol Chem* **278**, 21851–21859.

Noga, A.A., Zhao, Y., and Vance, D.E. (2002) An unexpected requirement for phosphatidylethanolamine N-methyltransferase in the secretion of very low density lipoproteins. *J Biol Chem* **277**, 42358–42365.

Ong, J.P. and Younossi, Z.M. (2007) Epidemiology and natural history of NAFLD and NASH. *Clin Liver Dis* **11**, 1–16, vii.

Ozarda Ilcol, Y., Uncu, G., and Ulus, I.H. (2002) Free and phospholipid-bound choline concentrations in serum during pregnancy, after delivery and in newborns. *Arch Physiol Biochem* **110**, 393–399.

Pardridge, W.M. (1986) Blood–brain transport of nutrients. Introduction. *Fed Proc* **45**, 2047–2049.

Park, E.I. and Garrow, T.A. (1999) Interaction between dietary methionine and methyl donor intake on rat liver betaine–homocysteine methyltransferase gene expression and organization of the human gene. *J Biol Chem* **274**, 7816–7824.

Pogribny, I.P., Tryndyak, V.P., Bagnyukova, T.V., *et al.* (2009) Hepatic epigenetic phenotype predetermines individual susceptibility to hepatic steatosis in mice fed a lipogenic methyl-deficient diet. *J Hepatol* **51,** 176–186.

Pomfret, E.A., da Costa, K., and Zeisel, S.H. (1990) Effects of choline deficiency and methotrexate treatment upon rat liver. *J Nutr Biochem* **1,** 533–541.

Pyapali, G., Turner, D., Williams, C., *et al.* (1998) Prenatal choline supplementation decreases the threshold for induction of long-term potentiation in young adult rats. *J. Neurophysiol* **79,** 1790–1796.

Resseguie, M., Song, J., Niculescu, M.D., *et al.* (2007) Phosphatidylethanolamine N-methyltransferase (PEMT) gene expression is induced by estrogen in human and mouse primary hepatocytes. *FASEB J* **21,** 2622–2632.

Savendahl, L., Mar, M.-H., Underwood, L., *et al.* (1997) Prolonged fasting results in diminished plasma choline concentration but does not cause liver dysfunction. *Am J Clin Nutr* **66,** 622–625.

Selhub, J., Seyoum, E., Pomfret, E.A., *et al.* (1991) Effects of choline deficiency and methotrexate treatment upon liver folate content and distribution. *Cancer Res* **51,** 16–21.

Seress, L., Abraham, H., Tornoczky, T., *et al.* (2001) Cell formation in the human hippocampal formation from mid-gestation to the late postnatal period. *Neuroscience* **105,** 831–843.

Sha, W., da Costa, K.A., Fischer, L.M., *et al.* (2010) Metabolomic profiling can predict which humans will develop liver dysfunction when deprived of dietary choline. *FASEB J* **24,** 2962–2975.

Shaw, G.M., Carmichael, S.L., Laurent, C., *et al.* (2006) Maternal nutrient intakes and risk of orofacial clefts. *Epidemiology* **17,** 285–291.

Shaw, G.M., Carmichael, S.L., Yang, W., *et al.* (2004) Periconceptional dietary intake of choline and betaine and neural tube defects in offspring. *Am J Epidemiol* **160,** 102–109.

Shaw, G.M., Finnell, R.H., Blom, H.J., *et al.* (2009) Choline and risk of neural tube defects in a folate-fortified population. *Epidemiology* **20,** 714–719.

Sheard, N.F., Tayek, J.A., Bistrian, B.R., *et al.* (1986) Plasma choline concentration in humans fed parenterally. *Am J Clin Nutr* **43,** 219–224.

Shin, W., Yan, J., Abratte, C.M., *et al.* (2010) Choline intake exceeding current dietary recommendations preserves markers of cellular methylation in a genetic subgroup of folate-compromised men. *J Nutr* **140,** 975–980.

Song, J., da Costa, K.A., Fischer, L.M., *et al.* (2005) Polymorphism of the PEMT gene and susceptibility to nonalcoholic fatty liver disease (NAFLD). *FASEB J* **19,** 1266–1271.

Sweiry, J.H., Page, K.R., Dacke, C.G., *et al.* (1986) Evidence of saturable uptake mechanisms at maternal and fetal sides of the perfused human placenta by rapid paired-tracer dilution: studies with calcium and choline. *J Dev Physiol* **8,** 435–445.

Teodoro, J.S., Rolo, A.P., Duarte, F.V., *et al.* (2008) Differential alterations in mitochondrial function induced by a choline-deficient diet: understanding fatty liver disease progression. *Mitochondrion* **8,** 367–376.

Thomas, J.D., Biane, J.S., O'Bryan, K.A., *et al.* (2007) Choline supplementation following third-trimester-equivalent alcohol exposure attenuates behavioral alterations in rats. *Behav Neurosci* **121,** 120–130.

van Praag, H., Kempermann, G., and Gage, F.H. (1999) Running increases cell proliferation and neurogenesis in the adult mouse dentate gyrus [see comments]. *Nat Neurosci* **2,** 266–270.

Vance, D.E., Walkey, C.J., and Cui, Z. (1997) Phosphatidylethanolamine N-methyltransferase from liver. *Biochim Biophys Acta* **1348,** 142–150.

Varela-Moreiras, G., Selhub, J., da Costa, K., *et al.* (1992) Effect of chronic choline deficiency in rats on liver folate content and distribution. *J Nutr Biochem* **3,** 519–522.

Vickroy, T.W., Roeske, W.R., and Yamamura, H.I. (1984) Sodium-dependent high-affinity binding of [3H]hemicholinium-3 in the rat brain: a potentially selective marker for presynaptic cholinergic sites. *Life Sci* **35,** 2335–2343.

Vrablic, A.S., Albright, C.D., Craciunescu, C.N., *et al.* (2001) Altered mitochondrial function and overgeneration of reactive oxygen species precede the induction of apoptosis by 1-O-octadecyl-2-methyl- rac-glycero-3-phosphocholine in p53-defective hepatocytes. *FASEB J* **15,** 1739–1744.

Wang, Z., Klipfell, E., Bennett, *et al.* (2011) Gut flora metabolism of phosphatidylcholine promotes cardiovascular disease. *Nature* **472,** 57–63.

Watkins, S.M., Zhu, X., and Zeisel, S.H. (2003) Phosphatidylethanolamine-N-methyltransferase activity and dietary choline regulate liver-plasma lipid flux and essential fatty acid metabolism in mice. *J Nutr* **133,** 3386–3391.

Williams, C.L., Meck, W.H., Heyer, D.D., *et al.* (1998) Hypertrophy of basal forebrain neurons and enhanced visuospatial memory in perinatally choline-supplemented rats. *Brain Res* **794,** 225–238.

Wong-Goodrich, S.J., Glenn, M.J., Mellott, T.J., *et al.* (2008) Spatial memory and hippocampal plasticity are differentially sensitive to the availability of choline in adulthood as a function of choline supply in utero. *Brain Res* **1237,** 153–166.

Xu, X., Gammon, M.D., Zeisel, S.H., *et al.* (2008) Choline metabolism and risk of breast cancer in a population-based study. *FASEB J* **22,** 2045–2052.

Xu, X., Gammon, M.D., Zeisel, S.H., *et al.* (2009) High intakes of choline and betaine reduce breast cancer mortality in a population-based study. *FASEB J* **23,** 4022–4028.

Yang, E.K., Blusztajn, J.K., Pomfret, E.A., *et al.* (1988) Rat and human mammary tissue can synthesize choline moiety via the methylation of phosphatidylethanolamine. *Biochem. J* **256,** 821–828.

Yang, W., Shaw, G.M., Carmichael, S.L., *et al.* (2008) Nutrient intakes in women and congenital diaphragmatic hernia in their offspring. *Birth Defects Res A Clin Mol Teratol* **82,** 131–138.

Yen, C.L., Mar, M.H., and Zeisel, S.H. (1999) Choline deficiency-induced apoptosis in PC12 cells is associated with diminished membrane phosphatidylcholine and sphingomyelin, accumulation of ceramide and diacylglycerol, and activation of a caspase. *FASEB J* **13,** 135–142.

Yuan, Z., Wagner, L., Poloumienko, A., *et al.* (2004) Identification and expression of a mouse muscle-specific CTL1 gene. *Gene* **341,** 305–312.

Zeisel, S.H. (2006a) Choline: critical role during fetal development and dietary requirements in adults. *Annu Rev Nutr* **26,** 229–250.

Zeisel, S.H. (2006b) The fetal origins of memory: the role of dietary choline in optimal brain development. *J Pediatr* **149**(5 Suppl), S131–136.

Zeisel, S.H. (2009) Epigenetic mechanisms for nutrition determinants of later health outcomes. *Am J Clin Nutr* **89,** 1488S–1493S.

Zeisel, S.H. and Blusztajn, J.K. (1994) Choline and human nutrition. *Annu Rev Nutr* **14,** 269–296.

Zeisel, S.H. and Wurtman, R.J. (1981) Developmental changes in rat blood choline concentration. *Biochem J* **198,** 565–570.

Zeisel, S.H., Albright, C.D., Shin, O.-K., *et al.* (1997) Choline deficiency selects for resistance to p53-independent apoptosis and causes tumorigenic transformation of rat hepatocytes. *Carcinogenesis* **18,** 731–738.

Zeisel, S.H., Char, D., and Sheard, N.F. (1986) Choline, phosphatidylcholine and sphingomyelin in human and bovine milk and infant formulas. *J Nutr* **116,** 50–58.

Zeisel, S.H., daCosta, K.-A., Franklin, P.D., *et al.* (1991) Choline, an essential nutrient for humans. *FASEB J* **5,** 2093–2098.

Zeisel, S.H., Epstein, M.F., and Wurtman, R.J. (1980a) Elevated choline concentration in neonatal plasma. *Life Sci* **26,** 1827–1831.

Zeisel, S.H., Growdon, R.J., Wurtman, J.H., *et al.* (1980b) Normal plasma choline responses to ingested lecithin. *Neurology* **30,** 1226–1229.

Zeisel, S.H., Mar, M.H., Howe, J.C., *et al.* (2003a) Concentrations of choline-containing compounds and betaine in common foods. *J Nutr* **133,** 1302–1307.

Zeisel, S.H., Mar, M.-H., Howe, J.C., *et al.* (2003b) Erratum: Concentrations of choline-containing compounds and betaine in common foods. *J Nutr* **133,** 2918–2919.

Zeisel, S.H., Mar, M.-H., Zhou, Z.-W., *et al.* (1995) Pregnancy and lactation are associated with diminished concentrations of choline and its metabolites in rat liver. *J Nutr* **125,** 3049–3054.

Zeisel, S.H., Story, D.L., Wurtman, R.J., *et al.* (1980c) Uptake of free choline by isolated perfused rat liver. *Proc Natl Acad Sci USA* **77,** 4417–4419.

Zeisel, S.H., Zola, T., daCosta, K., *et al.* (1989) Effect of choline deficiency on S-adenosylmethionine and methionine concentrations in rat liver. *Biochem J* **259,** 725–729.

Zhu, X., Song, J., Mar, M.H., *et al.* (2003) Phosphatidylethanolamine N-methyltransferase (PEMT) knockout mice have hepatic steatosis and abnormal hepatic choline metabolite concentrations despite ingesting a recommended dietary intake of choline. *Biochem J* **370,** 987–993.

27

DIETARY FLAVONOIDS

GARY WILLIAMSON, PhD

University of Leeds, Leeds, UK

Summary

Flavonoids are found in a wide variety of plant-based foods and beverages. Intake varies widely between individuals but is typically several hundred milligrams per day. The pathways of absorption are quite well understood and the amount absorbed and excreted for many flavonoids has been documented. For many flavonoids, a substantial percentage of the dose is absorbed, but is also rapidly metabolized and excreted within 24 hours. Some flavonoids such as proanthocyanidins and anthocyanins are poorly absorbed intact, but their catabolites are very efficiently absorbed after microbial biotransformation. Flavonoids are chemical antioxidants, but work in vivo primarily by indirect antioxidant mechanisms, such as inhibition of oxidative enzymes and induction of antioxidant defenses. Certain flavonoids modulate sugar metabolism, blood pressure, LDL cholesterol, and platelet function. Together, these mechanisms reduce the risk of cardiovascular disease, and possibly type 2 diabetes and inflammatory diseases, as supported by human intervention and epidemiological studies. Future work should focus on long-term dietary dose intervention studies and also consider the introduction of some form of recommended intake values for flavonoids.

Introduction

Flavonoids are present in all diets where plants, or foods or beverages derived from plants, are present. In plants, they protect against stress and excess ultraviolet light exposure. They also are responsible for the color of most fruits and flowers, and also contribute to the taste sensation of foods such as red wine, tea, coffee, and chocolate, as well as fruits. Flavonoids possess antioxidant activity in vitro and affect cellular and molecular processes to provide health benefits by reducing the risk of chronic diseases such as cardiovascular disease. Over the last 20 years there has been an enormous and growing interest in this class of compounds which have also been referred to as polyphenols, phytonutrients, non-nutrients, protective factors, dietary bioactives, and phytochemicals. Although there are many thousands of compounds in the plant kingdom, only a handful are present in significant amounts in the diet of most humans. This review will focus only on the flavonoids that are most abundant and important in the Western diet, and not on the minor or rare compounds, or those that are present in more exotic foods.

Present Knowledge in Nutrition, Tenth Edition. Edited by John W. Erdman Jr, Ian A. Macdonald and Steven H. Zeisel.
© 2012 International Life Sciences Institute. Published 2012 by John Wiley & Sons, Inc.

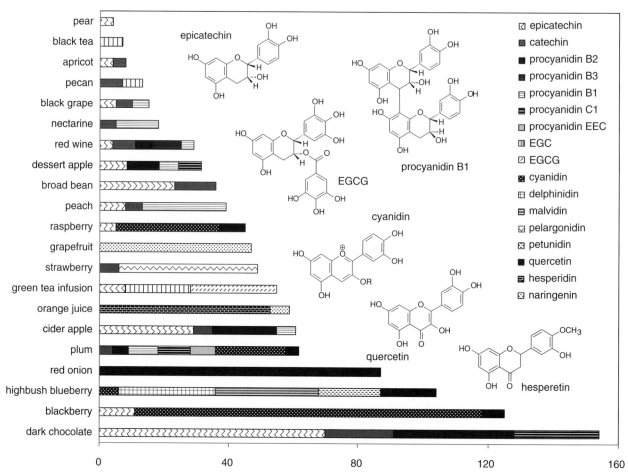

FIG. 27.1 Representative chemical structures and content of commonly occurring flavonoid-rich foods in mg per 100 g fresh weight: flavanols ([epi]catechin, procyanidins, epigallocatechin [EGC], and epigallocatechin gallate [EGCG]); anthocyanins (cyanidin, delphinidin, malvidin, pelargonidin, and petunidin); flavonols (quercetin); and flavanones (hesperidin and naringenin). All data are from the phenol explorer database (www.phenol-explorer.eu) and are in aglycone equivalents.

Catechins (including galloylated catechins and procyanidins), selected anthocyanins, quercetin, and citrus flavanones (hesperetin and naringenin) are covered, but not isoflavones (present only in soya), and phenolic compounds which are not flavonoids such as hydroxycinnamates (widely present in food and drinks, especially coffee, but less work has been done on these lower molecular weight compounds).

Classification and Distribution in Foods

Figure 27.1 shows the flavonoid content of foods and some representative chemical structures of the most abundant flavonoids. They can be considered as minor constituents

as the maximum amount in foods is always less than 1%, although the biological activity can be quite high. Figure 27.1 does not include the higher molecular weight tannins, which are not well defined at a molecular level, such as the thearubigens and theaflavins in black tea (Lewis *et al.*, 1998), and the larger procyanidins, which have only been measured in a limited range of foods such as apples (Huemmer *et al.*, 2008) and cocoa (Lazarus *et al.*, 1999). The foods highest in flavonoids are cocoa, berries, apples, onions, stone fruits, tea, citrus, and grapes. The intake of flavonoids is difficult to estimate, since the average intake will be very variable within the population. Estimates range from 26 mg/day of flavonols in the Dutch diet (Hertog *et al.*, 1993) to a median intake of total flavonoids of 239 mg/day, with a very wide range of 0.6 to 3524 mg/day among 34 708 US women (Cutler *et al.*, 2008). Mean pro(antho)cyanidin intake in the US population (>2 years old) was 58 mg/day, with the main contributions coming from consumption of apples (32%), chocolate (18%), and grapes (18%). The average consumption of 2- to 5-year-olds was 68 mg/day, for men >60 years old it was 71 mg/day, for 4- to 6-month-old infants 1.3 mg/day, and for 6- to 10-month-old infants 27 mg/day (Gu *et al.*, 2004). The mean intake of anthocyanins was also estimated in the United States to be 12.5 mg/day (Wu *et al.*, 2006). This value is surprisingly low and is subject to enormous inter-individual variation, since one portion of fresh blueberries contains 300–400 mg anthocyanins per 100 g fresh weight, but the stated "average" intake is only ~1 g blueberries per day. An individual consuming 100 g blueberries in a day will therefore consume ~30 times the average US consumption of anthocyanins (Wu *et al.*, 2006).

Absorption, Metabolism, and Excretion – Quantitative and Mechanistic Aspects

The principles controlling absorption and metabolism in the small intestine are now broadly understood for common flavonoids. After consumption of food, flavonoids are generally stable in the stomach (Rios *et al.*, 2002) and reach the small intestine unchanged. Figure 27.2 shows the metabolic pathways for quercetin, epicatechin, and hesperetin in the small intestine and liver, for which the mechanisms of uptake, conjugation, and export are now fairly well established. The pathways shown in Figure 27.2 are when the flavonoid is either unconjugated in the food or is glucosylated. When other sugars are present, this can affect dramatically the site of absorption. Other flavonoids, such as anthocyanins, procyanidins, and other flavonoids with a sugar attached which is not hydrolysable by mammalian enzymes such as rhamnose, are not absorbed in the small intestine, but pass through and enter the colon where they are absorbed after microbial metabolism into lower molecular weight compounds (Williamson and Clifford, 2010). Absorption into the blood is often measured as a pharmacokinetic profile after consumption of a single "dose," usually in the form of a flavonoid-rich food. For simplicity, this is often presented as a total of all forms (free plus unconjugated). The C_{max} (concentration at the time point corresponding to maximum concentration of a compound at any time point in a pharmacokinetic study) for various flavonoids has been reported in many papers

(Williamson and Manach, 2005), and an updated indication for various flavonoids is shown in Figure 27.3. The values are normalized for dose assuming a linear relationship, and indicate only the concentration of the parent compound (normally after deconjugation with β-glucuronidase and sulfatase). Quercetin and hesperetin glucosides are the most efficiently absorbed (but after deglycosylation since they are not present in plasma as glucosides [Day and Williamson, 2001]), and epicatechin and epigallocatechin are also well absorbed. These compounds are all absorbed in the small intestine and have a relatively rapid T_{max} (time point corresponding to maximum concentration of a compound at any time point in a pharmacokinetic study) of between 0.5 and 2 hours. Hesperidin, naringin, and rutin (hesperetin, naringenin, and quercetin, respectively, linked to glucose and rhamnose) are all absorbed less efficiently, and exhibit a higher T_{max} of ~6 hours, indicating absorption in the colon after removal of the rhamnose by microflora. Anthocyanins are very poorly absorbed in the intact form and appear to be the only flavonoid class which are absorbed and appear in plasma as the glucosylated form but at an extremely low level (Felgines *et al.*, 2007) in addition to some glucuronide forms (Mullen *et al.*, 2008). Intact procyanidins are only just detectable in plasma after consumption of large quantities of the compound (Holt *et al.*, 2002). After absorption, the flavonoids circulate in the blood as a mixture of conjugated forms, such as glucuronides, sulfates, or methylated forms (Williamson *et al.*, 2005). The amount of unconjugated forms is generally small, with some exceptions, such as epigallocatechin gallate where ~90% of the total plasma EGCG was unconjugated after consumption of green tea (Chow *et al.*, 2003).

Flavonoids can be excreted in the urine or bile. The amount in urine can be used as a biomarker of flavonoid intake (Perez-Jimenez *et al.*, 2010). The percentage excretion in urine is an indicator of the *minimum* amount that has been absorbed. Some flavonoids such as quercetin are well absorbed but only a few percent of the dose appears in urine, since the majority is excreted via the bile or catabolized by gut microflora. The food matrix has a substantial effect on the absorption of flavonoids, where factors such as fat content affect bioavailability (Scholz and Williamson, 2007). Many flavonoids are degraded during food processing, especially processes that involve alkaline pH conditions (Gil-Izquierdo *et al.*, 2003).

The amount absorbed in the small intestine has been estimated for some flavonoids using the ileostomy model.

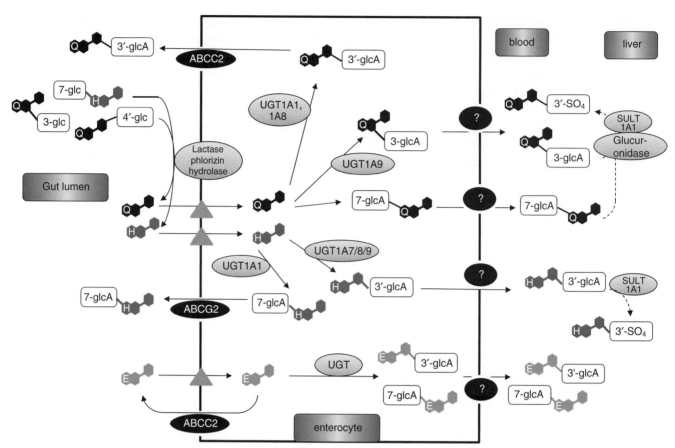

FIG. 27.2 Pathways of absorption of the flavonoids, quercetin, hesperetin, and epicatechin. Quercetin (Q) is glucosylated (glc) in some foods and is deglycosylated by lactase phlorizin hydrolase (Day *et al.*, 2000c; Sesink *et al.*, 2003). The resulting quercetin aglycone passively diffuses across the apical membrane of enterocytes. Hesperetin-7-*O*-glucoside also follows the same pathway (hesperetin aglycone is shown by the letter H). Once inside the cell, quercetin and hesperetin can be conjugated with glucuronic acid by the action of defined isoforms of UDP-glucuronosyl transferases (UGT): for hesperetin, 1A1 preferentially glucuronidates position 7, whereas isoforms 1A7, 1A8, and 1A9 favor position 3′; for quercetin, 1A9 is more active at the 3 and 7 positions (Chen *et al.*, 2005; Brand *et al.*, 2010). The resulting conjugates can be absorbed by as yet unknown transporters on the basolateral membrane, or effluxed back into the intestinal lumen via ABC transporters (Brand *et al.*, 2007, 2008). Epicatechin is not glycosylated and enters the cell by passive diffusion, whereupon it can be rapidly effluxed by ABCC2 transporter (Zhang *et al.*, 2004). Alternatively it can be glucuronidated and transported into the blood. It is likely that some sulfation and methylation also take place in the enterocytes. The absorbed compounds can be further processed in the liver to produce further conjugates (O'Leary *et al.*, 2003).

These are patients who have had their colon removed owing to a disease, and the contents of the small intestine are ejected into a pouch. The contents of this can be collected and analysed, and the amount compared with the original dose. For quercetin glucosides in onions, the amount absorbed was estimated to be 52%, but rutin absorption (for reasons stated above) was much lower (Hollman *et al.*, 1995). For flavonols administered in green tea, the amount absorbed in the small intestine was ~30% (Stalmach *et al.*, 2010). However, identification of metabolites shows that an additional ~37% of the dose was absorbed into the enterocyte and effluxed back into the gut lumen as conjugates. Less than 10% of procyanidins were apparently absorbed in the ileostomy model

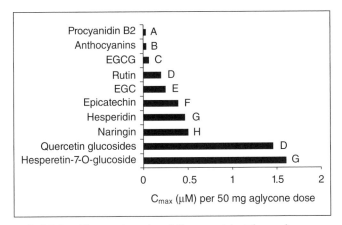

FIG. 27.3 Plasma levels of flavonoids. The values are presented as C_{max} values (μM) normalized to a 50 mg dose of aglycone (data from [Manach *et al.*, 2005]; except for hesperetin-7-*O*-glucoside [Nielsen *et al.*, 2005] and for EGCG/EGC [calculated as weighted averages from Henning *et al.* [2004], Stalmach *et al.* [2009], and Yang *et al.* [1998]). Form of flavonoids present in plasma: A, unknown free and conjugated procyanidin dimers (Holt *et al.*, 2002); B, anthocyanin glycosides, free and conjugated with glucuronic acid (Felgines *et al.*, 2003); C, EGCG, mainly unconjugated; D, quercetin-3-*O*-glucuronide, quercetin-3'-*O*-sulfate and some methylated derivatives (Day *et al.*, 2001; Mullen *et al.*, 2004); E, EGC conjugates, especially methylated EGC derivatives (Lee *et al.*, 2002; Stalmach *et al.*, 2009); F, epicatehin conjugates such as epicatechin-3'-*O*-glucuronide (Natsume *et al.*, 2003); G, hesperetin-3'-*O*-glucuronide and hesperetin-3'-*O*-sulfate, with some hesperetin-7-*O*-glucuronide (Brett *et al.*, 2008; Bredsdorff *et al.*, 2010a); H, naringenin-4'-*O*-glucuronide and naringenin-7-*O*-glucuronide (Brett *et al.*, 2008; Bredsdorff *et al.*, 2010b).

(Kahle *et al.*, 2007), and less than 15% for anthocyanins (Kahle *et al.*, 2006). However, some of the data indicated a higher level of absorption (Kahle *et al.*, 2006), but for anthocyanins such as cyanidin-3-*O*-glucoside this could be due to inherent instability of the compound at physiological pH (Kay *et al.*, 2009).

It is now considered that the microbial metabolites contribute to the biological effects of dietary flavonoids (Williamson and Clifford, 2010). Flavonoids which are not absorbed in the small intestine reach the colon and are subject to extensive catabolism. Reactions that occur are dehydroxylation, reduction, ring cleavage, and hydrol-

ysis of esters and sugars. Although intact procyanidins are hardly absorbed, radiolabel studies in rodents have shown that ~80% of the microbial metabolites are absorbed and appear in the urine (Stoupi *et al.*, 2010). Equol is a microbial metabolite of the isoflavone, daidzein, and has increased biological activity compared with the parent compound (Setchell *et al.*, 2002). The main products in the colon from flavonoid catabolism are benzoic acids including protocatechuic acid, phenylacetic acids, and phenylpropionic acids, where the latter are mainly in the dihydro form, especially dihydrocaffeic acid, dihydroferulic acid, phenylpropionic acid, and hydroxyphenylpropionic acid. Some of these compounds can each reach millimolar concentrations in fecal water (Jenner *et al.*, 2005). Although some biological activities of these breakdown products are known (Williamson and Clifford, 2010), the activity of these lower molecular weight phenolics deserves further research in the future.

Biological Effects of Flavonoids

There have now been several hundred human intervention studies on flavonoids and flavonoid-rich foods, and these have been the subject of several reviews (Manach *et al.*, 2005; Erdman *et al.*, 2007; Cooper *et al.*, 2008; Thielecke and Boschmann, 2009). The role of flavonoid-rich foods in health has also been supported by many epidemiological studies including meta-analyses comprising large total numbers of volunteers (Arab *et al.*, 2009). These studies support a general and consistent protection against heart disease and biomarkers of cardiovascular risk, although the evidence for protection against cancer is weaker. Intervention studies have generally been short term, high dose. However, health benefits of polyphenols in real life are likely due to long-term chronic exposure to relatively low doses, but these types of intervention studies are difficult to do. A 10% change in a biomarker for a year may be highly significant biologically, but a 10% measurement error is difficult to achieve for biomarker measurements. Therefore higher doses are used acutely and the data extrapolated to the longer term (Sies, 2010). In addition, inter-individual variation also contributes substantially to biomarker variability. For a flavonoid to exert a biological effect, it is necessary for the compound to reach the target site or to exert a secondary effect which in turn affects the target site. From bioavailability studies it is probable that flavonoids are not stored in the body. Studies on rodents have shown, for example, that radiolabeled quercetin is extensively metabolized (Graf *et al.*, 2005) and that 80% of metabolites of procyanidins are excreted in the urine (Stoupi *et al.*, 2010). Effects of polyphenols are more conceptually comparable to those of drugs, where an effect is produced and then the compound is excreted, rather than to those of vitamins or minerals, which are stored and can therefore be defined by a status measurement. Thus any effects measured in vitro only show a potential mechanism which must then be demonstrated in vivo. There are many thousands of studies on the action of flavonoids in vitro, utilizing a wide range of concentrations. Since flavonoids are at low micromolar concentrations in vivo, it is usually considered that an effect should be seen in vitro at <10 μM in order for it to have potential dietary relevance (Kroon *et al.*, 2004).

Direct Antioxidant Effects

Many biological activities of flavonoids have been reported in vitro. The most commonly reported in the last 20 years has been antioxidant activity, and there have been many papers describing this activity, including structure–function relationships (Rice-Evans *et al.*, 1995). Flavonoids can act as antioxidants by chelating iron, scavenging free radical species, donating an electron to an oxidant, scavenging peroxyl radicals, and inhibiting lipid peroxidation. These chemical characteristics led to the development of antioxidant assays to measure activity in vitro, such as TEAC (Trolox equivalent antioxidant capacity), TRAP (total reactive antioxidant potential), and ORAC (oxygen radical absorbance capacity). These assays measure a chemical aspect of the test compound (Huang *et al.*, 2005) such as the ORAC assay, which is based on a hydrogen atom transfer reaction mechanism. Many foods have been characterized by these methods (Wu *et al.*, 2004) and they are reasonably good indicators of total phenolic content. In addition, some of these methods, especially FRAP (ferric reducing ability of plasma), have also been used to measure the antioxidant activity of plasma (Romay *et al.*, 1996; Prior, 2004), and many studies have reported the effect of flavonoid consumption on plasma antioxidant activity (Cao *et al.*, 1998). However, endogenous antioxidants such as albumin, uric acid, and vitamin C, present at high concentrations, dominate the antioxidant activity of blood. Since the bioavailability of flavonoids is known, and concentrations are in the low micromolar range, these concentrations will not have a direct effect on the plasma

antioxidant activity, and the concept of using these assays in vivo has received major criticism (Sies, 2007). It is now considered that more specific biochemical measurements are useful in determining the effect of flavonoids in vivo rather than a global antioxidant estimation. The antioxidant assays are still useful for measuring total redox active compounds (dominated by flavonoids, phenolic acids, (ellagi)tannins, and comparable compounds) in foods (Wu *et al.*, 2004). The advantage of the global antioxidant effect is that the concept is simple. In fact the action of flavonoids is more complex than this, and it is unlikely that direct antioxidant effects are relevant in vivo. However, flavonoids in vivo can affect oxidative status, antioxidant enzymes, and oxidative processes, and so act as potent indirect antioxidants by influencing cell function. The overall effect of flavonoids in vivo can still be an antioxidant one, but by specific mechanisms rather than a generalized, global effect. Some of these more specific effects are discussed below. However, there is not enough space to discuss all effects, and so only certain well studied effects are considered that are most likely to be physiological.

Effects in the Gut Lumen

There is a high concentration of flavonoids in the lumen of the gastrointestinal tract after consumption of flavonoid-rich foods, and a high concentration of lower molecular weight phenolics, derived at least partly from flavonoid catabolism, in the colon (Jenner *et al.*, 2005). A portion (100 g) of blackberries might contain 120 mg of flavonoids (Figure 27.3). If consumed with a small drink of ~200 ml, then this equates to very approximately ~1 mM concentration of total flavonoids. This is of course diluted by digestive fluids but the exposure of the gut tissues can therefore be several hundred micromolar. This concentration would elicit responses in the various cells of the small intestine (Erlejman *et al.*, 2008; Romier-Crouzet *et al.*, 2009), and may also affect the action of digestive enzymes.

Effects in the Gut Lumen Related to Diabetes

The postprandial glucose spike, particularly influenced by the transporter GLUT2, can affect endothelial function (Ceriello *et al.*, 2008; Kellett *et al.*, 2008) and oxidative stress (Sies *et al.*, 2005), and is considered undesirable for diabetics and those with metabolic syndrome. Sugar absorption, also important for regulating many other physiological functions, is influenced by flavonoids, with effects on the glycemic index and blood glucose levels. In vitro studies have shown that certain flavonoids inhibit α-amylase (Lo *et al.*, 2008), interact with the sugar transporters SGLT1 (Gee *et al.*, 1998) and GLUT2 (Song *et al.*, 2002), and inhibit sucrose-isomaltase (Ramachandra *et al.*, 2005). This is supported by studies in vitro on volunteers, where effects on insulin are also seen, involving various flavonoid-rich foods such as cranberry (Wilson *et al.*, 2008), black tea (Bryans *et al.*, 2007), and dark chocolate (Grassi *et al.*, 2008). These effects have been reviewed (Cazarolli *et al.*, 2008) and may play an important role in the metabolic syndrome and type 2 diabetes. Flavonoids may also reduce reactive oxygen species in the gut (Halliwell, 2007), thereby protecting gut cells against oxidative damage (Erlejman *et al.*, 2006), and also affect barrier function through modification of tight junctions (Suzuki and Hara, 2009).

There is also evidence from intervention studies that certain flavonoids, such as grape seed extract, can affect markers of diabetes risk in type 2 diabetic patients (Kar *et al.*, 2009), and pycnogenol (a flavonoid-rich pine bark extract) can improve metabolic markers in diabetic patients (Zibadi *et al.*, 2008). Kuna Indians with very high flavonol intake have lower rates of diabetes and heart disease (Bayard *et al.*, 2007), although not all epidemiological studies show an effect of flavonoids at reducing diabetes risk (Song *et al.*, 2005).

Systemic Effects Related to Cardiovascular Disease

There is now a substantial body of evidence, both in vivo and mechanistic in vitro, to show that flavonoids affect risk factors for cardiovascular disease. Several mechanisms of action have been elucidated to explain the effects, with support from human intervention studies and epidemiology. One of the important indicators of cardiovascular risk is endothelial function (Widlansky *et al.*, 2003a) and this biomarker is disrupted by factors such as a high-fat diet (Vogel *et al.*, 1997). Protective effects on endothelial function by flavonoids have been widely reported, especially for the flavanol, epicatechin. Improvement of endothelial function is seen in vivo in volunteers from red wine (Cuevas *et al.*, 2000), tea (Vita, 2003), and cocoa (Heiss

et al., 2003), and by pure epicatechin (Schroeter *et al.*, 2006). The mechanism of modulation of endothelial function is summarized in Figure 27.4. Epicatechin, and especially its metabolite, methylepicatechin, inhibit NADPH oxidase (Steffen *et al.*, 2007), inhibit arginase (Schnorr *et al.*, 2008), and modulate nitric oxide concentration in endothelial cells. This affects cellular pathways resulting in vasodilatation and improvement of endothelial function. Other complementary mechanisms also operate within the cell. Xanthine oxidase produces superoxide and this enzyme is inhibited by quercetin metabolites found in vivo (Day *et al.*, 2000b). It has been shown that cyclooxygenase-2 (COX-2) inhibition improves endothelial function (Widlansky *et al.*, 2003b), and some flavonoids are potent COX-2 inhibitors at levels of both enzyme activity and transcription (Michihiro *et al.*, 2000; O'Leary *et al.*, 2004). Inhibition of COX-2 and NF-κB leads to reduced inflammation, improved platelet activity, and less vasoconstriction, thus leading to improved endothelial function. Flavanones, flavonols, and flavanols suppress NF-κB activity (Frei and Higdon, 2003; Kim *et al.*, 2006; Min *et al.*, 2007). Endothelial function has been shown to be improved by dark chocolate in many intervention studies including those on hypertensive patients (Grassi *et al.*, 2008), young soccer players (Fraga *et al.*, 2005), and smokers (Heiss *et al.*, 2005), and by green tea flavanols in healthy women (Lorenz *et al.*, 2007). A meta-analysis of 133 intervention studies (Hooper *et al.*, 2008) has supported these effects. It is concluded that many flavonoid-rich foods can improve endothelial function via subtle effects on several cellular targets.

Another parameter of cardiovascular disease risk, blood pressure (Bogers *et al.*, 2007), is decreased by flavonoids and flavonoid-rich foods in various subjects including glucose-intolerant, hypertensive patients (Hooper *et al.*, 2008; Grassi *et al.*, 2010). Part of this activity may be via inhibition of angiotensin converting enzyme (Actis-Goretta *et al.*, 2003). Platelet function is another risk factor and is affected by flavonoids (Vita, 2005), and there was a suppressive effect of cocoa flavanols on platelet reactivity in human subjects (Keevil *et al.*, 2000). Red grape juice has more effect than citrus juices on platelets in volunteers, suggesting that flavanols are more effective than flavanones (Rein *et al.*, 2000); flavonols (quercetin) are also active on platelets after oral consumption in vivo (Hubbard *et al.*, 2004). Cardiovascular disease is also influenced by lipid metabolism, and LDL oxidation and

Endothelial cell signaling

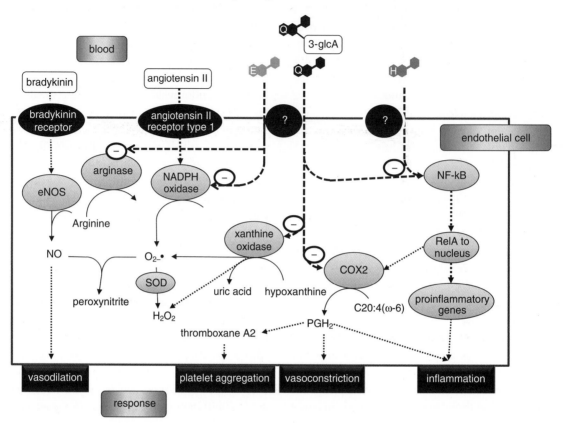

FIG. 27.4   Effect of flavonoids on endothelial cell signaling. Several compounds in blood can affect endothelial cell function. Flavonoids and their conjugates/metabolites can inhibit intracellular oxidative enzymes such as xanthine oxidase (Day *et al.*, 2000a), NADPH oxidase (Steffen *et al.*, 2007), NF-κB (Kim *et al.*, 2006), and cyclooxygenase 2 (COX2) (O'Leary *et al.*, 2004). Modification of these targets affects processes related to cardiovascular disease risk, such as vasodilation and endothelial function.

cholesterol levels are markers of risk (Verhoye and Langlois, 2009). Effects on lipid metabolism have been reported in vivo in rodents (Odbayar *et al.*, 2006), including beneficial effects on cholesterol and LDL oxidation in humans summarized in Williamson and Manach (2005). There is an improvement of lipid profile in hyperlipidemic patients (Esmaillzadeh *et al.*, 2004), and hesperidin reduces cholesterol levels in mice (Jeong *et al.*, 2003).

The protective effect of flavonoids is supported by epidemiological studies. For example, tea flavonoids protect against stroke in epidemiological meta-analyses (Arab *et al.*, 2009), and various flavonoids protected against risk of cardiovascular disease-induced death in 34400 postmenopausal women (Mink *et al.*, 2007).

Systemic Effects Related to Inflammation

Chronic inflammation is associated with obesity, arthritis, Crohn's disease, and ulcerative colitis, and may be influenced by diet, including flavonoids with anti-inflammatory effects (Pan *et al.*, 2010). Although many animal studies report an effect of flavonoids on acute inflammation, it is unlikely that acute inflammation would be affected by normal dietary levels in humans. However, some epidemiological studies support an effect against chronic inflammation, and there is an inverse association of flavonoid intake with C-reactive protein (a marker of inflammation) in a US population (Chun *et al.*, 2008). In animal models, microbial catabolites of flavanones are anti-inflammatory (Larrosa *et al.*, 2009), and grape-seed procyanidins modify cytokine expression in rats fed a high-fat diet (Terra *et al.*, 2009). Effect of flavonoids on inflammation in humans has been reviewed (Rahman *et al.*, 2006; Biesalski, 2007).

Detoxification and Carcinogenesis

Cells in vivo are continuously subject to stresses from endogenous metabolism as well as exogenous compounds, and many defense mechanisms are in place to protect the cell. Detoxification reactions are important defenses in this respect. Phase 2 enzymes catalyze the conjugation of xenobiotics (Prestera and Talalay, 1995) and hence improve their solubility and excretion. Phase 2 enzymes are also important as defense against carcinogens, and induction of these enzymes has been proposed to reduce the risk of carcinogenesis (Prestera *et al.*, 1993; Cornblatt *et al.*, 2007). Flavonoids, especially quercetin, affect detoxification mechanisms and modulate the effect of toxic insults (Uda *et al.*, 1997). In vitro, flavonols, especially quercetin, induce cellular antioxidant defenses via nrf2 and the ARE (Tanigawa *et al.*, 2007; Arredondo *et al.*, 2010). Other detoxification reactions have been observed including effects of some metabolites. For example, quercetin and quercetin 3′-sulfate opposed glyceryl trinitrate-induced tolerance in vitro, and quercetin selectively enhanced cyclic-GMP-dependent relaxation (Suri *et al.*, 2010). However, these effects have been demonstrated in rodents and cells, where protective effects against toxic insults are often observed (Anjaneyulu and Chopra, 2003; Dihal *et al.*, 2006), but very few human studies have been performed in this area. The consequence in vitro is lowered damage to DNA. This protection is observed by, for example, apple extracts (Bellion *et al.*, 2010). Other mechanisms have also been proposed, such as (−)-epigallocatechin-3-gallate inhibition of membrane receptor (Met) signaling, proliferation, and invasiveness in human colon cancer cells (Larsen and Dashwood, 2010), and protection by hesperetin against aberrant crypts in dimethylhydrazine-induced colon carcinogenesis in rats (Aranganathan *et al.*, 2008).

There are very few reported studies on flavonoids and carcinogenesis in human intervention studies, and these studies are often confounded by inter-individual variation (Wilms *et al.*, 2007). There are some epidemiological studies but the evidence for reduction in the risk of cancer is ambiguous (Neuhouser, 2004; Fink *et al.*, 2007; Arts, 2008; Wang and Stoner, 2008) or shows no effect (Wang *et al.*, 2009).

Effect of Flavonoids on Neurodegenerative Diseases

This is an area of much interest, but there is only limited data at the current time. Most research has been done on anthocyanin-rich foods such as berries (Joseph *et al.*, 2009; Spencer, 2009). Several mechanisms have been suggested, and it has been shown that quercetin and some metabolites affect cell signaling in neurons (Spencer *et al.*, 2003).

Future Directions

There is still a need for more human intervention studies, especially using equivalent experimental foods containing a high content and with an absence of flavonoids, and for human intervention studies using intermediate biomarkers of chronic exposure and effects. The field would be advanced by standardization of analytical methods for flavonoids in food and in biological samples, and by better designed in vitro experiments, especially using combinations that could occur and be found in vivo. An obvious gap in bioavailability is the possible role of active transporters in tissue uptake. The focus should be to better understand and develop the effects of flavonoids on the main targets of action. Finally, communication of nutritional issues to the public could be improved by the development of recommended intake values for flavonoids, perhaps based around the 5-a-day recommendation.

Suggestions for Further Reading

Andersen, O.M. and Markham, K.R. (2006) *Flavonoids – Chemistry, Biochemistry and Applications*. CRC Taylor & Francis: Boca Raton, FL.

Erdman, J.W., Jr, Balentine, D., Arab, L., *et al.* (2007) Flavonoids and Heart Health: Proceedings of the ILSI North America Flavonoids Workshop, May 31–June 1, 2005, Washington, DC. *J Nutr* **137**, 718S–737S.

Harborne, J.B. (1989) *Methods in Plant Biochemistry, Vol. 1, Plant Phenolics*. Academic Press, London.

Haslam, E. (1998) *Practical Polyphenolics – From Structure to Molecular Recognition and Physiological Action*. Cambridge University Press, Cambridge.

Kroon, P.A., Clifford, M.N., Crozier, A., *et al.* (2004) How should we assess the effects of exposure to dietary polyphenols in vitro? *Am J Clin Nutr* **80**, 15–21.

Manach, C., Williamson, G., Morand, C., *et al.* (2005) Bioavailability and bioefficacy of polyphenols in humans. I. Review of 97 bioavailability studies. *Am J Clin Nutr* **81**, 230S–242S.

Santos-Buelga, C. and Williamson, G. (2003) *Methods in Polyphenol Analysis.* The Royal Society of Chemistry, Cambridge.

Schewe, T., Steffen, Y., and Sies, H. (2008) How do dietary flavanols improve vascular function? A position paper. *Arch Biochem Biophys* **476**, 102–106.

Williamson, G. and Manach, C. (2005) Bioavailability and bioefficacy of polyphenols in humans. II. Review of 93 intervention studies. *Am J Clin Nutr* **81**, 243S–255S.

References

Actis-Goretta, L., Ottaviani, J.I., Keen, C.L., *et al.* (2003) Inhibition of angiotensin converting enzyme (ACE) activity by flavan-3-ols and procyanidins. *FEBS Lett* **555**, 597–600.

Anjaneyulu, M. and Chopra, K. (2003) Quercetin, a bioflavonoid, attenuates thermal hyperalgesia in a mouse model of diabetic neuropathic pain. *Progr Neuropsychopharmacol Biol Psychiatr* **27**, 1001–1005.

Arab, L., Liu, W., and Elashoff, D. (2009) Green and black tea consumption and risk of stroke: a meta-analysis. *Stroke* **40**, 1786–1792.

Aranganathan, S., Selvam, J.P., and Nalini, N. (2008) Effect of hesperetin, a citrus flavonoid, on bacterial enzymes and carcinogen-induced aberrant crypt foci in colon cancer rats: a dose-dependent study. *J Pharm Pharmacol* **60**, 1385–1392.

Arredondo, F., Echeverry, C., Abin-Carriquiry, J.A., *et al.* (2010) After cellular internalization, quercetin causes Nrf2 nuclear translocation, increases glutathione levels, and prevents neuronal death against an oxidative insult. *Free Radic Biol Med* **49**, 738–747.

Arts, I.C. (2008) A review of the epidemiological evidence on tea, flavonoids, and lung cancer. *J Nutr* **138**, 1561S–1566S.

Bayard, V., Chamorro, F., Motta, J., *et al.* (2007) Does flavanol intake influence mortality from nitric oxide-dependent processes? Ischemic heart disease, stroke, diabetes mellitus, and cancer in Panama. *Int J Med Sci* **4**, 53–58.

Bellion, P., Digles, J., Will, F., *et al.* (2010) Polyphenolic apple extracts: effects of raw material and production method on antioxidant effectiveness and reduction of DNA damage in Caco-2 cells. *J Agric Food Chem* **58**, 6636–6642.

Biesalski, H.K. (2007) Polyphenols and inflammation: basic interactions. *Curr Opin Clin Nutr Metab Care* **10**, 724–728.

Bogers, R.P., Bemelmans, W.J., Hoogenveen, R.T., *et al.* (2007) Association of overweight with increased risk of coronary heart disease partly independent of blood pressure and cholesterol levels: a meta-analysis of 21 cohort studies including more than 300 000 persons. *Arch Intern Med* **167**, 1720–1728.

Brand, W., Boersma, M.G., Bik, H., *et al.* (2010) Phase II metabolism of hesperetin by individual UDP-glucuronosyltransferases and sulfotransferases and rat and human tissue samples. *Drug Metab Dispos* **38**, 617–625.

Brand, W., van der Wel, P.A., Rein, M.J., *et al.* (2008) Metabolism and transport of the citrus flavonoid hesperetin in Caco-2 cell monolayers. *Drug Metab Dispos* **36**, 1794–1802.

Brand, W., van der Wel, P.A.I., Williamson, G., *et al.* (2007) Modulating hesperetin bioavailability at the level of its intestinal metabolism and ABC transporter mediated efflux studied in Caco-2 monolayers. *Chemico-Biol Interact* **169**, 132–133.

Bredsdorff, L., Nielsen, I.L., Rasmussen, S.E., *et al.* (2010a) Absorption, conjugation and excretion of the flavanones, naringenin and hesperetin from alpha-rhamnosidase-treated orange juice in human subjects. *Br J Nutr* **103**, 1602–1609.

Bredsdorff, L., Nielsen, I.L., Rasmussen, S.E., *et al.* (2010b) Absorption, conjugation and excretion of the flavanones, naringenin and hesperetin from alpha-rhamnosidase-treated orange juice in human subjects. *Br J Nutr* **103**, 1602–1609.

Brett, G.M., Hollands, W., Needs, P.W., *et al.* (2008) Absorption, metabolism and excretion of flavanones from single portions of orange fruit and juice and effects of anthropometric variables and contraceptive pill use on flavanone excretion. *Br J Nutr* **101**, 1–12.

Bryans, J.A., Judd, P.A., and Ellis, P.R. (2007) The effect of consuming instant black tea on postprandial plasma glucose and insulin concentrations in healthy humans. *J Am Coll Nutr* **26**, 471–477.

Cao, G.H., Russell, R.M., Lischner, N., *et al.* (1998) Serum antioxidant capacity is increased by consumption of strawberries, spinach, red wine or vitamin C in elderly women. *J Nutr* **128**, 2383–2390.

Cazarolli, L.H., Zanatta, L., Alberton, E.H., *et al.* (2008) Flavonoids: cellular and molecular mechanism of action in glucose homeostasis. *Mini Rev Med Chem* **8**, 1032–1038.

Ceriello, A., Esposito, K., Piconi, L., *et al.* (2008) Glucose "peak" and glucose "spike": impact on endothelial function and oxidative stress. *Diabetes Res Clin Pract* **82**, 262–267.

Chen, Y.K., Chen, S.Q., Li, X., *et al.* (2005) Quantitative regioselectivity of glucuronidation of quercetin by recombinant

UDP-glucuronosyltransferases 1A9 and 1A3 using enzymatic kinetic parameters. *Xenobiotica* **35**, 943–954.

Chow, H.H., Cai, Y., Hakim, I.A., *et al.* (2003) Pharmacokinetics and safety of green tea polyphenols after multiple-dose administration of epigallocatechin gallate and polyphenon E in healthy individuals. *Clin Cancer Res* **9**, 3312–3319.

Chun, O.K., Chung, S.J., Claycombe, K.J., *et al.* (2008) Serum C-reactive protein concentrations are inversely associated with dietary flavonoid intake in U.S. adults. *J Nutr* **138**, 753–760.

Cooper, K.A., Donovan, J.L., Waterhouse, A.L., *et al.* (2008) Cocoa and health: a decade of research. *Br J Nutr* **99**, 1–11.

Cornblatt, B.S., Ye, L., Dinkova-Kostova, A.T., *et al.* (2007) Preclinical and clinical evaluation of sulforaphane for chemoprevention in the breast. *Carcinogenesis* **28**, 1485–1490.

Cuevas, A.M., Guasch, V., Castillo, O., *et al.* (2000) A high-fat diet induces and red wine counteracts endothelial dysfunction in human volunteers. *Lipids* **35**, 143–148.

Cutler, G.J., Nettleton, J.A., Ross, J.A., *et al.* (2008) Dietary flavonoid intake and risk of cancer in postmenopausal women: the Iowa Women's Health Study. *Int. J Cancer* **123**, 664–671.

Day, A.J. and Williamson, G. (2001) Biomarkers for exposure to dietary flavonoids: a review of the current evidence for identification of quercetin glycosides in plasma. *Br J Nutr* **86**, S105–S110.

Day, A.J., Bao, Y., Morgan, M.R.A., *et al.* (2000a) Conjugation position of quercetin glucuronides and effect on biological activity. *Free Radic Biol Med* **29**, 1234–1243.

Day, A.J., Bao, Y.P., Morgan, M.R.A., *et al.* (2000b) Conjugation position of quercetin glucuronides and effect on biological activity. *Free Radic Biol Med* **29**, 1234–1243.

Day, A.J., Canada, F.J., Diaz, J.C., *et al.* (2000c) Dietary flavonoid and isoflavone glycosides are hydrolysed by the lactase site of lactase phlorizin hydrolase. *FEBS Lett* **468**, 166–170.

Day, A.J., Mellon, F.A., Barron, D., *et al.* (2001) Human metabolism of dietary flavonoids: identification of plasma metabolites of quercetin. *Free Radic Res* **212**, 941–952.

Dihal, A.A., de Boer, V.C., van der Woude, H., *et al.* (2006) Quercetin, but not its glycosidated conjugate rutin, inhibits azoxymethane-induced colorectal carcinogenesis in F344 rats. *J Nutr* **136**, 2862–2867.

Erdman, J.W., Jr, Balentine, D., Arab, L., *et al.* (2007) Flavonoids and Heart Health: Proceedings of the ILSI North America Flavonoids Workshop, May 31–June 1, 2005, Washington, DC. *J Nutr* **137**, 718S–737S.

Erlejman, A.G., Fraga, C.G., and Oteiza, P.I. (2006) Procyanidins protect Caco-2 cells from bile acid- and oxidant-induced damage. *Free Radic Biol Med* **41**, 1247–1256.

Erlejman, A.G., Jaggers, G., Fraga, C.G., *et al.* (2008) TNFalpha-induced NF-kappaB activation and cell oxidant production

are modulated by hexameric procyanidins in Caco-2 cells. *Arch Biochem Biophys* **476**, 186–195.

Esmaillzadeh, A., Tahbaz, F., Gaieni, I., *et al.* (2004) Concentrated pomegranate juice improves lipid profiles in diabetic patients with hyperlipidemia. *J Med Food* **7**, 305–308.

Felgines, C., Talavera, S., Gonthier, M.P., *et al.* (2003) Strawberry anthocyanins are recovered in urine as glucuro- and sulfoconjugates in humans. *J Nutr* **133**, 1296–1301.

Felgines, C., Texier, O., Besson, C., *et al.* (2007) Strawberry pelargonidin glycosides are excreted in urine as intact glycosides and glucuronidated pelargonidin derivatives in rats. *Br J Nutr* **98**, 1–6.

Fink, B.N., Steck, S.E., Wolff, M.S., *et al.* (2007) Dietary flavonoid intake and breast cancer risk among women on Long Island. *Am J Epidemiol* **165**, 514–523.

Fraga, C.G., Actis-Goretta, L., Ottaviani, J.I., *et al.* (2005) Regular consumption of a flavanol-rich chocolate can improve oxidant stress in young soccer players. *Clin Dev Immunol* **12**, 11–17.

Frei, B. and Higdon, J.V. (2003) Antioxidant activity of tea polyphenols in vivo: evidence from animal studies. *J Nutr* **133**, 3275S–3284S.

Gee, J.M., Dupont, M.S., Rhodes, M.J.C., *et al.* (1998) Quercetin glucosides interact with the intestinal glucose transport pathway. *Free Radic Biol Med* **25**, 19–25.

Gil-Izquierdo, A., Gil, M.I., Tomas-Barberan, F.A., *et al.* (2003) Influence of industrial processing on orange juice flavanone solubility and transformation to chalcones under gastrointestinal conditions. *J Agric Food Chem* **51**, 3024–3028.

Graf, B.A., Mullen, W., Caldwell, S.T., *et al.* (2005) Disposition and metabolism of [2-14C]quercetin-4′-glucoside in rats. *Drug Metab Dispos* **33**, 1036–1043.

Grassi, D., Desideri, G., and Ferri, C. (2010) Blood pressure and cardiovascular risk: what about cocoa and chocolate? *Arch Biochem Biophys* **501**, 112–115.

Grassi, D., Desideri, G., Necozione, S., *et al.* (2008) Blood pressure is reduced and insulin sensitivity increased in glucose-intolerant, hypertensive subjects after 15 days of consuming high-polyphenol dark chocolate. *J Nutr* **138**, 1671–1676.

Gu, L., Kelm, M.A., Hammerstone, J.F., *et al.* (2004) Concentrations of proanthocyanidins in common foods and estimations of normal consumption. *J Nutr* **134**, 613–617.

Halliwell, B. (2007) Dietary polyphenols: good, bad, or indifferent for your health? *Cardiovasc Res* **73**, 341–347.

Heiss, C., Dejam, A., Kleinbongard, P., *et al.* (2003) Vascular effects of cocoa rich in flavan-3-ols. *JAMA* **290**, 1030–1031.

Heiss, C., Kleinbongard, P., Dejam, A., *et al.* (2005) Acute consumption of flavanol-rich cocoa and the reversal of endothelial dysfunction in smokers. *J Am Coll Cardiol* **46**, 1276–1283.

Henning, S.M., Niu, Y., Lee, N.H., *et al.* (2004) Bioavailability and antioxidant activity of tea flavanols after consumption of green tea, black tea, or a green tea extract supplement. *Am J Clin Nutr* **80**, 1558–1564.

Hertog, M.G., Feskens, E.J., Hollman, P.C., *et al.* (1993) Dietary antioxidant flavonoids and risk of coronary heart disease: the Zutphen Elderly Study. *Lancet* **342**, 1007–1011.

Hollman, P.C., de Vries, J.H., van Leeuwen, S.D., *et al.* (1995) Absorption of dietary quercetin glycosides and quercetin in healthy ileostomy volunteers. *Am J Clin Nutr* **62**, 1276–1282.

Holt, R.R., Lazarus, S.A., Sullards, M.C., *et al.* (2002) Procyanidin dimer B2 [epicatechin-(4 beta-8)-epicatechin] in human plasma after the consumption of a flavanol-rich cocoa. *Am J Clin Nutr* **76**, 798–804.

Hooper, L., Kroon, P.A., Rimm, E.B., *et al.* (2008) Flavonoids, flavonoid-rich foods, and cardiovascular risk: a meta-analysis of randomized controlled trials. *Am J Clin Nutr* **88**, 38–50.

Huang, D., Ou, B., and Prior, R.L. (2005) The chemistry behind antioxidant capacity assays. *J Agric Food Chem* **53**, 1841–1856.

Hubbard, G.P., Wollfram, S., Lovegrove, J.A., *et al.* (2004) Ingestion of quercetin inhibits platelet aggregation and essential components of the collagen-stimulated platelet activation pathway in humans. *J Thromb Haemost* **2**, 2138–2145.

Huemmer, W., Dietrich, H., Will, F., *et al.* (2008) Content and mean polymerization degree of procyanidins in extracts obtained from clear and cloudy apple juices. *Biotechnol J* **3**, 234–243.

Jenner, A.M., Rafter, J., and Halliwell, B. (2005) Human fecal water content of phenolics: the extent of colonic exposure to aromatic compounds. *Free Radic Biol Med* **38**, 763–772.

Jeong, T.S., Kim, E.E., Lee, C.H., *et al.* (2003) Hypocholesterolemic activity of hesperetin derivatives. *Bioorg Med Chem Lett* **13**, 2663–2665.

Joseph, J., Cole, G., Head, E., *et al.* (2009) Nutrition, brain aging, and neurodegeneration. *J Neurosci* **29**, 12795–12801.

Kahle, K., Huemmer, W., Kempf, M., *et al.* (2007) Polyphenols are intensively metabolized in the human gastrointestinal tract after apple juice consumption. *J Agric Food Chem* **55**, 10605–10614.

Kahle, K., Kraus, M., Scheppach, W., *et al.* (2006) Studies on apple and blueberry fruit constituents: do the polyphenols reach the colon after ingestion? *Mol Nutr Food Res* **50**, 418–423.

Kar, P., Laight, D., Rooprai, H.K., *et al.* (2009) Effects of grape seed extract in Type 2 diabetic subjects at high cardiovascular risk: a double blind randomized placebo controlled trial examining metabolic markers, vascular tone, inflammation, oxidative stress and insulin sensitivity. *Diabet Med* **26**, 526–531.

Kay, C.D., Kroon, P.A., and Cassidy, A. (2009) The bioactivity of dietary anthocyanins is likely to be mediated by their degradation products. *Mol Nutr Food Res* **53**(Suppl 1), S92–101.

Keevil, J.G., Osman, H.E., Reed, J.D., *et al.* (2000) Grape juice, but not orange juice or grapefruit juice, inhibits human platelet aggregation. *J Nutr* **130**, 53–56.

Kellett, G.L., Brot-Laroche, E., Mace, O.J., *et al.* (2008) Sugar absorption in the intestine: the role of GLUT2. *Annu Rev Nutr* **28**, 35–54.

Kim, J.Y., Jung, K.J., Choi, J.S., *et al.* (2006) Modulation of the age-related nuclear factor-kappaB (NF-kappaB) pathway by hesperetin. *Aging Cell* **5**, 401–411.

Kroon, P.A., Clifford, M.N., Crozier, A., *et al.* (2004) How should we assess the effects of exposure to dietary polyphenols in vitro? *Am J Clin Nutr* **80**, 15–21.

Larrosa, M., Luceri, C., Vivoli, E., *et al.* (2009) Polyphenol metabolites from colonic microbiota exert anti-inflammatory activity on different inflammation models. *Mol Nutr Food Res* **53**, 1044–1054.

Larsen, C.A. and Dashwood, R.H. (2010) (-)-Epigallocatechin-3-gallate inhibits Met signaling, proliferation, and invasiveness in human colon cancer cells. *Arch Biochem Biophys* **501**, 52–57.

Lazarus, S.A., Adamson, G.E., Hammerstone, J.F., *et al.* (1999) High-performance liquid chromatography/mass spectrometry analysis of proanthocyanidins in foods and beverages. *J Agric Food Chem* **47**, 3693–3701.

Lee, M.J., Maliakal, P., Chen, L., *et al.* (2002) Pharmacokinetics of tea catechins after ingestion of green tea and (-)-epigallocatechin-3-gallate by humans: formation of different metabolites and individual variability. *Cancer Epidemiol Biomarkers Prev* **11**, 1025–1032.

Lewis, J.R., Davis, A.L., Cai, Y., *et al.* (1998) Theaflavate B, isotheaflavin-3′-O-gallate and neotheaflavin-3-O-gallate: three polyphenolic pigments from black tea. *Phytochemistry* **49**, 2511–2519.

Lo, P.E., Scheib, H., Frei, N., *et al.* (2008) Flavonoids for controlling starch digestion: structural requirements for inhibiting human alpha-amylase. *J Med Chem* **51**, 3555–3561.

Lorenz, M., Jochmann, N., von Krosigk, A., *et al.* (2007) Addition of milk prevents vascular protective effects of tea. *Eur Heart J* **28**, 219–223.

Manach, C., Williamson, G., Morand, C., *et al.* (2005) Bioavailability and bioefficacy of polyphenols in humans. I. Review of 97 bioavailability studies. *Am J Clin Nutr* **81**, 230S–242S.

Michihiro, M., Mami, T., Kazunori, F., *et al.* (2000) Suppression by flavonoids of cyclooxygenase-2 promoter-dependent transcriptional activity in colon cancer cells: structure–activity relationship. *J Cancer Res* **91**, 686–691.

Min, Y.D., Choi, C.H., Bark, H., et al. (2007) Quercetin inhibits expression of inflammatory cytokines through attenuation of NF-kappaB and p38 MAPK in HMC-1 human mast cell line. Inflamm Res 56, 210–215.

Mink, P.J., Scrafford, C.G., Barraj, L.M., et al. (2007) Flavonoid intake and cardiovascular disease mortality: a prospective study in postmenopausal women. Am J Clin Nutr 85, 895–909.

Mullen, W., Boitier, A., Stewart, A.J., et al. (2004) Flavonoid metabolites in human plasma and urine after the consumption of red onions: analysis by liquid chromatography with photodiode array and full scan tandem mass spectrometric detection. J Chromatogr A, 1058, 163–168.

Mullen, W., Edwards, C.A., Serafini, M., et al. (2008) Bioavailability of pelargonidin-3-O-glucoside and its metabolites in humans following the ingestion of strawberries with and without cream. J Agric Food Chem 56, 713–719.

Natsume, M., Osakabe, N., Oyama, M., et al. (2003) Structures of (−)-epicatechin glucuronide identified from plasma and urine after oral ingestion of (−)-epicatechin: differences between human and rat. Free Radic Biol Med 34, 840–849.

Neuhouser, M.L. (2004) Dietary flavonoids and cancer risk: evidence from human population studies. Nutr Cancer 50, 1–7.

Nielsen, I.L.F., Chee, W., Poulsen, L., et al. (2005) Increased bioavailability of the citrus antioxidant hesperidin: a randomized, double blind, cross-over trial. Second International Conference on Polyphenols and Health, Davis, CA, October, 2005.

O'Leary, K.A., Day, A.J., Needs, P.W., et al. (2003) Metabolism of quercetin-7- and quercetin-3-glucuronides by an in vitro hepatic model: the role of human beta-glucuronidase, sulfotransferase, catechol-O-methyltransferase and multi-resistant protein 2 (MRP2) in flavonoid metabolism. Biochem Pharmacol 65, 479–491.

O'Leary, K.A., De Pascual-Teresa, S., Needs, P.W., et al. (2004) Effect of flavonoids and vitamin E on cyclo-oxygenase (COX-2) transcription. Mutat Res 551, 245–254.

Odbayar, T.O., Badamhand, D., Kimura, T., et al. (2006) Comparative studies of some phenolic compounds (quercetin, rutin, and ferulic acid) affecting hepatic fatty acid synthesis in mice. J Agric Food Chem 54, 8261–8265.

Pan, M.H., Lai, C.S., and Ho, C.T. (2010) Anti-inflammatory activity of natural dietary flavonoids. Food Funct 1, 15–31.

Perez-Jimenez, J., Hubert, J., Hooper, L., et al. (2010) Urinary metabolites as biomarkers of polyphenol intake in humans: a systematic review. Am J Clin Nutr 92, 801–809.

Prestera, T. and Talalay, P. (1995) Electrophile and antioxidant regulation of enzymes that detoxify carcinogens. Proc Natl Acad Sci USA 92, 8965–8969.

Prestera, T., Holtzclaw, W.D., Zhang, Y., et al. (1993) Chemical and molecular regulation of enzymes that detoxify carcinogens. Proc Natl Acad Sci USA 90, 2965–2969.

Prior, R.L. (2004) Plasma antioxidant measurements. J Nutr 134, 3184S–3185S.

Rahman, I., Biswas, S.K., and Kirkham, P.A.(2006) Regulation of inflammation and redox signaling by dietary polyphenols. Biochem Pharmacol 72, 1439–1452.

Ramachandra, R., Shetty, A.K., and Salimath, P.V. (2005) Quercetin alleviates activities of intestinal and renal disaccharidases in streptozotocin-induced diabetic rats. Mol Nutr Food Res 49, 355–360.

Rein, D., Paglieroni, T.G., Pearson, et al. (2000) Cocoa and wine polyphenols modulate platelet activation and function. J Nutr 130, 2120S–2126S.

Rice-Evans, C.A., Miller, N.J., Bolwell, P.G., et al. (1995) The relative antioxidant activities of plant-derived polyphenolic flavonoids. Free Radic Res 22, 375–383.

Rios, L., Bennett, R.N., Lazarus, S.A., et al. (2002) Cocoa proanthocyanidins are stable during gastric transit in humans. Am J Clin Nutr 76, 1106–1110.

Romay, C., Pascual, C., and Lissi, E.A. (1996) The reaction between ABTS radical cation and antioxidants and its use to evaluate the antioxidant status of serum samples. Braz J Med. Biol Res 29, 175–183.

Romier-Crouzet, B., Van De Walle, J., During, A., et al. (2009) Inhibition of inflammatory mediators by polyphenolic plant extracts in human intestinal Caco-2 cells. Food Chem Toxicol 47, 1221–1230.

Schnorr, O., Brossette, T., Momma, T.Y., et al. (2008) Cocoa flavanols lower vascular arginase activity in human endothelial cells in vitro and in erythrocytes in vivo. Arch Biochem Biophys 476, 211–215.

Scholz, S. and Williamson, G. (2007) Interactions affecting the bioavailability of dietary polyphenols in vivo. Int J Vitam Nutr Res 77, 224–235.

Schroeter, H., Heiss, C., Balzer, J., et al. (2006) (−)-Epicatechin mediates beneficial effects of flavanol-rich cocoa on vascular function in humans. Proc Natl Acad Sci USA 103, 1024–1029.

Sesink, A.L., Arts, I.C., Faassen-Peters, M., et al. (2003) Intestinal uptake of quercetin-3-glucoside in rats involves hydrolysis by lactase phlorizin hydrolase. J Nutr 133, 773–776.

Setchell, K.D., Brown, N.M., and Lydeking-Olsen, E. (2002) The clinical importance of the metabolite equol – a clue to the effectiveness of soy and its isoflavones. J Nutr 132, 3577–3584.

Sies, H. (2007) Total antioxidant capacity: appraisal of a concept. J Nutr 137, 1493–1495.

Sies, H. (2010) Polyphenols and health: update and perspectives. *Arch Biochem Biophys* **501**, 2–5.

Sies, H., Stahl, W., and Sevanian, A. (2005) Nutritional, dietary and postprandial oxidative stress. *J Nutr* **135**, 969–972.

Song, J., Kwon, O., Chen, S., *et al.* (2002) Flavonoid inhibition of sodium-dependent vitamin C transporter 1 (SVCT1) and glucose transporter isoform 2 (GLUT2), intestinal transporters for vitamin C and Glucose. *J Biol Chem* **277**, 15252–15260.

Song, Y., Manson, J.E., Buring, J.E., *et al.* (2005) Associations of dietary flavonoids with risk of type 2 diabetes, and markers of insulin resistance and systemic inflammation in women: a prospective study and cross-sectional analysis. *J Am Coll Nutr* **24**, 376–384.

Spencer, J.P. (2009) Flavonoids and brain health: multiple effects underpinned by common mechanisms. *Genes Nutr* **4**, 243–250.

Spencer, J.P.E., Rice-Evans, C., and Williams, R.J. (2003) Modulation of pro-survival Akt/protein kinase B and ERK1/2 signaling cascades by quercetin and its in vivo metabolites underlie their action on neuronal viability. *J Biol Chem* **278**, 34783–34793.

Stalmach, A., Mullen, W., Steiling, H., *et al.* (2010) Absorption, metabolism, and excretion of green tea flavan-3-ols in humans with an ileostomy. *Mol NutrFood Res* **54**, 323–334.

Stalmach, A., Troufflard, S., Serafini, M., *et al.* (2009) Absorption, metabolism and excretion of Choladi green tea flavan-3-ols by humans. *Mol Nutr Food Res* **53**(Suppl 1), S44–53.

Steffen, Y., Schewe, T., and Sies, H. (2007) (-)-Epicatechin elevates nitric oxide in endothelial cells via inhibition of NADPH oxidase. *Biochem Biophys Res Commun* **359**, 828–833.

Stoupi, S., Williamson, G., Viton, F., *et al.* (2010) In vivo bioavailability, absorption, excretion, and pharmacokinetics of [14C] procyanidin B2 in male rats. *Drug Metab Dispos* **38**, 287–291.

Suri, S., Liu, X.H., Rayment, S., *et al.* (2010) Quercetin and its major metabolites selectively modulate cyclic GMP-dependent relaxations and associated tolerance in pig isolated coronary artery. *Br J Pharmacol* **159**, 566–575.

Suzuki, T. and Hara, H. (2009) Quercetin enhances intestinal barrier function through the assembly of zonula [corrected] occludens-2, occludin, and claudin-1 and the expression of claudin-4 in Caco-2 cells. *J Nutr* **139**, 965–974.

Tanigawa, S., Fujii, M., and Hou, D.X. (2007) Action of Nrf2 and Keap1 in ARE-mediated NQO1 expression by quercetin. *Free Radic Biol Med* **42**, 1690–1703.

Terra, X., Montagut, G., Bustos, M., *et al.* (2009) Grape-seed procyanidins prevent low-grade inflammation by modulating cytokine expression in rats fed a high-fat diet. *J Nutr Biochem* **20**, 210–218.

Thielecke, F. and Boschmann, M. (2009) The potential role of green tea catechins in the prevention of the metabolic syndrome – a review. *Phytochemistry* **70**, 11–24.

Uda, Y., Price, K.R., Williamson, J., *et al.* (1997) Induction of the anticarcinogenic marker enzyme, quinone reductase, in murine hepatoma cells in vitro by flavonoids. *Cancer Lett* **120**, 213–216.

Verhoye, E. and Langlois, M.R. (2009) Circulating oxidized low-density lipoprotein: a biomarker of atherosclerosis and cardiovascular risk? *Clin Chem Lab Med* **47**, 128–137.

Vita, J.A. (2003) Tea consumption and cardiovascular disease: effects on endothelial function. *J Nutr* **133**, 3293S–3297S.

Vita, J.A. (2005) Polyphenols and cardiovascular disease: effects on endothelial and platelet function. *Am J Clin Nutr* **81**, 292S–297S.

Vogel, R.A., Corretti, M.C., and Plotnick, G.D. (1997) Effect of a single high-fat meal on endothelial function in healthy subjects. *Am J Cardiol* **79**, 350–354.

Wang, L., Lee, I.M., Zhang, S.M., *et al.* (2009) Dietary intake of selected flavonols, flavones, and flavonoid-rich foods and risk of cancer in middle-aged and older women. *Am J Clin Nutr* **89**, 905–912.

Wang, L.S. and Stoner, G.D. (2008) Anthocyanins and their role in cancer prevention. *Cancer Lett* **269**, 281–290.

Widlansky, M.E., Gokce, N., Keaney, J.F., Jr, *et al.* (2003a) The clinical implications of endothelial dysfunction. *J Am Coll Cardiol* **42**, 1149–1160.

Widlansky, M.E., Price, D.T., Gokce, N., *et al.* (2003b) Short- and long-term COX-2 inhibition reverses endothelial dysfunction in patients with hypertension. *Hypertension* **42**, 310–315.

Williamson, G. and Clifford, M.N. (2010) Colonic metabolites of berry polyphenols: the missing link to biological activity? *Br J Nutr* **104**(Suppl 3), S48–S66.

Williamson, G. and Manach, C. (2005) Bioavailability and bioefficacy of polyphenols in humans. II. Review of 93 intervention studies. *Am J Clin Nutr* **81**, 243S–255S.

Williamson, G., Barron, D., Shimoi, K., *et al.* (2005) In vitro biological properties of flavonoid conjugates found in vivo. *Free Radic Res* **39**, 457–469.

Wilms, L.C., Boots, A.W., de Boer, V.C., *et al.* (2007) Impact of multiple genetic polymorphisms on effects of a 4-week blueberry juice intervention on ex vivo induced lymphocytic DNA damage in human volunteers. *Carcinogenesis* **28**, 1800–1806.

Wilson, T., Singh, A.P., Vorsa, N., *et al.* (2008) Human glycemic response and phenolic content of unsweetened cranberry juice. *J Med Food* **11**, 46–54.

Wu, X., Beecher, G.R., Holden, J.M., *et al.* (2004) Lipophilic and hydrophilic antioxidant capacities of common foods in the United States. *J Agric Food Chem* **52**, 4026–4037.

Wu, X., Beecher, G.R., Holden, J.M., *et al.* (2006) Concentrations of anthocyanins in common foods in the United States and estimation of normal consumption. *J Agric Food Chem* **54,** 4069–4075.

Yang, C.S., Chen, L.S., Lee, M.J., *et al.* (1998) Blood and urine levels of tea catechins after ingestion of different amounts of green tea by human volunteers. *Cancer Epidem Biomarker Prev* **7,** 351–354.

Zhang, L., Zheng, Y., and Chow, M.S. (2004) Investigation of intestinal absorption and disposition of green tea catechins by Caco-2 monolayer model. *Int J Pharm* **287,** 1–12.

Zibadi, S., Rohdewald, P.J., Park, D., *et al.* (2008) Reduction of cardiovascular risk factors in subjects with type 2 diabetes by pycnogenol supplementation. *Nutr Res* **28,** 315–320.

28

CALCIUM

CONNIE M. WEAVER, PhD

Purdue University, West Lafayette, Indiana, USA

Summary

Calcium is the most abundant mineral in the body, existing primarily in the skeleton where it serves a structure–function role but also serves as a reserve when dietary calcium is inadequate. All homeostatic mechanisms are evolved to maintain constant serum calcium levels to ensure cell signal transmission. Dietary calcium intakes around the world are below recommended intakes. Concern over risk of osteoporosis has public health messages and clinical guidelines calling for use of calcium supplements. Consequently, calcium intakes are increasing, but heavy supplement use is raising concerns for increased risk of adverse events. Yet, the incidence of osteoporosis continues to climb, with suboptimal development of peak bone mass during growth and loss of bone later in life, periods when diet and physical activity play important roles.

Introduction

Calcium is the most abundant mineral in the body, with >99% in the skeleton. The skeleton is a functional reserve that supports our mobility and can be drawn upon during periods of dietary inadequacy of calcium. Because essentially all body processes require calcium, finely tuned homeostatic control mechanisms to maintain constant blood levels of calcium have evolved, as have complex cellular mechanisms to control movement of intracellular calcium. Inadequate dietary calcium is associated with increased risk of a number of diseases.

Distribution

The whole body calcium of an adult female is 23–25 M (920–1000 g) and for adult males is 30 M (1200 g). Calcium occurs mainly in the skeleton as hydroxyapatite, $Ca_{10}(PO_4)_6(OH)_2$. The remaining calcium in the body is in soft tissue, primarily in extracellular fluids and in subcellular stores. Fluxes in intracellular calcium concentration are key signaling events. About half of the calcium in plasma exists in free ionized form and is functionally available. Most of the rest is bound to albumin; some to globulin; and <10% is complexed to phosphate, citrate, and other anions.

Present Knowledge in Nutrition, Tenth Edition. Edited by John W. Erdman Jr, Ian A. Macdonald and Steven H. Zeisel.
© 2012 International Life Sciences Institute. Published 2012 by John Wiley & Sons, Inc.

Chemistry and Function

Calcium is a divalent cation. It is the most abundant element in the body. Because calcium is of intermediate solubility, it exists in both solid form (bones) and in solution (plasma). Calcium binds to proteins through the oxygen atoms of glutamic and aspartic acid residues which fix the tertiary structures of proteins, thereby governing their activity and stability. In this capacity, calcium serves as the most common signal transmitter in cell biology. Calcium has only one oxidation state so it is not prone to be toxic at high concentrations.

Calcium is unusual in that the storage form is also functional. As part of hydroxyapatite, it forms a material strong enough to support our bodies for many decades but light enough to allow mobility. Lifelong cumulative calcium status can be assessed by measuring bone mineral content by bone densitometry because >99% of the body's calcium is in the skeleton and it is present in a constant ratio (36% of total body bone mineral content).

Bone remodeling occurs throughout life except in teeth. Bone resorption initiated by osteoclasts (bone-resorbing cells) results in microscopic pits on bone surfaces. This is necessary for modeling changes in bone size during growth, microarchitectural damage, and maintaining serum calcium levels as well as serving as a source of other minerals. Bone formation under the control of osteoblasts fills in the pits. It exceeds resorption during growth and often lags behind resorption later in life, resulting in age-related bone loss.

Extracellular Fluid Calcium

Calcium concentrations in blood and extracellular fluids are maintained under tight regulation at ~2.5 mM. Extracellular calcium levels can be perceived by a surface Ca^{2+} sensing receptor (CaR), a member of the superfamily of G-protein-coupled receptors in parathyroid, kidney, intestine, lung, brain, skin, bone marrow, osteoblasts, breast, and other cells (Brown, 1999). The CaR permits Ca^{2+} to act as an extracellular first messenger in the manner of a calciotropic hormone. For example, parathyroid glands detect small changes in extracellular concentrations of Ca^{2+}, which regulate the release of parathyroid hormone (PTH) into the circulation. Similarly, CaR allows minute-to-minute regulation of renal tubular calcium reabsorption. The role of these actions in calcium homeostasis is described below.

Extracellular calcium serves mainly as a source of Ca^{2+} to the skeleton and cells but fulfills essential functions in its own right including participating in blood clotting and intercellular adhesion.

Intracellular Calcium

Intracellular calcium concentrations, at 100 nmol/M, are >10 000-fold less than extracellular calcium concentrations. In response to a chemical, electrical, or physical stimulus interaction with a cell surface receptor, intracellular calcium concentrations rise from an influx of extracellular calcium or from intracellular calcium stores such as the endoplasmic or sarcoplasmic reticulum. The rise in intracellular calcium triggers a specific cellular response, usually through activating one or more kinases to phosphorylate one or more proteins. Thus, calcium acts as a second messenger to activate a wide range of physiological responses including muscle contractions, hormone release, neurotransmitter release, vision, glycogen metabolism, cellular differentiation, proliferation, and motility.

A number of enzymes are activated or stabilized by Ca^{2+}, a function unrelated to changes in intracellular calcium concentration. These include several proteases and dehydrogenases.

Calcium Absorption and Homeostasis

Blood calcium levels are almost invariant. Thus, serum calcium concentrations do not reflect nutritional status. The homeostatic regulation of serum calcium to ensure a constant supply to tissues is complex and incompletely understood. When calcium levels fall even slightly, levels are returned to normal by a PTH–vitamin D-controlled increase in calcium absorption, increase in renal tubular reabsorption, and bone resorption (Figure 28.1). Elevated levels of extracellular Ca^{2+} inhibit secretion of PTH and production of calcitriol (1,25-dihydroxy vitamin D) as well as stimulating secretion of calcitonin, a peptide hormone produced in the thyroid gland. This results in decreased calcium absorption, increased urinary calcium excretion, and decreased bone resorption. Extracellular Ca^{2+} binds to CaR on the surface of parathyroid cells, which stimulates a conformational change in the receptor leading to an inhibition of PTH secretion from the parathyroid (Pearce, 1999). CaR has also been located on the calcitonin-secreting c-cells of the thyroid gland, in the calcitriol-producing cells of the renal proximal tubule and the intestine, and in osteoblast cell lines (Brown, 1999) suggesting CaR plays a similar role in monitoring Ca^{2+}

levels at these sites in order to normalize serum calcium levels.

Calcium is not efficiently absorbed or retained in the body. The intestine is the dominant site of adaptation to dietary calcium deficiency. Calcium absorption efficiency (fractional absorption) is influenced by calcium status and physiological state (higher in adolescence, pregnancy, and lactation, and lower in aging). However, prolonged calcium deficiency is not completely corrected by an increase in absorption efficiency, so bone loss ensues to maintain serum calcium concentration. Calcium absorption occurs by two routes. The vitamin D–PTH-dependent transcellular route is saturable and subject to homeostatic regulation. Calcium absorption by this route is up-regulated with increased calcitriol due to reduced levels of serum calcium, as shown in Figure 28.1, which interacts with the vitamin D receptor in the enterocyte and stimulates the synthesis of calcium-binding proteins. Epithelial calcium channels, i.e. $TRPV_6$, mediate calcium entry into the cell, and calcium transporters, i.e. calbindin 9K, shuttle Ca^{2+} across the intestinal epithelial cell (Song *et al.*, 2003). Calcium absorption by the paracellular route (passive diffusion which occurs between cells) is largely dependent upon intestinal luminal calcium concentration.

For calcium intakes approaching 800 to 1000 mg/day, the saturable component of calcium absorption may account for half of total calcium absorption (Fleet and Schoch, 2010). Calcium absorption is also influenced by the calcium content of the meal. As the calcium load increases, absorption efficiency from the saturable pathway decreases (Heaney *et al.*, 1990) although net calcium absorbed increases as the non-saturable component becomes increasingly dominant (Figure 28.2). Practically, calcium absorption is more efficient if consumed in divided doses throughout the day.

Some dietary constituents have an important role in calcium retention. Urinary calcium excretion accounts for ~50% of the variability in calcium retention. Dietary sodium is the key dietary factor which influences urinary calcium loss. Every additional 43 mmol (1 g) sodium results in an additional loss of ~0.66 mmol (26.3 mg) calcium in adults (Weaver *et al.*, 1999). The effect of sodium on urinary calcium loss and net calcium retention is greater in white than black children (Wigertz *et al.*, 2005). A longitudinal study in postmenopausal women illustrated the negative consequences of high salt intakes on bone density (Devine *et al.*, 1995). No bone loss

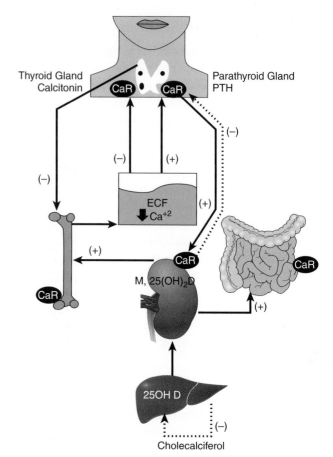

FIG. 28.1 Homeostatic regulation of calcium. The + and – signs indicate the stimulatory and inhibitory responses to a fall in serum or extracellular fluid (ECF) Ca^{2+} below 2.5 mM. The Ca^{2+}-sensing receptor, CaR, has been localized in each of the cells depicted, but its direct role in calcium homeostasis in the intestine has not been demonstrated.

occurred on calcium intakes as high as 44.2 mmol/day (1768 mg/day) or on urinary sodium excretion (reflecting dietary intakes) as low as 92 mmol/day (2115 mg/day). Dietary protein also increases urinary calcium loss, but does not decrease net calcium retention because of offsetting changes in endogenous secretion or calcium absorption (Kerstetter *et al.*, 2005). In fact, bone loss and fractures in the elderly are reduced by higher protein intakes (Dawson-Hughes, 2003). Calcium intake explains only 1 to 6% of the variation in urinary calcium (Jackman *et al.*, 1997).

Calcium Requirements

The 2010 DRIs for calcium relied on bone health as the indicator in setting calcium recommendations, as with previous recommendations (Institute of Medicine, 2011). Newer balance studies (Braun *et al.*, 2006, 2007; Hunt and Johnson, 2007; Lu *et al.*, 2010), meta-analyses of large-scale randomized trials (Tang *et al.*, 2007; Avenell *et al.*, 2009), and longitudinal calcium accretion reports (Vatanparast *et al.*, 2010) have been published giving sufficient confidence to set RDAs rather than AIs for all life stages except infants (Table 28.1). The only absolute values that changed for this transition from the 1997 DRIs was for young children. The 2010 RDAs for children aged 1–3 years increased from an AI of 500 mg/day to an RDA of 700 mg/day and for children aged 4–8 years the RDA increased from an AI of 800 mg/day to 1000 mg/day. The 2010 IOM DRI committee considered the interdependence of calcium and vitamin D and concluded that "calcium appears to be the more critical nutrient in the case of bone health" and "calcium, or lack thereof, 'drives' the need for vitamin D". In Western populations, vitamin D status appears to be sufficiently high so that supplementation has little benefit for calcium absorption.

The range in calcium recommendations around the world is large; for example, recommended calcium intakes for adolescents range between 500 and 1300 mg/day. In addition to assumed differences in peoples, differences in calcium requirements occur through aiming for the prevention of deficiencies vs. optimal health and preventing chronic disease, with different endpoints from maximal

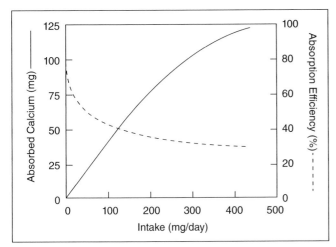

FIG. 28.2 Theoretical relationship between calcium intake and net calcium absorbed (solid line) and absorption efficiency (dashed line). To convert grams to moles, multiply by 0.023.

TABLE 28.1 Dietary reference intakes for calcium by life-stage group for the United States and Canada

Life-stage group	AI (mg)	EAR (mg)	RDA (mg)	UL (mg)
0–6 months	200	–	–	1000
7–12 months	260	–	–	1500
1–3 years	–	500	700	2500
4–8 years	–	800	1000	2500
9–13 years	–	1100	1300	3000
14–18 years	–	1100	1300	3000
19–30 years	–	800	1000	2500
31–50 years	–	800	1000	2500
51–70 years, male	–	800	1000	2000
51–70 years, female	–	1000	1200	2000
71+ years	–	1000	1200	2000
14–18 years pregnant	–	1100	1300	3000
19–30 years pregnant	–	800	1000	2500
31–50 years pregnant	–	800	1000	2500
14–18 years lactating	–	1100	1300	3000
19–30 years lactating	–	800	1000	2500
31–50 years lactating	–	800	1000	2500

AI, adequate intake; EAR, estimated average requirement; RDA, recommended dietary allowance; UL, tolerable upper intake level.
Data from Institute of Medicine (2011).

retention to replacing losses, and using different assumptions for absorption efficiency, losses, and safety margins. Many countries simply adopt the requirements determined by North America, the United Kingdom, or authoritative bodies such as the FAO or WHO.

Recommended calcium intakes for women in North America are not higher for pregnancy and lactation, in contrast to the increased requirement during lactation established by the United Kingdom (Department of Health, 1998). Calcium supplementation does not prevent lactation-induced bone loss, but the bone calcium is regained upon weaning (Kalkwarf *et al.*, 1997). Calcium absorption efficiency is enhanced by the second trimester of pregnancy and greatest during the third trimester, when fetal demand for calcium is greatest (Ritchie *et al.*, 1998). Generally, fetal skeletons are protected at all but exceptionally low calcium intakes of mothers and there is no association between pregnancy, lactation, and risk of fracture (Kalkwarf and Specker, 2002). A longitudinal study showed some compromise of pelvic and spine bone mineral density despite an increase in arm and leg bone mineral density during pregnancy (Naylor *et al.*, 2000). Low dairy intake was associated with decreased fetal femur length in pregnant African-American adolescents (Chang *et al.*, 2003). The need for calcium in breast milk to support neonatal development is met by maternal adaptation of increased bone resorption (Prentice *et al.*, 1995). The additional allowance for lactation (17.5 mmol for non-lactating women vs. 30 mmol for lactating women) by the United Kingdom brings their requirements closer to and even higher than the recommendation for adult women in North America.

Dietary Sources of Calcium

Calcium intakes declined when cultivated cereal grains became the staple plants in the diet of most of the world, as the calcium content of grains and fruits are typically quite low. Consequently, the major source of concentrated calcium from foods in most parts of the world is dairy products. A recent estimate in the United States is that 64% of food calcium comes from dairy products and mixed foods containing dairy ingredients (Institute of Medicine, 2011).

Sources of calcium should be evaluated for their calcium bioavailability as well as content. A summary of calcium bioavailability from a variety of foods and a comparison of the number of servings necessary to provide an amount of absorbable calcium equivalent to that from a glass of milk is given in Table 28.2.

TABLE 28.2 Comparing food sources for absorbable calcium

Food	Serving size (g)	Calcium content (mg)	Fractional absorption (%)	Estimated absorbable Ca/serving (mg)	Servings needed to = 1 cup milk
Milk	240	300	32.1	96.3	1.0
Beans, pinto	86	44.7	26.7	11.9	8.1
Beans, red	172	40.5	24.4	9.9	9.7
Beans, white	110	113	21.8	24.7	3.9
Bok choy	85	79	53.8	42.5	2.3
Broccoli	71	35	61.3	21.5	4.5
Cheddar cheese	42	303	32.1	97.2	1.0
Chinese mustard green	85	212	40.2	85.3	1.1
Juices fortified with					
most calcium salts	240	300	32.1	96.3	1.0
calcium citrate malate	240	300	52.0	15.6	0.62
Kale	85	61	49.3	30.1	3.2
Soy milk fortified with					
calcium carbonate	240	387	31.2	121	0.80
Spinach	85	115	5.1	5.9	16.3
Sweet potatoes	164	44	22.2	9.8	9.8
Rhubarb	120	174	8.54	10.1	9.5
Yogurt	240	300	32.1	96.3	1.0

Adapted from Weaver *et al.* (1999).

Typically, bioavailability of calcium is dictated by the ability of the cation to become free of its ligands or dissociated from the salt and then to remain soluble. However, calcium does not have to be dissociated from low-molecular-weight salts such as calcium carbonate or calcium oxalate to be absorbed, presumably by the paracellular route or by pinocytosis (Hanes et al., 1999). That low-molecular-weight calcium salts can be absorbed without the aid of a vitamin D-inducible calcium transporter, as is required in active calcium absorption, suggests possible treatments for individuals with impaired kidney function who cannot synthesize calcitriol. Solubility of calcium salts in water over the wide range of 0.1–10.0 mmol/L did not influence calcium absorption (Heaney et al., 1990). The condition of achlorhydria also does not reduce calcium absorption as long as the salt is consumed with food (Recker, 1985). Not considered by Recker (1985) is the possibility that appreciable quantities of calcium carbonate were absorbed intact in patients with achlorhydria. Thus, either the pH of the intestinal milieu is an important factor in calcium bioavailability or we need to revise our understanding of calcium absorption, because it appears that solubility of a calcium source may be less important than we have traditionally thought.

Calcium absorption can be inhibited by some ligands and enhanced by others. The strongest known inhibitor of calcium absorption, oxalate, forms a salt with calcium that has a solubility (0.04 mmol/L) considerably below the solubility range discussed above (Heaney et al., 1990). Other modest inhibitors to calcium absorption form salts that cannot be completely dissociated in the gut and are too large to be absorbed intact by the paracellular route. Phytic acid is such an inhibitor. A threefold difference in phytic acid content in soybeans reduced calcium absorption by 25% (Heaney et al., 1991). Although phytate is a more modest inhibitor of calcium absorption than oxalate, it is consumed in higher amounts. However, in developed countries, phytate consumption is less detrimental where bread is leavened and phytate complexes are hydrolyzed by enzymes in yeast during fermentation. Fiber was once thought to inhibit calcium absorption, but it is now considered to be more likely that the phytate associated with fibers in seeds is the inhibitor. Purified fibers have little effect on 5-hour calcium absorption (Heaney and Weaver, 1995). Enhanced calcium absorption can result from extremely soluble salts. Enhancers may work by preventing precipitation of calcium by phosphates in the gut or they

alter the calcium absorption capacity of the intestinal epithelium.

Calcium citrate malate, with a solubility of 80 mmol/L, is the best-studied example of a salt with superior calcium absorption (Heaney et al., 1990). Some casein and whey peptides prevent precipitation of calcium by phosphates (Mykkanen and Wasserman, 1980). Inulin and fructooligosaccharides have been shown to increase calcium absorption, suppress bone resorption, and improve accretion during growth and inhibit bone resorption later in life (Zafar et al., 2004; Abrams et al., 2005). As a rule, calcium absorption determined on the same calcium intake or load is similar for most dairy foods, salts used to fortify foods, and supplements which provide the major contributors of calcium to the diet. Consequently, when assessing dietary calcium, it is appropriate to ensure adequate total intake without undue focus on bioavailability. However, if alternatives to dairy products are selected as the primary source of calcium, it is important to ensure that nutrients other than calcium provided by dairy products – including magnesium, vitamin D (fluid milk), riboflavin, and vitamin B_{12} – are also adequate.

Calcium Deficiency

Calcium intakes of most populations, especially adolescent females, are below the calcium requirements of their country (Figure 28.3). Generally, calcium intakes are

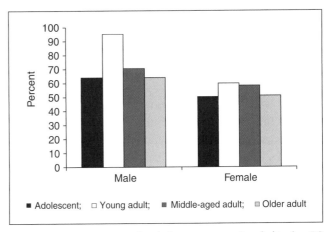

FIG. 28.3 Percent of adolescents and adults in 20 countries meeting country-specific calcium recommendations. Data from Looker (2006).

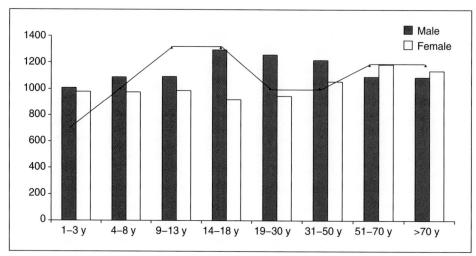

FIG. 28.4 RDAs for calcium with age (line) compared with mean intakes of calcium for men and women in the US (bars). Mean intakes for calcium are from the NHANES 2003–2006 data (Bailey *et al.*, 2010).

highest in Scandinavian countries and lowest in Asian countries. The current marketing trend of so many additional calcium-fortified foods and supplements has shifted total calcium intakes in the United States upward according to a recent analysis of NHANES 2003–2006 data (Figure 28.4). Most Americans older than 9 years of age still are not reaching the recommended calcium intakes, but the gap has decreased substantially since 1997 when the last DRIs were set and compared with intake data using CFS II food intake data (Institute of Medicine, 1997), although all sources of calcium were not included at that time. Adolescent and elderly males and most females over age 9 years are the age groups of most concern for inadequacy. Only 15% of females aged 9–13 years and 13% of females aged 14–18 years met the recommended intake for calcium (Bailey *et al.*, 2010).

Effects of Calcium Deficiency

Low calcium intake has been associated with a multitude of disorders. When the functional reserve (skeleton) is depleted chronically to maintain normal serum calcium levels, low bone mass ensues and can lead to osteoporosis. Low amounts of calcium reaching the lower bowel (unabsorbed calcium) can increase vulnerability to colon cancer and kidney stones. Failure to maintain extracellular calcium concentrations may increase risk of hypertension, preeclampsia, premenstrual syndrome, obesity, polycystic ovary syndrome, and hyperparathyroidism.

Osteoporosis

Of the relationships between dietary calcium and disease prevention, osteoporosis is the most studied (see Chapter 50). Connecting calcium intake to skeletal health is obvious given that 99% of the body's calcium resides in the skeleton. Osteoporosis is characterized by reduced bone mass resulting in increased skeletal fragility and susceptibility to fractures.

The benefit of calcium for skeletal health has been reviewed (Heaney, 2000; Cranney *et al.*, 2002; Chung *et al.*, 2009). Most guidelines recommend adequate calcium intake as an integral part of the prevention or treatment of osteoporosis (US DHHS, 2004; NOF, 2008). Calcium enhances skeletal strength, both as the principal constituent of mineralization and by lowering bone turnover rate through reduction of serum PTH (Heaney and Weaver, 2005). Calcium is not the only nutrient important to bone health, but it is the one most likely to be deficient. Good nutrition is not the only requisite for good bone health; also important are physical activity, especially weight-bearing exercise and not smoking. Hormonal sufficiency promotes bone maintenance, but estrogen therapy after menopause has also been associated with increased risk of breast cancer and stroke (Rossouw *et al.*, 2002). Adequate calcium intake can potentiate the advantage to bone of physical activity in growth (Iuliano-Burns *et al.*, 2003) and adulthood (Specker, 1996) and estrogen in postmenopausal women (Nieves *et al.*, 1998). The primary strategies for reducing the risk of osteoporosis are to maximize development of peak bone mass during growth and to reduce bone loss later in life. Adequate calcium intakes are important for both of these aims. Maximizing peak bone density protects against fracture at any age. Children who avoid milk had a fracture rate 1.75 times higher than expected from their birth cohort (Goulding et al., 2004). Milk may have skeletal benefits beyond adequate calcium. Rats provided calcium from non-fat dry milk solids during growth grew stronger bones than rats fed calcium from calcium carbonate, and the advantages were largely retained after switching to a low-calcium diet where all calcium came from calcium carbonate during maturity (Weaver et al., 2009). Whether the advantage of milk is due to bioactive constituents or simply to providing one or more nutrients such as phosphorus at higher levels requires further investigation.

In adults, systematic reviews have shown the strongest evidence for bone outcomes from trials of combined calcium and vitamin D (Craney et al., 2002; Tang et al., 2007; Chung et al., 2009). Response to supplementation depends in part on the nutrient status at the start of the intervention and the magnitude of change with the intervention. As with children, within populations, milk avoiders have a higher risk of fractures than milk consumers (Honkanen et al., 1997).

On cessation of calcium supplementation, the skeletal advantage gained during treatment in randomized, controlled trials disappears with follow-up in most trials (Dawson-Hughes et al., 2000) unless on low habitual calcium intakes when the trial began (Dodink-Gad et al., 2005). In children habitually consuming approximately 850 mg/day, skeletal advantages in the radius and total body BMD with calcium supplementation compared with the placebo group gained during puberty disappeared on average in spite of continued supplementation during postpuberty (Matkovic et al., 2005). However, the ability for girls to exhibit "catch up" skeletal growth was size dependent as those who were taller at peak bone mass had reduced bone accretion at the forearm if on placebo compared with calcium treatment from age 10 to 18. Furthermore, other skeletal sites such as the hip failed to exhibit complete catch-up growth (Matkovic et al., 2004). At this time, the best recommendation is to maintain adequate calcium intakes throughout life to optimize development of peak bone mass during growth and to minimize bone loss later in life.

Hypertension and Cardiovascular Disease

The ability of calcium supplementation to control hypertension has been controversial. High dietary calcium intake may reduce cardiovascular risk through decreasing blood lipid and cholesterol levels (Pereira et al., 2002; Reid et al., 2002). Lipids are less well absorbed and are therefore excreted in the stools when calcium binds fatty acids and forms insoluble soaps. Ensuring adequate calcium intake, particularly through dairy products, is a primary non-pharmacologic strategy for reduction of high blood pressure recommended by the Joint Committee on Prevention, Detection, Evaluation, and Treatment of High Blood Pressure (Chobanian et al., 2003). In 85 764 women participating in the Nurses' Health Study, those who had calcium intakes in the lowest quintile of calcium intake had a significantly greater incidence of ischemic stroke than those in the highest quintile of calcium intake (Iso et al., 1999). Meta-analyses of randomized-controlled calcium supplement trials show that blood pressure reduction is greater in persons with low habitual calcium intakes (Bucher et al., 1996a) and during pregnancy (Bucher et al., 1996b). However, a recent meta-analysis of RCTs of calcium supplementation with or without vitamin D found no relation to CVD (Wang et al., 2010).

The influence of dietary patterns rather than individual nutrients is more closely linked to disease prevention. The Dietary Approaches to Stop Hypertension (DASH) study showed an impressive and quick response of lowered blood pressure to a diet rich in fruits and vegetables and an even greater reduction if three servings of low-fat dairy foods were consumed daily (Appel et al., 1997). Approximately 70% of subjects who would have required antihypertension drug therapy experienced normalization of blood pressure on the DASH diet. Calcium may influence blood pressure by reducing sympathetic nervous system activity or through its role in intracellular signaling.

Cancer

Increasing calcium and dairy food intakes appears to reduce the risk of colon cancer, particularly of the distal colon (Wu et al., 2002; Chia and Newcomb, 2004). Calcium may lower fecal free bile acid and free fatty acid concentrations, thereby lowering cytotoxicity and/or it may have direct effects on the colorectum epithelium (Chia and Newcomb, 2004). Recurrent colorectal adenomas were decreased ~20% with calcium supplementation (Shaukat et al., 2005).

A systematic review (Chung *et al.*, 2009) found no association between calcium intake and risk for breast cancer. Nor was there an effect of calcium supplementation at 1000 mg/day on breast-cancer incidence or risk in the Woman's Health Initiative trial (Chelbowski *et al.*, 2008). A secondary analysis of calcium at 1400 mg/day plus vitamin D at 1000 IU/day in postmenopausal women showed a significant (p < 0.03) reduction in total cancer (Lappe *et al.*, 2007).

Kidney Stones

Observational studies suggest that adequate dietary calcium decreases incidence of kidney stones (Curhan *et al.*, 1993). A controlled trial demonstrated that increased calcium intake reduced kidney-stone incidence by half and was associated with a decreased urinary oxalate excretion (Borghi *et al.*, 2002). In the gut, calcium combines with oxalate from dietary sources. The rather insoluble calcium oxalate salt is poorly absorbed (Hanes *et al.*, 1999) and oxalic acid is less available for stone formation. However, when calcium supplements are not consumed with meals, they have no opportunity to bind with dietary oxalate and may increase urinary calcium levels which are often already high in people who form stones, further aggravating stone formation (Curhan *et al.*, 1997). People who form kidney stones are often characterized by a renal leak of calcium that reduces skeletal mass (Heller, 1999). Lowering calcium intake in such individuals would not likely correct their kidney-stone problem but would undoubtedly further compromise their skeletal health.

Other Disorders

Adequate calcium intake may be associated with protection against several other disorders. One multicenter trial showed that calcium supplementation at 30 mmol/day (1200 mg/day) of calcium for 3 months significantly reduced symptoms of premenstrual syndrome by 48% compared with 30% in the placebo group (Thys-Jacobs *et al.*, 1998). An observational study showed a protective effect of calcium and vitamin D against polycystic ovarian syndrome, a common cause of menstrual dysfunction and infertility (Thys-Jacobs *et al.*, 1999). All of these relationships may work through regulation of parathyroid hormone levels by dietary calcium.

Calcium Supplementation

Dietary supplements are popular in some populations. From an analysis of NHANES 2003–2006 data, 43% of Americans over age 1 and almost 70% of older women were found to use calcium supplements (Bailey *et al.*, 2010). Among users, 17% of women over age 70 years met the RDA for calcium simply through the use of dietary supplements.

Calcium absorption from calcium salts used in supplements is often comparable to that from milk, but adjuvants used in pharmaceutical preparations may reduce bioavailability of calcium (Weaver *et al.*, 1999). Choice of calcium supplement is dependent on cost and preference. Calcium citrate is recommended for some patients. Divided doses with meals can improve absorption and decrease risk of kidney stones.

Potential Problems of Excessive Calcium Intake

Tolerable upper intake levels (ULs) for calcium were established by the Food and Nutrition Board for North America for the first time in 1997 at 2500 mg/day. They were revised in 2010 (Table 28.1) to adjust for increased requirements for adequacy at various lifestages. An upper limit of 2500 mg/day for calcium has also been adopted by the European Community, Japan, the Nordic countries, and Taiwan. The prevalence of intake above UL is small on average (<2% exceeding 2500 mg/day except for 4% for adolescent males and females over age 50 years) (Bailey *et al.*, 2010).

The hallmark concern of excessive calcium intake is hypercalcemia where serum calcium levels exceed 10.5 mg/dL or 2.63 mmol/L, and hypercalciuria where urinary calcium exceeds 250 mg/day in women or 275–300 mg/day in men. This is rare in healthy people and is usually caused by conditions such as malignancy or urinary hyperparathyroidism but has been increasing, especially in postmenopausal and pregnant women with ingestion of large quantities of supplements (>3 g/day) together with alkali (Patel and Golfarb, 2010). This calcium alkali syndrome may be accompanied by renal insufficiency and is associated with hypophosphatemia (Patel and Golfarb, 2010). Symptoms of hypercalcemia include lax muscle tone, constipation, large urine volumes, anorexia, and, ultimately, confusion, coma, and death.

Concerns over prolonged calcium supplementation have been raised for risk of kidney stones, prostate cancer, myocardial infarction, and vascular calcification. There was a 17% increase in incidence of kidney stones in the Women's Health Initiative trial (Jackson *et al.*, 2006). However, as discussed earlier, obtaining calcium from food or by taking supplements with food to bind any oxalates minimizes risk of stones. Of recent concern is the observation that calcium supplements (without co-ingested vitamin D) increased myocardial infarction, stroke, and mortality (Bolland *et al.*, 2010) and vascular calcification (Daly and Ebeling, 2010). These observations are inconsistent with the reported benefits to cardiovascular health of high calcium intakes. The studies to date are secondary analyses and tend to be small with few events.

Risk of prostate cancer has been associated with calcium intake in observational studies. A twofold increased intake in prostate cancer was reported for milk consumption but not for other dairy products or dietary calcium (Raimonde *et al.*, 2010). Generally, risk for prostate cancer has been observed at calcium intakes associated with supplement use, i.e. >2000 mg/day, and the association lacks strong biological plausibility. Some concern about calcium supplementation and reduced absorption of trace elements has been raised, especially regarding iron. However, Minihane and Fairweather-Tate (1998) showed that although calcium at 10 mmol (400 mg) can significantly reduce iron absorption in a single meal, chronic calcium supplementation at 30 mmol/day (1200 mg/day) does not decrease iron status. Presumably, iron absorption is upregulated as stores decrease. Neither iron status nor zinc metabolism or retention was affected by 1 g calcium supplementation in girls (McKenna *et al.*, 1997; Ilich-Ernst *et al.*, 1998).

Individuals should avoid exceeding the ULs. However, at present, inadequate calcium intake is still the primary concern for optimizing calcium nutrition for most individuals.

Future Directions

More is known about the relationship between calcium and bone health than for any other disorder, yet several questions remain. The US Surgeon General's Report on Bone Health and Osteoporosis (US DHHS, 2004) emphasized the role of good nutrition, and calcium and vitamin D in particular, for normal bone growth and osteoporosis prevention and treatment. Important areas for future research include strategies to maximize peak bone mass in boys and girls in ethnically diverse populations. The prevention and reversibility of calcium and vitamin D deficiency and disease states need to be better understood. Can calcium protect the skeleton against low vitamin D status except for very low levels, i.e. <10 nmol/L? Future research should focus on more complex interactions that consider not only calcium and vitamin D, but also phosphorus.

For each of the other calcium nutrition-related disorders outlined above, additional research will clarify benefits of adequate calcium and risks of excess. We need to better understand the importance of calcium intake in late-stage cancers. A new area of active research stemming from increased incidence of obesity is the consequence of bone loss accompanying weight loss. The Surgeon General's report identified finding mechanisms and interventions to preserve bone during weight loss as an important area for future research. Adequate dietary calcium has been shown to be a useful countermeasure (Shapses *et al.*, 2004). Epidemiological studies would become more useful in identifying the relationship of calcium intake and disease once more accurate means for assessing calcium intake are developed. For each calcium-related disease and metabolic parameter, the interaction between diet and genetics will be a dominant area of investigation in the coming decades. Vitamin D polymorphisms have been associated with fractional calcium absorption (Ames *et al.*, 1999). Further insights into genetics and nutrition are likely to help explain racial and sex differences in calcium absorption as well as identify individuals who can benefit by rigorous interventions. Concern over excesses is a modern phenomenon as more people turn to supplements to meet their calcium needs. Still, we should understand the risks of this popular alternative to meeting calcium recommendations through food.

Suggestions for Further Reading

Weaver, C.M. (2008) Osteoporosis: the early years. In A.M. Coulston and C.J. Boushey (eds), *Nutrition in the Prevention and Treatment of Disease*, 2nd Edn. Elsevier Academic Press, Burlington, MA, pp. 833–851.

Weaver, C.M. and Heaney, R.P. (eds) (2006) *Calcium in Human Health*. Humana Press, Totowa, NJ.

Weaver, C.M. and Heaney, R.P. (2012) Calcium. In *Modern Nutrition in Health and Disease*. 11th Edn., Lippincott, Williams & Wilkins, Baltimore, MD, in press.

References

Abrams, S.A., Griffin, I.J., Hawthorne, K.M., *et al.* (2005) A combination of prebiotic short- and long-chain inulin type fructans enhances calcium absorption and bone mineralization in young adolescents. *Am J Clin Nutr* **85**, 471–476.

Ames, S.K., Ellis, K.J., Gunn, S.R., *et al.* (1999) Vitamin D receptor gene F_{ok1} polymorphism predicts calcium absorption and bone mineral density in children. *J Bone Min Res* **14**, 740–746.

Appel, L.J., Moore, T.J., Obarzanek, E., *et al.* (1997) A clinical trial of the effects of dietary patterns of blood pressure. *N Engl J Med* **336**, 1117–1124.

Avenell, A., Gillespie, W.J., Gillespie, L.D., *et al.* (2009) Vitamin D and vitamin D analogues for preventing fracture associated with involutional and post-menopausal osteoporosis. *Cochrane Database Syst Rev* (2), CD000227.

Bailey, R.L., Dodd, K.W., Goldman, J.A., *et al.* (2010) Estimation of total usual calcium and vitamin D intakes in the United States. *J Nutr* **140**, 817–822.

Bolland, M.J., Avenell, A., Baron, J.A., *et al.* (2010) Effect of calcium supplements on risk of myocardial infarction and cardiovascular events: meta-analysis. *Br Med J* **341**, 3691–3699.

Borghi, L., Schianchi, T., Meschi, T., *et al.* (2002) Comparison of two diets for the prevention of recurrent stones in idiopathic hypercalciuria. *N Engl J Med* **346**, 77–84.

Braun, M., Martin, B.R., Kern, M., *et al.* (2006) Calcium retention in adolescent boys on a range of controlled calcium intakes. *Am J Clin Nutr* **84**, 414–418.

Braun, M., Palacios, C., Wigertz, K., *et al.* (2007) Racial differences in skeletal calcium retention in adolescent girls on a range of controlled calcium intakes. *Am J Clin Nutr* **85**, 1657–1663.

Brown, E.M. (1999) Physiology and pathophysiology of the extra-cellular calcium-sensing receptor. *Am J Med* **106**, 238–253.

Bucher, H.C., Cook, R.J., Guyatt, G.H., *et al.* (1996a) Effects of dietary calcium supplementation on blood pressure: a meta-analysis of randomized controlled trials. *JAMA* **275**, 1016–1022.

Bucher, H.C., Guyatt, G.H., Cook, R.J., *et al.* (1996b) Effect of calcium supplementation on pregnancy-induced hypertension and preeclampsia: a meta-analysis of randomized clinical trials. *JAMA* **275**, 1113–1117.

Chang, S.C., O'Brien, K.O., Nathansen, M.S., *et al.* (2003) Fetal femur length is influenced by maternal dairy intake in pregnant African American adolescents. *Am J Clin Nutr* **77**, 1248–1254.

Chelbowski, R.T., Johnson, K.C., Kooperberg, C., *et al.* (2008) Calcium plus vitamin D supplementation and the risk of breast cancer. *J Natl Cancer Inst* **100**, 1581–1591.

Chia, V. and Newcomb, R.A. (2004) Calcium and colorectal cancer: some questions remain. *Nutr Rev* **62**, 115–120.

Chobanian, A.V., Bakris, G.L., Black, H.R., *et al.* (2003) The Seventh Report of the Joint National Committee for Prevention, Detection, Evaluation, and Treatment of High Blood Pressure: the JNC 7 report. *JAMA* **289**, 2560–2571.

Chung, M., Balk, E.M., Brendel, M., *et al.* (2009) Vitamin D and calcium: a systematic review of health outcomes. Evidence Report No. 183. Prepared by the Tufts Evidence-based Practice Center under Contract No. HHSA 290-2007-10055-I. AHRQ Publication No. 09-E015. Agency for Healthcare Research and Quality, Rockville, MD.

Cranney, A., Tugwell, P., Zytaruk, N., *et al.* (2002) Meta-analysis of therapies for postmenopausal osteoporosis. VI Meta-analysis of calcitonin for the treatment of postmenopausal osteoporosis. *Endocr Rev* **23**, 540–551.

Curhan, G.C., Willett, W.C., Rumm, E.B., *et al.* (1993) A protective study of dietary calcium and other nutrients and the risk of symptomatic kidney stones. *N Engl J Med* **328**, 833–838.

Curhan, G.C., Willett, W.C., Speizer, F.E., *et al.* (1997) Comparison of dietary calcium with supplemental calcium and other nutrients are factors affecting the risk of kidney stones in women. *Ann Int Med* **126**, 497–504.

Daly, R.M. and Ebeling, P.R. (2010) Is excess calcium harmful to health? *Nutrients* **2**, 505–522.

Dawson-Hughes, B. (2003) Interaction of dietary calcium and protein in bone health in humans. *J Nutr* **133**, 852S–854S.

Dawson-Hughes, B., Harris, S.S., Krall, E.A., *et al.* (2000) Effect of withdrawal of calcium and vitamin D supplements on bone mass in elderly men and women. *Am J Clin Nutr* **72**, 745–750.

Devine, A., Criddle, R.A., Dick, I.M., *et al.* (1995) A longitudinal study of the effect of sodium and calcium intakes on regional bone density in postmenopausal women. *Am J Clin Nutr* **62**, 740–745.

Dodink-Gad, R., Rozen, G.S., Reunert, G., *et al.* (2005) Sustained effect of short term calcium supplementation on bone mass in adolescent girls with low calcium intake. *Am J Clin Nutr* **81**, 168–174.

Fleet, J.C. and Schoch, R.D. (2010) Molecular mechanisms for regulation of intestinal calcium absorption by vitamin D and other factors. *Crit Rev Clin Lab Sci* **47**, 181–195.

Goulding, A., Rochell, J.E.P., Black, R.E., *et al.* (2004) Children who avoid drinking cow's milk are at increased risk for prepubertal bone fractures. *J Am Diet Assoc* **104**, 250–253.

Hanes, D.A., Weaver, C.M., Heaney, R.P., *et al.* (1999) Absorption of calcium oxalate does not require dissociation in rats. *J Nutr* **129**, 170–173.

Heaney, R.P. (2000) Calcium, dairy products, and osteoporosis. *J Am Coll Nutr* **19**, 83S–99S.

Heaney, R.P. and Weaver, C.M. (1995) Effect of psyllium on absorption of co-ingested calcium. *J Am Geriatr Soc* **43**, 1–3.

Heaney, R.P. and Weaver, C.M. (2005) Newer perspective on calcium nutrition and bone quality. *Am J Clin Nutr* **24**, 574S–581S.

Heaney, R.P., Recker, R.R., and Weaver, C.M. (1990) Absorbability of calcium sources: the limited role of solubility. *Calcif Tissue Int* **46**, 300–304.

Heaney, R.P., Weaver, C.M., and Fitzsimmons, M.L. (1990) Influence of calcium load on absorption fraction. *J Bone Miner Res* **5**, 1135–1138.

Heaney, R.P., Weaver, C.M., and Fitzsimmons, M.L. (1991) Soybean phytate content: effect and calcium absorption. *Am J Clin Nutr* **53**, 745–747.

Heller, J.H. (1999) The role of calcium in the prevention of kidney stones. *J Am Coll Nutr* **18**, 373S–378S.

Honkanen, R., Kroger, H., Alhava, E., *et al.* (1997) Lactose intolerance associated with fractures of weight bearing bones in Finnish women aged 38–57. *Bone* **21**, 473–477.

Hunt, C.D. and Johnson, L.K. (2007) Calcium requirements: new estimations for men and women by cross-sectional statistical analysis of calcium balance data from metabolic studies. *Am J Clin Nutr* **86**, 1054–1063.

Ilich-Ernst, J.Z., McKenna, A.A., Badenhop, N.E., *et al.* (1998) Iron status, menarche, and calcium supplementation in adolescent girls. *Am J Clin Nutr* **68**, 880–887.

Institute of Medicine (1997) *Dietary Reference Intakes for Calcium, Phosphorus, Magnesium, Vitamin D, and Fluoride.* National Academy Press, Washington, DC.

Institute of Medicine (2011) *Dietary Reference Intakes for Calcium and Vitamin D.* National Academies Press, Washington, DC.

Iso, H., Stampfer, M.J., Manson, J.E., *et al.* (1999) Prospective study of calcium, potassium, and magnesium intake and risk of stroke in women. *Stroke* **30**, 1772–1779.

Iuliano-Burns, S., Saxon, L., Naughton, G., *et al.* (2003) Regional specificity of exercise and calcium during skeletal growth in girls: A randomized controlled trial. *J Bone Miner Res* **18**, 156–162.

Jackman, L.A., Millane, S.S., Martin, B.R., *et al.* (1997) Calcium retention in relation to calcium intake and postmenarcheal age in adolescent females. *Am J Clin Nutr* **66**, 327–333.

Jackson, R.D., La Croix, A.Z., Gass, M., *et al.* for the Women's Health Initiative Investigators (2006) Calcium plus vitamin D supplementation and the risk of fractures. *N Engl J Med* **354**, 669–683.

Kalkwarf, H.J. and Specker, B.L. (2002) Bone mineral changes during pregnancy and lactation. *Endocrine* **17**, 49–53.

Kalkwarf, H.J., Specker, B.L., Bianchi, C., *et al.* (1997) The effect of calcium supplementation on bone density during lactation and after weaning. *N Engl J Med* **337**, 523–528.

Kerstetter, J.E., O'Brien, K.O., Caseria, D.M., *et al.* (2005) The impact of dietary protein on calcium absorption and kinetic measures of bone turnover in women. *J Clin Endocrinol Metab* **90**, 26–31.

Lappe, J.M., Travers-Gustafson, D., Davies, K.M., *et al.* (2007) Vitamin D and calcium supplementation reduced cancer risk: results of a randomized trial. *Am J Clin Nutr* **85**, 1586–1591.

Looker, A.C. (2006) Dietary calcium intake. In C.M. Weaver and R.P. Heaney (eds), *Calcium in Human Health.* Humana Press, Totawa, NJ, pp. 105–127.

Lu, W., Martin, B.R., Braun, M.M., *et al.* (2010) Calcium requirements and metabolism in Chinese American boys and girls. *J Bone Miner Res* **25**, 1842–1849.

Matkovic, V., Goel, P.K., Badenhop-Stevens, N.E., *et al.* (2005) Calcium supplementation and bone mineral density in females from childhood to young adulthood: a randomized controlled trial. *Am J Clin Nutr* **81**, 175–188.

Matkovic, V., Landoll, J.D., Badenhop-Stevens, N.E., *et al.* (2004) Nutrition influences skeletal development from childhood to adulthood: A study of hip, spine, and forearm in adolescent females. *J Nutr* **134**, 701S–705S.

McKenna, A.A., Ilich, J.Z., Andon, M.B., *et al.* (1997) Zinc balance in adolescent females consuming a low- or high-calcium diet. *Am J Clin Nutr* **65**, 1460–1464.

Minihane, A.M. and Fairweather-Tate, M. (1998) Effect of calcium supplementation on daily nonheme-iron absorption and long-term iron status. *Am J Clin Nutr* **68**, 96–102.

Mykkanen, H.M. and Wasserman, R.H. (1980) Enhanced absorption of calcium by casein phosphopeptides in rachitic and normal chicks. *J Nutr* **110**, 2141–2148.

Naylor, K.E., Igbal, P., Fledelius, C., *et al.* (2000) The effect of pregnancy on bone density and bone turnover. *J Bone Miner Res* **15**, 129–137.

Nieves, J.W., Komar, L., Cosman, F., *et al.* (1998) Calcium potentiates the effect of estrogen and calcitonin on bone mass: review and analysis. *Am J Clin Nutr* **67**, 18–24.

NOF (2008) *Physician's Guide to Prevention and Treatment of Osteoporosis.* National Osteoporosis Foundation, Washington, DC.

Patel, A.M. and Goldfarb, S. (2010) Got calcium? Welcome to the calcium–alkali syndrome. *J Am Soc Nephrol* **21**, 440–443.

Pearce, S. (1999) Extracellular "calcistat" in health and disease. *Lancet* **353**, 83–84.

Pereira, M.A., Jacobs, D.R., Van Horn, L., *et al.* (2002) Dairy consumption, obesity, and the insulin resistance syndrome in young adults. *JAMA* **287**, 2081–2089.

Prentice, A., Jarjou, L.M., Cole, T.J., *et al.* (1995) Calcium requirements of lactating Gambian mothers: effects of a calcium supplement on breast-milk calcium concentration, maternal bone mineral content, and urinary calcium excretion. *Am J Clin Nutr* **62**, 58–67.

Raimonde, S., Mabrook, J.B., Skatenstein, B., *et al.* (2010) Diet and prostate cancer risk with specific focus on dairy products and dairy calcium: a case-control study. *Prostate* **70**, 1054–1065.

Recker, R.R. (1985) Calcium absorption and achlorhydria. *N Engl J Med.* **313**, 70–73.

Reid, I.R., Mason, B., Horne, A., *et al.* (2002) Effects of calcium supplementation on serum lipid concentrations in normal older women: a randomized controlled trial. *Am J Med* **112**, 343–347.

Ritchie, L.D., Fung, E.B., Halloran, B.P., *et al.* (1998) A longitudinal study of calcium homeostasis during human pregnancy and lactation and after resumption of menses. *Am J Clin Nutr* **67**, 693–701.

Rossouw, J.E., Anderson, G.L., Prentice, R.L., *et al.* (Writing Group for the Women's Health Initiative Investigators) (2002) Risks and benefits of estrogen plus progestin in healthy postmenopausal women. *JAMA* **288**, 321–333.

Shapses, S.A., Heshka, S., and Heymsfield, S.B. (2004) Effect of calcium supplementation on weight and fat loss in women. *J Clin Endocrinol Metab* **89**, 632–637.

Shaukat, A., Scouras, N., and Schunemann, H.J. (2005) Role of supplemental calcium in the recurrence of colorectal adenomas: a metaanalysis of randomized controlled trials. *Am J Gastroenterol* **100**, 390–394.

Song, Y., Peng, X., Porta, A., *et al.* (2003) Calcium transporter and epithelial calcium channel messenger ribonucleic acid are differentially regulated by 1,25 dihydroxyvitamin D_3 in the intestine and kidney of mice. *Endocrinology* **144**, 3885–3894.

Specker, B.L. (1996) Evidence for an interaction between calcium intake and physical activity on changes in bone mineral density. *J Bone Miner Res* **11**, 1539–1544.

Tang, B.M., Eslick, G.D., Nowson, C., *et al.* (2007) Use of calcium or calcium in combination with vitamin D supplementation to prevent fractures and bone loss in people aged 50 years and older: a meta-analysis. *Lancet* **370**, 9588, 657–666.

Thys-Jacobs, S., Donovan, D., Papadopoulos, A., *et al.* (1999) Vitamin D and calcium dysregulation in the polycystic ovarian syndrome. *Steroids* **64**, 430–435.

Thys-Jacobs, S., Starhey, P., Bernstein, D., *et al.* (1998) Calcium carbonate and premenstrual syndrome: effects on premenstrual and menstrual symptoms. *Am J Obst Gynecol* **179**, 444–452.

US DHHS (2004) *Bone Health and Osteoporosis: A Report of the Surgeon General.* US Department of Health and Human Services, Office of the Surgeon General, Rockville, MD.

Vatanparast, H., Bailey, D.A., Baxter-Jones, A.D.G., *et al.* (2010) Calcium requirements for bone growth in Canadian boys and girls during adolescence. *Br J Nutr* **103**, 575–580.

Wang, L., Manson, J.E., Song, Y., *et al.* (2010) Systematic review: vitamin D and calcium supplementation in prevention of cardiovascular events. *Ann Int Med* **152**, 315–323.

Weaver, C.M., Janle, E., Martin, B., *et al.* (2009) Dairy versus calcium carbonate in promoting peak bone mass and bone maintenance during subsequent calcium deficiency. *J Bone Miner Res* **24**, 1411–1419.

Weaver, C.M., Proulx, W.R., and Heaney, R.P. (1999) Choices for achieving dietary calcium within a vegetarian diet. *Am J Clin Nutr* **70**, 543S–548S.

Wigertz, K., Palacios, C., Jackman, L.A., *et al.* (2005) Racial differences in calcium retention in response to dietary salt in adolescent girls. *Am J Clin Nutr* **81**, 845–850.

Wu, K., Willett, W.C., Fuchs, C.S., *et al.* (2002) Calcium intake and risk of colon cancer in women and men. *J Natl Cancer Inst* **94**, 437–446.

Zafar, T.A., Weaver, C.M., Zhao, Y., *et al.* (2004) Nondigestible oligosaccharides increase calcium absorption and suppress bone resorption in ovariectomized rats. *J Nutr* **123**, 399–402.

29

PHOSPHORUS

ROBERT P. HEANEY, MD

Creighton University Medical Center, Omaha, Nebraska, USA

Summary

Phosphorus, as phosphate, is essential for all life and is widely distributed in both plant and animal foods. A diet adequate in other nutrients, particularly calcium and protein, will automatically be adequate in phosphorus. ECF [P_i], which varies little with dietary phosphorus intake, is itself vital for normal physiological function in all the higher vertebrates, and the principal abnormalities of phosphate metabolism involve either excessively low or excessively high concentrations of this critical anion. ECF [P_i] is regulated by a feedback control loop in which fibroblast growth factor-23 (FGF-23) is the effector hormone. Low serum phosphorus is most commonly due to increased renal phosphorus clearance produced by high levels of parathyroid hormone or FGF-23. The result is rickets or osteomalacia as well as muscle weakness and general metabolic dysfunction of all body tissues and organs. High serum phosphorus is most commonly due to decreased renal clearance as a result of kidney failure. The results include extra-osseous calcification, especially of critical arterial systems.

Introduction

Phosphorus in the biosphere most commonly occurs in its pentavalent form, as phosphate (PO_4^{3-}), and it is in this form that it is found in living organisms. Phosphorus is a limiting nutrient in the sense that the mass of the biota in any given environment is determined strictly by phosphorus availability in that environment. As a reflection of that dependence, and with the exception of guano deposits, virtually all of the phosphorus in an environment will be tied up in its biota.

Phosphorus is an essential constituent of the fabric of all life. In addition to its role in the mineral component of the endoskeleton of vertebrates, phosphorus is involved, for example, in cell membrane structure as phospholipids, in information coding as DNA and RNA, in energy metabolism as ATP and GTP, and in enzymatic activation, by phosphorylation of catalytic proteins. Additionally, inorganic phosphate (P_i) concentration in the extracellular fluid (ECF) of higher vertebrates plays a vital role in supporting both mineralization of bone and the intermediary metabolism of all body tissues.

Phosphorus in the Human Body

Phosphorus is the sixth most abundant element in the human body, comprising in adults about 1.0–1.4% of

Present Knowledge in Nutrition, Tenth Edition. Edited by John W. Erdman Jr, Ian A. Macdonald and Steven H. Zeisel.
© 2012 International Life Sciences Institute. Published 2012 by John Wiley & Sons, Inc.

fat-free mass or ~12 g (0.4 mol) per kilogram. Of this total 85% is in the mineral of bones and teeth, with 15% distributed through the blood and soft tissues (especially myelin). Thus a 70-kg adult with 25% fat mass would have a total body phosphorus of ~630 g (~21 mol). ECF P_i makes up <0.1% of total body phosphorus, but it is into this virtual compartment that phosphorus is transferred from digestion of food in the gut and resorption of mineral from bone; and it is out of the phosphorus of this compartment that bone mineral is formed and urine phosphorus is derived. At physiological pH (7.4), ECF inorganic phosphorus exists as a mixture of $H_2PO_4^-$ and HPO_4^{2-}, with an effective valence of −1.8. While serum $[P_i]$ is not always a faithful reflection of tissue phosphate levels, it is nevertheless the case that most situations of phosphate deficiency or excess express themselves and are mediated through excessively low or high values of serum $[P_i]$.

Phosphorus in Foods

Phosphorus is found widely distributed in various foods, with a strong relation to protein content. This is simply a reflection of the fact that protein and phosphorus are each the stuff of which protoplasm is made, and most foods, plant or animal, come ultimately from living organisms. Although the phosphorus density of foods varies widely, depending mainly upon fat and carbohydrate content, the phosphorus to protein ratio is quite narrow (ranging typically from 0.25 to 0.65 mmol P per gram of protein in, for example, muscle meats).

Bioavailability

With the exception of seed foods and unleavened breads, most food phosphorus is in the form of readily hydrolyzable organic phosphate esters. Seed foods contain, in addition to such digestible, protoplasmic phosphorus, a storage form of phosphorus, phytic acid (hexainositol phosphate), needed to make up for the lack of phosphorus in most soils, and absolutely required in order for the plant embryos to increase their protoplasmic mass. The principal significance of phytic acid for human nutrition is that the human intestine lacks phytase and is hence unable to utilize most of the phytate phosphorus in any given diet. Colonic bacteria, which do possess phytase, are able to release some of that phosphorus for absorption. Additionally, yeasts can hydrolyze phytic acid, and hence leavened cereal-grain foods (e.g. many breads) exhibit good phosphorus availa-

TABLE 29.1 Usual phosphorus intakes (mg/day) for females (NHANES 2005–2006)[a]

Age	Percentiles						
	5	10	25	50	75	90	95
19–30	585[b]	681	864	1090	1344	1596	1753
31–50	623[b]	729	924	1166	1438	1704	1876
51–70	679[b]	758	899	1079	1279	1480	1605
71+	576[b]	648[b]	785	956	1163	1372	1502

[a]Moshfegh et al. (2009).
[b]Below the adult RDA (700 mg/day).

bility whereas unleavened products do not. Finally, diets high in phytate-containing foods can lead to iron, zinc, and calcium malabsorption, and hence to deficiencies of these minerals, because ingested phytate complexes with them and blocks their absorption. Aside from phytate, the principal factor influencing phosphorus bioavailability is not the food itself, but co-ingested calcium (see below, Phosphorus Absorption), which binds phosphorus in the digestate and prevents its absorption.

Human Diet Phosphorus

Table 29.1 sets forth the diet phosphorus distribution for adult women from NHANES 2005–2006 by age (Moshfegh et al., 2009). As can be seen, median diet phosphorus ranges from 1090 mg/day (35 mmol) for individuals in the age range 19–30, to 956 mg/day (31 mmol) for individuals 71 years and older. At any given age (e.g. 51–70), phosphorus intake ranges from 679 mg/day (22 mmol) at the 5th percentile to 1605 mg (52 mmol) at the 95th. The RDA for phosphorus (Institute of Medicine, 1997) in adult women (see below), is 700 mg/day (22.6 mmol), and, as Table 29.1 shows, by age 71 more than 10% of women have intakes below the RDA.

By contrast, various animal chows have relatively higher phosphorus densities. Table 29.2 sets forth the phosphorus nutrient densities of various standard lab chows based on their labeled nutrient contents. As can be seen, these diets, even those of the non-human primates, have substantially higher phosphorus densities (by factors of two to four times) than do even the most extreme of human diets. This is an important consideration in evaluating studies of the effect of raising phosphorus intakes in animals and then extrapolating the results thereof to humans.

For further information on the foregoing topics see the review by Nordin (1988), the introductory material in

TABLE 29.2 Diet phosphorus densities for various animals[a]

Animal	Phosphorus density (mmol P/100 kcal)
Human	2.0
Chimpanzees	4.6–5.4
Swine	6.0–6.5
Dogs	8.7
Cats	6.5
Rats and mice	4.2–6.6
Guinea pigs	5.6

[a]Calculated from labeled content values of standard laboratory chows.

TABLE 29.3 Prevalent serum phosphorus concentrations in healthy individuals, by age[a]

Age	Mean	SD
2	1.81 (5.61)	0.19 (0.59)
6	1.72 (5.33)	0.19 (0.59)
10	1.63 (5.05)	0.19 (0.59)
14	1.53 (4.74)	0.24 (0.74)
18	1.44 (4.46)	0.19 (0.59)
Adult	1.15 (3.59)	0.13 (0.40)

[a]Units are mmol/L (mg/dL).
Data from Institute of Medicine (1997).

Institute of Medicine (1997), and *Documenta Geigy* (any of several editions).

Phosphorus Metabolism

Because phosphorus, in contrast to calcium, is a trace element in the biosphere, the principal components of phosphorus homeostasis differ substantially from those regulating calcium homeostasis. For phosphorus, the regulatory apparatus is optimized to deal with environmental scarcity whereas for calcium the organism must deal with environmental surfeit. Increase in protoplasmic mass, as in generation and growth of new organisms or tissues, creates an obligatory requirement for phosphorus. In addition to the structural role of phosphorus in protoplasm, as inorganic phosphate, it buffers pH changes in the extracellular fluid, and is involved in the storage of intracellular energy (e.g. glycogen synthesis).

Extracellular Fluid Phosphorus

In complex vertebrate organisms, phosphorus availability is critically expressed in the concentration of inorganic phosphate (P_i) in the extracellular fluid (ECF) bathing all of the tissues and organs. Table 29.3 sets forth mean (± standard deviation [SD]) values for serum $[P_i]$ in healthy humans (Institute of Medicine, 1997). Note the higher values during growth. Maintenance of an adequate concentration of phosphate ($[P_i]$) in the ECF is a critical concern of the organism, and will be described in detail in what follows.

At physiological pH and pCO_2, the calcium phosphate salt that would likely precipitate from the ECF is $CaHPO_4$ (Nordin, 1988). Normally ECF is only about half saturated with respect to this product. However, ECF calcium and phosphorus concentrations are supersaturated with

respect to another crystal form, hydroxyapatite, and readily precipitate as such in the presence of a suitable crystal nucleus. Hence the ECF supports mineralization when and where the body creates a suitable crystal nucleus, but is indefinitely stable as it circulates and bathes the other tissues.

The concentrations of ionized calcium and phosphorus in serum (and ECF) of adults are typically 1.1–1.3 mmol/L for calcium and 0.9–1.4 mmol/L for phosphorus. These values produce a $Ca \times P$ ion product $\cong 1.3$ mmol²/L². Since serum calcium is typically held much more constant than is serum phosphorus, most of the clinically encountered variation in the $Ca \times P$ product is produced by variations in serum $[P_i]$.

There is a common misconception that ECF concentrations of calcium and phosphorus are reciprocally related by solubility product considerations. In other words, when one goes up, the other must go down. That would be true only if the ECF were saturated with respect to $CaHPO_4$, but, as just noted, it is not. For example, serum $[P_i]$ actually rises in response to an intravenous calcium infusion, and both concentrations fall in nutritional vitamin D deficiency. (The mechanisms underlying these changes will be described in what follows.) While sometimes the concentrations of these two ions do seem to vary inversely, that is through physiological regulation of their respective levels, not because of a physical chemical equilibrium.

When ECF $Ca \times P$ rises by a factor of about 2×, the solubility constant for $CaHPO_4$ is exceeded and spontaneous calcification of non-osseous tissues tends to develop. And when the ion product falls by a factor of about 0.5×, bone mineralization effectively stops. Thus metastatic calcification occurs when $[P_i]$ rises above 2.4–2.5 mmol/L, and rickets or osteomalacia occurs when serum $[P_i]$ falls below 0.5–0.6 mmol/L. However, even within the nominal normal range, the rate of bone mineralization is to some extent dependent upon the serum Ca × P product. It is not that a higher Ca × P product is inherently more mineralizing, but rather that, since blood flow past a mineralizing site is pulsatile, the blood in each pulse is more quickly depleted of its minerals at lower Ca × P values, and mineralization slows or stops until another pulse of blood comes by. During infancy, rapid skeletal growth requires a high ECF Ca × P, with serum $[P_i]$ reaching as high as 2.0–2.4 mmol/L. At such Ca × P values, there is simply more mineral in a pulse, facilitating greater transfer from blood to bone per unit time.

Regulation of ECF $[P_i]$ Concentration

The relatively small mass of phosphate in the ECF turns over many times each day. Phosphate traffic in and out of the ECF consists mainly, on the input side, of intestinal absorption of ingested phosphorus and release of bone mineral phosphorus in the resorptive phase of bone remodeling. On the output side, phosphate leaves the ECF mainly in the urine, in gastrointestinal secretions, and in the mineralization of newly forming bone (in the reconstruction phase of bone growth and remodeling).

While ECF $[P_i]$ is inevitably affected by this ion traffic, the actual *regulation* of this critical concentration, as is true also for calcium, is mainly through adjusting the kidney threshold for excretion. Approximately 200 mmol of phosphorus is filtered each day at the kidney, the vast majority of which is reabsorbed from the glomerular filtrate in the proximal tubule. This tubular reabsorption is mediated by sodium-dependent phosphate co-transporters in the brush border of the proximal tubular epithelium. This reabsorption has a limited capacity (termed the "tubular maximum" for phosphate [TmP]), which in turn is regulated up or down so as to adjust serum $[P_i]$ concentration. The two factors most involved in this regulation are parathyroid hormone (PTH) and several agents known collectively as phosphatonins, principally fibroblast growth factor-23 (FGF-23). Both FGF-23 and PTH lower the TmP and hence increase renal phosphorus clearance, i.e. the virtual volume of serum effectively cleared of its P_i per unit time. When the TmP decreases (i.e. serum phosphorus clearance rises), serum $[P_i]$ falls, and vice versa.

Long an enigma, the details of the regulation of ECF $[P_i]$ are just now becoming clearer (Ferrari *et al.*, 2005; White and Econs, 2008; Jüppner *et al.*, 2010). Following the general scheme of a classical negative feedback control

loop, the principal regulator is FGF-23, produced in bone by cells of the osteoblast lineage. The principal stimulus to FGF-23 production is a rise in ECF $[P_i]$, whether due to normal dietary absorption, or, with inability of the kidneys to clear absorbed phosphorus, to renal failure. By lowering the TmP, FGF-23 increases phosphorus clearance, leading to a fall in ECF $[P_i]$ and reducing the secretion of FGF-23. PTH, as noted, also lowers the TmP and reduces serum $[P_i]$, but this effect is not a direct part of the $[P_i]$ feedback control loop.

Not surprisingly, FGF-23 serum concentration is typically quite high in patients with end-stage renal disease (ESRD); whether sustained high levels of FGF-23 are themselves responsible, through "off-loop" effects, for some of the morbidity of this condition is uncertain (Jüppner *et al.*, 2010).

FGF-23 also directly regulates renal synthesis of $1,25(OH)_2D$ (calcitriol), but in a direction opposite to the effect of PTH. FGF-23 down-regulates and PTH up-regulates the expression of the renal 1-α-hydroxylase. This discordance is a direct reflection of the differing control systems for which these hormones are the effector molecules. PTH is responsive to ECF $[Ca^{2+}]$, and its up-regulation of calcitriol synthesis leads to increased calcium entry from the gut and decreased renal calcium clearance, thus raising ECF $[Ca^{2+}]$. FGF-23, for its part, is responsive to ECF $[P_i]$ and adjusts renal phosphorus clearance to keep $[P_i]$ from rising unduly (Ferrari *et al.*, 2005). PTH on the other hand, by lowering $[P_i]$, enhances osteoclastic release of bone mineral at pre-existing resorption loci (Raisz and Niemann, 1969), thereby raising ECF $[Ca^{2+}]$. Where the two control systems intersect is in their similar effect on the TmP and, accordingly, $[P_i]$.

Serum $[P_i]$ is itself active in this regulation, with low $[P_i]$ leading to independent up-regulation of renal calcitriol synthesis. By contrast, FGF-23, although it lowers serum $[P_i]$ as a consequence of increasing renal phosphorus clearance, does not lead to the expected increase in 1-α-hydroxylation of 25(OH)D. This is because, as just noted, FGF-23 itself down-regulates the 1-α-hydroxylase, thus preventing the increase in calcitriol synthesis that would otherwise have accompanied the drop in serum $[P_i]$.

The general relationship between absorbed phosphorus intake and plasma P_i in adults is set forth in Figure 29.1, derived by Nordin (1988) from the infusion studies of Bijovet (1969). (In Bijovet's studies, a neutral phosphate solution was infused intravenously at a steadily increasing rate, producing a controlled hyperphosphatemia.) The

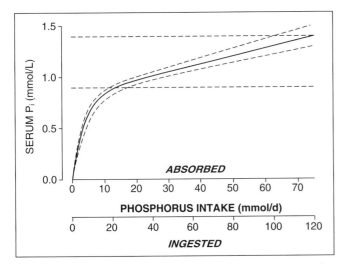

FIG. 29.1 Relation of serum [P_i] to absorbed intake in adults with normal renal function. (See Nordin [1988] for further details.) The lower row of values on the horizontal axis is for ingested intake, and the upper row for absorbed intake (estimated at 62.5% of ingested). The solid curve can be empirically approximated by the following equation:

$$P_i = 0.00765 \times \text{AbsP} + 0.8194 \times (1 - e^{(0.2635 \times \text{AbsP})}).$$

in which P_i = serum P_i (in mmol/liter), and AbsP = absorbed phosphorus intake (also in mmol). The dashed horizontal lines represent approximate upper and lower limits of the normal range, while the dashed curves reflect the relationship between serum P_i and ingested intake for absorption efficiencies about 15% higher and lower than average. Copyright Robert P. Heaney, 1996. Reproduced with permission.

achieved plasma P_i could thus be directly related to actual intakes. When intake is low, the filtered load will be below the TmP, and little of the infused/absorbed phosphorus will be lost in the urine. The steep, ascending portion of the curve in Figure 29.1 thus represents a filling up of the ECF with absorbed phosphate. At higher intakes, the TmP is exceeded and urinary excretion rises to match absorbed input and plasma levels change much more slowly.

The relationship shown in Figure 29.1 holds only in adult individuals with adequate renal function; that is, the slow rise of plasma [P_i] with rising phosphorus intake over most of the intake range applies only so long as excess absorbed phosphate can be spilled into the urine. As renal function is reduced, phosphorus clearance remains essentially normal so long as GFR is at least 20% of mean adult normal values. Below that level, excretion of absorbed phosphate requires higher and higher levels of plasma P_i to maintain a filtered load at least equal to the absorbed load. This is the reason for the hyperphosphatemia typically found in patients with ESRD.

Bone Mineralization

There are three main features of the relation of phosphorus to bone: (1) bone mineral is not just calcium but specifically a complex calcium phosphate salt (hydroxyapatite) comprising 85% of total body phosphorus; (2) adequate quantities of ingested phosphorus, expressed physiologically as a serum phosphate concentration of 1.5–2.0 mmol/L, are essential for bone building during growth; and (3) hypophosphatemia from whatever cause limits mineralization at new bone-forming sites at all ages, impairs osteoblast function, and enhances osteoclastic bone resorption. The amorphous calcium phosphate formed in the first stages of mineralization exhibits a Ca:P molar ratio of about 1.33:1, or very close to the molar ratio of Ca:P in adult ECF. At active bone-forming sites, ECF is depleted of both its calcium and its phosphate. Osteoblast function seems not to be appreciably affected by ECF [Ca^{2+}], but, like other tissues, the osteoblast needs a critical level of [P_i] in its bathing fluid for fully normal cellular functioning. Local P_i depletion both impairs osteoblast function and limits mineral deposition in previously deposited matrix.

Bone Resorption

[P_i] also affects the responsiveness of the osteoclast to PTH: for any given PTH level, resorption is higher when [P_i] is low (Raisz and Niemann, 1969), while high [P_i] values reduce bony responsiveness to PTH, leading to increased PTH secretion in order to maintain calcium homeostasis, and thereby to a lowering of ECF [P_i]. Similarly, high plasma [P_i] suppresses renal synthesis of 1,25(OH)$_2$D (Portale *et al.*, 1989), thereby slightly reducing net phosphorus absorption from the diet. Both mechanisms reduce phosphorus input into the ECF when [P_i] is high and augment it when [P_i] is low. However, in neither circumstance is the effect on plasma [P_i] more than modest. (See below for other special circumstances.)

Intestinal Absorption of Phosphorus

Most organisms get the phosphorus they need by consuming the tissues of other organisms (plant and animal), and they absorb that ingested phosphorus with high efficiency.

In adult humans, for example, net phosphorus absorption typically ranges from 55% to 80% of ingested intake, and in infants from 65% to 90%. The most active intestinal absorptive site is the jejunum.

Most protoplasmic phosphorus in ingested foods is quickly hydrolyzed by intestinal phosphatases, and hence most absorbed phosphorus is in the form of inorganic phosphate. The principal exception is the phosphorus in phytic acid (see above under "Bioavailability"). Otherwise intrinsic bioavailability of most food phosphorus sources is high.

Because phosphorus is intimately involved in virtually all of the functions and structures of living organisms, phosphorus content of most animal tissues varies little, ranging, as noted earlier, from 0.25 to 0.65 mmol per gram of protein. The resulting ubiquitous distribution of phosphorus in all natural foods makes it all but impossible to construct, for patients on renal dialysis, a diet that is low in phosphorus and at the same time nutritionally adequate.

Absorption of phosphorus, as for calcium, is considered to be by a combination of active transport and passive diffusion, with the former being the regulated component. It is widely held that active phosphorus absorption is influenced by vitamin D status. It is also true that the molecular apparatus for vitamin D-stimulated active absorption of phosphorus exists in the intestine (Fleet, 2011). Indeed, it is almost an article of faith that the canonical function of vitamin D is to promote absorption of calcium *and phosphorus*. In support of this effect, Ferrari *et al.* (2005) showed in 29 normal humans that large increases in phosphorus intake induced a decrease in serum $1,25(OH)_2D$ level, a change which, if associated with a reduction in phosphorus absorption, would suggest endocrine feedback regulation of phosphorus absorption (see also below). Ramirez *et al.* (1986), using an intestinal wash-out method, showed an appreciable effect of large daily doses of calcitriol on meal phosphorus absorption in five patients on chronic hemodialysis, producing essentially normal phosphorus absorption efficiency, and suggesting that the loss of renal synthesis of calcitriol reduced phosphorus absorption in patients with end-stage renal disease. Nevertheless, despite low calcitriol production, dietary phosphorus absorption in ESRD patients is higher than the body can handle – which is the rationale for use of intestinal phosphate binders.

Despite the foregoing evidence of a vitamin D effect, the net result is probably small. It is instructive to note that net phosphorus absorption in adults is approximately 65%, leaving relatively little room for vitamin D-mediated absorption to increase. (By contrast, net absorption of calcium is approximately 10%, leaving much room for further increases due to vitamin D.) Such vitamin D effects on phosphorus absorption as can be found in intact humans may be more indirect than direct, as the following data suggest.

Heaney and Nordin, pooling two large datasets of human metabolic balance studies (Heaney and Nordin, 2002), showed that, over a wide range of ingested calcium : phosphorus ratios, the principal determinant of fecal phosphorus (and therefore inversely of *absorbed* phosphorus) was fecal calcium, with phosphorus intake itself exerting a significant but weaker effect. Figure 29.2 is a plot of 470 measurements of net phosphorus absorption in adult women. Together, and altogether apart from vitamin D status, fecal calcium and diet phosphorus explained about 80% of the observed variance of phosphorus absorption. Each 10 mmol of ingested calcium, by complexing phosphate in the intestinal lumen, blocked the absorption of ~4 mmol of diet phosphorus. (As noted earlier, this phenomenon is the basis for the use of calcium salts as phosphate binders in patients with ESRD.) This very high correlation leaves little room for an effect of vitamin D status. However, as calcium absorption rises in response to vitamin D, less calcium is left behind in the intestinal lumen to bind still unabsorbed phosphorus, and hence phosphorus absorption would predictably rise under conditions of high vitamin D status. But that would not necessarily mean that vitamin D directly stimulated phosphorus absorption. Thus experiments such as those of Brown *et al.* (2002), in which calcitriol increased absorption of both calcium and phosphorus in rats, cannot be interpreted unambiguously. In brief, the actual effect of vitamin D on adult phosphorus absorption under usual conditions and in health remains unclear.

Endogenous Fecal Phosphorus

The emphasis in the foregoing section is on transfer of phosphorus from the gut lumen into the blood. But it should be noted that there is a substantial transfer in the opposite direction, i.e. from the mucosa into the chyme. The magnitude of this outward-directed flux has been estimated from studies involving systemic administration of a phosphorus isotope, with measurement of its appearance in the feces (Kierulf-Jensen, 1941; Nordin, 1988). Best current estimates for the magnitude of this flux lie in the range of 8–10 mmol/day (250–300 mg/day). Probably much of that total is in the form of sloughed-off gastroin-

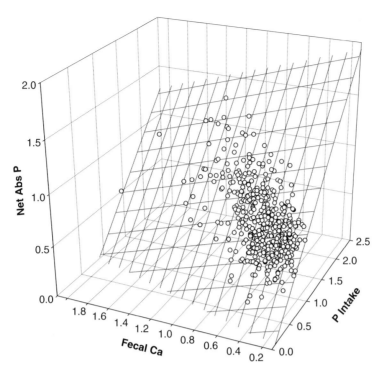

FIG. 29.2 Plot of net phosphorus absorption expressed as a function of diet phosphorus and fecal calcium. (Units on all three axes are grams.) See text for details. Copyright Robert P. Heaney, 2002. Reproduced with permission.

testinal mucosal cells (which typically turn over approximately every 5 days). This phosphorus source is digested just as is food phosphorus, and thereby becomes available for reabsorption. Using 8.8 mmol/day (275 mg/day) for intestinally secreted phosphorus, and 65% for net phosphorus absorption, and taking the median phosphorus intake for women aged 50–70 from NHANES, i.e. 34.8 mmol/day (1079 mg/day), one can easily compute that the total phosphorus load presented to the absorptive sites amounts to 43.6 mmol/day (1354 mg/day), with fecal phosphorus amounting to 12.2 mmol/day (378 mg/day). That means that gross absorption was 72%. This is but one indication of the avidity of the organism for ingested phosphorus.

Urinary Phosphorus Excretion

Normally, most phosphorus loss from the body is through the kidneys. Under steady-state conditions (neither building nor reducing tissue mass), 24-hour urine phosphorus excretion is equal to net intestinal absorption of phosphorus. The kidney capacity for excretion of phosphorus is

very great, as can be seen from Figure 29.1. Across a doubling of phosphorus intake, ECF $[P_i]$ rises very little, with essentially all the absorbed phosphorus being excreted. Very little elevation of the filtered load (as reflected in the serum $[P_i]$) is needed to clear the body of unneeded phosphorus.

Recommended Dietary Intake of Phosphorus

An adequate intake for any nutrient is one such that additional inputs of the same nutrient confer no further benefit. This concept is expressed in Figure 29.3A, which is a schematic plot of effect (or benefit) against intake. Intakes above the beginning of the plateau region are judged "adequate," in the sense that no further benefit accrues to further intake. Not everyone reaches the plateau at the same intake, and Figure 29.3B shows schematically a family of intake–effect curves for different individuals. The intake at the average of these inflection points is what is meant by the estimated average requirement (EAR); the

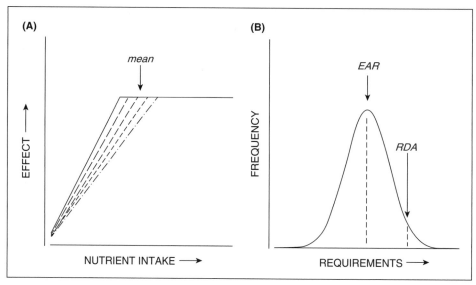

FIG. 29.3 Schematic intake–effect diagrams for a typical nutrient. (A) The basic plateau (or threshold) relationship for a typical nutrient, showing individual variation in approach to a plateau. (B) A frequency distribution of plateau intakes in a population, showing the position of two DRIs (i.e. the EAR and the RDA). Copyright Robert P. Heaney, 2010. Reproduced with permission.

TABLE 29.4 Dietary reference intakes for phosphorus[a]

Ages	EAR[b]	RDA[b]	UL[b]
1–3	380 (12.3)	460 (14.8)	3000 (96.8)
4–8	405 (13.1)	500 (16.1)	3000 (96.8)
9–18	1055 (34)	1250 (40.3)	4000 (130)
19–50	580 (18.7)	700 (22.6)	4000 (130)
51–70	580 (18.7)	700 (22.6)	4000 (130)

[a]Values given as mg/day (mmol/day).
[b]EAR, estimated average requirement; RDA, recommended dietary allowance; UL, tolerable upper intake level.
Data from Institute of Medicine (1997).

recommended dietary allowance (RDA) is the intake at which 97.5% of a population would have achieved their individual plateaus.

Table 29.4 sets forth the 1997 Institute of Medicine (IOM) dietary reference intakes (DRIs) for phosphorus by age (Institute of Medicine, 1997). (The DRIs for pregnancy and lactation are the same as for women of the same age.) The adult value for the EAR in Table 29.4 is based on the intake required to sustain ECF [P_i] at or above the lower limit of normal (see Figure 29.1). Interestingly, the 1997 DRIs were the first to use a functional indicator (i.e.

ECF [P_i]) as a basis for determining the phosphorus intake requirement.

The DRIs in Table 29.4 reflect the obvious need for higher intakes as body size is increasing, and particularly for periods of the greatest tissue accumulation (e.g. adolescence). However, the recommendations for children and adolescents, while reasonable, are not so firmly based as for the adult. The sole reflection of the diet which the tissues "see" is the serum [P_i], and, as Figure 29.1 shows, mean serum [P_i] rises by less than 0.2 mmol/L as intake increases from 20 to 40 mmol/day (620–1240 mg/day). Serum [P_i] in this range is generally considered "normal," and whether the higher end of that range would be more or less beneficial than the lower end is simply unknown.

There is a sense in which the phosphorus requirement is moot. The occurrence of an isolated dietary phosphorus deficiency is highly unlikely (except in low-birth-weight newborn infants). Individuals meeting even the modest published requirements for calcium and protein will automatically meet the phosphorus requirement. As a reflection of this tie between total nutrition and phosphorus status, the first seven editions of the US RDAs did not so much as list phosphorus, and, as recently as 20 years ago, most nations had not established an RDA for phosphorus.

Phosphorus-Related Human Disease

Deficiency

Phosphorus deficiency is expressed as hypophosphatemia. This only rarely occurs because of inadequate dietary phosphorus intake, and is almost always due to non-dietary metabolic disorders.

Only limited quantities of phosphate are stored within cells, and most tissues depend upon ECF $[P_i]$ for their metabolic phosphate. When ECF $[P_i]$ is low, the result is cellular dysfunction in all tissues. At a whole-organism level, the effects of hypophosphatemia include anorexia, anemia, muscle weakness, bone pain, rickets and osteomalacia, general debility, increased susceptibility to infection, paresthesias, ataxia, confusion, and even death. The muscle weakness involves especially proximal muscle groups, and when prolonged or severe can lead to muscle-fiber degeneration. The skeleton will exhibit either rickets or osteomalacia, depending upon growth status. In both, the disorder consists of a failure to mineralize forming growth plate cartilage or bone matrix, together with impairment of chondroblast and osteoblast function. This functional disturbance both slows osteoid deposition and disturbs the normal maturation process in the hypertrophic zone of the growth cartilage. Such severe manifestations are usually confined to situations in which ECF$[P_i]$ falls below ~0.3 mmol/L (~1 mg/dL). However, for reasons discussed above, when growth is rapid, beginning bone lesions may be found at $[P_i]$ values in the peripheral blood as high as 0.5–0.6 mmol/L (1.5–1.8 mg/dL).

This spectrum of dysfunction is common to all hypophosphatemia from any cause, whether nutritional or otherwise. Examples unrelated to dietary phosphorus intake include severe vitamin D deficiency rickets, in which the hypophosphatemia is due not so much to insufficient absorption of dietary phosphorus as to high levels of production of PTH (which lowers the TmP, and hence the plasma $[P_i]$). The same is true for renal tubular acidosis, familial hypophosphatemia, Fanconi's syndrome, or any condition in which tubular P_i reabsorption is reduced (directly or indirectly) and hence renal clearance of P_i is high. Examples include X-linked hypophosphatemia, autosomal dominant hypophosphatemic rickets, tumoral osteomalacia, and, in some cases, fibrous dysplasia. In the first, the defect is due to an inactivating mutation in an endopeptidase (PHEX), leading to increased synthesis of FGF-23 (and hence renal phosphate wasting). The second is due to an activating mutation of the FGF-23 gene, rendering FGF-23 resistant to proteolytic change. Tumoral osteomalacia comes about because of inappropriate secretion of FGF-23 (and other phosphatonins) by the neoplastic tissue (Strom and Jüppner, 2008).

As noted above, hypophosphatemia almost never occurs spontaneously for dietary reasons alone. However, with respiratory alkalosis or after major catabolic episodes, or recovery from alcoholic bouts, from diabetic ketoacidosis, or from similar situations, refeeding with calorie-rich sources without paying attention to phosphorus needs will usually produce serious and possibly fatal hypophosphatemia (Knochel, 1977, 1985; Bushe, 1986; Dale *et al.*, 1986). The so-called "refeeding syndrome" or "refeeding hypophosphatemia" is a well recognized problem following gut shut-down for any cause (Stein *et al.*, 1966; Travis *et al.*, 1972; Ritz, 1982; Knochel, 1985; Young *et al.*, 1985; Marik *et al.*, 1996). It is generally considered to be due to cellular uptake of phosphate as glucose moves into cells replenishing exhausted energy stores, and can occur following as little as 48 hours without oral feeding, particularly in previously malnourished individuals. Finally, aluminum-containing antacids, by binding diet phosphorus in the gut, can also produce hypophosphatemia in their own right, as well as aggravating phosphate deficiency related to these other problems (Lotz *et al.*, 1968).

Similarly, in infants, severe hypophosphatemia is likely to occur only in situations of parenteral nutrition, in which intakes of phosphate are inadequate, or with inappropriate administration of fluid and electrolyte therapy which causes excessive renal phosphorus loss, or with rapid refeeding after prolonged dietary restriction (Koo and Tsang, 1977; Weinsier and Krumdieck, 1981). In the case of severely malnourished infants, especially with accompanying severe diarrhea, hypophosphatemia has been reported with an associated hypokalemia and hypotonia (Freiman *et al.*, 1982).

Excess

In assessing the potential for harmful effects of increasing phosphorus intakes, it may be helpful to recall that phosphorus intakes by humans fall at the low end of the continuum of standard pet and laboratory animal chows (see Table 29.2). The published tolerable upper intake level (TUIL or, more commonly today, simply UL) for adult humans is 129 mmol (4000 mg)/day (Institute of Medicine, 1997). Few individuals ever even approach that level.

The adverse effects of hyperphosphatemia (and high Ca × P product values) include metastatic calcification, particularly of the kidney and the coronary arteries, and, in some species, increased porosity of the skeleton. The kidney effects have been studied mainly in rats and mice (McFarlane, 1941; Craig, 1959; Hamuro et al., 1970), have required very high phosphate loads in addition to the animals' already high basal phosphate intakes, and in several reports have required partial reduction of renal tissue mass for their expression. The bony lesions have been described in rabbits (Jowsey and Balasubramaniam, 1972) and bulls (Krook et al., 1975). As with kidney toxicity, the bony lesions required extremely large phosphate intakes – in rabbits about 40-fold human intakes (per kilogram), and in the bulls feeding of a ration designed to support milk production in cows. None of these situations has any evident relevance to human nutrition or to human dietary intake of phosphate.

In humans the most common cause of significant hyperphosphatemia is not high intake, but renal failure. With advanced kidney failure especially, even sharply reduced phosphorus diets may still be excessive (in the sense that they still lead to hyperphosphatemia). Moreover, serum $[P_i]$ is positively associated with coronary artery calcification and with cardiovascular disease risk in patients with ESRD. Management of serum $[P_i]$ is a major problem in patients with ESRD. Concern has been expressed that even individuals with normal renal function may exhibit the same sort of adverse association between serum $[P_i]$ values at the high end of the normal range and subsequent cardiac disease (Foley et al., 2008, 2009). The associations found to date are weak; nevertheless, it remains true that the upper end of the normal range for ECF $[P_i]$ is defined empirically, and it is not clear whether a value of, for example, 1.4 mmol/L is more or less salubrious than a value of 1.1 mmol/L.

While ECF in adults is less than half saturated with respect to $CaHPO_4$, elevation of plasma $[P_i]$, if extreme, can bring the ECF to the point of saturation. Under such conditions susceptible tissue matrices will begin to accumulate calcium phosphate crystals, particularly if local pH rises above 7.4. This almost never occurs in individuals with normal renal function, mainly because urine phosphate excretion rises in direct proportion to dietary intake. As Figure 29.1 shows, the upper limit of the nominal normal adult range for serum $[P_i]$ occurs at absorbed intakes above 70 mmol/day. At 62.5% absorption, that means ingested intakes of 114 mmol/day. The distributional data of NHANES (Table 29.1) indicate that, out of the total population, only a very few adolescent and young adult men consume close to this level (Moshfegh et al.,

2009). Hyperphosphatemia can also be a problem in such conditions as vitamin D intoxication.

There has also been concern expressed about apparently rising phosphorus intake in recent years, for example because of a presumed population-level increase in phosphorus intake through such sources as cola beverages and food phosphate additives (Calvo and Heath, 1988). A high-phosphorus diet inevitably produces a slightly higher level of plasma $[P_i]$, especially during the absorptive phase after eating. It has been speculated that any elevation of serum $[P_i]$, even within the usual normal range, could have adverse effects on the skeleton (Calvo and Heath, 1988; Calvo et al., 1988, 1990). In the animal studies cited above, increased bony porosity develops (Jowsey and Balasubramaniam, 1972; Krook et al., 1975). It is known that phosphate loads in humans lead acutely to very slight drops in ECF $[Ca^{2+}]$ and to elevated PTH levels (Calvo and Heath, 1988). However, these changes revert to normal by 5 days while still on the high-phosphorus intake (Silverberg et al., 1986). The acute, mild hypocalcemic effect is often attributed to the formation of calcium phosphate complexes in plasma, with a resultant reduction in $[Ca^{2+}]$. This in turn would lead to enhanced PTH release. However, as noted above, it is doubtful that this is the correct explanation. Rather, it is more likely that the initial fall in $[Ca^{2+}]$ following elevation of plasma P_i is produced by direct inhibition of PTH-mediated osteoclastic release of calcium from bone, cited earlier (Raisz and Niemann, 1969). (Thus, rather than harmful, this inhibition of bone resorption could actually be considered potentially beneficial to bone, since it amounts to a relative resistance to the bone-resorbing effects of PTH.)

Diets high in phosphorus and low in calcium produce a sustained rise in PTH (Calvo et al., 1988, 1990) which has been presumed to be harmful for bone; but diets low in calcium without extra phosphorus produce the same change (Silverberg et al., 1986) and for that reason it is unlikely that the high phosphorus component of the altered intake is the culprit in the first instance. More to the point, chronic administration of ~65 mmol phosphorus per day in men for at least 8 weeks produced no effect on calcium balance or calcium absorption relative to a diet containing only 26 mmol phosphorus (Spencer et al., 1965, 1978). Calcium intake (low, normal, or high) had no influence on this lack of effect, further underscoring the lack of physiological relevance of the dietary Ca:P ratio in adults. Further, calcium kinetic studies performed in adult women in whom phosphorus intake was doubled (from 37 mmol to 74.5 mmol – an intake well above the

95th percentile in NHANES) showed no effect whatsoever on bone turnover processes after 4 months of treatment (Spencer *et al.*, 1965). Thus it seems unlikely that phosphorus intakes, within the range currently experienced by the US population, adversely affect bone health.

Future Directions

The fundamental importance of phosphorus for life is well established, and, while more could be learned, no health policy decisions hinge on unresolved issues of basic phosphorus cell chemistry. On the other hand, four important areas of the understanding of phosphorus metabolism need elucidation:

- Better understanding of the role of the phosphatonins (and especially FGF-23), to include quantitative details of the endocrine feedback loop regulating serum [P$_i$].
- Elucidation of the consequences (if any) of variations in serum [Pi]; specifically, is there an optimal value within the nominal "normal" range, and, if so, does this optimum vary with age?
- Development of more effective means of controlling hyperphosphatemia in patients with end-stage renal disease.
- Determination of whether high FGF-23 levels, produced by hyperphosphatemia, exert adverse off-loop effects on various body systems.

Suggestions for Further Reading

Drezner, M.K. (2005) Clinical disorders of phosphate homeostasis. In D. Feldman, J.W. Pike, and F.H. Glorieux (eds), *Vitamin D*, Vol. II, 2nd Edn. Elsevier Academic Press, San Diego, pp. 1159–1187.

Econs, M.J. (2005) Disorders of phosphate metabolism: autosomal dominant hypophosphatemic rickets, tumor induced osteomalacia, fibrous dysplasia, and the pathophysiological relevance of FGF23. In D. Feldman, J.W. Pike, and F.H. Glorieux (eds), *Vitamin D*, Vol. II, 2nd Edn. Elsevier Academic Press, San Diego, pp. 1189–1195.

Institute of Medicine (1997) Phosphorus. In *Dietary Reference Intakes for Calcium, Magnesium, Phosphorus, Vitamin D, and Fluoride*. Food and Nutrition Board. National Academy Press, Washington, DC, pp. 146–189.

Nordin, B.E.C. (1988) Phosphorus. *J Food Nutr* **45**, 62–75.

References

Bijovet, O.L.M. (1969) Regulation of plasma phosphate concentration to renal tubular reabsorption of phosphate. *Clin Sci* **37**, 23–26.

Brown, A.J., Finch, J., and Slatopolsky, E. (2002) Differential effects of 19-nor-1,25-dihydroxyvitamin D(2) and 1,25-dihydroxyvitamin D(3) on intestinal calcium and phosphate transport. *J Lab Clin Med* **139**, 279–284.

Bushe, C.J. (1986) Profound hypophosphataemia in patients collapsing after a "fun run". *Br Med J* **292**, 898–899.

Calvo, M.S. and Heath, H., III (1988) Acute effects of oral phosphate-salt ingestion on serum phosphorus, serum ionized calcium, and parathyroid hormone in young adults. *Am J Clin Nutr* **47**, 1026–1029.

Calvo, M.S., Kumar, R., and Heath, H., III (1988) Elevated secretion and action of serum parathyroid hormone in young adults consuming high phosphorus, low calcium diets assembled from common foods. *J Clin Endocrinol Metab* **66**, 823–829.

Calvo, M.S., Kumar, R., and Heath, H., III (1990) Persistently elevated parathyroid hormone secretion and action in young women after four weeks of ingesting high phosphorus, low calcium diets. *J Clin Endocrinol Metab* **70**, 1334–1340.

Craig, J.M. (1959) Observations on the kidney after phosphate loading in the rat. *Arch Pathol* **68**, 306–315.

Dale, G., Fleetwood, J.A., Inkster, J.S., *et al.* (1986) Profound hypophosphataemia in patients collapsing after a "fun run". *Br Med J (Clin Res)* **292**, 447–448.

Ferrari, S.L., Bonjour, J.P., and Rizzoli, R. (2005) Fibroblast growth factor-23 relationship to dietary phosphate and renal phosphate handling in healthy young men. *J Clin Endocrinol Metab* **90**, 1519–1524.

Fleet, J. (2011) Molecular regulation of calcium/phosphate absorption. In D. Feldman, J. Adams, and W. Pike (eds), *Vitamin D*, 3rd Edn. Elsevier, San Diego, pp. 349–362.

Foley, R.N., Collins, A.J., Herzog, C.A., *et al.* (2009) Serum phosphorus levels associate with coronary atherosclerosis in young adults. *J Am Soc Nephrol* **20**, 397–404.

Foley, R.N., Collins, A.J., Ishani, A., *et al.* (2008) Calcium-phosphate levels and cardiovascular disease in community-dwelling adults: The Atherosclerotic Risk in Communities (ARIC) Study. *Am Heart J* **156**, 556–563.

Freiman, I., Pettifor, J.M., and Moodley, G.M. (1982) Serum phosphorus in protein energy malnutrition. *J Pediatr Gastroenterol Nutr* **1**, 547–550.

Hamuro, Y., Shino, A., and Suzuoki, Z. (1970) Acute induction of soft tissue calcification with transient hyperphosphatemia in the KK mouse by modification in dietary contents of calcium, phosphorus, and magnesium. *J Nutr* **100**, 404–412.

Heaney, R.P. and Nordin, B.E.C. (2002) Calcium effects on phosphorus absorption: implications for the prevention and co-therapy of osteoporosis. *J Am Coll Nutr* **21**, 239–244.

Institute of Medicine (1997) Phosphorus. In *Dietary Reference Intakes for Calcium, Phosphorus, Magnesium, Vitamin D, and Fluoride*. Food and Nutrition Board. National Academy Press, Washington, DC, pp.146–189.

Jowsey, J. and Balasubramaniam, P. (1972) Effect of phosphate supplements on soft-tissue calcification and bone turnover. *Clin Sci* **42**, 289–299.

Jüppner, H., Wolf, M., and Salusky, I.B. (2010) FGF-23: More than a regulator of renal phosphate handling? *J Bone Miner Res* **25**, 2091–2097.

Kjerulf-Jensen, K. (1941) Excretion of phosphorus by the bowel. *Acta Physiol Scand* **3**, 1–27.

Knochel, J.P. (1977) The pathophysiology and clinical characteristics of severe hypophosphatemia. *Arch Intern Med* **137**, 203–220.

Knochel, J.P. (1985) The clinical status of hypophosphatemia: an update. *N Engl J Med* **313**, 447–449.

Koo, W. and Tsang, R. (1997) Calcium, magnesium, phosphorus and vitamin D. In R.C. Tsang, S.H. Zlotkin, B.L. Nichols, *et al.* (eds), *Nutrition During Infancy: Principles and Practice*. Digital Education, Cincinnati, pp. 175–189.

Krook, L., Whalen, J.P., Lesser, G.V., *et al.* (1975) Experimental studies on osteoporosis. *Methods Achiev Exp Pathol* **7**, 72–108.

Lotz, M., Zisman, E., and Bartter, F.C. (1968) Evidence for a phosphorus-depletion syndrome in man. *N Engl J Med* **278**, 409–415.

Marik, P.E. and Bedigian, M.K. (1996) Refeeding hypophosphatemia in critically ill patients in an intensive care unit. *Arch Surg* **131**, 1043–1047.

McFarlane, D. (1941) Experimental phosphate nephritis in the rat. *J Pathol* **52**, 17–24.

Moshfegh, A., Goldman, J., Ahuja, J., *et al.* (2009) *What We Eat in America, NHANES 2005–2006: Usual Nutrient Intakes from Food and Water Compared to 1997 Dietary Reference Intakes for Vitamin D, Calcium, Phosphorus, and Magnesium*. US Department of Agriculture, Agricultural Research Service. http://www.ars.usda.gov/ba/bhnrc/fsrg (accessed July 2009).

Nordin, B.E.C. (1988) Phosphorus. *J Food Nutr* **45**, 62–75.

Portale, A.A., Halloran, B.P., and Morris, R.C., Jr (1989) Physiologic regulation of the serum concentration of 1,25-dihydroxyvitamin D by phosphorus in normal men. *J Clin Invest* **83**, 1494–1499.

Raisz, L.G. and Niemann, I. (1969) Effect of phosphate, calcium and magnesium on bone resorption and hormonal responses in tissue culture. *Endocrinology* **85**, 446–452.

Ramirez, J.A., Emmett, M., White, M.G., *et al.* (1986) The absorption of dietary phosphorus and calcium in hemodialysis patients. *Kidney Int* **30**, 753–759.

Ritz, E. (1982) Acute hypophosphatemia. *Kidney Int* **22**, 84–94.

Silverberg, S.J., Shane, E., Clemens, T.L., *et al.* (1986) The effect of oral phosphate administration on major indices of skeletal metabolism in normal subjects. *J Bone Miner Res* **1**, 383–388.

Spencer, H., Kramer, L., and Osis, D. (1978) Effect of a high protein (meat) intake on calcium metabolism in man. *Am J Clin Nutr* **31**, 2167–2180.

Spencer, H., Menczel, J., Lewin, I., *et al.* (1965) Effect of high phosphorus intake on calcium and phosphorus metabolism in man. *J Nutr* **86**, 125–132.

Stein, J.H., Smith, W.O., and Ginn, H.E. (1966) Hypophosphatemia in acute alcoholism. *Am J Med Sci* **252**, 78–83.

Strom, T.M. and Jüppner, H. (2008) PHEX, FGF23, DMP1 and beyond. *Curr Opin Nephrol Hypertens* **17**, 357–362.

Travis, S.F., Sugerman, H.J., Ruberg, R.L., *et al.* (1971) Alterations of red cell glycolytic intermediates and oxygen transport as a consequence of hypophosphatemia in patients receiving intravenous hyperalimentation. *N Engl J Med* **285**, 763–768.

Weinsier, R.L. and Krumdieck, C.L. (1981) Death resulting from overzealous total parenteral nutrition: the refeeding syndrome revisited. *Am J Clin Nutr* **34**, 393–399.

White, K.E. and Econs, M.J. (2008) Fibroblast growth factor-23. In C.J. Rosen, J.E. Compston, and J.B. Lian (eds), *Primer on the Metabolic Bone Diseases and Disorders of Mineral Metabolism*, 7th Edn. American Society for Bone and Mineral Research, Washington, DC, pp. 112–116.

Young, G.P., Thomas, R.J., Bourne, D.W., *et al.* (1985) Parenteral nutrition. *Med J Aust* **143**, 597–601.

30

MAGNESIUM

STELLA LUCIA VOLPE, PhD, RD, LDN, FACSM

Drexel University College of Nursing and Health Professions, Philadelphia, Pennsylvania, USA

Summary

Magnesium is a required mineral and cofactor for over 300 metabolic reactions in the body. The body consists of about 25 g of magnesium, with about 50–60% in the bone and the remainder in soft tissue. Magnesium (Mg^{2+}) is a divalent metal ion. It is the fourth most abundant cation in the body after calcium, potassium, and sodium. Food sources high in magnesium include green, leafy vegetables, unpolished grains, and nuts. Magnesium deficiency may lead to cardiovascular disease, hypertension, the metabolic syndrome, and type 2 diabetes mellitus.

Introduction

Magnesium (Mg) is a required mineral and a cofactor for over 300 enzymatic reactions in the body (Bohl and Volpe, 2002; Elin, 2010). These reactions include: deoxyribonucleic acid (DNA) and ribonucleic acid (RNA) synthesis, protein synthesis, cell growth and reproduction, adenylate cyclase synthesis, cellular energy production and storage, preservation of cellular electrolyte composition, and stabilization of mitochondrial membranes (Rude and Oldham, 1990; Newhouse and Finstad, 2000; Bohl and Volpe, 2002; Chubanov *et al.*, 2005; Elin, 2010). Magnesium plays a primary role in controlling nerve transmission, cardiac excitability, neuromuscular conduction, muscular contraction, vasomotor tone, and blood pressure (Rude and Oldham, 1990; Elin, 1994; Newhouse and Finstad, 2000; Bohl and Volpe, 2002; Chubanov *et al.*, 2005).

Magnesium deficiency has also been linked to the metabolic syndrome, insulin resistance, and diabetes mellitus in humans and animal models, and thus Mg plays a role in glucose metabolism (Rodriguez-Moran and Guerrero-Romero, 2003; Song *et al.*, 2004, 2005; Huerta *et al.*, 2005; Soltani *et al.*, 2005; Everett and King, 2006; He *et al.*, 2006; Mayer-Davis *et al.*, 2006).

Magnesium Concentration in the Body

The body consists of about 25 g of magnesium, with about 50–60% in the bone, and the remainder in soft tissue (Bohl and Volpe, 2002; Elin, 2010). Less than 1% of total body magnesium is in the blood (Elin, 2010). Note that most of the clinical laboratory data are derived from the assessment of serum magnesium concentrations (Elin,

Present Knowledge in Nutrition, Tenth Edition. Edited by John W. Erdman Jr, Ian A. Macdonald and Steven H. Zeisel.
© 2012 International Life Sciences Institute. Published 2012 by John Wiley & Sons, Inc.

TABLE 30.1   Distribution of magnesium in the body

Location	Concentration
Bone	0.5% of bone ash
Muscle	9 mmol/kg wet weight
Soft tissue	9 mmol/kg wet weight
Adipose tissue	0.8 mmol/kg wet weight
Serum magnesium (free)	~0.56 mmol/L
Saliva, gastric, bile	0.3–0.7 mmol/L
Sweat	0.3 mmol/L

Adapted from Elin (1994).

2010), though this has changed in the last several years as other methods of magnesium assessment have evolved such as evaluating plasma ionized magnesium, red blood cell magnesium, and, though more cumbersome, urinary magnesium via the magnesium loading test.

Approximately one-third of skeletal magnesium is exchangeable, acting as a pool for maintaining normal extracellular magnesium levels (Elin, 1994) (Table 30.1). Normal serum magnesium concentrations range from 1.8 to 2.3 mg/dL (Institute of Medicine, 1997), and this concentration is tightly regulated. Wary *et al.* (1999) reported that 30 healthy male volunteers showed no significant change in plasma magnesium levels after 1 month of supplementation with 12 mmol/day of magnesium lactate. Conversely, Day *et al.* (2010) reported significantly increased serum magnesium levels in post menopausal women after they consumed magnesium-supplemented water for 84 days (120 mg/L of magnesium as magnesium bicarbonate in spring water, compared with a control). Though serum magnesium concentrations are often used to evaluate magnesium status in clinical and research settings, recall that it may not be the best indicator of magnesium status.

Chemistry and Functions

Magnesium (Mg^{2+}) is a divalent metal ion. It is the fourth most abundant cation in the body after calcium, potassium, and sodium (Rude, 1998). Magnesium is the most prevalent intracellular divalent cation and the second most abundant intracellular cation after potassium (Elin, 1987; Rude, 1998). It is usually bound to ligands, and forms comparatively stable complexes (Frausto da Silva and Williams, 1991; Elin, 1994). Ionized magnesium represents the physiologically active form of the mineral;

however, protein-bound and chelated magnesium act as buffers for the ionized pool (Elin, 1994).

There are a minimum of three different body pools of magnesium in the human body: one with a quick turnover (from about 1.6 to 28 hours), largely comprised of extracellular magnesium; a second with a turnover rate of half the first pool, primarily consisting of intracellular magnesium (about 11 days); and a third pool containing skeletal magnesium with a slow turnover rate (>11 days) (Wester, 1987; Feillet-Coudray *et al.*, 2000, 2002).

Approximately 30% of serum magnesium is bound to protein, while the majority of the residual portion is ionized and filtered through the kidney. Intracellular magnesium is bound principally to protein and energy-rich phosphates (Frausto da Silva and Williams, 1991; Bohl and Volpe, 2002). The principal role of magnesium in the body is to complex highly charged anions, such as polyphosphates and nucleic acids, to support enzyme–substrate interactions, or stabilize the conformation of polymers (Wester, 1987; Bohl and Volpe, 2002).

Magnesium is required for a number of metabolic reactions including: aerobic and anaerobic metabolism; glycolysis, both directly as an enzyme activator, and indirectly as part of the magnesium–adenosine triphosphate (ATP) complex; and in oxidative phosphorylation (Elin, 1987, 2010). Magnesium is also required for the adequate supply of purines and pyrimidines for RNA and DNA synthesis. Magnesium may directly augment adenylate cyclase activity, as well as sodium-potassium-ATPase activity (Maguire, 1984), which is required for the active transport of potassium (Dorup and Clausen, 1993). Magnesium also plays a significant role in protein kinase activity.

Hekmat-Nejad *et al.* (2010) recently studied the steady-state kinetics of kinase activity and magnesium requirements of the interleukin-1 receptor-associated kinase-4. Interleukin-1 receptor-associated kinase-4 (IRAK-4) is a serine/threonine-specific protein kinase that plays a crucial role in intracellular signaling cascades that are mediated by interleukin-1 (IL-1) receptors. Hekmat-Nejad *et al.* (2010) reported that more than one Mg^{2+} ion interacts with the phosphoryl transfer activity of IRAK-4, and that the enzyme has its greatest activity in the presence of 5–10 mM of free Mg^{2+}. Furthermore, though one divalent metal is required for catalysis as part of a chelate complex with ATP, their kinetic evidence demonstrated that unbound Mg^{2+} further enhanced the catalytic activity of IRAK-4.

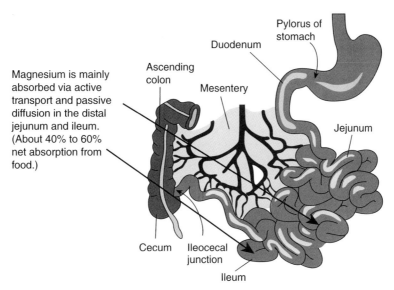

Magnesium is mainly absorbed via active transport and passive diffusion in the distal jejunum and ileum. (About 40% to 60% net absorption from food.)

FIG. 30.1 Magnesium absorption.

Magnesium has been called "nature's physiological calcium channel blocker" (Iseri and French, 1984; White and Hartzell, 1989; Schmid-Elsaesser *et al.*, 2006), because, during magnesium depletion, intracellular calcium increases. It has been well documented that calcium plays an important role in skeletal and smooth muscle contraction; therefore, magnesium depletion can lead to muscle cramps, hypertension, and coronary and cerebral vasospasms (Institute of Medicine, 1997). Schmid-Elsaesser *et al.* (2006) reported that magnesium prevented delayed ischemic neurological deficits in patients with aneurysmal subarachnoid hemorrhage equally as effectively as nimodipine (a calcium-channel blocker). Studies combining their use may be worth researching, because of the differences in their properties; however, magnesium has very few side-effects, and may be a promising treatment itself.

In addition, magnesium therapy may show promise as an important adjuvant therapy for acute myocardial infarction (Sadeh, 1989; Horner, 1992; Herzog *et al.*, 1995). Because magnesium is an inorganic calcium channel blocker (Iseri and French, 1984; White and Hartzell, 1989), its ability to decrease infarct size may be a result of magnesium's calcium channel blocking action at the level of the plasma membrane or an intracellular site (Sadeh, 1989).

Absorption and Homeostasis

Like most minerals, the amount of magnesium absorbed is inversely related to the amount consumed. Though magnesium is absorbed throughout the intestinal tract, the greatest amount of magnesium is absorbed in the distal jejunum and ileum (Rude, 1998), with about 40–60% net absorption rate from food (Figure 30.1). Magnesium is absorbed via active transport and passive diffusion; active transport accounts for a greater fractional absorption of magnesium at low dietary intakes, while passive diffusion occurs at higher dietary intakes, resulting in lower fractional absorption (Fine *et al.*, 1991; Kayne and Lee, 1993). Calbindin-D_{9k} may play a role in magnesium absorption (Institute of Medicine, 1997); however, its role has not been clearly defined.

The kidney is the primary organ regulating magnesium homeostasis (Quamme and Dirks, 1986). About 65% of filtered magnesium is reabsorbed at the loop of Henle via active transport (Quamme and Dirks, 1986) (Figure 30.2). Approximately 20–30% of magnesium is reabsorbed via passive diffusion in the proximal convoluted tubule of the kidney, which is associated with calcium, sodium and water transport (Schwartz *et al.*, 1984; Rude, 1998) (Figure 30.2). Though excessive magnesium is almost entirely excreted through the kidneys, this is not the case during

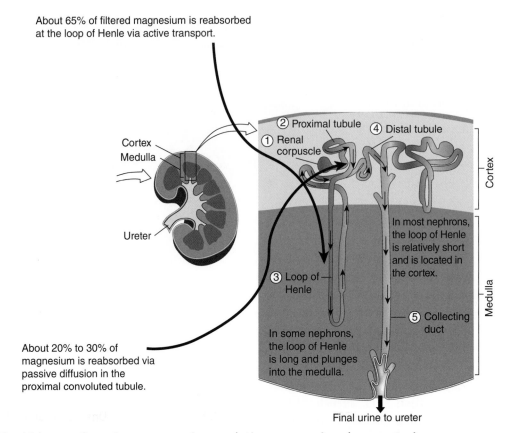

About 65% of filtered magnesium is reabsorbed at the loop of Henle via active transport.

Cortex
Medulla

Ureter

About 20% to 30% of magnesium is reabsorbed via passive diffusion in the proximal convoluted tubule.

② Proximal tubule   ④ Distal tubule
① Renal corpuscle

In most nephrons, the loop of Henle is relatively short and is located in the cortex.

③ Loop of Henle

In some nephrons, the loop of Henle is long and plunges into the medulla.

⑤ Collecting duct

Cortex

Medulla

Final urine to ureter

FIG. 30.2   The kidney – the primary organ in regulating magnesium homeostasis.

magnesium deficiency. During magnesium deficiency, the kidney prevent magnesium loss by excreting less than 12 to 24 mg/day of magnesium (Rude, 1998). Renal magnesium excretion is augmented by diets high in sodium, calcium, and protein, as well as caffeine and alcohol consumption (Mahalko *et al.*, 1983; Martinez *et al.*, 1985; Massey and Whiting, 1993). Although the method(s) of magnesium transport in the intestine and kidney have not been elucidated, at present, there have not been any specific hormones or other compounds that have been designated to play a major role (Rude, 1998).

Factors Affecting Absorption

A dietary intake averaging about 300 to 350 mg/day of magnesium will typically result in a fractional absorption rate between 30% and 50% (Schwartz *et al.*, 1984). A number of factors can decrease magnesium absorption, including fiber, phytates and oxalates from fruits, vegetables, and grains; excessive alcohol intake; and medications such as diuretics. Phosphorus, calcium, and protein have also been shown to decrease magnesium absorption. It

appears that the phytate in high-fiber foods results in the binding of magnesium to the phosphate groups on the phytates, leading to decreased magnesium absorption (Franz, 1989; Wisker *et al.*, 1991; Brink and Beynen, 1992; Greger, 1999).

Several researchers have reported no effects of either high-calcium diets (up to 2000 mg/day) on magnesium absorption, or high-magnesium intakes (up to 826 mg/day) on calcium absorption (Schwartz *et al.*, 1984; Abbott *et al.*, 1994). Nevertheless, because many calcium channels are reliant on magnesium, intracellular calcium levels increase with magnesium deficiency (Dacey, 2001). Moreover, persons who have low serum-magnesium concentrations and are also calcium deficient do not react to calcium supplementation until the magnesium deficiency has been corrected (Al-Ghamdi *et al.*, 1994; Dhupa and Proulx, 1998). Parathyroid hormone (PTH) is most likely the principal reason for this occurrence, because magnesium deficiency impairs PTH release and its uptake by bone (Estep *et al.*, 1969; Freitag and Martin, 1979; Al-Ghamdi *et al.*, 1994; Dhupa and Proulx, 1998).

Protein has also been linked with impaired magnesium status; magnesium absorption is lower when dietary protein is less than 30 g/day (Hunt and Schofield, 1969). Higher protein intakes of more than 94 g/day may result in increased renal magnesium excretion due to the increased acid load; however, magnesium retention remained the same on higher-protein diets (Mahalko *et al.*, 1983; Wong *et al.*, 1986). Others have reported that, when compared with lower protein intakes (43 g/day), magnesium absorption and maintenance were improved with higher protein intakes (93 g/day) (Schwartz *et al.*, 1973).

Though there is no definitive research on how boron may affect magnesium absorption, there does seem to be an interaction between boron and magnesium (Volpe *et al.*, 1993; Meacham *et al.*, 1994,1995). It appears that, when boron concentrations are low, magnesium may be the mineral called upon to take on boron's roles in the body (Volpe *et al.*, 1993). Furthermore, it appears that boron supplementation may increase serum magnesium concentrations over time (Meacham *et al.*, 1994, 1995).

Magnesium Transport

Magnesium transport in and out of cells requires carrier-mediated transport systems (Gunther, 1993; Romani *et al.*, 1993). Magnesium efflux from the cell is linked to sodium transport, while magnesium influx is associated with sodium and bicarbonate transport; however, it uses a different method than that of magnesium efflux (Gunther, 1993; Romani *et al.*, 1993; Institute of Medicine, 1997).

Magnesium Requirements

The United States dietary reference intakes (DRIs) for magnesium are listed in Table 30.2. These represent the

TABLE 30.2 Dietary reference intakes for magnesium

Age and sex	AI (mg/day)	RDA (mg/day)	UL[a] (mg/day)
Infants (boys and girls)			
0–6 months	30	NA	Unable to establish
7–12 months	75	NA	for magnesium
			supplementation
Children (boys and girls)			
1–3 years	NA	80	65
4–8 years	NA	130	110
9–13 years	NA	240	350
Males			
14–18 years	NA	410	350
19–30 years	NA	400	350
31–>70 years	NA	420	350
Females			
14–18 years	NA	360	350
19–30 years	NA	310	350
31–>70 years	NA	320	350
Pregnancy			
14–18 years	NA	400	350
19–30 years	NA	350	350
31–50 years	NA	360	350
Lactation			
14–18 years	NA	360	350
19–30 years	NA	310	350
31–50 years	NA	320	350

AI, adequate intake; EAR, estimated average requirement; RDA, recommended dietary allowance; UL, tolerable upper intake levels; NA, not applicable.
[a]Only includes intake from supplements, not food and water.
Adapted from Institute of Medicine (1997).

most recent DRIs for magnesium, which were last established in 1997. Though the requirements for the United States are slightly higher than some countries (e.g. England has a Recommended Daily Allowance of 300 mg/day, with an upper limit of 350 mg/day), in general, magnesium requirements are within 300 to 450 mg/day throughout the world.

The indicators used to establish the estimated average requirements (EAR) for magnesium were based upon magnesium balance studies, since there were not sufficient data to determine an advantage for maximal magnesium retention (Institute of Medicine, 1997). Because magnesium intake from foods has not been shown to result in adverse effects, the tolerable upper intake level (UL) of magnesium was established by assessing pharmacological doses of magnesium (e.g. magnesium salts) that resulted in adverse outcomes (Institute of Medicine, 1997). (Refer to later section entitled "Effects of magnesium excess" for examples of adverse outcomes with high levels of magnesium intake.)

Food Sources of Magnesium

Magnesium is a ubiquitous mineral, found in a number of foods. Food sources high in magnesium include green, leafy vegetables, unpolished grains, and nuts. Intermediate sources of magnesium include meats, starches, and milk. Refined foods are poor sources of magnesium. Table 30.3

TABLE 30.3 Food sources of magnesium

Food	Content (mg)
Halibut, cooked, 3 ounces	90
Almonds, dry roasted, 1 ounce	80
Cashews, dry roasted, 1 ounce	75
Soybeans, mature, cooked, ½ cup	75
Spinach, frozen, cooked, ½ cup	75
Nuts, mixed, dry roasted, 1 ounce	65
Cereal, shredded wheat, 2 rectangular biscuits	55
Oatmeal, instant, fortified, prepared with water, 1 cup	55
Potato, baked with skin, 1 medium	50
Peanuts, dry roasted, 1 ounce	50
Peanut butter, smooth, 2 tablespoons	50
Wheat bran, crude, 2 tablespoons	45
Black-eyed peas, cooked, ½ cup	45
Yogurt, plain, skim milk, 8 fluid ounces	45
Bran flakes, ½ cup	40
Vegetarian baked beans, ½ cup	40
Rice, brown, long-grained, cooked, ½ cup	40
Lentils, mature seeds, cooked, ½ cup	35
Avocado, California, ½ cup pureed	35
Kidney beans, canned, ½ cup	35
Pinto beans, cooked, ½ cup	35
Wheat germ, crude, 2 tablespoons	35
Chocolate milk, 1 cup	33
Banana, raw, 1 medium	30
Milk chocolate candy bar, 1.5 ounce bar	28
Milk, reduced fat (2%) or fat free, 1 cup	27
Bread, whole wheat, commercially prepared, 1 slice	25
Raisins, seedless, ½ cup packed	25
Whole milk, 1 cup	24
Chocolate pudding, 4-ounce ready-to-eat portion	24

More foods can be found at the following website (USDA website): http://www.nal.usda.gov/fnic/cgi-bin/nut_search.pl.
Adapted from http://ods.od.nih.gov/factsheets/magnesium.asp#en1 (retrieved September 10, 2010).

lists several sources of magnesium (US Department of Agriculture, 2003; National Institutes of Health, Office of Dietary Supplements, 2005).

Magnesium Deficiency

Though approximately 60% of adults in the United States do not consume the dietary reference intake for magnesium, the long-term effects of this low intake have not been adequately reported (Nielsen, 2010). In addition to lower dietary intakes of magnesium, magnesium deficiency may now be more common because of the increased incidence of the metabolic syndrome and type 2 diabetes mellitus, which increase magnesium excretion (or, perhaps, some of these chronic diseases may be a result of poor magnesium intake). "Marginal-to-moderate magnesium deficiency through exacerbating chronic inflammatory stress may be contributing significantly to the occurrence of chronic diseases such as atherosclerosis, hypertension, osteoporosis, diabetes mellitus, and cancer" (Nielsen, 2010).

In addition, many weight-loss diets do not provide the proper amount of micronutrients. Gardner *et al.* (2010) compared the micronutrient intake between overweight or obese women who had been randomly assigned to four popular diets that differed in their macronutrient distribution. They found that micronutrient intake decreased to inadequacy in a large proportion of the individuals in all the diets. Magnesium was one of the micronutrients found to be inadequate in intake. They suggested that there could be a "micronutrient advantage" to low-energy diets, which could positively affect health and weight loss.

Magnesium deficiency may be caused by excessive alcohol intake, certain medications (e.g. diuretics), malabsorption (typically resulting from short bowel syndrome, celiac disease [gluten-sensitive enteropathy], and Crohn's disease), and/or inadequate intake of magnesium (Institute of Medicine, 1997). Loss of appetite, nausea, vomiting, fatigue, and weakness are early signs of magnesium deficiency. As magnesium deficiency worsens, such symptoms as numbness, tingling, muscle contractions and cramps, seizures, personality changes, and coronary spasms (angina pectoris) can emerge (Institute of Medicine, 1997; Rude, 1998).

Magnesium deficiency has been shown to lead to hypocalcemia, neuromuscular excitability, osteoporosis, diabetes mellitus, and cardiac complications, such as hypertension, dysrhythmias, angina pectoris, acute myocardial infarc-

tion, and dyslipidemias (Gums, 2004; Shecter, 2010). Magnesium supplementation will reverse most of these conditions. Normen *et al.* (2005) assessed whether magnesium (and calcium and sulfate) would be absorbed from mineral water in subjects who had an ileostomy. The main purpose of conducting this randomized, controlled, crossover study was to assess if the mineral water would provide an alternative for individuals at risk for developing a deficiency due to low intakes. When compared with the control period, participants absorbed 30% more magnesium with the mineral water, with consumption during meals showing greater absorption (Normen *et al.*, 2005). Therefore, supplementation with magnesium in the form of mineral water appears to be a viable method of increasing intake and absorption.

Effects of Deficiency

Severe hypomagnesaemia (<12.3 mg/dL) has been associated with increased mortality rates (41%) in patients admitted to a postoperative intensive care unit (ICU) compared with patients in ICU with normal serum magnesium concentrations (13%) (Chernow *et al.*, 1989). The authors concluded that low serum magnesium levels, though not a sensitive or precise predictor of patient survival, was frequent among postoperative ICU patients, and that patients with severe hypomagnesemia had more cases of hypokalemia (which can lead to dysrhythmias) and greater mortality rates than patients with comparable illnesses who had normal serum magnesium concentrations (Chernow *et al.*, 1989).

Cardiovascular Disease

Magnesium may play a role in the management of acute myocardial infarction and atherosclerosis (Elin, 1994; Shecter, 2010). Because cardiovascular disease typically does not manifest itself until later in life, it is important that there is an improved understanding of ionized magnesium metabolism, which will lead to a better comprehension of the chronic changes in magnesium status that may be dormant (Elin, 1994). Rosenlund *et al.* (2005) did not find a protective effect against myocardial infarction in individuals who consumed drinking water that had higher levels of magnesium. Similarly, and more recently, Day *et al.* (2010) did not find positive effects of magnesium-supplemented spring water on cardiovascular risk markers in postmenopausal women, 50 to 70 years of age with a body mass index (BMI) of 20 to 35 kg/m^2.

Conversely, Hashimoto *et al.* (2010) measured 728 participants from the general Japanese population, with a mean age of 67 years (68.4% were women), to determine the risk of serum magnesium levels and cardiovascular disease risk. They reported that low serum magnesium concentrations were related to risk of carotid artery alteration.

Mathers and Beckstrand (2009) reviewed randomized controlled trials and prospective studies for the safety of magnesium supplementation in individuals with coronary heart disease or risk of coronary heart disease. They did not find any adverse events from magnesium supplementation in any of the published research. They reported, based on published work, a modest association between a lower risk of coronary heart disease in men and increased magnesium intake, and thus suggest diets higher in magnesium as a possible method for lowering the risk of cardiovascular disease. Furthermore, Shecter (2010) states as follows:

> there are theoretical potential benefits of magnesium supplementation as a cardioprotective agent in CAD [coronary artery disease] patients, as well as promising results from previous work in animal and humans. These studies are cost effective, easy to handle and are relatively free of adverse effects, which gives magnesium a role in treating CAD patients, especially high-risk groups such as CAD patients with heart failure, the elderly and hospitalized patients with hypomagnesemia. Furthermore, magnesium therapy is indicated in life-threatening ventricular arrhythmias such as Torsades de Pointes and intractable ventricular tachycardia.

As noted by Bobkowski *et al.* (2005), "Idiopathic mitral valve prolapse (IMVP) refers to the systolic displacement of one or both mitral leaflets into the left atrium, with or without mitral regurgitation." IMVP is most commonly seen among young women and may be caused by latent tetany due to magnesium deficiency (as a result of either insufficient intake or excessive urinary loss). Galland *et al.* (1986) reported that latent tetany due to magnesium deficiency is seen in 85% of IMVP cases. Because normal plasma magnesium levels are not indicative of magnesium deficiency, Bobkowski *et al.* (2005) recommend that laboratory evaluation should include assessment of plasma, and erythrocyte and urinary magnesium concentrations, as well as blood and urinary markers of calcium. Furthermore, correction of the symptoms by the oral magnesium load test (5 mg of magnesium/kg/day) is indicative of the cause being magnesium deficiency. Finally, the authors state that

it is necessary to combine magnesium-sparing diuretics or physiological doses of vitamin D with oral magnesium supplementation to sustain the positive results (Bobkowski *et al.*, 2005).

Blood Pressure

One of the recommendations from the Canadian Hypertension Education Program is to "follow a reduced fat, low cholesterol diet with an adequate intake of potassium, magnesium and calcium" (Khan *et al.*, 2005). It appears that diets high in calcium, magnesium, and potassium help to manage hypertension, though the results of epidemiological studies have provided stronger evidence for this (Ascherio *et al.*, 1992; Ma *et al.*, 1995) than magnesium supplementation trials (Sacks *et al.*, 1995; Yamamoto *et al.*, 1995). Nevertheless, as is often the case with nutritional studies, more than one nutrient may play a role. Appel *et al.* (1997) reported a significant reduction in blood pressure in non-hypertensive adults who increased their dietary intake of magnesium by approximately 247 mg/day through increased consumption of fruits and vegetables. These individuals also increased their potassium intake and calcium intake through non-fat dairy consumption (Appel *et al.*, 1997); both minerals positively influence blood pressure. More recently, the Dietary Approaches to Stop Hypertension (DASH) trial (essentially, a diet high in fruits, vegetables, and low-fat dairy, with reductions in fat and cholesterol intake), has led to significant reductions in hypertension (Chen *et al.*, 2010). Though magnesium cannot be singled out as the primary effect of the decrease in hypertension with the DASH diet, the increased intake of magnesium (and potassium) plays a role in decreasing hypertension. Furthermore, the DASH diet has been shown to decrease the risk of coronary heart disease (a decrease that has been reported over a 10-year period) (Chen *et al.*, 2010).

Research has shown that magnesium supplementation alone will decrease hypertension. In a 24-week, double-blind, placebo-controlled study by Baker *et al.* (2009), 50 patients with implantable cardioverter defibrillators, who also had hypertension, received either 504 mg of elemental magnesium per day (in the form of six tablets of magnesium L-lactate) or a placebo. They reported that 86% of the total sample had an intracellular magnesium deficiency at baseline. Systolic blood pressure was significantly lowered in patients who were supplemented with magnesium at 12 weeks and at 24 weeks. Additionally, intracellular magnesium levels were found to be a better indicator of magnesium status compared with serum magnesium concentrations.

Diabetes Mellitus and the Metabolic Syndrome

There is growing evidence that magnesium deficiency is related to diabetes mellitus and to the metabolic syndrome. Investigations have also shown the effectiveness of magnesium supplementation in reversing diabetes mellitus and the metabolic syndrome in individuals who are magnesium deficient (Guerrero-Romero and Rodríguez-Morán, 2006; Volpe, 2008; Guerrera et al., 2009; Davì et al., 2010).

Magnesium's effect on insulin sensitivity may be a result of insulin's regulation of the shift of magnesium from the extracellular to the intracellular space (Paolisso and Barbagallo, 1997). A sub-optimal magnesium concentration within the body, such as in a person with diabetes mellitus, may lead to malfunctioning tyrosine kinase activity at the insulin receptor level, leading to insulin resistance (Paolisso and Barbagallo, 1997).

Kirii et al. (2010) reported an inverse relationship between dietary intake of magnesium and age- and BMI-adjusted diabetes incidence in men and women 40 to 65 years of age. Evangelopoulos et al. (2008) reported a strong inverse association between serum magnesium concentrations and the metabolic syndrome. They also reported that, as serum magnesium levels decreased, the number of metabolic syndrome components increased. Furthermore, there was a relationship between serum magnesium concentrations and C-reactive protein levels, indicating the relationship between magnesium and inflammation, which could lead to the metabolic syndrome.

Afridi et al. (2008) evaluated the levels of potassium, calcium, magnesium, and sodium in blood, urine, and hair in individuals with hypertension and diabetes mellitus compared with those without hypertension who had diabetes mellitus. They found that individuals with diabetes mellitus who had hypertension and/or were normotensive had lower levels of potassium, calcium, and magnesium, but had higher levels of sodium compared with controls.

Guerrero-Romero et al. (2004) set out to establish whether oral magnesium supplementation would improve insulin sensitivity in individuals who had both insulin resistance (homeostasis model assessment of insulin resistance index [HOMA-IR] index >3.0) and hypomagnesemia, defined as serum magnesium concentrations <0.74 mmol/L (Guerrero-Romero and Rodríguez-Morán,

2002; Rodríguez-Morán and Guerrero-Romero, 2003). Participants were randomly assigned to receive either 2.5 g/day of magnesium chloride (12.5 mmol or 300 mg of magnesium) or a placebo. Individuals who were supplemented with magnesium significantly increased their serum magnesium concentrations compared with the control subjects. Individuals who were supplemented with magnesium also significantly reduced HOMA-IR index, with no change seen in the control subjects.

Prevention of type 2 diabetes mellitus is extremely important, but so is its treatment. Rodríguez-Morán and Guerrero-Romero (2003) evaluated whether oral magnesium supplementation (300 mg of magnesium) improved insulin sensitivity as well as metabolic control in individuals with both type 2 diabetes mellitus and decreased serum magnesium concentrations (<0.74 mmol/L). They studied 63 individuals who qualified for this 16-week, randomized, double-blind, placebo-controlled trial. At 16 weeks, those who received the magnesium supplementation had a significantly greater serum magnesium concentration than control subjects. Those who were supplemented also significantly improved insulin sensitivity and metabolic control, based on a lower HOMA-IR index, lower fasting blood glucose levels, and lower glycosylated hemoglobin concentrations compared with control subjects. These two prospective trials demonstrate that magnesium supplementation can be an effective agent in improving insulin sensitivity.

Diabetes mellitus can lead to long-term complications, such as angiopathy (cardiovascular disease), neuropathy (nerve damage), nephropathy (kidney disease), and retinopathy (retinal problems with the eye).

Because of the high rate of cardiovascular disease that occurs with diabetes mellitus, Soltani et al. (2005) examined whether oral magnesium administration would prevent vascular complications in rats with diabetes. The rats were separated into six groups: two groups received tap water for 8 weeks (control), two groups (made diabetic by injection of STZ) were treated with magnesium sulfate (10 g/L) added to the drinking water, and two groups (made diabetic by injection of STZ) received tap water only. Mean arterial blood pressure and mean perfusion pressure of the mesenteric vascular bed were significantly lower in the magnesium-treated rats than in the non-treated rats. The authors concluded that magnesium sulfate supplementation was effective in preventing vascular complications associated with diabetes mellitus (Soltani et al., 2005).

Body Mass Index

Though there is no direct association between magnesium and body mass index [BMI: weight (kg)/height (m²)], there may be a relationship between the two. Wang *et al.* (2005) assessed calcium, copper, iron, magnesium, potassium, sodium, and zinc concentrations in the hair samples of women 20 to 50 years of age (*n* = 392). The women were separated into four groups based upon their BMI: BMI <18 kg/m², BMI = 18 to 25 kg/m², BMI = 26 to 35 kg/m², and BMI >35 kg/m². The group with a BMI <18 kg/m² had the highest ratios for calcium:magnesium, iron:copper, and zinc:copper, but the lowest ratio for potassium:sodium (Wang *et al.*, 2005). In contrast, the group with a BMI >35 kg/m² had the highest ratio for potassium:sodium, but the lowest for iron:copper and zinc:copper (Wang *et al.*, 2005). There were significant differences between groups in hair magnesium concentrations. More research is required to evaluate if there is a direct link between obesity and magnesium deficiency. However, magnesium deficiency is related to the inflammatory response (e.g. increased C-reactive protein), and obesity is characterized by low-grade inflammation, thus there may be a stronger relationship between obesity and magnesium deficiency than is currently known (Nielsen, 2010; Rayssiguier *et al.*, 2010).

Osteoporosis

Osteoporosis is widespread chronic disease that results in 2 million fractures per year in the United States, costing more than $17 billion in health care (Rude *et al.*, 2009). Women are more affected than men by osteoporosis, and have an average magnesium intake in their diets of only about 68% of the recommended intake (Rude *et al.*, 2009). Magnesium deficiency has been shown to be a risk factor for osteoporosis (Saito *et al.*, 2004; Stendig-Lindberg *et al.*, 2004). Stendig-Linberg *et al.* (2004) reported a significant increase in radial bone mineral density in women after 750 mg/day of magnesium supplementation for 6 months, followed by 250 mg/day of magnesium for 18 months.

In more recent studies, Ohgitani *et al.* (2005) found a negative correlation between fingernail magnesium concentration and lumbar bone mineral density. Additionally, Day *et al.* (2010) did not find that magnesium-supplemented spring water improved biomarkers of bone in postmenopausal women.

None the less, there is a need for prospective clinical trials to elucidate the effects of magnesium intake (via supplementation and/or increased dietary intake) on the prevention of osteoporosis in humans (Rude *et al.*, 2009). Mechanisms that may explain how magnesium deficiency may result in osteoporosis include impaired production of PTH and 1,25-dihydroxyvitamin D₃; and a compound P-stimulated release of inflammatory cytokines (Rude *et al.*, 2009).

Calcium Stones

One of the effects of magnesium deficiency is hypocalcemia, which can then lead to calcium urolithiasis (calcium stones).

Magnesium has been shown to reduce calcium oxalate crystallization in human urine (Massey, 2005).

Johansson *et al.* (1980) reported that, in 56 individuals given magnesium hydroxide, 45 were free of recurrences of new calcium stones, and those who did have recurrences only had 0.03 stones per year during a 2-year follow-up period, compared with 0.8 stones per year prior to the magnesium treatment. Of the 34 individuals who had no prophylactic magnesium therapy, 15 had experienced calcium stones after 2 years.

Conversely, in a retrospective study of 7000 patients suffering from calcium oxalate stones, Schwartz *et al.* (2001) reported that calcium stone formation was slightly, but not significantly, increased in patients with hypomagnesuria. They stated that:

> The beneficial effects of urinary magnesium on stone formation may be less than previously reported. The role of oral magnesium supplementation and the subsequent increase in urinary magnesium in calcium urinary stone formation remains unknown . . . If magnesium has a protective effect, it may work through pathways that enhance citrate excretion.

Massey (2005) reported that clinical-trial evidence does not support the use of magnesium oxide or magnesium hydroxide as an exclusive therapy for calcium oxalate stones; however, when magnesium is added to potassium citrate therapy, there are better outcomes.

Magnesium Supplementation

Magnesium supplementation may be required in specific conditions that may decrease magnesium absorption, or result in excessive loss (Ladefoged *et al.*, 1996; Kelepouris and Agus, 1998; Vormann, 2003). As previously discussed, some medications may result in magnesium deficiency, such as some diuretics, antibiotics, and anti-cancer medications (Ramsey *et al.*, 1994; Lajer and Daugaard, 1999). Some examples of these medications are the diuretics Lasix, Bumex, Edecrin, and hydrochlorothiazide; antibiotics, e.g. gentamicin, amphotericin, and cyclosporin; and anti-cancer medication (cisplatin).

Hypomagnesemia occurs in approximately 30–60% of individuals with alcoholism (Abbott *et al.*, 1994; Elisaf *et al.*, 1998). Low serum magnesium concentrations occur in about 90% of individuals who are going through withdrawal from alcohol (Abbott *et al.*, 1994; Elisaf *et al.*, 1998).

Those with Crohn's disease, gluten-sensitive enteropathy (celiac disease) or regional enteritis, or who have had intestinal surgery, or have other chronic malabsorptive problems may lose magnesium through diarrhea and fat malabsorption (Rude and Olerich, 1996). These individuals may be candidates for magnesium supplementation.

It has been shown that individuals who have poorly managed diabetes mellitus may require supplementation. This is due to the fact that they have increased urinary magnesium excretion coupled with hyperglycemia (Volpe, 2008).

As previously stated, magnesium interacts with calcium and potassium. Therefore, persons with persistently low blood calcium and potassium concentrations may actually have a fundamental problem with magnesium deficiency. Supplements with magnesium may help to alleviate the calcium and potassium deficiencies.

There is emerging evidence that individuals with mild to moderate asthma may benefit from oral magnesium supplementation (Kazaks *et al.*, 2010). In a 6.5-month randomized, placebo-controlled trial (340 mg of magnesium per day versus a placebo), individuals who were supplemented with magnesium had improved objective measures of bronchial reactivity and improved subjective measures of asthma management and quality of life.

Another group of individuals who may require magnesium supplementation comprises older adults. The National Health and Nutrition Examination Surveys (NHANES, both 1999 to 2000 and 1998 to 1994) have shown that older individuals have lower dietary magnesium intakes than do younger individuals (Bialostosky *et al.*, 2002; Ford and Mokdad, 2003). Furthermore, older individuals have a greater rate of renal magnesium excretion and a lower rate of intestinal magnesium absorption, exacerbating the problem of a low intake (Institute of

Medicine, 1997). Many older adults are on multiple medications, possibly leading to a drug–magnesium interaction, further aggravating the decreased intake and absorption and increased renal excretion (Institute of Medicine, 1997).

Effects of Magnesium Excess

Magnesium intake from food substances has not been shown to be harmful; however, magnesium intake from excess supplement intakes has been shown to be harmful (Institute of Medicine, 1997). A UL for magnesium has been established by the Institute of Medicine (1997) (Table 30.2).

The main initial effect of excess magnesium intake is diarrhea; magnesium is known for its cathartic effect (Rude and Singer, 1980; Fine *et al.*, 1991). Nausea and abdominal cramping may also occur (Ricci *et al.*, 1991).

High serum magnesium concentrations can result in renal failure, which is typically accompanied by high intakes of non-food sources of magnesium (Randall *et al.*, 1964; Mordes and Wacker, 1978). For example, high doses of magnesium-containing laxatives and antacids have been shown to cause toxicity (Xing and Soffer, 2001).

Signs of excess magnesium can be similar to magnesium deficiency and include changes in mental status, nausea, diarrhea, appetite loss, muscle weakness, difficulty breathing, extremely low blood pressure, and irregular heartbeat (Ho *et al.*, 1995; Nordt *et al.*, 1996; Whang, 1997; Jaing *et al.*, 2002).

Methods for Assessing Magnesium Status in Individuals

Serum magnesium is perhaps the most common and straightforward method of assessing magnesium status. An atomic absorption spectrophotometer is used to evaluate magnesium concentration. A serum magnesium concentration of <1.8 mg/dL is indicative of magnesium depletion (Elin, 1987). However, Elin (2010) states:

> The traditional method to establish a reference interval for the SMC [serum magnesium concentration] is flawed by the large number of "normal" individuals who have a subtle chronic negative magnesium balance due to a significant decrease in magnesium intake over the past century. Evidence-based medicine should be used to establish the appropriate lower limit of the reference interval for health and I recommend 0.85 mmol/L based on current literature.

The decrease in magnesium in the diet has led to chronic latent magnesium deficiency in a large number of people since their SMC is still within the reference interval due to primarily the bone magnesium supplementing the SMC. These individuals need adjustment of their diet or magnesium supplementation to achieve a normal magnesium status for health.

Nevertheless, plasma ionized magnesium may be a better method of assessing magnesium status (Institute of Medicine, 1997). Other techniques to assess magnesium status include: clinical evaluation, blood mononuclear cells, magnesium excretion, intracellular magnesium assessment, red blood cell magnesium concentration determined by nuclear magnetic resonance, magnesium balance studies, magnesium tolerance test, and epidemiological studies and meta-analysis (Institute of Medicine, 1997). The magnesium tolerance test has been used for a number of years, and is considered the "gold standard" for assessing magnesium status in adults but not in infants and children (Institute of Medicine, 1997). In the magnesium tolerance test, the renal excretion of magnesium is assessed and is based on magnesium that has been supplied through a parenteral route (Institute of Medicine, 1997). Although the magnesium tolerance test may be a good indicator of hypomagnesemia, it does not appear to be sensitive enough to sense changes in magnesium status in healthy individuals who have been given magnesium supplementation (Institute of Medicine, 1997).

Approximately 99% of the body's magnesium is intracellular; thus, assessment of intracellular ionized magnesium is physiologically appropriate (Malon *et al.*, 2004). These authors examined ionized magnesium in erythrocytes to establish reliable methodology in the evaluation of functional magnesium status. Malon *et al.* also assessed ionized magnesium and total serum magnesium (by atomic absorption spectrometry). The measurements were conducted in critically ill postoperative patients. The authors reported hypomagnesemia in 15.9% of the patients using total serum magnesium, compared with 22.2% using ionized magnesium, and 36.5% using ionized magnesium in erythrocytes. Malon *et al.* concluded that ionized magnesium in erythrocytes may be the best method to detect hypo- or hypermagnesemia.

Future Directions

Given magnesium's role in many reactions in the body, there are a number of research areas that could be pursued,

especially those that may help to prevent disease. It is clear that magnesium may improve insulin resistance, but what is the mechanism behind its action? Many scientists connect the mechanism to magnesium's role with tyrosine kinase and in the inflammatory response. Basic scientific research needs to be conducted to ascertain the mechanisms involved. In addition, longitudinal studies in humans are required to evaluate the levels of magnesium necessary to prevent chronic disease. These need to be followed by magnesium supplementation studies to evaluate the effectiveness of supplementation on the prevention of disease, and the effects it may have on exercise performance.

Suggestions for Further Reading

Davì, G., Santilli, F., and Patrono, C. (2010) Nutraceuticals in diabetes and metabolic syndrome. *Cardiovasc Ther* **28**, 216–226.

Elin, R.J. (2010) Assessment of magnesium status for diagnosis and therapy. *Magnes Res* **23**, S194–198.

Guerrera, M.P., Mao, J.J., and Volpe, S.L. (2009) Therapeutic uses of magnesium. *Am Family Phys* **80**, 157–162.

Nielsen, F.H. (2010) Magnesium, inflammation, and obesity in chronic disease. *Nutr Rev* **68**, 333–340.

Rayssiguier, Y., Libako, P., Nowacki, W., et al. (2010) Magnesium deficiency and metabolic syndrome: stress and inflammation may reflect calcium activation. *Magnes Res* **23**, 73–80.

Rude, R.K., Singer, F.R., and Gruber, H.E. (2009) Skeletal and hormonal effects of magnesium deficiency. *J Am Coll Nutr* **28**, 131–141.

Shechter, M. (2010) Magnesium and cardiovascular system. *Magnes Res* **23**, 60–72.

Volpe, S.L. (2008) Magnesium, the metabolic syndrome, insulin resistance and type 2 diabetes mellitus. *Crit Rev Food Sci Nutr* **48**, 293–300.

References

Abbott, L., Nadler, J., and Rude, R.K. (1994) Magnesium deficiency in alcoholism: possible contribution to osteoporosis and cardiovascular disease in alcoholics. *Alcohol Clin Exp Res* **18**, 1076–1082.

Afridi, H.I., Kazi, T.G., Kazi, N., *et al.* (2008) Potassium, calcium, magnesium, and sodium levels in biological samples of hypertensive and nonhypertensive diabetes mellitus patients. *Biol Trace Elem Res* **124**, 206–224.

Al-Ghamdi, S.M., Cameron, E.C., and Sutton, R.A. (1994) Magnesium deficiency: pathophysiology and clinical overview. *Am J Kidney Dis* **24**, 737–752.

Appel, L.J., Moore, T.J., Obarzanek, E., *et al.* (1997) A clinical trial of the effects of the dietary patterns on blood pressure. *New Engl J Med* **336**, 1117–1124.

Ascherio, R., Rimm, E.B., Giovannucci, E.L., *et al.* (1992) A prospective study of nutritional factors and hypertension among US men. *Circulation* **86**, 1475–1484.

Baker, W.L., Kluger, J., White, C.M., *et al.* (2009) Effect of magnesium L-lactate on blood pressure in patients with an implantable cardioverter defibrillator. *Ann Pharmacol* **43**, 569–576.

Bialostosky, K., Wright, J.D., Kennedy-Stephenson, J., *et al.* (2002) Dietary intake of macronutrients, micronutrients and other dietary constituents: United States 1988–1994. *Vital Health Stat* **11**, 1–158.

Bobkowski, W., Nowak, A., and Durlach, J. (2005) The importance of magnesium status in the pathophysiology of mitral valve prolapse. *Magnes Res* **18**, 35–52.

Bohl, C.H. and Volpe, S.L. (2002) Magnesium and exercise. *Crit Rev Food Sci Nutr* **42**, 533–563.

Brink, E.J. and Beynen, A.C. (1992) Nutrition and magnesium absorption: a review. *Prog Food Nutr Sci* **16**, 125–162.

Chen, S.T., Maruthur, N.M., and Appel, L.J. (2010) The effect of dietary patterns on estimated coronary heart disease risk: results from the Dietary Approaches to Stop Hypertension (DASH) trial. *Circ Cardiovasc Qual Outcomes* **3**, 484–489.

Chernow, B., Bamberger, S., Stoiko, M., *et al.* (1989) Hypomagnesemia in patients in postoperative intensive care. *Chest* **95**, 391–397.

Chubanov, V., Gudermann, T., and Schlingmann, K.P. (2005) Essential role for TRPM6 in epithelial magnesium transport and body magnesium homeostasis. *Eur J Physiol* **451**, 228–234.

Dacey, M.J. (2001) Hypomagnesemic disorders. *Crit Care Clin* **17**, 155–173.

Davì, G., Santilli, F., and Patrono, C. (2010) Nutraceuticals in diabetes and metabolic syndrome. *Cardiovasc Therapeut* **28**, 216–226.

Day, R.O., Liauw, W., Tozer, L.M., *et al.* (2010) A double-blind, placebo-controlled study of the short term effects of a spring water supplemented with magnesium bicarbonate on acid/base balance, bone metabolism and cardiovascular risk factors in postmenopausal women. *BMC Res Notes* **3**, 180.

Dhupa, N. and Proulx, J. (1998) Hypocalcemia and hypomagnesemia. *Vet Clin North Am Small Anim Pract* **28**, 587–608.

Dorup, I. and Clausen, T. (1993) Correlation between magnesium and potassium contents in muscle: role of Na(+)-K(+)pump. *Am J Physiol* **264**, C457–C463.

Elin, R.J. (1987) Assessment of magnesium status. *Clin Chem Online* **33**, 1965–1970.

Elin, R.J. (1994) Magnesium: the fifth but forgotten electrolyte. *Am J Clin Pathol* **102**, 616–622.

Elin, R.J. (2010) Assessment of magnesium status for diagnosis and therapy. *Magnes Res* **23**, 194–198.

Elisaf, M., Bairaktari, E., Kalaitzidis, R., *et al.* (1998) Hypomagnesemia in alcoholic patients. *Alcohol Clin Exp Res* **22**, 244–246.

Estep, H., Shaw, W.A., Watlington, C., *et al.* (1969) Hypocalcemia due to hypomagnesemia and reversible parathyroid hormone unresponsiveness. *J Clin Endocrinol Metab* **29**, 842–848.

Evangelopoulos, A.A., Vallianou, N.G., Panagiotakos, D.B., *et al.* (2008) An inverse relationship between cumulating components of the metabolic syndrome and serum magnesium levels. *Nutr Res* **28**, 659–663.

Everett, C.J. and King, D.E. (2006) Serum magnesium and the development of diabetes. *Nutrition* **22**, 679.

Feillet-Coudray, C., Coudray, C., Brule, F., *et al.* (2000) Exchangeable magnesium pool masses reflect the magnesium status of rats. *J Nutr* **130**, 2306–2311.

Feillet-Coudray, C., Coudray, C., Tressol, J.C., *et al.* (2002) Exchangeable magnesium pool masses in healthy women: effects of magnesium supplementation. *Am J Clin Nutr* **75**, 72–78.

Fine, K.D., Santa Ana, C.A., Porter, J.L., *et al.* (1991) Intestinal absorption of magnesium from food and supplements. *J Clin Invest* **88**, 396–402.

Ford, E.S. and Mokdad, A.H. (2003) Dietary magnesium intake in a national sample of U.S. adults. *J Nutr* **133**, 2879–2882.

Franz, K.B. (1989) Influence of phosphorus on intestinal absorption of calcium and magnesium. In Y. Itokawa and J. Durlach (eds), *Magnesium in Health and Disease*. John Libbey and Co, London, pp. 71–78.

Frausto da Silva, J.J.R. and Williams, R.J.P. (1991) The biological chemistry of magnesium: phosphorus metabolism. *The Biological Chemistry of the Elements*. OUP, Oxford, pp. 241–267.

Freitag, J.J. and Martin, K.J. (1979) Evidence for skeletal resistance to parathyroid hormone in magnesium deficiency: studies in isolated perfused bone. *J Clin Invest* **264**, 1238–1244.

Galland, L.D., Baker, S.M., and McLellan, R.K (1986) Magnesium deficiency in the pathogenesis of mitral valve prolapse. *J Magnesium* **5**, 165–174.

Gardner, C.D., Kim, S., Bersamin, A., *et al.* (2010) Micronutrient quality of weight-loss diets that focus on macronutrients: results from the A to Z study. *Am J Clin Nutr* **92**, 304–312.

Greger, J.L. (1999) Nondigestible carbohydrates and mineral bioavailability. *J Nutr* **129**, 1434S–1435S.

Guerrera, M.P., Mao, J.J., and Volpe, S.L. (2009) Therapeutic uses of magnesium. *Am Family Phys* **80**, 157–162,

Guerrero-Romero, F. and Rodríguez-Morán, M. (2002) Low serum magnesium levels and metabolic syndrome. *Acta Diabetológica* **39**, 209–213.

Guerrero-Romero, F. and Rodríguez-Morán, M. (2006) Hypomagnesemia, oxidative stress, inflammation, and metabolic syndrome. *Diabetes Metab Res Rev* **22**, 471–476.

Guerrero-Romero, F., Tamez-Perez, H.E., Gonzalez-Gonzalez, G., et al. (2004) Oral magnesium supplementation improves insulin sensitivity in non-diabetic subjects with insulin resistance. A double-blind placebo-controlled randomized trial. *Diabetes Metab* **30**, 253–258.

Gums, J.G. (2004) Magnesium in cardiovascular and other disorders. *Am J Health Syst Pharm* **61**, 1569–1576.

Gunther, T. (1993) Mechanisms and regulation of Mg2+ efflux and Mg2+ influx. *Miner Electrolyte Metab* **19**, 259–265.

Hashimoto, T., Hara, A., Ohkubo, T., et al. (2010) Serum magnesium, ambulatory blood pressure, and carotid artery alteration: the Ohasama study. *Am J Hypertens* **23**, 1292–1298.

He, K., Liu, K., Daviglus, M.L., et al. (2006) Magnesium intake and incidence of metabolic syndrome among young adults. *Circulation* **113**, 1675–1682.

Hekmat-Nejad, M., Cai, T., and Swinney, D.C. (2010) Steady-state kinetic characterization of kinase activity and requirements for Mg2+ of interleukin-1 receptor associated kinase-4. *Biochemistry* **49**, 1495–1506.

Herzog, W.R., Schlossberg, M.L., MacMurdy, K.S., et al. (1995) Timing of magnesium therapy affects experimental infarct size. *Circulation* **92**, 2622–2626.

Ho, J., Moyer, T.P., and Phillips, S. (1995) Chronic diarrhea: the role of magnesium. *Mayo Clin Proc* **70**, 1091–1092.

Horner, S.M. (1992) Efficacy of intravenous magnesium in acute myocardial infarction in reducing arrhythmia and mortality. *Circulation* **86**, 774–779.

Huerta, M.G., Roemmich, J.N., Kington, M.L., et al. (2005) Magnesium deficiency is associated with insulin resistance in obese children. *Diabetes Care* **28**, 1175–1181.

Hunt, M.S. and Schofield, F.A. (1969) Magnesium balance and protein intake level in adult human female. *Am J Clin Nutr* **22**, 367–373.

Institute of Medicine (1997) Institute of Medicine Standing Committee on the Scientific Evaluation of Dietary Reference Intakes, Food and Nutrition Board. *Dietary Reference Intakes for Calcium, Phosphorus, Magnesium, Vitamin D, and Fluoride*. National Academy Press, Washington, DC.

Iseri, L.T. and French, J.H. (1984) Magnesium: Nature's physiologic calcium blocker. *Am Heart J* **108**, 188–193.

Jaing, T.H., Hung, I.J., Chung, H.T., et al. (2002) Acute hypermagnesemia: a rare complication of antacid administration after bone marrow transplantation. *Clin Chim Acta* **326**, 201–203.

Johansson, G., Backman, U., Danielson, B.G., et al. (1980) Biochemical and clinical effects of the prophylactic treatment of renal calcium stones with magnesium hydroxide. *J Urol* **124**, 770–774.

Kayne, L.H. and Lee, D.B.N. (1993) Intestinal magnesium absorption. *Miner Electrolyte Metab* **19**, 210–217.

Kazaks, A.G., Uriu-Adams, J.Y., Albertson, T.E., et al. (2010) Effect of oral magnesium supplementation on measures of airway resistance and subjective assessment of asthma control and quality of life in men and women with mild to moderate asthma: a randomized placebo controlled trial. *J Asthma* **47**, 83–92.

Kelepouris, E. and Agus, Z.S. (1998) Hypomagnesemia: renal magnesium handling. *Semin Nephrol* **18**, 58–73.

Khan, N.A., Lewanczuk, R.Z., McAlister, F.A., et al. (2005) The 2005 Canadian Hypertension Education Program recommendations for the management of hypertension: Part II – Therapy. *Can J Cardiol* **21**, 657–672.

Kirii, K., Iso, H., Date, C., et al. (2010) Magnesium intake and risk of self-reported type 2 diabetes among Japanese. *J Am Coll Nutr* **29**, 99–106.

Ladefoged, K., Hessov, I., and Jarnum, S. (1996) Nutrition in short-bowel syndrome. *Scand J Gastroenterol* **216**, 122–131.

Lajer, H. and Daugaard, G. (1999) Cisplatin and hypomagnesemia. *Cancer Treat Rev* **25**, 47–58.

Lopez-Ridaura, R., Willett, W.C., Rimm, E.B., et al. (2004) Magnesium intake and risk of type 2 diabetes in men and women. *Diabetes Care* **27**, 134–140.

Ma, J., Folsom, A.R., Melnick, S.L., et al. (1995) Associations of serum and dietary magnesium with cardiovascular disease, hypertension, diabetes, insulin, and carotid arterial wall thickness: the ARIC study. Atherosclerosis Risk in Community Study. *J Clin Epidemiol* **48**, 927–940.

Maguire, M.E. (1984) Hormone-sensitive magnesium transport and magnesium regulation of adenylate cyclase. *Trends Pharmacol Sci* **5**, 73–77.

Mahalko, J.R., Sandstead, H.H., Johnson, L.K., et al. (1983) Effect of a moderate increase in dietary protein on the retention and excretion of Ca, Cu, Fe, Mg, P, and Zn by adult males. *Am J Clin Nutr* **37**, 8–14.

Malon, A., Brockmann, C., Fijalkowska-Morawska, J., et al. (2004) Ionized magnesium in erythrocytes – the best magnesium parameter to observe hypo- or hypermagnesemia. *Clin Chim Acta* **349**, 67–73.

Martinez, M.E., Salinas, M., Miguel, J.L., et al. (1985) Magnesium excretion in idiopathic hypercalciuria. *Nephron* **40**, 446–450.

Massey, L. (2005) Magnesium therapy for nephrolithiasis. *Magnesium Res* **18**, 123–126.

Massey, L.K. and Whiting, S.J, (1993) Caffeine, urinary calcium, calcium metabolism and bone. *J Nutr* **123**, 1611–1614.

Mathers, T.W. and Beckstrand, R.L., (2009) Oral magnesium supplementation in adults with coronary heart disease or coronary heart disease risk. *J Am Acad Nurse Pract* **21**, 651–657.

Mayer-Davis, E.J., Nichols, M., Liese, A.D., *et al.* (2006) Dietary intake among youth with diabetes: the SEARCH for Diabetes in Youth Study. *J Am Diet Assoc* **106**, 689–697.

Meacham, S.L., Taper, L.J., and Volpe, S.L. (1994) Effects of boron supplementation on bone mineral density and dietary, blood and urinary calcium, phosphorus, magnesium, and boron in female athletes. *Environ Health Perspect* **102**, 79–82.

Meacham, S.L., Taper, L.J., and Volpe, S.L. (1995) The effect of boron supplementation on blood and urinary calcium, magnesium, phosphorus, and urinary boron in female athletes. *Am J Clin Nutr* **61**, 341–345.

Mordes, J.P. and Wacker, W.E.C. (1978) Excessive magnesium. *Pharmacol Rev* **29**, 273–300.

National Institutes of Health, Office of Dietary Supplements (2005) http://ods.od.nih.gov/factsheets/magnesium.asp (retrieved September 10 2010; updated January 30, 2005).

Newhouse, I.J. and Finstad, E.W. (2000) The effects of magnesium supplementation on exercise performance. *Clin J Sports Med* **10**, 195–200.

Nielsen, F.H. (2010) Magnesium, inflammation, and obesity in chronic disease. *Nutr Rev* **68**, 333–340.

Nordt, S., Williams, S.R., Turchen, S., *et al.* (1996) Hypermagnesemia following an acute ingestion of Epsom salt in a patient with normal renal function. *J Toxicol Clin Toxicol* **34**, 735–739.

Normen, L., Arnaud, M.J., Carlsson, N.G., *et al.* (2005) Small bowel absorption of magnesium and calcium sulphate from a natural mineral water in subjects with ileostomy. *Eur J Nutr* **45**, 105–112.

Ohgitani, S., Fujita, T., Fujii, Y., *et al.* (2005) Nail calcium and magnesium content in relation to age and bone mineral density. *J Bone Min Metab* **23**, 318–322.

Paolisso, G. and Barbagallo, M. (1997) Hypertension, diabetes mellitus, and insulin resistance: the role of intracellular magnesium. *Am J Hypertens* **10**, 346–355.

Paolisso, G., Passariello, N., Pizza, G., *et al.* (1989) Dietary magnesium supplements improve B-cell response to glucose and arginine in elderly non-insulin dependent diabetic subjects. *Acta Endocrinologica (Copenh)* **121**, 16–20.

Ramsay, L.E., Yeo, W.W., and Jackson, P.R. (1994) Metabolic effects of diuretics. *Cardiology* **84**, 48–56.

Randall, R.E., Cohen, D., Spray, C.C., *et al.* (1964) Hypermagnesemia in renal failure. *Ann Int Med* **61**, 73–88.

Rayssiguier, Y., Libako, P., Nowacki, W., *et al.* (2010) Magnesium deficiency and metabolic syndrome: stress and inflammation may reflect calcium activation. *Magnes Res* **23**, 73–80.

Ricci, J.M., Hariharan, S., and Helfott, A. (1991) Oral tocolysis with magnesium chloride: a randomized controlled prospective clinical trial. *Am J Obstet Gynecol* **165**, 603–610.

Rodríguez-Morán, M. and Guerrero-Romero, F. (2003) Oral magnesium supplementation improves insulin sensitivity and metabolic control in type 2 diabetic subjects. A randomized, double-blind controlled trial. *Diabetes Care* **26**, 1147–1152.

Romani, A., Marfella, C., and Scarpa, A. (1993) Cell magnesium transport and homeostasis: role of intracellular compartments. *Miner Electrolyte Metab* **19**, 282–289.

Rosenlund, M., Berglind, N., Hallqvist, J., *et al.* (2005) Daily intake of magnesium and calcium from drinking water in relation to myocardial infarction. *Epidemiology* **16**, 570–576.

Rude, R.K. (1998) Magnesium deficiency: a cause of heterogeneous disease in humans. *J Bone Min Res* **13**, 749–758.

Rude, R.K. and Oldham, S.B. (1990) Disorders of magnesium metabolism. In R.D. Cohen, B. Lewis, and K.G.M.M Alberti (eds), *The Metabolic and Molecular Basis of Acquired Disease*. Bailliere Tindall, London, pp. 1124–1148.

Rude, R.K. and Olerich, M. (1996) Magnesium deficiency: possible role in osteoporosis associated with gluten sensitive enteropathy. *Osteoporosis Int* **6**, 453–461.

Rude, R.K. and Singer, F.R. (1980) Magnesium deficiency and excess. *Ann Rev Med* **32**, 245–259.

Rude, R.K., Singer, F.R., and Gruber, H.E. (2009) Skeletal and hormonal effects of magnesium deficiency. *J Am Coll Nutr* **28**, 131–141.

Sacks, F.M., Brown, L.E., Appel, L., *et al.* (1995) Combinations of potassium, calcium, and magnesium supplements in hypertension. *Hypertension* **26**, 950–956.

Sadeh, M. (1989) Action of magnesium sulfate in the treatment of preeclampsia–eclampsia. *Stroke* **20**, 1273–1275.

Saito, N., Saito, S., Tabata, N., *et al.* (2004) Bone mineral density, serum albumin and serum magnesium. *J Am Coll Nutr* **23**, 701S–703S.

Schmid-Elsaesser, R., Kunz, M., Zausinger, S., *et al.* (2006) Intravenous magnesium versus nimodipine in the treatment of patients with aneurysmal subarachnoid hemorrhage: a randomized study. *Neurosurgery* **58**, 1054–1065.

Schwartz, B.F., Bruce, J., Leslie, S., *et al.* (2001) Rethinking the role of urinary magnesium in calcium urolithiasis. *J Endourol* **15**, 233–235.

Schwartz, R., Spencer, H., and Welsh, J.J. (1984) Magnesium absorption in human subjects from leafy vegetables, intrinsically labeled with stable 26Mg. *Am J Clin Nutr* **39**, 571–576.

Schwartz, R., Walker, G., Linz, M.D., *et al.* (1973) Metabolic responses of adolescent boys to two levels of dietary magnesium and protein. I. Magnesium and nitrogen retention. *Am J Clin Nutr* **26,** 510–518.

Shechter, M. (2010) Magnesium and cardiovascular system. *Magnes Res* **23,** 60–72.

Soltani, N., Keshavarz, M., Minaii, B., *et al.* (2005) Effects of administration of oral magnesium on plasma glucose and pathological changes in the aorta and pancreas of diabetic rats. *Clin Exp Pharmacol Physiol* **32,** 604–610.

Song, Y., Manson, J.E., Buring, J.E., *et al.* (2004) Dietary magnesium intake in relation to plasma insulin levels and risk of type 2 diabetes in women. *Diabetes Care* **27,** 59–65.

Song, Y., Ridker, P.M., Manson, J.E., *et al.* (2005) Magnesium intake, C-reactive protein, and the prevalence of metabolic syndrome in middle-aged and older U.S. women. *Diabetes Care* **28,** 1438–1444.

Stendig-Lindberg, G., Koeller, W., Bauer, A., *et al.* (2004) Prolonged magnesium deficiency causes osteoporosis in the rat. *J Am Coll Nutr* **23,** 704S–711S.

US Department of Agriculture, Agricultural Research Service (2003) USDA National Nutrient Database for Standard Reference, Release 16. http://www.ars.usda.gov/main/site_main.htm?modecode=12-35-45-00.

Volpe, S.L. (2008) Magnesium, the metabolic syndrome, insulin resistance and type 2 diabetes mellitus. *Crit Rev Food Sci Nutr* **48,** 293–300.

Volpe, S.L., Taper, L.J., and Meacham, S.L. (1993) The relationship between boron and magnesium status, and bone mineral density in humans: a review. *Magnes Res* **6,** 291–296.

Vormann, J. (2003) Magnesium: nutrition and metabolism. *Mol Aspects Med* **24,** 27–37.

Wang, C.T., Chang, W.T., Zeng, W.F., *et al.* (2005) Concentrations of calcium, copper, iron, magnesium, potassium, sodium and zinc in adult female hair with different body mass indexes in Taiwan. *Clin Chem Lab Med* **43,** 389–393.

Wary, C., Brillault-Salvat, C., Bloch, G., *et al.* (1999) Effect of chronic magnesium supplementation on magnesium distribution in healthy volunteers evaluated by 31P-NMRS and ion selective electrodes. *Br J Clin Pharmacol* **48,** 655–662.

Wester, P.O. (1987) Magnesium. *Am J Clin Nutr* **45**(Suppl), 1305–1312.

Whang, R. (1997) Clinical disorders of magnesium metabolism. *Compr Ther* **23,** 168–173.

White, R.E. and Hartzell, H.C. (1989) Magnesium ions in cardiac function. *Biochem Pharmacol* **38,** 859–867.

Wisker, E., Nagel, R., Tanudjaja, T.K., *et al.* (1991) Calcium, magnesium, zinc, and iron balances in young women: effects of a low-phytate barley-fiber concentrate. *Am J Clin Nutr* **54,** 553–559.

Wong, N.L., Quamme, G.A., and Dirks, J.H. (1986) Effects of acid–base disturbances on renal handling of magnesium in the dog. *Clin Sci* **70,** 277–284.

Xing, J.H. and Soffer, E.E. (2001) Adverse effects of laxatives. *Dis Colon Rectum* **44,** 1201–1209.

Yamamoto, M.E., Applegate, W.B., Klag, M.J., *et al.* (1995) Lack of blood pressure effect with calcium and magnesium supplementation in adults with high–normal blood pressure. Results from Phase I of the Trials of Hypertension Prevention (TOPH). Trials of Hypertension Prevention (TOPH) Research Group. *Ann Epidemiol* **5,** 96–107.

31

SODIUM, CHLORIDE, AND POTASSIUM

HARRY G. PREUSS[1], MD AND DALLAS L. CLOUATRE[2], PhD

[1]*Georgetown University Medical Center, Washington, DC, USA*
[2]*Glykon Technologies Group, LLC, Santa Monica, California, USA*

Summary

Although some limitations exist in interpreting earlier studies, most experts today commonly recommend decreasing the intake of sodium chloride (salt) while increasing that of potassium because these maneuvers could save lives and reduce health costs. Sodium is an essential mineral vital in the balance of bodily fluids, i.e. the amount of bodily sodium is directly correlated with fluid volume. Most people in the Western world ingest more sodium chloride than generally recommended, which can result in volume expansion, edema, and elevated blood pressure. In general, the INTERMAP study corroborated the findings of INTERSALT and most other epidemiological studies in finding higher sodium intakes associated with higher blood pressure leading to many cardiovascular perturbations. In contrast, too small a circulating volume emanating from low sodium ingestion can cause symptoms and signs ranging from tiredness and low blood pressure to outright disorientation and shock. In contrast to sodium, ingestion of adequate amounts of potassium is associated with lower blood pressures and better cardiovascular performance. Circulating potassium enters all tissues and has profound effects on the function of some organs, primarily depolarization and contraction of the heart. Too much potassium ingestion in the face of renal perturbations can lead to potassium overload and serious cardiovascular complications.

Introduction

Life and the Ancient Seas

Many scientists assume that the existence of ancient seas on Earth were essential for development of life (Follman and Brownson, 2009). Life is estimated to have begun 2 billion years ago in the Pre-Cambrian seas, which provided mobility, dissolved substances such as sodium, potassium, and chloride, and stable physico-chemical conditions (Conway, 1942, 1947; Smith, 1943; Elkinton and Danowsky, 1955; Battarbee and Meneely, 1978). The presence of seas on Earth is unique in the solar system (Encrenaz, 2008). No other planet possesses surface liquid water to the extent to which it occurs on Earth: >70% of its surface. The minute amount of water present elsewhere in the solar system exists as ice (Encrenaz, 2008).

Although life probably started in the sea billions of years ago, terrestrial forms are believed to have emerged only 360 million years ago (Battarbee and Meneely, 1978). Strengthening the contention that life began in seas is

Present Knowledge in Nutrition, Tenth Edition. Edited by John W. Erdman Jr, Ian A. Macdonald and Steven H. Zeisel.
© 2012 International Life Sciences Institute. Published 2012 by John Wiley & Sons, Inc.

TABLE 31.1   Ion concentrations (mmol/L) in the oceans at various geological periods and in vertebrate extracellular fluid

Ion	Pre-Cambrian sea[a]	Early Ordovician sea[b]	Ocean today	Human plasma	Human muscle[c]
Sodium	298	379	478	142	10
Potassium	104	51	10	4	160
Calcium	2	7	11	5	
Magnesium	11	38	55	3	18
Chloride	298	441	559	103	2
Sulfate	54	40	29	1	
Phosphate			Trace	2	140
Protein[d]				16	55

[a]Approximate time of the development of unicellular organisms.
[b]Period of emergence of vertebrates.
[c]Per liter of water.
[d]Expressed as mEq/L.
Data derived from Conway (1947), Smith (1953), and Elkinton and Danowski (1955).

knowledge that terrestrial life forms had to retain their own internal sea in the form of extracellular and intracellular body fluids containing electrolytes in order to live on land (Smith, 1953; Elkinton and Danowsky, 1955). Man probably came upon the scene 2 million years ago (Pitts, 1974).

The proportions of sodium, chloride, and potassium in ancient seas have been closely linked with life. Table 31.1 compares estimated concentrations of many constituents in seawater during various geological periods with that of human plasma and muscle water (Conway, 1947; Smith, 1953; Elkinton and Danowski, 1955). It is interesting to speculate on whether life could have evolved from ancient seas had they possessed the current distributions of electrolytes, which have changed significantly with time. Over many centuries, the concentrations of sodium and chloride have steadily increased, whereas that of potassium has decreased.

An interesting hypothesis concerning the evolution of life is based upon knowledge that potassium content in the Pre-Cambrian seas was much higher with respect to sodium than now. Many relate this observation to the high potassium concentrations within cells. Later, with emergence of life from seas having higher sodium content, this became the basis for the high levels of sodium in extracellular fluid (Macallum, 1926). Regardless of whether these suppositions are real, cells in the body could survive, grow, and function only by retaining a friendly environment via tight regulation of an internal sea.

Maintaining the Sea Within

Kidneys played a major role in the emergence of terrestrial life. Homer Smith (1943, 1953) and later Robert Pitts (1974) discussed the crucial role of kidneys in regulating ions and fluid in the body that allowed vertebrates to leave the sea. The renal regulation of sodium, chloride, and potassium in body spaces is especially crucial because the presence of these cations and anions dictates the size of the body fluid compartments via effects on osmolality, and they play a significant role in acid–base balance. A major difference between plasma and the past and current seas is the presence of proteins in the former. Proteins occupy ~6% of the blood plasma volume. Healthy kidneys protect the circulating concentrations of proteins by preventing renal losses.

In addition to renal regulation, oral intake of these micronutrients is also of paramount importance (Dahl, 1958). Dietary intake has changed over the years, and these changes play a prominent role in the overall health of numerous modern countries. Nutritional intake can strongly influence development of many prevalent current health perturbations (Suter *et al.*, 2002; Hooper *et al.*, 2003). With the emergence of the modern Western diet, cardiovascular and metabolic disorders have become relatively more common (Suter *et al.*, 2002; Hooper *et al.*, 2003). Cardiovascular diseases (CVD) account for approximately 50% of mortality beyond age 65 (Kotchen and Kotchen, 2003). Cordain *et al.* (2005) noted seven crucial areas in modern diets that may relate to the prevalence of modern diseases. Prominent among the listings is the sodium–potassium ratio.

Problems with the Modern Western Diet

Diets from earlier times and those from primitive areas of the world today compared with the modern Western diet contain(ed) higher proportions of potassium relative to sodium (Frassetto *et al.*, 2001). This reversal of potassium and sodium concentrations in the food supply may play a significant role in the development of many chronic diseases (Frassetto *et al.*, 2001; Cordain *et al.*, 2005; Brown *et al.*, 2009). Too much sodium consumption has the proclivity to raise blood pressure and create cardiovascular perturbations (Brown *et al.*, 2009). Differently put, Americans consume too little potassium, roughly one-half the recommended adequate intake. In contrast to sodium, potassium tends to benefit the cardiovascular system (Frassetto *et al.*, 2001). Frassetto *et al.* (2009) compared effects of changing from the modern diet to a Paleolithic one containing more potassium and fiber (Cordain, 2002). The Paleolithic diet includes lean meat, fruits, vegetables, and nuts, and excludes cereal grains, dairy, and legumes. Even short-term consumption (10 days) of a Paleolithic diet relative to the modern diet improved blood pressure and glucose tolerance, decreased insulin secretion, increased insulin sensitivity, and improved lipid profiles (Frassetto *et al.*, 2009).

General Lifestyle Recommendations Today

Although some limitations exist in interpreting earlier studies (Lackland and Egan, 2007), lowering sodium intake and raising potassium intake is commonly recommended by most experts (Appel, 2009b). Modest reduction of salt intake could save lives and reduce health costs (Asaria *et al.*, 2007; Bibbins-Domingo, 2010). To strengthen the reasoning behind consuming less sodium and more potassium, these two cations will be discussed in detail separately.

Sodium

Generalizations about Sodium and Salt

To gain better understanding of sodium balance, it is necessary to differentiate between sodium and salt (sodium chloride). Sodium is an essential mineral (micronutrient) vital in the balance of body fluids. Dietary sodium is usually measured in grams, and sometimes in milliequivalents or millimoles. The most common source of dietary sodium is table salt, sodium chloride. Because table salt is only 40% sodium, the remaining 60% being chloride, it is necessary to discern whether any reference to mass is discussing grams of sodium or salt. In the US, one teaspoonful of table salt contains 5.75 g of salt, equivalent to 2.3 g of sodium. A realistic average daily intake of salt by the general public in the United States today is roughly 6.0 g ± 1.0 (SEM) – close to a US teaspoonful – providing about 2.4 g ± 0.4 (SEM) of sodium.

Most people living in the Western world ingest more sodium than generally recommended and thus face consequences of an overload. For adolescents and adults of all ages (14 years and older), the Institute of Medicine (IOM) set the tolerable upper intake level (UL) at 2300 mg per day. The UL is the highest daily nutrient intake level that is likely to pose no risk of adverse health effects, for example, for sodium, increased blood pressure for almost all individuals in the general population. The IOM recognized that the association between sodium intake and blood pressure was continuous and without a threshold (i.e. a level below which the association no longer exists). The UL was based on several trials, including data from the Dietary Approaches to Stop Hypertension (DASH) sodium trial. The IOM noted that, in the DASH-sodium trial, blood pressure was lowered when target sodium intake was reduced to 2300 mg per day, and lowered even further when sodium was targeted to the level of 1200 mg/day (IOM, 2005). The United Kingdom recommended nutritional intake (RNI) advocates an upper limit of 1.6 g (http://wikipedia.org/wiki/Salt). The National Research Council of the National Academy of Sciences suggests a daily range of 1.1 to 3.3 g for adult intake. The American Heart Association recommends that intake of 2.3 g per day not be exceeded. It is wise to individualize recommendations to certain groups of individuals. People with hypertension as suggested above, African-Americans, and older adults tend to have a greater blood-pressure response to sodium challenge and should be advised appropriately. Many believe that an average daily intake should not exceed 1.5 g of sodium in individuals with hypertension.

In contrast to sodium overload, sodium deficiency is less common for it is hard to exclude salt from the modern diet, and normal kidneys are primed to prevent excessive losses in the urine. Table 31.2 lists the sodium content of some common foods. Harmful losses may nevertheless occur due to excess sweating during heavy exertion and/or may be associated with high external temperatures and

TABLE 31.2   Approximate values for sodium content in some common foods[a]

Foodstuff	Sodium	
	(mmol)	(mg)
Apple, raw, with skin (1 apple, 138 g)	0.04	1
Flounder/sole species, cooked, dry heat (3 oz, 85 g)	3.9	89
Banana, raw (1 cup, 150 g)	0.09	2
Beer, regular (12 oz, 355 g)	0.6	14
Bread, commercially prepared, white (1 slice, 25 g)	7.4	170
Cocoa, unsweetened powder (1 tbsp, 5.4 g)	0.04	1
Cocoa mix, powder (3 heaping tsp, 28.35 g)	6.2	143
Corn flakes (1 cup, 28 g)	8.8	202
Egg, scrambled (1 large, 61 g)	7.4	171
Lemon meringue pie, prepared (1 piece, 113 g)	7.2	165
Pancake, fast-food butter/syrup (2 pancakes, 232 g)	48	1104
Pizza, fast-food pepperoni (1 slice, 106 g)	29.1	670
Red wine (3.5 oz, 103 g)	0.17	4
Spaghetti, cooked, enriched, no salt (1 cup, 140 g)	0.04	1
Tuna, canned in oil, drained solids (3 oz, 85 g)	13.1	301

[a]Based on USDA National Nutrient Database for Standard Reference, Release 22, 2009.

require replacement (Sawka *et al.*, 2007). Too severe restriction of dietary sodium can also lead to harmful body depletion (Dahl *et al.*, 1955). Physicians treating renal patients with hypertension and congestive heart failure by reducing the body content of sodium via reduced intake and/or diuresis are not infrequently surprised by an elevation of blood urea (BUN), indicating too much removal. This may be a sign of too little blood flow to the kidneys and suggests that other organs are being poorly perfused as well. Subjective signs of sodium deficiency include thirst, nausea, weakness, fatigue, disorientation, and cramps.

Composition of Sodium and Chloride in the Body

The total body sodium of a normal adult averages ~60 mmol/kg body weight (Pitts, 1959). For the typical 70-kg person this is approximately 4200 mmol – almost 100 g of sodium as depicted in Figure 31.1, top. Bone contains roughly 1680 mmol, that is, about 40% of the total body sodium. Approximately 2520 mmol of the remaining sodium resides in the extracellular and intracellular fluid. In addition to that in bone, roughly 50% of total sodium is extracellular and 10% is intracellular.

Sodium stores can be classified as exchangeable and non-exchangeable (Pitts, 1959). Via measurements using radioactive isotopes, exchangeable sodium has been estimated at 42 mmol/kg body weight (Figure 31.1, bottom).

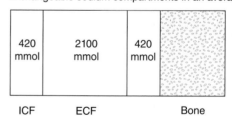

FIG. 31.1   Sodium compartments. ECF, Extracellular fluid; ICF, intracellular fluid.

Exchangeable sodium consists of all extracellular sodium, all intracellular sodium, and less than half the bone sodium. Essentially all non-exchangeable sodium is in bone, where it is buried within the bone structure. Exchangeable sodium is important because, when sodium is lost from the blood plasma into the urine or feces, it can be replaced rapidly from other compartments via diffusion. In turn, sodium retained in edema is also spread out among these various compartments.

Total body chloride averages 33 mmol/kg body weight – that is, a 70-kg person has 2310 mmol chloride (Pitts, 1959). The majority of the chloride, ~70%, is distributed in the extracellular fluid. Much of the remaining chloride is localized in the collagen of connective tissue and is largely exchangeable.

Sodium Homeostasis

Over 40 years ago Dahl (1958) remarked, "Widespread use of salt has received little attention from nutritionists." This certainly is not the case today. It is now generally recognized that a substance in such common use as salt might be noxious when consumed in amounts determined by dietary customs and tastes. It is further recognized that potential adverse effects from salt consumption are also influenced by genetic factors and the simultaneous intake of other nutrients, such as potassium, magnesium, and calcium (Nurminen et al., 1998).

As indicated above, the amount of sodium consumed (intake) must equal the amount of sodium lost (output) to maintain balance. Calculating intake is fairly simple. Sodium essentially is absorbed completely in the small intestine. Therefore, if 4 g sodium is ingested, 4 g is delivered to the body. Salt intake can be influenced by salt appetite, and the brain renin–angiotensin system is important in this respect. We know this because intracerebral injection of angiotensin II stimulates salt appetite whereas blocking formation of angiotensin II via central administration of captopril diminishes salt appetite (Fitzsimmons, 1980). Thirst also plays a significant role in the regulation of volume and body space size. Changes in osmolality related to sodium and chloride homeostasis influence the thirst mechanism and the release of vasopressin, which affects the handling of water in the renal collecting duct (Robertson, 1987).

In contrast to calculating input, calculating output can be difficult because a number of routes must be considered in the estimate. Normal losses of sodium occur through the skin, feces, and urine. In the absence of considerable physical effort or heat stress, only small amounts are lost via the skin, mainly by sweating with lesser losses through skin sloughing. In subjects who were ambulatory but not actively working or sweating, daily consumption of 100–150 mg sodium led to average daily losses of <25 mg sodium. The investigators attributed this small loss to desquamation of epithelial cells, sebaceous secretions, unnoticed sweat, and possibly some insensible perspiration (Dahl et al., 1955). Changing production of salt-retaining hormones such as aldosterone can regulate losses of sodium in sweat. Conn (1949) demonstrated that healthy individuals sweating as much as 5–9 L/day could decrease sodium concentrations in sweat to as little as 0.1 g/L after acclimatization. Under normal conditions, skin losses are small but substantial amounts of sodium can be removed through excess sweating.

Loss of sodium via feces is small even when sodium intake is high (Baldwin et al., 1960). On a daily sodium intake ranging widely from 0.05 to 4.1 g/day, only 10–125 mg appeared in stools (Dole et al., 1950). Cases of severe diarrhea may result in substantial losses. Potential losses via hair, nails, saliva, semen, and menstruation are too negligible in the overall picture to be considered.

It is safe to state that more than 90% of sodium output is via the kidneys. When sodium intake is acutely reduced to an extremely low value, urinary sodium excretion falls exponentially over 4–5 days; increased sodium intake above a certain level results in the excretion of an increased amount after a few days (Strauss et al., 1958). The intake of sodium is accurately estimated by the amount present in urine in the absence of gross sweating. Pragmatically, the small amounts in the sweat and feces can be ignored in the overall calculations of balance, because the amount of sodium in the modern Western diet is relatively large.

The overall control of body sodium homeostasis via the interplay of various factors on the kidneys is incompletely understood. Both intrarenal and extrarenal factors are involved. Associated with sodium homeostasis, extrarenal mechanisms working interdependently are plasma renin activity (Laragh et al., 1972); plasma angiotensin II (Brown et al., 1972); aldosterone production (Brown et al., 1972); atrial natriuretic peptide (Sagnella, 1987); catecholamines such as adrenaline, noradrenaline, and dopamine (Romoff et al., 1979); hormones such as vasoactive intestinal peptide (Duggan and Macdonald, 1987); and possible Na^+,K^+-ATPase inhibitors (deWardener and MacGregor, 1983; Blaustein, 1985).

To re-emphasize, the major control for sodium output is via renal excretion. In Figure 31.2 we depict an example of what generally happens when sodium intake suddenly increases. In our example, the usual daily dose of 4 g sodium is balanced by 4 g excreted (day 0). The body is in so-called homeostasis, since output matches input. On day 1, intake is doubled to 8 g, and the increased intake

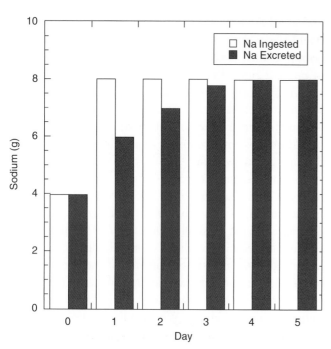

FIG. 31.2 Results of increasing dietary sodium intake. Daily sodium intake doubled from 4 g to 8 g on day 1. Sodium excretion initially does not equal the higher intake but over 3–4 days once more equals intake, never to exceed it. See body of text for more detailed explanation.

is continued over the ensuing period of time. On day 1, excretion rises more than the previous day when intake was less but falls short of actual intake that day. On days 2 and 3, sodium excretion continues to rise with the higher sodium challenge and eventually matches the daily intake. We are in balance with the increased intake as mentioned previously but at what cost? The crucial point here is that excretion does not exceed intake to overcome the earlier retention. Accordingly, it is apparent from the depiction that sodium consumed earlier is retained such that total body sodium has risen a percentage point or two. This in turn leads to a similar rise in the extracellular fluid volume. On the doubled sodium intake, we have once again reached a homeostatic point where output matches input but with a higher total body sodium and balance. Most physicians believe that this can be harmful over the long run and must be removed by lessening intake or increasing sodium excretion, perhaps via the use of diuretics. The lesson to be learned here is that cutting down intake of sodium should lead to lower total body

sodium, less fluid volume, and in general a healthier status – especially in terms of blood pressure and the cardiovascular system.

Maintenance of Body Fluid Compartments

The total body water content of an individual varies roughly between 45% and 70% of body weight, a range of 50–60% being most representative of normal adults (Pitts, 1959, 1974). Infants have proportionately more water, whereas the elderly have less. Females have proportionately less water than do males. As illustrated in Figure 31.3, body water is divided into extracellular and intracellular compartments: one-third extracellular and two-thirds intracellular. The extracellular compartment is further divided into plasma and interstitial fluid. The latter is roughly three times larger than the former, that is, one-twelfth and one-quarter of the total body water.

Sodium and chloride, being the most important electrolytes of the extracellular compartment, determine the extracellular volume to a great extent. Circulating proteins also influence the relationship between the plasma and interstitial fluid volumes. The endothelium of the capillaries allows rapid distribution of diffusible ions and water but restricts the passage of protein between the plasma and interstitial fluid. Interstitial fluid, therefore, is an ultrafiltrate of plasma. Because of the virtual absence of protein with its negative charge on one side of the capillary wall (1% vs. 6%), diffusible ions distribute themselves according to the Gibbs–Donnan rule, i.e. more anions such as chloride and bicarbonate will be on the relatively protein-free side of the membrane (interstitial space) (Pitts, 1974). Nevertheless, the sum of the cations and anions must be equal on each side of the membrane. The presence of the non-penetrable protein also causes a slight increase in oncotic pressure on the plasma side that is balanced by the hydrostatic pressure developed by the heart. Sodium is maintained in the extracellular compartment and potassium in the intracellular compartment mainly through the actions of the Na^+,K^+-ATPase exchange pump. Accordingly, sodium is the major cation in the extracellular fluid and the major osmotic particle outside the borders of the cell, whereas potassium is concentrated within the cells.

In the above discussion, sodium and chloride have been considered together. Total amounts of both sodium and chloride determine the size of the extracellular space. Restriction of dietary chloride without restriction of sodium prevents expansion whereas it is well recognized

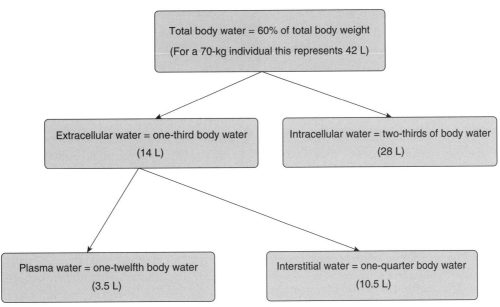

FIG. 31.3 Body fluid compartments. Total body water is broken down into extracellular and intracellular compartments. The extracellular water is broken down further into plasma and interstitial water.

that administration of sodium coupled to other anions such as bicarbonate has a negligible effect on expansion of the extracellular body space (Kotchen, 2005). The average concentration of sodium, estimated via specific electrodes or flame photometry, is 135–145 mmol/L, and of chloride, estimated by titration and specific electrodes, is 98–108 mmol/L. Because of various forces maintaining high sodium concentration in the extracellular fluid, infusions of normal saline result predominantly in expansion of the extracellular space. Infusions of dextrose solutions result in the fluid distribution between intracellular and extracellular water compartments.

Clinical Conditions Associated with Sodium Perturbations

Edema, the accumulation of excess fluid in the body, can lead to symptoms such as swelling of a part or all of the body (Michelis and Rakowski, 1988). Accumulation of fluid in the lungs leads to difficulty in breathing. Causes of generalized edema are listed in Box 31.1: the major causes relate to cardiac, renal, or hepatic perturbations. Sodium chloride retention may indicate a physiological response of the kidneys to what is perceived as inadequate arterial blood volume or may reflect an abnormal renal response to internal damage or hormonal imbalances. In

BOX 31.1   Causes of generalized edema

Cardiac
  Congestive heart failure
  Pericardial disease
Renal
  Nephrotic syndrome
  Renal insufficiency
Hepatic
  Cirrhosis
  Hepatic venous disease
Endocrine
  Myxedema
  Hyperaldosteronism
Pharmaceuticals that cause fluid retention
  Nonsteroidal anti-inflammatory drugs
  Chlorpropamide
  Tolbutamide
  Hormones
Protein malnutrition
Idiopathic edema

addition to treating the major cause of the edema, the excess fluid is often treated by limiting the intake of salt and/or removing excess sodium by using diuretics (Ellison, 1994). Too small a circulating volume can cause symptoms and signs ranging from tiredness and low blood pressure to outright disorientation and shock. Judicious replacement of salt and water often overcomes this status. Protein malnutrition may cause edema in a number of poor countries and can be overcome by including more protein in the diet.

The subject of hyponatremia (low serum sodium) and hypernatremia (high serum sodium) (Michaelis and Davis, 1988) is beyond the scope of this chapter. Suffice it to say that hyponatremia can be associated with an excess of total body sodium as well as with an excess of water, because the overall water volume is important in the disturbance. Thus, a patient with hyponatremia may not be depleted of body sodium but instead may have an excess of intravascular water (e.g. if an increase in water volume exceeds an increase in sodium, hyponatremia will develop despite the increase in total body sodium) (DeVita and Michaelis, 1993). Similarly, hypernatremia can occur in the face of low or normal body sodium if dehydration (i.e. water depletion) is present. In hospitalized patients the prevalence of hyponatremia (defined as sodium concentration <135 mmol/L) is commonly as high as 15–22%, but more severe dilutions of <130 mmol/L are seen in only 1–4% of patients (Verbalis, 1998). Symptoms may vary depending on the acuteness of the hyponatremia; slow decreases in sodium (nausea, lassitude, muscle cramps) are usually less severe than rapid decreases (confusion, coma, convulsions).

Sodium and Hypertension

Historical Perspective

Many observations and clinical studies over the past century implicate salt (sodium and chloride) intake in hypertension (Haddy and Pamnani, 1995). Around 1900, French workers proposed that hypertension arose from failure of kidneys to adapt to excess dietary salt (Ambard and Bedaujard, 1904). In support, Allen (1925) showed that severe restriction of dietary salt in many hypertensive patients reduced blood pressure, which he believed was due to an unknown renal defect in sodium excretion. The beneficial effects of the famous Kempner rice diet, an early low-sodium diet prescribed by many physicians, were attributed to low sodium content (Kempner, 1948). Hypertension in the elderly and blacks is generally characterized by low plasma renin activity, suggesting volume expansion and less sodium excretion when challenged with this cation (Haddy and Pamnani, 1995). Furthermore, the elevated blood pressure of blacks responds especially well

to treatment with diuretics (Fries, 1979). However, studies limited to industrialized societies have not always found a conclusive relationship between blood pressure and sodium excretion (Pickering, 1980; INTERSALT Cooperative Group, 1988).

What is known about the genetic component of sodium-induced hypertension? Laboratory studies provide evidence that Allen (1925) could be correct – that a genetic component works through kidneys. Dahl *et al.* (1962) developed two rat substrains, one exquisitely sensitive to salt and one very resistant, and showed that the expression of the genetic defect in salt-sensitive rats was in the kidneys. The salt-resistant rats were nephrectomized and then received kidneys from the salt-sensitive rats; hypertension developed when these rats ate high-salt diets (4–8% by weight). In contrast, nephrectomized salt-sensitive rats receiving kidneys from salt-resistant rats did not develop hypertension while eating high-salt diets. Experiments using isolated kidneys from the salt-sensitive rats confirmed an intrinsic renal defect that allows less sodium excretion compared with the salt-resistant rats at comparable inflow pressures (Tobian *et al.*, 1979). Tobian *et al.* (1979) also reported that thiazide diuretics overcame hypertension in the salt-sensitive rats.

Salt Sensitivity

As mentioned previously, not all studies have found a close relationship between salt and hypertension (Pickering, 1980). A plausible explanation for the difficulty in associating sodium consumption with blood pressure may be that the connection pertains only to those individuals that are "salt sensitive." Some individuals can eat large amounts of sodium without affecting blood pressure markedly, because they excrete excess sodium adequately. However, more than half of those with hypertension have a marked increase in blood pressure in response to a sodium challenge (Sullivan, 1991). These individuals tend to retain the sodium, because they excrete the sodium load more slowly. Normotensive relatives of hypertensive subjects, especially older individuals, show a blunted natriuretic effect. Supporting the contention that sodium retention is important in the pathogenesis of hypertension is that those individuals on a modern, Western diet have an extracellular fluid volume 15% greater than those on a more primitive diet who exhibit less hypertension (Haddy and Overbeck, 1976).

Many believe that blood pressure rises to compensate for sodium and water retention, because elevated blood pressure allows the kidney to excrete more sodium and water to maintain balance (Guyton *et al.*, 1972). In general, more blacks than whites have difficulty handling a sodium challenge, and hypertension is more prevalent in the black population, suggesting genetic predisposition. Inappropriate renal sodium handling can occur via many initiating causes: e.g. inheritance of inborn renal transport defects, presence of circulating factors influencing renal reabsorption, or decreasing renal mass. Other factors associated with salt sensitivity include female gender, aging, obesity, insulin resistance, and a positive history of hypertension (Suter *et al.*, 2002).

Perhaps the greatest ability of salt intake to elevate blood pressure occurs in those individuals said to have "resistant hypertension" (Appel, 2009a; Pimenta *et al.*, 2009). Resistant hypertension is defined as being present in patients with uncontrolled blood pressure despite therapeutic use of three or more medications generally accepted as being beneficial for pressure reduction (Pimenta *et al.*, 2009). Blood pressure of two different groups of patients with resistant hypertension were examined: one on low sodium (1.2 g per day), the other on high (5.7 g per day). Comparing blood pressures, the lower-level group showed a reduced average systolic blood pressure of 22.7 mm Hg and a diastolic of 9.1 mm Hg compared with the high-level group.

INTERSALT and INTERMAP

Two large epidemiological studies examined the role of salt in hypertension. These have been labeled INTERSALT and INTERMAP (INTERSALT Cooperative Research Group, 1988; Dennis *et al.*, 2003). In the INTERSALT study, sodium excretion data from 52 centers throughout the world were examined (INTERSALT Cooperative Research Group, 1988). The ranges of intake, adjusted for body mass index and alcohol intake, were roughly from 50 to 250 mmol (1.2 to 5.8 g) sodium over 24 hours. The INTERSALT Cooperative Research Group reported that the prevalence of hypertension was 1.7% in non-obese subjects consuming a low-sodium diet compared with 11.9% for non-obese subjects consuming a high-sodium diet. Interestingly, the four centers with the lowest sodium excretion also had the lowest average systolic and diastolic blood pressures. Although the INTERSALT study shows a positive correlation between blood pressure and sodium ingestion from the 52 participating centers, removal of data from the four centers reporting the lowest sodium intake lessens the significance of the correlation. One

assumption based on these and other data is that a sodium intake of <100 mmol/day (2.3 g/day) would lead to a healthful reduction in blood pressure even in individuals without hypertension.

The INTERSALT study was carried out between 1985 and 1987. Approximately 10 years later (1996–1999), the INTERMAP study was performed (Dennis *et al.*, 2003; Robertson *et al.*, 2005). INTERMAP followed measurements of dietary sodium intake and urinary sodium excretion in men and women aged 40–59 years, from 17 population samplings. Multiple samples from the number of population groups indicated were obtained: Japan (4), China (3), the United Kingdom (2), and the United States (8). Food recalls and timed urine specimens were used to estimate salt intake. In general, the INTERMAP study corroborated the findings of INTERSALT and most other epidemiologic studies in finding higher sodium intakes associated with higher blood pressures (Dennis *et al.*, 2003; Robertson *et al.*, 2005). In corroboration, the well-recognized studies with the Dietary Approach to Stop Hypertension (DASH) diet revealed that the lowest blood pressures were found with the lowest sodium intake: 500 mg/day (Sacks *et al.*, 2001).

Dietary Salt

Importance of Chloride

Early on, the chloride moiety was assumed to be responsible for the blood pressure disorders – possibly because the measurement of chloride was much more accurate than that of sodium and afforded better evaluation (Kaunitz, 1978). Later, the development of the flame photometer led to more emphasis on the sodium moiety as the major perturbation in the significant elevation of blood pressure by salt. However, the two ions seem to work together to control extracellular volume and blood pressure. It is worth repeating that the sodium coupled to chloride – not so much to other anions such as bicarbonate – affects fluid distribution in the extracellular compartment (Kotchen, 2005). Therefore, although most references here are to "sodium," it is important to remember that sodium and chloride are coupled most of the time in the actions, both good and bad.

Intake and Requirements

Primal herbivorous humans probably consumed ≤10 mmol/day (0.2–0.3 g/day) of sodium (Dahl, 1958; Meneely and

Dahl, 1961). On a successful hunting day, carnivorous humans might even have ingested as much as 60 mmol (1.4 g) sodium. Over the ensuing years, however, humans developed a significant salt appetite that brought about an estimated increase in sodium intake of 87–260 mmol/day (2.0–6.0 g/day). No doubt this increase has occurred because most individuals experience enhanced flavor and improved texture of foods with added salt. Also, salt serves as a preservative and thickener. The bottom line is that many who depend on food for a livelihood believe that salt makes cheap, unpalatable foods taste better at a low cost. Unfortunately, the ubiquitous nature of salt in foods has allowed the general public to become accustomed to high levels.

Sodium intake varies greatly among countries according to reports in the late 1980s (Simpson, 1988). At that time, daily intake was ≥300 mmol (6.9 g) by some Japanese men; 235 mmol (5.4 g) in Finland; 150–170 mmol (3.5–3.9 g) in the United States, Thailand, and New Zealand; 62 mmol (1.4 g) in a Polynesian island; and <30 mmol (0.69 g) in the Amazon Jungle, New Guinea Highlands, and the Kalahari Desert (Engstrom et al., 1997). The values for the United States are slightly higher than the average daily intake reported 10 years later by the United States Department of Agriculture (USDA, 1997). Between 1994 and 1996, the typical US diet had an average sodium content of 3.27 g/day that significantly exceeded the average potassium content of 2.62 g/day according to the Agriculture Department (USDA, 1997). Recent guidelines from the Institute of Medicine urge the FDA to set government standards for amount of salt added by manufacturers, restaurants, and food-service companies, because analysts estimate that population-wide reductions in sodium intake could prevent more than 100 000 deaths annually (Henney et al., 2010).

Japan in the late 1950s had the dubious distinction of having the highest death rate from strokes of any nation (He and MacGregor, 2009). In 1960, the Japanese government initiated a program to reduce salt intake from 13.5 to 12.1 g/day over 10 years. Paralleling this decrement were falls in blood pressure and an 80% reduction in stroke mortality despite increases in fat intake, cigarette smoking, alcohol consumption, and obesity. Since the 1970s, the Finnish Ministry of Social Affairs and Health has worked closely with food companies to decrease salt content of products and has educated physicians to lower sodium intake (Tuomilheto et al., 1984). Sodium intake decreased at least 40% during this period (Havas et al., 2007) and prevention of cardiovascular diseases was noted

(Puska et al., 1998). The British government's Food Standards Agency has a goal of reducing sodium consumption by 33% over 5 years. Why is this necessary? Lifetime probability of hypertension approaches 90%. Worldwide more than 26% of adults have hypertension. Virtually all reports on clinical trials examining the lessening of sodium in the diet found reduction in blood pressure, and lowered incidence of strokes and, to a lesser extent, coronary events (Strazzullo et al., 2009).

Brown et al. (2009) recently updated the information concerning salt intake throughout the world. In the 21st century, sodium intake around the world remains well in excess of physiological needs, i.e. intake may be five to 20 times above need. In part, the multiple sources of sodium contribute to the prevalence of sodium ingested worldwide. In North America and Europe, 75% of sodium intake is via manufactured foods, with cereals and baked goods being the largest contributors. In the Far East, salt added at home and in soy sauce proved to be the largest contributors.

Tackling the Problem

Concerning disturbances in the balance of sodium, the major problem usually lies with input, not output. Concerning output, healthy kidneys are amazing in their ability to compensate adequately under most circumstances for either too little or too much sodium intake. This is important to the average individual with normal renal function who from day to day pays little attention to sodium balance even though his intake varies markedly. An example of a usual balance of sodium chloride might be the following: 10.5 g/day in foods and a dietary output of 10.5 g/day (in urine [10.0 g/day], sweat [0.25 g/day], and feces [0.25 g/day]). In the case of too little intake, the healthy kidney conserves sodium at the expense of hydrogen and potassium (Pitts, 1974). The renal conservation of sodium is so efficient that, if necessary, a daily intake of only a few millimoles is required to balance the small non-urinary losses of sodium (Pitts, 1974).

Although the problem usually lies on the intake side, recent changes have started to take place because the public is becoming alarmingly aware of the consequences of "too much salt." The major effort to decrease sodium intake between 1980 and 1990 was via salt shakers (0.06 vs. 0.02 mmol]1.4 vs. 0.5 g]). Unfortunately, sodium intake emanating directly from foods, by far the major source, was not affected (Havas et al., 2007). Thus, overall sodium intake has not decreased enough to satisfy most health experts (He and MacGregor, 2007; Cook, 2008).

A decrease in sodium can often be accomplished successfully without affecting consumer enjoyment of food products if it is done in a stepwise process that systematically and gradually lowers sodium levels across the food supply (Henney *et al.*, 2010). In addition to hypertension, heavy consumption of salt-laden foods such as breads, grains, and cereal products increases the risk of strokes, osteoporosis, obesity, stomach cancer, and kidney stones, left ventricular hypertrophy, congestive heart failure, and severity of asthma (Mickleborough and Fogarty, 2006; Frassetto *et al.*, 2008; He *et al.*, 2008; Forrester *et al.*, 2010).

Potassium

General Background

Potassium is the major intracellular cation and plays a significant role in several physiological processes (Brown, 1986; Perez *et al.*, 1988; Latta *et al.*, 1993). Circulating potassium enters all tissues and has profound effects on the function of some organs, particularly depolarization and contraction of the heart. A number of organ systems are involved in maintaining potassium balance. Under usual circumstances, roughly 90% of ingested potassium is absorbed via the gastrointestinal tract for use in the body, leaving the remaining 10% to be excreted in stools (Figure 31.4). Potassium is readily absorbed in the small intestine in proportion to the presented load. Circulating concentrations are relatively stable, because cells immediately take up most potassium entering the body. Cellular uptake is facilitated by insulin, catecholamines, and aldosterone. Since the kidney is the principal excretory organ and decreased renal function from any cause may result in excess potassium retention, it usually takes from several days to as much as 3 weeks for the kidney to adapt to excess potassium intake. When kidneys cannot respond appropriately, the gastrointestinal tract can reestablish balance, at least in part, by eliminating increased amounts of potassium (i.e. 30–40% of daily intake) (Brown, 1986).

Facts about Potassium

The total body potassium of a normal adult male averages 45 mmol/kg body weight (Pitts, 1959), i.e. the body of a 70-kg person has 3150 mmol (120 g) potassium. Only 60 mmol or ~2% of potassium is distributed in the extracellular fluid. Virtually all the body's potassium is labile and exchangeable. A typical balance of potassium for an average 70-kg man is depicted in Figure 31.4. The circulating potassium concentrations are low, ~3.5–5.0 mmol/L, and the plasma concentration of potassium is often a poor indicator of tissue potassium stores. Intracellular potassium is maintained at 140–150 mmol/L (Hayslett and Binder, 1982). Potassium status not only depends on the intake and output of potassium but on its distribution as well (Perez *et al.*, 1988). Distribution depends on the energy-consuming processes at the cell membranes in which sodium extrusion is coupled to entry of potassium. Although the kidneys can adapt to high and low potassium intakes over a period of 2–3 weeks, the minimum rate of excretion is 5 mmol/day. Taken together with obligatory extra renal losses, this implies that potassium balance cannot be achieved on intakes <10–20 mmol/day (<0.4–0.8 g/day)(Perez *et al.*, 1988).

Functions of Potassium within the Body

A major function of potassium is membrane polarization. Membrane polarization depends on the concentrations of internal and external potassium (on either side of the membrane). The major clinical features of disordered potassium homeostasis relate to perturbations in membrane function, especially in the neuromuscular and cardiac conduction systems. Accordingly, both deficient and excessive circulating potassium concentrations can lead to disorders in cardiac, muscle, and neurological functions.

Sources

Because potassium is the principal cation of the intracellular fluid, the major source of dietary potassium is the cellular materials consumed in foodstuffs (Table 31.3). It is a major constituent of meats, vegetables, and fruits (Institute of Medicine, 2004). Consequently, a potassium-free diet is virtually impossible to devise. Since most foods

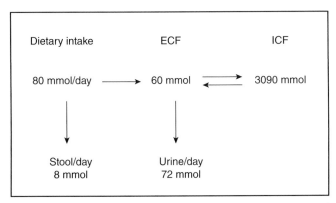

FIG. 31.4 Potassium distribution balance in a normal 70-kg man. ECF, Extracellular fluid; ICF, intracellular fluid.

TABLE 31.3 Approximate values for potassium content in some common foods[a]

Foodstuff	Potassium	
	(mmol)	(mg)
Apple, raw, with skin (1 apple, 138 g)	3.8	148
Asparagus, boiled no salt (4 spears, 60 g)	2.6	103
Avocado, raw California (1 oz, 28.35 g)	3.7	144
Banana, raw (1 banana, 118 g)	10.8	422
Beef patty, 75% lean/25% fat , broiled (3 oz, 85 g)	6.3	246
Beer, regular (12 oz, 355 g)	2.5	96
Butter, salted (1 tbsp, 14.2 g)	0.08	3
Celery, raw (1 stalk, 40 g)	2.7	104
Chicken, breast meat only, roasted (half breast, 86 g)	5.6	220
Egg, scrambled (1 large, 61 g)	2.1	84
Frankfurter, beef (1 frankfurter, 45 g)	1.8	70
Milk, whole, 3.25% milk fat (1 cup, 244 g)	8.9	349
Sweet potato, baked in skin (1 potato, 146 g)	17.7	694
Sweet potato, boiled without skin (1 potato, 156 g)	9.2	359
Tomato juice, canned, salt added (1 cup, 243 g)	14.2	556

[a]Based on USDA National Nutrient Database for Standard Reference, Release 21, 2008.

contain some potassium, mineral imbalances do not, as a rule, occur through dietary inadequacies but rather through excessive fluid losses from sweating, diarrhea, or the use of diuretics.

The potassium content of the average American diet ranges between 50 and 100 mmol/day (2.0–4.0 g/day). Foods containing high concentrations of potassium include avocado, apricots, cantaloupes, lima beans, oranges, and all meats, poultry, and fish. Milk and yogurt, as well as nuts, are recognized as being excellent sources of potassium (Institute of Medicine, 2004). Apple juice, asparagus beets, carrots, peas, and lettuce are considered to have moderate levels. Those often listed as low in potassium are blueberries, cabbage, beans, mushrooms, pineapples, and plums. The famous DASH (Dietary Approach to Stop Hypertension) diet to ameliorate elevated blood pressure is higher in potassium than the typical American diet (McGill *et al.*, 2008).

Only a small portion of oral potassium absorbed remains in the extracellular compartment. Normal rates of dietary intake cause only negligible changes in plasma levels. At high intakes of 200–300 mmol/day (8–12 g/day), patients unaccustomed to large loads may develop a significant elevation in circulating potassium despite normal renal function (Perez *et al.*, 1988). Potassium loads augment secretions of insulin, catecholamines, and aldosterone which help maintain balance.

Dietary Recommendations

Our ancestors consumed a diet relatively high in potassium in contrast to that consumed in modern societies. This recent lowering of intake is associated with the increasing consumption of processed foods low in potassium and a reduced intake of fruits and vegetables. The average potassium intake in the modern world has been estimated to be around 70 mmol/day or 2.8 g/day (Anderson *et al.*, 2010) – far from the current recommendation of 120 mmol/day (4.7 g/day). Most individuals who eat a reasonably healthy diet that includes fresh fruits and vegetables consume sufficient potassium.

The following dietary intakes of potassium according to age have been recommended by the Food and Nutrition Center of the Institute of Medicine (Institute of Medicine, 2004).

Infants
   0–6 months: 0.4 g/day
   7–12 months 0.7 g/day
Children and adolescents
   1–3 years: 3.0 g/day
   4–8 years: 3.8 g/day
   9–13 years: 4.5 g/day
   14–18 years: 4.7 g/day
Adults
   19-up: 4.7 g/day

Potassium and Blood Pressure

In contrast to deleterious effects of high sodium intake that frequently increase blood pressure, ingestion of more potassium may influence blood pressure favorably by lowering any elevations (Cappuccio and MacGregor, 1991; Bari and Wingo, 1997). Many studies have shown that potassium has a good blood-pressure-lowering effect, especially in salt-sensitive individuals (He and MacGregor, 2008). The beneficial effects of potassium (even magnesium and calcium) work, at least in part, through an effect on sodium balance: a greater sodium excretion despite no change in intake (Perez et al., 1988; Latta et al., 1993).

A high intake of potassium has been reported to protect against increased blood pressure and other cardiovascular risks (Cappuccio and MacGregor, 1991; Nowsom et al., 2003; He and MacGregor, 2008). Analysis of results from the INTERSALT study shows a lowering of systolic blood pressure at higher potassium excretory rates, presumably reflecting higher intakes (INTERSALT Cooperative Research Group, 1988). Various clinical trials suggest a lowering of blood pressure in persons taking potassium supplements (Siani et al., 1991). One meta-analysis reviewed 19 clinical trials involving a total of 586 participants (Cappuccio and MacGregor, 1991). Results showed that oral potassium supplements significantly lowered systolic blood pressure (−5.9 mm Hg) and diastolic blood pressure (−3.4 mm Hg). In mildly hypertensive individuals, a low-potassium diet can augment the already elevated systolic and diastolic pressures and also causes sodium retention (Krishna and Kapoor, 1991). In normal people, dietary potassium depletion can also cause sodium retention and augmented blood pressure (Krishna et al., 1987). Low intake of potassium rather than excess sodium consumption may be more important in the prominence of severe hypertension among blacks (Langford and Watson, 1990; Weinberger, 1993). In addition to benefiting hypertensive individuals, potassium supplementation of diabetics could appreciably check the negative effects of diabetic vascular disease by enhancing vascular perfusion and improving carbohydrate metabolism (Whang and Sims, 2000). Over and above the natriuretic effects of potassium, increased urinary kallikrein (Valdes et al., 1991) and stimulation of the Na$^+$, K$^+$-ATPase in vascular smooth muscle cells and adrenergic nerve terminals (Haddy, 1983, 1988) may be important in lowering blood pressure.

The DASH diet seems particularly effective in lowering blood pressure. Results from two DASH studies have been published (Appel et al., 1997; Sacks et al., 2001; Bray et al., 2004). The basic diet resulted in a marked reduction of blood pressure. Although many nutrients are responsible for the overall effect, potassium is probably most important in producing the beneficial effects. In the second DASH-sodium trial, salt intake was monitored at three different levels, with the greatest effects on blood pressure being seen with the lowest sodium intake. A 12-month follow-up study was instituted to determine the effects of the DASH diet with sodium reduction after discontinuation of the feeding intervention (Ard et al., 2004). Compared with control participants, DASH diet participants ate more fruit and vegetables and maintained reduced blood pressure even though their sodium intake increased. Organic forms of potassium may be more influential than inorganic forms in lowering blood pressure (Sebastian et al., 2006)

A recent report indicated that a higher sodium-to-potassium excretion ratio is associated with the increased risk of cardiovascular diseases (Cook et al., 2009). This association is stronger for the ratio than for sodium and potassium alone. Therefore, diets that lower the overall intake of sodium while increasing the intake of potassium are recommended for the best cardiovascular health.

Severe Disturbances in Potassium Balance

Total body potassium can be decreased and lead to decreased serum concentration of potassium, i.e. hypokalemia (Hayslett and Binder, 1982; Brown, 1986). However, hypokalemia can also result from shifts of potassium out of the blood and into the cells even though total body potassium is normal. Common causes of hypokalemia include increased renal excretion (poor renal tubular function, diuretic drugs), adrenal disorders (hyperaldosteronism), increased gastrointestinal losses (vomiting, diarrhea), increased uptake by cells (insulin, beta-adrenergic agonists), and decreased intake (chronic alcoholism, anorexia nervosa). Mild hypokalemia may be asymptomatic or present with muscle weakness, constipation, fatigue, and malaise. Patients with underlying cardiac diseases are prone to arrhythmias. Moderate hypokalemia may result in more severe constipation, an inability to concentrate urine accompanied by polyuria, and a tendency for the development of encephalopathy in patients with concomitant renal disease. Severe hypokalemia can result in muscular paralysis and even in poor respiration because of immobilization of the diaphragm and decreased blood pressure.

Diuretic usage is the most common cause of hypokalemia in the United States (Gennari, 1998). Elderly women using long-acting thiazides or loop diuretics are at increased risk. A low-sodium/high-potassium diet, lower doses of diuretic agents, and substitution of different antihypertensive drugs may ameliorate the problem. Patients with normal renal function who receive diuretics and digitalis-type compounds may need potassium supplementation or an agent that reduces potassium loss via the kidneys, e.g. aldactone, triamterene, or amiloride. Laxative abuse often leads to hypokalemia and can be overcome by ceasing to use the causative agent.

When high circulating concentrations of potassium are present (hyperkalemia), it is important to differentiate between pseudohyperkalemia and/or laboratory error and the actual increases in total body potassium. Pseudohyperkalemia is not a real increase in circulating potassium but rather a response to a condition that should be recognized. Pseudohyperkalemia may arise from hemolysis of red blood cells with potassium release into the serum or potassium release into serum from massive leukocytosis or thrombocytosis. In the case of true hyperkalemia, the most important clinical manifestation is cardiac arrest caused by perturbations in electrical (membrane) conduction. Various characteristic changes in the electrocardiogram assessment aid in the diagnosis. Neuromuscular symptoms of too much potassium include tingling, paresthesia, weakness, and flaccid paralysis. In addition to spurious hyperkalemia caused by hemolysis or too many blood cells in the specimen, other common causes of true hyperkalemia are decreased renal excretion; adrenal disorders; and the use of medications such as spironolactone, triamterene, amiloride, angiotensin-converting enzyme inhibitors, nonsteroidal anti-inflammatory drugs, and heparin.

Treatment for Severe Potassium Perturbations

Oral replacement in deficiency states is generally preferable to intravenous administration, and the amount given depends on the body deficit. A rough rule is that a 1 mmol/L decrease in circulating levels is equivalent to 200–300 mmol of body potassium stores. Oral or intravenous potassium at a dose of 40–120 mmol/day generally improves all symptoms of hypokalemia. Any intravenous fluid should contain ≤40 mmol/L and administration should be <10 mmol/hour. If more rapid administration is necessary, it should be performed with electrocardiogram monitoring.

Hyperkalemia is, of course, treated by eliminating excess intake and reversing the other causes mentioned above.

When the problem is severe and immediate action must be taken, several therapeutic choices exist. First, one can antagonize the membrane effects by giving calcium gluconate or hypertonic saline. Second, cellular uptake of potassium can be stimulated by giving sodium bicarbonate, glucose, or insulin. Finally, potassium can be removed from the body by using certain diuretics (thiazides), cation-exchange resins (Kayexalate), and dialysis (peritoneal or hemodialysis).

Chronic hyperkalemia is treated by eliminating excess potassium from the extracellular space and reversing the primary cause of the disturbance and any cofactors that would increase potassium retention. Many drugs and conditions accentuate potassium retention. Drugs causing hyperkalemia include β-adrenergic blocking agents, digitalis, arginine succinylcholine, potassium penicillin, potassium salts, angiotensin-converting enzyme inhibitors, and potassium-retaining diuretics (aldactone, triamterene, amiloride). Acidosis, insulinemia, low levels of catecholamines, and hypoaldosteronism may contribute to high levels of circulating potassium.

Hypokalemia is often associated with metabolic alkalosis. Therefore, replacement of potassium in the form of potassium chloride may ameliorate the alkalosis more effectively. Hypomagnesemia is somehow related to hypokalemia. The latter may prove resistant to replacement until the magnesium deficiency is corrected. Drugs causing hypokalemia include diuretics, antibiotics (carbenicillin, penicillin, polymyxin B, gentamicin), drugs causing magnesium wasting, and drugs causing metabolic alkalosis.

Contraindications

Potassium supplementation must be considered carefully in the face of evident renal failure because kidneys are the major regulator of potassium homeostasis. Because some potassium salts can be irritating to the gut lining, patients with severe gastrointestinal stress such as previous history of ulcers and bleeding should be considered carefully for oral potassium replacement.

Future Directions

It is important to note that when life emerged from the safe confines of the relatively stable seas, it became necessary to retain at all times a similar internal sea-like environment (extracellular and intracellular body fluid) within acceptable limits. Falling short or exceeding the acceptable range would lead to disaster. This meant that the daily intake of salts and electrolytes had to equal losses and vice versa, that is, the intake and output of sodium, potassium, and chloride over a finite period of time had to equal each other. It is obvious that any phenomenon necessary for life, such as maintaining the *correct* balance of electrolytes and fluids, has to be controlled by more than one mechanism: checks and balances regulating intake and output. Therefore, when symptoms occur because the acceptable limits for a healthy existence have not been maintained, more than one mechanism is involved. Of further note, adaptations to change often occur gradually. Accordingly, attempts to treat perturbations are more successful when they can be instituted gradually, either by correcting the major pathological processes involved or by carefully replacing deficits or correcting excesses of fluids and electrolytes. Diet-wise, the average individual would benefit from increasing his/her potassium intake while limiting the intake of sodium chloride (salt). A rational therapeutic approach to ameliorate or overcome perturbations in fluid and electrolyte balance mandates a solid knowledge of pertinent physiology and pathophysiology.

Suggestions for Further Reading

Appel, L.J. (2009) ASH position paper: dietary approaches to lower blood pressure. *J Clin Hypertens* **11**, 358–368.

Frassetto, L.A., Schloetter, M., Mietus-Synder, M., *et al.* (2009) Metabolic and physiologic improvements from consuming a Paleolithic, hunter-gatherer type diet. *Eur J Nutr* **63**, 947–955.

He, F.J. and MacGregor, G.A. (2008) Beneficial effects of potassium on human health. *Physiol Plant* **133**, 725–735.

He, F.J. and MacGregor, G.A. (2009) A comprehensive review on salt and health and current experience of worldwide salt reduction programs. *J Hum Hypertens* **23**, 363–384.

Sack, F.M., Svetkey, L.P., Vollmer, W.M., *et al.* (2001) DASH-Sodium Collaborative Research Group. Effects on blood pressure of reduced dietary sodium and the Dietary Approaches to Stop Hypertension (DASH) diet. DASH-Sodium Collaborative Research Group. *N Engl J Med* **344**, 3–10.

References

Allen, F.M. (1925) *Treatment of Kidney Disease and High Blood Pressure*. The Psychiatric Institute, Morristown, NJ.

Ambard, L. and Bedaujard, E. (1904) Causes de l'hypertension arterielle. *Arch Intern Med* **1**, 520–533.

Anderson, J., Young, L., and Long, E. (2010) Potassium and health. (http://www.ext.colostate.edu/pubs/foodnut/09355.html.)

Appel, L.J. (2009a) Another major role for dietary sodium reduction. Improving blood pressure control in patients with resistant hypertension. *Hypertension* **54**, 444–446.

Appel, L.J. (2009b) ASH position paper: dietary approaches to lower blood pressure. *J Clin Hypertens* **11**, 358–368.

Appel, L.J., Moore, T.J., Obarzanek, E., *et al.* (1997) A clinical trial of the effects of dietary patterns on blood pressure. DASH Collaborative Research Group. *N Engl J Med* **336**, 1117–1124.

Ard, J.D., Coffman, C.J., Lin, P.H., *et al.* (2004) One-year follow-up study of blood pressure and dietary patterns in dietary approaches to stop hypertension (DASH)-sodium participants. *Am J Hypertens* **17**, 1156–1162.

Asaria, P., Chisholm, C., Ezzati, M., *et al.* (2007) Chronic disease prevention: health effects and financial costs of strategies to reduce salt intake and control tobacco use. *Lancet* **370**, 2044–2053.

Baldwin, D., Alexander, R.W., and Warner, E.G., Jr (1960) Chronic sodium chloride challenge studies in man. *J Lab Clin Med* **55**, 362–375.

Bari, Y.M. and Wingo, C.S. (1997) The effects of potassium depletion and supplementation on blood pressure: a clinical review. *Am J Med Sci* **314**, 37–40.

Battarbee, H.D. and Meneely, G.R. (1978) Nutrient toxicities in animal and man: sodium. In M. Rechcigl Jr (ed.), *Handbook Series in Nutrition and Food*. CRC Press, West Palm Beach, FL, pp 119–140.

Bibbins-Domingo, K., Chertow, G.M., Coxson, P.G., *et al.* (2010) Projected effect of dietary salt reduction on future cardiovascular disease. *N Engl J Med* **362**, 590–599.

Blaustein, M.P. (1985) How salt causes hypertension: the natriuretic hormone–Na/Ca exchange–hypertension hypothesis. *Klin Wochenschr* **63**(Suppl III), 82–85.

Bray, G.A., Vollmer, V.M., Sack, F.M., *et al.* (2004) DASH Collaborative Research Group: a further subgroup analysis of the effects of the DASH diet and three dietary sodium levels on blood pressure: results of the DASH-sodium trial. *Am J Cardiol* **94**, 222–227.

Brown, I.J., Tzoulaki, I., Candeias, V., *et al.* (2009) Salt intakes around the world: implications for public health. *Int J Epidemiol* **38**, 791–813.

Brown, J.J., Lever, A.F., Morton, J.J., *et al.* (1972) Raised plasma angiotensin II and aldosterone during dietary sodium restriction in man. *Lancet* **ii**, 1106–1107.

Brown, R.S. (1986) Extrarenal potassium homeostasis. *Kidney Int* **30**, 116–127.

Cappuccio, F.P. and MacGregor G.A. (1991) Does potassium supplementation lower blood pressure? A meta-analysis of published trials. *J Hypertens* **9**, 465–473.

Conn, J.W. (1949) Mechanism of acclimatization to heat. *Adv Intern Med* **3**, 373–393.

Conway, E.J. (1942) Mean geochemical data in relation to oceanic evolution. *Proc R Irish Acad* **48**, 119–152.

Conway, E.J. (1947) Exchanges of K, Na and H ions between the cell and the environment. *Irish J Med Sci* **263**, 654–680.

Cook, N.R. (2008) Salt intake, blood pressure and clinical outcomes. *Curr Opin Hypertens* **17**, 310–314.

Cook, N.R., Obar-Zanek, E., and Cutler J.A. (2009) Joint effects of sodium and potassium intake on subsequent cardiovascular disease. *Arch Int Med* **169**, 32–40.

Cordain, L. (2002) The nutritional characteristics of a contemporary diet based upon Paleolithic food groups. *J Am Nutraceutical Assoc* **5**, 15–24.

Cordain, L., Eaton, S.B., Sebastian, A., *et al.* (2005) Origins and evolution of the Western diet: health implications for the 21st century. *Am J Clin Nutr* **81**, 341–354.

Dahl, L.K. (1958) Salt intake and salt need. *N Engl J Med* **258**, 1152–1157, 1205–1208.

Dahl, L.K., Heine, M., and Tassinari, L. (1962) Effects of chronic salt ingestion: evidence that genetic factors play an important role in susceptibility to experimental hypertension. *J Exp Med* **115**, 1173–1190.

Dahl, L.K., Stall, B.G., and Cotzias, G.C. (1955) Metabolic effects of marked sodium restriction in hypertensive patients: skin electrolyte losses. *J Clin Invest* **34**, 462–470.

Dennis, B., Stamler, J., Buzzard, M., *et al.* (2003) INTERMAP: the dietary data – process and quality control. *J Hum Hypertens* **17**, 609–622.

DeVita, M.V. and Michelis, M.F. (1993) Perturbations in sodium balance: hyponatremia and hypernatremia. In H.G. Preuss (ed.), *Clinics in Laboratory Medicine: Renal Function*. WB Saunders Co, Philadelphia, PA, pp 135–148.

deWardener, H.E. and Macgregor, G.A. (1983) The relation of a circulating sodium transport inhibitor (the natriuretic hormone?) to hypertension. *Medicine* **62**, 310–326.

Dole, V.P., Dahl, L.K., Cotzias, G.C., *et al.* (1950) Dietary treatment of hypertension: clinical and metabolic studies of patients on rice-fruit diets. *J Clin Invest* **29**, 1189–1206.

Duggan, K.A. and Macdonald, G.J. (1987) Vasoactive intestinal peptide: a direct natriuretic substance. *Clin Sci* **72**, 195–200.

Elkinton, J.R. and Danowsky, T.S. (1955) *The Body Fluids: Basic Physiology and Practical Therapeutics*. Williams and Wilkins Company, Baltimore, MD.

Ellison, D.H. (1994) Clinical use of diuretics: therapy of edema. In *Primer on Kidney Diseases*. Academic Press, San Diego, CA, pp. 324–332.

Encrenaz, T. (2008) Water in the solar system. *Ann Rev Astron Astrophys* **46**, 57–87.

Engstrom, A., Tobelmann, R.C., and Albertson, A.M. (1997) Sodium intake trends and food choices. *Am J Clin Nutr* **65**(Suppl), 704S–707S.

Fitzsimmons, J.T. (1980) Angiotensin stimulation of the central nervous system. *Rev Physiol Biochem Pharmacol* **87**, 117–167.

Follman, H. and Brownson, C. (2009) Darwin's warm little pond revisited: from molecules to the origin of life. *Naturwissenschaften* **96**, 1265–1292.

Forrester, D.L., Britton, J., Lewis, S.A., *et al.* (2010) Impact of adopting low sodium diet on biomarkers of inflammation and coagulation: a randomized controlled trial. *J Nephrol* **23**, 49–54.

Frassetto, L., Morris, R.C., Jr, Sellmeyer, D.E., *et al.* (2001) Diet, evolution and aging – the pathophysiologic effects of the post-agricultural inversion of the potassium-to-sodium and base-to-chloride ratios in the human diet. *Eur J Nutr* **40**, 200–213.

Frassetto, L.A., Morris, R.C., Jr, Sellmeyer, D.E., *et al.* (2008) Adverse effects of sodium chloride on bone in the aging human population resulting from habitual consumption of typical American diets. *J Nutr* **138**, 419S–422S.

Frassetto, L.A., Schloetter, M., Mietus-Synder, M., *et al.* (2009) Metabolic and physiologic improvements from consuming a Paleolithic, hunter-gatherer type diet. *Eur J Nutr* **63**, 947–955.

Fries, E.D. (1979) Salt in hypertension and the effects of diuretics. *Annu Rev Pharmacol Toxicol* **19**, 13–23.

Gennari, F.J. (1998) Hypokalemia. *N Engl J Med* **339**, 451–458.

Guyton, A.C., Coleman, T.G., Cowley, A.W., *et al.* (1972) Arterial pressure regulation: overriding dominance of the kidneys in long-term regulation and in hypertension. *Am J Med* **52**, 584–594.

Haddy, F.J. (1983) Potassium effects on contraction in arterial smooth muscle mediated by Na+,K+-ATPase. *Fed Proc* **42**, 239–245.

Haddy, F.J. (1988) Ionic control of vascular smooth muscle cells. *Kidney Int* **346**(Suppl 25), S2–S8.

Haddy, F.J. and Overbeck, H.W. (1976) The role of humoral agents in volume expanded hypertension. *Life Sci* **19**, 935–948.

Haddy, F.J. and Pamnani, M.B. (1995) Role of dietary salt in hypertension. *J Am Coll Nutr* **14**, 428–438.

Havas, S., Dickinson, B.D., and Wilson, M. (2007) The urgent need to reduce sodium consumption. *JAMA* **298**, 1439–1441.

Hayslett, J.P. and Binder, H.J. (1982) Mechanism of potassium adaptation. *Am J Physiol* **243**, F103–F112.

He, F.J. and MacGregor, G.A. (2007) Salt, blood pressure and cardiovascular disease. *Curr Opin Cardiol* **22**, 298–305.

He, F.J. and MacGregor, G.A. (2008) Beneficial effects of potassium on human health. *Physiol Plant* **133**, 725–735.

He, F.J. and MacGregor, G.A. (2009) A comprehensive review on salt and health and current experience of worldwide salt reduction programs. *J Hum Hypertens* **23**, 363–384.

He, F.J., Marrero, N.M., and MacGregor, G.A. (2008) Salt intake is related to soft drink consumption in children and adolescents: a link to obesity? *Hypertension* **51**, 629–634.

Henney, J.E., Taylor, C.L., and Boon, C.S. (eds) (2010) *Strategies to Reduce Sodium Intake in the United States*. National Academies Press, Washington, DC

Hooper, L., Bartlett, C., Davey, S.G., *et al.* (2003) Advice to reduce dietary salt for prevention of cardiovascular disease. *Cochrane Database Syst Rev* CD003656.

Institute of Medicine (2005) Panel on Dietary Reference Intakes for Electrolytes and Water. *Dietary Reference Intakes for Water, Potassium, Chloride and Sulfate*. National Academies Press, Washington, DC.

INTERSALT Cooperative Research Group (1988) Intersalt: an international study of electrolyte excretion and blood pressure. Results for 24 hour urinary sodium and potassium excretion. *BMJ* **297**, 319–328.

Kaunitz, H. (1978) Toxic and nontoxic effects of chloride in animals and man. In M. Rechcigl (ed.), *Handbook Series in Nutrition and Food*. CRC Press, West Palm Beach, FL, pp. 141–145.

Kempner, W. (1948) Treatment of hypertensive vascular disease with rice diet. *Am J Med* **4**, 545–577.

Kotchen, T.A. (2005) Contributions of sodium and chloride to NaCl-induced hypertension. *Hypertension* **45**, 849–850.

Kotchen, T.A. and Kotchen, J.M. (2003) Nutrition and cardiovascular health. In F. Bronner (ed.), *Nutritional Aspects and Clinical Management of Chronic Disorders and Diseases*. CRC Press, Boca Raton, FL, pp 23–43.

Krishna, G.G. and Kapoor, S.C. (1991) Potassium depletion exacerbates essential hypertension. *Ann Intern Med* **115**, 77–93.

Krishna, G.G., Cushid, P., and Hoeldtke, E.D. (1987) Mild potassium depletion provides renal sodium retention. *J Lab Clin Med* **109**, 724–730.

Lackland, D.T. and Egan, B.M. (2007) Dietary salt restriction and blood pressure in clinical trials. *Curr Hypertens Rep* **9**, 314–319.

Langford, H.C. and Watson, R.L. (1990) Potassium and calcium intake, excretion, and homeostasis in blacks and their relation to blood pressure. *Cardiovasc Drugs Ther* **4**(Suppl 2), 403–406.

Laragh, J.H., Baer, L., Brunner, H.R., *et al.* (1972) Renin, angiotensin, and aldosterone system in pathogenesis and management of hypertensive vascular disease. *Am J Med* **52**, 633–652.

Latta, K., Hisano, S., and Chan, J.C.M. (1993) Perturbations in potassium balance. In H.G. Preuss (ed.), *Clinics in Laboratory Medicine: Renal Function*. WB Saunders Co, Philadelphia, PA, pp. 149–156.

Macallum, A.B. (1926) The paleochemistry of the body fluids and tissues. *Physiol Rev* **6**, 316–357.

McGill, C.R., Fulgoni, V.L., III, diRienzo, D., *et al.* (2008) Contribution of dairy products to dietary potassium intake in the United States population. *J Am Coll Nutr* **27**, 44–50.

Meneely, G.R. and Dahl, L.K. (1961) Electrolytes in hypertension: the effects of sodium chloride. *Med Clin North Am* **45**, 271–283.

Michelis, M.F. and Davis, B.B. (1988) Hypo- and hypernatremia. In H.G. Preuss (ed.), *Management of Common Problems in Renal Disease*. Field and Wood, Philadelphia, PA, pp. 118–127.

Michelis, M.F. and Rakowski, T.A. (1988) Edema and diuretic therapy. In H.G. Preuss (ed.), *Management of Common Problems in Renal Disease*. Field and Wood, Philadelphia, PA, pp. 109–117.

Mickleborough, T.D. and Fogarty, A. (2006) Dietary sodium intake and asthma: an epidemiological and clinical review. *Int J Clin Pract* **60**, 1616–1624.

Nowsom, C.A., Morgan, T.O., and Gibbons, C. (2003) Decreasing dietary sodium while following a self-selected potassium-rich diet reduces blood pressure. *J Nutr* **133**, 4118–4123.

Nurminen, M.L., Korpela, R., and Vapaatalo, H. (1998) Dietary factors in the pathogenesis and treatment of hypertension. *Ann Med* **30**, 143–150.

Perez, G., Delaney, V.B., and Bourke, E. (1988) Hypo- and hyperkalemia. In H.G. Preuss (ed.), *Management of Common Problems in Renal Disease*. Field and Wood, Philadelphia, PA, pp. 109–117.

Pickering, G. (1980) Salt intake and essential hypertension. *Cardiovasc Rev Rep* **1**, 13–17.

Pimenta, E., Gaddam, K.K., Oparil, S., *et al.* (2009) Effect of dietary sodium reduction on blood pressure in subjects with resistant hypertension. Results from a randomized trial. *Hypertension* **54**, 475–481.

Pitts, R.F. (1959) Ionic composition of body fluids. In *The Physiological Basis of Diuretic Therapy*. Charles C. Thomas Publisher, Springfield, IL, pp. 11–29.

Pitts, R.F. (1974) *Physiology of the Kidney and Body Fluids*, 3rd Edn. Year Book Medical Publishers, Chicago, pp. 11–35

Puska, P., Vartiainen, E., Tuomilehto, J., *et al.* (1998) Changes in premature deaths in Finland: successful long-term prevention of cardiovascular diseases. *Bull World Health Org* **76**, 419–425.

Robertson, C., Conway, R., Dennis, B., *et al.* (2005) Attainment of precision in implementation of 24 h dietary recalls: INTERMAP UK. *Br J Nutr* **94**, 588–594.

Robertson, J.L.S. (1987) Salt, volume, and hypertension: causation or correlation. *Kidney Int* **32,** 590–602.

Romoff, M.S., Keusch, G., Campese, V.M., *et al.* (1979) Effect of sodium intake on plasma catecholamines in normal subjects. *J Clin Endocrinol Metab* **48,** 26–31.

Sacks, F.M., Svetkey, L.P., Vollmer, W.M., *et al.* (2001) DASH–Sodium Collaborative Research Group. Effects on blood pressure of reduced dietary sodium and the Dietary Approaches to Stop Hypertension (DASH) diet. DASH–Sodium Collaborative Research Group. *N Engl J Med* **344,** 3–10.

Sagnella, G.A., Markandu, N.D., Shore, A.C., *et al.* (1987) Plasma immunoreactive atrial natriuretic peptide and changes in dietary sodium intake in man. *Life Sci* **40,** 139–143.

Sawka, M.N., Burke, L.M., Eichner, E.R., *et al.* (2007) American College of Sports Medicine position stand. Exercise and fluid replacement. *Med Sci Sports Exerc* **39,** 377–390.

Sebastian, A., Frassetto, L.A., Sellmeyer, D.E., *et al.* (2006) The evolution-informed optimal dietary potassium intake of human beings greatly exceeds current and recommended intakes. *Semin Nephrol* **26,** 447–453.

Siani, A., Strazzullo, P., Giacco, A., *et al.* (1991) Increasing the dietary potassium intake reduces the need for antihypertensive medication. *Ann Intern Med* **115,** 753–759.

Simpson, F.O. (1988) Sodium intake, body sodium, and sodium excretion. *Lancet* **2,** 25–28.

Smith, H.W. (1943) The evolution of the kidney. In *Lectures on the Kidney, Porter Lectures, Series IX*. University of Kansas Press, Lawrence, Kansas, pp. 1–23.

Smith, H.W. (1974) *From Fish to Philosopher*. Little, Brown & Co, Boston, MA.

Strauss, M.B., Lamdin, E., Smith, W.P., *et al.* (1958) Surfeit and deficit of sodium. *Arch Intern Med* **102,** 527–536.

Strazzullo, P., D'Elia, L., Kandala, N.B., *et al.* (2009) Salt intake, stroke, and cardiovascular disease: meta-analysis of prospective studies. *BMJ* **24,** 339.

Sullivan, J.M. (1991) Salt sensitivity. *Hypertension* **17**(Suppl 1), 161–168.

Suter, P.M., Sierro, C., and Vetter, W. (2002) Nutritional factors in the control of blood pressure and hypertension. *Nutr Clin Care* **5,** 9–19.

Tobian, L., Pumper, M., Johnson, S., *et al.* (1979) A circulating humoral pressor agent in Dahl S rats with salt hypertension. *Clin Sci Mol Med* **57,** 345s–347s

Tuomilheto, J., Puska, P., Nissinen, A., *et al.* (1984) Community-based prevention of hypertension in North Karelia Finland. *Ann Clin Res* **16**(Suppl 43), 18–27.

USDA (1997) *Data tables: results from USDA's 1994–96 Continuing Survey of Food Intakes by Individuals and 1994–96 Diet and Health Knowledge Survey*. ARS Food Surveys Research Group.

Valdes, G., Bio, C.P., Montero, J., *et al.* (1991) Potassium supplementation lowers blood pressure and increases urinary kallikrein in essential hypertensives. *J Hum Hypertens* **5,** 91–96.

Verbalis, J.G. (1998) Hyponatremia and hypoosmolar disorders. In A. Greenberg (ed.), *Primer on Kidney Diseases*, 2nd Edn. Academic Press, San Diego, CA, pp. 57–63.

Weinberger, M.G. (1993) Racial differences in renal sodium excretion: relationship to hypertension. *Am J Kidney Dis* **21**(Suppl 1), 41–45.

Whang, R. and Sims, G. (2000) Magnesium and potassium supplementation in the prevention of diabetic vascular disease. *Med Hypoth* **55,** 263–265.

32

HUMAN WATER AND ELECTROLYTE BALANCE

ROBERT W. KENEFICK, PhD, SAMUEL N. CHEUVRONT, PhD,
SCOTT J. MONTAIN, PhD, ROBERT CARTER, III, PhD, AND
MICHAEL N. SAWKA, PhD

US Army Research Institute of Environmental Medicine, Natick, Massachusetts, USA

Summary

Among the greatest challenges to body water homeostasis is the imposition of prolonged exercise and environmental stress. Sweating results in water and electrolyte losses. Because sweat output often exceeds water intake, there is an acute water deficit that results in a hypertonic hypovolemia and intracellular and extracellular fluid contraction. Although water and electrolyte needs increase as a result of exercise, physiological and behavioral adaptations allow humans to regulate daily body water and electrolyte balance so long as food and fluid are readily available. Although there is presently no consensus for choosing one hydration assessment approach over another, deviations in daily fluid balance can be determined with the use of two or more markers, which should provide added diagnostic confidence when serial measures are made. Hypohydration increases heat storage by reducing sweating rate and skin blood-flow responses for a given core temperature. In addition, hypohydration increases the risk for heat exhaustion and is a risk factor for heat stroke. Aerobic exercise tasks can be adversely affected if hypohydration exceeds 2% of normal body mass, with the potential effect greater in warm environments and lesser in cool environments. Hyperhydration provides no thermoregulatory or exercise performance advantages over euhydration in the heat. Excessive consumption of hypotonic fluid over many hours can lead to hyponatremia. Marked electrolyte losses can accelerate the dilution and exacerbate the problem. Hyponatremia can be avoided by proper attention to diet and fluid needs.

Introduction

Humans typically maintain stable day-to-day body water and electrolyte balance so long as food and fluid are readily available (Institute of Medicine, 2005). The ability to detect and correct for water and electrolyte flux is essential considering the potential day-to-day imposition of physical activity and environmental stressors and the negative consequences of gross fluid and electrolyte imbalances on health and performance.

Water (total body water) plays many unique and vital roles within the body. Water is the principal chemical constituent of the human body and serves as the solvent for biochemical reactions supporting cellular homeostasis (Institute of Medicine, 2005). Water is also essential to sustain cardiovascular volume, and serves as the medium for transport within the body by supplying nutrients and removing waste. Water has unique properties, such as high specific heat, which allow it to absorb metabolic heat within the body, thus playing a vital role in thermoregulation. In addition, cell hydration is an important signal to regulate cell metabolism and gene expression (Haussinger and Gerok, 1994).

For an average young adult male, total body water is relatively constant and represents 50–70% of body weight (Sawka, 1988). The distribution of total body water is divided into intracellular fluid (ICF) and extracellular fluid (ECF) compartments. The ICF and ECF contain ~67% and ~33% of total body water, respectively. The ECF is further divided into the interstitial and plasma spaces (Sawka, 1988). Figure 32.1 depicts these fluid compartments and common mechanisms for compartmental fluid exchange.

The hydration of lean body mass is fairly constant (~73% water) across the lifespan and independent of sex and ethnicity. As a result, variability in total body water is primarily due to differences in body composition (Institute of Medicine, 2005). For example, using the equation, total body water $= 0.73 \times$ lean body mass $+ 0.1 \times$ fat mass (Institute of Medicine, 2005), two individuals of 90 kg and body compositions of 15% and 30% fat will have total body water values of 57.2 L and 48.7 L, respectively. Thus, similar absolute total body water losses would result in a greater percentage of total body water losses for individuals with more body fat.

Water balance represents the net difference between water intake and loss. However, when losses exceed intakes, total body water is decreased. Within the course of a day, it is not uncommon to see wide deviations in hydration status. The most common type of dehydration (hypertonic hypovolemia) is caused by a net loss of hypotonic body fluids such as sweat, e.g. during heavy physical labor or exercise. For example, individuals may dehydrate during physical activity or exposure to hot weather because of fluid non-availability or a mismatch between thirst and body water losses (Costill, 1977; Sawka, 1992). In these instances, the person begins the task with normal total body water and dehydrates over a prolonged period. A different type of dehydration (isotonic dehydration) occurs as a result of illness (diarrhea, vomiting), exposure to extreme environments (cold, high altitude), injury (hemorrhage, burns), or use of certain medications (diuretics).

Fluid replacement is encouraged during physical activity to avoid excessive dehydration, as water losses that exceed approximately 2% of initial body mass have been repeatedly shown to compromise endurance performance capability (Sawka *et al.*, 2007). However, indiscriminate drinking of water and other electrolyte-poor beverages without consideration of need can have negative consequences. Hyponatremia is a clinical example of the consequences of overdrinking and can be produced by drinking in excess of volume necessary to restore total body water, and by drinking in excess of what is necessary to preserve electrolyte balance (Vrijens and Rehrer, 1999; Montain *et al.*, 2001).

This chapter reviews the physiology, needs, and assessment of human water and electrolyte balance. The extent to which water and electrolyte imbalances affect temperature regulation and exercise performance are also considered. Throughout the chapter, euhydration refers to normal body water content, hypohydration refers to a body water deficit, and hyperhydration to increased body water content. Dehydration refers to the dynamic loss of body water.

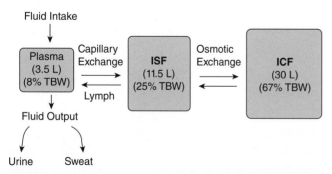

FIG. 32.1 Schematic of the approximate volume of water and mechanisms for exchange between plasma, interstitial fluid (ISF), and intracellular fluid (ICF) compartments. Example assumes total body water (TBW) of ~45 L for a 70-kg individual. Adapted from Sawka (1988).

Physiology of Water and Electrolyte Balance

Net body water balance (loss = gain) is generally regulated well as a result of thirst and hunger drives coupled with free access to food and beverage (Institute of Medicine, 2005). This is accomplished by neuroendocrine and renal responses (Andreoli *et al.*, 2000) to body water volume and tonicity changes, as well as non-regulatory social-behavioral factors (Rolls and Rolls, 1982). These homeostatic responses collectively ensure that small degrees of hyper- and hypohydration are readily compensated for in the short term. Using water balance studies, Adolph (Adolph and Dill, 1938; Adolph, 1943) found that daily body water varied narrowly between 0.22% and 0.48% in temperate and warm environments, respectively. However, exercise and environmental insult often pose a greater acute challenge to fluid balance homeostasis.

When body water deficits occur from sweat losses, a hypertonic hypovolemia generally results. Plasma volume decreases and plasma osmotic pressure increases in proportion to the decrease in total body water. Plasma volume decreases because it provides the fluid for sweat, and osmolality increases because sweat is ordinarily hypotonic relative to plasma (Costill, 1977). Resting plasma osmolality increases in a linear manner from about 288 mosmol/kg when euhydrated to more than 300 mosmol/kg when hypohydrated (Institute of Medicine, 2005). The increase in osmotic pressure is primarily due to increased plasma sodium and chloride with no consistent effect on potassium concentrations (Edelman *et al.*, 1958; Senay, 1968; Kubica *et al.*, 1983). Figure 32.2 shows the impact of hyperosmotic hypovolemia on fluid regulation, i.e. conservation of water at the site of the kidney and acquisition of water via the stimulation of thirst.

Incomplete fluid replacement decreases total body water and, as a consequence of free fluid exchange, affects each fluid space (Figure 32.1) (Costill *et al.*, 1976; Nose *et al.*, 1983; Durkot *et al.*, 1986; Singh *et al.*, 1993). For example, Costill *et al.* (1976) determined the distribution of body water loss among the fluid spaces as well as among different body organs during hypohydration. They dehydrated humans via exercise and heat exposure to a range of body mass losses from 2.2% to 5.8% of body mass and determined the fluid deficit apportioned between plasma and the intracellular and extracellular spaces. At a 2.2% body mass loss, 10% of total body water losses were from the plasma and 30% and 60% were from the intracellular and extracellular spaces, respectively. At 5.8% body mass loss, 11% of total body water losses were from the plasma, and 50% and 39% were from the intracellular and extracellular spaces, respectively. This demonstrates that hypohydration results in osmotic water redistribution from the intracellular to extracellular fluid space to maintain blood volume,

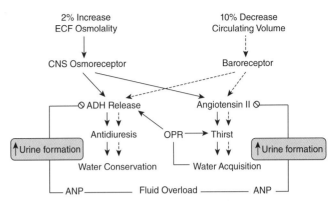

FIG. 32.2 Schematic diagram of fluid regulation in situations of fluid deficit and surfeit. Solid lines indicate the osmotically stimulated pathways (primary) and dashed lines indicate volume-stimulated pathways (secondary). ⊘ indicates negative feedback pathways; ANP, atrial natiuretic peptide; ADH, antidiuretic hormone; CNS, central nervous system; ECF, extracellular fluid; OPR, oropharyngeal reflex. Adapted from Reeves *et al.* (1998).

but it also underscores that body water losses are shared among all fluid compartments.

Different methods of dehydration are known or suspected to affect the partitioning of body water losses differently than those just described. For example, diuretics increase urine formation and generally result in the loss of both solutes and water. Diuretic-induced hypohydration generally results in an isotonic hypovolemia, with a much greater ratio of plasma loss to body water loss than either exercise or heat-induced hypohydration (Kubica *et al.*, 1983). As a result, relatively less intracellular fluid is lost after diuretic administration, since there is not an extracellular solute excess to stimulate redistribution of body water. Factors such as heat acclimatization status, posture, climate, and mode and intensity of exercise can also produce significant variability in the distribution of fluids throughout body fluid compartments.

Consequences of Fluid Imbalance

During prolonged physical exercise, profuse sweating coupled with the challenges of drinking enough often leads to dehydration by 2–6% of typical body mass (Sawka *et al.*, 2005). Although this is more common in hot environments, similar deficits are observed in cold climates when working in heavy clothing (O'Brien *et al.*, 1996). The mismatch between intakes and losses is due to physiological and behavioral factors. There are other situations where individuals purposefully dehydrate to gain a performance advantage. For example, boxers, power lifters, and wrestlers will dehydrate to compete in lower weight classes, presumably to improve their strength-to-mass ratio.

Water deficits increase the core temperature and heart-rate response to exercise and increase perception of effort to perform any given physical task (Sawka, 1992). In warm weather, the core temperature is typically increased an additional 0.1–0.2°C for every percent body weight lost due to water losses, whereas heart rate increases an additional 3–5 bpm (Sawka, 1992; Institute of Medicine, 2005). The magnitude of the penalty is of sufficient magnitude that it effectively negates the core temperature and cardiovascular advantages conferred by high aerobic fitness and heat acclimation (Sawka, 1992). In cooler weather, hypohydration induces a more modest impact on core temperature and heart rate (Cheuvront et al., 2005a).

The thermal and cardiovascular burden accompanying dehydration are regulated adjustments to compensate for the reduced ability to deliver heat from core to skin without compromising blood pressure. Consistent with this hypothesis are observed increases in the threshold core temperature for skin vasodilatation and commencement of sweating, and reduced sensitivity of each to changes in core temperature (Kenney and Johnson, 1992; Montain et al., 1995). Both the singular and combined effects of plasma hyperosmolality and hypovolemia have been implicated for mediating these thermoregulatory adjustments (Sawka, 1992). As mentioned earlier, the thermal and cardiovascular adjustment is tempered in cooler environments (Sawka et al., 1983; Kenefick et al., 2004; Cheuvront et al., 2005a).

A physiological consequence of hypohydration is deterioration in the ability to perform endurance-type physical activities. For example, McGregor et al. (1999) reported that semi-professional soccer players who were hypohydrated by >2% of body mass were less able to sprint during the later stages of a variable-intensity running protocol meant to simulate match play. They also took longer to complete an embedded soccer dribbling task. Hypohydration appears to have little or no effect on muscular strength (Greiwe et al., 1998; Evetovich et al., 2002) or anaerobic performance (Jacobs, 1980; Cheuvront et al., 2005a) but sometimes has been reported to reduce dynamic small-muscle endurance (Montain et al., 1998; Bigard et al., 2001) and tolerance to repeated bouts of high-

intensity work (Judelson et al., 2007). Hypohydration in excess of 2% body mass is, however, associated with deterioration in the ability to execute sport-specific skills (Dougherty et al., 2006; Baker et al., 2007). For example, Baker et al. (2007) reported that basketball players attempted fewer shots and were less able to make shots linked with movement (e.g. lay-up) when hypohydration had exceeded 3%, and shooting was further impaired when 4% hypohydrated. While the mechanism remains unresolved, it may be linked to changes in vestibular function and/or vestibular sensitivity as a consequence of water deficit (Lepers et al., 1997; Gauchard et al., 2002).

The threshold for performance decrements appears to be at or about >2% of body mass, at least in temperate–warm–hot environments (Cheuvront et al., 2003). As the level of dehydration increases, aerobic exercise performance is degraded proportionally (Institute of Medicine, 2005). It has previously been demonstrated that high levels of aerobic fitness and acclimatization status provide some thermoregulatory advantage. However, dehydration seems to cancel out this protective effect during exercise heat stress (Buskirk et al., 1958; Sawka et al., 1983; Merry et al., 2010). A review of studies (Cheuvront et al., 2003) that observed the specific effects of hypohydration (−2% body mass) on aerobic exercise performance found that, in environments of >30°C, aerobic exercise performance was decreased by anywhere from 7% to 60%. It also appears that the magnitude of the effect increases as exercise extends beyond 90 minutes. Overall what can be taken from this review is that the impact of hypohydration on prolonged work effort is magnified by hot environments and probably worsens as the level of hypohydration increases.

The performance penalty accompanying hypohydration may be dampened in cool weather. Cheuvront and Sawka (2005) observed an 8% reduction in total work during a 30-minute cycling time trial when hypohydrated by 3% of body mass in a 20°C environment. However, in a 2°C environment, no effect of hypohydration was observed. More recently, Kenefick et al. (2010) observed decrements in aerobic performance (15-minute cycling time trial) of −3%, −5%, −12%, and −23% in 10°C, 20°C, 30°C, and 40°C respectively, when volunteers were hypohydrated by 4% of body mass. Therefore, the temperature cusp at which dehydration altered aerobic exercise performance to an extent considered meaningful appears to be at 20°C.

The physiological factors that contribute to the hypohydration-mediated aerobic exercise performance

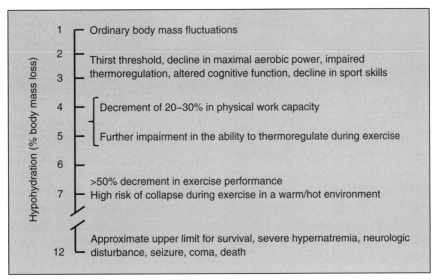

FIG. 32.3 The impact of dehydration on physiological function and ability to perform work/exercise relative to percent losses in body mass. Adapted from Greenleaf (1992).

decrements include increased body core temperature, increased cardiovascular strain, increased glycogen utilization, and perhaps altered central nervous system function (Montain *et al.*, 1998; Febbraio, 2000; Nybo and Nielsen, 2001; Cheuvront *et al.*, 2010b). Though each factor is unique, evidence suggests that they interact to contribute in concert, rather than in isolation, to degrade aerobic exercise performance (Cheuvront *et al.*, 2003). The relative contribution of each factor may differ depending on the specific activity, environmental conditions, heat acclimatization status, and athletic prowess, but elevated hyperthermia probably acts to accentuate the performance decrement. One explanation for the impact of hypohydration on exercise performance is a reduction in circulating blood and plasma volume. Cardiac filling is reduced and larger fractional utilization of oxygen is required at any given workload (Cheuvront *et al.*, 2010b). Ultimately, these responses have a negative impact on exercise/work performance, especially in warm/hot environments.

Hypohydration and hyperthermia have also been shown to degrade cognitive/mental performance when concentration, skilled tasks, and tactical issues are involved (Institute of Medicine, 2005). The evidence is stronger for a negative effect of hyperthermia than for mild hypohydration on degrading cognitive/mental performance (Cian *et al.*, 2000), but the two are closely linked when physically active in warm/hot weather. The impact of hypohydration on physiological function, ability to perform work/exercise and survivability are depicted in Figure 32.3.

Illnesses and Disease

In clinical medicine, disturbances of body fluid and electrolyte balance are associated with significant medical costs, morbidity, and mortality across the lifespan (Warren *et al.*, 1994; Black *et al.*, 2003). Fluid and electrolyte imbalances represent a common problematic complication of acute medical treatment scenarios (e.g. cardiovascular, renal, burns) and are also functionally linked to a number of acute and chronic diseases (Manz, 2007). The World Health Organization (1995) considers hypohydration of ≤5% of body mass to be mild on a life-threatening scale. When substantial solute (electrolyte) is lost in situations of long duration work and heat stress (profuse sweating), or during cold or high-altitude exposure, and in numerous illnesses and disorders (e.g. gastroenteritis, hyperemesis, diuretic treatment, dialysis), an isotonic or hypotonic hypovolemia is the result (World Health Organization, 1995; Mange *et al.*, 1997; Cheuvront *et al.*, 2005b; Sawka *et al.*, 2007). However, proper diagnosis of hypovolemia of isotonic or hypotonic origins, especially in austere environments, remains elusive because an accurate and reliable method for assessment has not yet been developed (McGee *et al.*, 1999).

It has been suggested that chronic plasma hypertonicity as a result of hypohydration may promote obesity and related metabolic dysregulation, and may play a role in chronic disease (Haussinger *et al.*, 1993; Keller *et al.*, 2003; Stookey *et al.*, 2004). Presently, support is limited, but there is increasing evidence that chronic mild hypohydration may account for various morbidities including urolithiasis (kidney stones), urinary tract infections, bladder and colon cancer, constipation, hypertension, venous thromboembolism, coronary artery disease, mitral valve prolapse, stroke, gallstones, glaucoma, and dental diseases (Manz, 2007). While further epidemiological studies will be needed to determine possible links between chronic hypohydration and these morbidities, the dangers of over-drinking (hyponatremia), are well known.

Hyponatremia

Hyperhydration is not easy to sustain since overdrinking of water or carbohydrate-electrolyte solution produces a fluid overload that is rapidly excreted by the kidneys (Figure 32.2) (Freund *et al.*, 1995). However, excessive intake of hypotonic fluid, especially over an extended time, can dilute plasma sodium to dangerously low levels (<135 mEq/L). Dilution of plasma sodium will induce movement of water from the extracellular fluid into cells. If it occurs rapidly and is of sufficient magnitude, this fluid shift can congest the lungs, swell the brain, and alter central nervous system function. The clinical signs and symptoms associated with hyponatremia include confusion, disorientation, mental obtundation, headache, nausea, vomiting, aphasia, incoordination, and muscle weakness with the severity of symptomatology related to the magnitude of decline in serum sodium and the rapidity with which it develops (Knochel, 1996). Complications of severe and rapidly evolving hyponatremia include seizures, coma, pulmonary edema, and cardiorespiratory arrest. Symptomatic hyponatremia arises during clinical care, but has developed in otherwise healthy individuals participating in marathon and ultramarathon competition (Davis *et al.*, 2001; Speedy *et al.*, 2001; Hew *et al.*, 2003), military training (Garigan and Ristedt, 1999; O'Brien *et al.*, 2001), and recreational activities (Backer *et al.*, 1993).

The hyponatremia associated with prolonged exercise most often occurs when individuals consume low-sodium drinks or sodium-free water in excess of sweat losses, either during or shortly after completing exercise (Garigan and Ristedt, 1999; Montain *et al.*, 2001; Speedy *et al.*, 2001). Unreplaced sodium losses contribute to the rate and magnitude of sodium dilution. In those individuals who produce a relatively salty sweat, there are situations where drinking sodium-free water at rates near to or slightly less than sweating rate can theoretically produce biochemical hyponatremia when coupled with the progressive loss of electrolytes (Montain *et al.*, 2001). As such, the mechanism that leads to exercise-associated hyponatremia is overdrinking in its absolute (volume-related) and relative forms (relative to sodium loss).

Exercise-associated hyponatremia can be prevented by not drinking in excess of sweating rate, and by consuming salt-containing fluids or foods when participating in exercise events that produce multiple hours of continuous or near-continuous sweating.

Hydration Assessment

Human hydration assessment is a key component for prevention and proper treatment of fluid and electrolyte imbalances (Mange *et al.*, 1997; Oppliger and Bartok, 2002; Cheuvront *et al.*, 2005). The efficacy of any assessment marker depends critically upon the nature of body fluid losses. In many clinical and most sports medicine situations, hypertonic hypovolemia occurs when there is net loss of hypotonic body fluids (Mange *et al.*, 1997; Cheuvront *et al.*, 2005; Sawka *et al.*, 2007). The rise in extracellular tonicity is a hallmark clinical feature that provides diagnostic distinction from isotonic or hypotonic hypovolemia (Feig and McCurdy, 1977; Mange *et al.*, 1997). Hypotonic fluid losses modulate renal function and urine composition in accordance with the body water deficit (Robertson and Mahr, 1971), thus providing the fundamental framework for using blood (osmolality, sodium, fluid regulatory hormones) and urine (osmolality, specific gravity, color) as principal body-fluid hydration assessment measures.

Although plasma osmolality is the criterion hydration assessment measure for large-scale fluid needs assessment surveys (Institute of Medicine, 2005), the optimal choice of method for assessing hydration is limited by the circumstances and intent of the measurement. Popular hydration assessment techniques vary greatly in their applicability to laboratory or field use because of methodological limitations which include the necessary circumstances for accurate measurement, ease of application, and sensitivity for detecting small but meaningful changes in hydration status (Table 32.1). Large population heterogeneity explains, in part, why there are presently few hydration

TABLE 32.1   Laboratory hydration assessment techniques summary

Technique	Advantages	Disadvantages
Complex markers		
Total body water (dilution)	Accurate, reliable	Analytically complex, expensive, requires baseline and serial measures
Plasma osmolality	Accurate, reliable (clinical standard)	Analytically complex, expensive, invasive
Simple markers		
Fluid input/output	Accurate, reliable (clinical standard)	Requires urinary catheter and serial measures
Urine concentration	Easy, rapid, screening tool	Easily confounded, timing critical, frequency and color subjective
Body mass	Easy, rapid, screening tool	Requires baseline; confounded by changes in body composition
Other markers		
Blood:		
Plasma volume	No advantages over	Analytically complex, expensive,
Plasma sodium	osmolality (except	invasive, multiple confounders
Fluid balance hormones	hyponatremia detection for plasma sodium)	
Bioimpedance	Easy, rapid	Requires baseline, multiple confounders
Saliva	Easy, rapid	Highly variable, multiple confounders
Physical signs	Easy, rapid	Too generalized, subjective
Tilt test (orthostatic challenge)	Rapid	Highly variable, insensitive, requires tilt table or ability to stand
Thirst	Positive symptomatology	Subjective and variable, develops late and is quenched early

Adapted from Institute of Medicine (2004) and Cheuvront *et al.* (2005).

TABLE 32.2   Biomarkers of hydration status

Measure	Euhydration	Population reference interval	Dehydration
Total body water (L)	<1%	N/A	≥3%(?)
Plasma osmolality (mmol/kg)	<290	285–295	≥297
Urine specific gravity (units)	<1.02	1.005–1.035	≥1.025
Urine osmolality (mmol/kg)	<700	300–900	≥831
Urine color (units)	<4	N/A	≥5.5
Body weight[a] (kg)	<1%	N/A	≥2%

[a]Potentially confounded by changes in body composition during very prolonged assessment periods.
Compiled from Kratz *et al.* (2004), Cheuvront *et al.* (2005, 2010a), and Sawka *et al.* (2007).

status markers that display potential for high nosological sensitivity from a practical, single measure (Cheuvront *et al.*, 2010a). Change measures can provide good diagnostic accuracy, but their usefulness also depends on the homogeneity of measures taken on the same person if day-to-day monitoring is desired (Cheuvront *et al.*, 2010a). More acute change measures (over hours) require a valid baseline and control over confounding variables. Table 32.2 provides definable thresholds which can be used as a guide to detect a negative body fluid balance stemming from hypertonic hypovolemia. Hydration should be considered adequate when any two assessment outcomes are consistent with euhydration (Table 32.2) (Cheuvront and Sawka, 2005; Sawka *et al.*, 2007). Values that occur between euhydration and hypohydration represent typical human variation (Kratz *et al.*, 2004) in homeostatic setpoints relating to biology as well as to social (diet) and environmental (exercise, climate) influences.

Water and Electrolyte Needs

Human water and electrolyte needs should not be based on a "minimal" intake, as this might eventually lead to a deficit and possible adverse performance and health consequences. The Food and Nutrition Board of the Institute of Medicine instead base the dietary recommended intake (DRI) for water needs on an adequate intake (AI). The AI is based on experimentally derived intake levels that are expected to meet nutritional adequacy for essentially all members of a healthy population. The AI level for water is 2.7 to 3.7 L/day for sedentary women and men over age 19, respectively (Institute of Medicine, 2005). These values represent total water intake from all fluids (80%) and foods (20%). The AI for sodium is 1.5 g/day, or 3.8 g/day sodium chloride (Institute of Medicine, 2005). It should be recognized, however, that endurance athletes and occupational laborers performing extended hours of work, particularly in warm climates, may greatly exceed the AI for water and sodium (Institute of Medicine, 2005).

Table 32.3 (Rehrer and Burke, 1996) illustrates the wide variability in hourly sweat losses observed both within and between sports and occupations. Depending upon the duration of activity and heat stress exposure, the impact of these elevated hourly sweat rates on daily water requirements will vary. Figure 32.4 depicts generalized modeling approximations for daily water and sodium requirements based upon calculated sweating rates as a function of daily energy expenditure (activity level) and air temperature (Institute of Medicine, 2005). Applying this prediction model, it is clear that daily water requirements can increase two- to six-fold from baseline by simple manipulation of either variable. For example, daily water requirements for any given energy expenditure in temperate climates (20°C) can triple in very hot weather (40°C). In addition to air temperature, other environmental factors also modify sweat losses to include relative humidity, air motion, solar

load, and choice of clothing for protection against environmental elements (Latzka and Montain, 1999). Therefore, water losses, and hence water needs, will vary considerably among moderately active people based on changing extraneous influences.

Sweat contains electrolytes, primarily sodium chloride and to a lesser extent potassium, calcium, and magnesium (Costill *et al.*, 1975; Costill, 1977; Verde *et al.*, 1982). Sweat sodium concentration averages ~35 mEq/L (range 10–70 mEq/L) and varies depending upon diet, sweating rate, hydration level, and heat acclimation state (Allan and WIlson, 1971; Costill *et al.*, 1975). Sweat potassium concentration averages 5 mEq/L (range 3–15 mEq/L), calcium averages 1 mEq/L (range 0.3–2 mEq/L), magnesium averages 0.8 mEq/L (range 0.2–1.5 mEq/L), and chloride averages 30 mEq/L (range 5–60 mEq/L) (Costill,1977). Neither gender, maturation nor aging seems to have marked effects on sweat electrolyte concentrations (Morimoto *et al.*, 1967; Meyer *et al.*, 1992). Sweat glands reabsorb sodium by active transport, but the ability to reabsorb sweat sodium does not increase proportionally with the sweating rate. As a result, the concentration of sweat sodium increases at high sweating rates (Allan and

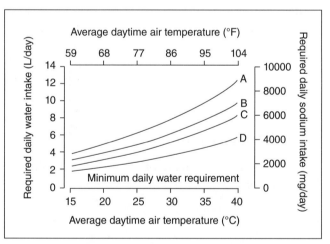

FIG. 32.4 Daily water needs and required daily sodium intake estimated from sweat-loss predictions as a result of changes in physical activity and air temperature. Daily energy expenditures of A = 3600 kcal/day, B = 2900 kcal/day, C = 2400 kcal/day, and D = 1900 kcal/day corresponds to very active, active, low activity, and sedentary. Adapted from Institute of Medicine (2005).

TABLE 32.3 Sweating rates for different sports

Sport	Mean (L/h)	Range (L/h)
Water polo	0.55	0.30–0.80
Cycling	0.80	0.29–1.25
Running	1.10	0.54–1.83
Basketball	1.11	0.70–1.60
Soccer	1.17	0.70–2.10

Data compiled from Rehrer and Burke (1996).

Wilson, 1971; Costill *et al.*, 1975; Buono *et al.*, 2008). Heat acclimation improves the ability to reabsorb sodium, thus heat-acclimated persons have lower sweat sodium concentrations (>50% reduction) for any given sweating rate (Allan and Wilson, 1971).

Generalized modeling approximations for daily sodium needs based upon calculated sweating rates as a function of daily energy expenditure (activity level) and air temperature (Institute of Medicine, 2005) are presented in Figure 32.4. This analysis assumes that persons are heat acclimated and have a sweat sodium concentration of 25 mEq/L (about 0.6 g/L). The average American diet contains ~4 g/day sodium (Institute of Medicine, 2005) but varies greatly depending upon ethnic preferences for food. Increases or decreases in sodium stores are usually corrected by adjustments in a person's salt appetite. In addition, when physical activity increases, the additional caloric intake associated with increased activity usually covers the additional sodium required (Institute of Medicine, 2005). Therefore, sodium supplementation is generally not necessary, as normal dietary sodium intake appears adequate to compensate for sweat sodium losses (Sawka *et al.*, 2007). There are two exceptions: first, prolonged heavy sweating can produce substantial salt losses, and secondly, for those unacclimatized to the weather, during the first few days of warm/hot weather as they will be secreting saltier than usual sweat. Salting food to taste is usually an adequate solution in these circumstances. Another strategy is to rehydrate with fluids containing ~20 mEq/L of sodium. Most commercial sports beverages approximate this concentration (Sawka *et al.*, 2007).

Fluid Replacement

The 2007 American College of Sports Medicine Position Statement on Exercise and Fluid Replacement (Sawka *et al.*, 2007) summarizes current knowledge regarding fluid and electrolyte needs and the impact of their imbalances on performance and health. This statement stresses the fact that individuals have varying sweat rates, and individual fluid needs can be very different despite performing a similar task in nearly identical environmental conditions. The ACSM Position Statement also provides recommendations in relation to hydration prior to, during, and following exercise/activity. Briefly, the objective is to begin physical activity euhydrated and with normal plasma electrolyte levels. If sufficient beverages are consumed with

meals and a protracted recovery period (8 to 12 hours) has elapsed since the last exercise session, then the person should already be close to being euhydrated (Institute of Medicine, 2005). During exercise the objective is to drink enough fluid to prevent excessive dehydration (>2% body mass loss) to accrue and compromise performance. The amount and rate of fluid replacement depends upon an individual's sweating rate, the exercise duration, and opportunities to drink. It is recommended that individuals should monitor body mass changes during training/activity to estimate their sweat lost during a particular exercise task with respect to the weather conditions.

Carbohydrate consumption can be beneficial to sustain exercise intensity during high-intensity exercise events of ~1 hour or longer, as well as less intense exercise/activity sustained for longer periods (Coyle and Montain, 1992). Carbohydrate-based sports beverages are used to meet carbohydrate needs, while attempting to replace sweat water and electrolyte losses. Carbohydrate solutions of 5–10% consumed at a rate of 1 L per hour would approximate a consumption rate of 1 g per minute, which has been demonstrated to maintain blood glucose levels and exercise performance (Coyle and Montain, 1992). The greatest rates of carbohydrate delivery have been achieved with a mixture of simple sugars (e.g. glucose, sucrose, fructose, maltodextrin).

The Institute of Medicine also provides general guidance for composition of "sports beverages" for persons performing prolonged physical activity in hot weather (Institute of Medicine, 1994). The need for these different components will depend on the specific exercise task (e.g. intensity and duration) and weather conditions, and can be met using non-fluid sources such as gels, energy bars, and other foods. Following activity, consumption of normal meals and snacks with a sufficient volume of plain water will restore euhydration, provided the food contains sufficient sodium to replace sweat losses (Institute of Medicine, 2005). If hypohydration is substantial (>2% body mass loss) with a relatively short recovery period (<4–6 hours), then an aggressive rehydration program may be merited (Maughan *et al.*, 1996).

In most cases of gastrointestinal tract disturbances that result in diarrhea and/or vomiting (~1 day), typical intake of food and fluid over the course of a few days will correct fluid and electrolyte losses. However, when these maladies are left untreated, prolonged bouts (>1 day) may require a unique fluid replacement strategy. Severe hypohydration of this type can require intravenous rehydration and hospitalization. However, when possible, oral rehydration with an oral electrolyte solution is the treatment of choice and is recommended by the World Health Organization (1995). While sport drinks contain carbohydrate and electrolytes, they are specifically designed for situations of hypertonic hypovolemia. The fluid and electrolyte losses resulting from diarrhea and/or vomiting (isotonic dehydration) can be more rapidly corrected with oral rehydration solutions containing 50–90 mEq per liter of sodium and ~20 mEq per liter of potassium, and ingested with complex carbohydrates (World Health Organization, 1995).

Future Directions

The ability to assess hydration state is vitally important in clinical, occupational, and sport settings. Further work is required to develop simple, accurate, non-invasive technologies or methods that can assess hydration state without the need for baseline or repeated measures.

A wide range in the percent decrement of aerobic exercise performance due to dehydration has been reported in the literature. Further work is needed to more precisely define the specific impacts of dehydration on aerobic exercise performance.

In the scientific literature a number of chronic health conditions have been suggested to be associated with hydration, including kidney stones, gallstones, bladder, colon and other cancers, arrhythmias, and blood clots among other conditions. Further work is required to determine if any link between hydration state and these and other conditions exists.

The etiology of skeletal muscle cramps has been debated in the scientific literature. Dehydration and sodium deficits have been proposed as a causal mechanism. Further work is required to determine the relationship between dehydration/sodium deficits and skeletal muscle cramps.

Acknowledgments

The authors would like to thank Kurt Sollanek for technical assistance in preparing this chapter. The views, opinions, and/or findings contained in this chapter are those of the authors and should not be construed as an official Department of the Army position, or decision, unless so designated by other official documentation. Approved for public release; distribution unlimited.

Suggestions for Further Reading

Adolph, E.F. (1947) *Physiology of Man in the Desert*. Interscience Publishers, New York.

Andreoli, T., Reeves, W., and Bichet, D. (2000) Endocrine control of water balance: endocrine regulation of water and electrolyte balance. In J. Fray and H. Goodman (eds), *Handbook of Physiology*. Oxford University Press, New York, pp. 530–569.

Edelman, I.S. and Leibman, J. (1959) Anatomy of body water and electrolytes. *Am J Med* **27**, 256–277.

Institute of Medicine (2005) *Dietary Reference Intakes for Water, Potassium, Sodium, Chloride, and Sulfate*. National Academies Press, Washington, DC.

Robertson, G.L. (1983) Thirst and vasopressin function in normal and disordered states of water balance. *J Lab Clin Med* **101**, 351–371.

Robertson, G.L. and Mahr, E. (1971) The importance of plasma osmolality in regulating antidiuretic hormone secretion in man. *Clin Res* **19**, 562.

References

Adolph, E.F. (1943) *Physiological Regulations*. Jacques Cattell Press, Lancaster, PA.

Adolph, E.F. and Dill, D.B. (1938) Observations on water metabolism in the desert. *Am J Physiol* **123**, 369–378.

Allan, J.R. and Wilson, C.G. (1971) Influence of acclimatization on sweat sodium concentration. *J Appl Physiol* **30**, 708–712.

Andreoli, T., Reeves, W., and Bichet, D. (2000) Endocrine control of water balance: endocrine regulation of water and electrolyte balance. In J. Fray and H. Goodman (eds), *Handbook of Physiology*. Oxford University Press, New York, pp. 530–569.

Backer, H.D., Shopes, E., and Collins, S.L. (1993) Hyponatremia in recreational hikers in Grand Canyon National Park. *J. Wilderness Med* **4**, 391–406.

Baker, L.B., Dougherty, K.A., Chow, M., *et al.* (2007) Progressive dehydration causes a progressive decline in basketball skill performance. *Med Sci Sports Exerc* **39**, 1114–1123.

Bigard, A.X., Sanchez, H., Claveyrolas, G., *et al.* (2001) Effects of dehydration and rehydration on EMG changes during fatiguing contractions. *Med Sci Sports Exerc* **33**, 1694–1700.

Black, R.E., Morris, S.S., and Bryce, J. (2003) Where and why are 10 million children dying every year? *Lancet* **361**, 2226–2234.

Buono, M.J., Claros, R., Deboer, T., *et al.* (2008) Na^+ secretion rate increases proportionally more than the Na^+ reabsorption rate with increases in sweat rate. *J Appl Physiol* **105**, 1044–1048.

Buskirk, E.R., Iampietro, P.F., and Bass, D.E. (1958) Work performance after dehydration: effects of physical conditioning and heat acclimatization. *J Appl Physiol* **12**, 189–194.

Cheuvront, S.N. and Sawka, M.N. (2005) Hydration assessment of athletes. *Sport Sci Exchange, Gatorade Sports Sci Inst* **18**, 1–5.

Cheuvront, S.N., Carter, R., Castellani, J.W., *et al.* (2005) Hypohydration impairs endurance exercise performance in temperate but not cold air. *J Appl Physiol* **99**, 1972–1976.

Cheuvront, S.N., Carter, R., and Sawka, M.N. (2003) Fluid balance and endurance exercise performance. *Curr Sports Med Rep* **2**, 202–208.

Cheuvront, S.N., Ely, B.R., Kenefick, R.W., *et al.* (2010a) Biological variation and diagnostic accuracy of dehydration assessment markers. *Am J Clin Nutr* **92**, 565–573.

Cheuvront, S.N., Kenefick, R.W., Montain, S.J., *et al.* (2010b) Mechanisms of aerobic performance impairment with heat stress and dehydration. *J Appl Physiol* **109**, 1989–1995.

Cian, C., Koulmann, N., Barraud, P.A., *et al.* (2000) Influence of variations in body hydration on cognitive function: effect of hyperhydration, heat stress, and exercise-induced dehydration. *J Psychophysiol* **14**, 29–36.

Costill, D.L. (1977) *Sweating: Its Composition and Effects on Body Fluids*. Academic Press, New York, pp. 160–174.

Costill, D.L., Cote, R., and Fink, W. (1976) Muscle water and electrolytes following varied levels of dehydration in man. *J Appl Physiol* **1**, 6–11.

Costill, D.L., Cote, R., Miller, E., *et al.* (1975) Water and electrolyte replacement during repeated days of work in the heat. *Aviat Space Environ Med* **46**, 795–800.

Coyle, E.F. and Montain, S.J. (1992) Carbohydrate and fluid ingestion during exercise: are there trade-offs? *Med Sci Sports Exerc* **24**, 671–678.

Davis, D.P., Videen, J.S., Marino, A., *et al.* (2001) Exercise-associated hyponatremia in marathon runners: a two-year experience. *J Emerg Med* **21**, 47–57.

Dougherty, K.A., Baker, L.B., Chow, M., *et al.* (2006) Two percent dehydration impairs and six percent carbohydrate drink improves boys' basketball skills. *Med Sci Sports Exerc* **38**, 1650–1658.

Durkot, M.J., Martinez, O., Brooks-McQuade, D., *et al.* (1986) Simultaneous determination of fluid shifts during thermal stress in a small animal model. *J Appl Physiol* **61**, 1031–1034.

Edelman, I.S., Leibman, J., O'Meara, M., *et al.* (1958) Interrelations between serum sodium concentration, serum osmolarity and total exchangeable sodium, total exchangeable potassium and total body water. *J Clin Invest* **37**, 1236–1256.

Evetovich, T.K., Boyd, J.C., Drake, S.M., *et al.* (2002) Effect of moderate dehydration on torque, electromyography, and mechanomyography. *Muscle Nerve* **26**, 225–231.

Febbraio, M.A. (2000) Does muscle function and metabolism affect exercise performance in the heat? *Exerc Sport Sci Rev* **28**, 171–176.

Feig, P.U. and McCurdy, D.K. (1977) The hypertonic state. *N Engl J Med* **297**, 1444–1454.

Freund, B.J., Montain, S.J., Young, A.J., *et al.* (1995) Glycerol hyperhydration: hormonal, renal, and vascular fluid responses. *J Appl Physiol* **6**, 2069–2077.

Garigan, T.P. and Ristedt, D.E. (1999) Death from hyponatremia as a result of acute water intoxication in an Army basic trainee. *Mil Med* **164**, 234–238.

Gauchard, G.C., Gangloff, P., Vouriot, A., *et al.* (2002) Effects of exercise-induced fatigue with and without hydration on static postural control in adult human subjects. *Int J Neurosci* **112**, 1191–1206.

Greenleaf, J.E. (1992) Problem: thirst, drinking behavior, and involuntary dehydration. *Med Sci Sports Exerc* **24**, 645–656.

Greiwe, J.S., Staffey, K.S., Melrose, D.R., *et al.* (1998) Effects of dehydration on isometric muscular strength and endurance. *Med Sci Sports Exerc* **30**, 284–288.

Haussinger, D. and Gerok, W. (1994) Role of the cellular hydration state for cellular function: physiological and pathophysiological aspects. *Adv Exp Med Biol* **368**, 33–44.

Haussinger, D., Roth, E., Lang, F., *et al.* (1993) Cellular hydration state: an important determinant of protein catabolism in health and disease. *Lancet* **341**, 1330–1332.

Hew, T.D., Chorley, J.N., Cianca, J.C., *et al.* (2003) The incidence, risk factors, and clinical manifestations of hyponatremia in marathon runners. *Clin J Sport Med* **13**, 41–47.

Institute of Medicine (1994) *Fluid Replacement and Heat Stress*. National Academy Press, Washington, DC.

Institute of Medicine (2004) Hydration status monitoring. In *Monitoring Metabolic Status: Predicting Decrements in Physiological and Cognitive Performance*. National Academy Press, Washington, DC, pp. 270–280.

Institute of Medicine (2005) *Dietary Reference Intakes for Water, Potassium, Sodium, Chloride, and Sulfate*. National Academies Press, Washington, DC.

Jacobs, I. (1980) The effects of thermal dehydration on performance of the Wingate anaerobic test. *Int J Sports Med* **1**, 21–24.

Judelson, D.A., Maresh, C.M., Anderson, J.M., *et al.* (2007) Hydration and muscular performance: does fluid balance affect strength, power and high-intensity endurance? *Sports Med* **37**, 907–921.

Keller, U., Szinnai, G., Bilz, S., *et al.* (2003) Effects of changes in hydration on protein, glucose and lipid metabolism in man: impact on health. *Eur J Clin Nutr* **57**(Suppl 2), S69–S74.

Kenefick, R.W., Cheuvront, S.N., Palombo, L.J., *et al.* (2010) Skin temperature modifies the impact of hypohydration on aerobic performance. *J Appl Physiol* **109**, 79–86.

Kenefick, R.W., Mahood, N.V., Hazzard, M.P., *et al.* (2004) Hypohydration effects on thermoregulation during moderate exercise in the cold. *Eur J Appl Physiol* **92**, 565–570.

Kenney, W.L. and Johnson, J.M. (1992) Control of skin blood flow during exercise. *Med Sci Sports Exerc* **4**, 303–312.

Knochel, J.P. (1996) Clinical complications of body fluid and electrolyte balance. In E.R. Buskirk and S.M. Puhl (eds), *Body Fluid Balance: Exercise and Sport*. CRC Press, Boca Raton, FL, pp. 297–317.

Kratz, A., Ferraro, M., Sluss, P.M., *et al.* (2004) Case records of the Massachusetts General Hospital. Weekly clinicopathological exercises. Laboratory reference values. *N Engl J Med* **351**, 1548–1563.

Kubica, R., Nielsen, B., Bonnesen, A., *et al.* (1983) Relationship between plasma volume reduction and plasma electrolyte changes after prolonged bicycle exercise, passive heating and diuretic dehydration. *Acta Physiol Polon* **34**, 569–579.

Latzka, W.A. and Montain, S.J. (1999) Water and electrolyte requirements for exercise. *Clin Sports Med* **18**, 513–524.

Lepers, R., Bigard, A.X., Diard, J.P., *et al.* (1997) Posture control after prolonged exercise. *Eur J Appl Physiol Occup Physiol* **76**, 55–61.

Mange, K., Matsuura, D., Cizman, B., *et al.* (1997) Language guiding therapy: the case of dehydration versus volume depletion. *Ann Intern Med* **127**, 848–853.

Manz, F. (2007) Hydration and disease. *J Am Coll Nutr* **26**(Suppl), 535S–541S.

Maughan, R.J., Leiper, J.B., and Shirreffs, S.M. (1996) Restoration of fluid balance after exercise-induced dehydration: effects of food and fluid intake. *Eur J Appl Physiol* **73**, 317–325.

McGee, S., Abernethy, W.B., III, and Simel, D.L. (1999) The rational clinical examination. Is this patient hypovolemic? *J Am Med Assoc* **281**, 1022–1029.

McGregor, S.J., Nicholas, C.W., Lakomy, H.K., *et al.* (1999) The influence of intermittent high-intensity shuttle running and fluid ingestion on the performance of a soccer skill. *J Sports Sci* **17**, 895–903.

Merry, T.L., Ainslie, P.N., and Cotter, J.D. (2010) Effects of aerobic fitness on hypohydration-induced physiological strain and exercise impairment. *Acta Physiol (Oxf)* **198**, 179–190.

Meyer, F., Bar-Or, O., MacDougal, D., *et al.* (1992) Sweat electrolyte loss during exercise in the heat: effects of gender and maturation. *Med Sci Sports Exerc* **24**, 776–781.

Montain, S.J., Latzka, W.A., and Sawka, M.N. (1995) Control of thermoregulatory sweating is altered by hydration level and exercise intensity. *J Appl Physiol* **79**, 1434–1439.

Montain, S.J., Sawka, M.N., and Wenger, C. B. (2001) Hyponatremia associated with exercise: risk factors and pathogenesis. *Exerc Sport Sci Rev* **29**, 113–117.

Montain, S.J., Smith, S.A., Matott, R.P., *et al.* (1998) Hypohydration effects on skeletal muscle performance and metabolism: a ^{31}P MRS study. *J Appl Physiol* **84**, 1889–1894.

Morimoto, T., Slabochova, Z., Naman, R.K., *et al.* (1967) Sex differences in physiological reactions to thermal stress. *J Appl Physiol* **22**, 526–532.

Nose, H., Morimoto, T., and Ogura, K. (1983) Distribution of water losses among fluid compartments of tissues under thermal dehydration in the rat. *Japanese J Physiol* **33**, 1019–1029.

Nybo, L. and Nielsen, B. (2001) Hyperthermia and central fatigue during prolonged exercise in humans. *J Appl Physiol* **91**, 1055–1060.

O'Brien, C., Freund, B.J., Sawka, M.N., *et al.* (1996) Hydration assessment during cold-weather military field training exercises. *Arctic Med Res* **55**, 20–26.

O'Brien, K.K., Montain, S.J., Corr, W.P., *et al.* (2001) Hyponatremia associated with overhydration in U.S. Army trainees. *Mil Med* **166**, 405–410.

Oppliger, R.A. and Bartok, C. (2002) Hydration testing of athletes. *Sports Med* **32**, 959–971.

Reeves, W.B., Bichet, D.G., and Andreoli, T.E. (1998) The posterior pituitary and water metabolism. In J.D. Wilson and D.W. Foster (eds), *Williams Textbook of Endocrinology*, 9th Edn. WB Saunders, Philadelphia, pp. 341–387.

Rehrer, N. and Burke, L. (1996) Sweat losses during various sports. *Aust J Nutr Diet* **53**, S13–S16.

Robertson, G.L. and Mahr, E. (1971) The importance of plasma osmolality in regulating antidiuretic hormone secretion in man. *Clin Res* **19**, 562.

Rolls, B. and Rolls, E (1982) *Thirst*. Cambridge University Press, Cambridge.

Sawka, M.N. (1988) Body fluid responses and hypohydration during exercise-heat stress. In K.B. Pandolf, M.N. Sawka, and R.R. Gonzalez (eds), *Human Performance Physiology and Environmental Medicine at Terrestrial Extremes*. Cooper Publishing Group, Indianapolis, IN, pp. 227–266.

Sawka, M.N. (1992) Physiological consequences of hydration: exercise performance and thermoregulation. *Med Sci Sports Exerc* **24**, 657–670.

Sawka, M.N., Burke, L.M., Eichner, E.R., *et al.* (2007) American College of Sports Medicine position stand. Exercise and fluid replacement. *Med Sci Sports Exerc* **39**, 377–390.

Sawka, M.N., Cheuvront, S.N., and Carter, R., III (2005) Human water needs. *Nutr Rev* **63,** S30–S39.

Sawka, M.N., Toner, M.M., Francesconi, R.P., *et al.* (1983) Hypohydration and exercise: effects of heat acclimation, gender, and environment. *J Appl Physiol* **55,** 1147–1153.

Senay, L.C., Jr (1968) Relationship of evaporative rates to serum [Na+], [K+], and osmolarity in acute heat stress. *J Appl Physiol* **25,** 149–152.

Singh, M.V., Rawal, S.B., Pichan, G., *et al.* (1993) Changes in body fluid compartments during hypohydration and rehydration in heat-acclimated tropical subjects. *Aviation Space Environ Med* **64,** 295–299.

Speedy, D.B., Noakes, T.D., and Schneider, C. (2001) Exercise-associated hyponatremia. *Emerg Med* **13,** 17–27.

Stookey, J.D., Pieper, C.F., and Cohen, H.J. (2004) Hypertonic hyperglycemia progresses to diabetes faster than normotonic hyperglycemia. *Eur J Epidemiol* **19,** 935–944.

Verde, T., Shephard, R.J., Corey, P., *et al.* (1982) Sweat composition in exercise and in heat. *J Appl Physiol* **53,** 1540–1545.

Vrijens, D.M. and Rehrer, N.J. (1999) Sodium-free fluid ingestion decreases plasma sodium during exercise in the heat. *J Appl Physiol* **86,** 1847–1851.

Warren, J.L., Bacon, W.E., Harris, T., *et al.* (1994) The burden and outcomes associated with dehydration among US elderly, 1991. *Am J Publ Health* **84,** 1265–1269.

World Health Organization (1995) *The Treatment of Diarrhoea: A Manual for Physicians and Other Senior Health Workers*. WHO, Geneva.

33

IRON

PETER J. AGGETT, MSc, FRCP, FRCPCH

Lancaster University, Lancaster, UK

Summary

Iron is essential for energy metabolism, mixed-function oxidase systems, neurodevelopment and function, connective-tissue synthesis, hormone synthesis, and antioxidant activity. Over 80% of systemic iron is involved in acquiring and delivering oxygen (hemoglobin), or storing it (myoglobin) to support systemic metabolism. Since iron has such diverse and fundamental roles, the effects of iron deficiency can be protean, subtle, and difficult to distinguish from other nutrient deficiencies; however, anemia and compromised physical performance, psychomotor development, and immune function are important consequences. The systemic trafficking and use of iron exploit its interchange between ferrous and ferric states, and protect tissues from the oxidative damage that ionic iron can cause. The protection involves minimizing the entry of iron into the body by down-regulating absorption of iron, and by a tight recycling of systemic iron. Iron needed to replace losses is gained by derepressing the absorption of iron. Any immune activation overrides iron-responsive homeostasis, and creates a functional iron deficiency called the anemia of chronic disease. This adaptation makes it difficult to assess iron deficiency and the efficiency of iron absorption from foods. Similar issues arise from the natural adaptations of iron turnover that occur in children and pregnant women. The causes of iron deficiency and the population groups at risk are the same as for other nutrients. Iron deficiency is likely to be accompanied by other deficiencies, and many studies inappropriately attribute anemia and its accompanying defects to iron deficiency alone. A major cause of such deficiencies is blood loss secondary to intestinal infestations. WHO reports have emphasized these points in relation to therapeutic and preventive strategies to reduce the prevalence of iron deficiency. If they were to be eradicated, there would be less need for concern about the quantity and availability of iron intakes.

Introduction

Sources for unreferenced material in this chapter can be found in the suggestions for further reading. Iron (atomic weight 55.85, atomic number 26) comprises 6.2% of the Earth's crust and is the fourth most common element, after oxygen, silicon, and aluminium. Iron binds strongly to oxygen, and its most abundant ores, magnetite and hematite, are both oxides (Earnshaw and Greenwood, 2010). Iron also complexes with sulfur and nitrogen, forming

Present Knowledge in Nutrition, Tenth Edition. Edited by John W. Erdman Jr, Ian A. Macdonald and Steven H. Zeisel.
© 2012 International Life Sciences Institute. Published 2012 by John Wiley & Sons, Inc.

iron–sulfur clusters (ISCs) comprising four-coordinated iron with four or fewer sulfur atoms, and heme, which is a six-coordinated iron within a porphyrin ring. These molecules may have contributed to the origin of life and to the subsequent genesis of atmospheric oxygen (Theil and Goss, 2010). Iron enters the food chain through its mobilization from geochemical sources by bacterial siderophores (Doherty, 2007).

Iron's oxidation states range from −2 to +6: ferrous (Fe^{2+}) and ferric (Fe^{3+}) are the most biologically relevant. Ferrous iron is easily oxidized by oxygen to ferric iron. However, the process, involving the Haber–Weiss–Fenton reactions:

$$Fe^{2+} + O_2 \rightleftarrows [Fe^{2+} - O_2 \rightleftarrows Fe3+ - O_2^{\cdot}] \rightleftarrows Fe3+ + O_2\bullet;$$
$$Fe^{2+} + H_2O_2 \rightarrow OH^{\cdot} + OH^{-} + Fe^{3+},$$

also produces oxidative radicals, which damage proteins, nucleic acids, lipids, and carbohydrates, and generate more reactive species including sulfur and nitrogen radicals. Organisms have evolved chains of carriers by which iron is distributed to its functional sites, with minimal risk of oxidative damage and simultaneously overcoming problems arising from the poor solubility of iron, particularly ferric iron, at physiological pH. The effectiveness of this system is evident in that the intracellular concentration of iron at 10^{-4} M is far higher than the aqueous solubility of ferric iron (10^{-18} M) (Theil and Goss, 2009), and intracellular free iron is restricted to 10^{-24} M (Doherty, 2007).

Functions of Iron

The biological functions of iron are achieved via four categories of metalloproteins: (1) the globin–heme, non-enzymatic ferroproteins (e.g. hemoglobin, myoglobin, and neuroglobin); (2) heme enzymes which are involved with electron transfer (e.g. cytochromes a, b, and c, cytochrome c oxidase) and oxidase activities (e.g. cytochrome P450 (mixed-function) oxidases, myeloperoxidase, peroxidases, catalase, and sulphite oxidase); (3) iron–sulfur clusters involved in electron transfer in energy production (succinate, isocitrate and NAPH dehydrogenases, and aconitase) and oxidoreductase activities (e.g. xanthine oxidase); and (4) activities that depend on iron as a cofactor (e.g. phenylalanine, tyrosine, and tryptophan hydroxylases, and proline and lysine hydroxylases).

Globin–hemes are transporters of oxygen, carbon dioxide, carbon monoxide, and nitric oxide (e.g. hemo-globin and neuroglobin), stores of oxygen (e.g. myoglobin and neuroglobin), and scavengers of free radicals (Brunore and Vallone, 2006). Heme is made in mitochondria where Fe^{2+} iron is inserted into protoporphyrin IX whose synthesis is completed in mitochondria. Most heme is incorporated into hemoglobin, but there are carriers which export heme to avoid its excess accumulation in mitochondria, or to support cytosolic production of heme enzymes. The reactivities of individual heme proteins are determined by interactions between the two components, e.g. in heme enzymes, iron switches between Fe^{2+} and Fe^{3+} whereas this does not happen with globin–heme proteins.

Hemoglobin is a tetramer comprising two pairs of α- and β-globin–heme units, each of which bind a molecule of oxygen; thus a molecule of hemoglobin transports four oxygen molecules which is 1.34 mL of oxygen per gram of hemoglobin, and as a result blood carries 50–70 times more oxygen than would plasma alone. Erythrocytic hemoglobin binds and releases oxygen, forming oxyhemoglobin and deoxyhemoglobin, respectively; the process depends on a histidine molecule in the globin which coordinates with the heme iron and controls its spin state. The iron is in a low spin state at the pulmonary alveolar–capillary interface, where, relative to the peripheral tissues, the pO_2 is high, the pCO_2 is low, and the pH is less acidic. This and a conformational change in the globin enable the unit to accommodate and bind oxygen without the ferrous iron becoming oxidized. In peripheral tissues, the higher pCO_2, lower pO_2, and more acidic milieu protonate the histidine, which switches the iron to a high spin state, reducing its affinity for oxygen, which is released. This phenomenon, including its enhancement by cooperativity between the hemoglobin subunits, is known as the Bohr effect. The release of oxygen is also facilitated by phosphate anions, higher temperature, and 2,3-diphosphoglycerate, a glycolytic product, which displaces oxygen from heme. Deoxyhemoglobin is able to transport carbon dioxide to the lungs, but because CO_2 is highly soluble in plasma this mechanism accounts for only 15–20% of carbon dioxide excretion. The fetus has a form of hemoglobin which has a higher affinity for oxygen than adult hemoglobin. This enables the fetus to acquire oxygen from maternal hemoglobin at the placenta and subsequently to release it in the low pO_2 in utero.

Myoglobin is a monomeric, mainly muscle, store of oxygen. It functions analogously to hemoglobin but the heme–globin complex is adapted to function in the ambient pO_2, pH, and pCO_2 of muscle.

Cytochrome P450 oxidase is not a single entity. There are over 11 000 activities involving a diverse range of metabolic pathways and substrates. These include phase I metabolism of xenobiotics, and the metabolism of endogenous substrates including organic acids, fatty acids, prostaglandins, steroids, and sterols including cholesterol, and vitamins A, D, and K.

The citric acid cycle and respiratory chain involves six different heme proteins and six iron–sulfur centers, as well as copper-based electron transfer from cytochrome c to cytochrome c oxidase at the ultimate transfer of electrons to molecular oxygen.

Iron: Systemic Distribution and Turnover

Adult women and men contain 3.5–4 g iron, which represents about 4.3×10^{22} atoms of iron to underpin its functions. The iron (see Figure 33.1) is distributed as hemoglobin: 3000–3500 mg; myoglobin: 400–500 mg;

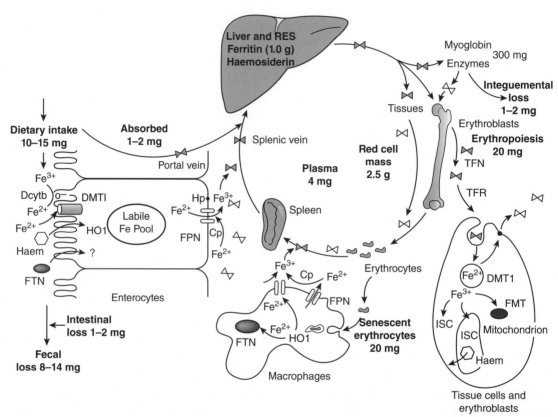

FIG. 33.1　Diagrammatic representation of iron turnover in the body: there is a cycle centered principally on the use and reuse of endogenous iron to sustain hemoglobin concentrations in the erythrocytes, alongside a smaller pool in other tissues which turns over as the tissues are renewed. The major depots of iron are in the liver and reticulo-endothelial system as ferritin and hemosiderin, muscle and other organs, and the red-cell hemoglobin. Iron is lost from the gut in shed enterocytes and minor blood loss, and from integumental loss which amounts to about 1–2 mg/day. This loss, and other needs to replace menstrual loss or to support the synthesis of new tissue, are replenished by intestinal uptake and transfer. Blood from the spleen mixes with that from the intestine in the portal circulation and enters the liver where the hepatocytes are able to sense the transferrin iron load and adjust the production of hepcidin secretion to control the absorption of iron. Cp, Ceruloplasmin; DcytB, duodenal cytochrome B reductase; DMT1, divalent metal transporter 1; FPN, ferroportin; FTN, ferritin; HO1, haemoxygenase 1; Hp, hephaestin; ISC, iron–sulfur cluster; TFR, transferrin receptor; ⋈, apotransferrin; ⋈, transferrin.

heme and non-heme enzymes: 100 mg; ferritin and hemo-siderin: 1000 mg; transferrin: 3 mg; and an intracellular or transit pool: 7 mg. The body cannot excrete iron; systemic iron is efficiently conserved and recycled, and basal losses, losses from menstruation, and the needs for the synthesis of new tissue are balanced by adjustments in gastrointestinal absorption. Thus only a small proportion of dietary iron needs to be absorbed.

Ferritin is an iron depot found in the cytosol and mitochondria of all cells. It is a hollow sphere of 24 apoferritin subunits with six channels through which iron can enter and leave the molecule. There are two types of subunits, heavy (H) and light (L), and the ratio of these influences the mobility of the iron and varies between organs. H chains predominate in the heart and brain, and L chains in the liver and spleen. H chains have ferroxidase activity which facilitates storage of iron as a ferric hydroxyphosphate. Each ferritin molecule can reversibly bind up to 4500 atoms of iron but usually only 20–50% of this capacity is occupied. Mitochondrial ferritin has a 75% homology to H ferritin and a smaller homology to L ferritin. Ferritin may be an iron reserve, but it also rapidly sequesters iron in response to inflammation, ionic iron, and the risk of oxidative damage. Hepatocytic ferritin is a depot to top up the systemic cycle and is the primary repository of excess iron. The other large ferritin pool, in the reticulo-endothelial system (RES), is part of the endogenous recycling pool of iron supporting the erythron. Ferritin is degraded by proteasomal lysis and the iron is recycled. However, with chronic iron excess or inflammation, accumulated ferritin is incompletely degraded, producing hemosiderin which contains iron that is not mobilizable but which may still cause oxidative damage.

Transferrin (TFN) is the main carrier of iron in the circulation and extracellular space, distributing iron to cell-surface transferrin receptors (TFRs) on erythroblasts and other tissues. It is synthesized principally in the liver as a sialylated glycoprotein, apotransferrin, which binds one or two ferric molecules. Its degree of sialylation affects its function; in pregnancy it is highly sialylated, favoring uptake of iron by the placenta, whereas, if there is less sialylation – as happens with infections or eclampsia – it binds TFRs less effectively.

The recycling of endogenous iron involves about 35 mg of iron daily and is at least 90% efficient; hence the body only needs to absorb enough iron to replace basal losses (~14 µg/kg body weight per day), which approximates to 1–2 mg/day.

The systemic turnover of iron recycles iron in tissues; the major focus is the salvage and recycling of the heme iron in the erythron. About 10^{11} senescent red cells are phagocytosed daily, mostly by macrophages in the spleen. The heme is degraded by macrophage hemoxygenase to iron, biliverdin, and carbon monoxide. One gram of hemoglobin contains 3.47 mg of iron, and the released iron is then either deposited in the macrophages' ferritin or exported as ferric iron by a membrane carrier, ferroportin (FPN), to apotransferrin for transit elsewhere. Heme is potentially toxic because, without the globin molecule to control it, heme iron is an active oxidant. However, there is a protein, hemopexin, which scavenges any free heme in the plasma and delivers it to hepatocytes for degradation.

There are two types of TFR. TFR1 is in all tissues, but is most dense on erythroblasts, lymphoid cells, and the neuroepithelium, and TFR2 is mainly located on the hepatocytic basolateral membrane and is a sensor for iron homeostasis.

The transferrin–TFR1 complexes are endocytosed. Any local cellular need for iron up-regulates both TFR1 and the cytoskeletal support for endocytosis. The endosome is acidified, and at pH 5.5 the ferric iron is released and reduced and the resultant ferrous iron is transported with a proton into the cytoplasm by a divalent metal transporter 1 (DMT1) located on the endosomal membrane. There is also a separate, DMT1-independent means (using transient receptor potential cation channel, mucolipin subfamily [TRPML.1] protein) of translocating iron across the endosomal membrane. The residual endosomal complex returns to the cell surface. It is not clear how iron is trafficked in the cytosol: it is part of a poorly characterized, labile iron pool. However, a chaperone, poly(rC)-binding protein 1 (PCBP1), has been identified which delivers ferrous iron to ferritin. Iron is also passed to sites for the synthesis of ISCs and enzymes, or is conveyed to mitochondria where it binds to a mitochondrial carrier, mitoferrin, and is distributed to mitochondrial ferritin, used to synthesize ISCs, or transferred to ferrochelatase which places ferrous iron into protoporphyrin IX to make heme (Richardson et al., 2010).

Iron Absorption: Gastrointestinal Mucosal Uptake and Transfer

Separate mechanisms exist for the mucosal uptake of non-heme iron, heme iron (mainly from meat), and ferritins. Lactoferrin and other ferrins are not significant dietary sources of iron. Gastroduodenal acidity and proteolysis may release non-heme iron from its matrix, but more extensive digestion might be needed to release heme and ferritin. It is possible therefore that the routes for the uptake of the three forms of iron are differently distributed along the intestine. Ferric and ferrous irons are most soluble in acid conditions, and non-heme iron is predominantly absorbed as ferrous iron in the proximal duodenum, i.e. before hepato-pancreatic secretions increase the luminal pH. None the less non-heme iron can be absorbed in the distal intestine.

Mucosal uptake of ferrous iron involves the aggregation of iron by the surface mucus and glycocalyx of the epithelial brush border. Any ferric iron is converted by a brush-border ferrireductase, duodenal cytochrome B reductase (DcytB), to ferrous iron which is then co-transported, with protons, across the brush-border membrane by an enterocytic DMT1. There may be another pathway for the uptake of ferric iron from mucin but this has not been fully characterized (Conrad and Umbreit, 2002).

Ferritin in an intact or partly degraded form is taken up by carrier-mediated endocytosis in the small intestine (Lönnerdal, 2009). Heme is only soluble at neutral or alkaline pHs such as those of the jejunum and ileum, but as yet a definitive carrier for its uptake has not been characterized. A candidate heme carrier protein, which is distributed throughout the small intestine, has been isolated, but it is probably a folate transporter, unless it has both functions. The relative importance of the uptake mechanisms is currently unclear, but it is noteworthy that DMT1-deficient mice absorb iron well.

Iron taken up in heme is released by an enterocytic hemoxygenase and joins a common transit pool of ferrous iron with non-heme iron, and, probably, that from ferritin. The ferrous iron is transported by an uncharacterized mechanism to the basolateral membrane where it is exported by FPN and oxidized either by plasma ceruloplasmin or by a related copper-dependent oxidase, hephaestin, which is co-located with ferroportin. The resultant ferric iron then binds to apoferritin and is distributed via the portal and systemic circulations. Eighty percent of transferrin iron is delivered for hemoglobin synthesis, and the half-life of the iron in plasma is about 75 minutes.

Iron Homeostasis: the Regulation of Iron Acquisition and Distribution

Iron homeostasis is controlled at cellular and systemic levels, and is sensitive to the need for iron, hypoxia, and inflammation. The response to inflammation can override adaptation to an inadequate iron supply.

Homeostasis of Cellular Iron

Cellular iron homeostasis is mediated by two iron-responsive proteins (IRP1 and IRP2) which bind to iron-responsive elements (IREs) on untranslated regions (UTRs) of mRNAs for proteins involved in iron kinetics. When iron supply is limited, IRP1 binds the 5'UTR and represses the translation of the mRNAs for the two apoferritin chains, ferroportin, hypoxia-inducible factor 2α and α-levulinic acid synthetase which is the initial and rate-limiting enzyme in heme synthesis. This stops ferritin sequestration of iron, and FPN export of iron, and reduces its use by inhibiting synthesis of erythropoietin and heme; simultaneously, IRP binding to the 3'UTR of the mRNAs for TFR1, DMT1, and an organizing molecule for the actin cytoskeleton necessary for endocytosis, prevents nucleolysis and sustains production of the cellular apparatus for the uptake of iron (Richardson et al., 2010; Ye and Rouault, 2010).

If cells have an adequate supply of iron, the IRPs dissociate from the IREs and their synthesis is reduced. IRP1 exists in two forms. In one, when iron supply is adequate, IRP1 binds a cytosolic ISC forming a complex that has aconitase activity. When there is a cellular lack of iron, the aconitase disaggregates and IRP1 binds to its IRE. IRP1 may also be controlled by the same mechanism as IRP2. This involves F-box/LRR-repeat protein 5 (FBXL5), a highly conserved protein analogous to an oxygen-binding non-heme protein, hemerythrin, found in invertebrates and bacteria. In iron-replete cells FBXL5 enables the proteasomal lysis of IRPs, but in the absence of iron FBXL5 is unstable and unable to stimulate proteolysis of IRP2 and IRP1, which are then available to bind to the IREs (Richardson et al., 2010; Ye and Rouault, 2010). This iron-responsive intracellular homeostasis of iron is disrupted by inflammation; reactive oxygen and nitrogen radicals, nitric oxide and phosphorylation inhibit the formation of cytosolic aconitase from IRP1, irrespective of any need for iron.

Homeostasis of Absorption and Systemic Turnover of Iron

The gastrointestinal absorption of iron is regulated in response to systemic needs for iron, and as part of the response of iron turnover to inflammation and some stressors. The intestinal mucosal uptake and transfer of all three forms of dietary iron are inversely related to systemic serum ferritin concentrations, particularly at values below a threshold of 60 μg/L. The elements of this control are achieved through transcriptional control of the carriers involved in iron acquisition and distribution during cell production. The expression of DMT1 and FPN would be set when macrophages are produced in the RES, or when enterocytes are produced by enteroblasts in the epithelial crypts. Further control is provided by a hormone, hepcidin, and by cellular mechanisms.

Hepcidin is synthesized by hepatocytes and, to a lesser extent, by monocytes, macrophages, and adipocytes, as an 84 amino acid prepropeptide, which is subsequently modified to a prohormone and then to the active hormone of 25 amino acids (Nemeth and Ganz, 2009). Hepcidin is down-regulated by increased iron needs and by hypoxia, and is up-regulated by inflammation. It blocks the export of iron from enterocytes and macrophages by inducing the degradation of FPN. It also reduces DMT1 activities. The iron retained in the cells is sequestered in ferritin and, in the case of enterocytes, the iron is subsequently lost into the gut lumen when the cells are shed. The hepatic sensory regulation of hepcidin expression involves an interaction of HFE (a membrane-bound protein which has long been known to be linked with hereditary hemochromatosis), TFR1, and TFR2: usually HFE is associated with TFR1, but it can be displaced by transferrin. If this happens, HFE binds instead to TFR2, and the HFE–TFR2 complex activates a membrane complex of a bone morphogenic protein (BMP6) and haemojuvelin (HJV), which co-stimulate phosphorylation and activation of a transcription factor for the expression of hepcidin. This stimulus is inhibited by proteolysis of HJV by a membrane-bound protease, matriptase, but it is not known how this is regulated. In hypoxic conditions, including iron deficiency and anemia, hypoxia-inducible factor (HIF) depresses hepcidin expression and stimulates erythropoiesis, thereby ensuring an iron supply for red cell production. In inflammatory states interleukins 1 and 6 stimulate hepcidin production.

The generic cellular control of iron homeostasis operates also in the enterocyte, and high levels of iron in the mature enterocyte induce ferritin by local control mechanisms. This sequesters iron and blocks its transfer to the portal circulation, thereby reducing the risk of systemic iron overload. Additionally, enterocytes have an isoform of FPN which is not down-regulated if the cells are iron deficient; this enables intestinal transfer of iron in iron deficiency.

Inborn Disorders of Iron Kinetics and Use

The hemochromatoses include at least five inherited overload syndromes arising from unregulated absorption of iron caused by defects in HFE, HJV, hepcidin, TFR2, and FPN (Pietrangelo 2004; OMIM, 2012). Dysregulation of iron turnover also results from loss of ceruloplasmin, martriptase, transferrin and defective sialylation of transferrin and from defects in proteins involved with the assembly of iron–sulfur clusters and intracellular trafficking of iron. The latter causes functional and structural defects of the heart, central nervous system (Friedrich's ataxia), muscle (myopathies), red cell formation (sideroblastic anemias), and mitochondrial function (Ye and Rouault, 2010; OMIM, 2012).

Influence of Inflammation on Iron Kinetics

Activation of the immune system by chronic and acute infections, malignancy, inflammatory conditions in the bowel, joints, and kidneys, and even low-grade inflammatory states such as obesity, induce an adaptive state called the anemia of chronic disease (ACD) (Weiss and Goodnough, 2005). ACD is manifest as a mild anemia (hemoglobin 80–95 g/L) that is unresponsive to iron, with normal red-cell indices and reduced erythropoiesis; a normal or elevated serum ferritin accompanied by subnormal serum values of iron; a normal or reduced serum value of transferrin, which has a low saturation with iron; normal values for TFR1; and a ratio of serum transferrin receptors/ log ferritin concentrations <1 (Weiss and Goodnough, 2005). These changes are mediated by inflammatory cytokines (interferon-γ, tumor necrosis factor-α, and interleukins) that up-regulate hepcidin, and by the cellular responses to reactive species. Collectively these increase the uptake and sequestration of iron by cells, especially macrophages, and block its export by FPN. The inflammatory mediators stimulate phagocytosis of senescent red cells and reduce erythropoietin production and effectiveness by direct actions on the kidneys and erythroblasts. Increased output of hepcidin reduces the absorption of iron and augments the signals for the retention of iron by macrophages. The adaptation may have evolved as a protection against damage caused by "free iron" liberated by tissue damage, and to deny pathogens access to iron (Doherty, 2007). ACD can become sustained and lead to a significant paradoxical functional iron deficiency syndrome despite there being appreciable amounts of iron in tissue depots (Weiss and Goodnough, 2005).

Iron and the Infant

Neonates have 150–250 mg of iron and hemoglobin levels of 160–180 g/L. They adapt to the higher pO_2 ex utero, by reducing synthesis of fetal haemoglobin, the levels of which fall to 90–110 g/L at 3–4 months. At 4–6 months of age, hemoglobin production resumes with the synthesis of adult hemoglobin. The degraded hemoglobin releases 50–60 mg of iron which is deposited in reticuloendothelial ferritin. In early infancy serum ferritin concentrations are as much as 400 μg/L; these fall to about 30 μg/L as the endogenous iron depot is used for new tissue synthesis. Therefore there is a risk of iron deficiency at 6–9 months; however, the iron reserve can be increased by 30–50 mg of iron if, at birth, the cord is not clamped until it has stopped pulsing, thereby letting these late pulsations transfer the 32% of the neonate's blood volume which is in the fetal circulation of the placenta back to the baby (McDonald and Middleton, 2008). Thus until 6 months of age, healthy babies have little if any need for iron from external sources (Ziegler et al., 2009). Compared with that available from its systemic depots, relatively little iron is received by babies from breast milk, the iron content (0.2–0.4 mg/L) of which is not altered by either maternal iron deficiency or supplementation. Intestinal absorption is down-regulated until 6 months of age when infants become more reliant on exogenous iron.

Iron and Women in Their Reproductive Years

The demands of menstruation, pregnancy, lactation, and, in adolescence, growth on iron homeostasis and iron requirements are uncertain. There are concerns that women may be at risk of inadequate iron supply because contemporary lifestyle and diets favor reduced energy expenditure and the consumption of diets with a lower iron density than those on which humans evolved (Hallberg and Hulthen, 2002).

Menstrual blood loss of adolescent girls is marginally less than that of older women, and in nutritional risk assessments of iron nutriture it is assumed that adolescent menstrual losses match those in adult women. There is little intra-individual variation in blood loss but considerable interindividual variation. Estimates of menstrual loss

in different countries are consistent in showing that 95% of women lose 118 mL or less per cycle with median and mean losses of 30 mL and 44 mL respectively: these equate to iron losses of 0.49 mg and 0.7 mg/day (Hallberg and Hulthen, 2002). Intrauterine devices increase menstrual blood loss two- to fourfold, whereas oral contraceptive users have smaller median menstrual blood and iron losses (e.g. 18 mL/cycle and 0.26 mg/day) with mean losses of 26 mL/cycle and 0.43 mg/day. There is an inverse correlation between menstrual blood loss and serum ferritin concentrations; on average an increase in menstrual iron loss of 1 mg/day is associated with a reduction in serum ferritin of 7 μg/L.

Measuring Iron Status

Adequate iron status (i.e. sufficiency) implies having normal erythropoiesis and iron functions that are not limited by iron supply, as well as having a reserve. There is no single unequivocal marker of iron deficiency or excess, except, perhaps, for serum ferritin at extreme deficiency or excess. Assessment of deficiency and excess relies on the use and interpretation of markers of (1) functional iron, i.e. hemoglobin concentrations (Table 33.1), and indices of reduced red-cell mean cell volume (MCV; 80–94 fL) and mean cell hemoglobin (MCH; 27–32 pg); (2) the adequacy of iron supply to tissues, serum iron (10–30 μmol/L), transferrin saturation (16–50%), red-cell zinc protoporphyrin (>80 μmol/mol Hb), and serum transferrin receptors; and (3) tissue depots, indicated by serum ferritin concentrations (males 15–300 μg/L, and females 15–200 μg/L). Each of these markers is subject to con-

TABLE 33.1 Hemoglobin thresholds used to define anemia at sea level

Group	Hemoglobin (g/L)
Children	
0.5–4.99 years	110
5–11.99 years	115
12–14.99 years	120
Non-pregnant women >15 years	120
Pregnant women	110
Men (>15 years)	130

Values for those of African heritage are 4–10 g/L lower than those of Caucasian origin. A further amendment used by the WHO classifies anemia as mild, moderate, or severe, according to whether the values are above 80%, 80–60%, or below 60% of the appropriate population threshold.

founding, particularly from coexistent infections and nutritional deficiencies (Gibson, 2005). An approach was developed for NHANES II using combinations of markers such as serum ferritin, transferrin saturation, and erythrocyte protoporphyrin, or MCV, transferrin saturation, and erythrocyte protoporphyrin: individuals with two or more abnormal values in either trio could be considered iron deficient. Other approaches use hemoglobin, serum ferritin values, and serum transferrin receptors coupled with C-reactive protein and alpha-1-acid glycoprotein as indicators of acute and chronic inflammatory disease (World Health Organization/Centers for Disease Control and Prevention, 2004). The STfR/log ferritin ratio may be a marker of iron depots; positive ratios indicate that stores are present whereas negative values do not. The ratio may be less influenced by inflammation, and an algorithm based on serum thresholds and sTfR/log ferritin ratios to differentiate iron-deficiency anemia and anemia of chronic disease, or a combination of the two, has been proposed (Weiss and Goodnough, 2005). Diagnosing iron deficiency on the basis of the response to an iron supplement is unreliable if ACD or additional nutrient deficiencies are present.

Each μg/L of serum ferritin in the circulation is equivalent to 7–10 mg of stored iron. Serum ferritin originates from the RES macrophages and not from hepatocytes; the value therefore underestimates total systemic ferritin iron, and since hepatocytes are the first tissue to accumulate any surplus iron, serum ferritin is a poor marker of early iron overload.

Dietary Sources of Iron

The proportions of non-heme iron, heme, and ferritin in the diet reflect the relative intakes of animal and plant material, and usually non-heme sources predominate. Generally meats and plants are similar sources of iron: the richest include cereals, pulses, vegetables, nuts, shellfish, fish, and meat. Cereal sources may contribute about 40% of iron intake, and about half of that may come from iron fortification of breakfast cereals. Additionally non-heme iron is acquired as fortification or restoration of iron lost during processing, and from contamination. The latter arises from extrusion processes and from cast-iron cooking utensils, particularly if citrate or similarly acidic ingredients are used.

Iron is present in many forms in plants, including complexes which may either enhance or reduce its availability

for mucosal uptake. The iron content of plant cultivars varies appreciably. An example is that of non-aromatic rice which contains about 11 mg/kg compared with 18 mg/kg in aromatic rice. The proportion of total iron coming from heme in meat is also variable. The heme content of foods is measured indirectly as the difference between an initial assay of inorganic iron content and a subsequent measurement of the total iron content of the sample. The proportion of total iron derived from heme in meat ranges in beef from 64% to 78% and between 52% and 83% in other red meats. Cooking reduces the water and fat content of meat, thereby increasing the iron content on a weight-for-weight basis.

The above points illustrate sources of uncertainty in food composition data on iron. Additionally composition reference data do not provide information from which the effect of the food matrix on the availability of iron could be assessed.

Bioavailability of Iron

The efficiency with which dietary iron is utilized in the body is influenced by (1) the physico-chemical form of iron; (2) dietary factors affecting the amount of luminal iron that is available for intestinal uptake, both of which are dietary factors (Hallberg and Hulthen, 2002; Hurrell and Egli, 2010); and (3) the homeostatic settings of the mucosa to take up and transfer iron to the body, both of which adapt to the body's need for iron, and to inflammation (i.e. ACD).

Non-heme iron compounds that are soluble in acid are most available in the proximal gut lumen. Inhibitors of non-heme iron's availability include phytates found in whole-grain cereals, legumes, nuts, and seeds, and other phosphates (e.g. caseins) whose effects may be exacerbated by calcium and magnesium. Polyphenols found in tea, particularly black tea, and coffee are more powerful inhibitors than those from herb teas, cocoa or red wine; perhaps because they have higher levels of galloyl esters and tannates. Adding milk to black tea or coffee does not improve the availability of iron.

Practices such as soaking, germination, or fermentation before cooking may enable intrinsic phytase to break down phytate. Cooking itself may improve the solubilization of iron by physically degrading phytate; this would be particularly appropriate for oats which have little phytase activity. It is difficult to predict the effect of processing on the bioavailability of iron; for instance, milling grain removes its husk which is rich in phytate, but also removes much of the iron content. Thus, although the processing may have improved availability, there may not be enough iron left for that to be of any benefit.

Bioavailability of non-heme iron is enhanced by organic acids such as ascorbic acid, malic acid, tartaric acid, lactic acid, and citric acid, which occur naturally in fruit and vegetables and in fermented products. Heat processing may destroy some of these. Meat improves the uptake of non-heme iron, but it is not clear how this is achieved.

Bioavailability enables dietary sources of iron to be ranked; however, quantitative values of availability cannot be extrapolated to a food or diet universally, partly because of uncertainties about the dietary characteristics, and importantly also because of systemic adaptation. The use of dietary characteristics to derive equations and models to predict the bioavailability of iron are of limited value (Beard et al., 2007).

The principal determinants of bioavailability of iron are usually the systemic need for the element and the homeostatic setting for the absorption of iron. The effects of inhibitors and enhancers on bioavailability are often overestimated because they have used single-meal studies, and have made no allowance for adaptation, which might take 3–7 days, or the iron status of the study subjects.

Fortunately, in the case of iron, it is possible to use isotopes differentially to correct for the subjects' iron status and gut adaptation. The dietary components of bioavailability are of particular importance when intestinal adaptation is not sufficient to acquire enough iron to meet systemic needs for the metal. This is important in planning management strategies for endemic iron deficiency, and in the assessment of intake reference values.

Iron Intake Reference Values

Table 33.2 gives two sets of reference dietary intake values for iron (European Commission Scientific Committee for Food, 1993; Institute of Medicine, 2001). The advisory groups involved explain the bases for their values, and describe the limitations of the data which they had available. The values support public health measures and are cautious, and although they support assessments of dietary intakes, they are not diagnostic of iron deficiency or excess. The discrepancies between the two sets of recommendations arise in the areas of most uncertainty, which are the needs of children and of menstruating, pregnant, and lactating women, and the impact of homeostatic adaptation on the bioavailability of iron. The uncertainties in the reference values, composition tables, and status determina-

TABLE 33.2   Dietary reference values developed for the USA and Canada, and for the European Union

USA and Canada[a] (recommended dietary allowance) (18% absorption)			European Union Population Reference Intake[b] (15% bioavailability)		
Age	mg/day		Age	mg/day	
0–6 months	0.27		0–6 months	–	
7–12 months	11.0		6–12 months	6.2	
1–3 years	7.0		1–3 years	3.9	
4–8 years	10.0		4–6 years	4.2	
			7–10 years	5.9	
	Male	Female		Male	Female
9–13 years	8.0	8.0	11–14 years	9.7	9.3 (21.8[c])
14–18 years	11.0	15.0	15–17 years	12.5	20.7
19–50 years	8.0	18.0	18+ years	9.1	19.6
50+ years	8.0	8.0	Postmenopausal	–	7.5
Pregnancy	–	27.0			
Lactation	–		Lactation		10.0
14–18 years		10.0			
18+ years		9.0			

[a]Institute of Medicine (2001).
[b]European Commission Scientific Committee for Food (1993).
[c]If menstruating.

tion are reflected in the lack of congruence between population surveillance data on iron intakes, the apparent prevalence of iron deficiency, and dietary reference values (Scientific Advisory Committee on Nutrition, 2011).

Iron Deficiency

Inadequate intakes of iron relative to needs may occur during periods of rapid growth, particularly in infancy, early childhood, and adolescence. Inappropriate diversification of diet, the use of cows' milk or of low-nutrient-density foods, or inappropriate vegetarian diets are common causes in late infancy and early childhood. Maldigestion and malabsorption as causes of reduced iron absorption arise from reduced gastroduodenal acidity, enteropathies (e.g. celiac disease), and intestinal mucosal damage. These conditions are also associated with malabsorption and systemic loss of protein and other nutrients, including iron. Similarly blood loss from the gastrointestinal, genito-urinary, and respiratory tracts entails the loss of other endogenous nutrients as well as iron. Globally the major causes of iron deficiency and anemia are probably the enteropathies and blood losses caused by gastrointestinal parasites such as *Helicobacter pylori*, *Necator americanus*, *Ancylostoma duodenale*, *Trichuris trichiura*, and schistosomes (which may also cause urinary blood loss) (Steketee, 2003). ACD would accompany these conditions, as it does with infectious causes of hemolytic anemias such as malaria (Doherty, 2007).

Features of Iron Deficiency

Iron deficiency, with or without anemia, is associated with numerous defects. Studies in animal models show inefficient energy metabolism, with altered glucose and lactate metabolism; and reduced muscle myoglobin content and impaired muscle strength and endurance. Reduced cytochrome oxidase activity has been found in muscle and the intestinal mucosa. Impaired collagen synthesis and associated osteoporosis have been noted, and the latter may also in part be secondary to interrupted hydroxylation of vitamin D. Vitamin A metabolism is also disturbed. Other defects include altered prostaglandin metabolism; impaired dopaminergic and serotonin neurotransmission, particularly in dopaminergic areas such as the substantia nigra, globus pallidus, cerebellar nuclei, and hippocampus; defective neuromyelination and synapse and dendrite development; and altered brain membrane fatty acid profiles with, for example, less docosahexaenoic acid (Georgieff, 2008).

Functional psychomotor defects include increased anxiety, impaired memory and spatial navigation, and delayed responses to auditory and visual stimuli. These phenomena provide plausible mechanistic bases for inferring that iron deficiency, both with and without anemia, has similar effects in humans, and show that tissues with a rapid turnover, a specialized function or high energy dependency, such as immunocytes, enterocytes, brain and muscle, are likely to have overt defects.

Iron Deficiency in Humans

Since the causes and effects of iron deficiency usually involve intakes and losses of other nutrients, and disruption of the utilization of other nutrients and substrates, it is often difficult to ascribe specific features to iron deficiency or even to expect that pure isolated iron deficiency exists, although it may do so in developed communities with inappropriate diets in young people. However, iron deficiency appears as a component of a broader and variable syndrome of nutritional deficiency. Thus classic features ascribed to iron deficiency such as koilonychia, soft nails, glossitis, cheilitis, mood changes, muscle weakness, and impaired immunity may be secondary to several other deficiencies. This is relevant to both clinical and public-health nutrition.

The hematological criteria for assessing iron adequacy are described above, but any coincidental ACD needs to be considered (Weiss and Goodnough, 2005).

Anemia reduces circulatory transport and supply of oxygen to muscle, impairing endurance capacity and energetic efficiency which are further compromised by reduced myoglobin content. In humans, reductions by phlebotomy of customary hemoglobin values to 100–110 g/L reduced aerobic capacity by 16–18%. In adults, iron-responsive fatigability and defects in endurance capacity of muscle during aerobic exercise training have been seen in groups without anemia but with subnormal serum ferritin concentrations (Brownlie *et al.*, 2004). Although data are inconclusive, there is a risk that iron deficiency, or even mild anemia, or both, reduce voluntary activity and work productivity.

Iron deficiency reduces the proportion of circulating T lymphocytes and impairs T-cell lymphocyte proliferative responses. Impairments also affect neutrophil activity, phagocytosis, and microbiocidal activity with a weakened neutrophil respiratory burst, free radical production and myeloperoxidase activity, and secretion of interleukin-2. However, B-cell functions are little affected.

Iron Deficiency and Cognitive, Motor, and Behavioral Development

Iron is transported across the blood–brain barrier (BBB) by mechanisms analogous to those in other tissues (Moos et al., 2007). The BBB is an effective boundary and it protects the CNS from systemic iron overload as in the hemochromatoses. Ferric iron is delivered by transferrin to neurones and oligodendrocytes. The CNS accumulates iron until early adulthood. Undoubtedly iron deficiency in animal models compromises neurological and psychomotor development with critical periods, particularly in infancy and early childhood, when the defects are irredeemable. Furthermore, models suggest that in young animals iron is preferentially distributed to erythroid tissues rather than the brain and other organs, implying that deficiencies of iron might occur in the brain unaccompanied by anemia. Iron-deficient and anemic infants and children have delayed attention, poor recognition memory, and reduced reward-seeking behaviors, and are more withdrawn and have poor social interactions. However, research in this area is confounded by concomitant nutrient deficiencies, socioeconomic factors, infections, and, not least, difficulties in standardizing outcomes, and characterizing the causes and degree of iron deficiency; many studies only consider the degree of anemia and assume that it is caused by iron deficiency (McCann and Ames, 2007).

It is difficult to identify thresholds of iron-deficiency anemia, or ages at which defects may occur, because most studies have not been designed to address these public health risk assessment issues. Existing studies imply that iron-responsive defects occur at hemoglobin values below 80, 95, and 110 g/L, and that early-life deficiencies may persist. However, children from poor environments may be more vulnerable to the long-term cognitive deficits than those from more affluent backgrounds. There is some evidence that adolescent girls who were anemic as toddlers have altered memory and that maternal iron deficiency impairs their responsiveness to their children. Additionally, iron therapy normalizes cognitive function in young, iron-deficient, anemic women.

There are other conditions that have a variable and unpredictable response to iron therapy. These include sleep disturbances, disturbed thermal regulation, breath-holding attacks in early childhood (Zehetner et al., 2010), and restless-leg syndrome in adults (Connor et al., 2009). Any primary role of altered iron supply in the pathogenesis of these is unclear.

Iron in Pregnancy and Lactation

Red cell mass increases until 32–34 weeks' gestation in response to a two- to fourfold increase in erythropoietin production; the usual inverse relationship between erythropoietin and red cell mass is lost but it reappears later in pregnancy if the hemoglobin falls below 90 g/L. Transferrin production also increases with a more dense sialylation which favors its binding to placental receptors. However, the hematocrit, hemoglobin, and serum iron, ferritin, and transferrin fall because at the same time the plasma volume expands by about 1.3 L. This increase is independent of the preceding non-pregnant plasma volume, which is about 2.7 L. The increase is larger for multiple pregnancies and multigravida. Thus the declining values reflect the physiological hemodilution of pregnancy, and are not necessarily indicative of iron deficiency or anemia. The plasma volume expansion stops at the end of the second trimester, and decreases near term.

The efficiency of iron absorption increases during pregnancy and is sustained during lactation; iron bioavailability has been shown to increase from 7% at 12 weeks' gestation to 66% at 30 weeks. This of course contradicts ideas that women who become pregnant need to increase their iron intakes, and is consistent with observations that women do not increase their intakes during pregnancy.

The risk of adverse outcomes such as low birth weight and premature delivery is increased at hemoglobin values below 90 g/L or above 130 g/L. This range reflects the healthy range of hemoglobin in pregnancy: lower values may indicate a degree of anemia whereas values above the range indicate failure of normal adaptation, possibly secondary to other causes of failed pregnancy. The limits are not well defined; the lower limits from various studies vary between 86 and 105 g/L, at least in part because the values were not taken at the same stage of pregnancy. The most predictive values are those determined in early pregnancy; later values, particularly those from the last trimester, correlate poorly with outcomes. Interpreting such data in populations beset by infections and nutritional deficiencies is further complicated by the possible effects of ACD and because infections, especially parasitism, are independent causes of impaired placental perfusion and function, intra-uterine growth retardation, and early onset of labour (Steketee, 2003). Iron supplements may improve women's hematological parameters in pregnancy, but have little impact in reducing adverse outcomes in women with normal levels of hemoglobin. Some studies suggest beneficial effects of iron supplementation on reducing the incidence of low birth weight if it is initiated early in pregnancy. There are few data to enable a confident risk assessment of the influence of birth spacing on iron requirements in pregnancy. There is no general agreement on the need for increased reference intakes of iron during pregnancy and lactation. Extra iron is needed, but whereas some advisory bodies (European Commission Scientific Committee for Food, 1993; Scientific Advisory Committee on Nutrition, 2010) think that this can be acquired from the customary diet by physiological adaptation, others do not rely on this and advise higher reference values (Institute of Medicine, 2001). None the less, many agencies no longer advise regular iron supplements during pregnancy, recommending them only for women with hemoglobin values less than 110 g/L in the first trimester and 105 g/L at 28 weeks' gestation.

Treatment and Prevention of Iron Deficiency

For both populations and individuals it is important to treat the cause of the iron deficiency and any coexisting nutritional deficiencies; more often than not, as in nutritional rehabilitation from pan-malnutrition, it is best to do this before giving any iron. This applies particularly to clinical management. Iron salts used to treat iron deficiency include orally taken ferrous sulphate (60 mg of iron/300 mg of the salt), ferrous fumarate (65 mg of iron/200 mg of the salt), and ferrous gluconate (35 mg of iron/300 mg of the salt), although other preparations are available for oral and parenteral use. The response to iron should be monitored, and if this is not possible or practical, then dosage should be cautious.

At a population level, iron fortification of foods can be undertaken and has been thoroughly considered (World Health Organization/Food and Agricultural Organization of the United Nations, 2006). Strategies for the selection of fortificants have to consider the oxidative effects of inorganic iron salts on the organoleptic properties, and shelf-life of the products. Preferred fortificants are ferrous sulphate or ferrous fumarate, either as simple salts or encapsulated within shells of vegetable oils or stearates; electrolytic iron; and sodium iron EDTA. Recent innovations include microencapsulated ferrous fumarate "sprinkles" that can be sprinkled over food, and a micronutrient powder containing a phytase (Troesch et al., 2009). The latter is used to fortify complementary feeds and to optimize the availability of the intrinsic iron, thereby minimizing the risks of high exposure to iron (see next section). Strategies involving multi-micronutrient supplements are increasingly being applied to address coincident deficiencies and to assuage uncertainty about the identity of the limiting nutrients other than iron (Allen et al., 2009).

Iron Overload

The risk of iron overload from dietary sources is negligible with normal intestinal function (European Food Safety Authority, 2004) and there are insufficient data to inform a risk assessment to set upper safe limits for iron consumption. In the UK, for adults without medical supervision, a guidance level of 17 mg iron/day for supplemental iron was set based on gastrointestinal effects, and in North America a tolerable upper intake level of iron intake from all sources of 45 mg/day was advised based on interactions with other transition elements (Institute of Medicine, 2001). Acute intakes of iron solutions without food induce gastritis, nausea, abdominal pain, vomiting, and faintness. Large intakes of 20 mg elemental iron per kilogram body weight, or more, cause corrosive hemorrhagic necrosis of the intestine with loose stools and blood loss, hypovolemic shock, damage and failure of systemic organs, and death.

Chronic iron overload with hemochromatoses has an increased incidence of systemic cancer, cardiovascular disease, neurological disease, arthropathies, and diabetes mellitus, but there is no evidence in the general population, including heterozygotes for hemochromatoses, that these or colorectal cancer are associated with dietary intakes of iron. However, there is a probable positive correlation of the incidence of colorectal cancer with exposure to meat and processed meat products (World Health Organization/Food and Agricultural Organization of the United Nations, 2006).

African iron overload, previously called Bantu siderosis, is an ecogenetic disorder arising from a combination of a genetic defect and increased exposure to iron from food and beer that have been prepared or stored in iron utensils. The abnormal iron overload is distributed in the Kupffer (RES) cells of the liver in contrast to the hemochromatoses in which the excess iron is in the hepatocytes.

There are unresolved concerns about the significance of interactions between iron, zinc, and copper along their kinetic pathways; for example, they all may use DMT1, and all bind to transferrin. Iron can inhibit the utilization of zinc and copper with adverse effects on growth (Sachdev et al., 2006), immune function, and ceruloplasmin concentrations. However, the circumstances in which these phenomena occur and their significance are fully characterized, and it is not clear which components of bioavailability are involved.

The acute-phase recompartmentation of iron might be a host defense mechanism to restrict the availability of iron to pathogens. Bacterial pathogens need iron, and to acquire it they create local tissue redox and acid conditions that cause release of iron from its binding sites, and they release siderophores that can strip iron from iron-proteins and from heme. If iron is freely available, for example from iron overload or haemolysis as in malaria, bacteremias, commonly with enteric organisms, may arise. Thus the effect of iron supplements on malaria may depend on more subtle interactions than a direct one between the metal and the plasmodium. The same point probably applies to interactions between iron supply and its homeostasis with HIV and tuberculosis, for which at the population level there are few data on whether they are exacerbated by iron supplementation (Doherty, 2007). The avidity of enteric bacteria for iron may explain why iron supplements and fortification have been considered to increase the incidence of diarrheal disease but not that of non-diarrheal or respiratory disease. The WHO has advised that, in areas of high risk of malarial transmission, "folic acid supplementation should be targeted at children who are anemic and at risk of iron deficiency and that they should also receive concurrent protection from malaria and other infectious diseases" (World Health Organization/UNICEF, 2006).

Public Health and Preventive Measures to Combat Iron Deficiency

The data on the effects of iron deficiency are not as good as those on the association of defects with anemia, which suggest that, irrespective of their pathogenesis, hemoglobin values of less than 110 g/L have adverse effects. Thus it is understandable that public health measures should address anemia and its several causes, rather than iron deficiency per se. The latter would anyway be addressed by measures to reduce blood loss and improve nutritional intake as a general measure.

The elements of preventing iron deficiency are similar in both developed and developing countries, although appropriate cultural and locale-specific emphases need to be applied. The key components at all ages involve minimizing iron loss from intestinal and other parasites, ensuring access to adequate diets, and being aware that

multi-nutrient supplements are probably needed to ensure adequate nutrition in general and effective use of dietary and supplemental iron. In children, delayed clamping of the cord at birth and sustaining breastfeeding are additionally important (Lutter, 2008). It needs governmental interventions to support the infrastructural interventions to achieve these measures, which would have a broader benefit because they would break the infection–malnutrition cycle. National, regional, and local governments need to appreciate the socioeconomic benefits of reducing the prevalence of iron deficiency (Hunt, 2002). The political will to act on this could be generated by an increased engagement and empowerment of the citizenry who themselves could undertake some of the basic public-health and sanitary measures which would control some of the causes of iron deficiency.

Future Directions

Uncertainties persist about how much iron we need, how to determine iron status, and how to ensure adequate iron status in individuals and populations. The assessment and management of iron deficiency and anemia will probably continue to be conflated and conservative. The challenge lies in how to use new knowledge in cell biology to address these core issues. Part of this strategy will entail refining our current approaches by using improved understanding of iron trafficking and use to appraise critically our current practice and investigative approaches. It is particularly important to appreciate the difference between iron deficiency and anemia, and to be able to consider, in the context of risk assessment and management, whether the differentiation matters or not. Assessment of requirements and of status will benefit from applying improved awareness of how iron homeostasis interacts with that of other nutrients, and possibly more importantly with other systemic phenomena such as any degree of inflammation. This should also influence the use of iron supplementation and fortification programs, bearing in mind concerns about trace-element interactions causing other deficiencies, impaired growth, and activation of infections, in which regard the role of enteric pathogens is probably important. It is unlikely that new markers of iron status will emerge, but it may be possible using cell biology to better validate existing markers or to evolve algorithms to assess the adequacy of dietary intakes, systemic iron supply and function. Overall it is important that iron should be considered in a broad nutritional and health context.

Suggestions for Further Reading

Andrews, N.C. (2008) Forging a field: the golden age of iron biology. *Blood* **112**, 219–230.

Bothwell, T.H., Charlton, R.W., Cook, J.D., *et al.* (1979) *Iron Metabolism in Man*. Blackwell Scientific, Oxford.

Hallberg, L. and Hulthen, L. (2002) Perspectives on iron absorption. *Blood Cells Mol Dis* **29**, 562–573.

Institute of Medicine (2001) *Dietary Reference Intakes for Vitamin A, Vitamin K, Arsenic, Boron, Chromium, Copper, Iodine, Iron, Manganese, Molybdenum, Nickel, Silicon, Vanadium, and Zinc*. National Academy Press, Washington, DC.

Online Mendelian Inheritance in Man (OMIM). www.omim.org.

Scientific Advisory Committee on Nutrition (2010) *Iron and Health*. The Stationery Office London. www.sacn.gov.uk/pdfs/sacn_iron_and_health_report_web.pdf.

References

Allen, L.H., Peerson, J.M., and Olney, D.K. (2009) Provision of multiple rather than two or fewer micronutrients more effectively improves growth and other outcomes in micronutrient deficient children and adults. *J Nutr* **139**, 1022–1030.

Beard, J.L., Murray-Kolb, L.E., Haas, J.D., *et al.* (2007) Iron absorption prediction equations lack agreement and underestimate iron absorption. *J Nutr* **137**, 1741–1746.

Brownlie, T., Utermohlen, V., Hinton, P.S. *et al.* (2004) Tissue iron deficiency without anemia impairs adaptation in endurance capacity after aerobic training in previously untrained women. *Am J Clin Nutr* **79**, 437–443.

Brunore, M. and Vallone, B. (2006) A globin for the brain. *FASEB J* **20**, 2192–2197.

Connor, J.R., Wang, X-S., Allen, R.P., *et al.* (2009) Altered dopaminergic profile in the putamen and substantia nigra in restless leg syndrome. *Brain* **132**, 2403–2412.

Conrad, M.E. and Umbriet, J.N. (2002) Pathways of iron absorption *Blood Cells Mol Dis* **29**, 336–355.

Doherty, C.P. (2007) Host–pathogen interactions: the role of iron. *J Nutr* **137**, 1341–1344.

Earnshaw, A.A. and Greenwood, N.N. (2010) Iron, ruthenium and osmium. In *Chemistry of the Elements*, 2nd Edn. Butterworth Heinemann, Oxford, pp 1070–1112.

European Commission Scientific Committee for Food (1993) *Reports of the Scientific Committee for Food (Thirty-first series). Nutrient and Energy Intakes for the European Community* 1993. http://ec.europa.eu/food/fs/sc/scf/out89.pdf.

European Food Safety Authority (2004) Opinion of the Scientific Panel on Dietetic Products, Nutrition and Allergies on a request from the Commission related to the Tolerable Upper Intake Level of Iron. *EFSA J* **125**, 1–34.

Georgieff, M.K. (2008) The role of iron in neurodevelopment: fetal iron deficiency and the developing hippocampus. *Biochem Soc Trans* **36**, 1267–1271.

Gibson, R.S. (2005) Assessment of iron status. In *Principles of Nutritional Assessment*, 2nd Edn. Oxford University Press, Oxford, pp. 443–476.

Hallberg, L. and Hulthen, L. (2002) Perspectives on iron absorption. *Blood Cells Mol Dis* **29**, 562–573.

Hunt, J.M. (2002) Reversing productivity losses from iron deficiency: the economic case. *J Nutr* **132**, 794–801.

Hurrell, R. and Egli, I. (2010) Iron bioavailability and dietary reference values. *Am J Nutr* **91**, 1461S–1467S.

Institute of Medicine (2001) *Dietary Reference Intakes for Vitamin A, Vitamin K, Arsenic, Boron, Chromium, Copper, Iodine, Iron, Manganese, Molybdenum, Nickel, Silicon, Vanadium, and Zinc*. National Academy Press, Washington, DC.

Lönnerdal, B. (2009) Soybean ferritin: implications for iron status of vegetarians. *Am J Clin Nutr* **89**, 1680S–1685S.

Lutter, C.K. (2008) Iron deficiency in young children in low-income countries and new approaches for its prevention. *J Nutr* **138**, 2523–2528.

McCann, J.C. and Ames, B.N. (2007) An overview of evidence for a causal relation between iron deficiency during development and deficits in cognitive or behavioral function. *Am J Clin Nutr* **85**, 931–945.

McDonald, S.J. and Middleton, P. (2008) Effect of timing of umbilical cord clamping of term infants on maternal and neonatal outcomes. *Cochrane Database Syst Rev* (2) CD004074.

Moos, T., Rosengren, N.T., Skjorringe, T., *et al.* (2007) Iron trafficking inside the brain. *J Neurochem* **103**, 1730–1740.

Nemeth, E. and Ganz, T. (2009) The role of hepcidin in iron metabolism. *Acta Haematol* **122**, 78–86.

OMIM (2012) Online Mendelian Inheritance in Man. www.omim.org.

Pietrangelo, A. (2004) Heriditary hemochromatosis – a new look at an old disease. *N Engl J Med* **350**, 2383–2397.

Richardson, D.R., Lane, D.J.R., Becker, E.M., *et al.* (2010) Mitochondrial iron trafficking and the integration of iron metabolism between the mitochondrion and cytosol. *Proc Natl Acad Sci* **107**, 10775–10782.

Sachdev, H., Gera, T., and Nestel, P. (2006) Effect of iron supplementation on physical growth in children: systematic review of randomised controlled trials. *Publ Health Nutr* **9**, 904–920.

Scientific Advisory Committee on Nutrition (2010) *Iron and Health*. The Stationery Office, London. http://

www.sacn.gov.uk/pdfs/sacn_iron_and_health_report_
web.pdf.

Steketee, R.W. (2003) Pregnancy, nutrition and parasitic diseases. *J Nutr* **133,** 1661S–1667S.

Theil, E.C. and Goss, D.J. (2009) Living with iron (and oxygen): questions and answers about iron homeostasis. *Chem Rev* **109,** 4568–4579.

Troesch, B., Egli, I., Zeder, C., *et al.* (2009) Optimization of a phytase-containing micronutrient powder with low amounts of highly bioavailable iron for in-home fortification of complementary foods. *Am J Clin Nutr* **89,** 539–544.

Weiss, G. and Goodnough, L.T. (2005) Anemia of chronic disease. *N Engl J Med* **35,** 1011–1023.

World Cancer Research Fund/American Institute for Cancer Research (2007) *Food, Nutrition, Physical Activity and the Prevention of Cancer: a Global Perspective.* AICR, Washington, DC.

World Health Organization/Centers for Disease Control and Prevention (2004) *Assessing the Iron Status of Populations.* WHO, Geneva.

World Health Organization/Food and Agricultural Organization of the United Nations (2006) *Guidelines on Food Fortification with Micronutrients.* WHO, Geneva.

World Health Organization/UNICEF (2006) Joint Statement: Iron supplementation of young children in regions where malaria transmission is intense and infectious disease highly prevalent. www.who.int/nutrition/publications/WHOStatement_%20 iron%20suppl.pdf.

Ye, H. and Rouault, T.A (2010) Human iron–sulfur cluster assembly, cellular iron homeostasis and disease. *Biochemistry* **49,** 4945–4956.

Zehetner, A.A., Orr, N., Buckmaster, A., *et al.* (2010) Iron supplementation for breath-holding attacks in children. *Cochrane Database Syst Rev* CD008132.

Ziegler, E.E., Nelson, S.E., and Jeter, J.M. (2009) Iron supplementation of breastfed infants from an early age. *Am J Clin Nutr* **89,** 525–532.

34

ZINC

ROBERTA R. HOLT, BSc, JANET Y. URIU-ADAMS, PhD, AND CARL L. KEEN, PhD

University of California, Davis, California, USA

Summary

The trace element zinc is essential to a diverse array of structural, catalytic, and regulatory functions in mammals. With no known storage form of this element, zinc deficiency is rapidly induced in animal models, and, in humans, zinc deficiency contributes to reduced growth and immune function. While severe zinc deficiency is not common in the developed world, marginal zinc deficiency could contribute to a number of disease states. Current research is focused on understanding the cellular regulation of zinc including intracellular transporters that shuttle zinc within organelles, and between cells and the extracellular space, and the role of zinc in human health.

Introduction

The importance of zinc has long been recognized; zinc ores being used in the making of brass as early as 1000 AD. Zinc was recognized as a distinct element in 1509, and evidence of its essentiality was demonstrated in plants in 1869 and in experimental animals in 1933 (Todd *et al.*, 1933). Approximately 10% of proteins encoded in the mammalian genome require zinc for their proper structure and function (Andreini *et al.*, 2006). Most physiological processes are dependent on zinc, and the metabolism and regulatory roles of zinc are areas of considerable research. Given its wide prevalence in foodstuffs, naturally occurring zinc deficiency was long considered to be unlikely; however, in 1961, zinc deficiency was reported to be a problem in parts of the Middle East. In 2002, the World Health Organization estimated that nearly half of the world's population had suboptimal zinc status, and that, globally, zinc deficiency is a major risk factor for disease mortality and morbidity (WHO, 2002). Conversely, zinc toxicity can also represent a public health risk.

Chemistry

Zinc has an atomic number of 30 and an atomic weight of 65.37. Zinc is a period 4, group 12 d-block element with a complete d subshell and an oxidation state of 2. Zinc is a strong Lewis acid and has an affinity for thiol and hydroxyl groups and for ligands containing electron-rich nitrogen as a donor (Vallee and Auld, 1990). In biological systems, zinc is virtually always in the divalent state, and as such does not exhibit direct redox chemistry; however, when coupled as a zinc–thiol complex, as seen

Present Knowledge in Nutrition, Tenth Edition. Edited by John W. Erdman Jr, Ian A. Macdonald and Steven H. Zeisel.
© 2012 International Life Sciences Institute. Published 2012 by John Wiley & Sons, Inc.

with cysteine ligands, zinc is key to redox signaling (Foster and Samman, 2010). Zinc has a coordination geometry of 4, which, as will later be described, is important structurally for gene regulation (Maret and Li, 2009).

Zinc can be measured using a variety of methodologies. Zinc radioisotopes are routinely measured using gamma-ray spectrometry, liquid scintillation spectrometry, and autoradiography. Stable isotopes of zinc are typically measured using thermal ionization mass spectrometry, fast atom bombardment mass spectrometry, and inductively coupled mass spectrometry. Zinc occurs as five stable isotopes with the following natural abundances: ^{64}Zn, 48.89%; ^{66}Zn, 27.91%; ^{67}Zn, 4.11%; ^{68}Zn, 18.57%; and ^{70}Zn, 0.62%.

Atomic absorption spectrophotometry (AAS) is the most common method used to measure total zinc concentrations. Samples analyzed for zinc by AAS typically need to either undergo dry ashing (approximately 500°C) or wet ashing, with the latter often accomplished with the use of nitric or other acids. Fluorescent probes (e.g. Zinquin [(2-methyl-8-p-toluenesulphonamido-6-quinolyloxy) acetic acid] and protein biosensors that can measure free zinc concentrations within cells are increasingly being used to further our understanding of zinc metabolism and its regulatory roles (Tomat and Lippard, 2010).

Metabolism

The homeostatic regulation of zinc metabolism is still being elucidated; however, it is generally understood as the balance between absorption of dietary or endogenous zinc and the excretion of endogenous zinc. With regard to dietary zinc, the net delivery of zinc to the organism is a function of the total amount of zinc in the diet and its bioavailability. As with most minerals, zinc absorption typically exceeds the amount actually utilized; therefore, to maintain zinc homeostasis the excess zinc needs to be excreted. The exact mechanism of this regulation is the focus of a number of ongoing research programs.

Tissue Zinc

Zinc is present in all organs, tissues, fluids, and secretions of the body, with total body zinc content in the adult ranging from 1.5 g in women to 2.5 g in men. Zinc is primarily an intracellular ion, with well over 95% of the total body zinc found within cells (Jackson, 1989). The largest percentage of zinc can be found in the skeletal muscle (57%), followed by bone (29%), with remaining tissues and blood contributing approximately 14% (Jackson, 1989). In most species, plasma zinc represents approximately 0.1% of total body zinc, with typical concentrations being on the order of 1 µg/mL. Approximately 75% of plasma zinc is associated with albumin, with the remainder bound to α2-macroglobulin (15–30%) and amino acids (~1%; primarily cysteine and histidine) (Tapiero and Tew, 2003). The zinc concentration in erythrocytes is an order of magnitude higher than that of plasma (~1 ng/10^6 cells). The majority of erythrocyte zinc (~85%) is associated with carbonic anhydrase, and approximately 5% is associated with superoxide dismutase (SOD). As plasma zinc is commonly analyzed as a biomarker for zinc status (see below), it should be noted that the use of hemolyzed blood samples can yield artificially high plasma zinc concentrations. Circulating mononuclear and polynuclear cells can contain appreciable amounts of zinc (~5 ng/10^6 cells), and they are sometimes used to assess zinc status (Milne et al., 1985; Gibson et al., 2008).

Absorption

Pre-Absorption Factors

The bioavailability of zinc is largely a function of the presence or absence of substances in the food matrices that influence the absorption of zinc. These include food components that form insoluble zinc complexes that inhibit zinc absorption, or elements that compete with zinc at absorption sites thereby inhibiting zinc uptake. For example, phytate (myoinositol hexaphosphate), which is found in plant foods such as seeds, roots, and tubers, can significantly inhibit zinc absorption in many species, including humans, by forming insoluble complexes. The consumption of high-phytate diets has been linked to the induction of zinc deficiency in humans, particularly in situations where the overall diet is marginal in zinc content (Hambidge et al., 2010). A ratio of phytate to zinc above 10 increases the risk of poor zinc utilization. Removal of phytate from a food such as soy protein can significantly increase zinc availability from the product. Fermentation of bread can reduce its phytic acid content and significantly improve zinc absorption. The selection of low phytate variants of certain crops, such as maize, barley, and rice, may also represent an approach to improving the zinc bioavailability from these foods (Lonnerdal et al., 2011). Extrusion cooking, which is used for breakfast cereals, can inhibit the degradation of phytic acid in the gut and cause less efficient absorption of zinc (Sandstrom and Lonnerdal, 1989).

In contrast to inhibitory factors, some dietary factors can enhance zinc availability. For example, meats, liver, eggs, and seafood are considered to be good sources of zinc because of the relative absence of chemical constituents that inhibit zinc absorption and because of the presence of certain amino acids that improve zinc solubility. Several amino acids can form zinc complexes with high stability constants, which may facilitate zinc uptake (Krebs, 2000; Lonnerdal, 2000).

Within the intestinal lumen, pH does not seem to influence zinc uptake; rather, after a meal, digestive enzymes release zinc from food matrices. Zinc available for absorption is a combination of that provided by diet as well as from endogenous sources of zinc, such as biliary and pancreatic secretions (Krebs, 2000; Lonnerdal, 2000). The free zinc is able to form coordination complexes with amino acids, phosphates, and other organic acids, which can further influence zinc bioavailability. For example, zinc preferentially binds to the amino acid ligands histidine and cysteine forming a stable complex that enhances absorption (Scholmerich et al., 1987). Evidence indicates that a zinc–histidine complex is absorbed 30–40% more efficiently than zinc–sulfate complexes (Scholmerich et al., 1987).

Intestinal Absorption
In monogastric animals, zinc is mainly absorbed from the duodenum, jejunum, and ileum, with very little being absorbed from the stomach. Zinc absorption has been estimated at 20–40% (Tapiero and Tew, 2003), with maximal absorption occurring in either the distal duodenum or proximal jejunum (Lee et al., 1989; Krebs, 2000). These areas of the small intestine are characterized by increased expression of specific zinc transporters, such as Zrt/Irt-like protein (Zip)4 and Zinc Transporter (ZnT)1, which are involved in apical and basolateral enterocyte zinc flux, respectively (Yu et al., 2007; Cousins, 2010; Wang and Zhou, 2010).

Zinc transport across the brush border occurs by both a saturable carrier and a non-saturable transport mechanism that appears to be energy-independent. At low to normal luminal concentrations of zinc (0.1–1.8 mM), the active transport carrier mechanism predominates (Hoadley et al., 1987; Lee et al., 1989). With high zinc intakes (luminal concentration >1.8 mM), the non-saturable mechanism for zinc absorption becomes prominent and

may involve paracellular passive zinc diffusion. The precise mechanisms underlying the regulation of zinc absorption have remained elusive despite intensive investigation. A number of zinc transporters have now been described and are classified into two families, the ZnT (SLC30) family, and the Zip (SLC39) family (Lichten and Cousins, 2009; Wang and Zhou, 2010). Ten ZnTs and 14 Zips have been identified, with dietary zinc currently known to influence about eight of these (Lichten and Cousins, 2009). Zip4, found on the enterocyte apical membrane, is known to be regulated by zinc intake, and is a major contributor to the saturable kinetics of zinc absorption (Wang and Zhou, 2010). Individuals with the genetic disorder acrodermatitis enteropathica (AE), who have a mutation in the Zip4 gene, can develop signs of severe zinc deficiency if supplementary dietary zinc is not provided (Lichten and Cousins, 2009).

The ileum is the major site for ZnT-1. It is localized to the basolateral membrane and appears to regulate the export of zinc across the enterocyte into the mesenteric capillary where it is carried by the portal blood to the liver (Wang and Zhou, 2010). ZnT-2 is found in acidic vesicles that accumulate zinc in the duodenum and jejunum. ZnT-4 is found in all parts of the small intestine. ZnT-2 and ZnT-4 are involved in the flux of zinc in the endosomes, possibly regulating intracellular trafficking of zinc (Cousins et al., 2006; Sekler et al., 2007; Wang and Zhou, 2010). All of these transporters are found primarily in villus cells, and much less frequently in crypt cells. A superfamily of human zinc transport proteins has been identified (zinc importer proteins, ZIP1 and ZIP2) that are involved in cellular zinc uptake. These proteins are localized in the plasma membrane and have structural characteristics typical of other transport proteins (e.g. permeable membrane domains, a transport channel, and high-affinity binding domains). Within the cell, the disposition of zinc is diverse. Zinc trapped within the enterocyte is eventually lost in the feces in the normal course of mucosal cell turnover. In all cell types, intracellular zinc may be used for zinc-dependent processes, become bound firmly to metallothionein (MT) and held within the cell, or pass through the cell. Low-molecular-weight cellular proteins, such as MT, can bind zinc, as well as other divalent metals such as copper and cadmium. Zinc induces MT in mucosal cells, but only at relatively high dietary intakes.

The bioavailability of zinc is determined from the amount of zinc that is available from the food matrix and the total amount of zinc in the food (Hambidge *et al.*, 2010; King, 2010). As discussed above, a number of food components, such as phytate, can interfere with zinc absorption; therefore, stable isotope studies are often employed in order to determine the fraction or percent of zinc absorbed from the diet (i.e. fractional zinc absorbed), which is subsequently multiplied by the total dietary zinc to determine the bioavailable quantity of zinc (i.e. total zinc absorbed) (King, 2010). Short-term, controlled, dietary human intervention trials have determined that total zinc absorbed is associated with zinc intake and not status (Chung *et al.*, 2008; King, 2010), with an inverse association between intake and fractional zinc absorption which is representative of the known saturation kinetics of zinc absorption (Hambidge *et al.*, 2010). Therefore, a diet that is low in zinc will have an increased fractional zinc absorption, but reduced total zinc absorbed, compared with a diet that is zinc adequate (Chung *et al.*, 2008).

It is also well recognized that select divalent metal ions, such as iron, can compete with zinc for mucosal cell binding sites and transporters such as divalent metal transporter 1 (DMT1), although the significance of this interaction with respect to overall zinc balance can be questioned. Zinc and copper can also compete for cell transporters; however, while secondary copper deficiencies can clearly arise as a consequence of excessive zinc intakes (see below), high levels of dietary copper have not been reported to be a significant issue with respect to zinc absorption. Presumably this is due to the fact that dietary copper intakes are normally much lower than those of zinc. In animals, high-calcium diets can impair zinc absorption (Sandstrom and Lonnerdal, 1989) whereas, in humans, zinc balance is not affected by the addition of calcium salts unless the diet is also high in phytate (Lonnerdal, 2000). Early studies suggested that folic acid supplementation could also interfere with zinc homeostasis; however, subsequent studies with either short- or long-term folic acid supplementation demonstrated no effect on zinc absorption or homeostasis (Campbell, 1996).

Excretion

Approximately 2.6–4.6 mg of zinc is secreted into the duodenum following a meal, mainly from pancreatic secretions. Additional sources of endogenous zinc include bile and gastroduodenum secretions, zinc from transepithelial flux from mucosal cells, and mucosal cells that are sloughed into the gut (Hambidge *et al.*, 1986). An intact enteropancreatic zinc circulation is important for mainte-

nance of body zinc as much of the zinc secreted into the gut is reabsorbed. The amount of zinc secreted into the gut is affected by zinc intake. In humans, extremely low zinc intakes are associated with low endogenous fecal zinc losses (<1 mg/day) while extremely high zinc intakes can result in losses of over 5 mg/day (Baer and King, 1984; Jackson *et al.*, 1984). Fecal excretion is the major route of unabsorbed dietary zinc and endogenous zinc excretion (Hambidge *et al.*, 2010). An increase in the fecal excretion of endogenous zinc provides the "fine control" needed to balance the net retention of zinc with metabolic needs. Endogenous fecal zinc losses can be increased several-fold to maintain zinc homeostasis with high intake of zinc (Coppen and Davies, 1987). Data from zinc tracer studies show that 90–98% is lost in the feces while only 2–10% is recovered in the urine (Hambidge *et al.*, 1986). Typical urinary excretion rates are about 400–600 µg zinc/day arising largely from the low molecular weight zinc pool (Hambidge *et al.*, 1986). Except in extreme zinc deficiency or supplementation conditions, dietary zinc does not have a major impact on urinary zinc excretion. Typically, 95% of zinc that is filtered by the glomerulus will be reabsorbed (Victery *et al.*, 1981). Several factors can affect urinary zinc excretion including the rate of urine production (or the urine volume) and creatinine excretion. Urinary zinc losses are also significantly elevated when catabolism is increased such as in severe burn cases, trauma/surgery, starvation, or under treatment with chelating agents such as ethylenediaminetetraacetic acid (EDTA) (Hambidge *et al.*, 1986). Loss of zinc up to 1 mg/day also occurs via surface loss (desquamation of skin, hair outgrowth, and sweat), which can be affected by marked changes in dietary zinc intake (Milne *et al.*, 1984). Semen secretions can contribute up to 1 mg and menstrual secretions can account for 0.1–5 mg of endogenous zinc losses (Hess *et al.*, 1977).

Zinc excretion can be increased when supplements of tin are given (50 mg) (Johnson *et al.*, 1982); however, this is not thought to be a common problem as dietary tin intake is typically low (<1 mg/day). High levels of dietary cadmium do not appear to impact zinc absorption, but can alter zinc distribution in the body via competition for MT binding sites (Goyer, 1997).

Homeostasis

To date, specific zinc "stores" that are homeostatically controlled have not been identified. In all species studied, signs of zinc deficiency occur quickly after the individual consumes a zinc-deficient diet, indicating that zinc stores are not readily available. Total body zinc is maintained by the regulation of intestinal absorption, intracellular and tissue distribution, and the excretion of endogenous zinc pools (King *et al.*, 2000). This is possibly achieved by changes in the expression of zinc transporters (Tapiero and Tew, 2003; Cragg *et al.*, 2005; Wang and Zhou, 2010; Fukada *et al.*, 2011). For example, in the enterocyte, apically located Zip4 is down-regulated with high zinc intake and up-regulated when zinc intake is reduced (Wang and Zhou, 2010). Similarly, as intracellular zinc rises, transporters such as ZnT-1 are up-regulated, thereby increasing zinc efflux into intracellular vesicles (Wang and Zhou, 2010).

As noted above, long-term storage pools of zinc have not been identified. However, it can be argued that MT-bound zinc may be a short-term zinc pool. In favor of this idea is the observation that MT is inducible by dietary zinc via the metal response element (MRE) and metal-binding transcription factor (MTF-1) (see below). Furthermore, it is known that acute and chronic changes in tissue MT concentrations can result in marked alterations in plasma zinc concentrations as well as the intracellular distribution of zinc. Interestingly, MT-null mice have been reported to have relatively normal lifespans, and they do not show marked alterations in zinc metabolism (Wastney and House, 2008). An exception to the above is when zinc metabolism is studied in MT-null mice exposed to certain acute challenges, such as high concentrations of inflammatory cytokines like interleukin 1, interleukin 6, and tumor necrosis factor-alpha. The typical hypozincemia that is observed in cytokine-challenged animals is not evident in the MT-null mice. Whether this represents a benefit or a risk to the animal has yet to be defined.

Albumin has a low association constant for zinc, thus albumin zinc represents a highly exchangeable pool of zinc for tissue uptake. The kidneys are able to filter amino acid-bound zinc. Because the pool of zinc in tissues is large relative to plasma, small variations in the zinc content of tissues can markedly affect plasma zinc. For example, a stress-induced increase in zinc retention in the liver can result in a 40% reduction in plasma zinc. In contrast, even minor muscle catabolism can release enough zinc to increase plasma levels. This issue should be considered when blood samples are taken from individuals following a prolonged fast. In contrast, plasma zinc levels fall following a meal (Kiilerich *et al.*, 1980; McMillan and Rowe, 1982). Together, these data show that the use of plasma zinc concentrations to assess zinc status can be complicated.

Considerable information about zinc pools and their turnover has been obtained from kinetic modeling studies using zinc stable isotopes. Elimination of absorbed zinc from the body is best described by a two-component model (Hambidge *et al.*, 1986). The initial rapid phase, thought to primarily represent the initial uptake and release of zinc from the liver, has a half-life in humans of approximately 12.5 days. The slower turnover phase reflects differing rates of zinc turnover in various extrahepatic tissues and has a half-life of approximately 300 days (Hambidge *et al.*, 1986). The uptake and turnover of zinc can be relatively slow, as observed in the central nervous system and bones, or relatively fast as observed in the pancreas, liver, kidney, and spleen. Uptake and exchange of zinc in red blood cells and muscle are slower than in the viscera. In rats, dietary zinc restriction enhances zinc retention in soft tissues and organs by reducing zinc turnover (Coppen and Davies, 1987). These homeostatic adjustments protect tissue zinc concentration from marked decline. In humans, daily loading with 100 mg of zinc can increase the turnover of the slower zinc pool (Aamodt *et al.*, 1982).

A number of factors can influence zinc homeostatic regulation. The age of the individual can influence absorptive capacity. Suboptimal zinc status has been reported to be common in the elderly; whether or not zinc absorption is reduced in the elderly is a subject of debate (Fairweather-Tait *et al.*, 2008). Increased fractional zinc absorption has been reported to occur in women during pregnancy and lactation (Donangelo *et al.*, 2005). In addition, changes in zinc transport may regulate absorption and deposition into milk (Kelleher and Lonnerdal, 2009).

Physiological (Biochemical) Function

Data mining of potential metal–protein binding domains has identified over 3000 putative zinc proteins in humans. Zinc has a role in a multitude of catalytic, structural, and regulatory functions (Andreini *et al.*, 2006; Cousins *et al.*, 2006; Tuerk and Fazel, 2009). Given its multitude of functions, it is not surprising that a deficit of this element can pose serious, and diverse, physiological challenges. A brief outline of some of the biochemical and physiological functions of zinc is presented below.

Zinc has been confirmed as an important component of over 50 enzymes representing all six International Union of Biochemistry (IUB) classes (Vallee, 1983; Hambidge *et al.*, 1986). With respect to these metalloenzymes, zinc can function in a catalytic, co-catalytic or structural fashion (Clegg *et al.*, 2005; Stefanidou *et al.*, 2006). The catalytic site of enzymes such as carbonic anhydrase, alcohol dehydrogenase, and carboxypeptidase form and break bonds via Lewis acid–base chemistry through the coordination of zinc to three amino acid side chains of histidine, glutamate, aspartate or cysteine and water (McCall *et al.*, 2000; Clegg *et al.*, 2005; Stefanidou *et al.*, 2006). Two or more zinc ions plus other metals, such as magnesium, serve in a co-catalytic role within alkaline phosphatase and phospholipase C (McCall *et al.*, 2000).

In addition, zinc serves to stabilize the tertiary structure of a number of proteins, including those involved in DNA replication and reverse transcription, through the coordination of side chains from amino acids such as cysteine (Stefanidou *et al.*, 2006). Moreover, transcription factors known as "Zn-finger" regions contain repeated cysteine and histidine domains that bind zinc in a tetrahedral configuration. These Zn-finger domains mediate the interaction of proteins to other proteins, DNA, RNA, and lipids (Matthews and Sunde, 2002; Klug, 2010). Transcription factors can contain several Zn-fingers, each with a set of triplet amino acid sequences involved in DNA base recognition, allowing for specificity to a DNA sequence (Hartwig, 2001). Members of the nuclear receptor family including glucocorticoid, retinoic acid and vitamin D_3 receptors utilize Zn-fingers to recognize their DNA binding domain. Zn-finger binding domains also exist in enzymes involved in DNA repair, cell cycle control, and apoptosis (Hartwig, 2001). Given the widespread occurrence of Zn-finger binding domains, it would be reasonable to speculate that this function of zinc would be highly protected; however, there are reports that severe zinc deficiency can influence Zn-finger-dependent transcription factors (Duffy *et al.*, 2004).

While the zinc ion itself is not redox active, zinc-coordinated to the sulfur of cysteine within catalytic sites or structural proteins allows for the potential of redox regulation (Maret, 2006). Similarly, zinc can help to ensure biomembrane structure and function, due in part to its ability to: (1) interact with and stabilize thiol groups of antioxidant enzymes and membrane channel proteins; (2) displace redox active transition metals, such as iron; and (3) reduce production of transition metal-induced reactive oxygen species (ROS) through the induction of MT (Willson, 1989; O'Dell, 2000; Laity and Andrews, 2007).

Indeed, one of the primary regulatory roles of zinc is through the activation of MTF-1, a six-Zn-finger-containing transcription factor, which after complexing zinc, binds to the MT promoter as well as to the promoters for ZnT-1 and γ-glutamylcysteine synthase (Beyersmann and Haase, 2001; Maret, 2006; Laity and Andrews, 2007).

Zinc Deficiency

Deficits of zinc can affect a multitude of systems, including the central nervous, reproductive, integumentary, skeletal, gastrointestinal, and immune systems (Tuerk and Fazel, 2009). Zinc deficiency can be both inherited and acquired. As stated above, AE is a rare, inherited, autosomal recessive disease (Aggett, 1989). In AE, the intestinal uptake and transfer of zinc across the apical membrane is impaired due to a defect in the Zip4 gene (Lichten and Cousins, 2009). An increased risk of an acquired zinc deficiency has also been reported for patients receiving total parenteral nutrition (TPN) solutions that are low in zinc, or who are treated with divalent metal chelating agents and drugs (e.g. the use of penicillamine therapy for Wilson's disease). In addition, zinc deficiency can be the result of malabsorption syndromes, chronic alcoholism, and, as discussed above, the consumption of diets high in phytate (Tuerk and Fazel, 2009).

The expression of zinc deficiency in an individual depends on the severity of the deficiency and other factors, but classic signs of severe zinc deficiency include growth retardation, diarrhea, skin and eye lesions, neuropsychiatric changes, and alopecia (Aggett, 1989). Dwarfism, hypogonadism, and delayed sexual maturation were initially observed in Middle Eastern adolescents consuming diets high in phytate (Prasad *et al.*, 1961). Skin lesions found on the extremities and near body orifices that are often erythematous and pustular in nature, and increased loss of hair, which may become hypopigmented with a reddish hue, are common to severe forms of zinc deficiency (Hambidge *et al.*, 1986; Aggett, 1989). Zinc is particularly concentrated in the retina and other eye structures, and severe zinc deficiency has been reported to alter vision (Grahn *et al.*, 2001). A synergistic relationship between zinc and vitamin A status has been postulated that could be detrimentally altered with a zinc deficiency (Christian and West, 1998).

The major pathophysiological abnormalities contributing to secondary zinc deficiency are zinc malabsorption and excessive urinary zinc losses. Therefore, any disease or condition that increases transit time for absorption or alters the integrity of the gastrointestinal mucosa, such as is the case with enteric infections and inflammation, can affect zinc absorption. Patients who become zinc deficient often have conditions that predispose them to the problem, such as diarrhea, inflammatory bowel disease, and other malabsorptive conditions such as Crohn's disease, sprue, and short bowel syndrome. Recently, there has been increasing concern that zinc deficiency might be a common complication of gastric bypass surgery (Salle *et al.*, 2010). Specifically, surgical procedures that promote malabsorption, such as Roux-en-Y gastric bypass (RYGB) and duodenal switch, have been reported to produce a zinc deficiency in 40% and 91% of patients, respectively, 12 months post-surgery (Salle *et al.*, 2010). Significantly, it has been estimated that over 350 000 gastric bypass surgeries were performed globally in 2008, with 40% of these using RYGB (Padwal *et al.*, 2011); therefore, it could be predicted that up to 56 000 of these individuals could have been zinc deficient as late as a year post-surgery. Alarmingly, if one considers the increasing prevalence of severe obesity in many countries and the associated use of bypass surgery, the potential is there for literally millions of new cases of marginal zinc deficiency over the next decade.

Diarrhea is a complication of AE, in those receiving TPN, and in those with intestinal infection. Zinc supplementation has been shown to be an effective treatment for acute diarrhea, especially in children (Berni Canani *et al.*, 2010; Yakoob *et al.*, 2011). Enteric pathogens promote diarrhea by enhancing secretion of chloride ion, with subsequent loss of water, through a number of species-specific pathways. In in vitro model systems, zinc supplementation has been shown to inhibit three out of four key signaling pathways involved in chloride ion secretion including inhibition of cyclic AMP, the inducible isoform of nitric oxide synthase (iNOS), and transactivator factor peptide (Tat)-induced Ca^{2+}-dependent chloride ion secretion (Berni Canani *et al.*, 2010).

A number of potential mechanisms underlying zinc deficiency-induced pathology have been advanced based on cell culture and animal model systems. In animals, zinc deficiency during early development is highly teratogenic. Typical malformations associated with severe zinc deficiency in experimental animals include brain and eye defects, spina bifida, cleft lip and palate, and numerous malformations of the heart, lung, skeleton, and urogenital system (Keen and Hurley, 1989). In addition to the gross structural defects evident at birth, biochemical alterations from developmental zinc deficiency can persist into adulthood. Illustrative of this, Beach and co-workers (Beach *et al.*, 1982) reported that offspring of mouse dams who were fed moderately low-zinc diets (5 μg zinc/g diet) during pregnancy had immunological abnormalities that persisted over several generations, despite dams and offspring receiving adequate zinc diets after birth. Similarly, recent reports show that developmental zinc deficiency in rats can result in persistent alterations in nitric oxide pools that can be associated with elevated blood pressure (Tomat *et al.*, 2010, 2011). As outlined below, the mechanisms leading to zinc-deficiency-associated abnormal development are multifactorial in nature. Biochemical lesions proposed to contribute to the teratogenicity of zinc deficiency include altered DNA and protein synthesis, alterations in cell proliferation and survival, impairment in tubulin polymerization with resultant reductions in cell motility and division, chromosomal defects, altered cell signaling, and excessive peroxidation of cell membrane lipids (Keen and Hurley, 1989; Uriu-Adams and Keen, 2010). In addition to its impact on the fetus, zinc deficiency during late gestation can result in parturition difficulties with delayed deliveries and excessive bleeding (Apgar, 1985; Keen and Hurley, 1989).

When dietary zinc intake is insufficient, the first response is to conserve tissue zinc by reducing endogenous losses. Tissue zinc loss is not uniform: plasma, liver, bone, and testicle zinc concentrations decrease, with apparent conservation of tissue zinc concentrations in hair, skin, heart and skeletal muscle (King *et al.*, 2000). If the dietary deficiency is mild, zinc homeostasis may be re-established and no further functional or biochemical changes occur. However, with a markedly deficient diet, the organism cannot reestablish homeostasis through adjustments in endogenous losses and growth. As a consequence, an increase in tissue catabolism occurs, and a generalized tissue dysfunction develops quickly. Zinc deficiency can be induced rapidly in some species. For example, within 24 hours of consuming a zinc-deficient diet, plasma zinc concentrations in the rat can be decreased by as much as 50% (Hurley *et al.*, 1982). That this reduction in plasma zinc can be functionally significant is illustrated by the observation that the feeding of a zinc-deficient diet to pregnant rats for only a few days during the first trimester is sufficient to cause embryonic abnormalities (Uriu-Adams and Keen, 2010). Although all species may not respond to a zinc-deficient diet as rapidly as the rat, the lack of any appreciable zinc stores under homeostatic control is a consistent finding for all mammalian species to date.

Early effects of zinc deficiency for many species include anorexia and cyclic feeding. In rats, it has been suggested that dietary zinc stimulates food intake via the activation of vagal afferents, which subsequently stimulates the release of the hypothalamic orexigenic peptides orexin and neuropeptide Y (Ohinata *et al.*, 2009). Regardless of the biochemical explanation for the anorexia, the cyclic food intake pattern of zinc-deficient animals may represent an adaptation of the animal to increase muscle catabolism and release zinc into the plasma pool for zinc-dependent processes used by hepatic and extrahepatic tissues including the embryo and fetus. For example, in pregnant animals fed a zinc-deficient diet, increased fetal apoptosis is observed during periods of increased maternal food intake (relatively low plasma zinc), versus those time periods where food intake is low (relatively high plasma zinc) (Uriu-Adams and Keen, 2010). Impaired growth is also associated with zinc deficiency, which, like cyclic food intake, has been suggested to represent an accommodation of the animal to the zinc deficit by increasing zinc availability for zinc-dependent metabolic processes. An alternative explanation for the slower rate of growth is that it is secondary to the anorexia and the concomitant reduction in food intake. However, animals fed diets adequate in zinc, in amounts equivalent to those consumed by zinc-deficient animals, gain considerably more weight than the zinc-deficient animals. Thus, the lower weight gain observed with zinc deficiency cannot be ascribed solely to reduced food intake (O'Dell and Reeves, 1989).

As stated above, zinc is essential for a number of biological processes including enzyme function and protein structure. In addition, zinc deficiency alters DNA and protein expression. Zinc deficiency has been shown to affect DNA integrity in humans (Song *et al.*, 2009) as well as experimental animals (Song *et al.*, 2010). Alterations in cell proliferation and survival pathways are also induced with zinc deficiency. These include a number of downstream events regulated by growth factors through receptor tyrosine kinase signaling, such as insulin-like growth factor (IGF), which functions to inhibit apoptosis and promote cell differentiation to increase growth. For example, in zinc-deficient cell culture systems, a reduced phosphorylation of Ras-dependent extracellular-signal-regulated kinase (ERK 1/2), as well as the serine/threonine protein kinase, AKT, results in a dephosphorylation of the Bcl-2-associated death promoter protein (BAD); leaving BAD to form het-

erodimers with anti-apoptotic factors Bcl-2 and Bcl-XL, and with pro-apoptotic Bcl-2-associated X protein (BAX). The BAD/BAX heterodimer can then proceed to permeabilize mitochondrial membranes, resulting in cytochrome C release and subsequent caspase activation, leading to apoptosis (Clegg *et al.*, 2005; Uriu-Adams and Keen, 2010) (Figure 34.1). The increase in oxidative stress that is observed during zinc deficiency can induce cell cycle arrest and apoptosis through oxidation of proteins, lipids and DNA. The tumor suppressor protein p53 is involved in the detection and repair of DNA or in triggering apoptosis. The DNA binding region of p53 contains zinc. In zinc-deficient cells p53 expression is increased, but its DNA binding ability can be reduced. Zinc prevents the oxidation of redox-sensitive thiol groups in cysteine, and can reduce ROS production by displacing redox active transition metals. Zinc deficiency activates NADPH oxidase and the inducible isoform of nitric oxide synthase (NOS), which can increase both ROS and reactive nitrogen species (RNS). Finally, zinc plays a role in cytoskeletal function, which is involved in the translocation to the nucleus of transcription factors such as nuclear factor kappa B (NFκB) and nuclear factor of activated T-cells (NFAT) (Mackenzie *et al.*, 2002; Aimo *et al.*, 2010; Uriu-Adams and Keen, 2010) (Figure 34.1).

A potential consequence of zinc-deficiency-induced changes in cell signaling is marked alterations in several components of the immune system (Table 34.1). In animals and humans, zinc deficiency can result in thymic atrophy and reduced cell-mediated and humoral immune responses (Fraker and King, 2004). Zinc deficiency induces apoptosis in susceptible cells during key stages of lymphopoiesis. For example, Pro- and Pre-B cells maturing within the bone marrow have reduced levels of anti-apoptotic Bcl-2 compared with mature B cells. A reduction of Pre-B cell numbers is observed with zinc deficiency; whereas zinc deficiency has little effect on the mature B cell (Fraker and King, 2004). Similar effects are observed with double-positive T-cells, which could account for the reduction of thymic size observed with zinc deficiency. Mature T-helper and cytotoxic cells are not affected by a reduction in zinc (Fraker and King, 2004), but an increase in the number of myeloid cells (i.e. neutrophils and monocytes) is observed with zinc deficiency (Tuerk and Fazel, 2009).

In addition to effects on cellular number, zinc influences immune cell activity. Natural killer (NK) cell activity is zinc dependent. Zinc is required for the interaction of the

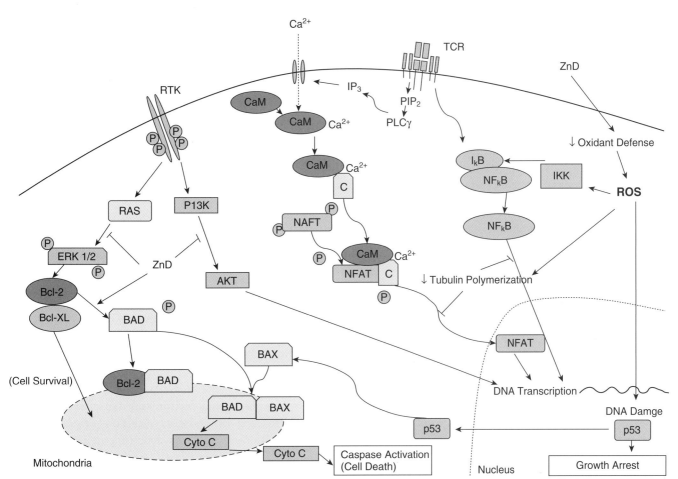

FIG. 34.1 Zinc deficiency and cellular signaling. Depending on the cell type, zinc deficiency influences a number of signaling pathways involved in cell proliferation, cell survival, and death. For example, a number of growth hormones activate receptor tyrosine kinases (RTK); zinc deficiency reduces extracellular signal-regulated kinase (ERK 1/2) phosphorylation by RAS and promotes dimerization of pro-apoptotic Bcl-2-associated death promoter (BAD), with anti-apoptotic Bcl-2, thereby reducing functional mitochondrial Bcl-2. Zinc-deficiency-induced increases in reactive oxygen species (ROS) affect nuclear factor of activated T-cells (NFAT); nuclear factor kappa beta (NFκB); and AKT gene expression through a reduction of tubulin polymerization and translocation of these transcription factors to the nucleus. In addition, zinc-deficiency-induced increases in ROS result in DNA damage and activation of p53 signaling, leading to growth arrest. Further signaling by p53 can facilitate Bcl-2-associated X protein (BAX) translocation to the mitochondria and dimerization with BAD, increasing mitochondrial permeability, cytochrome C (Cyto C) release, and subsequent activation of caspases that initiate apoptosis (cell death). TCR, T-cell receptor; CaM, calmodulin; C, calcineurin; IκB, inhibitor of κB; IKK, IκB kinase; PIP$_2$, phosphatidylinositol 3,4-bisphosphate; PLCγ, phospholipase C-γ; PI3K, phosphatidylinositol 3-OH kinase; IP$_3$, inositol triphosphate.

killer cell immunoglobulin-like receptors (KIRs) of the NK cell with major histocompatibility complex (MHC)-I molecules. Therefore, zinc deficiency increases non-specific lytic activity of the NK cell, as well as reducing NK activity (Rink and Gabriel, 2001). In addition to reduced T-cell numbers, a reduction in Th1 cytokines (interferon-(IFN)-

γ and interleukin (IL)-2) is observed whereas Th2 cytokines are unaffected (IL-4, IL-6, IL-10) (Ibs and Rink, 2003). Recently, it has been proposed that ionic zinc in lozenges reduces the severity of cold symptoms by enhancing IFN-γ production and inhibiting intracellular adhesion molecule-1 (ICAM-1), resulting in overall antiviral

TABLE 34.1 Zinc deficiency and immune function

Immune effect	Reference
Decreased epithelial barrier functions (i.e. gastrointestinal, skin, respiratory)	Fraker and King (2004)
Increased susceptibility of infection	Keen and Gershwin (1990)
Suppression of oral tolerance	Finamore et al. (2003)
Suppression of delayed-type hypersensitivity reactions	Keen and Gershwin (1990)
Increased Pre- and Pro-B cell apoptosis	Fraker and King (2004)
Increased thymic atrophy	Fraker and King (2004)
Reduced thymulin	Rink and Gabriel (2001)
Increased double-positive T-cell apoptosis	Fraker and King (2004)
Altered T-cell receptor (TCR) signaling	Haase and Rink (2009)
Decreased T helper (Th1) cytokines	Ibs and Rink (2003)
Increased myeloid cell (i.e. neutrophils and monocyte) numbers	Tuerk and Fazel (2009)
Increased non-specific natural killer (NK) cell lytic activity	Rink and Gabriel (2001)

response (Eby, 2010; Singh and Das, 2011). Several aspects of T-cell receptor (TCR) signaling are influenced by zinc. Activation of the TCR complex involves the recruitment and dimerization of lymphocyte protein tyrosine kinases (Lck) by zinc-dependent mechanisms (Haase and Rink, 2009). Further downstream, zinc affects the activation of signaling pathways and transcription factors, such as NFAT, NFκB, and MAPK kinases, that regulate cytokine gene expression (Haase and Rink, 2009; Honscheid et al., 2011; Yu et al., 2011). With its diverse influence over immune signaling, the trafficking of intracellular zinc via the expression of specific zinc transporters and MT is an active area of research (Cousins et al., 2006; Eide, 2006; Nishida et al., 2009; Overbeck et al., 2008; Yu et al., 2011). MT expression is induced by the pro-inflammatory cytokines IL-1, IL-6, and TNF-α, and hormones such as the glucocorticoids, epinephrine, and glucagon (Schroeder and Cousins, 1990; Mocchegiani et al., 2009; Takeda and Tamano, 2010). It has been postulated that the pro-inflammatory cytokines can increase glucocorticoid release, resulting in an induction of MT synthesis via the glucocorticoid response element on the MT promoter (Schroeder and Cousins, 1990). In addition, IL-6 has been demonstrated to increase hepatocyte Zip14 expression, therefore increasing intracellular zinc which can induce MT synthesis via MTF-1 (Liuzzi et al., 2005). The end result is a redistribution of zinc to the liver during stress and an inflammation-induced acute phase response, resulting in hypozincemia (Schroeder and Cousins, 1990; Liuzzi et al., 2005). Therefore, perturbation of intracellular MT expression may have profound implications for a number of inflammatory conditions and chronic disease states.

Mild-to-marginal states of zinc deficiency may go undetected as individuals at risk may not display the specific clinical features of zinc depletion. Although the occurrence of severe zinc deficiency in humans is well documented, whether a physiologically significant mild zinc deficiency exists in humans is controversial. Currently, research in this area is hampered by the lack of reliable, sensitive biomarkers for zinc status (Gibson et al., 2008). Demonstration of mild zinc deficiency in humans is not as straightforward as in experimental animals. If one is to use impaired growth velocity as the primary clinical feature of mild zinc deficiency, several studies have provided convincing evidence that zinc supplementation reverses this trend (Hambidge, 2000). Moreover, meta-analyses of well controlled trials examining the effects of zinc supplementation in children show improved growth (Hambidge, 2000; Brown et al., 2002).

A marginal zinc deficiency may occur in those with an increased utilization of zinc, such as during periods of increased growth or in pregnancy, particularly if their dietary zinc intake is also low. Women with AE first provided evidence that a severe zinc deficiency results in poor pregnancy outcomes (King, 2000; Uriu-Adams and Keen, 2010). Subsequently, Jameson was the first to associate a low maternal serum zinc status in the first trimester of pregnancy with congenital malformations, fetal dysmaturity, prematurity, and maternal complications in otherwise healthy women (Jameson, 1976). That report stimulated further research examining the relationship between zinc status and pregnancy outcome. Detailed reviews of this topic are available (Apgar, 1985; Swanson and King, 1987; Keen and Hurley, 1989; King, 2000; Uriu-Adams and

Keen, 2010). Several groups have reported that mothers of infants with congenital anomalies, or who suffer from pregnancy complications, have lower plasma zinc concentrations than other mothers; however, this is an inconsistent finding (King, 2000; Uriu-Adams and Keen, 2010).

Numerous clinical situations can result in reduced absorption, increased loss, or increased need for zinc. Cadmium from sources such as cigarette smoke competes with zinc for transport mechanisms, such as Zip8 and MT (He *et al.*, 2009); thus, zinc deficiency could increase the risk for cadmium toxicity, and potentially lead to an individual's susceptibility to the development of chronic diseases including cardiovascular disease (Messner *et al.*, 2009; Afridi *et al.*, 2011) and cancer (Kazi *et al.*, 2010). Patients with alcoholic liver disease are often characterized by hyperzincuria, hypozincemia, and low liver zinc concentrations compared with controls or with patients without cirrhosis (Kang and Zhou, 2005). Because the teratogenic expression of zinc deficiency is similar to that of fetal alcohol spectrum disorders (FASD), alcohol-induced zinc deficiency has been proposed as a mechanism underlying the development of FASD (Keen *et al.*, 2010). It has been estimated that half of the elderly do not meet the recommended dietary allowance (RDA) for zinc (Hodkinson *et al.*, 2007), potentially placing them at risk for osteoporosis and impaired cognitive and immune function (Meunier *et al.*, 2005; Yamaguchi, 2010). Finally, epidemiology studies have shown an association between reduced zinc status in those with diabetes (Islam and Loots, 2007; Jansen *et al.*, 2009). Alterations in zinc

metabolism have been shown to occur in both diabetic humans and experimental animals. Adult rats with genetically or chemically induced diabetes are characterized by zinc accumulation in the liver and kidney and by hyperzincuria (Failla and Kiser, 1983; Uriu-Hare *et al.*, 1989). Both type I and type 2 diabetic patients can exhibit hyperzincuria, which increases with the severity of the diabetes (Walter *et al.*, 1991). It has been postulated that the hyperzincuria can result in a conditioned zinc deficiency in some individuals, and hypozincemia is a relatively common finding in diabetics (Walter *et al.*, 1991). However, randomized controlled zinc supplementation trials for the prevention of type 2 diabetes have failed to show a benefit (Beletate *et al.*, 2007).

Requirements, Recommended Dietary Allowance, Upper Limits, and Evaluation of Zinc Status

Age, sex, pregnancy, and lactation are all factors that were used by the US Institute of Medicine for the dietary zinc recommendations in 2001. The suggested values were based on a combination of factors including balance and isotopic zinc tracer studies, and a mix of zinc supplementation studies (Table 34.2) (Institute of Medicine, 2001). The factors and underlying principles that were used to estimate the RDA, estimated average requirement (EAR), average intake (AI) and tolerable upper intake levels (UL) for zinc are described in detail in the committee's

TABLE 34.2 Dietary reference intakes

Life stage	Age	AI (mg/day)		EAR (mg/day)		RDA (mg/day)		UL (mg/day)	
		Male	Female	Male	Female	Male	Female	Male	Female
Infants	0–6 months	2.0	2.0					4.0	4.0
	7–12 months			2.5	2.5	3.0	3.0	5.0	5.0
Children	1–3 years			2.5	2.5	3.0	3.0	7.0	7.0
	4–8 years			4.0	4.0	5.0	5.0	12.0	12.0
	9–13 years			7.0	7.0	8.0	8.0	23.0	23.0
	14–18 years			8.5	7.3	11.0	9.0	34.0	34.0
Adults	>19 years			9.4	6.8	11.0	8.0	40.0	40.0
Pregnancy	14–18 years				10.0		12.0		34.0
	19–50 years				9.5		11.0		40.0
Lactation	14–18 years				10.9		13.0		34.0
	19–50 years				10.4		12.0		40.0

AI, adequate intake; EAR, estimated average requirement; RDA, recommended dietary allowance; UL, tolerable upper intake level.
Data from Institute of Medicine (2001).

report. A key question facing the field today is to what extent zinc intake levels below the suggested RDA represent a true health risk.

At present, a major impediment to the identification of the extent and severity of suboptimal zinc status in select populations is the lack of sensitive, specific, and agreed-upon biomarkers for zinc status (King, 2011). As noted above, while an assessment of zinc status is often based on an analysis of plasma zinc concentrations, this approach can be fraught with difficulties as plasma zinc values can be affected by numerous factors including acute meal-related changes, circadian variations, fasting, and cytokine-induced changes in tissue zinc stores (Hurley et al., 1982; King, 2011). It is generally agreed that plasma zinc concentrations can be a poor indicator of whole-body zinc status for the above reasons. It can also be argued that, with respect to humans, plasma zinc concentrations do not significantly decrease until dietary zinc levels are so low that homeostasis cannot be reestablished. Thus, while plasma zinc measurements may have potential value in the identification of individuals with severe deficiencies, they may be of limited value with respect to the identification of cases of marginal deficiency. In all cases, it should be stressed that, when plasma zinc measurements are used as predictors of zinc status, it is important to control for other metabolic factors that can influence the concentrations of this element (e.g. stress, fasting, diurnal considerations, hormonal state, etc.) (Institute of Medicine, 2001). As a complement to plasma zinc concentrations, the measurement of zinc in leukocytes, erythrocytes, saliva, and hair have all been advanced as possible approaches to the assessment of zinc status (Gibson et al., 2008; Cummings and Kovacic, 2009); however, similar to plasma zinc, none of the above measurements are thought to be sensitive with respect to the identification of marginal zinc deficiency (Institute of Medicine, 2001).

A different approach to the assessment of zinc status has been the measurement of the activity of zinc-dependent enzymes such as angiotensin converting enzyme (ACE) or extracellular SOD. However, similar to plasma zinc concentrations, measurements of the above enzyme activities have not been shown to be sensitive to conditions of marginal zinc status. Zinc-regulated genes have also been proposed to be useful as indices of zinc status. In this regard the assessment of MT concentrations, as well as MT mRNA concentrations, in circulating cells (erythrocytes, reticulocytes, and monocytes) have shown promise;

however, the widespread use of this approach has been limited by difficulties in developing assays that can be easily employed (Cao and Cousins, 2000; Liuzzi and Cousins, 2004). The concentrations of certain hormones and growth factors, such as growth hormone and IGF, have also been proposed to be sensitive to zinc status; however, these markers show little specificity.

Given the above, a suite of markers, as opposed to single markers, may more accurately reflect zinc status (Lowe et al., 2009). As an example of this, it is known that zinc deficiency can result in hypogeusia (taste impairment). A report by Takeda et al. (2004) found that, in patients with zinc-deficiency-related hypogeusia, serum zinc concentrations were within the normal range; however, the ratio of ACE activity (apo-ACE/holo-ACE) was a more sensitive indicator of zinc status than serum zinc. The discovery of the ZnT (SLC30/CDF) and ZIP (Zrt/IRT-like proteins) families of zinc transporters involved in the regulation, export, and import of zinc in a variety of tissues prompts the question of whether the protein or mRNA of a suite of these proteins can be used as biomarkers for zinc status. Using quantitative real-time polymerase chain reaction (RT-PCR), it has been shown that modest dietary zinc supplementation in humans (15 mg zinc/day for 10 days) increased MT and ZnT1 mRNA, and decreased Zip3 mRNA in dried spots of whole blood, indicating that these targets were responsive to zinc supplementation (Aydemir et al., 2006).

Food and Other Sources of Zinc

Foods can differ widely in their zinc content. For example, zinc concentrations range from 0.03 mg/100 g egg white, to 1 mg/100 g chicken meat, to 75 mg/100 g oysters. Shellfish, beef, and other red meats are good zinc sources, as are nuts and legumes (USDA, 2010). Whole-grain cereals are relatively rich in zinc, and are the primary plant source of zinc (USDA, 2010). Zinc is mostly contained in the bran and germ portions, thus, nearly 80% of the total zinc in these foodstuffs can be lost in the wheat milling process (Hambidge et al., 1986). There is no standard enrichment policy for zinc but some breakfast cereal manufacturers fortify the zinc content of their product in amounts ranging from 25% to 100% of the United States RDA, depending on the end consumer. Apart from fortification, other strategies include enhancing agricultural practices so that the ratio of zinc to phytate is increased. For example, plant zinc concentrations may be enhanced if grown in zinc-rich soil or treated with zinc-rich fertilizers (Cakmak, 2008).

The availability of zinc in the United States food supply has been estimated at 16.2 mg per capita per day (USDA 2005). As noted above, total dietary zinc intakes will be influenced greatly by an individual's food choices. Animal products, especially meat, provide about 70% of the zinc consumed by the average individual in the United States. Frequently, zinc intakes are correlated with protein intake, but the exact relationship is influenced by protein source. For example, diets consisting primarily of eggs, milk, poultry, and fish have a lower zinc to protein ratio than those composed of shellfish, beef, and other red meats. Similar variations occur in vegetarian diets in that diets with a high zinc to protein ratio contain liberal quantities of legumes, whole grains, nuts, and cheese, whereas diets that are based on fruits and vegetables have relatively low zinc to protein ratios. Mean intakes from adult self-selected mixed diets in the United States have been reported to range from 9.5 to 15.4 mg zinc/day (Institute of Medicine, 2001). During the first 6 months of life, zinc intake varies with the mode of feeding. Zinc intake in breast-fed infants tends to decline over the first year of life from 2.3 mg/day at 1 month of age to 0.94 mg/day at 6 months (Institute of Medicine, 2001); formula-fed infants consume approximately 5.5 mg/day between 2 and 11 months of age (Briefel et al., 2000). The zinc content of commercial infant formulas depends on the fortification policy of the manufacturer, but still contributes substantially to daily zinc intake (Arsenault and Brown, 2003). Children 1 to 8 years old consume 6.9 to 9 mg/day and girls and boys (9–13 years old) report daily intakes of about 9.6 to 11.8 mg; the daily intake of adolescents (14 to 18 years) is reported as approximately 9.3 mg for girls and 15.1 mg for boys. The range of intake for elderly populations is 8.6 to 13.8 mg/day (Briefel et al., 2000; Institute of Medicine, 2001). Due to supplement use by pregnant and lactating women, zinc intakes are often higher in these groups, 9.2 mg and 10.4 mg, respectively, than the reported 8.5 mg/day for adult women (Briefel et al., 2000; Institute of Medicine, 2001) .

The bioavailability of zinc can be significantly affected by other diet constituents, thus it is important to note that simple calculations of dietary zinc intakes can be misleading with respect to the prediction of the zinc status of an individual. Such calculations are of value, however, with respect to the identification of potential at-risk populations. As an example, in a diet survey of pregnant Hispanic women living in an agricultural region of California, it was estimated that approximately 45% of the women surveyed had dietary zinc intakes that were below the EAR for this population group (9.5 mg zinc/day) (Harley et al., 2005). Based on this finding, one interpretation is that marginal zinc deficiency is a significant health problem in many countries, including the United States, and that studies aimed at the assessment of zinc status in such population groups would clearly be warranted. However, as part of their survey, the above investigators also collected information regarding supplement use. When the zinc provided by the supplements was added to the estimated zinc intake from food, the percentage of women who had combined zinc intakes from food and supplements below the EAR fell to 4.5% (Harley et al., 2005). The above illustrates the importance of considering the zinc intake from supplements, as well as the potential use of fortified functional food products.

Excess and Toxicity

Although rare, cases of acute zinc toxicity in humans resulting from exposure to excessive amounts of zinc have been reported. Exposure to zinc can occur through three routes: through the skin, by inhalation, and by ingestion. Dermal exposure to zinc is not thought to represent a significant toxicological risk. Metal fume fever is considered to be the most common form of zinc toxicosis through inhalation. This disease occurs as a consequence of the inhalation of zinc-containing smoke, which typically contains zinc oxide. Signs can develop within 8 hours and include hyperpnoea, profuse sweating, and general weakness. Signs of acute zinc toxicity have been reported to disappear within 1–4 days after the individual is removed from the zinc-contaminated environment (Plum et al., 2010).

With respect to zinc toxicity due to excessive ingestion of zinc in the diet, or the ingestion of non-food zinc-containing products, isolated outbreaks of zinc toxicity have occurred as a result of the consumption of foods and beverages contaminated with zinc released from galvanized containers. Typical signs of acute zinc toxicosis include abdominal pain, diarrhea, nausea, and vomiting (Fosmire, 1990; Plum et al., 2010). Doses of zinc in excess of 200 mg/day are typically emetic. A fatal outcome was reported in a woman who was inadvertently given 1.5 g of zinc intravenously over a 3-day period. It can be noted that, in companion animals, zinc toxicity can result from the consumption of zinc-galvanized nuts and bolts or die-cast toys, and of coins, specifically, US and Canadian pennies minted after 1987 and between 1997 and 2001, respectively (Cummings and Kovacic, 2009).

The long-term consumption of zinc supplements in excess of 150 mg/day has been reported to result in low serum HDL levels, gastric erosion, and depressed immune function (Fosmire, 1990; Plum *et al.*, 2010). The major reported consequence of the long-term excessive ingestion of zinc supplements is the induction of secondary copper deficiency, which is thought to be due to the competitive interaction between these elements with regard to intestinal absorption (Plum *et al.*, 2010). Relatively low levels of dietary zinc can interfere with copper absorption. An intake of 18.5 mg/day for 2 weeks was reported to increase copper excretion in the feces (Festa *et al.*, 1985). Ten weeks of zinc supplementation at 50 mg/day was reported to result in reductions in erythrocyte copper–zinc SOD activity (Yadrick *et al.*, 1989). Sickle cell patients given zinc supplements of 150 mg/day were reported to be characterized by hypocupremia (Prasad *et al.*, 1978). Based on the ability of zinc to reduce the gastrointestinal uptake of copper, in 1997, zinc acetate was approved by the US Food and Drug Administration for the treatment of Wilson's disease, an inborn error of copper metabolism that causes excessive tissue accumulation of copper (Anderson *et al.*, 1998). It is important to note that over-aggressive use of zinc supplements in the treatment of Wilson's disease can result in a copper deficiency (Horvath *et al.*, 2010).

Recently, additional potential sources of excessive zinc in the environment have been identified. Several investigators have suggested that the excessive use of denture creams that contain zinc may represent a toxicological risk as they may contribute to the development of a copper deficiency (Nations *et al.*, 2008; Tezvergil-Mutluay *et al.*, 2010; Barton *et al.*, 2011). Given the significant number of individuals who use denture cream, the above hypothesis merits investigation. Similar concerns potentially exist for the use of zinc lozenges for colds. While current recommendations are for a brief period of use (Singh and Das, 2011) at a total recommended daily dose (i.e. 80 mg/day for 3–7 days), a number of side-effects have been reported in studies, including nausea (Das and Singh, 2011; Singh and Das, 2011). As with the excessive use of denture creams, there is the potential for a reduction in copper status if zinc lozenges are consumed in large amounts for

a prolonged period of time, such as might occur if an individual takes them prophylactically during the cold season, or if an individual consumes lozenges in amounts that exceed what is recommended. Another potential source of excessive zinc in the environment that has been identified is zinc oxide nanoparticles, which are used in a number of industries. Preliminary data suggest that these particles are occurring at increasing concentrations in several foodstuffs and water sources and have been shown to be cytotoxic in some in vitro models (Croteau *et al.*, 2011; Som *et al.*, 2011). Given their widespread use, the potential human health risks of zinc nanoparticles are an area that also demands research.

Observations that high amounts of zinc in the diet can result in reductions in copper uptake, and potentially copper deficiency, were critical in the setting of the current UL values for zinc in the United States and Canada. Based on the report by Yadrick *et al.* (1989) that young women who had daily dietary zinc intakes over a period of 10 weeks of the order of 60 mg (50 mg provided through the consumption of zinc supplements and approximately 10 mg provided by the foods typically consumed by the individuals) were characterized by reductions in erythrocyte SOD activity, a lowest observed adverse effect level (LOAEL) of 60 mg/day for dietary zinc was determined. After using an uncertainty factor of 1.5, a UL of 40 mg/day was identified for adult men and women.

While the logic that drove the current UL for zinc is certainly reasonable, it is critical to note that the UL value was in essence derived from a study in which the majority of "dietary" zinc was obtained from a dietary supplement. There is a need for additional studies that can provide more information on LOAELs for zinc when different types of zinc supplements are used, or when naturally occurring high zinc foods, as well as zinc-fortified foods, are included in the diet. Underscoring the need for such studies is the observation that the use of dietary supplements is widespread in many developed countries (Bailey *et al.*, 2011). Zinc-containing supplements in particular are being widely used for multiple purposes ranging from the desire to improve athletic performance or cognitive skills, to the perceived need to reduce the onset and progression of a vast array of chronic diseases as well as the common cold. When coupled with the observation that suboptimal zinc status may represent a significant public health concern in select populations, there is a clear need for more work aimed at the evaluation of what constitutes a "safe and appropriate" intake of zinc. Of critical importance in such studies will be the need also to better define the extent to which an individual's dietary copper intake, and copper status, influence their response to "high" zinc diets.

Future Directions

Our knowledge of the metabolism of zinc and its physiological roles has been significantly advanced over the past decade. However, there are still major gaps in our understanding of zinc metabolism on several fronts. The homeostatic mechanisms that help regulate tissue and cellular zinc concentrations are still not well characterized. Similarly, there is minimal information regarding how subtle changes in intracellular and extracellular zinc pools contribute to metabolic regulation. In contrast to early literature that suggested that zinc deficiency, as well as zinc toxicity, were relatively rare events, recent literature suggests that zinc deficiency may be common in certain populations, and there is emerging evidence that zinc toxicity may also increasingly be a public health concern. The above has resulted in a stimulation of research that is focused on better defining the short- and long-term consequences of not just severe zinc deficiency and toxicity, but also the effects associated with marginal deficits or excesses of this essential nutrient. Critical to the above work will be the identification of suites of biomarkers that, when combined, can give an accurate indication of zinc status.

Suggestions for Further Reading

Lichten, L.A. and Cousins, R.J. (2009) Mammalian zinc transporters: nutritional and physiologic regulation. *Annu Rev Nutr* **29**, 153–176.

Lowe, N.M., Fekete, K., and Decsi, T. (2009) Methods of assessment of zinc status in humans: a systematic review. *Am J Clin Nutr* **89**, 2040S–2051S.

Plum, L.M., Rink, L., and Haase, H. (2010) The essential toxin: impact of zinc on human health. *Int J Environ Res Public Health* **7**, 1342–1365.

Uriu-Adams, J.Y. and Keen, C.L. (2010) Zinc and reproduction: effects of zinc deficiency on prenatal and early postnatal development. *Birth Defects Res B Dev Reprod Toxicol* **89**, 313–325.

References

Aamodt, R.L., Rumble, W.F., Babcock, A.K., *et al.* (1982) Effects of oral zinc loading on zinc metabolism in humans—I: Experimental studies. *Metabolism* **31**, 326–334.

Afridi, H.I., Kazi, T.G., Kazi, N., *et al.* (2011) Interactions between cadmium and zinc in the biological samples of Pakistani smokers and nonsmokers cardiovascular disease patients. *Biol Trace Elem Res* **139**, 257–268.

Aggett, P.J. (1989) Severe zinc deficiency. In C.F. Mills (ed.), *Zinc in Human Biology*. International Life Sciences Institute, London, pp. 259–279.

Aimo, L., Mackenzie, G.G., Keenan, A.H., *et al.* (2010) Gestational zinc deficiency affects the regulation of transcription factors AP-1, NF-kappaB and NFAT in fetal brain. *J Nutr Biochem* **11**, 1069–1075.

Anderson, L.A., Hakojarvi, S.L., and Boudreaux, S.K. (1998) Zinc acetate treatment in Wilson's disease. *Ann Pharmacother* **32**, 78–87.

Andreini, C., Banci, L., Bertini, I., *et al.* (2006) Counting the zinc-proteins encoded in the human genome. *J Proteome Res* **5**, 196–201.

Apgar, J. (1985) Zinc and reproduction. *Annu Rev Nutr* **5**, 43–68.

Arsenault, J.E. and Brown, K.H. (2003) Zinc intake of US preschool children exceeds new dietary reference intakes. *Am J Clin Nutr* **78**, 1011–1017.

Aydemir, T.B., Blanchard, R.K., and Cousins, R.J. (2006) Zinc supplementation of young men alters metallothionein, zinc transporter, and cytokine gene expression in leukocyte populations. *Proc Natl Acad Sci USA* **103**, 1699–1704.

Baer, M.T. and King, J.C. (1984) Tissue zinc levels and zinc excretion during experimental zinc depletion in young men. *Am J Clin Nutr* **39**, 556–570.

Bailey, R.L., Gahche, J.J., Lentino, C.V., *et al.* (2011) Dietary supplement use in the United States, 2003–2006. *J Nutr* **141**, 261–266.

Barton, A.L., Fisher, R.A., and Smith, G.D. (2011) Zinc poisoning from excessive denture fixative use masquerading as myelopolyneuropathy and hypocupraemia. *Ann Clin Biochem* **48**, 383–385

Beach, R.S., Gershwin, M.E., and Hurley, L.S. (1982) Gestational zinc deprivation in mice: persistence of immunodeficiency for three generations. *Science* **218**, 469–471.

Beletate, V., El Dib, R.P., and Atallah, A.N. (2007) Zinc supplementation for the prevention of type 2 diabetes mellitus. *Cochrane Database Syst Rev* CD005525.

Berni Canani, R., Buccigrossi, V., and Passariello, A. (2010) Mechanisms of action of zinc in acute diarrhea. *Curr Opin Gastroenterol* **27**, 8–12.

Beyersmann, D. and Haase, H. (2001) Functions of zinc in signaling, proliferation and differentiation of mammalian cells. *Biometals* **14**, 331–341.

Briefel, R.R., Bialostosky, K., Kennedy-Stephenson, J., *et al.* (2000) Zinc intake of the US population: findings from the third National Health and Nutrition Examination Survey, 1988–1994. *J Nutr* **130**, 1367S–1373S.

Brown, K.H., Peerson, J.M., Rivera, J., *et al.*. (2002) Effect of supplemental zinc on the growth and serum zinc concentrations of prepubertal children: a meta-analysis of randomized controlled trials. *Am J Clin Nutr* **75**, 1062–1071.

Cakmak, I. (2008) Enrichment of cereal grains with zinc: agronomic or genetic biofortification? *Plant Soil* **302**, 1–17.

Campbell, N.R. (1996) How safe are folic acid supplements? *Arch Intern Med* **156**, 1638–1644.

Cao, J. and Cousins, R.J. (2000) Metallothionein mRNA in monocytes and peripheral blood mononuclear cells and in cells from dried blood spots increases after zinc supplementation of men. *J Nutr* **130**, 2180–2187.

Christian, P. and West, K.P., Jr (1998) Interactions between zinc and vitamin A: an update. *Am J Clin Nutr* **68**, 435S–441S.

Chung, C.S., Stookey, J., Dare, D., *et al.* (2008) Current dietary zinc intake has a greater effect on fractional zinc absorption than does longer term zinc consumption in healthy adult men. *Am J Clin Nutr* **87**, 1224–1229.

Clegg, M.S., Hanna, L.A., Niles, B.J., *et al.* (2005) Zinc deficiency-induced cell death. *IUBMB Life* **57**, 661–669.

Coppen, D.E. and Davies, N.T. (1987) Studies on the effects of dietary zinc dose on 65Zn absorption in vivo and on the effects of Zn status on 65Zn absorption and body loss in young rats. *Br J Nutr* **57**, 35–44.

Cousins, R.J. (2010) Gastrointestinal factors influencing zinc absorption and homeostasis. *Int J Vitam Nutr Res* **80**, 243–248.

Cousins, R.J., Liuzzi, J.P., and Lichten, L.A. (2006) Mammalian zinc transport, trafficking, and signals. *J Biol Chem* **281**, 24085–24089.

Cragg, R.A., Phillips, S.R., Piper, J.M., *et al.* (2005) Homeostatic regulation of zinc transporters in the human small intestine by dietary zinc supplementation. *Gut* **54**, 469–478.

Croteau, M.N., Dybowska, A.D., Luoma, S.N., *et al.* (2011) A novel approach reveals that zinc oxide nanoparticles are bioavailable and toxic after dietary exposures. *Nanotoxicology*, **5**, 79–90.

Cummings, J.E. and Kovacic, J.P. (2009) The ubiquitous role of zinc in health and disease. *J Vet Emerg Crit Care (San Antonio)* **19**, 215–240.

Das, R.R. and Singh, M. (2011) Zinc lozenges for the common cold: should we ignore the side-effects? *Med Hypotheses* **77**, 308–309.

Donangelo, C.M., Zapata, C.L., Woodhouse, L.R., *et al.* (2005) Zinc absorption and kinetics during pregnancy and lactation in Brazilian women. *Am J Clin Nutr* **82**, 118–124.

Duffy, J.Y., Overmann, G.J., Keen, C.L., *et al.* (2004) Cardiac abnormalities induced by zinc deficiency are associated with alterations in the expression of genes regulated by the zinc-finger transcription factor GATA-4. *Birth Defects Res B Dev Reprod Toxicol* **71**, 102–109.

Eby, G.A., 3rd (2010) Zinc lozenges as cure for the common cold – a review and hypothesis. *Med Hypotheses* **74**, 482–492.

Eide, D.J. (2006) Zinc transporters and the cellular trafficking of zinc. *Biochim Biophys Acta* **1763**, 711–722.

Failla, M.L. and Kiser, R.A. (1983) Hepatic and renal metabolism of copper and zinc in the diabetic rat. *Am J Physiol* **244**, E115–121.

Fairweather-Tait, S.J., Harvey, L.J., and Ford, D. (2008) Does ageing affect zinc homeostasis and dietary requirements? *Exp Gerontol* **43**, 382–388.

Festa, M.D., Anderson, H.L., Dowdy, R.P., *et al.* (1985) Effect of zinc intake on copper excretion and retention in men. *Am J Clin Nutr* **41**, 285–292.

Finamore, A., Roselli, M., Merendino, N., *et al.* (2003) Zinc deficiency suppresses the development of oral tolerance in rats. *J Nutr* **133**, 191–198.

Fosmire, G.J. (1990) Zinc toxicity. *Am J Clin Nutr* **51**, 225–227.

Foster, M. and Samman, S. (2010) Zinc and redox signaling: perturbations associated with cardiovascular disease and diabetes mellitus. *Antioxid Redox Signal* **13**, 1549–1573.

Fraker, P.J. and King, L.E. (2004) Reprogramming of the immune system during zinc deficiency. *Annu Rev Nutr* **24**, 277–298.

Fukada, T., Yamasaki, S., Nishida, K., *et al.* (2011) Zinc homeostasis and signaling in health and diseases : zinc signaling. *J Biol Inorg Chem* PMID 21660546.

Gibson, R.S., Hess, S.Y., Hotz, C., *et al.* (2008) Indicators of zinc status at the population level: a review of the evidence. *Br J Nutr* **99** (Suppl 3), S14–23.

Goyer, R.A. (1997) Toxic and essential metal interactions. *Annu Rev Nutr* **17**, 37–50.

Grahn, B.H., Paterson, P.G., Gottschall-Pass, K.T., *et al.* (2001) Zinc and the eye. *J Am Coll Nutr* **20**, 106–118.

Haase, H. and Rink, L. (2009) Functional significance of zinc-related signaling pathways in immune cells. *Annu Rev Nutr* **29**, 133–152.

Hambidge, K.M., Casey, C.E., and Krebs, N.F. (1986) *Zinc*. Academic Press, Orlando, FL.

Hambidge, K.M., Miller, L.V., Westcott, J.E., *et al.* (2010) Zinc bioavailability and homeostasis. *Am J Clin Nutr* **91**, 1478S–1483S.

Hambidge, M. (2000) Human zinc deficiency. *J Nutr* **130**, 1344S–139S.

Harley, K., Eskenazi, B., and Block, G. (2005) The association of time in the US and diet during pregnancy in low-income women of Mexican descent. *Paediatr Perinat Epidemiol* **19**, 125–134.

Hartwig, A. (2001) Zinc finger proteins as potential targets for toxic metal ions: differential effects on structure and function. *Antioxid Redox Signal* **3**, 625–634.

He, L., Wang, B., Hay, E.B., *et al.* (2009) Discovery of ZIP transporters that participate in cadmium damage to testis and kidney. *Toxicol Appl Pharmacol* **238**, 250–257.

Hess, F.M., King, J.C., and Margen, S. (1977) Zinc excretion in young women on low zinc intakes and oral contraceptive agents. *J Nutr* **107**, 1610–1620.

Hoadley, J.E., Leinart, A.S., and Cousins, R.J. (1987) Kinetic analysis of zinc uptake and serosal transfer by vascularly perfused rat intestine. *Am J Physiol* **252**, G825–831.

Hodkinson, C.F., Kelly, M., Alexander, H.D., *et al.* (2007) Effect of zinc supplementation on the immune status of healthy older individuals aged 55–70 years: the ZENITH Study. *J Gerontol A Biol Sci Med Sci* **62**, 598–608.

Honscheid, A., Dubben, S., Rink, L., *et al.* (2011) Zinc differentially regulates mitogen-activated protein kinases in human T cells. *J Nutr Biochem*. PMID 21333516

Horvath, J., Beris, P., Giostra, E., *et al.* (2010) Zinc-induced copper deficiency in Wilson disease. *J Neurol Neurosurg Psychiatry* **81**, 1410–1411.

Hurley, L.S., Gordon, P., Keen, C.L., *et al.* (1982) Circadian variation in rat plasma zinc and rapid effect of dietary zinc deficiency. *Proc Soc Exp Biol Med* **170**, 48–52.

Ibs, K.H. and Rink, L. (2003) Zinc-altered immune function. *J Nutr* **133**, 1452S–1456S.

Institute of Medicine (2001) *Dietary Reference Intakes for Vitamin A, Vitamin K, Arsenic, Boron, Chromium, Copper, Iodine, Iron, Manganese, Molybdenum, Nickel, Silicon, Vanadium, and Zinc.* National Academy Press, Washington, DC.

Islam, M.S. and Loots, D.T. (2007) Diabetes, metallothionein, and zinc interactions: a review. *Biofactors* **29**, 203–212.

Jackson, M. (1989) Physiology of zinc: general aspects. In C.F. Mills (ed.), *Zinc in Human Biology*. Springer-Verlag, New York, pp. 1–14.

Jackson, M.J., Jones, D.A., Edwards, R.H., *et al.* (1984) Zinc homeostasis in man: studies using a new stable isotope-dilution technique. *Br J Nutr* **51**, 199–208.

Jameson, S. (1976) Variations in maternal serum zinc during pregnancy and correlation to congenital malformations, dysmaturity, and abnormal parturition. *Acta Med Scand (Suppl)* **593**, 21–37.

Jansen, J., Karges, W., and Rink, L. (2009) Zinc and diabetes – clinical links and molecular mechanisms. *J Nutr Biochem* **20**, 399–417.

Johnson, M.A., Baier, M.J., and Greger, J.L. (1982) Effects of dietary tin on zinc, copper, iron, manganese, and magnesium metabolism of adult males. *Am J Clin Nutr* **35**, 1332–1338.

Kang, Y.J. and Zhou, Z. (2005) Zinc prevention and treatment of alcoholic liver disease. *Mol Aspects Med* **26**, 391–404.

Kazi, T.G., Wadhwa, S.K., Afridi, H.I., *et al.* (2010) Interaction of cadmium and zinc in biological samples of smokers and chewing tobacco female mouth cancer patients. *J Hazard Mater* **176**, 985–991.

Keen, C.L. and Gershwin, M.E. (1990) Zinc deficiency and immune function. *Ann Rev Nutr* **10**, 415–431.

Keen, C.L. and Hurley, L.S. (1989) Zinc and reproduction: effects of deficiency on fetal and postnatal development. In C.F. Mills (ed.), *Zinc in Human Biology*. Springer-Verlag, New York, pp. 183–220.

Keen, C.L., Uriu-Adams, J.Y., Skalny, A., *et al.* (2010) The plausibility of maternal nutritional status being a contributing factor to the risk for fetal alcohol spectrum disorders: the potential influence of zinc status as an example. *Biofactors* **36**, 125–35.

Kelleher, S.L. and Lonnerdal, B. (2009) Nutrient transfer: mammary gland regulation. *Adv Exp Med Biol* **639**, 15–27.

Kiilerich, S., Christensen, M.S., Naestoft, J., *et al.* (1980) Determination of zinc in serum and urine by atomic absorption spectrophotometry; relationship between serum levels of zinc and proteins in 104 normal subjects. *Clin Chim Acta* **105**, 231–239.

King, J.C. (2000) Determinants of maternal zinc status during pregnancy. *Am J Clin Nutr* **71**, 1334S–1343S.

King, J.C. (2010) Does zinc absorption reflect zinc status? *Int J Vitam Nutr Res* **80**, 300–306.

King, J.C. (2011) Zinc: an essential but elusive nutrient. *Am J Clin Nutr* **94**, 679S–684S

King, J.C., Shames, D.M., and Woodhouse, L.R. (2000) Zinc homeostasis in humans. *J Nutr* **130**, 1360S–1366S.

Klug, A. (2010) The discovery of zinc fingers and their applications in gene regulation and genome manipulation. *Annu Rev Biochem* **79**, 213–231.

Krebs, N.F. (2000) Overview of zinc absorption and excretion in the human gastrointestinal tract. *J Nutr* **130**, 1374S–1377S.

Laity, J.H. and Andrews, G.K. (2007) Understanding the mechanisms of zinc-sensing by metal-response element binding transcription factor-1 (MTF-1). *Arch Biochem Biophys* **463**, 201–210.

Lee, H.H., Prasad, A.S., Brewer, G.J., *et al.* (1989) Zinc absorption in human small intestine. *Am J Physiol* **256**, G87–91.

Lichten, L.A. and Cousins, R.J. (2009) Mammalian zinc transporters: nutritional and physiologic regulation. *Annu Rev Nutr* **29**, 153–176.

Liuzzi, J.P. and Cousins, R.J. (2004) Mammalian zinc transporters. *Annu Rev Nutr* **24**, 151–172.

Liuzzi, J.P., Lichten, L.A., Rivera, S., *et al.* (2005) Interleukin-6 regulates the zinc transporter Zip14 in liver and contributes to the hypozincemia of the acute-phase response. *Proc Natl Acad Sci USA* **102**, 6843–6848.

Lonnerdal, B. (2000) Dietary factors influencing zinc absorption. *J Nutr* **130**, 1378S–1383S.

Lonnerdal, B., Mendoza, C., Brown, K.H., *et al.* (2011) Zinc absorption from low phytic acid genotypes of maize (*Zea mays* L.), barley (*Hordeum vulgare* L.), and rice (*Oryza sativa* L.) assessed in a suckling rat pup model. *J Agric Food Chem* **59**, 4755–4762.

Lowe, N.M., Fekete, K., and Decsi, T. (2009) Methods of assessment of zinc status in humans: a systematic review. *Am J Clin Nutr* **89**, 2040S–2051S.

Mackenzie, G.G., Keen, C.L., and Oteiza, P. I. (2002) Zinc status of human IMR-32 neuroblastoma cells influences their susceptibility to iron-induced oxidative stress. *Dev Neurosci* **24**, 125–133.

Maret, W. (2006) Zinc coordination environments in proteins as redox sensors and signal transducers. *Antioxid Redox Signal* **8**, 1419–1441.

Maret, W. and Li, Y. (2009) Coordination dynamics of zinc in proteins. *Chem Rev* **109**, 4682–4707.

Matthews, J.M. and Sunde, M. (2002) Zinc fingers—folds for many occasions. *IUBMB Life* **54**, 351–355.

McCall, K.A., Huang, C., and Fierke, C.A. (2000) Function and mechanism of zinc metalloenzymes. *J Nutr* **130**, 1437S–1446S.

McMillan, E.M. and Rowe, D.J. (1982) Clinical significance of diurnal variation in the estimation of plasma zinc. *Clin Exp Dermatol* **7**, 629–632.

Messner, B., Knoflach, M., Seubert, A., *et al.* (2009) Cadmium is a novel and independent risk factor for early atherosclerosis mechanisms and in vivo relevance. *Arterioscler Thromb Vasc Biol* **29**, 1392–1398.

Meunier, N., O'Connor, J.M., Maiani, G., *et al.* (2005) Importance of zinc in the elderly: the ZENITH study. *Eur J Clin Nutr* **59** (Suppl 2), S1–4.

Milne, D.B., Canfield, W.K., Mahalko, J.R., *et al.* (1984) Effect of oral folic acid supplements on zinc, copper, and iron absorption and excretion. *Am J Clin Nutr* **39**, 535–539.

Milne, D.B., Ralston, N.V., and Wallwork, J.C. (1985) Zinc content of cellular components of blood: methods for cell separation and analysis evaluated. *Clin Chem* **31**, 65–69.

Mocchegiani, E., Giacconi, R., Cipriano, C., *et al.* (2009) NK and NKT cells in aging and longevity: role of zinc and metallothioneins. *J Clin Immunol* **29**, 416–425.

Nations, S.P., Boyer, P.J., Love, L.A., *et al.* (2008) Denture cream: an unusual source of excess zinc, leading to hypocupremia and neurologic disease. *Neurology* **71**, 639–643.

Nishida, K., Hasegawa, A., Nakae, S., *et al.* (2009) Zinc transporter Znt5/Slc30a5 is required for the mast cell-mediated delayed-type allergic reaction but not the immediate-type reaction. *J Exp Med* **206**, 1351–1364.

O'Dell, B.L. (2000) Role of zinc in plasma membrane function. *J Nutr* **130**, 1432S–1436S.

O'Dell, B.L. and Reeves, P. (1989) Zinc status and food intake. In C. F. Mills (ed.), *Zinc in Human Biology.* International Life Sciences Institute, London, pp. 173–182.

Ohinata, K., Takemoto, M., Kawanago, M., *et al.* (2009) Orally administered zinc increases food intake via vagal stimulation in rats. *J Nutr* **139**, 611–616.

Overbeck, S., Uciechowski, P., Ackland, M.L., *et al.* (2008) Intracellular zinc homeostasis in leukocyte subsets is regulated by different expression of zinc exporters ZnT-1 to ZnT-9. *J Leukoc Biol* **83**, 368–380.

Padwal, R., Klarenbach, S., Wiebe, N., *et al.* (2011) Bariatric surgery: a systematic review of the clinical and economic evidence. *J Gen Intern Med* PMID 21538168.

Plum, L.M., Rink, L., and Haase, H. (2010) The essential toxin: impact of zinc on human health. *Int J Environ Res Public Health* **7**, 1342–1365.

Prasad, A.S., Brewer, G.J., Schoomaker, E.B., *et al.* (1978) Hypocupremia induced by zinc therapy in adults. *JAMA* **240**, 2166–2168.

Prasad, A.S., Halsted, J.A., and Nadimi, M. (1961) Syndrome of iron deficiency anemia, hepatosplenomegaly, hypogonadism, dwarfism and geophagia. *Am J Med* **31**, 532–546.

Rink, L. and Gabriel, P. (2001) Extracellular and immunological actions of zinc. *Biometals* **14**, 367–383.

Salle, A., Demarsy, D., Poirier, A.L., *et al.* (2010) Zinc deficiency: a frequent and underestimated complication after bariatric surgery. *Obes Surg* **20**, 1660–1670.

Sandstrom, B. and Lonnerdal, B. (1989) Promoters and antagonists of zinc absorption. In C.F. Mills (ed.), *Zinc in Human Biology.* International Life Sciences Institute, London, pp. 57–78.

Scholmerich, J., Freudemann, A., Kottgen, E., *et al.* (1987) Bioavailability of zinc from zinc–histidine complexes. I. Comparison with zinc sulfate in healthy men. *Am J Clin Nutr* **45**, 1480–1486.

Schroeder, J.J. and Cousins, R.J. (1990) Interleukin 6 regulates metallothionein gene expression and zinc metabolism in hepatocyte monolayer cultures. *Proc Natl Acad Sci USA* **87**, 3137–3141.

Sekler, I., Sensi, S.L., Hershfinkel, M., *et al.* (2007) Mechanism and regulation of cellular zinc transport. *Mol Med* **13**, 337–343.

Singh, M. and Das, R.R. (2011) Zinc for the common cold. *Cochrane Database Syst Rev* CD001364.

Som, C., Wick, P., Krug, H., *et al.* (2011) Environmental and health effects of nanomaterials in nanotextiles and facade coatings. *Environ Int* **37**, 1131–1142

Song, Y., Chung, C.S., Bruno, R.S., *et al.* (2009) Dietary zinc restriction and repletion affects DNA integrity in healthy men. *Am J Clin Nutr* **90**, 321–328.

Song, Y., Elias, V., Loban, A., *et al.* (2010.) Marginal zinc deficiency increases oxidative DNA damage in the prostate after chronic exercise. *Free Radic Biol Med* **48**, 82–88.

Stefanidou, M., Maravelias, C., Dona, A., *et al.* (2006) Zinc: a multipurpose trace element. *Arch Toxicol* **80**, 1–9.

Swanson, C.A. and King, J.C. (1987) Zinc and pregnancy outcome. *Am J Clin Nutr* **46,** 763–771.

Takeda, A. and Tamano, H. (2010) Zinc signaling through glucocorticoid and glutamate signaling in stressful circumstances. *J Neurosci Res* **88**, 3002–3010.

Takeda, N., Takaoka, T., Ueda, C., *et al.* (2004) Zinc deficiency in patients with idiopathic taste impairment with regard to angiotensin converting enzyme activity. *Auris Nasus Larynx* **31**, 425–428.

Tapiero, H. and Tew, K.D. (2003) Trace elements in human physiology and pathology: zinc and metallothioneins. *Biomed Pharmacother* **57**, 399–411.

Tezvergil-Mutluay, A., Carvalho, R.M., and Pashley, D.H. (2010) Hyperzincemia from ingestion of denture adhesives. *J Prosthet Dent* **103**, 380–383.

Todd, W.R., Elvehjem, C.A., and Hart, E.B. (1933) Zinc in the nutrition of the rat. *Am J Physiol* **107**, 146–156.

Tomat, E. and Lippard, S.J. (2010) Imaging mobile zinc in biology. *Curr Opin Chem Biol* **14**, 225–230.

Tomat, A., Elesgaray, R., Zago, V., *et al.* (2010) Exposure to zinc deficiency in fetal and postnatal life determines nitric oxide system activity and arterial blood pressure levels in adult rats. *Br J Nutr* **104**, 382–389.

Tomat, A.L., Costa, L., and Arranz, C.T. (2011) Zinc restriction during different periods of life: influence in renal and cardiovascular diseases. *Nutrition* **27**, 392–398.

Tuerk, M.J. and Fazel, N. (2009) Zinc deficiency. *Curr Opin Gastroenterol* **25**, 136–143.

Uriu-Adams, J.Y. and Keen, C.L. (2010) Zinc and reproduction: effects of zinc deficiency on prenatal and early postnatal development. *Birth Defects Res B Dev Reprod Toxicol* **89**, 313–325.

Uriu-Hare, J.Y., Stern, J.S., and Keen, C.L. (1989) Influence of maternal dietary Zn intake on expression of diabetes-induced teratogenicity in rats. *Diabetes* **38**, 1282–1290.

US Department of Agriculture (2010) Agricultural Research Service, USDA National Nutrient Database for Standard Reference, Release 23. http://www.ars.usda.gov/ba/bhnrc/ndl.

US Department of Agriculture (2005) Center for Nutrition Policy and Promotion, Nutrient Content of the US Food Supply. http://www.cnpp.usda.gov/Publications/FoodSupply/FoodSupply2005Report.pdf.

Vallee, B. (1983) Zinc in biology and biochemistry. In T. Spiro (ed.), *Zinc Enzymes.* John Wiley, New York, pp. 1–24.

Vallee, B.L. and Auld, D.S. (1990) Zinc coordination, function, and structure of zinc enzymes and other proteins. *Biochemistry* **29**, 5647–5659.

Victery, W., Smith, J.M., and Vander, A.J. (1981) Renal tubular handling of zinc in the dog. *Am J Physiol* **241**, F532–539.

Walter, R.M., Uriu-Hare, J.Y., Olin, K.L., *et al.* (1991) Copper, zinc, manganese, and magnesium status and complications of diabetes mellitus. *Diabetes Care* **14**, 1050–1056.

Wang, X. and Zhou, B. (2010) Dietary zinc absorption: a play of Zips and ZnTs in the gut. *IUBMB Life* **62**, 176–182.

Wastney, M.E. and House, W.A. (2008) Development of a compartmental model of zinc kinetics in mice. *J Nutr* **138**, 2148–2155.

WHO (2002) *The World Health Report: Reducing Risks, Promoting Healthy Life.* World Health Organization, Geneva.

Willson, R.L. (1989) Zinc and iron in free radical pathology and cellular control. In C.F. Mills (ed.), *Zinc in Human Biology.* Springer-Verlag, New York, pp. 147–172.

Yadrick, M.K., Kenney, M.A., and Winterfeldt, E.A. (1989) Iron, copper, and zinc status: response to supplementation with zinc or zinc and iron in adult females. *Am J Clin Nutr* **49**, 145–150.

Yakoob, M.Y., Theodoratou, E., Jabeen, A., *et al.* (2011) Preventive zinc supplementation in developing countries: impact on mortality and morbidity due to diarrhea, pneumonia and malaria. *BMC Public Health* **11** (Suppl 3)**,** S23.

Yamaguchi, M. (2010) Role of nutritional zinc in the prevention of osteoporosis. *Mol Cell Biochem* **338**, 241–254.

Yu, M., Lee, W.W., Tomar, D., *et al.* (2011) Regulation of T cell receptor signaling by activation-induced zinc influx. *J Exp Med* **208**, 775–785.

Yu, Y.Y., Kirschke, C.P., and Huang, L. (2007) Immunohistochemical analysis of ZnT1, 4, 5, 6, and 7 in the mouse gastrointestinal tract. *J Histochem Cytochem* **55**, 223–234.

35

COPPER

JOSEPH R. PROHASKA, PhD

University of Minnesota Medical School Duluth, Duluth, Minnesota, USA

Summary

Research during the past five years has provided new and exciting insights about copper home-ostasis at the cellular level. Ongoing investigations employing the tools of molecular genetics and confocal microscopy are certain to identify additional genes and proteins required for the transport of copper across membranes and its utilization within various cellular compartments. Elucidation of the direct and indirect roles of copper in the development and degeneration of the nervous system, the integrity of the cardiovascular and skeletal systems, and the activities of the immune system will certainly be facilitated by judicious use of molecular techniques such as gene knockout, overexpression, functional genomics, and proteomics. Stable isotope tech-nology has provided an understanding of whole-body copper metabolism in healthy adults. Continued application of this methodology and increased use of mathematical modeling are expected to provide new information about copper metabolism and requirements for selected populations, and especially those likely to be at higher risk of developing copper deficiency. These include premature and term infants, pregnant malnourished adolescents, the institution-alized elderly, and individuals with chronic diseases such as cystic fibrosis, Crohn's disease and other malabsorption syndromes. Studies in animals suggest the possibility that marginal copper deficiency, though difficult to diagnose, may compromise our ability to adapt metabolically to various physiological, pathophysiological, and emotional stresses. Development of a panel of sensitive biochemical and functional indices for the accurate assessment of copper status rep-resents an important challenge for investigators interested in the biology and nutrition of copper.

Introduction

Copper was thought essential for humans as early as the middle of the nineteenth century but was proven to be required through careful experimental work in plants and rodents in the 1920s. Organisms use protein-bound oxi-dized cupric ion (Cu^{2+}) or reduced cuprous ion (Cu^+) for a number of single-electron transfer reactions involving oxygen. Sophisticated mechanisms for the regulated acqui-sition, tissue distribution, utilization, and excretion exist so as to prevent deleterious reactions from copper excess. Major advances in our understanding of copper homeos-

Present Knowledge in Nutrition, Tenth Edition. Edited by John W. Erdman Jr, Ian A. Macdonald and Steven H. Zeisel.
© 2012 International Life Sciences Institute. Published 2012 by John Wiley & Sons, Inc.

tasis have evolved through the use of molecular genetics which may impact human health and disease and impact the Dietary Recommended Intakes.

Biological Functions of Copper

Humans contain about 1 mg copper/kg body weight. Copper has no known structural role, nor is there a major copper storage reservoir; rather, copper serves as an essential catalytic cofactor for many mammalian cuproenzymes (Table 35.1). The metal centers in these proteins bind oxygen and produce water, superoxide, or hydrogen peroxide in addition to various organic products. These cuproenzymes are involved in fundamental processes in energy production, iron utilization, maturation of the extracellular matrix, activation of neuropeptides, and neurotransmitter synthesis. The physical properties of these enzymes have been reviewed elsewhere (Linder and Hazegh-Azam, 1996).

Mammalian copper-dependent amine oxidases (EC 1.4.3.6) include a group of enzymes found in plasma and tissues as dimers. They deaminate monoamines and diamines, releasing aldehydes, ammonia, and hydrogen peroxide. They are inhibited by semicarbazide and contain the cofactor 2,4,5-trihydroxyphenylalanine quinone (TPQ) whose synthesis is also copper-dependent (Brazeau et al., 2004). They may function in metabolism of certain amines or may be involved in intracellular signaling by generation of hydrogen peroxide. An example is vascular adhesion protein-1 (VAP-1), a copper amine oxidase that

TABLE 35.1 Mammalian copper-dependent enzymes

Enzyme	Function
Amine oxidases	Oxidative deamination
Ceruloplasmin	Fe^{2+} oxidation
Cytochrome c oxidase	Oxygen electron transfer
Dopamine-β-monooxygenase	Norepinephrine synthesis
Extracellular superoxide dismutase	Superoxide disproportionation
Hephaestin	Fe^{2+} oxidation
Lysyl oxidase	Elastin cross-linking
Peptidylglycine α-amidating monooxygenase	Peptide C-terminal α-amidation
Superoxide dismutase 1	Superoxide disproportionation
Tyrosinase	DOPA quinone synthesis
Zyklopen	Fe2+ oxidation

is involved in leukocyte trafficking (Salmi and Jalkanen, 2001). Absence of the protein, also called amine oxidase, copper-containing-3 (AOC3), decreased both leukocyte and lymphocyte homing and attenuated inflammatory responses (Stolen et al., 2005).

Ceruloplasmin (Cp) is blue multicopper oxidase, also known as ferroxidase, which oxidizes ferrous iron thought to be important in loading transferrin, the ferric iron transport protein. Cp is an abundant 132-kD plasma glycoprotein made and secreted mainly by liver. Brain and other organs such as spleen, kidney, and heart express a splice variant GPI-anchored form of Cp (Mostad and Prohaska, 2011). Individuals with aceruloplasminemia clearly demonstrate an essential function of Cp as they are characterized by low serum iron, high iron deposits in liver, brain and pancreas, and the development of insulin-dependent diabetes (Hellman and Gitlin, 2002). However, copper metabolism is normal in aceruloplasminemic patients. Studies with Cp-null mice confirmed the impairment in iron mobilization and normal copper metabolism (Meyer et al., 2001). Thus, former hypotheses suggesting that the main function of Cp was to transport copper are likely false.

Cytochrome c oxidase (CCO), also known as mitochondrial complex IV, contains 13 protein subunits, two heme groups, zinc, magnesium, and three copper ions. CCO catalyzes the reduction of molecular oxygen to water and generates a proton gradient that is necessary for ATP synthesis. The assembly of CCO is dependent on additional accessory proteins, some of which are involved in copper delivery and insertion into subunits I and II. Adequate dietary copper is necessary to support the activity and stability of CCO. Mutations resulting in total loss of CCO are likely lethal. Mutations in the assembly proteins affect CCO and result in pathophysiology (Hamza and Gitlin, 2002).

Dopamine-β-monooxygenase (DBM) requires copper in each of its four subunits and ascorbate as a cosubstrate to convert dopamine to norepinephrine. DBM is expressed in adrenal medulla, sympathetic neurons of the peripheral nervous system, and noradrenergic and adrenergic neurons in brain. Deletion of the DBM gene is lethal for mouse embryos, suggesting a critical role of norepinephrine during development (Thomas et al., 1995).

Mammals have three separate genes that produce proteins that catalyze dismutation of superoxide, the univalent reduction product of molecular oxygen. Two of these proteins, Cu,Zn-superoxide dismutase (SOD1) and extracellular superoxide dismutase (EC-SOD) require copper. The other protein is located in the mitochondrial matrix, manganese superoxide dismutase (SOD2). Both SOD1 and EC-SOD also contain zinc as a cofactor. SOD1 is a homodimer of subunit size 16 kD. EC-SOD is a tetramer of subunit size 135 kD that functions as an antioxidant in the extracellular matrix and is the predominant dismutase in extracellular fluids such as lymph, synovial fluid, and plasma (Fattman *et al.*, 2003). Studies with EC-SOD knockout mice support a role for this protein and extracellular superoxide in modulating vascular tone by interacting with nitric oxide (Jung *et al.*, 2003).

Hephaestin is multicopper oxidase that is 50% identical to Cp. It was discovered as the defective gene product in sex-linked anemia in mice. The mutation resulted in iron retention in the intestine, suggesting an iron efflux function similar to Cp (Kuo *et al.*, 2004). Recently another Cp homolog, zyklopen, was described that may function in placental iron efflux (Chen *et al.*, 2010).

Lysyl oxidase (LO) (EC 1.4.3.13), a copper-dependent amine oxidase, contains a unique cofactor, lysyl tyrosyl quinone (LTQ), required for the oxidative deamination of specific lysine residues in the extracellular matrix (Kagan and Li, 2003). This reaction initiates the formation of cross-links that stabilize elastin and collagen. Discovery of at least four additional genes expressing proteins related to LO (LOXL1-4), with conserved catalytic domain, copper and cofactor binding sites, that are highly expressed in specific tissues, is opening a new chapter for investigation and function of these cuproenzymes (Molnar *et al.*, 2003).

Peptidylglycine α-amidating monooxygenase (PAM), like DBM, requires both copper and ascorbate as cofactors. PAM is required for post-translational modification of many peptides to their bioactive forms. Copper and ascorbate are required for monooxygenase activity to convert C-terminal glycine residues to hydroxyglycyl residues that are subsequently hydrolyzed by a lyase domain to produce α-amidated peptides and glyoxylate (Eipper *et al.*, 1992). PAM is especially enriched in the nervous and endocrine system with very high levels in the pituitary and cardiac atria. The importance of PAM has recently been documented by demonstrating embryonic lethality in mice following gene ablation (Czyzyk *et al.*, 2003). Importantly, PAM heterozygote mice have impaired thermoregulation and enhanced sensitivity to seizures (Bousquet-Moore *et al.*, 2010). More than half of all neuropeptides require PAM for activation and underscore this important role of copper in biology. Examples of these

neuropeptides include: adrenomedullin, calcitonin, cholecystokinin, gastrin, neuropeptide Y, oxytocin, substance P, thyrotropic hormone-releasing hormone (TRH), vasoactive intestinal peptide (VIP), and vasopressin (Bousquet-Moore *et al.*, 2010).

Tyrosinase, monophenol oxidase, performs a highly specialized function in melanin biosynthesis in melanocytes. Mutational loss of catalytic function leads to albinism. Copper restriction confirms an important role of tyrosinase in pigmentation as achromotrichia is observed in domestic and laboratory animals consuming diets low in copper.

In response to changes in nutritional copper intake, there are a number of enzymes whose activity either increases or decreases; however, these changes do not necessarily mean these are cuproenzymes (Prohaska, 1988). There are other proteins that may have catalytic properties dependent on copper but are less well established, including clotting factors V and VIII, S-adenosylhomocysteine hydrolase, prion protein, and others (Prohaska, 1988).

There are a number of copper-binding proteins in mammals that function as transport proteins and copper chaperones to maintain copper homeostasis (Bertinato and L'Abbé, 2004; Prohaska and Gybina, 2004). Additional roles for these copper binding proteins continue to be elucidated (Table 35.2). CCS and COMMD1 both impact

TABLE 35.2   Mammalian copper-binding proteins

Protein	Putative copper function
Albumin	Plasma transport
Amyloid precursor protein	Transport
Atox1	Chaperone, transcription factor
ATP7A	Efflux, metallation
ATP7B	Efflux, Cp metallation
CCS	SOD1 chaperone, HIF-1α activity
Clotting factors V, VIII	Unknown
COMMD1	Biliary excretion, SOD1 assembly
Cox11	CCO chaperone
Cox17	CCO chaperone
Ctr1	Transport
Ctr2	Transport
α2-Macroglobulin	Plasma transport
Metallothionein	Storage
Prion protein	Unknown
Sco1	CCO chaperone
Sco2	CCO chaperone
XIAP	Ubiquitination of COMMD1 and CCS

FIG. 35.1 Cellular copper transport and excretion – intestine to liver. Cu$^+$ is transferred across the enterocyte plasma membrane by Ctr1. Copper binds to chaperones (Atox1, Cox17, and CCS) that deliver copper to targeted cuproenzymes (CCO and SOD1) or copper-translocating ATPases (ATP7A and ATP7B). ATPases move copper into the trans Golgi network for incorporation into apo-cuproenzymes (e.g. intestine Heph and liver aCp) or to cytoplasmic vesicles near plasma membranes to mediate copper efflux. Copper pools are also associated with mitochondria (MT). Specialized copper binding proteins function in liver (COMMD1 and XIAP) to regulate ATP7B and copper efflux. They also regulate SOD1 and CCS. Mitochondria possess several chaperones needed to deliver copper to CCO.

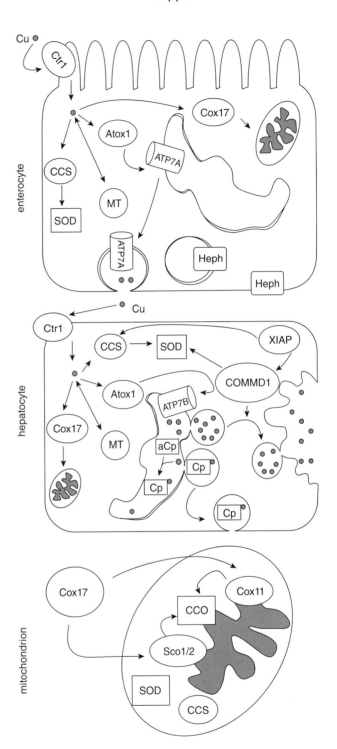

HIF-1α function (van de Sluis *et al.*, 2007; Feng *et al.*, 2009). ATOX1 appears to be a transcription factor in cell cycle regulation (Itoh *et al.*, 2008). X-linked inhibitor of apoptosis (XIAP) is a copper binding protein that regulates survival of both CCS and COMMD1 (Brady *et al.*, 2010). COMMD1 regulates dimerization of SOD1 (Vonk *et al.*, 2010).

Copper Homeostasis

Whole-Body Metabolism

Tracer studies have contributed markedly to our present understanding of mammalian copper metabolism. Ingested food and digestive secretory fluids (salivary, pancreatic, and biliary) all contribute to the copper pool present in the intestinal lumen. Copper likely enters small intestinal epithelial cells by a facilitated process that involves a specific cuprous ion carrier, Ctr1, located on the brush-border surface (Figure 35.1) The tissue acquisition of newly absorbed copper occurs in two phases. The first involves vectorial transport of copper across the basolateral membrane of the enterocyte into portal circulation where it is transported to liver in association with albumin and α2-macroglobulin. Newly arrived copper is secreted into plasma bound to Cp; however, the lack of disturbances in copper metabolism in aceruloplasminemia patients and mice clearly demonstrates that plasma Cp does not mediate cellular acquisition of copper. Plasma has a small non-Cp component, likely amino acid complexes; however, the mechanisms by which protein-bound or amino-acid-

bound copper is transported from plasma into cells remain unknown.

Copper concentration varies with tissue (Linder and Hazegh-Azam, 1996). Generally, copper is not stored in tissues, suggesting that differences in concentrations of the metal may reflect relative quantities of cuproenzymes. Transport of copper from the liver into the bile represents the primary route for excretion of endogenous copper. This pathway is immature in fetal and neonatal liver, thereby accounting for the storage of hepatic copper at these early stages of development. Likewise, cholestasis can result in accumulation of hepatic copper after the neonatal period. Copper of biliary origin and non-absorbed oral copper are eliminated from the body in feces. Daily losses of copper in urine are minimal in healthy individuals.

Stable isotope studies with healthy human subjects under controlled conditions have shown that both absorption and retention of copper readily respond to wide fluctuations in dietary copper intake. Under normal copper intake conditions it has been estimated that true copper absorption is about 10% since there is a 30% loss of newly absorbed copper via the endogenous secretion pathway involving active biliary excretion (Harvey *et al.*, 2005). Absorption of ingested copper appears to increase when dietary intakes are low (Turnlund *et al.*, 1998). Likewise, copper retention in many organs, particularly in brain and heart, is markedly increased in response to restricted copper intake in the rat (Levenson and Janghorbani, 1994). However, the ability of these adaptive mechanisms to maintain normal copper status in humans is exceeded when chronic dietary copper intake is less than 0.7 mg/day below that present in typical western diets, which average about 1.2 mg/day in the USA (Milne and Nielsen, 1996; Turnlund *et al.*, 1997).

Cellular Homeostasis

Cells adapt to obtain adequate but not excessive amounts of copper using a complex set of transporters and metallochaperones (Figure 35.1, Table 35.2). Luminal copper must be reduced to cuprous ion for uptake by Ctr1. This reduction process has not been elucidated but may be provided by Dcytb or Steap2, two putative reductases reviewed elsewhere (Collins *et al.*, 2010). Ctr1 is a transmembrane protein essential for copper distribution to the organism as deletion is lethal to embryos and surviving heterozygous knockout mice *Ctr1* +/− have reduced copper content and function in selected organs (Kuo *et al.*, 2001; Lee *et al.*, 2001). If a redundant copper transport system does exist, as suggested from in vitro cell culture studies with immortalized cell lines and studies in Caco-2 cells, it must be weak since it cannot replace Ctr1 function in the whole animal.

Imported cytoplasmic copper binds to a group of ubiquitous copper chaperone proteins and perhaps other copper binding species such as metallothioneins I and II (MT). Metallothioneins are cysteine-rich proteins with high affinity for heavy metal ions. They provide cells with a secondary system of detoxification when the copper efflux process is either not operational (e.g. during early stages of development and when efflux is defective) or when activity of the efflux pump becomes inadequate during acute exposure to high amounts of copper. Chaperones directly deliver copper to target proteins in cytoplasm and in membranes of organelles for incorporation of copper to apo-cuproproteins (Prohaska and Gybina, 2004).

The copper chaperone for superoxide dismutase, CCS, transfers copper to cytoplasmic and intermitochondrial membrane space SOD1. Deletion of CCS results in low SOD1 activity, a phenotype similar to SOD1 knockout mice (Wong *et al.*, 2000). Cox17 is necessary to deliver copper to the mitochondria for CCO assembly. Deletion of Cox17 results in embryonic lethality in a temporal pattern similar to Ctr1 knockout mice (Takahashi *et al.*, 2002). Within the mitochondria additional chaperones (Cox11, Sco1 and Sco2) are necessary to deliver copper to CCO subunits I and II (Hamza and Gitlin, 2002). Atox1 delivers copper to P-type ATPases that mediate energy-dependent transport of the metal to the lumen of the trans-Golgi network for incorporation of the metal into secretory copper-dependent proteins such as Cp, DBM, LO, PAM, and tyrosinase. Deletion of Atox1 results in perinatal mortality with symptoms consistent with copper deficiency (Hamza *et al.*, 2001).

Two distinct copper-translocating, P-type ATPases have been identified (Lutsenko, 2010). Hepatocytes, mammary tissue, and certain neurons express the copper translocating ATPase, ATP7B, whereas other cells have a highly homologous ATPase, ATP7A. It is now recognized that ATP7A and ATP7B cycle between the trans-Golgi network and cytoplasmic vesicles. ATP7A is the protein missing or mutated in humans with Menkes' disease that results in copper deficiency. ATP7B is the protein mutated in Wilson's disease and leads to hepatic copper overload toxicity. When intracellular copper is low or normal, copper ATPases are localized predominantly in the trans-Golgi network to facilitate the delivery of the metal to secretory apo-cuproproteins. As cellular copper increases, the ATPases are redistributed into cytoplasmic vesicles

(Lutsenko and Petris, 2003). Fusion of copper-loaded cytoplasmic vesicles with the canicular membrane of the hepatocyte is required for biliary copper excretion (Figure 35.1). This process requires another protein, COMDD1, that interacts with ATP7B and is missing in canine copper toxicosis, a disorder of liver copper overload (Tao et al., 2003). Fusion of copper-loaded vesicles with the basolateral surface of enterocyte and placental trophoblast are likely to facilitate copper efflux to plasma and transfer of placental copper to the fetal compartment, respectively. The high efficiency of the copper efflux pathway is supported by minimal binding of copper to cytoplasmic MT after weaning.

Some have suggested that MT might be a copper storage pool or provide a buffer for copper during times when the metal is limiting (Suzuki et al., 2002). Perhaps copper is stored in a vesicular compartment and transported by Ctr2, a protein homologous to Ctr1 that provides this function in budding yeast and that has been shown to impact copper uptake (van den Berghe et al., 2007).

There are many copper binding proteins whose functions remain unknown (Prohaska, 1988). Recent candidates include prion protein PrP^C and amyloid precursor protein APP. Some suggest a function of PrP^C is to transport copper into brain and serve as another superoxide dismutase or chaperone for SOD1 (Brown, 2001). However, others found no changes in brain copper or SOD1 activity in PrP^C knockout mice or transgenic mice overexpressing this protein 10-fold (Waggoner et al., 2000). Stronger evidence exists for amyloid precursor protein APP. APP-null mice have increased brain copper levels (White et al., 1999). In contrast, mice overexpressing APP have reduced brain copper levels (Maynard et al., 2002). These observations suggest a role for APP in regulation of brain copper content. Since APP is expressed in all major tissues, it may function elsewhere in modulating copper homeostasis. Some studies indicate that APP mRNA expression may be regulated by copper (Bellingham et al., 2004).

Factors Affecting Copper Status

When thresholds of copper exposure exceed adaptive responses, development of copper deficiency or toxicity can occur. In addition to copper intake, other dietary components and physiological factors can affect the bioavailability and tissue exposure to copper.

Copper Intake

The copper content of the typical diet in the United States provides the majority of adults with a slight excess of intake over the current RDA, 0.9 mg (Pennington and Schoen, 1996). However, certain gender and age groups appear to consume less than the RDA levels (Hunt and Meacham, 2001). Absorption efficiency can range between 50% and 25% when diets contain 1–7 mg of copper, respectively. The richest food sources of copper include shellfish, nuts, seeds, organ meats, wheat-bran cereals, whole-grain products, and chocolate foods. Vegetarian diets generally contain a generous supply of copper, though the efficiency of copper absorption seems lower (Hunt et al., 1998). Multi-mineral and vitamin supplements represent another potential source of copper intake, although copper is often present in adult, pediatric, and prenatal formations as cupric oxide which is very poorly absorbed (Baker, 1999). Drinking water can be an additional source of copper. Although fresh drinking water generally contains very low levels of copper, regional variability and leaching from copper pipes leads to exposure differences.

Copper Bioavailability

Adverse effects of certain proteins, zinc, iron, molybdenum, ascorbic acid, certain amino acids, and certain saccharides on copper absorption and utilization have been reported (Lonnerdal, 1998). It is clear that administration of high doses of zinc will induce copper-deficient signs in both infants and adults. Recently, this has become an issue in subjects exposed to high zinc via denture cream (Hedera et al., 2009). Perhaps low intake of dietary zinc can impact copper status of humans (Milne et al., 2001). Dietary fiber appears to have minimal impact on copper absorption by adults in contrast to effects on zinc and iron availability. Infants may be more sensitive to bioavailability perturbations since digestive processes and the regulation of copper absorption and excretion are not fully mature.

Physiological Conditions

Gender, age, and pregnancy may impact copper absorption and retention (Johnson et al., 1992). Hepatic levels of copper bound to MT are elevated markedly during the final trimester of fetal development, presumably as a copper storage pool to provide the rapidly growing newborn with a supply of copper. However, adequate copper during lactation is necessary to prevent its deficiency. Plasma levels of copper increase transiently during episodes of inflammation and infection since Cp synthesis and secretion are stimulated by proinflammatory cytokines. Similarly, plasma copper and Cp are elevated in response to increased plasma estrogen (Linder and Hazegh-Azam, 1996). The significance, if any, of changes in plasma copper on whole body metabolism, utilization, and requirement is unknown. Studies in rats following copper injection show that lactation markedly enhances the avidity of the mammary gland for copper (Donley *et al.*, 2002). These studies collectively illustrate that copper requirements and metabolism are impacted by physiological state.

Genetic Factors

Human copper requirements will be influenced by genetic factors that determine the expression of copper homeostatic genes. In elegant studies in fungi, many of the genetic and transcriptional details of copper homeostasis have been worked out (Rutherford and Bird, 2004). Thus far, no copper-responsive mammalian transcription factors have been discovered with the possible exception of ATOX1 (Itoh *et al.*, 2008). Steady-state mRNA levels of Ctr1, ATP7A, and ATP7B are not altered by dietary copper deficiency in mammals (Prohaska and Gybina, 2004). Rather, transport and efflux are regulated by copper-dependent post-translational trafficking (van den Berghe and Klomp, 2010). Genetic aberrations in copper metabolism in humans are evident due to mutations of ATP7A (Menkes' disease) or ATP7B (Wilson's disease), two genes coding for copper efflux transporters.

Copper Requirement

Dietary reference intakes (DRIs) for copper were established in 2001 (Trumbo *et al.*, 2001). Recommended dietary allowance (RDA) for adult males and females was set at 0.9 mg. This is approximately a 1.8 mg/kg copper diet based on a 2000 kcal and 500 g dry weight estimate. Prior to 2001, the recommended Estimated Safe and Adequate Daily Dietary Intake of copper for adults was 1.5–3.0 mg/day. The RDA for pregnancy is 1 mg and for lactation 1.3 mg. Work with mice suggests the possibility that the human RDA for pregnancy/lactation may be set too low (Prohaska and Brokate, 2002). The same dietary level of copper that was lethal to pups during mid-lactation produced no discernible changes in copper status to non-lactating adult females. The tolerable upper intake level

(UL) for copper is 10 mg. Using a categorical regression model with many published data sets, a value of 2.6 mg was estimated to provide the best intake to avoid deficiency and minimize toxicity (Chambers *et al.*, 2010). This level of intake is approximately two times higher than the reported level of copper intake in North America.

Copper Deficiency

Common characteristics of severe copper deficiency in mammals include hypochromic anemia (refractory to iron supplementation), neutropenia, thrombocytopenia, hypopigmentation, plus anatomical and functional abnormalities in the skeletal, cardiovascular, and immune systems (Uauy *et al.*, 1998). Copper deprivation during the fetal and neonatal periods also causes neurological abnormalities. Although many of these diverse effects seem associated with decreased activities of known cuproenzymes (Table 35.1), unequivocal evidence that the decline in catalytic activity actually alters the metabolic flux and generation of products in specific pathways remains somewhat elusive.

Inadequate tissue levels of copper result from insufficient absorption of exogenous copper and excessive losses of endogenous copper. The pleiotropic effects of defective cellular copper transport in individuals with Menkes' disease are consistent with tissue copper deficiency observed in experimental animals. Acquired copper deficiency is relatively rare in humans, although reports of copper deficiency in infants, children, and adults continue to appear in the clinical literature. Groups that are susceptible to developing copper deficiency include the following: individuals at any age receiving total parenteral nutrition without supplemental copper for extended periods; preterm infants fed milk-based formula without adequate copper; infants recovering from malnutrition or chronic diarrhea, patients undergoing chronic peritoneal dialysis; severe burn patients; ambulatory renal dialysis patients; and individuals consuming excessive doses of zinc, antacids, or copper chelators.

Copper deficiency can also develop in humans with malabsorption syndromes. Examples of conditions that can compromise copper status include: celiac disease, cystic fibrosis, and sprue. Recently, the intervention of surgical resection of the short bowel to manage obesity has surfaced as a major factor in adult onset copper deficiency that is only partially corrected by supplementation (Griffith *et al.*, 2009). An RDA intake of copper may be too low under these conditions. Impact of copper deficiency, regardless of its etiology, can have a major impact on several biological systems.

Cardiovascular System

Anatomical, electrical, mechanical, and biochemical abnormalities are evident in hearts of young animals fed diets severely restricted in copper. Severely copper-deficient young rats often die of ventricular rupture. Many of the defects are generally assumed to result from decreased activities of various cardiac cuproenzymes, including CCO, DBM, LO, PAM, or SOD1 as reviewed elsewhere (Medeiros and Wildman, 1997). Notable observations are that cardiac hypertrophy in copper-deficient rats is not dependent on anemia; marginally copper-deficient diets also induce cardiac abnormalities; and adult rats fed a copper-deficient diet develop cardiovascular defects, but not hypertrophy. Exciting new data in mice with cardiac deletion of Ctr1 suggest that development of hypertrophy is intrinsic to the heart and requires no systemic disturbance (Kim et al., 2010).

Development of cardiovascular abnormalities in animals fed low copper diets provides the conceptual basis for speculation that copper deficiency contributes to the incidence of ischemic heart disease in humans. Although cardiac arrhythmias were experienced by several subjects ingesting low-copper diets in metabolic trials, healthy adults in other studies, in which low-copper diets were fed for extended periods, had normal cardiac function. Individuals with Menkes' disease exhibit pathology in major vessels but not the heart (Danks, 1988).

Copper status can also impact the circulatory system. Proper cross-linking in large vessels, as well as vasoactivity in arterioles, capillaries, and venules, are copper dependent (Saari and Schuschke, 1999). Dietary copper deficiency increases histamine-mediated protein leakage in venules by increasing numbers of localized mast-cells, inhibits platelet interactions that lead to thrombogenesis, and decreases nitric oxide-induced relaxation of arteriolar smooth muscle cells. Copper status also has an impact on the acute inflammatory response including vasodilation, protein extravasation from microvascular leakage, and neutrophil adhesion and diapedesis. These lines of investigation are expected to uncover specific roles for copper in the regulation of peripheral blood flow and hemostasis.

Altered blood lipid profiles, blood pressure, and anemia can all impact the cardiovascular system and are known to be impacted by copper status. Hypertriglyceridemia and hypercholesterolemia are frequently observed in severe copper deficiency, and involve alteration in thiol status (Kim et al., 1992). Copper deficiency also increases plasma HDL protein levels in rats. This change appears to be due to enhanced transcription of apolipoprotein A-I gene in liver (Wu et al., 1997). Gel shift assay suggested that binding of hepatocyte nuclear factor 4 and other undefined nuclear proteins to oligonucleotides containing one of the regulatory sites in the promoter of apoA-I gene is enhanced by copper deficiency.

Hemopoietic System

It is likely that copper plays a fundamental role in myeloid progenitor cell differentiation, as a prominent feature of copper deficiency is alteration in erythrocyte (lower), neutrophil (lower), and platelet (higher) levels. The anemia of copper deficiency is a consequence of fewer red blood cells and also of a lower hemoglobin content per cell. Some believe the primary determinant of anemia is a failure to absorb and retain dietary iron following dietary copper deficiency (Reeves et al., 2005). Others believe it is related to a failure to mobilize iron from tissue stores such as liver because Cp (ferroxidase) is copper dependent. However, Cp-null mice and aceruloplasminemia in humans do not result in pronounced anemia. The role of copper in iron biology is quite complex (Collins et al., 2010). It would appear that the anemia associated with copper deficiency is the result of failure to utilize iron properly rather than of a failure to deliver iron to bone marrow (Prohaska, 2011).

Immune System

Clinical and experimental reports indicate that inherited and acquired copper deficiencies often are associated with increased risk of infection (Prohaska and Failla, 1993). Severe copper deficiency generally changes the phenotypic profiles of immune cells in blood, bone marrow, and lymphoid tissues, and suppresses a number of activities of lymphocytes and phagocytic cells. In vitro DNA synthesis and IL-2 secretion by mitogen-treated splenic T-lymphocytes and respiratory burst activity of neutrophils were markedly impaired in cells from animals fed diet marginal in low copper (Hopkins and Failla, 1995). Recently a role for copper in macrophage function has emerged (White et al., 2009).

Neutropenia is a hallmark of copper deficiency in humans. Several recent studies have suggested that moderate and even marginal copper deficiency also affect some activities of T-lymphocytes and phagocytic cells adversely. In vitro responsiveness of T-lymphocytes to mitogenic activation was decreased after adult males were fed a diet with 0.38 mg copper per day for 6 weeks. This alteration was associated with a reduction in plasma copper and activities of several cuproenzymes, but not hematologic indices (Kelley *et al.*, 1995). Similarly, IL-2 synthesis by a human T-cell line and bactericidal activity and secretion of proinflammatory cytokines TNF-alpha, IL-1, and IL-6 by a human monocytic cell line were decreased after inducing moderate copper deficiency with a copper chelator (Hopkins and Failla, 1999). These changes were eliminated by supplementation of medium with copper, but not iron or zinc, and were not associated with alterations in cellular iron status or general metabolic activities.

The decreased synthesis of IL-2 in low-copper T-cells results from decreased transcription of the IL-2 gene in activated cells. Although these results support a direct role for copper in the ability of defense cells to respond to stimuli, unique roles that copper plays in the maturation, activation, and effector activities of immune cells remain unknown. Likewise, the link between suppressed activities of immune cells in copper-deficient humans and increased susceptibility to infection remains weak, partly because of the inability to accurately assess marginal and moderate deficiencies of this micronutrient.

Nervous System

The essentiality of adequate copper intake and utilization for the normal development of the brain is well recognized (Lutsenko *et al.*, 2010). Domestic animals grazing on pastures low in copper produced offspring that exhibited ataxia and severe neuronal pathology (Smith, 1983). Neuronal pathology is a salient feature of infants who die of Menkes' disease. Copper accumulates in brain during late gestation and lactation. Thus, restricted intake of copper by pregnant and lactating individuals has severe consequences for offspring. In fact, rats that experienced copper deficiency during the perinatal period exhibited permanent behavioral abnormalities, even after ingesting a copper-adequate diet for 6 months (Prohaska and Hoffman, 1996; Penland and Prohaska, 2004). Even marginal copper deficiency can impact the brain. Brain copper was significantly lower in rats fed a diet containing moderate copper (2.8 mg/kg) than in those fed adequate copper (6.7 mg/kg); whereas growth and copper concentration in liver, lung, and bone were similar for the two dietary groups (Hopkins and Failla, 1995). Similarly maturation of hippocampus and dentate gyrus was impaired in rats

subjected to moderate copper deficiency during gestation and lactation (Hunt and Idso, 1995). These studies underscore the importance of adequate copper during perinatal development.

The neurochemical functions of copper are thought to be associated with the cuproenzymes that are present in most tissues (Table 35.1) and several unique cuproproteins. Copper deficiency alters the enzyme activity and protein level of rodent brain CCO, DBM, SOD1, and PAM (Prohaska *et al.*, 2005). Perhaps altered enzyme activity and levels are responsible for the altered neuropathology and behavior. Transfer of copper from plasma to neurons and delivery to cuproenzymes require Ctr1, Atox1, ATP7A, and perhaps ATP7B. Ctr1 +/− mice and Atox1 −/− mice have lower brain copper levels and decreased CCO activity (Hamza *et al.*, 2001; Lee *et al.*, 2001). Brindled mice that contain a non-functional ATP7A protein have altered PAM activity as evidenced by peptide amidation defects (Steveson *et al.*, 2003). A glycosylphosphatidylinositol-anchored form of Cp that is synthesized from an alternatively spliced RNA variant has been identified in brain (Patel *et al.*, 2002). Ablation of the Cp gene in mice is associated with iron overload in brain. In contrast, dietary copper deficiency, and lower Cp activity, are associated with lower brain iron (Prohaska and Gybina, 2005). Judicious use of gene knockout techniques are expected to reveal unique neurochemical roles of copper and to elucidate mechanisms of neuronal pathology that accompany imbalances in copper homeostasis.

Although it is generally believed that copper is most critical during brain development, other neurological functions depend on adequate copper throughout life. Recently, several cases of adult myelopathy have been characterized and associated with low serum copper and Cp, implying a relationship to a copper-deficient state (Kumar *et al.*, 2004).

Skeletal and Integumentary System

There is a well established association between decreased LO activity, connective tissue disorders, generalized osteoporosis, and bone defects that occur in dietary and inherited copper deficiency in humans and other species (Danks, 1988). LO and perhaps LOXL proteins are involved in cross-linking of collagen.

Bone abnormalities are common in copper-deficient infants and resemble features observed following vitamin C deficiency (Uauy *et al.*, 1998). Changes include osteoporosis, bone fractures, spur formation, and subperiosteal new bone formation. Relationships between copper and bone health exist in adults as well. Long-term studies suggest that copper supplementation may decrease bone loss. Reduction of copper intake from 1.6 to 0.7 mg/day for 8 weeks increased the rate of bone resorption as assessed by urinary excretion of pyridinium cross-links in healthy adult males; this change was reversed after restoration of dietary copper to 1.6 mg/day (Baker et al., 1999). However, supplementation of healthy males and females aged 22–46 years with 3 and 6 mg copper/day for 6 weeks did not affect biochemical markers of bone formation or resorption. The possibility that long-term supplementation of aging males and females with copper may retard net losses of bone merits further investigation.

Copper Toxicity

It is not surprising that the incidence of copper toxicity is quite low in the general population considering the homeostatic regulation of copper absorption and excretion. Copper, like inorganic iron, can participate in Fenton chemistry and generate reactive oxygen species (Prohaska, 1997). Symptoms associated with the ingestion of fluids and foods contaminated with large quantities of copper usually include metallic taste and gastrointestinal distress. Copper was used historically to induce vomiting. The recent North American UL for copper is 10 mg. Results from a multicenter (Chile, Northern Ireland, USA) study indicate the No Adverse Effect Level (NOAEL) in drinking water was about 5 mg copper per liter. Taste of copper in water was detected at about half this level (Araya et al., 2003). WHO guidelines indicate a provisional safety of 2 mg copper per liter. The safety of copper in drinking water is controversial (Brewer et al., 2010).

Inclusion of copper in micronutrient and complete nutritional supplements does not seem to pose any adverse effects. Supplementation of adults with 10 mg copper daily as cupric gluconate for 12 weeks did not cause gastrointestinal difficulties or liver damage in a double-blind study (Pratt et al., 1985). Immaturity of biliary excretion and increased efficiency of copper absorption suggest potential risk of copper toxicity in infants. Accumulation of toxic levels of copper in livers of children diagnosed with Indian childhood cirrhosis, certain infants in the Austrian Tyrol, and those with idiopathic copper toxicosis is often associated with use of copper-contaminated water to prepare infant formula and other foods that were stored or prepared in brass vessels (Araya et al., 2003). Public health programs aimed at changing practices associated with infant feeding and genetic dilution have largely eliminated the incidence of these diseases. Obviously, individuals with Wilson's disease and other inherited or acquired disorders that impair elimination of excess copper via the biliary route should avoid ingestion of copper-fortified products and copper-contaminated water.

Assessment of Copper Status

Identification of copper-status biomarkers that are sensitive, non-invasive, and reliable indicators continues to be problematic (Harvey et al., 2009). Experimental studies with young animals show that moderate to severe reductions of the copper content of standard formulations of nutritionally adequate, semi-purified diets usually induces a relatively rapid decline in plasma copper and Cp activity. The impact of dietary treatment on the concentration of the metal and cuproenzyme activities in cells and tissues is dependent on numerous factors, including severity of the reduction in dietary copper, species, strain, organ, and gender. The traditional approach in human studies has been to examine the level of copper and activities of cuproenzymes in plasma and blood cells. Reductions of plasma copper and Cp are often observed in individuals with diagnosed copper deficiency. However, estrogen status and conditions such as pregnancy, infection, inflammation, and some cancers increase plasma Cp and copper levels, thereby compromising their utility as reliable indicators for screening copper status. Even under well-controlled conditions, dietary copper must be reduced to 0.6 mg copper/day or less for periods of at least 6 weeks for healthy adults before markers decline. Other potential markers that have been monitored in various human studies include copper content in platelets and mononuclear cells, and activities of SOD1 in erythrocytes and CCO in platelets and mononuclear cells. Influences of factors other than copper, required sample volume, wide variations within individuals, and technical difficulties represent difficulties for using these markers as reliable indicators for assessing copper status.

Other cuproenzymes deserve further evaluation as possible indicators of copper status. Serum and tissue activity of PAM in rats are correlated with dietary copper intake (Prohaska et al., 2005). A study using plasma from several subjects with a mild variant of Menkes' disease and an individual with acquired copper deficiency suggested that the assay may be a useful marker of copper status in humans (Prohaska et al., 1997). Studies in an adult subject with acquired copper deficiency and response to copper supplementation suggest activity of plasma diamine oxidase as a biomarker (DiSilvestro *et al.*, 1997; Kehoe *et al.*, 2000). The utility of this enzyme as a marker of copper status may be limited, since a number of pathological conditions of the intestine or kidney, and pregnancy, affect plasma activity (Failla, 1999). Another potential assessment tool has recently been proposed. In rodents following copper deficiency the immunoreactive content of SOD1 is lower and that of its specific chaperone, CCS, is markedly higher (Bertinato *et al.*, 2003; Prohaska *et al.*, 2003). Thus the ratio of CCS to SOD1 protein is markedly higher in copper-deficient tissues including erythrocytes (West and Prohaska, 2004). CCS mRNA in peripheral blood mononuclear cells seems responsive to copper supplementation (Suazo *et al.*, 2008).

Although functional and behavioral activities in animals and in vitro cellular assays have been shown to be quite responsive to marginal and moderate reductions in copper, their potential utility for evaluating copper status in humans remains unknown currently.

Future Directions

Continued use of novel genetic and dietary investigations will reveal exciting clarification of the mechanisms responsible for copper homeostasis. It is very clear that the cellular copper binding proteins do more than chaperone for metallation. Elucidation of robust biomarkers will help establish copper needs for special groups and for special clinical circumstances. Reevaluation of the current copper DRI levels will require solid experimental and clinical data on subjects of various ages and physiological states.

Acknowledgment

Several in-press manuscripts were shared by my colleagues in the copper-research field.

Suggestions for Further Reading
Human copper homeostasis: (Lutsenko, 2010).
Copper chaperones (Robinson and Winge, 2010).
Copper and development (Uriu-Adams *et al.*, 2010).
Biomarkers (Bertinato and Zouzoulas, 2009).

References

Araya, M., Koletzko, B., and Uauy, R. (2003) Copper deficiency and excess in infancy: developing a research agenda. *J Pediatr Gastroenterol Nutr* **37**, 422–429.

Baker, A., Harvey, L., Majask-Newman, G., *et al.* (1999) Effect of dietary copper intakes on biochemical markers of bone metabolism in healthy adult males. *Eur J Clin Nutr* **53**, 408–412.

Baker, D.H. (1999) Cupric oxide should not be used as a copper supplement for either animals or humans. *J Nutr* **129**, 2278–2279.

Bellingham, S.A., Lahiri, D.K., Maloney, B., *et al.* (2004) Copper depletion down-regulates expression of the Alzheimer's disease amyloid-beta precursor protein gene. *J Biol Chem* **279**, 20378–20386.

Bertinato, J. and L'Abbé, M.R. (2004) Maintaining copper homeostasis: regulation of copper-trafficking proteins in response to copper deficiency or overload. *J Nutr Biochem* **15**, 316–322.

Bertinato, J. and Zouzoulas, A. (2009) Considerations in the development of biomarkers of copper status. *J AOAC Int* **92**, 1541–1550.

Bertinato, J., Iskandar, M., and L'Abbé, M.R. (2003) Copper deficiency induces the upregulation of the copper chaperone for Cu/Zn superoxide dismutase in weanling male rats. *J Nutr* **133**, 28–31.

Bousquet-Moore, D., Mains, R.E., and Eipper, B.A. (2010) Peptidylglycine alpha-amidating monooxygenase and copper: a gene–nutrient interaction critical to nervous system function. *J Neurosci Res* **88**, 2535–2545.

Brady, G.F., Galban, S., Liu, X., *et al.* (2010) Regulation of the copper chaperone CCS by XIAP-mediated ubiquitination. *Mol Cell Biol* **30**, 1923–1936.

Brazeau, B.J., Johnson, B.J., and Wilmot, C.M. (2004) Copper-containing amine oxidases. Biogenesis and catalysis; a structural perspective. *Arch Biochem Biophys* **428**, 22–31.

Brewer, G.J., Danzeisen, R., Stern, B.R., *et al.* (2010) Letter to the editor and reply: toxicity of copper in drinking water. *J Toxicol Environ Health B Crit Rev* **13**, 449–459.

Brown, D.R. (2001) Copper and prion disease. *Brain Res Bull* **55**, 165–173.

Chambers, A., Krewski, D., Birkett, N., *et al.* (2010) An exposure-response curve for copper excess and deficiency. *J Toxicol Environ Health* **13**, 546–578.

Chen, H., Attieh, Z.K., Syed, B.A., *et al.* (2010) Identification of zyklopen, a new member of the vertebrate multicopper ferroxidase family, and characterization in rodents and human cells. *J Nutr* **140**, 1728–1735.

Collins, J.F., Prohaska, J.R., and Knutson, M.D. (2010) Metabolic crossroads of iron and copper. *Nutr Rev* **68**, 133–147.

Czyzyk, T.A., Morgan, D.J., Peng, B., *et al.* (2003) Targeted mutagenesis of processing enzymes and regulators: implications for development and physiology. *J Neurosci Res* **74**, 446–455.

Danks, D.M. (1988) Copper deficiency in humans. *Annu Rev Nutr* **8**, 235–257.

DiSilvestro, R.A., Jones, A.A., Smith, D., *et al.* (1997) Plasma diamine oxidase activities in renal dialysis patients, a human with spontaneous copper deficiency and marginally copper deficient rats. *Clin Biochem* **30**, 559–563.

Donley, S.A., Ilagan, B.J., Rim, H., *et al.* (2002) Copper transport to mammary gland and milk during lactation in rats. *Am J Physiol Endocrinol Metab* **283**, E667–E675.

Eipper, B.A., Stoffers, D.A., and Mains, R.E. (1992) The biosynthesis of neuropeptides: peptide alpha-amidation. *Annu Rev Neurosci* **15**, 57–85.

Failla, M.L. (1999) Considerations for determining "optimal nutrition" for copper, zinc, manganese and molybdenum. *Proc Nutr Soc* **58**, 497–505.

Fattman, C.L., Schaefer, L.M., and Oury, T.D. (2003) Extracellular superoxide dismutase in biology and medicine. *Free Radic Biol Med* **35**, 236–256.

Feng, W., Ye, F., Xue, W., *et al.* (2009) Copper regulation of hypoxia-inducible factor-1 activity. *Mol Pharmacol* **75**, 174–182.

Griffith, D.P., Liff, D.A., Ziegler, T.R., *et al.* (2009) Acquired copper deficiency: a potentially serious and preventable complication following gastric bypass surgery. *Obesity* **17**, 827–831.

Hamza, I. and Gitlin, J. D. (2002) Copper chaperones for cytochrome c oxidase and human disease. *J Bioenerg Biomembr* **34**, 381–388.

Hamza, I., Faisst, A., Prohaska, J., *et al.* (2001) The metallochaperone Atox1 plays a critical role in perinatal copper homeostasis. *Proc Natl Acad Sci USA* **98**, 6848–6852.

Harvey, L.J., Ashton, K., Hooper, L., *et al.* (2009) Methods of assessment of copper status in humans: a systematic review. *Am J Clin Nutr* **89**, 2009S–2024S.

Harvey, L.J., Dainty, J.R., Hollands, W.J., *et al.* (2005) Use of mathematical modeling to study copper metabolism in humans. *Am J Clin Nutr* **81**, 807–813.

Hedera, P., Peltier, A., Fink, J.K., *et al.* (2009) Myelopolyneuropathy and pancytopenia due to copper deficiency and high zinc levels of unknown origin II. The denture cream is a primary source of excessive zinc. *Neurotoxicology* **30**, 996–999.

Hellman, N.E. and Gitlin, J.D. (2002) Ceruloplasmin metabolism and function. *Annu Rev Nutr* **22**, 439–458.

Hopkins, R.G. and Failla, M.L. (1995) Chronic intake of a marginally low copper diet impairs in vitro activities of lymphocytes and neutrophils from male rats despite minimal impact on conventional indicators of copper status. *J Nutr* **125**, 2658–2668.

Hopkins, R.G. and Failla, M.L. (1999) Transcriptional regulation of interleukin-2 gene expression is impaired by copper deficiency in Jurkat human T lymphocytes. *J Nutr* **129**, 596–601.

Hunt, C.D. and Idso, J.P. (1995) Moderate copper deprivation during gestation and lactation affects dentate gyrus and hippocampal maturation in immature male rats. *J Nutr* **125**, 2700–2710.

Hunt, C.D. and Meacham, S.L. (2001) Aluminum, boron, calcium, copper, iron, magnesium, manganese, molybdenum, phosphorus, potassium, sodium, and zinc: concentrations in common western foods and estimated daily intakes by infants; toddlers; and male and female adolescents, adults, and seniors in the United States. *J Am Diet Assoc* **101**, 1058–1060.

Hunt, J.R., Matthys, L.A., and Johnson, L.K. (1998) Zinc absorption, mineral balance, and blood lipids in women consuming controlled lactoovovegetarian and omnivorous diets for 8 wk. *Am J Clin Nutr* **67**, 421–430.

Itoh, S., Kim, H.W., Nakagawa, O., *et al.* (2008) Novel role of antioxidant-1 (Atox1) as a copper-dependent transcription factor involved in cell proliferation. *J Biol Chem* **283**, 9157–9167.

Johnson, P.E., Milne, D.B., and Lykken, G.I. (1992) Effects of age and sex on copper absorption, biological half-life, and status in humans. *Am J Clin Nutr* **56**, 917–925.

Jung, O., Marklund, S.L., Geiger, H., *et al.* (2003) Extracellular superoxide dismutase is a major determinant of nitric oxide bioavailability: in vivo and ex vivo evidence from ecSOD-deficient mice. *Circ Res* **93**, 622–629.

Kagan, H.M. and Li, W. (2003) Lysyl oxidase: properties, specificity, and biological roles inside and outside of the cell. *J. Cell Biochem* **88**, 660–672.

Kehoe, C.A., Turley, E., Bonham, M.P., *et al.* (2000) Response of putative indices of copper status to copper supplementation in human subjects. *Br J Nutr* **84**, 151–156.

Kelley, D.S., Daudu, P.A., Taylor, P.C., *et al.* (1995) Effects of low-copper diets on human immune response. *Am J Clin Nutr* **62**, 412–416.

Kim, B.E., Turski, M.L., Nose, Y., *et al.* (2010) Cardiac copper deficiency activates a systemic signaling mechanism that communicates with the copper acquisition and storage organs. *Cell Metab* **11**, 353–363.

Kim, S., Chao, P.Y., and Allen, K.G. (1992) Inhibition of elevated hepatic glutathione abolishes copper deficiency cholesterolemia. *FASEB J* **6**, 2467–2471.

Kumar, N., Crum, B., Petersen, R.C., *et al.* (2004) Copper deficiency myelopathy. *Arch Neurol* **61**, 762–766.

Kuo, Y.M., Su, T., Chen, H., *et al.* (2004) Mislocalisation of hephaestin, a multicopper ferroxidase involved in basolateral intestinal iron transport, in the sex linked anaemia mouse. *Gut* **53**, 201–206.

Kuo, Y.M., Zhou, B., Cosco, D., *et al.* (2001) The copper transporter CTR1 provides an essential function in mammalian embryonic development. *Proc Natl Acad Sci USA* **98**, 6836–6841.

Lee, J., Prohaska, J.R., and Thiele, D.J. (2001) Essential role for mammalian copper transporter Ctr1 in copper homeostasis and embryonic development. *Proc Natl Acad Sci USA* **98**, 6842–6847.

Levenson, C.W. and Janghorbani, M. (1994) Long-term measurement of organ copper turnover in rats by continuous feeding of a stable isotope. *Anal Biochem* **221**, 243–249.

Linder, M.C. and Hazegh-Azam, M. (1996) Copper biochemistry and molecular biology. *Am J Clin Nutr* **63**, 797S–811S.

Lonnerdal, B. (1998) Copper nutrition during infancy and childhood. *Am J Clin Nutr* **67**, 1046S–1053S.

Lutsenko, S. (2010) Human copper homeostasis: a network of interconnected pathways. *Curr Opin Chem Biol* **14**, 211–217.

Lutsenko, S. and Petris, M.J. (2003) Function and regulation of the mammalian copper-transporting ATPases: insights from biochemical and cell biological approaches. *J Membr Biol* **191**, 1–12.

Lutsenko, S., Bhattacharjee, A., and Hubbard, A.L. (2010) Copper handling machinery of the brain. *Metallomics* **2**, 596–608.

Maynard, C.J., Cappai, R., Volitakis, I., *et al.* (2002) Overexpression of Alzheimer's disease amyloid-beta opposes the age-dependent elevations of brain copper and iron. *J Biol Chem* **277**, 44670–44676.

Medeiros, D.M. and Wildman, R.E. (1997) Newer findings on a unified perspective of copper restriction and cardiomyopathy. *Proc Soc Exp Biol Med* **215**, 299–313.

Meyer, L.A., Durley, A.P., Prohaska, J.R., *et al.* (2001) Copper transport and metabolism are normal in aceruloplasminemic mice. *J Biol Chem* **276**, 36857–36861.

Milne, D.B. and Nielsen, F.H. (1996) Effects of a diet low in copper on copper-status indicators in postmenopausal women. *Am J Clin Nutr* **63**, 358–364.

Milne, D.B., Davis, C.D., and Nielsen, F.H. (2001) Low dietary zinc alters indices of copper function and status in postmenopausal women. *Nutrition* **17**, 701–708.

Molnar, J., Fong, K.S., He, Q.P., *et al.* (2003) Structural and functional diversity of lysyl oxidase and the LOX-like proteins. *Biochim Biophys Acta* **1647**, 220–224.

Mostad, E. and Prohaska, J. R. (2011) Glycosylphosphatidylinositol-linked ceruloplasmin is expressed in multiple rodent organs and is lower following dietary copper deficiency. *Exp Biol Med* **236**, 298–308.

Patel, B.N., Dunn, R.J., Jeong, S.Y., *et al.* (2002) Ceruloplasmin regulates iron levels in the CNS and prevents free radical injury. *J Neurosci* **22**, 6578–6586.

Penland, J.G. and Prohaska, J.R. (2004) Abnormal motor function persists following recovery from perinatal copper deficiency in rats. *J Nutr* **134**, 1984–1988.

Pennington, J.A. and Schoen, S.A. (1996) Total diet study: estimated dietary intakes of nutritional elements, 1982–1991. *Int J Vitam Nutr Res* **66**, 350–362.

Pratt, W.B., Omdahl, J.L., and Sorenson, J.R. (1985) Lack of effects of copper gluconate supplementation. *Am J Clin Nutr* **42**, 681–682.

Prohaska, J.R. (1988) Biochemical functions of copper in animals. In A.S. Prasad (ed.), *Essential and Toxic Trace Elements in Human Health and Disease*. Alan R. Liss, New York, pp. 105–124.

Prohaska, J.R. (1997) Neurochemical roles of copper as antioxidant or prooxidant. In J.R. Connor (ed.), *Metals and Oxidative Damage in Neurological Disorders*. Plenum Press, New York, pp. 57–75.

Prohaska, J.R. (2011) Impact of copper limitation on expression and function of multicopper oxidases (ferroxidases). *Adv Nutr* **2**, 129–137.

Prohaska, J.R. and Brokate, B. (2002) The timing of perinatal copper deficiency in mice influences offspring survival. *J Nutr* **132**, 3142–3145.

Prohaska, J.R. and Failla, M.L. (1993) Copper and immunity. In D.M. Klurfield (ed.), *Human Nutrition—A Comprehensive Treatise*. Plenum Press, New York, pp. 309–332.

Prohaska, J.R. and Gybina, A.A. (2004) Intracellular copper transport in mammals. *J Nutr* **134**, 1003–1006.

Prohaska, J.R. and Gybina, A.A. (2005) Rat brain iron concentration is lower following perinatal copper deficiency. *J Neurochem* **93**, 698–705.

Prohaska, J.R. and Hoffman, R.G. (1996) Auditory startle response is diminished in rats after recovery from perinatal copper deficiency. *J Nutr* **126**, 618–627.

Prohaska, J.R., Broderius, M., and Brokate, B. (2003) Metallochaperone for Cu,Zn-superoxide dismutase (CCS) protein but not mRNA is higher in organs from copper-deficient mice and rats. *Arch Biochem Biophys* **417**, 227–234.

Prohaska, J.R., Gybina, A.A., Broderius, M., *et al.* (2005) Peptidylglycine-alpha-amidating monooxygenase activity and protein are lower in copper-deficient rats and suckling copper-deficient mice. *Arch Biochem Biophys* **434**, 212–220.

Prohaska, J.R., Tamura, T., Percy, A.K., *et al.* (1997) In vitro copper stimulation of plasma peptidylglycine alpha-amidating monooxygenase in Menkes' disease variant with occipital horns. *Pediatr Res* **42**, 862–865.

Reeves, P.G., Demars, L.C., Johnson, W.T., *et al.* (2005) Dietary copper deficiency reduces iron absorption and duodenal enterocyte hephaestin protein in male and female rats. *J Nutr* **135**, 92–98.

Robinson, N.J. and Winge, D.R. (2010) Copper metallochaperones. *Annu Rev Biochem* **79**, 537–562.

Rutherford, J.C. and Bird, A.J. (2004) Metal-responsive transcription factors that regulate iron, zinc, and copper homeostasis in eukaryotic cells. *Eukaryot Cell* **3**, 1–13.

Saari, J.T. and Schuschke, D.A. (1999) Cardiovascular effects of dietary copper deficiency. *Biofactors* **10**, 359–375.

Salmi, M. and Jalkanen, S. (2001) VAP-1: an adhesin and an enzyme. *Trends Immunol* **22**, 211–216.

Smith, R.M. (1983) Copper and the developing brain. In I.E. Dreosti and R.M. Smith (eds), *Neurobiology of the Trace Elements*. Humana Press, Clifton, NJ, pp. 1–40.

Steveson, T.C., Ciccotosto, G.D., Ma, X.M., *et al.* (2003) Menkes protein contributes to the function of peptidylglycine alpha-amidating monooxygenase. *Endocrinology* **144**, 188–200.

Stolen, C.M., Marttila-Ichihara, F., Koskinen, K., *et al.* (2005) Absence of the endothelial oxidase AOC3 leads to abnormal leukocyte traffic in vivo. *Immunity* **22**, 105–115.

Suazo, M., Olivares, F., Mendez, M.A., *et al.* (2008) CCS and SOD1 mRNA are reduced after copper supplementation in peripheral mononuclear cells of individuals with high serum ceruloplasmin concentration. *J Nutr Biochem* **19**, 269–274.

Suzuki, K.T., Someya, A., Komada, Y., *et al.* (2002) Roles of metallothionein in copper homeostasis: responses to Cu-deficient diets in mice. *J Inorg Biochem* **88**, 173–182.

Takahashi, Y., Kako, K., Kashiwabara, S., *et al.* (2002) Mammalian copper chaperone Cox17p has an essential role in activation of cytochrome C oxidase and embryonic development. *Mol Cell Biol* **22**, 7614–7621.

Tao, T.Y., Liu, F., Klomp, L., *et al.* (2003) The copper toxicosis gene product Murr1 directly interacts with the Wilson disease protein. *J Biol Chem* **278**, 41593–41596.

Thomas, S.A., Matsumoto, A.M., and Palmiter, R.D. (1995) Noradrenaline is essential for mouse fetal development. *Nature* **374**, 643–646.

Trumbo, P., Yates, A.A., Schlicker, S., *et al.* (2001) Dietary reference intakes: vitamin A, vitamin K, arsenic, boron, chromium, copper, iodine, iron, manganese, molybdenum, nickel, silicon, vanadium, and zinc. *J Am Diet Assoc* **101**, 294–301.

Turnlund, J.R., Keyes, W.R., Peiffer, G.L., *et al.* (1998) Copper absorption, excretion, and retention by young men consuming low dietary copper determined by using the stable isotope 65Cu. *Am J Clin Nutr* **67**, 1219–1225.

Turnlund, J.R., Scott, K.C., Peiffer, G.L., *et al.* (1997) Copper status of young men consuming a low-copper diet. *Am J Clin Nutr* **65**, 72–78.

Uauy, R., Olivares, M., and Gonzalez, M. (1998) Essentiality of copper in humans. *Am J Clin Nutr* **67**, 952S–959S.

Uriu-Adams, J.Y., Scherr, R.E., Lanoue, L., *et al.* (2010) Influence of copper on early development: prenatal and postnatal considerations. *Biofactors* **36**, 136–152.

Van de Sluis, B., Muller, P., Duran, K., *et al.* (2007) Increased activity of hypoxia-inducible factor 1 is associated with early embryonic lethality in Commd1 null mice. *Mol Cell Biol* **27**, 4142–4156.

Van den Berghe, P.V. and Klomp, L.W. (2010) Posttranslational regulation of copper transporters. *J Biol Inorg Chem* **15**, 37–46.

Van den Berghe, P.V., Folmer, D.E., Malingre, H.E., *et al.* (2007) Human copper transporter 2 is localized in late endosomes and lysosomes and facilitates cellular copper uptake. *Biochem J* **407**, 49–59.

Vonk, W.I., Wijmenga, C., Berger, R., *et al.* (2010) Cu/Zn superoxide dismutase maturation and activity are regulated by COMMD1. *J Biol Chem* **285**, 28991–29000.

Waggoner, D.J., Drisaldi, B., Bartnikas, T.B., *et al.* (2000) Brain copper content and cuproenzyme activity do not vary with prion protein expression level. *J Biol Chem* **275**, 7455–7458.

West, E.C. and Prohaska, J.R. (2004) Cu,Zn-superoxide dismutase is lower and copper chaperone CCS is higher in erythrocytes of copper-deficient rats and mice. *Exp Biol Med* **229**, 756–764.

White, A.R., Reyes, R., Mercer, J.F., *et al.* (1999) Copper levels are increased in the cerebral cortex and liver of APP and APLP2 knockout mice. *Brain Res* **842**, 439–444.

White, C., Lee, J., Kambe, T., *et al.* (2009) A role for the ATP7A copper-transporting ATPase in macrophage bactericidal activity. *J Biol Chem* **284**, 33949–33956.

Wong, P.C., Waggoner, D., Subramaniam, J.R., *et al.* (2000) Copper chaperone for superoxide dismutase is essential to activate mammalian Cu/Zn superoxide dismutase. *Proc Natl Acad Sci USA* **97**, 2886–2891.

Wu, J.Y., Zhang, J.J., Wang, Y., *et al.* (1997) Regulation of apolipoprotein A-I gene expression in Hep G2 cells depleted of Cu by cupruretic tetramine. *Am J Physiol* **273**, C1362–C1370.

36

IODINE AND IODINE DEFICIENCY DISORDERS

MICHAEL B. ZIMMERMANN, MD

Swiss Federal Institute of Technology, Zürich, Switzerland

Summary

Iodine is an essential component of hormones produced by the thyroid gland. Thyroid hormones, and therefore iodine, are essential for mammalian life. Optimal dietary iodine intakes for healthy adults are 150–250 μg/day. In regions where iodine in soils and drinking water is low, humans and animals may become iodine deficient. Iodine deficiency has multiple adverse effects in humans due to inadequate thyroid hormone production that are termed the iodine deficiency disorders. Assessment methods for iodine deficiency include urinary iodine concentration, goiter, newborn thyroid-stimulating hormone, and blood thyroglobulin. Globally, it is estimated that 2 billion individuals have an insufficient iodine intake, many in developing countries. However, iodine deficiency also affects industrialized countries: ~50% of continental Europe remains mildly iodine deficient, and iodine intakes in other industrialized countries, including the United States, the United Kingdom and Australia, have fallen sharply in recent years. Iodine deficiency during pregnancy and infancy may impair growth and neurodevelopment of the offspring and increase infant mortality. Deficiency during childhood reduces somatic growth and cognitive and motor function. In most countries, the best strategy to control iodine deficiency in populations is carefully monitored iodization of salt, one of the most cost-effective ways to contribute to economic and social development.

Introduction

In 1811, Courtois discovered iodine as a violet vapour arising from seaweed ash while manufacturing gunpowder for Napoleon's army. Gay-Lussac identified it as a new element, and named it iodine (atomic weight 126.9 g/atom), from the Greek word meaning "violet" (Zimmermann, 2008b). The Swiss physician Coindet, in 1813, hypothesized that the traditional treatment of goiter with seaweed was effective because of its iodine content, and successfully treated goitrous patients with iodine. In 1851, the French chemist Chatin published the hypothesis that iodine deficiency was the cause of goiter, and, in 1896, Baumann and Roos discovered iodine in the thyroid

Present Knowledge in Nutrition, Tenth Edition. Edited by John W. Erdman Jr, Ian A. Macdonald and Steven H. Zeisel.
© 2012 International Life Sciences Institute. Published 2012 by John Wiley & Sons, Inc.

(Zimmermann, 2008b). In the first two decades of the twentieth century, pioneering studies by Swiss and American physicians demonstrated the efficacy of iodine prophylaxis in the prevention of goiter and cretinism. Today, control of the iodine deficiency disorders is an integral part of most national nutrition strategies.

> I am satisfied. I have seen the principal features of Swiss scenery – Mount Blanc and the goiter – and now for home.
> Mark Twain, 1880

Ecology and Dietary Sources

Iodine (as iodide) is widely but unevenly distributed in the Earth's environment. In many regions, leaching from glaciation, flooding, and erosion have depleted surface soils of iodide, and most iodide is found in the oceans. The concentration of iodide in seawater is ~50 µg/L. Iodide ions in seawater are oxidized to elemental iodine, which volatilizes into the atmosphere and is returned to the soil by rain, completing the cycle (Küpper et al., 2011). However, iodine cycling in many regions is slow and incomplete, leaving soils and drinking-water iodine depleted. Crops grown in these soils will be low in iodine, and humans and animals consuming food grown in these soils become iodine deficient. In plant foods grown in deficient soils, iodine concentration may be as low as 10 µg/kg dry weight, compared with ~1 mg/kg dry weight in plants from iodine-sufficient soils.

Iodine-deficient soils are common in mountainous areas (e.g. the Alps, Andes, Atlas, and Himalaya ranges) and areas of frequent flooding, especially in South and Southeast Asia (for example, the Ganges River plain of north-eastern India). Many inland areas, including central Asia and Africa, the Midwestern Region of North America, and central and eastern Europe, are iodine deficient. Iodine deficiency in populations residing in these areas will persist until iodine enters the food chain through addition of iodine to foods (e.g. by iodization of salt) or through dietary diversification via introduction of foods produced outside the iodine-deficient area.

The native iodine content of most foods and beverages is low. In general, commonly consumed foods provide 3–80 µg per serving (Pearce et al., 2004; Haldimann et al., 2005). Foods of marine origin have higher iodine content because marine plants and animals concentrate iodine from seawater. Iodine in organic form occurs at high levels in certain seaweeds. Inhabitants of the coastal regions of Japan, whose diets contain large amounts of seaweed, have remarkably high iodine intakes amounting to 50–80 mg/day. In the United States the median intake of iodine from food in the mid-1990s was estimated to be 240–300 µg/day for men and 190–210 µg/day for women (Institute of Medicine, 2001). Major dietary sources of iodine in the United States are bread and milk (Pearce et al., 2004). In Switzerland, based on direct food analysis, mean intake of dietary iodine is ~140 µg/day, mainly from bread and dairy products (Haldimann et al., 2005). In many countries, use of iodized salt in households for cooking and at the table provides additional iodine. Boiling, baking, and canning of foods containing iodized salt cause only small losses (≤10%) of iodine content (Chavasit et al., 2002).

Iodine content in foods is also influenced by iodine-containing compounds used in irrigation, fertilizers, and livestock feed. Iodophors used for cleaning milking machines and transport containers can increase the native iodine content of dairy products. Traditionally, iodate was used in bread making as a dough conditioner, but it is being replaced by non-iodine-containing conditioners. Erythrosine is a red coloring agent high in iodine that is widely used in foods, cosmetics, and pharmaceuticals. Dietary supplements often contain iodine. Based on data from the Third National Health and Nutrition Examination Survey (NHANES III), 12% of men and 15% of non-pregnant women took a dietary supplement that contained iodine, and the median intake of iodine from supplements was ~140 µg/day for adults (Institute of Medicine, 2001). Other sources of iodine include water purification tablets, radiographic contrast media, medicines (e.g. amiodarone, an antiarrhythmic drug, contains 75 mg/tablet), and skin disinfectants (e.g. povidone-iodine contains ~10 mg/mL).

Absorption, Metabolism, and Excretion

Iodine is ingested in several chemical forms. Iodide is rapidly and nearly completely absorbed in the stomach and duodenum. The sodium/iodide symporter (NIS), a transmembrane protein on the apical surface of enterocytes, mediates active iodine absorption (Nicola et al., 2009). Iodate, widely used in salt iodization, is reduced in the gut and absorbed as iodide. In healthy adults, the absorption of iodide is >90% (Institute of Medicine, 2001). Organically bound iodine is typically digested and the released iodide absorbed, but some forms may be absorbed intact. For example, ≈75% of an oral dose of thyroxine, the thyroid hormone, is absorbed intact.

Iodine deficiency is the main cause of endemic goiter (see later in this chapter), but other dietary substances that interfere with thyroid metabolism can aggravate the effect and they are termed goitrogens (Gaitan, 1990). A well-known example is linamarin, a thioglycoside found in cassava, which is a staple food in many developing counties. If cassava is not adequately soaked or cooked to remove the linamarin, it is hydrolyzed in the gut to release cyanide, which is metabolized to thiocyanate. Thiocyanate blocks thyroidal uptake of iodine. Other goitrogenic substances are found in millet, sweet potato, beans, and cruciferous vegetables (e.g. cabbage). Unclean drinking water may contain humic substances that block thyroidal iodination. Industrial pollutants, including resorcinol, perchlorate, and phthalic acid, may also be goitrogenic. Most of these substances do not have a major clinical effect unless there is coexisting iodine deficiency.

Deficiencies of selenium, iron, and vitamin A exacerbate the effects of iodine deficiency. Glutathione peroxidase and the deoidinases are selenium-dependent enzymes. In selenium deficiency, accumulated peroxides may damage the thyroid, and deiodinase deficiency impairs thyroid hormone synthesis (Zimmermann and Kohrle, 2002). These effects have been implicated in the etiology of myxedematous cretinism (see next section). Iron deficiency reduces heme-dependent thyroperoxidase activity in the thyroid and impairs production of thyroid hormone. In goitrous children, iron deficiency anemia blunts the efficacy of iodine prophylaxis while iron supplementation improves the efficacy of iodized oil and iodized salt (Zimmermann, 2006). Vitamin A deficiency in iodine-deficient children increases TSH stimulation and risk for goiter, probably through decreased vitamin A-mediated suppression of the pituitary TSHβ gene (Zimmermann et al., 2007).

The distribution space of absorbed iodine in the body is nearly equal to the extracellular fluid volume. Iodine is cleared from the circulation mainly by the thyroid and kidney (Figure 36.1), and whereas renal iodine clearance is fairly constant, thyroid clearance varies with iodine intake. In conditions of adequate iodine supply, ≤10% of absorbed iodine is taken up by the thyroid. In chronic iodine deficiency, this fraction can exceed 80%. During lactation, the mammary gland concentrates iodine and secretes it into breast milk to provide for the newborn. Iodine in the blood is turned over rapidly; under normal circumstances, plasma iodine has a half-life of ~10 hours,

but this is shortened if the thyroid is overactive as in iodine deficiency or hyperthyroidism.

The body of a healthy adult contains up to 20 mg of iodine, of which 70–80% is in the thyroid. In chronic iodine deficiency, the iodine content of the thyroid may fall to <1 mg. In iodine-sufficient areas, the adult thyroid traps 60–80 μg of iodine per day to balance losses and maintain thyroid hormone synthesis. An NIS in the basolateral membrane transfers iodide into the thyroid at a concentration gradient 20 to 50 times that of plasma (Eskandari et al., 1997). The NIS concentrates iodine by an active transport process that couples the energy released by the inward translocation of sodium down its electrochemical gradient to the simultaneous inward translocation of iodine against its electrochemical gradient.

Thyroglobulin (Tg), a large glycoprotein (molecular weight 660 000), is the carrier of iodine in the thyroid. At the apical surface of the thyrocyte, the enzymes thyroperoxidase (TPO) and hydrogen peroxide oxidize iodide and attach it to tyrosyl residues on Tg, to produce monoiodotyrosine (MIT) and diiodotyrosine (DIT), the precursors of thyroid hormone (Figure 36.2). TPO then catalyzes the coupling of the phenyl groups of the iodotyrosines through a di-ether bridge to form the thyroid hormones. Linkage of two DIT molecules produces tetraiodothyronine or thyroxine (T4), and linkage of an MIT and a DIT produces triiodothyronine (T3). Thus, T3 is structurally identical to T4 but has one less iodine (at the 5′ position on the outer ring) (Figure 36.3). Iodine comprises 65% and 59% of the weights of T4 and T3, respectively. In the thyroid, mature Tg, containing 0.1 to 1.0% of its weight as iodine, is stored extracellularly in the luminal colloid of the thyroid follicle. After endocytosis, endosomal and lysosomal proteases digest Tg and release T4 and T3 into the circulation. MIT and DIT are not normally released into the blood. Iodine is removed from their tyrosines by a selenium-dependent deiodinase and is then recycled for use within the thyroid, conserving iodine (Kohrle and Gartner, 2009).

In the circulation, thyroid hormone is bound noncovalently to carrier proteins, mainly thyroxine-binding globulin, but also to transthyretin and albumin. In target tissues – liver, kidney, heart, muscle, pituitary, and the developing brain – T4 is deiodinated to T3. T3 is the main physiologically active form of thyroid hormone and binds to nuclear receptors. The thyroid hormone receptors have been cloned and regulatory DNA elements identified in thyroid hormone responsive genes (Yen,

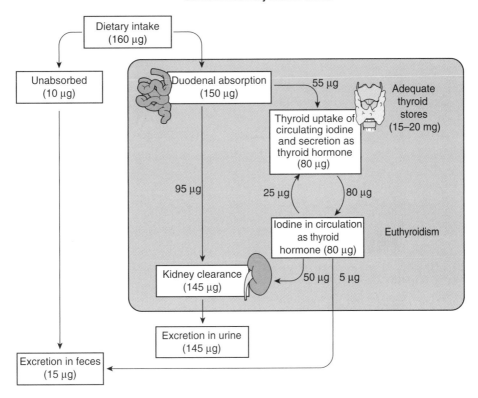

Sufficient dietary iodine intake

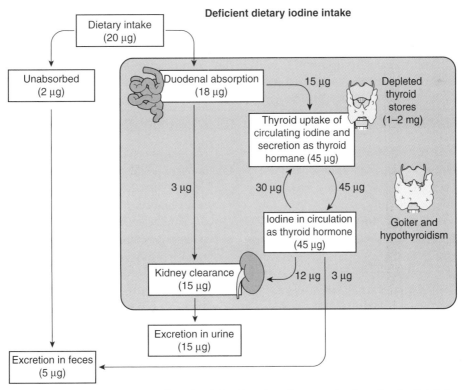

Deficient dietary iodine intake

FIG. 36.1 Over 90% of dietary iodine is absorbed in the duodenum. Iodine (as iodide) is cleared from the circulation mainly by the thyroid and kidney. Thyroid clearance varies with iodine intake. Above: in iodine-sufficient individuals with adequate thyroid iodine stores, about 35% of circulating iodide is taken up by the thyroid to balance losses and maintain thyroid hormone synthesis. Below: in chronic iodine deficiency, the fraction of circulating iodide cleared by the thyroid increases to about 65% but the iodine content of the thyroid is depleted and hypothyroidism develops.

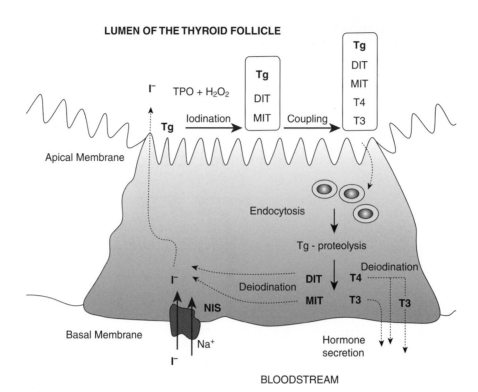

FIG. 36.2 Iodine pathway in the thyroid cell. Iodide (I⁻) is transported into the thyrocyte by the sodium iodide symporter (NIS) at the basal membrane and migrates to the apical membrane. The I⁻ is oxidized by the enzymes thyroperoxidase (TPO) and hydrogen peroxidase (H_2O_2), and attached to tyrosyl residues in thyroglobulin (Tg) to produce the hormone precursors iodotyrosine (MIT) and diiodotyrosine (DIT). The residues then couple to form thyroxine (T4) and triiodothyronine (T3) within the Tg molecule in the follicular lumen. Tg enters the cell by endocytosis and is digested. T4 and T3 are released into the circulation, and non-hormonal iodine on MIT and DIT is recycled within the thyrocyte.

2001). Hormone–receptor interactions stimulate several pathways, including the adenosine triphosphate (ATP) and inositol phosphate–Ca^{2+} cascades, which in turn stimulate or inhibit protein synthesis.

Both T4 and T3 are degraded through a complex series of pathways, and their turnover is relatively slow: the half-lives of T4 and T3 are ~5 days and 1.5–3 days (Oppenheimer *et al.*, 1975). The released iodine enters the plasma iodine pool and can be taken up again by the thyroid or excreted by the kidney. More than 90% of ingested iodine is ultimately excreted in the urine, with only a small amount appearing in the feces.

The principal regulator of thyroid hormone metabolism is thyroid-stimulating hormone (TSH), a protein hormone (molecular weight ~28 000) secreted by the pituitary. TSH secretion is controlled through negative feedback by the level of circulating thyroid hormone, modulated by TSH-releasing hormone from the hypothalamus. In the thyroid,

TSH increases iodine uptake through stimulation of NIS expression. TSH exerts its action at the transcription level of the NIS gene through a thyroid-specific enhancer that contains binding sites for the transcription factor Pax8 and a cAMP response element-like sequence (Taki *et al.*, 2002). TSH also stimulates breakdown of Tg and release of thyroid hormone into the blood. Because the primary stimulus to TSH secretion is circulating thyroid hormone, an elevated serum TSH concentration generally indicates primary hypothyroidism, while a low concentration indicates primary hyperthyroidism.

Physiologic Function and Deficiency Disorders

Thyroid hormone regulates a variety of physiologic processes, including reproductive function, growth, and development. During pregnancy, thyroid hormone crosses the

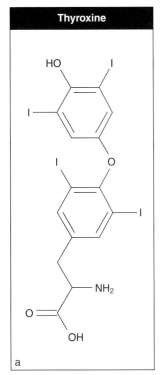

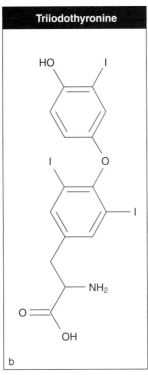

FIG. 36.3 Iodine is an essential component of the thyroid hormones, thyroxine (T4) and triiodotyrosine (T3).

TABLE 36.1 Iodine deficiency disorders by age group

Age group	Health consequences of iodine deficiency
All ages	Goiter
	Increased susceptibility of the thyroid gland to nuclear radiation
Fetus	Abortion
	Stillbirth
	Congenital anomalies
	Perinatal mortality
Neonate	Infant mortality
	Endemic cretinism
Child and adolescent	Impaired mental function
	Delayed physical development
Adults	Impaired mental function
	Reduced work productivity
	Toxic nodular goiter; iodine-induced hyperthyroidism
	Hypothyroidism in moderate-to-severe iodine deficiency

Adapted from World Health Organization (2007).

placenta to the fetus early in the first trimester, before the fetal thyroid is functioning. In the developing brain, it influences cell growth and migration (Morreale de Escobar *et al.*, 2004). It also promotes growth and maturation of peripheral tissues and the skeleton. Thyroid hormone increases energy metabolism in most tissues, and raises the basal metabolic rate.

Iodine deficiency has multiple adverse effects on growth and development in animals and humans. These are collectively termed the iodine deficiency disorders (IDD) (Table 36.1), and are one of the most important and common human diseases (World Health Organization, 2007). They result from inadequate thyroid hormone production due to lack of sufficient iodine.

Thyroid enlargement (goiter) is the classic sign of iodine deficiency (Figure 36.4A). It is a physiologic adaptation to chronic iodine deficiency. As iodine intake falls, secretion of TSH increases in an effort to maximize uptake of available iodine, and TSH stimulates thyroid hypertrophy and hyperplasia. Initially, goiters are characterized by diffuse, homogeneous enlargement, but over time thyroid follicles may fuse and become encapsulated, a condition termed nodular goiter. Large goiters may be cosmetically unattractive, can obstruct the trachea and esophagus, and may damage the recurrent laryngeal nerves and cause hoarseness.

Although goiter is the most visible effect of iodine deficiency, the most serious adverse effect is damage to the developing brain. Severe iodine deficiency during pregnancy is associated with a greater incidence of stillbirths, abortions, and congenital abnormalities. Iodine prophylaxis with iodized oil in pregnant women in areas of severe iodine deficiency reduces fetal and perinatal mortality (Zimmermann, 2009). The fetal brain is particularly vulnerable to iodine deficiency. Normal levels of thyroid hormones are required for neuronal migration and myelination of the central nervous system (Auso *et al.*, 2004). The most severe form of neurological damage from fetal hypothyroidism is termed cretinism. It is characterized by gross mental retardation along with varying degrees of short stature, deaf mutism, and spasticity (Zimmermann *et al.*, 2008) (Figure 36.4B). Up to 10% of populations with severe iodine deficiency may be cretinous. Iodine prophylaxis has completely eliminated the appearance of new cases of cretinism in previously severely iodine-deficient Alpine regions in Switzerland, Austria, and Italy.

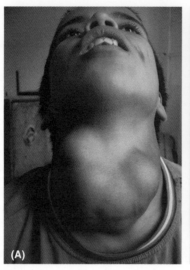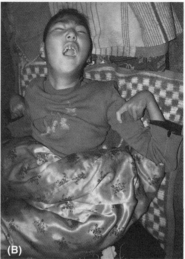

© MB Zimmermann

FIG. 36.4. (A) Large nodular goiter in a 14-year-old boy in northern Morocco, with tracheal and esophageal compression and hoarseness, likely due to damage to the recurrent laryngeal nerves. (B) This 9-year-old girl from western China demonstrates the three characteristic features of neurological cretinism: severe mental deficiency together with squint, deaf mutism, and motor spasticity of the arms and legs. Reproduced with permission from Michael B. Zimmermann.

Although new cases of cretinism are now rare, iodine deficiency still affects approximately one-third of the global population (see later) and can impair cognitive development. A meta-analysis concluded that moderate-to-severe iodine deficiency (severity of iodine deficiency was defined by the cut-off values for median urinary iodine concentrations shown in Table 36.4) reduces mean IQ scores by 13.5 points (Bleichrodt *et al.*, 1996). Iodine deficiency is one of the most common causes of preventable mental impairment worldwide. Even in areas of mild to moderate iodine deficiency, cognitive impairment in school-age children is at least partly reversible by administration of iodine (Zimmermann *et al.*, 2006a; Gordon *et al.*, 2009).

Only a few countries – Switzerland, the Scandinavian countries, Australia, the United States, and Canada – were completely iodine sufficient before 1990. Since then, widespread introduction of iodized salt has produced dramatic reductions in iodine deficiency. The World Health Organization recently estimated the worldwide prevalence of iodine deficiency. Defined as a UI <100 μg/L, just over 2 billion individuals have inadequate iodine nutrition, of whom 266 million are school-age children (Table 36.2). The prevalence of iodine deficiency in school-age children is 31.5% (de Benoist *et al.*, 2008). In Australia, the United

TABLE 36.2 Prevalence of iodine deficiency in general population (all age groups) and in school-age children (6–12 years), by WHO region, in 2007

WHO region[a]	Population[b] (millions) with urinary iodine <100 μg/L (%)	
	General population	School-age children
Africa	312.9 [41.5%]	57.7 [40.8%]
Americas	98.6 [11.0%]	11.6 [10.6%]
Eastern Mediterranean	259.3 [47.2%]	43.3 [48.8%]
Europe	459.7 [52.0%]	38.7 [52.4%]
Southeast Asia	503.6 [30.0%]	73.1 [30.3%]
Western Pacific	374.7 [21.2%]	41.6 [22.7%]
Total	2008.8 [30.6%]	266.0 [31.5%]

[a]193 WHO Member States.
[b]Based on population estimates for 2006 (see also United Nations, 2011). Data from de Benoist *et al.* (2008).

Kingdom, and the United States, three countries previously iodine sufficient, iodine intakes are falling. Australia and the United Kingdom are now mildly iodine deficient, and in the United States the median UI in women is 130 μg/L, still adequate but less than half the median value of 321 μg/L found in the 1970s (Perrine *et al.*, 2010).

Dairy products are an important iodine source in US diets, and women who do not consume dairy products may be at risk for iodine deficiency (Perrine *et al.*, 2010). These changes emphasize the importance of regular monitoring of iodine status in countries throughout the world.

Requirements and Status Assessment

The US Food and Nutrition Board of the National Academy of Sciences has set an adequate intake (AI) for iodine in infancy and a recommended dietary allowance (RDA) for children, adults and pregnant and lactating women (Institute of Medicine, 2001) (Table 36.3). The WHO has established recommended nutrient intakes for iodine (World Health Organization, 2007) (Table 36.3). Iodine requirements for different age and population groups have been established based on studies of radio-iodine uptake by the thyroid, balance studies, and factorial estimates (Institute of Medicine, 2001).

Several methods are available for assessment of iodine status. The most commonly used are measurement of thyroid size and concentration of urinary iodine (UI) (World Health Organization, 2007). Additional indicators include newborn thyrotropin (TSH), and blood concentrations of thyroglobulin, thyroxine (T4) or triiodothyronine (T3). As discussed below, UI is a sensitive indicator of recent iodine intake (days), and serum Tg shows an intermediate response (weeks to months), whereas changes in the goiter rate reflect long-term iodine nutrition (months to years).

Two methods are available for measuring goiter: neck inspection and palpation, and thyroid ultrasonography. Goiter surveys are usually done in school-age children. By palpation, a thyroid is considered goitrous when each lateral lobe has a volume greater than the terminal phalanx of the thumbs of the subject being examined. In the classification system of WHO, grade 0 is defined as a thyroid that is not palpable or visible, grade 1 is a goiter that is palpable but not visible when the neck is in the normal position (i.e. the thyroid is not visibly enlarged), and grade 2 goiter is a thyroid that is clearly visible when the neck is in a normal position.

In areas of mild to moderate iodine deficiency, where goiters are small, measurement of thyroid size by ultrasonography is a more objective and precise method and is preferable to palpation. Portable ultrasound equipment can be used in the field, and goiter classified according to international reference criteria for iodine-sufficient children by age, gender, and body surface area (Zimmermann *et al.*, 2004a). The total goiter rate is used to define severity using the following criteria: <5%, iodine sufficiency; 5.0–19.9%, mild deficiency; 20.0–-29.9%, moderate deficiency; and >30%, severe deficiency (World Health Organization, 2007).

In areas of endemic goiter, although thyroid size predictably decreases in response to increases in iodine intake, thyroid size may not return to normal for months or years after correction of iodine deficiency (Zimmermann *et al.*, 2003a). During this transition period, the goiter rate is difficult to interpret because it reflects both a population's history of iodine nutrition and its present status. Despite this lag period, a sustained salt iodization program will decrease the goiter rate to <5% in school-age children, and this indicates disappearance of iodine deficiency as a significant public health problem (World Health Organization, 2007).

TABLE 36.3 Recommendations for iodine intake (μg/day) by age or population group

Age or population group	US Institute of Medicine[a]		Age or population group	World Health Organization[b]
	EAR	AI or RDA		RNI
Infants 0–12 months	–	110–130	Children 0–5 years	90
Children 1–8 years	65	90	Children 6–12 years	120
Children 9–13 years	73	120		
Adults ≥14 years	95	150	Adults >12 years	150
Pregnancy	160	220	Pregnancy	250
Lactation	200	290	Lactation	250

AI, adequate intake; EAR, estimated average requirement; RDA, recommended daily allowance; RNI, recommended nutrient intake.
[a]Data from Institute of Medicine (2001).
[b]Data from World Health Organization (2007).

Because >90% of ingested iodine is excreted in the urine, UI is an excellent indicator of recent iodine intake. Most methods of measuring UI are based on the Sandell-Kolthoff reaction, in which iodide catalyzes the reduction of yellow ceric ammonium sulfate to the colorless cerous form in the presence of arsenious acid (Bier *et al.*, 1998). UI can be expressed as a concentration (μg/L), in relation to creatinine excretion (μg iodine/g creatinine), or as 24-hour excretion (μg/day). To estimate iodine intakes in individuals, 24-hour collections may be preferable. For populations, because it is impractical to collect 24-hour samples in field studies, UI can be measured in spot urine specimens from a representative sample of the target group, and expressed as the median, in μg/L (World Health Organization, 2007) (Table 36.4). Variations in hydration among individuals generally even out in a large number of samples, so that the median UI in spot samples correlates well with that from 24-hour samples. Creatinine may be unreliable for estimating daily iodine excretion from spot samples, especially in malnourished subjects where creatinine concentration is low. Spot UI measurements in population studies are often misinterpreted. Although the median UI is a population indicator, it is a common mistake to assume that all subjects with a spot UI <100 μg/L are iodine deficient, but, even in iodine-sufficient regions where intrathyroidal iodine stores are adequate, individual spot UI concentrations are highly variable from day to day.

Daily iodine intake for population estimates can be extrapolated from UI, using estimates of mean 24-hour urine volume and assuming an average iodine bioavailability of 92%. This can be done using the following formula (Institute of Medicine, 2001):

$$\text{Urinary iodine (μg/L)} \times 0.0235 \times \text{body weight (kg)}$$
$$= \text{daily iodine intake}$$

TABLE 36.4 Epidemiological criteria from the World Health Organization for assessment of iodine nutrition in a population based on median or range of urinary iodine concentrations

Population group	Iodine intake	Iodine nutrition
School-age children		
<20 μg/L	Insufficient	Severe iodine deficiency
20–49 μg/L	Insufficient	Moderate iodine deficiency
50–99 μg/L	Insufficient	Mild iodine deficiency
100–199 μg/L	Adequate	Optimum
200–299 μg/L	More than adequate	Risk of iodine-induced hyperthyroidism in susceptible groups
>300 μg/L	Excessive	Risk of adverse health consequences (iodine-induced hyperthyroidism, autoimmune thyroid disease)
Pregnant women		
<150 μg/L	Insufficient	
150–249 μg/L	Adequate	
250–499 μg/L	More than adequate	
≥500 μg/L[a]	Excessive	
Lactating women[b]		
<100 μg/L	Insufficient	
≥100 μg/L	Adequate	
Children less than 2 years of age		
<100 μg/L	Insufficient	
≥100 μg/L	Adequate	

[a]The term "excessive" means in excess of the amount needed to prevent and control iodine deficiency. There may be an increased risk of adverse effects at this level of intake.
[b]In lactating women, the numbers for median urinary iodine are lower than the iodine requirements, because of the iodine excreted in breast milk.
Data from World Health Organization (2007).

Using this formula, a UI of 100 µg/L in an average adult corresponds roughly to a daily intake of 150 µg.

Because serum TSH is determined mainly by the level of circulating thyroid hormone, which in turn reflects iodine intake, TSH can be used as an indicator of iodine nutrition. However, in older children and adults, although serum TSH may be slightly increased by iodine deficiency, values often remain within the normal range. TSH is therefore a relatively insensitive indicator of iodine nutrition in adults. In contrast, TSH is a sensitive indicator of iodine status in the newborn period. Compared with the adult, the newborn thyroid contains less iodine but has higher rates of iodine turnover. Particularly when iodine supply is low, maintaining high iodine turnover requires increased TSH stimulation. Serum TSH concentrations are therefore increased in iodine-deficient infants for the first few weeks of life, a condition termed transient newborn hypothyroidism. In areas of iodine deficiency, an increase in transient newborn hypothyroidism, indicated by >3 % of newborn TSH values above the threshold of 5 mU/L whole blood, suggests iodine deficiency in the population (Zimmermann et al., 2005a). TSH is used in many countries for routine newborn screening to detect congenital hypothyroidism. If already in place, such screening offers a sensitive indicator of iodine nutrition. Newborn TSH is an important measure because it reflects iodine status during a period when the developing brain is particularly sensitive to iodine deficiency.

Thyroglobulin (Tg) is synthesized only in the thyroid, and is the most abundant intrathyroidal protein. In iodine sufficiency, small amounts of Tg are secreted into the circulation, and serum Tg is normally <10 µg/L. In areas of endemic goiter, serum Tg increases due to greater thyroid cell mass and TSH stimulation, and is a sensitive indicator of iodine status (Zimmermann et al., 2003b; Vejbjerg et al., 2009). Tg can also be assayed on dried blood spots taken by a finger prick, simplifying collection and transport (Zimmermann et al., 2006b), and Tg in school-age children is now recommended to assess iodine status in populations (World Health Organization, 2007). In contrast, thyroid hormone concentrations are poor indicators of iodine status. In iodine-deficient populations, serum T3 increases or remains unchanged, and serum T4 usually decreases. However, these changes are often within the normal range, and the overlap with iodine-sufficient populations is large enough to make thyroid hormone levels an insensitive measure of iodine nutrition.

Prophylaxis and Treatment

There are two methods commonly used to correct iodine deficiency in a population: iodized oil and iodized salt. In nearly all regions affected by iodine deficiency, the most effective way to control iodine deficiency is through salt iodization (World Health Organization, 2007). All salt for human consumption, including salt used in the food industry, should be continuously iodized. In Switzerland, previously affected by endemic goiter and cretinism, a monitored national program, in place for over half a century, has effectively eliminated iodine deficiency (Zimmermann et al., 2005a). Iodine can be added to salt in the form of potassium iodide (KI) or potassium iodate (KIO$_3$). Because KIO$_3$ has higher stability in the presence of salt impurities, humidity, and porous packaging (Diosady and Mannar, 2000), it is the recommended form. Iodine is usually added at a level of 20–40 mg iodine/kg salt, depending on local salt intake(World Health Organization, 2007). But in industrialized countries, because 80–90% of salt consumption is from purchased processed foods (Sanchez-Castillo et al., 1987; Andersen et al., 2009), if only household salt is iodized it will not supply adequate iodine. Thus, although it is critical that the food industry use iodized salt, in many countries it is not added to processed foods. Food producers are often reluctant to add iodized salt because of the widespread misperception that iodine can precipitate adverse sensory changes in their products. However, this does not occur, as the iodine is added in only minute amounts; fortified salt has only parts-per-million concentrations. The current push to reduce salt consumption to prevent chronic diseases and the policy of salt iodization to eliminate iodine deficiency do not conflict: iodization methods can fortify salt to provide recommended iodine intakes even if per capita salt intakes are reduced to <5 g/day (World Health Organization, 2008).

As a result of a major international effort led by WHO, the United Nations Children's Fund (UNICEF) and the International Council for the Control of Iodine Deficiency Disorders (ICCIDD), more than 120 countries have implemented salt iodization programs and ~70% of people worldwide have access to iodized salt in 2006, compared with <10% in 1990 (United Nations Children's Fund, 2008). However, when coverage is not complete, iodized salt use is often lowest in the poorest socioeconomic classes, typically the population most affected by iodine deficiency. For a national program to succeed, ≥95% of salt for human consumption should be iodized according to government standards at the production or importation site. Worldwide, sustainability of iodized salt programs has become a major focus. These programs are fragile, and require a long-term commitment from national governments, donors, consumers, and the salt industry. In several countries where iodine deficiency had been eliminated, salt iodization programs fell apart, and iodine deficiency recurred (Dunn, 2000). Children in iodine-deficient areas are vulnerable to even short-term lapses in iodized salt programs (Zimmermann *et al.*, 2004b).

In some regions, iodization of salt may not be practical for control of iodine deficiency, at least in the short term. This may occur in remote areas where communications are poor or where there are numerous very small-scale salt producers. In these areas, other options for correction of iodine deficiency should be considered, such as iodized oil (World Health Organization, 2007). Iodized oil is prepared by esterification of the unsaturated fatty acids in seed or vegetable oils, and addition of iodine to the double bonds. It can be given orally or by intramuscular injection. The intramuscular route has a longer duration of action (up to 2 years), but oral administration is more common because it is simpler. Iodized oil is recommended for populations with moderate to severe iodine deficiencies that do not have access to iodized salt, and may be targeted at women of child-bearing age, pregnant women, and children. The recommended dose is 400 mg iodine per year for women and 200 mg iodine per year for children 7–24 months of age (World Health Organization, 2007). Iodine can also be given as potassium iodide or iodate as drops or tablets, and in drinking or irrigation water (Squatrito *et al.*, 1986). Iodine supplements (~150 μg/day) are recommended for pregnant and lactating women residing in areas of mild to moderate iodine deficiency. In the United States, because it is uncertain if dietary iodine intakes are adequate in pregnancy, expert groups have recently called for iodine supplementation of this group (Becker *et al.*, 2006). In countries where iodized salt programs supply sufficient iodine to older children and pregnant women, weaning infants, particularly those not receiving iodine-containing infant formula milk, may be at risk of iodine deficiency (Andersson *et al.*, 2010).

Excess and Toxicity

Acute iodine poisoning caused by ingestion of many grams causes gastrointestinal irritation, abdominal pain, nausea, vomiting, and diarrhea, as well as cardiovascular symptoms, coma, and cyanosis (Pennington, 1990). Most people are remarkably tolerant of high dietary intakes of iodine. The US Food and Nutrition Board of the National Academy of Sciences has set a tolerable upper intake level (UL) for iodine (Institute of Medicine, 2001). The UL is the highest level of daily intake that is likely to pose no risk of adverse health effects in almost all individuals. The UL is 200 μg/day for ages 1–3 years, 300 μg/day for ages 4–8 years, 600 μg/day for ages 9–13 years, 900 μg/day for ages 14–18 years, and 1100 μg/day thereafter. Individuals with autoimmune thyroid disease or chronic iodine deficiency may respond adversely to intakes lower than these (Zimmermann, 2008a).

In iodine-sufficient individuals, the earliest effect of high iodine intakes is typically an increase in serum TSH without a decrease in serum T4 or T3, a condition termed subclinical hypothyroidism. Large excesses of iodine inhibit thyroid hormone production, leading to increased TSH stimulation, thyroid growth, and goiter. A clinical trial in healthy adults found TSH concentrations were increased by total iodine intakes of ≥750 μg/day (Chow *et al.*, 1991). In children, chronic intakes of ≥500 μg/day are associated with increased thyroid volume, an early sign of thyroid dysfunction (Zimmermann *et al.*, 2005b). Iodine-induced goiter and hypothyroidism can occur in newborns due to high maternal intakes, or through exposure to excess iodine at delivery from the use of antiseptics containing beta-iodine (Nishiyama *et al.*, 2004). Prospective studies in China have suggested chronic excess iodine intakes are associated with a small increase in subclinical hypothyroidism and autoimmune thyroiditis, but not overt hypo- or hyperthyroidism (Teng *et al.*, 2006).

A rapid increase in iodine intake of populations with chronic iodine deficiency may precipitate iodine-induced hyperthyroidism (IIH) (Delange *et al.*, 1999). This is more likely to occur if the iodine is given in excess, e.g. if the iodine content of iodized salt is too high, or when iodine-containing medication is given. IIH occurs mainly in older people with nodular goiter. Thyrocytes in nodules often become insensitive to TSH control, and, if iodine supply is suddenly increased, these autonomous nodules may overproduce thyroid hormone (Corvilain *et al.*, 1998). Symptoms of IIH include weight loss, tachycardia, muscle weakness, and skin warmth, without the ophthalmopathy of Graves' disease. IIH is dangerous when superimposed on underlying heart disease, and may be lethal. Introduction of iodine prophylaxis has been associated with increased hospitalizations for IIH in Europe, the United States, and several African countries. The incidence tends to gradually abate, but may rise again when the level of iodine in salt is increased. Its occurrence should not be an argument against salt iodization, as the underlying cause of most autonomous nodules and IIH is chronic iodine deficiency. To reduce risk for IIH, the iodine level in salt should be monitored and reduced if too high.

Future Directions

Future research priorities in iodine nutrition should include correlation of community iodine intake with thyroid disease, the potential role of iodine in fibrocystic breast disease and the immune response, and interactions with other nutrients, particularly vitamin A, iron, and selenium. In the field of IDD, efforts should focus on ensuring adequate iodine during pregnancy and infancy. Monitoring indicators for these key target populations need to be developed and tested. More research on the effects of high intakes of iodine from iodized salt and/or other sources could lead to better estimates of the UL for iodine in different ages and populations. Globally, the elimination of iodine deficiency is within reach, but effort is needed to cover the remaining populations at risk and to ensure quality control and sustainability of existing iodized salt programs.

Suggestions for Further Reading

World Health Organization, United Nations Children's Fund, International Council for Control of Iodine Deficiency Disorders (2007) *Assessment of Iodine Deficiency Disorders and Monitoring Their Elimination: A Guide for Programme Managers*, 3rd Edn. World Health Organization, Geneva.

Zimmermann, M.B. (2009) Iodine deficiency. *Endocr Rev* **30**, 376–408.

Zimmermann, M.B., Jooste, P.L., and Pandav C.S. (2008) Iodine-deficiency disorders. *Lancet* **372**, 1251–1262.

References

Andersen, L., Rasmussen, L.B., Larsen, E.H., *et al.* (2009) Intake of household salt in a Danish population. *Eur J Clin Nutr* **63**, 598–604.

Andersson, M., Aeberli, I., Wüst, N., *et al.* (2010) The Swiss iodized salt program provides adequate iodine for school children and pregnant women but weaning infants not receiving iodine-containing complementary foods are iodine deficient. *J Clin Endocrinol Metab* **95**, 5217–5224.

Auso, E., Lavado-Autric, R., Cuevas, E., *et al.* (2004) A moderate and transient deficiency of maternal thyroid function at the beginning of fetal neocorticogenesis alters neuronal migration. *Endocrinology* **145**, 4037–4047.

Becker, D.V., Braverman, L.E., Delange, F., *et al.* (2006) Iodine supplementation for pregnancy and lactation – United States and Canada: recommendations of the American Thyroid Association. *Thyroid* **16**, 949–951.

Bier, D., Rendl, J., Ziemann, M., *et al.* (1998) Methodological and analytical aspects of simple methods for measuring iodine in urine. Comparison with HPLC and Technicon Autoanalyzer II. *Exp Clin Endocrinol Diabetes* **106**(Suppl 3), S27–31.

Bleichrodt, N., Shrestha, R.M., West, C.E., *et al.* (1996) The benefits of adequate iodine intake. *Nutr Rev* **54**, S72–78.

Chavasit, V., Malaivongse, P., and Judprasong, K. (2002) Study on stability of iodine in iodated salt by use of different cooking model conditions. *J Food Comp Anal* **15**, 265–276.

Chow, C.C., Phillips, D.I., Lazarus, J.H., *et al.* (1991) Effect of low dose iodide supplementation on thyroid function in potentially susceptible subjects: are dietary iodide levels in Britain acceptable? *Clin Endocrinol (Oxf)* **34**, 413–416.

Corvilain, B., Van Sande, J., Dumont, J.E., *et al.* (1998) Autonomy in endemic goiter. *Thyroid* **8**, 107–113.

de Benoist, B., McLean, E., Andersson, M., *et al.* (2008) Iodine deficiency in 2007: global progress since 2003. *Food Nutr Bull* **29**, 195–202.

Delange, F., de Benoist, B., and Alnwick, D. (1999) Risks of iodine-induced hyperthyroidism after correction of iodine deficiency by iodized salt. *Thyroid* **9**, 545–556.

Diosady, L.L. and Mannar, M.G.V. (2000) Stability of iodine in iodized salt. *8th World Salt Symposium*, Vols **1 and 2**, pp. 977–982

Dunn, J.T. (2000) Complacency: the most dangerous enemy in the war against iodine deficiency. *Thyroid* **10**, 681–683.

Eskandari, S., Loo, D.D., Dai, G.O., *et al.* (1997) Thyroid Na+/I- symporter. Mechanism, stoichiometry, and specificity. *J Biol Chem* **272**, 27230–27238.

Gaitan, E. (1990) Goitrogens in food and water. *Annu Rev Nutr* **10**, 21–39.

Gordon, R.C., Rose, M.C., Skeaff, S.A., *et al.* (2009) Iodine supplementation improves cognition in mildly iodine-deficient children. *Am J Clin Nutr* **90**, 1264–1271.

Haldimann, M., Alt, A., Blanc, A., *et al.* (2005) Iodine content of food groups. *J Food Comp Anal* **18**, 461–471.

Institute of Medicine (2001) Iodine. In *Dietary Reference Intakes for Vitamin A, Vitamin K, Arsenic, Boron, Chromium, Copper, Iodine, Iron, Manganese, Molybdenum, Nickel, Silicon, Vanadium and Zinc.* National Academy Press, Washington, DC.

Kohrle, J. and Gartner, R. (2009) Selenium and thyroid. *Best Pract Res Clin Endocrinol Metab* **23**, 815–827.

Küpper, F.C., Feiters, M.C., Olofsson, B., *et al.* (2011) Commemorating two centuries of iodine research: an interdisciplinary overview of current research. *Angew Chem Int Ed Engl* **50** (49), 11598–11620.

Morreale de Escobar, G., Obregon, M.J., and Escobar del Rey, F. (2004) Role of thyroid hormone during early brain development. *Eur J Endocrinol* **151**(Suppl 3), U25–37.

Nicola, J.P., Basquin, C., Portulano, C., *et al.* (2009) The Na+/I-symporter mediates active iodide uptake in the intestine. *Am J Physiol Cell Physiol* **296**, C654–662.

Nishiyama, S., Mikeda, T., Okada, T., *et al.* (2004) Transient hypothyroidism or persistent hyperthyrotropinemia in neonates born to mothers with excessive iodine intake. *Thyroid* **14**, 1077–1083.

Oppenheimer, J.H., Schwartz, H.L., and Surks, M.I. (1975) Determination of common parameters for iodothyronine metabolism and distribution in man by noncompartmental analysis. *J Clin Endocrinol Metab* **41**, 319–324.

Pearce, E.N., Pino, S., He, X., *et al.* (2004) Sources of dietary iodine: bread, cows' milk, and infant formula in the Boston area. *J Clin Endocrinol Metab* **89**, 3421–3424.

Pennington, J.A. (1990) A review of iodine toxicity reports. *J Am Diet Assoc* **90**, 1571–1581.

Perrine, C.G., Herrick, K., Serdula, M.K., *et al.* (2010) Some subgroups of reproductive age women in the United States may be at risk for iodine deficiency. *J Nutr.* **140**, 1489–1494

Sanchez-Castillo, C.P., Warrender, S., Whitehead, T.P., *et al.* (1987) An assessment of the sources of dietary salt in a British population. *Clin Sci (Lond)* **72**, 95–102.

Squatrito, S., Vigneri, R., Runello, F., *et al.* (1986) Prevention and treatment of endemic iodine-deficiency goiter by iodination of a municipal water supply. *J Clin Endocrinol Metab* **63**, 368–375.

Taki, K., Kogai, T., Kanamoto, Y., *et al.* (2002) A thyroid-specific far-upstream enhancer in the human sodium/iodide symporter gene requires Pax-8 binding and cyclic adenosine 3',5'-monophosphate response element-like sequence binding proteins for full activity and is differentially regulated in normal and thyroid cancer cells. *Mol Endocrinol* **16**, 2266–2282.

Teng, W., Shan, Z., Teng, X., *et al.* (2006) Effect of iodine intake on thyroid diseases in China. *N Engl J Med* **354**, 2783–2793.

United Nations (2011) Population Division of the Department of Economic and Social Affairs of the United Nations Secretariat. *World Population Prospects: The 2004 Revision.* United Nations, New York. Available at: http://esa.un.org/unpd/wpp/index.htm.

United Nations Children's Fund (2008) *Sustainable Elimination of Iodine Deficiency.* UNICEF, New York.

Vejbjerg, P., Knudsen, N., Perrild, H., *et al.* (2009) Thyroglobulin as a marker of iodine nutrition status in the general population. *Eur J Endocrinol* **161**, 475–481.

World Health Organization (2007) *Assessment of Iodine Deficiency Disorders and Monitoring Their Elimination: a Guide for Programme Managers*, 3rd Edn. World Health Organization, Geneva

World Health Organization(2008) *WHO expert consultation on salt as a vehicle for fortification, Luxembourg, March 21–22, 2007.* World Health Organization, Geneva.

Yen, P.M. (2001) Physiological and molecular basis of thyroid hormone action. *Physiol Rev* **81**, 1097–1142.

Zimmermann, M.B. (2006) The influence of iron status on iodine utilization and thyroid function. *Annu Rev Nutr* **26**, 367–389.

Zimmermann, M.B. (2008a) Iodine requirements and the risks and benefits of correcting iodine deficiency in populations. *J Trace Elem Med Biol* **22**, 81–92.

Zimmermann, M.B. (2008b) Research on iodine deficiency and goiter in the 19th and early 20th centuries. *J Nutr* **138**, 2060–2063.

Zimmermann, M.B. (2009) Iodine deficiency in pregnancy and the effects of maternal iodine supplementation on the offspring: a review. *Am J Clin Nutr* **89**, 668S–672S.

Zimmermann, M.B. and Kohrle, J. (2002) The impact of iron and selenium deficiencies on iodine and thyroid metabolism: biochemistry and relevance to public health. *Thyroid* **12**, 867–878.

Zimmermann, M.B., Aeberli, I., Torresani, T., *et al.* (2005a) Increasing the iodine concentration in the Swiss iodized salt program markedly improved iodine status in pregnant women and children: a 5-y prospective national study. *Am J Clin Nutr* **82**, 388–392.

Zimmermann, M.B., Connolly, K., Bozo, M., *et al.* (2006a) Iodine supplementation improves cognition in iodine-deficient schoolchildren in Albania: a randomized, controlled, double-blind study. *Am J Clin Nutr* **83**, 108–114.

Zimmermann, M.B., de Benoist, B., Corigliano, S., *et al.* (2006b) Assessment of iodine status using dried blood spot thyroglobulin: development of reference material and establishment of an international reference range in iodine-sufficient children. *J Clin Endocrinol Metab* **91**, 4881–4887.

Zimmermann, M.B., Hess, S.Y., Adou, P.T., *et al.* (2003a) Thyroid size and goiter prevalence after introduction of iodized salt: a 5-y prospective study in schoolchildren in Cote d'Ivoire. *Am J Clin Nutr* **77,** 663–667.

Zimmermann, M.B., Hess, S.Y., Molinari, L., *et al.* (2004a) New reference values for thyroid volume by ultrasound in iodine-sufficient schoolchildren: a World Health Organization/Nutrition for Health and Development Iodine Deficiency Study Group Report. *Am J Clin Nutr* **79,** 231–237.

Zimmermann, M.B., Ito, Y., Hess, S.Y., *et al.* (2005b) High thyroid volume in children with excess dietary iodine intakes. *Am J Clin Nutr* **81,** 840–844.

Zimmermann, M.B., Jooste, P.L., Mabapa, N.S., *et al.* (2007) Vitamin A supplementation in iodine-deficient African children decreases thyrotropin stimulation of the thyroid and reduces the goiter rate. *Am J Clin Nutr* **86,** 1040–1044.

Zimmermann, M.B., Jooste, P.L., and Pandav C.S. (2008) Iodine-deficiency disorders. *Lancet* **372,** 1251–1262.

Zimmermann, M.B., Moretti, D., Chaouki, N., *et al.* (2003b) Development of a dried whole-blood spot thyroglobulin assay and its evaluation as an indicator of thyroid status in goitrous children receiving iodized salt. *Am J Clin Nutr* **77,** 1453–1458.

Zimmermann, M.B., Wegmuller, R., Zeder, C., *et al.* (2004b) Rapid relapse of thyroid dysfunction and goiter in school-age children after discontinuation of salt iodization. *Am J Clin Nutr* **79,** 642–645.

37

SELENIUM

EMILY N. TERRY, MS AND ALAN M. DIAMOND, PhD

University of Illinois at Chicago, Chicago, Illinois, USA

Summary

The essential trace element selenium has been a focus of attention due to its impact on human health, with there being consequences to both its deficiency and excess. While there is considerable knowledge of selenium's metabolic pathways, the means whereby it impacts immunity, and susceptibility to viral infection and a host of human diseases, remain under investigation. Many of the biological consequences of selenium status are likely to be mediated by its role as a constituent of selenium-containing proteins, one class of which includes selenium as the amino acid selenocysteine, which is encoded by the UGA codon within selenoprotein mRNAs. Future efforts to better appreciate how selenium impacts health and disease will likely result in a better understanding of selenium's biology and an improved basis from which to make recommendations about the optimal amount that should be included in the diet.

Introduction

Selenium is a trace element that was discovered in 1817 by Jons Jacob Berzelius following analysis of a red deposit on a lead wall of a sulfuric acid plant in Sweden. Following examination of its properties, and finding a similarity to tellurium, named as a reference to earth, this new element was named selenium after the moon goddess, Selene. In the late 1930s and into the 1940s, selenium was mostly known for its toxicity in farm animals. Acute poisoning in horses, for example, was referred to as "blind staggers" and was characterized by blindness, excessive perspiration, abdominal pain, colic, diarrhea, increased heart and respiration rates, and lethargy. Chronic toxicity in these animals was referred to as "alkali disease" and resulted in symptoms including alopecia and cracked hooves. In contrast, insufficient intake of selenium in animals can result in a variety of symptoms, such as nutritional muscular dystrophy, which appears as muscle weakness, loss of weight, diarrhea, and decreased fertility (reviewed in Koller and Exon, 1986). As a consequence, it became common practice to supplement feed with selenium to ensure adequate dietary intake. The essentiality of selenium to good health rather than being a toxin was established by Schwarz and Foltz in 1957 following their description of the prevention of liver necrosis in vitamin E-deficient rats given selenium supplementation (Schwarz and Foltz, 1958). A major breakthrough in understanding the biology of selenium occurred when its incorporation into protein was reported by Rotruck *et al.* (1973) and Flohe *et al.* (1973), and it later became apparent that there was an entire family of proteins in which selenium was present in the form of selenocysteine. In this chapter, we describe the nutritional aspects of selenium biology, ranging from its metabolism to its impact on human health and with an emphasis on the family of proteins that include selenium as a critical component.

Dietary Selenium, Recommended Daily Allowance, and Assessment

The accumulation of selenium in foods begins with its uptake by plants from the soil, the resulting concentration of which varies dramatically by region throughout the world. Since the amount of selenium in the soil affects its availability in feeds for livestock, standard supplementation strategies for animals in selenium-poor areas has been implemented (Ullrey, 1992; Ellison, 2002). The form of selenium taken up by plants is typically inorganic selenate (SeO_4^2) or selenite (SeO_3^{2-}), which is then ultimately used to produce selenomethionine, the predominant form found in plants, through the sulfur assimilation pathway (reviewed in Terry et al. (2000) and Li et al. (2008a)). More than 50% of the selenium found in plants is selenomethionine or its methylated forms, although selenocysteine is also significantly present. Uptake of selenium may also be influenced by additional variables such as acidity, oxygen levels, amount of rainfall, and sulfur levels (Zayed and Terry, 1994; Haygarth et al., 1995; Miladinovic et al., 1998; Li et al., 2008a).

The content of selenium in the diet is influenced by where the food is grown; the impact of growth location is less in places where a sizable portion of the diet is obtained from varied locations. Selenium intake in humans is principally from the consumption of meat, fish, and egg, which contain high levels of selenium in relation to other foods, ranging from 180 to 800 ng/g (http://www.ars.usda.gov/main/site_main.htm?modecode=12-35-45-00). Most plants do not accumulate high levels of selenium, but a few noted exceptions include members of the *Brassica* genus, which includes broccoli and kale, and garlic and mushrooms (~300 μg/g) (reviewed in Dumont et al., 2006), and brazil nuts, which contain the highest levels of bioavailable selenium (Thomson and Robinson, 1990; Ip and Lisk, 1994; Thomson et al., 2008). How food is processed may also affect selenium dietary availability; for example, heating food during preparation may decrease selenium content by volatilization (Thomson and Robinson, 1990).

As a consequence of the geological distribution of selenium and regional dietary customs, selenium intake levels vary greatly among populations. In areas such as parts of China which are associated with diseases attributed to selenium deficiency, intake has been reported to be as low as 7–11 μg per person per day. In other parts of China which are associated with selenosis, intake ranges from 750 to 4990 μg per person per day. Countries where dietary selenium levels are generally low include Croatia, Germany, Sweden, and New Zealand, and countries with higher selenium intake include Canada, Greece, the United States, and Venezuela (Combs, 2001). A comprehensive compilation of worldwide selenium intake levels as well as blood and plasma selenium contents was published in 2001 (Combs, 2001) and the levels of plasma selenium in populations of the world are displayed in Figure 37.1.

Tissue Distribution

The amount of total body selenium is typically dependent upon the region one lives in, with the population of the United States exhibiting high total body selenium levels of over 13 mg, whereas others, such as people living in New Zealand, contain approximately 6 mg (Zachara et al., 2001). The major site of selenium storage in the body is skeletal muscle, accounting for approximately 28–46% of the total selenium pool depending on the population analyzed (Oster et al., 1988; Zachara et al., 2001). The kidneys contain the highest amount of selenium on a per-weight basis, with 470 ng/g wet tissue, as compared with skeletal muscle which contains only 51 ng/g wet tissue as determined in a cohort of Polish individuals (Zachara et al., 2001). Liver selenium levels fall midway between those of kidney and muscle. The typical distribution of selenium in human organs generally lies in the order kidney > liver > spleen > pancreas > heart > brain > lung > bone > skeletal muscle.

Assessment of Selenium Status

In order to appreciate the impact of selenium on human health, there needs to be a reliable means of determining the status of individuals and populations and of relating these data to health outcomes. However, multiple methods are currently employed to assess selenium status, and which is the most appropriate is a complicated issue. One consideration is the source of the biological material from which the measurements are being made. Different tissues and body fluids can be utilized, with the most commonly used being whole blood, plasma, serum, erythrocytes,

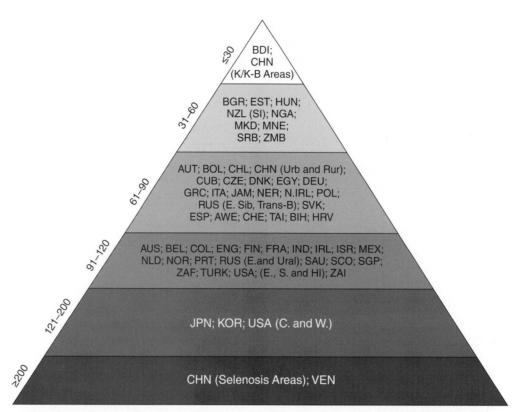

FIG. 37.1 Levels of plasma/serum selenium (µg/L) in distinct global populations. Specific regions of countries are indicated, where available. Data represents an average of plasma/serum selenium concentrations as presented in Combs (2001). AUS, Australia; AUT, Austria; BDI, Burundi; BEL, Belgium; BGR, Bulgaria; BIH, Bosnia and Herzegovina; BOL, Bolivia; CHE, Switzerland; CHL, Chile; CHN, China; COL, Colombia; CUB, Cuba; CZE, Czech Republic; DEU, Germany; DNK, Denmark; EGY, Egypt; ENG, England; E. Sib., Eastern Siberia; ESP, Spain; EST, Estonia; FIN, Finland; FRA, France; HI, Hawaii; HRV, Croatia; HUN, Hungary; IND, India; IRL, Ireland; ISR, Israel; ITA, Italy; JAM, Jamaica; JPN, Japan; K/K-B Areas, Keshan/Kaschin-Beck Areas; KOR, Korea; MEX, Mexico; MKD, Macedonia; MNE, Montenegro; NER, Niger; NGA, Nigeria; NLD, Netherlands; NOR, Norway; NZL, New Zealand; POL, Poland; PRT, Portugal; Rur, rural, non-Keshan; RUS, Russia; SAU, Saudi Arabia; SCO, Scotland; SGP, Singapore; SI, South Island; SRB, Serbia; SVK, Slovakia; SWE, Sweden; TAI, Taiwan; Trans-B, Trans-Baikal; TUR, Turkey; Urb, Urban; USA, United States; VEN, Venezuela; ZAF, South Africa; ZAI, Zaire; C, Central; E, eastern; S, southern; W, western.

urine, hair, and nails (reviewed in Gibson, 1989; Salbe and Levander, 1990). Measurements of plasma selenium are most often cited but may not be the most reliable (Burk *et al.*, 2006), while blood and urine provide an indication of short-term selenium intake. Analysis of hair and nails is more typically used as a measure of long-term intake over months and years. Plasma and serum samples may provide the best result for immediate changes in selenium status, whereas whole blood can provide longer-term status (reviewed in Thomson, 2004). Analysis of selenium in

urine generally provides information on recent intake, typically within the most recent days (reviewed in Thomson, 2004).

The use of blood or urine is relatively non-invasive, and samples are easy to process and store, while the analysis of hair or toenails may be even more convenient and typically provides a more reliable assessment of long-term status. However, hair can be contaminated by common grooming and cleansing products which often contain selenium, and the growth rate of hair, which may influence selenium accumulation, is variable among individuals and can be dependent on their health status (Morris *et al.*, 1983; LeBlanc *et al.*, 1999). Nails have a more consistent growth rate and are less prone to contamination (reviewed in Thomson, 2004). Urine selenium levels were more closely correlated with predicted intake as assessed through food frequency questionnaires and duplicate food samples. Selenium levels are directly quantified by mass spectrometry of blood and urine (Reamer and Veillon, 1983) and by neutron activation analysis of nails or hair (Morris *et al.*, 1983).

Indirect measures of selenium status by quantification of selenium-containing proteins can also be used. One approach is to use the measured activity of the selenoprotein glutathione peroxidase (GPx), either in plasma or erythrocytes, using a coupled spectrophotometric assay. However, this approach may be most applicable in determining selenium deficiency as individuals with what are often considered adequate selenium levels are likely to have maximized GPx activity and therefore this approach may not be appropriate for assessment of higher intakes (Brown *et al.*, 2000). More recently, the quantification of selenoprotein P (SEPP1), the major selenoprotein in plasma, has also been considered for these purposes. SEPP1 levels were shown to be optimized at 75 μg/day of selenium intake as compared with GPx in the serum which was said to have a maximal activity at 35 mg/day (Xia *et al.*, 2005). An evaluation of the different methods used to determine selenium status has been published (Ashton *et al.*, 2009).

Selenium RDA

The recommended daily allowance (RDA) for selenium indicated by the Food and Nutrition Board of the Institute of Medicine is 55 μg/day (0.7 μmol/day) for healthy adults over age 13; a higher intake is suggested during pregnancy (60 μg/day) and lactation (70 μg/day). These values are based on the expected intake of selenium that would maximize the activity of the glutathione peroxidase (GPx-3) selenoprotein, which is found in the highest concentration in the plasma (Institute of Medicine, 2000). This RDA is clearly below that required to reach maximal levels of all of the selenoproteins. For example, a population in a region in China showed maximal activity of GPx-3 when supplemented with 37 μg/day selenomethionine, and twice that amount of selenite (Xia *et al.*, 2005). However, SEPP1 levels did not reach maximal activity at either of these doses, or at the highest doses administered (61 μg/day selenomethionine or 66 μg/day selenite). There

continues to be significant debate as to what an appropriate selenium RDA should be and the basis for making the decision. Clearly, higher intake than the RDA would be required to maximize the levels of all of the selenoproteins, and, using an additional criterion of need, it was suggested that men required 80 μg/day and women 57 μg/day to maintain selenium balance, and these values were dependent on lean body mass and historical selenium intake (Levander, 1984).

Diseases of Excess and Deficiency

The interest in the possible benefits of selenium supplementation follows a long history in which selenium was given more attention because of its associated toxicity. Thousands of animals were killed by selenium overdose and the adverse effects associated with high-level selenium intake which are referred to as selenosis. Selenosis has also been reported in humans, most often in regions of the world where there are very high levels of selenium in the soil and consequently in the plants grown in that soil (Yang *et al.*, 1983). Symptoms of selenosis include hair loss, brittle and discolored nails, dermatitis if exposure was topical, peripheral neuropathy, nausea, diarrhea, fatigue, and irritability (reviewed in Nuttall, 2006). One of the additional signs of selenosis is an odor on the breath resembling garlic. Selenosis can occur due to exposure to selenium from industrial sources, and several cases of individuals overdosing on selenium appear in the literature. A striking example of selenium toxicity occurred in a 2008 outbreak of selenosis affecting 201 individuals in nine different states in the United States (MacFarquhar *et al.*, 2010). These individuals suffered from the classical signs of selenosis, over 70% reporting diarrhea, fatigue, and hair loss. Each was taking a multivitamin supplement that was labeled to contain 200 μg of selenium in the form of sodium selenite per ounce of supplement, the recommended dose. Subsequent analysis of the product revealed that it in fact contained 40 800 μg per ounce, approximately 200 times the level indicated on the label.

The exact causes for the symptoms associated with selenium toxicity are likely to be multifactorial and to include the erroneous substitution of selenium for sulfur in the sulfur-containing amino acids cysteine and methionine, as well as the induction of selenium-associated oxidative stress. Exposure of either cells in culture to high levels of selenium or of animals given excessive selenium supplements led to enhanced mutagenesis, the induction of chromosomal abnormalities such as micronuclei forma-tion, and the induction of cell-cycle arrest and apoptosis (reviewed in Valdiglesias *et al.*, 2010). Examples of seleno-sis continue to be reported but they are rare, and perhaps a greater concern is the adverse consequences of selenium supplementation resulting from taking the recommended doses, concerns that emerged following the results of sele-nium supplementation clinical trials.

The best known disease associated with selenium defi-ciency is Keshan disease, a serious cardiomyopathy first described in Keshan County in north-east China. The disease is endemic among the poor population of the region, being most prevalent among younger women and children, and results in myocardial necrosis and eventually congestive heart failure. Given the low selenium status of the afflicted population, the Chinese government initiated an oral selenium supplementation program that greatly reduced the disease incidence (Xia *et al.*, 1989). However, the disease cannot be fully prevented by selenium sup-plementation, which indicates that there are additional likely etiological factors. Evidence has been presented that infection with a Coxsackie B virus (Li *et al.*, 2000) and increased risk found in association with a polymor-phism in the glutathione peroxidase 1 (GPx-1) selenium-containing protein (Lei *et al.*, 2009; Xiong *et al.*, 2010) are contributing factors. Kashin-Beck disease is an osteo-arthropathy also endemic to China and is associated with joint destruction and possibly dwarfism (Schepman *et al.*, 2011). Selenium deficiency also occurs in Kashin-Beck endemic regions, and a recent meta-analysis of 15 trials with selenium supplementation has supported the benefits of intervening with selenium supplementation in prevent-ing the disease (Zou *et al.*, 2009). As with Keshan disease, increased risk of Kashin-Beck disease is found in associa-tion with a polymorphism in GPx-1 (Xiong *et al.*, 2010). Myxedematous cretinism is endemic in a region of both selenium and iodine deficiency in central Africa (Dumont *et al.*, 1994), and the deficiency of these elements in the diet is likely to contribute to the thyroid pathology seen in these cases (Kohrle *et al.*, 2005).

Metabolism

Ingestion, Absorption, and Transport

The bioavailability of selenium depends on the form ingested, such as whether the forms are organic or inor-ganic, as well as other dietary components that might inhibit uptake such as heavy metals, and varies between species (reviewed in Thomson, 1998). Organic selenium is predominantly found as selenomethionine, although selenocysteine and methylated forms of selenomethionine are also ingested (reviewed in Rayman, 2008). Inorganic forms include selenite and selenate salts. Selenomethionine is the most readily absorbed form of dietary selenium, and is metabolized following active transport from the small intestine by a sodium-dependent transporter (Wolffram *et al.*, 1989). After absorption, selenomethionine is found bound to hemoglobin and then accumulates in liver and muscle (Beilstein and Whanger, 1986; Yeh *et al.*, 1997). Selenocysteine is also taken up in the intestine, but at a less efficient rate than selenomethionine, as shown in a simulated digestion experiment (Shen *et al.*, 1997). Selenocysteine is absorbed by red blood cells by an unknown transporter (Imai *et al.*, 2009). The inorganic selenium is absorbed passively and is stored less efficiently than organic forms (reviewed in Fairweather-Tait *et al.*, 2010). Selenite is more bioavailable than selenate, and can be seen in erythrocytes within minutes of intravenous administration in rats (Suzuki *et al.*, 1998). Selenite is metabolized to selenide following reduction by glutath-ione, and then can be found bound to albumin or hemo-globin and is transported to the liver for further processing (Haratake *et al.*, 2008). Conversely, selenate is taken up in plasma and transported, unmetabolized, to the liver where it is metabolized or is excreted in urine (Kobayashi *et al.*, 2001). Selenide is then used for conversion to seleno-cysteine for selenoprotein incorporation (reviewed in Rayman, 2000). The major metabolic steps in selenium processing are presented in Figure 37.2.

The major organ for controlling selenium levels in the body is the liver where it is designated for excretion or for further processing for use in selenoproteins, which include the major transport selenium-containing protein, Sepp1 (Burk and Hill, 2009). Sepp1 is an extracellular protein containing 10 selenocysteines and comprises the major form of selenium in plasma. Sepp1 accounts for approxi-mately 44% of the selenium in plasma, whereas GPx3 accounts for approximately 30%; the remaining 37% is associated with albumin (Janghorbani *et al.*, 1999). The major means of selenium supply to the brain and testes is by uptake of Sepp1 via the apolipoprotein E Receptor-2 (ApoER2) (Olson *et al.*, 2007), and via megalin, another member of the lipoprotein receptor family, in kidney prox-imal tubule epithelial cells (Olson *et al.*, 2008). Sepp1

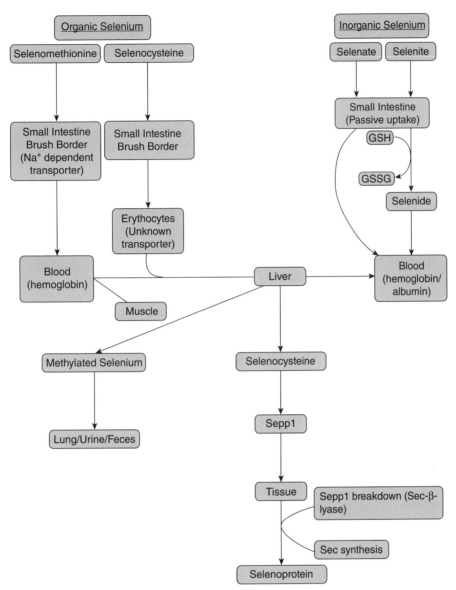

FIG. 37.2 The major steps of selenium metabolism ranging from ingestion to excretion. GSH, Glutathione; GSSG, reduced glutathione; Sec, selenocysteine.

enters the tissue where the protein is catabolized by Sec-β-lyase and the products are funneled into selenium metabolism (Esaki *et al.*, 1982).

Excretion

Selenium for excretion is metabolized in the liver to trimethylselonium by S-adenosylmethionine methylation or to selenosugars, with evidence that selenosugars are the predominant form excreted (Suzuki *et al.*, 2005).

Metabolized selenium is primarily excreted via the kidneys in urine either as selenosugars or as methylated selenide, which, together with absorption, function to regulate homeostasis. In cases of excess selenium intake, selenium is not trimethylated, and is excreted from the lung as dimethyl selenide (Kremer *et al.*, 2005). Rats injected with high doses of selenium (2 mg/kg) demonstrated excretion via the lungs of up to 26% of the initial dose after 24 hours, as compared with 14% excreted via the kidneys as trimethylselenonium (Vadhanavikit *et al.*, 1987). Intestinal excretion of selenium was thought to be a minor method of excretion with most of it being excreted by this route unabsorbed; however, evidence points to intestinal excretion being a form of homeostatic control (Hawkes *et al.*, 2003). In men given supranutritional levels of selenium, approximately half of the detected selenium excreted was in the feces (Bugel *et al.*, 2008).

Selenium and Human Health

Selenium, Viral Infectivity, and Immunity

Dietary intake of selenium may have an effect on immune function in humans. Most of the data in support of this comes from studies examining the physiological consequences of selenium deficiency. Reduced intake of selenium has been shown to negatively affect the components of the innate immune system, such as B- and T-lymphocytes and neutrophils that participate in the response to infectious challenge, and these effects are likely to be mediated through the action of selenoproteins (reviewed in Arthur *et al.*, 2003). Animal studies have indicated that selenium status could adversely affect interleukin-2, its high-affinity receptor, interferon γ, and CD40 ligand levels (Hoffmann *et al.*, 2010). Given the possible role of selenium in inflammation, it is noteworthy that selenium levels may have an impact on both the risk and severity of asthma. Conflicting data regarding the impact of selenium levels and asthma in humans as well as animal data indicate a bimodal response where lower or higher levels of selenium are associated with increased asthma (reviewed in Hoffmann and Berry, 2008). The authors suggest that the complexity of the issue may result from the ability of selenium to both stimulate the immune system and enhance the levels of antioxidant selenoproteins that might provide protection to the lung.

In addition to the possible role of selenium in influencing immune function, its levels may have an impact on viral infectivity and the consequential impact on the diseases associated with those infections. This may be most apparent in the case of the pediatric cardiomyopathy associated with selenium deficiency, Keshan's disease (see earlier in this chapter). In spite of the success of the vast selenium supplementation program that dramatically reduced disease incidence, the seasonal pattern of incidence indicated the likely involvement of another etiological determinant, and the detection of the coxsackie virus (a picornavirus), in Keshan tissue prompted further

examination. Animal studies support the role for this virus in this disease as it was shown that mice fed a selenium-deficient diet developed cardiac disease following infection with a relatively benign CVB3 coxsackie virus whereas mice with adequate selenium levels did not develop myocarditis (Beck *et al.*, 1994). It was subsequently shown that the pathology observed in the selenium-deficient mice was associated with the acquisition of six point mutations in the CVB30 genome that accounted for the change in virulence (Beck *et al.*, 1995) and that this effect may have been mediated by the reduced levels of the GPx-1 selenoprotein that occur during selenium deficiency (Beck *et al.*, 1998). Selenium deficiency has also been shown to exacerbate the disease induced by influenza viruses (Beck *et al.*, 2001), including H1N1 (Yu *et al.*, 2010). Although there was an indication that low selenium levels might be a contributor to HIV-associated mortality (Baum *et al.*, 1997), the results of randomized placebo-controlled selenium intervention trials have not yielded a clear answer to the question of the nutrient's benefits in the management of AIDS (Pitney *et al.*, 2009).

Selenium and Cancer

Much of the attention directed towards evaluating the role of selenium in human health has centered on its potential use in reducing cancer incidence. This focus can be traced back over 40 years ago when inverse associations between dietary selenium intake and cancer mortality were first realized (Shamberger and Frost, 1969). Since then, there have been a significant number of epidemiological studies investigating the relationship between selenium intake and cancer incidence, and many but certainly not all have revealed an inverse association for a diverse list of cancer types (reviewed in Whanger, 2004). Perhaps the strongest data in this regard are for cancers of the colon and prostate. For example, a case-control study in Montreal involving 402 incidence cases of colon cancer from a cohort of 1048 incidence cases and 688 population-based controls indicated a statistically significant inverse correlation between toenail selenium levels and the risk of colon cancer for both genders (OR = 0.42 at p = 0.009) (Ghadirian *et al.*, 2000). A significant inverse association between selenium levels and the incidence of large adenomatous polyps, after adjusting for confounding variables in patients less than 60 years of age (OR = 0.17, p = 0.029), has also been reported (Fernandez-Banares *et al.*, 2002). These conclusions were substantiated by an analysis of pooled data from three independent studies (Jacobs *et al.*, 2004) and a recent study similarly showing the inverse association between serum selenium levels and the risk of advanced colorectal adenoma (Peters *et al.*, 2006).

Research involving animal models has also indicated that selenium supplementation may be a useful strategy to reduce cancer risk. Hundreds of independent reports have shown that providing rodents with selenium at non-toxic doses can reduce tumor incidence, being protective for most organs and against a wide range of carcinogens (El-Bayoumy, 1991). Selenium supplementation studies in humans are few, and the Nutritional Prevention of Cancer (NPC) trial conducted by Clark *et al.* in 1991 received considerable attention. The study (Clark *et al.*, 1996) was a double-blind trial to examine the efficacy of providing 200 μg a day of selenium as selenized yeast on the recurrence of non-melanoma skin cancer as compared with placebo. The results of this study indicated that selenium supplementation did not protect against skin cancer, but long-term follow-up revealed that there was protection against prostate cancer for those men with lowest baseline selenium status (Duffield-Lillico *et al.*, 2003). Encouraged by the collective data indicating a possible protective effect of selenium on prostate cancer incidence, the Selenium and Vitamin E Cancer Prevention Trial (SELECT), a double-blind placebo-controlled supplementation study began in 2001 involving over 35 000 men from the United States, Canada, and Puerto Rico randomized to selenium, vitamin E, both or placebo (Lippman *et al.*, 2005). Unlike the NPC trial, men were given selenium in the form of selenomethionine. The SELECT trial was terminated ahead of schedule in 2008 for an apparent lack of efficacy of the supplements (Lippman *et al.*, 2009). There have been several commentaries offering explanations of the apparent contradictions between the animal, epidemiological and supplementation results on selenium efficacy in reducing cancer risk (El-Bayoumy, 2009; Hatfield and Gladyshev, 2009; Rayman, 2009; Schrauzer, 2009).

Mechanism of Cancer Prevention

While the animal and human epidemiological data indicate a likely role for selenium in cancer prevention, the mechanisms involved remain elusive and controversial. It is attractive to assume that many of the beneficial effects of selenium are due to its consequential effects on selenoproteins because many of these are regulated by selenium intake, several have clear antioxidant functions, and there is a significant amount of data indicating that genetic variants of selenoproteins are associated with disease risk and outcome (Rayman, 2009; Zhuo and Diamond, 2009). In support of this concept, mice genetically engineered to express reduced selenoprotein levels are predisposed to develop premalignant lesions linked to both colon and prostate cancer (Diwadkar-Navsariwala *et al.*, 2006; Irons *et al.*, 2006). In the case of the colon cancer study, it was shown that selenoprotein-dependent and -independent mechanisms of cancer prevention were accounting for the effects (Irons *et al.*, 2006). This is consistent with a large body of evidence indicating that non-protein selenium metabolites can exert an anti-cancer effect by targeting tumor cells, although this typically requires relatively high concentrations of selenium. The use of such non-protein forms of selenium in cancer prevention and control have recently been reviewed (Nadiminty and Gao, 2008).

Whatever the mechanism, it appears as if selenium may be exerting its beneficial function, at least in part, by preventing mutations. The evidence that selenium protects DNA from damage comes from studies beginning in the 1980s that used both yeast and mammalian systems (Rosin, 1981; Diamond *et al.*, 1996). Supplementation of the culture media of Chinese hamster ovary cells with low levels of selenium (30 nM) in the form of sodium selenite significantly reduces the mutation frequency following exposure to X-rays (Diamond *et al.*, 1996). Selenium can also increase the repair of N-nitrosobis(2-oxopropyl) amine-induced single-strand breaks, even when provided 2 days post-carcinogen exposure (Lawson and Birt, 1983; Lawson, 1989), and induce DNA repair synthesis in an isolated rat liver cell system (Russell *et al.*, 1980); also, selenomethionine induced a DNA repair response in human fibroblasts (Seo *et al.*, 2002). Both p53 and BRCA1 may be involved in the mechanism by which selenium reduces DNA damage (Fischer *et al.*, 2006). In this regard, the observation that genomic instability in cells of women who were BRCA1 mutation carriers, as measured by chromosome breakage in cultured lymphocytes from these patients, could be complemented by oral selenium supplementation is particularly interesting (Kowalska *et al.*, 2005). Additionally, in a different cohort of women also carrying the BRCA1 mutation, supplementation was shown to reduce the formation of 8-oxo-7,8-dihydro-2′-deoxyguanosine (8-OH-dG), a DNA adduct caused by increased reactive oxygen species in cells (Dziaman, 2009). A subsequent increase in urinary 8-OH-dG levels was noted, which indicates that selenium could be protecting against mutation by actually increasing the role of repair by base excision.

Selenium and Diabetes

The results of the NPC trial were encouraging and generated enthusiasm for the continued development of selenium for use in cancer prevention. A secondary analysis of the NPC trial was conducted to assess whether selenium supplementation would reduce the incidence of type 2 diabetes (Stranges *et al.*, 2007). Surprisingly, there was a higher incidence of type 2 diabetes in the selenium-supplemented group (HR = 1.55, 95% CI 1.03–2.33). In addition, the data indicated a statistically significant dose–response gradient with the greatest risk for type 2 diabetes occurring in the supplemented group within the highest tertile of baseline selenium levels (HR = 2.7, CI 1.30–5.61). As discussed in the paper, the determination of an association between selenium supplementation and diabetes had significant limitations, including the use of self-reported data, diabetes not being the primary endpoint, and the absence of significant data on diabetes-associated risk factors. Furthermore, sampling was from a subset population that was relatively older and from a low-selenium region.

The SELECT selenium supplementation trial was terminated early for apparent lack of efficacy of the test compounds and, of note, a non-significant increase in the risk of diabetes in the group receiving selenium was observed (RR = 1.07, 99% CI 0.94–1.22; p = 0.16) (Lippman *et al.*, 2009). The possibility that selenium might increase the risk of diabetes therefore appeared in two independent clinical supplementation trials, conducted in two different populations and with different forms of selenium, raising concerns over the possible risks of selenium supplementation especially among those with higher baseline levels.

Human epidemiological data also indicated a possible risk of diabetes associated with higher selenium intake. An examination of NHANES data on US populations indicated an increased risk of type 2 diabetes among those with the highest selenium levels, as well as associations with adverse serum-lipid profiles and arterial disease (Bleys *et al.*, 2007; Laclaustra *et al.*, 2009). A similar report indicating an association between higher selenium levels, poor lipid profiles, and arterial disease among British citizens was also published (Stranges *et al.*, 2010). Bleys *et al.* (2008) also investigated the relationship between serum selenium levels and all causes of death, also using NHANES data. They reported a non-linear association between serum selenium levels and deaths by all causes, and specifically those due to cancer. Below a baseline serum concentration of 130 ng/mL, increased selenium levels were associated with a reduced risk of all-cause mortality and cancer-associated deaths; there was no effect of selenium within the range 130–150 ng/mL; and there was evidence for increased risk of death from all causes as well as cancer mortality above 150 ng/mL. Thus, the results of supplementation/epidemiological studies might indicate that there are individuals, such as those with adequate or relatively high levels of selenium, who may be at greater risk of disease were they to supplement their diets with selenium. Such a response to selenium supplementation, where low or high levels of selenium may be detrimental with the optimal levels lying somewhere in between, is supported by research in dogs indicating a U-shaped dose–response curve between the levels of selenium in toenails and DNA damage in prostatic tissue (Waters *et al.*, 2005) and these data have recently been discussed in comparison with what has been observed in humans (Chiang *et al.*, 2009).

Selenoproteins

Selenium-containing proteins generally fall into one of three categories (reviewed in Behne and Kyriakopoulos, 2001; Kryukov *et al.*, 2003). One of these classes includes those proteins containing selenomethionine in which selenium, due to its structural similarity to sulfur, incorporates non-specifically into the sulfur-containing amino acids (Gladyshev and Hatfield, 2001). The most common and best studied class of selenium-containing proteins includes those that contain the amino acid selenocysteine (Sec). Throughout evolution, from bacteria to man, Sec is incorporated co-translationally by its insertion in response to UGA codons that otherwise would serve as translational termination signals. In eukaryotes, the recognition of UGA as Sec requires a regulatory sequence, called a SECIS element, in the 3′-untranslated region of the selenoprotein mRNA (Berry *et al.*, 1991). All in-frame UGA codons contained in a SECIS-including mRNA are recognized as encoding Sec, which is incorporated into the elongating peptide by a unique translational machinery that includes a highly unusual tRNA (Lee *et al.*, 1989), an elongation factor, as well as other proteins required for selenoprotein synthesis (reviewed in Driscoll and Copeland, 2003; Bellinger *et al.*, 2009).

Based on in silico analyses, there are 25 human Sec-containing selenoprotein genes and 24 in the mouse (Kryukov *et al.*, 2003). Most of the selenoproteins can be classified by the position of the Sec residue: either those that contain Sec in the carboxy-terminus of the protein or those that contain Sec in the amino-terminus as part of the CxxC motif (reviewed in Lobanov *et al.*, 2009). Human selenoproteins can be considered to belong to seven functional classes: antioxidant enzymes (GPx-1, GPx-2, GPx-3, GPx-4, GPx-6, SelK, SelR, SelW), redox signaling (TrxR1, TrxR2, TrxR3), thyroid hormone metabolism (DIO1, DIO2, DIO3), selenocysteine biosynthesis (SBP2), selenium transport (SelP), protein folding (Sep15, SelN, SelM, SelS), and others of unknown function (reviewed in Gromer *et al.*, 2005; Papp *et al.*, 2007). The biological roles of many of these proteins, even when their enzymatic functions have been resolved, continue to be investigated and a description of each of them, including their biochemical functions, biological roles, and chromosome locations, can be found in the literature (reviewed in Gromer *et al.*, 2005; Papp *et al.*, 2007; Bellinger

et al., 2009). Table 37.1 provides a list of selenoproteins implicated in human disease by genetic evidence. As a protein class, selenoproteins are critical for normal tissue function as has been extensively investigated using mice in which selenoprotein synthesis is selectively inhibited in individual organ systems. These studies and the resulting pathology have been reviewed (Moustafa *et al.*, 2003).

The third class of selenium-containing proteins includes those proteins in which selenium is bound but not incorporated into an amino acid. One such protein is the selenium binding protein 1 (SBP1) (Bansal *et al.*, 1989). The human selenium-binding protein gene (SBP1, SELENBP1, or hSP56) (Chang *et al.*, 1997) is located on chromosome 1 at q21–22, and is the homolog of the mouse SP56 gene which was originally reported as a 56-kDa mouse protein that stably bound ^{75}selenium (Bansal *et al.*, 1989). The

TABLE 37.1 Selenoproteins implicated in disease risk and etiology by genetic evidence[a]

Selenoprotein	Disease	Genetic factor	Reference
GPx-1	Cardiovascular disease	Variable Ala codon repeats N-terminus	Winter *et al.* (2003)
	Cancer	Pro198Leu Ala repeats	Reviewed in Zhuo and Diamond, (2009)
	Metabolic syndrome (men)	Pro198Leu	Kuzuya *et al.* (2008)
	Keshan's disease	Pro198Leu	Lei *et al.* (2009)
	Intracerebral hemorrhage	Pro198Leu	Pera *et al.* (2008)
GPx3	Arterial ischemic stroke	Six polymorphisms forming two haplotypes	Voetsch *et al.* (2007)
GPx4	Cancer	C718T	Udler *et al.* (2007)
SepP	Cancer	Ala234Thr (in conjunction with MN-SOD Ala16Val) A/G 3'UTR C/T 3'UTR C/G 5'UTR	Cooper *et al.* (2008) Peters *et al.* (2008)
SepN	SePN1 related myopathies	Multiple polymorphisms	Reviewed in Arbogast and Ferreiro, (2010)
SepS	Cardiovascular disease/stroke	Multiple polymorphisms	Alanne *et al.* (2007)
	Pre-eclampsia	G-105A[b]	Moses *et al.* (2008)
	Rheumatoid arthritis	G-105A[b]	Marinou *et al.* (2009)
	Cancer	G-105A[b]	Shibata *et al.* (2009)
SBP2	Cancer	T/G interaction with GPx4 and SOD2	Meplan *et al.* (2010)
Sep15	Cancer	C811T G1125A	Apostolou *et al.* (2004) Penney *et al.* (2010)

[a]These examples do not include situations where specific selenoproteins are implicated in cancer progression due to observed loss of heterozygosity (LOH) in DNA obtained from tumor samples. Examples of LOH at selenoprotein loci can be found in Zhuo and Diamond (2009).
[b]"-" indicates a position 5' of the start codon.

human cDNA contains a 472 amino acid encoding open reading frame (Chang *et al.*, 1997) and protein resides in both the nucleus and the cytoplasm (Chen *et al.*, 2004). It is expressed in a variety of tissue types, including the heart, lung, kidney, and tissues of the digestive tract. The form of selenium in SBP1 is unknown as is the nature of its association: the selenium remains bound to the protein when electrophoresed in SDS acrylamide gels but dissociates at extremes of pH (Bansal *et al.*, 1989). The function of SBP1 is unknown although it may be involved in intra-Golgi transport (Porat *et al.*, 2000), and its reported association with the von Hippel–Lindau protein-interacting deubiquitinating enzyme 1 indicates SBP1 may function in protein degradation (Jeong *et al.*, 2009). SBP1 levels inversely correlate with poor clinical outcome in patients with lung, ovarian, and colon carcinoma (Yang and Sytkowski, 1998; Chen *et al.*, 2004; Huang *et al.*, 2006; Kim *et al.*, 2006; Li *et al.*, 2008b). More recently SBP1 was found to become silenced by methylation in colon cancers, and it can influence sensitivity to oxidative stress, cell migration, and tumorigenesis (Pohl *et al.*, 2009).

Selenoproteins and Thyroid Hormone Function

Among the selenoproteins with more clearly defined functions are the three iodothyronine deiodinases (DIO), types I, II, and III, that activate or deactivate thyroid hormone by the removal of specific iodine atoms (reviewed in Bianco *et al.*, 2002; Bianco and Kim, 2006). Reduced levels of selenium in the diet can result in thyroid dysfunction as a result of consequential reduction in DIO, and this has been extensively reviewed (Schomburg and Kohrle, 2008). In addition, mutations in the gene for SECIS Binding Protein 2 (SBP2), a protein that recognizes the SECIS element to facilitate the appropriate recognition of in-frame UGA codons (Copeland and Driscoll, 1999), were shown in 2005 to be associated with abnormal thyroid tests (Dumitrescu *et al.*, 2005), and this association was subsequently reported again among additional families (Dumitrescu *et al.*, 2010). These effects are likely to be mediated, at least in part, by the consequences of altered DIO regulation.

Selenoprotein N

Selenoprotein N (SelN) was discovered following an in silico scan of nucleotide sequence databases in search of SECIS elements (Lescure *et al.*, 1999). SelN contains one Sec residue and is a glycoprotein found within the endoplasmic reticulum. This protein is localized in skeletal muscle and implicated as a causative factor in "Rigid Spine Muscular Dystrophy" (RSMD), which now belongs to a family of SelN-related myopathies (Moghadaszadeh *et al.*, 2001; Arbogast and Ferreiro, 2010). Linkage disequilibrium indicated SelN's involvement in RSMD and other SelN-related myopathies, which are characterized by weak neck and trunk musculature, hypotonia, scoliosis, and elevated creatine kinase levels (Arbogast and Ferreiro, 2010). SelN mRNA is highly expressed in fetal tissue, with a subsequent reduction into adulthood (Moghadaszadeh *et al.*, 2001). There are multiple different mutations involved in SelN-related myopathies, the most common of which mutates the Sec codon (TGA) to TAA, inserting a stop codon and truncating the mRNA (Moghadaszadeh *et al.*, 2001; Tajsharghi *et al.*, 2005). Other forms of SelN-related myopathies exhibit mutations within the SECIS element, but with more mild effects than in those carrying the truncated mRNA.

The Glutathione Peroxidases

The glutathione peroxidases (GPx1-7) represent a conserved group of five selenium-containing enzymes (GPx1-4, GPx6) as well as three others in which cysteine is substituted for selenocysteine. GPx have been studied extensively, using reducing equivalents from glutathione to detoxify peroxides. The least studied of the selenium-containing GPx is GPx6, expressed in the olfactory epithelium (Kryukov *et al.*, 2003). The non-selenium-containing enzymes include GPx5 which is expressed in the epididymis (Vernet *et al.*, 1996) and considered to be involved in protecting that organ from oxidative stress (Chabory *et al.*, 2009) and GPx7 which was detected by in silico analysis (Kryukov *et al.*, 2003) and considered to be involved in antioxidant defenses in breast cancer cells (Utomo *et al.*, 2004). GPx1 is the oldest and best studied of the family, being ubiquitously expressed in most tissues. GPx2 (also known as the gastrointestinal GPx) has a more restricted expression pattern, being highest in the liver and gastrointestinal tract (Chu *et al.*, 1993; Florian *et al.*, 2001). The plasma glutathione peroxidase, GPx3, is produced by the proximal tubule of the kidney and is abundant in the plasma (Tham *et al.*, 1998) where its biological role is still unclear. The phospholipid/cholesterol hydroperoxide detoxifying glutathione peroxidase, GPx4, is highly unusual as not only does it function as a peroxidase (Zhang *et al.*, 1989), but it also undergoes polymerization and fills a major structural role in the midpiece of mature spermatozoa (Ursini *et al.*, 1999).

A strong indication of the impact of any of the seleno-proteins on human health is the association of polymorphic variants of the gene that encode for a particular selenoprotein and increased risk for specific disease. For the GPx1 gene, a polymorphism resulting in either a leucine or proline at position 198 of the protein has been shown to be associated with increased risk of cancers of the lung, breast, bladder, prostate, liver, and lymphomas (reviewed in Rayman, 2009, and Zhuo and Diamond, 2009). In addition to data indicating that polymorphisms in selenoprotein genes are associated with increased cancer risk, loss of one of two copies of the genes for GPx1 is also associated with cancers of the lung, breast, colon, and the head and neck (Ratnasinghe *et al.*, 2000; Hu *et al.*, 2005). Clonal expansion of cells that lose one of two copies of a particular gene is often taken as an indication that the gene provides a protective function and that loss either unmasks a recessive mutation or reduces the amount of a protective enzyme.

Selenoprotein Genetics and Disease

Polymorphisms in the genes for other selenoproteins (GPx-4, SePP, Sep15, and TRR) have also been associated with cancer risk or mortality of cancer (reviewed in Rayman, 2009; Zhuo and Diamond, 2009). In the case of Sep15, a protein believed to function in the quality control of protein folding (Korotkov *et al.*, 2001), functional allelic variants of this protein associated with cancer risk have been implicated in cancers of the breast (Hu *et al.*, 2001) and lung (Jablonska *et al.*, 2008), and in malignant mesothelioma (Apostolou *et al.*, 2004). More recently, an association between a Sep15 polymorphism and prostate cancer-associated mortality was reported (Penney *et al.*, 2010). SEPS1 (SelS, selenoprotein S) is an endoplasmic reticulum-associated protein implicated in inflammation, and polymorphisms of this gene have been associated with both coronary heart disease (Alanne *et al.*, 2007) and preeclampsia, a condition of pregnancy-associated hypertension (Moses *et al.*, 2008).

Future Directions

The interest in selenium and its impact on human health began with concerns over its toxicity. The focus has shifted to better understanding how individuals who receive adequate dietary levels benefit through the resultant prevention of disease. This will necessitate a continued effort to define the level of selenium intake that will enhance its

health-promoting effects, requiring improved methods of assessment and evaluation that are based on research findings. This challenge is perhaps best exemplified by the recent lack of efficacy of selenium supplementation in reducing the incidence of prostate cancer in the SELECT prostate cancer trial. This large study proceeded as a result of a substantial body of evidence that selenium could prevent cancer of several types in animal models and that selenium levels in the diet are inversely correlated with prostate cancer risk. However, there remains a large gap in the understanding of how different forms of selenium are eventually used by the body; of the mechanisms by which selenium prevents disease; and of the biological roles for most of the 25 selenocysteine-containing proteins. Similarly, the functions of other proteins that bind selenium remain to be clarified. Such information, partnered with a better appreciation of the impact of individualized genetic diversity among humans on selenium-influenced health outcomes, should be gathered prior to the launch of large supplementation studies. Furthermore, increased knowledge of selenium biology will be critical to understanding the risks and benefits of enhancing dietary selenium intake, perhaps based on a particular person's baseline levels, and thus making revised recommendations as to how much selenium to consume in order to reduce disease incidence.

Suggestions for Further Reading

Dumont, E., Vanhaeecke, F., and Canelis, R. (2006) Selenium speciation from food source to metabolites: a critical review. *Anal Bioanal Chem* **385**, 1304–1323.

Flohé, L. (2009) The labour pains of biochemical selenology: the history of selenoprotein biosynthesis. *Biochem Biophys Acta* **1790**, 1389–1403.

Mueller, A.S., Mueller, K., Wolf, N.M., *et al.* (2009) Selenium and diabetes: an enigma? *Free Rad Res* **43**, 1029–1059.

References

Alanne, M., Kristiansson, K., Auro, K., *et al.* (2007) Variation in the selenoprotein S gene locus is associated with coronary heart disease and ischemic stroke in two independent Finnish cohorts. *Hum Genet* **122**, 355–365.

Apostolou, S., Klein, J.O., Mitsuuchi, Y., *et al.* (2004) Growth inhibition and induction of apoptosis in mesothelioma cells by selenium and dependence on selenoprotein SEP15 genotype. *Oncogene* **23**, 1–9.

Arbogast, S. and Ferreiro, A. (2010) Selenoproteins and protection against oxidative stress: selenoprotein N as a novel player at the crossroads of redox signaling and calcium homeostasis. *Antioxid Redox Signal* **12**, 893–904.

Arthur, J.R., McKenzie, R.C., and Beckett, G.J. (2003) Selenium in the immune system. *J Nutr* **133**, 1457S–1459S.

Ashton, K., Hooper, L., Harvey, L.J., *et al.* (2009) Methods of assessment of selenium status in humans: a systematic review. *Am J Clin Nutr* **89**, 2025S–2039S.

Bansal, M.P., Oborn, C.J., Danielson, K.G., *et al.* (1989) Evidence for two selenium-binding proteins distinct from glutathione peroxidase in mouse liver. *Carcinogenesis* **10**, 541–546.

Baum, M.K., Shor-Posner, G., Lai, S., *et al.* (1997) High risk of HIV-related mortality is associated with selenium deficiency. *J Acquir Immune Defic Syndr Hum Retrovirol* **15**, 370–374.

Beck, M.A., Esworthy, R.S., Ho, Y.S., *et al.* (1998) Glutathione peroxidase protects mice from viral-induced myocarditis. *FASEB J* **12**, 1143–1149.

Beck, M.A., Kolbeck, P.C., Rohr, L.H., *et al.* (1994) Benign human enterovirus becomes virulent in selenium-deficient mice. *J Med Virol* **43**, 166–170.

Beck, M.A., Nelson, H.K., Shi, Q., *et al.* (2001) Selenium deficiency increases the pathology of an influenza virus infection. *FASEB J* **15**, 1481–1483.

Beck, M.A., Shi, Q., Morris, V.C., *et al.* (1995) Rapid genomic evolution of a non-virulent coxsackievirus B3 in selenium-deficient mice results in selection of identical virulent isolates. *Nat Med* **1**, 433–436.

Behne, D. and Kyriakopoulos, A. (2001) Mammalian selenium-containing proteins. *Annu Rev Nutr* **21**, 453–473.

Beilstein, M.A. and Whanger, P.D. (1986) Chemical forms of selenium in rat tissues after administration of selenite or selenomethionine. *J Nutr* **116**, 1711–1719.

Bellinger, F.P., Raman, A.V., Reeves, M.A., *et al.* (2009) Regulation and function of selenoproteins in human disease. *Biochem J* **422**, 11–22.

Berry, M.J., Banu, L., Chen, Y., *et al.* (1991) Recognition of UGA as a selenocysteine codon in Type I deiodinase requires sequences in the 3′ untranslated region. *Nature* **353**, 273–276.

Bianco, A.C. and Kim, B.W. (2006) Deiodinases: implications of the local control of thyroid hormone action. *J Clin Invest* **116**, 2571–2579.

Bianco, A.C., Salvatore, D., Gereben, B., *et al.* (2002) Biochemistry, cellular and molecular biology, and physiological roles of the iodothyronine selenodeiodinases. *Endocrinol Rev* **23**, 38–89.

Bleys, J., Navas-Acien, A., and Guallar, E. (2007) Serum selenium and diabetes in US adults. *Diabetes Care* **30**, 829–834.

Bleys, J., Navas-Acien, A., and Guallar, E. (2008) Serum selenium levels and all-cause, cancer, and cardiovascular mortality among US adults. *Arch Intern Med* **168**, 404–410.

Brown, K.M., Pickard, K., Nicol, F., *et al.* (2000) Effects of organic and inorganic selenium supplementation on selenoenzyme activity in blood lymphocytes, granulocytes, platelets and erythrocytes. *Clin Sci (Lond)* **98**, 593–539.

Bugel, S., Larsen, E.H., Sloth, J.J., *et al.* (2008) Absorption, excretion, and retention of selenium from a high selenium yeast in men with a high intake of selenium. *Food Nutr Res* **52**. PMID 19109661.

Burk, R.F. and Hill, K.E. (2009) Selenoprotein P-expression, functions, and roles in mammals. *Biochim Biophys Acta* **1790**, 1441–1447.

Burk, R.F., Norsworthy, B.K., Hill, K.E., *et al.* (2006) Effects of chemical form of selenium on plasma biomarkers in a high-dose human supplementation trial. *Cancer Epidemiol Biomarkers Prev* **15**, 804–810.

Chabory, E., Damon, C., Lenoir, A., *et al.* (2009) Epididymis seleno-independent glutathione peroxidase 5 maintains sperm DNA integrity in mice. *J Clin Invest* **119**, 2074–2085.

Chang, P.W., Tsui, S.K., Liew, C., *et al.* (1997) Isolation, characterization, and chromosomal mapping of a novel cDNA clone encoding human selenium binding protein. *J Cell Biochem* **64**, 217–224.

Chen, G., Wang, H., Miller, C.T., *et al.* (2004) Reduced selenium-binding protein 1 expression is associated with poor outcome in lung adenocarcinomas. *J Pathol* **202**, 321–329.

Chiang, E.C., Shen, S., Kengery, S.S., *et al.* (2009) Defining the optimal selenium dose for prostate cancer risk reduction: insights from the U-shaped relationship between selenium status, DNA damage, and apoptosis. *Dose Response* **8**, 285–300.

Chu, F.F., Doroshow, J.H., and Esworthy, R.S. (1993) Expression, characterization, and tissue distribution of a new cellular selenium-dependent glutathione peroxidase, GSHPx-GI. *J Biol Chem* **268**, 2571–2576.

Clark, L.C., Combs, G.F.J., Turnbull, B.W., *et al.* (1996) Effects of selenium supplementation for cancer prevention in patients with carcinoma of the skin. A randomized controlled trial. *J Am Med Assoc* **276**, 1957–1963.

Combs, G.F., Jr (2001) Selenium in global food systems. *Br J Nutr* **85**, 517–547.

Cooper, M.L., Adami, H.O., Gronberg, H., *et al.* (2008) Interaction between single nucleotide polymorphisms in selenoprotein P and mitochondrial superoxide dismutase determines prostate cancer risk. *Cancer Res* **68**, 10171–10177.

Copeland, P.R. and Driscoll, D.M. (1999) Purification, redox sensitivity, and RNA binding properties of SECIS-binding protein 2, a protein involved in selenoprotein biosynthesis. *J Biol Chem* **274**, 25447–25454.

Diamond, A.M., Dale, P., Murray, J.L., *et al.* (1996) The inhibition of radiation-induced mutagenesis by the combined effects of selenium and the aminothiol WR-1065. *Mutat Res* **356**, 147–154.

Diwadkar-Navsariwala, V., Prins, G.S., Swanson, S.M., *et al.* (2006) Selenoprotein deficiency accelerates prostate carcinogenesis in a transgenic model. *Proc Natl Acad Sci USA* **103**, 8179–8184.

Driscoll, D.M. and Copeland, P.R. (2003) Mechanism and regulation of selenoprotein synthesis. *Annu Rev Nutr* **23**, 17–40.

Duffield-Lillico, A.J., Dalkin, B.L., Reid, M.E., *et al.* (2003) Selenium supplementation, baseline plasma selenium status and incidence of prostate cancer: an analysis of the complete treatment period of the Nutritional Prevention of Cancer Trial. *BJU Int* **91**, 608–612.

Dumitrescu, A.M., Di Cosmo, C., Liao, X.H., *et al.* (2010) The syndrome of inherited partial SBP2 deficiency in humans. *Antioxid Redox Signal* **12**, 905–920.

Dumitrescu, A.M., Liao, X.H., Abdullah, M.S., *et al.* (2005) Mutations in SECISBP2 result in abnormal thyroid hormone metabolism. *Nat Genet* **37**, 1247–1252.

Dumont, E., Vanhaecke, F., and Cornelis, R. (2006) Selenium speciation from food source to metabolites: a critical review. *Anal Bioanal Chem* **385**, 1304–1323.

Dumont, J.E., Corvilain, B., and Contempre, B. (1994) The biochemistry of endemic cretinism: roles of iodine and selenium deficiency and goitrogens. *Mol Cell Endocrinol* **100**, 163–166.

Dziaman, T., Huzarski, T., Gackowski, D., *et al.* (2009) Selenium supplementation reduced oxidative DNA damage in adnexectomized BRCA1 mutations carriers. *Cancer Epidemiol Biomarkers Prev* **18**, 2923–2928.

El-Bayoumy, K. (Ed.) (1991) *The Role of Selenium in Cancer Prevention*. J.B. Lippincott, Philadelphia.

El-Bayoumy, K. (2009) The negative results of the SELECT study do not necessarily discredit the selenium–cancer prevention hypothesis. *Nutr Cancer* **61**, 285–286.

Ellison, R.S. (2002) Major trace elements limiting livestock performance in New Zealand. *N Z Vet J* **50**, 35–40.

Esaki, N., Nakamura, T., Tanaka, H., *et al.* (1982) Selenocysteine lyase, a novel enzyme that specifically acts on selenocysteine. Mammalian distribution and purification and properties of pig liver enzyme. *J Biol Chem* **257**, 4386–4391.

Fairweather-Tait, S.J., Collings, R., and Hurst, R. (2010) Selenium bioavailability: current knowledge and future research requirements. *Am J Clin Nutr* **91**, 1484S–1491S.

Fernandez-Banares, F., Cabre, E., Esteve, M., *et al.* (2002) Serum selenium and risk of large size colorectal adenomas in a geographical area with a low selenium status. *Am J Gastroenterol* **97**, 2103–2108.

Fischer, J.L., Lancia, J.K., Mathur, A., *et al.* (2006) Selenium protection from DNA damage involves a Ref1/p53/Brca1 protein complex. *Anticancer Res* **26**, 899–904.

Flohe, L., Gunzler, W.A., and Schock, H.H. (1973) Glutathione peroxidase: a selenoenzyme. *FEBS Lett* **32**, 132–134.

Florian, S., Wingler, K., Schmehl, K., *et al.* (2001) Cellular and subcellular localization of gastrointestinal glutathione peroxidase in normal and malignant human intestinal tissue. *Free Radic Res* **35**, 655–663.

Ghadirian, P., Maisonneuve, P., Perret, C., *et al.* (2000) A case-control study of toenail selenium and cancer of the breast, colon, and prostate. *Cancer Detect Prev* **24**, 305–313.

Gibson, R.S. (1989) Assessment of trace element status in humans. *Prog Food Nutr Sci* **13**, 67–111.

Gladyshev, V.N. and Hatfield, D.L. (2001) Analysis of selenocysteine-containing proteins. *Curr Protoc Protein Sci* Chapter 3, Unit 3.8.

Gromer, S., Eubel, J.K., Lee, B.L., *et al.* (2005) Human selenoproteins at a glance. *Cell Mol Life Sci* **62**, 2414–2437.

Haratake, M., Hongoh, M., Miyauchi, M., *et al.* (2008) Albumin-mediated selenium transfer by a selenotrisulfide relay mechanism. *Inorg Chem* **47**, 6273–6280.

Hatfield, D.L. and Gladyshev, V.N. (2009) The outcome of Selenium and Vitamin E Cancer Prevention Trial (SELECT) reveals the need for better understanding of selenium biology. *Mol Interv* **9**, 18–21.

Hawkes, W.C., Alkan, F.Z., and Oehler, L. (2003) Absorption, distribution and excretion of selenium from beef and rice in healthy North American men. *J Nutr* **133**, 3434–3442.

Haygarth, P.M., Harrison, A.F., and Jones, K.C. (1995) Plant selenium from soil and the atmosphere. *J Environ Qual* **24**, 768–771.

Hoffmann, F.W., Hashimoto, A.C., Shafer, L.A., *et al.* (2010) Dietary selenium modulates activation and differentiation of CD4+ T cells in mice through a mechanism involving cellular free thiols. *J Nutr* **140**, 1155–1161.

Hoffmann, P.R. and Berry, M.J. (2008) The influence of selenium on immune responses. *Mol Nutr Food Res* **52**, 1273–1280.

Hu, Y., Benya, R.V., Carroll, R.E., *et al.* (2005) Allelic loss of the gene for the GPX1 selenium-containing protein is a common event in cancer. *J Nutr* **135**, 3021S–3024S.

Hu, Y.J., Korotkov, K.V., Mehta, R., *et al.* (2001) Distribution and functional consequences of nucleotide polymorphisms in the 3′-untranslated region of the human Sep15 gene. *Cancer Res* **61**, 2307–2310.

Huang, K.C., Park, D.C., Ng, S.K., *et al.* (2006) Selenium binding protein 1 in ovarian cancer. *Int J Cancer* **118**, 2433–2440.

Imai, T., Mihara, H., Kurihara, T., *et al.* (2009) Selenocysteine is selectively taken up by red blood cells. *Biosci Biotechnol Biochem* **73**, 2746–2748.

Institute of Medicine (2000) *Dietary Reference Intakes for Vitamin C, Vitamin E, Selenium and Carotenoids.* National Academy Press, Washington, DC.

Ip, C. and Lisk, D.J. (1994) Bioactivity of selenium from Brazil nut for cancer prevention and selenoenzyme maintenance. *Nutr Cancer* **21**, 203–212.

Irons, R., Carlson, B.A., Hatfield, D.L., *et al.* (2006) Both selenoproteins and low molecular weight selenocompounds reduce colon cancer risk in mice with genetically impaired selenoprotein expression. *J Nutr* **136**, 1311–1317.

Jablonska, E., Gromadzinska, J., Sobala, W., *et al.* (2008) Lung cancer risk associated with selenium status is modified in smoking individuals by Sep15 polymorphism. *Eur J Nutr* **47**, 47–54.

Jacobs, E.T., Jiang, R., Alberts, D.S., *et al.* (2004) Selenium and colorectal adenoma: results of a pooled analysis. *J Natl Cancer Inst* **96**, 1669–1675.

Janghorbani, M., Xia, Y., Ha, P., *et al.* (1999) Effect of dietary selenium restriction on selected parameters of selenium status in men with high life-long intake. *J Nutr Biochem* **10**, 564–572.

Jeong, J.Y., Wang, Y., and Sytkowski, A.J. (2009) Human selenium binding protein-1 (hSP56) interacts with VDU1 in a selenium-dependent manner. *Biochem Biophys Res Commun* **379**, 583–588.

Kim, H., Kang, H.J., You, K.T., *et al.* (2006) Suppression of human selenium-binding protein 1 is a late event in colorectal carcinogenesis and is associated with poor survival. *Proteomics* **6**, 3466–3476.

Kobayashi, Y., Ogra, Y., and Suzuki, K.T. (2001) Speciation and metabolism of selenium injected with 82Se-enriched selenite and selenate in rats. *J Chromatogr B Biomed Sci Appl* **760**, 73–81.

Kohrle, J., Jakob, F., Contempre, B., *et al.* (2005) Selenium, the thyroid, and the endocrine system. *Endocrinol Rev* **26**, 944–984.

Koller, L.D. and Exon, J.H. (1986) The two faces of selenium – deficiency and toxicity – are similar in animals and man. *Can J Vet Res* **50**, 297–306.

Korotkov, K.V., Kumaraswamy, E., Zhou, Y., *et al.* (2001) Association between the 15-kDa selenoprotein and UDP-glucose:glycoprotein glucosyltransferase in the endoplasmic reticulum of mammalian cells. *J Biol Chem* **276**, 15330–15336.

Kowalska, E., Narod, S.A., Huzarski, T., *et al.* (2005) Increased rates of chromosomal breakage in BRCA1 carriers are normalized by oral selenium supplementation. *Cancer Epidemiol Biomarkers Prev* **14**, 1302–1306.

Kremer, D., Ilgen, G., and Feldmann, J. (2005) GC-ICP-MS determination of dimethylselenide in human breath after ingestion of (77)Se-enriched selenite: monitoring of in-vivo methylation of selenium. *Anal Bioanal Chem* **383**, 509–515.

Kryukov, G.V., Castellano, S., Novoselov, S.V., *et al.* (2003) Characterization of mammalian selenoproteomes. *Science* **300**, 1439–1443.

Kuzuya, M., Ando, F., Iguchi, A., *et al.* (2008) Glutathione peroxidase 1 Pro198Leu variant contributes to the metabolic syndrome in men in a large Japanese cohort. *Am J Clin Nutr* **87**, 1939–1944.

Laclaustra, M., Navas-Acien, A., Stranges, S., *et al.* (2009) Serum selenium concentrations and diabetes in US adults: National Health and Nutrition Examination Survey (NHANES) 2003–2004. *Environ Health Perspect* **117**, 1409–1413.

Lawson, T. (1989) Nicotinamide and selenium stimulate the repair of DNA damage produced by N-nitrosobis(2-oxopropyl) amine. *Anticancer Res* **9**, 483–486.

Lawson, T. and Birt, D.F. (1983) Enhancement of the repair of carcinogen-induced DNA damage in the hamster pancreas by dietary selenium. *Chem Biol Interact* **45**, 95–104.

LeBlanc, A., Dumas, P., and Lefebvre, L. (1999) Trace element content of commercial shampoos: impact on trace element levels in hair. *Sci Total Environ* **229**, 121–124.

Lee, B.J., Worland, P.J., Davis, J.N., *et al.* (1989) Identification of a selenocysteyl-tRNA(Ser) in mammalian cells that recognizes the nonsense codon, UGA. *J Biol Chem* **264**, 9724–9727.

Lei, C., Niu, X., Wei, J., *et al.* (2009) Interaction of glutathione peroxidase-1 and selenium in endemic dilated cardiomyopathy. *Clin Chim Acta* **399**, 102–108.

Lescure, A., Gautheret, D., Carbon, P., *et al.* (1999) Novel selenoproteins identified in silico and in vivo by using a conserved RNA structural motif. *J Biol Chem* **274**, 38147–38154.

Levander, O.A. (1984) The importance of selenium in total parenteral nutrition. *Bull NY Acad Med* **60**, 144–155.

Li, H.F., McGrath, S.P., and Zhao, F.J. (2008a) Selenium uptake, translocation and speciation in wheat supplied with selenate or selenite. *New Phytol* **178**, 92–102.

Li, T., Yang, W., Li, M., *et al.* (2008b) Expression of selenium-binding protein 1 characterizes intestinal cell maturation and predicts survival for patients with colorectal cancer. *Mol Nutr Food Res* **52**, 1289–1299.

Li, Y., Peng, T., Yang, Y., *et al.* (2000) High prevalence of enteroviral genomic sequences in myocardium from cases of endemic cardiomyopathy (Keshan disease) in China. *Heart* **83**, 696–701.

Lippman, S.M., Goodman, P.J., Klein, E.A., *et al.* (2005) Designing the Selenium and Vitamin E Cancer Prevention Trial (SELECT). *J Nat Cancer Inst* **97**, 94–102.

Lippman, S.M., Klein, E.A., Goodman, P.J., *et al.* (2009) Effect of selenium and vitamin E on risk of prostate cancer and other cancers: the Selenium and Vitamin E Cancer Prevention Trial (SELECT). *JAMA* **301**, 39–51.

Lobanov, A.V., Hatfield, D.L., and Gladyshev, V.N. (2009) Eukaryotic selenoproteins and selenoproteomes. *Biochim Biophys Acta* **1790**, 1424–1428.

MacFarquhar, J.K., Broussard, D.L., Melstrom, P., *et al.* (2010) Acute selenium toxicity associated with a dietary supplement. *Arch Intern Med* **170**, 256–261.

Marinou, I., Walters, K., Dickson, M.C., *et al.* (2009) Evidence of epistasis between interleukin 1 and selenoprotein-S with susceptibility to rheumatoid arthritis. *Ann Rheumatic Dis* **68**, 1494–1497.

Meplan, C., Hughes, D.J., Pardini, B., *et al.* (2010) Genetic variants in selenoprotein genes increase risk of colorectal cancer. *Carcinogenesis* **31**, 1074–1079.

Miladinovic, D., Djujic, I., and Stankovic, S. (1998) Variation of selenium content in growing wild plants during vegetative period. *J Environ Pathol Toxicol Oncol* **17**, 217–220.

Moghadaszadeh, B., Petit, N., Jaillard, C., *et al.* (2001) Mutations in SEPN1 cause congenital muscular dystrophy with spinal rigidity and restrictive respiratory syndrome. *Nat Genet* **29**, 17–18.

Morris, J.S., Stampfer, M., and Willett, W. (1983) Dietary selenium in human toenails as an indicator. *Biol Trace Elem Res* **5**, 529–537.

Moses, E.K., Johnson, M.P., Tommerdal, L., *et al.* (2008) Genetic association of preeclampsia to the inflammatory response gene SEPS1. *Am J Obstet Gynecol* **198**, e1–5.

Moustafa, M.E., Kumaraswamy, E., Zhong, N., *et al.* (2003) Models for assessing the role of selenoproteins in health. *J Nutr* **133**, 2494S–2496S.

Nadiminty, N. and Gao, A.C. (2008) Mechanisms of selenium chemoprevention and therapy in prostate cancer. *Mol Nutr Food Res* **52**, 1247–1260.

Nuttall, K.L. (2006) Evaluating selenium poisoning. *Ann Clin Lab Sci* **36**, 409–420.

Olson, G.E., Winfrey, V.P., Hill, K.E., *et al.* (2008) Megalin mediates selenoprotein P uptake by kidney proximal tubule epithelial cells. *J Biol Chem* **283**, 6854–6860.

Olson, G.E., Winfrey, V.P., Nagdas, S.K., *et al.* (2007) Apolipoprotein E receptor-2 (ApoER2) mediates selenium uptake from selenoprotein P by the mouse testis. *J Biol Chem* **282**, 12290–12297.

Oster, O., Schmiedel, G., and Prellwitz, W. (1988) The organ distribution of selenium in German adults. *Biol Trace Elem Res* **15**, 23–45.

Papp, L.V., Lu, J., Holmgren, A., *et al.* (2007) From selenium to selenoproteins: synthesis, identity, and their role in human health. *Antioxid Redox Signal* **9**, 775–806.

Penney, K.L., Schumacher, F.R., Li, H., *et al.* (2010) A large prospective study of SEP15 genetic variation, interaction with plasma selenium levels, and prostate cancer risk and survival. *Cancer Prev Res (Phila)* **3**, 604–610.

Pera, J., Slowik, A., Dziedzic, T., *et al.* (2008) Glutathione peroxidase 1 C593T polymorphism is associated with lobar intracerebral hemorrhage. *Cerebrovasc Dis* **25**, 445–449.

Peters, U., Chatterjee, N., Church, T.R., *et al.* (2006) High serum selenium and reduced risk of advanced colorectal adenoma in a colorectal cancer early detection program. *Cancer Epidemiol Biomarkers Prev* **15**, 315–320.

Peters, U., Chatterjee, N., Hayes, R.B., *et al.* (2008) Variation in the selenoenzyme genes and risk of advanced distal colorectal adenoma. *Cancer Epidemiol Biomarkers Prev* **17**, 1144–1154.

Pitney, C.L., Royal, M., and Klebert, M. (2009) Selenium supplementation in HIV-infected patients: is there any potential clinical benefit? *J Assoc Nurses AIDS Care* **20**, 326–333.

Pohl, N.M., Tong, C., Fang, W., *et al.* (2009) Transcriptional regulation and biological functions of selenium-binding protein 1 in colorectal cancer in vitro and in nude mouse xenografts. *PLoS One* **4**, e7774.

Porat, A., Sagiv, Y., and Elazar, Z. (2000) A 56-kDa selenium-binding protein participates in intra-Golgi protein transport. *J Biol Chem* **275**, 14457–14465.

Ratnasinghe, D., Tangrea, J.A., Andersen, M.R., *et al.* (2000) Glutathione peroxidase codon 198 polymorphism variant increases lung cancer risk. *Cancer Res* **60**, 6381–6383.

Rayman, M.P. (2000) The importance of selenium to human health. *Lancet* **356**, 233–241.

Rayman, M.P. (2008) Food-chain selenium and human health: emphasis on intake. *Br J Nutr* **100**, 254–268.

Rayman, M.P. (2009) Selenoproteins and human health: insights from epidemiological data. *Biochim Biophys Acta* **1790**, 1533–1540.

Reamer, D.C. and Veillon, C. (1983) A double isotope dilution method for using stable selenium isotopes in metabolic tracer studies: analysis by gas chromatography/mass spectrometry (GC/MS). *J Nutr* **113**, 786–792.

Rosin, M.P. (1981) Inhibition of spontaneous mutagenesis in yeast cultures by selenite, selenate and selenide. *Cancer Lett* **13**, 7–14.

Rotruck, J.T., Pope, A.L., Ganther, H.E., *et al.* (1973) Selenium: biochemical role as a component of glutathione peroxidase. *Science* **179**, 588–590.

Russell, G.R., Nader, C.J., and Partick, E.J. (1980) Induction of DNA repair by some selenium compounds. *Cancer Lett* **10**, 75–81.

Salbe, A.D. and Levander, O.A. (1990) Effect of various dietary factors on the deposition of selenium in the hair and nails of rats. *J Nutr* **120**, 200–206.

Schepman, K., Engelbert, R.H., Visser, M.M., *et al.* (2011) Kashin Beck Disease: more than just osteoarthrosis: a cross-sectional study regarding the influence of body function-structures and activities on level of participation. *Int Orthop* **35**, 767–776.

Schomburg, L. and Kohrle, J. (2008) On the importance of selenium and iodine metabolism for thyroid hormone biosynthesis and human health. *Mol Nutr Food Res* **52**, 1235–1246.

Schrauzer, G.N. (2009) RE: Lessons from the selenium and vitamin E cancer prevention trial (SELECT). *Crit Rev Biotechnol* **29**, 81.

Schwarz, K. and Foltz, C.M. (1958) Factor 3 activity of selenium compounds. *J Biol Chem* **233**, 245–251.

Seo, Y.R., Sweeney, C., and Smith, M.L. (2002) Selenomethionine induction of DNA repair response in human fibroblasts. *Oncogene* **21**, 3663–3669.

Shamberger, R.J. and Frost, D.V. (1969) Possible protective effect of selenium against human cancer. *Can Med Assoc J* **100**, 682.

Shen, L., Van Dyck, K., Luten, J., *et al.* (1997) Diffusibility of selenate, selenite, seleno-methionine, and seleno-cystine during simulated gastrointestinal digestion. *Biol Trace Elem Res* **58**, 55–63.

Shibata, T., Arisawa, T., Tahara, T., *et al.* (2009) Selenoprotein S (SEPS1) gene −105G>A promoter polymorphism influences the susceptibility to gastric cancer in the Japanese population. *BMC Gastroenterol* **9**, 2.

Stranges, S., Laclaustra, M., Ji, C., *et al.* (2010) Higher selenium status is associated with adverse blood lipid profile in British adults. *J Nutr* **140**, 81–87.

Stranges, S., Marshall, J.R., Natarajan, R., *et al.* (2007) Effects of long-term selenium supplementation on the incidence of type 2 diabetes: a randomized trial. *Ann Intern Med* **147**, 217–223.

Suzuki, K.T., Kurasaki, K., Okazaki, N., *et al.* (2005) Selenosugar and trimethylselenonium among urinary Se metabolites: dose- and age-related changes. *Toxicol Appl Pharmacol* **206**, 1–8.

Suzuki, K.T., Shiobara, Y., Itoh, M., *et al.* (1998) Selective uptake of selenite by red blood cells. *Analyst* **123**, 63–67.

Tajsharghi, H., Darin, N., Tulinius, M., *et al.* (2005) Early onset myopathy with a novel mutation in the selenoprotein N gene (SEPN1). *Neuromuscul Disord* **15**, 299–302.

Terry, N., Zayed, A.M., De Souza, M.P., *et al.* (2000) Selenium in higher plants. *Annu Rev Plant Physiol Plant Mol Biol* **51**, 401–432.

Tham, D.M., Whitin, J.C., Kim, K.K., *et al.* (1998) Expression of extracellular glutathione peroxidase in human and mouse gastrointestinal tract. *Am J Physiol* **275**, G1463–1471.

Thomson, C.D. (1998) Selenium speciation in human body fluids. *Analyst* **123**, 827–831.

Thomson, C.D. (2004) Assessment of requirements for selenium and adequacy of selenium status: a review. *Eur J Clin Nutr* **58**, 391–402.

Thomson, C.D. and Robinson, M.F. (1990) Selenium content of foods consumed in Otago, New Zealand. *NZ Med J* **103**, 130–135.

Thomson, C.D., Chisholm, A., McLachlan, S.K., *et al.* (2008) Brazil nuts: an effective way to improve selenium status. *Am J Clin Nutr* **87**, 379–384.

Udler, M., Maia, A.T., Cebrian, A., *et al.* (2007) Common germline genetic variation in antioxidant defense genes and survival after diagnosis of breast cancer. *J Clin Oncol* **25**, 3015–3023.

Ullrey, D.E. (1992) Basis for regulation of selenium supplements in animal diets. *J Anim Sci* **70**, 3922–3927.

Ursini, F., Heim, S., Kiess, M., *et al.* (1999) Dual function of the selenoprotein PHGPx during sperm maturation. *Science* **285**, 1393–1396.

Utomo, A., Jiang, X., Furuta, S., *et al.* (2004) Identification of a novel putative non-selenocysteine containing phospholipid hydroperoxide glutathione peroxidase (NPGPx) essential for alleviating oxidative stress generated from polyunsaturated fatty acids in breast cancer cells. *J Biol Chem* **279**, 43522–43529.

Vadhanavikit, S., Kraus, R.J., and Ganther, H.E. (1987) Metabolism of selenocyanate in the rat. *Arch Biochem Biophys* **258**, 1–6.

Valdiglesias, V., Pasaro, E., Mendez, J., *et al.* (2010) In vitro evaluation of selenium genotoxic, cytotoxic, and protective effects: a review. *Arch Toxicol* **84**, 337–351.

Vernet, P., Rigaudiere, N., Ghyselinck, N., *et al.* (1996) In vitro expression of a mouse tissue specific glutathione-peroxidase-like protein lacking the selenocysteine can protect stably transfected mammalian cells against oxidative damage. *Biochem Cell Biol* **74**, 125–131.

Voetsch, B., Jin, R.C., Bierl, C., *et al.* (2007) Promoter polymorphisms in the plasma glutathione peroxidase (GPx-3) gene: a novel risk factor for arterial ischemic stroke among young adults and children. *Stroke* **38**, 41–49.

Waters, D.J., Shen, S., Glickman, L.T., *et al.* (2005) Prostate cancer risk and DNA damage: translational significance of selenium supplementation in a canine model. *Carcinogenesis* **26,** 1256–1262.

Whanger, P.D. (2004) Selenium and its relationship to cancer: an update. *Br J Nutr* **91,** 11–28.

Winter, J.P., Gong, Y., Grant, P.J., *et al.* (2003) Glutathione peroxidase 1 genotype is associated with an increased risk of coronary artery disease. *Coron Artery Dis* **14,** 149–153.

Wolffram, S., Berger, B., Grenacher, B., *et al.* (1989) Transport of selenoamino acids and their sulfur analogues across the intestinal brush border membrane of pigs. *J Nutr* **119,** 706–712.

Xia, Y., Hill, K.E., Byrne, D.W., *et al.* (2005) Effectiveness of selenium supplements in a low-selenium area of China. *Am J Clin Nutr* **81,** 829–834.

Xia, Y.M., Hill, K.E., and Burk, R.F. (1989) Biochemical studies of a selenium-deficient population in China: measurement of selenium, glutathione peroxidase and other oxidant defense indices in blood. *J Nutr* **119,** 1318–1326.

Xiong, Y.M., Mo, X.Y., Zou, X.Z., *et al.* (2010) Association study between polymorphisms in selenoprotein genes and susceptibility to Kashin-Beck disease. *Osteoarthritis Cartilage* **18,** 817–824.

Yang, G., Wang, S., Zhou, R., *et al.* (1983) Endemic selenium intoxication of humans in China. *Am J Clin Nutr* **37,** 872–881.

Yang, M. and Sytkowski, A.J. (1998) Differential expression and androgen regulation of the human selenium-binding protein gene hSP56 in prostate cancer cells. *Cancer Res* **58,** 3150–3153.

Yeh, J., Vendeland, S.C., Gu, Q., *et al.* (1997) Dietary selenium increases selenoprotein W levels in rat tissues. *J Nutr* **127,** 2165–2172.

Yu, L., Sun, L., Nan, Y., *et al.* (2010) Protection from H1N1 influenza virus infections in mice by supplementation with selenium: a comparison with selenium-deficient mice. *Biol Trace Elem Res* **141,** 254–261

Zachara, B.A., Pawluk, H., Bloch-Boguslawska, E., *et al.* (2001) Tissue level, distribution, and total body selenium content in healthy and diseased humans in Poland. *Arch Environ Health* **56,** 461–466.

Zayed, A.M. and Terry, N. (1994) Selenium volatilization in roots and shoots – effects of shoot removal and sulfate level. *J Plant Physiol* **143,** 8–14.

Zhang, L.P., Maiorino, M., Roveri, A., *et al.* (1989) Phospholipid hydroperoxide glutathione peroxidase: specific activity in tissues of rats of different age and comparison with other glutathione peroxidases. *Biochim Biophys Acta* **1006,** 140–143.

Zhuo, P. and Diamond, A.M. (2009) Molecular mechanisms by which selenoproteins affect cancer risk and progression. *Biochim Biophys Acta* **1790,** 1546–1554

Zou, K., Liu, G., Wu, T., *et al.* (2009) Selenium for preventing Kashin-Beck osteoarthropathy in children: a meta-analysis. *Osteoarthritis Cartilage* **17,** 144–151.

38

MANGANESE, MOLYBDENUM, BORON, CHROMIUM, AND OTHER TRACE ELEMENTS

FORREST H. NIELSEN, PhD

Grand Forks Human Nutrition Research Center, USDA-ARS-NPA, Grand Forks, North Dakota, USA

Summary

This review presents current knowledge about the essentiality, biochemical function, beneficial actions, deficiency signs, absorption, transport, retention, excretion, and nutritional importance of the trace and ultra trace elements manganese, molybdenum, boron, chromium, arsenic, fluoride, nickel, silicon, strontium, and vanadium in human nutrition. Although the nutritional importance of each of the elements covered in this chapter is limited, unclear, or speculative, emerging evidence indicates that some of these elements have beneficial bioactivity in nutritional or reasonable supra-nutritional amounts. They may become recognized in a manner similar to other essential nutrients provided in supra-nutritional amounts, or phytonutrients and omega-3 fatty acids in nutritional amounts, in promoting health and preventing chronic disease in humans. Therefore, future studies are needed to determine the mechanisms behind the beneficial effects, whether some effects reflect an essential function, and the dietary intakes that give optimal response.

Introduction

If the lack of a mineral element cannot be shown to cause death or interrupt the life cycle, then that element is not generally considered essential unless it has a defined biochemical function. On this basis, two elements, manganese and molybdenum, discussed in this chapter, are well established essential elements because they are known

enzyme cofactors. Genetic defects eliminating some of these cofactor functions result in death in humans. Currently, however, human excessive or high intakes of manganese and molybdenum causing pathological or pharmacological effects receive more attention than low intakes because their nutritional deficiencies have not been clearly identified in the general population. Boron and chromium have not been firmly established as nutrition-

Present Knowledge in Nutrition, Tenth Edition. Edited by John W. Erdman Jr, Ian A. Macdonald and Steven H. Zeisel.
© 2012 International Life Sciences Institute. Published 2012 by John Wiley & Sons, Inc.

ally essential because they lack clearly defined biochemical functions. However, numerous human studies have shown that boron in nutritional amounts and chromium in supra-nutritional amounts may influence health and disease by directly or indirectly producing beneficial functional outcomes. Thus, boron and chromium will receive significant attention in this review. Numerous other elements have been suggested to be of nutritional importance because of some promising physiological or clinical finding, most often in an animal model or special human situation. Of these elements, arsenic, fluorine, nickel, silicon, strontium, and vanadium have received the most research attention focused on their nutritional and pharmacological properties, and thus will be briefly discussed. Possible nutritional importance of elements other than those above will be only summarized in a table because there is limited recent evidence that provides further support for them having significant beneficial effects in humans. (Note: To achieve the guideline limit for the number of references for this review, other review articles instead of original reports often will be cited.)

Essential Trace Elements

Manganese

Essentiality Basis and Biochemical Function

The essentiality of manganese has been known for about 80 years. Manganese deficiency has been induced in many animal species (Freeland-Graves and Llanes, 1994). However, because manganese deficiency has been difficult to induce or identify in humans, it is considered to be of limited nutritional concern. None the less, manganese is an established essential nutrient for humans because it activates numerous enzymes and is a constituent of several metalloenzymes (Leach and Harris, 1997). Enzymes that are activated by manganese include oxidoreductases, lyases, ligases, hydrolases, kinases, decarboxylases, and transferases. Most enzymes activated by manganese in higher animals and humans also are activated by other metals, especially magnesium; exceptions are the manganese-specific activation of glycosyltransferases, glutamine synthetase, farnesyl pyrophosphate synthetase, and phosphoenolpyruvate carboxykinase. Arginase, pyruvate carboxylase, and manganese superoxide dismutase (MnSOD or SOD2) are manganese metalloenzymes found in humans and animals. MnSOD is essential for life; a deletion mutation in mice results in death within 5–21 days of birth (Macmillan-Crow and Cruthirds, 2001). The neonatal mice exhibit myocardial injury, neurodegeneration, lipid peroxidation, fatty liver, anemia, and severe mitochondrial damage. The essentiality of MnSOD contrasts with cytosolic and extracellular Cu, Zn SOD; gene deletions for these enzymes are not lethal.

Deficiency Signs and Beneficial and Toxicological Actions

Manganese deficiency causes a variety of effects depending on the animal species (Freeland-Graves and Llanes, 1994). Deficiency causes depressed growth, testicular degeneration, and seizures in rats; slipped tendons or perosis in chicks; osteodystrophy and severe glucose intolerance in guinea pigs; and ataxia in mice and mink. Signs of nutritional manganese deficiency in humans have not been firmly established. Perhaps the most convincing case of manganese deficiency is that of a child on long-term parenteral nutrition who exhibited diffuse bone demineralization and poor growth that were corrected by manganese supplementation (Norose and Arai, 1987). In another study, men fed a purified diet supplying only 0.11 mg/day of manganese for 39 days developed a finely scaling minimally erythematous rash, decreased serum cholesterol, and increased serum alkaline phosphatase activity (Freeland-Graves and Llanes, 1994).

A low manganese status, however, may contribute to disease processes. Low dietary manganese has been associated with osteoporosis, diabetes, epilepsy, atherosclerosis, impaired wound healing, and cataracts (Klimis-Tavantzis, 1994). Recently, decreased plasma manganese and associated increased nitric oxide have been associated with childhood asthma (Kocyigit et al., 2004) and Alzheimer's disease (Vural et al., 2009). In addition, low maternal blood manganese concentration has been associated with increased risk of low birth weight and fetal intrauterine growth retardation (Wood, 2009). Animal findings providing support for some of these associations have been described previously (Nielsen, 2006a). These findings probably reflect the participation of manganese-activated enzymes or metalloenzymes in carbohydrate metabolism, arginine metabolism, antioxidant action, and proteoglycan synthesis. None the less, direct evidence of dietary manganese deficiency inducing a pathological condition in humans is lacking.

Because documented human manganese deficiency is so rare and manganese was considered one of the least toxic of the essential trace elements, manganese in the past was perceived mostly as an irrelevant nutritional concern for humans. However, manganese is now receiving significant attention as a toxicological concern for individuals whose normal homeostatic mechanisms are undeveloped, bypassed, or ill-functioning. High retention of manganese in tissues, especially in brain, has been reported for individuals receiving parenteral nutrition high in manganese (Dickerson, 2001; Hardy, 2009) and for individuals undergoing hemodialysis (da Silva et al., 2007; Klein et al., 2008), especially when normal excretion via the hepatobiliary system is impaired. In addition, biliary excretion of manganese is poor in neonates (Aschner and Aschner, 2005); thus, high intakes of manganese may result in increased tissue and brain levels in infants. Manganese toxicity has clinical features similar to those of idiopathic Parkinson disease, including disequilibrium, tremor, muscle spasms, tinnitus, and hearing loss (da Silva et al., 2007). Iron deficiency may exacerbate manganese toxicity because it enhances manganese absorption (Finley, 2004) and animal experiments suggest that iron deficiency may increase retention of manganese by the brain (Garcia et al., 2007). Low magnesium status may be another manganese toxicity concern. Pigs fed diets containing only 25% of the dietary recommendation for magnesium died suddenly and showed heart changes when the diet was high in manganese (52 mg/kg) (Miller et al., 2000).

Absorption, Transport, Retention, and Excretion

Adult human absorption of manganese from diets apparently ranges from about 1% to 5% (Aschner and Aschner, 2005). Arriving at this range was difficult because endogenous manganese is mostly excreted through biliary, pancreatic, and intestinal secretions (Aschner and Aschner, 2005; Buchman, 2006). If manganese status is adequate, endogenous excretion of absorbed manganese into the gut is so rapid that it is difficult to determine the portion of fecal manganese not absorbed from the diet and the portion endogenously excreted. In addition, manganese absorption decreases as manganese intake increases and increases with low manganese and/or iron status (Finley, 2004; Aschner and Aschner, 2005). Iron status apparently affects manganese absorption because the primary non-heme iron transporter, divalent metal transporter 1 (DMT 1), in the intestine also transports manganese (Hansen et al., 2009). Infants during the neonatal period are apparently much more efficient than adults in absorbing and retaining manganese (about 20% contained in formula) (Aschner and Aschner, 2005).

Absorption of manganese apparently occurs equally well throughout the small intestine. Manganese apparently is absorbed by an active transport system that most likely involves DMT 1 (Buchman, 2006). Diffusion has also been implicated in manganese absorption; it especially may come into play when manganese intakes are high (Nielsen, 2006a).

Both Mn^{2+} bound to plasma α-2-macroglobulin and Mn^{2+} bound to albumin have been suggested to be the form of manganese in blood (Buchman, 2006). Regardless of form, manganese is rapidly removed from the blood by the liver, and more than 90% of absorbed manganese is excreted in the bile (Hardy, 2009). A fraction of absorbed manganese is oxidized to Mn^{3+}, perhaps by ceruloplasmin, and is transported in plasma bound to transferrin, albumin, and β-globulin transmanganin (Buchman, 2006).

Metabolically active organs with high numbers of mitochondria, where manganese is predominantly found (such as liver, kidney, and pancreas), have relatively high manganese concentrations. Manganese is present in extremely low concentrations in whole blood (7.7–12.1 μg/L) and serum (0.38–1.1 μg/L) (Hardy, 2009). The range of manganese concentrations in mammalian tissues generally range between 0.3 and 2.9 μg/g (Aschner and Aschner, 2005). About 25% of the estimated 10–20 mg of manganese in the body is in bone (Buchman, 2006).

Excretion of manganese occurs mainly via the bile and thus in the feces. Very little manganese is excreted in the urine, and urinary excretion does not correlate with dietary intake (Hansen et al., 2009).

Dietary Guidance

The Food and Nutrition Board (Institute of Medicine, 2001) has set adequate intakes (AI) and tolerable upper intake levels (UL) for manganese, which are shown in Table 38.1. Although the manganese AI for adult females is 1.8 mg/day and for adult males is 2.3 mg/day, adults fed a diet containing 0.8 to 1.0 mg/day under carefully controlled experimental conditions did not exhibit any obvious differences from those fed amounts of manganese ≥AI (Finley, 2004; Nielsen, 2006a). Also, under carefully controlled experimental conditions, normal healthy adults fed amounts of manganese higher than the UL (20 mg/day) were not adversely affected (Finley, 2004). Good food sources of manganese include unrefined grains, nuts, and leafy vegetables.

TABLE 38.1 Dietary reference intakes (DRIs): recommended dietary allowances (RDAs), adequate intakes (AIs) and tolerable upper levels (ULs) for boron, manganese, molybdenum, and other trace elements

Element (mg/day)	Boron UL	Chromium	Fluoride AI	Fluoride UL	Manganese AI	Manganese UL	Molybdenum RDA	Molybdenum UL	Nickel UL	Vanadium UL
Life-stage group										
Infants										
0–6 months	ND[a]	0.0002	0.01	0.7	0.003	ND	0.002(AI)	ND	ND	ND
7–12 months	ND	0.0055	0.5	0.9	0.6	ND	0.003(AI)	ND	ND	ND
Children										
1–3 years	3	0.011	0.7	1.3	1.2	2	0.017	0.3	0.2	ND
4–8 years	6	0.015	1	2.2	1.5	3	0.022	0.6	0.3	ND
Males										
9–13 years	11	0.025	2	10	1.9	6	0.034	1.1	0.6	ND
14–18 years	17	0.035	3	10	2.2	9	0.043	1.7	1.0	ND
19–50 years	20	0.035	4	10	2.3	11	0.045	2.0	1.0	1.8
>50 years	20	0.030	4	10	2.3	11	0.045	2.0	1.0	1.8
Females										
9–13 years	11	0.021	2	10	1.6	6	0.034	1.1	0.6	ND
14–18 years	17	0.024	3	10	1.6	9	0.043	1.7	1.0	ND
19–50 years	20	0.025	4	10	1.6	11	0.045	2.0	1.0	1.8
>50 years	20	0.020	4	10	1.6	11	0.045	2.0	1.0	1.8
Pregnant females										
≤18 years	17	0.029	3	10	2.0	9	0.050	1.7	1.0	ND
19–50 years	20	0.030	3	10	2.0	11	0.050	2.0	1.0	ND
Lactating females										
≤18 years	17	0.044	3	10	2.6	9	0.050	1.7	1.0	ND
19–50 years	20	0.045	3	10	2.6	11	0.050	2.0	1.0	ND

[a]ND, not determined.
Data from Institute of Medicine (1997, 2001).

Molybdenum

Essentiality Basis and Biochemical Function

Molybdenum is an established essential nutrient based on its need for a cofactor containing a pterin nucleus that is required for the activity of sulfite oxidase, xanthine dehydrogenase, and aldehyde oxidase in mammals (Johnson, 1997). Sulfite oxidase apparently is most critical for human health. The lack of this enzyme because of a defect in the gene coding for it or a genetic mutation resulting in molybdenum cofactor deficiency results in death in early childhood; some children survive only a few days (Johnson, 1997; Reiss and Johnson, 2003). The lack of xanthine dehydrogenase or deficiency in aldehyde oxidase does not have such dire consequences.

Deficiency Signs and Beneficial Actions

There has been no further expansion in the characterization of molybdenum deficiency in animals beyond that described in previous reviews (Mills and Davis, 1987; Nielsen, 2006a). In rats and chicks, molybdenum deficiency aggravated by excessive dietary tungsten results in the depression of molybdenum enzymes, disturbances in uric acid metabolism, and increased susceptibility to sulfite toxicity. Deficiency uncomplicated by high dietary tungsten or copper in goats resulted in depressed food consumption and growth, and impaired reproduction, characterized by infertility and elevated mortality in both mothers and offspring.

Nutritional molybdenum deficiency has not been unequivocally identified in humans other than in one individual with Crohn's disease and a short bowel; he was nourished by total parenteral nutrition for 18 months (Abumrad *et al.*, 1981). After 12 months, this patient developed hypermethioninemia, hypouricemia, hyperoxypurinemia, hypouricosuria, and very low sulfate excretion; these changes were exacerbated by methionine administration. In addition, the patient suffered mental disturbances that progressed to coma. Supplementation with ammonium molybdate improved the clinical condition, reversed the sulfur-handling defect, and normalized uric acid production.

No beneficial effects of molybdenum supplementation in nutritional amounts have been reported. However, some beneficial effects have been reported for supra-nutritional or pharmacological amounts of tetrathiomolybdate and sodium molybdate. Tetrathiomolybdate inhibits metal transfer functions between copper trafficking proteins (Alvarez *et al.*, 2010). Copper-lowering therapy by tetrathiomolybdate has been found to inhibit cancer growth in five rodent models, and in advanced and metastatic cancer in dogs and humans (Brewer, 2003). In animal studies, tetrathiomolybdate inhibited pulmonary fibrosis induced by bleomycin, hepatitis induced by concanavalin A, cirrhosis induced by carbon tetrachloride (Brewer, 2003), and hyperglycemia induced by streptozotocin (Zeng *et al.*, 2008). Sodium molybdate was found to prevent hyperinsulinemia and hypertension induced by fructose in rats (Güner *et al.*, 2001).

Absorption, Transport, Retention, and Excretion

Documented cases of molybdenum deficiency and toxicity may be rare because the body is able to adapt to a wide range of intakes. Molybdenum is readily absorbed, with food-bound molybdenum about 16% less bioavailable than soluble complexes (e.g. ammonium molybdate) over a broad range of intakes. Men absorbed 90–94% of daily intakes of molybdenum ranging from 22 to 1490 µg (Novotny and Turnland, 2006, 2007). Animal studies indicate that the absorption of molybdenum can be reduced by diets or foods high in sulfur; the sulfate anion is a competitive inhibitor of molybdenum absorption (Mills and Davis, 1987).

Molybdate is transported loosely attached to erythrocytes in blood (Johnson, 1997). Concentrations of molybdenum in tissues, blood, and milk vary with molybdenum intake. For example, reported plasma concentration for men with an intake of 22 µg/day was 0.51 µg/L; with an intake of 121 µg/day it was 1.17 µg/L; and with an intake of 1490 µg/day it was 6.22 µg/L (Novotny and Turnland, 2007). Highest concentrations of molybdenum are found in liver, kidney, and bone (normally >1 mg/kg dry weight) (Johnson, 1997). The concentration of molybdenum in other tissues is usually between 0.14 and 0.20 mg/kg dry weight. The molybdenum in liver is entirely present in macromolecular association, partly as known molybdoenzymes and the remainder as the molybdenum cofactor.

After absorption, most molybdenum is turned over rapidly and eliminated as molybdate through the kidney (Johnson, 1997; Novotny and Turnland, 2006, 2007). Urinary excretion is increased with increasing molybdenum intake. Thus, excretion rather than regulated absorption is the major homeostatic mechanism for molybdenum.

Dietary Guidance

The Food and Nutrition Board (Institute of Medicine, 2001) has set a molybdenum AI for infants, recommended dietary allowances (RDA) for adults, and ULs, which are listed in Table 38.1. Many people do not achieve the estimated average requirement (EAR) of 34 μg/day or the RDA of 45 μg/day. According to NHANES III (1988–1994) data, median molybdenum intakes for adult females and males were 22.7 and 23.9 μg/day, respectively (Institute of Medicine, 2001). The lack of documented cases of nutritional molybdenum deficiency suggests that the EAR and RDA may be too high, or that a search for molybdenum-responsive syndromes in humans may be warranted. Good food sources of molybdenum include milk and milk products, pulses, organ meats (liver and kidney), and cereals.

Beneficial Bioactive Trace Elements

Boron

Essentiality Status and Biochemical Function

Boron has been shown to be essential for the completion of the life cycle (i.e. deficiency causes impaired growth, development, or maturation such that procreation is prevented) for organisms in all phylogenetic kingdoms (Hunt, 2002; Nielsen, 2008). In the animal kingdom, boron deprivation prevented procreation in both the African clawed frog (*Xenopus laevis*) and zebrafish (*Brachydanio rerio*). However, because a biochemical function has not been clearly defined for boron in higher animals, it is only considered a beneficial bioactive element for humans.

The diverse responses reported for low intakes of boron in higher animals have made it difficult to identify a primary mechanism responsible for the bioactivity of boron. The wide range of responses is probably secondary to boron influencing a cell signaling system, or the formation and/or activity of an entity that is involved in many biochemical processes.

At the pH of most biological fluids, boron exists mainly as boric acid, which reacts with biomolecules with hydroxyl groups to form boron esters. This reaction occurs best when the groups are adjacent and *cis* (same side of the molecule), such as ribose (Hunt, 2002; Ricardo *et al.*, 2004), which is a component of adenosine. Boron might influence cellular activity by reacting with signaling molecules containing adenosine or formed from an adenosine-containing precursor. *S*-Adenosylmethionine and diadenosine phosphates (signaling nucleotides) have higher affinities for boron than any other currently recognized boron ligands present in animal tissues (Hunt, 2002). About 95% *S*-adenosylmethionine is used for methylation of DNA, RNA, proteins, phospholipids, hormones, and neurotransmitters, which yield *S*-adenosylhomocysteine that can be hydrolyzed to homocysteine and used to form cysteine. Boron deprivation increased plasma cysteine and homocysteine, and decreased liver *S*-adenosylmethionine and *S*-adenosylhomocysteine in rats (Nielsen, 2009a). The bacterial quorum-sensing signal molecule, auto-inducer AI-2, is a furanosyl borate ester synthesized from *S*-adenosylmethionine (Chen *et al.*, 2002). Quorum sensing is the cell-to-cell communication between bacteria accomplished through exchange of extracellular signaling molecules (auto-inducers). These findings suggest that boron may influence *S*-adenosylmethionine formation or utilization.

Boron also strongly binds oxidized nicotinamide adenine dinucleotide (NAD^+). Extracellular NAD^+ binds to the plasma membrane receptor, CD38 (an adenosine diphosphate (ADP)-ribosyl cyclase), which converts NAD^+ to cyclic ADP ribose (ADPR) that is released intracellularly (Eckhert, 2006). ADPR binds to the ryanodine receptor and releases Ca^{2+} from the endoplasmic reticulum (Eckhert, 2006). Thus, boron may be bioactive through binding NAD^+ and ADPR and inhibiting the release of Ca^{2+}. Ca^{2+} is a signal ion for many processes in which boron has been shown to have an effect, including insulin release, bone formation, immune response, and brain function.

Boron also may be bioactive through forming diester borate complexes with phosphoinositides, glycoproteins, and glycolipids, which contain *cis*-hydroxyl groups, in membranes. The finding that boron changes the ability of some hormones to express their actions supports the suggestion of a role affecting membrane receptors or signal transduction. Boron deprivation apparently decreases insulin sensitivity in chicks and rats (Hunt, 2008), increases the requirement for vitamin D to prevent gross bone abnormalities in chicks and rats (Nielsen, 2008), results in the need for exogenous thyroxine for tail resorption, and makes oocytes not responsive to progesterone in frogs (Fort *et al.*, 2002). The finding that the borate transporter NaBC1 conducts Na^+ and OH^- across cell membranes in the absence of boron (Park *et al.*, 2004) suggests that boron may affect the transduction of regulatory ions across cell membranes.

Beneficial Actions and Deficiency Signs

Boron and Bone. Microcomputed tomography (μCT) of the fourth lumbar vertebrae found that boron deprivation (0.1 vs. 3 mg/kg diet) decreased bone volume fraction and trabecular thickness, and increased trabecular separation and structural model index (a lower value or more plate-like structure is preferable) in rats (Nielsen and Stoecker, 2009). Boron deprivation (0.07 vs. 3 mg/kg diet) in rats also has been shown to decrease alveolar bone (primary support structure for teeth) repair in rats (Gorustovich et al., 2009), and growth in mice (Gorustovich et al., 2008). Histological examination revealed that boron deprivation decreased osteoblast surface and increased quiescent bone-forming surface in the alveolus. These findings, in addition to boron deprivation impairing the maturation of the bone growth plate in chicks (Nielsen, 2008), and inducing limb teratogenesis in frogs (Fort et al., 2002), suggest that boron is beneficial to bone growth and maintenance through affecting osteoblast and/or osteoclast presence or activity and not through affecting bone calcium concentrations.

Boron and Brain. Findings showing that nutritional intakes of boron have beneficial effects on central nervous function are among the most supportive in demonstrating that boron is a beneficial bioactive element for humans (Nielsen, 2008). Boron deprivation of older men and women altered electroencephalograms (EEG) such that they suggested states of reduced behavioral activation (i.e. drowsiness) and mental alertness. The EEG changes may have been responsible for the finding that boron deprivation impaired cognitive processes of attention, encoding skills and memory, and psychomotor measures of manual dexterity and fatigue. Boron-deprived (0.1 mg vs. 3.1 mg/kg diet) rats were found to be less active based on reduced number, distance, and time of horizontal movements, front entries, margin distance, and vertical breaks and jumps in a spontaneous activity evaluation (Nielsen and Penland, 2006).

Boron and the Inflammatory or Immune Response. The suggestion that boron may influence the inflammatory or immune response is supported by a study of mice infected with the nematode *H. bakeri* (Bourgeois et al., 2007). Boron deprivation down-regulated 30 of 31 cytokines or chemokines associated with the inflammatory response 6 days post-primary infection. An opposite pattern was found at 21 days post-challenge; mice consuming boron-low diets had >100% increases in 23 of 31 cytokines

determined. These findings are consistent with lower serum tumor necrosis factor-α (TNF-α) and interferon-γ after lipopolysaccharide injection in pigs fed a boron-low diet than a diet supplemented with nutritional amounts of boron (Spears and Armstrong, 2007). When injected with an antigen (*Mycobacterium butyricum*) to induce arthritis, boron-supplemented (2.0 mg/kg diet) rats had less swelling of the paws and lower circulating concentrations of natural killer cells and CD8a$^+$/CD4$^-$ cells than did boron-deprived (0.1 mg/kg diet) rats (Hunt, 2007).

Boron and Cancer. Based on a study of 95 cases and 8720 controls, low dietary boron was associated with increased prostate cancer risk (Cui et al., 2004). Boric acid in concentrations similar to that in blood was found to inhibit the proliferation of some human prostate cancer cell lines in vitro (Barranco and Eckhert, 2004). Cervical smears of 472 women with a high mean boron intake (8.41 mg/day) and 587 with marginal mean boron intake (1.26 mg/day) identified 15 cases of cytopathological indications of cervical cancer in boron-low women and none in the boron-high women (Korkmaz et al., 2007). In a study of 763 women with lung cancer and 838 matched healthy controls, boron intake was inversely associated with the incidence of cancer; odds increased substantially if they were not on hormone replacement therapy (Mahabir et al., 2008). In a study of 124 premenopausal breast-cancer patients, boron was associated with decreased number of estrogen-receptor negative tumors relative to estrogen-receptor positive tumors (Touillaud et al., 2005). Unidentified confounders may have an impact on the association between boron and cancer.

Boron Deficiency Signs. As indicated above, boron has been found to be essential for frogs (*Xenopus*) and zebrafish (Nielsen, 2008). Boron-deficient male frogs exhibit atrophied testes, decreased sperm counts, and sperm dysmorphology; female frogs exhibit atrophied ovaries and impaired oocyte maturation. Most embryos from boron-deprived frogs die before 96 hours of development. The early cleavage stage of zebrafish development was found to be most sensitive to boron deficiency; 46% of fertilized boron-deficient embryos did not complete the blastula stage compared with 2% for boron-adequate embryos. Adult F$_1$ boron-deficient zebrafish exhibited photophobia. The critical experiment demonstrating that boron is essential to complete the life cycle or has a defined biochemical role in mammals is lacking. However, boron deficiency signs in higher animals and humans may be deduced from beneficial effects (described above) of nutritional amounts of boron.

Absorption, Transport, Retention, and Excretion

About 85% of ingested boron is absorbed and then efficiently excreted via the urine mainly as boric acid (Nielsen, 2006a, 2008). As a result, urinary boron mirrors boron intake. During transport in the body, boron most likely is weakly attached to organic molecules containing *cis*-hydroxyl groups. A mammalian boron transporter (Park *et al.*, 2004) that has substantial homology to the plant boron transporter AtBor1 discovered in *Arabidopsis thaliana* (Takano *et al.*, 2005) and yeast (*Saccharomyces cerevisiae*) (Kaya *et al.*, 2009) has been identified. NaBC1 is essential for boron homeostasis, growth, and proliferation of mammalian HEK293 cells (Park *et al.*, 2004). A boron transporter may have been responsible for the observation that RAW264.7 and HL60 cells accumulate boron against a concentration gradient (Ralston and Hunt, 2004).

Boron is distributed throughout soft tissues at concentrations mostly between 1.39 and 1.85 μmol/kg fresh tissue (0.015–2.0 μg/g) (World Health Organization, 1998). Based on studies with postmenopausal women, normal fasting plasma boron concentrations range from 3.14 to 8.79 mmol/L (34–95 ng/mL) (Nielsen, 2006a).

Dietary Guidance

The Food and Nutrition Board of the National Academy of Sciences (Institute of Medicine, 2001) set ULs, which are shown in Table 38.1, but did not set an RDA for boron. Both animal and human data were used by the World Health Organization (1996) to suggest that an acceptable safe range of population mean intakes of boron for adults could be 1–13 mg/day. Many people apparently have boron intakes of less than 1 mg/day. The Continuing Survey of Food Intakes by Individuals (CSFII), 1994–1996, indicated that boron intakes ranged from a low of about 0.35 mg/day to a high of about 3.0 mg/day for adults (Institute of Medicine, 2001). Rich food sources of boron are fruits, leafy vegetables, nuts, legumes, and pulses.

Chromium

Essentiality Status and Biochemical Function

Approximately 50 years ago, trivalent chromium was reported to be the active component of the "glucose tolerance factor" that alleviated glucose tolerance in rats fed torula yeast–sucrose diets (Moukarzel, 2009). This finding was accepted as proof for chromium essentiality for higher animals. Essentiality for humans gained acceptance when it was reported between 1977 and 1986 that chromium supplementation alleviated glucose intolerance and/or neuropathy exhibited by three patients on long-term total parenteral nutrition (Moukarzel, 2009). Since then, no reports of chromium supplementation helping patients on long-term parenteral nutrition have appeared. In addition, efforts to induce consistent signs of chromium deficiency in animals have not produced convincing findings. Nutritional, metabolic, physiological, or hormonal stressors generally had to be employed to induce experimental animals to apparently respond to chromium deprivation (Vincent and Stallings, 2007). In most cases, the responses were not remarkable. Thus, after decades of effort that has produced no consistent deprivation signs or conclusive, specific, defined, biochemical functions, the essentiality of chromium has become uncertain and a controversial issue.

Cr^{3+} is the most stable oxidation state of this element and most likely the form of importance in biological systems. In aqueous solutions, Cr^{3+} complexes are relatively inert kinetically such that ligand-displacement reactions have half-times in the range of several hours. Therefore, chromium is unlikely to be involved as a metal catalyst at the active site of enzymes where the rate of exchange needs to be rapid. However, chromium may have a structural role such as in the tertiary structure of a protein or nucleic acid. In addition, chromium may bind ligands in the proper orientation to facilitate enzymatic catalysis; this may be the role of chromodulin (Vincent and Bennett, 2007), which was previously called low-molecular-weight chromium-binding substance. Chromodulin has been described as a naturally occurring mammalian oligopeptide with a mass of about 1.5 kDa that is composed of glycine, cysteine, aspartate, and glutamate and that binds four chromic ions tightly and cooperatively ($K_a \sim 10^{21} M^{-4}$) (Vincent and Bennett, 2007). Apochromodulin (apparently the predominant form in vivo) can accept chromic ions from other biological molecules such as transferrin, which may serve as a transporter of chromium (Vincent and Bennett, 2007).

Two potential functions have been described for chromodulin. Because chromodulin carries chromium into the urine after a large dose is given, it has been suggested that this oligopeptide is nothing more than a vehicle for the detoxification and excretion of chromium (Stearns, 2007).

However, substantial evidence suggests that chromodulin potentiates insulin's effects by amplifying insulin-dependent protein tyrsosine kinase activity of the insulin receptor; this stimulation apparently is dependent upon the chromium content of chromodulin (Vincent and Bennett, 2007). It is hypothesized that the binding of insulin to its receptor on an insulin-sensitive cell causes a conformational change resulting in the autophosphorylation of tyrosine residues on the internal side of the receptor. The receptor becomes an active tyrosine kinase that transmits the insulin signal into the cell. In response to insulin, chromium also moves into insulin-sensitive cells, which contain apochromodulin, to form holochromodulin. The holochromodulin then binds to the receptor to assist in maintaining it in an active form, thus amplifying the receptor's kinase activity. When blood insulin decreases, a change in the conformation of the insulin receptor causes a release of holochromodulin from the cell to blood and excretion in the urine.

Chromium up-regulates mRNA levels of insulin receptor GLUT 4 (glucose transporter), glycogen synthase, and uncoupling protein-3 in cultured skeletal muscle cells (Qiao et al., 2009). This up-regulation, however, may be occurring through the amplification of insulin, which also increases mRNA for those metabolic substances. None the less, chromium, or a biologically active form of chromium, might have a role in regulating gene expression of a critical substance in glucose metabolism. This is supported by the finding that RNA synthesis directed by free DNA in vitro has been shown to be enhanced by the binding of chromium to the template.

Another possible role suggested for chromium is the activation of GLUT 4 trafficking via a cholesterol-dependent mechanism (Chen et al., 2006). Chromium was found to alter plasma membrane cholesterol and mobilized GLUT 4 to the plasma membrane in cultured cells. It was suggested that chromium may have reduced membrane cholesterol through an effect on AMP-activated protein kinase.

Beneficial Actions and Deficiency Signs

Substantial evidence exists to indicate that chromium has beneficial bioactivity under certain circumstances. Numerous reports from various research groups have described beneficial effects provided by chromium supplementation in subjects with varying degrees of glucose intolerance, ranging from hypoglycemia to insulin-dependent diabetes (Anderson, 1998). A systematic review of randomized controlled trials found that chromium supplementation slightly but significantly improved glycemia in patients with diabetes (Balk et al., 2007). The review found no significant effects of chromium on lipid or glucose metabolism in people without diabetes. In addition, numerous other studies have found that chromium supplementation did not improve carbohydrate metabolism in individuals with metabolic syndrome, impaired glucose tolerance, or type 2 diabetes (Cefalu and Hu, 2004). Patient selection and chromium dosage may have been responsible for the inconsistent findings. A clinical response to chromium (i.e. decreased glucose and improved insulin sensitivity) apparently is most likely in insulin-resistant individuals with type 2 diabetes and highly elevated fasting plasma glucose and hemoglobin A_{1c} concentrations (Cefalu et al., 2010). Supra-nutritional amounts of chromium generally were needed to be therapeutically effective, which could mean that chromium was acting pharmacologically, not nutritionally.

Chromium supplementation has also been hypothesized to decrease body fat (weight loss) and to increase muscle or lean body mass. These hypotheses were based on the assumption that chromium would amplify the action of insulin under all circumstances, and this amplification would result in less glucose being converted into fat and in an up-regulation of protein synthesis for muscle gain. Findings indicating that chromium does not affect glucose metabolism or insulin action in people without insulin resistance and diabetes (Balk et al., 2007; Cefalu et al., 2010) explain why well-conducted randomized controlled trials showed no effect of supplemental chromium on weight and body composition (Lukaski and Scrimgeour, 2009).

Low toenail-chromium concentration has been associated with cardiovascular disease (Rajpathak et al., 2004; Guallar et al., 2005). However, these epidemiological findings are unable to determine whether the low concentrations indicate a cause or effect of cardiovascular disease. Long-term supplementation trials are needed to ascertain whether chromium supplementation would be beneficial to cardiovascular health.

Absorption, Transport, Retention, and Excretion

Estimates of Cr^{3+} absorption, based on metabolic balance studies or on urinary excretion during physiological intakes, range from 0.4% to 2.5% (Institute of Medicine, 2001). Most ingested chromium is excreted unabsorbed in the feces. Most absorbed chromium is excreted rapidly in the urine. Cr^{3+} competes for one of the binding sites on transferrin, and most of the chromium in blood (about 2–3 nmol/L) apparently is found bound to transferrin. The highest levels of chromium in human tissues are found in liver, spleen, and bone (Institute of Medicine, 2001).

Dietary Guidance

In the absence of a functional criterion for assessing chromium status or need, the Food and Nutrition Board (Institute of Medicine, 2001) set AIs for chromium rather than EARs and RDAs. The AIs shown in Table 38.1 are based on the mean chromium content of well-balanced daily diets (13.4 μg/1000 kcal) and estimated energy intakes for each group. No UL was set for dietary chromium (Cr^{3+}) because of insufficient data and little evidence for adverse effects. The toxicity of Cr^{3+} is minimized by its propensity to form complexes with oxygen-based ligands that are usually electrochemically inactive and have poor ability to cross cell membranes.

Chromium is widely distributed throughout the food supply, but the chromium content is highly variable among different lots of the same food. Chromium content in foods can be subject to significant decreases or increases during processing. Whole grains, pulses, some vegetables (e.g. broccoli and mushrooms), liver, processed meats, ready-to-eat cereals, spices, and beer are generally good sources of chromium.

Other Nutritionally Bioactive Trace Elements

Arsenic

Beneficial Actions and Possible Basis for Bioactivity

Arsenic is unquestionably a bioactive element in higher animals and humans. However, most studies of this bioactivity have been directed towards demonstrating that amounts sometimes found in food and water are toxic. High amounts of inorganic arsenic in drinking water have been associated with a number of pathological conditions including cardiovascular disease, dermatological changes, developmental abnormalities, neurologic and neurobehavioral disorders, diabetes, hematological disorders, renal damage, respiratory problems, and various types of cancer, including bladder, colon, kidney, liver, lung and skin cancer (Abernathy et al., 2003). Interestingly, the disorders found vary between areas that report high amounts of arsenic in drinking water, which suggests some other factors may be involved in the arsenic toxicity. The numerous reports appearing in the past five years on arsenic toxicity are beyond the scope of this review. Emphasis will be placed on discussing the concept that homeostatic mechanisms exist for arsenic, and thus there may be intakes that have beneficial effects.

Several animal studies suggest that arsenic ingested in low microgram or nanogram quantities is beneficial in higher animals. Reports between the years 1975 and 1995 indicated that arsenic deprivation (e.g. <12 ng/g diet for rats and chicks; <35 ng/g diet for goats) induced physiological changes in higher animals (Anke, 2005; Nielsen, 2006a). In the goat, pig, and rat, the most consistent signs of apparent arsenic deprivation were depressed growth and abnormal reproduction characterized by impaired fertility and increased perinatal mortality. Death with myocardial damage occurred in arsenic-deprived goats.

Limited epidemiological and animal findings also have suggested that arsenic can have beneficial effects at appropriate low exposures. Compared with exposure to drinking water containing about 50 μg/L, both low exposure (<50 μg/L) and high exposure (>100 μg/L resulted in a higher number of cancers (Kayajanian, 2003). A similar response was seen in an animal study that determined the effects of arsenic on dimethylhydrazine-induced aberrant crypts (Uthus and Davis, 2005). Arsenic in pharmacological amounts as arsenic trioxide has been found to be an effective treatment for some forms of cancer, especially promyelocytic leukemia, through apoptotic, not necrotic, mechanisms (Huang et al., 1999; Murgo, 2001).

Arsenic may be bioactive through affecting the methylation of metabolically or genetically important molecules. Low and excessive arsenic had similar effects on global DNA methylation in cultured Caco-2 cells. When the culture contained low (25 μg/L) or high (175 μg/L) arsenic, global methylation of DNA was significantly decreased from that of cells grown in culture containing 100 μg/L (Davis et al., 2000).

Absorption, Transport, Retention, and Excretion

In humans and most laboratory animals, more than 90% of inorganic arsenate and arsenite in water, and about 60–70% ingested with food, is absorbed by the gastrointestinal tract mainly by simple diffusion (Nielsen, 2006a). Once absorbed, inorganic arsenic is transferred to various tissues, including the liver, where it is methylated with S-adenosylmethionine as the methyl donor (Thomas et al., 2007). Before arsenate is methylated, it is reduced to arsenite; this reduction is facilitated by glutathione.

Arsenite methyltransferase methylates arsenite to form monomethylarsonic acid, which is then reduced to monomethylarsonous acid. Monomethylarsonous acid, a relatively toxic form of arsenic, is rapidly methylated by a methyltransferase to form dimethylarsinic acid. In humans, monomethylarsonous acid is found in urine only when excessive inorganic arsenic is consumed. If excessive amounts of inorganic arsenic are being methylated, dimethylarsinic acid can be reduced to dimethylarsinous acid, which also is a relatively toxic form of arsenic. However, with non-toxic or nutritional intakes of arsenic, dimethylarsinic acid is the final step in the metabolism of arsenic in humans and most animals, and thus is the major form of arsenic in urine, which is the major excretory route for arsenic.

Some foods, especially seafood, contain trimethylated forms of arsenic (arsenobetaine and arsenocholine), which are highly absorbed and rapidly excreted in the urine (Nielsen, 2006a). Most arsenocholine is transformed into arsenobetaine before being excreted in the urine. Arsenosugars, which are found in seaweed, are poorly absorbed. They apparently must be metabolized to a methylated form, which may be facilitated by intestinal bacteria, before the arsenic can be absorbed (Nielsen, 2006a).

Because mechanisms exist for ridding the body of arsenic, no tissue significantly accumulates this element if low or physiological amounts are ingested. Tissue analyses indicate that retained arsenic in most animals and humans is widely distributed in low concentrations ($<1.0 \mu g/g$ fresh weight) under normal conditions (National Research Council, 2005a). The highest amounts of arsenic are usually found in skin, hair, and nails, probably because inorganic arsenic binds to SH groups of proteins that are relatively plentiful in these tissues.

Excretion of ingested arsenic is rapid, principally in the urine (Nielsen, 2006a). The usual proportions of the forms of arsenic in human urine are about 20% inorganic arsenic, 15% monomethylarsonic acid, and 65% dimethylarsinic acid. The proportions are quite different with the consumption of organic arsenic in forms found in seafood; then trimethylated arsenic such as arsenobetaine predominates.

Dietary Guidance

The Food and Nutrition Board (2001) set no Dietary Reference Intakes for arsenic. The Total Diet Study (1991–1997) indicated that the median intake of arsenic from foods was only about 2.0 and 2.6 μg/day for women and men 19–70 years of age, respectively (Institute of Medicine, 2001). Another report gave an estimated mean total arsenic intake in the United States from all food, excluding shellfish, of 30 μg/day (Adams et al., 1994). This intake is similar to intakes of arsenic that were found to be beneficial in animals and in epidemiological studies.

Fluoride

Beneficial Actions and Possible Basis for Essentiality

Fluoride (the ionic form of fluorine) cannot be considered an essential nutrient because the critical experiment showing that it is required to complete the life cycle, or defining a biochemical role for fluoride necessary for life, is lacking. However, one research group found that intrauterine fluoride deprivation over 11 generations in goats resulted in intrauterine and postnatal growth depression, increased kid mortality, and skeletal and joint deformities in older animals (Anke et al., 2005a). These findings need confirmation or evidence of similar signs in another animal model before they will be accepted as evidence that fluoride might be essential.

Although evidence for essentiality is limited, fluoride certainly has beneficial bioactivity in pharmacological or supra-nutritional amounts. In humans, fluoride protects against pathological demineralization of calcified tissues. Fluoride inhibits tooth enamel degradation by two separate mechanisms (Whitford, 2006). Uptake of fluoride to form fluorohydroxyapatite during tooth development reduces the risk of caries because fluorohydroxyapatite is more acid-resistant than normal hydroxyapatite. After tooth development, fluoride protects enamel by inhibiting acid production by plaque bacteria and enhancing the rate of enamel remineralization during an acidogenic challenge. However, an average daily fluoride intake of 0.05 mg/kg body weight while teeth are developing is associated with mild tooth mottling; this is an intake found when water fluoride concentration is optimal (1.0 mg/L) (Whitford, 2006). Moderate mottling may occur at an average daily intake of 0.1 mg/kg body weight (Whitford, 2006). A recent report indicated that dental fluorosis ranged from 41% among adolescents aged 12–15 to 9% among adults aged 40–49 (Beltrán-Aguilar et al., 2010). Sodium fluoride has been shown repeatedly and reproducibly to increase spinal bone mass in a dose-dependent manner (Ringe, 2004). There has not, however, been a convincing demonstration that fluoride consistently reduces vertebral fracture rate in established spinal osteoporosis (Kleerekoper and Mendlovic, 1993; Ringe, 2004).

Moreover, the therapeutic dosages for osteoporosis (10–30 mg/day) (Whitford, 2006) meet or exceed the tolerable upper intake level (UL) of 10 mg/day for adults (Institute of Medicine, 1997). In animals, high or supra-nutritional amounts of fluoride prevented anemia and infertility caused by iron deficiency, improved suboptimal growth induced by an unbalanced diet, and alleviated nephrocalcinosis induced by phosphorus feeding and soft-tissue calcification caused by magnesium deprivation (Cerklewski, 1997; Nielsen, 2006a).

Absorption, Transport, Retention, and Excretion

Essentially 100% of fluoride ingested in the fasted state as fluoridated water, and 50% to 80% of fluoride ingested in food, are absorbed from the gastrointestinal tract (Nielsen, 1998a). Absorption of fluoride is rapid with about 50% of a moderate soluble dose absorbed in 30 minutes; complete absorption occurs in 90 minutes. The rapidity of absorption indicates that a significant portion (about 40%) is absorbed from the stomach as HF; the rest is absorbed throughout the small intestine.

Fluoride concentrations in plasma and most soft tissues are low, generally between 0.01 and 0.05 μg/g (Whitford, 2006). About 99% of body fluoride is found in the skeleton and teeth, where it exists mainly as hydroxyfluorapatite (Whitford, 2006). Approximately 50% of fluoride absorbed each day is deposited in calcified tissue (bone and developing teeth) and the rest is cleared by the kidney (Whitford, 2006). The rate of uptake by bone is affected by the stage of skeletal development. Urinary excretion of fluoride is directly related to urinary pH. When renal tubular fluid pH is high, less fluoride exists as hydrogen fluoride (HF), the form that is reabsorbed well, so clearance is high; when the pH is acidic, more HF is formed and reabsorbed, which results in lower clearance (Whitford, 2006). Thus, factors that affect urinary pH, such as diet, drugs, metabolic or respiratory disorders, and altitude of residence, can affect how much absorbed fluoride is excreted.

Dietary Guidance

The Food and Nutrition Board (Institute of Medicine, 1997) set AIs and ULs for fluoride, which are shown in Table 38.1. The major source of orally ingested fluoride is drinking water. Over 50% of the population in the United States uses water with fluoride adjusted to between 0.7 and 1.2 mg/L (37–63 nmol). Fluoride is ubiquitous in foods, but similar products can vary greatly with source. Thus,

estimating fluoride intakes is difficult. Estimated daily intakes range from 1.4 to 3.4 mg/day for adult males residing in a community with fluoridated water, and 0.3 to 1.0 mg/day in areas without fluoridation (Nielsen, 1998a).

Nickel

Beneficial Actions and Possible Basis for Bioactivity

Nickel is generally acknowledged as being essential for plants and some bacteria. Nickel in these lower forms of life has been identified as an essential component of enzymes whose substrates or products are dissolved gases: hydrogen, carbon monoxide, carbon dioxide, methane, oxygen, and ammonia. Details about these enzymes are given in another review (Nielsen, 2006b).

Nickel is not generally accepted as an essential nutrient for higher animals and humans, apparently because of the lack of a clearly defined specific biochemical function in these species. However, nutritional amounts of nickel prevent several physiological and biochemical changes induced by nickel deprivation in higher animals. Changes induced by nickel deprivation described in a previous review (Nielsen, 2006a) included impaired reproduction (decreased conception rate and sperm production and motility), impaired bone health (decreased strength and altered composition), altered carbohydrate and lipid metabolism (increased plasma lipids and decreased serum glucose), decreased iron status or utilization, and altered thyroid hormone metabolism. Other beneficial effects of nutritional amounts of nickel that have been described include improved bone strength in rats (Nielsen, 2006c) and chicks (Wilson et al., 2001), alleviation of renal damage and high blood pressure induced by a high salt diet in rats (Nielsen et al., 2002), and alleviation of vitamin B$_{12}$ deficiency and high blood homocysteine concentrations in pigs (Stangl et al., 2000). The nutritional importance of nickel for humans remains largely unstudied. However, in hemodialysis patients, serum nickel was negatively correlated with plasma total homocysteine (Katko et al., 2008).

Nickel is another element whose diverse beneficial effects at nutritional amounts under a variety of conditions (e.g. stressors that affect methionine and arginine metabolism) have made it difficult to identify a primary mechanism responsible for its bioactivity. Nickel bioactivity might involve the function of gaseous molecules such as oxygen (O$_2$), nitric oxide (NO), or carbon monoxide (CO). In most tissues, the molecular and cellular response to a low O$_2$ tension is the activation of the transcription factor hypoxia-inducible factor 1 (HIF-1). Nickel has the ability to stabilize HIF-1α protein and to activate hypoxia-inducible expression of genes (Kang *et al.*, 2006). These genes are involved in angiogenesis, glucose transport, glycolysis, erythropoiesis, and catecholamine metabolism. Activation of the HIF-1α pathway also increases osteogenesis (Wang et *al.*, 2007). NO synthesis inhibition promotes the renal production of CO by heme oxygenase, which is potently induced by nickel. CO inhibits NO synthase activity and activates guanyl cyclase which results in the production of cGMP. The cGMP signal transduction system has crucial roles in vision, taste, smell, blood pressure control, kidney function, and sperm motility, all of which are affected by nickel (Gordon and Zagotta, 1995; Nielsen *et al.*, 2002).

Nickel also may be bioactive through altering methyl metabolism. The lack of vitamin B_{12}, which is involved in methyl metabolism, inhibits the response of rats to nickel supplementation when dietary nickel is low (Nielsen, 2006a) and nickel can alleviate vitamin B_{12} deficiency in pigs (Stangl *et al.*, 2000). In addition, nickel ameliorated an increase in serum homocysteine in vitamin B_{12}-deficient pigs (Stangl *et al.*, 2000) and decreased homocysteine, cysteine, and *S*-adenosylhomocysteine production by human peripheral monocytes (Katko *et al.*, 2008).

Absorption, Transport, Retention, and Excretion
Knowledge about the metabolism of nickel has essentially remained unchanged since a previous review of the subject (Nielsen, 2006a). Less than 10% of nickel ingested with food is absorbed by animals and humans. When soluble nickel in water is ingested after an overnight fast, as much as 50%, but usually closer to 20% to 25%, of the dose is absorbed. Nickel absorption is heightened by iron deficiency, pregnancy, and lactation. The mechanism through which nickel is transported through the gut has not been clearly defined, but some studies indicate some nickel is absorbed through an iron-transport system.

Nickel is transported in blood principally bound to serum albumin. Small amounts of nickel in serum are associated with the amino acids histidine and aspartic acid, and with α_2-macroglobulin (nickeloplasmin). The transport of nickel into tissues may involve magnesium and/or iron transport mechanisms. Nickel is widely distributed in tissues in concentrations between 0.01 and 0.2 mg/kg wet weight (National Research Council, 2005b).

Fecal nickel excretion (mostly unabsorbed nickel) is 10 to 100 times higher than urinary excretion. Most of the small fraction of absorbed nickel is rapidly and efficiently excreted as urinary low-molecular-weight complexes in concentrations generally ranging from 0.1 to 1.3 μg nickel/L (Nielsen, 2006a).

Dietary Guidance
The Food and Nutrition Board (Institute of Medicine, 2001) set no RDA or AI for nickel, but did set ULs, which are shown in Table 38.1. Based on animal studies, a beneficial intake of nickel for humans might be near 50 μg/day (Nielsen, 1998a). Typical daily dietary intakes for nickel are 70–260 μg/day (Nielsen, 2006a).

Silicon
Beneficial Actions and Possible Basis for Bioactivity
Silicon is nutritionally essential for some lower forms of life (Carlisle, 1997; Nielsen, 2006a; Řezanka and Sigler, 2007). Silicon has a structural role in diatoms, radiolarians, and some sponges. Diatoms, which are unicellular microscopic plants, have an absolute requirement for silicon as monomeric silicic acid for normal cell growth. Silicon also may be essential for some higher plants (e.g. rice).

Silicon is not generally accepted as a confirmed essential nutrient for higher animals and humans because of the lack of a defined specific biochemical function. However, nutritional (10–35 mg/kg diet) and supra-nutritional (e.g. 100–500 mg/kg diet as a soluble salt) levels prevent several physiological and biochemical abnormalities observed in animals fed diets low in silicon (<5 mg/kg diet). Among the first changes reported to be alleviated by silicon (most experiments used supra-nutritional amounts) were abnormal bone structure and strength in chicks and rats, abnormal bone cartilage characterized by decreased hexosamine and increased collagen in chicks, and decreased collagen and prolylhydroxylase activity in chick skull bones from cultured chick embryos (Carlisle, 1997; Nielsen, 2006a). Subsequent experiments showed that nutritional amounts of silicon alleviated abnormal bone, hexosamine, and collagen metabolism found in animals fed diets low in silicon (Nielsen, 2006a). A subsequent experiment also found that silicon deprivation reduced bone growth plate thickness and increased chondrocyte density in rats (Jugdaohsingh *et al.*, 2008). Supra-nutritional amounts of silicon also alleviate bone loss in ovariectomized rats (Jugdaohsingh, 2007; Kim *et al.*, 2009), and stimulated gene expression of factors involved in osteoblastogenesis and suppressed expression of factors involved in osteoclastogenesis in mice (Maehira *et al.*, 2009).

Epidemiological, supplementation, and cell-culture studies have suggested that nutritional intakes of silicon are beneficially bioactive in humans. Dietary silicon was positively associated with bone mineral density in men and premenopausal women of the Framingham Offspring cohort of 1251 men and 1596 women (Jugdaohsingh, 2007). In the same cohort, the beneficial effect of a moderate consumption of beer on hip and spine bone-mineral density was associated with the silicon in the beer (Tucker *et al.*, 2009). Silicon intake also was positively associated with bone mineral density at the spine and femur in premenopausal women and postmenopausal women on hormone replacement therapy in the Aberdeen Prospective Osteoporosis Screening Study (Jugdaohsingh, 2007). Limited findings from supplementation trials suggest that silicon supplementation may increase bone mineral density in women with low bone mass (Jugdaohsingh, 2007). Silicon was found to stimulate collagen type 1 synthesis and osteoblastic differentiation in human osteoblast-like cells in vitro (Jugdaohsingh, 2007). The silicon in silica-based bioactive glass and ceramics has been implicated in the in vivo efficiency of bone implants through involvement in gene up-regulation, osteoblast proliferation and differentiation, type 1 collagen synthesis, and apatite formation (Jugdaohsingh, 2007). In other human-oriented studies, supplementation with choline-stabilized orthosilicic acid significantly improved photodamaged skin surface and mechanical properties and decreased hair and nail brittleness in women (Barel *et al.*, 2005), and increased silicon in drinking water has been associated with decreased incidence of Alzheimer's disease and associated disorders (Gillette-Guyonnet *et al.*, 2007).

The mechanism of action for the beneficial bioactivity of silicon has not been identified. Silicon may have some type of structural or binding role in connective tissue where it is strongly bound in significant concentrations. Silicon easily forms stable complexes with polyols that have at least four hydroxyl groups (Kinrade *et al.*, 1999). Tissue concentrations of polyol compounds, such as hexosamines and ascorbate, used to form the glycosaminoglycans, mucopolysaccharides, and collagen involved in connective tissue stabilization or formation, are affected by silicon status (Carlisle, 1997).

Silicon also may be beneficial by altering the absorption or utilization of other mineral elements (Nielsen, 2006a). Experimental and epidemiological findings suggest that silicon alleviates the toxic actions of aluminum (Gillette-Guyonnet *et al.*, 2007). This has resulted in the hypothesis that an interaction between silicon (as silicic acid) and aluminum compounds (e.g. $Al[OH]^{2+}$) forms an aluminosilicate. This interaction prevents aluminum from competing for iron-binding sites (e.g. in prolyl hydroxylase), which results in decreased functions requiring iron. Supranutritional amounts of silicon also facilitate the absorption, retention, or utilization of copper, iron, and magnesium (Nielsen, 2006a).

Absorption, Transport, Retention, and Excretion
Early balance studies with animals, and studies with silicate compounds used as additives to food and drugs, indicated that almost all ingested silicon was unabsorbed (Nielsen, 2006a). Recent findings indicate that silicon can be relatively well absorbed when consumed in low or milligram quantities in various foods and drinks. One study found an average of 41% of silicon in food was excreted in urine (an indicator of absorption) (Jugdaohsingh, 2007); another study found 64% of silicon absorbed from alcohol-free beer (Sripanyakorn *et al.*, 2009).

Silicon is not protein-bound in plasma, where it is believed to exist mainly as a neutral orthosilicic acid species that readily diffuses into erythrocytes and other tissues (Jugdaohsingh, 2007). Evidence that silicon entering the bloodstream is efficiently transferred to tissues and urine is that the silicon concentration in blood remains relatively constant over a range of dietary intakes. Human serum normally contains between 11 and 31 μg/dL (Nielsen, 2009b). Connective tissues, including aorta, bone, skin, tendon, trachea, and fingernails, contain much of the silicon that is retained in the body (Carlisle, 1997).

Absorbed silicon is rapidly excreted (Jugdaohsingh, 2007), mainly in the urine, where it probably exists as orthosilicic acid and/or magnesium orthosilicate (Nielsen, 2006a). The upper limits of urinary excretion apparently are set by the rate and extent of silicon absorption and not by the excretory ability of the kidney, because peritoneal injection of silicon can elevate urinary excretion above the upper limit achieved by dietary intake (Nielsen, 2006a, 2009b). This indicates that silicon homeostasis is controlled by both absorption and excretory mechanisms.

Dietary Guidance
The Food and Nutrition Board (Institute of Medicine, 2001) judged that animal and human data were too limited for the setting of any DRIs for silicon. On the basis of

extrapolations from animal data, weak balance data from humans, and the usual amount of silicon excreted daily by humans, it has been suggested that a daily minimum requirement for silicon might be near 10–25 mg/day (Nielsen, 2006a, 2009b). The dietary intake of silicon is between 15 and 50 mg/day for most Western populations (Nielsen, 2006a; Jugdaohsingh, 2007). Foods rich in silicon include unrefined grains, some vegetables, and seafood (Jugdaohsingh, 2007). The silicon in barley and hops is solubilized during the beer-making process, which makes this beverage a rich source of silicon (Jugdaohsingh, 2007).

Strontium
Beneficial Actions and Possible Basis for Bioactivity
There is no conclusive evidence that strontium is essential for higher animals and humans, but strontium in supra-nutritional or pharmacological amounts unquestionably has beneficial effects on teeth and bones (Nielsen, 1986, 2006a). In 1949, it was reported that rats and guinea pigs fed diets with no added strontium instead of 3 g of strontium sulfate per kilogram exhibited depressed growth, impaired calcification of bones and teeth, and increased dental caries incidence. More recently, it was found that moderate doses of strontium (e.g. 315–525 mg/L drinking water) stimulated bone formation and volume in rats (Marie et al., 2001), and a supplemental 50 mg strontium per kilogram to a corn–soybean-based diet enhanced breaking strength, mineral content, and mineral density of metatarsals and femurs in young pigs (Pagano et al., 2007).

In 1993, it was found that strontium ranelate (a compound containing the organic acid, ranelic acid, and two atoms of strontium) depressed bone resorption and maintained bone formation in ovariectomized rats (Marie et al., 2001). Since then, strontium ranelate has become a promising pharmaceutical for the treatment of postmenopausal osteoporosis (Marie et al., 2001; Boivin, 2010). Strontium ranelate at 2 g/day has been found to prevent fractures in both spine and hip and to increase bone mineral density in the spine and femur (Boivin, 2010). Similar findings have been obtained with animals supplemented with strontium ranelate in amounts that correspond to the therapeutic dose given to humans (Marie et al., 2001; Boivin, 2010).

The mechanism of action for the beneficial bioactivity of strontium has not been firmly established. In vitro studies suggest that strontium ranelate both increases bone formation by osteoblasts and decreases bone resorption by osteoclasts (Marie et al., 2001). A suggested mechanism for the anti-catabolic effect of strontium is that it acts upon the calcium-sensing receptor such that osteoclast apoptosis is induced through a signaling pathway similar to but different in some ways from the action of calcium (Hurtel-Lemaire et al., 2009). It has also been suggested that the stimulation of osteoblast replication by strontium ranelate occurs because it activates the calcium-sensing receptor and thus extracellular signal-regulated kinase 1/2 phosphorylation (Marie, 2007).

Absorption, Transport, Retention, and Excretion
The metabolism of strontium is similar but not identical to that of calcium. However, wherever there is a metabolically controlled passage of ions across a membrane (e.g. gastrointestinal absorption, renal excretion), calcium is transported better than strontium. Intestinal absorption by adults of various mammalian species ranges from 5 to 25% (Nielsen, 1986). Strontium is absorbed by both passive diffusion and active processes (Marie et al., 2001). The active process is vitamin D-dependent, and is depressed by aging and high dietary calcium and phosphorus (Marie, 2007).

Absorbed strontium is transported in blood with a plasma concentration normally in the range 10–27 µg (0.11–0.31 µmol)/L (Marie et al., 2001). Only a limited amount of strontium is retained, most being preferentially deposited by two distinct processes in bones and teeth. These processes are fairly rapid surface absorption by ionic exchange, and a slow incorporation into bone crystals during their formation (Nielsen, 1986; Marie et al., 2001). Most of the strontium absorbed daily is excreted mainly in the urine, but some is excreted in the bile and sweat.

Dietary Guidance
It is difficult to provide dietary guidance for strontium, because most studies of its beneficial bioactivity have used non-nutritional amounts of the element. However, because strontium is associated with improved bone and tooth health, increased intakes of foods that are relatively rich sources of strontium, such as whole grains, and unpeeled fruits and vegetables, would be a prudent recommendation. The typical daily dietary intake of strontium is 1.5–3 mg (Nielsen, 1986).

Vanadium

Beneficial Actions and Possible Basis for Bioactivity

Vanadium is essential for some lower forms of life (algae, seaweeds, a lichen, and a fungus) where it is a component of various haloperoxidases (Nielsen, 2006b). Vanadium is generally not accepted as an essential nutrient for higher animals and humans, but it does have beneficial actions in supra-nutritional and perhaps nutritional intakes. Beneficial activity at nutritional intakes is indicated by findings from vanadium deprivation studies (Nielsen, 1998b). As described in previous reviews (Nielsen, 1998b; Anke *et al.*, 2005b), vanadium deprivation resulted in swollen joints, skeletal deformations, and decreased lifespan in goats. Also, an increased death rate, sometimes preceded by convulsions, occurred in kids of vanadium-deprived goats. Vanadium deprivation altered thyroid hormone metabolism, impaired reproduction, and altered bone morphology in rats.

Vanadium in pharmacological or supra-nutritional amounts has been repeatedly found to have beneficial bioactivity. Its ability to selectively inhibit protein tyrosine phosphatases probably explains the broad range of effects reported for vanadium. High intakes of vanadium result in elevated tissue vanadium concentrations that affect cellular regulatory or signaling cascades that modulate gene expression, metabolite flow, and the switch between proliferation and differentiation (Hulley and Davison, 2003). Among the beneficial effects of vanadium are insulin-mimetic action and promotion of bone strength, mineralization, and formation. The insulin-like actions of vanadium have been well reviewed (Marzban and McNeill, 2003; Sakurai, 2007). Early studies showing insulin-mimetic actions of vanadium in animals used extremely high amounts of vanadium that were sometimes toxic (Nielsen, 2006a). The vanadium doses in human experiments were about 100-fold lower than those used in many animal studies, but were an order of magnitude greater (i.e. 100 mg vanadyl sulfate or 125 mg sodium metavanadate/day) than possible nutritional need (Nielsen, 2006a). Efforts are continuing in the hope of finding vanadium insulin-mimetic and anti-diabetic compounds that are non-toxic and thus clinically useful (Sakurai, 2007).

Absorption, Transport, Retention, and Excretion

Because urine vanadium is usually <0.8 µg/L and the estimated daily intake of vanadium is 12–30 µg, apparently <5% of vanadium ingested normally is absorbed with the remainder being excreted in the feces (Nielsen, 1995). Vanadate is absorbed three to five times more effectively than vanadyl. The different absorbability rates for vanadate and vanadyl, the rate at which vanadate is transformed to vanadyl, and the effects of other dietary components (e.g. chromium, protein, ferrous ion, chloride, aluminum hydroxide) on this transformation and binding influence the percentage of ingested vanadium absorbed.

When vanadate appears in the blood, it is quickly converted into the vanadyl cation (Nielsen, 1995). Vanadyl is bound and transported by transferrin and albumin (Nielsen, 1995). Vanadyl also forms complexes with ferritin in plasma and body fluids. Whether vanadyl-transferrin can transfer vanadium into cells through the transferrin receptor, or whether ferritin is a storage vehicle for vanadium has not been determined. Vanadium is rapidly removed from plasma and is generally retained in tissues under normal conditions at concentrations less than 10 ng/g fresh weight (Nielsen, 1995). Bone apparently is a major sink for excessive retained vanadium. Excretion patterns after parenteral administration indicate that urine is the major excretory route for absorbed vanadium (Nielsen, 1995).

Dietary Guidance

No RDA or AI was set for vanadium by the Food and Nutrition Board (Institute of Medicine, 2001). Based on animal experiments, any requirement for vanadium would be small; a daily dietary intake of 10 µg would probably meet any postulated requirement (Nielsen, 1998b). Typical intakes of vanadium from foods are 6–18 µg for adults (Nielsen, 2006a). A daily beer (contains about 28 µg/L) can significantly increase the intake (Anke *et al.*, 2005b).

Other Elements

In a previous review (Nielsen, 2006a), reports indicating that aluminum, bromide, cadmium, germanium, lead, lithium, rubidium, and tin have beneficial effects in higher animals and/or humans were briefly discussed. Since then, essentially no relevant evidence has appeared that further strengthens the suggestion of beneficial bioactivity for any of these elements. Thus, the findings presented in the previous review are briefly summarized in Table 38.2.

TABLE 38.2   Reported beneficial bioactivity of aluminum, bromine, cadmium, germanium, lead, lithium, rubidium, and tin

Element	Reported deprivation signs	Reported beneficial bioactivity	Typical daily intake and food sources
Aluminum	*Goat:* ↑spontaneous abortions, ↓growth, ↓lifespan, leg weakness and incoordination *Chick:* ↓growth	Stimulates osteoblasts to form bone in vitro by activating a putative G-protein-coupled system	2–25 mg; processed cheese, foods containing baking powder, grains, vegetables, herbs, tea
Bromine	*Goat:* ↑spontaneous abortions, ↓growth, ↓fertility, ↓lifespan ↓hematocrit, ↓hemoglobin *Humans:* insomnia	Alleviate ↓growth caused by hyperthyroidism in mice and chicks; substitute for chloride requirement of chicks	2–5 mg; grains, nuts, fish
Cadmium	*Rat:* ↓growth *Goat:* ↓growth	Stimulates growth of cells in soft agar; mostly a toxicological concern	10–20 μg; shellfish, grains grown in high cadmium soils
Germanium	*Rat:* alters bone and liver mineral content, ↓tibial DNA, ↓growth *Chick:* ↓growth	Anti-tumor and immune-enhancing action in animals; ↑bone strength and mineral density in osteoporotic rats	0.4–1.5 mg; wheat bran, vegetables, pulses
Lead	*Rat:* ↓growth, anemia, altered iron and lipid metabolism *Pig:* ↓growth, ↑serum cholesterol and phospholipids	Alleviates iron deficiency in young rats and depressed growth in rats fed unbalanced diet; mostly a toxicological concern	5–50 μg; seafood, foods grown on high-lead soils
Lithium	*Goat:* ↓fertility, ↓birth weight, ↓lifespan *Rat:* ↓fertility, ↓birth weight, ↓litter size, ↓weaning weight	↑Growth of some cultured cells; insulin-mimetic and immune-modulating actions; ↓status associated with violent crime, learning disability, and heart disease; anti-manic action	0.2–0.6 mg; eggs, meat, fish, milk, potatoes, vegetables (content varies with geographic origin)
Rubidium	*Goat:* ↓food intake, ↓growth, ↓lifespan, ↑increased spontaneous abortions *Rat:* altered tissue mineral concentrations	None found	1–5 mg; fruits, vegetables —especially asparagus, fish, poultry, black tea, coffee
Tin	*Rat:* ↓growth, ↓response to sound, ↓feed efficiency, altered tissue mineral composition, alopecia	Associated with thymus immune function	1–40 mg; canned foods

Data from Nielsen (2000).

Future Directions

Because the elements reviewed in this chapter may have unrecognized nutritional importance in promoting health and well-being, further studies about their beneficial intakes are warranted. These studies could include work to:

- Determine why low manganese intakes are associated with chronic diseases such as osteoporosis, atherosclerosis, cataracts, and diabetes.
- Reassess the DRIs for manganese including the validity of the AI and establishment of intakes and conditions under which manganese may be harmful to heart and brain health.
- Determine the mechanisms through which boron apparently promotes bone health, brain function, and immune function, and has anti-cancer activity.
- Define standards for intakes of boron that assure maximal beneficial activity.
- Determine whether nutritional intakes of silicon provide beneficial effects on bone and connective tissue health.
- Establish the conditions under which chromium is beneficial to carbohydrate and lipid metabolism.
- Determine whether low intakes of arsenic are without harm, and whether, at appropriate low intakes, arsenic may be beneficial through an effect on methyl metabolism.
- Determine the mechanism behind the bioactivity of nutritional amounts of nickel that affects methyl metabolism, sensory functions, and kidney function.
- Determine whether strontium has beneficial effects on calcium and bone metabolism in nutritional amounts.

Suggestions for Further Reading

Nielsen, F.H. (2006a) Boron, manganese, molybdenum, and other trace elements. In B.A. Bowman and R.M. Russell (eds), *Present Knowledge in Nutrition*, Vol. 1, 9th Edn. ILSI Press, Washington, DC, pp. 506–526.

Nielsen, F.H. (2006b) The ultratrace elements. In M.H. Stipanuk (ed.), *Biochemical, Physiological, Molecular Aspects of Human Nutrition*. Saunders Elsevier, St. Louis, pp. 1143–1163.

References

Abernathy, C.O., Thomas, D.J., and Calderon, R.L. (2003) Health effects and risk assessment of arsenic. *J Nutr* **133,** 1536S–1538S.

Abumrad, N.N., Schneider, A.J., Steel, D., *et al.* (1981) Amino acid intolerance during prolonged total parenteral nutrition reversed by molybdate therapy. *Am J Clin Nutr* **34,** 2551–2559.

Adams, M.A., Bolger, P.M., and Gunderson, E.L. (1994) Dietary intake and hazards of arsenic. In W.R. Chappell, C.O. Abernathy, and C.R. Cothern (eds), *Arsenic. Exposure and Health*. Science and Technology Letters, Northwood, pp. 41–49.

Alvarez, H.M., Xue, Y., and Robinson, C.D., *et al.* (2010) Tetrathiomolybdate inhibits copper trafficking proteins through metal cluster formation. *Science*, **327,** 331–334.

Anderson, R.A. (1998) Chromium, glucose intolerance and diabetes. *J Am Coll Nutr* **17,** 548–555.

Anke, M. (2005) Recent progress in exploring the essentiality of the non-metallic ultratrace element arsenic to the nutrition of animals and man. *Biomed Res Trace Elem* **16,** 188–197.

Anke, M., Groppel, B., and Masaoka, T. (2005a) Recent progress in exploring the essentiality of the non metallic ultratrace elements fluorine and bromine to the nutrition of animals and man. *Biomed Res Trace Elem* **16,** 177–182.

Anke, M., Illing-Günther, H., and Schäfer, U. (2005b) Recent progress on essentiality of the ultratrace element vanadium in the nutrition of animal and man. *Biomed Res Trace Elem* **16,** 208–214.

Aschner, J.L. and Aschner, M. (2005) Nutritional aspects of manganese homeostasis. *Mol Aspects Med* **26,** 353–362.

Balk, E., Tatsioni, A., Lichtenstein, A., *et al.* (2007) Effect of chromium supplementation on glucose metabolism and lipids: a systematic review of randomized controlled diets. *Diabetes Care* **8,** 2154–2163.

Barel, A., Calomme, M., Timchenko, A., *et al.* (2005) Effect of oral intake of choline-stabilized orthosilicic acid on skin, nails and hair in women with photodamaged skin. *Arch Dermatol Res* **297,** 147–153.

Barranco, W.T. and Eckhert, C.D. (2004) Boric acid inhibits human prostate cancer cell proliferation. *Cancer Lett* **216,** 21–29.

Beltrán-Aguilar, E.D., Barker, L., and Dye, B.A. (2010) Prevalence and severity of dental fluorosis in the United States, 1999–2004. *NCHS Data Brief, No 53*. National Center for Health Statistics, Hyattsville, MD.

Boivin, G. (2010) Bone quality and strontium ranelate. *IBMS BoneKey* **7,** 103–107.

Bourgeois, A.-C., Scott, M.E., Sabally, K., *et al.* (2007) Low dietary boron reduces parasite (Nematoda) survival and alters cytokine profiles but the infection modifies liver minerals in mice. *J Nutr* **137**, 2080–2086.

Brewer, G.J. (2003) Copper-lowering therapy with tetrathiomolybdate for cancer and diseases of fibrosis and inflammation. *J Trace Elem Exp Med* **16**, 191–199.

Buchman, A.L. (2006) Manganese. In M.E. Shils, M. Shike, B. Caballero, *et al.* (eds), *Modern Nutrition in Health and Disease*, 10th Edn. Lippincott Williams and Wilkins, Philadelphia, pp. 326–331.

Carlisle, E.M. (1997) Silicon. In B.L. O'Dell and R.A. Sunde (eds), *Handbook of Nutritionally Essential Minerals*. Marcel Dekker, New York, pp. 603–618.

Cefalu, W.T. and Hu, F.B. (2004) Role of chromium in human health and in diabetes. *Diabetes Care* **27**, 2741–2751.

Cefalu, W.T., Rood, J., Pinsonat, P., *et al.* (2010) Characterization of the metabolic and physiologic response to chromium supplementation in subjects with type 2 diabetes mellitus. *Metabolism* **59**, 755–762.

Cerklewski, F.L. (1997) Fluorine. In B.L. O'Dell and R.A. Sunde (eds), *Handbook of Nutritionally Essential Mineral Elements*. Academic Press, New York, pp. 583–602.

Chen, G., Liu, P., Pattar, G.R., *et al.* (2006) Chromium activates glucose transporter 4 trafficking and enhances insulin-stimulated glucose transport in 3T3-L1 adipocytes via a cholesterol-dependent mechanism. *Mol Endocrinol* **20**, 857–870.

Chen, X., Schauder, S., Potier, N., *et al.* (2002) Structural identification of a bacterial quorum-sensing signal containing boron. *Nature* **415**, 545–549.

Cui, Y., Winton, M.I., Zhang, Z.F., *et al.* (2004) Dietary boron intake and prostate cancer cell risk. *Oncol Rep* **11**, 887–892.

da Silva, C.J., da Rocha, A.J., Jeronymo, S., *et al.* (2007) A preliminary study revealing a new association in patients undergoing maintenance hemodialysis: manganism symptoms and T1 hyperintense changes in the basal ganglia. *Am J Neuroradiol* **28**, 1474–1479.

Davis, C.D., Uthus, E.O., and Finley, J.W. (2000) Dietary selenium and arsenic affect DNA methylation in vitro in Caco-2 cells and in vivo in rat liver and colon. *J Nutr* **130**, 2903–2909.

Dickerson, R.N. (2001) Manganese intoxication and parenteral nutrition. *Nutrition* **17**, 689–693.

Eckhert, C.D. (2006) Other trace elements. In M.E. Shils, M. Shike, B. Caballero, *et al.* (eds), *Modern Nutrition in Health and Disease*, 10th Edn. Lippincott Williams and Wilkins, Philadelphia, pp. 338–350.

Finley, J.W. (2004) Does environmental exposure to manganese pose a health risk to healthy adults? *Nutr Rev* **62**, 148–153

Fort, D.J., Rogers, R.L., McLaughlin, D.W., *et al.* (2002) Impact of boron deficiency on *Xenopus laevis*. A summary of biological

effects and potential biochemical roles. *Biol Trace Elem Res* **90**, 117–142.

Freeland-Graves, J. and Llanes, C. (1994) Models to study manganese deficiency. In D.J. Klimis-Tavantzis (ed.), *Manganese in Health and Disease*. CRC Press, Boca Raton, FL, pp. 59–86.

Garcia, S.J., Gellein, K., Syversen, T. *et al.* (2007) Iron deficient and manganese supplemented diets alter metals and transporters in the developing rat brain. *Toxicol Sci* **95**, 205–217.

Gillette-Guyonnet, S., Andrieu, S., and Vellas, B. (2007) The potential influence of silica present in drinking water on Alzheimer's disease and associated disorders. *J Nutr Health Aging* **11**, 119–124.

Gordon, S.E. and Zagotta, W.N. (1995) Subunit interactions in coordination of Ni^{2+} in cyclic nucleotide-gated channels. *Proc Natl Acad Sci USA* **92**, 10222–10226.

Gorustovich, A.A., Steimetz, T., Nielsen, F.H., *et al.* (2008) A histomorphometric study of alveolar bone modeling and remodeling in mice fed a boron-deficient diet. *Arch Oral Biol* **53**, 677–682.

Gorustovich, A.A., Steimetz, T., Nielsen, F.H., *et al.* (2009) Histomorphometric study of alveolar bone healing in rats fed a boron-deficient diet. *Anat Rec* **291**, 441–447.

Guallar, E., Jiménez, F. J., van't Veer, P., *et al.* (2005) Low toenail chromium concentration and increased risk of nonfatal myocardial infarction. *Am J Epidemiol* **162**, 157–164.

Güner, S., Tay, A., Altan, V.M., *et al.* (2001) Effect of sodium molybdate on fructose-induced hyperinsulinemia and hypertension in rats. *Trace Elem Electrolytes* **18**, 39–46.

Hansen, S. L., Trakooljul, N., Liu, H.-C., *et al.* (2009) Iron transporters are differentially regulated by dietary iron, and modifications are associated with changes in manganese metabolism in young pigs. *J Nutr* **139**, 1272–1479.

Hardy, G. (2009) Manganese in parenteral nutrition: who, when, and why should we supplement? *Gastroenterology* **137**, S29–S35.

Huang, C., Ma, W., Li, J., *et al.* (1999) Arsenic induces apoptosis through a c-Jun NH_2-terminal kinase- dependent, p53-independent pathway. *Cancer Res* **59**, 3053–3058.

Hulley, P. and Davison, A. (2003) Regulation of tyrosine phosphorylation cascades by phosphatases; what the actions of vanadium teach us. *J Trace Elem Exp Med* **16**, 281–290.

Hunt, C.D. (2002) Boron-binding-biomolecules: a key to understanding the beneficial physiologic effects of dietary boron from prokaryotes to humans. In H.E. Goldbach, B. Rerkasem, M.A. Wimmer, *et al.* (eds), *Boron in Plant and Animal Nutrition*. Kluwer Academic/Plenum Publishers, New York, pp. 21–36.

Hunt, C.D. (2007) Dietary boron: evidence for essentiality and homeostatic control in humans and animals. In F. Xu, H.E.

Goldbach, P.H. Brown, *et al.* (eds), *Advances in Plant and Animal Boron Nutrition* (eds), pp. 251–267. Springer, Dordrecht.

Hunt, C. (2008) Dietary boron: possible roles in human and animal physiology. *Biomed Trace Elem Res*, **19**, 243–253.

Hurtel-Lemaire, A.S., Mentaverri, R., Caudrillier, A., *et al.* (2009) The calcium-sensing receptor is involved in strontium ranelate-induced osteoclast apoptosis. New insights into the associated signaling pathways. *J Biol Chem* **284**, 575–584.

Institute of Medicine (1997) *Dietary Reference Intakes for Calcium, Phosphorus, Magnesium, Vitamin D, and Fluoride.* National Academy Press, Washington, DC.

Institute of Medicine (2001) *Dietary Reference Intakes for Vitamin A, Vitamin K, Arsenic, Boron, Chromium, Copper, Iodine, Iron, Manganese, Molybdenum, Nickel, Silicon, Vanadium, and Zinc.* National Academy Press, Washington, DC.

Johnson, J.L. (1997) Molybdenum. In B.L. O'Dell and R.A. Sunde (eds) *Handbook of Nutritionally Essential Mineral Elements.* Marcel Dekker, New York, pp. 413–438.

Jugdaohsingh, R. (2007) Silicon and bone health. *J Nutr Health Aging* **11**, 99–110.

Jugdaohsingh, R., Calomme, M.R., Robinson, K., *et al.* (2008) Increased longitudinal growth in rats on a silicon-depleted diet. *Bone*, **43**, 596–606.

Kang, G.S., Li, Q., Chen, H., *et al.* (2006) Effect of metal ions on HIF-1α and Fe homeostasis in human A549 cells. *Mutat Res* **610**, 48–55.

Katko, M., Liss, I., Karpati, I., *et al.* (2008) Relationship between serum nickel and homocysteine concentration in hemodialysis patients. *Biol Trace Elem Res* **124**, 195–205.

Kaya, A., Karakaya, H., Fomenko, D.E., *et al.* (2009) Identification of a novel system for boron transport: Atr 1 is a main boron exporter in yeast. *Mol Cell Biol* **29**, 3665–3674.

Kayajanian, G. (2003) Arsenic, cancer, and thoughtless policy. *Ecotoxicol Environ Saf* **55**, 139–142.

Kim, M.-H., Bae, Y.-J., Choi, M.-K., *et al.* (2009) Silicon supplementation improves bone mineral density of calcium-deficient ovariectomized rats by reducing bone resorption. *Biol Trace Elem Res* **128**, 239–247.

Kinrade, S., Del Nin, J.W., Schach, A.S., *et al.* (1999) Stable five- and six-coordinated silicate anions in aqueous solution. *Science* **285**, 1542–1545.

Kleerekoper, M. and Mendlovic, B. (1993) Sodium fluoride therapy of postmenopausal osteoporosis. *Endocr Rev* **14**, 312–323.

Klein, C.J., Nielsen, F.H., and Moser-Veillon, P.B. (2008) Trace element loss in urine and effluent following traumatic injury. *JPEN J Parenter Enteral Nutr* **32**, 129–139.

Klimis-Tavantzis, D.J. (1994) *Manganese in Health and Disease.* CRC Press, Boca Raton, FL.

Kocyigit, A., Zeyrek, D., Keles, H., *et al.* (2004) Relationship among manganese, arginase, and nitric oxide in childhood asthma. *Biol Trace Elem Res* **102**, 11–18

Korkmaz, M., Uzgören, E., Bakirdere, S., *et al.* (2007) Effects of dietary boron on cervical cytopathology and on micronucleus frequency in exfoliated buccal cells. *Environ Toxicol* **22**, 17–25.

Leach, R.M., Jr, and Harris, E.D. (1997) Manganese. In B.L. O'Dell and R.A. Sunde (eds), *Handbook of Nutritionally Essential Minerals.* Marcel Dekker, New York, pp. 335–355.

Lukaski, H.C. and Scrimgeour, A.G. (2009) Trace elements excluding iron – chromium and zinc. In J.A. Driskell (ed.), *Nutrition and Exercise Concerns of Middle Age.* CRC Press, Taylor and Francis Group, Boca Raton, FL, pp. 233–250.

Macmillan-Crow, L.A. and Cruthirds, D.L. (2001) Invited review. Manganese superoxide dismutase in disease. *Free Radic Res* **34**, 325–336.

Maehira, F., Miyagi, I., and Eguchi, Y. (2009) Effects of calcium sources and soluble silicate on bone metabolism and the related gene expression in mice. *Nutrition* **25**, 581–589.

Mahabir, S., Spitz, M.R., Barrera, S.L, *et al.* (2008) Dietary boron and hormone replacement therapy as risk factors for lung cancer in women. *Am J Epidemiol* **167**, 1070–1080.

Marie, P.J. (2007) Strontium ranelate: new insights into its dual mode of action. *Bone* **40**, S5–S8.

Marie, P.J., Ammann, P., Boivin, G., *et al.* (2001) Mechanisms of action and therapeutic potential of strontium in bone. *Calcif Tissue Int* **69**, 121–129.

Marzban, L. and McNeill, J.H. (2003) Insulin-like actions of vanadium: potential as a therapeutic agent. *J Trace Elem Exp Med* **16**, 253–267.

Miller, K.B., Caton, J.S., Schafer, D.M., *et al.* (2000) High dietary manganese lowers heart magnesium in pigs fed a low-magnesium diet. *J Nutr* **130**, 2032–2035.

Mills, C.F. and Davis, G.K. (1987) Molybdenum. In W. Mertz (ed.), *Trace Elements in Human and Animal Nutrition*, vol. 1. Academic Press, San Diego, pp. 429–463.

Moukarzel, A. (2009) Chromium in parenteral nutrition: too little or too much? *Gastroenterology* **137**, S18–S28.

Murgo, A.J. (2001) Clinical trials of arsenic trioxide in hematologic and solid tumors: overview of the National Cancer Institute Cooperative Research and Development Studies. *Oncologist* **6** (Suppl 2), 22–28.

National Research Council (2005a) Arsenic. In *Mineral Tolerance of Animals*, 2nd Edn. National Academies Press, Washington, DC, pp. 31–45.

National Research Council (2005b) Nickel. In *Mineral Tolerance of Animals*, 2nd Edn. National Academies Press, Washington, DC, pp. 276–289.

Nielsen, F.H. (1986) Other elements: Sb, Ba, B, Br, Cs, Ge, Rb, Ag, Sr, Sn, Ti, Zr, Be, Bi, Ga, Au, In, Nb, Sc, Te, Tl, W. In W. Mertz (ed.), *Trace Elements in Human and Animal Nutrition*, 5th Edn. Academic Press, New York, pp. 415–463.

Nielsen, F.H. (1995) Vanadium in mammalian physiology and nutrition. In H. Sigel and A. Sigel (eds), *Metal Ions in Biological Systems, Vanadium and Its Role in Life*, Vol. 31. Marcel Dekker, New York, pp. 543–573.

Nielsen, F.H. (1998a) Ultratrace elements in nutrition: current knowledge and speculation. *J Trace Elem Exp Med* **11**, 251–274.

Nielsen, F.H. (1998b) The nutritional essentiality and physiological metabolism of vanadium in higher animals. In A.S. Tracey and D.C. Crans (eds), *Vanadium Compounds. Chemistry, Biochemistry, and Therapeutic Applications*. ACS Symposium Series 711, American Chemical Society, Washington, DC, pp. 297–307.

Nielsen, F.H. (2000) Possibly essential trace elements. In J.D. Bogden and L.M. Klevay (eds), *Clinical Nutrition of the Essential Trace Elements and Minerals*. Humana Press, Totowa, NJ, pp. 11–36.

Nielsen, F.H. (2006a) Boron, manganese, molybdenum, and other trace elements. In B.A. Bowman and R.M. Russell (eds), *Present Knowledge in Nutrition*, Vol. 1, 9th Edn. ILSI Press, Washington, DC, pp. 506–526.

Nielsen, F.H. (2006b) The ultratrace elements. In M.H. Stipanuk (ed.), *Biochemical, Physiological, Molecular Aspects of Human Nutrition*. Saunders Elsevier, St. Louis, pp. 1143–1163.

Nielsen, F.H. (2006c) A mild magnesium deprivation affects calcium excretion but not bone strength and shape, including changes induced by nickel deprivation, in the rat. *Biol Trace Elem Res* **110**, 133–149.

Nielsen, F.H. (2008) Is boron nutritionally relevant? *Nutr Rev* **66**, 183–191.

Nielsen, F.H. (2009a) Boron deprivation decreases liver S-adenosylmethionine and spermidine and increases plasma homocysteine and cysteine in rats. *J Trace Elem Med Biol* **23**, 204–213.

Nielsen, F.H. (2009b) Micronutrients in parenteral nutrition: boron, silicon, and fluoride. *Gastroenterology* **137**, S55–S60.

Nielsen, F.H. and Penland, J.G. (2006) Boron deprivation alters rat behavior and brain mineral composition differently when fish oil instead of safflower oil is the diet fat source. *Nutr Neurosci* **9**, 105–112.

Nielsen, F.H. and Stoecker, B.J. (2009) Boron and fish oil have different beneficial effects on strength and trabecular microarchitecture of bone. *J Trace Elem Med Biol* **23**, 195–203.

Nielsen, F.H., Yokoi, K., and Uthus, E.O. (2002) The essential role of nickel affects physiological functions regulated by the cyclic-GMP signal transduction system. In L. Khassavova, P. Collery, I. Maymard, *et al.* (eds), *Metal Ions in Biology and Medicine*, Vol. 7. John Libbey Eurotext, Paris, pp. 29–33.

Norose, N. and Arai, K. (1987) Manganese deficiency due to long-term total parenteral nutrition in an infant. *JPEN J Parenter Enteral Nutr* **9**, 978–981.

Novotny, J.A. and Turnland, J.R. (2006) Molybdenum kinetics in men differs during molybdenum depletion and repletion. *J Nutr* **136**, 953–957.

Novotny, J.A. and Turnland, J.R. (2007) Molybdenum intake influences molybdenum kinetics in men. *J Nutr* **137**, 37–42.

Pagano, A.R., Yasuda, K., Roneker, K.R., *et al.* (2007) Supplemental *Escherichia coli* phytase and strontium enhance bone strength of young pigs fed a phosphorus-adequate diet. *J Nutr* **137**, 1795–1801.

Park, M., Li, Q., Shcheynikov, N., *et al.* (2004) NaBC1 is ubiquitous electrogenic Na$^+$-coupled borate transporter essential for cellular boron homeostasis and cell growth and proliferation. *Mol Cell* **16**, 331–341.

Qiao, W., Peng, Z., Wang, Z., *et al.* (2009) Chromium improves glucose uptake and metabolism through upregulating the mRNA levels of IR, Glut 4, GS, and UCP3 in skeletal muscle cells. *Biol Trace Elem Res* **131**, 133–142.

Rajpathak, S., Rimm, E.B., Li, T., *et al.* (2004) Lower toenail chromium in men with diabetes and cardiovascular disease compared with healthy men. *Diabetes Care* **27**, 2211–2216.

Ralston, N.V. and Hunt, C.D. (2004) Transmembrane partitioning of boron and other elements in RAW 264.7 and HL60 cell cultures. *Biol Trace Elem Res* **98**, 181–192.

Reiss, J. and Johnson, J.L. (2003) Mutations in the molybdenum cofactor biosynthetic genes MOCS1, MOCS2, and GEPH. *Hum Mutat* **21**, 569–576.

Řezanka, T. and Sigler, K. (2007) Biologically active compounds of semi-metals. *Phytochemistry* **69**, 585–606.

Ricardo, A., Carriagan, M.A., Olcott, A.N., *et al.* (2004) Borate minerals stabilize ribose. *Science* **303**, 196.

Ringe, J.D. (2004) Fluoride and bone health. In M.F. Holick and B. Dawson-Hughes (eds), *Nutrition and Bone Health*. Humana Press, Totowa, NJ, pp. 345–362.

Sakurai, H. (2007) Medicinal aspects of vanadium complexes: treatment of diabetes mellitus in model animals. *Biomed Res Trace Elem* **18**, 241–248.

Spears, J.W. and Armstrong, T.A. (2007) Dietary boron: evidence for a role in immune function. In F. Xu, H.E. Goldbach, P.H. Brown, *et al.* (eds) *Advances in Plant and Animal Boron Nutrition*. Springer, Dordrecht, pp.269–276.

Sripanyakorn, S., Jugdaohsingh, R., Dissayabutr, W., *et al.* (2009) The comparative absorption of silicon from different foods and food supplements. *Br J Nutr* **102**, 825–834.

Stangl, G.I., Roth-Maier, D.A., and Kirchgessner, M. (2000) Vitamin B-12 deficiency and hyperhomocysteinemia are partly ameliorated by cobalt and nickel supplementation in pigs. *J Nutr* **130,** 3038–3044.

Stearns, D.M. (2007) Multiple hypotheses for chromium (III) biochemistry: why the essentiality of chromium (III) is still questioned. In J.B. Vincent (ed.), *The Nutritional Biochemistry of Chromium (III).* Elsevier, Amsterdam, pp. 57–70.

Takano, J., Miwa, K., Yuan, L., *et al.* (2005) Endocytosis and degradation of BOR1, a boron transporter of *Arabidopsis thaliana,* regulated by boron availability. *Proc Natl Acad Sci USA* **102,** 12276–12281.

Thomas, D.J., Li, J., Waters, S.B., *et al.* (2007) Arsenic (+3 oxidation state) methyltransferases and the methylation of arsenicals. *Exp Biol Med (Maywood)* **232,** 3–13.

Touillaud, M.S., Pillow, P.C., Jakovljevic, J., *et al.* (2005) Effect of dietary intake of phytoestrogens on estrogen receptor status in premenopausal women with breast cancer. *Nutr Cancer* **51,** 162–169.

Tucker, K.L., Jugdaohsingh, R., Powell, J.J., *et al.* (2009) Effects of beer, wine, and liquor intakes on bone mineral density in older men and women. *Am J Clin Nutr* **89,** 1188–1196.

Uthus, E.O. and Davis, C.D. (2005) Dietary arsenic affects dimethylhydrazine-induced aberrant crypt formation and hepatic global DNA methylation and DNA methytransferase activity in rats. *Biol Trace Elem Res* **103,** 133–146.

Vincent, J.B. and Bennett, R. (2007) Potential and purported roles for chromium in insulin signaling: the search for the Holy Grail. In J.B. Vincent (ed.), *The Nutritional Biochemistry of Chromium (III).* Elsevier, Amsterdam, pp. 139–160.

Vincent, J.B. and Stallings, D. (2007) Introduction: a history of chromium studies. In J.B. Vincent (ed.), *The Nutritional Biochemistry of Chromium (III).* Elsevier, Amsterdam, pp. 1–40.

Vural, H., Sirin, B., Yilmaz, N., *et al.* (2009) The role of arginine-nitric oxide pathway in patients with Alzheimer disease. *Biol Trace Elem Res* **129,** 58–64.

Wang, Y., Wan, C., Deng, L., *et al.* (2007) The hypoxia-inducible factor α pathway couples angiogenesis to osteogenesis during skeletal development. *J Clin Invest* **117,** 1616–1626.

Whitford, G.M. (2006) Fluoride. In M.H. Stipanuk (ed.), *Biochemical, Physiological, and Molecular Aspects of Human Nutrition.* Saunders Elsevier, St. Louis, pp. 1127–1142.

Wilson, J.H., Wilson, E.J., and Ruszler, P.L. (2001) Dietary nickel improves male broiler (*Gallus domesticus*) bone strength. *Biol Trace Elem Res* **83,** 239–249.

Wood, R.J. (2009) Manganese and birth outcome. *Nutr Rev* **67,** 416–420.

World Health Organization (1996) Boron. In *Trace Elements in Human Nutrition and Health.* World Health Organization, Geneva, pp. 175–179.

World Health Organization, International Programme on Chemical Safety (1998) *Boron Environmental Health Criteria 204.* World Health Organization, Geneva.

Zeng, C., Hou, G., Dick, R., *et al.* (2008) Tetrathiomolybdate is partially protective against hyperglycemia in rodent models of diabetes. *Exp Biol Med* **233,** 1021–1025.

39

MATERNAL NUTRIENT METABOLISM AND REQUIREMENTS IN PREGNANCY AND LACTATION

LINDSAY H. ALLEN, PhD

USDA-ARS Western Human Nutrition Research Center, Davis, California, USA

Summary

This chapter describes how the additional nutrient requirements of the mother and her fetus during pregnancy are met by a combination of physiological events that affect maternal nutrient utilization and fetal nutrient transfer, and increased dietary intakes. The physiological changes complicate the interpretation of nutritional status measures in pregnancy. It is clear that the body composition of the mother in the periconceptional period affects pregnancy weight gain, so the newly revised weight-gain recommendations continue to be based on maternal body mass index (BMI) at conception. The adverse effects of consuming an inadequate amount of most vitamins and minerals during pregnancy are partially understood, often from research in developing country populations, but little is known about subclinical or long-term effects of deficiencies or their role in specific adverse pregnancy outcomes. Randomized controlled supplementation trials provide most of the information on this issue. After adjustments during the first postpartum weeks, maternal physiology is much less affected by lactation than by pregnancy. Most nutrient requirements are increased to provide for secretion in milk, but women consuming poor diets or who are depleted in specific nutrients may secrete low amounts of those nutrients. Maternal and/or infant supplementation can sometimes improve this situation.

Introduction

Enabling pregnant women to meet their nutrient needs has long been a public health priority in the United States and most other countries. This priority is based on evidence that undernutrition prior to and during the period of reproduction can have serious, short- and long-term adverse effects on the mother and child. Programs designed to improve maternal undernutrition are very cost-effective. In wealthier countries there is increasing information about how variability in diet, nutrient metabolism and requirements of individuals affects pregnancy weight gain, the risk of preterm delivery, birth defects, and other pregnancy outcomes. Well-designed studies on undernourished women in developing countries have revealed the impact that improved maternal nutrition can have on maternal and infant health. However, rates of preterm delivery, low birth weight, birth defects, and other pregnancy complications are still unacceptably high even in wealthier countries, and there is much to be learned about optimal maternal nutrient requirements during pregnancy and lactation.

Changes in Maternal Physiology during Pregnancy

Hormonal Changes

In pregnancy larger amounts of nutrients are required for the growth and metabolism of maternal and fetal tissues, and for storage in the fetus. Some of this additional need is met by increased maternal food intake, but regardless of dietary intake there are enormous metabolic adjustments in nutrient utilization that support the development of the fetus. Some of the most important changes in serum hormone concentrations, and in tissue deposition and metabolism, are summarized in Table 39.1.

Human chorionic gonadotropin (hCG) and human placental lactogen (hPL) concentrations increase a few days after implantation and maintain the corpus luteum. HPL stimulates placental and fetal growth, modulates fetal intrauterine growth factor (IGF) production, and helps to direct nutrients to the fetus by stimulating maternal fat breakdown and antagonizing the action of maternal insulin. It also stimulates mammary-gland development in preparation for lactation.

Estrogen synthesis is increased from early in pregnancy, and its functions include altering carbohydrate and lipid metabolism, increasing the rate of maternal bone turnover, and stimulating conversion of somatotroph cells in the maternal pituitary to prolactin-secreting mammotrophs

TABLE 39.1 Changes in hormone concentrations, and in tissue and nutrient deposition during pregnancy

Serum hormones, tissues, and metabolic processes	Week of gestation			
	10	20	30	40
Serum placental hormones				
Human chorionic gonadotropin (10^4 U/L)	1.3	4.0	3.0	2.5
Human placental lactogen (nmol/L)	23	139	255	394
Estradiol (pmol/L)	5	22	55	66
Products of conception				
Fetus (g)	5	300	1500	3400
Placenta (g)	20	170	430	650
Amniotic fluid (g)	30	250	750	800
Maternal tissue gain				
Uterus (g)	140	320	600	970
Mammary gland (g)	45	180	360	405
Plasma volume (mL)	50	800	1200	1500
Nutrient metabolism and accretion in mother + fetus				
Increase in basal metabolism/day	80[a]	170	260	400
	0.19[b]	0.41	0.62	0.95
Fat deposition (g)	328	2064	3594	3825
Protein deposition (g)	36	165	498	925
Iron accretion (mg)				565
Calcium accretion (g)				30
Zinc accretion (mg)				100
Hemoglobin (g/L)	125	117	119	130

[a] kcal.
[b] MJ.
Data from King (2000a).

required for the initiation and maintenance of lactation. Progesterone relaxes the smooth muscle cells of the gastrointestinal tract and uterus, stimulates maternal respiration, promotes development of mammary-gland lobules, and prevents milk secretion from occurring during pregnancy.

In general pregnancy is a period of increasing resistance of pancreatic β cells to insulin. This occurs in parallel with the higher secretion of hCG, progesterone, cortisol, and prolactin, and serves to permit glucose, very-low-density lipoproteins, and amino acids to flow to the fetus rather than being deposited in maternal tissues.

Although the weight of the fetus increases throughout pregnancy, about 90% of its ponderal growth occurs in the last 20 weeks (Table 39.1). Fetal growth is accompanied by expansion of the placenta, uterus, and mammary glands. The additional tissues cause maternal metabolic rate to be 60% higher during the last half of pregnancy, creating a need for additional dietary energy. The protein, fat, minerals, and vitamins deposited in fetal and maternal tissues come from increased maternal food intake and/or more efficient intestinal absorption or renal reabsorption, depending on the specific nutrient.

Changes in Blood and Other Fluids

Plasma volume increases by ~50% (1.5 L) by late pregnancy but red cell mass increases by only 15–20%. This "hemodilution of pregnancy" means that hemoglobin and hematocrit concentrations fall, especially during the second trimester when there is the largest rise in plasma volume (Table 39.1), and recommended cut-off values that signify anemia vary by trimester. Concentrations of serum albumin and most nutrients are also lower in pregnancy, because of hemodilution and alterations in turnover. In contrast there is a higher level of most globulins, lipids (especially triacylglycerol), and vitamin E. Renal plasma flow increases by 75% and glomerular filtration rate by 50%, accompanied by higher urinary glucose, amino acids, and water-soluble vitamins.

Weight Gain During Pregnancy

Guidelines for pregnancy weight gain in the United States were revised by the Institute of Medicine (IOM) in 2009 (Institute of Medicine, 2009); revision was needed because women are becoming pregnant when older and heavier, and are more likely to have multiple pregnancies and to gain too much weight in pregnancy. The guidelines con-

TABLE 39.2 Pregnancy weight gain recommendations

Body mass index category	Recommended weight gain kg (lb)	Rate of weight gain in second and third trimester Mean (range), lb/wk
Low (BMI <18.5)	12.5–18 (28–40)	1 (1–1.3)
Normal (BMI 18.5–24.9)	11.5–16 (25–35)	1 (0.8–1)
Overweight (BMI >25.0–29.9)	7–11.5 (15–25)	0.6 (0.5–0.7)
Obese (BMI ≥30.0)	≥6.0 (11–20)	0.5 (0.4–0.6)

Reproduced with permission from National Academies Press, Washington, DC.

tinue to recognize that pregnancy weight gain is inversely related to the fatness (body mass index, BMI, weight/height^2) of the woman at conception. The new recommended weight gains (Table 39.2) are associated with the lowest prevalence of cesarean delivery, excess postpartum weight retention, prematurity, low or high birth weight, and childhood obesity in each BMI category. BMI categories were changed to World Health Organization values.

Obese women tend to gain relatively low amounts of weight and yet produce a normal-birth-weight infant. For this reason, and to minimize excessive postpartum weight retention, it is recommended that they gain much less weight but at least 11 lb (5 kg). It is important for women to enter pregnancy with as normal a BMI as possible; overweight and obesity increase the risk for gestational diabetes and preeclampsia. Recommended weight gain does not differ by maternal age, height or ethnicity. While conception less than 2 years after menarche is associated with increased risk of preterm delivery, low birth weight, and infant mortality, recommended weight gains are the same for adolescent and adult women. Recommendations are higher for women bearing twins; for normal BMI women, 37–54 lb (16.8–24.5 kg); overweight, 16–25 lb (7.3–11.3 kg); and obese, 14–22 lb (6.4–10 kg). Because risk of low birth weight is highest for thin women who gain low amounts of weight during pregnancy, this group should be a priority for targeting nutrition counseling and support. Charts should be used to plot weight gain of individual women and compare it with recommended ranges (North Carolina State Department of Health and Human Services, 2010).

Metabolism and Recommended Intakes of Nutrients

The profound physiological changes that cause hemodilution, changes in the ratio of free to bound forms of nutrients, and alterations in nutrient turnover and homeostasis, affect our ability to assess nutritional status and requirements during pregnancy. For most nutrients the recommended intake is calculated using a factorial approach. This involves adding estimates of the amount of the nutrient deposited in the mother and fetus, and a factor to cover the inefficiency of utilization for tissue growth, to the requirements for non-pregnant women. For a few nutrients, including folate, some experimental data exist so recommendations can be based on the amount needed to maintain tissue levels and nutrient-dependent function. A summary of recommended nutrient intakes for pregnancy is provided in Table 39.3.

Energy

Energy requirements are increased to cover energy deposited in the mother and fetus (~180 kcal/day, as a total of 3.8 kg fat and 925 g protein over pregnancy) (Institute of Medicine, 2002/2005). In addition, energy expenditure increases by 8 kcal/week owing to the cost of additional

TABLE 39.3 Recommended intakes of nutrients for non-reproducing, pregnant, and lactating women[a]

Nutrient	Adult woman	Pregnancy	Lactation
Energy (kcal)	2000–2200[b]	+340[c], +452[d]	+330[e], +400[f]
Energy (MJ)	8.37–9.21[b]	+1.42[c], +1.89[d]	+1.38[e], +1.67[f]
Protein (g)	46[g]	71	71
Vitamin A (µg RE)	700	770	1300
Vitamin D (µg)	600 IU (15 µg)	600 IU (15 µg)	600 IU (15 µg)
Vitamin E (mg α-tocopherol)	15	15	19
Vitamin C (mg)	75	85	120
Thiamin (mg)	1.1	1.4	1.4
Riboflavin (mg)	1.1	1.4	1.6
Vitamin B_6 (mg)	1.3	1.9	2.0
Niacin (mg NE)	14	18	17
Folate (µg dietary folate equivalents)	400	600	500
Vitamin B_{12} (µg)	2.4	2.6	2.8
Pantothenic acid (mg)	5	6	7
Biotin (µg)	30	30	35
Choline (mg)	425	450	550
Calcium (mg)	1000	1000	1000
Phosphorus (mg)	700	700	700
Magnesium (mg)	320	350	310
Iron (mg)	18	27	9
Zinc (mg)	8	11	12
Iodine (µg)	150	220	290
Selenium (µg)	55	60	70
Fluoride (mg)	3	3	3

[a]Recommended dietary allowances for pregnant women age 19–30 years (for energy and protein from Institute of Medicine, 2002/2005; for vitamin A, iodine, iron, and zinc from Institute of Medicine, 2001; for calcium and vitamin D from Institute of Medicine, 2011; for vitamin E, vitamin C, and selenium from Institute of Medicine, 2000; for B vitamins from Institute of Medicine, 1999). Values are recommended dietary intakes (RDAs) except for pantothenic acid, biotin, and choline, where value is an adequate intake.
[b]Assuming moderately active woman.
[c]Trimester 2.
[d]Trimester 3.
[e]First 6 months.
[f]Second 6 months.
[g]Based on 0.8 g/kg.

fetal and maternal metabolism. These increased needs start primarily in the second trimester, when the estimated energy requirement (EER) is the non-pregnant requirement + (8 kcal/week × 20 weeks). In the third trimester (8 kcal/week × 34 weeks) is added to the non-pregnant requirement + 180 kcal/day. The actual amount of energy required varies greatly among women because of differences in the amount of weight and fat gain, and energy expenditure. One study of ten healthy North American women reported that the cumulative energy costs of tissue metabolism and deposition ranged from 60 000 to 170 000 kcal (252–714 MJ) (Bronstein et al., 1996). It is unclear how this variability in energy deposition translates into recommended energy intakes. Higher energy intakes given during pregnancy to underweight, energy-restricted women can improve birth weight and length, and reduce stillbirths and perinatal mortality (Ceesay et al., 1997; Moore, 1998). A higher energy intake causes more maternal fat deposition as well as a higher metabolic rate, across well and poorly nourished populations (Prentice and Goldberg, 2000). In The Gambia, the mid-pregnancy resting metabolic rate of undernourished women actually fell below pre-pregnancy values, but was significantly increased by energy supplementation. It is evident that although there are adaptations in energy expenditure and deposition depending on energy availability, they do not necessarily enable optimal fetal development. It has been hypothesized that an individual who suffered nutritional restriction in utero has a "thrifty genotype" or "thrifty phenotype," which may help survival in conditions of nutrient restriction, but may also increase the risk of obesity and type 2 diabetes when the food supply is plentiful. However, this hypothesis is the subject of ongoing debate (Prentice et al., 2005; Wells, 2010). Risk of coronary heart disease, hypercholesterolemia, and hypertension is higher for adults who were born small (Godfrey and Barker, 2000). In utero nutrition may also adversely affect later adult immunocompetence. Also in The Gambia, adults who had been born during the hungry season had an 11-fold higher risk of dying prematurely of infectious diseases than those born during the rest of the year (Moore, 1998). It is becoming increasingly evident that undernutrition in utero has serious long-term consequences for poor health (Langley-Evans, 2006).

At present the best strategy may be to monitor weight gain closely and counsel women to either consume more dietary energy or consume less as needed. Because the requirement for most nutrients increases substantially more than that for energy, however, recommendations of lower intake must be made with caution. Advice to improve dietary quality and to obtain sufficient exercise is usually appropriate. Excessive weight gain in pregnancy tends to cause excessive weight retention postpartum. Exclusive breastfeeding for at least 6 months reduces the risk of long-term retention of this weight.

Essential Fatty Acids

Essential polyunsaturated fatty acids (PUFAs), which must be consumed in the diet, include the parent essential fatty acids, linoleic acid (LA, 18:2n-6) and α-linolenic acid (ALA, 18:3n-3) found mainly in seed oils, and their longer-chain more unsaturated derivatives called long-chain polyenes (LCPs). Important LCPs derived from linoleic acid include arachidonic acid and dihomo-γ-linolenic acid. Those derived from linolenic acid include eicosapentaenoic acid (EPA) and docosahexanoic acid (DHA). The LA-derived LCPs and EPA are precursors of prostanoids, AA is a structural fatty acid in the brain, and DHA and AA can be converted to biologically active hydroxy fatty acids. The fetal supply of PUFAs depends on maternal PUFA status, which declines as pregnancy progresses. Indeed a review concluded that there is evidence that the PUFA status of some pregnant women is inadequate to support optimal neonatal status especially if there are multiple births (Hornstra, 2000). Neonatal DHA status is associated with their head circumference, birth length and weight, and DHA supplementation of preterm infants caused more rapid visual information processing and attention, and affected retinal function. Research is ongoing to resolve the long-term consequences of neonatal EFA status for function. The major sources of AA are egg yolk and lean meat. DHA is found in meat and fatty fish. The adequate intake (AI) recommendation for linoleic acid is increased from 12 to 13 g/day, and for linolenic acid from 1.1 to 1.4 g/day, based on usual population intakes. Higher intakes of *trans* fatty acids are associated with poorer maternal and neonatal PUFA status so it may be beneficial to consume less of these during pregnancy.

Protein

From very early in pregnancy there are adaptations in maternal nitrogen metabolism that increase nitrogen and protein deposition in the mother and fetus. These include lower urea production and excretion, lower plasma α-amino nitrogen, and a lower rate of branched chain amino acid transamination (Kalhan, 2000). The RDAs provide for an additional 925 g of protein deposited in the mother and fetus, of which ~8 g/day are needed during the second trimester and ~17 g/day during the third (Institute of Medicine, 2002/2005). Thus the total RDA is 1.1 g/kg/day or +25 g/day additional protein. Most pregnant women in industrialized countries, and probably the majority in developing countries, consume at least the recommended intake of protein.

Vitamin A

Vitamin A deficiency during pregnancy and lactation is not a public health problem in industrialized countries. There is more concern about the dangers of excessive supplementation with retinol or the analog isotretinoin which is used to treat severe cystic acne. Ingestion of large amounts of retinol has been associated with birth defects including abnormalities of the central nervous system, craniofacial and cardiovascular defects, and thymus malformations (Rothman et al., 1995). The first trimester is most critical because the malformations are derived from cranial neural crest cells. There are about 20 case reports of retinol toxicity during pregnancy although their interpretation is confounded by the fact that the retinol was usually consumed as part of a multinutrient supplement (Azaïs-Braesco and Pascal, 2000). Nevertheless, animal studies are clearly consistent with the teratogenic effects of even a single high dose of retinol. The upper safe limit has been set at 3000 μg daily for women of reproductive age and in pregnancy (World Health Organization, 1998). Large intakes of β-carotene do not have a teratogenic effect.

Vitamin A deficiency is highly prevalent in developing countries. Weekly supplementation of pregnant women in Nepal, where vitamin A deficiency is endemic, reduced maternal mortality by about 44% (West et al., 1999) and an equivalent amount of β-carotene had a similar effect. However, a follow-up trial in Bangladesh by the same investigators found no such benefit, possibly due to the better vitamin A status of that population.

Vitamin D

In both pregnant and non-pregnant individuals the serum concentration of 25-hydroxyvitamin D, the main circulating form of the vitamin, is a good indicator of tissue stores of vitamin D. It crosses the placenta and is converted to the active form, 1,25-dihydroxyvitamin D, by the neonate. The placenta synthesizes 1,25-dihydroxyvitamin D; maternal serum levels are more than doubled by late pregnancy, and calcium absorption is increased several-fold. Maternal and fetal concentrations of free 1,25-dihydroxycholecalciferol are correlated at term. The main predictors of maternal vitamin D status in Northern California, where low serum concentrations are common, are season of delivery (i.e. the amount synthesized in the skin through the action of ultraviolet light), vitamin D intake from fortified milk and supplements, and skin pigmentation (less being synthesized in darker skin) (Dror et al., 2011). When fortified dairy product intake is low, seasonal fluctuations in serum 25-hydroxyvitamin D are more evident, with little synthesized in the skin during winter in more northern latitudes. In France, about 24% of infants born to unsupplemented mothers in the winter or spring had signs of vitamin D deficiency (Zeghoud et al., 1997). In China, the bones of infants born in the spring were less developed than those born after the summer (Specker et al., 1992). Many other possible adverse outcomes of vitamin D deficiency in pregnancy remain to be confirmed (Dror and Allen, 2010). The RDA is 600 IU (15 μg), the same as for non-pregnant women (Institute of Medicine, 2011). While not all countries recommend routine vitamin D supplements in pregnancy, in the UK, for example, there are now recommendations that these should be taken by women at high risk of deficiency.

Vitamin B₆

Although plasma concentrations of pyridoxal and pyridoxal phosphate decline more than can be accounted for by hemodilution, this is probably caused by hormonal changes rather than by poorer vitamin status (Institute of Medicine, 1999). Pyridoxal is transferred by active diffusion to the placenta which converts it to pyridoxal phosphate (Schenker et al., 1992). In the United States non-pregnant women's intakes of vitamin B_6 average about 1.5 mg per day but there is no evidence of a significant vitamin B_6 deficiency problem. In Japan, a maternal supplement of 2 mg per day of the vitamin improved vitamin B_6 status and growth of the newborn (Chang, 1999).

Folate

There is a marked increase in folate utilization during pregnancy as a result of the acceleration of reactions requiring single-carbon transfer, the rapid rate of cell division in maternal and fetal tissues, and deposition in the fetus. The recommended intakes for pregnancy are based on the amount that maintained erythrocyte concentrations in clinical trials.

Randomized controlled trials have proven that taking folic acid supplements before conception and through about the first 4 weeks of pregnancy lowers the risk of genetically predisposed women having a baby with a neural tube defect (NTD) (Heseker *et al.*, 2009). Unfortunately most women are unaware that they are pregnant at this stage. NTDs occur in about 5.5/10000 births in the United States and up to 40/10000 in other countries, and tend to recur in subsequent pregnancies. A lower intake of folate from diet plus supplements (Werler *et al.*, 1993; Shaw *et al.*, 1995) or higher erythrocyte folate concentrations (Daly *et al.*, 1995) is inversely related to NTD risk. The metabolic defect that causes NTD, and the mechanisms by which folic acid lowers NTD risk, are not fully understood although disruption of the folate-metabolizing enzyme, serine hydroxymethyltransferase 1, has been implicated most recently (Beaudin *et al.*, 2011). Maternal supplements of 400 μg folic acid/day reduced the occurrence of NTDs in Northern China by up to 80% (Berry *et al.*, 1999), and by 70% in N England, 35% in California, and 28% overall in the USA; the percent reduction is higher in populations with a higher initial prevalence of NTDs (Heseker *et al.*, 2009). The policy of fortifying flour with folic acid has increased folate status substantially in the USA and Canada and elsewhere in the world, and also reduced the prevalence of NTDs (USDA, 2010). This policy improves maternal folate status prior to conception, although some concerns about its safety, especially in combination with use of folic acid supplements, still need to be resolved (Crider *et al.*, 2011). For this reason folic acid fortification of flour is not practiced in Europe.

Pregnant women are recommended to consume 200 μg/day of synthetic folic acid in addition to the non-pregnant RDA of 400 μg per day of dietary folate. The 200 μg of folic acid is equivalent to 400 μg of dietary folate, because food folates have only about half the bioavailability of the synthetic form. This amount of folate will maintain normal folate status in pregnancy and prevent elevated plasma homocysteine concentrations (Institute of Medicine, 1999). Orange juice, dark-green leafy vegetables, and legumes average ~75–100 μg folate per serving, and many commercial fortified breakfast cereals provide 100 μg folic acid (about 170 dietary folate equivalents, DFE).

Folic acid supplementation, even when started later in pregnancy, may lower the risk of other birth defects since low serum or red blood cell folate and elevated plasma total homocysteine concentrations (tHcy) are often associated with other pregnancy complications (Scholl *et al.*, 1997). For example, in a large, retrospective, Norwegian study, women in the upper quartile of plasma tHcy compared with the lower had a 32% greater risk of preeclampsia, 38% more risk of preterm delivery, and 101% more risk of a very low-birth-weight infant (Vollset *et al.*, 2000). A meta-analysis showed that of all vitamin and mineral supplements tested, only folic acid lowered the risk of preterm delivery (Gülmezoglu *et al.*, 1997).

Calcium

Additional calcium is made available to the fetus by the substantial increase in the efficiency of maternal calcium absorption starting early in pregnancy. Calcium is carried across the placenta by active transport involving calcium binding protein and 1,25-dihydroxyvitamin D. Although maternal bone resorption increases during pregnancy, there is no detectable change in bone mineral content between conception and parturition (Ritchie *et al.*, 1998). There is little need for additional dietary calcium during pregnancy, and calcium supplements do not improve maternal bone calcium or infant bone in the first year of life, even when maternal intakes are very low (Jarjou *et al.*, 2006). Recommended intakes are 1000 mg/day, the same as for non-pregnant women (Institute of Medicine, 2011).

Pregnancy-induced hypertension (PIH) affects about 10% of all pregnancies in the United States, and increases risk of maternal morbidity and mortality. PIH includes preeclampsia, eclampsia, and hypertension. Based on epidemiologic and experimental evidence of a link between calcium intake and PIH, several clinical trials tested whether calcium supplements could reduce this condition. A meta-analysis of 14 randomized controlled trials showed that supplements providing 375–2000 mg calcium reduced maternal blood pressure and lowered risk of gestational hypertension and preeclampsia to 30–40% of controls (Bucher *et al.*, 1996). The risk of preeclampsia was more reduced in six populations with low-calcium diets than in four groups with higher calcium intakes (Villar and Belizán, 2000). In contrast, the multicenter Calcium for Preeclampsia Prevention (CPEP) trial on 4589 pregnant women in the United States found no effect of 2000 mg/day on blood pressure, PIH or preeclampsia (Levine *et al.*, 1997), possibly because their usual dietary calcium intake averaged ~1100 mg/day.

Iron

On average an additional 6 mg iron per day needs to be absorbed during pregnancy (Hallberg, 1988). Iron is retained by the fetus (300 mg), deposited in the placenta (60 mg), used for the synthesis of additional maternal red blood cells (450 mg), lost in blood during delivery (200 mg), and retained by the mother's increased red cell mass after parturition (200 mg). Serum iron is carried on transferrin to transferrin receptors on the placenta, holotransferrin is endocytosed, iron is released, and apotransferrin is returned to the maternal circulation (Harris, 1992). Iron absorption increases several-fold during the second and third trimesters, and it has been calculated based on absorption data that good maternal diets can supply sufficient iron for pregnancy (Barrett et al., 1994). However, WHO estimates that ~18% of women in industrialized countries and from 35% to 75% of those in developing countries are anemic (ACC/SCN, 2000). The Centers for Disease Control and Prevention estimated that about 10% of low-income women are anemic in the first trimester, 14% in the second and 33% in the third (Kim et al., 1992). In another study, rates of iron deficiency anemia among low-income and minority women were 1.8%, 8.2%, and 27.4%, in the first, second, and third trimester, respectively (Iannotti et al., 2005). A much higher percentage of women become iron depleted by the end of pregnancy. Because of hemodilution the hemoglobin cut-offs that signify anemia are 110 g/L in trimesters 1 and 3 and 105 g/L in trimester 2. Serum ferritin concentrations fall, often to barely detectable levels, but transferrin concentrations are almost doubled.

In many countries, including the United States, iron supplementation is routinely recommended for all pregnant women; they should take an additional 30 mg/day starting at ~12 weeks, since not enough can be readily obtained in food (Institute of Medicine, 2001). Attaining adequate iron status prior to conception is important because it is more difficult to replenish stores during pregnancy when iron requirements are higher. Supplements are better absorbed if taken between meals and without coffee or tea (Institute of Medicine, 1993). Anemic women with low plasma ferritin (<30 μg/L) should take 60 to 120 mg of supplemental iron per day until hemoglobin values become normal. Taking iron once a week can also improve hemoglobin and iron status although 60 mg daily is more effective than 120 mg weekly because of the difficulty of consuming enough during the relatively short period of gestation (Beaton et al., 1992).

The advantages of routine maternal iron supplementation, regardless of iron status, are somewhat controversial (Ziaei et al., 2007) so supplements are not given routinely in some countries, including many in Europe. However, benefits include improved maternal hemoglobin and less risk of anemia and iron depletion in late pregnancy, even in industrialized countries (Allen, 2000; Beard, 2000). Also iron supplementation during pregnancy increases iron stores of the infant for ~6 months, which is an advantage especially in developing countries where complementary foods are low in available iron (Preziosi et al., 1997). Infants are at greatest risk of iron deficiency anemia if they were low birth weight and their mother was anemic (de Pee et al., 2002). Severe anemia probably increases the risk of maternal mortality but whether this is true for moderate anemia is uncertain (Brabin, 2001). Numerous studies report an association between preterm delivery and maternal anemia but this relationship has not been proven to be causal (Rasmussen, 2001).

Zinc

The estimated additional zinc required for pregnancy is ~100 mg, equivalent to 5–7% of the mother's body zinc (Swanson and King, 1987). About half of this zinc is deposited in the fetus, and one-quarter in the uterus. The recommendation is to increase zinc intake by an additional 3 mg/day to a total of 15 mg/day (Institute of Medicine, 2001). Average intakes of pregnant women in the United States are ~10 mg/day with vegetarians consuming much less (Apgar, 1992). Zinc deficiency is more prevalent in populations consuming low amounts of animal-source foods and high amounts of phytate, which inhibits its absorption.

Maternal zinc retention is increased primarily through greater intestinal absorption (King, 2000b). Zinc plays critical roles in cell division, hormone metabolism, protein and carbohydrate metabolism and immunocompetence. Zinc deficiency during pregnancy in animals causes birth defects and intrauterine growth retardation. Of 41 studies that described an association between maternal zinc status and birth weight, 17 found a positive association (Goldenberg et al., 1995; King, 2000b), 10 from industrialized countries and seven from developing countries. Sometimes different studies from the same country found different results. Of 12 randomized, controlled intervention trials, two (in the United States and India) found an increase in birth weight, and six found no effect. There was no impact of 15 or 30 mg zinc daily on gestational age or size at birth in well-designed, controlled studies in Peru and Bangladesh (Caulfield *et al.*, 1999; Osendarp *et al.*, 2000). However, it is prudent to ensure adequate zinc intake for women at higher risk of zinc deficiency; those with low intakes, on high-fiber diets, with high intakes of supplemental calcium, or iron (>30 mg per dose), and with gastrointestinal diseases that lower zinc absorption (King, 2000b).

Iodine

Iodine deficiency during pregnancy causes cretinism and has permanent adverse effects on the growth, development, and cognitive function of the infant. In areas of severe iodine deficiency iodized oil injection prior to midpregnancy produced a marked reduction in cretinism and a 30% reduction in neonatal mortality (Thilly *et al.*, 1978). In the United States and many other countries, iodized salt provides sufficient iodine for pregnant women. The World Health Organization has increased the recommended iodine intake for pregnancy from 200 μg/day to 250 μg/day and states that a urinary iodine excretion of 150–249 μg/L indicates an adequate intake (World Health Organization, 2007). In iodine-depleted populations, i.e. where <90% of households use iodized salt and the median urinary iodine concentration in school-age children is <100 μg/L, the World Health Organization recommends that both pregnant women and their infants be given iodine supplements.

Other Nutrition-Related Conditions

Pregnancy in the Obese Woman

There is general agreement that even moderate degrees of overweight increase the risk of pregnancy complications. Overweight women (BMI ≥25) have about two to six (increasing with higher BMI) times the risk of gestational diabetes, pregnancy hypertension and preeclampsia, diabetes, preterm delivery, and cesarean section compared with those with normal weight (Abenhaim *et al.*, 2007). Their infants are more likely to have low Apgar scores, macrosomia, about three times more perinatal mortality, a higher risk of NTDs, and difficulty in initiating breastfeeding (Hilson *et al.*, 1997). Macrosomic infants are more likely to become obese in later years. Many of these problems are probably caused by the relatively higher plasma insulin concentrations in obese women. Preconceptional counseling about the risks of obesity during pregnancy, followed by dietary counseling and exercise for weight

reduction, is clearly the best preventive strategy. Once they become pregnant, obese women need careful monitoring for diabetes and hypertension, and should be advised to gain lower amounts of weight (see Table 39.2) and to increase exercise.

Gestational Diabetes and Preeclampsia

Gestational diabetes is defined as intolerance to carbohydrate that appears during pregnancy, characterized by higher fasting and postprandial plasma glucose, amino acids (especially branched-chain), and lipids (fatty acids and especially triacylglycerol) (Butte, 2000). Associated risks include large infant birth weight (macrosomia), preeclampsia, and cesarean birth. It may be an extreme manifestation of the normal insulin resistance of pregnancy or reflect a predisposition to type 2 diabetes. Postprandial, but not fasting, concentrations of plasma glucose predict large birth weight. To improve insulin sensitivity and reduce the risk of infant macrosomia, the American College of Obstetricians and Gynecologists recommends spreading snacks and meals across the day, a healthy diet, self-monitoring of glucose and urinary ketones, and exercise (American College of Obstetricians and Gynecologists, 2001). Individuals vary in their needs for insulin therapy and specific dietary changes depending on their weight, blood glucose levels and fluctuations, so consultation with a qualified health-care provider is essential (National Institute of Child Health and Human Development, 2004).

Preeclampsia is a leading cause of maternal and perinatal mortality. Symptoms are the new development of hypertension with proteinuria, edema or both, usually during the third trimester, which can end in eclampsia or severe and potentially fatal seizures. The syndrome involves reduced placental perfusion and maternal endothelial dysfunction. Trials with antioxidant supplements did not reduce risk. Both vitamin D and selenium deficiency have been associated with greater risk but further trials are needed for confirmation. Although the causes of preeclampsia are not yet understood, several risk factors are nutrition-related: maternal obesity, diabetes, hypertension, and hyperhomocysteinemia. Salt restriction is not advised.

Alcohol and Caffeine Abuse

Heavy alcohol consumption in pregnancy has teratogenic effects. Fetal alcohol syndrome affects about 1200 infants annually in the United States. Infants with this condition are typically growth retarded with facial defects, and have abnormalities of the central nervous, cardiac and genitourinary systems. This syndrome affects 10% of women taking 1.5 to 8 alcoholic drinks per week [0.6 oz (15 mL) of absolute alcohol per drink], and 30–40% of those taking >8 drinks a week. The Surgeon General and the March of Dimes advise that no alcohol be consumed during pregnancy. Alcoholic drinks also displace other dietary items and can alter the absorption and metabolism of nutrients. While there is little evidence that multivitamin–mineral supplements counteract the effects of alcohol, it is prudent to advise these supplements for women who continue to abuse alcohol when pregnant.

Caffeine crosses the placenta and affects fetal heart rate and respiration. Large amounts of caffeine are teratogenic in animals. There is limited evidence that moderate coffee intake lowers birth weight in humans. It has not been proven without doubt that caffeine is safe for pregnant women, so the FDA recommends avoiding or limiting coffee in pregnancy. Caffeine consumption should be limited to <300 mg/day, equivalent to two to three cups of coffee, or four cups of tea, or six cola drinks.

Physiology of Lactation

At parturition, major hormonal changes lead to the onset of lactation. Estrogen and progesterone secretion fall markedly while the elevated prolactin concentrations are maintained. Prolactin causes the breasts to begin milk secretion. During the first 2 to 7 days postpartum, colostrum is secreted, a thick yellow fluid containing large amounts of immune factors, protein, minerals, and carotenoids. Colostrum can provide the newborn infant with large amounts of maternal antibodies, important because the immune system does not develop fully for some months. Between about 7 and 21 days postpartum the milk is transitional, and after 21 days mature milk is secreted. Suckling is required to empty the breast, which stimulates continued synthesis of prolactin and maintenance of milk production; once lactation is established suckling once a day can sustain milk production but synthesis stops within a few days of suckling cessation. Continued suckling inhibits release of luteinizing hormone and gonadotropin releasing hormone so the return of ovulation and menses is delayed, providing very effective birth control.

The volume of breast milk secreted increases rapidly to about 500 mL on day 5, 650 mL at 1 month, and 700 mL at 3 months (Neville et al., 1991; Brown et al., 1998). Subsequently the volume is relatively stable but falls during weaning. Although the infant grows continuously larger, its rate of growth declines markedly during the period of lactation, causing a fall in nutrient requirements per unit body weight. Thus, breast-milk production is usually adequate to meet energy and protein requirements of the infant until at least 6 months of age. Mothers can easily produce the amount of milk demanded by their infant, and can feed two or more infants adequately. Exclusive breast feeding is recommended until 6 months of life, and no other fluids or foods should be given. Introducing other liquids or foods introduces sources of infection and contamination, can lower the quantity of nutrients consumed (especially if special infant foods are not used), and may cause premature disruption of milk production. The latest international (WHO) standards for infant growth are based on infants predominantly breastfed for the first 4 to 6 months of life.

Milk Composition

For the purpose of estimating maternal and infant nutrient requirements the IOM estimates that the average volume of milk produced is 780 mL/day during the first 6 months and 600 mL for the second 6 months. Maternal malnutrition must be very severe before milk volume is affected adversely: production is still normal at a BMI of 18.5 kg/m^2. Milk fat content may be reduced by less severe malnutrition, however (Prentice et al., 1994).

The protein content of human milk is about 8–9 g/L, and contains roughly equal amounts (about 25%) of lactalbumin and casein, and substantial quantities of lactoferrin and IgA. It is not affected by maternal undernutrition. Cow's milk contains about 35 g/L protein, mostly casein. Feeding undiluted cow's milk to young infants is inadvisable because of the large osmotic load from protein and other solutes, and the risk of occult fecal blood loss and subsequent iron deficiency (Ziegler et al., 1999). About 25% of the total nitrogen in milk is non-protein nitrogen, mainly urea. Lactose concentrations tend to increase throughout lactation, providing an osmotic balance as the content of protein and monovalent items falls slightly. Lactose provides energy, galactose for central nervous system development, and enhanced growth of beneficial lactobacilli in the infant intestine. Fat provides about half of the energy in breast milk. The average fat content is about 3.8%, but hind milk contains substantially more fat than fore milk. The fatty acid content of the mother's diet affects the amount of fatty acids in her milk.

Vitamins and Minerals

The concentration of several vitamins and minerals in human milk is influenced by maternal diet and/or vitamin status. Table 39.4 summarizes the concentrations of these nutrients in normal milk, and the effect of maternal deficiency and supplementation on milk content and the infant. To predict risks caused by infant or maternal micronutrient deficiencies in lactation, and for planning interventions, it is useful to categorize nutrient deficiencies based on their effect on the nutrient in milk (Allen, 1994). Priority nutrients include vitamin A, thiamin, riboflavin, vitamins B_6 and B_{12}, iodine, and selenium. These nutrients are of most concern because low maternal intake or stores reduces their content in milk, which affects the infant adversely. However, the concentration in milk can be restored rapidly by maternal supplementation. Also infant stores of these nutrients are more readily depleted, increasing the infant's dependence on an adequate supply from breast milk or complementary foods. Lower-priority nutrients include folate, calcium, iron, copper, and zinc. Maternal intake and stores of these nutrients have little or no effect on breast-milk concentrations or infant status, or on the amount required from complementary foods. Consequently the mother is less likely to become depleted, and maternal supplementation is more likely to benefit herself than her infant. Milk vitamin D may be low if women are very deficient but their infants will respond readily to vitamin D supplements.

The deficiencies described in Table 39.4 occur predominantly in developing countries (Allen and Graham, 2003) but several do occur in the United States. Examples include low milk vitamin B_{12} and subsequent infant deficiency as a result of strict maternal vegetarianism (Specker et al., 1990), and low milk vitamin D and abnormal vitamin D status of infants receiving insufficient exposure to sunlight (Specker, 1994). The American Academy of Pediatrics recommends that all infants who are breastfed should receive 400 IU vitamin D per day as a supplement (Wagner et al., 2008). Infants fed formula but drinking <1 L (1 quart) per day should also receive supplemental vitamin D.

Low concentrations of nutrients in breast milk imply that maternal and/or infant supplementation is needed; breastfeeding is always the best way to feed young infants. Vitamin A in breast milk is adequate in industrialized countries, but high-dose (200 000 to 300 000 IU) vitamin A supplementation during the first 6 weeks postpartum, while there is minimal chance of conception, is recommended by WHO for increasing breast milk retinol and improving infant vitamin A status in developing countries (Stoltzfus et al., 1993). Vitamin B_{12} concentrations in milk from Guatemalan women were one-tenth of those in California, and correlated with both maternal and infant serum B_{12} with both groups having a high prevalence of deficiency (Allen et al., 2009). Human milk provides sufficient fluoride for the first 6 months of life, but the infant should be given 0.05 mg/kg/day starting at age 6 months. Iodine can be very low in breast milk in populations with endemic iodine deficiency, and infants and young children consume little iodized salt. Even in Switzerland, for example, weaning infants are at risk of iodine deficiency, especially if they are not consuming infant formulas (Andersson et al., 2010).

Maternal Nutrient Requirements During Lactation

The daily nutrient requirements of the lactating woman are higher than requirements during pregnancy. The higher recommended intakes are based primarily on the amounts secreted in milk. The most recent RDAs assume that the mother secretes about 500 kcal/day in milk, including about 5% as protein, more than 50% as fat, and 38% as lactose (Institute of Medicine, 2002/2005). This falls to 400 kcal/day in the second 6 months. In the first 6 months about 170 kcal/day are obtained from maternal weight loss. Thus the energy requirements in lactation are higher than those of the non-pregnant woman by 330 kcal/day in the first 6 months and 400 kcal/day in the second 6 months. Energy restriction to induce weight loss should not be attempted while breast feeding due to the risk of inadequate intakes of other nutrients in the diet. Exclusive breastfeeding and exercise, combined with a high quality diet, should lead to gradual weight loss during the postpartum period. Recommended protein intakes are increased from 0.8 g/kg/day in the non-lactating woman to 1.3 g/kg in lactation, or by 25 g/day.

The recommended intake of most micronutrients is also increased to cover the amounts secreted in milk (Table 39.3). The only nutrient that is needed in lower amounts during lactation is iron, except for women who need to synthesize large amounts of blood to replace major blood losses during delivery. Bone mineral content

TABLE 39.4 Effects of maternal micronutrient deficiencies and supplements during lactation on breast milk and infant micronutrient status

Nutrient	Normal milk concentration	Effect of maternal deficiency on milk content	Effect of maternal deficiency on infant	Effect of maternal supplementation on milk content	Effect of maternal supplementation on infant
Vitamin A, µg RE/L	500	↓ to 170–500	Low serum retinol, depletion	↑	↑Serum retinol and liver stores for 2–3 months after massive dose
Vitamin D, µg/L	0.55	↓ to 0.25	↑Risk of rickets depending on UV light exposure	↑	↑Serum 25(OH)D if dose >2000IU/day
Thiamin, mg/L	0.21	↓ to 0.11	Beri-beri	↑ to normal	↓Infant beri-beri
Riboflavin, mg/L	0.35	↓ to 0.2	High EGRAC[a]	↑	↓EGRAC in mother and infant
Vitamin B6, mg/L	0.93	↓ to 0.9	Neurological problems	↑	↓Neurological problems
Folate, µg/L	85	No change	Unknown		None, but ↑ maternal status
Vitamin B12, µg/L	0.97	↓ to <0.5	↑Urine MMA[b], neurological problems, developmental delays	↑	↓MMA
Ascorbic acid, mg/L	40	↓ to 25	Unknown	↑(small)	?
Calcium, mg/L	280	↓ to 215	↓Bone mineral but relative in utero vs. postpartum influence unclear	None	None
Iron, mg/L	0.3	No change	None	None	None
Zinc, mg/L	1.2	No change	None	None	None
Copper, mg/L	0.25	No change	None	None	None
Iodine, µg/L	110	No change/slight ↓	Uncertain; deficiency in pregnancy more important	↑	Unknown
Selenium, µg/L	20	↓ to ≤10	↓Plasma and RBC content	↑	Unknown

[a]EGRAC, erythrocyte glutathione reductase activity coefficient.
[b]MMA, methylmalonic acid.
Adapted from Allen (1994) and Allen and Graham (2003).

and urinary calcium fall during lactation to meet the additional calcium requirements for milk production (Prentice, 2000). The loss in mineral content is temporary, and it is gradually regained by about 3 months after weaning. Higher intakes of calcium than the recommended 1000 mg/day do not affect these lactation-associated changes in maternal bone turnover, bone mineral content, or the amount of calcium in breast milk (Institute of Medicine, 2011).

Future Directions

Although the risk for many adverse pregnancy outcomes are clearly higher in women who are undernourished or consume poor diets, much work remains to be done to confirm observed or hypothesized links between the importance of specific nutrients in causing or preventing (when supplemented) outcomes such as low birth weight, preeclampsia, and preterm delivery. In lactation, one important question is the extent to which the concentration of nutrients in breast milk from undernourished women is inadequate to support optimum infant growth and development, and whether and when maternal supplementation can prevent this potential problem.

Suggestions for Further Reading

Bhatia, J. (2005) *Perinatal Nutrition. Optimizing Infant Health and Development*. Marcel Dekker, New York.

Institute of Medicine (2009) *Weight Gain During Pregnancy: Reexamining the Guidelines*. National Academies Press, Washington, DC.

Kaiser, L.L and Allen, L.H. (2002) Position of the American Dietetic Association: nutrition and lifestyle for a healthy pregnancy outcome. *J Am Diet Assoc* **102**, 1479–1490.

References

Abenhaim, H.A., Kinch, R.A., Morin, L., *et al.* (2007) Effect of prepregnancy body mass index categories on obstetrical and neonatal outcomes. *Arch Gynecol Obstet* **275**, 39–43.

ACC/SCN (2000) *Fourth Report on the World Nutrition Situation*. Geneva.

Allen, L.H. (1994) Maternal micronutrient malnutrition: Effects on breast milk and infant nutrition, and priorities for intervention. *ACC/SCN Second Report on the World Nutrition Situation* **1**, 21–24.

Allen, L.H. (2000) Anemia and iron deficiency: effects on pregnancy outcome. *Am J Clin Nutr* **71**(Suppl), 1280S–1284S.

Allen, L.H. and Graham, J.M. (2003) Assuring micronutrient adequacy in the diets of young infants. In. F.M. Delange and K.P.J. West (eds), *Micronutrient Deficiencies in the First Six Months of Life*. S. Karger AG, Basel, pp. 55–88.

Allen, L.H., Deegan, K.L., Jones, K.M., *et al.* (2009) Breast milk vitamin B$_{12}$ concentrations in Guatemala: relationship to maternal and infant intake and status. *FASEB J* **23**, 344.3.

American College of Obstetricians and Gynecologists Committee on Practice Bulletins – Obstetrics (2001) ACOG Practice Bulletin. Clinical management guidelines for obstetrician-gynecologists. Number 30, September 2001 (replaces Technical Bulletin Number 200, December 1994). Gestational diabetes. *Obstet Gynecol* **98**, 525–538.

Andersson, M., Aeberli, I., Wüst, N., *et al.* (2010) The Swiss Iodized Salt Program provides adequate iodine for school children and pregnant women, but weaning infants not receiving iodine-containing complementary foods as well as their mothers are iodine deficient. *J Clin Endocrinol Metab* **95**, 5217–5224.

Apgar, J. (1992) Zinc and reproduction: an update. *J Nutr Biochem* **3**, 266–278.

Azaïs-Braesco, V. and Pascal, G. (2000) Vitamin A in pregnancy: requirements and safety limits. *Am J Clin Nutr* **71**, 1325S–1333S.

Barrett, J.F., Whittaker, P.G., and Williams, J.G. (1994) Absorption of non-haem iron from food during normal pregnancy. *BMJ* **309**, 79–82.

Beard, J.L. (2000) Effectiveness and strategies of iron supplementation during pregnancy. *Am J Clin Nutr* **71**, 1288S–1294S.

Beaton, G.H., Martorell, R., L'Abbé, K.A., *et al.* (1992) *Effectiveness of Vitamin A Supplementation in the Control of Young Child Morbidity and Mortality in Developing Countries*. University of Toronto, Toronto.

Beaudin, A.E., Abarinov, E.V., Noden, D.M. *et al.* (2011) Shmt1 and de novo thymidylate biosynthesis underlie folate-responsive neural tube defects in mice. *Am J Clin Nutr* **93**, 789–798.

Berry, R.J., Li, Z., Erickson, J.D., *et al.* (1999) Prevention of neural-tube defects with folic acid in China. China–U.S. Collaborative Project for Neural Tube Defect Prevention. *N Engl J Med* **341**, 1485–1490.

Brabin, B.J. (2001) An analysis of anemia and pregnancy-related maternal mortality. *J Nutr* **131**, 604S–614S.

Bronstein, M.N., Mak, R.P., and King, J.C. (1996) Unexpected relationship between fat mass and basal metabolic rate in pregnant women. *Br J Nutr* **75**, 659–668.

Brown, K.H., Dewey, K.G., and Allen, L.H. (1998) *Complementary Feeding of Young Children in Developing Countries: A Review of Current Scientific Knowledge*. World Health Organization, Geneva.

Bucher, H.C., Cook, R.J., Guyatt, G.H., *et al.* (1996) Effects of dietary calcium supplementation on blood pressure. A meta-analysis of randomized controlled trials. *JAMA* **275**, 1016–1022.

Butte, N.F. (2000) Carbohydrate and lipid metabolism in pregnancy: normal compared with gestational diabetes mellitus. *Am J Clin Nutr* **71**, 1256S–1261S.

Caulfield, L.E., Zavaleta, N., Figueroa, A., *et al.* (1999) Maternal zinc supplementation does not affect size at birth or pregnancy duration in Peru. *J Nutr* **129**, 1563–1568.

Ceesay, S.M., Prentice, A.M., Cole, T.J., *et al.* (1997) Effects on birth weight and perinatal mortality of maternal dietary supplements in rural Gambia: 5 year randomised controlled trial. *BMJ* **315**, 786–790.

Chang, S.J. (1999) Adequacy of maternal pyridoxine supplementation during pregnancy in relation to the vitamin B6 status and growth of neonates at birth. *J Nutr Sci Vitaminol* **45**, 449–458.

Crider, K.S., Bailey, L.B., and Berry, R.J. (2011) Folic acid fortification – its history, effect, concerns, and future directions. *Nutrients* **3**, 370–374.

Daly, L.E., Kirke, P.N., Molloy, A., *et al.* (1995) Folate levels and neural tube defects. Implications for prevention. *JAMA* **274**, 1698–1702.

de Pee, S., Bloem, M.W., Sari, M., *et al.* (2002) The high prevalence of low hemoglobin concentration among Indonesian infants aged 3–5 months is related to maternal anemia. *J Nutr* **132**, 2215–2221.

Dror, D., King, J.C., Durand, D.J., *et al.* (2011) Association of modifiable and nonmodifiable factors with vitamin D status in pregnant women and neonates in Oakland, CA. *J Am Diet Assoc* **111**, 111–116.

Dror, D.K. and Allen, L.H. (2010) Vitamin D adequacy in pregnancy: biology, outcomes, and interventions. *Nutr Rev* **68**, 465–477.

Godfrey, K.M. and Barker, D.J. (2000) Fetal nutrition and adult disease. *Am J Clin Nutr* **71**, 1344S–1352S.

Goldenberg, R.L., Tamura, T., Neggers, Y., *et al.* (1995) The effect of zinc supplementation on pregnancy outcome. *JAMA* **274**, 463–468.

Gülmezoglu, M., de Onis, M., and Villar, J. (1997) Effectiveness of interventions to prevent or treat impaired fetal growth. *Obstet Gynecol Surv* **52**, 139–149.

Hallberg, L. (1988) Iron balance in pregnancy. In H. Berger (ed.), *Vitamins and Minerals in Pregnancy and Lactation*. Raven Press, New York, pp. 115–127.

Harris, E.D. (1992) New insights into placental iron transport. *Nutr Rev* **50**, 329–331.

Heseker, H.B., Mason, J.B., Selhub, J., *et al.* (2009) Not all cases of neural tube defect can be prevented by increasing the intake of folic acid. *Br J Nutr* **102**, 173–180.

Hilson J. A., Rasmussen, K.M., Kjolhede, C.L. (1997) Maternal obesity and breast-feeding success in a rural population of white women. *Am J Clin Nutr* **66**, 1371–1378.

Hornstra, G. (2000) Essential fatty acids in mothers and their neonates. *Am J Clin Nutr* **71**, 1262S–1269S.

Iannotti, L.L., O'Brien, K.O., Chang, S.-H., *et al.* (2005) Iron deficiency anemia and depleted body iron reserves are prevalent among African-American adolescents. *J Nutr* **135**, 2572–2577.

Institute of Medicine (1993) *Iron Deficiency Anemia: Recommended Guidelines for the Prevention, Detection, and Management among US Children and Women of Child Bearing Age*. National Academies Press, Washington, DC.

Institute of Medicine (1999) *Dietary Reference Intakes. Thiamin, Riboflavin, Niacin, Vitamin B6, Folate, Vitamin B12, Pantothenic Acid, Biotin, and Choline*. National Academies Press, Washington, DC.

Institute of Medicine (2000) *Dietary Reference Intakes for Vitamin C, Vitamin E, Selenium, and Carotenoids*. National Academies Press, Washington, DC.

Institute of Medicine (2001) *Dietary Reference Intakes for Vitamin A, Vitamin K, Arsenic, Boron, Chromium, Copper, Iodine, Iron, Manganese, Molybdenum, Nickel, Silicon, Vanadium, and Zinc*. National Academies Press, Washington, DC.

Institute of Medicine (2002/2005) *Dietary Reference Intakes for Energy, Carbohydrate, Fiber, Fat, Fatty Acids, Cholesterol, Protein, and Amino Acids*. National Academies Press, Washington, DC.

Institute of Medicine (2009) *Weight Gain During Pregnancy: Reexamining the Guidelines*. National Academies Press, Washington, DC.

Institute of Medicine (2011) *Dietary Reference Intakes for Calcium and Vitamin D*. National Academies Press, Washington, DC.

Jarjou, L.M.A., Prentice, A., Sawo, Y., *et al.* (2006) Randomized, placebo-controlled, calcium supplementation study in pregnant Gambian women: effects on breast milk calcium concentrations and infant birth weight, growth, and bone mineral accretion in the first year of life. *Am J Clin Nutr* **83**, 657–666.

Kalhan, S.C. (2000) Protein metabolism in pregnancy. *Am J Clin Nutr* **71**, 1249S–1255S.

Kim, I., Hungerford, R., and Yip, R. (1992) Pregnancy nutrition surveillance system–United States, 1979–1990. *MMWR CDC Surveill Summ* **41**, 25–41.

King, J.C. (2000a) Physiology of pregnancy and nutrient metabolism. *Am J Clin Nutr* **71**, 1218S–1225S.

King, J.C. (2000b) Determinants of maternal zinc status during pregnancy. *Am J Clin Nutr* **71**, 1334S–1343S.

Langley-Evans, S.C. (2006) *Fetal Programming and Adult Disease. Programming of Chronic Disease through Fetal Exposure to Undernutrition.* CABI Publishing, Wallingford.

Levine, R.J., Hauth, J.C., Curet, L.B., *et al.* (1997) Trial of calcium to prevent preeclampsia. *N Engl J Med* **337**, 69–76.

Moore, S.E. (1998) Nutrition, immunity and the fetal and infant origins of disease hypothesis in developing countries. *Proc Nutr Soc* **57**, 241–247.

National Institute of Child Health and Human Development (2004) *Managing Gestational Diabetes.* Washington, DC.

Neville, M.C., Allen, J.C., Archer, P.C., *et al.* (1991) Studies in human lactation: milk volume and nutrient composition during weaning and lactogenesis. *Am J Clin Nutr* **54**, 81–92.

North Carolina State Department of Health and Human Services (2010) *Prenatal Weight Gain Charts.* http://www.nal.usda.gov/wicworks/Sharing_Center/NY/prenatalwt_charts.pdf

Osendarp, S.J., van Raaij, J.M., Arifeen, S.E., *et al.* (2000) A randomized, placebo-controlled trial of the effect of zinc supplementation during pregnancy on pregnancy outcome in Bangladeshi urban poor. *Am J Clin Nutr* **71**, 114–119.

Prentice, A. (2000) Maternal calcium metabolism and bone mineral status. *Am J Clin Nutr* **71**, 1312S–1316S.

Prentice, A.M. and Goldberg, G.R. (2000) Energy adaptations in human pregnancy: limits and long-term consequences. *Am J Clin Nutr* **71**, 1226S–1232S.

Prentice, A.M., Goldberg, G.R., and Prentice, A. (1994) Body mass index and lactation performance. *Eur J Clin Nutr* **48**(Suppl 3), S78–S86.

Prentice, A.M., Rayco-Solon, P. and Moore, S.E. (2005) Insights from the developing world: thrifty genotypes and thrifty phenotypes. *Proc Nutr Soc* **64**, 153–161.

Preziosi, P., Prual, A., Galan, P., *et al.* (1997) Effect of iron supplementation on the iron status of pregnant women: consequences for newborns. *Am J Clin Nutr* **66**, 1178–1182.

Rasmussen, K.M. (2001) Is there a causal relationship between iron deficiency or iron-deficiency anemia and weight at birth, length of gestation and perinatal mortality? *J Nutr* **131**, 590S–603S.

Ritchie, L.D., Fung, E.B., Halloran, B.P., *et al.* (1998) A longitudinal study of calcium homeostasis during human pregnancy and lactation and after resumption of menses. *Am J Clin Nutr* **67**, 693–701.

Rothman, K.J., Moore, L.L., Singer, M.R., *et al.* (1995) Teratogenicity of high vitamin A intake. *N Engl J Med* **333**, 1369–1373.

Schenker, S., Johnson, R.F., Mahuren, J.D., *et al.* (1992) Human placental vitamin B6 (pyridoxal) transport: normal characteristics and effects of ethanol. *Am J Physiol* **262**, R966–974.

Scholl, T.O., Hediger, M.L., Bendich, A., *et al.* (1997) Use of multivitamin/mineral prenatal supplements: influence on the outcome of pregnancy. *Am J Epidemiol* **146**, 134–141.

Shaw, G.M., Schaffer, D., Velie, E.M., *et al.* (1995) Periconceptional vitamin use, dietary folate, and the occurrence of neural tube defects. *Epidemiology* **6**, 219–226.

Specker, B.L. (1994) Do North American women need supplemental vitamin D during pregnancy or lactation? *Am J Clin Nutr* **59**, 490S–491S.

Specker, B.L., Black, A., Allen, L.H., *et al.* (1990) Vitamin B-12: low milk concentrations are related to low serum concentrations in vegetarian women and to methylmalonic aciduria in their infants. *Am J Clin Nutr* **52**, 1073–1076.

Specker, B.L., Ho, M.L., Oestreich, A., *et al.* (1992) Prospective study of vitamin D supplementation and rickets in China. *J Pediatr* **120**, 733–739.

Stoltzfus, R.J., Hakimi, M., Miller, K.W., *et al.* (1993) High dose vitamin A supplementation of breast-feeding Indonesian mothers: effects on the vitamin A status of mother and infant. *J Nutr* **123**, 666–675.

Swanson, C.A. and King, J.C. (1987) Zinc and pregnancy outcome. *Am J Clin Nutr* **46**, 763–771.

Thilly, C.H., Delange, F., Lagasse, R., *et al.* (1978) Fetal hypothyroidism and maternal thyroid status in severe endemic goiter. *J Clin Endocrinol Metab* **47**, 354–360.

USDA Nutrition Evidence Library (2010) What effect has folic acid fortification policy had on serum folate, plasma and/or red blood cell folate status of US and Canadian men, women, and children? http://www.nel.gov/evidence.cfm?evidence_summary_id=250078.

Villar, J. and Belizán, J.M. (2000) Same nutrient, different hypotheses: disparities in trials of calcium supplementation during pregnancy. *Am J Clin Nutr* **71**, 1375S–1379S.

Vollset, S.E., Refsum, H., Irgens, L.M., *et al.* (2000) Plasma total homocysteine, pregnancy complications, and adverse pregnancy outcomes: the Hordaland homocysteine study. *Am J Clin Nutr* **71**, 962–968.

Wagner, C.L., Greer, F., and the Section on Breastfeeding and Committee on Nutrition. (2008). Prevention of rickets and vitamin D deficiency in infants, children, and adolescents. *Pediatrics* **122**, 1142–1152.

Wells, J.C. (2010) The thrifty phenotype: an adaptation in growth or metabolism? *Am J Hum Biol* **23**, 65–75.

Werler, M.M., Shapiro, S., and Mitchell, A.A. (1993) Periconceptional folic acid exposure and risk of occurrent neural tube defects. *JAMA* **269,** 1257–1261.

West, K.P., Jr, Katz, J., Khatry, S.K., *et al.* (1999) Double blind, cluster randomised trial of low dose supplementation with vitamin A or beta carotene on mortality related to pregnancy in Nepal. The NNIPS-2 Study Group. *BMJ* **318,** 570–575.

World Health Organization (1998) *Safe Vitamin A Dosage during Pregnancy and Lactation. Recommendations and Report from a Consultation.* World Health Organization, Geneva.

World Health Organization (2007) *United Nations Children's Fund and International Council for the Control of Iodine Deficiency Disorders. Assessment of Iodine Deficiency Disorders and Monitoring their Elimination,* 2nd Edn. World Health Organization, Geneva.

Zeghoud, F., Vervel, C., Guillozo, H., *et al.* (1997) Subclinical vitamin D deficiency in neonates: definition and response to vitamin D supplements. *Am J Clin Nutr* **65,** 771–778.

Ziaei, S., Norrozi, M., Faghihzadeh, S., *et al.* (2007) A randomised placebo-controlled trial to determine the effect of iron supplementation on pregnancy outcome in pregnant women with haemoglobin = 13.2 g/dl. *BJOG* **114,** 684–688.

Ziegler, E.E., Jiang, T., Romero, E., *et al.* (1999) Cow's milk and intestinal blood loss in late infancy. *J Pediatr* **135,** 720–726.

40

INFANT NUTRITION

WILLIAM C. HEIRD, MD

Baylor College of Medicine, Houston, Texas, USA

Summary

The normal infant experiences a three-fold increase in weight and a two-fold increase in length during the first year of life, and also experiences dramatic developmental changes in organ function and body composition. These rapid rates of growth and development are superimposed on relatively high maintenance needs incident to the higher metabolic and nutrient turnover rates of infants vs. adults. Despite these unique nutritional needs, reference nutrient intakes for the 0- to 6- and the 7- to 12-month-old infant have been established. Some of these as well as specific issues relevant to infant nutrition, e.g. breast vs. formula feeding, introduction of complementary foods, use of formula vs. bovine milk, and the need for preformed long-chain polyunsaturated fatty acids (LC-PUFA), are discussed in this chapter. These discussions are preceded by a discussion of the differences among requirement, recommended intake, and reference intake.

Introduction

The "requirement" of a specific nutrient is the amount of that nutrient that results in some predetermined physiological endpoint. In infants, this endpoint is usually maintenance of satisfactory rates of growth and development and/or prevention of specific signs of deficiency. The requirement of a specific nutrient is usually defined experimentally, often in a relatively small study population. Thus, the mean requirement of a specific nutrient estimated in this way (the estimated average requirement, or EAR) usually meets the needs of roughly half the population. For some, it may be inadequate whereas, for others, it may be excessive.

In contrast, the recommended daily allowance (RDA) of a specific nutrient is the intake of that nutrient deemed by a scientifically knowledgeable group to meet the "requirement" of most healthy members of a population. If the EAR of a specific nutrient is normally distributed within the population, the RDA usually is set at the EAR of the population plus 2 standard deviations (SD). Since the EARs of many nutrients are not normally distributed, other considerations of population variability frequently are necessary. For example, if the EAR appears to be adequate for most of the population, the RDA may be less than the requirement plus 2 SD.

RDAs are useful guides for nutrient intakes of individuals but they are not useful for ascertaining the adequacy

Present Knowledge in Nutrition, Tenth Edition. Edited by John W. Erdman Jr, Ian A. Macdonald and Steven H. Zeisel.

or inadequacy of an individual's intake of a specific nutrient. Moreover, since the EAR of many nutrients is not known with certainty, it is often difficult to establish an RDA.

Because of the difficulties in establishing an EAR and the uncertainty of an RDA based on limited information concerning requirement, the Food and Nutrition Board, Institute of Medicine (USA) has established dietary reference intakes (DRIs). These include RDAs for the few nutrients for which an RDA can be established as well as other "reference intakes" such as adequate intake (AI) and tolerable upper intake level (UL).

AI, used when an RDA cannot be determined, is the observed or approximated daily intake of a specific nutrient by a group of healthy individuals, e.g. the intake of the breast-fed infant which is the basis of the most recent DRIs for infants under 6 months of age.

The UL is the highest intake of a specific nutrient likely to pose no risk. The UL is not a recommended level of intake but, rather, an aid in avoiding adverse effects secondary to excessive intake.

The DRIs established by the Food and Nutrition Board of the Institute of Medicine (Institute of Medicine, 1998, 2000, 2001, 2002, 2004, 2011a,b), for 0- to 6-month-old and 7- to 12-month-old infants are summarized in Table 40.1.

Dietary Reference Intakes of Specific Nutrients

Energy

Since an energy intake that is adequate for almost all individuals will result in excessive weight gain by individuals with a low or average requirement, the reference energy intakes reflect the "estimated" energy requirement (EER), i.e. the energy intake predicted to maintain energy balance in a healthy individual of a defined age, gender, weight, height, and level of physical activity. The EERs are based on predictive equations for normal-weight individuals that include daily energy expenditure measured by the doubly labeled water method plus an allowance for energy deposition. Since an RDA will exceed the EER of many individuals and result in excessive weight gain, setting an RDA for energy would only contribute to the growing prevalence of overweight and obesity. Similarly, the UL is not appropriate for energy because any intake above the EER will result in excessive weight gain.

TABLE 40.1 Reference intakes of nutrients for normal infants

Nutrient[a]	Intake per day	
	0–6 months	7–12 months
Energy [kcal (kJ)][b]		
Males	570 (2385)	743 (3109)
Females	520 (2176)	676 (2829)
Fat (g)	31	30
Carbohydrate	60	95
Protein (g) +	9.1	13.5
Electrolytes and minerals		
Calcium (mg)	210	270
Phosphorus (mg)	100	275
Magnesium (mg)	30	75
Sodium (mg)	115	368
Chloride (mg)	178	568
Potassium (mg)	390	702
Iron (mg)	0.27	11[c] (5)
Zinc (mg)	2	3[c] (5)
Copper (µg)	200	220
Iodine (µg)	110	130
Selenium (µg)	15	20
Manganese (mg)	0.003	0.6
Fluoride (mg)	0.01	0.5
Chromium (µg)	0.2	5.5
Molybdenum (µg)	2	3
Vitamins		
Vitamin A (µg)	400	500
Vitamin D (µg)	5	5
Vitamin E (mg α-TE)	4	6
Vitamin K (µg)	2.0	2.5
Vitamin C (mg)	40	50
Thiamine (mg)	0.2	0.3
Riboflavin (mg)	0.3	0.4
Niacin (mg NE)	2	4
Vitamin B_6 (µg)	0.1	0.3
Folate (µg)	65	80
Vitamin B_{12} (µg)	0.4	0.5
Biotin (µg)	5	6
Pantothenic acid (mg)	1.7	1.8
Choline (mg)	125	150

[a]Unless indicated otherwise, values are adequate intake (AI) (e.g. mean intake of normal breast-fed infants 0–6 months of age or mean intake of 7- to 12-month-old infants from human milk plus complementary foods).
[b]Estimated energy requirement.
[c]RDA.
Data from Institute of Medicine (1998, 2000, 2001, 2002, 2004, 2011).

Expressed per unit of body weight, the EER of the normal newborn infant is about twice that of the normal adult. The greater energy requirement reflects primarily the higher metabolic rate of the infant and the special needs for growth and development. The inefficient intestinal absorption of the infant vs. the adult contributes only minimally to the higher energy requirement of infants fed human milk or modern infant formula.

There is no evidence that either carbohydrate or fat is a superior source of energy. Sufficient carbohydrate to prevent ketosis and/or hypoglycemia is necessary (~5.0 g/kg/day) as is enough fat to provide essential fatty acid requirements (0.5–1.0 g/kg/day of linoleic acid [LA] plus a smaller amount of α-linolenic acid [ALA]). As discussed below, there is concern that infants may require long-chain polyunsaturated omega-3 and, perhaps, omega-6 fatty acids.

In toto, the minimum needs for carbohydrate and fat amount to no more than ~30 kcal (125.5 kJ)/kg/day, or only approximately a third of the infant's total energy need. Whether the remainder should be comprised of fat or equicaloric amounts of fat and carbohydrate is not known. The acceptable macronutrient distribution range (AMDR) for carbohydrate and fat specified by the Food and Nutrition Board, Institute of Medicine (2002), is 20–25% of total energy as fat and 45–65% of total energy as carbohydrate. While appropriate for older children and adults, the "acceptable" range for fat is lower than conventional intake for infants. Human milk and most currently available formulas contain equicaloric amounts of fat and carbohydrate. This distribution, ~45% of total energy as carbohydrate and ~45% as fat, seems appropriate.

The AI for omega-6 fatty acids (linoleic acid) is 4.4 g/day and 4.6 g/day, respectively, for the 0- to 6-month-old and the 7- to 12-month-old infant. The AI for omega-3 fatty acids (α-linolenic acid) is 0.5 g/day for both age groups. These reference intakes are based on the intake of these fatty acids in the average volume of human milk ingested from 4 to 6 months of age and the average intake from human milk plus complementary foods from 7 to 12 months of age.

Protein

The protein requirement of the normal infant also is greater per unit of body weight than that of the adult. In addition, it is thought that the infant requires a higher proportion of essential amino acids than the adult. These include the amino acids recognized as essential (or indis-

pensable) for the adult (i.e. leucine, isoleucine, valine, threonine, methionine, phenylalanine, tryptophan, lysine, and histidine) as well as cysteine and tyrosine. The need for cysteine is thought to reflect the fact that the hepatic activity of cystathionase, a key enzyme in conversion of methionine to cysteine, does not reach adult levels until at least 4 months of age (Sturman *et al.*, 1970; Gaull *et al.*, 1972). The reason for the infant's apparent need for tyrosine is not clear. Recent studies show that even preterm infants can convert phenylalanine to tyrosine (Räihä, 1973; Kilani *et al.*, 1995; Denne *et al.*, 1996).

Human milk protein and all proteins currently used in infant formulas contain adequate amounts of all essential amino acids, i.e. the amounts of each in the volume of human milk necessary to provide the AI for protein intake of the 0- to 6-month-old infant and the RDA for protein intake of the 7- to 12-month-old infant, which is set at the amount deposited in body protein by infants of this age corrected for efficiency plus the same maintenance needs as the adult (Institute of Medicine, 2002).

The required intake of a specific protein depends upon how closely its amino acid pattern resembles that of human milk. Further, the overall quality of a specific protein can be improved by supplementing it with the essential amino acid(s) that result(s) in its quality being low, i.e. the limiting amino acid. Native soy protein, for example, has insufficient methionine but, when fortified with methionine, the quality approaches or equals that of bovine milk protein (Fomon *et al.*, 1973).

The protein sources of most infant formulas, i.e. bovine milk protein and modern preparations of soy protein, like human milk protein, are very high quality proteins. Further, if properly processed, these proteins are utilized nearly as well as human milk protein. Thus, the amounts of these proteins needed are not much higher than the amount of human milk protein needed (Räihä, 1985). The recent DRIs for protein are considerably lower than previous RDAs (i.e. ~1.5 vs. 2.2 g/kg/day) throughout the first year of life.

Electrolytes, Minerals, and Vitamins

The normal infant's needs for electrolytes, minerals, and vitamins are not as well defined as those for energy and protein. Reference intakes, therefore, are usually the mean intake of each by normally growing 0- to 6-month-old, breast-fed infants or the mean intake of each from human milk and complementary food by the 7- to 12-month-old infant (Table 40.1).

Although the normal newborn infant is thought to have sufficient stores of iron to meet requirements for 4 to 6 months, iron deficiency remains the most common nutrient deficiency syndrome in infancy. This reflects the fact that iron stores at birth as well as the absorption of iron are quite variable. Interestingly, although human milk contains less iron than most formulas, iron deficiency is less common in breast-fed infants. To prevent iron deficiency, routine iron supplementation of breast-fed infants and use of iron-fortified formulas for formula-fed infants is recommended (Committee on Nutrition, AAP, 2009a). The use of iron-fortified formulas in recent decades has dramatically reduced the incidence of iron deficiency and resultant neurodevelopmental delay.

If protein intake is adequate, vitamin deficiencies are rare; if not, deficiencies of nicotinic acid and choline, which are synthesized, respectively, from tryptophan and methionine, may develop. In contrast, if bovine milk and bovine milk formulas were not supplemented with vitamin D, hypovitaminosis D would be endemic among formula-fed infants, particularly those with limited exposure to sunlight. Since breast-fed infants may be as susceptible to development of vitamin D deficiency, routine vitamin D supplementation of breast-fed infants is recommended, particularly if exposure to sunlight is limited (Committee on Nutrition, AAP, 2009b; Institute of Medicine, 2011b).

Routine perinatal administration of vitamin K is recommended as prophylaxis against hemorrhagic disease of the newborn. Thereafter, deficiency of this vitamin is uncommon except in infants with conditions associated with fat malabsorption.

Water

The normal infant's absolute requirement for water probably is considerably less than the DRIs, i.e. 700 mL/day for the 0- to 6-month-old and 800 mL/day for the 7- to 12-month-old. These are the amounts provided by the mean human milk intake of the 0- to 6-month-old and the mean intake of the 7- to 12-month-old from human milk plus complementary food. Because of higher obligate renal, pulmonary and dermal water losses as well as a higher overall metabolic rate, the infant is more susceptible to development of dehydration, with vomiting and/or diarrhea, particularly if solute intake is high. Thus, intake of high-solute foods (e.g. bovine milk) before a year of age is discouraged. The typical breast-fed infant or formula-fed infant usually consumes at least 150 mL/kg/day for the first several weeks of life. Although somewhat higher than the AI, there is no reason to believe that a fluid intake of this amount is excessive.

Feeding in the Second 6 Months of Life

By 6 months of age, the infant's capacity to digest and absorb a variety of dietary components as well as to metabolize, utilize, and excrete the absorbed products of digestion is near the capacity of the adult (Montgomery, 1991). Moreover, the infant is more active and beginning to explore his/her surroundings. With the eruption of teeth, the role of dietary carbohydrate in development of dental caries must be considered (Mandel, 1991). Consideration of the long-term effects of inadequate or excessive intake during infancy also assumes greater importance as does the psychosocial role of foods.

These latter considerations, rather than concerns about adequate amounts of nutrients, are the basis for many feeding practices advocated for the formula-fed infant during the second 6 months of life. While it is clear that all nutrient needs during this period can be met with reasonable amounts of currently available infant formulas, addition of other foods after 6 months of age is recommended. In contrast, the volume of milk produced by many women does not meet all nutrient needs of the breast-fed infant beyond 6 months of age. Thus, for these infants, complementary foods are an important source of nutrients.

By approximately 12 months of age, most infants have graduated successfully to table food and are content with three meals plus two to three snacks daily. Once a few teeth have erupted and tolerance of solid foods has been demonstrated, weaning can be completed.

Weaning or "follow-on" formulas are popular in many countries. These contain somewhat more protein than standard infant formulas. They also may have a lower fat content and a somewhat higher carbohydrate content. The types of fat and carbohydrate present are similar to those of standard infant formulas (vegetable oils and lactose plus corn-syrup solids). There is no convincing evidence that these formulas are superior to standard infant formulas or bovine milk.

Aside from the association of bottle feeding with dental caries (Mandel, 1991), little is known about either the potential hazards or the non-nutritional role of diet during the latter half of the first year of life. Thus, feeding practices during this period vary widely. None the less, recent surveys indicate that infants fed according to current practices in the United States receive the reference intakes for most nutrients (Devaney *et al.*, 2004).

Human Milk vs. Artificial Formula

The ready availability and safety of human milk coupled with the possibility that it may enhance intestinal development, resistance to infection and bonding between the mother and infant make human milk the perfect food for the normal infant. Thus, exclusive breastfeeding for the first 6 months of life with continued breastfeeding throughout the first year of life or longer is recommended (World Health Organization, 1995; Work Group on Breastfeeding, AAP, 1997). This recommendation is supported by evidence that breast-fed infants in both affluent and developing societies have fewer infections during early life than formula-fed infants (Kovar *et al.*, 1984; Brown *et al.*, 1989).

Despite this, it cannot automatically be assumed that maternal milk supply will be adequate and/or constant. Thus, it is essential that breast-fed infants, particularly first-born infants, be followed closely over the first few days to weeks of life to ensure that growth and development are proceeding normally. With proper counseling, most problems with breastfeeding can be corrected and/or avoided.

In large part, the historical problems associated with artificial feeding have been solved. The safety and easy digestibility of modern infant formulas approach the safety and digestibility of breast milk. Further, the clear economic advantages and microbiological safety of breastfeeding are of lesser importance for affluent, developed societies with ready access to clean water and refrigeration than for less developed, less affluent societies. Thus, as advocated by Fomon (1993), a reasonable and conservative approach is to allow the mother to make an informed choice of how she wishes to feed her infant and support her in that decision. As stated by Fomon (1993):

> . . . any woman with the least inclination toward breast feeding should be encouraged to do so, and all assistance possible should be provided by nurses, physicians, nutritionists and other health workers. At the same time, there is little justification for attempts to coerce women to breast feed. No woman in an industrialized country should be made to feel guilty because she elects not to breast feed her infant.

Several formulas are available for feeding the infant who is not breast-fed. All contain the DRIs recommended by the Life Sciences Research Organization (LSRO) (Raiten *et al.*, 1998) and the European Society of Gastroenterology, Hepatology and Nutrition (Koletzko *et al.*, 2005). Some of these are shown in Table 40.2. Most are available in both a "ready-to-use" and a concentrated liquid form. Powdered products also are available and are being used with increasing frequency. These products usually are the only ones available in many parts of the world.

The most commonly used infant formulas contain mixtures of bovine whey proteins and caseins at a total protein concentration of about 1.5 g/dL. Thus, the infant who receives from 150 to 180 ml/kg/day receives a protein intake of between 2.25 and 2.7 g/kg/day, or as much as 50% more than the intake of the breast-fed infant and, hence, the recent DRI for protein.

At one time, unmodified bovine milk protein, which has a whey:casein ratio of 18:82, was the protein source of all bovine milk formulas. Today, however, the majority of bovine milk formulas available in the United States contain mixtures of bovine milk protein and bovine whey proteins or mixtures of bovine whey proteins and caseins. The casein- and whey-predominant bovine milk formulas are equally efficacious for the normal-term infant.

Formulas containing soy protein as the protein source are available. These are intended for feeding infants who are intolerant of bovine milk protein. (Note: this is different from "soy milk.") Formulas containing partially hydrolyzed bovine milk protein are also available as are formulas containing only amino acids. These are intended for infants who are intolerant of both bovine milk and/or soy protein.

The major carbohydrate of most bovine milk formulas is lactose. Soy protein formulas usually contain either sucrose or a glucose polymer. Thus, these formulas are useful for the infant with either transient or congenital lactase deficiency.

The fat content of both bovine milk and soy protein formulas accounts for about 50% of the non-protein energy, and the blend of vegetable oils present in most formulas results in absorption of at least 90% of the ingested fat. Most formulas provide adequate intakes of the essential fatty acids, linoleic and α-linolenic acid. Many also contain the longer-chain, more unsaturated derivatives of these fatty acids (long-chain polyunsaturated fatty acids, or LC-PUFA) that are thought by some to contribute to the better neurodevelopmental outcome of breast-fed vs. formula-fed infants (see below).

The electrolyte, mineral, and vitamin contents of most formulas are similar and, when fed in adequate amounts

TABLE 40.2 Recommended composition (amount/100 kcal) of term infant formulas

Component	ESPGHAN[a]		LSRO[b]	
	Minimum	Maximum	Minimum	Maximum
Energy	60	70	63	71
Proteins				
Cow's milk protein (g)	1.8	3.0	1.7	3.4
Soy protein isolates (g)	2.25	3.0	–	–
Hydrolyzed cow's milk protein	1.8	3.0	–	–
Lipids				
Total fat (g)	4.4	6.0	4.4	6.4
Linoleic acid (g)	0.3	1.2	8.0	35
α-Linolenic acid (mg)	50	NS	1.75	4.0
Ratio linoleic/α-linolenic acids	5:1	15:1	6:1	16:1
Lauric + myristic acids (% of fat)	NS	20	–	–
Trans fatty acids (% of fat)	NS	3.0	–	–
Erucic acid (% of fat)	NS	1.0	–	–
Carbohydrates				
Total carbohydrates (g)	9.0	14.0	9.0	13
Vitamins				
Vitamin A (IU)	60	180	200	500
Vitamin D_3 (IU)	1.0	2.5	40	100
Vitamin E (mg α-TE/100 kcal)	0.5	5.0	0.5	5.0
Vitamin K (μg)	4.0	25	1.0	25
Thiamin (μg)	60	300	30	200
Riboflavin (μg)	80	400	80	300
Niacin (μg)	300	1500	550	2000
Vitamin B_6 (μg)	35	175	30	130
Vitamin B_{12} (μg)	0.1	0.5	0.08	0.7
Pantothenic acid (μg)	400	2000	300	1200
Folic acid (μg)	10	50	11	40
Vitamin C (mg)	10	30	6.0	15
Biotin (μg)	1.5	7.5	1.0	15
Minerals and trace elements				
Iron (formula based on cow's milk protein and protein hydrolysate) (mg)	0.3	1.3	0.2	1.65
Iron (formula based on soy protein isolate) (mg)	0.45	2.0	–	–
Calcium (mg)	50	140	50	140
Phosphorus (formula based on cow's milk protein and protein hydrolysate) (mg)	25	90	20	70
Phosphorus (formula based on soy protein isolate) (mg)	30	100	–	–
Ratio calcium/phosphorus (mg/mg)	1:1	2:1	–	–
Magnesium (mg)	5.0	15	4.0	17
Sodium (mg)	20	60	25	50
Chloride (mg)	50	160	50	160
Potassium (mg)	60	160	60	160
Manganese (μg)	1.0	50	1.0	100
Fluoride (mg)	NS	60	NS	60
Iodine (μg)	10	50	8.0	35
Selenium (μg)	1.0	9.0	1.5	5.0
Copper (μg)	35	80	60	160
Zinc (mg)	0.5	1.5	0.4	1.0
Other substances				
Choline (mg)	7.0	50	7.0	30
Myo-inositol (mg)	4.0	40	4.0	40
L-Carnitine (mg)	1.2	NS	1.2	2.0

[a]European Society for Pediatric Gastroenterology, Hepatology and Nutrition (Koletzko, 2005).
[b]Life Sciences Research Organization (Raiten et al., 1998).

TABLE 40.3 Composition (amount/100 kcal) of soy and hydrolyzed protein formulas

Component	Isomil[a]	Alimentum[a]
Protein (g)	2.45 (Soy protein isolate)	2.75 (Casein hydrolysate; cystine; tyrosine and tryptophan)
Fat (g)	5.46 (Soy and coconut oils)	5.54 (Medium-chain and triglycerides; safflower soy oils)
Carbohydrate (g)	10.3 (Corn syrup; sucrose)[b]	10.2 (Sucrose, modified tapioca starch)
Electrolytes and minerals		
Calcium (mg)	106	105
Phosphorus (mg)	75	75
Magnesium (mg)	7.5	7.5
Iron (mg)	1.8	1.8
Zinc (mg)	0.75	0.75
Manganese (μg)	25	8
Copper (μg)	75	75
Iodine (μg)	15	15
Selenium (μg)	–	2.8
Sodium (mg)	44	44
Potassium (mg)	108	118
Chloride	62	80
Vitamins		
Vitamin A (IU)	300	300
Vitamin D (IU)	60	45
Vitamin E (IU)	3	3.0
Vitamin K (IU)	11	15
Thiamine (μg)	60	60
Riboflavin (μg)	90	90
Vitamin B_6 (μg)	60	60
Vitamin B_{12} (μg)	0.45	0.45
Niacin (μg)	1350	1350
Folic acid (μg)	15	15
Pantothenic acid (μg)	750	750
Biotin (μg)	4.5	4.5
Vitamin C (mg)	9	9.0
Choline (mg)	8	8
Inositol (mg)	5	5

[a]Ross Laboratories, Columbus, Ohio.
[b]Isomil-SF (sucrose-free) has similar composition with the exception that glucose polymers are substituted for corn syrup and sucrose.

(150–180 mL/kg/day), provide the DRIs of these nutrients (Table 40.3). Both iron-supplemented (~12 mg/L) and non-supplemented (~1 mg/L) formulas are available; as mentioned above, iron-supplemented formulas are recommended. Many, in fact, favor making non-supplemented formulas unavailable.

The goal of both breastfeeding and formula-feeding is to deliver enough nutrients to support normal growth and development. As a rule of thumb, the normal-term infant's weight should double by 4–5 months of age and triple by 12 months of age. In general, unless an infant has other problems, normal growth is accompanied by normal development. Demand feeding is considered preferable, particularly during the early weeks of life. However, most infants easily adjust to roughly an every 3- or 4-hour schedule and, after 2 months of age, rarely demand night feedings.

Complementary Feeding

Although all nutrient needs for the first year of life can be met with reasonable amounts of currently available infant formulas, addition of other foods after about 6 months of age is recommended. In contrast, the volume of milk produced by many women may not be adequate to meet all nutrient needs beyond 6 months of age. This is particularly true for iron. Thus, for breast-fed infants, complementary foods are an important source of nutrients.

These foods should be introduced in a stepwise fashion to both breast-fed and formula-fed infants, beginning about the time the infant is able to sit without support. In the United States, rice cereal is usually the first such food given. It and other cereals are good sources of iron but rice cereal is less allergenic and unlikely to cause problems unless there is a family history of food and other allergies. Vegetables and fruits are usually introduced next, followed shortly by meats and, finally, eggs. Increasingly, meats are recommended as among the first foods. These are a good source of iron and zinc.

The order in which complementary foods are introduced is not crucial unless there is a family history of food and/or other allergies. However, it is recommended that only one new food be introduced at a time and that additional new foods should be spaced by at least 3 days to allow detection of adverse reactions to each newly introduced food.

Either home-prepared or manufactured complementary foods are available. The latter are convenient and also likely to contain less salt. Many such products also have supplemental nutrients (e.g. iron) and are available in different consistencies to match the infant's ability to tolerate larger size particles as he or she matures.

Prepared dinners and soups containing a meat and one or more vegetables are quite popular. However, the protein content of these products is not as high as that of strained meat. Puddings and desserts also are popular but, aside from their milk and egg content, are poor sources of nutrients other than energy; thus, intakes of these should be limited. Moreover, intake of egg-containing products should be delayed, especially if there is a family history of food and/or other allergies, until after the infant has demonstrated tolerance to eggs (either a mashed hard boiled egg yolk or a commercial egg yolk preparation).

Infant Formula vs. Bovine Milk

Although current recommendations are to limit the intake of bovine milk and to avoid low-fat or skimmed milk prior to a year of age (Committee on Nutrition, AAP, 1992), recent surveys show that some 6- to 12-month-old infants, albeit fewer than two decades ago (Martinez et al., 1985;

Ryan et al., 1987), are fed bovine milk rather than infant formula (Fox et al., 2004). More important, many of these infants are fed low-fat or skimmed milk – often, interestingly, on the advice of their physician.

The consequences of this practice, if any, are not known. However, infants fed bovine milk ingest three to four times the DRI of protein and considerably more sodium than the DRI of this electrolyte but less iron and linoleic acid than the DRIs of these nutrients. Ingestion of bovine milk also increases intestinal blood loss and, hence, contributes to development of iron-deficiency anemia (Ziegler et al., 1990).

The protein and sodium intakes of infants fed skimmed rather than whole bovine milk are even higher, the iron intake is equally low, and the intake of linoleic acid is very low. Ironically, while the most common reason for substituting low-fat or skimmed milk for whole milk or formula is to reduce fat and energy intakes, the total energy intake of infants fed skimmed milk is not lower than that of infants fed whole milk or formula (Martinez et al., 1985). This suggests that the infants compensate for the lower energy density of low-fat milk by taking more of it and/or increasing intake of other foods.

Whether the protein and sodium intakes of infants fed whole or skimmed bovine milk warrant concern is not certain. The low iron intake, clearly, is undesirable and may be accompanied by neurodevelopmental delay but medicinal iron supplementation should prevent development of iron deficiency. The low intake of linoleic acid may be more problematical. While signs and/or symptoms of essential fatty acid deficiency appear to be uncommon in infants fed whole or skimmed milk, an exhaustive search for such symptoms has not been made. Moreover, since essential fatty acid deficiency develops in both younger and older infants fed a low content of linoleic acid (Pettei et al., 1991), it is likely that such a search would reveal a reasonably high incidence of biochemical deficiency. On the other hand, infants who were breast-fed or fed formulas with high linoleic acid content early in life may have sufficient body stores to limit the consequences of a low intake later. Since essential fatty acid deficiency in animals is associated with long-term deleterious effects on development (Crawford et al., 1981), it is not wise to assume that biochemical essential fatty acid deficiency without clinically detectable symptoms is without consequences.

Resolving the issues concerning the use of bovine milk is important for economic as well as health reasons. Since the cost of bovine milk is less than half that of infant formula, replacing formula with homogenized bovine milk obviously would have important economic advantages for many families. In addition, if the Federal Food Assistance programs could provide homogenized bovine milk rather than formula to infants over 6 months of age, the current funds allocated to these programs would permit expansion of benefits to many more needy infants. Clearly, this cannot be considered without further data concerning the consequences of feeding bovine milk.

The practice of substituting skimmed or low-fat milk for whole milk or formula raises a number of more complex questions. For example, the suggestion that infants fed skimmed milk increase their intake of milk and/or other foods to maintain energy intake raises the important question of whether the amount of food intake during infancy may, in some way, imprint intake patterns throughout life. If so, this attempt to improve longevity, or at least cardiovascular health, paradoxically is likely to be more detrimental than a less prudent diet during infancy.

Long-Chain Polyunsaturated Fatty Acids

Long-chain polyunsaturated fatty acids, by definition, are more than 18 carbons in length and have more than two double bonds. There are several such fatty acids but those that are most relevant to infant nutrition are arachidonic acid (ARA; 20:4n-6) and docosahexaenoic acid (DHA; 22:6n-3). These fatty acids are the most prevalent n-6 and n-3 fatty acids, respectively, in the central nervous system and the latter comprises up to 40% of the fatty acid content of retinal photoreceptor membranes (Martinez, 1992).

Both ARA and DHA can be synthesized, respectively, from the essential fatty acids, linoleic acid (LA; 18:2n-6) and α-linolenic acid (ALA; 18:3n-3). These fatty acids undergo a series of desaturation and elongation reactions. Thus, the two families compete with each other for the desaturases and elongases involved. These enzymes prefer the n-3 fatty acids but the ratio of the two fatty acids in the diet can be an important determinant of the amount of each LC-PUFA synthesized.

Both term and preterm infants can convert LA and ALA, respectively, to ARA and DHA (Demmelmair et al., 1995; Carnielli et al., 1996; Salem et al., 1996; Sauerwald et al., 1996; Uauy et al., 2000). However, the content of ARA and DHA in plasma and erythrocyte lipids of infants fed unsupplemented formulas is lower than in plasma and erythrocyte lipids of breast-fed infants (Putnam et al., 1982). In addition, autopsy studies show that the low erythrocyte lipid content of DHA, but not ARA, is accompanied by a lower concentration in brain (Makrides et al., 1994). These differences probably reflect the presence of both fatty acids in human milk but not unsupplemented formula, suggesting that the synthetic pathway does not synthesize enough DHA. The better cognitive development of breast-fed vs. formula-fed infants also has been attributed to the presence of ARA and DHA in human milk (Rogan and Gladen, 1993; Pollock, 1994). In addition, since studies in both rodents and primates have shown that deficiency of n-3 fatty acids compromises visual function (Benolken et al., 1973; Neuringer et al., 1986), a number of studies have addressed differences in visual function of breast-fed vs. formula-fed infants.

Human milk contains a number of factors other than LC-PUFA that are important for development. Thus, the specific role of LC-PUFA in visual and cognitive development cannot be determined by studies of breast-fed vs. formula-fed infants. Moreover, there are major psychosocial and socioeconomic differences between mothers who choose to breast feed rather than formula feed their infants. Thus, many studies have addressed differences in visual function and/or neurodevelopmental status of infants fed LC-PUFA-supplemented vs. unsupplemented formulas. Some of these have shown distinct advantages of LC-PUFA supplementation but others have not. These are discussed more fully by Heird and Lapillonne (2005). The magnitude of the advantage of LC-PUFA supplementation of formulas for visual function in term infants equates to no more than one line on the Snellen chart and this advantage is not apparent at all ages.

Data concerning the effects of LC-PUFA on neurodevelopmental outcome are equally unclear. Some studies have shown up to a ~0.5 standard deviation advantage in the Bailey MDI at 18 months of age in infants fed DHA-supplemented vs. unsupplemented formula for the first 4 months of life (Birch et al., 2000). Others, however, have shown no advantages of DHA supplementation (Makrides et al., 2000; Auestad et al., 2001). None, however, has shown disadvantages.

Because of uncertainty concerning the functional effects of LC-PUFA, criticisms of methods used in studies to assess visual function and neurodevelopmental status, and concern about the safety of many of the sources available for supplementation of formulas, a panel of experts chosen by the LSRO to make recommendations for the nutrient content of term infant formulas failed to recommend addition of LC-PUFA to formulas manufactured and marketed in the United States (Raiten *et al.*, 1998). On the other hand, panels appointed by other agencies evaluating the same data recommend that formulas for term and, particularly, preterm infants be supplemented with LC-PUFA (British Nutrition Foundation, 1992; Food and Agriculture Organization, 1994) and such formulas have been available for more than a decade. Whether they are efficacious remains to be determined.

Future Directions

Although most infants in modern industrialized countries, whether breast-fed or formula-fed, grow and develop normally, a number of important issues relative to infant nutrition remain unresolved. Some of these are discussed briefly in the preceding sections. Others have been mentioned but not discussed, and still others have not been mentioned. Since it clearly is impossible to discuss all the relevant issues, only those that the author feels should receive the highest priority are discussed.

One such issue is the impact of size at birth and later on subsequent cardiovascular health. Epidemiological studies show a strong relationship between low birth weight as well as low weight at 1 year of age and the incidence of obesity, hypertension, diabetes, and/or cardiovascular disease in adolescence and adulthood (Barker, 1992; Eriksson *et al.*, 1993). Subsequent studies suggested that the risk of adult disease may be greater in those who are small at birth or a year of age but grow rapidly thereafter (Hales and Ozanne, 2003). Studies showing that preterm infants fed formulas that promote more rapid growth for only 4 weeks prior to hospital discharge have higher neurodevelopmental scores at 18 months (Lucas *et al.*, 1990) and 7 years (Lucas *et al.*, 1998) than those fed a less nutrient-dense formula during initial hospitalization. However, the former group has a higher incidence of risk factors for cardiovascular health at 14 to 16 years of age (Singhal *et al.*, 2004). Unraveling these issues obviously will yield important insights concerning optimal nutrition and, hence, growth during early life.

A related issue concerns the effect of intake during early life and intake thereafter. For example, do infants who are overfed tend to eat excessively once they begin feeding themselves? If so, could this contribute to the current epidemic of obesity in children as well as adults?

A final issue of particular relevance is the low prevalence of exclusive breastfeeding for the first 4 to 6 months of life and the even lower prevalence of breastfeeding for a year or longer, as currently recommended (World Health Organization, 1995; Work Group on Breastfeeding, AAP, 1997). While more than 75% of mothers in the United States begin breastfeeding, fewer than half are still doing so 3 months later. One reason for this may be that many modern mothers work outside the home, many of economic necessity, and today's maternity-leave policies in the United States and other countries make it necessary for many to return to work before the infant is 4 months old. The lack of facilities for collecting breast milk at work and the scarcity of on-site child-care facilities are additional factors making it difficult for women to continue breast feeding after returning to work.

While the need to return to work and the difficulty of continuing to breastfeed after doing so is a logical explanation for the low prevalence of breastfeeding, definitive proof for this explanation is lacking. This is unfortunate since business executives and government officials are unlikely to be enthusiastic about supporting expensive changes in maternity leave and child-care policies that may not increase the prevalence of breastfeeding. These officials also are likely to want data substantiating the advantages of exclusive breastfeeding for the first 6 months of life and continued breastfeeding for the next 6 months, or longer. Such advantages are easy to substantiate in developing countries, where alternatives to breastfeeding are prohibitively expensive or hazardous; however, they are much more difficult to substantiate in more affluent societies. None the less, until this is done, it is unlikely that the expensive social changes that might increase the duration of breastfeeding will be instituted, or that the prevalence of breastfeeding as currently recommended will increase.

Acknowledgments

This work is a publication of the USDA/ARS Children's Nutrition Research Center, Department of Pediatrics, Baylor College of Medicine, Houston, Texas, and has been funded, in part, with federal funds from the US Department of Agriculture, Agricultural Research Service under Cooperative Agreement No. 38-6250-1-003. The contents of this publication do not necessarily reflect the views or policies of the US Department of Agriculture, nor does the mention of trade names, commercial products, or organizations imply endorsement by the United States Government.

Suggestions for Further Reading

Devaney, B., Ziegler, P., Pac, S., *et al.* (2004) Nutrient intakes of infants and toddlers. *J Am Diet Assoc* **104**(Suppl 1), S14–S21.

Fomon, S.J. (ed.) (1993) Recommendation for feeding normal infants. In *Nutrition of Normal Infants*. Mosby, St. Louis. pp. 455–458.

Fox, M.K., Pac, S., Devaney, B., *et al.* (2004) Feeding infants and toddlers study: what foods are infants and toddlers eating? *J Am Diet Assoc* **104**(Suppl 1), S22–S30.

Heird, C. and Lapillonne, A. (2005) The role of essential fatty acids in development. *Annu Rev Nutr* **25**, 549–571.

World Health Organization (1995) The World Health Organization's infant feeding recommendations. *WHO Weekly Epidemiological Record* **70**, 119–120.

References

Auestad, N., Halter, R., Hall, R.T., *et al.* (2001) Growth and development in term infants fed long-chain polyunsaturated fatty acids: a double-masked, randomized, parallel, prospective, multivariate study. *Pediatrics* **108**, 372–381.

Barker, D.J.P. (ed.) (1992) *Fetal and Infant Origins of Adult Disease*. BJM Publishing, London.

Benolken, R.M., Anderson, R.E., and Wheeler, T.G. (1973) Membrane fatty acids associated with the electrical response in visual excitation. *Science* **182**, 1253–1254.

Birch, E.E., Garfield, S., Hoffman, D.R., *et al.* (2000) A randomized controlled trial of early dietary supply of long-chain polyunsaturated fatty acids and mental development in term infants. *Dev Med Child Neurol* **42**, 174–181.

British Nutrition Foundation (1992) Recommendation for intakes of unsaturated fatty acids. In *Unsaturated Fatty Acids: Nutritional and Physiological Significance*. Chapman and Hall, London, pp.152–163.

Brown, K.H., Black, R.E., Lopez de Romana, G., *et al.* (1989) Infant-feeding practices and their relationship with diarrheal and other diseases in Hauscar (Lima), Peru. *Pediatrics* **83**, 31–40.

Carnielli, V.P., Wattimena, D.J., Luijendijk, I.H., *et al.* (1996) The very low birth weight premature infant is capable of synthesizing arachidonic and docosahexaenoic acids from linoleic and linolenic acids. *Pediatr Res* **40**, 169–174.

Committee on Nutrition, American Academy of Pediatrics (1992) The use of whole cow's milk in infancy [policy statement]. *AAP News* **8**, 8–22.

Committee on Nutrition, American Academy of Pediatrics (2009a) Iron deficiency. In R.E. Kleinman (ed.), *Pediatric Nutrition Handbook*, 6th Edn. American Academy of Pediatrics, Elk Grove, IL, Chapter 18.

Committee on Nutrition, American Academy of Pediatrics (2009b) Fat soluble vitamins, vitamin D. In R.E. Kleinman (ed.), *Pediatric Nutrition Handbook*, 6th Edn. American Academy of Pediatrics, Elk Grove, IL, Chapters 20 and 21.

Crawford, M.A., Hassam, A.G., and Stevens, P.A. (1981) Essential fatty acid requirements in pregnancy and lactation with special reference to brain development. *Progr Lipid Res* **20**, 31–40.

Demmelmair, H., von Schenck, U., Behrendt, E., *et al.* (1995) Estimation of arachidonic acid synthesis in full term neonates using natural variation of ^{13}C content. *J Pediatr Gastroenterol Nutr* **21**, 31–36.

Denne, S.C., Karn, C.A., Ahlrichs, J.A., *et al.* (1996) Proteolysis and phenylalanine hydroxylation in response to parenteral nutrition in extremely premature and normal newborns. *J Clin Invest* **97**, 746–754.

Devaney, B., Ziegler, P., Pac, S., *et al.* (2004) Nutrient intakes of infants and toddlers. *J Am Diet Assoc* **104**(Suppl 1), S14–S21.

Eriksson, J.G., Forsén, T., Tuomilehto, J., *et al.* (1993) Catch-up growth in childhood and death from coronary heart disease: longitudinal study. *BMJ* **318**, 427–431.

Fomon, S.J. (ed.) (1993) Recommendation for feeding normal infants. In *Nutrition of Normal Infants*. Mosby, St. Louis, pp. 455–458.

Fomon, S.J., Thomas, L.N., Filer, L.J. Jr, *et al.* (1973) Requirements of protein and essential amino acids in early infancy: studies with a soy-isolate formula. *Acta Paediatr Scand* **62**, 33–45.

Food and Agriculture Organization/World Health Organization Expert Committee (1994) *Fats and Oils in Human Nutrition*. Report of a Joint Expert Consultation. FAO Food and Nutrition Paper No. 57. FAO, Rome.

Fox, M.K., Pac, S., Devaney, B., *et al.* (2004) Feeding infants and toddlers study: what foods are infants and toddlers eating? *J Am Diet Assoc* **104**, S22–S30.

Gaull, G.E., Sturman, G.A., and Räihä, N.C. (1972) Development of mammalian sulfur metabolism: absence of cystathionase in human fetal tissues. *Pediatr Res* **6**, 538–547.

Hales, C.N. and Ozanne, S.E. (2003) The dangerous road of catch-up growth. *J Physiol* **547**, 5–10.

Heird, C. and Lapillonne, A. (2005) The role of essential fatty acids in development. *Annu Rev Nutr* **25**, 549–571.

Institute of Medicine (1998) *Dietary Reference Intakes for Thiamin, Riboflavin, Niacin, Vitamin B_6, Folate, Vitamin B_{12},*

Pantothenic Acid, Biotin and Choline. National Academy Press, Washington, DC.

Institute of Medicine (2000) *Dietary Reference Intakes for Vitamin C, Vitamin E, Selenium and Carotenoids.* National Academy Press, Washington, DC.

Institute of Medicine (2001) *Dietary Reference Intakes for Vitamin A, Vitamin K, Arsenic Boron, Chromium, Copper, Iodine, Iron, Manganese, Molybdenum, Nickel, Silicon, Vanadium, and Zinc.* National Academy Press, Washington, DC.

Institute of Medicine (2002) *Dietary Reference Intakes for Energy, Carbohydrate, Fiber, Fat, Fatty Acids, Cholesterol, Protein and Amino Acids.* National Academy Press, Washington, DC.

Institute of Medicine (2011a) *Dietary Reference Intakes for Water, Potassium, Sodium, Chloride, and Sulfate.* National Academy Press, Washington, DC.

Institute of Medicine (2011b) *Dietary Reference Intakes for Calcium, Phosphorus, Magnesium, Vitamin D, and Fluoride.* National Academy Press, Washington, DC.

Kilani, R.A., Cole, F.S., and Bier, D.M. (1995) Phenylalanine hydroxylase activity in preterm infants: is tyrosine a conditionally essential amino acid? *Am J Clin Nutr* **61**, 1218–1223.

Koletzko, B., Baker, S., Cleghorn, G., *et al.* (2005) Global standard for the composition of infant formula: recommendations of an ESPGHAN coordinated international expert group. *J Pediatr Gastroenterol Nutr* **41**, 584–599.

Kovar, M.G., Serdula, M.K., Marks, J.S., *et al.* (1984) Review of the epidemiologic evidence for an association between infant feeding and infant health. *Pediatrics* **74**, S615–S638.

Lucas, A., Morley, R., and Cole, T.J. (1998) Randomised trial of early diet in preterm babies and later intelligence quotient. *BMJ* **317**, 1481–1487.

Lucas, A., Morley, R., Cole, T.J., *et al.* (1990) Early diet in preterm babies and developmental status at 18 months. *Lancet* **335**, 1477–1481.

Makrides, M., Neumann, M.A., Byard, R.W., *et al.* (1994) Fatty acid composition of brain, retina, and erythrocytes in breast- and formula-fed infants. *Am J Clin Nutr* **60**, 189–194.

Makrides, M., Neumann, M.A., Simmer, K., *et al.* (2000) A critical appraisal of the role of dietary long-chain polyunsaturated fatty acids on neural indices of term infants: a randomized, controlled trial. *Pediatrics* **105**, 32–38.

Mandel, I.D. (1991) The nutritional impact on dental caries. In W.C. Heird (ed.), *Nutritional Needs of the Six- to Twelve-Month-Old Infant.* Raven Press, New York, pp. 89–107.

Martinez, M. (1992) Tissue levels of polyunsaturated fatty acids during early human development. *J Pediatr* **120**, S129–S138.

Martinez, G.A., Ryan, A.S., and Malec, D.J. (1985) Nutrient intakes of American infants and children fed cow's milk or infant formula. *Am J Dis Child* **139**, 1010–1018.

Montgomery, R.K. (1991) Functional development of the gastrointestinal tract: the small intestine. In W.C. Heird (ed.), *Nutritional Needs of the Six- to Twelve-Month-Old Infant.* Raven Press, New York, pp. 1–17.

Neuringer, M., Connor, W.E., Lin, D.S., *et al.* (1986) Biochemical and functional effects of prenatal and postnatal ω3 fatty acid deficiency on retina and brain in rhesus monkeys. *Proc Natl Acad Sci USA* **83**, 4021–4025.

Pettei, M.J., Daftary, S., and Levine, J.J. (1991) Essential fatty acid deficiency associated with the use of a medium-chain-triglyceride infant formula in pediatric hepatobiliary disease. *Am J Clin Nutr* **53**, 1217–1221.

Pollock, J.I. (1994) Long-term associations with infant feeding in a clinically advantaged population of babies. *Dev Med Child Neurol* **36**, 429–440.

Putnam, J.C., Carlson, S.E., DeVoe, P.W., *et al.* (1982) The effect of variations in dietary fatty acids on the fatty acid composition of erythrocyte phosphatidylcholine and phosphatidylethanolamine in human infants. *Am J Clin Nutr* **36**, 106–114.

Räihä, N.C. (1973) Phenylalanine hydroxylase in human liver during development. *Pediatr Res* **7**, 1–4.

Räihä, N.C. (1985) Nutritional proteins in milk and the protein requirements of normal infants. *Pediatrics* **75**, 136–141.

Raiten, D.J., Talbot, J.M., and Waters, J.H. (1998) Assessment of nutrient requirements for infant formulas. *J Nutr* **128**(Suppl 11), 2059S–2293S.

Rogan, W.J. and Gladen, B.C. (1993) Breast-feeding and cognitive development. *Early Hum Dev* **31**, 181–193.

Ryan, A.S., Martinez, G.A., and Kreiger, F.W. (1987) Feeding low-fat milk during infancy. *Am J Phys Anthropol* **73**, 539–548.

Salem, N. Jr, Wegher, B., Mena, P., *et al.* (1996) Arachidonic and docosahexaenoic acids are biosynthesized from their 18-carbon precursors in human infants. *Proc Natl Acad Sci USA* **93**, 49–54.

Sauerwald, T.U., Hachey, D.L., Jensen, C.L., *et al.* (1996) Effect of dietary α-linolenic acid intake on incorporation of docosahexaenoic and arachidonic acids into plasma phospholipids of term infants. *Lipids* **31**(Suppl), S131–S135.

Singhal, A., Cole, T.J., Fewtrell, M., *et al.* (2004) Is slower early growth beneficial for long-term cardiovascular health? *Circulation* **109**, 1108–1113.

Sturman, J.A., Gaull, G.A., and Räihä, N.C. (1970) Absence of cystathionase in human liver: is cystine essential? *Science* **169**, 74–76.

Uauy, R., Mena, P., Wegher, B., *et al.* (2000) Long chain polyunsaturated fatty acid formation in neonates: effect of gestational
age and intrauterine growth. *Pediatr Res* **47,** 127–135.

Work Group on Breastfeeding, American Academy of Pediatrics
(1997) Breastfeeding and the use of human milk. *Pediatrics*
100, 1035–1039.

World Health Organization (1995) The World Health Organization's
Infant Feeding Recommendations. *WHO Weekly Epidemiological
Record* **70,** 119–120.

Ziegler, E.E., Fomon, S.J., Nelson, S.E., *et al.* (1990) Cow milk
feeding in infancy: further observations on blood loss from the
gastrointestinal tract. *J Pediatr* **116,** 11–18.

41

ADOLESCENCE

ASIM MAQBOOL, MD, KELLY A. DOUGHERTY, PhD,
ELIZABETH P. PARKS, MD, MSCE, AND VIRGINIA A. STALLINGS, MD

University of Pennsylvania, Perelman School of Medicine, Philadelphia, Pennsylvania, USA

Summary

Adolescence represents an important period of growth and development, for which there are specific nutritional needs and considerations. Accrual of bone mass is critical during this stage. Gender-based divergence of specific micronutrient needs emerge during this period. Macronutrient intake, energy requirements and expenditure also change at this age, and hydration status for physically active adolescents is emerging as a very important consideration for health status. Eating behaviors and disorders also frequently emerge at this age. Adolescents are prone to develop eating disorders, and may be at risk for malnutrition from anorexia, bulimia, obesity, and dyslipidemias, which may carry lifelong consequences for health and disease. Preconceptional nutritional status is key to all females of childbearing age, and unique to the adolescent pregnancy are the nutritional and growth needs of both mother and fetus, which may pose specific nutritional concerns and risks.

Introduction

Adolescence is an important period during which major biological, social, physiological, and cognitive changes take place. Adolescents have special nutritional needs as a result of rapid growth (lean body mass, fat mass, bone mineralization) and maturational changes associated with the onset of puberty. Dietary surveys show that most adolescents do not meet age and gender nutrient recommendations and have inadequate dietary intake of calcium, iron, thiamin, riboflavin, and vitamins A and C (Skiba *et al.*, 1997). Despite their poor dietary intakes, the only clinical nutrient deficiency commonly seen among adolescents is iron-deficiency anemia. Iron deficiency is the most common

nutritional deficiency worldwide, and per the 1999–2000 United States National Health and Nutrition Examination Survey (NHANES) has a prevalence of 5% for males 12–15 years of age, and of 12% for females 12–15 years of age (Centers for Disease Control and Prevention [CDC], 2002). Women of childbearing age may be at the highest risk for iron-deficiency anemia. The global prevalence of anemia is estimated to be 30% in non-pregnant women, rising to 47% during pregnancy (de Benoist, 2008). Iron deficiency during pregnancy bears fetal consequences (low birth weight, preterm delivery) and affects cognitive and physical development of infants, children, and adolescents, and also has an effect on work capacity (Haas and Brownlie, 2001; Rasmussen, 2001). This data

Present Knowledge in Nutrition, Tenth Edition. Edited by John W. Erdman Jr, Ian A. Macdonald and Steven H. Zeisel.
© 2012 International Life Sciences Institute. Published 2012 by John Wiley & Sons, Inc.

underlies the importance of the nutritional status of adolescent females of childbearing age in particular, as preconceptional nutritional status is critical to their health and that of their babies.

An increasing number of adolescents have problems with excess food intake and obesity. In the United States, obesity prevalence in youths aged 12–19 has increased dramatically from 5% to 18% when comparing NHANES data from 1976–1980 with data in 2007–2008 (Ogden and Carroll, 2010). Obesity is a global concern. The prevalence is increasing worldwide, often in parallel with the nutrition transition from traditional to the modern western diet, with obesity now coexisting in communities where malnutrition from calorie and nutrient deficits had been prevalent (Caballero and Popkin, 2002).

In this chapter we will discuss growth changes, nutritional needs, nutritional assessment, and nutrition-related issues applicable to adolescence. Most of the material presented reflects data emanating from the United States and Canadian populations. The Dietary Reference Intakes published by the Food and Nutrition Board of the Institute of Medicine form the basis for many of the recommendations provided therein, with some global references also provided from the World Health Organization.

Growth during Adolescence

The age at onset and rate of progression through puberty varies considerably among children (Tanner, 1962). Driven by hormonal changes, resulting alterations in body size, body composition (muscle, fat, bone), and sexual maturation are the basis for increased dietary requirements for energy, protein, and most micronutrients. Boys and girls of similar age differ in some nutritional requirements due to the male adolescent growth spurt occurring approximately 2 years later. Chronic disease and undernutrition can delay the onset of puberty (Zemel and Jenkins, 1989; Ramakrishan et al., 1999; Zeitler et al., 1999). In addition, growth is not a continuous process, but rather a series of small growth spurts varying in amplitude and frequency (Lampl et al., 1993). All of these factors influence an adolescent's nutritional requirements, which will vary within and among individuals over the age range. Adequate nutritional intake is necessary to support a normal pattern of growth and maturation.

The onset of puberty varies by ethnicity. In a national sample of US boys and girls (National Health and Nutrition Examination Survey – NHANES III 1988–1994) evaluated at 8 to 19 years of age (Sun et al., 2002), the median ages of onset of pubic hair development were 11.2, 12.0, and 12.3 years for Non-Hispanic Black, Non-Hispanic White, and Mexican-American boys, respectively, and 9.4, 10.6, and 10.4 years for Non-Hispanic Black, Non-Hispanic White, and Mexican-American girls, respectively.

A comparison of NHANES III 1988–1994 with NHANES 1999–2002 indicates a decline in the age at menarche from 12.53 to 12.34 years (Anderson and Must, 2005). Higher relative weight was associated with increased likelihood of menarche, suggesting the US obesity epidemic may play a role in the trend for younger menarche. Menarche usually occurs just after the adolescent linear growth spurt. At peak adolescent linear growth velocity, the rate of increase in height is about 10.3 cm/year for boys (range 7.2–13.4) and 9.0 cm/year for girls (range 7.0–11.0) (Tanner, 1962). From the onset of the adolescent growth spurt to the attainment of adult stature, both boys and girls gain about 17% of their final height (Abbassi et al., 1998).

During and following the adolescent growth spurt there is a rapid accrual of bone mass. Peak bone mass is achieved by the end of adolescence or early adulthood (Matkovic, 1992; Theintz et al., 1992). Higher peak bone mass is associated with both greater dietary calcium intake and lower rates of hip fracture later in life (Matkovic, 1992). Thus, adequate calcium intake to ensure optimal accrual of bone mass during childhood and adolescence may have important lifelong health implications (Weaver et al., 1999). To accommodate rapid gains, calcium requirements are higher for adolescents than for children or adults. The recommended dietary allowance (RDA) for calcium and intake data from two NHANES surveys is shown in Table 41.1. The RDA is defined as the average daily dietary nutrient intake level sufficient to meet the nutrient requirement of nearly all healthy individuals (97–98%) in a particular life stage and gender group (Institute of Medicine, 2006).

Nutritional Needs of Adolescents

Nutritional needs of adolescents are higher than those of children because of rapid growth, sexual maturation, changes in body composition, skeletal mineralization, and changes in physical activity. Physical activity is not necessarily increased, but total energy needs are increased because of larger body size and, in particular, fat-free mass. Unlike children, adolescent males and females differ in their nutritional needs, and some of these sex-based dif-

TABLE 41.1 Calcium intake (mg/day) for males and females from the National Health and Nutrition Examination 1988–1991 and 1999–2000 surveys

Population group	Males		Females	
1988–1992[a]	6–11 years	12–15 years	6–11 years	12–15 years
Non-Hispanic white	994	822	822	744
Non-Hispanic black	761	688	688	613
Mexican-American	986	890	890	790
1999–2000[b]	6–11 years	12–19 years	6–11 years	12–19 years
All race/ethnic groups	843	956	812	661

Recommended dietary allowance of calcium for 4- to 8-year-old children is 1000 mg/day, and 1300 mg/day for children 9–18 years of age (Institute of Medicine, 2010a).
[a]Data from Alaimo *et al.* (1994).
[b]Data from Ervin *et al.* (2004a).

ferences continue into adulthood. Substantial differences in body composition occur, with relatively increased body fat for females and increased lean body mass for males. Nutrient needs are increased for protein, energy, calcium, iron, and zinc. Importantly, preconceptional nutritional considerations are key for females of child-bearing age. Recommended dietary intakes for adolescents (Institute of Medicine, 1998) often represent interpolations based on known requirements for children and adults rather than evidence from adolescent subjects. Nutrient requirements are usually greater for males than for females and for pregnant and lactating females than for non-pregnant females. Review of the Dietary Reference Intakes by age and gender reflect and illustrate the divergent needs for specific nutrients by age and gender.

Often, adolescents' dietary habits differ from those of children and adults. Adolescents tend to skip meals, eat more meals outside their home, and eat snacks (especially soda, candy, and diet and fast foods): up to 20% of adolescents skip breakfast (Videon and Manning, 2003). Some develop strongly held food beliefs, adopt food fads, or become vegetarians. These diet patterns may reflect an expression of independence, a busy lifestyle, alterations of body image perception, or an expression of self-identity, or they may be secondary to peer and social pressures.

Typically, intake of calcium, iron, and vitamins A and C are insufficient in the diets of US adolescents, with boys having somewhat better intake than girls. Adolescents often have high intakes of soda, coffee, tea, and alcohol, and low intakes of milk and juice (Dwyer, 1996). In a large survey of 12 500 children aged 11–18 years, Cavadini and colleagues showed that total energy intake, as well as the proportion of total fat and saturated fat, unexpectedly decreased from 1965 to 1996 (Cavadini *et al.*, 2000). Total milk consumption decreased, accompanied by an increase

in intake of soft drinks and non-citrus juices. Among US high-school students surveyed between 1999 and 2003, only about 17% reported drinking more than three glasses of milk daily (Centers for Disease Control and Prevention, 2005). Fruit and vegetable intake was lower than the recommended five servings per day, and folate, iron, and calcium intakes were lower than stipulated in the recommendations (Institute of Medicine, 1997, 1998, 2001; Cavadini *et al.*, 2000). In adolescent females and low-income youth in general, vitamins B_6, A, E, iron, calcium, and zinc intakes were low (Story and Alton, 1996). In the typical American adolescent's diet, french fried white potatoes make up 25% of all vegetables consumed; intake of simple sugars exceeds the intake of complex carbohydrates; and more than a third of the dietary fat is saturated fat (Krebs-Smith *et al.*, 1996; Munoz *et al.*, 1997). Additionally, foods with high added simple-sugar content (which in general have fewer nutrients than foods with naturally occurring sugars, have limited nutritional value beyond providing calories, and are commonly referred to as "junk food") and high-fat fast food account for >33% of the daily caloric intake (USDA, 2005).

About 23% of high-school students surveyed between 1999 and 2003 in the National Youth Risk Behavior Survey (Eaton *et al.*, 2010) ate the recommended ≥5 servings of fruits and vegetables per day. In an earlier survey, fruit and vegetable intake was found to be higher in whites than in adolescents from other ethnic groups (Dwyer, 1996).

Recommendations for adolescent nutrient intake from various sources stress the need for the following: increased intake of calcium-rich and iron-containing foods in adolescent girls; limitation of foods high in simple sugars; decrease in the intake of complex carbohydrate foods that could be retained in the mouth and contribute to dental

TABLE 41.2   Equations for estimating energy requirement (EER) for adolescents and physical activity level (PAL)

Adolescent group and activity level	Equation
EER by gender	EER (kcal/day) = Total energy expenditure + Energy deposition
Males	
9–18 years	EER = 88.5 − (61.9 × age [years]) + PAL × [(26.7 × weight [kg]) + (903 × height [m]) + 25
Females	
9–18 years	EER = 135.3 − (30.8 × age [years]) + PAL × [(10.0 × weight [kg]) + (934 × height [m]) + 25
Pregnancy EER by trimester	EER (kcal /day) = Non-pregnant EER + Pregnancy energy deposition
1st trimester	EER = Non-pregnant EER; needs are not increased
2nd trimester	EER = Non-pregnant EER + 340
3rd trimester	EER = Non-pregnant EER + 452
Lactation EER	EER (kcal/day) = Non-pregnant EER + milk energy output − weight loss
0–6 months postpartum	EER = non-pregnant EER + 500 − 170
7–12 months postpartum	EER = non-pregnant EER + 400 − 0
Physical activity level (PAL)	
Sedentary	PAL >1.0 <1.4
Low active	PAL >1.4 <1.6
Active	PAL >1.6 <1.9
Very active	PAL >1.9 <2.5

Adapted from Institute of Medicine (2006).

caries; use of fluoridated water, dentifrices, topical treatments, and rinses to prevent dental caries; limitation of fat intake to <30% of energy intake, with saturated fat intake <10% and cholesterol <300 mg/day; limitation of salt intake to <6 g/day and daily protein intake more than twice the RDA. The American Academy of Pediatrics recommends that 20–30% of total energy intake should be from dietary fat for this period of rapid adolescent growth (American Academy of Pediatrics, 2004).

Energy

The exact energy requirement of the individual is difficult to determine (Gong and Heald, 1999). The Dietary Reference Intakes (DRI) issued by the Food and Nutrition Board of the Institute of Medicine provide a method for estimating the requirement for energy as a set of Estimated Energy Requirements (EER, kcal/day) prediction equations (Table 41.2) (Institute of Medicine, 2002). Specifically, the EER for adolescents estimates dietary energy needs by age, gender, weight, and height, and for growth and development changes (as energy deposition for

the accretion of new tissue) and a range of physical activity levels (PAL). The four PAL categories are: sedentary, low active, active, and very active (Table 41.2). Determining the appropriate PAL for individuals remains a challenge. In general, peak energy requirements occur in girls at about 15 to 16 years of age and in boys at about 18 years of age. Active adolescent females require about 2300 kcal/day, whereas males require 2600–3300 kcal/day. Energy needs increase during the second and third trimester of pregnancy and during the first and second 6 months of lactation (Institute of Medicine, 2002). EER are available to estimate energy needs for obese adolescent females and males (Institute of Medicine, 2002).

The NHANES III Survey showed that energy intakes were higher for males than for females, and intakes peaked in late adolescence (Bialostosky *et al.*, 2002). Despite a trend toward decreasing dietary fat intake, fat intake is still higher than recommended (Dwyer, 1996). The dietary reference intakes provide guidance regarding macronutrient distribution, with total fat intake to provide 25–35%, carbohydrates 45–65%, and protein 10–30% of caloric

TABLE 41.3 Dietary reference intakes (DRI) for total protein for adolescents by life stage and gender

Life-stage group	DRI values (g/kg/day)			
	Estimated average requirement[a]		Recommended dietary allowance[b]	
	Males	Females	Males	Females
9–13 years	0.76	0.76	0.95	0.95
14–18 years	0.73	0.71	0.85	0.85
Pregnancy	–	0.88	–	1.1
Lactation	–	1.05	–	1.3

[a]The average daily nutrient intake level estimated to meet the requirements of half of the healthy individuals in a group.
[b]The average daily intake level to meet the nutrient requirements of 97–98% of healthy individuals in a group.
Adapted from Institute of Medicine (2006).

intake. With respect to type of dietary fat intake, reducing intake of dietary cholesterol, *trans* fats, and saturated fats as much as possible while maintaining 5–10% of linoleic acid and 0.6–1.2% of α-linoleic acid is recommended. Added sugars, such as those provided in carbonated soda beverages, have little nutritive value (Institute of Medicine, 2006).

Protein

Protein recommendations are shown in Table 41.3. Most adolescents easily achieve these levels in the United States (Bialostosky *et al.*, 2002). Peak protein requirement coincides with peak energy needs, and corresponds to peak growth rates as opposed to chronological age: protein should account for 12–14% of energy intake. Adolescents at risk for low protein intake are those with eating disorders, malabsorption, chronic disease with anorexia, and socioeconomic limitations resulting in food insecurity. In the event of substantially inadequate energy intake, protein is used for energy, resulting in both protein and energy malnutrition.

Micronutrients
Minerals

Many adolescents have inadequate micronutrient intakes, including calcium, iron, zinc, and magnesium. Calcium and phosphorus are essential for bone health. The former is required for bone mass accretion. Peak bone mass is usually attained by the age of 25, and calcium intake during adolescence is key for lifelong bone health. Though

dietary phosphorus intake is usually adequate, calcium intake is often inadequate in adolescents. National surveys show that calcium intake is less than recommended, and has generally declined over the last 20-plus years. For example, among girls aged 15–18 years, the average calcium intake dropped from 680 mg/day in 1980 to 600 mg/day in 1990 (Albertson *et al.*, 1997). Among girls aged 12–19 years in the NHANES 1999–2000 dietary survey (Ervin *et al.*, 2004a), median calcium intake was 611 mg/day, which is about 51% of the currently recommended 1300 mg/day (Institute of Medicine, 1997). The 2003–2006 NHANES survey suggested that approximately 22% of males 9–13 years of age and 40% of males between 14 and 18 years of age exceeded the adequate intake (AI; the adequate intake of the dietary reference intakes is a recommended intake value based on observed or experimentally determined approximations or estimates of nutrient intake by a group [or groups] of healthy people that are assumed to be adequate, and is used when an RDA cannot be determined) (Institute of Medicine, 2010a). In contrast, only 13% of females between 9 and 13 years of age and 9.5% of females 14–18 years of age had a calcium intake in excess of the AI. Ethnic differences are also noteworthy: calcium intake is lower in Non-Hispanic Black compared with Non-Hispanic White and Mexican-American children and adolescents (Alaimo *et al.*, 1994). Net calcium absorption is highest in infancy and adolescence (Matkovic, 1991). However, it is unlikely that increased efficiency with inadequate intake is sufficient to optimize peak bone mass. Calcium is more efficiently absorbed in combination with lactose in foods, and dairy products provide about 55% of the calcium intake in the US diet. Calcium from other dietary sources is important, however, especially in communities where dairy products are not culturally preferred and for adolescents who have lactose intolerance. Calcium supplementation can increase bone mineral density in children (Johnston *et al.*, 1992), a finding that underscores the importance of adequate calcium intake from all sources.

Despite the iron fortification of many cereal grains, iron deficiency remains common. Iron needs are higher during adolescence because of increases in blood volume and muscle mass for both males and females. In females, needs are further increased by menstrual losses. Groups of adolescent females who are at increased risk for iron deficiency are older, pregnant or athletes. Median iron intake for 12- to 19-year-old girls in the NHANES 1999–2000 survey was 11.7 mg/day, about 78% of the 15 mg/day recommended for girls aged 14–18 years (Institute of Medicine, 2001; Ervin *et al.*, 2004a). Iron deficiency during pregnancy results in an increased risk of preterm birth and low-birth-weight infants. Young pubertal boys are also at risk for iron-deficiency anemia and then iron needs decrease with slower growth after puberty. Iron deficiency is more common among low-income youth and is seen more often in adolescent females than in adolescent males (Dwyer, 1996). The prevalence of iron deficiency has increased for males 12–15 years of age from 1% (NHANES 1988–1994) to 5% (NHANES 1999–2000) but has remained stable for females at 9% in the United States across the same surveys (Centers for Disease Control and Prevention, 2002). Globally, approximately a quarter of the world's population has iron-deficiency anemia. The highest risk group for iron-deficiency anemia is non-pregnant women of child-bearing age – approximately 470 million of them, and the greatest prevalence by numbers occurs in Africa and Southeast Asia (de Benoist *et al.*, 2008).

Increased zinc is needed for growth and puberty, and zinc intake is often low in adolescents. Zinc deficiency is associated with growth retardation and hypogonadism, and zinc supplementation treats these clinical manifestations.

Sodium Chloride

Sodium chloride (table salt) intake is excessive in the United States. NHANES III indicated more than 95% of men and 75% of women consumed more than the upper limit for salt. The sodium recommended for adolescents is 1500 mg/day, and the upper limit is 2300 mg/day; excess sodium intake is associated with risk for hypertension and cardiovascular disease. One teaspoon of table salt contains 2300 mg of sodium. Sodium is high in processed food (such as in hot dogs, processed lunch meats, canned soups, and some condiments), which provides an estimated 80% of intake. Reduction of sodium chloride intake is an important public health initiative (USDA, 2005). Conversely, potassium intake is most likely suboptimal (but not in the range to be associated with clinical findings such as cardiac arrhythmias, muscle weakness, and glucose intolerance). An increase in potassium supports lower blood pressure and reduces the negative health effect of sodium. The current recommended potassium intake for adolescents and adults is 4700 mg/day. While potassium chloride may be a useful and available substitute for sodium chloride, the current US recommendations are that potassium intake should come from food sources, not supplements (USDA, 2005; Institute of Medicine, 2006).

Vitamins

Adolescents' diets are low in vitamins A, B_6, E, D, C and folic acid. Because girls have lower food intakes than boys, dietary deficiencies are more common in girls (Institute of Medicine, 1998, 2001; Ervin *et al.*, 2004b). Folic acid is a key preconception micronutrient for females of child-bearing age. Folic acid deficiency is associated with increased risk for neural tube defects in the fetus, and ensuring adequate folic acid status before pregnancy by increasing dietary and supplement-based folic acid intake reduces this risk (Centers for Disease Control and Prevention, 1992). Therefore a key concept for all females of childbearing age is to establish optimal nutritional status prior to becoming pregnant.

Vitamin D is essential for bone health as well as many other functions. Vitamin D status is suboptimal among children and adolescents. Lower 25-hydroxyvitamin D levels are more common during the winter season, in individuals with a higher body mass index, and by race, with black race/ethnicity at higher risk than other groups (Rovner and O'Brien, 2008). Vitamin D is obtained via photoconversion of provitamin D at the dermal level by UVB exposure, and by food and supplement intake. Although daily sunlight exposure to the hands and face is sufficient to achieve adequate vitamin D levels in healthy adolescents (Holick, 1997), seasonal fluctuations in sunlight exposure, skin pigment, and health status may affect vitamin D status (Docio *et al.*, 1998). Inadequate intake may be greater in adolescent females than in males (Moore *et al.*, 2004). Adequate vitamin D levels are necessary to facilitate calcium absorption in the gut and for bone health. Newer data suggest that vitamin D influences health status in a myriad of ways, and, as such, the paradigm of optimal vitamin D status and blood concentration is now based on optimal health outcomes. Serum vitamin D status is now considered as a predictor of risk for chronic diseases, including susceptibility to infections, inflammation autoimmune disorders, cardiovascular and neurological disease, and some cancers. There are two important points to note here: first, the nature of the association, i.e. causality between vitamin D status and some of these diseases has not been established; secondly, optimal serum levels with respect to improved health outcomes are in the process of being established.

Fiber

Adolescents ingest much less than recommended amounts of fiber (Williams *et al.*, 1995; Bialostosky *et al.*, 2002). Average fiber intake is about 12 g/day in comparison to the 25 g/day recommended by the American Heart Association for blood cholesterol reduction and the 35–45 g/day recommended for reduction of colon cancer risk (Nicklas *et al.*, 1995). The DRI (Institute of Medicine, 2002) recommendations are for males aged 9–13 years to consume 31 g/day, and aged 14–18 years to consume 38 g/day. Female recommended intake is 26 g/day for ages 9–18 years.

Nutritional Assessment

During the adolescent years, nutritional status assessment is complicated by the influence of puberty on weight, height, and body composition. In addition to standard growth charts (Kuczmarski *et al.*, 2000), height and height-velocity growth charts (Tanner and Davies, 1985), which include a classification for early and late onset of maturation, are useful to assess height growth relative to maturity status. For early- or late-maturing children whose growth deviates from the standard growth curve, these charts are important for the interpretation of growth velocity and patterns. Assessment of sexual maturity is classified according to the stages described by Tanner (1962) for both pubic hair and genital development in boys and for breast development in girls. A self-assessment pictorial questionnaire can be used to establish puberty stage (Morris and Udry, 1980). For assessment of weight-for-height status, the body mass index (BMI; expressed in kg/m²) is commonly used. With the use of BMI charts, a sex- and age-specific BMI percentile or z scores can be plotted in the same manner as for weight and height. BMI ≤5th percentile is considered underweight, ≥5th percentile to 84.9th percentile is considered normal weight range, ≥85th percentile is considered overweight, and ≥95th percentile is considered to be obese. Caution should be taken to interpret overweight children using only BMI for age and gender as some children may have relatively high weights primarily because of high lean mass rather than high body fat levels, especially in adolescent boys (Krebs *et al.*, 2007)

Special Nutrition-related Issues

Obesity

Obesity (defined as a BMI ≥95th percentile) (Kuczmarski *et al.*, 2002) is caused by an energy imbalance in which individuals expend less energy than they consume. A chronic, small energy surplus can have a large effect on weight gain over time and makes the prevention and treatment of obesity challenging.

TABLE 41.4 Prevalence of obesity (≥95th percentile BMI) in adolescents (ages 12–19 years)

Time frame	Ethnic group		
	Non-Hispanic white	Non-Hispanic black	Mexican
Boys			
1976–1980	3.8	6.1	7.7
1988–1994	11.6	10.7	14.1
1999–2002	14.6	18.7	24.7
2007–2008	16.7	19.8	25.5
Girls			
1976–1980	4.6	10.7	8.8
1988–1994	8.9	16.3	13.4
1999–2002	12.7	23.6	19.6
2007–2008	14.5	29.2	17.5

Data from Hedley *et al.* (2004) and Ogden and Carroll (2010).

As previously stated, the prevalence of obesity in adolescence is increasing internationally (Caballero and Popkin, 2002). According to NHANES data the prevalence of obesity in children and adolescents in the United States has tripled between the 1960s and 2000 but has stabilized in 2003–2006 in children aged 2–19 years (Ogden *et al.*, 2008). (See Table 41.4.) Even with this stabilization, according to the NHANES 2007–2008 surveys, 34.3% of adolescents between the ages of 12–19 years are overweight (BMI ≥85th percentile), and 18.1% are obese (BMI ≥95th percentile) (Ogden and Carroll, 2010). The prevalence of US adolescents in the severe obesity category continues to rise. In 2007 there were 12.5% of adolescents classified as severely obese (BMI ≥97th percentile) as opposed to 4.8% in 2004 (Ogden *et al.*, 2008; Skelton *et al.*, 2009; Ogden and Carroll, 2010). Similarly, childhood obesity prevalence rates although still elevated appear to have stabilized after 2000 in France, and in 2004 in Germany, Poland, Switzerland, and England (Bluher *et al.*, 2009; Salanave *et al.*, 2009; Aeberli *et al.*, 2010; Stamatakis *et al.*, 2010).

The risk of becoming obese as a child and remaining obese as an adult is influenced by family history and by the child's age of onset. There is an 80% chance of an obese adolescent becoming an obese adult (Whitaker *et al.*, 1997). The risk associated with parental obesity is evidenced by the fact that 80% of children with two overweight parents were overweight, 40% of children with one overweight parent are overweight, and only 10% of children with no overweight parents become overweight. Additionally, it has been noted that children with obese grandparents are about 18 times more likely to be obese than those with non-obese grandparents (Davis *et al.*, 2008). The risk of becoming an obese adult increases seven-fold for adolescents compared with preschool-aged children (Whitaker *et al.*, 1997). This age of obesity onset relationship reinforces the need to prevent and treat obesity in adolescence.

Adolescent physiologic and social challenges lend themselves to increased risk/exacerbation of obesity. The transition from the pubertal stages Tanner stage 1 to Tanner stage 3 is associated with increased fat deposition which is more pronounced in adolescent females who experience early menarche (<11.9 years of age) (Remsberg *et al.*, 2005). Additionally, increased independent food choices and decreased physical activity provide opportunities and challenges for adolescent weight management. Physical activity, dietary factors, sedentary activity, and other environmental influences are variables in adolescent obesity. Obese adolescents are less likely to participate in sports (Levin *et al.*, 2003). With regard to diet, for every additional serving of a sugar-sweetened beverage there is a six-fold increase in the odds of being obese (Ludwig *et al.*, 2001). Similarly, pre-adolescents and young adolescents were 5.5 times as likely to be overweight if they watched television >5 hours/day (Renna *et al.*, 2008). Other common environmental influences include supermarket availability, fast food restaurants and convenience store use, neighborhood safety, presence of a television in the bedroom, eating meals as a family, and family socioeconomic status (Kumanyika, 2008).

Health Consequences of Obesity

Medical conditions that require immediate intervention (e.g. sleep apnea, type 2 diabetes, hypertension, non-alcoholic fatty liver disease) are increasingly common in obese adolescents (Box 41.1). Whereas at one point diabetes in children was almost entirely type 1, type 2 diabetes now accounts for 44% of all cases of diabetes in children (Nadeau and Dabelea, 2008) as opposed to 95% of diabetes in adults (Campbell, 2009) Eight-four percent of children diagnosed with type 2 diabetes are overweight or obese. The high prevalence of obesity in children with type 2 diabetes emphasizes the importance of glucose screening for diabetes in overweight and obese children (American Diabetes Association, 2000; Barlow, 2007).

Obesity is often associated with psychosocial complications for children and adolescents, including low self-esteem, poor body image, depression, and learning

---

BOX 41.1   Medical conditions associated with obesity in adolescents

Hypertension
Lipid disorders (especially hypertriglyceridemia and low HDL)
Insulin resistance and type 2 diabetes
Acanthosis nigricans
Metabolic syndrome
Orthopedic problems
  Slipped capital femoral epiphysis
  Blount's disease
Cholelithiasis
Non-alcoholic steatohepatitis
Obstructive sleep apnea
Polycystic ovary syndrome and menstrual irregularities
Pseudotumor cerebri
Psychosocial dysfunction

Adapted from Spear *et al.* (2007).

---

problems. Obese individuals are frequently the targets of social discrimination and stigmatization (Wang *et al.*, 2009). Obese adolescents suffer more frequently from low self-esteem than do overweight pre-adolescents, perhaps because of the greater influence of peers on self-esteem for adolescents (Wang *et al.*, 2009).

Evaluation and Treatment

The assessment of an obese adolescent should include a routine history and physical examination, which includes a review for signs of obesity-related syndromes or conditions. Screening for associated conditions (e.g. hyperlipidemia, insulin resistance) or contributing processes (e.g. hypothyroidism) should be considered. Additionally, significant family dysfunction or adolescent psychological problems should also be evaluated (Barlow, 2007).

Behavioral Treatment. Lifestyle behavioral management should involve the family and others who are key to the adolescent's support. Target behaviors that have been demonstrated to be effective in obesity prevention and treatment include the limiting of sweetened beverages, energy-dense foods, portion sizes, and eating out in restaurants; restricting screen time (TV, computer, and videogames) to ≤2 hours daily; eating breakfast daily; eating as a family; and encouraging 1 hour of physical activity of a

TABLE 41.5 Screening guidelines for hypercholesterolemia in adolescents

Indication for screening	Screening test
Total cholesterol >240 mg/dL (6.2 mmol/L) in parents	Non-fasting total cholesterol
Family history of premature heart disease; or total cholesterol >200 mg/dL (5.2 mmol/L)	Two fasting lipid profiles (total cholesterol, triglycerides, HDL, calculated LDL); average the results
Total cholesterol >170–199 mg/dL (4.4–5.2 mmol/L) in patient	Repeat total cholesterol; if average >170 mg/dL (4.4 mmol/L), proceed with lipid profile screening

To convert mg/dl to mmol/L, multiply by 0.02586. 1 lb = 454 g.
Adapted from American Academy of Pediatrics (1992).

level equal to or greater than moderate on a daily basis (Barlow, 2007).

Surgical Treatment. Adolescents with a BMI ≥50 without co-morbidities or ≥40 with one or more co-morbidities who are Tanner stage 4 or 5 and have failed lifestyle behavioral management may be eligible for bariatric surgery. Compliance with postsurgical nutritional supplementation and weight management can be particularly challenging with adolescent patients. Bariatric surgery patients are susceptible to developing protein malnutrition, and thiamine, iron, vitamin B_{12}, and fat-soluble-vitamin deficiencies (Woo, 2009).

Hyperlipidemia

Adult cardiovascular disease has its roots in childhood and adolescence. The Bogalusa Heart Study and the Pathobiological Determinants of Atherosclerosis in Youth Research Group found correlations between early atherosclerotic changes seen at autopsy and both total and LDL cholesterol levels (Strong, 1986). These and other studies suggest that adolescents at risk of developing premature atherosclerosis should be identified to effect risk reduction for premature heart disease. Adolescents with cholesterol levels >75th percentile are considered hypercholesterolemic and potentially at risk for adult heart disease (Daniels and Greer, 2008; American Society for Bariatric Surgery, 2010).

Blood cholesterol levels track over time. Thus, adolescents with high cholesterol levels tend to have high levels as young adults. However, tracking is not perfect as cholesterol levels vary between genders and fluctuate with sexual maturation, growth, percentage body fat, and age (Daniels and Greer, 2008; American Society for Bariatric Surgery, 2010). These differences are reflected in the NHANES age- and gender-specific lipoprotein distri-

butions (Jolliffe and Janssen, 2008). Adolescents may have elevated cholesterol levels for a variety of reasons. Primary genetic defects, familial hyperlipidemia, and secondary medical causes of hyperlipoproteinemia should be considered. Inappropriate dietary habits, by themselves or by interaction with any of the above factors, can contribute to moderately raised cholesterol levels. Although a few children have a well defined familial hyperlipidemia, most individuals with hyperlipidemia do not have specific syndromes.

Screening for Hypercholesterolemia

Adolescents with unavailable or positive family histories for dyslipidemia, or premature cardiovascular disease (≤55 years of age for men and ≤65 years of age for women in a first-degree relative) or those with other risk factors for coronary heart disease such as hypertension (blood pressure ≥95th percentile), diabetes mellitus, BMI ≥85th percentile, cigarette smoking, or oral contraceptive use should be screened for hypercholesterolemia using a fasting lipid profile (Table 41.5) (Daniels and Greer, 2008).

Treatment of Hyperlipidemia

Dietary modification is the hallmark for hypercholesterolemia treatment. Dietary goals are similar to those of adults (see Chapter 48, which looks at atherosclerotic disease). Diet modification in adolescents should include supervision by a registered pediatric dietitian in order to ensure a balanced diet that promotes normal growth and development. Besides dietary modification, other cardiovascular disease risk factors such as sedentary lifestyle, obesity, diabetes, hypertension, and smoking should be evaluated and minimized (Daniels and Greer, 2008).

Some adolescents require drug therapy. Children over the age of 8 with "pure" hyperlipidemia (specifically, increased LDL only) (based on the same guidelines as adults) can be treated with cholestyramine and statins [3-hydroxy-3-methylglutaryl-coenzyme A (HMG-CoA) reductase inhibitors]. Although considered safe, cholestyramine has considerable gastrointestinal-related side-effects, and dosage commonly makes long-term compliance unsuccessful (Daniels and Greer, 2008).

Unhealthy Eating Practices and Eating Disorders

Concomitant with puberty are a heightened awareness and preoccupation with body image and size. In the western world, the epitome of beauty is for girls to be tall and thin and for boys to be tall and muscular, and many adolescents are dissatisfied with their body image (American Academy of Pediatrics, 2003). Data from the 2008–2009 National Youth Risk Behavior Survey (Eaton et al., 2010) showed that 28% of high-school students described themselves as overweight, with 44% actively trying to lose weight, the prevalence being higher in females (53%) compared with males (31%). By race, the prevalence was higher among white (61%), black (47%), and Hispanic (62%) female students compared with white (28%), black (26%), and Hispanic (42%) male students, respectively. Most students employed healthy measures to achieve weight loss such as eating less food overall or less calories or fat in their meals (28–52%) or exercising more frequently (62%). Yet a surprising proportion reported using increasingly less healthy methods to achieve weight loss such as not eating for more than 24 hours at least once within the 30 days prior to the survey (11%) or vomiting and using laxatives at least once within the past month (4–5%) (Eaton et al., 2010). Complications associated with dieting and decreased energy intake include weight loss, delayed sexual maturation, menstrual irregularities, constipation, weakness, irritability, sleep problems, poor concentration, and impulses to binge eat (American Academy of Pediatrics, 2003).

The number of adolescents with eating disorders (anorexia nervosa and bulimia) has increased steadily since 1950 (Lukas, et al., 1991; Hsu, 1996). Psychosocial issues such as environmental problems, low self-esteem, abnormal family dynamics, and depression are often associated with eating disorders (Rome et al., 2003). Anorexia nervosa is characterized by a persistent, progressive, and severe restriction of food intake, often combined with excessive physical activity. Bulimia is characterized by binge eating that is followed by purging, induced vomiting, diuretic use, exercise, or fasting. While patients with eating disorders usually belong to the middle- or upper-income group,

eating disorders also occur in other economic groups (Kreipe and Dukarm, 1999). Biological factors include a familial increased incidence of eating disorders and neurotransmitter imbalance of serotonin and other neurotransmitters. Groups at risk for developing eating disorders include gymnasts, runners, ballet dancers, and some other athletes. Societal factors include stereotypical and unrealistic body images, women's role in society, and media pressure. The nutritional changes seen with eating disorders are those of malnutrition and starvation. Though most patients with binge-eating disorders are thin, some may be obese. Amenorrhea is usually seen in anorexia nervosa. In the malnourished patient, bradycardia, orthostatic hypotension, hypothermia, wasting, thin pale-colored hair, dry skin, alopecia, acrocyanosis, and poor capillary refill may be evident. Parotid gland enlargement, erosion of dental enamel, and abrasions over the metacarpophalangeal joints (Russell's sign) may be related to induced vomiting. Laboratory evaluation reveals electrolyte abnormalities (hypokalemic alkalosis), anemia, and mildly elevated liver enzymes (consistent with fatty infiltration of the liver seen with malnutrition).

Pregnancy

Sexual activity among American adolescents has increased over the past decades. Predictive factors for sexual activity in early adolescent years include early puberty, poverty, history of sexual abuse, cultural and family patterns of early sexual experience, poor school performance, lack of school goals, and lack of attentive and nurturing parents (Felice et al., 1999). Approximately 1 million teenagers become pregnant every year in the United States (Felice et al., 1999) and the United States has the highest adolescent birth rate of all developed countries. Poverty is a significant factor in adolescent pregnancy (Felice et al., 1999). Accompanying these adolescent pregnancies are challenges and concerns that differ from those that relate to the grown adult. These concerns are associated in the adolescent with increased risk for medical complications including intrauterine growth retardation, neonatal and maternal morbidity and mortality. Micronutrient-associated deficiencies may have consequences such as iron deficiency and anemia, which may have profound implications for the fetus. Intrauterine growth retardation and neonatal demise are greater risks for adolescents less than 14 years of age, and in the African-American population. Prenatal care has improved infant and maternal health and reduced morbidity and mortality.

Nutritional considerations must be borne in mind at the preconception stage, and since many of these pregnancies are unplanned, the considerations are those that are critical for all females at or near childbearing age, for example folic acid intake, and risk reduction for neural tube defects (American Academy of Pediatrics, 1999). Because many adolescent females who get pregnant are psychosocially at risk, efforts to optimize the nutritional support of pregnant teens may have long-term positive health effects on their children (Kleinman, 2009).

Prepregnancy weight is one of the major predictors of birth weight of the child. Both being underweight and overweight increases risk of poor reproductive health outcomes. Underweight females are at risk for preterm delivery, and intrauterine growth retardation is increased, with maternal height a predictor of the fetus's length. Overweight pregnant females are at increased risk for gestational diabetes, pregnancy-induced hypertension, and cesarean-section deliveries. Body mass index (BMI) classification may predict these risks and identify higher-risk individuals for interventions, ideally in the preconception stage but also for the purpose of providing prenatal guidelines. The Institute of Medicine has published new guidelines for total weight gain and rates of weight gain during pregnancy (specifically for the second and third trimesters of pregnancy) based on prepregnancy BMI (Institute of Medicine, 2010b). This information, in addition to weight gain by pediatric BMI classification schema, is summarized in Table 41.6. Weight gain in the first and second trimesters is related to improved birth weight (Hediger et al., 1997). Nutrition and weight gain during the second and third trimester are of particular importance, as maternal deprivation during these critical periods of neonatal development may confer increased risk for chronic conditions including diabetes and cardiovascular disease (Barker, 1995).

Pregnancy energy requirements are based on increased basal metabolic rate as well as energy deposition for accretion of maternal and fetal tissues. Energy requirements increase most in the third trimester. Evidence indicates that adolescent mothers continue to grow in stature and fat-free and bone mass during pregnancy. This growth may occur at the expense of the fetus and result in decreased birth weight despite maternal weight gain, or in suboptimal maternal nutritional status and growth. For this subset of pregnancies, requirements may vary by nutrient; for example, maternal calcium intake may influence bone loss in expectant adolescent females and their growth, as well as bone growth and development in their offspring. Additionally, reduced maternal ferritin, cord blood ferritin, and folate blood levels have been noted in the adolescents who grew during pregnancy (Scholl and Hediger, 1993; Scholl et al., 1997). The fact that pregnant adolescents still grow implies that their nutrient needs are even greater than those for non-adolescent pregnant women. To accommodate the potential growth of the pregnant adolescent, recommendations for gestational weight gain are based on adult prepregnancy BMI, which, when applied to adolescents, results in them being categorized in a lighter weight group. The rationale here is that young teens require more weight gain than their adult counterparts to have infants born at the same size (Scholl, 2008; Institute of Medicine 2010b). Please refer to Chapter 39 of this book for further energy requirements and for macro- and micronutrient needs.

Other micronutrients may pose adverse risks to the fetus if ingested in excess. For example, although vitamin A is important for pregnancy, excessive exposure during the

TABLE 41.6 New recommendations for total and rate of weight gain during pregnancy, by prepregnancy BMI

Prepregnancy BMI	BMI (kg/m²)	Pediatric BMI classification (percentiles)	Total weight gain (lb)	Rates of weight gain (lb/week) during the 2nd and 3rd trimester
Underweight	<18.5	<25th	28–40	1.0 (1–1.3)
Normal weight	18.5–24.9	25th–85th	25–35	1.0 (0.8–1)
Overweight	25.0–29.9	85th–95th	15–25	0.6 (0.5–0.7)
Obese	≥30.0	>95th	11–20	0.5 (0.4–0.6)

Adapted from Institute of Medicine (2010b).

first trimester poses teratogenic risks. Topical acne treatments, which contain synthetic retinol compounds, for example, pose specific increased risks. Exposure to alcohol and tobacco also causes adverse effects on the fetus, and adolescents may be particularly at risk for use of alcohol and tobacco. Glycemic control in adolescents with diabetes may reduce the risk of pregnancy complications and fetal loss as well as birth defects.

In summary, preconceptional as well as prenatal nutritional considerations in the growing adolescent have profound implications for maternal and child health. An underlying understanding of the weight and body-mass issues in adolescent growth and pregnancy, and establishing energy and macronutrient requirements and micronutrients at risk for deficiency or excess at key gestational stages are important determinants of health outcomes for mother and child. Nutritional education and counseling are an important part of pregnant adolescents' prenatal care. Pregnant teens should gain weight at the upper end of the recommended range for their prepregnancy weight (Institute of Medicine, 2010b). Weight gain in the first and second trimesters is related to improved birth weight (Hediger *et al.*, 1997). Pregnant and lactating teens also need additional calories (Institute of Medicine, 2002) and protein (Table 41.3), calcium, iron, vitamins B_6, C, A, D, and folate. A prenatal supplement that contains vitamins A and D, zinc, calcium, folate, and iron is recommended.

Vegetarianism

Adolescents may become vegetarians for many reasons including peer pressure, religious expression, humanitarian feelings, weight control, and self-expression, and these decisions for the most part should be respected. According to the American Dietetic Association, vegetarian diets that are appropriately planned and monitored are healthful and nutritionally adequate, and may provide health benefits in disease prevention and treatment (Craig and Mangels, 2009). It is important to know which type of vegetarianism the adolescent is practicing in order to assess the different nutritional risks (Table 41.7). The most common deficiencies include: vitamins B_{12} and D, protein, calcium, iron, zinc, iodine, riboflavin, and essential fatty acids. The high fiber and low fat content of vegetarian foods are beneficial, and can result in decreased energy intake. Dietary protein may be used for energy, thus negatively affecting protein status. Because a purely vegetarian diet is deficient in vitamin B_{12}, a supplement is needed. High intakes of grains can decrease intestinal absorption of iron,

TABLE 41.7 Categories of vegetarianism and the associated nutritional risks

Category	Food allowances	Nutritional deficiency risk
Semi-vegetarian	Fish, chicken, milk, eggs	No additional nutritional risks
Lacto-ovo-vegetarian	Milk and eggs	Iron deficiency
Lacto-vegetarian	Milk products only	Iron deficiency
Vegan	No milk, eggs, fish, or meat of any kind	Vitamin B_{12}, Vitamin D, zinc, calcium, essential fatty acids, and protein

Adapted from Craig and Mangels (2009).

calcium, and zinc. The vegetarian adolescent should learn about the core dietary principles, and plan a diet that is sufficient in energy, protein, and micronutrients. A daily multivitamin supplement may be beneficial.

Adolescent vegetarian diets are low in energy, with cereals being a major energy source. A study examining whether vegetarian adolescents meet the Healthy People 2010 objectives (Perry *et al.*, 2002) found that they were less likely to consume fast food, sugar-sweetened beverages, and cholesterol. Vegetarian adolescents consumed more folate and iron, and were more likely to consume less than 30% of calories from fat and to consume ≥5 servings of vegetables and fruit per day (Perry *et al.*, 2002). Vegetarians were more likely to engage in disordered eating behaviors such as binge eating, taking diet pills, intentional vomiting, and the use of laxatives and diuretics than non-vegetarians (Robinson-O'Brien *et al.*, 2009). Thus it is important to explore the reason for choosing a vegetarian diet as for some adolescents the practice of vegetarianism may mask an underlying eating disorder. With appropriate knowledge and guidance, a vegetarian diet for growing adolescents can be designed to meet their nutritional needs and to fit into the complex set of changes in their social, economic, and biological environments.

Physical Activity and Sports Medicine

For adolescents, current physical activity recommendations include 60 minutes or more per day of moderate to vigorous physical activity (Physical Activity Guidelines

Steering Committee, 2008). Unfortunately, hypokinesis is prevalent among American adolescents, with most not meeting the prescribed intensity or duration of physical activity. From 2008 to 2009 only 18% of students in grades 9 to 12 engaged in physical activity that increased their heart rate and made them breathe hard for at least 60 minutes per day for all 7 days (Eaton et al., 2010). The benefits of regular physical activity, including improved cardiorespiratory fitness, muscle strength, bone and mental health, and reductions in adiposity and disease risk factors are well documented (Physical Activity Guidelines Steering Committee, 2008). Thus, increasing physical activity levels among adolescents is vital for overall health and well-being.

Adequate energy intake for the adolescent is important to ensure proper growth, development, and maturation. Due to the greater energy expenditure from physical activity, the adolescent athlete will have additional nutritional needs. The onset of the adolescent growth spurt and concomitant increased energy requirements is variable. Thus, the estimated energy requirement is based upon equations that consider the adolescent's age, height, weight, and physical activity level classified as sedentary, moderately active, active or very active (Institute of Medicine, 2002, and see Table 41.2). Carbohydrate, fat, and protein in adequate amounts are important to support overall growth and development. Specific to physical activity, the glycolytic capacity of an adolescent may not be fully developed (Eriksson et al., 1973; Eriksson and Saltin, 1974). Therefore fat may play as important a role as carbohydrate in supporting performance and endurance. Competitive athletes' diets commonly are deficient in calcium and iron. Iron needs are higher because of the decreased absorption during strenuous activity and increased losses in sweat and stool. Iron deficiency can lead to anemia with decreased endurance (Petrie et al., 2004).

Adolescent athletes become progressively dehydrated when voluntary fluid intake is insufficient to match sweat losses. Dehydration is common in adolescents during team sports, with children routinely losing 1–3% body weight (Broad et al., 1996; Casa et al., 2005; Decher et al., 2005). Compared with euhydration during exercise, dehydration as low as 2% of initial body weight in adolescents results in an elevated heart rate (Allen et al., 1977) and body core temperature (Bar-Or et al., 1980), suggesting that even low levels of dehydration result in greater physiological stress during exercise in this age group. Few studies have examined the impact of dehydration or pos-

sible performance-enhancing effects of various nutritional products (drinks, bars, gels) on sport-specific performance in adolescent athletes. Dougherty et al. (2006) showed that in skilled 12- to 15-year-old boys, basketball performance was impaired by 2% dehydration. Additionally, euhydration with a 6% carbohydrate electrolyte solution significantly improves shooting skill performance and on-court sprinting over euhydration with water alone. It is interesting to note that in this study, as in others (Walker et al., 2004), although encouraged to stay well hydrated, adolescents often arrived for sports competitions already dehydrated by 1 to 2%. Previous studies suggest that, compared with water, flavoring a beverage attenuates the dehydration incurred during exercise in the heat whereas adding flavor plus 6% carbohydrates and 18 mmol/L NaCl prevents dehydration altogether (Wilk and Bar-Or, 1996; Wilk et al., 1998). Thus, it appears that, to enhance drinking behavior in adolescents, beverages should be flavored and contain electrolytes and simple carbohydrates when used as true rehydration fluids in dehydrated young athletes.

Future Directions

Many food and food-related products, advertising, and popular culture will continue to focus on adolescents as consumers. They have significant freedom in food choices and meal settings, and often are responsible for arranging their meals within a complex family, school, and social environment. With new guidelines for federally supported school meals and the snacks available in school settings, more healthful food and beverage choices and portion sizes will be a part of the adolescent experience. The adolescent obesity epidemic must call attention to the changes needed in nutrition and health awareness at the individual adolescent, family, clinical, and community level. The future direction for nutrition and adolescent health will be to support healthful food and activity choices to maintain a healthy weight. Emphasis will also be placed on ensuring that adolescent females enter young adulthood in optimal nutritional status to support the health and development of the children they may have in their third and fourth decades of life.

Acknowledgments

Maria R. Mascarenhas, Babette Zemel and Andrew M. Tershakovec contributed to the Adolescence chapter in the eighth edition of this chapter. Joan I. Schall contributed to the updates for the chapter in the ninth edition.

Suggestions for Further Reading

American Academy of Pediatrics, Committee on Nutrition (2004) *Adolescent Nutrition*. AAP, Elk Grove Village, IL.

Institute of Medicine (2006) *Dietary Reference Intakes: The Essential Guide to Nutritional Requirements*. National Academy Press, Washington, DC.

Kleinman, R.E. (2009) Adolescent nutrition. In *Pediatric Nutrition Handbook*, 6th edn. American Academy of Pediatrics, Elk Grove Village, IL, pp. 175–182.

United States Department of Agriculture. (2005). *Dietary Guidelines for Americans*, Washington DC. http://www.cnpp.usda.gov/DGAs2005Guidelines.htm.

References

Abbassi, V., Bailey, D.A., McKay, H.A., *et al.* (1998) Growth and normal puberty. *Pediatrics* **102**, 507–511.

Aeberli, I., Henschen, I., Molinari, L., *et al.* (2010) Stabilization of the prevalence of childhood obesity in Switzerland. *Swiss Med Wkly* **140**, w13046.

Alaimo, K., McDowell, M.A., Briefel, R.R., *et al.* (1994) Dietary intake of vitamins, minerals, and fiber of persons aged 2 months and over in the United States: Third National Health and Nutrition Examination Survey, Phase 1, 1988–91. *Adv Data* 1–28.

Albertson, A.M., Tobelmann, R.C., and Marquart, L. (1997) Estimated dietary calcium intake and food sources for adolescent females: 1980–92. *J Adolesc Health* **20**, 20–26.

Allen, T.E., Smith, D.P., and Miller, D.K. (1977) Hemodynamic response to submaximal exercise after dehydration and rehydration in high school wrestlers. *Med Sci Sports* **9**, 159–163.

American Academy of Pediatrics (1992) National cholesterol education program: report of the expert panel on blood cholesterol levels in children and adolescents. *Pediatrics* **89**, 525–584.

American Academy of Pediatrics (1999) Folic acid for the prevention of neural tube defects. American Academy of Pediatrics. Committee on Genetics. *Pediatrics* **104**, 325–327.

American Academy of Pediatrics (2003) Identifying and treating eating disorders. *Pediatrics* **111**, 204–211.

American Academy of Pediatrics, Committee on Nutrition (2004) *Adolescent Nutrition*. AAP, Elk Grove Village, IL.

American Diabetes Association (2000) Type 2 diabetes in children and adolescents. *J Pediatr* **105**, 671–680.

American Society for Bariatric Surgery (2010) Updated position statement on sleeve gastrectomy as a bariatric procedure. *Surg Obes Relat Dis* **6**, 1–5.

Anderson, S.E. and Must, A. (2005) Interpreting the continued decline in the average age at menarche: results from two nationally representative surveys of US girls studied 10 years apart. *J Pediatr* **147**, 753–760.

Bar-Or, O., Dotan, R., Inbar, O., *et al.* (1980) Voluntary hypohydration in 10- to 12-year-old boys. *J Appl Physiol* **48**, 104–108.

Barker, D.J. (1995) The fetal and infant origins of disease. *Eur J Clin Invest* **25**, 457–463.

Barlow, S.E. (2007) Expert committee recommendations regarding the prevention, assessment, and treatment of child and adolescent overweight and obesity: summary report. *Pediatrics* **120**(Suppl 4), S164–192.

Bialostosky, K., Wright, J.D., Kennedy-Stephenson, J., *et al.* (2002) Dietary intake of macronutrients, micronutrients, and other dietary constituents: United States 1988–94. *Vital Health Stat* **11**, 1–158.

Bluher, S., Meigen, C., Gausche, R., *et al.* (2009) Prevalence of childhood obesity is levelling off in Germany. *Horm Res* **72**, 338.

Broad, E.M., Burke, L.M., Cox, G.R., *et al.* (1996) Body weight changes and voluntary fluid intakes during training and competition sessions in team sports. *Int J Sport Nutr* **6**, 307–320.

Caballero, B. and Popkin, B.M. (2002) *The Nutrition Transition*. Academic Press, San Diego.

Campbell, R.K. (2009) Type 2 diabetes: where we are today: an overview of disease burden, current treatments, and treatment strategies. *J Am Pharm Assoc* **49**(Suppl 1), 3–9

Casa, D.J., Yeargin, S.W, Decher, N.R, *et al.* (2005) Incidence and degree of dehydration and attitudes regarding hydration in adolescents at summer football camp. *Med Sci Sports Exerc* **37**, S463.

Cavadini, C., Siega-Riz, A.M., and Popkin, B.M. (2000) US adolescent food intake trends from 1965 to 1996. *Arch Dis Child* **83**, 18–24.

Centers for Disease Control and Prevention (1992) Recommendations for the use of folic acid to reduce the number of cases of spina bifida and other neural tube defects. MMWR 41, RR-14. http://www.cdc.gov/mmwr/preview/mmwrhtml/00019479.htm. [Accessed 02/01/2011.]

Centers for Disease Control and Prevention (2002) Iron deficiency– United States, 1999–2000. *MMWR Morb Mortal Wkly Rep* **51**, 897–899.

Centers for Disease Control and Prevention (2005) *Trends in the Prevalence of Dietary Behaviors and Weight Control Practices 1991–2003*. http://www.cdc.gov/yrbss.

Craig, W.J. and Mangels, A.R. (2009) Position of the American Dietetic Association: vegetarian diets. *J Am Diet Assoc* **109**, 1266–1282.

Daniels, S.R. and Greer, F.R. (2008) Lipid screening and cardiovascular health in childhood. *Pediatrics* **122**, 198–208.

Davis, M.M., McGonagle, K., Schoeni, R.F., *et al.* (2008) Grandparental and parental obesity influences on childhood overweight: implications for primary care practice. *J Am Board Fam Med* **21**, 549–554.

De Benoist, B., McLean, E., Egli, I., *et al.* (eds) (2008) *Worldwide Prevalence of Anaemia 1993–2005. WHO Global Database on Anaemia*. World Health Organization, Geneva.

Decher, N.R., Casa, D.J., Yeargin, S.W., *et al.* (2005) Attitudes towards hydration and incidence of dehydration in youths at summer soccer camp. *Med Sci Sports Exerc* **37**, S463.

Docio, S., Riancho, J.A., Perez, A., *et al.* (1998) Seasonal deficiency of vitamin D in children: a potential target for osteoporosis-preventing strategies? *J Bone Miner Res* **13**, 544–548.

Dougherty, K.A., Baker, L.B., Chow, M., *et al.* (2006) Two percent dehydration impairs and six percent carbohydrate drink improves boys' basketball skills. *Med Sci Sports Exerc* **38**, 1650–1658.

Dwyer, J.T. (1996) *Adolescence*. ILSI Press, Washington, DC.

Eaton, D.K., Kann, L., Kinchen, S., *et al.* (2010) Youth risk behavior surveillance – United States, 2009. *MMWR Surveill Summ* **59**, 1–142.

Eriksson, B.O., Gollnick, P.D., and Saltin, B. (1973) Muscle metabolism and enzyme activities after training in boys 11–13 years old. *Acta Physiol Scand* **87**, 485–497.

Eriksson, O. and Saltin, B. (1974) Muscle metabolism during exercise in boys aged 11 to 16 years compared to adults. *Acta Paediatr Belg* **28**(Suppl), 257–265.

Ervin, R.B., Wang, C.Y., Wright, J.D., *et al.* (2004a) Dietary intake of selected minerals for the United States population: 1999–2000. *Adv Data* 1–5.

Ervin, R.B., Wright, J.D., Wang, C.Y., *et al.* (2004b) Dietary intake of selected vitamins for the United States population: 1999–2000. *Adv Data* 1–4.

Felice, M.E., Feinstein, R.A., Fisher, M.M., *et al.* (1999) Adolescent pregnancy – current trends and issues: 1998 American Academy of Pediatrics Committee on Adolescence, 1998–1999. *Pediatrics* **103**, 516–520.

Gong, E.J. and Heald, F.P. (1999) Diet, nutrition and adolescence. In M.E. Shils, J.A. Olson, and M. Shike (eds), *Modern Nutrition in Health and Disease*. Lea & Febiger, Philadelphia, pp. 759–769.

Haas, J.D. and Brownlie, T.T. (2001) Iron deficiency and reduced work capacity: a critical review of the research to determine a causal relationship. *J Nutr* **131**, 676S–688S; Discussion 688S–690S.

Hediger, M.L., Scholl, T.O., and Schall, J.I. (1997) Implications of the Camden Study of adolescent pregnancy: interactions among maternal growth, nutritional status, and body composition. *Ann NY Acad Sci* **817**, 281–291.

Hedley, A.A., Ogden, C.L., Johnson, C.L., *et al.* (2004) Prevalence of overweight and obesity among US children, adolescents, and adults, 1999–2002. *JAMA* **291**, 2847–2850.

Holick, M.F. (1997) *Photobiology of Vitamin D*. Academic Press, San Diego.

Hsu, L.K. (1996) Epidemiology of the eating disorders. *Psychiatr Clin North Am* **19**, 681–700.

Institute of Medicine (1990) *Nutrition during Pregnancy*. National Academy Press, Washington, DC.

Institute of Medicine (1997) *Dietary Reference Intakes for Calcium, Phosphorus, Magnesium, Vitamin D and Fluoride*, National Academy Press, Washington, DC.

Institute of Medicine (1998) *Dietary Reference Intakes for Thiamin, Riboflavin, Niacin, Vitamin B6, Folate, Vitamin B12, Pantothenic Acid, Biotin and Choline*. National Academy Press, Washington, DC.

Institute of Medicine (2001) *Dietary Reference Intakes for Vitamin A, Vitamin K, Boron, Chromium, Copper, Iodine, Iron, Manganese, Molybdenum, Nickel, Vanadium and Zinc*. National Academy Press, Washington, DC.

Institute of Medicine (2002) *Dietary Reference Intakes for Energy, Carbohydrate, Fiber, Fat, Fatty Acids, Cholesterol, Protein and Amino Acids*. National Academy Press, Washington, DC.

Institute of Medicine (2006) *Dietary Reference Intakes: The Essential Guide to Nutritional Requirements*. National Academy Press, Washington, DC.

Institute of Medicine (2010a) *Dietary Reference Intakes for Calcium and Vitamin D*. National Academy Press, Washington, DC. http://www.iom.edu/Reports/2010/Dietary-Reference-Intakes-for-Calcium-and-Vitamin-D.aspx. [Accessed: 01/01/2011.]

Institute of Medicine (2010b) *Weight Gain during Pregnancy: Re-examining the Guidelines*. National Academies of Sciences, Washington, DC.

Johnston, C.C., Jr, Miller, J.Z., Slemenda, C.W., *et al.* (1992) Calcium supplementation and increases in bone mineral density in children. *N Engl J Med*, **327**, 82–87.

Jolliffe, C.J. and Janssen, I. (2008). Age-specific lipid and lipoprotein thresholds for adolescents. *J Cardiovasc Nurs* **23**, 56–60.

Kleinman, R.E. (ed.) (2009) Nutrition in pregnancy. In *Pediatric Nutrition Handbook*, 6th Edn. American Academy of Pediatrics, Elk Grove Village, IL, pp. 249–274.

Krebs, N.F., Himes, J.H., Jacobson, D., *et al.* (2007) Assessment of child and adolescent overweight and obesity. *Pediatrics* **120**(Suppl 4), S193–228.

Krebs-Smith, S.M., Cook, A., Subar, A.F., et al. (1996) Fruit and vegetable intakes of children and adolescents in the United States. *Arch Pediatr Adolesc Med* **150**, 81–86.

Kreipe, R.E. and Dukarm, C.P. (1999) Eating disorders in adolescents and older children. *Pediatr Rev* **20**, 410–421.

Kuczmarski, R.J., Ogden, C.L., Grummer-Strawn, L.M., et al. (2000) CDC growth charts: United States. *Adv Data* 1–27.

Kuczmarski, R.J., Ogden, C.L., Guo, S.S., et al. (2002) 2000 CDC growth charts for the United States: methods and development. *Vital Health Stat* **11**, 1–190.

Kumanyika, S.K. (2008) Environmental influences on childhood obesity: ethnic and cultural influences in context. *Physiol Behav* **94**, 61–70.

Lampl, M., Johnson, M.L., Sun, S.S., et al. (1993) A case study of daily growth during adolescence: a single spurt or changes in the dynamics of saltatory growth? *Ann Hum Biol* **20**, 595–603.

Levin, S., Lowry, R., Brown, D.R., et al. (2003) Physical activity and body mass index among US adolescents: youth risk behavior survey, 1999. *Arch Pediatr Adolesc Med* **157**, 816–820.

Lucas, A.R., Beard, C.M., O'Fallon, W.M., et al. (1991) 50-year trends in the incidence of anorexia nervosa in Rochester, Minn.: a population-based study. *Am J Psychiatry* **148**, 917–922.

Ludwig, D.S., Peterson, K.E., and Gortmaker, S.L. (2001) Relation between consumption of sugar-sweetened drinks and childhood obesity: a prospective, observational analysis. *Lancet* **357**, 505–508.

Matkovic, V. (1991) Calcium metabolism and calcium requirements during skeletal modeling and consolidation of bone mass. *Am J Clin Nutr* **54**, 245S–260S.

Matkovic, V. (1992) Calcium and peak bone mass. *J Intern Med* **231**, 151–160.

Moore, C., Murphy, M.M., Keast, D.R., et al. (2004). Vitamin D intake in the United States. *J Am Diet Assoc* **104**, 980–983.

Morris, N.M. and Udry, J.R. (1980) Validation of a self-administered instrument to assess stage of adolescent development. *J Youth Adolesc* **9**, 271–280.

Munoz, K.A., Krebs-Smith, S.M., Ballard-Barbash, R., et al. (1997). Food intakes of US children and adolescents compared with recommendations. *Pediatrics* **100**, 323–329.

Nadeau, K. and Dabelea, D. (2008) Epidemiology of type 2 diabetes in children and adolescents. *Endocrinol Res* **33**, 35–58.

Nicklas, T.A., Myers, L., and Berenson, G.S. (1995) Dietary fiber intake of children: the Bogalusa Heart Study. *Pediatrics* **96**, 988–994.

Ogden, C.L. and Carroll, M. (2010) Prevalence of Obesity Among Children and Adolescents: United States, Trends 1963–1965 Through 2007–2008. National Center for Health Statistics, Centers for Disease Control. http://www.cdc.gov/nchs/data/hestat/obesity_child_07_08/obesity_child_07_08.htm.

Ogden, C.L., Carroll, M.D., and Flegal, K.M. (2008) High body mass index for age among US children and adolescents, 2003–2006. *JAMA* **299**, 2401–2405.

Perry, C.L., McGuire, M.T., Neumark-Sztainer, D., et al. (2002) Adolescent vegetarians: how well do their dietary patterns meet the Healthy People 2010 objectives? *Arch Pediatr Adolesc Med* **156**, 431–437.

Petrie, H.J., Stover, E.A., and Horswill, C.A. (2004) Nutritional concerns for the child and adolescent competitor. *Nutrition* **20**, 620–631.

Physical Activity Guidelines Steering Committee (2008) Physical activity guidelines for Americans. www.health.gov/paguidelines/default.aspx.

Ramakrishnan, U., Barnhart, H., Schroeder, D.G., et al. (1999) Early childhood nutrition, education and fertility milestones in Guatemala. *J Nutr* **129**, 2196–2202.

Rasmussen, K. (2001) Is there a causal relationship between iron deficiency or iron-deficiency anemia and weight at birth, length of gestation and perinatal mortality? *J Nutr* **131**, 590S–601S; Discussion, 601S–603S.

Remsberg, K.E., Demerath, E.W., Schubert, C.M., et al. (2005) Early menarche and the development of cardiovascular disease risk factors in adolescent girls: the Fels Longitudinal Study. *J Clin Endocrinol Metab* **90**, 2718–2724.

Renna, F., Grafova, I.B., and Thakur, N. (2008) The effect of friends on adolescent body weight. *Econ Hum Biol* **6**, 377–387.

Robinson-O'Brien, R., Perry, C.L., Wall, M.M., et al. (2009) Adolescent and young adult vegetarianism: better dietary intake and weight outcomes but increased risk of disordered eating behaviors. *J Am Diet Assoc* **109**, 648–655.

Rome, E.S., Ammerman, S., Rosen, D.S., et al. (2003) Children and adolescents with eating disorders: the state of the art. *Pediatrics* **111**, e98–108.

Rovner, A.J. and O'Brien, K.O. (2008) Hypovitaminosis D among healthy children in the United States: a review of the current evidence. *Arch Pediatr Adolesc Med* **162**, 513–519.

Salanave, B., Peneau, S., Rolland-Cachera, M.F., et al. (2009) Stabilization of overweight prevalence in French children between 2000 and 2007. *Int J Pediatr Obes* **4**, 66–72.

Scholl, T.O. (2008) Biological determinants of gestational weight gain. Presentation at the Workshop on Implications of Weight Gain for Pregnancy Outcomes: Issues and Evidence, March 10, 2008, Washington, DC. http://www.iom.edu/Activities/Women/PregWeightGain/2008-MAR-10.aspx. Accessed September 30, 2011.

Scholl, T.O. and Hediger, M.L. (1993) A review of the epidemiology of nutrition and adolescent pregnancy: maternal growth during pregnancy and its effect on the fetus. *J Am Coll Nutr* **12,** 101–107.

Scholl, T.O., Hediger, M.L., and Schall, J.I. (1997) Maternal growth and fetal growth: pregnancy course and outcome in the Camden Study. *Ann NY Acad Sci* **817,** 292–301.

Skelton, J.A., Cook, S.R., Auinger, P., *et al.* (2009) Prevalence and trends of severe obesity among US children and adolescents. *Acad Pediatr* **9,** 322–329.

Skiba, A., Loghmani, E., and Orr, D.P. (1997) Nutritional screening and guidance for adolescents. *Adol Health Update* **9,** 1–8.

Spear, B.A., Barlow, S.E., Ervin, C., *et al.* (2007) Recommendations for treatment of child and adolescent overweight and obesity. *Pediatrics* **120**(Suppl 4), S254–288.

Stamatakis, E., Zaninotto, P., Falaschetti, E., *et al.* (2010) Time trends in childhood and adolescent obesity in England from 1995 to 2007 and projections of prevalence to 2015. *J Epidemiol Community Health* **64,** 167–174.

Story, M. and Alton, I. (1996) Adolescent nutrition: current trends and critical issues. *Top Clin Nutr* **11,** 56–69.

Strong, J.P. (1986) Landmark perspective: coronary atherosclerosis in soldiers. A clue to the natural history of atherosclerosis in the young. *JAMA* **256,** 2863–2866.

Sun, S.S., Schubert, C.M., Chumlea, W.C., *et al.* (2002) National estimates of the timing of sexual maturation and racial differences among US children. *Pediatrics* **110,** 911–919.

Tanner, J.M. (1962) *Growth at Adolescence*, 2nd Edn. Blackwell, Oxford, pp. 28–39.

Tanner, J.M. and Davies, P.S. (1985) Clinical longitudinal standards for height and weight velocity for North American children. *J Pediatr* **107,** 317–329.

Theintz, G., Buchs, B., Rizzoli, R., *et al.* (1992) Longitudinal monitoring of bone mass accumulation in healthy adolescents: evidence for a marked reduction after 16 years of age at the levels of lumbar spine and femoral neck in female subjects. *J Clin Endocrinol Metab* **75,** 1060–1065.

United States Department of Agriculture (2005) *Dietary Guidelines for Americans*, Washington DC. http://www.cnpp.usda.gov/DGAs2005Guidelines.htm.

Videon, T.M. and Manning, C.K. (2003) Influences on adolescent eating patterns: the importance of family meals. *J Adolesc Health* **32,** 365–373.

Walker, S.M., Casa, D.J., Levreault, M.L., *et al.* (2004) Children participating in summer soccer camps are chronically dehydrated. *Med Sci Sports Exerc* **36,** S180–181.

Wang, F., Wild, T.C., Kipp, W., *et al.* (2009) The influence of childhood obesity on the development of self-esteem. *Health Reports/Statistics Canada, Canadian Centre for Health Information – Rapports sur la santé. Statistique Canada, Centre canadien d'information sur la santé*, vol. 20, no. 2, pp. 21–27.

Weaver, C.M., Peacock, M., and Johnston, C.C., Jr (1999) Adolescent nutrition in the prevention of postmenopausal osteoporosis. *J Clin Endocrinol Metab* **84,** 1839–1843.

Whitaker, R.C., Wright, J.A., Pepe, M.S., *et al.* (1997) Predicting obesity in young adulthood from childhood and parental obesity. *N Engl J Med* **337,** 869–873.

Wilk, B. and Bar-Or, O. (1996) Effect of drink flavor and NaCl on voluntary drinking and hydration in boys exercising in the heat. *J Appl Physiol* **80,** 1112–1117.

Wilk, B., Kriemler, S., Keller, H., *et al.* (1998) Consistency in preventing voluntary dehydration in boys who drink a flavored carbohydrate–NaCl beverage during exercise in the heat. *Int J Sport Nutr* **8,** 1–9.

Williams, C.L., Bollella, M., and Wynder, E.L. (1995) A new recommendation for dietary fiber in childhood. *Pediatrics* **96,** 985–988.

Woo, T. (2009) Pharmacotherapy and surgery treatment for the severely obese adolescent. *J Pediatr Health Care* **23,** 206–212; Quiz, 213–215.

Zeitler, P.S., Travers, S., Kappy, M.D., *et al.* (1999) Advances in the recognition and treatment of endocrine complications in children with chronic illness. *Adv Padiatr* **46,** 101–149.

Zemel, B.S. and Jenkins, C. (1989) Dietary change and adolescent growth among the Bundi (Gende-speaking) people of Papua New Guinea. *Am J Human Biol* **1,** 709–718.

Zemel, B. S., Kawchak, D.A., Cnaan, A., *et al.* (1996) Prospective evaluation of resting energy expenditure, nutritional status, pulmonary function, and genotype in children with cystic fibrosis. *Pediatr Res* **40,** 578–586.

42

NUTRITION AND AGING

MARION SECHER, MD, PATRICK RITZ, MD, PhD, AND BRUNO VELLAS, MD, PhD

Gérontopôle de Toulouse, Toulouse, France

Summary

In the first part of this chapter, we present the effects of aging on nutritional status. We discuss the specificity of the evaluation of nutritional status in the older population, and then present four pathologies illustrating abnormal nutritional status: malnutrition, obesity, sarcopenia, and hydration disorders.

The second part of the chapter considers the effects of nutritional deficiencies on the older population. These are illustrated by three situations: frailty, osteoporosis, and cognitive decline and Alzheimer's disease.

Introduction

The average age and the proportion of the population which is older increase every year: around the world the number of people aged 60 years and over was estimated at 600 million in 2000, a figure that is expected to rise to 1.2 billion by 2025 and 2 billion by 2050 (WHO, 2009).

Many of the physiological changes associated with aging can be slowed down to some extent by eating a healthy diet and taking physical exercise, and many of the chronic diseases prevalent in older adults are either preventable or modifiable with healthy lifestyle habits. Thus, older adults can experience successful aging that allows them to achieve physical, social and mental well-being over the life course and to participate in society.

Much research has been conducted in recent years to determine how to keep older adults fully functional, physically, mentally, and socially. This chapter examines some of the areas of aging research currently being conducted, and addresses promising areas of research for the future.

Effects of Aging on Nutritional Status

Evaluation of Nutritional Status in the Older Population

Many geriatric assessment instruments have been developed to diagnose and treat high-risk situations in elderly patients. The major components of a geriatric assessment are:

- measurements of the functional status using Activities of Daily Living (ADL) (Katz, 1983) and Instrumental Activities of Daily Living (IADL) (Lawton and Brody, 1969);
- cognitive status using Mini-Mental State Examination (MMSE) (Folstein *et al.*, 1975);

Present Knowledge in Nutrition, Tenth Edition. Edited by John W. Erdman Jr, Ian A. Macdonald and Steven H. Zeisel.
© 2012 International Life Sciences Institute. Published 2012 by John Wiley & Sons, Inc.

- psychological health using Geriatric Depression Scale (GDS) (Yesavage *et al.*, 1982);
- physical status using Tinetti Balance and Gait Evaluation (Tinetti, 1986);
- a nutritional evaluation.

Nutritional status in the elderly can be best evaluated with a combination of several approaches using anthropometric, dietary, and biological parameters. Nutritional screening and assessment tools such as the Mini Nutritional Assessment (MNA®), which is an example of this combination of measurement systems, can also be used. This nutritional evaluation has to be repeated at times appropriate to the rhythm determined by the clinical setting (geriatric hospital, nursing home, community-dwelling) (Bauer *et al.*, 2010).

The single most important clinical aspect leading to diagnosis of malnutrition is weight change and especially unintentional weight loss. Weight loss is expressed as a percentage of a patient's usual weight or previous value. An able patient should be weighed in underwear or with light clothing, standing on a calibrated scale. Obtaining body weight may be challenging, particularly in frail patients or those with a disability. A calibrated chair or lifting scale should be used for patients who are unable to stand. When assessing body weight, some conditions such as the presence of edema or ascites have to be taken into account because they may lead to an overestimation of weight.

The calculation of Body Mass Index (BMI) (weight (kg)/height (m²)) requires measurement of patient's height. In dependent patients or those with kyphosis, stature can be estimated from knee height using Chumlea's formulae (Chumlea *et al.*, 1985). The patient must be able to fold the knee and the ankle to an angle of 90°. The knee-height caliper is used to measure length of the leg from the bottom of the foot to the top of the patella. Then, knee height is inserted into a mathematical formula and converted to stature. To estimate a patient's height, the measure of distance between the sternal notch to the finger roots can also be used (called demispan). Height is then calculated from a standard formula. Alternatively, instead of BMI, a Demiquet index can be computed directly from the demispan (Lehmann *et al.*, 1991). Nevertheless, BMI does not reflect the body composition (fat and muscle mass), and like weight it can be unreliable in the presence of confounding factors such as edema or ascites.

Skinfold measurement can be used as a reflection of fat mass (Frisancho and Flegel, 1982), but it is not an easy tool to use in clinical practice and it cannot be used to assess changes in body-fat mass because of age-related fat redistribution (Hughes *et al.*, 2004). Nevertheless, it could be used in serial measures of an individual over a defined, relatively short-term period. The use of parameters that reflect muscle mass, such as mid-calf or mid-arm circumference, is more appropriate in the elderly because of the relevance of muscle mass in relation to functionality (Portero-McLellan *et al.*, 2010).

A number of screening tools have been developed for identifying older adults at risk of poor nutrition (Bauer *et al.*, 2010). The Simplified Nutrition Assessment Questionnaire (SNAQ), a four-item screening test, has a sensitivity of 88.2% and a specificity of 83.5% for the identification of older persons at risk of a 10% weight loss (Wilson *et al.*, 2005). More recently developed, the Mini Nutritional Assessment (MNA®) represents the most widely accepted and validated nutritional assessment tool for older people, regardless of setting, with clearly defined thresholds (Guigoz, 2006). The MNA® aims to evaluate the risk of malnutrition without the need for specialized personnel and so permits early nutritional intervention when needed. The MNA® instrument is composed of simple measurements and questions to be completed in less than 15 minutes. It consists of 18 self-reported questions derived from four parameters of assessment, anthropometric, general, dietary, and self assessment, administered in two steps (see Figure 42.1). The MNA-SF® (Short Form) is a screening tool composed of the first six items that allows the detection of a decline in ingestion over the past 3 months (loss of appetite, decline in food intake, digestive problems, chewing or swallowing difficulties); weight loss during the past 3 months; current mobility impairment; an acute illness or major stress over the past 3 months; a neuropsychological problem (dementia or depression); and a decrease in BMI. The maximum score for this part of the MNA® is 14. A score of 12 points or more indicates that the patient has an acceptable nutritional status and that it is not necessary to complete the full MNA®. At this stage, it is important to give nutritional advice, to follow the patient's weight regularly (usually every month) and to complete the MNA-SF® at regular intervals (every 3 or 6 months) (Secher *et al.*, 2007). A score of 11 points or below is an indication to proceed with the complete version of the MNA® (see Figure 42.2). The full MNA® evaluates living arrangements, number of

Nestlé Nutrition Institute

Mini Nutritional Assessment
MNA®

Last name: _____   First name: _____

Sex: _____   Age: _____   Weight, kg: _____   Height, cm: _____   Date: _____

Complete the screen by filling in the boxes with the appropriate numbers. Add the numbers for the screen. If score is 11 or less, continue with the assessment to gain a Malnutrition Indicator Score.

Screening

A   Has food intake declined over the past 3 months due to loss of appetite, digestive problems, chewing or swallowing difficulties?
0 = severe decrease in food intake
1 = moderate decrease in food intake
2 = no decrease in food intake ☐

B   Weight loss during the last 3 months
0 = weight loss greater than 3kg (6.6lbs)
1 = does not know
2 = weight loss between 1 and 3kg (2.2 and 6.6 lbs)
3 = no weight loss ☐

C   Mobility
0 = bed or chair bound
1 = able to get out of bed / chair but does not go out
2 = goes out ☐

D   Has suffered psychological stress or acute disease in the past 3 months?
0 = yes   2 = no ☐

E   Neuropsychological problems
0 = severe dementia or depression
1 = mild dementia
2 = no psychological problems ☐

F   Body Mass Index (BMI) (weight in kg) / (height in m²)
0 = BMI less than 19
1 = BMI 19 to less than 21
2 = BMI 21 to less than 23
3 = BMI 23 or greater ☐

Screening score ☐☐
(subtotal max. 14 points)

12-14 points: Normal nutritional status
8-11 points: At risk of malnutrition
0-7 points: Malnourished

For a more in-depth assessment, continue with questions G-R

G   Lives independently (not in nursing home or hospital)
1 = yes   0 = no ☐

H   Takes more than 3 prescription drugs per day
0 = yes   1 = no ☐

I   Pressure sores or skin ulcers
0 = yes   1 = no ☐

J   How many full meals does the patient eat daily?
0 = 1 meal
1 = 2 meals
2 = 3 meals ☐

K   Selected consumption markers for protein intake
• At least one serving of dairy products (milk, cheese, yoghurt) per day   yes ☐   no ☐
• Two or more servings of legumes or eggs per week   yes ☐   no ☐
• Meat, fish or poultry every day   yes ☐   ☐
0.0 = if 0 or 1 yes
0.5 = if 2 yes
1.0 = if 3 yes ☐.☐

L   Consumes two or more servings of fruit or vegetables per day?
0 = no   1 = yes ☐

M   How much fluid (water, juice, coffee, tea, milk...) is consumed per day?
0.0 = less than 3 cups
0.5 = 3 to 5 cups
1.0 = more than 5 cups ☐.☐

N   Mode of feeding
0 = unable to eat without assistance
1 = self-fed with some difficulty
2 = self-fed without any problem ☐

O   Self view of nutritional status
0 = views self as being malnourished
1 = is uncertain of nutritional state
2 = views self as having no nutritional problem ☐

P   In comparison with other people of the same age, how does the patient consider his / her health status?
0.0 = not as good
0.5 = does not know
1.0 = as good
2.0 = better ☐.☐

Q   Mid-arm circumference (MAC) in cm
0.0 = MAC less than 21
0.5 = MAC 21 to 22
1.0 = MAC 22 or greater ☐.☐

R   Calf circumference (CC) in cm
0 = CC less than 31
1 = CC 31 or greater ☐

Assessment (max. 16 points) ☐☐.☐

Screening score ☐☐.☐

Total Assessment (max. 30 points) ☐☐.☐

Ref.   Vellas B, Villars H, Abellan G, et al. *Overview of MNA® - Its History and Challenges.* J Nut Health Aging 2006; 10: 456-465.
Rubenstein LZ, Harker JO, Salva A, Guigoz Y, Vellas B. Screening for Undernutrition in Geriatric Practice: *Developing the Short-Form Mini Nutritional Assessment (MNA-SF).* J. Geront 2001; 56A: M366-377.
Guigoz Y. The Mini-Nutritional Assessment (MNA®) *Review of the Literature – What does it tell us?* J Nutr Health Aging 2006; 10: 466-487.
® Société des Produits Nestlé, S.A., Vevey, Switzerland, Trademark Owners
© Nestlé, 1994, Revision 2006. N67200 12/99 10M
For more information: www.mna-elderly.com

Malnutrition Indicator Score

24 to 30 points   ☐   normal nutritional status

17 to 23.5 points   ☐   at risk of malnutrition

Less than 17 points   ☐   malnourished

FIG. 42.1   The MNA® Long Form. Reproduced with permission from Nestlé Nutrition. Available online at http://www.mna-elderly.com/.

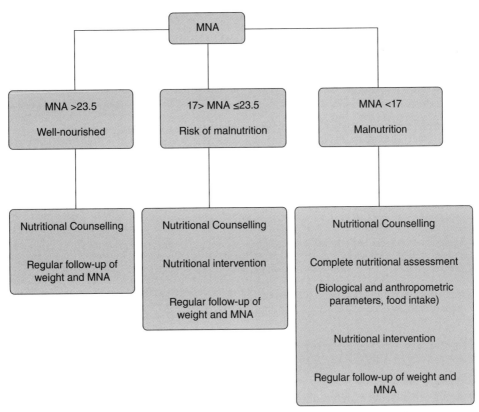

FIG. 42.2 The MNA® as a tool for the diagnosis of malnutrition and a guide for nutritional intervention. Adapted from Secher *et al.* (2007).

medications, presence of pressure ulcers, number of full meals eaten daily, amount and frequency of specific foods and fluids, and mode of feeding. The patient reports nutritional and health status, and the practitioner must determine mid-arm and mid-calf circumferences. The maximum score of the second part of the MNA® is 16. The scores of the two parts must be added to obtain the malnutrition indicator score, which has a maximum of 30. A score of 23.5 or higher classifies an individual as well-nourished. No specific follow-up is needed except to measure the person's weight regularly at routine visits, complete the MNA® at regular intervals, and provide general nutritional counselling based upon reminders about the basic rules of balanced food (e.g. recommended daily intake frequencies of fruits and vegetables, starchy foods, dairy products, meats, fish, seafood, and eggs, and reminders about not exceeding recommended intakes of fat and sweetened products); about taking regular daily physical exercise; and about ensuring good hydration. A score between 17 and 23.5 indicates risk of malnutrition. A specific nutritional

intervention program should be implemented, based on the impairments found after assessment by the MNA® (items leading to loss of points). The use of concentrated formulas increasing total intake of calories, proteins or micronutrients is a common strategy for improving nutritional status. Nutritional counselling, as just discussed, should always be provided. A score of less than 17 indicates protein-calorie malnutrition. At this stage it is important to quantify the severity of the malnutrition by complete nutritional assessment (biological and anthropometric parameters and food intakes). Nutritional intervention should be started, with specific and reasonable goals set in advance. It is necessary to support the oral route for as long as possible by improving total intake of calories and prescribing oral supplementation.

Assessment of dietary intakes can identify elderly people at risk of malnutrition by quantifying energy and nutrient intake. There is no easy method to assess dietary intakes in clinical practice. The quality of the data depends on the patient, the time of collection, and the tool used. Food composition tables are required to convert information gathered regarding food intake to consumption of energy and nutrients. One of the most accurate tools is keeping a food diary in which dietary intakes are collected prospectively over several days. Nevertheless, this method is cumbersome to implement. Another method is the 24-hour recall. It is a faster and easier method which retrospectively lists all dietary intakes over the past 24 hours, but it requires a good memory on the part of the patient which is sometimes difficult with the elderly.

Finally, various serum proteins are considered as markers of nutritional status such as albumin and transthyretin (prealbumin). They are not specific for malnutrition because their concentration may be influenced by a wide variety of acute and chronic inflammatory conditions (Baron *et al.*, 2010). Transthyretin is preferred to albumin because of its shorter half-life which means that its concentration more closely reflects recent dietary intakes (Shenkin, 2006).

Malnutrition

Malnutrition is a dynamic phenomenon that starts when nutritional intakes are insufficient to match requirements. Most commonly, malnutrition is used to refer to inadequate intakes of energy and protein, but the same reasoning can be applied to other nutrients (e.g. specific lipids such as long-chain polyunsaturated fatty acids, vitamins, and micronutrients).

Several studies have shown that aging is associated with an increasing prevalence of malnutrition (Bauer and Volkert, 2007). Nevertheless, the prevalence of malnutrition in the elderly varies depending on the parameters used for the diagnosis and on the setting considered: 5–10% of community-dwelling elderly people suffer from malnutrition, a level that increases to 30–60% in nursing-home residents and hospitalized older people (Vellas *et al.*, 2001).

There is no universally accepted clinical definition of malnutrition. However, recent French recommendations (Haute Autorité de Santé, 2007) suggest that malnutrition can be diagnosed when weight loss is 5% or greater within 6 months or when BMI is less than $21 \, kg/m^2$, or when MNA score is less than 17 or when albumin concentration is less than $35 \, g/L$ (without inflammation). Malnutrition is considered severe when weight loss is 10% or greater within 1 month or 15%, or greater within 6 months, or when albumin concentration is less than $30 \, g/L$. It is important to distinguish severe forms of malnutrition because they are associated with a considerable increase in morbidity and mortality and therefore require rapid nutritional management.

The American Society for Parenteral and Enteral Nutrition summarizes the selected nutrition screening and assessment instrument parameters (Mueller *et al.*, 2011).

Many studies have demonstrated that malnutrition is associated with increased mortality (Milne *et al.*, 2009), especially in neurodegenerative disease (Vellas *et al.*, 2005) and chronic diseases (Norman *et al.*, 2008). Even in populations who appear healthy, a weight loss of 4% or more multiplies the risk of death by 2.7 (Wallace *et al.*, 1995). Malnutrition is also associated with increased morbidity, for example significant impaired immunity (Chandra, 2002); an increased risk of infections (Paillaud *et al.*, 2005); impaired healing after surgical procedures and an increased risk of pressure sores (Dambach *et al.*, 2005); and an increased risk of cognitive decline (see later in this chapter). The economic consequences of malnutrition in elderly people are also considerable, especially in hospital, mainly due to increased length of stay and associated disease and treatment (Elia, 2005). In the elderly, and even more so in catabolic situations, weight loss affects lean mass (mainly muscle) and water reserves more than fat mass (Schneider *et al.*, 2002). This is of particular concern because these are also affected by natural aging (see "Sarcopenia" and "Hydration Disorders" later in this chapter).

Aging is associated with a physiological anorexia (Hays and Roberts, 2006) that is an independent predictor of poor outcomes (Cornali *et al.*, 2005). Food intake gradually diminishes with age: between the ages of 20 and 80 years, the decrease in food intake is approximately 1200 kcal/day for men and 800 kcal/day for women (Bales and Ritchie, 2002). This decrease in appetite is influenced by multiple physiological changes. Much of the intake decrease in early old age is an appropriate response to decreased energy needs due to reduced physical activity and loss of lean body mass (Blanc *et al.*, 2004). Furthermore, following a period of underfeeding, elderly people do not recover their usual intake as efficiently as young people do, and do not regain the total amount of weight lost (Irvine *et al.*, 2004). Other physiological changes associated with aging promote anorexia: changes in taste and smell lead to a decreased desire to eat; early satiety develops with age, related to gastrointestinal changes (delayed gastric emptying and altered gastric distension) and gastric hormone changes; and increased cytokine activity (Ahmed and Haboubi, 2010).

Multiple non-physiological causes can explain the inadequate nutrient intakes. These include social issues such as financial difficulty in buying food, and isolation. Several studies have demonstrated that the presence of others increased food intake in older adults (Locher *et al.*, 2005). Other causes include medical factors such as malignancy, and psychiatric factors such as depression (Wilson *et al.*, 1998); dental conditions, which may impair the ability to eat (Ritchie *et al.*, 2000); various handicaps such as paralysis from stroke or severe arthritis, which may limit the ability to prepare food and lead to a need for feeding assistance from others; and polymedication and medication side-effects which may affect appetite regulation.

Obesity

The prevalence of obesity decreases in extreme old age, but remains a common problem in the elderly. Aging is accompanied by an increase in fat mass and a decrease in lean mass (Kyle *et al.*, 2001). There are several explanations of increased fat mass: reduced physical activity and energy expenditure, reduced growth hormone secretion, diminished sex hormones, and decreased resting metabolic rate due to reduction of lean mass. Moreover, fat-mass distribution changes with aging: there is an increased central distribution of fat (intra-hepatic and intra-abdominal), which is associated with insulin resistance and non-insulin-dependent diabetes mellitus (Ahmed and Haboubi, 2010). Overweight and obese older adults are also affected by the problem of decrease in muscle mass with aging (sarcopenic obesity), which is a major determinant of physical function (see the next section).

For the population as a whole, overweight and obesity are associated with increase in all-cause mortality, as well as morbidity related to diseases for which overweight and obesity are risk factors (such as hypertension, dyslipidemia, diabetes, coronary heart disease, stroke, osteoarthritis, sleep apnea, some cancers). Several studies suggest that the relationship of overweight and obesity to mortality declines over time (Flegal *et al.*, 2007; Kulminski *et al.*, 2008). However, a few studies suggest that overweight in old age is associated with increased mortality (Sui *et al.*, 2007; Wannamethee *et al.*, 2007).

Although the mortality risk of obesity may lessen with age, there are still potential metabolic and functional benefits to weight loss in the obese elderly. Weight loss can improve physical function and quality of life for many older people (Villareal *et al.*, 2011). Nevertheless, negative outcomes are associated with weight loss in overweight older people, such as loss of muscle mass and decrease in bone mineral density (Villareal *et al.*, 2006a,b). Methods of achieving and maintaining weight loss in older adults are the same as in younger adults (Han *et al.*, 2011). Weight loss should be encouraged using moderate caloric restriction with appropriate calcium and vitamin D supplementation and a regular exercise program (see "Sarcopenia" and "Osteoporosis" in this chapter).

Sarcopenia

Sarcopenia has been defined as the loss of muscle mass and strength that occurs with advancing age (Morley *et al.*, 2001).

Sarcopenia is a complex, multifactorial process facilitated by a combination of voluntary and involuntary factors. These include: the aging process over the life course, less than optimal diet in older age, sedentary lifestyle, chronic diseases, and some drug treatments (Rolland *et al.*, 2008).

Aging leads to intrinsic muscle impairment related to a combination of the reduction in both absolute and relative amounts of type II fibers (glycolytic and mostly used during intense and acute exercise), fatty infiltration and muscular sclerosis within the sarcopenic muscle, a decrease in muscle protein synthesis (myofibrillar and mitochondrial proteins), and impaired postprandial fate of amino acids (Doherty, 2003).

Aging is associated with a gradual chronic increase in the production of proinflammatory cytokines, particularly interleukins (IL-1 and IL-6), leading to a hypercatabolic state (Roubenoff *et al.*, 1998). However, there is little evidence to support the hypothesis that cytokines predict sarcopenia in prospective studies (Schaap *et al.*, 2006).

An age-related decrease in the synthesis of testosterone and oestrogen appears to accelerate the sarcopenia process by causing a decrease in muscle anabolic potential. Testosterone treatment increases muscle mass in young subjects and is accompanied by an increase in strength. This effect is potentiated by exercise. In elderly persons free of disease, things are less clear. It seems that hormonal treatment only mildly increases plasma testosterone concentration and muscle mass, and has a weak effect on muscle strength (Emmelot-Vonk *et al.*, 2008). Moreover, sex-steroid treatment in the elderly is limited by the risk of prostate cancer and cardiovascular events.

Insulin, which also has an anabolic effect on muscle protein metabolism, seems to play a role in the onset of sarcopenia. With aging, increased fat mass promotes insulin resistance. This is characterized by a decline in the anabolic effect of insulin, potentially predisposing to sarcopenia (Roubenoff, 2003).

Sarcopenia is a risk factor for adverse outcomes such as mobility disorders; falls and fractures; impaired ability to perform ADL; disabilities; loss of independence; poor quality of life and increased risk of death (Delmonico et al., 2007; Rolland et al., 2008). A study by Janssen et al. (2004) showed that the estimate of the direct health cost attributable to sarcopenia in the United States was $18.5 billion in 2000, which represented about 1.5% of total health-care expenditures for that year. A 10% reduction in sarcopenia prevalence would result in savings of $1.1 billion (dollars adjusted to 2000 rate) per year in US health-care costs (Janssen et al., 2004).

Prevalence of sarcopenia varies greatly depending on the definition used for the diagnosis: in 60- to 70-year-old people, prevalence ranges from 5% to 13%, whereas it ranges from 11% to 50% in people older than 80 years (Morley, 2008). A report of the European Working Group on Sarcopenia in Older People (EWGSOP) has recently been published (Cruz-Jentoft et al., 2010) and recommends using the combination of both low muscle mass and low muscle function (strength or performance) for the diagnosis of sarcopenia. Tomography and magnetic resonance imaging are considered to be gold standards for estimating muscle mass in research. Nevertheless, high cost and limited access limit the use of these methods for routine clinical practice. Dual energy X-ray absorptiometry (DEXA) is an attractive alternative method for both research and clinical use to distinguish fat, bone mineral, and lean tissues. There are few well-validated techniques to measure muscle strength, including the widely used handgrip strength. To assess physical performance, several tests are available including the Short Physical Performance Battery (SPPB), usual gait speed, 6-minute walk test, and stair climb power test. The report of the EWGSOP proposed an algorithm in order to identify subjects with sarcopenia based on gait speed measurement, considered to be the easiest and most reliable way to screen sarcopenia in clinical practice. A cut-off point of more than 0.8 m/s identifies patients at risk for sarcopenia (Abellan van Kan et al., 2009).

Sarcopenia could benefit from intervention trials especially if based on physical activity and nutrition. Inadequate protein intake contributes to the development of sarcopenia. Because elderly people often present multiple pathologies that represent a risk of protein-energy malnutrition, some studies suggest that the recommended protein intakes of 1 g/kg/day are inadequate (Wolfe et al., 2008). In a 3-year prospective follow-up study, authors showed that subjects in the highest quintile of protein intake (1.2 g/kg/day ± 0.4) lost 40% less lean mass than subjects in the lowest quintile (0.8 g/kg/day ± 0.3) (Houston et al., 2008). For patients identified as malnourished or at risk of malnutrition, some studies have shown that increased protein intake seems to slow down the sarcopenia process (Morais et al., 2006). However, randomized controlled trials (RCTs) in the healthy elderly showed no benefit from protein supplementation (Roth et al., 2000). New approaches are evaluated such as specific essential amino acids (leucine) supplementation, which plays a major role in the control of protein anabolism (Fujita and Volpi, 2006). Data also suggest a role for vitamin D in the development of sarcopenia. Several studies have shown that reduced serum levels of vitamin D were associated with decreased muscle strength and gait speed, impaired equilibrium, and increased risk of falls and fractures (Gerdhem et al., 2005).

Physical activity decreases with aging, promoting muscle-mass loss and decreased muscle strength. Resistance exercise (when muscle works against an external force) increases muscle strength at all ages, but in a heterogeneous manner. A systematic review of 27 RCTs (Latham et al., 2004) showed that functional improvement is modest (number of falls, capacity to stand up from a chair), as is the favorable effect on autonomy. The American College of Sport Medicine suggested that training at a 70–90% of 1 RM (repetition maximum) on two or more non-consecutive days per week was the appropriate training intensity to produce gains in muscle size and strength, even in frail elderly people (Nelson et al., 2007).

Hydration Disorders

Water is the largest component of body mass. The total body water ranges between 45% and 70% of body mass. This proportion varies according to several factors, for example age, hydration, weight, and disease, and is a difficult component to measure. Because of the dramatic consequences of severe dehydration (both for individual health outcomes and for the health-care system, estimated to be responsible for 5% of hospital expenditure), diagnosis and treatment of hydration disorders should be a priority. A recent study showed that, since the 2003 heatwave in France, there has been a significant reduction in the prevalence of intracellular hydration disorders, indicating behavioral changes with a positive impact on hydration status (Kettaneh *et al.*, 2010).

Elderly people are more susceptible to dehydration than younger people for many reasons (Thomas *et al.*, 2008; Schols *et al.*, 2009).

With aging there is a decline in total body water. Two-thirds of the water in the body is intracellular, predominantly in lean mass. It is because of the decrease in lean mass that total body water decreases with aging.

Elderly people display reduced thirst sensations. In young adults the osmolarity threshold for thirst is approximately 294 mOsm/L. It increases to 297–300 mOsm/L in the healthy elderly, whereas the amount to be drunk to quench thirst is lower in the elderly. In the case of mild dehydration, elderly people are therefore less able to compensate with adequate fluid intake. These modifications in thirst are minimal in healthy elderly people but are always present in patients with neurologic disorders (such as dementia or stroke).

Furthermore, elderly people often have various disabilities and/or handicaps, such as visual and cognitive impairments and swallowing disorders, which create difficulties in accessing fluids. They also tend to use numerous medications such as diuretics which increase liquid losses. In addition, fear of incontinence may lead some elderly people to limit their liquid intake.

Low dietary intakes also decrease the water intake. It is estimated that 1000 kcal provides 400 mL of water, whereas oxidation of macronutrients produces a significant amount of metabolic water (1.4 g/g of fat and 0.6 g/g of glucose). It is therefore obvious that a reduction in appetite is a risk factor for dehydration.

The physiological decline in renal function associated with aging increases the risk of dehydration. There is an age-related decrease in renal ability to concentrate urine. After a 12-hour period of water deprivation, urine osmolarity is approximately 1200 mOsm/L in the young adult, whereas it is only 800 mOsm/L in a healthy elderly person. The number of active nephrons decreases with aging, leading to a decrease in glomerular filtration rate by half between 20 and 70 years of age. Aging is also associated with relative resistance of the kidney to antidiuretic hormone, diminution of renin activity, and low secretion of aldosterone, all parameters increasing the risk of dehydration.

Dehydration increases the risk of falls, kidney stones, and urinary infections in the elderly (Jequier and Constant, 2009).

Because water spaces are difficult to measure, it is difficult to accurately diagnose hydration disorders. Diagnosis still relies on clinical symptoms that are neither specific nor precise (Thomas *et al.*, 2008). Indeed, dehydration presents in atypical ways such as delirium (Flaherty *et al.*, 2007). The state-of-the-art technique for the measurement of water spaces is tracer dilution (with a minimum of 4–5 hours' equilibration for total body water), which is not compatible with the necessity to treat patients in a timely manner. Bioelectrical impedance analysis is an easy means of assessment, and valid equations have been proposed in the elderly (healthy and with disease) (Ritz *et al.*, 2008). Despite the accuracy of the measurements, there is no database of theoretical values for comparison. In the final analysis, the diagnosis of dehydration is biochemical (Thomas *et al.*, 2008).

Simple interventions such as regularly offering fluids to elderly people have been shown to significantly decrease the frequency with which dehydration develops (Simmons *et al.*, 2001).

Effects of Nutritional Deficiencies on the Older Population

Frailty

Frailty is a recent concept, and publications in this domain have increased exponentially over the last 20 years. It is defined as a syndrome resulting from multisystem impairments. Frailty is not part of the normal aging process. It increases the risk of poor outcomes such as the development of disabilities, dementia, falls, institutionalization, hospitalization, and increased mortality.

Although there is a universal, intuitive recognition of frailty by most physicians caring for older people, there is a lack of both consensus definition and of a standardized assessment tool to be used in clinical practice and research. The concept of frailty differs between working groups, and many investigators have treated it as synonymous with disability or dependence whereas others have attempted to describe frailty as a distinct concept.

A recent review of the literature explored trends in research into the concept of frailty and the different frailty models (Abellan Van Kan *et al.*, 2010). Nowadays, there are two main frailty phenotypes coexisting in literature: the physical phenotype, and the multidomain phenotype, which includes cognitive, functional, and social circumstances.

The phenotype of physical frailty was presented by Fried and colleagues in 2001 and was based on a specific list of five items (exhaustion, weight loss, weak grip strength, slow walking speed, and low energy expenditure). Subjects were considered as frail if they met three or more of the five criteria. The concept of frailty is very difficult to understand, and there is actually no consensual definition. To simplify, there are two phenotypes of frailty: the phenotype of physical frailty proposed by Fried *et al.* (2001), and the multidomain one which considers additional components as part of the syndrome including, for example, cognitive impairment, disability, or poor social conditions.

Even if the physical phenotype could be considered as a gold standard when assessing frailty, controversies still exist in relation to the definition of the frailty components. Many investigators considered additional components such as cognitive impairment, mood disorders, sensory impairment, poor social conditions and support, chronic diseases, and disability as part of the frailty syndrome. This is the concept of the multidomain phenotype. Most of the work performed on this phenotype model is based on comprehensive geriatric assessments, with frailty measures reflecting the accumulation of identified deficits in various domains such as cognition, autonomy, nutrition, mood or social resources. Similarly to sarcopenia, frailty has an ambiguous definition, with many working groups proposing different criteria to define it.

Cognitive Decline and Alzheimer's Disease

Among the complications of Alzheimer's Disease (AD), weight loss is frequent and contributes to adverse outcomes such as mortality, institutionalization, progression of cognitive impairment, and loss of functional autonomy (Gillette-Guyonnet *et al.*, 2005; Vellas *et al.*, 2005; Spaccavento *et al.*, 2009). Some studies have even suggested that weight loss was present before a formal diagnosis has been made (Knopman *et al.*, 2007; Inelmen *et al.*, 2010).

Recent studies suggested that age has a modifying effect on the association between body weight and risk of dementia: being overweight in middle age (40–45 years) increases risk of dementia in later life (Whitmer *et al.*, 2007), while the relation between body weight and risk of dementia in older age (65–75 years) appears to be U-shaped (Luchsinger *et al.*, 2007). In older subjects (76 years old and over), a higher BMI is associated with a decreased risk of dementia

(Luchsinger *et al.*, 2007; Naderali *et al.*, 2009). Furthermore, there is evidence that high adiposity is related to AD, particularly in the middle-aged and in the younger elderly (Luchsinger and Gustafson, 2009).

The onset of dementia is insidious, and the underlying pathologies are believed to be active for many years before the cognitive loss becomes apparent. Cognitive impairment can be influenced by a number of factors, and the potential effect of nutrition has become a topic of increasing scientific and public interest. In particular, various arguments suggest that nutrients (food and/or supplements) can affect the risk of cognitive decline and dementia, especially in frail elderly people at risk of deficiencies.

Experimental, clinical, neuropathological, and epidemiological investigations have implicated oxidative stress as a possible factor in the pathogenesis of cognitive decline and dementia. Antioxidants (such as vitamin E and C) may reduce neuronal damage and cellular death from oxidative reactions by decreasing beta-amyloid toxicity. Several RCTs looking at vitamin E and cognitive decline have been published, but none has found an association between supplementation and decreased risk of cognitive decline. A recent RCT on an antioxidants complex supplementation (including 34 elements) has shown increased cognitive performance during the 4 months of follow-up compared with the placebo group (Summers *et al.*, 2010). A long-term supplementation with β-carotene (50 mg every other day for 18 years) showed a beneficial effect compared with the placebo group (Grodstein *et al.*, 2007). However, a recent meta-analysis (Bjelakovic *et al.*, 2007), studying the effect of antioxidant supplements on mortality in randomized primary and secondary prevention trials, showed that treatment with β-carotene, vitamin A, or vitamin E might increase mortality. According to the authors, the potential impact of vitamin C and selenium on mortality needs further study.

It is now proved that deficiency of vitamin B_6, vitamin B_{12}, and vitamin B_9 (folate), co-factors in the methylation of homocysteine (Hcy), are associated with increased Hcy concentration. Supraphysiological levels of Hcy or deficits in folate and vitamin B_{12} should promote amyloid and tau protein accumulation and neuronal death, and also have a direct effect on cognitive decline. Several RCTs tested effects of supplementation with one or more supplementations with folate, vitamin B_{12} or vitamin B_6 in healthy individuals or cognitively impaired and demented older individuals. Only one trial has shown a positive effect on cognition: a 3-year folate supplementation (800 mg/day) significantly improved memory, sensorimotor speed and information processing speed compared with placebo (Durga *et al.*, 2007).

Prevalence of vitamin D deficiency seems to be more frequent in patients with AD (Evatt *et al.*, 2008) than in the general population. Moreover, some studies have found a positive association between decreased vitamin D serum concentrations and decreased cognitive performances (Annweiler *et al.*, 2010; Slinin *et al.*, 2010). However, no RCT on vitamin D supplementation in the prevention of cognitive decline has been published.

Among the macronutrients, fatty acids have been suggested to play a role in modulating the risk of cognitive impairment and dementia based on observational studies. Polyunsaturated fats (PUFA) comprise two major classes: the n-6 class (e.g. linoleic acid and arachidonic acid) and the n-3 class (e.g. α-linolenic acid, eicosapentaenoic acid [EPA] and docosahexaenoic acid [DHA]). In addition to their role in the composition and fluidity of neuron membranes and their vascular properties, PUFA have a modulating effect on neuro-inflammation, pro- (n-6) versus anti-inflammatory (n-3). Fatty fish is the primary dietary source of longer chain n-3 fatty acids, EPA and DHA. The main sources of n-6 PUFA are vegetable oils. Data associating dietary fat and cognitive decline or dementia are obtained mainly from observational studies. High intakes of saturated and *trans*-unsaturated (hydrogenated) fats were generally positively associated with increased risk of AD, whereas high intakes of PUFA and monounsaturated fats (MUFA) were protective against cognitive decline in the elderly. Moreover, several studies have found that regular fish consumption (at least once a week) was associated with lower risk of AD. Only one RCT has shown positive results: it examined the effect of n-3 fatty acid supplementation on cognitive functions in patients with mild to moderate AD. However, positive effects were observed in a small group of patients with very mild AD (MMSE >27 points) (Freund-Levi *et al.*, 2006).

Epidemiological analysis of the relationship between nutrient intake and cognitive decline is complex. It is necessary to focus both on food groups and on dietary patterns. One study suggested that undiversified diet increased the risk of dementia (Barberger-Gateau *et al.*, 2007). In this study, daily consumption of fruits and vegetables and regular consumption of n-3 PUFA-rich oils or fish was associated with decreased risk for dementia, and regular consumption of n-6 PUFA-rich oils with increased risk for AD and dementia. A recent paper showed that higher adherence to a diet approaching the Mediterranean diet is associated with reduced risk for AD (Feart *et al.*, 2010). The Mediterranean diet is characterized by a high intake of vegetables, legumes, fruits, and cereals; a high intake of unsaturated fats (mostly in the form of olive oil), but low intake of saturated fatty acids; moderately high intake of fish; low to moderate intake of dairy products; low intake of meat and poultry; and regular but moderate amount of ethanol (primarily in the form of wine during meals). A recent study suggested a synergistic action of Mediterranean diet and physical activity in the prevention of dementia (Scarmeas *et al.*, 2009).

An RCT on the association between physical activity and risk of dementia included subjects with a cognitive complaint but who did not meet criteria for dementia (hence without cognitive impairment). The intervention group received a program of physical activity at home (at least 150 minutes of moderate activity per week). After 24 weeks, patients of the intervention group improved their cognitive performance compared with patients in the placebo group. After 18 months, results were similar (Lautenschlager *et al.*, 2008). In another RCT, the intervention group received a program of aerobic physical activity (treadmill, stationary bike or elliptical, 45–60 minutes/day four times a week). The results showed an improvement in executive functions at 6 months among women of the intervention group (Baker *et al.*, 2010). An RCT testing the effectiveness of multidomain intervention (physical activity, cognitive and social activities, DHA supplementation) on cognitive function in frail elderly people is under way (the Multidomain Alzheimer Preventive Trial, MAPT).

Large studies are necessary to show whether nutritional intervention has an impact on cognitive decline. A policy of nutritional advice similar to that proposed for patients at risk of cardiovascular disease could then be envisaged.

Osteoporosis

Osteoporosis is defined as a systemic skeletal disorder characterized by low bone mass and microarchitectural deterioration of bone tissue. Osteoporosis diagnosis is based on the bone mineral density (BMD) measured by DEXA. A patient is osteoporotic based on a BMD measurement that is 2.5 standard deviations below the mean of the young healthy population. BMD is determined by bone capital accumulated during childhood and especially during growth (peak bone mass) and bone density loss, which begins for women during perimenopause.

Nowadays, osteoporosis is a public health issue because of the increased incidence of fractures related to osteoporosis.

There were an estimated 9 million osteoporotic fractures worldwide in 2000 (Johnell and Kanis, 2006) and some estimates predict a continued increase in the number of hip fractures over the next 40 years (Gullberg *et al.*, 1997). Hip and spine fractures are associated with increased mortality (Ioannidis *et al.*, 2009). Fractures may result in loss of independence, depression, and chronic pain (Poole and Compston, 2006; Adachi *et al.*, 2010).

Increase in and loss of bone density are influenced by genetic and environmental factors over the life course. Among these factors, calcium and vitamin D intakes are determinants because of their role in bone homeostasis: calcium from the bones can be mobilized to maintain calcium plasma concentration, and vitamin D synthesis promotes intestinal calcium absorption and bone mineralization.

In postmenopausal women, and also in aging men, several RCTs have shown a positive association between calcium with and without vitamin D supplementation, by means of increased dietary calcium intake (Daly *et al.*, 2006) or medication (calcium supplements) (Jackson *et al.*, 2006), and increased BMD.

Current data about the benefits of such supplementation in the prevention of osteoporotic fractures are equivocal. In fact it seems difficult to differentiate the respective effects of calcium and vitamin D. A current meta-analysis published results of 45 RCTs (84 585 subjects) with calcium with and without vitamin D supplementation (Avenell *et al.*, 2009). Results have shown that vitamin D supplementation alone is inefficient. Only the supplementation with both calcium and vitamin D was associated with a decrease in hip fractures, particularly in elderly people living in institutions. A recent review of the literature (Marian and Sacks, 2009) provides important information about micronutrients (vitamins and minerals) for older people. Some studies suggested that current vitamin D intakes are low in the majority of older people (Orwoll *et al.*, 2009). Many nutrition experts recommended a daily intake of 800–1000 IU/day to maintain an adequate serum level of 25-hydroxyvitamin D, the best laboratory indicator of vitamin D status (Avenell *et al.*, 2009). Routine monitoring of 25-hydroxyvitamin D levels in high-risk individuals is recommended with the goal of achieving levels ≥30 ng/mL. Increased sun exposure during summer months and consumption of vitamin D fortified food and/or supplements may help to improve overall vitamin D intakes. Recommendations for calcium (diet plus supplements) in postmenopausal women are now higher than in the past, approaching 1200–1500 mg/day.

Physical activity has positive effects on BMD in perimenopausal women, especially walking (Bonaiuti *et al.*, 2002). There is no scientific evidence showing that high-intensity exercises (such as running) are more beneficial than moderate-intensity exercises (e.g. walking). For adults, regular physical activity should decrease the risk of hip fractures. In a prospective study in which 61 000 postmenopausal women were included, those walking 4 hours or more per week had 40% less risk of being affected by hip fracture than women walking less than 1 hour per week (Feskanich *et al.*, 2002). It is currently recommended that adults take moderate-intensity activity (ideally walking) at least 30 minutes per day.

Future Directions

There are attractive hypotheses to support research on the relationships between nutrition and age-related diseases. Research identifying the role of certain nutrients, certain foods or certain dietary behaviors is an indispensable step if we are to propose specific recommendations in the future. The impact of the standard social and cultural determinants of food habits, such as regional cultures, social status and educational level, will obviously need to be considered. It would be of great value to adapt communication strategies and nutritional advice to eating habits and to the stage of aging.

Suggestions for Further Reading

Bauer, J.M., Kaiser, M.J., and Sieber, C.C. (2010) Evaluation of nutritional status in older persons: nutritional screening and assessment. *Curr Opin Clin Nutr Metab Care* **13**, 8–13.

Huang, T.L (2010) Omega-3 fatty acids, cognitive decline, and Alzheimer's disease: a critical review and evaluation of the literature. *J Alzheimers Dis* **21**, 673–690.

Marian, M. and Sacks, G. (2009) Micronutrients and older adults. *Nutr Clin Pract* **24**, 179–195.

Rolland, Y., Dupuy, C., Abellan Van Kan, G., *et al.* (2011) Treatment strategies for sarcopenia and frailty. *Med Clin North Am* **95**, 427–438.

Rolland, Y., Onder, G., Morley, J.E, *et al.* (2011) Current and future pharmacologic treatment of sarcopenia. *Clin Geriatr Med* **27**, 423–447.

References

Abellan Van Kan, G., Rolland, Y., Andrieu, S., *et al.* (2009) Gait speed at usual pace as a predictor of adverse outcomes in community-dwelling older people an International Academy on Nutrition and Aging (IANA) Task Force. *J Nutr Health Aging* **13**, 881–889.

Abellan Van Kan, G., Rolland, Y., Houles, M., *et al.* (2010) The assessment of frailty in older adults. *Clin Geriatr Med* **26**, 275–286

Adachi, J.D., Adami, S., Gehlbach, S., *et al.* (2010) Impact of prevalent fractures on quality of life: baseline results from the global longitudinal study of osteoporosis in women. *Mayo Clin Proc* **85**, 806–813.

Ahmed, T. and Haboubi, N. (2010) Assessment and management of nutrition in older people and its importance to health. *Clin Interv Aging* **5**, 207–216.

Annweiler, C., Schott, A.M., Allali, G., *et al.* (2010) Association of vitamin D deficiency with cognitive impairment in older women: cross-sectional study. *Neurology* **74**, 27–32.

Avenell, A., Gillespie, W.J., Gillespie, L.D., *et al.* (2009) Vitamin D and vitamin D analogues for preventing fractures associated with involutional and post-menopausal osteoporosis. *Cochrane Database Syst Rev* CD000227.

Baker, L.D., Frank, L.L., Foster-Schubert, K., *et al.* (2010) Effects of aerobic exercise on mild cognitive impairment: a controlled trial. *Arch Neurol* **67**, 71–79.

Bales, C.W. and Ritchie, C.S. (2002) Sarcopenia, weight loss, and nutritional frailty in the elderly. *Annu Rev Nutr* **22**, 309–323.

Barberger-Gateau, P., Raffaitin, C., Letenneur, L., *et al.* (2007) Dietary patterns and risk of dementia: the Three-City cohort study. *Neurology* **69**, 1921–1930.

Baron, M., Hudson, M., and Steele, R. (2010) Is serum albumin a marker of malnutrition in chronic disease? The scleroderma paradigm. *J Am Coll Nutr* **29**, 144–151.

Bauer, J.M., Kaiser, M.J., and Sieber, C.C. (2010) Evaluation of nutritional status in older persons: nutritional screening and assessment. *Curr Opin Clin Nutr Metab Care* **13**, 8–13.

Bauer, J.M. and Volkert, D. (2007) *Nutritional Assessment in the European Community.* CRC Press, Boca Raton, FL.

Bjelakovic, G., Nikolova, D., Gluud, L.L., *et al.* (2007) Mortality in randomized trials of antioxidant supplements for primary and secondary prevention: systematic review and meta-analysis. *JAMA* **297**, 842–857.

Blanc, S., Schoeller, D.A., Bauer, D., *et al.* (2004) Energy requirements in the eighth decade of life. *Am J Clin Nutr* **79**, 303–310.

Bonaiuti, D., Shea, B., Iovine, R., *et al.* (2002) Exercise for preventing and treating osteoporosis in postmenopausal women. *Cochrane Database Syst Rev* CD000333.

Chandra, R.K. (2002) Nutrition and the immune system from birth to old age. *Eur J Clin Nutr* **56** (Suppl 3), S73–76.

Chumlea, W.C., Roche, A.F., and Steinbaugh, M.L. (1985) Estimating stature from knee height for persons 60 to 90 years of age. *J Am Geriatr Soc* **33**, 116–120.

Cornali, C., Franzoni, S., Frisoni, G.B., *et al.* (2005) Anorexia as an independent predictor of mortality. *J Am Geriatr Soc* **53**, 354–355.

Cruz-Jentoft, A.J., Baeyens, J.P., Bauer, J.M., *et al.* (2010) Sarcopenia: European consensus on definition and diagnosis: Report of the European Working Group on Sarcopenia in Older People. *Age Ageing* **39**, 412–423.

Daly, R.M., Brown, M., Bass, S., *et al.* (2006) Calcium- and vitamin D3-fortified milk reduces bone loss at clinically relevant skeletal sites in older men: a 2-year randomized controlled trial. *J Bone Miner Res* **21**, 397–405.

Dambach, B., Salle, A., Marteau, C., *et al.* (2005) Energy requirements are not greater in elderly patients suffering from pressure ulcers. *J Am Geriatr Soc* **53**, 478–482.

Delmonico, M.J., Harris, T.B., Lee, J.S., *et al.* (2007) Alternative definitions of sarcopenia, lower extremity performance, and functional impairment with aging in older men and women. *J Am Geriatr Soc* **55**, 769–774.

Doherty, T.J. (2003) Invited review: aging and sarcopenia. *J Appl Physiol* **95**, 1717–1727.

Durga, J., Van Boxtel, M.P., Schouten, E.G., *et al.* (2007) Effect of 3-year folic acid supplementation on cognitive function in older adults in the FACIT trial: a randomised, double blind, controlled trial. *Lancet* **369**, 208–216.

Elia, M., Stratton, R., Russell, C., *et al.* (2005) *The Cost of Disease-Related Malnutrition in the UK and Economic Considerations for the Use of Oral Nutrition Supplements (ONS) in Adults.* British Association for Parenteral and Enteral Nutrition, Redditch.

Emmelot-Vonk, M.H., Verhaar, H.J., Nakhai Pour, H.R., *et al.* (2008) Effect of testosterone supplementation on functional mobility, cognition, and other parameters in older men: a randomized controlled trial. *JAMA* **299**, 39–52.

Evatt, M.L., Delong, M.R., Khazai, N., *et al.* (2008) Prevalence of vitamin D insufficiency in patients with Parkinson disease and Alzheimer disease. *Arch Neurol* **65**, 1348–1352.

Feart, C., Samieri, C., and Barberger-Gateau, P. (2010) Mediterranean diet and cognitive function in older adults. *Curr Opin Clin Nutr Metab Care* **13**, 14–18.

Feskanich, D., Willett, W., and Colditz, G. (2002) Walking and leisure-time activity and risk of hip fracture in postmenopausal women. *JAMA* **288**, 2300–2306.

Flaherty, J.H., Rudolph, J., Shay, K., *et al.* (2007) Delirium is a serious and under-recognized problem: why assessment of mental status should be the sixth vital sign. *J Am Med Dir Assoc* **8**, 273–275.

Flegal, K.M., Graubard, B.I., Williamson, D.F., *et al.* (2007) Cause-specific excess deaths associated with underweight, overweight, and obesity. *JAMA* **298**, 2028–2037.

Folstein, M.F., Folstein, S.E., and McHugh, P.R. (1975) "Mini-mental state". A practical method for grading the cognitive state of patients for the clinician. *J Psychiatr Res* **12**, 189–198.

Freund-Levi, Y., Eriksdotter-Jonhagen, M., Cederholm, T., *et al.* (2006) Omega-3 fatty acid treatment in 174 patients with mild to moderate Alzheimer disease: OmegAD study: a randomized double-blind trial. *Arch Neurol* **63**, 1402–1408.

Fried, L.P., Tangen, C.M., Walston, J., *et al.* (2001) Frailty in older adults. *J Gerontol A Biol Sci Med Sci* **56**, M146–156.

Frisancho, A.R. and Flegel, P.N. (1982) Relative merits of old and new indices of body mass with reference to skinfold thickness. *Am J Clin Nutr* **36**, 697–699.

Fujita, S. and Volpi, E. (2006) Amino acids and muscle loss with aging. *J Nutr* **136**, 277S–280S.

Gerdhem, P., Ringsberg, K.A., Obrant, K.J., *et al.* (2005) Association between 25-hydroxy vitamin D levels, physical activity, muscle strength and fractures in the prospective population-based OPRA Study of Elderly Women. *Osteoporos Int* **16**, 1425–1431.

Gillette-Guyonnet, S., Cortes, F., Cantet, C., *et al.* (2005) Long-term cholinergic treatment is not associated with greater risk of weight loss during Alzheimer's disease: data from the French REAL.FR cohort. *J Nutr Health Aging* **9**, 69–73.

Grodstein, F., Kang, J.H., Glynn, R.J., *et al.* (2007) A randomized trial of beta carotene supplementation and cognitive function in men: the Physicians' Health Study II. *Arch Intern Med* **167**, 2184–2190.

Guigoz, Y. (2006) The Mini Nutritional Assessment (MNA) review of the literature – what does it tell us? *J Nutr Health Aging* **10**, 466–85; discussion 485–487.

Gullberg, B., Johnell, O., and Kanis, J.A. (1997) World-wide projections for hip fracture. *Osteoporos Int* **7**, 407–413.

Han, T.S., Tajar, A., and Lean, M.E. (2011) Obesity and weight management in the elderly. *Br Med Bull* **97**, 169–196.

Haute Autorité de Santé (2007) Nutritional support strategy for protein-energy malnutrition in the elderly. French Professional Recommendations. http://www.has-sante.fr/portail/jcms/c_546549/strategie-de-prise-en-charge-en-cas-de-denutrition-proteino-energetique-chez-la-personne-agee.

Hays, N.P. and Roberts, S.B. (2006) The anorexia of aging in humans. *Physiol Behav* **88**, 257–266.

Houston, D.K., Nicklas, B.J., Ding, J., *et al.* (2008) Dietary protein intake is associated with lean mass change in older, community-

dwelling adults: the Health, Aging, and Body Composition (Health ABC) Study. *Am J Clin Nutr* **87**, 150–155.

Hughes, V.A., Roubenoff, R., Wood, M., *et al.* (2004) Anthropometric assessment of 10-y changes in body composition in the elderly. *Am J Clin Nutr* **80**, 475–482.

Inelmen, E.M., Sergi, G., Coin, A., *et al.* (2010) An open-ended question: Alzheimer's disease and involuntary weight loss: which comes first? *Aging Clin Exp Res* **22**, 192–197.

Ioannidis, G., Papaioannou, A., Hopman, W.M., *et al.* (2009) Relation between fractures and mortality: results from the Canadian Multicentre Osteoporosis Study. *CMAJ* **181**, 265–271.

Irvine, P., Mouzet, J.B., Marteau, C., *et al.* (2004) Short-term effect of a protein load on appetite and food intake in diseased mildly undernourished elderly people. *Clin Nutr* **23**, 1146–1152.

Jackson, R.D., Lacroix, A.Z., Gass, M., *et al.* (2006) Calcium plus vitamin D supplementation and the risk of fractures. *N Engl J Med* **354**, 669–683.

Janssen, I., Shepard, D.S., Katzmarzyk, P.T., *et al.* (2004) The healthcare costs of sarcopenia in the United States. *J Am Geriatr Soc* **52**, 80–85.

Jequier, E. and Constant, F. (2009) Water as an essential nutrient: the physiological basis of hydration. *Eur J Clin Nutr* **64**, 115–123.

Johnell, O. and Kanis, J.A. (2006) An estimate of the worldwide prevalence and disability associated with osteoporotic fractures. *Osteoporos Int* **17**, 1726–1733.

Katz, S. (1983) Assessing self-maintenance: activities of daily living, mobility, and instrumental activities of daily living. *J Am Geriatr Soc* **31**, 721–727.

Kettaneh, A., Fardet, L., Mario, N., *et al.* (2010) The 2003 heat wave in France: hydration status changes in older inpatients. *Eur J Epidemiol* **25**, 517–524.

Knopman, D.S., Edland, S.D., Cha, R.H., *et al.* (2007) Incident dementia in women is preceded by weight loss by at least a decade. *Neurology* **69**, 739–746.

Kulminski, A.M., Arbeev, K.G., Kulminskaya, I.V., *et al.* (2008) Body mass index and nine-year mortality in disabled and nondisabled older U.S. individuals. *J Am Geriatr Soc* **56**, 105–110.

Kyle, U.G., Genton, L., Slosman, D.O., *et al.* (2001) Fat-free and fat mass percentiles in 5225 healthy subjects aged 15 to 98 years. *Nutrition* **17**, 534–541.

Latham, N.K., Bennett, D.A., Stretton, C.M., *et al.* (2004) Systematic review of progressive resistance strength training in older adults. *J Gerontol A Biol Sci Med Sci* **59**, 48–61.

Lautenschlager, N.T., Cox, K.L., Flicker, L., *et al.* (2008) Effect of physical activity on cognitive function in older adults at risk for Alzheimer disease: a randomized trial. *JAMA* **300**, 1027–1037.

Lawton, M.P. and Brody, E.M. (1969) Assessment of older people: self-maintaining and instrumental activities of daily living. *Gerontologist* **9**, 179–186.

Lehmann, A.B., Bassey, E.J., Morgan, K., et al. (1991) Normal values for weight, skeletal size and body mass indices in 890 men and women aged over 65 years. *Clin Nutr* **10**, 18–22.

Locher, J.L., Robinson, C.O., Roth, D.L., et al. (2005) The effect of the presence of others on caloric intake in homebound older adults. *J Gerontol A Biol Sci Med Sci* **60**, 1475–1478.

Luchsinger, J.A. and Gustafson, D.R. (2009) Adiposity and Alzheimer's disease. *Curr Opin Clin Nutr Metab Care* **12**, 15–21.

Luchsinger, J.A., Patel, B., Tang, M.X., et al. (2007) Measures of adiposity and dementia risk in elderly persons. *Arch Neurol* **64**, 392–398.

Marian, M. and Sacks, G. (2009) Micronutrients and older adults. *Nutr Clin Pract* **24**, 179–195.

Milne, A.C., Potter, J., Vivanti, A., et al. (2009) Protein and energy supplementation in elderly people at risk from malnutrition. *Cochrane Database Syst Rev* CD003288.

Morais, J.A., Chevalier, S., and Gougeon, R. (2006) Protein turnover and requirements in the healthy and frail elderly. *J Nutr Health Aging* **10**, 272–283.

Morley, J.E. (2008) Sarcopenia: diagnosis and treatment. *J Nutr Health Aging* **12**, 452–456.

Morley, J.E., Baumgartner, R.N., Roubenoff, R., et al. (2001) Sarcopenia. *J Lab Clin Med* **137**, 231–243.

Mueller, C., Compher, C., and Ellen, D.M. (2011) A.S.P.E.N. clinical guidelines: nutrition screening, assessment, and intervention in adults. *JPEN J Parenter Enteral Nutr* **35**, 16–24.

Naderali, E.K., Ratcliffe, S.H., and Dale, M.C. (2009) Obesity and Alzheimer's disease: a link between body weight and cognitive function in old age. *Am J Alzheimers Dis Other Demen* **24**, 445–449.

Nelson, M.E., Rejeski, W.J., Blair, S.N., et al. (2007) Physical activity and public health in older adults: recommendation from the American College of Sports Medicine and the American Heart Association. *Circulation* **116**, 1094–1105.

Norman, K., Pichard, C., Lochs, H., et al. (2008) Prognostic impact of disease-related malnutrition. *Clin Nutr* **27**, 5–15.

Orwoll, E., Nielson, C.M., Marshall, L.M., et al. (2009) Vitamin D deficiency in older men. *J Clin Endocrinol Metab* **94**, 1214–1222.

Paillaud, E., Herbaud, S., Caillet, P., et al. (2005) Relations between undernutrition and nosocomial infections in elderly patients. *Age Ageing* **34**, 619–625.

Poole, K.E. and Compston, J.E. (2006) Osteoporosis and its management. *BMJ* **333**, 1251–1256.

Portero-McLellan, K.C., Staudt, C., Silva, F.R., et al. (2010) The use of calf circumference measurement as an anthropometric tool to monitor nutritional status in elderly inpatients. *J Nutr Health Aging* **14**, 266–270.

Ritchie, C.S., Joshipura, K., Silliman, R.A., et al. (2000) Oral health problems and significant weight loss among community-dwelling older adults. *J Gerontol A Biol Sci Med Sci* **55**, M366–371.

Ritz, P., Vol, S., Berrut, G., et al. (2008) Influence of gender and body composition on hydration and body water spaces. *Clin Nutr* **27**, 740–746.

Rolland, Y., Czerwinski, S., Abellan Van Kan, G., et al. (2008) Sarcopenia: its assessment, etiology, pathogenesis, consequences and future perspectives. *J Nutr Health Aging* **12**, 433–450.

Roth, S.M., Ferrell, R.F., and Hurley, B.F. (2000) Strength training for the prevention and treatment of sarcopenia. *J Nutr Health Aging* **4**, 143–155.

Roubenoff, R. (2003) Catabolism of aging: is it an inflammatory process? *Curr Opin Clin Nutr Metab Care* **6**, 295–299.

Roubenoff, R., Harris, T.B., Abad, L.W., et al. (1998) Monocyte cytokine production in an elderly population: effect of age and inflammation. *J Gerontol A Biol Sci Med Sci* **53**, M20–26.

Scarmeas, N., Luchsinger, J.A., Schupf, N., et al. (2009) Physical activity, diet, and risk of Alzheimer disease. *JAMA* **302**, 627–637.

Schaap, L.A., Pluijm, S.M., Deeg, D.J., et al. (2006) Inflammatory markers and loss of muscle mass (sarcopenia) and strength. *Am J Med* **119**, 526 e9–17.

Schneider, S.M., Al-Jaouni, R., Pivot, X., et al. (2002) Lack of adaptation to severe malnutrition in elderly patients. *Clin Nutr* **21**, 499–504.

Schols, J.M., De Groot, C.P., Van der Cammen, T.J., et al. (2009) Preventing and treating dehydration in the elderly during periods of illness and warm weather. *J Nutr Health Aging* **13**, 150–157.

Secher, M., Soto, M.E., Villars, H., et al. (2007) The Mini Nutritional Assessment (MNA) after 20 years of research and clinical practice. *Rev Clin Gerontol* **17**, 293–310.

Shenkin, A. (2006) Serum prealbumin: Is it a marker of nutritional status or of risk of malnutrition? *Clin Chem* **52**, 2177–2179.

Simmons, S.F., Alessi, C., and Schnelle, J.F. (2001) An intervention to increase fluid intake in nursing home residents: prompting and preference compliance. *J Am Geriatr Soc* **49**, 926–933.

Slinin, Y., Paudel, M.L., Taylor, B.C., et al. (2010) 25-Hydroxyvitamin D levels and cognitive performance and decline in elderly men. *Neurology* **74**, 33–41.

Spaccavento, S., Del Prete, M., Craca, A., et al. (2009) Influence of nutritional status on cognitive, functional and neuropsychiatric deficits in Alzheimer's disease. *Arch Gerontol Geriatr* **48**, 356–360.

Sui, X., Lamonte, M.J., Laditka, J.N., *et al.* (2007) Cardiorespiratory fitness and adiposity as mortality predictors in older adults. *JAMA* **298**, 2507–2516.

Summers, W.K., Martin, R.L., Cunningham, M., *et al.* (2010) Complex antioxidant blend improves memory in community-dwelling seniors. *J Alzheimers Dis* **19**, 429–439.

Thomas, D.R., Cote, T.R., Lawhorne, L., *et al.* (2008) Understanding clinical dehydration and its treatment. *J Am Med Dir Assoc* **9**, 292–301.

Tinetti, M.E. (1986) Performance-oriented assessment of mobility problems in elderly patients. *J Am Geriatr Soc* **34**, 119–126.

Vellas, B., Lauque, S., Andrieu, S., *et al.* (2001) Nutrition assessment in the elderly. *Curr Opin Clin Nutr Metab Care* **4**, 5–8.

Vellas, B., Lauque, S., Gillette-Guyonnet, S., *et al.* (2005) Impact of nutritional status on the evolution of Alzheimer's disease and on response to acetylcholinesterase inhibitor treatment. *J Nutr Health Aging* **9**, 75–80.

Villareal, D.T., Banks, M., Sinacore, D.R., *et al.* (2006a) Effect of weight loss and exercise on frailty in obese older adults. *Arch Intern Med* **166**, 860–866.

Villareal, D.T., Chode, S., Parimi, N., *et al.* (2011) Weight loss, exercise, or both and physical function in obese older adults. *N Engl J Med* **364**, 1218–1229.

Villareal, D.T., Fontana, L., Weiss, E.P., *et al.* (2006b) Bone mineral density response to caloric restriction-induced weight loss or exercise-induced weight loss: a randomized controlled trial. *Arch Intern Med* **166**, 2502–2510.

Wallace, J.I., Schwartz, R.S., Lacroix, A.Z., *et al.* (1995) Involuntary weight loss in older outpatients: incidence and clinical significance. *J Am Geriatr Soc* **43**, 329–337.

Wannamethee, S.G., Shaper, A.G., Lennon, L., *et al.* (2007) Decreased muscle mass and increased central adiposity are independently related to mortality in older men. *Am J Clin Nutr* **86**, 1339–1346.

Whitmer, R.A., Gunderson, E.P., Quesenberry, C.P., Jr, *et al.* (2007) Body mass index in midlife and risk of Alzheimer disease and vascular dementia. *Curr Alzheimer Res* **4**, 103–109.

WHO (2009) *Ageing and the Life Course.* World Health Organization, Geneva.

Wilson, M.M., Thomas, D.R., Rubenstein, L.Z., *et al.* (2005) Appetite assessment: simple appetite questionnaire predicts weight loss in community-dwelling adults and nursing home residents. *Am J Clin Nutr* **82**, 1074–1081.

Wilson, M.M., Vaswani, S., Liu, D., *et al.* (1998) Prevalence and causes of undernutrition in medical outpatients. *Am J Med* **104**, 56–63.

Wolfe, R.R., Miller, S.L., and Miller, K.B. (2008) Optimal protein intake in the elderly. *Clin Nutr* **27**, 675–684.

Yesavage, J.A., Brink, T.L., Rose, T.L., *et al.* (1982) Development and validation of a geriatric depression screening scale: a preliminary report. *J Psychiatr Res* **17**, 37–49.

43

SPORTS NUTRITION

LOUISE M. BURKE, OAM, PhD, APD

Australian Institute of Sport, Belconnen, ACT, Australia

Summary

Despite the range of physiological challenges and practical considerations that arise between and within sports, there are some common themes shared by all athletes. During training, the athlete needs to eat to achieve an ideal physique for their event, to stay healthy and injury free, and to be able to train hard and recover optimally from each session. Each competitive event involves a physiological challenge; in many cases, nutritional strategies undertaken before and during the event, or in the recovery between games or heats and the final, can help to reduce or delay fatigue and allow the athlete to perform optimally. The practical needs of sports also create special challenges: these include finding opportunities to eat well while travelling, having access to suitable foods and fluids at the strategic times around workouts or competition, and making good decisions regarding supplements and sports foods.

Introduction

The demands of sport vary greatly according to the type of event, the phase of training or competition, and the individual characteristics of each athlete. However, there are some common threads to the nutritional goals of sport. The aim of this chapter is to provide a summary of these key goals of sports nutrition, and to provide recommendations and strategies that will help the athlete achieve some of these goals. It will also identify emerging or controversial ideas in sports nutrition from which new recommendations in sports nutrition will evolve. Given the breadth of topics that will be covered, it is impossible to provide the depth of information that would allow adequate coverage of any single area. To counter this problem, efforts will be made to cite recent papers in which a more sophisti-

cated review of the current knowledge on a specific area is provided, with particular reference to applications in sport. This is not meant to show disrespect to the pioneers of sports nutrition and the original or seminal papers. Rather, the aim is to provide a connection to literature from which both the historical and current perspectives can be gained.

Goal 1: Eat Adequate Energy and Fuel to Cover Your Individual Needs, Tracking Changes in Needs over Different Times of the Sporting Year

Energy intake provides an important focus for an athlete's training diet since it must provide the carbohydrate cost

Present Knowledge in Nutrition, Tenth Edition. Edited by John W. Erdman Jr, Ian A. Macdonald and Steven H. Zeisel.
© 2012 International Life Sciences Institute. Published 2012 by John Wiley & Sons, Inc.

of training and recovery, protein needs for growth, repair and adaptation, and sufficient foods to supply any additional requirements for micronutrients and phytonutrients that arise from the commitment to daily exercise. It also plays a direct role in physique changes, and can influence health and injury risks. Energy requirements vary between sports, between athletes in the same sport, and across various times in an individual athlete's periodized training program. Extremes in energy intake and energy demand can be demonstrated. At the low end of the energy spectrum are athletes in sports focused on brief moments of skill/technique rather than prolonged movement (such as archery or shooting), those who need to achieve or maintain a low body mass/fat level (e.g. athletes in weight-division sports or physique-conscious sports), and those in which these two characteristics are combined (e.g. gymnastics, horse-racing). At the high end of the energy range are athletes in sports involving prolonged sessions of high-intensity exercise (e.g. cyclists undertaking a stage race), those supporting growth, large muscle mass or intentional muscle-gain programs (e.g. adolescent basketball players, American football players), and combinations of these (e.g. heavyweight rowers).

High energy needs often require athletes to consume energy in greater amounts than would be provided in culturally determined eating patterns, or dictated by their appetite and hunger. They may also need to consume energy during and after exercise when the availability of foods and fluids, or opportunities to consume them, are limited. Practical issues interfering with the achievement of energy intake goals during post-exercise recovery include loss of appetite and fatigue, poor access to suitable foods, and distraction from other activities. Specialized advice from a sports dietitian is useful in the development of a plan to address the energy intake challenges faced by individual athletes. Valuable strategies include a pattern of frequent eating occasions, good organization in order to ensure access to suitable foods and drinks in a busy day, and a focus on choices that are low in bulk and high in energy density including high-energy fluids and specialized sports foods (Burke, 2001). Alternatively, the athlete with reduced energy needs faces their own practical challenges to meet their nutritional goals and appetite with a smaller energy budget. General principles that may assist in this scenario include behavior modification to reduce unnecessary eating, focus on choices that are high in bulk or satiety, and choosing nutrient-rich foods that can meet nutritional goals with a lower energy cost (Burke, 2001).

Recent updates to sports nutrition guidelines include the recognition that an athlete's energy requirements change from day to day, and across various parts of the sporting calendar, particularly with changes in the energy demands of an athlete's training (or competition) program or strategies to alter physique. There are several advantages in trying to track energy intake with energy needs. For example, a consistently high energy intake is needed during periods of extremely high energy demands since it may be beyond the absorptive capacity of the gut to play "catch up" once a significant energy deficit has accumulated (Saris et al., 1989). Furthermore, a new concept of energy availability has been developed to assess the suitability of an athlete's energy intake. Defined operationally as the energy cost of the athlete's exercise program subtracted from their total energy intake (see Table 43.1), energy availability provides an approximation of the amount of energy that the body can utilize for everyday activities required for good health (Loucks, 2004). Energy availability may be low when an athlete restricts their energy intake to achieve or maintain a light or lean physique, or when they fail to increase their energy intake sufficiently to meet a strenuous exercise load. When energy availability drops below about 30 kcal (125 kJ) per kilogram of the athlete's fat-free mass for as little as 3–5 days, there is impairment of homeostasis and function, including impaired hormone and bone function (Loucks et al., 1998). Therefore, it makes sense for the athlete to adjust their daily energy intake in reasonable harmony with fluctuations in training load. A strategy that can assist with this goal is to consume food and drinks before, during, and after each exercise session. As will be discussed under the heading "Goal 4," this will help to support performance and recovery around the workout or event. However, it is also a practical way to allow energy intake to increase as sessions are increased in duration or frequency, and to remove unnecessary intake when the training load is reduced, especially during injuries or the off-season. Table 43.1 summarizes various levels of energy availability with examples of situations in which it has been increased to allow gain of body mass, as well as scenarios depicting both a healthy and suboptimal approach to energy restriction for weight loss.

Goal 2: Achieve and Maintain a Physique That Is Associated with Good Performance

Physical characteristics such as height, body mass (BM), lean mass (LBM), and body fat play a role in the perform-

TABLE 43.1 Calculating energy availability in sport

Situation	Energy availability (= energy intake – energy cost of exercise)	Examples
Weight gain, growth, hypertrophy, etc.	>45 kcal (189 kJ) per kg fat-free mass (FFM)	Swimmer A: 65 kg (20% body fat = 80% FFM); weekly training = 5600 kcal (23.5 MJ); daily energy intake = 3520 kcal (14.7 MJ) energy availability = (3520 – 800)/(0.8*65) = 52 kcal/kg FFM (219 kJ)
Weight/physique maintenance	~45 kcal (189 kJ) per kg FFM	Swimmer B: 65 kg (15% body fat = 85% FFM); weekly training = 5600 kcal (2.35 MJ) daily energy intake = 3285 kcal (13.8 MJ) energy availability = (3285 – 800)/ (0.85 * 65) = 45 kcal/kg FFM (189 kJ)
Healthy weight loss (or weight maintenance at reduced metabolic rate)	30–45 kcal (125–189 kJ) per kg FFM	Runner C: 55 kg (20% body fat = 80% FFM); weekly training = 5600 kcal (23.5 MJ); daily energy intake = 2340 kcal (9.8 MJ) energy availability = (2340 – 800)/(0.8 * 55) = 35 kcal/kg FFM (164 kJ)
Low energy availability – health implications	<30 kcal (125 kJ) per kg FFM	Runner D: 55 kg (25% body fat = 75% FFM); weekly training = 5600 kcal (2.35 MJ) daily energy intake = 1980 kcal (8.3 MJ) energy availability = (1980 – 800)/(0.75 * 55) = 29 kcal/kg FFM (120 kJ)

ance of many sports (O'Connor *et al.*, 2007). For example, a large BM and LBM are linked with strength, power, and momentum and are important in many football codes, throwing and lifting events, rowing, and track cycling. By contrast, low BM and body fat levels offer biomechanical and "power to weight" advantages to allow athletes to move their bodies over distances, against gravity or in a small space (e.g. distance running, uphill cycling, diving, and gymnastics). Esthetic considerations are important for the subjectively biased outcomes of sports such as gymnastics, figure skating, and bodybuilding; however, many athletes are also motivated by a personal desire to look good in a skimpy or figure-hugging sporting uniform. In combative events (e.g. boxing, wrestling, judo), weight-lifting, and light-weight rowing, athletes compete in weight divisions which attempt to match competitors based on size, strength, and reach. Eligibility for competition is decided at a weigh-in undertaken just before the event, according to specific roles of the sport.

Elite competitors typically reach the optimal physique for their event via the genetic predispositions that have helped to determine their sporting interests and the conditioning effects of nutrition and training. While some appear to achieve this physique easily, others need to manipulate their training and dietary programs to achieve their desired size and shape. Unfortunately, some athletes embark on extreme weight-loss schemes, often involving excessive training, chronic low energy and nutrient intake, and psychological distress (Beals *et al.*, 2010; O'Connor and Caterson, 2010). Problems arising from these activities include fatigue, inadequate intake of protein and micronutrients (especially iron and calcium), reduced immune status, altered hormonal balance, disordered eating, and poor body image. "Making weight" is another common activity undertaken in weight-division sports whereby athletes, many of whom are already lean, shed kilograms in the hours or days prior to the weigh-in to qualify for a division lighter than their normal BM (Walberg Rankin, 2010). Although this strategy is used to gain advantage in strength or reach over a smaller opponent, it brings disadvantages in terms of dehydration or suboptimal nutritional status resulting from rapid weight-loss techniques. Medical committees and governing organizations have issued guidelines warning against extreme "making weight" activities (Burke, 2007).

Targets for "ideal" BM and body fat should be set in terms of ranges, with each athlete setting individual targets that are compatible with long-term health and performance, rather than short-term benefits alone. Where it is warranted, loss of body fat should be achieved by a gradual program of sustained and moderate energy deficit. Each athlete should be able to achieve targets while eating a diet adequate in energy and nutrients, and free of unreasonable food-related stress (O'Connor and Caterson, 2010). Most importantly, athletes should not strive for minimal levels of body fat per se, and the characteristics of elite athletes should not be considered natural or necessary for recreational and sub-elite performers. Even then, most elite athletes periodize their body mass and body fat levels, achieving their "race weight" only for times they are at their competition peak. Special nutrition support should be given to athletes in weight-making sports to assist them to choose an appropriate weight division, and to adopt the diet and exercise strategies that achieve their weigh-in targets with minimal negative effects (Burke, 2007).

At the other end of the spectrum are athletes who wish to gain muscle mass. These athletes often focus dietary interests on excessive protein intake and special supplements that make extravagant claims. However, emerging evidence suggests that the key nutritional support for a resistance-training program is well-timed intake of nutrition (Burd et al., 2009). Modest amounts (15–25 g) of high-quality protein (particularly from dairy, eggs or animal sources) consumed close to the workout promote maximal protein synthesis during the immediate recovery period (Moore et al., 2009). Total protein requirements are generally easily met within the high energy intakes typical of athletes undertaking heavy training. Meanwhile, carbohydrate may be needed to fuel training sessions and recovery, and an energy surplus may be needed to promote optimal gain in BM or general growth.

Goal 3: Eat to Stay Healthy and Injury Free

Staying healthy and injury free is a key ingredient in a sporting career since it supports consistent training and ensures that the athlete can be at their peak for important competitions. However, the intensive exercise programs undertaken by many athletes straddle the fine line between providing the maximum stimulus for performance improvements and increasing the risk of illness and injury. Although we do not have sufficient evidence to set recommendations for nutritional practices that will guarantee good health and minimum down-time due to injury, some

nutritional risk factors for the opposite outcome can be identified.

There is a somewhat contentious belief that athletes are at increased risk of succumbing to infectious illnesses, particularly upper respiratory tract infections, during periods of high-volume training or after strenuous competitive events (Walsh et al., 2011a). However, there is evidence of suppression of markers of acquired immune function during the acute response to a bout of exercise, and it is intuitive that an exacerbation of the duration or severity of such effects could lead to chronic immunosuppression and compromised resistance to common infections (Walsh et al., 2011a). Nutritional factors that may exacerbate this risk include inadequate fuelling (low carbohydrate availability) around exercise sessions, and poor energy availability. Athletes are advised to follow nutritional practices that avoid such deficiencies. Meanwhile, nutritional supplements have been promoted to offer protection with mixed support; there is limited evidence of benefits from supplementation with vitamin C, and from herbal products such as echinacea and glutamine, mixed support for colostrum and probiotics, and some apparent potential associated with polyphenolic compounds such as quercetin (Walsh et al., 2011b).

Injuries generally occur via two mechanisms: acute problems occurring following a collision or contact impact, or chronic problems that arise from inadequate resilience to continual impact. Nutritional factors may be indirectly involved with some aspects of acute injury if inadequate nutrition contributes to the fatigue that facilitates poor concentration and technique or an increased risk of accidents (Brouns et al., 1986). Nutritional factors are often involved in the development of stress fractures since low bone density is a risk factor in the development of this chronic injury (Bennell et al., 1996). Reduced bone density in athletes seems contradictory, since exercise is an important protector of bone health. However, a serious consequence of low energy availability and menstrual disturbances frequently observed in female athletes is the high risk of either direct loss of bone density, or failure to optimize the gaining of peak bone mass that should occur during the 10–15 years after the onset of puberty (Kerr et al., 2010). The female athlete triad is a term first coined to describe the coincidental presence of eating disorders, amenorrhea, and osteoporosis in female athletes, and the relationships between these problems (Otis et al., 1997). However, the syndrome has been updated to describe the interrelatedness of three issues of energy availability, menstrual health and bone health in female athletes (Nattiv *et al.*, 2007). Each of these factors is seen to exist in a continuum between optimal function and a clinical disorder (as in the previous definition). However, female athletes are now encouraged to regard movement toward the negative end of any of these spectra as unwelcome, and to seek early intervention for such changes.

The reduced "medicalization" of the triad may be important in encouraging athletes to recognize and address problematic nutrition at an early stage; for example, we now know that low energy availability can arise through the lack of recognition of increased energy requirements when energy expenditure is high rather than requiring the stigma of the label of eating disorder/disordered eating (Loucks, 2004). Healthy bones require an environment of adequate energy availability, hormone function and adequate calcium intake, with suggestions that calcium recommendations be increased to 1300–1500 mg/day in female athletes with impaired menstrual function, as is the case for post menopausal women (Kerr *et al.*, 2010). Where adequate calcium intake cannot be met through dietary means, usually through use of low-fat dairy foods or calcium-enriched soy alternatives, a calcium supplement may be considered. Low bone density is also seen in male athletes, with high-risk groups including elite cyclists; this presumably results from the low energy availability associated with heavy energy expenditure and a desire for low body fat levels, but may be exacerbated by the lack of bone loading during cycling activities (Campion *et al.*, 2010).

Vitamin D deficiency or insufficiency is now recognized as a community health problem with consequences including impairment of bone health, muscle function, and immune status. Education campaigns target people at high risk to seek assessment and reversal of inadequate vitamin D status. Some athletes may be vulnerable to such problems (Larson-Meyer and Willis, 2010); risk factors include indoor training (e.g. gymnasts, swimmers), residing at latitudes greater than 35 degrees, training in the early morning or late evening thus avoiding sunlight exposure, wearing protective clothing or sunscreen, and consuming a diet low in vitamin D. Athletes with these characteristics should seek professional advice and have their vitamin D status monitored. Although there is dispute over optimal vitamin D status, vitamin D supplementation may be required to prevent or treat insufficiency (Larson-Meyer and Willis, 2010).

Goal 4: Understand the Physiological Limitations to Performance in an Event, and Eat Before and During the Event to Reduce or Delay the Onset of Such Fatigue

To achieve optimal performance, an athlete should identify potentially preventable factors that contribute to fatigue during an exercise task and undertake nutritional strategies before, during, and after the event that minimize or delay the onset of this fatigue. This is obviously important during competition, but athletes should also practice such strategies during key training sessions, both to support technique and intensity during the workout as well as to fine-tune the nutritional plan for a specific event. The nutritional challenges of competition vary according to length and intensity of the event, the environment, and factors that influence the recovery between events or the opportunity to eat and drink during the event itself (see Table 43.2).

Carbohydrate reserves for the muscle and central nervous system limit the performance of prolonged (>90 minutes) submaximal or intermittent high-intensity exercise, and play a permissive role in the performance of brief or sustained high-intensity work (Coyle, 2004). Competition eating should target strategies to consume carbohydrate before and during such events so as to meet these fuel needs. Carbohydrate should be consumed over the day(s) leading up to an event commensurate with the muscle glycogen requirements of the task. The trained muscle is able to normalize its high resting stores with as little as 24 hours of rest and carbohydrate intake (see Table 43.3), and extending the time and carbohydrate ingestion to 24–48 hours can achieve a super-compensation of muscle glycogen commonly known as carbohydrate loading and improve performance of events of more than 90 minutes' duration (Hawley *et al.*, 1997). Carbohydrate eaten in the hours prior to an event can also ensure adequate liver glycogen, especially for events undertaken after an overnight fast (Hargreaves *et al.*, 2004). Although general recommendations can be provided for the pre-event meal (Table 43.3), the type, timing, and amount of carbohydrate-rich foods and drinks will need to be chosen with consideration of practical issues such as gastrointestinal comfort, individual preferences, and catering arrangements in the competition environment. Sustained-release (low-glycemic-index) carbohydrate sources, or foods

TABLE 43.2 Factors related to nutrition that could produce fatigue or suboptimal performance during sports competition

Factor	Description	Examples of high risk/common occurrence in sports
Dehydration	Mismatch between sweat losses and fluid intake during an event. May be exacerbated if an athlete begins the event in fluid deficit	Events undertaken in hot conditions, particularly involving high-intensity activity patterns and/or heavy protective garments. Repeated competitions (e.g. tournaments) may increase risk of compounding dehydration from one event to the next. Athletes in weight-making sports may deliberately dehydrate themselves to achieve their weigh-in target, with insufficient time between weigh-in and the start of their event to restore fluid levels
Muscle glycogen depletion	Depletion of key muscle fuel due to high utilization in a single event and/or poor recovery of stores from previous activity/event. Typically occurs in events longer than 90 minutes of sustained or intermittent high-intensity exercise	Occurs in endurance events such as marathon and distance running, road cycling, and Ironman triathlons. May occur in some team sports in "running" players with large total distances covered at high intensities (e.g. midfield players in soccer, Australian Rules football). Repeated competitions (e.g. tournaments) may increase risk of poor refueling from one match to the next
Hypoglycemia	Reduction in blood glucose concentrations due to poor carbohydrate availability. However, not all athletes are susceptible to feeling fatigue when blood glucose concentrations become low Note that even when the central nervous system is not fuel deprived, intake of carbohydrate can promote a "happy brain," allowing the muscle to work at a higher power output	Low blood-glucose concentrations may occur in athletes with high carbohydrate requirements (see above) who fail to consume carbohydrate during their event Events of 45–75 minutes' duration may benefit from intake of even small amounts of carbohydrate which stimulate the brain and central nervous system. This includes half-marathons, 40-km cycling time trial, many team sports
Disturbance of muscle acid–base balance	High rates of H^+ production via anaerobic glycolytic power system	Prolonged high-intensity activities lasting 1–8 minutes, e.g. rowing events, middle-distance running, 200–800 m swimming, track cycling team pursuit. May also occur in events with repeated sustained periods of high-intensity activity – perhaps in some team games, racquet sports

TABLE 43.2 *(Continued)*

Factor	Description	Examples of high risk/common occurrence in sports
Depletion of phosphocreatine	Inadequate recovery of phosphocreatine system of ATP regeneration leading to gradual decline in power output in subsequent efforts	Occurs in events with repeated efforts of high-intensity activity with short recovery intervals – perhaps in some team games, racquet sports
Gastrointestinal disturbances	These include vomiting and diarrhea which directly reduce performance as well as interfering with nutritional strategies aimed at managing fluid and fuel status	Poorly chosen intake of food and fluid before and/or during event. Risks included consuming a large amount of fat or fibre in pre-event meal, consuming excessive amounts of single carbohydrates during the event or becoming significantly dehydrated
Salt depletion(?)	Inadequate replacement of sodium lost in sweat. There is anecdotal evidence that salt depletion may increase the risk of a specific type of whole-body muscle cramp	Salty sweaters: individuals with high sweat rates and high sweat sodium concentrations who may acutely or chronically deplete exchangeable sodium pools
Water intoxication/ hyponatremia (low blood sodium)	Excessive intake of fluids leading to hyponatremia ranging from mild (often asymptomatic) to severe (can be fatal). While this problem is more of a medical concern than a cause of fatigue, symptoms can include headache and disorientation, which can be mistaken as signs of dehydration	Athletes with low sweat losses (e.g. low-intensity exercise in cool weather) who overzealously consume fluid before and during the event. This has most often been seen during marathons, ultra-endurance sports, and hiking

Adapted from Burke (2011).

TABLE 43.3 Summary of recommendations for carbohydrate intake by athletes

	Situation	Carbohydrate targets	Comments on type and timing of carbohydrate intake
Daily needs for fuel and recovery: these general recommendations should be fine-tuned with individual consideration of total energy needs, specific training needs, and feedback from training performance			
Light	Low-intensity or skill-based activities	3–5 g/kg of athlete's body mass (BM)/ day	• Timing of intake may be chosen to promote speedy refuelling, or to provide fuel intake around training sessions in the day. Otherwise, as long as total fuel needs are provided, the pattern of intake may simply be guided by convenience and individual choice

(Continued)

TABLE 43.3   *(Continued)*

	Situation	Carbohydrate targets	Comments on type and timing of carbohydrate intake
Moderate	Moderate-exercise program (i.e. ~1 hour/day)	5–7 g/kg/day	• Protein- and nutrient-rich carbohydrate foods or meal combinations will allow the athlete to meet other acute or chronic sports nutrition goals
High	Endurance program (e.g. 1–3 hours/day moderate- to high-intensity exercise)	6–10 g/kg/day	
Very high	Extreme commitment (i.e. >4–5 hours/day moderate- to high-intensity exercise	8–12 g/kg/day	

Acute fuelling strategies: these recommendations promote high carbohydrate availability to promote optimal performance in competition or key training sessions

General fuelling up	Preparation for events <90 minutes' exercise	7–12 g/kg per 24 hours as for daily fuel needs	• Athletes may choose compact carbohydrate-rich sources that are low in fiber/residue and easily consumed to ensure that fuel targets are met, and to meet goals for gut comfort or lighter "racing weight"
Carbohydrate loading	Preparation for events >90 minutes' sustained/ intermittent exercise	36–48 hours of 10–12 g/kg BM per 24 hours	
Speedy refuelling	<8 hours' recovery between two fuel-demanding sessions	1–1.2 g/kg/hour for first 4 hours then resume daily fuel needs	• There may be benefits in consuming small, regular snacks • Compact carbohydrate-rich foods and drink may help to ensure that fuel targets are met
Pre-event fuelling	Before exercise >60 minutes	1–4 g/kg consumed 1–4 hours before exercise	• Timing, amount and type of carbohydrate foods and drinks should be chosen to suit the practical needs of the event and individual preferences/experiences • Choices high in fat/protein/fiber may need to be avoided to reduce risk of gastrointestinal issues during the event • Low glycemic index choices may provide a more sustained source of fuel for situations where carbohydrate cannot be consumed during exercise
During brief exercise	<45 minutes	Not needed	

TABLE 43.3 *(Continued)*

	Situation	Carbohydrate targets	Comments on type and timing of carbohydrate intake
During sustained high-intensity exercise	45–75 minutes	Small amounts including mouth rinse	• A range of drinks and sports products can provide easily consumed carbohydrate
During endurance exercise including "stop and start" sports	1–2.5 hours	30–60 g/hour	• Opportunities to consume foods and drinks vary according to the rules and nature of each sport • A range of everyday dietary choices and specialized sports products ranging in form from liquid to solid may be useful • The athlete should practice to find a refueling plan that suits their individual goals including hydration needs and gut comfort
During ultra-endurance exercise	>2.5–3 hours	Up to 90 g/hour	• As above • Higher intakes of carbohydrate are associated with better performance • Products providing multiple transportable carbohydrates (glucose/fructose mixtures) will achieve high rates of oxidation of carbohydrate consumed during exercise

Reproduced with permission from Burke (2011).

consumed just prior to the start of the competition will also provide an ongoing source of glucose from the gut during exercise (O'Reilly *et al.*, 2010).

According to the specific logistics and culture of a sport, athletes can continue to consume carbohydrate during an event from a range of specialized sports products (e.g. carbohydrate-electrolyte sports drinks, gels, bars) or everyday foods (soft drinks, fruit, confectionery). Until recently, refuelling recommendations for athletes during exercise encouraged the development of a personalized nutrition plan for events of >60 minutes that combined carbohydrate intake of 30–60 g/hour and adequate rehydration with the practical opportunities for intake during the session (Sawka *et al.*, 2007). Opportunities for a more systematic approach to specific carbohydrate needs for different types of situations were, however, discouraged by prevailing beliefs including the capping of the oxidation rate of exogenous carbohydrate at 60 g/hour, the concern that larger intakes might cause gastrointestinal distress, and the lack of evidence of a dose response to carbohydrate

intake during exercise (Burke *et al.*, 2011). New information has allowed a differentiation of strategies for both non-endurance (45–75 minutes) and ultra-endurance (>3–4 hours) events.

There is now robust evidence that intestinal absorption provides the limits to the provision of an exogenous supply of carbohydrate to the working muscle, and that this can be overcome by consuming a mixture of carbohydrate sources that use different intestinal transport mechanisms, such as fructose and glucose (Jeukendrup, 2010). Such mixes allow better gastrointestinal comfort and higher rates of oxidation of ingested carbohydrate with higher rates of intake. The emerging evidence of a dose response between carbohydrate intake and performance benefits in ultra-endurance exercise (Smith *et al.*, 2010a,b) has led to separate recommendations for such events (Table 43.3). The optimal feeding rates may be up to 80–90 g/hour with these carbohydrate targets provided in absolute amounts since the absorptive capacity of the gut appears to be independent of body size (Jeukendrup, 2010). Athletes are also encouraged to practice intake during training sessions, since this may also be associated with an adaptation of the gut to promote greater exogenous fuel use (Cox *et al.*, 2010).

Events of ~60 minutes' duration are not associated with limitations of muscle fuel supply when adequate preparation has been achieved. However, new research has shown that intake of small amounts of carbohydrate, even in the form of frequent rinsing of the mouth with a carbohydrate-solution, are associated with better performance in such protocols (Jeukendrup and Chambers, 2010). It appears that there is communication between receptors in the mouth/throat and centres of reward and motor control in the central nervous system (Chambers *et al.*, 2009). These findings have been incorporated into new recommendations for athletes (Table 43.3) although further work is required to investigate whether the effect is dampened by the consumption of a pre-event carbohydrate-rich meal (Jeukendrup and Chambers, 2010).

Other major nutritional strategies during exercise involve replacement of the fluid and electrolytes lost in sweat (see Figure 43.1). Sweat losses vary during exercise according to such factors as the duration and intensity of exercise, environmental conditions, and the acclimatization of the athlete, but typically range between 500 and 2000 mL/hour (O'Reilly *et al.*, 2010). As the resulting fluid deficit increases, however, it gradually increases the stress associated with exercise such as the drifting increase in heart rate and perception of effort (Montain and Coyle,

1992) The point at which this causes a noticeable or significant impairment of exercise capacity and performance will depend on the individual, their environment (effects are greater in the heat or at altitude), and the type of exercise (Cheuvront *et al.*, 2003; Goulet *et al.*, 2008) In events lasting longer than ~45 minutes there may be opportunities to consume fluids during the session and advantages in doing so. The general recommendations are that athletes use the opportunities that are specific to their sport to replace as much of their sweat loss as is practical during the event, and particularly to keep the fluid deficit below 2% of body mass in stressful environments (Sawka *et al.*, 2007; Shirreffs and Sawka, 2011). Depending on the event, there may be opportunities to drink during breaks in play (i.e. half time, substitutions or time-outs in team games) or during the exercise itself (from aid stations, handlers or self-carried supplies). Checking body mass before and after the session, then accounting for the weight of drinks and foods consumed during the session, will allow the athlete to calculate sweat rates, rates of fluid replacement, and the total sweat deficit over the session (Maughan and Shirreffs, 2008). This can be useful in developing and fine-tuning an individualized hydration plan that is specific to an event and its conditions (Cheuvront *et al.*, 2003; Goulet *et al.*, 2008).

The need to replace sodium losses during exercise is debated. The inclusion of modest amounts of salt in commercial carbohydrate–electrolyte beverages (sports drinks) improves the taste and voluntary intake of a beverage.

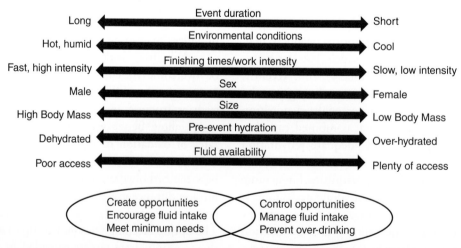

FIG. 43.1 Considerations for managing fluid balance during an exercise session of >1 hour's duration. Adapted from Burke and Cox (2011).

Large salt losses are documented in the case of athletes who experience large losses of sweat during prolonged sessions of exercise in the heat (Godek *et al.*, 2005) and/or excrete "salty sweat" (Godek *et al.*, 2010). There is anecdotal evidence that pro-active replacement of salt during and between exercise sessions may prevent the development of whole body cramps during exercise in the heat in some individuals (Eichner, 2007), but this hypothesis is disputed by others (Schwellnus, 2009). Similarly, the contribution of large salt losses to the development of hyponatremia or low plasma salt concentrations has been a contentious topic. Modeling of salt and fluid changes during exercise shows that sodium losses can contribute to a worsening of plasma sodium homeostasis for any given level of dehydration/fluid replacement (Montain *et al.*, 2006). However, we now recognize that the most important risk factor for the development of this potentially fatal syndrome is excessive intake of fluids compared with fluid losses (Almond *et al.*, 2005; Noakes *et al.*, 2005). This has created scrutiny (Noakes and Speedy, 2007c) and continual evolution (Shirreffs *et al.*, 2004; Sawka *et al.*, 2007) of the recommendations for hydration during exercise (see controversy 1 below).

Other strategies to attenuate the physiological factors causing fatigue during sport include the use of ergogenic aids such as caffeine, the buffering agents beta-alanine and bicarbonate, and creatine (see Goal 6).

Goal 5: Eat Strategically After Training and Competition Sessions to Recover Optimally

Recovery is a major challenge for the elite athlete, who undertakes two or even three workouts each day during certain phases of the training cycle with 4 to 24 hours between each session. But it can also be a concern for recreational athletes who train once or twice a day in preparation for a special endurance event such as a marathon or triathlon. Recovery may also be important in determining the outcome of multi-bout or multi-day competitions such as tournaments, stage races, and events with heats and finals. Recovery involves a complex range of processes of restoration of homeostasis and adaptation to the physiological stress of exercise, including factors related to the maintenance of health and function covered in Goal 4. Other recovery goals include the restoration of fluid balance following the loss of fluid and electrolytes in sweat (Shirreffs *et al.*, 2004), replacement of fuel stores including

muscle and liver glycogen and intramuscular triglycerides (Burke *et al.*, 2004), and the synthesis of new protein for muscular development, adaptation, and repair (Burd *et al.*, 2009). A relatively robust research base allows recommendations to be provided for each of these goals, and each athlete needs to individualize recovery eating strategies after each workout based on the nutritional stress or challenges of the specific session, the recovery period until the next session, and their "bigger picture" nutrition goals such as physique management. In all cases, there may be practical impediments to consuming the foods and drinks needed to achieve recovery eating goals, such as loss of appetite after intense exercise, lack of availability of suitable choices, and distraction from other post-competition activities (e.g. performance debriefs, drug tests, equipment management, and media commitments).

Recommendations for carbohydrate intake in the everyday diets and specific recovery eating strategies of athletes have evolved over the past decade. While early sports nutrition recommendations proposed a seemingly ubiquitous "high carbohydrate diet" for athletes (Coyle, 1991), later refinements discouraged the terminology of expressing carbohydrate intake as a percentage of energy intake in favour of guidelines scaled to the size of the athlete and the fuel cost of their exercise program (Burke *et al.*, 2004). An athlete's carbohydrate status is best considered in terms of whether their total daily intake and the timing of its consumption in relation to exercise maintain an adequate supply of carbohydrate substrate for the muscle and central nervous system ("high carbohydrate availability") or whether carbohydrate fuel sources are depleted or limiting for the daily exercise program ("low carbohydrate availability") (Burke *et al.*, 2011). While high carbohydrate availability is important for situations where the athlete needs to perform optimally, especially with exercise of high intensities, in real life there may be practical reasons why athletes undertake some training sessions with low carbohydrate availability. Whether there may be some advantages gained by deliberately training in this way is a topical question (see Controversy 2).

Table 43.3 summarizes the current recommendations for carbohydrate intake in the athlete's everyday recovery diet including strategies to enhance post-exercise refueling by commencing intake soon after the completion of the exercise bout. Another remodeling of key messages regarding everyday carbohydrate intake is that the athlete's needs are not static, but rather move between these categories according to changes in the daily, weekly, or seasonal goals and exercise commitments in a periodized training program (Burke *et al.*, 2011). It can be useful to adjust an athlete's carbohydrate intake by strategically consuming meals/snacks providing carbohydrate and other nutrients around important exercise sessions. This allows nutrient and energy intake to track with the needs of the athlete's exercise commitments as well as specifically promoting the potential for high carbohydrate availability to enhance performance and recovery at key times (Burke *et al.*, 2011).

Recommendations regarding rehydration and consumption of protein to promote muscular development, adaptation, and repair are provided in Table 43.4. New insights into protein needs in response to exercise are a particularly fertile area of current sports nutrition research (Phillips and van Loon, 2011). Many of the adaptations to training result from the synthesis of new proteins during the recovery from each individual exercise bout (Hawley *et al.*, 2011), with the various types of protein (myofibrillar, sarcolemmal, mitochondrial, cytosolic, etc.) being determined by the characteristics of the exercise stimulus. To maximize the functional output of training (i.e. growth in muscle size and strength, enhancement of aerobic or anaerobic metabolism), the athlete needs to enhance the protein synthetic response to the exercise stimulus; recent studies show, at least with regard to resistance exercise, that muscle protein synthesis is optimized with the intake of 20–25 g of high-quality protein close in time to the exercise bout (Moore *et al.*, 2009).

TABLE 43.4   Recommendations for rehydration and repair/adaptation following exercise

Issue	Summary of current recommendations

Rehydration	• Fluid intake equal to 125–150% of a post-exercise fluid deficit will be needed to accommodate further sweat and urine losses and restore fluid balance
	• Thirst may not guarantee adequate fluid intake: when the fluid deficit is >2% body mass, an athlete should have a fluid plan and access to a supply of palatable beverages
	  ◦ Sweetened, cool drinks encourage voluntary intake of fluids
	• Rehydration requires replacement of the electrolytes lost in sweat, especially sodium. Fluid intake in the absence of electrolyte replacement will reduce plasma osmolarity and result in large urine losses
	  ◦ Sodium can be replaced via special drinks such as oral rehydration solutions (50–80 mmol/L) or higher-salt-containing sports drinks (30–35 mmol/L)
	  ◦ Alternatively, sodium can be consumed in foods or added to the meals eaten in conjunction with fluid intake
	• Where possible, it is better to space fluid intake over a period rather than consuming large volumes at a single time: this pattern will reduce urine losses and maximize fluid retention

Repair and adaptation (protein synthesis)	• Protein should be consumed soon after an exercise session to promote the synthesis of new proteins as dictated by the specific exercise stimulus
	  ◦ An intake of 20–25 g of protein is sufficient to optimize the response to exercise
	  ◦ Protein intake should include high-quality proteins such as animal sources (e.g. dairy, eggs, meats)
	• Although previous discussions on increased protein requirements for athletes remain unresolved, it is likely that all needs can be met from intake of 1.2–1.6 g/kg/day
	  ◦ Recommendations for the spread of protein over the day are not yet available, but there is logic in consuming protein in modest amounts (20–25 g) spread over a number of eating occasions to take advantage of the increased potential for muscle protein synthesis in the 24 hours after an exercise bout

Adapted from Burke (2010b).

Should I use this supplement/sports food?

PROs

Issue	Questions to consider
EFFICACY	• Does this product provide a practical way to meet nutritional goals? • Is there evidence that this product produces a direct ergogenic effect to my specific situation and type of exercise? • Can I benefit from the power of positive thinking (placebo effect)

Versus

CONs

Issue	Questions to consider
SAFETY	• Could this product cause side-effects? • Could this product be contaminated with substances that are harmful?
ETHICS/LEGALITY	• Could this product be contaminated with substances that are banned by anti-doping codes in sport • Does this product contain substances that are not approved/legal in my country and by purchasing it via Internet or mail order, am I in breach of customs laws • Could public knowledge of my use of this product (i.e. role modeling) lend undeserved credibility to the product?
EXPENSE	• Can I afford this product? • Is there some other strategy to enhance performance or meet my nutritional goals that is better value?

FIG. 43.2 Balance sheet for considering the use of commercially available sports foods and sports drinks.

Goal 6: Make Good Choices Regarding Specialized Sports Foods and Supplements

Given that the podium places at important sporting competitions are decided by milliseconds and millimeters, it is understandable that elite athletes are in constant search for any product or intervention that might improve performance by even a small margin. However, even recreational athletes are seduced by the multitude of sports foods and supplements that promise to enhance speed, increase endurance, improve recovery, reduce body fat levels, increase muscle mass, or otherwise make them a better athlete. Some of these products target the provision of known nutrient needs in a practical form to suit intake around exercise or in an athlete's busy lifestyle, while others contain special ingredients that are claimed to directly achieve performance-enhancing effects. The commercial market for these products is both crowded and lucrative, and provides a challenge to stay abreast of the number of products, the marketing claims, and the evidence base for their real contribution to an athlete's sporting goals. There is potential for both positive and negative outcomes related to the use of supplements and sports foods, and each athlete is encouraged to make a well-considered decision based on consideration of their specific situation and issues (see Figure 43.2).

The Australian Institute of Sport has developed a system to provide guidance about the efficacy of products or supplement ingredients which is continually updated based on evolving knowledge (see Table 43.5). Nutritional ergogenic aids that are supported by clear evidence of performance benefits include caffeine for delaying the perception of fatigue (Burke, 2008), bicarbonate as an extracellular buffering agent (McNaughton *et al.*, 2008), and creatine as a fuel for repeated sprint efforts with short recovery intervals (Mujika and Padilla, 1997; Hespel and Derave, 2007). Meanwhile products with emerging evidence include nitrate (including dietary sources such as beetroot juice) (Bailey *et al.*, 2009) and beta-alanine as an intracellular buffer (Derave *et al.*, 2010). Athletes and coaches should, however, be aware that these benefits are limited

TABLE 43.5 Overview of Australian Institute of Sport (AIS) Sports Supplement Program (www.ausport.gov.au/ais/nutrition/supplements)

Supplement category	Supplement characteristics	Examples of products included in category
Group A – supported for use by athletes	• Provide a useful and timely source of energy and nutrients in the athlete's diet • Or have been shown in scientific trials to provide a performance benefit, when used according to a specific protocol in a specific situation in sport	• Sport drinks (carbohydrate–electrolyte drinks) • Protein supplements (especially whey-based products) • Liquid meal supplements • Sport gels and jellies • Sport bars • Caffeine • Creatine • Bicarbonate • Multivitamin and mineral supplement • Iron supplement • Calcium supplement • Probiotics used for gut protection • Vitamin D
Group B – considered for use by AIS athletes only under a research trial	• Have received some scientific attention, sometimes in populations other than highly trained athletes, or have preliminary data which suggest possible benefits to performance • Are of topical interest to athletes and coaches	• β-Alanine • Carnitine • Hydroxy-methylbutyrate (HMB) • Nitrate/beetroot juice • NO stimulators • Fish oils • Antioxidant vitamins C and E • Quercetin and other polyphenols/phytonutrients • Probiotics used for immune system protection
Group C – little proof of benefits	• This category includes the majority of supplements and sports products promoted to athletes • These supplements, despite enjoying a cyclical pattern of popularity and widespread use, have not been proven to provide a worthwhile enhancement of sports performance. Although we can't categorically state that they don't "work," current scientific evidence shows that either the likelihood of benefits is very small or that any benefits that occur are too small to be useful • In fact, in some cases, these supplements have been shown to impair sports performance, with a clear mechanism to explain these results	• Chromium picolinate • Coenzyme Q10 • Cordyceps • Cytochrome C • Gamma-oryzanol and ferulic acid • Ginseng • Inosine • Lactaway • Oxygenated waters • Pyruvate • Rhodiola rosea • Vitamin supplements and free-form amino acids when used in situations other than summarized in Group A • Zinc monomethionine aspartate (ZMA)

TABLE 43.5 *(Continued)*

Supplement category	Supplement characteristics	Examples of products included in category
Group D – should not be used	• We have named a few of the products that belong in this category, but others that have not been named in our supplement system more than likely belong here • These supplements are either directly banned by the World Anti-Doping Agency code or provide a high risk of producing a positive doping outcome due to the potential for contamination with banned substances	• Androstenedione and related compounds • DHEA • 19-norandrostenedione and 19-norandrostenediol • Tribulus terristris and other herbal testosterone supplements • Ephedra • Strychnine • Methylhexaneamine • Glycerol used for hyperhydration (has recently been added to WADA List of Banned Substances as a plasma expander)

to specific situations. Furthermore, the range of disadvantages associated with the use of supplements includes, for elite athletes who compete in sports governed by an anti-doping code, the possibility of ingestion of contaminants including prohibited substances that can lead to an inadvertent doping outcome (Geyer *et al.*, 2008).

Future Directions

Controversy 1: "Train Low" for Optimal Training Adaptations

Although current recommendations promote exercise under conditions of high carbohydrate availability to enhance performance, increase capacity at high intensity, or improve technique, there is recent interest in the potential advantages of training with low carbohydrate availability. Many of the signaling cascades that drive the adaptation to training appear to be up-regulated when an exercise stimulus is applied in a low-carbohydrate environment (low glycogen and/or low exogenous carbohydrate availability) (Philp *et al.*, 2011). Several studies have shown

that this can enhance the increase in proteins associated with exercise metabolism (e.g. oxidative enzymes and regulatory proteins such as transcription factors), even in well-trained individuals (Hawley and Burke, 2010; Philp *et al.*, 2011). However, to date, only one study has shown that this translates into better exercise capacity, with this investigation involving previously untrained subjects (Hansen *et al.*, 2005). There are some caveats to apply to the interest among athletes and coaches in "training low." The first is to note that these benefits have not been achieved by exposing the exercising individual to chronic periods of a low-carbohydrate diet. In fact, the favorable protocols involve a short period of carbohydrate depletion in an otherwise carbohydrate-replete daily environment: either by undertaking exercise in an overnight fasted situation without carbohydrate intake during the session, or by scheduling two sessions of exercise close together such that the second bout is undertaken with reduced glycogen stores due to the lack of refuelling from the first bout (Burke, 2010a). This limits the total exposure of the body to the disadvantages of low carbohydrate availability and could allow the athlete to periodize their training so that only some workouts are undertaken with the "train low" stimulus. The potential disadvantages of "training low" (Burke, 2010a) include an increase in the perception of effort and a reduction in training intensity (e.g. speed, power outputs), a potential for down-regulation of metabolic pathways promoting carbohydrate utilization and high power outputs during exercise, and an increased risk of injury, illness, and over-reaching. "Training low" may have greater application to populations who exercise to overcome problems of metabolic syndrome and metabolic inflexibility, allowing such individuals to "train smarter" (derive greater benefits from the same exercise stimulus). However, as noted previously (Burke, 2010a), it may already occur in the periodized training and nutritional programs practiced by athletes in real life, and deliberate implementation of such strategies requires further study.

Controversy 2: Are Fluid Guidelines Useful or Harmful?

Fluid mismatches during competitive events mostly err on the side of a fluid deficit (Sawka et al., 2007). However, it is possible for some athletes to overhydrate if they drink excessively during events in which sweat rates are actually low (Almond et al., 2005). This situation is generally unnecessary and may even be dangerous if it leads to the potentially fatal condition of hyponatremia (low blood sodium concentration; often known as water intoxication) (Noakes, 2003; Noakes and Speedy, 2007b). The recognition of this problem and the justifiable publicity surrounding deaths in some community participation events has led some sports scientists to blame guidelines for fluid intake or the marketing of sports drinks as a contributing cause (Noakes and Speedy, 2007a,c). Indeed, there has been a gradual evolution of recommendations for fluid intake over the past 30 years in view of the recognition of the unsuitability of prescriptive advice and the implication from previous guidelines that athletes should drink as much as possible during exercise (Casa et al., 2000; Sawka et al., 2007). As stated above, the current guidelines warn against overdrinking but encourage an individualized fluid plan that keeps the fluid deficit to an acceptable level.

It should be noted that even these recommendations have been subjected to the criticism of being unnecessary, complicated and still capable of leading to hyponatremia (Noakes, 2003; Noakes and Speedy, 2007c). Instead, it has been argued that athletes should simply drink according to their thirst (Noakes and Speedy, 2007c). The opinion of this author is that thirst or ad libitum intake of fluid

provides a reasonable starting point for developing a fluid plan. However, there are often good reasons to improve on these subjective dictates. For example, in sports where opportunities for fluid intake are limited, the athlete may need to drink at the available opportunities early in an event (i.e. "ahead of their thirst") to better pace total fluid intake over the session. In addition, as long as it does not require an excessive fluid intake, athletes may consume beverages such as sports drinks to meet carbohydrate refueling targets. Finally, it is possible that some individuals have poor judgment of portion control or thirst response and may need some guidance regarding appropriate fluid volumes.

Controversy 3. Anti-oxidants: Friend or Foe?

Exercise is known to increase the production of free oxygen and nitrogen radical species (RNOS) which in excess are thought to contribute to acute impairment of the muscle's ability to produce force as well as longer-term inflammation, damage and soreness (Konig et al., 2001). While increasing cellular antioxidant capacity via supplementary intake of antioxidants seems a logical approach to counteract the negative effects of RNOS on muscle force capability, the results of studies of supplementation with antioxidant vitamins in association with acute or chronic exercise models have been unclear with respect to muscle damage or performance outcomes (Fisher-Wellman and Bloomer, 2009). Newer insights now find that it is only excessive oxidative damage that is problematic, and that small and confined oxidative changes in the muscle fulfil an important role in the adaptation to exercise; for example, inducing signaling cascades and up-regulating the endogenous oxidative defense system, which consists of complex interactions of compartmentalized antioxidants (Hawley et al., 2011). In fact, some recent studies have found that supplementation with isolated antioxidants such as vitamin C and/or E can actually reduce the benefits of exercise training (Gomez-Cabrera et al., 2008; Ristow et al., 2009). The most recent recommendations for athletes promote the benefits of a varied diet including a range of antioxidant- and phytochemical-containing fruits and vegetables, although research continues to investigate potential benefits from the specific consumption of polyphenols such as quercetin and epigallocatechin-3-gallate (EGCG), which may contribute a range of functions including effects on the immune system, the anti-inflammatory response, and mitochondrial biogenesis (Hawley et al., 2011).

Suggestions for Further Reading

Burke, L.M. (2007) *Practical Sports Nutrition*. Human Kinetics, Champaign, IL.

Burke, L.M. and Cox, G. (2011) *The Complete Guide to Food for Sports Performance*, 3rd Edn. Allen and Unwin, Sydney.

Maughan, R.J. (ed.) (2011) Foods, nutrition and exercise III. *J Sports Sci* (Special Issue) (in press).

References

Almond, C.S.D., Shin, A.Y., Fortescue, E.B., *et al.* (2005) Hyponatremia among runners in the Boston marathon. *N Engl J Med* **352,** 1550–1556.

Bailey, S.J., Winyard, P., Vanhatalo, A., *et al.* (2009) Dietary nitrate supplementation reduces the O2 cost of low-intensity exercise and enhances tolerance to high-intensity exercise in humans. *J Appl Physiol* **107,** 1144–1155.

Beals, K.A., Houtkooper, L., and Dalton, B. (2010) Disordered eating in athletes. In L. Burke and V. Deakin (eds), *Clinical Sports Nutrition*, 4th Edn. McGraw-Hill, Sydney, pp. 171–192.

Bennell, K.L., Malcolm, S.A., Wark, J.D., *et al.* (1996) Models for the pathogenesis of stress fractures in athletes. *Br J Sports Med* **30,** 200–204.

Brouns, F.J.P.H., Saris, W.H.M., and Ten Hoor, F. (1986) Dietary problems in the case of strenuous exertion. *J Sports Med* **26,** 306–319.

Burd, N.A., Tang, J.E., Moore, D.R., *et al.* (2009) Exercise training and protein metabolism: influences of contraction, protein intake, and sex-based differences. *J Appl Physiol* **106,** 1692–1701.

Burke, L.M. (2001) Energy needs of athletes. *Can J Appl Physiol* **26,** S202–S219.

Burke, L.M. (2007) Weight-making sports. In *Practical Sports Nutrition*. Human Kinetics, Champaign, IL, pp. 289–312.

Burke, L.M. (2008) Caffeine and sports performance. *Appl Physiol Nutr Metab* **33,** 1319–1334.

Burke, L.M. (2010a) Fueling strategies to optimize performance: training high or training low? *Scand J Med Sci Sports* **20** (Suppl 2), 48–58.

Burke, L.M.(2010b) Fasting and recovery from exercise. *Br J Sports Med* **44,** 502–508.

Burke, LM. (2011) Nutrition for competition. In S. Stear and S.M. Shirreffs (eds), *Sport and Exercise Nutrition*. Wiley, London, pp. 200–216.

Burke, L.M. and Cox, G. (2011) *The Complete Guide to Food for Sports Performance*, 3rd Edn. Allen and Unwin, Sydney.

Burke, L.M., Hawley, J.A., Wong, S., *et al.* (2011) Carbohydrates for training and competition, *J Sports Sci* PMID 21660838.

Burke, L.M., Kiens, B., and Ivy, J.L. (2004) Carbohydrates and fat for training and recovery. *J Sports Sci* **22,** 15–30.

Campion, F., Nevill, A.M., Karlsson, M.K., *et al.* (2010) Bone status in professional cyclists. *Int J Sports Med* **31,** 511–515.

Casa, D.J., Armstrong, L.E., Hillman, S.K., *et al.* (2000) National Athletic Trainers' Association position statement: fluid replacement for athletes. *J Athl Train* **35,** 212–224.

Chambers, E.S., Bridge, M.W., and Jones, D.A. (2009) Carbohydrate sensing in the human mouth: effects on exercise performance and brain activity. *J Physiol* **587,** 1779–1794.

Cheuvront, S.N., Carter, R., Sawka, M.N. (2003) Fluid balance and endurance exercise performance. *Curr Sports Med Rep* **2,** 202–208.

Cox, G.R., Clark, S.A., Cox, A.J., *et al.* (2010) Daily training with high carbohydrate availability increases exogenous carbohydrate oxidation during endurance cycling. *J Appl Physiol* **109,** 126–134.

Coyle, E.F. (1991) Timing and method of increased carbohydrate intake to cope with heavy training, competition and recovery. *J Sports Sci* **9,** 29–52.

Coyle, E.F. (2004) Fluid and fuel intake during exercise. *J Sports Sci* **22,** 39–55.

Derave, W., Everaert, I., Beeckman, S., *et al.* (2010) Muscle carnosine metabolism and beta-alanine supplementation in relation to exercise and training. *Sports Med* **40,** 247–263.

Eichner, E.R. (2007) The role of sodium in "heat cramping". *Sports Med* **37,** 368–370.

Fisher-Wellman, K. and Bloomer, R.L. (2009) Acute exercise and oxidative stress: a 30 year history. *Dyn Med* **8,** 1.

Geyer, H., Parr, M.K., Koehler, K., *et al.* (2008) Nutritional supplements cross-contaminated and faked with doping substances. *J Mass Spectrom* **43,** 892–902.

Godek, S.F., Bartolozzi, A.R., and Godek, J.J. (2005) Sweat rate and fluid turnover in American football players compared with runners in a hot and humid environment. *Br J Sports Med* **39,** 205–11.

Godek, S.F., Peduzzi, C., Burkholder, R., *et al.* (2010) Sweat rates, sweat sodium concentrations, and sodium losses in 3 groups of professional football players. *J Athl Train* **4,** 364–371.

Gomez-Cabrera, M.C., Domenech, E., and Romagnoli, M. (2008) Oral administration of vitamin C decreases muscle mitochondrial biogenesis and hampers training-induced adaptations in endurance performance. *Am J Clin Nutr* **87,** 142–149.

Goulet, E.D., Mélançon, M.O., and Madjar, K. (2008) Meta-analysis of the effect of exercise-induced dehydration on endurance performance (abstr). *Med Sci Sports Exerc* **40** (5 Suppl), S396.

Hansen, A.K., Fischer, C.P., Plomgaard, P., et al. (2005) Skeletal muscle adaptation: training twice every second day vs. training once daily. J Appl Physiol **98**, 93–99.

Hargreaves, M., Hawley, J.A., and Jeukendrup, A.E. (2004) Pre-exercise carbohydrate and fat ingestion: effects on metabolism and performance. J Sports Sci **22**, 31–38.

Hawley, J.A. and Burke, L.M. (2010) Carbohydrate availability and training adaptation: effects on cell metabolism. Exerc Sport Sci Rev **38**, 152–160.

Hawley, J.A., Burke, L.M., Phillips, S.M., et al. (2011) Nutritional modulation of training-induced skeletal muscle adaptation. J Appl Physiol **110**, 834–845.

Hawley, J.A., Schabort, E.J., Noakes, T.D., et al. (1997) Carbohydrate-loading and exercise performance: an update. Sports Med **24**, 73–81.

Hespel, P. and Derave, W. (2007) Ergogenic effects of creatine in sports and rehabilitation. Subcell Biochem **46**, 245–259.

Jeukendrup, A.E. (2010) Carbohydrate and exercise performance: the role of multiple transportable carbohydrates. Curr Opin Clin Nutr Metabol Care **13**, 452–457.

Jeukendrup, A.E. and Chambers, E.S. (2010) Oral carbohydrate sensing and exercise performance. Curr Opin Clin Nutr Metabol Care **13**, 447–451.

Kerr, D., Khan, K., and Bennell, K. (2010) Bone, exercise and nutrition. In L. Burke and V. Deakin (eds), Clinical Sports Nutrition, 4th Edn. McGraw-Hill, Sydney, pp. 200–221.

Konig, D., Wagner, K.H., Elmadfa, I., et al. (2001) Exercise and oxidative stress: significance of antioxidants with reference to inflammatory, muscular, and systemic stress. Exerc Immunol Rev **7**, 108–133.

Larson-Meyer, D.E. and Willis, K.S. (2010) Vitamin D and athletes. Curr Sports Med Rep **9**, 220–226.

Loucks, A.B. (2004) Energy balance and body composition in sports and exercise. J Sports Sci **22**, 1–14.

Loucks, A.B., Verdun, M., and Heath, E.M. (1998) Low energy availability, not stress of exercise, alters LH pulsatility in exercising women. J Appl Physiol **84**, 37–46.

Maughan, R.J. and Shirreffs, S.M. (2008) Development of individual hydration strategies for athletes. Int J Sport Nutr Exerc Metab **18**, 457–472.

McNaughton, L.R., Siegler, J., and Midgley, A. (2008) Ergogenic effects of sodium bicarbonate. Curr Sports Med Rep **7**, 230–236.

Montain, S.J. and Coyle, E.F. (1992) Influence of graded dehydration on hyperthermia and cardiovascular drift during exercise. J Appl Physiol **73**, 1340–1350.

Montain, S.J., Cheuvront, S.N., and Sawka, M.N. (2006) Exercise associated hyponatraemia: quantitative analysis to understand the aetiology. Br J Sports Med **40**, 98–105.

Moore, D.R., Robinson, M.J., Fry, J.L., et al. (2009) Ingested protein dose response of muscle and albumin protein synthesis after resistance exercise in young men. Am J Clin Nutr **89**, 161–168.

Mujika, I. and Padilla, S. (1997) Creatine supplementation as an ergogenic aid for sports performance in highly trained athletes: a critical review. Int J Sports Med **18**, 491–496.

Nattiv, A., Loucks, A.B., Manore, M.M., et al. (2007) American College of Sports Medicine position stand. The female athlete triad. Med Sci Sports Exerc **39**, 1867–1882.

Noakes, T.D. (2003) Overconsumption of fluid by athletes. Br Med J **327**, 113–114.

Noakes, T.D. and Speedy, D.B. (2007a) Lobbyists for the sports drink industry: an example of the rise of "contrarianism" in modern scientific debate. Br J Sports Med **41**, 107–109.

Noakes, T.D. and Speedy, D.B. (2007b) The aetiology of exercise-associated hyponatraemia is established and is not "mythical". Br J Sports Med **41**, 111–113.

Noakes, T.D. and Speedy, D.B. (2007c) Time for the American College of Sports Medicine to acknowledge that humans, like all other earthly creatures, do not need to be told how much to drink during exercise. Br J Sports Med **41**, 109–111.

Noakes, T.D., Sharwood, K., Speedy, D., et al. (2005) Three independent biological mechanisms cause exercise-associated hyponatremia: evidence from 2,135 weighed competitive athletic performances. Proc Natl Acad Sci **102**, 18550–18555.

O'Connor, H. and Caterson, I. (2010) Weight loss and the athlete. In L. Burke and V. Deakin (eds), Clinical Sports Nutrition, 4th Edn. McGraw-Hill, Sydney, pp. 116–148.

O'Connor, H., Olds, T., and Maughan, R.J. (2007) Physique and performance for track and field events. J Sports Sci **25** (1 Suppl), 49S–60S.

O'Reilly, J., Wong, S.H., and Chen, Y. (2010) Glycaemic index, glycaemic load and exercise performance. Sports Med **40**, 27–39.

Otis, C.L., Drinkwater, B., Johnson, M., et al. (1997) American College of Sports Medicine position stand. The female athlete triad. Med Sci Sports Exerc **29**, i–ix.

Phillips, S.M. and van Loon, L. (2011) Dietary protein for athletes: from requirements to optimal adaptation. J Sports Sci in press.

Philp, A., Burke, L.M., and Baar, K. (2011) Altering endogenous carbohydrate availability to support training adaptations. In R. Maughan and L.M. Burke (eds), Sports Nutrition: More than Just Calories – Triggers for Adaptation. Nestlé Nutrition Series **69** (in press).

Powers, S.P., Nelson, W.B., and Enette-Larsen, E. (2011) Antioxidant and vitamin D supplements for athletes: sense or nonsense? J Sports Sci PMID 21830999.

Ristow, M., Zarse, K., Oberbach, A., *et al.* (2009) Antioxidants prevent healthpromoting effects of physical exercise in humans. *Proc Natl Acad Sci USA* **106,** 8665–8670.

Saris, W.H.M., Van Erp-Baart, M.A., Brouns, F., *et al.* (1989) Study on food intake and energy expenditure during extreme sustained exercise: the Tour de France. *Int J Sports Med* **10,** S26–S31.

Sawka, M.N., Burke, L.M., Eichner, E.R., *et al.* (2007) American College of Sports Medicine position stand. Exercise and fluid replacement. *Med Sci Sports Exerc* **39,** 377–390.

Schwellnus, M.P. (2009) Cause of exercise associated muscle cramps (EAMC)–altered neuromuscular control, dehydration or electrolyte depletion? *Br J Sports Med* **43,** 401–408.

Shirreffs, S.M. and Sawka, M.N. (2011) Fluid needs during and after exercise. *J Sports Sci* 2011 (in press).

Shirreffs, S.M., Armstrong, L.E., and Cheuvront, S.N. (2004) Fluid and electrolyte needs for preparation and recovery from training and competition. *J Sports Sci* **22,** 57–63.

Smith, J.W., Zachwieja, J.J., Horswill, C.A., *et al.* (2010a) Evidence of a carbohydrate dose and prolonged exercise performance relationship [abstr]. *Med Sci Sports Exerc* **42**(5 Suppl), 84.

Smith, J.W., Zachwieja, J.J., Peronnet, F., *et al.* (2010b) Fuel selection and cycling endurance performance with ingestion of [13C]glucose: evidence for a carbohydrate dose response. *J Appl Physiol* **108,** 1520–1529.

Walberg Rankin, J. (2010) Making weight in sports. In L. Burke and V. Deakin (eds), *Clinical Sports Nutrition,* 4th Edn. McGraw-Hill, Sydney, pp. 149–170.

Walsh, N.P., Gleeson, M., Shephard, R.J., *et al.* (2011a) Position Statement Part one: Immune function and exercise. *Exerc Immunol Rev* **17,** 6–63.

Walsh, N.P., Gleeson, M., Pyne, D.B., *et al.* (2011b) Position Statement Part two: Maintaining immune health *Exerc Immunol Rev* **17,** 64–103.

44

NUTRIENT REGULATION OF THE IMMUNE RESPONSE

PHILIP C. CALDER[1], PhD, DPHIL, RNUTR AND PARVEEN YAQOOB[2], MA, DPHIL, RNUTR

[1]University of Southampton Faculty of Medicine, Southampton, UK
[2]University of Reading, Reading, UK

Summary

There is a bidirectional interaction between nutrition, infection, and immunity: undernutrition decreases immune defenses, making an individual more susceptible to infection, but the immune response to an infection can itself impair nutritional status and alter body composition. Practically all forms of immunity are affected by protein–energy malnutrition, but non-specific defenses and cell-mediated immunity are more severely affected than humoral (antibody) responses. Micronutrients are required for an efficient immune response, and deficiencies in one or more micronutrients diminish immune function, providing a window of opportunity for infectious agents. Essential fatty acids play a role in the regulation of immune responses since they provide precursors for the synthesis of eicosanoids. Deficiencies in essential amino acids impair immune function, but some non-essential amino acids (e.g. arginine and glutamine) may become conditionally essential in stressful situations. Probiotic bacteria enhance immune function in laboratory animals and may do so in humans. Prebiotics may also have these effects but research in this area is not conclusive. Breast milk has a composition that promotes the development of the neonatal immune response and may protect against infectious diseases.

Introduction

Associations between famine and epidemics of infectious disease have been noted throughout history: as early as 370 BC Hippocrates recognized that poorly nourished people are more susceptible to infectious disease. In general, undernutrition impairs the immune system, suppressing immune functions that are fundamental to host protection against pathogenic organisms (Chandra, 1991; Scrimshaw and SanGiovanni, 1997; Calder and Jackson, 2000). Undernutrition leading to impairment of immune function can be due to insufficient intake of energy and macronutrients and/or due to deficiencies in specific micronutrients. These may occur in combination. The

Present Knowledge in Nutrition, Tenth Edition. Edited by John W. Erdman Jr, Ian A. Macdonald and Steven H. Zeisel.

impact of undernutrition is greatest in developing countries, but it is also important in developed countries, especially among the elderly, individuals with eating disorders, alcoholics, patients with certain diseases, premature babies and those born small for gestational age. Although it has proven difficult to identify the precise effects of individual nutrients on different aspects of immune function, it is now clear that many nutrients have an important role in maintaining the immune response. Thus, the functioning of the immune system is influenced by nutrients consumed as normal components of the diet, and appropriate nutrition is required for the host to maintain adequate immune defenses towards bacteria, viruses, fungi, and parasites. This chapter begins with an overview of the key components of the immune system, concentrating on the cells that participate in immune responses and the mechanisms by which they communicate. The role of nutrients in the immune system is examined using specific examples, and the cyclic relationship between infection and nutritional status is discussed. The main body of the chapter is devoted to an evaluation of the influence of individual micronutrients and macronutrients on immune function. The content of this chapter is based on Yaqoob and Calder (2011).

The Immune System

The immune response acts to protect the host from infectious agents that exist in the environment (bacteria, viruses, fungi, parasites) and from other noxious insults. It is a complex system involving various cells that are distributed in many locations throughout the body and that move between these locations in the lymph and the bloodstream. In some locations the cells are organized into discrete lymphoid organs. These can be classified as primary lymphoid organs where immune cells arise and mature (bone marrow and thymus) and secondary lymphoid organs (lymph nodes, spleen, gut-associated lymphoid tissue) where mature immune cells interact and respond to antigens. The immune system has two functional divisions: the innate (or natural) immune system and the acquired (also termed specific or adaptive) immune system (see Figure 44.1).

Innate Immunity

Innate immunity consists of physical barriers, soluble factors and phagocytic cells, which include granulocytes (neutrophils, basophils, eosinophils), monocytes, and macrophages (Table 44.1). Innate immunity has no memory and is therefore not influenced by prior exposure to an organism. Phagocytic cells, the main effectors of innate immunity, express surface receptors that recognize certain structures on bacteria; the receptors are termed pattern recognition receptors and the bacterial structures are termed microbe-associated molecular patterns. Binding of bacteria to the receptors triggers phagocytosis (engulfing) and subsequent destruction of the pathogenic microorganism by toxic chemicals, such as superoxide radicals and hydrogen peroxide. Natural killer cells also possess surface receptors and destroy their target cells by the release of cytotoxic proteins. In this way, innate immunity provides a first line of defense against invading pathogens. However, an immune response often requires the coordinated actions of both innate immunity and the more powerful and flexible acquired immunity.

Acquired Immunity

Acquired immunity involves the specific recognition of molecules (termed antigens) on an invading pathogen which distinguish it as being foreign to the host. Lymphocytes, which are classified into T- and B-lymphocytes (also called T-cells and B-cells), are responsible for this form of immunity (Figure 44.1). All lymphocytes (indeed all cells of the immune system) originate in the bone marrow. B-lymphocytes undergo further development and maturation in the bone marrow before being released into the circulation, while T-lymphocytes mature in the thymus. From the bloodstream, lymphocytes can enter peripheral lymphoid organs, which include lymph nodes, the spleen, tonsils, and gut-associated lymphoid tissue. Immune responses occur largely in these lymphoid organs, which are highly organized to promote the interaction of cells and invading pathogens.

Since each lymphocyte carries surface receptors for a single antigen, the acquired immune system is highly specific. However, acquired immunity is extremely diverse; the lymphocyte repertoire in humans has been estimated at recognition of approximately 10^{11} antigens. The high degree of specificity, combined with the huge lymphocyte repertoire, means that only a relatively small number of lymphocytes will be able to recognize any given antigen. The acquired immune system has developed the ability for clonal expansion to deal with this. Clonal expansion involves the proliferation of a lymphocyte once an interaction with its specific antigen has occurred, so that a single lymphocyte gives rise to a clone of lymphocytes, all of

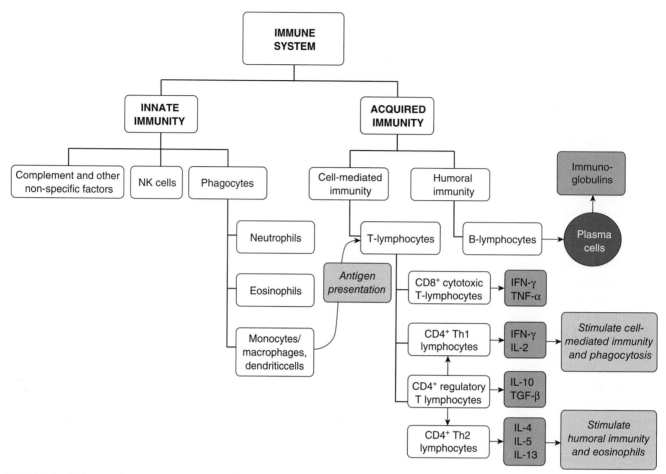

FIG. 44.1   Schematic representation of the immune system. IFN, interferon; IL, interleukin; NK, natural killer; TGF, transforming growth factor; Th1, type 1 helper; Th2, type 2 helper; TNF, tumor necrosis factor.

TABLE 44.1   Components of innate and acquired immunity

	Innate	Acquired
Physicochemical barriers	Skin	Cutaneous and mucosal immune systems
	Mucous membranes	Antibodies in mucosal secretions
	Lysozyme	
	Stomach acid	
	Commensal bacteria	
Circulating molecules	Complement	Antibodies
Cells	Granulocytes	Lymphocytes (T and B)
	Monocytes/macrophages	
	Natural killer cells	
Soluble mediators	Macrophage-derived cytokines	Lymphocyte-derived cytokines

which have the ability to recognize the antigen causing the initial response. The acquired immune response becomes effective over several days after the initial activation, but it also persists for some time after the removal of the initiating antigen. This persistence gives rise to immunological memory, which is also a characteristic feature of acquired immunity. It is the basis for the stronger, more effective, immune response to re-exposure to an antigen (i.e. reinfection with the same pathogen) and is the rationale for vaccination. Eventually, the immune system will re-establish homeostasis using self-regulatory mechanisms which involve communication between cells.

B- and T-Lymphocytes

B-lymphocytes are characterized by their ability to produce antibodies (these are soluble antigen-specific immunoglobulins). This form of protection is termed humoral immunity. B-lymphocytes also carry immunoglobulins, which are capable of binding an antigen, on their cell surface (Figure 44.1). Binding of immunoglobulin with antigen causes proliferation of the B-lymphocytes and subsequent transformation into plasma cells, which secrete large amounts of antibody with the same specificity as the parent cell.

There are five major classes of immunoglobulin (IgA, IgD, IgG, IgM, and IgE), each of which elicits different components of the humoral immune response. Antibodies work in several ways to combat invading pathogens. They can "neutralize" toxins or microorganisms by binding to them and preventing their attachment to host-cells, and they can activate complement proteins in plasma, which in turn promote the destruction of bacteria by phagocytes. Since they have binding sites for both an antigen and for receptors on phagocytic cells, antibodies can also promote the interaction of the two components by forming physical "bridges," a process known as opsonization. The type of phagocytic cell bound by the antibody will be determined by the antibody class; macrophages and neutrophils are specific for IgM and IgG, while eosinophils are specific for IgE. In this way, antibodies are a form of communication between the acquired and the innate immune response; although they are elicited through highly specific mechanisms, they are ultimately translated to a form that can be interpreted by the innate immune system, enabling it to destroy the pathogen.

Humoral immunity deals with extracellular pathogens. However, some pathogens, particularly viruses, but also certain bacteria, infect individuals by entering cells. These pathogens will escape humoral immunity and are instead dealt with by cell-mediated immunity, which is conferred by T-lymphocytes. T-lymphocytes express antigen-specific T-cell receptors (TCR) on their surface, which have an enormous antigen repertoire. However, unlike B-lymphocytes, they are only able to recognize antigens that are presented to them on a cell surface (the cell presenting the antigen to the T-lymphocyte is termed an antigen presenting cell); this is the distinguishing feature between humoral and cell-mediated immunity. Activation of the TCR results in entry of T-lymphocytes into the cell cycle and, ultimately, proliferation. Activated T-lymphocytes also begin to synthesize and secrete the cytokine interleukin-2 (IL-2), which further promotes proliferation and differentiation. Thus, the expansion of T-lymphocytes builds up an army of antigen-specific T-lymphocytes in much the same way as that of B-lymphocytes. Effector T-lymphocytes have the ability to migrate to sites of infection, injury, or tissue damage. There are three principal types of T-lymphocytes; cytotoxic T-cells, helper T-cells, and regulatory T-cells. Cytotoxic T-lymphocytes carry the surface protein marker CD8 and kill infected cells and tumor cells by secretion of cytotoxic enzymes, which cause lysis of the target cell. Helper T-lymphocytes carry the surface protein marker CD4 and eliminate pathogens by stimulating the phagocytic activity of macrophages and the proliferation of, and antibody secretion by, B-lymphocytes. Helper T-lymphocytes have traditionally been subdivided into two broad categories according to the pattern of cytokines they produce, although new categories have recently been identified (Figure 44.2). Helper T-cells that have not previously encountered antigen produce mainly IL-2 upon the initial encounter with an antigen. These cells may differentiate into a population, sometimes referred to as Th0 cells, which differentiate further into either Th1 or Th2 cells. This differentiation is regulated by cytokines: IL-12 and interferon-gamma (IFN–γ) promote the development of Th1 cells, while IL-4 promotes the development of Th2 cells. Th1 and Th2 cells have relatively restricted profiles of cytokine production: Th1 cells produce IL-2 and IFN-γ, which activate macrophages, natural killer cells, and cytotoxic T-lymphocytes and are the principal effectors of cell-mediated immunity. Interactions with bacteria, viruses, and fungi tend to induce Th1 activity. Th2 cells produce IL-4, which stimulates IgE production, and IL-5, an eosinophil-activating factor. Th2 cells are responsible for defense against helminthic parasites, which is due to IgE-mediated activation of

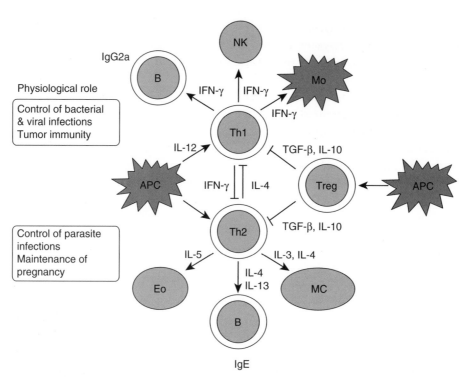

FIG. 44.2 Schematic representation of the roles of helper T-cells in regulating immune responses. APC, antigen presenting cell; B, B-cell; Eo, eosinophil; IFN, interferon; Ig, immunoglobulin; IL, interleukin; MC, mast cell; NK, natural killer cell; TGF, transforming growth factor; Th1, type 1 helper T-cell; Th2, type 2 helper T-cell; Treg, regulatory T-cell. Adapted from Calder *et al.* (2006).

mast-cells and basophils. The patterns of cytokine secretion by Th1 and Th2 lymphocytes were first demonstrated in mice. Human helper T-lymphocytes do show differences in cytokine profile, the divisions are not as clear, with the majority secreting a mixture of Th1 and Th2 cytokines in differing proportions. Thus, the terms "Th1 dominant" and "Th2 dominant" are commonly used to describe the cytokine profiles of these cells. More recently characterized categories of helper T-cells include Th17 cells, which appear to play an important role in autoimmunity (where the immune system attacks host tissues inappropriately). However, the range of activities of these new categories of helper T-cells is not yet fully understood. Regulatory T-cells (CD4+CD25+FoxP3+) produce IL-10 and transforming growth factor-β and suppress the activities of B-cells and other T-cells, preventing inappropriate activation.

The Gut-associated Immune System

The immune system of the gut (sometimes termed the gut-associated lymphoid tissue) is extensive and includes the physical barrier of the intestine as well as components of innate and adaptive immune responses (Mowat, 2003). The physical barrier includes acid in the stomach, peristalsis, mucus secretion, and tightly connected epithelial cells, which collectively prevent the entry of pathogens. The cells of the immune system are organized into specialized lymphoid tissue, termed Peyer's patches, which are located directly beneath the epithelium in the lamina propria (Mowat, 2003). This also contains M cells, which sample small particles from the gut lumen. Other lymphocytes are also present in the lamina propria, as well as associated with the epithelium itself. Because the gut-associated immune system of humans is inaccessible and requires invasive techniques for study, it is relatively poorly understood and much of our understanding of the influence of nutrition on this aspect of immunity comes from animal studies.

The Immune System in Health and Disease

Clearly, a well-functioning immune system is essential to health and serves to protect the host from the effects of ever-present pathogenic organisms. Cells of the immune system also have a role in identifying and eliminating cancer cells. There are, however, some undesirable features of immune responses. First, in developing the ability to recognize and eliminate foreign antigens effectively, the immune system is responsible for the rejection of transplanted tissues. Secondly, the ability to discriminate between "self" and "non-self" is an essential requirement of the immune system and is normally achieved by the destruction of self-recognizing T- and B-lymphocytes before their maturation. However, since lymphocytes are unlikely to be exposed to all possible self-antigens in this way, a second mechanism termed "clonal anergy" exists, which ensures that an encounter with a self-antigen induces tolerance. In some individuals there is a breakdown of the mechanisms that normally preserve tolerance; a number of factors contribute to this, including a range of immunological abnormalities and a genetic predisposition in some individuals. As a result, an inappropriate immune response to host tissues or to normally benign environmental antigens is generated and this can lead to autoimmune and inflammatory diseases, which are typified by ongoing chronic inflammation and a dysregulated T-cell response.

Factors Influencing Immune Function

Many factors influence immune function and resistance to infection, leading to great variability in immune responses within the population (Calder and Kew, 2002; Cummings *et al.*, 2004). These factors include genetics, sex, early life events, age, and hormonal status. Immunological "history" also plays a role in the form of previous exposure to pathogens, vaccination history, and chronic disease burden (accumulating conditions over time). Other factors influencing immune function include stress (environmental, physiological, and psychological), exercise (acute and chronic), obesity (see below), smoking, alcohol consumption, gut microbiota, and nutritional status. In a newborn baby, immunologic competence is gained as the immune system encounters new antigens and so matures and expands. Some of these early encounters with antigens play an important role in ensuring tolerance, and a breakdown in this system can lead to increased likelihood of childhood atopic diseases and perhaps also to certain inflammatory conditions later in life (Calder *et al.*, 2006). At the other end of the lifecycle, older people experience a progressive dysregulation of the immune system, leading to decreased

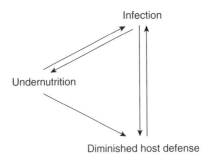

FIG. 44.3 The interrelationship between undernutrition and infection. Adapted from Calder and Jackson (2000).

cell-mediated immunity and a greater susceptibility to infection (Castle, 2000; Burns and Goodwin, 2004; Agarwal and Busse, 2010). Innate immunity appears to be less affected by aging; indeed, there is a progressive increase in chronic inflammation during aging.

Impact of Infection on Nutrient Status

Undernutrition decreases immune defenses against invading pathogens and makes an individual more susceptible to infections. However, the immune response to an infection can itself impair nutritional status and alter body composition (Scrimshaw and SanGiovanni, 1997; Calder and Jackson, 2000). Thus, there is a bidirectional interaction between nutrition, infection and immunity (Figure 44.3).

Infection impairs nutritional status and body composition in the following ways:

- Infection is characterized by anorexia. Reduction in food intake (anorexia) can range from as little as 5% to almost complete loss of appetite. This can lead to nutrient deficiencies even if the host is not deficient before the infection and may make apparent existing borderline deficiencies.
- Infection is characterized by nutrient malabsorption and loss. The range of infections associated with nutrient malabsorption is wide and includes bacteria, viruses, protozoa, and intestinal helminths. Infections that cause diarrhea or vomiting will result in nutrient loss. Apart from malabsorption, nutrients may also be lost through the feces as a result of damage to the intestinal wall caused by some infectious agents.

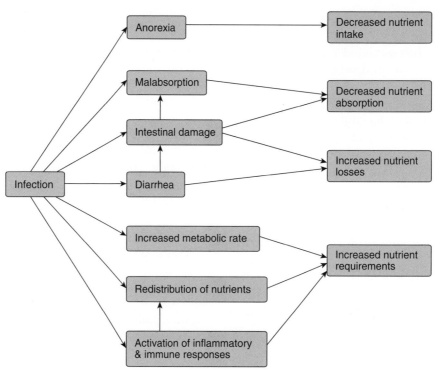

FIG. 44.4 Effects of infection on the host which can decrease nutrient status. Adapted from Calder and Jackson (2000).

- Infection is characterized by increased resting energy expenditure. Infection increases the basal metabolic rate during fever: each 1°C increase in body temperature is associated with a 13% increase in metabolic rate, which significantly increases energy requirements. This places a significant demand on nutrient supply, particularly when coupled with anorexia, diarrhea, and other nutrient losses (e.g. in urine and sweat).
- Infection is characterized by altered metabolism and redistribution of nutrients. The "acute-phase response" is the name given to the metabolic response to infections, and it includes the onset of fever and anorexia, the production of specific acute-phase reactants, and the activation and proliferation of immune cells. This catabolic response occurs with all infections, even when they are subclinical, and serves to bring about a redistribution of nutrients away from skeletal muscle and adipose tissue and towards the host immune system. This redistribution is mediated by the production of proinflammatory cytokines by leukocytes and associated endocrine changes. Amino acids, mobilized from skeletal muscle, are used by the liver for the synthesis of acute-phase

proteins (e.g. C-reactive protein) and by leukocytes for the synthesis of immunoglobulin and cytokines. The average loss of protein over a range of infections has been estimated to be 0.6–1.2 g/kg body weight per day.

It is clear that the inflammatory cytokines mediate many of the effects that lead to compromised nutritional status following an infection, including anorexia, increased energy expenditure, and redistribution of nutrients, while malabsorption and maldigestion are brought about by the pathogen itself. The result is that an increased nutrient requirement coincides with reduced nutrient intake, reduced nutrient absorption, and nutrient losses (Figure 44.4).

Why Should Nutrients Affect Immune Function?

Although the immune system is functioning at all times, specific immunity becomes activated when the host is challenged by pathogens. This activation is associated with a marked increase in the demand of the immune system for substrates and nutrients to provide a ready source of energy, which can be supplied from exogenous sources (i.e. from the diet) and/or from endogenous pools. The cells of the immune system are metabolically active and are able to utilize glucose, amino acids, and fatty acids as fuels (Calder, 1995). Energy generation involves electron carriers and a range of coenzymes, which are usually derivatives of vitamins. The final component of the pathway for energy generation (the mitochondrial electron transfer chain) includes electron carriers that have iron or copper at their active site. Activation of the immune response gives rise to the production of proteins (immunoglobulins, cytokines, cytokine receptors, adhesion molecules, acute-phase proteins) and lipid-derived mediators (prostaglandins, leukotrienes). To respond optimally there must be the appropriate enzymic machinery in place (for RNA synthesis and protein synthesis and their regulation) and ample substrate available (nucleotides for RNA synthesis, the correct mix of amino acids for protein synthesis, polyunsaturated fatty acids [PUFAs] for eicosanoid synthesis). An important component of the immune response is oxidative burst, during which superoxide anion radicals are produced from oxygen in a reaction linked to the oxidation of NADPH. The reactive oxygen species produced can be damaging to host tissues and thus antioxidant protective mechanisms are necessary. Among these are the classic antioxidant vitamins (vitamins E and C), glutathione, the antioxidant enzymes superoxide dismutase and catalase, and the glutathione recycling enzyme glutathione peroxidase. The antioxidant enzymes all have metal ions at their active site (manganese, copper, zinc, iron, selenium). Cellular proliferation is a key component of the immune response, providing amplification and memory: before division there must be replication of DNA and then of all cellular components (proteins, membranes, intracellular organelles, etc.). In addition to energy, this clearly needs a supply of nucleotides (for DNA and RNA synthesis), amino acids (for protein synthesis), fatty acids, bases, and phosphate (for phospholipid synthesis), and other lipids (e.g. cholesterol) and cellular components. Although nucleotides are synthesized mainly from amino acids, some of the cellular building blocks cannot be synthesized in mammalian cells and must come from the diet (e.g. essential fatty acids, essential amino acids, minerals). Amino acids (e.g. arginine) are precursors for the synthesis of polyamines, which have roles in the regulation of DNA replication and cell division. Various micronutrients (e.g. iron, folic acid, zinc, magnesium) are also involved in nucleotide and nucleic acid synthesis. Thus, the roles for nutrients in immune function are many and varied, and it is easy to appreciate that an adequate and balanced supply of these is essential if an appropriate immune response is to be mounted.

Assessment of the Effect of Nutrition on Immune Function

There is a wide range of methodologies by which to assess the impact of nutrients on immune function (Cummings et al., 2004; Albers et al., 2005; Calder, 2007a). Assessments can be made of cell functions ex vivo (i.e. of the cells isolated from animals or humans subjected to dietary manipulation and studied in short- or long-term culture) or of indicators of immune function in vivo (e.g. by measuring the concentrations of proteins relevant to immune function in the bloodstream or the response to an immunological challenge). Box 44.1 lists some examples of approaches used for the assessment of immune function. However, the biological relevance of these markers of immune function remains unclear, and there is no single marker that can be used to draw conclusions about modulation of the immune system as a whole, apart from infection as a clinical outcome. An expert group identified measures of delayed-type hypersensitivity (DTH; the cell-mediated immune response to controlled application of an antigen usually through the skin), the response to vaccination, and the production of secretory IgA as the most suitable assessments of immune function in humans (Albers et al., 2005).

Obesity and Immune Function

Comparisons between lean and obese individuals suggest that obesity is associated with impairments of the bacterial killing capacity of granulocytes, T-lymphocyte proliferation, natural killer cell activity, and delayed-type hypersensitivity, with increased susceptibility to infection, and with poorer outcome from infection (Marti et al., 2001). Obesity was identified as one of the major co-morbidities associated with death from H1N1 influenza infection during the 2009–2010 pandemic (Lucas, 2010). Factors derived from adipose tissue, such as the cytokine-like hormone leptin, may play a role in immune regulation and may explain some of the effects of obesity on immunity (Matarese et al., 2010). Adipose tissue is infiltrated with immune cells, notably, but not exclusively, macrophages, and releases a range of inflammatory mediators (Tilg and Moschen, 2006). As such, obesity is a state of chronic low-grade inflammation.

Protein–Energy Malnutrition and Immune Function

Protein–energy malnutrition, although often considered a problem solely of developing countries, has been described in even the most affluent nations. It is important to recognize that protein–energy malnutrition often coexists with micronutrient deficiencies, and poor outcome of intervention can result from a lack of awareness of multi-ple deficiencies. Practically all forms of immunity may be affected by protein–energy malnutrition, but non-specific defenses and cell-mediated immunity are more severely affected than humoral (antibody) responses (Chandra, 1991; Kuvibidila *et al.*, 1993; Woodward, 1998, 2001). Protein–energy malnutrition causes atrophy of the lymphoid organs (thymus, spleen, lymph nodes, tonsils) in laboratory animals and humans. There is a decline in the number of circulating lymphocytes, which is proportional to the extent of malnutrition, and the proliferative responses of T-lymphocytes to mitogens and antigens is decreased by malnutrition as is the synthesis of IL-2 and IFN-γ and the activity of natural killer cells. Production of cytokines by monocytes (TNF-α, IL-6, and IL-1β) is also decreased by malnutrition, although their phagocytic capacity appears to be unaffected. The in vivo skin DTH response to challenge with specific antigens is reduced by malnutrition. However, numbers of circulating B-lymphocytes and immunoglobulin levels do not seem to be affected or may even be increased by malnutrition; underlying infections may influence these latter observations.

The Influence of Individual Micronutrients on Immune Function

Much of what is known about the impact of single nutrients on immune function comes from studies of deficiency states in animals and humans, and from controlled animal studies in which the nutrients are included in the diet at known levels. There is now overwhelming evidence from these studies that particular nutrients are required for an efficient immune response and that deficiencies in one or more of these nutrients diminish immune function and provide a window of opportunity for infectious agents. It is logical that multiple nutrient deficiencies might have a more significant impact on immune function, and therefore resistance to infection, than a single nutrient deficiency. What is also apparent is that excess amounts of some nutrients also impair immune function and decrease resistance to pathogens. Thus, for some nutrients, there may be a relatively narrow range of intake that is associated with optimal immune function.

Vitamin A
The vitamin A (or retinoid) family includes retinol, retinal, retinoic acid, and esters of retinoic acid. There is a transi-

tory decrease in serum retinol during the acute-phase response which follows infection, which is likely to be due to decreased synthesis of retinol binding protein (RBP) by the liver, and therefore decreased release of retinol–RBP by the liver, and also to increased vascular permeability at sites of inflammation, allowing leakage into the extravascular space. For these reasons, serum retinol cannot be used as an indicator of vitamin A status in individuals with an active acute-phase response.

Vitamin A is essential for maintaining epidermal and mucosal integrity; vitamin A-deficient mice have histopathological changes in the gut mucosa consistent with a breakdown in gut barrier integrity and impaired mucus secretion, both of which would facilitate entry of pathogens through this route. One of the key changes caused by vitamin A deficiency is the loss of mucus-producing goblet cells; the resulting lack of mucus diminishes resistance to infection by pathogens that would otherwise be trapped and washed away. Vitamin A regulates keratinocyte differentiation, and vitamin A deficiency induces changes in skin keratinization, which may explain the observed increased incidence of skin infection. Many aspects of innate immunity, in addition to barrier function, are affected by vitamin A (Semba, 1998, 1999, 2002; Stephensen, 2001; Villamor and Fawzi, 2005). It modulates gene expression to control the maturation of neutrophils; in vitamin A deficiency there are increased neutrophil numbers, but decreased phagocytic function. Macrophage-mediated inflammation is increased by vitamin A deficiency, but the ability to ingest and kill bacteria is impaired. Vitamin A deficiency may therefore lead to more severe infections, coupled with excessive inflammation. Natural killer cell activity is diminished by vitamin A deficiency. The impact of vitamin A on acquired immunity is less clear, but there is some evidence that vitamin A deficiency alters the Th1/Th2 balance, decreasing the Th2 response, but often without affecting the Th1 response (Stephensen, 2001). This area requires further research.

The impact of vitamin A deficiency on infectious disease has been studied widely in the developing world (Scrimshaw and SanGiovanni, 1997; Semba, 1999; Calder and Jackson, 2000; Stephensen, 2001; Villamor and Fawzi, 2005). Vitamin A deficiency is associated with increased morbidity and mortality in children, and appears to predispose to respiratory infections, diarrhea, and severe measles. Although vitamin A deficiency increases the risk of infectious disease, the interaction is bidirectional such that infections can lead to vitamin A deficiency: diarrhea, respiratory infections, measles, chickenpox, and human immunodeficiency virus infection are all associated with the development of vitamin A deficiency.

Replenishment of vitamin A in deficient children by provision of supplements decreases mortality in areas of the world where deficiency is a problem. In general, frequent small doses tend to decrease mortality more dramatically than infrequent high doses. Vitamin A supplements improve recovery from measles and decrease the duration, risk of complications, and mortality from the disease. Because measles is an acute, immunosuppressive viral infection, it is often associated with secondary opportunistic bacterial infections, and it is not clear whether vitamin A improves recovery from the measles itself, the secondary infection, or both. The ability of vitamin A to promote the regeneration of damaged mucosal epithelium and phagocytic activity of neutrophils and macrophages results in a reduction in the incidence and duration of diarrhea, which may be of particular benefit to infants who are not breast-fed.

B Vitamins

B vitamins participate as coenzymes in the synthesis of nucleic acids and proteins, pathways which are crucial for many aspects of immune function. There is some suggestion that folate supplementation of elderly individuals improves immune function, and, in particular, natural killer cell activity, although this is not conclusive (Troen et al., 2006). Elderly subjects supplemented for 4 months with a combination of folic acid (400 µg/day), vitamin E (120 IU/day), and vitamin B_{12} (3.8 µg/day) were reported to have increased natural killer cell activity and fewer infections in one study (Bunout et al., 2004). Elderly individiuals tend to be at risk of vitamin B_{12} deficiency, and studies have shown that subjects >65 years with low serum vitamin B_{12} concentrations have impaired antibody responses to vaccination (Fata et al., 1996). Patients with vitamin B_{12} deficiency also have decreased numbers of lymphocytes and suppressed natural killer cell activity, which may be reversed with supplementation (Tamura et al., 1999). Vitamin B_6 deficiency in laboratory animals causes thymus and spleen atrophy, and decreases lymphocyte proliferation and the DTH response. In a study in healthy elderly humans, a vitamin B_6-deficient diet (3 µg/kg body weight per day or about 0.17 and 0.1

mg/day for men and women, respectively) for 21 days resulted in a decreased percentage and total number of circulating lymphocytes, decreased T- and B-cell proliferation in response to mitogens, and decreased IL-2 production (Meydani *et al.*, 1991). Repletion at 15 or 22.5 μg/kg body weight per day for 21 days did not return the immune functions to starting values; however, repletion at 33.75 μg/kg body weight per day (about 1.9 and 1.1 mg/day for men and women, respectively) returned immune parameters to starting values. This comprehensive study indicates that vitamin B_6 deficiency impairs human immune function, and that the impairment is reversible by repletion.

Vitamin C

Vitamin C is a water-soluble antioxidant found in high concentrations in circulating leukocytes and appears to be utilized during infections. High circulating levels of vitamin C are associated with enhanced antibody responses, neutrophil function, and antiviral activity in animal studies. In humans, supplementation studies have often been conducted in athletes. The interest in athletes is due to the fact that exercise induces an increase in the numbers of neutrophils and their capacity to produce reactive oxygen species, which, if prolonged, can be immunosuppressive and reduce neutrophil activity in the recovery period following exercise. Since neutrophils form an important part of the defense against viruses, the suppression of neutrophil activity after strenuous exercise may explain why upper respiratory tract infections are often noted to coincide with this. Because of its antioxidant capacity, vitamin C could potentially counteract the exercise-induced generation of reactive oxygen species and limit the post-exercise immunosuppression. However, randomized controlled trials (RCTs) have often been limited by lack of statistical power and do not conclusively show an effect of vitamin C on cell numbers, neutrophil function, or reactive oxygen species production (Wintergerst *et al.*, 2007).

Several studies suggest a modest benefit of vitamin C supplementation at doses ranging between 1000 and 8000 mg/day in reducing the duration, but not the incidence, of respiratory infections (Douglas *et al.*, 2007). However, the incidence of common colds and pneumonia has been shown to be reduced by vitamin C in those individuals who regularly engage in strenuous physical activity, and also in those who live in crowded conditions. The potential benefits and risks of vitamin C supple-

mentation at doses above 8000 mg/day, and the role of vitamin C in non-respiratory infections, have not been investigated.

Vitamin D

The active form of vitamin D (1,25-dihydroxyvitamin D_3) is referred to here as vitamin D. Vitamin D receptors have been identified in most immune cells, and some cells of the immune system can synthesize the active form of vitamin D from its precursor, suggesting that vitamin D is likely to have immunoregulatory properties. Some reports suggest immune defects in vitamin D-deficient patients and experimental animals, and there is anecdotal evidence that individuals with rickets are particularly prone to infection. A recent study reported that individuals with low vitamin D status had a higher risk of viral respiratory tract infections (Sabetta *et al.*, 2010). Supplementation of Japanese schoolchildren with vitamin D (1200 U/day) for 4 months during winter decreased by about 40% the risk of influenza (Urashima *et al.*, 2010). These studies suggest that vitamin D acts to improve immune function. However, there is, paradoxically, a large body of literature supporting an immunosuppressive role for vitamin D and related analogs (Griffin *et al.*, 2003; Hayes *et al.*, 2003; Cantorna *et al.*, 2004; van Etten and Mathieu, 2005; Bruce *et al.*, 2010). The current view is that under physiological conditions vitamin D probably facilitates immune responses, but that it may also play an active role in the prevention of autoimmunity and that there may be a therapeutic role for vitamin D in some immune-mediated diseases. Vitamin D acts by binding to its receptor and regulating gene expression in target cells. Its effects include promotion of phagocytosis, superoxide synthesis, and bacterial killing, but it is also reported to inhibit T-cell proliferation, production of Th1 cytokines, and B-cell antibody production, highlighting the paradoxical nature of its effects. The role of vitamin D in autoimmunity is particularly interesting: there is increasing evidence, mainly from animal studies, that vitamin D deficiency is linked with autoimmune diseases such as multiple sclerosis, rheumatoid arthritis, and inflammatory bowel disease. The inhibition by vitamin D of Th1-type immune activity, which underlies many autoimmune conditions, is thought to be key to this link (Lemire *et al.*, 1995; Bruce *et al.*, 2010). In addition, a polymorphism in the vitamin D receptor gene has been associated with increased risk of Crohn's disease. Taken together, the evidence suggests that vitamin D is a selective regulator of immune function and the effects of vitamin D deficiency, vitamin D receptor deficiency or vitamin D supplementation depend on the immunological situation (e.g. health, infectious disease, autoimmune disease).

Vitamin E

Vitamin E is the major lipid-soluble antioxidant in the body and is required for protection of membrane lipids from peroxidation. Free radicals and lipid peroxidation are immunosuppressive; thus, it is considered that vitamin E should act to optimize and even enhance the immune response (Meydani and Beharka, 1998; Meydani et al., 2005). Indeed, a positive association exists between plasma vitamin E levels and DTH responses, and a negative association has been demonstrated between plasma vitamin E levels and the incidence of infections in healthy adults over 60 years of age (Chavance et al., 1989). There appears to be particular benefit of vitamin E supplementation for the elderly (Meydani et al., 1990; Pallast et al., 1999), with studies demonstrating enhanced Th1 cell-mediated immunity at high doses. A comprehensive study demonstrated increased DTH responses in elderly subjects supplemented with 60, 200, and 800 mg/day of vitamin E, with maximal effect at a dose of 200 mg/day (Meydani et al., 1997). This dose also increased the antibody responses to hepatitis B, tetanus toxoid and pneumococcus vaccinations. This "optimal" dose of 200 mg/day of vitamin E is well in excess of the recommended dietary intake; thus, it appears that adding vitamin E to the diet at levels beyond those normally recommended may enhance some immune functions above normal, and it has even been argued that the recommended intake for vitamin E is not adequate for optimal immune function. However, RCTs do not consistently support a role for vitamin E supplementation in reducing the incidence, duration or severity of respiratory infections in elderly populations (Graat et al., 2002), although one large study did show benefit specifically for upper respiratory tract infections (Meydani et al., 2004).

Zinc

Zinc is important for DNA synthesis and in cellular growth and differentiation and antioxidant defense. Zinc deficiency impairs many aspects of innate immunity, including phagocytosis by macrophages and neutrophils, natural killer cell activity, and respiratory burst and complement activity, all of which could be important contributors to increased susceptibility to infection (Fraker et al., 1993; Scrimshaw and SanGiovanni, 1997; Shankar and Prasad, 1998; Calder and Jackson, 2000; Prasad, 2002, 2008; Fraker and King, 2004). Zinc deficiency has a marked impact on bone marrow, decreasing the number of nucleated cells and the number and proportion of cells that are lymphoid precursors (Fraker and King, 2004). In patients with zinc deficiency related to sickle-cell disease, natural killer cell activity is decreased, but can be returned to normal by zinc supplementation. In acrodermatitis enteropathica, which is characterized by reduced intestinal zinc absorption, thymic atrophy, impaired lymphocyte development, and reduced lymphocyte responsiveness and DTH are observed (Shankar and Prasad, 1998). Moderate or mild zinc deficiency or experimental zinc deficiency (induced by consumption of <3.5 mg zinc/day) in humans results in decreased thymulin activity, natural killer cell activity, lymphocyte proliferation, IL-2 production, and DTH response; all can be corrected by zinc repletion (Beck et al., 1997).

Low plasma zinc levels can be used to predict the subsequent development of lower respiratory tract infections and diarrhea in malnourished populations (Calder and Jackson, 2000; Prasad, 2002; Fischer Walker and Black, 2004). Indeed, diarrhea is considered a symptom of zinc deficiency and several studies show that zinc supplementation decreases the incidence, duration, and severity of childhood diarrhea. Effects of zinc on respiratory tract infections are less clear. Most (but not all) studies fail to show a benefit of zinc supplementation in respiratory disease in malnourished populations, and available trials on the effect of zinc on the common cold in non-malnourished populations report conflicting results (Marshall, 2000; Turner and Cetnarowski, 2000). Very high zinc intakes can result in copper depletion, and copper deficiency impairs immune function and increases susceptibility to infection (Failla and Hopkins, 1998; Percival, 1998).

Iron

Iron deficiency has multiple effects on immune function in laboratory animals and humans (Sherman and Spear, 1993; Kuvibidila and Baliga, 2002; Weiss, 2002). However, the relationship between iron deficiency and susceptibility to infection remains controversial (Oppenheimer, 2001; Weiss, 2002; Schaible and Kaufmann, 2004). Furthermore, evidence suggests that infections caused by organisms that spend part of their life cycle intracellularly, such as plasmodia, mycobacteria, and invasive salmonellae, may actually be enhanced by iron therapy. In the tropics in children of all ages, at doses of >2 mg/kg/day, iron has been associated with increased risk of malaria and other infections, including pneumonia. For these reasons, iron intervention in malaria-endemic areas is not advised, particularly high doses in the young, those with compromised immunity (e.g. HIV infection), and during the peak malaria transmission season. Iron treatment for anemia in a malarious area must be preceded by effective antimalarial therapy and should be oral rather than parenteral. The detrimental effects of iron administration may occur because microorganisms require iron and providing it may favor the growth and replication of the pathogen. Indeed, it has been argued that the decline in circulating iron concentrations that accompanies infection is an attempt by the host to "starve" the infectious agent of iron. There are several mechanisms for withholding iron from a pathogen in this way. Lactoferrin has a higher binding affinity for iron than do bacterial siderospores, making bound iron unavailable to the pathogen. Furthermore, once lactoferrin reaches 40% saturation with iron, it is sequestered by macrophages. It is notable that breast milk contains lactoferrin, which may protect against the use of free iron by pathogens transferred to an infant. It is important to note that oral iron supplementation has not been shown to increase risk of infection in non-malarious countries (Oppenheimer, 2001).

Selenium

Selenium is essential for an effectively functioning immune system. Deficiency in laboratory animals affects both innate and adaptive immunity, particularly neutrophil function (Stabel and Spears, 1993; McKenzie *et al.*, 1998). It also increases susceptibility to bacterial, viral, fungal, and parasitic challenges. Lower selenium concentrations in humans have also been linked with increased virulence, diminished natural killer cell activity, increased mycobacterial disease, and HIV progression. Selenium supplementation has been shown to improve various aspects of immune function in humans (Kiremidjian-Schumacher *et al.*, 1994; Roy *et al.*, 1994; Hawkes *et al.*, 2001), including the elderly (Peretz *et al.*, 1991; Roy *et al.*, 1995). Selenium supplementation (50 or 100 μg/day) in adults with low selenium status improved some aspects of their immune response to a poliovirus vaccination (Broome *et al.*, 2004).

Dietary Fat and Immune Function

Eicosanoids: A Link between Fatty Acids and the Immune System

Fatty acids can affect immune function through a variety of actions, including alterations in membrane structure, cell signalling mechanisms, and gene expression (Calder, 2008). However, the best described mechanism of action of polyunsaturated fatty acids (PUFAs) is through influencing the production of a class of lipid mediators termed eicosanoids that play important roles in regulating immunity and inflammation (Tilley *et al.*, 2001). The membranes of most immune cells contain large amounts of arachidonic acid, which is the principal precursor for eicosanoid synthesis. Arachidonic acid in cell membranes can be mobilized by various phospholipase enzymes, most notably phospholipase A_2, and the free arachidonic acid can subsequently act as a substrate for cyclooxygenase enzymes (COX), forming prostaglandins (PGs) and related compounds, or, for one of the lipoxygenase (LOX) enzymes, forming leukotrienes (LTs) and related compounds. Di-homo-γ-linolenic acid and eicosapentaenoic acid are also precursors for eicosanoid synthesis, and the mediators produced from each different substrate have different structures and different biological potencies. Eicosanoids are formed in a cell-specific manner and may have opposing effects to one another, so the overall physiological or pathophysiological effect will be governed by the nature of the cells producing the eicosanoids, the concentrations of the different eicosanoids, the timing of their production, and the sensitivities of target cells to their effects.

Essential Fatty Acid Deficiency and Immune Function

Animal studies have shown that deficiencies in both linoleic and α-linolenic acids result in decreased thymus and spleen weight, and reduced lymphocyte proliferation, neutrophil chemotaxis, macrophage-mediated cytotoxicity, and DTH response. Thus, the immunological effects of essential fatty acid deficiency appear to be similar to the effects of single micronutrient deficiencies, although there are no human studies to confirm this (essential fatty acid deficiency is very rare in humans). Essential fatty acid deficiency probably has its effects because cells of the immune system require PUFAs for membrane synthesis and as precursors for the synthesis of eicosanoids.

Amount of Dietary Fat and Immune Function

High-fat diets have been reported to result in diminished immune cell functions (both natural and cell-mediated immunity) compared with low-fat diets in both humans (Barone *et al.*, 1989; Kelley *et al.*, 1992; Han *et al.*, 2003) and experimental animals, but the precise effect depends on the exact level of fat used in the high-fat diet and its source.

Effect of Specific Fatty Acids or Fatty Acid Families on Immune Function

Saturated fatty acids appear to have little impact on humoral or cell-mediated immune function, but cell culture, animal model, and human epidemiological studies all indicate that some saturated fatty acids promote inflammation. N-6 PUFAs are also believed to promote inflammation through the actions of eicosanoids, but human studies do not fully support this contention. Cell culture and animal model studies have shown that marine n-3 PUFAs (eicosapentaenoic acid [EPA] and docosahexaenoic acid [DHA]) suppress both inflammation and cell-mediated immune responses (Calder, 2003, 2006), acting through a variety of mechanisms including altered:

- membrane structure;
- membrane and intracellular signalling processes;
- gene expression profiles;
- production of eicosanoids.

EPA and DHA also give rise to resolvins and related lipid mediators that have potent anti-inflammatory and inflammation-resolving activities (Serhan *et al.*, 2008).

Epidemiological studies in humans, and studies in which human subjects are given marine n-3 PUFAs, demonstrate that these fatty acids are anti-inflammatory, but less consistent effects of cell-mediated immunity are demonstrated. Consistent with their anti-inflammatory effects, marine n-3 PUFAs have some treatment efficacy in certain chronic inflammatory conditions (Calder, 2009a,b). Animal studies show variable effects of marine n-3 PUFAs (and indeed other fatty acids) on the ability to handle pathogens (Anderson and Fritsche, 2002) and there is little information on fatty acids and infection in humans.

Dietary Amino Acids and Immune Function

Sulfur Amino Acids

Sulfur amino acids are essential in humans. Deficiency in methionine and cysteine results in atrophy of the thymus,

spleen and lymph nodes, and prevents recovery from protein–energy malnutrition (Gross and Newberne, 1980; Grimble and Grimble, 1998; Grimble, 2002). When combined with a deficiency of isoleucine and valine, also essential amino acids, sulfur amino acid deficiency results in severe depletion of gut lymphoid tissue, very similar to the effect of protein deprivation (Gross and Newberne, 1980). Glutathione is a tripeptide that consists of glycine, cysteine, and glutamate. It is recognized to have antioxidant properties. Glutathione concentrations in the liver, lung, small intestine, and immune cells fall in response to inflammatory stimuli (probably as a result of oxidative stress), and this fall can be prevented in some organs by the provision of cysteine in the diet. Although the limiting precursor for glutathione biosynthesis is usually cysteine, the ability of sulfur amino acids to replete glutathione stores is related to the protein level of the diet. Glutathione can enhance the activity of cytotoxic T-cells, while depletion of intracellular glutathione diminishes lymphocyte proliferation and the generation of cytotoxic T-lymphocytes (Peterson *et al.*, 1998).

Arginine

Arginine is a non-essential amino acid in humans and is involved in protein, urea, and nucleotide synthesis, and adenosine triphosphate (ATP) generation. It also serves as the precursor of nitric oxide, a potent immunoregulatory mediator that is cytotoxic to tumor cells and to some microorganisms. In laboratory animals arginine decreases the thymus involution associated with trauma, promotes thymus repopulation and cellularity, increases lymphocyte proliferation, natural killer cell activity, and macrophage cytotoxicity, improves DTH, increases resistance to bacterial infections, increases survival to sepsis and burns, and promotes wound healing (Evoy *et al.*, 1998; Duff and Daly, 2002). There are indications that arginine may have similar effects in humans, although these have not been tested thoroughly.

Glutamine

Glutamine is the most abundant amino acid in the blood and in the free amino acid pool in the body; skeletal muscle is considered to be the most important glutamine producer in the body. Once released from skeletal muscle, glutamine acts as an inter-organ nitrogen transporter. One important user of glutamine is the immune system. Plasma glutamine levels are lowered (by up to 50%) by sepsis, injury, and burns, and following surgery. Furthermore, the skeletal muscle glutamine concentration is lowered by more than 50% in at least some of these situations. These observations indicate that a significant depletion of the skeletal muscle glutamine pool is characteristic of trauma. The lowered plasma glutamine concentrations that occur are likely to be the result of demand for glutamine (by the liver, kidney, gut, and immune system) exceeding the supply, and it has been suggested that the lowered plasma glutamine contributes, at least in part, to the impaired immune function that accompanies such situations. It has been argued that restoring plasma glutamine concentrations in these situations should restore immune function. As with arginine, there are animal studies to support this (Calder and Yaqoob, 1999; Calder and Newsholme, 2002). Clinical studies, mainly using intravenous infusions of solutions containing glutamine, have also reported beneficial effects for patients undergoing bone marrow transplantation and colorectal surgery, patients in intensive care, and low-birth-weight babies, all of whom are at risk from infection and sepsis (Calder, 2007b). In some of these studies, improved outcome was associated with improved immune function. In addition to a direct immunological effect, glutamine, even provided intravenously, improves gut barrier function in patients at risk of infection. This would have the benefit of decreasing the translocation of bacteria from the gut and eliminating a key source of infection.

Probiotics, Prebiotics and Immune Function

Indigenous bacteria are believed to contribute to the immunological protection of the host by creating a barrier against colonization by pathogenic bacteria. This barrier can be disrupted by disease and by the use of antibiotics, so allowing easier access to the host gut by pathogens. It is now believed that this barrier can be maintained by providing supplements containing live "desirable" bacteria; such supplements are termed probiotics. Probiotic organisms are found in fermented foods including traditionally cultured dairy products and some fermented milks. The organisms used commercially as probiotics are typically lactobacilli or bifidobacteria. These organisms only colonize the gut temporarily, making regular consumption necessary. In addition to creating a barrier effect, some of the metabolic products of probiotic bacteria (e.g. lactic acid and a class of antibiotic proteins termed bacteriocins produced by some bacteria) may inhibit the growth of pathogenic organisms. Probiotic bacteria may also compete with pathogenic bacteria for nutrients and may enhance the gut immune response to pathogenic bacteria. Probiotics have various routes for internalization by the gut epithelium and contact with underlying immune tissues; it is through these interactions that probiotics are thought to be able to influence immune function. However, the nature of this regulation is not very well understood. A number of studies have examined the influence of various probiotic organisms, either alone or in combination, on immune function, infection and inflammatory conditions in humans (Lomax and Calder, 2009a). Probiotics appear to enhance innate immunity (particularly phagocytosis and natural killer cell activity), but have lesser effects on adaptive immunity. In children, probiotics have been shown to reduce the incidence and duration of diarrhea, although the effects depend on the nature of the condition. In adults, some studies demonstrate a reduction in the risk of traveller's diarrhea. The effect on other infectious outcomes is much less clear. There is some evidence that probiotics could be beneficial in ulcerative colitis, irritable bowel syndrome, and allergy. One of the difficulties in interpreting results is that there may be significant species and strain differences in the effects of probiotics, as well as differences in doses used, duration of treatment, and subject characteristics.

Prebiotics are typically, though not exclusively, carbohydrates which are not digestible by mammalian enzymes but which are selectively fermented by gut microbiota, leading to increased numbers of beneficial bacteria within the gut. Although there is growing evidence for potential immunomodulatory effects of prebiotics (Lomax and Calder, 2009b), it is not clear whether they are direct effects, or manifested through alteration of the gut microbiota.

Breastfeeding and Immune Function

The Composition of Breast Milk

Breast milk is the best example of a foodstuff with immune-enhancing properties. Breast milk contains a wide range of immunologically active components, including cells (macrophages, T- and B-lymphocytes, neutrophils), immunoglobulins (IgG, IgM, IgD, sIgA), lysozyme (which has direct antibacterial action), lactoferrin (which binds iron, so preventing its uptake by bacteria), cytokines (IL-1, IL-6, IL-10, IFN-γ, TNF-α, transforming growth factor-β), growth factors (epidermal growth factor, insulin-like growth factor), hormones (thyroxin), fat-soluble vitamins

(vitamins A, D, E), amino acids (taurine, glutamine), fatty acids, amino sugars, nucleotides, gangliosides, and prebiotic oligosaccharides (Emmett and Rogers, 1997; Bernt and Walker, 1999). Breast milk also contains factors that prevent the adhesion of some microorganisms to the gastrointestinal tract and so prevents bacterial colonization. Human breast milk contains factors that promote the growth of useful bacteria (e.g. bifidobacteria) in the gut. The content of many factors varies among milks of different species, and is different between human breast milk and infant formulas.

Breastfeeding and Infection

Breastfeeding is thought to play a key role in the prevention of infectious disease, particularly diarrhea and gastrointestinal and lower respiratory infections, in both developing and developed countries (Golding *et al.*, 1997a,b,c). In addition to preventing infectious disease, breastfeeding enhances the antibody responses to vaccination. A meta-analysis of studies that examined the effect of breastfeeding versus formula-feeding on risk of death due to infectious diseases in developing countries identified that infants who are not breast-fed have a six-fold greater risk of dying from infectious diseases in the first 2 months of life than those who are breast-fed. However, it appears that this protection decreases steadily with age, as infants begin complementary feeding, so that, by 6–11 months, the protection afforded by breastfeeding is no longer apparent. Breastfeeding may provide better protection against diarrhea (up to 6 months of age) than against deaths due to respiratory infections. There are also geographical influences on the protection afforded by breastfeeding; in some continents, protection can be observed throughout the first year of life, whereas in others it is much more short-lived.

Other Considerations

Deficiencies of total energy or of one or more essential nutrients, including vitamins A, B_6, B_{12}, C, and E, folic acid, zinc, iron, copper, selenium, essential amino acids, and essential fatty acids, impair immune function and increase susceptibility to infectious pathogens. This occurs because each of these nutrients is involved in the molecular and cellular responses to challenge of the immune system. Providing these nutrients to deficient individuals restores immune function and improves resistance to infection. For

some nutrients the dietary intakes that result in greatest enhancement of immune function are greater than recommended intakes. However, excessive intake of some nutrients also impairs immune responses. It is often assumed, when considering the relationship between nutrient intake and immune function, that all components of the immune system will respond in the same dose-dependent fashion to a given nutrient. This is not correct, at least as far as some nutrients are concerned, and it appears likely that different components of the immune system show an individual dose–response relationship to the availability of a given nutrient, meaning that the overall impact of the nutrient is difficult to predict.

Although outside the scope of this chapter, it is important to consider the role of hormones in regulating immune function during malnutrition. An inadequate supply of nutrients to the body may cause physiological stress, leading to an elevation in the circulating concentrations of glucocorticoids and catecholamines. Both classes of hormones have an inhibitory effect on immune function and may therefore be important factors when considering the relationship between nutrient supply and immunological outcome.

It is now appreciated that the supply of nutrients that are not considered to be essential according to traditional criteria may also influence immune function; this is particularly notable for the amino acids glutamine and arginine, and may indicate that a re-evaluation of the definitions of essentiality, nutrient requirements, and nutrient status is required for some dietary components.

Finally, an early point of contact between nutrients and the immune system occurs within the intestinal tract. Relatively little is known about the relationship between nutrient status and the function of the gut-associated immune system. This is of particular relevance when considering adverse reactions to foods: the role of immunoregulatory nutrients in responses to food components and in sensitization to food-borne allergens is largely unknown. An understanding of the interaction between nutrients, the types of bacteria that inhabit the gut, and gut-associated and systemic immune responses is only now beginning to emerge.

The term "optimal immune function" is often used in the literature without careful thought about its definition. An optimal immune response to any given nutrient measured by one marker will not necessarily be optimal according to a second marker of immune function. Furthermore, the effect of a given nutrient on immune response may be altered by levels of other nutrients. For these reasons, the desire to "optimize" the immune response may not be realistic. At best, it is reasonable to expect that correction of marginal deficiencies will improve immunity, but further enhancement using supplements cannot be guaranteed and in excessive doses is likely to be detrimental. At the other extreme, there is interest in the potential therapeutic effect of nutrients in diseases involving dysregulation of the immune system (e.g. n-3 fatty acids in rheumatoid arthritis). In some but by no means all cases, there is supportive evidence for this approach. Between these extremes there are many unanswered questions, but it is clear that the modulation of immune function by nutrients has important implications in both developing and developed countries.

Future Directions

Impaired immunity, in part related to poor nutrition, remains a major public health problem (Calder and Jackson, 2000). Diseases involving dysregulated immunity are of great clinical significance, with evidence that certain dietary components may have some influence on these conditions (Calder et al., 2009). Thus, it is highly likely that significant research activity in the area of nutritional immunology will continue for the foreseeable future, that advances in identifying the effects of individual nutrients, combinations of nutrients, and particular foodstuffs will be made, and that these will be coupled with advances in the understanding of mechanisms of action involved (Calder et al., 2002) and of the determinants that confer an individual's sensitivity to the immunomodulating activity of particular nutrients (Calder and Kew, 2002). The discovery of new immune cell subtypes (e.g. regulatory T-cells, Th17 cells) and new mediators of immunity and inflammation (e.g. resolvins) is opening new avenues of research that will aid our understanding of the nutrition–immunity axis. Recognition of the chronology of events and of the factors that contribute to the acquisition of immune competence early in life (Calder et al., 2006) and to the decline in immune competence with aging (Castle, 2000; Burns and Goodwin, 2004; Agarwal and Busse, 2010) will provide opportunities for studying and then targeting nutrition towards vulnerable periods of the life cycle. Awareness of immune impairments associated with obesity (Marti et al., 2001) and that obesity and chronic diseases of aging such as cardiovascular disease have an

inflammatory component (Calder et al., 2009) will focus attention on the interaction between nutrition, the immuno-inflammatory response, and other lifestyle, as well as genetic, factors. Finally the role of the gut microbiota in shaping host immune maturation and immune responses is beginning to be defined (Calder et al., 2006), but the exact nature of the bacteria–host interaction is not yet well described; it is likely that this area will become a focus of research in nutritional immunology, and it is anticipated that great advances will be made fairly quickly (Saulnier et al., 2009).

Suggestions for Further Reading

Albers, R., Antoine, J.M., Bourdet-Sicard, R., et al. (2005) Markers to measure immunomodulation in human nutrition intervention studies. Br J Nutr 94, 452–481.

Calder, P.C. (2007) Immunological parameters: what do they mean? J Nutr 137, 773S–780S.

Calder, P.C. and Jackson, A.A. (2000) Undernutrition, infection and immune function. Nutr Res Rev 13, 3–29.

Calder, P.C. and Kew, S. (2002) The immune system: a target for functional foods? Br J Nutr 88, S165–S177.

Calder, P.C., Albers, R., Antoine, J.M., et al. (2009) Inflammatory disease processes and interactions with nutrition. Br J Nutr 101, S1–S45.

Calder, P.C., Field, C.J., and Gill, H.S. (2002) Nutrition and Immune Function. CAB International, Wallingford.

Calder, P.C., Krauss-Etschmann, S., de Jong, E.C., et al. (2006) Early nutrition and immunity – progress and perspectives. Br J Nutr 96, 774–790.

Chandra, R.K. (1991) 1990 McCollum Award lecture. Nutrition and immunity: lessons from the past and new insights into the future. Am J Clin Nutr 53, 1087–1101.

Scrimshaw, N.S. and SanGiovanni, J.P. (1997) Synergism of nutrition, infection, and immunity: an overview. Am J Clin Nutr 66, 464S–477S.

Yaqoob, P. and Calder, P.C. (2011) The immune and inflammatory systems. In S. Lanham-New, H.M. Roche, and I.A. MacDonald (eds), Nutrition and Metabolism, 2nd Edn. Wiley-Blackwell, Chichester, pp. 312–338.

References

Agarwal, S. and Busse, P.J. (2010) Innate and adaptive immunosenescence. *Ann Allergy Asthma Immunol* **104**, 183–190.

Albers, R., Antoine, J.M., Bourdet-Sicard, R., *et al.* (2005) Markers to measure immunomodulation in human nutrition intervention studies. *Br J Nutr* **94**, 452–481.

Anderson, M. and Fritsche, K.L. (2002) (n-3) Fatty acids and infectious disease resistance. *J Nutr* **132**, 3566–3576.

Barone, J., Hebert, J.R., and Reddy, M.M. (1989) Dietary fat and natural-killer-cell activity. *Am J Clin Nutr* **50**, 861–867.

Beck, F.W., Prasad, A.S., Kaplan, J., *et al.* (1997) Changes in cytokine production and T cell subpopulations in experimentally induced zinc-deficient humans. *Am J Physiol* **272**, E1002–E1007.

Bernt, K.M. and Walker, W.A. (1999) Human milk as a carrier of biochemical messages. *Acta Paediatr Suppl* **88**, 27–41.

Broome, C.S., McArdle, F., Kyle, J.A., *et al.* (2004) An increase in selenium intake improves immune function and poliovirus handling in adults with marginal selenium status. *Am J Clin Nutr* **80**, 154–162.

Bruce, D., Ooi, J.H., Yu, S.H., *et al.* (2010) Vitamin D and host resistance to infection? Putting the cart in front of the horse. *Exp Biol Med* **235**, 921–927.

Bunout, D., Barrera, G., Hirsch, S., *et al.* (2004) Effects of a nutritional supplement on the immune response and cytokine production in free-living Chilean elderly. *JPEN J Parenter Enteral Nutr* **28**, 348–354.

Burns, E.A. and Goodwin, J.S. (2004) Effect of aging on immune function. *J Nutr Health Aging* **8**, 9–18.

Calder, P.C. (1995) Fuel utilisation by cells of the immune system. *Proc Nutr Soc* **54**, 65–82.

Calder, P.C. (2003) N-3 polyunsaturated fatty acids and inflammation: from molecular biology to the clinic. *Lipids* **38**, 343–352.

Calder, P.C. (2006) n-3 polyunsaturated fatty acids, inflammation, and inflammatory diseases. *Am J Clin Nutr* **83**, 1505S–1519S.

Calder, P.C. (2007a) Immunological parameters: what do they mean? *J Nutr* **137**, 773S–780S.

Calder, P.C. (2007b) Immunonutrition in surgical and critically ill patients. *Br J Nutr* **98**, S133–S139.

Calder, P.C. (2008) The relationship between the fatty acid composition of immune cells and their function. *Prostaglandins Leukot Essent Fatty Acids* **79**, 101–108.

Calder, P.C. (2009a) Polyunsaturated fatty acids and inflammation: therapeutic potential in rheumatoid arthritis. *Curr Rheumatol Rev* **5**, 214–225.

Calder, P.C. (2009b) Fatty acids and immune function: relevance to inflammatory bowel diseases. *Int Rev Immunol* **28**, 506–534.

Calder, P.C. and Jackson, A.A. (2000) Undernutrition, infection and immune function. *Nutr Res Rev* **13**, 3–29.

Calder, P.C. and Kew, S. (2002) The immune system: a target for functional foods? *Br J Nutr* **88**, S165–S177.

Calder, P.C. and Newsholme, P. (2002) Glutamine and the immune system. In P.C. Calder, C.J. Field, and H.S. Gill (eds), *Nutrition and Immune Function*. CAB International, Wallingford, pp. 109–132.

Calder, P.C. and Yaqoob, P. (1999) Glutamine and the immune system. *Amino Acids* **17**, 227–241.

Calder, P.C., Albers, R., Antoine, J.M., *et al.* (2009) Inflammatory disease processes and interactions with nutrition. *Br J Nutr* **101**, S1–S45.

Calder, P.C., Field, C.J., and Gill, H.S. (2002) *Nutrition and Immune Function*. CAB International, Wallingford.

Calder, P.C., Krauss-Etschmann, S., de Jong, E.C., *et al.* (2006) Early nutrition and immunity – progress and perspectives. *Br J Nutr* **96**, 774–790.

Cantorna, M.T., Zhu, Y., Froicu, M., *et al.* (2004) Vitamin D status, 1,25-dihydroxyvitamin D3, and the immune system. *Am J Clin Nutr* **80**, 1717S–1720S.

Castle, S.C. (2000) Clinical relevance of age-related immune dysfunction. *Clin Infect Dis* **31**, 578–585.

Chandra, R.K. (1991) 1990 McCollum Award lecture. Nutrition and immunity: lessons from the past and new insights into the future. *Am J Clin Nutr* **53**, 1087–1101.

Chavance, M., Herbeth, B., Fournier, C., *et al.* (1989) Vitamin status, immunity and infections in an elderly population. *Eur J Clin Nutr* **43**, 827–835.

Cummings, J.H., Antoine, J.M., Azpiroz, F., *et al.* (2004) PASSCLAIM – gut health and immunity. *Eur J Nutr* **43**, II118–II173.

Douglas, R.M., Hemilä, H., Chalker, E., *et al.* (2007) Vitamin C for preventing and treating the common cold. *Cochrane Database Syst Rev* CD000980.

Duff, M.D. and Daly, J.M. (2002) Arginine and immune function. In P.C. Calder, C.J. Field, and H.S. Gill (eds), *Nutrition and Immune Function*. CAB International, Wallingford, pp. 93–108.

Emmett, P.M. and Rogers, I.S. (1997) Properties of human milk and their relationship with maternal nutrition. *Early Hum Dev* **49**, S7–28.

Evoy, D., Lieberman, M.D., Fahey, T.J., *et al.* (1998) Immunonutrition: the role of arginine. *Nutrition* **14**, 611–617.

Failla, M.L. and Hopkins, R.G. (1998) Is low copper status immunosuppressive? *Nutr Rev* **56**, S59–S64.

Fata, F.T., Herzlich, B.C., Schiffman, G., *et al.* (1996) Impaired antibody responses to pneumococcal polysaccharide in elderly patients with low serum vitamin B12 levels. *Ann Int Med* **124,** 299–304.

Fischer Walker, C. and Black, R.E. (2004) Zinc and the risk for infectious disease. *Annu Rev Nutr* **24,** 255–275.

Fraker, P.J. and King, L.E. (2004) Reprogramming of the immune system during zinc deficiency. *Annu Rev Nutr* **24,** 277–298.

Fraker, P.J., King, L.E., Garvy, B.A., *et al.* (1993) The immunopathology of zinc deficiency in humans and rodents: a possible role for programmed cell death. In D.M. Klurfeld (ed.), *Nutrition and Immunology.* Plenum Press, New York, pp. 267–283.

Golding, J., Emmett, P.M., and Rogers, I.S. (1997a) Gastroenteritis, diarrhoea and breast feeding. *Early Hum Dev* **49,** S83–103.

Golding, J., Emmett, P.M., and Rogers, I.S. (1997b) Does breast feeding protect against non-gastric infections? *Early Hum Dev* **49,** S105–120.

Golding, J., Emmett, P.M., and Rogers, I.S. (1997c) Breast feeding and infant mortality. *Early Hum Dev* **49,** S143–155.

Graat, J.M., Schouten, E.G., and Kok, F.J. (2002) Effect of daily vitamin E and multivitamin–mineral supplementation on acute respiratory tract infections in elderly persons: a randomized controlled trial. *JAMA* **288,** 715–721.

Griffin, M.D., Xing, N., and Kumar, R. (2003) Vitamin D and its analogs as regulators of immune activation and antigen presentation. *Annu Rev Nutr* **23,** 117–145.

Grimble, R.F. (2002) Sulphur amino acids, glutathione and immune function. In P.C. Calder, C.J. Field, and H.S. Gill (eds), *Nutrition and Immune Function.* CAB International, Wallingford, pp. 133–150.

Grimble, R.F. and Grimble, G.K. (1998) Immunonutrition: the role of sulfur amino acids, related amino acids and polyamines. *Nutrition* **14,** 605–610.

Gross, R.L. and Newberne, P.M. (1980) Role of nutrition in immunologic function. *Physiol Rev* **60,** 188–302.

Han, S.N., Leka, L.S., Lichtenstein, A.H., *et al.* (2003) Effect of a therapeutic lifestyle change diet on immune functions of moderately hypercholesterolemic humans. *J Lipid Res* **44,** 2304–2310.

Hawkes, W.C., Kelley, D.S., and Taylor, P.C. (2001) The effects of dietary selenium on the immune system in healthy men. *Biol Trace Elem Res* **81,** 189–213.

Hayes, C.E., Nashold, F.E., Spach, K.M., *et al.* (2003) The immunological functions of the vitamin D endocrine system. *Cell Mol Biol* **49,** 277–300.

Kelley, D.S., Dougherty, R.M., Branch, L.B., *et al.* (1992) Concentration of dietary N-6 polyunsaturated fatty acids and

the human immune status. *Clin Immunol Immunopathol* **62,** 240–244.

Kiremidjian-Schumacher, L., Roy, M., Wishe, H.I., *et al.* (1994) Supplementation with selenium and human immune cell functions. II. Effect on cytotoxic lymphocytes and natural killer cells. *Biol Trace Elem Res* **41,** 115–127.

Kuvibidila, S. and Baliga, B.S. (2002) Role of iron in immunity and infection. In P.C. Calder, C.J. Field, and H.S. Gill (eds), *Nutrition and Immune Function.* CAB International, Wallingford, pp. 209–228.

Kuvibidila, S., Yu, L., Ode, D., *et al.* (1993) The immune response in protein-energy malnutrition and single nutrient deficiency. In D.M. Klurfeld (ed.), *Nutrition and Immunology.* Plenum Press, New York, pp. 121–155.

Lemire, J.M., Archer, D.C., Beck, L., *et al.* (1995) Immunosuppressive actions of 1,25-dihydroxyvitamin D3: preferential inhibition of Th1 functions. *J Nutr* **125,** 1704S–1708S.

Lomax, A.R. and Calder, P.C. (2009a) Probiotics, immune function, infection and inflammation: a review of the evidence from studies conducted in humans. *Curr Pharm Des* **15,** 1428–1518.

Lomax, A.R. and Calder, P.C. (2009b) Prebiotics, immune function, infection and inflammation: a review of the evidence. *Br J Nutr* **101,** 633–658.

Lucas, S. (2010) Predictive clinicopathological features derived from systematic autopsy examination of patients who died with A/H1N1 influenza infection in the UK 2009–10 pandemic. *Health Technol Assess* **14,** 83–114.

Marshall, I. (2000) Zinc for the common cold. *Cochrane Database Syst Rev* CD001364.

Marti, A., Marcos, A., and Martinez, J.A. (2001) Obesity and immune function relationships. *Obes Rev* **2,** 131–140.

Matarese, G., Procaccini, C., De Rosa, V., *et al.* (2010) Regulatory T cells in obesity: the leptin connection. *Trends Mol Med* **16,** 247–256.

McKenzie, R.C., Rafferty, T.S., and Beckett, G.J. (1998) Selenium: an essential element for immune function. *Immunol Today* **19,** 342–345.

Meydani, S.N. and Beharka, A.A. (1998) Recent developments in vitamin E and immune response. *Nutr Rev* **56,** S49–S58.

Meydani, S.N., Barklund, M.P., Liu, S., *et al.* (1990) Vitamin E supplementation enhances cell-mediated immunity in healthy elderly subjects. *Am J Clin Nutr* **52,** 557–563.

Meydani, S.N., Han, S.N., and Wu, D. (2005) Vitamin E and immune response in the aged: mechanisms and clinical implications. *Immunol Rev* **205,** 269–284

Meydani, S.N., Leka, L.S., Fine, B.C., *et al.* (2004) Vitamin E and respiratory tract infections in elderly nursing home residents: a randomized controlled trial. *JAMA* **292,** 828–836.

Meydani, S.N., Meydani, M., Blumberg, J.B., *et al.* (1997) Vitamin E supplementation and in vivo immune response in healthy subjects. *JAMA* **277**, 1380–1386.

Meydani, S.N., Ribaya-Mercado, J.D., Russell, R.M., *et al.* (1991) Vitamin B6 deficiency impairs interleukin-2 production and lymphocyte proliferation in elderly adults. *Am J Clin Nutr* **53**, 1275–1280.

Mowat, A.M. (2003) Anatomical basis of tolerance and immunity to intestinal antigens. *Nat Rev Immunol* **3**, 331–341.

Oppenheimer, S.J. (2001) Iron and its relation to immunity and infectious disease. *J Nutr* **131**, 616S–635S.

Pallast, E.G., Schouten, E.G., de Waart, F.G., *et al.* (1999) Effect of 50- and 100-mg vitamin E supplements on cellular immune function in noninstitutionalized elderly persons. *Am J Clin Nutr* **69**, 1273–1281.

Percival, S.S. (1998) Copper and immunity. *Am J Clin Nutr* **67**, 1064S–1068S.

Peretz, A., Nève, J., Desmedt, J., *et al.* (1991) Lymphocyte response is enhanced by supplementation of elderly subjects with selenium-enriched yeast. *Am J Clin Nutr* **53**, 1323–1328.

Peterson, J.D., Herzenberg, L.A., Vasquez, K., *et al.* (1998) Glutathione levels in antigen-presenting cells modulate Th1 versus Th2 response patterns. *Proc Natl Acad Sci USA* **95**, 3071–3076.

Prasad, A.S. (2002) Zinc, infection and immune function. In P.C. Calder, C.J. Field, and H.S. Gill (eds), *Nutrition and Immune Function*. CAB International, Wallingford, pp. 193–207.

Prasad, A.S. (2008) Zinc in human health: effect of zinc on immune cells. *Mol Med* **14**, 353–357.

Roy, M., Kiremidjian-Schumacher, L., Wishe, H.I., *et al.* (1994) Supplementation with selenium and human immune cell functions. I. Effect on lymphocyte proliferation and interleukin 2 receptor expression. *Biol Trace Elem Res* **41**, 103–114.

Roy, M., Kiremidjian-Schumacher, L., Wishe, H.I., *et al.* (1995) Supplementation with selenium restores age-related decline in immune cell function. *Proc Soc Exp Biol Med* **209**, 369–375.

Sabetta, J.R., DePetrillo, P., Cipriani, R.J., *et al.* (2010) Serum 25-hydroxyvitamin D and the incidence of acute viral respiratory tract infections in healthy adults. *PLoS One* **5**, e11088.

Saulnier, D.M., Spinler, J.K., Gibson, G.R., *et al.* (2009) Mechanisms of probiosis and prebiosis: considerations for enhanced functional foods. *Curr Opin Biotechnol* **20**, 135–141.

Schaible, U.E. and Kaufmann, S.H. (2004) Iron and microbial infection. *Nat Rev Microbiol* **2**, 946–953.

Scrimshaw, N.S. and SanGiovanni, J.P. (1997) Synergism of nutrition, infection, and immunity: an overview. *Am J Clin Nutr* **66**, 464S–477S.

Semba, R.D. (1998) The role of vitamin A and related retinoids in immune function. *Nutr Rev* **56**, S38–S48.

Semba, R.D. (1999) Vitamin A and immunity to viral, bacterial and protozoan infections. *Proc Nutr Soc* **58**, 719–727.

Semba, R.D. (2002) Vitamin A, infection and immune function. In P.C. Calder, C.J. Field, and H.S. Gill (eds), *Nutrition and Immune Function*. CAB International, Wallingford, pp. 151–169.

Serhan, C.N., Chiang, N., and Van Dyke, T.E. (2008) Resolving inflammation: dual anti-inflammatory and pro-resolution lipid mediators. *Nat Rev Immunol* **8**, 349–361.

Shankar, A.H. and Prasad, A.S. (1998) Zinc and immune function: the biological basis of altered resistance to infection. *Am J Clin Nutr* **68**, 447S–463S.

Sherman, A.R. and Spear, A.T. (1993) Iron and immunity. In D.M. Klurfeld (ed.), *Nutrition and Immunology*. Plenum Press, New York, pp. 285–307.

Stabel, J.R. and Spears, J.W. (1993) Role of selenium in immune responsiveness and disease resistance. In D.M. Klurfeld (ed.), *Nutrition and Immunology*. Plenum Press, New York, pp. 333–356.

Stephensen, C.B. (2001) Vitamin A, infection, and immune function. *Annu Rev Nutr* **21**, 167–192.

Tamura, J., Kubota, K., Murakami, H., *et al.* (1999) Immunomodulation by vitamin B12: augmentation of CD8+ T lymphocytes and natural killer (NK) cell activity in vitamin B12-deficient patients by methyl-B12 treatment. *Clin Exp Immunol* **116**, 28–32.

Tilg, H. and Moschen, A.R. (2006) Adipocytokines: mediators linking adipose tissue, inflammation and immunity. *Nat Rev Immunol* **6**, 772–783.

Tilley, S.L., Coffman, T.M., and Koller, B.H. (2001) Mixed messages: modulation of inflammation and immune responses by prostaglandins and thromboxanes. *J Clin Invest* **108**, 15–23.

Troen, A.M., Mitchell, B., Sorensen, B., *et al.* (2006) Unmetabolized folic acid in plasma is associated with reduced natural killer cell cytotoxicity among postmenopausal women. *J Nutr* **136**, 189–194.

Turner, R.B. and Cetnarowski, W.E. (2000) Effect of treatment with zinc gluconate or zinc acetate on experimental and natural colds. *Clin Infect Dis* **31**, 1202–1208.

Urashima, M., Segawa, T., Okazaki, M., *et al.* (2010) Randomized trial of vitamin D supplementation to prevent seasonal influenza A in schoolchildren. *Am J Clin Nutr* **91**, 1255–1260.

van Etten, E. and Mathieu, C. (2005) Immunoregulation by 1,25-dihydroxyvitamin D3: basic concepts. *J Steroid Biochem Mol Biol* **97**, 93–101.

Villamor, E. and Fawzi, W.W. (2005) Effects of vitamin A supplementation on immune responses and correlation with clinical outcomes. *Clin Microbiol Rev* **18**, 446–464.

Weiss, G. (2002) Iron and immunity: a double-edged sword. *Eur J Clin Invest* **32**(Suppl 1)**,** 70–78.

Wintergerst, E.S., Maggini, S., and Hornig, D.H. (2007) Contribution of selected vitamins and trace elements to immune function. *Ann Nutr Metab* **51,** 301–323.

Woodward, B. (1998) Protein, calories and immune defences. *Nutr Rev* **56,** S84–S92.

Woodward, B. (2001) The effect of protein-energy malnutrition on immune competence. In R.M. Suskind and K. Tontisirin (eds), *Nutrition, Immunity and Infection in Infants and Children.* Lippincott Williams and Wilkins, Philadelphia, pp. 89–120.

Yaqoob, P. and Calder, P.C. (2011) The immune and inflammatory systems. In S. Lanham-New, H.M. Roche, and I.A. MacDonald (eds), *Nutrition and Metabolism,* 2nd Edn. Wiley-Blackwell, Chichester, pp. 312–338.

45

OBESITY AS A HEALTH RISK

SUE D. PEDERSEN[1], MD, FRCPC, ANDERS SJÖDIN[2], MD, DMSc, AND ARNE ASTRUP[2], MD, DMSc

[1]LMC Endocrinology Centre, Calgary, Alberta, Canada
[2]University of Copenhagen, Frederiksburg, Denmark

Summary

Obesity is defined as a state of excess body fat and is classified by body mass index, though body fat distribution should also be taken into consideration. The prevalence of obesity has reached epidemic proportions globally. The etiology of most cases of obesity rests in a complex interplay between environmental, genetic, and psychosocial contributors, with endocrinological causes of obesity being responsible for only a minority of cases. Obesity carries with it many medical co-morbidities, including diabetes mellitus, several cardiac risk factors, an increased risk of malignancy, obstructive sleep apnea, osteoarthritis, and several psychosocial issues. Through these co-morbidities, obesity has a pronounced impact on disability and mortality. While an effective means of obesity prevention continues to evade us on a population level, a hypocaloric diet, a sustained commitment to physical activity, and attention to individual psychosocial and environmental contributors to obesity can be successful in weight reduction and maintenance of a healthy body weight.

Introduction

Obesity has become the major nutrition-related disease of this century, and is defined as a condition of excessive body fat accumulation to an extent that increases the risk of complicating diseases. Overweight and obesity are responsible for the majority of new cases of type 2 diabetes, and contribute to high blood pressure, adverse blood lipid profile, infertility, birth complications, arthritis, and several cancers, and can amplify asthma and generally worsen overall health status. Although obesity should theoretically be preventable through changes in lifestyle, especially diet, physical activity, sleep, and psychological stress, there are many powerful environmental and genetic drivers of obesity that can make effecting these changes and successfully preventing the disease exquisitely challenging.

Epidemiology of Obesity

Definition and Measurement of Obesity

Obesity is not a single entity, but it is most commonly classified by a single measure, the body mass index (BMI), a ratio of weight and height (BMI = weight (kg)/height² (m²)). The World Health Organization (WHO) classifies

Present Knowledge in Nutrition, Tenth Edition. Edited by John W. Erdman Jr, Ian A. Macdonald and Steven H. Zeisel.
© 2012 International Life Sciences Institute. Published 2012 by John Wiley & Sons, Inc.

TABLE 45.1 The international classification of adult underweight, overweight and obesity according to body mass index (BMI)

Classification	BMI (kg/m²)
Underweight	<18.5
Normal range	18.5–24.9
Overweight	≥25
Obese	≥30
Class I	30–34.9
Class II	35–39.9
Class III	≥40

underweight, normal weight, overweight and obesity according to categories of BMI (Table 45.1). This height-independent measure of weight allows comparisons to be made more readily within and between populations of the same ethnic origin. The definition of the "normal" range of BMI is based on Caucasian mortality data. For Asian populations the categories are: $18.5\,kg/m^2$ underweight; $18.5–23\,kg/m^2$, increasing but acceptable risk; $23–27.5\,kg/m^2$, increased risk; and $27.5\,kg/m^2$ or higher, high risk.

The body mass index has limitations, however, as it does not distinguish fat from lean tissue or water, nor does it identify whether the fat is accumulated in particular sites such as the abdomen, where it has more serious metabolic consequences. Techniques such as bioelectric impedance to estimate body fat, and DEXA (dual energy X-ray absorptiometry) scans to separate body mass into fat-free mass and fat mass, are increasingly used. DEXA, MR (magnetic resonance), and CT (computer tomography) scans are used for an accurate assessment of intra-abdominal adipose tissue, although BMI in combination with simple waist circumference is increasingly recognized as an easy and valid measure of overall cardiovascular risk. Waist to hip ratio and skinfold thickness may also be used to verify fatness in individuals.

Prevalence and Time Trends of Overweight and Obesity

The prevalence of the problem of excess body weight is staggering, with over 1.5 billion overweight or obese adults worldwide. The steep increase in the prevalence of obesity that has been seen in recent decades has prompted this development to be called an epidemic, and, because it is worldwide, a pandemic. In 2010, 15% of adult men and 18% of women in Denmark were obese, and in the UK,

21% of men and 24% of women were obese, and a further 47% of men and 33% of women were overweight (BMI $25–30\,kg/m^2$). Rates of overweight and obesity range from 10% to 20% in northern Europe and are higher still in southern Europe – from 20% to as high as 36% in parts of southern Italy. There is a higher than expected level of obesity among certain ethnic groups living in Europe, probably due to increased genetic susceptibility to the European lifestyle. Obesity rates are highest among people of Indian, Pakistani, and black Caribbean origin, and the prevalence of obesity in young people of Asian origin is three to four times higher than among Caucasians.

In the United States, the situation is even more extreme. In 2010, the prevalence there of obesity was 34%, though this obesity prevalence may now represent a plateau (Flegal et al., 2010). Europe is following the track of the USA, but is about 10 years behind, so in 10 years can expect to reach the same level of obesity that exists in the USA today.

Obesity is now apparent in even some of the poorest countries of the world. Normally the obesity problem first appears in a country in the more affluent parts of the population, but in recent decades obesity is characteristically higher among groups with low levels of education, low income, and low social class.

The proportion of obese people increases with age until around the age of retirement. Beyond this age, the impact of obesity-related premature death and disease-related weight loss leads to a modest decline in the proportion of obese adults. People who today are in their 60s or older were born at a time of austerity and limited food supplies. Younger people have largely grown up in a world where a greater variety of food than ever before has become available, and at relatively low cost, and so they are more prone to develop obesity at a younger age.

Attention is increasingly focused on young people, where the problem of overweight and obesity has become more pronounced. Among young Danish males attending draft boards, there has been a dramatic increase in the prevalence of obesity, from 0.1% in 1955 to about 8% in 2000, corresponding to an 80-fold increase. In the United Kingdom in 1997, among 4- to 18-year-olds 4% were obese and a further 15% were overweight, with a higher rate of obesity among young people in Scotland and Wales relative to England. Childhood obesity was first recognized as a major problem in industrialized countries, but a sharp increase in the number of obese children in subpopulations of developing countries has more recently been observed, particularly in urban areas. In heavily populated countries such as India and China, this poses a huge future health challenge unless the present trend is effectively halted. The decrease in the age of onset of obesity that is currently being observed is likely to lead to an increase in the number of years that subjects suffer from obesity-related morbidity and disability.

Childhood Obesity

Obesity in children is one of the most important health challenges of our time. Even in young children, obesity is associated with higher blood pressure and LDL-cholesterol, in addition to an increased risk of steatohepatitis, type 2 diabetes, and psychosocial and musculoskeletal problems (Lobstein and Jackson-Leach, 2006; Puder and Munsch, 2010). However, for the majority of moderately obese children, the negative health consequences are mainly related to the risk of ongoing obesity into later life, and the concomitant risk of serious associated diseases (e.g. diabetes, cardiovascular disease, and cancer) (Adair, 2008). Appropriate strategies for identification of children at risk, coupled with effective treatment and prevention, are therefore of utmost importance, given the alarming increase in the prevalence of childhood obesity over the last 20 to 30 years.

Defining overweight and obesity in a meaningful way in the growing child is a particular challenge due to normal growth, which affects the BMI calculation. BMI normally increases sharply during the first 9–12 months after which it falls until around the age of 6–7 years, when it again increases through childhood and continues to do so during puberty, though with some gender differences. Overweight and obesity in children are therefore better assessed using BMI percentile curves (see www.cdc.gov/growthcharts/cdc_charts.htm). From these curves, age- and sex-specific cut-off values are generally used to assess obesity prevalence, though many different methods are utilized clinically around the world. A slightly different pattern of adiposity compared with BMI is also seen when measured by skinfold thickness. Early on, fat is predominantly found subcutaneously, whereas intra-abdominal fat depots increase with age.

Interestingly, longitudinal studies have shown that an early rise in BMI before the age of 5 years, after the initial fall during the preschool years (i.e. adiposity rebound), is a risk factor for later obesity (Rolland-Cachera et al.,

2006). The combination of early growth retardation and later fatness, a condition typical in many developing countries, may be especially dangerous with regard to the risk of developing cardiovascular disease later in life.

Genetic factors alone, rare diseases such as Prader-Willi syndrome, and endocrine disorders can only explain a minority of the present obesity prevalence seen among children, though common genetic allelic variants may set the stage for obesity within an obesogenic environment. A cluster of factors linked to psychosocial and environmental contributors is most likely to be blamed for the recent development of obesity in the vast majority of affected children (see next section).

Etiology

Environmental Contributors to Obesity

It is a truism that the development of obesity results from excess energy intake that is not balanced by sufficient energy expenditure. Thus, lack of physical activity and increased consumption of foods rich in fat and sugar are easy to blame for the development of obesity. However, meta-analyses exploring the effects of dietary fat content and physical exercise suggest that these two conventional factors are likely to explain only a limited amount of weight gain, and it has become increasingly clear that obesity is a multifactorial condition with a complex and diverse pathogenesis. For instance, it has been shown that the risk of being overweight or obese is clearly higher for both children and adults who have a number of non-traditional risk factors (e.g. short sleep duration and less calcium in the diet) compared with those reporting traditional risk factors such as high-fat diets and lack of physical exercise (Chaput et al., 2006, 2010a). It is therefore important to look beyond the traditional risk factors in order to develop successful strategies to counteract the increasing prevalence of obesity and its co-morbidities.

Recent studies have emphasized the importance of other dietary factors than fat, and there is solid evidence that demonstrates that sugar-rich soft drinks and a diet rich in total carbohydrates (instead of protein) and refined carbohydrates (instead of whole-grain and low-glycemic-index carbohydrates) promotes weight gain, as well as weight regain following weight loss (Larsen et al., 2010).

Perhaps no other demographic group in history has undergone such significant transformation in lifestyle than our younger generations over recent decades. This transition coincides with a sharp increase in body weight that has resulted in an *obesity epidemic*. The typical sedentary lifestyle, which is a result of our modern environment and way of living, is problematic in regard to the maintenance of energy balance. Physical activity is no longer a natural component of work and transportation for most people; rather, it is limited to those who are engaged in structured physical exercise in their leisure time. The problem of positive energy balance is not, however, only a matter of the low amount of calories expended, but also that many of the sedentary activities that we are involved in seem to promote overconsumption of food (Chaput *et al.*, 2010b). In a sedentary environment characterized by an abundance of affordable, easily accessible, highly palatable, energy-dense foods and beverages served in large portion sizes and intensively marketed, such stimuli are likely to have substantial effects on energy balance. In childhood, the number of hours of TV and computer time is positively associated with a high consumption of calorie-dense, low-fiber foods, and with less time spent physically active.

Mainly based on associations found in epidemiological studies, a number of environmental factors with hypothesized mechanisms that may directly or indirectly affect both sides of the energy balance equation have been identified. The term *obesogenic environment* is often used to describe this cluster of factors. The potential causative effects of these factors are often difficult to validate in experimental studies, and these factors often have a very complex, multifaceted association with obesity. Confounding and reverse causality may therefore easily confuse our understanding of their actual contribution to obesity. However, recent studies have given us a better understanding of this emerging research field.

The effects of short sleep duration and mental stress on the predisposition to obesity are two novel areas of investigation. According to the US National Sleep Foundation, the prevalence of young adults sleeping less than 7 hours per night has risen from 16% to 37% in 40 years, while obesity has increased from 13% to 32% during the same time period (Kutson *et al.*, 2010). Several epidemiological studies have described a strong association between short sleep and obesity (Chaput *et al.*, 2010c). Additionally, short-term partial sleep restriction has been shown to negatively affect glucose metabolism and regulation of food intake in young adults (Grandner *et al.*, 2010).

Mental stress has been shown to result in increased energy intake. This has been demonstrated in the absence of alteration in perceived hunger or changes in appetite hormones, suggesting an influence on the hedonic aspects of regulation of food intake (Chaput *et al.*, 2010b). It could be speculated that there may be common mechanisms explaining the effects of stress on food intake and the associations between obesity and attention disorders, depression, and psychosocial issues. In an environment characterized by high cognitive demands rather than physical challenges, this is important knowledge needed to develop effective strategies for prevention of obesity, but represents a challenging area of study.

The environment in which we eat has also been shown to affect how much we eat. Distractors such as watching TV or playing computer games while eating increase food intake and attenuate the development of feelings of fullness during that meal. Interestingly, engaging in these activities (particularly playing video games) also leads to more snacking later on. Other distractors such as music can also affect our eating depending on rhythm and volume, while our eating company affects us as well. We generally tend to eat more with friends than alone or with strangers, and we tend to eat more or less in order to mimic our mealtime companions.

Finally, it should be noted that the present trend in overweight and obesity is not limited to humans but is also present in a number of animals, ranging from domesticated dogs and cats to wild rats living in close contact with us, suggesting that they may be affected by many of the same factors as humans (Klimentidis *et al.*, 2010). This trend also holds true for laboratory animals that have not been feeding from our leftovers, but fed with strictly controlled ad libitum diets with constant composition for decades, and without any obvious concomitant changes in physical activity habits. These observations suggest the possibility of additional obesogenic factors in our common environment. Several studies have shown a positive correlation between accumulation of lipid-soluble organochlorines in our bodies and BMI, suggesting that these environmental pollutants may play a role (Major *et al.*, 2007). Increases in plasma organochlorine levels found during weight loss have been shown to decrease energy expenditure, potentially via a decrease in thyroid hormone levels.

Genetics

In only a minority of cases is obesity caused by a chromosome abnormality or a mutation in a single gene. However, there exists a complex genetic predisposition towards obesity in each individual, with pathogenetic mechanisms that operate within this genetic framework to affect both body-fat content and body-fat distribution.

The increasing activity within the field of genome-wide association studies for disease susceptibility genes has led to the identification of approximately 30 loci influencing body mass index, one of the most well known being the fat mass and obesity-associated (FTO) gene. The effect of each gene on body weight is small, though it may be as much as 2–3 kg for certain genes identified. At least 15 loci influencing visceral patterns of fat distribution have also been identified, many showing stronger associations in women than in men (McCarthy, 2010). Epigenetic influences during pregnancy may have a significant role in the etiology of obesity as well; chemicals or hormones transferred from mother to fetus during pregnancy may program the offspring to be susceptible to obesity and the metabolic syndrome.

The genetic contribution to common obesity is not such that obesity is fixed in the genes from the outset and not amenable to change. Rather, the genetic component is perceived as a predisposition, which is expressed only when certain environmental factors are favorable. The most important obesity-triggering environmental factors that are generally acknowledged are a diet high in fat and refined carbohydrate, and a low level of physical activity. It is still not precisely known how the genetic component is expressed physiologically, although a number of studies suggest that abnormal lipid metabolism, altered appetite regulation or taste preference, and a reduced ability to spontaneously increase physical activity during periods of overeating, are the most important candidates.

Prader-Willi syndrome is the most common (though still very rare) chromosomal obesity disorder, caused by either a deletion or a double maternally derived region of chromosome 15, and manifest by hyperphagia, cognitive impairment, and several dysmorphic features. Other less common congenital disorders include Bardet-Biedl, Alström, and Cohen's syndromes.

Single gene mutations that cause obesity in humans are extremely rare. A deficit of the satiety hormone leptin is characterized by severe hyperphagia, and responds with considerable weight loss when treated with leptin injections. The most common form of obesity due to a single gene mutation involves mutations in the melanocortin-4 receptor, which occur in 3–4% of children with severe obesity. Other mutations, such as in the proopiomelano-

cortin and the prohormone convertase 1 genes, are similarly associated with obesity.

Medical Conditions

Although several endocrine disorders can cause weight gain, these conditions are responsible for only a minority of cases of obesity. Hypothyroidism is often accompanied by weight gain, which can be attributed to the fact that energy expenditure falls proportional to the degree of hypothyroidism. Despite effective treatment, it is often difficult to shed the excess pounds and return to baseline body weight. With thyrotoxicosis, weight loss is most commonly seen, but increase in weight often occurs with treatment and return to a euthyroid state. Return to a euthyroid state can result in a weight gain of 5–7 kg within a year, or more if the patient becomes transiently hypothyroid as a consequence of treatment. This weight gain may be exacerbated if treatment is targeted to render the patient biochemically euthyroid in the lower end of the normal range, as this may result in a subnormal energy expenditure (Jacobsen et al., 2006).

Cushing's syndrome, which is a condition of excess cortisol production, often results in weight gain, particularly in the abdominal fat distribution. Other features of Cushing's syndrome include type 2 diabetes, hypertension, dyslipidemia, and oligomenorrhea. It can be challenging clinically to distinguish Cushing's syndrome from a patient with visceral obesity and the metabolic syndrome, as many of the clinical features overlap. However, it is crucial to make this distinction clinically, as the treatment of Cushing's syndrome is directed at the cause of the excess cortisol production (usually a tumor of the pituitary or adrenal gland).

Growth hormone deficiency is an uncommon condition, usually caused by a pathologic disturbance of the pituitary gland, such as a tumor, damage from radiation therapy, or infiltrative disease. Lean body mass is decreased, and fat mass (particularly visceral fat) is increased in untreated adults who are deficient in growth hormone, compared with those who have normal growth hormone secretion. These parameters improve with growth hormone therapy.

There are several medications which may provide an iatrogenic contribution to obesity (Box 45.1), and the use of alternative agents should be considered carefully by the prescribing physician (Leslie et al., 2007). For example, in the realm of antidepressive agents, tricyclic antidepressants are associated with significant weight gain, whereas some

BOX 45.1   Etiologic contributors to obesity

Environmental contributors
- Increased availability of highly processed, calorie-dense food sources
- Increased portion sizes
- Sedentary modern lifestyle
- Decreased sleep
- Increased mental/cognitive stressors
- Environmental pollutants

Genetic factors
- Common genetic polymorphisms (e.g. FTO gene variations)
- Epigenetic factors
- Genetic syndromes (e.g. Prader-Willi syndrome)
- Rare single gene mutations (e.g. leptin deficiency)

Medical conditions
- Hypothyroidism
- Cushing's syndrome
- Growth hormone deficiency

Iatrogenic
- Oral hypoglycemic agents
- Insulin
- Tricyclic antidepressants
- Glucocorticoids
- Antipsychotic agents
- Antiepileptic agents
- Beta blockers

Psychosocial contributors
- Depression
- Binge eating disorder
- Low socioeconomic status

selective serotonin reuptake inhibitors have been associated with weight loss. The antiepileptic drugs valproate and carbamazepine are associated with weight gain, whereas the antiepileptic drug topiramate is currently under study in combination with an amphetamine, phentermine, as a potential combination weight-loss agent. First-generation antipsychotic agents have been shown to cause several kilograms of weight gain after only a few months of therapy. Glucocorticoids, which are used to treat a wide array of conditions, cause weight gain and a Cushing's phenotype.

Co-Morbidities of Obesity

Diabetes Mellitus

Type 2 Diabetes mellitus is a condition that arises when the pancreas does not produce enough insulin to overcome the insulin resistance in the peripheral tissues, leading to hyperglycemia. Type 2 diabetes is distinguished from type 1 diabetes, which is an autoimmune disease characterized by absolute failure of pancreatic insulin production. Overweight and obesity are the major causes of the development of type 2 diabetes, though individuals with normal body weight but a high genetic susceptibility towards insulin resistance can develop type 2 diabetes as well. The genetic predisposition is an important determinant as to whether an obese individual develops type 2 diabetes or not, and many morbidly obese subjects without the genetic predisposition maintain normoglycemia throughout life.

The health impact of diabetes is serious, and may arguably be the most important medical consequence of obesity. Diabetes is a common condition, affecting over 8% of the US population, and accounts for almost 14% of American health-care expenditures. Chronic hyperglycemia is associated with microvascular complications affecting the eyes (retinopathy), kidneys (nephropathy), and nerves (neuropathy), and macrovascular complications affecting the heart, brain, and peripheral circulation. Diabetes is a leading cause of myocardial infarction, stroke, kidney failure, blindness, and amputation, and may reduce life expectancy by as much as 8–10 years.

The foundation of diabetes prevention and treatment among overweight individuals is weight loss. It is possible to put diabetes into remission with weight loss in some cases, though this is less likely if the genetic predisposition to type 2 diabetes is strong, or the diabetes has persisted for too long a time with irreversible damage to the insulin secretory capacity of pancreatic β cells (Harder *et al.*, 2004). In those cases, there is still an improvement in the severity of type 2 diabetes with weight loss, by virtue of a concomitant decrease in the degree of peripheral insulin resistance. In patients with prediabetes, which can be manifest as impaired glucose tolerance or impaired fasting glucose, weight loss can prevent or delay development of type 2 diabetes.

In the treatment of a patient with type 2 diabetes, consideration should be given to the effect of various treatment agents on weight. Metformin, which is the first-line therapy for type 2 diabetes, is often associated with mild to moderate weight loss, whereas other commonly utilized oral hypoglycemic agents, such as sulfonylureas and thiazolidinediones, cause weight gain. While insulin causes weight gain, it is often a necessary treatment agent in type 2 diabetes, particularly in later stages or more severe cases of the disease. The incretin-based therapies represent newer

BOX 45.2 International Diabetes Federation definition of metabolic syndrome

Waist ≥94 cm (men) or ≥80 cm (women)[a] plus two or more of:

- Blood glucose ≥5.6 mmol/L, or diagnosed diabetes
- HDL cholesterol <1.0 mmol/L (men); <1.3 mmol/L (women), or on drug treatment for low HDL
- Triglycerides ≥1.7 mmol/L, or on drug treatment for high triglycerides
- Blood pressure ≥130/85 mm Hg or drug treatment for hypertension

[a]For South Asia and Chinese patients, waist ≥90 cm (men) or ≥80 cm (women); for Japanese patients, waist ≥90 cm (men) or ≥80 cm (women).

treatment options for type 2 diabetes which are associated with weight loss (in the case of GLP-1 agonists) or weight neutrality (in the case of DPP-IV enzyme inhibitors).

Other Cardiovascular Risk Factors

An abundance of literature points to the existence of a particular metabolic syndrome encompassing insulin resistance, hypertension, dyslipidemia, and abdominal obesity. This syndrome is also known as insulin resistance syndrome, since the underlying pathophysiology is that of reduced sensitivity to the action of insulin. A variety of risk factors for the development of cardiovascular disease appear to be associated with this syndrome, which links obesity with the most significant health complications (type 2 diabetes, atherosclerosis, and hypertension). In addition to the degree of obesity, other factors are significantly associated with the metabolic syndrome: pattern of body-fat distribution, level of physical activity, and genetic disposition. The International Diabetes Federation has proposed a definition of the syndrome (Box 45.2).

The way in which overweight and obesity contribute to the metabolic syndrome is not entirely clear, but hormones and substrates secreted by the adipose tissue are thought to be the main cause. Reduced secretion of the hormone adiponectin from fat tissue, increased metabolism of free fatty acids, as well as increased secretion of cytokines and inflammatory mediators such as tumor necrosis factor alpha and interleukin 6, appear to play an important role in the development of insulin resistance and the accompanying metabolic disturbances. Treatment of the meta-

bolic syndrome includes weight loss and physical activity, with close attention to cardiovascular risk reduction.

The risk of developing hypertension is several-fold greater in an obese individual compared with non-obese individuals, and can be seen with or without other manifestations of the metabolic syndrome. Blood pressure is positively correlated with both abdominal circumference and with the degree of obesity. Insulin resistance and hyperinsulinemia appear to be the underlying pathophysiological mechanisms responsible for the hypertension in most cases. Insulin has an anti-natriuretic effect that results in an increase of both extracellular and intravascular volume. Hyperinsulinemia may also have a direct trophic effect on the smooth muscle cells of the arterioles, which can lead to increased vascular tone and arterial vascular resistance.

The hypertension associated with obesity has the same potential consequences as hypertension from other causes, including increased risk of myocardial infarction, stroke, renal damage, and retinal damage. As such it is imperative that blood pressure be managed and controlled to the same targets as in the normal-weight patient. Weight loss is a key component of management of hypertension as even a small weight loss can result in a marked drop in blood pressure.

Following the discussion above, it should come as no surprise that obesity, and abdominal obesity in particular, are associated with a significant increased risk of atherosclerotic complications. The risk of developing ischemic heart disease or stroke is 2.5 and 6 times greater, respectively, with a predominantly abdominal fat distribution compared with individuals with a more even fat distribution. The increased risk portended by abdominal obesity is multifactorial, including a predisposition towards an unfavorable lipid profile, hypertension, insulin resistance and type 2 diabetes, an increase in inflammatory markers such as fibrinogen and C-reactive protein, and reduced fibrinolytic activity. A recent large study has suggested that BMI and waist circumference do not improve cardiovascular risk prediction when blood pressure, diabetes status, and lipid profiles are known, illustrating that the cardiovascular risk of obesity is mediated by these parameters (The Emerging Risk Factors Collaboration, 2011).

Obesity is associated with congestive heart failure, which may be secondary to ischemic heart disease, or may be related to increased cardiac work with subsequent myocardial hypertrophy and dysfunction, severe insulin resistance, excessive fat accumulation in the myocardium, pulmonary hypertension, or any combination of these factors. Obesity is associated with an increased risk of atrial fibrillation compared with normal-weight individuals (52% and 46% increased risk for men and women, respectively) (Wang et al., 2004).

Malignancy

Obesity is responsible for an increased risk of several types of malignancy, including cancer of solid organs including colon, esophagus, endometrium, kidney, female breast, pancreas, liver, gallbladder, and stomach, as well as hematologic malignancies such as non-Hodgkin's lymphoma and multiple myeloma. It is estimated that overweight and obesity may be responsible for 3% of cancers in men, and 9% of cancers in women.

The mechanisms by which obesity promote tumorigenesis are complex, and vary by site (Darren et al., 2010). Chronic hyperinsulinemia may increase availability of bioactive IGF-1, which can stimulate tumor growth and development. Epidemiologic studies have linked high levels of insulin secretion with increased risk of breast, colon, pancreatic, and endometrial cancer, and these high levels are an adverse prognostic factor for cancer-related mortality. Increased bioavailability of estrogen due to aromatization in adipose tissue is an important mechanism predisposing to an increased risk of breast and endometrial cancer. Polypeptides derived from adipocytes, such as leptin and adiponectin, as well as inflammatory mediators, also play an important and complex role.

The impact of obesity on the risk of death from cancer is even more profound. In men and women with a BMI ≥40, the relative risk of dying from cancer compared with normal-weight subjects is 1.5 and 1.6, respectively (Calle et al., 2003). In the United States, it is estimated that overweight and obesity may be responsible for 14% of all cancer deaths in men, and 20% in women. Major weight loss reduces the risk of cancer-specific mortality.

Obstructive Sleep Apnea

Obstructive sleep apnea (OSA) is a disorder that is characterized by obstructive pauses in breathing during sleep, caused by repetitive collapse of the upper airway. Clinical features include restlessness and snoring during sleep, waking feeling unrested, frequent morning headaches, poor concentration, and daytime somnolence. OSA is associated with an increased risk of hypertension, diabetes, myocardial infarction, cardiac arrhythmias, congestive heart failure, and accidental injury. Patients with untreated severe OSA are at a 3 to 6 times increased risk of death compared with patients without OSA (Marshal et al., 2008; Young et al., 2008).

Obesity is the most well documented risk factor for OSA. The prevalence of OSA progressively increases as the body mass index, neck circumference, and waist-to-hip ratio increase. Inflammatory mediators which are increased in both OSA and obesity, and which contribute to the atherosclerotic complications of OSA, may have an etiologic role in OSA as well.

Other alterations may occur in pulmonary function in the setting of obesity, including a restrictive component with lower lung volumes due to increased chest-wall impedance, and reduced endurance of respiratory muscles.

Osteoarthritis

The risk of osteoarthritis increases with increasing BMI, and accounts for a significant proportion of the total health-care expenditures associated with obesity. Weight-bearing joints are at the highest risk, but non-weight-bearing joints are affected as well, suggesting alterations in the cartilage and/or bone in the setting of metabolic syndrome and obesity that are independent of weight-related trauma. Weight loss is linearly associated with a decreased risk of developing osteoarthritis; one study demonstrated that a BMI reduction of $2 \, kg/m^2$ or more among women in the preceding 10 years decreased the odds of developing osteoarthritis of the knee by 50% (Felson, 1992). Weight loss of even a modest degree can improve joint pain and function in patients with established osteoarthritis.

Other Medical Co-Morbidities

As the physical and metabolic alterations seen with excess weight impact every body system, there are many other medical conditions associated with obesity.

Obesity can have an important impact on the gastrointestinal and hepatobiliary system. Accumulation of fat in the liver can lead to steatohepatitis, which is increasingly recognized as an important cause of liver cirrhosis. There is an increased risk of gallstone formation in obesity. Interestingly, the risk of gallstones increases with weight loss as well, particularly if the weight loss is rapid (>1–1.5 kg per week), as the flux of cholesterol through the biliary system increases in this setting. Obesity is also a risk factor for gastroesophageal reflux disease, and several gastrointestinal cancers (see earlier section on Malignancy).

There is an association between obesity and deep vein thrombosis, which can be life threatening as it can lead to potentially fatal pulmonary embolism. This risk is particularly high in patients with additional risk factors for thromboembolic disease, such as smokers, passengers on long-haul flights, and oral contraceptive users.

Fertility can be significantly impaired in obese patients, often in the context of polycystic ovary syndrome (PCOS). The underlying pathophysiologic defect in PCOS is insulin resistance, which leads to increased testosterone production by the ovaries, resulting in impairment of ovulation, irregular, infrequent, or absent menses, hirsutism, and acne. Although PCOS can occur in normal-weight women, the PCOS symptom complex does worsen with weight gain as this exacerbates the underlying insulin resistance. Treatment is focused on decreasing the insulin resistance, primarily by weight loss in obese or overweight women. For any pregnant woman with obesity, there is an increased risk of several complications, including pregnancy-induced hypertension, gestational diabetes, and delivery by cesarean section.

From a genitourinary perspective, the most important obesity-related complication is renal impairment, which is in turn related to the increased risk of diseases known to cause renal dysfunction, including diabetes and hypertension. There is an increased risk of kidney stones with obesity and with weight gain. Urinary incontinence is an important obesity-related issue for many women as well.

Other conditions associated with obesity include gout, which is characterized by increased serum urate concentrations, leading to precipitation in joints with both acute and chronic sequelae. Excess body weight has been associated with dementia and psoriasis, though a causal association has not been established.

Psychosocial Issues

A number of studies have examined the relationship between BMI and various aspects of quality of life. A robust finding across these studies has been the negative impact of obesity on physical functioning, such as general health perception and vitality, as well as psychological functioning and social well-being. Obesity was associated with more reports of poor body image, stigmatization, discrimination, diminished social interactions, depression, increased absence from the workplace, and lower socioeconomic status. Physical fitness was, however, shown to be a strong modifier, attenuating the negative effects of obesity (Castres *et al.*, 2010; Griffiths *et al.*, 2010).

The direction of causality has often been discussed regarding these associations. The interrelatedness between obesity and psychological problems seems in many cases to be bidirectional, potentially adding to the severity and complexity of the problem. It is therefore of critical importance to address not only the weight problem, but also the psychosocial co-morbidities of obesity.

In children as well as adults, psychological distress may foster weight gain at the same time as obesity may lead to psychosocial problems. In a meta-analysis of longitudinal studies including close to 60,000 subjects, it was shown that obese people had a 55% increased risk of developing depression over time, whereas depressed individuals had a 58% increased risk of becoming obese (Luppino *et al.*, 2010). Somewhat weaker associations are also found between overweight and depression.

In terms of the treatment of obesity, a concomitant reduction in co-morbidities, including an improvement in psychosocial aspects, is one important defining aspect of treatment success. Psychosocial factors should be part of pretreatment evaluation of the patient, prior to selection of the most appropriate management strategy (Palmeira *et al.*, 2010).

Weight loss is often, though not uniformly, found to be accompanied by improvement in most aspects of quality of life. An improvement in quality of life is often seen with initial weight loss, regardless of treatment mechanism, but this may regress once a plateau in weight is reached; psychological and physiological mechanisms are hypothesized to be involved. Anecdotal observations also describe frustration when patients realize that life did not "become perfect" following a very successful weight loss, even with achievement of a normal body weight.

The effect of obesity and weight loss on different psychosocial issues may differ considerably, depending on the individual and the context (i.e. different populations and subcultures), and particular consideration for patient-specific factors is therefore of the utmost importance.

Co-morbidities associated with obesity are summarized in Box 45.3.

Mortality

The complications of obesity and abdominal overweight are poorly recognized, but are responsible for a major

BOX 45.3 Co-morbidities associated with obesity

Type 2 diabetes mellitus
Cardiovascular disease
• Atherosclerotic heart disease
• Congestive heart failure
• Stroke
• Hypertension
• Peripheral vascular disease
• Deep vein thrombosis/pulmonary embolism
• Atrial fibrillation
Malignancy
Respiratory disease
• Obstructive sleep apnea
• Restrictive lung disease
Musculoskeletal
• Osteoarthritis
• Gout
Gastrointestinal
• Steatohepatitis
• Gallstones
• Gastroesophageal reflux
Genitourinary
• Renal failure
• Kidney stones
• Urinary incontinence
Reproductive
• Polycystic ovary syndrome
• Pregnancy-induced hypertension
• Gestational diabetes mellitus
• Increased cesarean-section risk
Psychosocial
• Depression
• Societal discrimination
• Loss of work days
• Medical costs

burden on the health system, accounting for an increasing proportion of all health-cost expenditures. Even a normal BMI, but with abdominal fat accumulation, can be responsible for hypertension, hyperlipidemia, type 2 diabetes, and cardiovascular disease, which makes it important to identify increased adiposity as the underlying cause of the condition or disease. The increase in obesity rates has an important impact on the global incidence of cardiovascular disease, type 2 diabetes mellitus, cancer, osteoarthritis, infertility, birth complications, work disability, and sleep apnea. By virtue of these effects, obesity has a pronounced impact on mortality (Berrington de Gonzalez et al., 2010). Obesity amongst 40-year-old non-smokers is estimated to shorten life expectancy by 5.8 years and 7.1 years for males

and females, respectively. For smokers, obesity has an even more profound effect, shortening lifespan by 13.3 years for females, and 13.7 years for males (Peeters et al., 2003). In the United States, obesity is responsible for more deaths than smoking.

Obesity Prevention

In light of the obesity epidemic that grips the globe, a wealth of research studies have attempted to find an effective means by which to prevent obesity. On a population level, an effective means of obesity prevention continues to evade us.

Numerous popular diets promote changing diet composition in accordance with principles that are claimed to have a favorable impact on weight maintenance. These claims are generally unsubstantiated, and some may even promote nutritionally insufficient diets. A diet abundant in fiber, vegetables, fruits, and whole grains, which are more satiating for fewer calories, are beneficial in weight maintenance. A large body of experimental human data suggests that protein possesses a higher satiating power per calorie than carbohydrate and fat. A recent large randomized clinical trial in eight European countries demonstrated that both a modestly higher-protein and lower-glycemic-index diet is beneficial in weight maintenance, confirming findings of smaller studies (Larsen et al., 2010). Overall, the balance of the evidence suggests that a low-fat higher-protein, moderate complex-carbohydrate diet seems to be more effective for long-term weight maintenance.

Daily physical activity and exercise are important components of weight maintenance. The impact of exercise for weight control is based on the ability of patients to engage in adequate levels of activity. The minimal level that should be recommended is at least 45–60 minutes of moderate intensity physical activity on most days of the week (Saris et al., 2003). This level of physical activity not only helps to prevent obesity, but also improves health-related factors. A sustained commitment to physical activity is an important part of a lifelong commitment to health.

Future Directions

In a world in which obesity has reached epidemic proportions, the impact on morbidity and mortality of our populations, as well as the health-care expenditures associated with managing these co-morbidities, are staggering. Successful strategies are desperately needed to both treat and prevent obesity. Societal strategies are needed that address unhealthy eating tendencies, promote healthier eating habits, and encourage more active lifestyles in an otherwise permissively sedentary environment. New therapies that modify the interplay of satiety and hunger hormones and cues, such as the incretin-based therapies, show promise as medical treatment options for obesity, and research on these and related compounds is ongoing. Bariatric surgery is currently the only treatment of obesity that has been shown to be effective and sustainable in the long term; it may be the most appropriate treatment option for more extreme and refractory cases of obesity, or those cases of refractory obesity associated with significant co-morbidities, particularly type 2 diabetes. Bariatric surgery is associated with variable degrees of success and improvement of co-morbidities, but also carries a variable profile of complications and risks, depending on the type of surgery performed. Further research is needed to determine which type of bariatric surgery provides the optimum balance of benefit in the context of associated risk of complications, and to gain a better understanding of the long-term outcomes of these procedures.

Suggestions for Further Reading

Abete, I., Astrup, A., Martínez, J.A., *et al.* (2010) Obesity and the metabolic syndrome: role of different dietary macronutrients distribution patterns and specific nutritional components on weight loss and maintenance. *Nutr Rev* **68**, 214–231.

Astrup, A. (2004) Treatment of obesity. In E. Ferrannini, P. Zimmet, R.A. De Fronzo, *et al.* (eds), *International Textbook of Diabetes Mellitus*, 3rd Edn. John Wiley, Chichester.

Astrup, A. (2008) Dietary management of obesity. *JPEN J Parenter Enteral Nutr* **32**, 575–577.

Astrup, A., Kristensen, M., Gregersen, N.T., *et al.* (2010) Can bioactive foods affect obesity? *Ann NY Acad Sci* **1190**, 25–41.

Melanson, E.L., Astrup, A., and Donahoo, W.T. (2009) The relationship between dietary fat and fatty acid intake and body weight, diabetes, and the metabolic syndrome. *Ann Nutr Metab* **55**, 229–243.

Paddon-Jones, D., Westman, E., Mattes, R.D., *et al.* (2008) Protein, weight management, and satiety. *Am J Clin Nutr* **87**, 1558S–1561S.

Aller, E., Abete I., Astrup A., *et al.* (2011) Starches, sugars and obesity. *Nutrients* **3**, 341–369.

References

Adair, L.S. (2008) Children and adolescent obesity: epidemiology and development perspectives. *Physiol Behav* **94**, 8–16.

Berrington de Gonzalez, A., Hartge, P., Cerhan, J.R., *et al.* (2010) Body-mass index and mortality among 1.46 million white adults. *N Engl J Med* **363**, 2211–2219.

Calle, E.E., Rodriguez, C., Walker-Thurmond, K., *et al.* (2003) Overweight, obesity, and mortality from cancer in a prospectively studied cohort of U.S. adults. *N Engl J Med* **348**, 1625–1638.

Castres, I., Folope, V., Dechelotte, P., *et al.* (2010) Quality of life and obesity class relationships. *Int J Sports Med* **31**, 773–778.

Chaput, J.P., Brunet, M., and Tremblay, A. (2006) Relationship between short sleeping hours and childhood overweight/obesity: results from the "Quebec en Form" project. *Int J Obes Relat Metab Disord* **30**, 1080–1085.

Chaput, J.P., Klingenberg, L., Astrup, A., *et al.* (2010b) Modern sedentary activities promote overconsumption of food in our current obesogenic environment. *Obes Rev* PMID 20576006

Chaput, J.P., Klingenberg, L., and Sjödin, A. (2010c) Do all sedentary activities lead to weight gain: sleep does not. *Curr Opin Clin Nutr Metab Care* **13**, 601–607.

Chaput, J.P., Sjödin, A.M., Astrup, A., *et al.* (2010a) Risk factors for adult overweight and obesity: the importance of looking beyond the "Big Two". *Obes Facts* **3**, 320–327.

Darren, L., Roberts, D.L., Dive, C., *et al.* (2010) Biological mechanisms linking obesity and cancer risk: new perspectives. *Ann Rev Med* **61**, 301–316.

Felson, D.T., Zhang, Y., Anthony, J.M., *et al.* (1992) Weight loss reduces the risk for symptomatic knee osteoarthritis in women. The Framingham Study. *Ann Int Med* **116**, 535–539.

Flegal, K., Carroll, M.D., Ogden, C.L., *et al.* (2010) Prevalence and trends in obesity among US adults, 1999–2008. *JAMA* **303**, 235–241.

Grandner, M.A., Patel, N.P., Gehrman, P.R., *et al.* (2010) Problems associated with short sleep: bridging the gap between laboratory and epidemiological studies. *Sleep Med Rev* **14**, 239–247.

Griffiths, L.J., Parson, T.J., and Hill, A.J. (2010) Self-esteem and quality of life in obese children and adolescents: a systematic review. *Int J Pediatr Obes* **5**, 282–304.

Harder, H., Dinesen, B., and Astrup, A. (2004) The effect of a rapid weight loss on lipid profile and glycemic control in obese type 2 diabetic patients. *Int J Obes Relat Metab Disord* **28**, 180–182.

Jacobsen, R., Lundsgaard, C., Lorenzen, J., *et al.* (2006) Subnormal energy expenditure: a putative causal factor in the weight gain induced by treatment of hyperthyroidism. *Diabetes Obes Metab* **8**, 220–227.

Klimentidis, Y.C., Beasly, T.M., Lin, H.Y., *et al.* (2010) Canaries in the coalmine: a cross-species analysis of the plurality of obesity epidemics. *Proc R Soc Biol Sci* **278**, 1626–1632.

Kutson, K.L., Van Kauter, E., Rathouz, P.J., *et al.* (2010) Trends in the prevalence of short sleepers in USA 1975–2006. *Sleep* **33**, 37–45.

Larsen, T.M., Dalskov, S.M., van Baak, M., *et al.* (2010) Diets with high or low protein content and glycemic index for weight-loss maintenance. *N Engl J Med* **363**, 2102–2113.

Leslie, W.S., Hankey, C.R., and Lean, M.E. (2007) Weight gain as an adverse effect of some commonly prescribed drugs: a systematic review. *QJM* **100**, 395–404.

Lobstein, T. and Jackson-Leach, R. (2006) Estimated burden of pediatric obesity and co-morbidities in Europe. Part 2. Number of children with indicators of obesity related disease. *Int J Pediatr Obes* **1**, 33–41.

Luppino, F.S., de Wit, L.M., Bouvy, P.F., *et al.* (2010) Overweight, obesity, and depression: a systematic review and meta-analysis of longitudinal studies. *Arch Gen Psychiatry* **67**, 220–229.

Major, G.C., Doucet, E., Trayhurn, P., *et al.* (2007) Clinical significance of adaptive thermogenesis. *Int J Obes Relat Metab Disord* **31**, 204–212.

Marshall, N.S., Wong, K.K., Liu, P.Y., *et al.* (2008) Sleep apnea as an independent risk factor for all-cause mortality: the Busselton Health Study. *Sleep* **31**, 1079–1085.

McCarthy, W.I. (2010) Genomics, type 2 diabetes, and obesity. *N Engl J Med* **363**, 2339–2350.

Palmeira, A.L., Branco, T.L., Martins, S.C., *et al.* (2010) Changes in body image and psychosocial well-being during behavioural obesity treatment: associations with weight loss and maintenance. *Body Image* **7**, 187–193.

Peeters, A., Barendregt, J.J., Willekens, F., *et al.* (2003) Obesity in adulthood and its consequences for life expectancy: a life-table analysis. *Ann Int Med* **138**, 24–32.

Puder, J.J. and Munsch, S. (2010) Psychological correlates of childhood obesity. *Int J Obes Relat Metab Disord* **34**(Suppl 2), S37–S43.

Rolland-Cachera, M.F., Deheeger, M., Malliot, M., *et al.* (2006) Early adiposity rebound: causes and consequences for obesity in children and adults. *Int J Obes Relat Metab Disord* **30**(Suppl 4), S11–S17.

Saris, W.H., Blair, S.N., van Baak, M.A., *et al.* (2003) How much physical activity is enough to prevent unhealthy weight gain? Outcome of the IASO 1st Stock Conference and consensus statement. *Obes Rev* **4**, 101–114.

The Emerging Risk Factors Collaboration (2011) Separate and combined associations of body-mass index and abdominal adiposity with cardiovascular disease: collaborative analysis of 58 prospective studies. *Lancet* **377**, 1085–1095.

Wang, T.J., Parise, H., Levy, D., *et al.* (2004) Obesity and the risk of new-onset atrial fibrillation. *JAMA* **292**, 2471–2477.

Young, T., Finn, L., Peppard, P.E., *et al.* (2008) Sleep disordered breathing and mortality: eighteen-year follow-up of the Wisconsin sleep cohort. *Sleep* **31**, 1071–1078.

46

HYPERTENSION

THOMAS A.B. SANDERS, PhD, DSc

King's College London, London, UK

Summary

Hypertension is an established and independent risk factor for stroke, coronary heart disease, and heart and kidney failure. The relationship between blood pressure and cardiovascular risk is continuous with no threshold. Blood pressure increases with age and is on average higher in men than in women. The cause of elevated blood pressure in most cases is unknown but it is a self-amplifying condition that is more amenable to treatment in its early stages. Consequently, lowering blood pressure in the whole population including normotensive individuals contributes to lowering the burden of cardiovascular disease. Convincing evidence exists for the effects of overweight/obesity and of high intakes of alcohol and salt on increasing blood pressure. Pharmacologically high intakes (>3 g/day) of long-chain n-3 polyunsaturated fatty acids lower blood pressure but not intakes within the range of normal dietary intakes (up to 2 g/day). There is probable evidence to show that the consumption of low-fat milk products is associated with lower blood pressure and for an increased intake of calcium to be associated with a reduced risk of hypertension. There is a probable relationship between low potassium intake and increased blood pressure, and possible relationships with the intakes of nitrate. Low birth weight and poor growth in early life are associated with an increased risk of developing hypertension. Meta-analyses of randomized controlled trials show convincing evidence that salt reduction, moderation of alcohol intake, and weight loss in the overweight/obese lower blood pressure. An integrated dietary approach involving a global change in dietary pattern appears to be more effective in lowering blood pressure than single dietary interventions.

Introduction

High blood pressure or hypertension is classified as systolic blood pressure of 140 mm Hg or above and diastolic blood pressure of 90 mm Hg or above, or being on specific treatment (Table 46.1). Elevated blood pressure is a major modifiable risk factor for cardiovascular disease, and especially stroke. Severe hypertension results in end-organ damage, particularly to the microvasculature of the retina, brain, and kidney, and is an important cause of blindness, dementia, and chronic renal failure (Box 46.1). However, the hazards of cardiovascular disease associated with blood

Present Knowledge in Nutrition, Tenth Edition. Edited by John W. Erdman Jr, Ian A. Macdonald and Steven H. Zeisel.
© 2012 International Life Sciences Institute. Published 2012 by John Wiley & Sons, Inc.

TABLE 46.1 Classification of blood pressure (mm Hg) based on seated clinic blood pressure

Condition	Systolic BP	Diastolic BP
Ideal	<120	<80
Pre-hypertension	120–139	80–89
Hypertension	140–159	90–99
Grade 1	140–159	90–99
Grade 2	160–179	100–109
Grade 3	>180	>110

BOX 46.1   Major hazards of hypertension

Cardiovascular disease
  Stroke
  Coronary heart disease
  Peripheral vascular disease
Renal failure
Retinal damage

pressure extend well into the normal range, and the hazards are greater in the presence of other risk factors (increasing age, high blood cholesterol, smoking, diabetes mellitus, and target organ damage). Data from the analysis of prospective cohort studies (Lewington *et al.*, 2002) show that all-cause mortality, stroke, and coronary heart disease (CHD) incidence increase on a doubling scale (log-linear) with increasing blood pressure. This has led to the conclusion that the relationship of blood pressure and risk of cardiovascular disease has no threshold. There is convincing evidence that lowering raised blood pressure using drugs reduces mortality, especially from stroke but also from CHD (Czernichow *et al.*, 2011). It has been difficult to demonstrate benefit from lowering blood pressure below 120/80 mm Hg in high-risk groups such as people with type 2 diabetes (Cushman *et al.*, 2010).

The prevalence of hypertension increases with age so that the majority of people over the age of 50 are at risk or are already hypertensive in economically developed areas of the world; this age group carries the greatest population attributable risk of cardiovascular disease (Lewington *et al.*, 2002). Measuring blood pressure is subject to substantial measurement error and bias. The use of automated sphygmomanometers reduces bias such as digit preference and cut-offs for diastolic blood pressure. However, equipment needs to be regularly calibrated, and elevated readings may be obtained when subjects are stressed ("white-coat hypertension"). Ambulatory blood pressure monitoring devices provide more robust measures of blood pressure, but give values that are 5 mm Hg lower than clinic seated blood pressure (O'Brien *et al.*, 2005). The techniques used to measure blood pressure and appropriate placebos are crucial issues when evaluating diet and lifestyle effects on blood pressure.

Nationwide cross-sectional studies tend to overestimate the prevalence of hypertension because they are made on measurements on a single occasion. It is well known that blood pressure falls in response to repeat measurement, regressing towards the mean. The association of blood pressure with risk of cardiovascular disease tends to be underestimated because of resulting regression dilution bias. Adjusting for regression dilution bias by using multiple measures of blood pressure on different days gives a better estimate of true blood pressure and strengthens the relationship with risk. The absolute risk of hypertension increases markedly with age and it is in the older age groups that the benefits of treating hypertension are greatest because their absolute risk is greatest (Lewington *et al.*, 2002).

High blood pressure usually results from increased resistance to blood flow by small arterioles (resistance vessels). It is a self-amplifying process in which the arterioles develop thicker, more muscular walls in response to the increased pressure which further increases peripheral resistance when stimulated by vasoconstrictor substances or by sympathetic stimulation. Systolic blood pressure (SBP) increases with age whereas diastolic blood pressure (DBP) tends to increase in line with SBP until the sixth decade and then tends to fall. Stiffening of the large arteries occurs with aging and this contributes to hypertension and is emerging as a powerful predictor of vascular events, at least in older people. Women on average have lower blood pressure than men. However, blood pressure rises around/following the menopause, indicating that ovarian hormones, especially oestrogen, have a protective effect. Drug treatment of hypertension becomes warranted when the absolute annual risk of cardiovascular events is greater than 2% or where there is severe elevation of blood pressure (Williams *et al.*, 2004; Jessani *et al.*, 2006). It also takes several years for the full effects of blood pressure lowering treatments to have their maximal effects, as was demonstrated in the ALLHAT study (ALLHAT Investigators, 2002). A high proportion of the population has "pre-hypertension" or "mild hypertension" where the risk profile does not favor drug treatment. Diet and lifestyle are considered to have their most important influence on the prevention of high blood pressure rather than on the management of established hypertension, and early intervention in the hypertensive process almost certainly helps prevent blood pressure becoming severely elevated. Accelerated hypertension has dramatically reduced in frequency over the last few decades in countries with reasonable health services where high blood pressure detection occurs.

International comparisons show large variations in the prevalence of hypertension and the rate of increase in blood pressure with age. Hypertension is more common in groups of African compared with white European ethnic origin. Early epidemiological studies which were predominantly cross-sectional ecological comparisons showed marked geographical variations in the prevalence of hypertension within countries and within populations that were related to lifestyle. For example, migrants from rural areas of Kenya were found to show large increases in blood pressure when they moved into cities (Poulter et al., 1990). The INTERSALT investigators (Elliott et al., 1996) showed that the age-related increase in blood pressure across a large number of different communities was independently related to body mass index, alcohol intake, and the urinary ratio of sodium/potassium. Later analyses from the INTERSALT group (Elliott et al., 2006) reported an inverse association between vegetable protein intake and blood pressure. As these studies were cross-sectional, they are limited in their ability to adjust for confounding factors. More robust evidence is provided by prospective cohort studies. These consistently show a relationship between hypertension, increased body mass index, and change in body weight. Prospective studies have revealed mixed conclusions regarding salt intake and raised blood pressure. However, estimates of salt intake from dietary records are generally unreliable compared with measures of intake based on the collection of 24-hour urine samples.

Over the past decade, evidence has emerged that blood pressure is falling in many countries (Tunstall-Pedoe et al., 2006), which cannot be attributed to more effective drug management of hypertension. The reason for this decline is unknown. Yet there is some evidence to suggest that early growth development may affect susceptibility to hypertension. Barker et al. (2005), in a follow-up of birth and growth records of children born in Hertfordshire, UK, showed a strong relationship between low birth weight, low weight gain in the first year of life, and adult blood

pressure. They went on to show that infants who have low birth weight and have a low body mass index at the age of 2 years but who subsequently gain weight and have a high body mass index at age 11 years are more prone to develop hypertension (Barker et al., 2005). Children in a subsequent longitudinal study who had been small at birth but who gained weight rapidly during early childhood (1 to 5 years) had the highest adult blood pressure at age 22 years. The US Collaborative Perinatal Project (1959–1974) studied 55 908 pregnancies and showed that each 1-kg increase in birth weight increased the odds by 2.19 for raised SBP at 7 years of age and confirmed the finding that those who crossed growth centiles were most at risk (Hemachandra et al., 2007).

Role of Adult Diet and Lifestyle in Influencing Blood Pressure

Several dietary factors in adult life have been linked to elevated blood pressure, including stress, lack of physical activity, high alcohol intake, high salt intake, obesity, and low dairy and fruit and vegetable intake. Stress acutely influences blood pressure, and this is why measurements need to be made in subjects in a relaxed situation. However, stress management does not appear to be a useful strategy for lowering blood pressure. The population approach to controlling blood pressure focuses on lowering the average population blood pressure, not just in those with hypertension. It aims to decrease exposure to factors that increase risk and to empower individuals to make healthier lifestyle choices. Frost et al. (1991) argue that lowering the blood pressure of the whole population is likely to have a greater impact on cardiovascular mortality than focusing on individuals with high blood pressure. In practice a combination of a population approach and a high-risk approach is needed as it would be unethical to deny drug treatment to individuals at high risk. Guidelines (Jessani et al., 2006; Mancia et al., 2007) have been developed to stratify individuals according to their risk of cardiovascular disease where risk is greater than 20% over the next 10 years or if blood pressure is severely elevated. At levels of 160/100 mm Hg, drug treatment is recommended. A healthy diet and lifestyle is advocated for all.

Body Weight and Blood Pressure

There is a convincing relationship between body mass index and usual blood pressure from the meta-analysis of prospective cohort studies (Whitlock et al., 2009). Results from a meta-analysis of 25 studies indicates (Neter *et al.*, 2003) that net weight reduction of 5 kg, by means of energy restriction, increased physical activity, or both, reduced SBP/DBP by 4.4/3.6 mm Hg. In this respect a reduction of total fat intake that results in lower energy intake and weight loss lowered blood pressure. However, there is no clear evidence to indicate the superiority of low-calorie diets which contain a higher proportion of fat than carbohydrate. Thus, for each kilogram of weight lost, blood pressure falls by about 1 mm Hg over a range of weight loss of 1–5 kg. The effects of overweight and obesity on blood pressure are associated with changes in insulin sensitivity. How systemic vascular resistance is increased is uncertain, but sympathetic nervous system activation plays a major role linking obesity to the development of hypertension. Part of this effect appears to be mediated via the melanocortin 4 receptor independent of insulin (Greenfield, 2011). The accumulation of fat itself may result in changes in small vessel reactivity (Greenstein *et al.*, 2009; Withers *et al.*, 2011).

Dietary Lipids and Blood Pressure

The INTERMAP study (Ueshima *et al.*, 2007; Miura *et al.*, 2008) has provided some evidence for a relationship between fatty acid intake and blood pressure by using four 24-hour dietary recalls to assess dietary intake and eight clinic BP measurements over 3 weeks in 17 populations in Japan, China, the United Kingdom, and the United States ($n = 4680$). This study concluded that dietary linoleic acid intake may contribute to prevention and control of adverse blood pressure levels in the general population. It was estimated that the systolic/diastolic blood pressure differences with 2 SD higher linoleic acid intake (3.77% kcal) were −1.42/−0.91 mm Hg ($p < 0.05$ for both) for participants not being treated for hypertension. Similar findings were made for total polyunsaturated fatty acids intake. The same study reported small effects <1 mm Hg for n-3 PUFA, especially those derived from oily fish.

A number of randomized dietary intervention trials have examined the effect on blood pressure of modifying the type of fat and the intake level. However, most studies have not been of sufficient size to detect small variations in blood pressure, and few have used ambulatory blood pressure monitoring, which is a more robust measure of blood pressure. Some studies have reported falls in blood pressure when moving from a diet high in saturated fatty acids to one low in saturated fatty acids. However, a major

criticism of these studies is that they have failed to randomize treatment order. This introduces bias, with the diet rich in saturated fatty acids being administered first in the sequence. This is particularly important as blood pressure tends to regress towards the mean. Some well controlled studies such as the DASH (Appel *et al.*, 1997) and Premier Studies (Appel *et al.*, 2003) discussed below have used a reduced saturated fatty acid intake as part of a multifaceted intervention to lower blood pressure. However, the nature of these studies often resulted in weight loss, making it difficult to attribute changes to a lower saturated fatty acid intake. The OMNIHEART study (Appel *et al.*, 2005) provided evidence to suggest that replacement of carbohydrate with unsaturated fatty acids or protein lowers SBP by 1.3 and 1.4 mm Hg, respectively, compared with carbohydrate, without any change in body weight. A meta-analysis comparing diets high in monounsaturated fatty acids vs. ones high in carbohydrates was unable to demonstrate superiority of monounsaturated fatty acids (Shah *et al.*, 2007). A recent large randomized multicenter controlled trial was unable to show any effect of replacing saturated fatty acids with MUFA or carbohydrate (either of high or low glycemic index) on clinic blood pressure (Jebb *et al.*, 2010).

The blood-pressure-lowering effect of a high intake of long-chain n-3 polyunsaturated fatty acids, usually provided as fish oil supplements, is more consistent, at least at high intakes. Meta-analyses of randomized controlled trials (Geleijnse *et al.*, 2002) indicated that intakes in the region of 2–5 g/day of long-chain n-3 polyunsaturated fatty acids as fish oil lowered both SBP and DBP, particularly in subjects over the age of 45. They concluded, however, that the effects of lower intakes were uncertain; the average fall in SBP/DBP was 2.3/1.5 mm Hg. Most of the studies provided relatively high intakes, and there were insufficient numbers of subjects treated to come to any conclusions regarding lower intakes, i.e. below 2 g/day. Several randomized controlled trials using doses in the range of 0.4–1.8 g/day in participants with pre-existing cardiovascular disease, many receiving blood-pressure-lowering medication, did not report changes in blood pressure (Yokoyama *et al.*, 2007; GISSI-HF Investigators *et al.*, 2008; Kromhout *et al.*, 2010). A recent 12-month double-blind randomized controlled trail in 312 nonsmoking adults aged 45–70 years found no effect of doses ranging from 0.45 g/day to 1.8 g/day long-chain polyunsaturated fatty acids using ambulatory blood pressure monitoring (Sanders *et al.*, 2011). Overall it appears that dietary fat composition has minimal effects on population blood pressure within the normal ranges of dietary intake.

Salt

There is compelling evidence to show an association between dietary salt (sodium chloride) intake and the prevalence of raised blood pressure. In particular, the age-related increase in blood pressure is greater in populations with a high salt intake. The INTERSALT study (Elliott et al., 1996) concluded that an increase in sodium intake of 100 mmol/day was associated with an increase in SBP/DBP of 3–6/0–3 mm Hg. This relationship was found to be true for both men and women, young and old people, and hypertensive and normotensive subjects. Research in chimpanzees has also shown the potent blood pressure raising effects of salt in the diet (Denton et al., 1995). It has been demonstrated that long-term modest salt restriction achieved with dietary advice can yield significant benefits. A meta-analysis concluded that a reduction of 3 g/day of salt predicts a fall in SBP/DBP of 3.6–5.6/1.9–3.2 mm Hg in hypertensives and 1.8–3.5/0.8–1.8 mm Hg in normotensives (He and MacGregor, 2004). The blood pressure lowering effect is likely to be greater in individuals where the renin–angiotensin system is less active. Low renin concentrations are more prevalent in people of black African origin (He et al., 2009), who are more likely to benefit from salt reduction as are people over the age of 50 years. While sodium retention and increased plasma volume are a plausible mechanism for raised blood pressure in older people, it does not readily explain the effects of salt in younger people. There is some emerging evidence to indicate that salt intake may adversely influence endothelial function (Dickinson et al., 2011) and that low birth weight may increase sensitivity to salt intake (Perala et al., 2011). While the relationship between salt intake and blood pressure is well established, there is no clear relationship between measures of salt intake by 24-hour sodium excretion and subsequent cardiovascular mortality. However, a systematic review of prospective cohort studies found a 23% increase in risk of stroke in participants with the highest intake of salt compared with those with the lowest intake (Strazzullo et al., 2009).

Salt intakes have fallen in many developed countries as the consumption of salted and pickled foods has declined while the consumption of fresh, chilled, and frozen food has increased. This is most notable in Japan, where both blood pressure and stroke incidence have fallen (Ueda et al., 1988). In practice a meta-analysis of dietary advice (Hooper et al., 2004) suggested that lower salt intake leads to only a small reduction in blood pressure (SBP-1/DBP-0.6) with an average reduction in 24-hour urinary sodium excretion of 35.5 mmol/day (about 2 g/day). Providing advice to cut down on salt intake is generally limited in its efficacy as salt in the diet is mainly provided by processed foods such as bread, rather than being added at table or during cooking. Consequently, it has often been argued that it is more important to focus on reducing the levels of salt in commercially processed foods (Anderson et al., 2010). However, there are large cultural differences with regard to the use of salt in domestic food preparation, and in some communities large amounts of salt are added at home.

The UK Government's Food Standards Agency embarked on a policy to persuade food manufacturers to reduce the salt content of processed foods, particularly bread and ready prepared meals, and launched a media campaign to make consumers aware of the salt in processed food. There is some evidence from measurement of 24-hour urine sodium excretion to suggest that salt intakes have fallen in the UK. In contrast a review of measures of salt intake by 24-hour urinary excretion in the USA showed little change in salt intake over the past 50 years (Bernstein and Willett, 2010). Current dietary guidelines advocate that salt intakes should not exceed 6 g/day (100 mmol) for adults in Europe, levels that are achievable. However, in the United States there is a more stringent target of less than 4 g/day (65 mmol/day) in adults over 51 years of age and those with hypertension.

Alcohol

Alcohol intake increases blood pressure acutely in young subjects, and binge drinking can lead to large increases in blood pressure. Heavy alcohol intake is a well known cause of hypertension. Binge drinking is also an important cause of hemorrhagic stroke and sudden cardiac death. The blood-pressure-raising effects of alcohol may decrease with increasing age, and the effect of low to moderate alcohol intake may lower blood pressure. Alcohol acutely suppresses vasopressin (antidiuretic hormone) secretion, thereby having a diuretic effect, but this is followed by a transient increase in renin secretion. It is believed that plasma renin activity is increased as a compensatory reaction to the vasodilatation and diuresis caused by alcohol. Renin catalyzes the conversion of angiotensinogen into angiotensin I. Angiotensin I is subsequently converted into angiotensin II by the action of angiotensin converting enzyme (ACE) which is expressed in endothelial cells, especially in the lung. Angiotensin II causes vasoconstriction of resistance arterioles and acutely elevates blood pressure. The blood pressure raising effect of alcohol is rapidly reversible and can be inhibited by alpha-adrenergic blockade. Randomized controlled trials have shown that moderation of alcohol intake results in a reduction in blood pressure. A meta-analysis of 15 randomized controlled clinical trials of hypertensive and normotensive heavy drinkers (>3 drinks daily) found that alcohol reduction was associated with a significant reduction in mean systolic BP of 3.3 mm Hg and diastolic BP of 2.0 mm Hg (Xin et al., 2001).

Fruit and Vegetable Consumption

Prospective cohort studies show an association between reported increased intake of fruit and vegetables and lower risk of stroke and CHD (He et al., 2006, 2007). It is widely assumed that this difference may be due to an effect on blood pressure. However, it is not possible to exclude residual confounding caused by the association of a healthy lifestyle with higher intakes of fruit and vegetables. For example, plasma vitamin C concentration is a biomarker of fruit and vegetable intake but is also lowered by tobacco use. Higher plasma vitamin C concentrations are also associated with a lower risk of stroke (Myint et al., 2008) but there is no good evidence from randomized controlled trials to indicate that vitamin C supplementation lowers blood pressure. Advice to increase fruit and vegetable consumption to five portions a day in a general-practice setting was found to lower SBP by 4 mm Hg compared with the control group (John et al., 2002). However, this was an incidental finding and not the planned primary outcome of the study. Furthermore, the intervention was a single session of dietary advice, and the blood pressure measurements were done in clinic. This finding was not confirmed in a randomized controlled trial specifically designed to address this question and using ambulatory blood pressure monitoring (Berry et al., 2010). It had been argued that the beneficial effects of increased fruit and vegetable intake can be at least partly attributed to the resultant increased intake of potassium. However, potatoes are an important source of dietary potassium but are generally not regarded as qualifying as "fruit and vegetables" in many food-based dietary guidelines.

Potassium Intake

Prospective epidemiological studies consistently show a consistent relationship between low potassium intake and increased risk of stroke. A meta-analysis of 33 randomized controlled trials of oral potassium supplements (Whelton et al., 1997) revealed significant heterogeneity between studies, and post hoc analyses indicate a reduction in blood pressure that was only apparent when salt intakes were high (>165 mmol/day). Potassium supplementation lowered SBP in China by about 5 mm Hg (Gu et al., 2001). However, salt intakes are high, and habitual intake of potassium is low in the UK. Two recent randomized controlled trials using ambulatory blood pressure monitoring (Berry et al., 2010; He et al., 2010) failed to show any benefit from potassium supplementation in UK subjects with early hypertension. These findings are in agreement with a Cochrane Review (Dickinson et al., 2006) which found no benefit of potassium supplementation for the treatment of hypertension. It is also possible that there is a threshold effect of potassium intake around 40 mmol/day at which increases in potassium intake may lower blood pressure.

Plant Bioactive Materials

Caffeine has a short-term blood-pressure-raising effect which is mainly a consequence of its effect on heart rate. A meta-analysis of chronic caffeine/coffee intake in randomized controlled trials (Noordzij et al., 2005) found that caffeine intake increased SBP by 2.04 mm Hg (95% CI, 1.10–2.99) and DBP by 0.73 mm Hg (95% CI, 0.14–1.31) without affecting heart rate. A meta-analysis (Ried et al., 2010) of cocoa flavonoids suggests a reduction of SBP/DBP by 3.2/2.0 mm Hg. However, a recent well-controlled trial using theobromine-enriched cocoa resulted in a 3.2 mm Hg higher 24-hour ambulatory SBP (van den Bogaard et al., 2010).

The soy isoflavone genistein when infused into the forearm has a similar effect to estradiol on forearm blood flow, which could be attributed to differences in nitric oxide bioavailability (Walker et al., 2001). A meta-analysis of soy isoflavones and blood pressure reported a 1.92 mm lower SBP with intakes ranging between 25 and 375 mg soy isoflavones (Taku et al., 2010). However, this level of isoflavone intake is well above the exposure of people consuming Western diets. There is a lack of reliable data to support claims for a blood-pressure-lowering effect of other flavonoids and anthocyanins.

Arginine and Nitrate

Nitric oxide (NO) produced by the vascular endothelium from arginine causes vasodilation and plays an important role in the regulation of vascular tone. Impaired NO-dependent vasodilation is associated with the development of hypertension (Weil *et al.*, 2011); arginine supplements acutely lower blood pressure (Vasdev and Gill, 2008) and conversely inhibitors of arginine metabolism such as N^G-monomethyl-L-arginine (L-NMMA) raise blood pressure. Dietary intake of arginine is dependent on the level and type of protein consumed. A systematic review (Altorf-van der Kuil *et al.*, 2010) of the effect of protein intake on blood pressure in observational prospective cohort studies and randomized intervention trials indicated a small blood-pressure-lowering effect, especially in the case of plant protein. Plant foods have a higher non-protein nitrogen content than foods of animal origin, and this is mainly due to the presence of nitrate which is well known to lower blood pressure in animals. The blood-pressure-lowering effects of organic nitrates are well established, but recently evidence has emerged to show that dietary inorganic nitrate can acutely lower blood pressure by generating NO (Webb *et al.*, 2008). This effect is apparently a consequence of some bacterial conversion of nitrate to nitrite in the mouth that subsequently results in increased NO (Lundberg *et al.*, 2009; Kapil *et al.*, 2010). In a randomized controlled trial of beetroot juice a reduction in SBP of 5.4 mm Hg was demonstrated. The effects, however, appear to last only a few hours. Currently, there is a lack of evidence from randomized controlled trials of more widely consumed vegetables with an increased nitrate content, and further research in this area in required.

Dairy Products

A meta-analysis of prospective cohort studies supports the inverse association between low-fat dairy foods and fluid dairy foods and the risk of elevated blood pressure (Ralston *et al.*, 2011). No relationship was found with cheese. As milk products are a major source of dietary calcium, it is not surprising that a similar relationship has been found with calcium intake and blood pressure. It has also been proposed that vitamin D status may influence blood pressure but the few randomized controlled trials to date provide no clear evidence (Geleijnse, 2011). However, a systematic review of combined vitamin D and calcium supplementation (Chung *et al.*, 2009) concluded that supplementation lowered SBP but not DBP by 2–4 mm Hg.

Furthermore a meta-analysis also concluded that calcium supplementation had a beneficial effect in pregnancy on preventing hypertensive disorders (Hofmeyr *et al.*, 2010).

Peptides produced through the fermentation of dairy products with *Lactobacillus helveticus* have blood-pressure-lowering properties (Seppo *et al.*, 2003). These peptides appear to partially inhibit angiotensin converting enzyme and thereby reduce blood pressure. Foods containing these peptides were first marketed in Japan, then Finland and some other European countries. However, using ambulatory blood pressure monitoring as outcomes, two large multicenter studies were unable to confirm the blood-pressure-lowering effects of dairy peptides (van Mierlo *et al.*, 2009). At present, the evidence suggests a possible beneficial effect of reduced-fat liquid milk products in protecting against hypertension, but this requires further investigation because of possible residual confounding.

An Integrated Dietary Approach to Prevent Hypertension

From the above it can be seen that several dietary factors can influence blood pressure, and in most cases the effects on SBP are in the range of 1–3 mm Hg (Table 46.2). However, these small differences may have additive or synergistic effects when combined. The Dietary Approaches to Stop Hypertension (DASH) study (Appel *et al.*, 1997) compared three diets: a control diet that was low in fruit, vegetables, and dairy products with a fat content typical of the American diet; a diet rich in fruit and vegetables; and a "combination diet" rich in fruits and vegetables and low in saturated fats and added sugars (the diet comprised whole grains, low-fat dairy products, fish, and poultry, with restrictions on the consumption of red meat, sugary drinks, cakes, and biscuits). Blood pressure was measured using ambulatory monitoring on multiple occasions, and the study was statistically well powered. SBP was

TABLE 46.2 Summary of well-established individual dietary effects on blood pressure (mm Hg)

Dietary factor	Systolic BP	Diastolic BP
5 kg overweight	4.4	3.3
Salt	2.5	1.3
Alcohol	3.3	2
Caffeine	2	0.7

BOX 46.2   The DASH eating plan

Emphasizes fruit, vegetables, and low-fat dairy foods
Includes whole grains, poultry, fish, and nuts
Contains less red meat, sweets, and sugar-containing beverages
Minimizes the use of salt
Alcohol allowed only in moderation
Aims at maintaining a healthy weight

3–4 mm Hg lower for the high fruit and vegetable group compared with the control group, and a much greater reduction in blood pressure was obtained with the "combination diet." Since the initial DASH study, several further studies have examined the effects of a DASH-style eating plan in combination with other lifestyle interventions. The DASH-2 study (Sacks *et al.*, 2001) examined the effects of different levels of dietary salt reduction in conjunction with the DASH diet. The benefits of the DASH diet for blood pressure reduction were enhanced with a reduction in salt intake. Combined effects on blood pressure of a low salt intake and the DASH diet were greater than the effects of either intervention alone. The combined effect of the DASH diet with a low salt intake resulted in a reduction in SBP of 7.1 mmHg in normotensives and 11.5 mmHg in hypertensives. The modified DASH eating plan is shown in Box 46.2.

The DASH studies, however, were tightly controlled dietary interventions as opposed to tests of the effectiveness of dietary advice. The PREMIER study (Appel *et al.*, 2003) was designed for this purpose and compared the effect of lifestyle advice with and without behavioral therapy on blood pressure in free-living subjects after 6 months of intervention. Participants were given the lifestyle advice with the DASH diet alone or with behavioral therapy, a third group received standard dietary advice (reduce salt intake, lose weight, and cut back on alcohol intake) and behavioral therapy. Dietary advice alone resulted in a reduction in SBP/DBP of 3.7/1.7 mm Hg. However, if advice was accompanied by behavioral therapy, reductions in SBP/DBP of 8/4.3 mm Hg were observed. In this study similar reductions in blood pressure were obtained with standard advice (reduce salt intake, lose weight, and cut back on alcohol intake) compared with the DASH diet. Most of the changes in blood pressure in the groups that received behavioral intervention could be attributed to changes in weight (4–5 kg difference compared with advice alone) as intakes of alcohol were low at baseline and sodium intake as estimated from urinary excretion of sodium was only 10 mmol/day lower. The approach adopted by the DASH investigators has been replicated in other countries, and currently appears to be the most effective dietary intervention.

Conclusions

Blood pressure shows a continuous relationship with risk of stroke and coronary heart disease. Small reductions in the population average blood pressure translate into a significant reduction in the number of deaths from cardiovascular disease. Decreasing the intake of salt, alcohol, and saturated fat, increasing the intake of fruit and vegetables, and losing weight can lower SBP/DBP by up to 8/4 mmHg. However, lifestyle changes tend to be difficult to adopt, and so in practice dietary advice alone is only likely to result in a 3–4 mm Hg change in blood pressure in the short term. Even such small changes in blood pressure can translate into greater reductions in the long term and are likely to substantially reduce the burden of cardiovascular disease in the population. The genesis of hypertension is likely to be during fetal development and early life. Consequently, the prevention of hypertension also needs to consider optimum maternal and infant nutrition.

Future Directions

Arterial stiffening is emerging as a major predictor of vascular mortality and contributes to increases in SBP in older people. Further research is needed to understand whether dietary factors such as vitamins D and K are involved in arterial stiffening. The mechanisms by which blood pressure is programmed in early life require further attention, and there is a need for trials in pregnancy to see if risk of hypertension in offspring can be reduced. Confirmation of the blood-pressure-lowering effects of dairy products is required by appropriately powered randomized controlled trials. The role of nitric oxide and dietary nitrate in the regulation of blood pressure continues to be a topic that deserves further research, as are the mechanisms by which the central nervous system influences peripheral vascular resistance.

Suggestions for Further Reading

Appel, L.J. (2009) ASH position paper: dietary approaches to lower blood pressure. *J Am Soc Hypertens* **3**, 321–331.

Lundberg, J.O., Gladwin, M.T., Ahluwalia, A., *et al.* (2009) Nitrate and nitrite in biology, nutrition and therapeutics. *Nat Chem Biol* **5**, 865–869.

Nuyt, A.M. (2008) Mechanisms underlying developmental programming of elevated blood pressure and vascular dysfunction: evidence from human studies and experimental animal models. *Clin Sci (Lond)* **114**, 1–17.

References

ALLHAT Investigators (2002) Major outcomes in high-risk hypertensive patients randomized to angiotensin-converting enzyme inhibitor or calcium channel blocker vs diuretic: The Antihypertensive and Lipid-Lowering Treatment to Prevent Heart Attack Trial (ALLHAT). *JAMA* **288**, 2981–2997.

Altorf-van der Kuil, W., Engberink, M.F., Brink, E.J., *et al.* (2010) Dietary protein and blood pressure: a systematic review. *PLoS One* **5**, e12102.

Anderson, C.A., Appel, L.J., Okuda, N., *et al.* (2010) Dietary sources of sodium in China, Japan, the United Kingdom, and the United States, women and men aged 40 to 59 years: the INTERMAP study. *J Am Diet Assoc* **110**, 736–745.

Appel, L.J., Champagne, C.M., Harsha, D.W., *et al.* (2003) Effects of comprehensive lifestyle modification on blood pressure control: main results of the PREMIER clinical trial. *JAMA* **289**, 2083–2093.

Appel, L.J., Moore, T.J., Obarzanek, E., *et al.* (1997) A clinical trial of the effects of dietary patterns on blood pressure. DASH Collaborative Research Group. *N Engl J Med* **336**, 1117–1124.

Appel, L.J., Sacks, F.M., Carey, V.J., *et al.* (2005) Effects of protein, monounsaturated fat, and carbohydrate intake on blood pressure and serum lipids: results of the OmniHeart randomized trial. *JAMA* **294**, 2455–2464.

Barker, D.J., Osmond, C., Forsen, T.J., *et al.* (2005) Trajectories of growth among children who have coronary events as adults. *N Engl J Med* **353**, 1802–1809.

Bernstein, A.M. and Willett, W.C. (2010) Trends in 24-h urinary sodium excretion in the United States, 1957–2003: a systematic review. *Am J Clin Nutr* **92**, 1172–1180.

Berry, S.E., Mulla, U.Z., Chowienczyk, P.J., *et al.* (2010) Increased potassium intake from fruit and vegetables or supplements does not lower blood pressure or improve vascular function in UK men and women with early hypertension: a randomised controlled trial. *Br J Nutr* **104**, 1839–1847.

Chung, M., Balk, E.M., Brendel, M., *et al.* (2009) Vitamin D and calcium: a systematic review of health outcomes. *Evid Rep Technol Assess (Full Rep)* **183**, 1–420.

Cushman, W.C., Evans, G.W., Byington, R.P., *et al.* (2010) Effects of intensive blood-pressure control in type 2 diabetes mellitus. *N Engl J Med* **362**, 1575–1585.

Czernichow, S., Zanchetti, A., Turnbull, F., *et al.* (2011) The effects of blood pressure reduction and of different blood pressure-lowering regimens on major cardiovascular events according to baseline blood pressure: meta-analysis of randomized trials. *J Hypertens* **29**, 4–16.

Denton, D., Weisinger, R., Mundy, N.I., *et al.* (1995) The effect of increased salt intake on blood pressure of chimpanzees. *Nat Med* **1**, 1009–1016.

Dickinson, H.O., Nicolson, D.J., Campbell, F., *et al.* (2006) Potassium supplementation for the management of primary hypertension in adults. *Cochrane Database Syst Rev* CD004641.

Dickinson, K.M., Clifton, P.M., and Keogh, J.B. (2011) Endothelial function is impaired after a high-salt meal in healthy subjects. *Am J Clin Nutr* **93**, 500–505.

Elliott, P., Stamler, J., Dyer, A.R., *et al.* (2006) Association between protein intake and blood pressure: the INTERMAP Study. *Arch Intern Med* **166**, 79–87.

Elliott, P., Stamler, J., Nichols, R., *et al.* (1996) Intersalt revisited: further analyses of 24 hour sodium excretion and blood pressure within and across populations. Intersalt Cooperative Research Group. *BMJ* **312**, 1249–1253.

Frost, C.D., Law, M.R., and Wald, N.J. (1991) By how much does dietary salt reduction lower blood pressure? II – Analysis of observational data within populations. *BMJ* **302**, 815–818.

Geleijnse, J.M. (2011) Vitamin D and the prevention of hypertension and cardiovascular diseases: a review of the current evidence. *Am J Hypertens* **24**, 253–262.

Geleijnse, J.M., Giltay, E.J., Grobbee, D.E., *et al.* (2002) Blood pressure response to fish oil supplementation: metaregression analysis of randomized trials. *J Hypertens* **20**, 1493–1499.

GISSI-HF Investigators, Tavazzi, L., Maggioni, A.P., *et al.* (2008) Effect of n-3 polyunsaturated fatty acids in patients with chronic heart failure (the GISSI-HF trial): a randomised, double-blind, placebo-controlled trial. *Lancet* **372**, 1223–1230.

Greenfield, J.R. (2011) Melanocortin signalling and the regulation of blood pressure in human obesity. *J Neuroendocrinol* **23**, 186–193.

Greenstein, A.S., Khavandi, K., Withers, S.B., *et al.* (2009) Local inflammation and hypoxia abolish the protective anticontractile properties of perivascular fat in obese patients. *Circulation* **119**, 1661–1670.

Gu, D., He, J., Wu, X., *et al.* (2001) Effect of potassium supplementation on blood pressure in Chinese: a randomized, placebo-controlled trial. *J Hypertens* **19**, 1325–1331.

He, F.J. and MacGregor, G.A. (2004) Effect of longer-term modest salt reduction on blood pressure. *Cochrane Database Syst Rev* CD004937.

He, F.J., Marciniak, M., Carney, C., *et al.* (2010) Effects of potassium chloride and potassium bicarbonate on endothelial function, cardiovascular risk factors, and bone turnover in mild hypertensives. *Hypertension* **55**, 681–688.

He, F.J., Marciniak, M., Visagie, E., *et al.* (2009) Effect of modest salt reduction on blood pressure, urinary albumin, and pulse wave velocity in white, black, and Asian mild hypertensives. *Hypertension* **54**, 482–488.

He, F.J., Nowson, C.A., Lucas, M., *et al.* (2007) Increased consumption of fruit and vegetables is related to a reduced risk of coronary heart disease: meta-analysis of cohort studies. *J Hum Hypertens* **21**, 717–728.

He, F.J., Nowson, C.A., and MacGregor, G.A. (2006) Fruit and vegetable consumption and stroke: meta-analysis of cohort studies. *Lancet* **367**, 320–326.

Hemachandra, A.H., Howards, P.P., Furth, S.L., *et al.* (2007) Birth weight, postnatal growth, and risk for high blood pressure at 7 years of age: results from the Collaborative Perinatal Project. *Pediatrics* **119**, e1264–e1270.

Hofmeyr, G.J., Lawrie, T.A., Atallah, A.N., *et al.* (2010) Calcium supplementation during pregnancy for preventing hypertensive disorders and related problems. *Cochrane Database Syst Rev* CD001059.

Hooper, L., Bartlett, C., Davey, S.G., *et al.* (2004) Advice to reduce dietary salt for prevention of cardiovascular disease. *Cochrane Database Syst Rev* CD003656.

Jebb, S.A., Lovegrove, J.A., Griffin, B.A., *et al.* (2010) Effect of changing the amount and type of fat and carbohydrate on insulin sensitivity and cardiovascular risk: the RISCK (Reading, Imperial, Surrey, Cambridge, and Kings) trial. *Am J Clin Nutr* **92**, 748–758.

Jessani, S., Watson, T., Cappuccio, F.P., *et al.* (2006) Prevention of cardiovascular disease in clinical practice: The Joint British Societies' (JBS 2) guidelines. *J Hum Hypertens* **20**, 641–645.

John, J.H., Ziebland, S., Yudkin, P., *et al.* (2002) Effects of fruit and vegetable consumption on plasma antioxidant concentrations and blood pressure: a randomised controlled trial. *Lancet* **359**, 1969–1974.

Kapil, V., Milsom, A.B., Okorie, M., *et al.* (2010) Inorganic nitrate supplementation lowers blood pressure in humans: role for nitrite-derived NO. *Hypertension* **56**, 274–281.

Kromhout, D., Giltay, E.J., and Geleijnse, J.M. (2010) n-3 fatty acids and cardiovascular events after myocardial infarction. *N Engl J Med* **363**, 2015–2026.

Lewington, S., Clarke, R., Qizilbash, N., *et al.* (2002) Age-specific relevance of usual blood pressure to vascular mortality: a meta-analysis of individual data for one million adults in 61 prospective studies. *Lancet* **360**, 1903–1913.

Lundberg, J.O., Gladwin, M.T., Ahluwalia, A., *et al.* (2009) Nitrate and nitrite in biology, nutrition and therapeutics. *Nat Chem Biol* **5**, 865–869.

Mancia, G., De Backer, G., Dominiczak, A., *et al.* (2007) 2007 Guidelines for the Management of Arterial Hypertension: The Task Force for the Management of Arterial Hypertension of the European Society of Hypertension (ESH) and of the European Society of Cardiology (ESC). *J Hypertens* **25**, 1105–1187.

Miura, K., Stamler, J., Nakagawa, H., *et al.* (2008) Relationship of dietary linoleic acid to blood pressure. The International Study of Macro-Micronutrients and Blood Pressure Study [corrected]. *Hypertension* **52**, 408–414.

Myint, P.K., Luben, R.N., Welch, A.A., *et al.* (2008) Plasma vitamin C concentrations predict risk of incident stroke over 10 y in 20649 participants of the European Prospective Investigation into Cancer Norfolk prospective population study. *Am J Clin Nutr* **87**, 64–69.

Neter, J.E., Stam, B.E., Kok, F.J., *et al.* (2003) Influence of weight reduction on blood pressure: a meta-analysis of randomized controlled trials. *Hypertension* **42**, 878–884.

Noordzij, M., Uiterwaal, C.S., Arends, L.R., *et al.* (2005) Blood pressure response to chronic intake of coffee and caffeine: a meta-analysis of randomized controlled trials. *J Hypertens* **23**, 921–928.

O'Brien, E., Asmar, R., Beilin, L., *et al.* (2005) Practice guidelines of the European Society of Hypertension for clinic, ambulatory and self blood pressure measurement. *J Hypertens* **23**, 697–701.

Perala, M.M., Moltchanova, E., Kaartinen, N.E., *et al.* (2011) The association between salt intake and adult systolic blood pressure is modified by birth weight. *Am J Clin Nutr* **93**, 422–426.

Poulter, N.R., Khaw, K.T., Hopwood, B.E., *et al.* (1990) The Kenyan Luo migration study: observations on the initiation of a rise in blood pressure. *BMJ* **300**, 967–972.

Ralston, R.A., Lee, J.H., Truby, H., *et al.* (2011) A systematic review and meta-analysis of elevated blood pressure and consumption of dairy foods. *J Hum Hypertens* PMID 21307883.

Ried, K., Sullivan, T., Fakler, P., *et al.* (2010) Does chocolate reduce blood pressure? A meta-analysis. *BMC Med* **8**, 39.

Sacks, F.M., Svetkey, L.P., Vollmer, W.M., *et al.* (2001) Effects on blood pressure of reduced dietary sodium and the Dietary Approaches to Stop Hypertension (DASH) diet. DASH-Sodium Collaborative Research Group. *N Engl J Med* **344**, 3–10.

Sanders, T.A.B., Hall, W.L., Maniou, Z., *et al.* (2011) Effect of low doses of long chain n-3 polyunsaturated fatty acids on endothelial function and arterial stiffness: a randomized, controlled trial. *Am J Clin Nutr* **94**, 973–980.

Seppo, L., Jauhiainen, T., Poussa, T., *et al.* (2003) A fermented milk high in bioactive peptides has a blood pressure-lowering effect in hypertensive subjects. *Am J Clin Nutr* **77**, 326–330.

Shah, M., dams-Huet, B., and Garg, A. (2007) Effect of high-carbohydrate or high-cis-monounsaturated fat diets on blood pressure: a meta-analysis of intervention trials. *Am J Clin Nutr* **85**, 1251–1256.

Strazzullo, P., D'Elia, L., Kandala, N.B., *et al.* (2009) Salt intake, stroke, and cardiovascular disease: meta-analysis of prospective studies. *BMJ* **339**, b4567.

Taku, K., Lin, N., Cai, D., *et al.* (2010) Effects of soy isoflavone extract supplements on blood pressure in adult humans: systematic review and meta-analysis of randomized placebo-controlled trials. *J Hypertens* **28**, 1971–1982.

Tunstall-Pedoe, H., Connaghan, J., Woodward, M., *et al.* (2006) Pattern of declining blood pressure across replicate population surveys of the WHO MONICA project, mid-1980s to mid-1990s, and the role of medication. *BMJ* **332**, 629–635.

Ueda, K., Hasuo, Y., Kiyohara, Y., *et al.* (1988) Intracerebral hemorrhage in a Japanese community, Hisayama: incidence, changing pattern during long-term follow-up, and related factors. *Stroke* **19**, 48–52.

Ueshima, H., Stamler, J., Elliott, P., *et al.* (2007) Food omega-3 fatty acid intake of individuals (total, linolenic acid, long-chain) and their blood pressure: INTERMAP study. *Hypertension* **50**, 313–319.

van den Bogaard, B., Draijer, R., Westerhof, B.E., *et al.* (2010) Effects on peripheral and central blood pressure of cocoa with natural or high-dose theobromine: a randomized, double-blind crossover trial. *Hypertension* **56**, 839–846.

van Mierlo, L.A., Koning, M.M., van der Zander, K., *et al.* (2009) Lactotripeptides do not lower ambulatory blood pressure in untreated whites: results from 2 controlled multicenter crossover studies. *Am J Clin .Nutr* **89**, 617–623.

Vasdev, S. and Gill, V. (2008) The antihypertensive effect of arginine. *Int J Angiol* **17**, 7–22.

Walker, H.A., Dean, T.S., Sanders, T.A., *et al.* (2001) The phytoestrogen genistein produces acute nitric oxide-dependent dilation of human forearm vasculature with similar potency to 17beta-estradiol. *Circulation* **103**, 258–262.

Webb, A.J., Patel, N., Loukogeorgakis, S., *et al.* (2008) Acute blood pressure lowering, vasoprotective, and antiplatelet properties of dietary nitrate via bioconversion to nitrite. *Hypertension* **51**, 784–790.

Weil, B.R., Stauffer, B.L., Greiner, J.J., *et al.* (2011) Prehypertension is associated with impaired nitric oxide-mediated endothelium-dependent vasodilation in sedentary adults. *Am J Hypertens* **24**, 976–981.

Whelton, P.K., He, J., Cutler, J.A., *et al.* (1997) Effects of oral potassium on blood pressure. Meta-analysis of randomized controlled clinical trials. *JAMA* **277**, 1624–1632.

Whitlock, G., Lewington, S., Sherliker, P., *et al.* (2009) Body-mass index and cause-specific mortality in 900,000 adults: collaborative analyses of 57 prospective studies. *Lancet* **373**, 1083–1096.

Williams, B., Poulter, N.R., Brown, M.J., *et al.* (2004) British Hypertension Society guidelines for hypertension management 2004 (BHS-IV): summary. *BMJ* **328**, 634–640.

Withers, S.B., Agabiti-Rosei, C., Livingstone, D.M., *et al.* (2011) Macrophage activation is responsible for loss of anticontractile function in inflamed perivascular fat. *Arterioscler Thromb Vasc Biol* **31**, 908–913.

Xin, X., He, J., Frontini, M.G., *et al.* (2001) Effects of alcohol reduction on blood pressure: a meta-analysis of controlled trials. *Hypertension* **38**, 1112–1117.

Yokoyama, M., Origasa, H., Matsuzaki, M., *et al.* (2007) Effects of eicosapentaenoic acid on major coronary events in hypercholesterolaemic patients (JELIS): a randomised open-label, blinded endpoint analysis. *Lancet* **369**, 1090–1098.

47

INSULIN RESISTANCE AND THE METABOLIC SYNDROME

JENNIE BRAND-MILLER, PhD, FAIFST, FNSA AND STEPHEN COLAGIURI, MD

University of Sydney, Sydney, New South Wales, Australia

Summary

Insulin resistance is a physiological phenomenon that describes impairments or weakness in insulin action. Insulin resistance occurs naturally at puberty and during pregnancy and is usually severe in overweight and obese individuals and those with type 2 diabetes and cardiovascular disease. The "metabolic syndrome" is now a widely recognized yet controversial concept that refers to a clustering of metabolic risk factors, such as raised blood pressure, dyslipidemia (raised triglycerides and lowered high-density lipoprotein cholesterol), raised fasting glucose, and central obesity in the one individual. Insulin resistance is the most accepted unifying theory explaining the origins of the metabolic syndrome. Prevention and management of the metabolic syndrome by lifestyle interventions, including weight loss, a healthy diet, and increased physical activity, represent the best chance of reducing the personal, societal, and economic burden of chronic disease. The molecular basis of insulin resistance, its role in health and disease, and the optimal diet composition for improving insulin sensitivity present continuing challenges to research scientists around the world.

Introduction

In 1936, Harold Himsworth introduced the concept of "insulin sensitivity," separating diabetes into two main types, an insulin-sensitive and an insulin-resistant phenotype (Himsworth, 1936). He developed the first method for measuring insulin resistance and began studies to show that diet might influence glucose tolerance by altering insulin sensitivity. Today, being insulin-sensitive is considered instrumental to good health and the prevention of

chronic diseases such as type 2 diabetes and cardiovascular disease. Insulin resistance, the opposite of insulin sensitivity, is a physiological phenomenon that describes impairments of insulin action, usually in respect of glucose metabolism rather than fatty acids or amino acids (Draznin, 2008). Compared with insulin-sensitive individuals, those with insulin resistance require higher concentrations of insulin to facilitate the disposal of glucose in tissues. Insulin-resistant humans and animals therefore develop compensatory hyperinsulinemia in order to ensure normal

Present Knowledge in Nutrition, Tenth Edition. Edited by John W. Erdman Jr, Ian A. Macdonald and Steven H. Zeisel.

utilization of glucose by the insulin target tissues. As a consequence, hyperinsulinemia and insulin resistance go hand in hand (DeFronzo *et al.*, 1992).

Insulin resistance can be a normal, physiological state or pathologically severe. Insulin resistance increases naturally at puberty (Goran and Gower, 2001) and during pregnancy (Butte, 2000), but it is more extreme in overweight and obese individuals, in people with type 2 diabetes and pre-diabetes, and in those with cardiovascular disease (Facchini *et al.*, 2001). Recent research links insulin resistance to many conditions, including fatty liver disease, polycystic ovarian syndrome, sleep apnea, and cancer. Insulin resistance is the most accepted unifying theory explaining the origins of the "metabolic syndrome" (Mikhail, 2009).

The metabolic syndrome is now a widely recognized yet controversial concept that refers to a clustering of metabolic risk factors, such as high waist circumference, low HDL-cholesterol, high serum triglycerides, hypertension, and impaired glucose tolerance, in the one individual. There is a lack of consensus on its practical utility either as a diagnostic or a management tool, and even its definition and diagnostic criteria vary around the world (Table 47.1). While there is general agreement on four of the central components, there is disagreement on waist circumference and how this should be adjusted for use in different ethnic groups. A recent WHO Expert Consultation concluded that it was a premorbid condition rather than a clinical diagnosis and should exclude individuals with established diabetes or known cardiovascular disease (Simmons *et al.*, 2010).

The clustering of metabolic risk factors with diabetes and cardiovascular disease has been recognized for more than 80 years, but the modern concept of the metabolic syndrome began when Gerald Reaven proposed that apparently unrelated biological parameters were part of a single physiological condition (Reaven, 1988). He argued that insulin resistance provided a common mechanism to link the abnormalities although this remains a subject of debate. The parallel presence of compensatory hyperinsulinemia may well have effects that are distinct from those of insulin resistance *per se*, stimulating or even overstimulating certain aspects of insulin action in various cells and tissues (Low *et al.*, 2004). It is therefore difficult to distinguish between causes and consequences of insulin resistance.

Prevalence of the Metabolic Syndrome

The prevalence of the metabolic syndrome varies markedly around the world. It has strong lifestyle determinants, which are in turn influenced by socioeconomic status, culture, and education. Depending on the definition, approximately one in four or five adults in industrialized countries meet the criteria for the metabolic syndrome (Ford *et al.*, 2004). It is increasingly common in younger age groups and in developing nations.

Insulin resistance by itself may be a normal physiological response to changes in metabolic circumstances. Both energy restriction and energy surplus cause a decline in insulin sensitivity. Indeed, insulin resistance in one set of tissues may facilitate the redirection of fuels around the body to the tissues in greater need. During lactation, the mammary glands become exquisitely insulin-sensitive, while muscles remain insulin resistant, thus driving uptake of glucose for the synthesis of lactose (Vernon, 1989). Insulin resistance also appears at birth in infants born small or large for gestational age (McMillen and Robinson, 2005).

Insulin resistance is associated with excess visceral fat in the abdomen but not excess subcutaneous fat (Cnop *et al.*, 2002). Surgical removal of visceral fat immediately restores insulin sensitivity. Because skeletal muscle is the largest insulin-sensitive tissue, higher proportions of lean mass are associated with greater insulin sensitivity.

TABLE 47.1 International Diabetes Federation definition of the metabolic syndrome

Measure	Categorical cut-points[a]
Elevated waist circumference	Population and country-specific definitions (e.g. Europid ≥94 cm in males, and ≥80 cm in females or China ≥85 cm in males, ≥80 cm in females)
Elevated triglycerides	>150 mg/dL or 1.7 mmol/L
Reduced HDL-cholesterol	<40 mg/dL or 1.0 mmol/L in males, <50 mg/dL or <1.3 mmol/L in females
Elevated blood pressure	Systolic ≥130 and/or diastolic ≥85 mm Hg
Elevated fasting glucose	≥100 mg/dL or 5.5 mmol/L

[a]Drug treatment for any specific parameter is an alternative indicator.
Data from Alberti *et al.* (2009).

Within healthy European populations, the amount of physical activity is the main determinant of insulin sensitivity, accounting for a two-fold range (Balkau *et al.*, 2008; Helmerhorst *et al.*, 2009). Both resistance exercise and aerobic exercise increase insulin sensitivity whereas total time in sedentary activities reduces insulin sensitivity.

Insulin sensitivity also varies from one ethnic group to another. Pima Indians, distinguished by having the highest recorded rate of type 2 diabetes in the world, are among the most insulin resistant even when young and lean (Bogardus, 1993). In some studies, European Caucasians were twice as insulin sensitive as BMI-matched individuals of African-American or Asian origin (Osei and Schuster, 1994; Dickinson *et al.*, 2002) (Figure 47.1). Profound compensatory hyperinsulinemia is evident in response to a realistic carbohydrate meal in lean young adults of Asian origin (Figure 47.2).

Insulin resistance is also influenced by perinatal factors (Hales and Barker, 2001). Young adults who were born prematurely with a very low birth weight are more likely to have insulin resistance, glucose intolerance, and the metabolic syndrome than those who were born with normal birth weight (Hovi *et al.*, 2007). Higher body fat at birth is also associated with greater insulin resistance and type 2 diabetes later in life (Wei *et al.*, 2003). Maternal glucose intolerance, in particular, promotes excess fetal growth and fetal insulin resistance (Luo *et al.*, 2010).

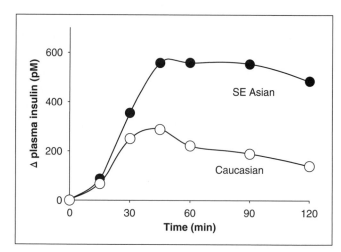

FIG. 47.2 Postprandial insulin responses to a 75-g carbohydrate portion of white bread in lean young healthy subjects of Southeast Asian origin ($n = 10$) and European Caucasian origin ($n = 10$). The higher insulin response in Asians reflects compensatory hyperinsulinemia stemming from intrinsic insulin resistance (Dickinson *et al.*, 2002).

Together, these effects produce a vicious cycle that promotes higher risk of chronic disease in children and young adults.

Normal Actions of Insulin

Insulin, the most potent anabolic hormone in the body, exerts a multitude of effects on carbohydrate, lipid and protein metabolism, ion and amino acid transport, nitric oxide (NO) synthesis, and cell proliferation and differentiation (Draznin, 2008). At the onset of eating, insulin is released from the pancreatic beta-cells in order to re-establish euglycemia. Insulin promotes glucose uptake in skeletal muscle by stimulating translocation of glucose transporter 4 (GLUT 4) from the cytosol to the plasma membrane where it facilitates glucose transport into the cell. Concomitantly, insulin stimulates intracellular utilization of glucose by many other tissues as well. In the fasting state, the main physiological function of insulin is to suppress glucose production by the liver and prevent uncontrolled lipolysis and ketogenesis, without which diabetic ketoacidosis would quickly develop. Hence, if either of these aspects of insulin action is impaired, then peripheral or liver hepatic insulin resistance or both are said to be present.

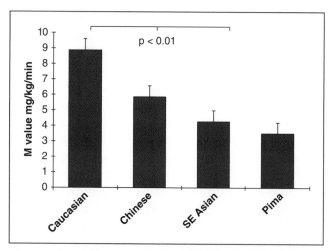

FIG. 47.1 Differences in insulin sensitivity assessed by the euglycemic–hyperinsulinemic clamp procedure in lean young healthy individuals from four ethnic groups. Drawn from Dickinson *et al.* (2002) and Lillioja *et al.* (1988).

On a cellular level, insulin stimulates glycogen, protein, and lipid synthesis while also inhibiting glycogenolysis, lipolysis, protein degradation and apoptosis. But selective insulin resistance is usually present, affecting one tissue more than others. Insulin resistance usually defines an inadequate strength of insulin signalling from the insulin receptor downstream to the final substrates of insulin action involved in metabolic aspects of cellular function.

Molecular Mechanisms of Insulin Resistance

Although great strides are being made in our understanding, the molecular mechanisms still remain unclear. The defect in most people appears to lie *downstream* of the insulin receptor. Numerous studies show that the number and function (tyrosine kinase activity) of insulin receptors are usually normal in people with type 2 diabetes. Magnetic resonance spectroscopy studies in vivo indicate that there is a defect in insulin-stimulated glucose transport into skeletal muscle. Recent studies consistently show reduced strength in the insulin receptor substrate-1/phosphotidylinositol 3-kinase (IRS-1/PI 3-kinase) pathway (i.e. the pathway responsible for most, if not all, of the metabolic effects of insulin), resulting in diminished glucose uptake and utilization in target tissues (Draznin, 2008) However, the culprit that initiates and sustains the impaired insulin signaling is not known.

Two complementary mechanisms have been suggested to explain reduced strength in this pathway. In the first, increased activity of several serine kinases diminishes insulin signal transduction by phosphorylating serine residues on IRS-1. Excessive phosphorylation interferes with normal conductance of the insulin signal. The trigger could be hyperinsulinemia or hyperglycemia, occurring under conditions of nutrient saturation or nutritional excess. Activation of the transcription factor NF-kappa B in response to oxidative stress or proinflammatory molecules, including hyperglycemia, also produces insulin resistance via this mechanism. The second molecular mechanism that could lead to insulin resistance is a disruption in the balance between the amounts of the two PI-3 kinase subunits (Draznin, 2008). The regulatory subunit, p85, is tightly associated with the catalytic subunit, p110. Insulin-resistant states could be associated with decreases in the expression of the p85 monomer, causing decreased PI-3 kinase activity. Pregnancy appears to be associated with increased expression of skeletal muscle p85 in response to increasing concentrations of human placental growth hormone.

Another hypothesis gaining ground is that insulin resistance is caused by mitochondrial dysfunction or reduced numbers of mitochondria with decreased fatty acid oxidation and accumulation of fatty acid acyl CoA and diacylglycerol (Lowell and Shulman, 2005). The mechanism in this case is thought to be activation of novel protein kinase C (PKC), which leads to increased serine phosphorylation of IRS-1. Insulin resistance may therefore be an appropriate response to nutrient excess, i.e. a cellular antioxidant defense mechanism. Indeed, mitochondrial superoxide production has been shown to be a common feature of many different models of insulin resistance in isolated adipocytes, myotubes, and animal models (Hoehn *et al.*, 2009). Insulin resistance can be rapidly reversed by agents that act as mitochondrial uncouplers or inhibitors of the electronic transport chain. In fact, artificial induction of mitochondrial superoxide production causes rapid impairments in insulin action independently of changes in the PI-3 kinase pathway (Hoehn *et al.*, 2009). Mitochondrial superoxide could be described as a metabolic sensor of energy excess.

Techniques Used to Assess Insulin Action

In healthy, normal individuals, blood glucose concentration is maintained within a narrow range. After an overnight fast or between meals, blood glucose normally falls within the range of 3.5–5.5 mM. Immediately after a meal containing carbohydrate, blood glucose concentration rises to a peak of 6–10 mM followed by a sharp decline back to baseline within 60 minutes. This exquisite control is achieved by a fine balance between glucose absorption from the gut, glucose production by the liver, and glucose extraction from the blood into the cells and tissues.

Insulin plays a central role in the regulation of blood glucose concentration by suppressing hepatic glucose production and stimulating peripheral glucose uptake. Most methods used to measure any impairment in insulin action (i.e. insulin resistance) therefore assess the quantitative relationship between a given plasma insulin concentration and some measurable insulin-dependent process, usually at the whole body level. A simple and common marker of insulin resistance is called HOMA–IR (homeostasis modelling assessment–insulin resistance), simply calculated as the product of the fasting glucose in mmol/L and the fasting insulin in µU/mL divided by 22.5 (Matthews *et al.*, 1985). In lean, young, healthy individuals, this value approximates 1, but the range within the normal adult population is around 1 to 4. The top quartile is regarded as being relatively insulin resistant. Obese people and individuals with type 2 diabetes show values in the range 4 to 8. Since HOMA is calculated using fasting glucose and insulin, it reflects mostly hepatic insulin resistance and not the ability to metabolize a large carbohydrate challenge. Others have endeavoured to improve on HOMA–IR by using the quantitative insulin sensitivity check index (QUICKI), and the fasting glucose-to-insulin ratio (FG insulin resistance). Techniques such as the frequently sampled intravenous glucose tolerance test (FSIGTT) or Bergman minimal model, endeavor to measure how quickly blood glucose levels return to normal after injection of a given amount of insulin (Bergman *et al.*, 2003). The "gold standard" method for measuring insulin resistance is the euglycemic–hyperinsulinemic clamp (Matthews, 1985), in which a constant intravenous infusion of insulin is balanced by a simultaneous infusion of glucose in a clinical research setting. Because of the invasive, time-consuming nature of the clamp procedure, it is difficult to use in routine clinical practice or in large epidemiological studies.

How Does Insulin Resistance Cause Cardiovascular Disease and Type 2 Diabetes?

Under normal circumstances, insulin exerts anti-atherogenic and anti-inflammatory actions in the endothelial cells and vascular smooth muscle cells lining the blood vessels (Wang *et al.*, 2004). Insulin inhibits the expression of adhesion molecules, monocyte chemo-attractant protein-1, and the inflammatory transcription factor, NF-kappa B. However, in the presence of insulin resistance (i.e. with impaired PI 3-kinase signaling), hyperinsulinemia appears to exert adverse effects on the arterial wall. Compensatory hyperinsulinemia becomes pro-atherogenic by stimulating both the MAP-kinase signaling pathway and excessive prenylation of Ras and Rho proteins (Figure 47.3). Hence, management of insulin-resistant individuals must include effective measures to improve insulin sensitivity as well as decrease ambient insulinemia. The metabolic stages in the transition from normal glucose tolerance

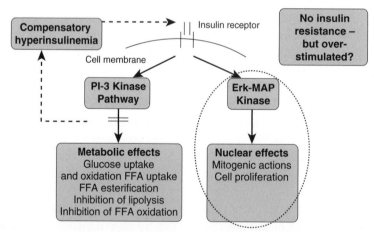

FIG. 47.3 Two major pathways are stimulated when insulin binds to insulin receptors on cell membranes of insulin-sensitive tissues: phosphatidyl inositol-3 kinase and MAP-kinase. Insulin resistance appears to originate downstream of the insulin receptor in the PI-3 kinase pathway involved in the metabolism of carbohydrates, fats, and proteins but not in the MAP-kinase pathway. Compensatory hyperinsulinemia resulting from insulin resistance in the PI-3 kinase pathway can mean overstimulation of the MAP-kinase pathway, with implications for cell growth, multiplication, and differentiation. Modified from Draznin (2008).

BOX 47.1   How insulin resistance causes type 2 diabetes

Stage 1. Normal glucose tolerance, mild insulin resistance, compensatory hyperinsulinemia

Stage 2. Glucose tolerance begins to deteriorate; postprandial hyperglycemia becomes common

Stage 3. Impaired glucose tolerance worsens, marked fasting and postprandial hyperinsulinemia

Stage 4. Beta-cells begin to fail, fasting and postprandial insulinemia declines, marked fasting and postprandial hyperglycemia

Stage 5. Beta-cell mass declines, insulin replacement may be necessary

to beta-cell failure and type 2 diabetes are described in Box 47.1.

What Can We Do to Maximize Insulin Sensitivity?

The most important environmental and modifiable factors that worsen insulin resistance are excessive body weight, physical inactivity, unhealthy diet, and smoking. Increased muscle mass and lower abdominal fat mass each markedly improve insulin sensitivity. Hence a combination of weight loss and physical activity, particularly resistance exercise, is the ideal lifestyle intervention to reduce the risk of type 2 diabetes and cardiovascular disease.

However, diet composition has been shown to have a separate additional effect. Observational studies and intervention trials have shown that the macronutrient distribution (i.e. the ratio of fat:carbohydrate:protein energy) and the quality of individual macronutrients directly influence insulin sensitivity. In particular, the amount and quality of fat and carbohydrate are factors involved in the development of insulin resistance and type 2 diabetes.

Diet Composition and Insulin Resistance

The effect of dietary fat and carbohydrate on insulin sensitivity have been debated for decades. Some of the controversy stems from divergent findings in animals vs. humans and in differing study designs. Insulin resistance can be induced in animal models by diets high in fat, sucrose, or fructose. However, a single bout of exercise or a high-starch meal can completely reverse the defect. In humans, some studies suggest that a high intake of fat is associated with impaired insulin sensitivity but this may be modified by the type of fat and by the type of subject. Several studies indicate that a diet high in saturated fat may be especially deleterious in physically inactive, sedentary individuals.

Free fatty acids (FFA) are thought to be involved in the early stages of insulin resistance when subjects are still normoglycemic. In skeletal muscle, FFA inhibit insulin-stimulated glucose uptake at the level of glucose transport and/or phosphorylation through mechanisms that involve intramyocellular accumulation of diacylglycerol and long-chain acyl-CoA, activation of protein kinase C (PKC), and decreased tyrosine phosphorylation of insulin receptor substrate 1/2 (Boden, 2004). In liver, plasma FFA within the physiological range cause insulin resistance along with increased liver diacylglycerol content and higher activity of serine/threonine kinases. Expression of proinflammatory nuclear factors and cytokines is also increased (Boden *et al.*, 2005).

Using clamp studies in humans, Vessby (2000) was the first to show that insulin resistance could be related to the fatty acid composition of the diet. High proportions of saturated fatty acids and low proportions of unsaturated fatty acids characterized the serum cholesterol esters of healthy 50-year-old men who later developed type 2 diabetes. Later, fatty acid composition of the phospholipids in the skeletal muscle cell membranes was found to be directly related to insulin sensitivity in healthy men (Borkman *et al.*, 1993). Specifically, the sum of the proportions of long-chain fatty acids with 20–22 carbohydrate atoms correlated strongly with insulin sensitivity. Unfortunately, the fatty acid pattern of skeletal muscle is influenced not just by diet but also by the degree of physical activity and by muscle fiber composition. None the less, the implication is that if dietary fat composition is changed from more saturated to more unsaturated under strictly controlled isoenergetic conditions, then insulin sensitivity should improve.

Unfortunately, nutrition science is not that simple. Well-designed, but short (usually 3–4 weeks) studies in lean, healthy subjects comparing the effects of changes in dietary fatty acids on insulin sensitivity have uniformly shown negative results (Vessby, 2000). Similarly, placebo-controlled studies on supplementation with fish oil or n-3 fatty acids have shown no effect. Animal studies, however, suggest that n-3 fatty acids improve insulin sensitivity, and it is conceivable that longer timeframes are needed to cause a change in human skeletal muscle phospholipids.

Two well-designed longer-term studies stand out. The KANWU study included 162 healthy subjects who received isoenergetic diets for 3 months containing either a high proportion of saturated fatty acids (SAFA) or monounsaturated (MUFA) acids (Vessby *et al.*, 2001). Within each group there was a second assignment to fish oil supplements or placebo. Insulin sensitivity as assessed by the frequently sampled intravenous glucose tolerance test (FSIVGTT) was significantly impaired by the SAFA diet (−10%) but did not change on the MUFA diet. However, the beneficial effects of MUFA were *not* seen when total fat intake exceeded 37%E (the median level of participants). Addition of n-3 fatty acids did not influence insulin sensitivity, and neither diet altered insulin secretion.

The second study (Due *et al.*, 2008) compared three diets over 6 months. Forty-six obese individuals were randomly assigned to one of three diets after ≥8% weight loss: a diet high in MUFA (40%E as fat, 45% as carbohydrate), a low-fat diet (25%E as fat, 60% as carbohydrate), and a control diet with 35% energy as fat (>15% as saturated fat, 50% as carbohydrate). Protein accounted for 15% of energy in all three diets. At the end of the 6 months, the high-fat/high-MUFA diet had improved insulin resistance (according to the HOMA score) by 12%, while the control diet and the low-fat diet had worsened insulin resistance (by 23% and 16% respectively). This study therefore clearly indicated that both high-carbohydrate and high-saturated-fat diets were each capable of worsening insulin resistance. Taken together, these and other findings suggest that, at fat intake close to average in industrialized nations (i.e. 32–37%E), it is preferable to maintain higher fat intake but increase the proportion of MUFA or PUFA fatty acids, rather than increase the percentage energy derived from carbohydrate.

Dietary Carbohydrates and Insulin Sensitivity

Like fat, the quantity and quality of carbohydrate can influence insulin sensitivity. In a cross-sectional analysis of ~3000 individuals in the Framingham Offspring Study, whole grains, total fiber from all sources, as well as fiber from cereals and fruit, were inversely related to HOMA–insulin resistance (McKeown *et al.*, 2004). There was no relationship with total carbohydrate intake or intake of refined grains. Dietary glycemic index (GI) and glycemic load (GL) were also directly related to insulin resistance, with approximately 10% more insulin resistance in the highest quintile of GI than in the lowest.

Some high-carbohydrate diets appear to have beneficial effects on insulin sensitivity. In healthy, young persons, isoenergetic substitution of high-fibre carbohydrate foods (to 57%E as carbohydrate) for saturated fatty acids improved insulin sensitivity within 4 weeks (Perez-Jimenez *et al.*, 2001). In this instance, the proportions of whole grains, simple sugars and dietary GI of this high-carbohydrate diet may have been critical, each with independent effects on insulin sensitivity. Indeed, carbohydrates consumed without fiber may produce detrimental effects (Due *et al.*, 2008). In individuals with diabetes, higher carbohydrate intake has the potential to raise postprandial glucose and increase insulin demand, an effect that might worsen insulin resistance. However, under metabolic ward conditions for 21 days, Garg *et al.* (1988) showed that hepatic and peripheral insulin sensitivity as assessed by the glucose clamp remained unchanged in 10 type 2 patients on either a high-carbohydrate (60%E) or low-carbohydrate (35%E) diet, matched for fiber. The patients in this study were treated with insulin, a factor that may fundamentally affect the ability to metabolize a high-carbohydrate meal.

Higher whole-grain intake has been directly correlated with insulin sensitivity in cross-sectional studies in which insulin sensitivity was assessed by the FSIVGTT (Liese *et al.*, 2003). A well-designed but small intervention study incorporated 6–10 servings of breakfast cereal, bread, rice, pasta, muffins, cookies, and snacks from either whole or refined grains (in both cases mostly ground to flour) in a diet containing 55%E from carbohydrate and 30%E from fat. Using the glucose clamp, insulin sensitivity was higher after 6 weeks on the whole-grain diet compared with a similar period on the refined-grain diet (Pereira *et al.*, 2002). Unfortunately, this finding was not confirmed in the larger WHOLEheart Study in which 60–120 g/day whole-grain foods were ingested for up to 16 weeks (Brownlee *et al.*, 2010). However, the modified QUICKI method used to assess insulin sensitivity may not have been sensitive enough to detect any difference.

Sucrose and Fructose

The effect of fructose and sucrose on insulin sensitivity remains controversial. Studies in animals, often fed extremely high intakes (e.g. 70% of total energy) or in solution in place of water, have shown a detrimental effect of fructose and sucrose compared with starch or glucose (Daly *et al.*, 1997). When fructose and glucose were compared directly, fructose was found to be the culpable moiety.

The evidence in humans, however, suggests that fructose and sucrose in realistic amounts might have beneficial effects on insulin sensitivity. In lean, young, healthy males, a diet containing 25% sucrose produced higher insulin sensitivity as assessed in a two-step clamp procedure than a diet containing 1% sucrose (Kiens and Richter, 1996). Similarly, a study in people with type 2 diabetes showed that a diet with 10% fructose produced a 34% improvement in insulin sensitivity measured by the euglycemic–hyperinsulinemic clamp (Koivisto and Yki-Jarvinen, 1993). In this study, patients lived in a hospital environment and all food was provided. Finally, using the glucose clamp, no effects on insulin sensitivity were noted after 3 months of a 13% fructose vs. sucrose diet (Thorburn et al., 1988). It is conceivable, however, that at very high intakes (>30%E), sucrose and fructose have adverse effects on insulin sensitivity.

Low-Glycemic-Index Diets

Low-glycemic-index (GI) diets in which the carbohydrates are more slowly digested and absorbed, resulting in lower postprandial glycemia, have been associated with improved insulin sensitivity in some studies but not others. Glucose uptake was 45% higher during the clamp procedure in people with type 2 diabetes who ate a low-GI diet for 4 weeks compared with a macronutrient-matched high-GI diet (Rizkalla et al., 2004). The alpha-glucosidase inhibitor, Acarbose, which slows carbohydrate digestion but is not absorbed into the systemic circulation, also produces improvements in insulin sensitivity (Holman et al., 1999). Low-GI diets improved insulin sensitivity in women with polycystic ovary syndrome as judged by the glucose tolerance test-based insulin sensitivity index (Marsh et al., 2010). Low-GI diets did not improve insulin sensitivity as judged by the glucose clamp in lean, active, young males (Kiens and Richter, 1996). In older, obese individuals a 7-day low-GI diet combined with exercise training improved clamp-derived insulin sensitivity just as well as a high-GI diet + exercise although there were greater benefits of the low-GI diet on systolic blood pressure and VO$_2$ max (Solomon et al., 2010).

Micronutrients and Insulin Sensitivity

Insulin sensitivity has also been related to intake of specific micronutrients. Magnesium is an important co-factor for enzymes involved in carbohydrate metabolism, and magnesium deficiency as judged by serum and dietary magnesium concentration is associated with insulin resistance and increased risk of type 2 diabetes (Huerta et al., 2005). In randomized controlled trials, magnesium supplements given to deficient subjects with type 2 diabetes improved HOMA–insulin resistance (Rodriguez-Moran and Guerrero-Romero, 2003).

The ability of chromium to improve insulin sensitivity remains controversial. Chromium is clearly essential for carbohydrate metabolism but it is widely available in the diet and deficiency states are rare. There is growing evidence that chromium supplementation, particularly at higher doses (1000 µg/day) in the form of chromium picolinate, is safe and may improve insulin sensitivity and glucose tolerance (Cefalu and Hu, 2004).

Vitamin intake and status may also play a role in maintenance of insulin sensitivity. Lipid oxidation, for example, might be a mechanism contributing to impaired mitochondrial function. Variations in insulin-mediated glucose disposal were observed in healthy individuals according to plasma concentrations of lipid-soluble antioxidant vitamins including lutein, carotenoids, and tocopherols (Facchini et al., 2000). But in other cross-sectional studies, antioxidant vitamins E and C, showed no relationship to insulin sensitivity as judged by the FSIVGTT (Sanchez-Lugo et al., 1997). The concentration of 25(OH)vitamin D correlated independently with clamp-derived insulin sensitivity in a study of 126 healthy, glucose-tolerant individuals living in California (Chiu et al., 2004). Those with hypovitaminosis D were also three times more likely to have the metabolic syndrome. Salt sensitivity of blood pressure, as judged by the difference in blood pressure after a high vs. low sodium diet, was also strongly associated with insulin resistance in lean essential hypertensive patients (Yatabe et al., 2010).

Diet and the Metabolic Syndrome

The best evidence that dietary changes can improve the metabolic syndrome comes from landmark studies in which intensive lifestyle interventions prevented or delayed progression from impaired glucose tolerance to type 2 diabetes mellitus (Tuomilehto et al., 2001; Diabetes Prevention Program Research Group, 2002). Both studies employed low-fat, high-carbohydrate diets (30% of energy from fat, 10% from saturated fat) in combination with physical activity to achieve the goal of weight loss. These findings have since been perceived as a rational basis for recommending low-fat, high-carbohydrate diets. Unfortunately, weight loss per se likely played the most important role, and the superiority of low-fat diets for those with the metabolic syndrome is questionable.

In intervention trials, increased carbohydrate intake is well known to increase serum triglycerides and lower HDL, two markers of the metabolic syndrome (Garg, 1998). Indeed the similarity implies that high-carbohydrate diets of a certain nature play an etiological role in the metabolic syndrome. Several meta-analyses and reviews have concluded that low-carbohydrate, high-protein diets (Halton and Hu, 2004), low-glycemic-index (GI) or low-glycemic-load (GL) diets (Thomas *et al.*, 2007; Livesey *et al.*, 2008; Thomas and Elliott, 2009), and Mediterranean-style diets (Shai *et al.*, 2008) may be more effective (or just as effective) for improving components of the insulin resistance syndrome as traditional low-fat, high-carbohydrate diets. This higher effectiveness holds true over both the shorter and the longer term. Some studies suggest that these alternative dietary approaches may also be more successful for preventing weight regain than low-fat, high-carbohydrate diets.

In prospective observational studies, carbohydrate intake (whether high or low) is not usually an independent predictor of the development of type 2 diabetes or cardiovascular disease. In meta-analyses, however, quality of carbohydrate intake as assessed as the GI or GL shows a consistent positive relationship to the risk of type 2 diabetes and CVD despite non-significant findings in some individual prospective studies (Barclay *et al.*, 2008). The highest relative risks (>2) were observed among those with both a higher dietary GI or GL and lower (cereal) fiber intake. Recently, some prospective cohort studies have demonstrated that higher intake of high-GI carbohydrates, but not low-GI carbohydrates, is associated with greater risk of developing CVD (Sieri *et al.*, 2010). Similarly, there is increased risk of type 2 diabetes and overweight associated with dietary patterns that are characterized by higher intakes of refined grains or white bread, ready-to-eat breakfast cereals, sugar-sweetened beverages, potatoes or French fries, sweets or sweet bakery products (Buyken *et al.*, 2010). In contrast, a protective pattern commonly included carbohydrate choices such as fruits, vegetables, legumes, wholemeal or whole-grain bread, and high-fiber breakfast cereals. Finally, greater adherence to the "Alternative Healthy Eating Index," a set of dietary guidelines which targets fruits, vegetables, the ratio of white to red meat, the ratio of polyunsaturated to saturated fat, fiber, nuts, soy, and alcohol intake, was associated with reversion of the metabolic syndrome over a 5-year period

of study in participants in the Whitehall II Study (Akbaraly *et al.*, 2010).

Taken together, these studies imply that dietary approaches that reduce the risk of developing type 2 diabetes or CVD share a unifying mechanism of reduced postprandial glycemia and insulinemia despite variable macronutrient distribution. It is possible that a diet that facilitates reduced glycemia without increasing dyslipidemia is likely to improve insulin sensitivity and the metabolic syndrome, and relieve the burden on the beta-cell The least effective (or even most damaging) diet would be one that increased postprandial glycemia and placed extra demands on beta-cell function (Figure 47.4). These adverse effects will be most detrimental for individuals with insulin resistance. Conventional low-fat, high-carbohydrate diets may therefore not be the optimal dietary approach for persons at risk of developing the metabolic syndrome and its sequelae.

Implications for Management

The triad of metabolic syndrome, insulin resistance, and overweight/obesity are strongly associated. Reducing weight in people who are overweight/obese compared with their population norm results in improvement in insulin resistance and the clinical manifestations of the metabolic syndrome. Therefore the aim of management should be weight reduction and sustained weight-loss maintenance through increased physical activity and dietary modification. Reduction in total energy intake is usually required to achieve weight loss. While research continues into other specific dietary recommendations, some general conclusions can be drawn from the literature. Salt reduction will assist with blood-pressure lowering. Reducing saturated fat and total carbohydrate intake will assist with controlling the typical lipid abnormalities seen in the metabolic syndrome. Avoiding high total carbohydrate intake, increasing fiber intake, and preferentially consuming low-GI carbohydrates will assist with controlling the glucose intolerance associated with the metabolic syndrome and help prevent progression to type 2 diabetes.

Future Directions

The molecular basis of insulin resistance, its role in health and disease, and the role of diet composition in worsening or improving insulin sensitivity present continuing challenges to research scientists the world over. The recogni-

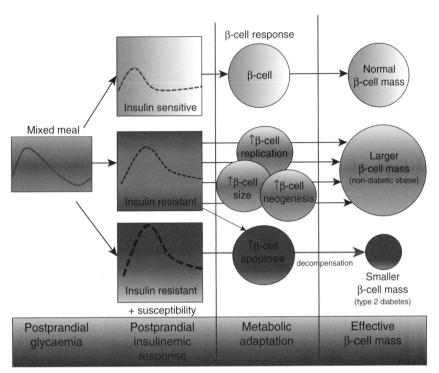

FIG. 47.4 A tenuous balance exists between insulin resistance and an effective beta-cell mass. For the most part, the beta-cell mass adapts adequately to compensate for changes in the metabolic load. However, beta-cells can be pushed too far in susceptible individuals. Poor diets can worsen insulin resistance and contribute to an overwhelming metabolic load. Eventually the beta-cell mass fails to compensate for insulin resistance, and type 2 diabetes ensues. This failure may be caused by a marked increase in beta-cell apoptosis, most likely induced by a combination of chronic postprandial hyperglycemia and hyperlipidemia, and/or cytokines that interfere with the signaling pathways that maintain normal beta-cell growth and survival. Of all tissues, the beta-cells in particular are especially sensitive to endoplasmic reticulum and oxidative stress caused by high throughput through the mitochondrial chain. The net effect is a reduction in functional beta-cell mass in the type 2 diabetic state. Data from Rhodes (2005). Adapted from Buyken *et al.* (2010).

tion of a "metabolic syndrome" might prompt some health professionals to assess related risk factors when one risk factor is detected. However, a recent WHO Expert Consultation (Simmons *et al.*, 2010) recommended that the metabolic syndrome not be applied as a clinical diagnosis. Rather, it should be considered as a premorbid condition, and individuals with established diabetes and known CVD should be excluded.

Suggestions for Further Reading

Alberti, K.G.M.M., Eckel, R.H., Grundy, S.M., *et al.* (2009) Harmonizing the Metabolic Syndrome: A Joint Interim Statement of the International Diabetes Federation Task Force on Epidemiology and Prevention; National Heart, Lung, and Blood Institute; American Heart Association; World Heart Federation; International Atherosclerosis Society; and International Association for the Study of Obesity. *Circulation* **120**, 1640–1645.

Buyken, A., Mitchell, P., Ceriello, A., *et al.* (2010) Optimal dietary approaches for prevention of type 2 diabetes: a lifecourse perspective. *Diabetologia* **53**, 406–418.

Simmons, R., Alberti, K., Gale, E., *et al.* (2010) The metabolic syndrome: useful concept or clinical tool? Report of a WHO Expert Consultation. *Diabetologia* **53**, 600–605.

Zeitler, P.S. and Nadeau, K.J. (2008) *Insulin Resistance. Childhood Precursors and Adult Disease*. Humana Press, Totowa, NJ.

References

Akbaraly, T.N., Singh-Manoux, A., Tabak, A.G., *et al.* (2010) Overall diet history and reversibility of the metabolic syndrome over 5 years: the Whitehall II Prospective Cohort Study. *Diabetes Care* **33**, 2339–2341.

Alberti, K.G.M.M., Eckel, R.H., Grundy, S.M., *et al.* (2009) Harmonizing the Metabolic Syndrome: A Joint Interim Statement of the International Diabetes Federation Task Force on Epidemiology and Prevention; National Heart, Lung, and Blood Institute; American Heart Association; World Heart Federation; International Atherosclerosis Society; and International Association for the Study of Obesity. *Circulation* **120**, 1640–1645.

Balkau, B., Mhamdi, L., Oppert, J.-M., *et al.* (2008) Physical activity and insulin sensitivity. *Diabetes* **57**, 2613–2618.

Barclay, A., Petocz, P., McMillan-Price, J., *et al.* (2008) Glycemic index, glycemic load and chronic disease risk – a meta-analysis of observational studies. *Am J Clin Nutr* **87**, 627–637.

Bergman, R.N., Zaccaro, D.J., Watanabe, R.M., *et al.* (2003) Minimal model-based insulin sensitivity has greater heritability and a different genetic basis than homeostasis model assessment or fasting insulin. *Diabetes* **52**, 2168–2174.

Boden, G. (2004) Free fatty acids as target for therapy. *Curr Opin Endocrinol Diabetes Obes* **11**, 258–263.

Boden, G., She, P., Mozzoli, M., *et al.* (2005) Free fatty acids produce insulin resistance and activate the proinflammatory nuclear factor-kappaB pathway in rat liver. *Diabetes* **54**, 3458–3465.

Bogardus, C. (1993) Insulin resistance in the pathogenesis of NIDDM in Pima Indians. *Diabetes Care* **16**, 228–231.

Borkman, M., Storlien, L., Pan, D., *et al.* (1993) The relationship between insulin sensitivity and the fatty acid composition of skeletal-muscle phospholipids. *N Engl J Med* **328**, 238–244.

Brownlee, I.A., Moore, C., Chatfield, M., *et al.* (2010) Markers of cardiovascular risk are not changed by increased whole-grain intake: the WHOLEheart study, a randomised, controlled dietary intervention. *Br J Nutr* **104**, 125–134.

Butte, N. (2000) Carbohydrate and lipid metabolism in pregnancy: normal compared with gestational diabetes mellitus. *Am J Clin Nutr* **71**, 1256S–1261S.

Buyken, A., Mitchell, P., Ceriello, A., *et al.* (2010) Optimal dietary approaches for prevention of type 2 diabetes: a lifecourse perspective. *Diabetologia* **53**, 406–418.

Cefalu, W.T. and Hu, F.B. (2004) Role of chromium in human health and in diabetes. *Diabetes Care* **27**, 2741–2751.

Chiu, K.C., Chu, A., Go, V.L.W., *et al.* (2004) Hypovitaminosis D is associated with insulin resistance and {beta} cell dysfunction. *Am J Clin Nutr* **79**, 820–825.

Cnop, M., Landchild, M.J., Vidal, J., *et al.* (2002) The concurrent accumulation of intra-abdominal and subcutaneous fat explains the association between insulin resistance and plasma leptin concentrations. *Diabetes* **51**, 1005–1015.

Daly, M.E., Vale, C., and Walker, M. (1997) Dietary carbohydrates and insulin sensitivity. *Am J Clin Nutr* **66**, 1072–1085.

DeFronzo, R.A., Bonadonna, R.C., and Ferrannini, E. (1992) Pathogenesis of NIDDM: a balanced overview. *Diabetes Care* **15**, 318–368.

Diabetes Prevention Program Research Group (2002) Reduction in the incidence of type 2 diabetes with lifestyle intervention or metformin. *N Engl J Med* **346**, 393–403.

Dickinson, S., Colagiuri, S., Faramus, E., *et al.* (2002) Postprandial hyperglycemia and insulin sensitivity differ among lean young adults of different ethnicities. *J Nutr* **132**, 2574–2579.

Draznin, B. (2008) Molecular mechanisms of insulin resistance. In P. Zeitler and K. Nadeau (eds), *Insulin Resistance. Childhood Precursors and Adult Disease.* Humana Press, Totowa, NJ, pp. 95–108.

Due, A., Larsen, T.M., Mu, H., *et al.* (2008) Comparison of 3 ad libitum diets for weight-loss maintenance, risk of cardiovascular disease, and diabetes: a 6-mo randomized, controlled trial. *Am J Clin Nutr* **88**, 1232–1241.

Facchini, F., Hua, N., Abbasi, F., *et al.* (2001) Insulin resistance as a predictor of age-related diseases. *J Clin Endocrinol Metab* **86**, 3574–3578.

Facchini, F.S., Humphreys, M.H., Donascimento, C.A., *et al.* (2000) Relation between insulin resistance and plasma concentrations of lipid hydroperoxides, carotenoids, and tocopherols. *Am J Clin Nutr* **72**, 776–779.

Ford, E., Giles, W., and Mokdad, A. (2004) Increasing prevalence of the metabolic syndrome among U.S. adults. *Diabetes Care* **27**, 2444–2449.

Garg, A. (1998) High-monounsaturated-fat diets for patients with diabetes mellitus: a meta-analysis. *Am J Clin Nutr* **67**, 577S–582S.

Garg, A., Bonanome, A., Grundy, S.M., *et al.* (1988) Comparison of a high-carbohydrate diet with a high-monounsaturated-fat diet in patients with non-insulin-dependent diabetes mellitus. *N Engl J Med* **319**, 829–834.

Goran, M. and Gower, B. (2001) Longitudinal study on pubertal insulin resistance. *Diabetes* **50**, 2444–-2450.

Hales, C.N. and Barker, D.J.P. (2001) The thrifty phenotype hypothesis. *Br Med Bull* **60**, 5–20.

Halton, T.L. and Hu, F.B. (2004) The effects of high protein diets on thermogenesis, satiety and weight loss: a critical review. *J Am Coll Nutr* **23**, 373–385.

Helmerhorst, H.J.F., Wijndaele, K., Brage, S.R., *et al.* (2009) Objectively measured sedentary time may predict insulin resistance independent of moderate- and vigorous-intensity physical activity. *Diabetes* **58**, 1776–1779.

Himsworth, H. (1936) Diabetes mellitus: its differentiation into insulin-sensitive and insulin-insensitive sub-types. *Lancet* **227,** 127–130.

Hoehn, K.L., Salmon, A.B., Hohnen-Behrens, C., *et al.* (2009) Insulin resistance is a cellular antioxidant defense mechanism. *Proc Natl Acad Sci USA* **106,** 17787–17792.

Holman, R.R., Cull, C.A., and Turner, R.C. (1999) A randomized double-blind trial of acarbose in type 2 diabetes shows improved glycemic control over 3 years (UKPDS 44). *Diabetes Care* **22,** 960–964.

Hovi, P., Andersson, S., Eriksson, J.G., *et al.* (2007) Glucose regulation in young adults with very low birth weight. *N Engl J Med* **356,** 2053–2063.

Huerta, M.G., Roemmich, J.N., Kington, M.L., *et al.* (2005) Magnesium deficiency is associated with insulin resistance in obese children. *Diabetes Care* **28,** 1175–1181.

Kiens, B. and Richter, E. (1996) Types of carbohydrate in an ordinary diet affect insulin action and muscle substrates in humans. *Am J Clin Nutr* **63,** 47–53.

Koivisto, V.A. and Yki-Jarvinen, H. (1993) Fructose and insulin sensitivity in patients with type 2 diabetes. *J Intern Med* **233,** 145–153.

Liese, A.D., Roach, A.K., Sparks, K.C., *et al.* (2003) Whole-grain intake and insulin sensitivity: the Insulin Resistance Atherosclerosis Study. *Am J Clin Nutr* **78,** 965–971.

Lillioja, S., Mott, D.M., Howard, B.V., *et al.* (1988) Impaired glucose tolerance as a disorder of insulin action. *N Engl J Med* **318,** 1217–1225.

Livesey, G., Taylor, R., Hulshof, T., *et al.* (2008) Glycemic response and health – a systematic review and meta-analysis: relations between dietary glycemic properties and health outcomes. *Am J Clin Nutr* **87,** 258S–268S.

Low, C., Wang, L., Goalstone, M., *et al.* (2004) Molecular mechanisms of insulin resistance that impact cardiovascular biology. *Diabetes* **53,** 2735–2740.

Lowell, B. and Shulman, G. (2005) Mitochondrial dysfunction and type 2 diabetes. *Science* **307,** 384–387.

Luo, Z.-C., Delvin, E., Fraser, W.D., *et al.* (2010) Maternal glucose tolerance in pregnancy affects fetal insulin sensitivity. *Diabetes Care* **33,** 2055–2061.

Marsh, K.A., Steinbeck, K.S., Atkinson, F.S., *et al.* (2010) Effect of a low glycemic index compared with a conventional healthy diet on polycystic ovary syndrome. *Am J Clin Nutr* **92,** 83–92.

Matthews, D.R., Hosker, J., Redenski, A., *et al.* (1985) Homeostasis model assessment: insulin resistance and beta-cell function from fasting plasma glucose and insulin concentrations in man. *Diabetologia* **28,** 412–419.

McKeown, N., Meigs, J., Liu, S., *et al.* (2004) Carbohydrate nutrition, insulin resistance, and the prevalence of the metabolic syndrome in the Framingham offspring cohort. *Diabetes Care* **27,** 538–546.

McMillen, I. and Robinson, J. (2005) Developmental origins of the metabolic syndrome: prediction, plasticity, and programming. *Physiol Rev* **85,** 571–633.

Mikhail, N. (2009) The metabolic syndrome: insulin resistance. *Curr Hypertens Rep* **11,** 156–158.

Osei, K. and Schuster, D.P. (1994) Ethnic differences in secretion, sensitivity, and hepatic extraction of insulin in black and white Americans. *Diabet Med* **11,** 755–762.

Pereira, M., Jacobs, D., Pins, J., *et al.* (2002) Effect of whole grains on insulin sensitivity in overweight hyperinsulinemic adults. *Am J Clin Nutr* **75,** 848–855.

Perez-Jimenez, F., Lopez-Miranda, J., Pinillos, M., *et al.* (2001) A Mediterranean and a high carbohydrate diet improve glucose metabolism in healthy young persons. *Diabetologia* **44,** 2038–2043.

Reaven, G.M. (1988) Banting Lecture 1988. Role of insulin resistance in human disease. *Diabetes* **37,** 1595–1607.

Rhodes, C.J. (2005) Type 2 diabetes – a matter of beta-cell life and death? *Science* **307,** 380–384.

Rizkalla, S., Taghrid, L., Laromiguiere, M., *et al.* (2004) Improved plasma glucose control, whole-body glucose utilization, and lipid profile on a low-glycemic index diet in type 2 diabetic men: a randomized controlled trial. *Diab Care* **27,** 1866–1872.

Rodriguez-Moran, M. and Guerrero-Romero, F. (2003) Oral magnesium supplementation improves insulin sensitivity and metabolic control in type 2 diabetic subjects. *Diabetes Care* **26,** 1147–1152.

Sanchez-Lugo, L., Mayer-Davis, E., Howard, G., *et al.* (1997) Insulin sensitivity and intake of vitamins E and C in African American, Hispanic, and non-Hispanic white men and women: the Insulin Resistance and Atherosclerosis Study (IRAS). *Am J Clin Nutr* **66,** 1224–1231.

Shai, I., Schwarzfuchs, D., Henkin, Y., *et al.* (2008) Weight loss with a low-carbohydrate, Mediterranean, or low-fat diet. *N Engl J Med* **359,** 229–241.

Sieri, S., Krogh, V., Berrino, F., *et al.* (2010) Dietary glycemic load and index and risk of coronary heart disease in a large Italian cohort: the EPICOR study. *Arch Intern Med* **170,** 640–647.

Simmons, R., Alberti, K., Gale, E., *et al.* (2010) The metabolic syndrome: useful concept or clinical tool? Report of a WHO Expert Consultation. *Diabetologia* **53,** 600–605.

Solomon, T.P., Haus, J.M., Kelly, K.R., *et al.* (2010) A low, glycemic index diet combined with exercise reduces insulin resistance, postprandial hyperinsulinemia, and glucose-dependent insulinotropic polypeptide responses in obese, prediabetic humans. *The Am J Clin Nutr* **92** (6), 1359–1368.

Thomas, D. and Elliott, E. (2009) Low glycaemic index, or low glycaemic load, diets for diabetes mellitus. *Cochrane Database Syst Rev* CD006296.

Thomas, D., Elliott, E., and Baur, L. (2007) Low glycaemic index or low glycaemic load diets for overweight and obesity. *Cochrane Database Syst Rev* CD005105.

Thorburn, A., Crapo, P., Griver, K., *et al.* (1988) Insulin action and triglyceride turnover after long-term fructose feeding in subjects with non-insulin dependent diabetes-mellitus (NIDDM). *FASEB J* **2**, A1201–A1201.

Tuomilehto, J., Lindstrom, J., Eriksson, J.G., *et al.* (2001) Prevention of type 2 diabetes mellitus by changes in lifestyle among subjects with impaired glucose tolerance. *N Engl J Med* **344**, 1343–1350.

Vernon, R. (1989) Endocrine control of metabolic adaptation during lactation. *Proc Nutr Soc* **48**, 23–32.

Vessby, B. (2000) Dietary fat and insulin action in humans. *Br J Nutr* **83**, S91–S96.

Vessby, B., Uusitupa, M., Hermansen, K., *et al.* (2001) Insulin sensitivity in healthy men and women: the Kanwu study. *Diabetologia* **44**, 312–319.

Wang, C.C.L., Goalstone, M.L., and Draznin, B. (2004) Molecular mechanisms of insulin resistance that impact cardiovascular biology. *Diabetes* **53**, 2735–2740.

Wei, J.-N., Sung, F.-C., Li, C.-Y., *et al.* (2003) Low birth weight and high birth weight infants are both at an increased risk to have type 2 diabetes among schoolchildren in Taiwan. *Diabetes Care* **26**, 343–348.

Yatabe, M.S., Yatabe, J., Yoneda, M., *et al.* (2010) Salt sensitivity is associated with insulin resistance, sympathetic overactivity, and decreased suppression of circulating renin activity in lean patients with essential hypertension. *Am J Clin Nutr* **92**, 77–82.

48

ATHEROSCLEROTIC CARDIOVASCULAR DISEASE

SIMONE D. HOLLIGAN, BSc, MSc, CLAIRE E. BERRYMAN, BSc, LI WANG, BM,
MICHAEL R. FLOCK, BSc, KRISTINA A. HARRIS, BSc, AND
PENNY M. KRIS-ETHERTON, PhD, RD

The Pennsylvania State University, University Park, Pennsylvania, USA

Summary

Atherosclerotic cardiovascular disease (CVD) is initiated by a non-resolving inflammatory response, and later develops into a chronic disease in which genetic predisposition, diet, and lifestyle promote onset and progression. Modifiable CVD risk factors include overweight/obesity, elevated total cholesterol, low-density-lipoprotein (LDL) cholesterol and triglycerides, and low high-density-lipoprotein (HDL) cholesterol, elevated blood pressure, hyperglycemia, physical inactivity, cigarette smoking, stress, and an unhealthy dietary pattern. Effects of the macronutrients and selected vitamins, minerals, and antioxidants on CVD risk are reviewed. Combinations of various nutrients significantly reduce CVD risk factors. Furthermore, modifications in dietary patterns have been shown to reduce CVD risk by as much as 40%. Food-based dietary guidelines for reducing CVD risk are presented from various national and global health organizations. Efforts to manage co-morbidities such as obesity and diabetes also significantly impact disease risk. The need for population-wide strategies to curtail incidence of this epidemic is briefly discussed.

Introduction

Atherosclerotic cardiovascular disease is a leading cause of mortality, resulting in a third of all deaths globally, with 85% of the disease burden and mortality currently borne by low- and middle-income countries (WHO, 2004a). It is a multifactorial, chronic disease in which genetic predisposition, diet, and lifestyle are instrumental in its onset and disease progression. The term *atherosclerosis*, derived from the Greek words "*athere*" for gruel and "*skleros*" for

hard, was first coined by the German physician Felix Marchand in a paper he presented at the 21st Congress for Internal Medicine in 1904. More than a century later, this term is used to define the build-up of waxy plaque in an artery that leads to the occlusion of blood flow. Atherosclerosis is a "maladaptive, nonresolving inflammatory response" (Moore and Tabas, 2011) produced by the interactions among modified lipoproteins, monocyte-derived macrophages, and T-lymphocytes in the arterial wall (Glass and Witztum, 2001). The thrombus that is

Present Knowledge in Nutrition, Tenth Edition. Edited by John W. Erdman Jr, Ian A. Macdonald and Steven H. Zeisel.
© 2012 International Life Sciences Institute. Published 2012 by John Wiley & Sons, Inc.

formed in response to a ruptured or eroded atherosclerotic plaque leads to the progression of cardiovascular disease (CVD) and can result in a myocardial infarction or a stroke (Naghavi *et al.*, 2003a,b; Spagnoli *et al.*, 2004).

The role of nutrition in the initiation, progression, and reversal of CVD is well established. A heart-healthy diet has long been a focal point in prevention and treatment of CVD. As our knowledge base has expanded, it has become evident that nutrition affects CVD in a multitude of ways by targeting important risk factors. Moreover, although our understanding of the mechanisms by which diet affects CVD has increased impressively, there still are many frontiers of inquiry that remain to be resolved. In addition, the combination of nutrition and lifestyle changes also has proven beneficial. The purpose of this chapter is to review our current understanding of the role that nutrition plays in the prevention and treatment of CVD, and to provide an overview of the lifestyle behaviors that are recommended to decrease the risk of CVD.

Pathophysiology of Atherosclerotic Cardiovascular Disease (CVD)

Atherosclerotic Disease Progression

CVD is a chronic inflammatory disease mediated by endothelial damage and circulating blood lipids. An elevated cholesterol level is a contributing factor in atherogenesis (atherosclerotic plaque development) (Glass and Witztum, 2001). Low-density lipoprotein (LDL) modification, particularly by oxidation, contributes importantly to atherogenesis. Intrinsic factors such as antioxidant content, fatty acid composition, and particle size (small and dense sub-fractions of LDL are more susceptible to oxidation), and extrinsic factors including the surrounding pH, local antioxidant concentrations, and transition metal availability, increase the susceptibility of LDL to oxidation (Young and McEneny, 2001). LDL modification allows for its cellular uptake via the scavenger receptor and consequent promotion of atherogenesis. LDL oxidation is mediated in part by 15-lipoxygenase, myeloperoxidase, or nitric oxide synthase (NOS) (Glass and Witztum, 2001; Yoshida and Kisugi, 2010). Oxidized LDL (OxLDL) is atherogenic and is a direct and indirect chemoattractant for circulating monocytes (Quinn *et al.*, 1987), with the latter occurring via the release of monocyte chemoattractant protein-1 (MCP-1) from the endothelium (Cushing *et al.*, 1990). OxLDL inhibits the movement of the resident macrophages (Quinn *et al.*, 1987) and in turn

promotes the differentiation of monocytes into tissue macrophages via the release of macrophage colony-stimulating factor from the endothelial cells (Rajavashisth *et al.*, 1990). It also is a chemoattractant for T-lymphocytes (McMurray *et al.*, 1993) and is immunogenic, unlike its native form (Palinski *et al.*, 1989), in that it is cytotoxic to several cell types such as endothelial cells (Hessler *et al.*, 1983) and consequently may promote the loss of endothelial integrity (Young and McEneny, 2001). OxLDL also stimulates the release of interleukin-1β from macrophages (Thomas *et al.*, 1994), inhibits tumor necrosis factor expression (Hamilton *et al.*, 1990), inhibits endothelial cell-dependent arterial relaxation (Ohgushi *et al.*, 1993), and activates matrix-digesting enzymes that promote plaque instability (Xu *et al.*, 1999).

Endothelial Injury

Figure 48.1a shows the initiation of arterial plaque accumulation. Several events occur during the development of an atherosclerotic plaque and its progression towards a thrombotic event. The endothelium is sensitive to shear stress and the various hemodynamic conditions including branching, reverse flow, and low and oscillating shear stress which promote atherogenesis (Cunningham and Gotlieb, 2005). Susceptible blood vessels may contain lesion-prone regions consisting of leaky, activated, and dysfunctional endothelium (Davies *et al.*, 1988), where atherosclerotic lesions may develop. De-endothelialized or denuded areas may appear over advanced lesions as a result of the loss of endothelial cells, resulting in exposed sub-endothelial tissue with or without platelets adhering to the surface (Davies *et al.*, 1988). Lipoprotein particles (i.e. LDL) and other plasma molecules traverse the damaged endothelium into the intima or sub-endothelial space (Falk, 2006). Within the intima the lipoproteins are sequestered and modified, thereby contributing to their chemotaxic, pro-inflammatory, cytotoxic, and pro-atherogenic properties (Falk, 2006), thus initiating atherogenesis.

Inflammatory Response

The endothelium is activated by several atherogenic and pro-inflammatory particles (Falk, 2006) found in the circulation (Figure 48.1b). The endothelium in turn has increased expression of various cell adhesion molecules, such as the vascular cell adhesion molecule-1 (VCAM-1), which results in the recruitment of monocytes and T-lymphocytes (Falk, 2006). Other molecules also participate in the recruitment of blood-borne cells to the

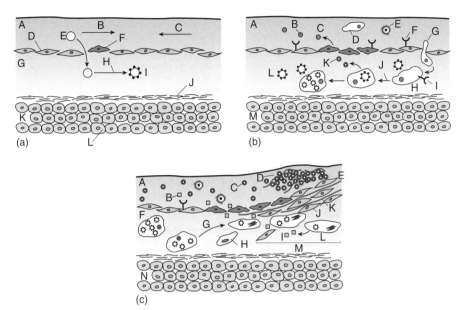

FIG. 48.1 **(a) Endothelial injury**. The endothelium is sensitive to shear stress and varying hemodynamic conditions. Susceptible regions of the endothelium contain lesion-prone areas with leaky, activated, and dysfunctional endothelial cells. Lipoprotein particles extravasate through the defective endothelium into the intima or sub-endothelial space. Within the intima the lipoproteins are retained and oxidized. Oxidization occurs via 15-lipoxygenase, myeloperoxidase, or nitric oxide synthase (NOS). OxLDL is highly chemotactic, cytotoxic, pro-inflammatory, and pro-atherogenic. **A** – lumen, **B** – blood flow, **C** – reverse flow, **D** – endothelial cell, **E** – LDL particle, **F** – dysfunctional endothelial cell, **G** – intima, **H** – 15-lipoxygenase, myeloperoxidase, nitric oxide synthase (NOS), **I** – oxidized LDL (OxLDL), **J** – internal elastic lamina, **K** – media, **L** – smooth muscle cell. **(b) Inflammatory response**. The activated endothelium increases its expression of vascular cell adhesion molecule-1 (VCAM-1) and the release of monocyte chemoattractant protein-1 (MCP-1) to enable the recruitment of monocytes and T-lymphocytes. Adhesion to the endothelium is followed by trans-endothelial migration into the intima. OxLDL and MCP-1 are the most potent atherogenic chemoattractants. Monocytes within the intima differentiate into macrophages and undergo receptor-mediated endocytosis of oxLDL via their scavenger receptors. These LDL-laden macrophages further release the pro-inflammatory cytokine known as interleukin 1-β and later develop into foam cells; foam cells are white in appearance due to the presence of several lipid-containing vacuoles. **A** – lumen, **B** – monocyte chemotactic protein-1 (MCP-1), **C**- release of MCP-1, **D** – monocyte, **E** – T-lymphocyte, **F** – vascular cell adhesion molecule -1 (VCAM-1), **G** – monocyte extravasation, **H** – macrophage, **I** – scavenger receptor, **J** – receptor-mediated endocytosis, **K** – interleukin-1β, **L** – OxLDL, **M** – intima. **(c) Fatty streak development and thrombosis**. Foam cells endocytose until death by either apoptosis or necrosis. Death of the foam cells forms a soft, unstable, lipid-rich core and results in the release of tissue factor and various matrix-degrading, proteolytic enzymes. The smooth muscle cells respond to the injury by migrating to form a collagen-rich matrix to stabilize the lipid-rich core or fatty streak. Release of tissue factor into the bloodstream initiates coagulation by the rapid recruitment of platelets and clotting factors to result in the formation of a fibrin-rich cap over the damaged endothelium and fatty streak. This fibro-proliferative process eventually leads to thrombosis, with an obstruction of blood flow within the arterial lumen. **A** – lumen, **B** – tissue factor, **C** – platelet, **D** – aggregation, **E** – fibrin, **F** – intima, **G** – necrosis or apoptosis, **H** – migrated smooth muscle cell, **I** – tissue factor, **J** – smooth muscle cell, **K** – collagen, **L** – necrotic foam cell, **M** – fatty streak, **N** – media.

atherosclerotic lesion, including intercellular adhesion molecule-1 (ICAM-1), E selectin, and P selectin (Libby, 2002; Hansson, 2005). Adhesion to the endothelium is followed by trans-endothelial migration mediated via one or more chemotactic cytokines (Falk, 2006). OxLDL and MCP-1 are the most potent atherogenic chemoattractants (Libby, 2002). In the intima the monocytes differentiate into macrophages and undergo receptor-mediated endocytosis of the atherogenic lipoproteins through their scavenger receptors and develop into foam cells. These scavenger receptors differ from the native LDL receptor in that their expression is not down-regulated with an increased cholesterol accumulation (Falk, 2006). In an abundance of atherogenic lipoproteins the activated macrophages or foam cells endocytose until death by either apoptosis or necrosis. Death of the foam cells leads to the formation of a soft and unstable lipid-rich core within the atherosclerotic plaque (Falk, 2006). In conditions of low LDL and high HDL levels, the foam cells may shrink through the efflux of cellular cholesterol to extracellular HDL mediated by membrane transporters (Glass and Witztum, 2001; Lewis and Rader, 2005), creating the initial step in reverse cholesterol transport (RCT). This process was first described by Glomset in 1968 in relation to the shuttling of peripheral cholesterol (Cuchel and Rader, 2006). Moderate to high levels of HDL have been found to be cardioprotective since the risk of atherosclerosis is inversely related to HDL levels (Tall *et al.*, 2000) with the protective effect due to the mediation of RCT by HDL (Burgess *et al.*, 2006). In this process HDL particles remove free cholesterol from the macrophages and transport these to the liver for excretion in the bile (Burgess *et al.*, 2006). Since HDL-mediated RCT contributes to a decrease in tissue cholesterol levels, increased RCT stimulates atheroregression and decreases the risk of atherosclerotic plaque development.

Fatty Streak and Plaque Formation

Progression of atherosclerosis occurs as the result of the development of a foam-cell lesion known as a fatty streak (Falk, 2006), as shown in Figure 48.1c. This is accompanied by a fibro-proliferative response mediated by the intimal smooth muscle cells (Falk, 2006). The smooth muscle cells produce a collagen-rich matrix that stabilizes the atherosclerotic plaques. With further progression, endothelial cells, macrophages, and smooth muscle cells die by either apoptosis or necrosis, and it is the breakdown

of the foam cells and the smooth muscle cells that leads to the development of a destabilized lipid-rich core with a fragile, fibrous cap (Geng and Libby, 2002). Breakdown of foam cells also is detrimental in that tissue factor is released and several matrix-degrading (proteolytic) enzymes are expressed, such as matrix metalloproteinases, which further destabilize the plaque and induce thrombogenesis (Libby, 2002). A relatively large atherosclerotic plaque is prone to plaque rupture where a defect or gap occurs in the fibrous cap leading to the loss of the separation between its lipid-rich core and the circulating blood (Schaar *et al.*, 2004). This results in a cascade of events beginning with plaque rupture followed by platelet aggregation to the exposed sub-endothelial tissue and fibrin formation over the ruptured plaque. The rapid onset of platelet aggregation creates an obstruction leading to a decrease in blood flow (Falk, 2006). Plaque rupture is the cause of about 76% of all fatal heart attacks worldwide that are caused by coronary thrombosis (Falk *et al.*, 2004).

Coronary Heart Disease, Stroke, and Peripheral Vascular Disease

Cardiovascular disease is defined as any disease plaguing the heart and its associated blood vessels. These include a variety of diseases including coronary heart disease, stroke, and peripheral vascular disease.

Coronary heart disease (CHD), also known as coronary artery disease (CAD), is disease of the coronary arteries, which provide the heart's oxygen and nutrient requirements (Morrow and Gersh, 2007). These arteries are at high risk for narrowing when cholesterol deposits (i.e. plaques) build up inside the artery. With significant narrowing of the coronary arteries the heart's blood supply is significantly decreased, resulting in pain or angina. If the plaque ruptures, a thrombus (blood clot) forms and may obstruct the artery, thereby decreasing blood flow and frequently causing a myocardial infarction or stroke. The stoppage of blood flow to the heart also causes the affected muscle to die, resulting in diminished function of the heart.

Stroke, also known as a cerebrovascular accident, is another form of cardiovascular disease that exists in two forms. Ischemic stroke results when the formation of a plaque blocks the blood flow within the artery leading to the brain, while hemorrhagic stroke results after the rupture of a blood vessel, and is characterized by uncontrolled bleeding into the surrounding tissue; ischemic and

TABLE 48.1 Modifiable and non-modifiable risk factors for atherosclerosis

Non-modifiable	Modifiable	Goals for modifiable risk factors
Age	Weight	BMI: 18.5–24.9 kg/m²
Sex	Lipid profile	Total cholesterol: <200 mg/dl (5.2 mmol/L)
Family history/ genetics		LDL-C[a]: Very high-risk individuals, <70 mg/dl (1.8 mmol/L) High-risk individuals, <100 mg/dl (2.6 mmol/L) with optional goal of <70 mg/dl (1.8 mmol/L) Moderate-risk individuals, <130 mg/dl (3.4 mmol/L) with optional goal of <100 mg/dl (2.6 mmol/L)
Race/ethnicity		
		HDL-C: Men: ≥40 mg/dl (1.0 mmol/L) Women: ≥50 mg/dl (1.3 mmol/L)
		Triglycerides: <150 mg/dl (1.7 mmol/L)
	Blood pressure	Systolic: <120 mmHg Diastolic: <80 mmHg
	Glycemic control	Fasting blood glucose: <100 mg/dl (5.6 mmol/L)
	Physical activity	150 minutes of moderate activity or 75 minutes of vigorous activity per week
	Smoking	Stop smoking
	Diet	Follow a healthy diet
	Stress	Keep stress as low as possible

[a]Goals for LDL-C levels are those recommended by the National Cholesterol Education Program Adult Treatment Panel III (Grundy et al., 2004). Very high-risk individuals are persons with established CHD, who also have diabetes, metabolic syndrome or other poorly controlled CVD risk factors. Individuals at high risk are those with established CHD, diabetes, or with two or more CVD risk factors which cause a greater than 20% risk of developing CHD within a 10-year period. Individuals at moderate risk refer to those with two or more risk factors for CHD, giving a 10–20% risk of developing CHD within a 10-year period.

hemorrhagic stroke represent ~80% and ~20% of all global cases respectively (World Health Organization, 2004b). Stoppage of blood flow for more than a few seconds leads to the loss of oxygen to cells within the brain, causing cell death and permanent brain damage.

Peripheral vascular disease is disease of the blood vessels outside of the brain and heart (World Health Organization, 2004b). Inflammation, tissue damage, and plaque accumulation cause narrowing of the blood vessels leading to the periphery – the arms, legs, stomach, and kidneys – and results in damage to these organs and tissues.

Risk Factors for Atherosclerosis

Atherosclerosis is affected by abnormal blood lipid and lipoprotein levels, elevated blood pressure, and smoking,

as well as other risk factors (Glass and Witztum, 2001). Approximately 20–25% of initial vascular events occur in patients with one major CVD risk factor, with about one-half of those having elevated LDL cholesterol (LDL-C) (Ridker et al., 2004). Recommended nutrition and medical interventions target modifiable risk factors and can significantly reduce the progression of atherosclerosis and CVD. These modifiable and non-modifiable risk factors are presented in Table 48.1 (Glass and Witztum, 2001; Sacco, 2011).

Persons diagnosed with metabolic syndrome (MetS) are at increased risk for developing cardiovascular disease. An individual with MetS, also known as insulin resistance syndrome, is classified by the International Diabetes Federation (IDF, 2006) as having central obesity, defined as a waist circumference of ≥94 cm for Europid men and ≥80 cm for Europid women, and any two of the four

TABLE 48.2   Inclusion criteria for metabolic syndrome diagnosis

International Diabetes Federation	World Health Organization	American Heart Association and National Heart, Lung, and Blood Institute
Individual must have central obesity classified as having a waist circumference of ≥94 cm (37 in) for Europid men or ≥80 cm (32 in) for Europid women[a], plus any two of the following factors:	Large waist circumference: ≥94 cm (37 in) in men and women Waist-to-hip ratio >0.9 BMI ≥30 g/m²	Large waist circumference: Men ≥40 in Women ≥35 in
Blood pressure ≥130/85 mm Hg or treatment for previously diagnosed hypertension	Blood pressure ≥140/90 mm Hg	Blood pressure ≥130/85 mm Hg
Triglycerides ≥150 mg/dL (1.7 mmol/L) or treatment for this lipid abnormality	Triglycerides ≥150 mg/dL	Triglycerides ≥150 mg/dL
HDL-cholesterol <40 mg/dL (1.03 mmol/L) for men and <50 mg/dL (1.29 mmol/L) for women or treatment for this lipid abnormality	HDL-cholesterol: <35 mg/dL for men and women	HDL-cholesterol: <40 mg/dL for men <50 mg/dL for women
Fasting plasma glucose ≥100 mg/dL (5.6 mmol/L) or previously diagnosed type 2 diabetes	Fasting blood glucose ≥100 mg/dL	Fasting blood glucose ≥100 mg/dL

[a]Specific values for waist circumference are provided for other ethnic groups (International Diabetes Federation, 2006).

criteria listed in the left panel in Table 48.2. The World Health Organization classifies a person with metabolic syndrome as having either high insulin levels, an elevated fasting blood glucose level or an elevated post-meal glucose level alone, along with at least two of the criteria listed in Table 48.2 in the center panel (Alberti and Zimmet, 1998). The American Heart Association (AHA) and the National Heart, Lung and Blood Institute (US Department of Human and Health Services) classify individuals with MetS as having three or more of the following factors shown in Table 48.2 in the right-hand column (Grundy et al., 2005).

High levels of LDL-C, as well as elevated total cholesterol concentrations, are potent contributors to atherogenesis (Glass and Witztum, 2001). The risk of atherosclerosis is inversely related to HDL levels (Tall et al., 2000); the protective effect is due to the mediation of reverse cholesterol transport (Burgess et al., 2006). Cigarette smoking is a major risk factor for the development of atherosclerosis; the main mechanisms involve endothelial dysfunction, inflammation, and an unfavorable lipid profile (CDC, 2010). Smoking is associated with increased triglyceride and decreased HDL-C concentrations (CDC, 2010). Another major risk factor for atherosclerosis, high blood pressure, causes endothelial injury through shear stress and micro-tears in the artery wall

(AHA, 2011). Other risk factors, such as weight, blood glucose, physical inactivity, and diet, play a major role in the progression of atherosclerosis. A chronic state of inflammation presented as elevated levels of C-reactive protein and other pro-inflammatory cytokines, along with decreased levels of anti-inflammatory cytokines, also has been found to promote atherosclerotic plaque development (Falk, 2006). Targeting these risk factors is central to reducing coronary artery disease (CAD). Table 48.3 shows the effects of targeted lifestyle and dietary changes on mortality risk in persons with CAD. Beneficial effects on reducing mortality risk are also achievable within the general population via combined dietary changes (−45%), incorporation of moderate-intensity physical activity at 40–60% VO₂ max for at least 30 minutes per day on at least 5 days per week (−25%), moderation of alcohol intake to 2 drinks per day for women and 3 drinks per day for men (−20%), and cessation of smoking (−45%) (Iestra et al., 2005). The aforementioned combined dietary changes include two or more of the following factors: limiting saturated (≤10% E) and *trans* fatty acid intake (≤1% E), consumption of 1–2 portions of oily fish per week, regular fruit and vegetable intake (>400 g/day), sufficient intake of fiber-containing grain products, legumes and/or nuts (≥3 U/day), and decreased salt intake (<2,400 mg/day).

TABLE 48.3 Effects of targeted diet and lifestyle interventions on mortality risk in individuals with coronary artery disease (CAD): evidence from prospective cohort studies and randomized controlled trials. Adapted from Iestra and colleagues, 2005

Intervention	Reduction in mortality risk for individuals with CAD
Combined dietary changes[a]	45%
Moderate-intensity physical activity[b]	25%
Moderation of alcohol intake[c]	20%
Smoking cessation	45%

[a]Represents a combination of ≥2 of the following factors: limiting saturated fat intake (≤10% E) and trans fatty acid intake (≤1% E); regular consumption of fish (1–2 portions of oily fish per week); regular fruit and vegetable intake (≥400 g/day); sufficient intake of fiber-containing grain products, legumes and/or nuts (≥3 U/day); reduction of salt intake (≤2,400 mg/day).
[b]Moderate-intensity physical activity (40–60% of VO$_2$ max) for at least 30 minutes per day on at least 5 days per week.
[c]A maximum of 2 drinks per day for women and 3 drinks per day for men (Iestra et al., 2005). Adapted with permission from Iestra et al. (2005).

Ranking of the Strength of the Scientific Evidence

There has been extensive primary research conducted on the effect of various nutrients on CVD risk factors as well as several evidence-based reviews on their overall mechanisms of action for reducing CVD risk. Expert panels rank such evidence to create national-policy public-health recommendations. Table 48.4 presents the 2010 Dietary Guidelines for Americans conclusion and grading system used by the expert panel to determine the strength of the current evidence. Specifically this system was used for the macronutrients, sodium and potassium. For the reader, this conclusion and grading system is also applicable to the strength of the evidence provided by the Institute of Medicine (IOM) and the American Heart Association (AHA) for magnesium, the B-vitamins, vitamin D, and the antioxidant vitamins C and E.

Role of the Macronutrients in Atherosclerosis

The macronutrient composition of dietary patterns affects lipids and lipoproteins and, consequently, CVD risk. A key question that has been addressed by many researchers concerns which macronutrient should replace calories provided by saturated fats. A meta-analysis of 60 controlled trials by Mensink and colleagues (2003) found that, rela-

tive to carbohydrates (CHO), SFAs increased LDL-C and HDL-C. Monounsaturated fatty acids (MUFAs) were associated with increasing HDL-C levels while significantly lowering LDL-C levels relative to CHO. Polyunsaturated fatty acids (PUFAs) resulted in the greatest LDL-C reduction with a slight but significant increase in HDL-C. The total cholesterol:HDL-C (TC:HDL-C) ratio did not change when SFA was replaced with CHO; however, the ratio decreased when SFA was replaced with MUFA or PUFA. In contrast, *trans* fatty acid (TFA) did not increase HDL-C relative to carbohydrate, but produced the greatest increase in LDL-C, resulting in the most detrimental TC:HDL-C ratio. Lastly, replacing carbohydrates with any type of fatty acid resulted in a lower triglyceride (TG) level. Additional dietary factors, including omega-3 (n-3) and omega-6 (n-6) fatty acids, the glycemic index, fiber content, and protein intake, also affect CVD risk through a variety of mechanisms that will be discussed in the following sections.

Saturated Fatty Acids

Strong evidence indicates a positive association between dietary SFA intake and increased total cholesterol and LDL-C, as well as increased CVD risk (DGAC, 2010b). As such, reducing SFA intake is a primary focus of dietary interventions to lower LDL-C (Lichtenstein *et al.*, 2006a). Regression analyses indicate that for every 1% increase in energy from SFAs, LDL-C increases by 0.033–0.045 mmol/L and HDL-C by 0.011–0.013 mmol/L (Mensink and Katan, 1992; Hegsted *et al.*, 1993; Clarke *et al.*, 1997). A meta-analysis of randomized controlled trials reported that all long-chain SFAs with the exception of stearic acid (18:0) increase LDL-C and HDL-C relative to carbohydrate (Mensink *et al.*, 2003). Stearic acid has been excluded from the category of cholesterol-raising fatty acids since it does not increase LDL-C compared with the other long-chain SFAs (DGAC, 2010a). Consequently, high stearic acid vegetable oils have been developed as a source of solid fat that is considered a healthy alternative in food applications requiring solid fat (Hunter *et al.*, 2010).

Reducing dietary SFAs typically is associated with an increase in some other macronutrient. The nutrient(s) replacing SFA(s) will differentially affect blood lipid levels and therefore influence the risk of atherosclerosis and CVD. Clinical evidence has consistently shown that replacing SFA with unsaturated fat improves lipid levels and decreases CVD risk. Consumption of PUFA (Chung

TABLE 48.4 Guidelines for determining the strength of evidence

Elements	Strong	Moderate	Limited	Expert opinion only	Grade not assignable
Quality: Scientific rigor and validity Study design and execution	Studies of strong design Free from design flaws, bias, and execution problems	Studies of strong design with minor methodological concerns Or only studies of weaker design for question	Studies of weak design for answering the question Or inconclusive findings due to design flaws, bias, or execution problems	No studies available Conclusion based on usual practice, expert consensus, clinical experience, opinion, or extrapolation from basic research	No evidence that pertains to question being addressed
Consistency: Consistency of findings across studies	Findings generally consistent in direction and size of effect or degree of association, and statistical significance with very minor exceptions	Inconsistency among results of studies with strong design Or consistency with minor exceptions across studies of weaker design	Unexplained inconsistency among results from different studies Or single study unconfirmed by other studies	Conclusion supported solely by statements of informed nutrition or medical commentators	NA
Quantity: Number of studies Number of study participants	One large study with a diverse population or several good quality studies Large number of subjects studied Studies with negative results have sufficiently large sample size for adequate statistical power	Several studies by independent investigators Doubts about adequacy of sample size to avoid Type I and Type II errors	Limited number of studies Low number of subjects studied and/or inadequate sample size within studies	Unsubstantiated by published research studies	Relevant studies have not been done
Impact: Importance of studied outcomes Magnitude of effect	Studied outcome relates directly to the question Size of effect is clinically meaningful Significant (statistical) difference is large	Some doubt about the statistical or clinical significance of the effect	Studied outcome is an intermediate outcome or surrogate for the true outcome of interest Or size of effect is small or lacks statistical and/or clinical significance	Objective data unavailable	Indicates area for future research
Generalizability: Generalizability to population of interest	Studied population, intervention and outcomes are free from serious doubts about generalizability	Minor doubts about generalizability	Serious doubts about generalizability due to narrow or different study population, intervention or outcomes studied	Generalizability limited to scope of experience	NA

Reproduced with permission from DGAC (2010b).

et al., 2004; Lichtenstein *et al.*, 2006b; Kralova Lesna, 2008) and MUFA (Yu-Poth *et al.*, 2000; Lichtenstein *et al.*, 2006b; Berglund *et al.*, 2007) in place of SFA decreases LDL-C. Replacing SFA with carbohydrate also lowers LDL-C; however, TG increases and HDL-C decreases compared with PUFA and MUFA replacement (Mensink *et al.*, 2003; Berglund *et al.*, 2007). Also, the type of carbohydrate replacing SFA contributes to the overall CVD risk. For example, replacing SFA with refined carbohydrate may increase the number of small LDL particles, another CVD risk factor, even though total LDL-C may be lowered slightly (Mensink *et al.*, 2003; Krauss *et al.*, 2006; Siri-Tarino *et al.*, 2010). Small, dense LDL particles are more atherogenic due to a greater ability to penetrate the endothelial wall and initiate foam cell formation (Gardner *et al.*, 1996; Stampfer *et al.*, 1996; Lamarche *et al.*, 1997).

Previous epidemiological evidence reported adverse associations between SFA and lipid and lipoprotein levels (Skeaff and Miller, 2009). SFAs were positively correlated with total cholesterol, as well as CVD incidence in different populations (Posner *et al.*, 1991; Hu *et al.*, 1997). However, recent epidemiological studies challenge these results and suggest that SFAs may not be associated with CVD risk. Skeaff and Miller (2009) conducted a meta-analysis using results from prospective cohorts to evaluate the associations between fatty acids and CVD risk. SFAs were not significantly associated with CHD events (RR 0.93 [95% CI: 0.83–1.05]) or CHD death (RR 1.14 [95% CI: 0.82–1.60]). However, the authors stated that the evidence available was unsatisfactory and unreliable. Many of the studies included in the analysis used a 24-hour recall to assess dietary intake, a particularly imprecise method for determining long-term dietary habits (Beaton *et al.*, 1979). Another recent meta-analysis of prospective studies by Siri-Tarino and colleagues (2010) also found that SFAs were not significantly related to CHD (RR 1.07 [95% CI: 0.96–1.19]). Only six of the 16 studies included in this analysis reported a positive association with CHD. However, the authors did not define CHD or separate CHD into events versus fatalities. Not unlike Skeaff and Miller (2009), many of the studies that were included (more than half) used 24-hour recalls or some other dietary assessment method with known limitations. The use of 24-hour recalls to assess long-term dietary habits raises questions about the reliability of the results, and through regression dilution bias may reduce the strength of association (Katan *et al.*, 2010).

Jakobsen and colleagues (2009) conducted a pooled analysis of prospective cohort studies from both Europe and the United States reporting that the substitution of PUFA for SFA was associated with a decreased risk of CHD events (HR 0.87 [CI: 0.77–0.97]) and CHD death (HR 0.74 [95% CI: 0.61–0.89]). In contrast, substitution of MUFA or carbohydrate for SFA was associated with an increased risk of CHD events (HR 1.19 [CI: 1.00–1.42] and HR 1.07 [CI: 1.01–1.14]), but not CHD death. These results suggest that PUFAs are the preferred substitute for SFAs over MUFAs or carbohydrate, in order to reduce CHD risk. The authors pointed out that no differentiation was made between carbohydrate sources of different glycemic indexes, which significantly influence CHD risk (Jakobsen *et al.*, 2009). Also, adjustments for TFA in the foods may have been incomplete and, in fact, possibly included in the hazard ratio estimations for MUFA intake. In contrast, Mente and colleagues (2009) pooled prospective cohort studies and found strong evidence for an inverse relationship between MUFA and CHD risk (RR 0.80 [CI: 0.67–0.930]), and a positive relationship between TFA and CHD risk (RR 1.32 [95% CI: 1.16–1.48]). These investigators also reported no significant relationship for SFAs (RR 1.06 [CI: 0.96–1.15]) and CHD. However, unlike the other recent studies, PUFAs (RR 1.02 [CI: 0.81–1.23]) were not related to CHD.

The inconsistencies among recent epidemiological studies may indeed be due to differences in the method of assessment of dietary SFA intake. As well, more clinical and observational studies may be used to determine why epidemiological evidence varies from that seen in clinical trials. None the less, strong clinical evidence indicates an association between SFA intake and increased CVD risk.

Monounsaturated Fatty Acids

There is strong evidence in support of MUFA replacement of SFA for an improvement in blood lipids (DGAC, 2010b). Clinical evidence has shown that MUFA substitution for SFA decreases LDL-C (Yu-Poth *et al.*, 2000; Lichtenstein *et al.*, 2006b; Berglund *et al.*, 2007). When replacing SFA with MUFA, compared with PUFA or carbohydrate, HDL-C is either less reduced or unchanged (Rudel *et al.*, 1998; Mensink *et al.*, 2003). Both MUFA and carbohydrate lower LDL-C levels when replacing SFA, but MUFA can increase HDL-C levels versus carbohydrate, lower the TC:HDL-C ratio, and potentially decrease apolipoprotein B levels (apo B), the main apolipoprotein in LDL-C (Garg, 1998; Mensink *et al.*, 2003). Evidence demonstrates that diets high in MUFAs versus PUFAs also may protect against LDL oxidation (Garg, 1998). MUFAs have a lower susceptibility to spontaneous oxidation compared with PUFAs and are less likely to form oxidative derivatives in the circulation (Ashton *et al.*, 2001; Hargrove *et al.*, 2001; Ahuja *et al.*, 2003). Therefore, MUFAs may protect against smooth muscle cell proliferation and oxidative stress (Colette *et al.*, 2003).

Primate studies have shown that MUFAs are more atherogenic than PUFAs, eliciting effects similar to SFAs (Rudel *et al.*, 1995, 1998). Rudel and colleagues (1995) fed atherogenic diets (35% fat, 0.8 mg cholesterol/kcal) high in SFAs, PUFAs, or MUFAs to adult male African green monkeys for 5 years to assess the effects on plasma lipoproteins and coronary artery atherosclerosis (CAA); CAA is the development of atheroscleroic plaques within the coronary arteries. Monkeys fed the PUFA and MUFA diets had significantly lower LDL-C levels than the monkeys fed the SFA diet, whereas HDL-C levels, while similar for the SFA and MUFA groups, were significantly lower in monkeys fed the PUFA diet. CAA was comparable in the MUFA and SFA groups, but significantly less in monkeys fed the PUFA diet. The authors concluded that the SFA and MUFA diets were more atherogenic than the PUFA diet. Interestingly, the diets high in SFA and MUFA elicited similar atherogenic effects. Unlike the group fed PUFA, cholesteryl oleate was the primary cholesterol ester accumulating in the coronary arteries in the SFA and MUFA groups. It was noted that LDL in animals fed MUFA was significantly enriched in cholesteryl oleate, which shifted the melting point of LDL above body temperature (Rudel *et al.*, 1995). This shift may have decreased the ability to hydrolyze and clear cholesterol ester droplets, thereby contributing to CAA. However, clinical studies have not shown MUFA consumption to be harmful, and the 2010 Dietary Guidelines for Americans state that PUFA or MUFA in place of SFA reduces CVD risk (DGAC, 2010a).

A recent meta-analysis by Cao and colleagues (2009) reported that moderate-fat (MF; average 23.6% of total kcal as MUFA) and low-fat (LF; average containing 11.4% of total kilocalories as MUFA) diets both lowered TC and LDL-C similarly. However, MF diets increased HDL-C [2.28 mg/dL (95% CI: 1.66–2.90) p < 0.0001] and decreased TG [−9.36 mg/dL [CI: −12.16, −6.08] p < 0.00001) vs. LF diets. Thus, the TC:HDL-C ratio was significantly reduced after MF diets (−0.36, p < 0.0001)

with a −0.30 ± 0.09 (p < 0.001) difference between MF and LF diets. Predicted changes in CVD risk estimated that MF diets led to greater reductions in CVD risk compared with LF diets for both men and women (−6.37% and −9.34%, respectively). Additional research is needed to explain why animal studies (in particular, those involving non-human primates) and human studies differ in how MUFAs affect CVD risk.

Epidemiological evidence for substituting MUFA in place of SFA has also been inconsistent with regard to CVD risk, as previously discussed. A recent pooled analysis of prospective cohort studies reported a positive association between substitution of MUFA for SFA and CHD events (HR: 1.19 [95% CI: 1.00–1.42]). In contrast, another pooled analysis of prospective cohort studies reported an inverse relationship between MUFA and CHD risk (RR 0.80 [CI: 0.67–0.93]). Further research is needed to clarify discrepancies associated with MUFA and CVD risk. The DGAC report states that a 5% energy replacement of SFA with MUFA can decrease the risk of CVD and type 2 diabetes (DGAC, 2010b). Therefore, substituting MUFA for SFA, TFA, and/or carbohydrate can improve the lipid and lipoprotein levels and other biomarkers of CVD risk.

Polyunsaturated Fatty Acids

There is strong and consistent evidence in support of the association between intake of polyunsaturated fatty acids (PUFAs) and an improvement in blood lipids, particularly when PUFAs replace SFAs and TFAs in the diet (DGAC, 2010b). PUFAs have multiple double bonds and consequently are more fluid than saturated fatty acids. Omega-3 (n-3) and omega-6 (n-6) PUFAs have their first double bond at 3 and 6 carbons from the omega end of the fatty acid, respectively. These are essential nutrients that cannot be synthesized by humans due to the lack of an enzyme required to insert a *cis* double bond into a carbon backbone (Institute of Medicine, 2002). Humans can synthesize long-chain (LC) n-3 or n-6 fatty acids from the essential, parent fatty acids obtained from the diet, albeit at a low rate. The parent fatty acid for the n-3 series is α-linolenic acid (ALA; 18:3n-3), and the parent fatty acid for the n-6 series is linoleic acid (LA; 18:2n-6). Bioconversion of these PUFAs leads to the production of several LC fatty acids including eicosapentaenoic acid (EPA; 20:5n-3) and docosahexaenoic acid (DHA; 22:4n-6) in the n-3 series, and arachidonic acid (AA; 20:4n-6) in the n-6 series. However, the bioconversion of the n-3

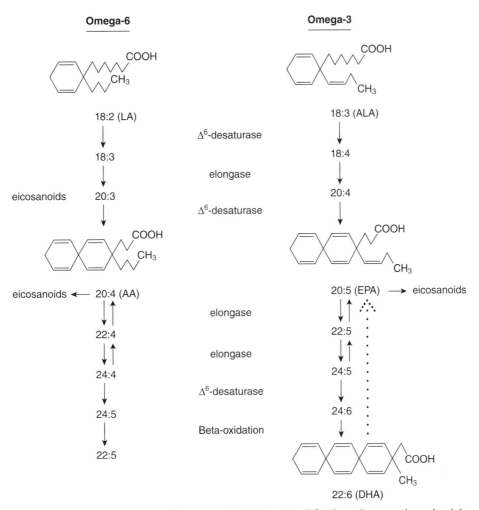

FIG. 48.2 The metabolism of omega-3 and omega-6 PUFAs. Modified and reproduced with permission from Harris *et al.* (2008). Questions remain about whether DHA is retroconverted to EPA, as shown by the dotted arrow.

series to these very long-chain FAs is low (Hussein *et al.*, 2005; Goyens *et al.*, 2006).

Figure 48.2 displays the metabolism of both n-3 and n-6 FAs, which primarily includes desaturase enzymes that remove hydrogen atoms to create a double bond, and elongase enzymes that add carbons to the backbone of the fatty acid. n-3 and n-6 FAs utilize the same enzymes for elongation and desaturation, and consequently there is competition between the fatty acid groups for these rate-limiting enzymes, most notably for the Δ^6-desaturases. Enzymatic competition is part of the basis for recommending decreased n-6 FA intake to improve the metabolism of short-chain dietary n-3 fatty acids (FAs) and to theoretically increase blood levels of EPA and DHA. Liou and colleagues (2007) addressed the effects of lowering the

n-6:n-3 ratio in a randomized cross-over study in men ($n = 22$). They compared two diets given for 4 weeks: a high-LA diet (7.0–15.8% total energy; approximately 10:1 LA/ALA ratio) with a low-LA diet (2.9–5.2% energy; 4:1 ratio) and found a decrease in phospholipid EPA and an increase in the AA:EPA ratio when participants consumed the high-LA diet, but no increase in phospholipid AA (Liou *et al.*, 2007). This suggests that the n-3 FA content in cell membranes may be affected by a high intake of n-6 FA, but perhaps only when consuming primarily shorter chain n-3 PUFAs.

The cardioprotective benefits of marine n-3 fatty acids were discovered in the 1970s by Danish researchers assessing the fish-rich diet and low CVD occurrence of Greenland Inuits (Dyerberg and Bang, 1979). Since this ecological observation, population, clinical, and basic investigations have confirmed the protective effect of both marine- and plant-derived n-3 FAs against CVD (Agency for Healthcare Research and Quality, 2004). The evidence for plant-based n-3 FAs (rich in ALA) is less conclusive than that for marine-based, longer-chain, n-3 FAs, EPA, and DHA (Wang *et al.*, 2006). Flaxseed, walnuts, flaxseed oil, walnut oil, and canola oil are sources of ALA, and cold-water fish such as salmon, mackerel, herring, and sardines are the species of seafood that are the richest sources of EPA and DHA (Harris *et al.*, 2008; DGAC, 2010a).

Plant-Based n-3 Fatty Acids: α-Linolenic Acid.

There is limited but supportive evidence that a higher intake of n-3 FAs from plant sources reduces CVD-related mortality among persons with existing CVD (DGAC, 2010b). Based on epidemiological studies, an intake of between 1.5 and 3 g/day of ALA is considered cardioprotective (Albert *et al.*, 2005; Mozaffarian *et al.*, 2005). In an 18-year follow-up of women (30–55 years at baseline) in the Nurses' Health Study ($n = 76\,723$), women in the top two quintiles for ALA intake (median: 1.16 and 1.39 g/day) had a 38–40% lower risk of sudden cardiac death vs. women in the lowest quintile (median: 0.66 g/day) (Albert *et al.*, 2005). This trial, however, showed no relationship between ALA intake and other types of fatal CHD or non-fatal myocardial infarction. After 14 years of follow-up, male participants in the Health Professionals Follow-Up Study ($n = 45\,722$) with little or low EPA and DHA intake (<100 mg/day) had a 47% reduction in the risk of CHD incidence for every 1 g/day increase in ALA intake (Mozaffarian *et al.*, 2005); however, this association was not seen in participants with higher EPA and DHA intakes (≥100 mg/day). Several clinical studies have investigated the effects of high ALA intake on CVD and mortality but the results have not been conclusive (Natvig *et al.*, 1968; de Lorgeril *et al.*, 1999; Harris, 2005). The Mediterranean (Lyon) Diet Heart Study demonstrated a 50% reduction in CHD risk over 4 years of follow-up in a secondary prevention population when the diet followed was increased in ALA (≈1 g/day). However, causality could not be determined because there were multiple dietary components that were altered between diets, including breads, fruits, vegetables, legumes, deli and regular meats, butter, cream, and margarine (de Lorgeril *et al.*, 1999). Natvig and colleagues (1968) supplemented middle-aged men ($n = 13\,578$; 50–59 years) with 5.5 g/day ALA or sunflower seed oil for 1 year and did not find any differences

in CVD endpoints between groups. The death rate in this study was lower than anticipated (0.4%), which decreased statistical power to detect a difference between groups (Natvig *et al.*, 1968).

Although ALA can be converted to long-chain FAs such as EPA and DHA, these rates are very low in humans, with values between 0.01 and 8% for EPA and less for DHA (Brenna, 2002; Plourde and Cunnane, 2007). The ALA conversion rate also is affected by age, gender, genetics, and overall dietary intake, as well as competition for enzymes catalyzing the conversion of LA to arachidonic acid (AA) as previously described. Due to the high intake of LA in the average American diet, a greater conversion of LA to AA often occurs, blunting the conversion of ALA to EPA and DHA (Chan *et al.*, 1993). Therefore, the recommendation to increase EPA + DHA levels by dietary ALA often includes the simultaneous recommendation to decrease LA intake. Recent studies have shown that daily supplementation of between 2.4 and 3.7 g of ALA for 12 weeks significantly increased erythrocyte EPA and docosapentaenoic acid (DPA), but not levels of DHA (Brenna, 2002; Harper *et al.*, 2006; Barcelo-Coblijn *et al.*, 2008). Despite the studies that show lower conversion rates of ALA to longer chain n-3 fatty acids (principally EPA) when LA is high, it is generally accepted that, if consumption of EPA and DHA meets current recommendations, modifications in LA intake (as well as ALA) are not necessary for the purposes of increasing production of longer chain n-3 fatty acids. The DGAC 2010 report concludes that the evidence currently available on ALA is insufficient to make recommendations for increasing intake of this n-3 fatty acid to reduce CVD risk (DGAC, 2010b). The adequate intake recommendation for ALA made by the Institute of Medicine is based on nutrient adequacy and is 1.6 and 1.1 g/day for men and women, respectively (Institute of Medicine, 2005).

Marine-Derived n-3 Fatty Acids: EPA and DHA.

There is a moderate body of evidence for an association between the consumption of two 4-oz (113 g) servings of seafood per week, providing a total of 250 mg/day of long-chain n-3 FAs, and reduced mortality from CHD or sudden death in persons with and without CVD (DGAC, 2010b). The association between CHD mortality and fish intake was assessed in a meta-analysis of over 220 000 persons who were followed for an average of 11.8 years (He *et al.*, 2004b). In contrast to non-fish-eating individuals, persons who consumed fish ≥5 times per week had a 38% decrease in CHD mortality risk. In addition, for every 20 g/day increase in fish intake there was a 7% decrease in risk of mortality due to coronary events. Also, a moderate intake of 1–3 servings of fish each month significantly reduced the risk of stroke (9%) and CHD mortality (11%) (He et al., 2004a,b). The Diet and Reinfarction Trial (DART) reported that male myocardial infarction survivors who consumed 200–400 g/week of fatty fish, which provided an additional 500–800 mg/day of n-3 FAs, had a 29% reduction in 2-year, all-cause mortality (Burr et al., 1989). However, in their study in men with angina, Burr and colleagues (2003) found that, in the group advised to eat oily fish (2 servings/week) and those supplied with fish-oil capsules (3 capsules/day), there was a higher risk of cardiac death (HR: 1.26 [95% CI: 1.00–1.58], p = 0.047), indicating possibilities for adverse events in particular subgroups of the population. Results from this study were unexpected given previous clinical and epidemiological findings. There were major concerns about the levels of compliance given that participants received dietary advice only. Participants were seen at baseline and at 6 months, but use of plasma EPA levels as a direct measure of compliance was only determined in 68 of the 3114 participants. Mailings and phone follow-up contacts were used for subsequent measures of compliance, but these are indirect and there may have been over-reporting of the capsules taken or the amount of fish consumed over time (Kris-Etherton and Harris, 2004). Mortality was determined after 3–9 years using National Health Service records, but it must be noted that, with any effectiveness trial of long duration, there is a tendency for participants to adopt high-risk behaviors if they view the intervention as preventive (Kris-Etherton and Harris, 2004). Several variables may have influenced the mortality rate, and, given the weak study design, only replication of these results in more controlled clinical studies would prompt revision of current recommendations for fish and fish-oil intake specifically for patients with angina.

Indeed, many intervention trials that have utilized fish-oil capsules instead of fish have noted significant reductions in CHD risk. The GISSI Prevention Study was a large prospective clinical trial that tested the efficacy of n-3 FAs for secondary prevention of CHD (GISSI-Prevenzione Investigators, 1999). Subjects randomized to the EPA + DHA supplement group (850 mg/day of n-3 ethyl esters) experienced a 15% reduction in the primary endpoint of death, non-fatal myocardial infarction and non-fatal stroke (p < 0.02). All-cause mortality was reduced by 20% (p = 0.01), and sudden death was reduced by 45% (p < 0.001) compared with the control group. Compared with baseline, no significant changes among groups were reported for TC, LDL-C, or HDL-C levels after 6 months; compared with controls, however, TG levels significantly decreased in patients receiving the EPA + DHA supplement (GISSI-Prevenzione Investigators, 1999). More recently, the Japan EPA Lipid Intervention Study (JELIS) (Yokoyama et al., 2007), a primary prevention study investigating the effects of EPA on CHD, assigned patients (n = 18 645) with elevated TC (>6.5 mmol/L) to receive treatment of either a statin alone or together with 1800 mg/day of EPA (no DHA). At mean follow-up of 4.6 years, EPA in combination with statin therapy reduced coronary events by 19% compared with statin alone (P = 0.011). Non-fatal coronary events and unstable angina also were significantly reduced in the EPA group (19% and 24%, respectively); however, the reduced risk did not apply to coronary death or sudden cardiac death. In addition, the reduced risk of coronary events in the EPA group was similar at different LDL-C levels, indicating that EPA benefits are independent of LDL-C reduction.

Recent trials on n-3 FAs have reported results inconsistent with previous findings. A Cochrane meta-analysis of 48 randomized controlled studies (RCTs) and 41 cohort studies reported no evidence that dietary or supplemental n-3 FAs reduce CVD events or total mortality (Hooper et al., 2004). However, there have been many concerns regarding the analysis. The Cochrane report included a study of questionable science (DART 2), omitted many relevant cohort and biomarker-based studies, and used contradictory search criteria. Not surprisingly, the DGAC 2010 report did not include this analysis in their evidence-based review of n-3 fatty acids. More recently, the Alpha Omega Trial (Kromhout et al., 2010) tested the effect of EPA + DHA in addition to ALA on the rate of CHD events in post-myocardial infarction patients. A low dose of EPA + DHA (mean: 376 mg/day), ALA (mean: 1.9 g/day), or both, in margarines had no significant effect on the occurrence of CVD events after 40 months of supplementation. Factors responsible for the lack of effect may include the low treatment dose and improvements in cardioprotective drug treatments, particularly statin therapy. Similarly, the addition of 1 g/day of EPA + DHA ethyl esters to current guideline-adjusted treatment (revascularization, clopidogrel, beta-blockers, statins and ACE-inhibitors, and rehabilitation lifestyle changes) for 1 year in a secondary prevention population (n = 3851) did not decrease mortality by sudden cardiac death (Rauch *et al.*, 2010). The potency of the current guideline-adjusted treatment for secondary prevention affected these results by decreasing the number of deaths and the statistical power to detect the effect of the EPA + DHA supplement. A higher dose of n-3 ethyl esters (8 g/day for 1 week; 3 g/day for 24 weeks) was not effective in treating atrial fibrillation as compared with a placebo in an adult population (n = 258) with atrial fibrillation but no structural heart disease (Kowey *et al.*, 2010). Finally, there was no effect of daily EPA + DHA supplements (600 mg) or B-vitamins (folate, 560 µg; vitamin B_6, 3 mg; vitamin B_{12}, 20 µg) on secondary prevention of myocardial infarction in a 5-year, double-blind, placebo-controlled, randomized controlled trial (Galan *et al.*, 2010). However, the dose of EPA + DHA in this trial did not meet the recommended amount for secondary prevention, and the death rate was lower than expected, thereby decreasing the statistical power of the intervention. While these results may raise uncertainties about the expectations for EPA + DHA supplements as preventative treatments for CVD patients, they do not disprove the previous studies, and have limitations that affected their ability to assess the efficacy of the intervention. The 2010 DGAC report concludes that "moderate evidence shows that consumption of about 8 ounces per week of a variety of seafood, which provide an average consumption of 250 mg per day of EPA and DHA, is associated with reduced cardiac deaths among individuals with and without pre-existing cardiovascular disease" (DGAC, 2010b).

The mechanism(s) of action for EPA + DHA in preventing cardiac events have been studied intensely in both animal models and randomized controlled clinical trials. EPA + DHA have been shown to reduce the susceptibility for cardiac arrhythmias (Campbell *et al.*, 1981; Stevenson *et al.*, 1993; Billman *et al.*, 1999; Leaf *et al.*, 2003; Schrepf *et al.*, 2004; Christensen *et al.*, 2005; Raitt *et al.*, 2005), stabilize atherosclerotic plaques (Thies *et al.*, 2003), favorably affect serum lipid levels and cholesterol, especially triglycerides (Stevenson *et al.*, 1993; Roche and Gibney, 1996; Nestel, 2000), modestly reduce blood pressure (Shimokawa and Vanhoutte, 1989; Yin *et al.*, 1991; Chu *et al.*, 1992; McVeigh *et al.*, 1994; Geleijnse *et al.*, 2002), produce less aggregatory eicosanoids compared with those from the n-6 FA family (Goodnight *et al.*, 1981; Sanders *et al.*, 1981; von Schacky *et al.*, 1985; Calder, 2004; Mori and Beilin, 2004), and decrease markers of systemic inflammation and oxidative stress (Chinetti *et al.*, 1998; Finstad *et al.*, 1998; Marx *et al.*, 1998; Baumann *et al.*, 1999; Massaro *et al.*, 2002; Lopez-Garcia *et al.*, 2004; Zampelas *et al.*, 2005; Zhao *et al.*, 2005; Richard *et al.*, 2008; Ambrozova *et al.*, 2010; Calzada *et al.*, 2010). The mechanisms by which EPA + DHA exert their effects relate mainly to their structure; they contain multiple double bonds that increase membrane fluidity. The specific conformations of EPA and DHA make them suitable ligands for many receptors, i.e. PPAR, that inhibit proinflammatory, cell-signaling cascades for subsequent production of inflammatory molecules, and EPA metabolites (eicosanoids) are known to have a vast number of beneficial functions in the body.

New avenues of research include measuring blood levels of n-3 FAs in clinical practice, determining the individual effects of EPA and DHA, and discovering sustainable and non-marine sources of longer-chain n-3 FAs. The omega-3 index is a novel biomarker of CHD risk that is currently used in both clinical and research settings. It represents long-term n-3 FA status and is measured as the percentage of EPA + DHA on the basis of total fatty acid content in erythrocyte membranes (Harris, 2008). An omega-3 index ≥8% has the greatest cardioprotective effect, while an index ≤4% is associated with a ten-fold increase in risk for sudden cardiac death. Since the development of purified EPA and DHA oils, new avenues of research also have focused on studying the separate mechanisms of action for EPA and DHA. Currently, DHA has been found to decrease blood pressure, heart rate and the number of total and small dense LDL particles, while EPA is known as the source for most eicosanoids and their action (Adkins and Kelley, 2010). Higher doses (8–14 g/day) of ALA have reportedly reduced inflammatory markers and adhesion molecules, but these amounts are 6 to 11 times greater than commonly consumed levels (Harris, 2005). It is not known as to whether there is a specific mechanism by which ALA may reduce CHD risk, independent of its conversion to EPA + DHA. In addition, stearidonic acid (SDA) has attracted much attention because it is a plant-derived n-3 FA that is more easily converted to EPA than ALA. This is because it is the product of ALA and the Δ^6-desaturase, and therefore bypasses the rate-limiting step during conversion. In a randomized, double-blind, placebo-controlled study (n = 252), 4.2 g/day of SDA raised EPA levels in erythrocyte membranes to a similar extent as 1 g/day of EPA during 12 weeks of supplementation and oil use (Lemke *et al.*, 2010).

n-6 Fatty Acids: Linoleic and Arachidonic Acid. Linoleic acid (LA) is the primary n-6 FA in the diet, accounting for 85–90% of n-6 PUFA intake (Harris *et al.*, 2009). It is metabolically converted to arachidonic acid (AA); however, the amount of AA in cell membranes is tightly regulated so that only about 0.2% of LA is converted (Hussein *et al.*, 2005). AA is provided by meat, poultry, eggs, and some species of fish, while LA is found in vegetable oils such as corn, soybean and safflower oil, as well as many seeds and nuts.

Results from a meta-analysis of 60 feeding studies indicated that substituting PUFAs (between 0.6% and 28.8% energy from n-6 FAs) for carbohydrate produced favorable effects on the ratio of total to HDL cholesterol in comparison with other fatty acids (Mensink *et al.*, 2003). When n-6 FAs replace 10% of calories from SFAs, there is an 18 mg/dL decrease in LDL-C (Mensink and Katan, 1992). Other improvements in CVD risk factors can be attributed to both higher serum LA levels, such as decreased blood pressure (Grimsgaard *et al.*, 1999), and increased LA intake, as well as improved insulin sensitivity (Summers *et al.*, 2002) and reduced incidence of diabetes mellitus (Salmeron *et al.*, 2001). Overall, results from metabolic studies, studies in non-human primates, and randomized controlled trials have shown that an n-6 FA intake between 10% and 21% of energy reduces CHD risk without adverse events (Harris *et al.*, 2009).

Suggestions to decrease LA intake have been based on the inflammatory nature of CHD and the fact that AA is a major substrate for the production of several pro-inflammatory molecules (Libby, 2006). While many eicosanoids derived from AA are pro-inflammatory, vasoconstrictive and pro-aggregatory, several other metabolic products of AA have anti-inflammatory and anti-aggregatory properties (Node *et al.*, 1999; Serhan, 2005). In addition, the conversion from LA to AA in cell membranes is tightly regulated, independent of the amount of LA consumed, as previously mentioned. Despite this, diets high in LA have been found to increase the ex vivo susceptibility of LDL to oxidation (Tsimikas *et al.*, 1999). Moreover, results from an angiographic study have shown a relationship between PUFA intake and luminal narrowing in women with CHD (Mozaffarian *et al.*, 2004b). In summary, the evidence for the benefits of n-6 FA intake and CHD risk is greater than the evidence to prove otherwise. Currently, there is limited evidence in support of a net pro-inflammatory or pro-atherogenic effect of n-6 intake, with greater evidence suggesting that decreasing current recommended levels of intake (5–10% energy) may increase, rather than decrease, CVD risk (Harris *et al.*, 2009). The American Heart Association (AHA) recommends a daily n-6 PUFA intake of 5% to 10% of total energy, along with other AHA dietary and lifestyle recommendations (Harris *et al.*, 2009).

The n-3 : n-6 Ratio. Estimates show that the ratio of n-6 to n-3 FAs in the human diet has changed over time from a ratio of 1:1 to 10:1 or greater, the latter of which is representative of that found in a typical Western diet (Simopoulos *et al.*, 2000; Kris-Etherton *et al.*, 2002). This switch is thought to be due to the combination of decreased fish consumption, since fish is a potent source of n-3 FAs, and an increased use of vegetable oils rich in n-6 FAs (Simopoulos, 1999). Proponents for reducing n-6 intakes, namely that of LA, assume that, since the n-6 FA, arachidonic acid (AA), is a substrate for the synthesis of many pro-inflammatory molecules, higher levels would contribute to the inflammatory state found in CVD (Harris *et al.*, 2009). However, AA also serves as a substrate for many anti-inflammatory and anti-aggregatory molecules (Node *et al.*, 1999), indicating its wide array of functions within the body. In addition, it is well established that the metabolic pathways for n-3 and n-6 FAs utilize the same enzymes, and intake of a large amount of n-6 FAs has been shown to decrease the rate of conversion of short- to long-chain n-3 FAs in those with a low intake of long-chain n-3 FAs (Liou *et al.*, 2007). However, there are multiple factors that affect the conversion of ALA to EPA and DHA besides n-6 FA intake, and tracer studies have shown that the extent of LA conversion to AA is only ≈0.2% (Hussein *et al.*, 2005). Results from human trials are intriguing. Increased levels of n-6 PUFAs, particularly AA, have been associated with decreased levels of pro-inflammatory markers and increased levels of anti-inflammatory markers (Ferrucci *et al.*, 2006). In another study by Kusumoto and colleagues (2007), daily supplementation of AA (840 mg/day) for 4 weeks had no effect on inflammatory markers or platelet aggregation (Kusumoto *et al.*, 2007). Results from observational studies in US adults showed that increased n-6 PUFA intake was associated with either lower or unaltered levels of inflammatory molecules (Pischon *et al.*, 2003).

In a European epidemiological study, participants (*n* = 4902) were classified as fish-eaters, meat-eaters, vegetarians, or vegans, based on a 7-day dietary record (Welch *et al.*, 2010). Intakes of ALA, EPA, DHA, and LA, as well as the circulating blood levels of these and their precursor-product ratios as an estimate of conversion, were compared between the groups. Not surprisingly, the fish-eaters consumed the most EPA + DHA, and the vegans ate high levels of LA and no EPA + DHA. Yet, the blood levels of total EPA + DHA in vegan women were higher than in female fish-eaters, and the difference between male fish-eaters and vegans was smaller than expected, albeit statistically significant. Women with the highest LA intake and lowest EPA + DHA intake still had the highest blood levels of EPA + DHA; the sample of vegan women was, however, very small ($n = 5$). Still, estrogen has been shown to promote the gene expression of Δ^5- and Δ^6-desaturases, increasing the efficiency of conversion to EPA + DHA. Indeed, the factors affecting the bioconversion of shorter-chain n-3 and n-6 FAs to longer-chain FAs and their effects on each other are beyond our current knowledge. The Joint FAO/WHO Expert Consultation on Fats and Fatty Acids in Human Nutrition (2008) concludes that "there is no rationale for a scientific recommendation for n-6:n-3 ratio, or LA to ALA ratio, if intakes of n-6 and n-3 fatty acids lie within the recommendation established in this report," referring to acceptable macronutrient distribution ranges (AMDR) of 2.5–9% total energy for n-6, and 0.5–2% total energy for n-3 PUFAs (Joint FAO/WHO Expert Consultation, 2008).

When recommending a decrease in one macronutrient, it is important to specify the foods or nutrients that should replace it. PUFAs generally are recommended as a replacement for SFAs and some CHO. Intake of long-chain n-3 FAs is still the most efficient way to increase blood levels of EPA + DHA and thereby decrease risk for CHD, regardless of LA intake. Reducing the amount of n-6 FAs available to improve n-3 conversion in the blood will not attain levels of EPA and DHA that have been shown to achieve cardiovascular benefits. Thus, increasing long-chain n-3 FAs rather than reducing n-6 FAs is recommended (Harris, 2006). Indeed, the vast majority of the clinical trials have proven the benefit of increased n-3 FA consumption over n-6 FA reduction. Nevertheless, populations that consume low levels of EPA + DHA, such as vegans and vegetarians, may benefit from decreasing LA intakes in order to improve their n-3 FA metabolism (Liou et al., 2007).

The body of evidence indicates that the type of fat and what it replaces in the diet affect CVD risk. Consumption of SFAs and TFAs is associated with an unfavorable lipid profile that increases CVD risk, while unsaturated fatty acids, namely MUFAs and PUFAs, are protective against CVD. Isocaloric substitution of SFAs and TFAs by MUFAs and PUFAs provides the greatest cardiometabolic benefits.

Trans Fatty Acids

Trans fatty acids are classified as unsaturated fatty acids containing at least one unsaturated, non-conjugated, double bond in the *trans* configuration. Industrial TFAs are produced during partial hydrogenation of vegetable oils. Conjugated fatty acids, formed as intermediates or by-products from the biohydrogenation of linoleic acid by ruminal microbes, are found within the tissues of ruminants and in the meat and dairy products they provide (Bauman et al., 2003). Vaccenic acid, the most commonly occurring TFA isomer in ruminant fats, represents 30–50% of the *trans*-isomers (Mozaffarian et al., 2009). Humans metabolize vaccenic acid to 9c,11t conjugated linoleic acid (CLA), a *trans* fat with two double bonds separated by a single, conjugated bond (Tricon et al., 2006). TFA consumption is of particular concern given the range of its effects on CVD risk. Observational studies and RCTs have shown adverse effects on lipids such as increased LDL-C levels, reduced HDL-C levels, and increased TC:HDL-C ratio, a pro-inflammatory response with elevated IL-6 and CRP levels, and TNF-α activity, as well as endothelial dysfunction (Mozaffarian et al., 2009).

Epidemiological and clinical studies have shown consistently that TFAs increase cardiovascular risk and adversely affect blood lipids (Ascherio et al., 1999), and there is strong and consistent evidence for improving blood lipids by substituting PUFAs for TFAs (DGAC, 2010b). TFAs have the most detrimental effects on blood lipid levels compared with all other dietary fatty acids, including SFAs. Saturated and TFAs similarly increase LDL-C; however, TFAs lower HDL-C compared with SFAs (Ascherio et al., 1999). Meta-regression analysis of randomized clinical trials has shown that a 2% increase in TFA raises the ratio of LDL to HDL cholesterol (LDL-C:HDL-C) by 0.1 unit, which corresponds to a 53% increase in CHD risk (Ascherio et al., 1999). In addition, compared with an equivalent amount of SFAs, a diet enriched in TFAs doubles the ratio of LDL-C:HDL-C, which demonstrates their highly atherogenic properties (Ascherio et al., 1999). Studies also have shown that high TFA intakes are associated with increased CHD incidence (Oomen et al., 2001; Oh et al., 2005b), increased levels of inflammatory markers, and impaired endothelial function (de Roos *et al.*, 2003; Mozaffarian *et al.*, 2004a). Recognition of the detrimental health effects of TFA led to demands for their removal from the food supply and resulted in the Food and Drug Administration mandating that all manufacturers of conventional and functional foods list all non-conjugated TFAs on the nutrition facts panel. Nutrition labeling provides consumers with knowledge of the TFAs in foods so they can make informed purchasing decisions in order to decrease TFA intake and lower their risk of CHD. In addition, food manufacturers are motivated to decrease TFAs in their products as a result of TFA labeling regulations.

Previous experimental animal studies indicated that CLA not only lowered total cholesterol, LDL-C and triglyceride levels, but also reduced the LDL-C:HDL-C and TC:HDL-C ratios (Lee *et al.*, 1994). Using cholesterol-fed hamsters, Lock and colleagues (2005) found that supplementation with vaccenic acid and CLA significantly altered the plasma cholesterol profile by reducing total cholesterol, LDL-C and very-low-density lipoprotein (VLDL), as well as lowering the ratio of atherogenic to anti-atherogenic plasma lipoproteins. However, meta-analyses by Brouwer and colleagues (2010) have shown that all TFAs, including CLA, had the same effect on raising the LDL-C to HDL-C ratio in humans. The authors reviewed 39 studies for their analyses that evaluated the effects on the LDL-C:HDL-C ratio due to industrial TFAs and ruminant fatty acids, as well as CLA. Industrial TFAs were found to increase the LDL-C:HDL-C ratio by 0.055 for every 1% dietary energy replacement of *cis*-monounsaturated fat. In addition, with every 1% energy replacement of *cis*-MUFA, industrial TFAs increased LDL-C by 0.048 mmol/L and decreased HDL by −0.01 mmol/L. Replacement of 1% dietary energy from *cis*-MUFA with ruminant fatty acids also increased the LDL to HDL ratio by 0.038, increase LDL levels by 0.045 mmol/L, and decrease HDL by −0.009 mmol/L. Replacement of 1% dietary energy from *cis*-MUFA by CLA increased the LDL to HDL ratio by 0.043, as well as LDL levels by 0.038 mmol/L, and reduced HDL levels by −0.008 mmol/L. These analyses demonstrate an increase in the LDL to HDL ratio by all three classes of TFA, with a modest increase in response to CLA intake, to result in an increased risk for coronary heart disease (Brouwer *et al.*, 2010). However, given that ruminant TFAs are consumed in low levels within the population (≈1–2 g/day) representing <0.5% total energy intake (DGAC, 2010b), and the fact that they cannot be entirely removed from the diet, their associated risk with CHD is

viewed as low (Mozaffarian *et al.*, 2009). There is currently a limited body of evidence to support a prominent biological difference in adverse health effects between ruminant and industrial TFAs when ruminant TFAs are consumed at levels between 7 to 10 times higher than the average level of intake (DGAC, 2010b). The differences in chemical structure also present a need for more studies on their metabolic effects. The stance of the European Food Safety Authority is that there is "no convincing evidence that any of the conjugated linoleic acid isomers in the diet play a role in prevention or promotion of diet-related diseases" (EFSA Panel on Dietetic Products Nutrition and Allergies, 2010b), while the FAO's Expert Consultation on Fats and Fatty Acids in Human Nutrition concludes that there should be an upper limit of <1% dietary energy from TFAs to reduce the risk of chronic disease. All non-conjugated TFAs are required to be listed on food labels, including the naturally occurring vaccenic acid (Joint FAO/WHO Expert Consultation, 2008). There is currently no requirement by the Food and Drug Administration (FDA) to list amounts of the conjugated *trans* fatty acid CLA on food labels.

Dietary Cholesterol
A moderate body of evidence from epidemiological studies shows a relationship between dietary cholesterol and several clinical markers for CVD (DGAC, 2010b). Dietary cholesterol generally increases blood cholesterol levels; however, the effect of dietary cholesterol on lipid levels and CVD risk varies as a function of diet response to cholesterol. Randomized clinical trials on dietary cholesterol often use eggs as the dietary source (DGAC, 2010b), as reduction in egg consumption is a common method for lowering cholesterol intake. Typically, dietary cholesterol suppresses the activity of LDL receptors, thereby inhibiting cholesterol clearance from plasma and increasing LDL-C levels (Katan, 2006). However, individuals known as hyper-responders are likely to have greater increases in LDL-C levels following the intake of dietary cholesterol than others who are hypo-responders (Katan *et al.*, 1986). An overview of epidemiological studies reported no association between eating one egg a day (≈200 mg cholesterol) and CVD risk in non-diabetic men and women (Kritchevsky and Kritchevsky, 2000). In contrast, several cohort studies have shown that persons with type 2 diabetes who consume one or more eggs a day have up to a two-fold increase in CVD risk over type 2 diabetics who consume less than one egg per week (Hu *et al.*, 1999;

Tanasescu *et al.*, 2004; Djousse and Gaziano, 2008b). Furthermore, consumption of two or more eggs a day has been associated with a greater risk of heart failure among male physicians [1.64 (95 % CI: 1.08–2.49), p < 0.006 for trend] (Djousse and Gaziano, 2008a). The DGAC 2010 report states that one egg per day (≤7 eggs per week) does not adversely affect lipid/lipoprotein levels or increase CVD risk in healthy adults, but does increase CVD risk in individuals with type 2 diabetes (DGAC, 2010b). Therefore, recommended dietary cholesterol intake is lower (<200 mg/day vs. 300 mg/day) for persons with or at high risk for CVD or type 2 diabetes (DGAC, 2010b).

Carbohydrate

The proportion of total fat and carbohydrate (CHO) intake in isocaloric diets can be tailored to target certain CVD risk factors, such as overweight and obesity, central obesity, glycemic control, and plasma lipids, especially TG. In clinical studies, an increase in dietary energy from carbohydrates usually is associated with a moderate increase in fasting plasma TG levels, a reduction in HDL cholesterol levels, and an increased fraction of small, dense LDL, all of which impact adversely on CVD risk. However, no clear evidence has shown that the quantity of dietary carbohydrates alters the risk of CVD independently.

The Ornish diet (<10% energy from fat) and the Atkins diet (<20 g CHO/day) represent very low-fat and very low-carbohydrate diets respectively, and both have beneficial effects on CVD risk factors with weight loss (Ornish *et al.*, 1998, 1990; Samaha *et al.*, 2003; Seshadri *et al.*, 2004; Dansinger *et al.*, 2005). Generally, very low-carbohydrate diets restrict energy from carbohydrate to <20–30 g/day, while very low-fat diets restrict total fat intake to <10–20% of energy. A number of weight-loss studies have shown that carbohydrate-restricted diets improve metabolic syndrome characteristics more effectively than low-fat diets (Sharman *et al.*, 2004; Shai *et al.*, 2008; Volek *et al.*, 2008, 2009). A meta-analysis of five randomized controlled trials found that very low-carbohydrate diets were more effective than very low-fat diets only for short-term weight loss (≈6 months), and induced more favorable changes in TG and HDL-C levels compared with low-fat diets, but low-fat diets elicited greater reductions in total cholesterol and LDL-C levels overall (Nordmann *et al.*, 2006). Results from the Pounds Lost study showed that, when macronutrients were kept within the recommended ranges (except for total fat for which an upper level was tested) and used in reduced-calorie diets of either low fat

(20%) or high fat (40%), average protein (15%) or high protein (25%), or a range of carbohydrate levels (35%, 45%, 55%, and 65%), weight loss was similar with each diet after 2 years (Sacks *et al.*, 2009). All diets decreased CVD risk factors at 2 years, and lowered TG levels by similar amounts ranging between −12% and −17% (Sacks *et al.*, 2009), indicating cardioprotection in the long term. After 2 years, LDL-C levels were significantly (p < 0.05) lowered by the low-fat (−5%) and high-carbohydrate (−6%) diets over the high-fat (−1%) and low-carbohydrate diets (−1%) respectively, while there was a significant increase in HDL levels by the lowest carbohydrate diet (9%) over the highest carbohydrate diet (1%). All diets but the highest carbohydrate diet decreased serum insulin levels by −6% to −12%, and blood pressure was lowered by −1 mm Hg to −2 mm Hg for all diets (Sacks *et al.*, 2009).

In addition to weight-loss studies on low-carbohydrate diets, an isocaloric weight-maintenance study (the OmniHeart Randomized Trial) showed that partial substitution of carbohydrate (about 10% of energy substitution, from 58% to 48%) with either protein or MUFA further lowered blood pressure, improved lipid levels, and reduced estimated CVD risk (Appel *et al.*, 2005). These results are consistent with evidence showing that high-carbohydrate weight-maintenance diets can induce atherogenic dyslipidemia, traditionally characterized by higher TGs, decreased HDL-C levels, and smaller LDL particle size (Cuchel and Rader, 2006). The potential adverse effects of low-fat, high-carbohydrate diets are supported by data from 16 clinical trials reporting that, for every 5% decrease in total fat, there would be a decrease in HDL-C by −2.2% and an increase in TGs by 6% (Trumbo *et al.*, 2002). A recent meta-analysis also shows that moderate-fat diets had greater estimated reductions in predicted CHD risk in men (−6.37%) and women (−9.34%) compared with low-fat, higher-carbohydrate diets, of −6.37% and −9.34%, respectively (Cao *et al.*, 2009).

Although low-carbohydrate diets have risen in popularity, evidence from intervention trials on the benefits and risks of low-carbohydrate diets to achieve weight loss and modify CVD risk factors is limited. Furthermore, little is known about the long-term health effects of these diets; micronutrient inadequacy may occur when carbohydrate intake is very low (Bolton-Smith and Woodward, 1995). In conclusion, consuming a diet too high or too low in either fat or carbohydrate may result in adverse health effects, and the relative proportions of the two within the diet should target specific CVD risk factors and personal preferences within current dietary recommendations. The acceptable macronutrient distribution range (AMDR) for carbohydrate (45–65 % of energy) promotes achieving nutrient adequacy and attaining a healthy lipid and lipoprotein profile.

Glycemic Index and Glycemic Load

A question of interest with respect to carbohydrate research is the determination and characterization of the most healthful types for inclusion in the diet. Examples of health-based classifications include the glycemic index or glycemic load, fiber-rich carbohydrates, available and resistant carbohydrates, and rapidly versus slowly digested starch. Use of health-based characterization versus structural characterization including starch, sugar, monosaccharides, and oligosaccharides, may convey more effective public-health messages.

Glycemic index (GI) and glycemic load (GL) quantify the postprandial blood glucose response to foods containing carbohydrate (Jenkins et al., 1981). Specifically, glycemic index is used to compare the potential of foods with the same carbohydrate content to increase blood glucose levels (Ludwig, 2002), while the glycemic load is obtained by multiplying the glycemic index of a food by the amount of carbohydrate it contains in grams, and dividing this product by 100 (Liu and Willett, 2002). A high-GI diet may lead to postprandial hyperglycemia and hyperinsulinemia, which are found to increase CVD risk by producing oxidative stress (Lefebvre and Scheen, 1998). Hyperinsulinemia and insulin resistance are predictors of CHD risk (Pyorala et al., 1998a,b), but the role of insulin as an independent CVD risk factor is uncertain. The evidence for an association between high GI or GL and CVD risk remains limited and inconclusive (DGAC, 2010b). Dietary recommendations currently do not include advice on GI or GL (DGAC, 2010a).

Recently, three reports from the Nurses' Health Study demonstrated positive associations between high GL and CVD, but two of them found positive associations only in women with BMIs greater than 23 kg/m^2 and 25 kg/m^2 (Liu et al., 2000; Oh et al., 2005a; Halton et al., 2006). In another follow-up study on middle-aged women, a positive association between GL and stroke was found, but the positive association between GI or GL and CHD was found only in women with a BMI greater than 25 kg/m^2 (Beulens et al., 2007). A prospective cohort study of 36 246 Swedish, middle-aged men found that GI and GL were not associated with ischemic cardiovascular disease or

mortality, but that GL was associated with a greater risk of stroke after 5 years of follow-up (Levitan et al., 2007). Two other observational studies found no significant association between GI or GL with CVD (Van Dam et al., 2000; Levitan et al., 2007). One case-control study reported no significant association between GI and GL and the risk of non-fatal acute myocardial infarction (Tavani et al., 2003). Discrepancies between these findings may be due to differences in the populations studied, short-term follow-up in some studies, and variations in the dietary contributions to GI and GL. Furthermore, assigning a GI or GL value to a food is difficult because of the large variability in glycemic response to carbohydrate between individuals (Vega-López et al., 2007). Based on recent evidence, the DGAC 2010 report concludes that the GI or GL values of a food do not meaningfully improve carbohydrate selection, and suggests that consumers ultimately focus on caloric intake, caloric density, and fiber content (DGAC, 2010b).

Fiber and Whole Grains

Dietary fiber is defined as non-digestible carbohydrate and lignin that are intrinsic in plants (Trumbo et al., 2002). The DGAC 2010 report states that there is a moderate body of evidence for a protective effect of dietary fiber from whole foods, and therefore recommends consumption of 14 g dietary fiber per 1000 kcal, or 25 g for adult women and 38 g for adult men per day (DGAC, 2010b). Observational and intervention studies have shown that dietary fiber lowers blood pressure, improves serum lipid levels, and reduces inflammation (Brown et al., 1999; Ajani et al., 2004; Pereira et al., 2004; Streppel et al., 2005; Whelton et al., 2005; Ma et al., 2006; King et al., 2007). However, the food source of fiber (cereal, fruits and vegetables, or functional foods) related to CVD risk is not clear. For example, the NIH-AARP Diet and Health Study found that high intake of dietary fiber significantly reduced risk of all-cause death after 9-year follow up in 567 169 men and women in the United States (Park et al., 2011). Upon further analysis, only fiber from grains and not that from other sources (fruits, vegetables, and beans) was significantly and inversely related to both total and CVD mortality (Park et al., 2011). Similarly, Wolk and colleagues (1999) found that women with the highest fiber intake (22.9 g/day) had a 47% reduction in risk for CVD events compared with women with the lowest intakes (11.5 g/day) (RR: 0.53, 95% CI: 0.40–0.69). Again, when sources of fiber were analyzed, only cereal fiber was associated with a reduction in CVD risk (RR: 0.63, 95% CI: 0.49–0.81) (Wolk *et al.*, 1999).

Cereal fiber is traditionally equated with whole grains and is distinct from refined grain products. However, Jacobs and colleagues (2000) found this assumption to be faulty after assessing the relationship between cereal fiber intake from either refined or whole grains and overall mortality in 11 040 postmenopausal women over 11 years of follow-up (Jacobs *et al.*, 2000). Despite matching total cereal fiber intake, the women consuming whole grains had a 17% lower mortality rate as compared with those eating refined grains. The synergy of nutritional components in whole grains, such as lignin, sterols, and phenolic compounds, is thought to account for the protective effects that extend beyond cereal fiber. Indeed, there is great variability among various grains in their nutrient content and bioactive components, and grain is not necessarily an excellent source of fiber (De Moura *et al.*, 2009). De Moura and colleagues (2009) found that broadening the concept of whole grain beyond the FDA's definition would provide more convincing evidence for the current CVD health claim through support from 14 observational and 15 interventional studies. However, the variability of individual grains used in these studies (oat bran, oatmeal, oat cereal, wheat, rice, barley) makes it difficult to dissociate the effects of various grain components. Currently there is moderate evidence from prospective cohort studies for a protective effect of whole-grain intake against CVD (DGAC, 2010b). Further investigations on the assessment of fiber in whole grains, as well as the health benefits of whole grains contributed by different grain components, are needed.

There is sufficient evidence showing beneficial effects of dietary fiber and whole-grain intake on CVD risk factors. However, questions on the differences in physiological effects between fiber from cereal vs. other sources, as well as other nutritional factors in whole grains found to provide these protective effects, still remain.

Resistant and Available Carbohydrate

Measurements of resistant and available CHO are used to characterize CHO bioavailability within the small intestine (Englyst *et al.*, 2007). Resistant CHO has chemical bonds that are not accessible to digestive enzymes and therefore is not absorbed in the small intestine, i.e. fiber and resistant starch. Available CHO is digested easily and absorbed in the small intestine because of its bond structure, i.e. sugars and starch. The concept of resistant and available starch is consistent with the GI and GL concepts of characterizing CHO by the glucose response they elicit in the body. Englyst and colleagues (2003) found that the GI value may be explained by the content of rapidly or slowly available glucose, which measures the rate of glucose release from foods. The resistant starch or slowly digested starch content in food also contributes to a lower GI value (Goni *et al.*, 1997). Although several studies have evaluated the physical effects of starches as categorized by their digestion rates, the structural properties and potential health benefits of slowly digested starches are not well understood. It must be noted that this classification scheme is determined under laboratory-controlled conditions and is related to the structure of the carbohydrate, making the characterization more consistent and reliable than GI values. In addition to defining carbohydrates by their digestibility, their source should also be considered, since evidence for the health effects of plant-based fiber in comparison with industrially processed fiber is not available.

Regardless of how carbohydrates will be characterized in the future, minimally processed plant sources of carbohydrate, such as whole grains, legumes, fruits, and vegetables, are an integral part of the dietary recommendations to reduce CVD risk.

Protein

High-protein diets ($\approx$34% of energy) have consistently been shown to lower CVD risk through weight reduction, which favorably affects blood lipids, glucose, insulin, and other CVD risk factors (Clifton *et al.*, 2008). In a study conducted to investigate the short-term (4-month) effects of a calorie-restricted, reduced-carbohydrate ($\approx$40% of energy), higher-protein ($\approx$30% of energy) diet compared with a higher-carbohydrate ($\approx$55% of energy), moderate-protein ($\approx$15% of energy) diet, there was no difference in total weight loss between diets, but a greater reduction in fat mass of −22% with the high-protein diet (Layman *et al.*, 2009). The same study evaluated the sustained long-term (8-month) effects of adherence to the two diets without calorie restriction. Both diets sustained long-term weight loss, but the high-protein diet had significantly greater improvements in body composition, TG, HDL-C, and the TG:HDL-C ratio (Layman *et al.*, 2009). Moderate- to high-protein (22–90% of energy) diets tend to increase energy expenditure, maintain lean body mass, and increase satiety, all of which are important factors for weight maintenance, energy balance, and the prevention of co-morbidities associated with weight gain (Westerterp-Plantenga *et al.*, 1999; Mikkelsen *et al.*, 2000; Feinman and Fine, 2003). Although higher-protein diets, such as the Atkins and Zone diets, commonly induce quick weight loss, the American Heart Association does not endorse high-protein diets that severely restrict carbohydrates and limit food choices (St. Jeor *et al.*, 2001). The current acceptable macronutrient distribution range (AMDR) for protein, set forth in the dietary reference intakes (DRIs), is 10–35% of calories from protein (Institute of Medicine, 2005). The AHA Science Advisory takes a more modest stance, and recommends that diets contain 15–20% of calories from protein (St. Jeor *et al.*, 2001). Higher-protein diets must be planned carefully to incorporate important nutrients found in fruits, vegetables, and whole grains and to avoid protein-rich foods excessively high in total fat, saturated fat, and dietary cholesterol.

Evidence suggests that isocaloric diets higher in protein (22–25% of energy), at the expense of carbohydrates, have beneficial effects on CVD risk factors in both normolipidemic and hypercholesterolemic individuals (Wolfe and Giovannetti, 1991; Appel *et al.*, 2005). A diet with 25% of energy from protein (half from plant sources) and 48% energy from carbohydrates, compared with a diet with 15% energy from protein and 58% energy from carbohydrates, significantly decreased total cholesterol (−7.8 mg/dL), LDL-C (−3.3 mg/dL), TG (−15.7 mg/dL), and HDL-C (−1.3 mg/dL), as well as systolic (−1.4 mm Hg) and diastolic (−1.2 mm Hg) blood pressure (Appel *et al.*, 2005).

There has been much discussion about the health effects of plant protein versus animal protein. There is limited and inconsistent evidence from prospective cohort studies for an association between intake of animal protein products and CVD; however, there has been more supportive evidence for an association between processed meat intake and CVD (DGAC, 2010b). A moderate body of evidence from prospective cohort studies has provided inconsistent results on a relationship between animal product intake and blood pressure (DGAC, 2010b). On the other hand, a moderate body of evidence from both cross-sectional and cohort studies has linked vegetable protein intake with lower blood pressure; due to inconsistent results, there is limited evidence suggesting a protective effect of vegetable protein against CVD (DGAC, 2010b). Additionally, vegetarians who consume all protein from plant sources tend to have lower mortality from CHD compared with non-vegetarians (Key *et al.*, 1999;

Fraser, 2009). In accordance with this observation, the lysine:arginine (Lys:Arg) ratio has been a popular topic of research because animal protein is high in lysine whereas plant protein is typically high in arginine. Studies investigating the cholesterol-lowering effects associated with substituting plant protein (soy) for casein and other animal proteins indicate a small but significant TC-lowering (−2.5%) and LDL-C-lowering (−3.0%) effect in humans (Balk *et al.*, 2005). In a 5-week, crossover, controlled-feeding trial of individuals ($n = 12$) fed a moderate-fat (30% of energy), low-cholesterol (<100 mg/day) diet supplemented with either arginine (1.2 g/day) or placebo, arginine supplementation resulted in a significant reduction in both serum cholesterol and LDL-C (Kohls *et al.*, 1987). In contrast, a 35-day, randomized, controlled, cross-over trial evaluating a low-Lys:Arg (0.70) diet vs. a high-Lys:Arg (1.41) diet reported no reduction in cholesterol or LDL-C with a low-Lys:Arg ratio diet (Vega-López *et al.*, 2010). Given these inconsistencies, further clinical studies on the applicability of the Lys:Arg ratio are needed.

In a trial investigating the effects of protein supplementation (40 g/day) in pre-hypertensive and hypertensive individuals (mean BP: 126.7/82.4 mm Hg), using either soy or milk protein and a high-GI carbohydrate control, there was a significant reduction (p < 0.01) in systolic blood pressure of −2.0 mm Hg and −2.3 mm Hg due to the soy and milk protein supplementation, respectively, with no difference between the protein interventions (He *et al.*, 2011). A reduction in diastolic blood pressure due to the protein supplementation also was demonstrated, but was not statistically significant (He *et al.*, 2011). In this study, He and colleagues (2011) demonstrated a blood-pressure-lowering effect of substituting carbohydrate with protein (via supplementation), whether plant or animal based, in pre-hypertensive and hypertensive individuals.

Higher-protein diets (22–34% of energy), both isocaloric and calorie-restricted, have demonstrated favorable effects on body composition and CVD risk factors. Further intervention studies are needed to investigate the safety, efficacy, and feasibility of long-term adherence to high-protein/low-carbohydrate diets.

Roles of Select Micronutrients and Antioxidants in Atherosclerosis

Some micronutrient deficiencies have been shown to increase the risk of atherosclerotic cardiovascular disease.

These nutrients act through gene–nutrient pathways to influence CVD risk and progression (Houston, 2010). There are several mechanisms by which micronutrients reduce CVD risk. Sodium, potassium, and magnesium have blood-pressure-lowering effects; magnesium also increases insulin sensitivity. Vitamin D lowers CVD risk via several mechanisms including down-regulation of the renin–angiotensin system and preservation of endothelial cell function. A recent cross-sectional study also has shown an independent association of vitamin D with blood pressure levels and with hypertension and pre-hypertension. The mechanisms by which vitamins B_6, B_{12} and folate beneficially affect CVD risk (i.e. by decreasing homocysteine levels) are unclear based on findings from large clinical trials. Niacin is, however, used therapeutically to improve the lipid and lipoprotein profile, and reduce CVD risk. Clinical studies have not demonstrated the efficacy of the antioxidant vitamins C and E.

Sodium

Sodium is an essential nutrient, and a strong body of evidence indicates that decreases in sodium intake decrease blood pressure in adults (DGAC, 2010b). Changes in sodium intake influence blood volume; increased sodium levels cause an increase in water retention resulting in an increase in blood volume and blood pressure (Sheng, 2000; Institute of Medicine, 2004). As summarized in the 2010 DGAC report, reduced sodium intake results in fewer strokes and CVD events and in decreased mortality. In the Dietary Approaches to Stop Hypertension (DASH) trial, a multicenter randomized controlled-feeding study, researchers evaluated the effects of a diet high in fruits and vegetables, and low-fat dairy products on blood pressure (Appel et al., 1997). In hypertensive (Stage 1) participants fed the DASH diet, high in fruits and vegetables (8–10 servings per day; 75th percentile of US consumption) and low-fat dairy products (2–3 servings per day) and low in saturated fat (6%) and total fat (27%), there was a decrease in systolic (−5.5 mm Hg) and diastolic (−3.0 mm Hg) blood pressure. In the DASH-Sodium trial, three levels of sodium were evaluated in the context of the DASH diet; a high target of 150 mmol/L (150 mEq/L), an intermediate target of 100 mmol/L (100 mEq/L), and a low target of 50 mmol/L (50 mEq/L) (Sacks et al., 2001). The combination of the DASH diet and sodium reduction (<5 g/day) resulted in a larger decrease in systolic (−11.5 mm Hg) and diastolic (−6.3 mm Hg) blood pressure (Sacks et al., 2001). A meta-analysis of 13 cohort studies by Strazzullo and colleagues

(2009) reported that an increased sodium intake increased risk for stroke and cardiovascular disease, a 2000 mg/day increase in intake resulting in a 23% higher risk for stroke (Strazzullo et al., 2009). Other evidence, however, has shown that a restricted sodium intake (1840 mg/day) in persons with heart failure significantly increased hospitalization and mortality when compared with persons on an intake of 2760 mg/day (Cohen et al., 2008), indicating that restriction may be harmful in certain populations (Jessup et al., 2009). Researchers have questioned these results since sodium intake was assessed by a single 24-hour recall. Despite these latter findings, there is general agreement that increasing sodium intake is accompanied by an increase in blood pressure, which increases risk for stroke and coronary heart disease. Results from the DASH and DASH-Sodium trials contributed importantly to the current dietary recommendations for sodium as well as fruits and vegetables, and low-fat dairy products for normotensive and hypertensive individuals. The DGAC 2010 guidelines recommend a daily sodium intake of less than 2300 mg and less than 1500 mg for persons at high risk including those over the age of 51, African-Americans, and persons with hypertension, diabetes or chronic kidney disease.

Potassium

There is a moderate body of evidence for an association between potassium intake and blood pressure levels (DGAC, 2010b). A higher potassium intake has been associated with lower blood pressure in adults (Cappuccio and MacGregor, 1991; Whelton et al., 1997; Whelton and He, 1999; Geleijnse et al., 2003; Houston and Harper, 2008), and several observational studies have shown that an increase in potassium intake decreases the risk of stroke and coronary heart disease (DGAC, 2010a). Meta-analyses of clinical and cohort studies showed that an increase in potassium intake, for an average supplemental level between 44 and 86 mmol/day, significantly lowered systolic (−2.4 to −5.9 mm Hg) and diastolic (−1.5 to −3.4 mm Hg) blood pressure (Cappuccio and MacGregor, 1991; Geleijnse et al., 2003). A meta-analysis by Whelton and colleagues (1997) showed average net systolic/diastolic blood pressure reductions of −4.4/−2.5 mm Hg for hypertensive persons and −1.8/−1.0 mm Hg for non-hypertensives from a 2 g/day increase in urinary potassium excretion. Increased potassium intake also may attenuate the adverse effects of sodium on blood pressure (DGAC, 2010a), as seen in the DASH trial where a diet rich in vegetables and fruits and low-fat dairy products, and therefore rich in potassium, lowered blood pressure (Appel *et al.*, 1997). Many trials have evaluated the effects of supplemental potassium (mostly as potassium chloride) and potassium provided by food. The blood-pressure-lowering effects of potassium are greater when sodium intake is high versus when it is low (DGAC, 2010a). A response in blood pressure due to a change in sodium chloride intake has been shown to vary between individuals, with the concept of "salt sensitivity" used to describe blood pressure that is directly associated with sodium chloride intake (Weinberger, 1996; Morris *et al.*, 1999). This "salt sensitivity" was shown to be a risk for hypertension and mortality due to CVD, even in non-hypertensive persons (Morimoto *et al.*, 1997; Weinberger *et al.*, 2001), and its expression was found to be modulated by the intake of dietary potassium (Morris *et al.*, 1999; Schmidlin *et al.*, 1999). Potassium, irrespective of the accompanying anion (van Buren *et al.*, 1992), acts on the renal tubule to increase urinary sodium chloride excretion (Brandis *et al.*, 1972; Stokes, 1982). Thus, evidence exists for the mitigation of the pressor effect of sodium chloride by potassium supplementation (Iimura *et al.*, 1981; Morgan *et al.*, 1984). The current Institute of Medicine recommendation is 4700 mg/day for an adult.

Magnesium

Epidemiological evidence has reported that populations with a low intake of magnesium have an increased incidence of hypertension (McCarron, 1983; Joffres *et al.*, 1987; Witteman *et al.*, 1989; Ascherio *et al.*, 1992; Ma *et al.*, 1995). Low magnesium status is associated with cardiac arrhythmias, electrocardiographic changes, and increased sensitivity to cardiac glycosides (Rude, 1993). The anti-arrhythmic effect of magnesium sufficiency is related to its role in maintaining intracellular potassium levels (Matsuda, 1991a,b). Magnesium competes with sodium for binding sites on vascular smooth muscle cells to induce vasodilatation and reduce blood pressure (DGAC, 2010a). Some epidemiological, observational, and clinical trials have shown that dietary magnesium ranging from 500 to 1000 mg/day is associated with lower blood pressure, but the evidence has not been as consistent as that for sodium and for potassium (Widman *et al.*, 1993; Houston and Harper, 2008). A diet rich in fruits and vegetables that increased dietary magnesium from around 176 mg/day to 423 mg/day significantly lowered blood pressure in non-hypertensive adults (systolic blood pressure <140 mm Hg/diastolic blood pressure <95 mm Hg) (Appel *et al.*, 1997). However, foods with high levels of magne-

sium often have high levels of potassium and fiber, making the determination of an independent blood-pressure-lowering effect of magnesium difficult (Institute of Medicine, 1997). Results from intervention studies with hypertensive patients on magnesium therapy also are not conclusive. Whereas several studies have reported a blood-pressure-lowering effect with magnesium supplementation (Dyckner and Wester, 1983; Motoyama *et al.*, 1989; Widman *et al.*, 1993; Geleijnse *et al.*, 1994; Witteman *et al.*, 1994), other studies have not (Cappuccio *et al.*, 1985; Wallach and Verch, 1986; Zemel *et al.*, 1990; Sacks *et al.*, 1995; Yamamoto *et al.*, 1995). The evidence for an effect of magnesium supplementation on reducing CVD risk is supportive but limited; more research on the relationships between markers of magnesium status, magnesium intake, and CVD is needed (Institute of Medicine, 1997).

Magnesium also influences insulin sensitivity (DGAC, 2010a); a decrease in insulin sensitivity has been associated with low magnesium status (Ma *et al.*, 1995). This is of particular interest as CVD is a common complication of type 2 diabetes. Results from the Framingham Offspring Cohort study ($n = 2708$) indicated that higher magnesium intake was associated with lower fasting insulin levels as well as post-glucose challenge plasma insulin levels and improved insulin sensitivity after adjusting for potential risk factors for type 2 diabetes mellitus and insulin resistance (McKeown, 2004). Clinical studies also have shown that insulin sensitivity in patients with type 2 diabetes is improved by magnesium supplementation (Paolisso *et al.*, 1989, 1992), which would decrease CVD risk. In a 1999 recommendation by the American Diabetes Association (ADA) "routine evaluation of blood magnesium level is recommended only in patients at high risk for magnesium deficiency. Levels of magnesium should be repleted [replaced] only if hypomagnesemia can be demonstrated" (ADA, 1999). Recommended dietary allowances by the Institute of Medicine range between 310 and 320 mg/day for women and between 400 and 420 mg/day for men.

Vitamin D

Prospective observational studies and randomized controlled clinical trials have shown that moderate to high doses of vitamin D supplementation (≈ 1000 IU/day) may reduce CVD risk (Wang *et al.*, 2010). Epidemiological studies in particular have shown an association between low serum 25-hydroxyvitamin D levels and higher rates of CVD morbidity (Giovannucci *et al.*, 2008; Wang *et al.*, 2008b) and mortality (Wolf *et al.*, 2007; Dobnig *et al.*, 2008; Melamed *et al.*, 2008; Pilz *et al.*, 2008; Wang *et al.*, 2008a). A recent cross-sectional study (*n* = 7228) also has shown that serum concentrations of 25-hydroxyvitamin D (22.3–22.9 ng/mL) and parathyroid hormone (42.7–49.8 pg/mL) were independently associated with blood pressure, hypertension, and pre-hypertension (Zhao *et al.*, 2010). Vitamin D preserves endothelial cell function (Levin and Li, 2005), down-regulates the renin–angiotensin system (Li *et al.*, 2004; Rammos *et al.*, 2008), inhibits proliferation of vascular smooth muscle cells (Carthy *et al.*, 1989), and improves insulin sensitivity and secretion (Maestro *et al.*, 2000; Chiu *et al.*, 2004). Randomized trials using vitamin D supplements versus a placebo have shown a statistically non-significant reduction in CVD risk due to vitamin D supplementation at moderate doses (100 000 IU every 4 months) (Trivedi *et al.*, 2003) and high doses (1000 IU/day) (Prince *et al.*, 2008). Other randomized trials evaluating the effects of vitamin D supplementation in conjunction with calcium supplementation did not show changes in CVD event risk (Brazier *et al.*, 2005; Hsia *et al.*, 2007). Renal disease patients tend to have a compromised vitamin D status and typically are treated with vitamin D supplements (Wang *et al.*, 2010). While not representative of the population at large, the association between vitamin D supplementation and CVD mortality in these patients has been evaluated (Marco *et al.*, 2003; Shoji *et al.*, 2004; Teng *et al.*, 2005; Wolf *et al.*, 2007; Naves-Diaz *et al.*, 2008). Reductions in CVD mortality with vitamin D supplementation have been reported in prospective studies of dialysis patients (Wang *et al.*, 2010). The pooled relative risk of CVD in these randomized trials was 0.90 (CI: 0.77–1.05) (Wang *et al.*, 2010). These findings suggest a protective effect of moderate to high doses of vitamin D on CVD risk (Wang *et al.*, 2010). However, given these limited and inconclusive findings, further intervention trials are needed to confirm causality and to determine the efficacy of vitamin D supplementation at different doses in various subpopulations. The 2010 DGAC report, assuming minimal sun exposure, recommends 600 IU/day of vitamin D for children and adults, and 800 IU per day for adults over age 70 (DGAC, 2010b). The Food and Nutrition Board of the Institute of Medicine issued dietary reference intakes of 600 IU/day (15 μg cholecalciferol) for children and adults, with a recommended intake of 800 IU/day (15–20 μg cholecalciferol) for persons over age 70, and an upper limit of 4000 IU/day (Institute of Medicine, 2010). This Institute of Medicine review was

jointly commissioned by the US and Canadian governments, with Health Canada (Ottawa) recommending intakes of 600 IU/day for children and adults, 800 IU/day for persons over 70, daily supplemental intake of 400 IU/day (10 μg cholecalciferol) for persons over 50, and an upper limit of 4000 IU/day (Health Canada, 2010).

B-Vitamins

Elevated plasma homocysteine levels are associated with increased risk of atherosclerosis (Gerhard and Duell, 1999; Marti-Carvajal *et al.*, 2009). Homocysteine levels are affected by vitamins B_6, B_{12}, and folate. Folate coenzymes catalyze the synthesis of methionine from homocysteine; homocysteine levels increase in folate deficiency (Gerhard and Duell, 1999). Homocysteine levels also are under the control of vitamins B_6 and B_{12}. Vitamin B_{12} acts as a co-factor for methionine synthase, an enzyme that catalyzes the conversion of homocysteine to methionine (Homocysteine Lowering Trialists, 1998). Vitamin B_6 is a cofactor for two enzymes involved in an alternative homocysteine pathway involving the conversion of homocysteine to cysteine (Folsom *et al.*, 1998). Each of the pathways involves the utilization of homocysteine, thus regulating plasma levels. Consequently, supplementation of these vitamins was hypothesized to lower homocysteine levels and decrease CVD risk (Folsom *et al.*, 1998; Gerhard and Duell, 1999). Martí-Carvajal and colleagues (2009) reviewed eight randomized controlled trials (*n* = 24 210) to determine the effects of B_6, folate, and B_{12} supplementation in either primary or secondary prevention interventions. The authors found no evidence that a decrease in homocysteine levels in response to B-vitamin supplementation decreased stroke or myocardial infarction, or reduced mortality in individuals with CVD (Marti-Carvajal *et al.*, 2009). Despite the inverse association between homocysteine concentration and folate intake, the body of evidence for an association between homocysteine concentration and CVD risk is inconsistent (Institute of Medicine, 1998). The American Heart Association Nutrition Committee concluded that there is inadequate evidence in support of the use of the B-vitamins for lowering CVD risk (Lichtenstein *et al.*, 2006a).

Therapeutic doses of niacin, or nicotinic acid, are prescribed primarily for TG-lowering and increasing HDL-C. Pharmacological doses of nicotinic acid (3 g/day) result in a global improvement in the lipid profile (Chapman *et al.*, 2010) including a reduction in total cholesterol and triglycerides, and a decreased risk of cardiovascular events

(Canner *et al.*, 1986). Niacin and derivatives decreased plasma triglyceride levels by −35% and LDL-C by −15%, and increased HDL-C by 25% (Chapman *et al.*, 2010). In addition, nicotinic acid (1–3 g/day) shifted the size and density of LDL particles from being small and dense to large and buoyant (Guyton and Capuzzi, 1998). The modulation of the lipid profile by niacin was reported to be dose-dependent, with 1.5 g/day providing the most tolerable and efficacious dose (Watts and Karpe, 2011). However, in their study on an antioxidant combination of vitamin E, vitamin C, selenium, and β-carotene, Cheung and colleagues (2001) found that the use of this antioxidant supplement cocktail blunted the effects of simvastatin–niacin therapy on HDL-C in persons with CAD and decreased HDL-C levels, indicating potential adverse antagonistic effects (Cheung *et al.*, 2001). In another study on CHD prevention, Brown and colleagues (2001) showed that, when an antioxidant cocktail (vitamin E, vitamin C, β-carotene, selenium) was administered with simvastatin and niacin, the clinical benefits of the lipid therapy (simvastatin and niacin alone), including a lowered frequency of occurrence for a first cardiovascular event, were no longer evident. In addition, this combination caused a significant reduction in HDL sub-fraction levels including one of the main fractions involved in reverse cholesterol transport, indicating a blunting of the main cardioprotective effect of the statin–niacin therapy (Brown *et al.*, 2001). People should be under the care of a health-care provider when taking therapeutic doses of niacin for the management of lipid disorders, and should avoid taking antioxidant supplements. The Institute of Medicine recommends 14 mg/day of niacin equivalents (NEs) for women and 16 mg/day NEs for men to achieve nutrient adequacy.

The Antioxidant Vitamins—Vitamins C and E

A diet high in fruits and vegetables has been found to be protective against CVD, and so the bioactive compounds that offer this cardioprotection are of great interest. Since CVD development and progression are influenced in large part by oxidative stress, the potential action of the antioxidant vitamins has been a major area of study. Vitamin C (ascorbic acid) and vitamin E (α-tocopherol) have been shown to protect against free radical production *in vitro* (Bagchi *et al.*, 1997) and may consequently reduce lipid peroxidation and formation of oxidized LDL (Knekt *et al.*, 2004). In addition, vitamin C may facilitate the regeneration of oxidized vitamin E (Knekt *et al.*, 2004), providing a synergistic scavenger effect. Generally, studies of these antioxidants have focused on both their dietary and supplemental forms and their effects on CVD risk.

Clinical evidence of cardioprotective roles of vitamins C and E have been limited and inconclusive. In a review of 67 ($n = 232\,550$) randomized controlled trials, Bjelakovic and colleagues (2008) assessed the effects of antioxidant supplements on overall mortality in primary and secondary prevention clinical trials. The authors found no evidence in support of antioxidant supplements in primary or secondary prevention measures for lowered mortality due to CVD. When a selection of 47 trials ($n = 180\,938$) with low risk for bias was used, there was a significant increase in relative risk for total mortality due to vitamin E of 1.04 (CI: 1.01–1.07), and a non-significant increase in relative risk for total mortality due to vitamin C of 1.06 (CI: 0.94–1.20) (Bjelakovic *et al.*, 2008).

In an analysis of nine prospective cohort studies ($n = 293\,172$), Knekt and colleagues (2004) found that persons with no pre-existing CHD, who were on supplemental vitamin C regimens (>700 mg/day), had a lower relative risk for CHD incidence of 0.75 (CI: 0.60–0.93) vs. persons not taking these supplements. Ye and Song (2008) also conducted a meta-analysis of 15 cohort studies ($n = 374\,488$) to evaluate the relationship between intakes of vitamin C and CHD risk. Their results showed that dietary intake of vitamin C, but not supplemental vitamin C, had an inverse relationship with CHD risk (Ye and Song, 2008). In another randomized controlled trial, using over 14 000 men who took part in the Physician's Health Study II, daily vitamin C supplementation (500 mg/day) had no significant effect on CVD events, myocardial infarction or mortality due to CVD (Sesso *et al.*, 2008). However, this study was limited in that all participants were 50 years or older, with about 5% having pre-existing heart disease, which probably resulted in a diminished preventive effect against CVD progression. Several studies also have shown improved vasodilation with supplemental vitamin C (500 mg) (Carr and Frei, 1999; Gokce *et al.*, 1999; Frikke-Schmidt and Lykkesfeldt, 2009; Versari *et al.*, 2009), and some, but not all, studies have shown a blood-pressure-lowering effect with supplemental vitamin C (Ness *et al.*, 1997). In their study with 69 hypertensive individuals supplemented for 6 weeks with vitamin C (500 mg/day), Ward and colleagues (2005) found a significant ($p < 0.05$) decrease in systolic blood pressure (−1.8 mm Hg) in comparison with a placebo (Ward *et al.*, 2005). Given the inconsistencies in the evidence, further replication in larger, controlled clinical trials is needed.

In their meta-analysis of nine prospective cohort studies ($n = 293\,172$), Knekt and colleagues (2004) also found that high dietary vitamin E intakes (100–249 mg/day) were associated with a lower CHD risk after accounting for age and energy intake. In the meta-analysis of 15 cohort studies ($n = 374\,488$) by Ye and Song (2008), both dietary and supplemental intake of vitamin E were inversely associated with CHD risk. In the Alpha-Tocopherol–Beta-Carotene Cancer Prevention study ($n = 299\,133$), vitamin E supplementation (50 mg/day) in a group of Finnish male smokers slightly lowered mortality of CHD (ischemic heart disease by −4% and ischemic stroke by −1.3%), but had no effect on incidence of non-fatal myocardial infarction (Alpha-Tocopherol–Beta Carotene Cancer Prevention Study Group, 1994). The Cambridge Heart Antioxidant Study (CHAOS) on secondary prevention by vitamin E supplementation (400 or 800 IU per day for 1.5 years) in patients with CHD ($n = 2002$) showed a significant reduction in risk for recurrent myocardial infarction (−77%), but no effect on CVD mortality, and a non-significant increase in total mortality (Stephens *et al.*, 1996). Other large-scale clinical trials in patients with established CHD also have not shown protective effects of vitamin E supplementation on future CVD events (GISSI-Prevenzione Investigators, 1999; Yusuf *et al.*, 2000), indicating the need for further study in different populations before conclusions are drawn.

Discrepancies between these studies have been attributed to the overall healthy lifestyles of persons on antioxidant vitamin regimens; for example, high serum ascorbic acid levels may be associated with high fruit and vegetable intake (Ye and Song, 2008). There also may have been discrepancies in CHD risk between persons in randomized controlled trials versus those in cohort studies, since the latter tend to recruit younger persons who are fairly healthy whereas controlled trials often study persons at high risk (Ye and Song, 2008). Toxicity with increased levels of supplement intake in smokers or persons with pre-existing CHD also is possible. Poor study design and distinct methods of analysis also may have contributed to the discrepancies in the overall findings (Traber *et al.*, 2008).

The Institute of Medicine (2000) states that data on the preventive effects of vitamins C and E, either dietary or supplemental, on CVD risk are both inconsistent and insufficient; the Academy of Nutrition and Dietetics provides no recommendation for routine supplementation

of either vitamin due to the lack of strong evidence at this time.

Dietary Prevention and Treatment of Cardiovascular Disease

Current Dietary Guidelines for the prevention of CVD

Over the years, specific nutrient recommendations have been issued in dietary guidelines reports from health-related institutions worldwide. More recently, with growing evidence on the role of dietary patterns and specific foods and food groups on health, there has been a transition from nutrient-based to food-based recommendations (Mozaffarian and Ludwig, 2010), as evidenced in the food-based dietary guidelines from several countries. A basic premise of these dietary guidelines is that nutrient needs should be met primarily through foods.

Food-Based Dietary Guidelines for Worldwide Application

The Department of Nutrition for Health and Development of the WHO (World Health Organization), in collaboration with the FAO (Food and Agriculture Organization of the United Nations), continually reviews new research and information from around the world on human nutrient requirements. The results of this work provide the foundation for all countries to develop food-based dietary guidelines for their populations. Food-based dietary guidelines from different countries share basic recommendations that are consistent with WHO guidelines. However, national dietary guidelines often contain unique features, which are designed to address the priorities of each country. A selection of food-based guidelines by region and country is given in Box 48.1. A summary of the recommendations, both shared and differing between countries, is shown in Box 48.2. Common recommendations include limiting salt intake, eating fruit and vegetables daily, eating foods rich in starch and fiber, and maintaining a healthy body weight.

For promoting cardiovascular health, the Joint WHO/FAO Expert Consultation published a technical report on Diet, Nutrition and the Prevention of Chronic Diseases in 2002 which provides general diet recommendations for the prevention of death and disability from major nutrition-related chronic diseases, including obesity, diabetes, several forms of cancer, osteoporosis, dental disease, and cardiovascular disease (Joint FAO/WHO Expert

BOX 48.1   Summary of a selection of food-based dietary guidelines by region (FAO)

Africa	Namibia	Eat a variety of foods; Eat vegetables and fruit every day; Eat more fish; Eat beans or meat regularly; Use whole-grain products; Use only iodized salt, but use less salt; Eat at least three meals a day; Avoid drinking alcohol; Consume clean and safe water and food; Achieve and maintain a healthy body weight. *(Ministry of Health and Social Services, Namibia)*
	Nigeria	Total food intake should be balanced with the level of physical activity; Individuals who do manual work need to consume more food than those who do sedentary work; Limit fat intake from animal foods; The diet should consist of as wide a variety of foods as possible, e.g. cereals, legumes, roots/tubers, fruits, vegetables, fish, lean meat, local cheese (wara); Limit intake of salt, bouillon cubes and sugar; Liberal consumption of whatever fruit is in season is encouraged. *(Ministry of Health, Abuja, Nigeria)*
	South Africa	Enjoy a variety of foods; Be active; Make starchy foods the basis of most meals; Eat dry beans, split peas, lentils and soya regularly; Chicken, fish, milk, meat or eggs can be eaten daily; Drink lots of clean, safe water; Eat plenty of vegetables and fruits every day; Eat fats sparingly; Use salt sparingly; Use food and drinks containing sugar sparingly and not between meals; If you drink alcohol, drink sensibly. *(Department of Health, Directorate: Nutrition, Pretoria, South Africa)*
Asia and the Pacific	China	Eat a variety of foods, with cereals as the staple; Consume plenty of vegetables, fruits and tubers; Consume milk, beans, or dairy or bean products every day; Consume appropriate amounts of fish, poultry, eggs, and lean meat; Reduce fatty meat and animal fat in the diet; Balance food intake with physical activity to maintain a healthy body weight; Choose a light diet that is also low in salt; If you drink alcoholic beverages, do so in limited amounts; Avoid unsanitary and spoiled foods. *(Chinese Nutrition Society)*
	India	Eat a variety of foods to ensure a balanced diet; Ensure provision of extra food and health care to pregnant and lactating women; Promote exclusive breastfeeding for 6 months and encourage breastfeeding until 2 years; Feed home-based, semi-solid foods to infants after 6 months; Ensure adequate and appropriate diets for children and adolescents both in health and sickness; Ensure moderate use of edible oils and animal foods and very much less use of ghee/butter/vanaspati; Overeating should be avoided to prevent overweight and obesity; Use salt in moderation/Restrict salt intake to minimum; Ensure the use of safe and clean foods; Practice good cooking methods and healthy eating habits; Drink plenty of water and take beverages in moderation; Minimize the use of processed foods rich in salt, sugar and fats; Include micronutrient-rich foods in the diets of elderly persons to enable them to be fit and active. *(National Institute of Nutrition, Indian Council of Medical Research, India)*
	Japan	Enjoy your meals; Establish a healthy rhythm by keeping regular hours for meals; Eat well-balanced meals with staple foods, as well as main and side dishes; Eat enough grains such as rice and other cereals; Combine vegetables, fruits, milk products, beans, and fish in your diet; Avoid too much salt and fat; Learn your healthy body weight and balance the calories you eat with physical activity. *(Japan Dietetic Association)*

(Continued)

	Singapore	Achieve and maintain body weight within the normal range; Eat sufficient amounts of grains, especially whole grains; Eat more fruits and vegetables every day; Choose and prepare food with less fat, especially SFA; Choose and prepare foods with less salt and sauces; Choose beverages and food with less sugar; If you drink alcoholic beverages, do so in moderation. *(Health Promotion Board, Singapore)*
	Thailand	Eat a variety of foods from each of the five food groups and maintain proper weight; Eat adequate amounts of rice or alternative carbohydrate sources; Eat plenty of vegetables and fruits regularly; Eat fish, lean meat, eggs, and legumes and pulses regularly; Drink milk in appropriate quality and quantity for one's age; Eat a diet containing appropriate amounts of fat; Avoid sweet and salty foods; Eat clean and safe foods; Avoid or reduce the consumption of alcoholic beverages. *(Department of Health, Thailand)*
Europe	Bulgaria	Eat a nutritious diet with a variety of foods; Do eat regularly, take enough time and enjoy your food in a friendly environment; Consume cereals as an important source of energy; Choose whole-grain bread and other whole-grain products; Eat a variety of vegetables and fruits, more than 400 g every day, preferably raw; Choose milk and dairy products with low fat and salt content; Choose lean meat, replace meat and meat products often with fish, poultry or pulses; Limit total fat intake, especially animal fat; Replace animal fats with vegetable oils when cooking; Limit the consumption of sugar, sweets and confectionery, avoid sugar-containing soft drinks; Reduce intake of salt and salty foods; If you drink alcoholic beverages, you should consume moderate quantities; Maintain a healthy body weight and be physically active every day; Drink plenty of water every day; Prepare and store food in a way to ensure its quality and safety. *(Ministry of Health, Bulgaria)*
	France	Increase consumption of fruits and vegetables, regardless of its form (fresh, frozen, canned, cooked), in order to achieve consumption of at least 5 fruits and vegetables daily; Consume food sources of calcium in sufficient quantity to achieve the recommended dietary allowances, or 3 dairy products per day; Limit consumption of fat, especially saturated fat; Increase intake of starch, including food grains, potatoes, legumes, etc. – have these with every meal; Eat meat, fish, seafood or eggs 1–2 times a day on alternate days; Choose meat with less fat and consume fish at least twice a week; Limit salt intake and always choose iodized salt; Limit alcohol consumption to a maximum of 2 glasses per day for women and a maximum of 3 glasses a day for men; Increase daily physical activity to at least 30 minutes of brisk walking or equivalent and reduce sedentary time, especially in children; Enjoy the benefits of sunlight without excess and monitor weight regularly. *(The Ministry of Health, Family and the Disabled, France)*
	Ireland	Enjoy your food; Eat a variety of foods, using the Food Pyramid as a guide; Eat the right amount of food to be a healthy weight, and exercise regularly; Eat 4 or more portions of fruit and vegetables every day; Eat more foods rich in starch – breads, cereals, potatoes, pasta, and rice – aim for at least 6 servings a day; Eat plenty of foods rich in fibers – breads and cereals (especially whole grain), potatoes, pasta and rice, fruit and vegetables; Reduce the amounts of fatty foods you eat, especially saturated fats – grill, boil, oven-bake or stir-fry in very little fat instead of deep-frying; If you drink alcohol, keep within sensible limits; Use a variety of seasonings, try not to always rely on salt to flavor foods – use herbs, spices and black pepper as alternatives. *(The Irish Nutrition and Dietetic Institute)*

	The Netherlands	Eat a variety of foods; Be moderate with fat; Eat plenty of carbohydrates and fiber; Have 3 meals a day and do not snack more than 4 times in-between meals; Be careful with salt; Drink 1.5 L of fluid daily, but be moderate with alcohol; Keep body weight at its correct level; Prevent food-borne infections by good hygiene; Keep in mind the presence of harmful substances in foods; Read the information on the food label. *(The Netherlands Bureau for Food and Nutrition Education)*
	Poland	Ensure you eat a variety of foods; Beware of overweight and obesity – be physically active; Cereal products should be the main source of calories; Drink at least 2 large glasses of low-fat milk daily – milk could be substituted for yogurt, kefir and partly for cheese also; Eat in moderation; Eat a lot of vegetables and fruits every day; Limit intake of fats, particularly of animal ones, and all foods containing cholesterol; Be moderate in intake of sugar and sweets; Limit salt intake; Avoid alcohol. *(Ministry of Health, Poland)*
	United Kingdom	Enjoy your food; Eat a variety of different foods; Eat the right amount to be a healthy weight; Eat plenty of foods rich in starch and fiber; Eat plenty of fruits and vegetables; Don't eat too many foods that contain a lot of fat; Don't have sugary foods and drinks too often; If you drink alcohol, drink sensibly. *(Health Education Authority, London, UK)*
Latin America and the Caribbean	Chile	Consume dairy products like milk, yogurt or cheese 3 times daily, preferably as low- or non-fat versions; Eat at least 2 dishes of vegetables, and 3 fruit of different colors each day; Eat beans, chickpeas, lentils or split peas at least 2 times per week as a replacement for meat; Eat fish at least 2 times per week cooked either by baking, steaming or grilling; Choose foods with less saturated fat and cholesterol; Reduce your intake of sugar and salt; Consume 6–9 glasses of water a day. *(Ministry of Health, Chile)*
	Cuba	A varied diet during the day is enjoyable and necessary for your health; Eat vegetables every day – fill your life; Eat fresh fruit to increase vitality; Choose vegetable oils – butter is more costly to your health; Fish and chicken are the healthiest of meats; Reduce sugar intake; Reduce salt intake – start by not adding it at the table; A good day starts with breakfast; Find a healthy weight for your height – stay in shape. *(Ministry of Public Health, Cuba)*
	Commonwealth of Dominica	Start the day with breakfast; Always try to eat a variety of foods every day; Eat more vegetables and fruits daily; Reduce fat and oil intake; Choose less sweet foods and drinks; Use less salt, salted foods, seasonings, and salty snacks; Make physical activity a part of your daily life; Drink water several times a day; If you use alcohol, do so in moderation. *(Ministry of Health and Social Security, Dominica)*
	Grenada	Eat a variety of foods; Eat larger amounts of fruits and colored vegetables; Eat less fatty, oily, greasy, and barbecued foods; Choose to use less sweet foods and drinks; Use less salt, salty foods, salty seasonings and salty snacks; Drink more water – it's the healthier choice; Drink little or no alcohol; Be more physically active every day – get moving. *(Grenada Food and Nutrition Council)*

(Continued)

	Mexico	Try to eat healthily, accompanied by family and/or friends, and make eating an enjoyable time; Eat raw vegetables and fruits in season; Have moderate consumption of fats (margarine, vegetable oils, and mayonnaise among others), sugars (soft drinks, honey, jam, sweets and table sugar) and salt; Eat according to your needs and conditions, neither more nor less; Eat moderate amounts of animal foods, choose legumes; Combine grains (tortillas, bread or pasta) with legumes such as beans, peas, or lentils; Try to choose whole grains such as corn tortillas, bread, oatmeal, and amaranth instead of refined versions; Try eating fish twice a week and skinless chicken instead of red meat; If using eggs, keep it in moderation; Avoid alcoholic beverages or consume them only sporadically since, among other factors, they are high in calories. *(National Institute of Medical and Nutrition Science, Mexico)*
	St. Vincent and the Grenadines	Eat a variety of foods; Eat more fruits and vegetables everyday; Reduce fats and oils by cutting back on fatty, oily, and greasy foods; Reduce the intake of sugar – use less sugar, sweet foods and drinks; When cooking, use less salt and salted seasonings – eat less salted foods and snacks; Water is essential – drink it several times a day; If you use alcohol, do so sparingly, both in drinking and in food preparation; Get moving – increase physical activity daily. *(Ministry of Health and the Environment, St. Vincent and the Grenadines)*
	Venezuela	Eat foods from all the basic groups; Breast milk is the only irreplaceable food for children under 6 months; Increase consumption of vegetables, fruits, legumes and cereals; Moderate your intake of sugar, salt, and alcohol; Eat foods of animal origin in moderation; Practice hygienic habits during food preparation; Water maintains health and is essential for life; Manage your money well during the selection and purchase of food; Take 30 minutes of physical activity daily. *(National Institute of Nutrition, Bolivarian Republic of Venezuela)*
Near East	Egypt	Limit red meat and dairy products; Use low fat milk; Do not fry; Consume plenty of fruits, vegetables, legumes and whole grains; Consume olive oil, nuts, plant proteins, and fish; Limit candies and soft drinks; Avoid salty, canned, preserved, and fast food; Establish and maintain at least 30 minutes of moderate-intensity physical activity on 5 or more days per week. *(The Egyptian Hypertension Society)*
	Oman	Vary your diet by making it healthy and balanced; Choose whole grains and cereals, and consume potatoes with their skin; Consume 3–5 servings of vegetables daily; Consume 2–4 servings of fruits daily; Consume fish, poultry, eggs or lean meat; Consume 1 serving of legumes daily; Consume milk or dairy products daily; Limit your fat intake and choose snacks wisely; Follow the five keys to safer food: keep everything clean, separate raw and cooked foods, cook foods thoroughly, keep food at safe temperatures, and use safe water and raw materials; Be active, exercise regularly and drink plenty of water. *(Ministry of Health, Oman)*

North America	Canada	Eat at least one dark green and one orange vegetable each day; Choose vegetables and fruit prepared with little or no added fat, sugar, or salt; Have vegetables and fruit more often than juice; Make at least half of your grain products whole grain each day; Choose grain products that are lower in fat, sugar, or salt; Drink skim, 1% or 2% milk each day; Select lower fat alternatives; Have meat alternatives such as beans, lentils, and tofu often; Eat at least 2 servings of fish each week; Select lean meat and alternatives prepared with little or no added fat or salt; Include a small amount (2 to 3 tbsp) of unsaturated fat each day; Use vegetable oils such as canola, olive and soybean; Choose soft margarines that are low in saturated and *trans* fats; Limit butter, hard margarine, lard and shortening; Drink water regularly; Build 30 to 60 minutes of moderate physical activity into daily life; Enjoy eating with family and friends. *(Health Canada)* **For First Nations, Inuit, and Métis**: Eat at least one dark green and one orange vegetable each day; Choose vegetables and fruit prepared with little or no added fat, sugar or salt; Have vegetables and fruit more often than juice; Make at least half of your grain products whole grain each day; Choose grains that are lower in fat, sugar or salt; Drink 2 cups (500 mL) of skim, 1% or 2% milk each day; Select lower fat milk alternatives – drink fortified soy beverages if you do not drink milk; Have meat alternatives such as beans, lentils, and tofu often; Eat at least 2 servings of fish each week; Select lean meat and alternatives prepared with little or no added fat or salt; Most of the time, use vegetable oils with unsaturated fats, including canola, olive and soybean oils – aim for a small amount (2 to 3 tbsp) each day; Traditional fats that are liquid at room temperature such as seal and whale oil, or ooligan grease, also contain unsaturated fats – these can be used as all or part of the recommended 2 to 3 tbsp per day; Choose soft margarines that are low in saturated and *trans* fats; Limit butter, hard margarine, lard, shortening and bacon fat; For strong body, mind and spirit, be active every day. *(Health Canada)*

BOX 48.2   Summary of global food-based dietary guidelines

Basic dietary recommendations shared among many countries
Eat a variety of foods
Eat vegetables and fruit every day
Limit salt intake
Moderate fat intake, reduce cholesterol intake
Eat poultry, fish, beans, and dairy products regularly
Eat plenty of foods rich in starch and fiber
Limit consumption of foods containing added sugars
Avoid drinking alcohol or, if alcohol is consumed, do so responsibly
Achieve and maintain a healthy body weight

Unique features
Consume clean and safe water and food (some developing countries)
Use only iodized salt (some developing countries)
Eat soya regularly (some African and Asian countries)
Eat eggs regularly (South Africa, China)
Drink plenty of liquids every day (South Africa, Bulgaria)
Consume iron-rich foods (some developing countries)
Eat breakfast every day (some developing countries)

TABLE 48.5   Joint WHO/FAO Expert Consultation dietary recommendations for CVD prevention

Recommendations	How to achieve
Fat intake (%E): SFA <7%; TFA <1%; 6–10% of PUFAs (n-6: 5–8%, n-3: 1–2%); MUFAs ≈15–30% *Dietary cholesterol*: <300 mg/day	Limit intake of fat from dairy and meat sources; avoid use of hydrogenated oils and fats in cooking and manufacturing of food products; using appropriate edible vegetable oils in moderation; regular intake of fish (1–2 times per week) and/or plant sources of ALA (n-3 PUFAs); utilize non-frying food preparation methods
Fruits and vegetables: 400–500 g/day is recommended to reduce the risk of CHD, stroke and high blood pressure	Daily intake of fresh fruit and vegetables (including berries, green leafy and cruciferous vegetables, legumes) in adequate quantities
Sodium: 1.7 g of sodium per day (equivalent to a daily sodium chloride intake of 4 g/day) is beneficial in reducing blood pressure and is not associated with adverse effects	Restrict daily salt (sodium chloride) intake to less than 5 g/day; minimize other forms of sodium consumption through food additives and preservatives, such as monosodium glutamate (MSG)
Potassium: Dietary intake sufficient to maintain sodium: potassium ratio close to 1, i.e. at daily potassium intake levels of 70–80 mmol/day	Adequate daily consumption of fruits and vegetables
Fish: Consumption of fish and other marine foods should provide over 200 mg/day of DHA and EPA	Regular fish consumption, as consumed on a weekly basis
Dietary fiber: Increase intake.	Adequate intake of fruits, vegetables and whole-grain cereals
Alcohol: Moderate consumption.	Regular low to moderate consumption of alcohol

Consultation, 2002). The primary aim of this report was to provide "effective and sustainable policies and strategies to deal with the increasing public health challenges related to diet and health." A summary of the recommendations specifically focused on CVD prevention is shown in Table 48.5.

Dietary Guidelines for Americans 2010

The first edition of *Nutrition and Your Health: Dietary Guidelines for Americans*, issued in 1980, provided guidance on total fat, saturated fat, cholesterol, sodium, sugar, starch, and fiber intake, as well as the maintenance of an ideal body weight and appropriate alcohol consumption, all of which are related to CVD risk. The most recent Dietary Guidelines for Americans 2010 (DGAC 2010a) continues to promote CVD prevention by providing food-based recommendations.

Generally, a healthy eating pattern limits the intake of sodium, solid fats, added sugars, and refined grains, and emphasizes nutrient-dense foods. The DGAC 2010 Report identified certain foods and food components that are consumed in excessive amounts and should be reduced in order to decrease the risk of overweight and certain chronic diseases, including major sources of sodium, SFAs, added sugar, solid fats, dietary cholesterol, refined grains, and alcohol (Box 48.3). Besides limiting these foods, the Dietary Guidelines for Americans (2010) also make recommendations for certain foods that should be increased, including vegetables and fruits, whole grains, fat-free or low-fat dairy products, seafood, lean meat and poultry, eggs, beans and peas, soy products, unsalted nuts and seeds, plant oils, and foods that provide more potassium, calcium, vitamin D, and dietary fiber. Of these foods and food groups that the DGAC recommends be increased or

---

BOX 48.3   Dietary components currently over- and underconsumed by the American population (DGAC, 2010a)

Overconsumed	Adults	Total energy intake, particularly energy intake from solid fats and added sugars; sodium; percentage of total energy from saturated fats; total cholesterol (in men); and refined grains
	Children	Energy intake from solid fats and added sugars; sodium; percentage of total energy from saturated fats; total cholesterol (only in boys, aged 12–19 years); and refined grains
Underconsumed	Entire population, on average	Americans of all ages consume too few vegetables, fruits, high-fiber whole grains, low-fat milk and milk products, seafood, and oils, and have low intakes of fiber, potassium, calcium, and vitamin D

---

decreased, most are related to a reduced risk of CVD; see Table 48.6 (DGAC, 2010a).

American Heart Association (AHA) Diet and Lifestyle Recommendations and 2020 Impact Goals

In 2006, the American Heart Association (AHA) released the Diet and Lifestyle Recommendations Revision for reducing CVD risk (Lichtenstein *et al.*, 2006a); overall, these diet and lifestyle recommendations are similar to those provided by the WHO and FAO. In 2010, the American Heart Association (AHA) issued the 2020 Impact Goals to achieve the following: "By 2020, to improve the cardiovascular health of all Americans by 20% while reducing deaths from cardiovascular diseases and stroke by 20%" (Lloyd-Jones *et al.*, 2010). The dietary intake goals are "in the context of a diet that is appropriate in energy balance, pursuing an overall dietary pattern that is consistent with a DASH-type eating plan" (Lloyd-Jones *et al.*, 2010). Specific food and nutrient recommendations to achieve the AHA 2020 Impact Goals are summarized in Table 48.7.

European Food Safety Authority (EFSA) Panel on Dietetic Products, Nutrition and Allergies (NDA) Scientific Opinion on Dietary Reference Values

In 2009 the EFSA Panel on Dietetic Products, Nutrition and Allergies issued reports to the European Commission on the Population Reference Intakes for the European population. The primary goal of these reports was to update the first dietary reference intake values set in 1993. Reference intakes for carbohydrate, dietary fiber, and water were assessed, as well as those for fat, the latter of which

included SFAs, MUFAs, PUFAs, *trans* fats and cholesterol (EFSA Panel on Dietetic Products Nutrition and Allergies, 2010a,b). These recommendations are shown in Tables 48.8 and 48.9. Advice on the reference intakes for protein, energy, vitamins, and minerals is forthcoming.

The EFSA's review of the literature and subsequent recommendations provide a model for countries and regions with very distinct food patterns. Recommendations could be made that are more sensitive to the culture and geographical region of interest in order to present the most cost-effective measures for the maintenance of overall health.

Dietary Patterns for Prevention

Both the DGAC 2010 and global recommendations focus on three dietary patterns designed for the prevention of chronic diseases, specifically CVD. Clinical and epidemiological evidence shows that the Dietary Approaches to Stop Hypertension (DASH) diet, a Mediterranean-style diet, and a vegetarian diet all reduce risk factors associated with CHD (DGAC, 2010a). The American Heart Association's Therapeutic Lifestyle Changes (TLC) diet is designed for the prevention and treatment of CHD, other cardiovascular diseases, diabetes, insulin resistance, metabolic syndrome, and elevated LDL-C (Expert Panel on Detection, Evaluation, and Treatment of High Blood Cholesterol in Adults, 2001). With these healthful dietary patterns, there are many options to accommodate individual preferences to enhance adherence to current guidelines for reducing CVD risk.

TABLE 48.6 Foods and food components recommended for increased or reduced consumption in the diet by the 2010 Dietary Guidelines for Americans (DGAC, 2010a)

Food	Recommended amount	Reduces risk of:
Increase:		
Vegetables and fruits	At least 2½ cups per day	CVD, cancer
Whole grains	At least half of recommended total grain intake or 3 oz equivalents per day	CVD, overweight, type 2 diabetes
Milk and milk products	3 cups per day of fat-free or low-fat milk and milk products for adults and children and adolescents ages 9–18 years, 2½ cups per day for children ages 4–8 years, and 2 cups for children ages 2–3 years	CVD, high blood pressure, type 2 diabetes
Protein foods	Consume a balanced variety of protein foods	CVD
Seafood	An intake of 8 oz or more per week (less for young children), which provide an average consumption of 250 mg per day of EPA and DHA	CVD
Oils	Replace solid fats with oils, rather than add oil to the diet, and use oils in small amounts	CVD
Reduce:		
Sodium	Less than 2300 mg and further reduce to 1500 mg among persons who are 51 and older and those of any age who are African-American or have hypertension, diabetes, or chronic kidney disease	High blood pressure, CVD, congestive heart failure, kidney disease
Saturated fat intake	Consume less than 10% and further reduce to 7% of calories from saturated fat (for persons at increased risk) and replace these with monounsaturated and/or polyunsaturated fat	Elevated LDL cholesterol, CVD
Trans fatty acids	As low as possible (<1% calories)	Elevated LDL cholesterol, CVD
Cholesterol	Less than 300 mg per day of cholesterol and further reduce to 200 mg per day for individuals at high risk of CVD	Elevated LDL cholesterol, CVD
Solid fats	Reducing sources of excess solid fats in the diet results in reduced intake of saturated fats, *trans* fats, and calories	Excess caloric intake, colorectal cancer, CVD
Added sugars	Reducing consumption of sources of added sugars lowers the calorie content of the diet without compromising its nutrient adequacy	Excess caloric intake
Refined grains	No more than 3 oz equivalents per day; at least half of all grains eaten as whole grains; reduce consumption of refined grain products that also are high in solid fats and/or added sugars, such as cakes, cookies, donuts, and other desserts	Excess caloric intake
Alcohol	Moderate alcohol consumption recommended for persons who consume alcohol; this is defined as up to 1 drink per day for women and up to 2 drinks per day for men	Cirrhosis of the liver, hypertension, stroke, type 2 diabetes, cancer of the upper gastrointestinal tract and colon, increased body weight, impairment of cognitive function, injury, and violence

TABLE 48.7 Food and nutrient recommendations to achieve the American Heart Association (AHA) 2020 Impact Goals; these are based on a 2000-calorie/day diet

Food goals and metrics	Recommended servings
Primary dietary metrics	
Fruits and vegetables	≥4.5 cups per day
Fish (preferably oily fish)	≥Two 3.5-oz servings per week
Fiber-rich whole grains (≥1.1 g of fiber per 10 g of carbohydrate)	≥Three 1-oz-equivalent servings
Sodium	<1500 mg per day
Sugar-sweetened beverages	≤450 kcal (36 oz) per week
Secondary dietary metrics	
Nuts, legumes, and seeds	≥4 servings per week
Processed meats	None or ≤2 servings per week
Saturated fat	<7% of total energy intake

TABLE 48.8 European Food Safety Authority (EFSA) reference intakes for carbohydrate, dietary fiber and water

Nutrient	Recommendation	Rationale
Carbohydrate	45–60% of energy intake for adults and children	To promote energy balance
Dietary fiber	25 g/day for adults	Promotes normal bowel function
		Evidence for reduced risk of CVD and type 2 diabetes and promotion of weight maintenance with higher levels
Water	Adequate intakes of 2 L/day for women and 2.5 L/day for men.	To ensure adequate hydration and to prevent water intoxication

Dietary Approaches to Stop Hypertension (DASH) Dietary Pattern

The DASH dietary pattern emphasizes fruits, vegetables, and low-fat dairy products; incorporates whole grains, fish, nuts, and poultry; and reduces intake of red meats, sweets, and sugar-sweetened beverages (Appel *et al.*, 1997).

Consequently, nutrient targets are higher for potassium (4700 mg/day), magnesium (500 mg/day), and calcium (1240 mg/day) and lower for total fat (27% total energy), saturated fat (6% total energy), and cholesterol (150 mg/day) in a diet providing 2100 kcal/day; carbohydrate and protein comprise 55% and 18% of total energy, respectively (Appel *et al.*, 1997). Other DASH-style dietary patterns have been evaluated with higher unsaturated fat content and higher protein content (Appel *et al.*, 2005).

The DASH diet has been shown to decrease CVD risk factors, including: systolic and diastolic blood pressure (−5.5 and −3.0 mm Hg, respectively), total cholesterol (−13 mg/dL), and LDL-C (−10.7 mg/dL) compared with a typical American diet (Appel *et al.*, 1997; Obarzanek *et al.*, 2001). The blood-pressure-lowering effect of the DASH dietary pattern compared with typical US dietary intake was significant in all populations studied, with this effect being greater in persons with stage 1 hypertension over those who were normotensive (Appel *et al.*, 1997). The total and LDL-cholesterol-lowering effects of the diet did not differ by race or baseline lipid concentration; however, the net reduction in total and LDL-cholesterol ware several units greater for men over women (a further −10.3 and −11.2 mg/dL reduction for total and LDL-cholesterol respectively in men over women) (Obarzanek *et al.*, 2001). Overall, the DASH diet decreased 10-year CHD risk by −18% compared with the control diet, i.e. the typical American diet (Chen *et al.*, 2010).

In a study that evaluated the original DASH diet, a higher-unsaturated-fat DASH diet (37% fat, 15% protein, 48% carbohydrate), and a higher-protein DASH diet (27% fat, 25% protein, 48% carbohydrate), all three diets reduced systolic (−8.2 to −9.5 mm Hg) and diastolic (−4.1 to −5.2 mm Hg) blood pressure and total (−12.4 to −19.9 mg/dL) and LDL-cholesterol (−11.6 to −14.2 mg/dL) concentrations in pre-hypertensive and stage 1 hypertensive individuals (Appel *et al.*, 2005). HDL-C significantly decreased in both the original DASH diet (−1.4 mg/dL) and the higher-protein DASH diet (−2.6 mg/dL), while HDL-C remained unchanged during the higher-fat DASH diet (Appel *et al.*, 2005). The higher-protein and higher-fat DASH diets both significantly decreased triglycerides (Appel *et al.*, 2005). Another study evaluating various DASH dietary sodium levels found that a low sodium intake of 1150 mg/day (50 mmol/day) compared with a high sodium intake of 3450 mg/day (150 mmol/day), the latter of which represents an average American diet, reduced systolic and diastolic blood pressure by −3.0 mm Hg and

TABLE 48.9 European Food Safety Authority (EFSA) reference intakes for fat and cholesterol

Nutrient	Recommendation	Rationale
Total fat	20–35% energy intake for adults	For maintenance of good health, body weight and for proper absorption of fat-soluble dietary components such as vitamins
Saturated fats	Intake should be as low as possible within a nutritionally adequate diet	SFAs are synthesized in the body and are not required in the diet
cis-MUFAs	No reference value set	MUFAs are synthesized in the body and have no specific role in either the prevention or promotion of diet-related diseases
n-3 PUFAs	Adequate intake levels of 250 mg/day of EPA + DHA as a primary preventive measure for healthy adults	n-3 PUFA supplementation or oily fish consumption (1–2 meals per week) decrease risk of mortality from CHD and sudden cardiac death
	Adequate intake levels of 0.5% energy for ALA	ALA is considered an essential fatty acid as it cannot be synthesized in the body and is required for the maintenance of metabolic integrity
n-6 PUFAs	Adequate intake level of 4% energy from LA	LA is an essential fatty acid that cannot be synthesized in the body and is required to maintain metabolic integrity
	No dietary reference intake value set for AA	AA is not an essential fatty acid and there is no consistent evidence for its promotion of diet-related diseases
Trans fatty acids	Intake should be as low as possible within a nutritionally adequate diet.	TFAs are not synthesized by the body and are not required in the diet
		High intakes increase risk of CHD
		TFA intake increases total cholesterol and LDL-C levels in a dose-dependent manner
		TFAs also decrease HDL levels and increase the total cholesterol: HDL ratio
		Evidence indicates that TFAs from ruminant sources have similar adverse effects as those from industrial sources when consumed in equivalent amounts
Conjugated linoleic acid	No dietary reference intake value set	No convincing evidence that CLA isomers are important in either the prevention or promotion of a diet-related disease
Cholesterol	No dietary reference value set	Cholesterol is synthesized in the body and is not required in the diet
		Positive dose-dependent association is seen with cholesterol intake and LDL-C levels; however, main determinant of LDL-C levels is SFA intake
		Most foods containing cholesterol are also significant sources of SFAs. Therefore, reference intake value for SFAs should first be considered

−1.6 mm Hg, respectively (Sacks *et al.*, 2001). Sacks and colleagues (2001) also showed that, when the low-sodium DASH diet was compared with the high-sodium average American diet (control), there was a significant reduction in systolic blood pressure of −7.1 mm Hg in pre-hypertensive individuals, with an even greater reduction of −11.5 mm Hg in hypertensive individuals. However, there is also evidence to suggest that humans self-regulate dietary sodium intake via hormonal and central nervous system mechanisms, leading some scientists to argue that current guidelines for sodium intake are below the physiologic set-point of 2.7 to 4.9 g/day, and are impractical for long-term adherence to recommendations (McCarron *et al.*, 2009). Overall, the original DASH dietary pattern, the higher-protein DASH diet, the higher-unsaturated-fat DASH diet, and the DASH diet with reduced sodium all favorably affect blood pressure, blood lipids, and CVD risk (DGAC, 2010a).

Mediterranean-Style Eating Patterns

The Mediterranean-style eating pattern represents the unique dietary patterns of many countries surrounding the Mediterranean Sea. Some common attributes of the Mediterranean diet include: increased consumption of fruits, vegetables (specifically root vegetables), whole grains, legumes, nuts, seeds, and olive oil; low to moderate consumption of wine (non-Islamic countries), fish, poultry, and dairy products; and decreased consumption of red meat (Kris-Etherton *et al.*, 2001). Diets from the Mediterranean area tend to be higher in monounsaturated fat and lower in saturated fat. Due to the diversity of the Mediterranean diet, scoring indices have been developed based on dietary components that are inherent to all variations of the diet; higher scores indicate greater adherence to the Mediterranean-style diet (Kourlaba and Panagiotakos, 2009).

Epidemiological and clinical evidence both show benefits of a Mediterranean-style diet for CVD risk factors. In a prospective cohort study of a Greek population, greater adherence to a Mediterranean diet was associated with decreased total mortality, CHD death, and cancer death (Trichopoulou *et al.*, 2003). In the Nurses' Health Study, women who followed a Mediterranean diet most closely were at a lower relative risk for CHD (RR 0.71 [95% CI: 0.62–0.82]) and stroke incidence (RR 0.87 [95% CI: 0.73–1.02]) and total CVD mortality (RR 0.61 [95% CI: 0.49–0.76]) compared with women with the lowest adherence (Fung *et al.*, 2009). A recent meta-analysis confirmed these results, reporting decreased total

mortality (RR 0.92 [95% CI: 0.90–0.94]) and CVD-related incidence or mortality (RR 0.90 [95% CI: 0.87–0.93]) with a 2-point increase in the Mediterranean diet scoring index (Sofi *et al.*, 2010).

The PREDIMED (Mediterranean Diet in the Primary Prevention of Cardiovascular Disease) clinical trial implemented a nutrition education intervention in free-living participants to evaluate the difference between a low-fat diet and a Mediterranean diet; subjects in the Mediterranean diet group were supplemented with either virgin olive oil (1 L/week) or nuts (30 g/day). Results after 3 months indicated that a Mediterranean diet supplemented with nuts (hazelnuts, almonds, and walnuts) significantly reduced fasting glucose (−5.4 mg/dL), systolic (−7.1 mm Hg) and diastolic (−2.6 mm Hg) blood pressure, total cholesterol (−6.2 mg/dL), triglyceride concentration (−13.0 mg/dL), and the total cholesterol : HDL-C ratio (−0.26), and increased HDL-C (1.6 mg/dL) compared with a low-fat diet (Estruch *et al.*, 2006). The Mediterranean diet supplemented with olive oil significantly reduced fasting glucose (−7.0 mg/dL), systolic (−5.9 mm Hg) and diastolic (−1.6 mm Hg) blood pressure, and the total cholesterol : HDL-C ratio (−0.38), and increased HDL-C (2.9 mg/dL) compared with a low-fat diet (Estruch *et al.*, 2006). The same trial reported that a Mediterranean diet, supplemented with olive oil or nuts, reduced the incidence of diabetes by −52% compared with a low-fat diet in individuals with high cardiovascular risk after 4 years of follow-up (Salas-Salvadó *et al.*, 2011). As summarized by the DGAC 2010 report, individuals with a higher Mediterranean diet scoring index tend to have reduced total mortality, CVD risk factors, and CVD incidence (DGAC, 2010a).

Vegetarian Dietary Pattern

Vegetarian dietary patterns represent a spectrum of food intake practices. "Vegetarian" is a broadly encompassing term used for a variety of different categories: ovo-lactovegetarians do not consume meat or fish; ovo-vegetarians do not consume meat, fish, or dairy products; lacto-vegetarians do not consume meat, fish, or eggs; vegans do not consume any animal products; while raw vegans, Su vegetarians, and fruitarians do not consume any animal products or vegetables in the *Allium* family (e.g. onions, garlic) (Li, 2011).

Vegetarian diets emphasize fruits, vegetables, whole grains, legumes, nuts, seeds, and soy foods and include little or no animal products. Vegetarians typically consume increased fiber, carbohydrates, potassium, magnesium, folic acid, n-6 PUFAs, non-heme iron (the less biologically absorbable form of iron found predominantly in plants) and vitamin C, and have decreased total calories, total fat, SFAs, cholesterol, and sodium compared with non-vegetarians (Duo *et al.*, 2000; DGAC, 2010a). Important nutrients that vegetarian diets may lack include: heme iron (the more biologically absorbable form of iron found in animal products), zinc, vitamin B_{12}, vitamin A, vitamin D, and n-3 PUFAs (Li *et al.*, 2000).

Vegetarians tend to have lower mortality from CHD, specifically, a −24% decrease in mortality from ischemic heart disease (IHD) compared with non-vegetarians (Key *et al.*, 1999; Fraser, 2009). In a group of Seventh Day Adventists, risk of fatal IHD was 2.31-fold greater in men who consumed beef ≥3 times per week as compared with vegetarian men, but this trend was not observed in women (Fraser, 1999). A recent British prospective trial reported no significant differences in mortality rates for ischemic heart disease and cerebrovascular disease between vegetarians and non-vegetarians (Key *et al.*, 2009). The authors attribute this discrepancy to the recruitment of relatively health-conscious non-vegetarians. Epidemiological data indicate that vegetarians have a decreased prevalence of diabetes and hypertension (Fraser, 1999, 2009) and a significantly lower BMI than non-vegetarians (Fraser, 1999, 2009; Haddad *et al.*, 1999; Li *et al.*, 2000). Cross-sectional studies consistently show decreased total cholesterol and LDL-C in individuals consuming plant-based diets as compared with the general population, with vegans experiencing the lowest cholesterol levels (Ferdowsian and Barnard, 2009).

Clinical interventions show decreased total cholesterol (−7.6 to −26.6%) and LDL-cholesterol (−9.2 to −37.4%) in participants randomized to a plant-based diet versus a typical Western diet (Ferdowsian and Barnard, 2009). A vegan combination diet (plant sterols 1.2 g/1000 kcal, soy protein 16.2 g/1000 kcal, viscous fiber 8.3 g/1000 kcal, almonds 16.6 g/1000 kcal) has been shown to decrease total cholesterol (−26.6% vs. −9.9%), LDL-C (−35.0% vs. −12.1%), the total cholesterol : HDL-C ratio (−20.8 vs. −2.6), and the LDL : HDL-C ratio (−30.0 vs. −5.1) compared with a low-fat control diet and similarly to first-generation statin drug therapy (Jenkins *et al.*, 2003). The improved lipid and lipoprotein profile may account for the −31.7% decrease in CHD mortality witnessed in individuals who follow plant-based, vegetarian, and vegan diets (Jenkins *et al.*, 2003).

A concern for vegetarians, especially vegans, is that they typically have lower levels of circulating serum ferritin and vitamin B_{12} and decreased phospholipid-incorporated n-3 PUFAs (Haddad *et al.*, 1999; Li *et al.*, 2000; Elmadfa and Singer, 2009). Vegetarians also show elevated blood homocysteine levels (Elmadfa and Singer, 2009) which have been associated with increased risk of atherosclerosis (Gerhard and Duell, 1999). Individuals consuming vegetarian diets should therefore monitor their B_{12} levels, consume B_{12}-fortified foods, and consider taking a B_{12} supplement. In addition, decreased intake of dietary n-3 PUFAs (especially longer-chain n-3 fatty acids) in vegetarians may contribute to platelet aggregation and platelet structural changes, which may be associated with an increased tendency for thrombosis (Li, 2011).

The CHD-related benefits of plant-based, vegetarian, and vegan diets have been demonstrated repeatedly in epidemiological and clinical trials and are endorsed by the US Department of Agriculture (USDA) as one of several healthy diets. Specialized food-guide pyramids for vegetarian and vegan diets also have been developed. Well-planned, plant-based diets can provide sufficient macronutrients and micronutrients to meet current dietary recommendations for all stages of life.

Therapeutic Lifestyle Changes (TLC)

The National Cholesterol Education Program TLC diet is designed for individuals with elevated LDL-C, lipid disorders, cardiovascular disease, diabetes, insulin resistance, and/or metabolic syndrome. The diet emphasizes decreased saturated fat (<7% of calories) and cholesterol (<200 mg) intake, and provides two therapeutic options of increasing soluble fiber (10–25 g/day) and plant sterol/stanol (2 g/day) intake to further reduce LDL-C. Macronutrient intake recommendations are as follows: total fat (25–35%), MUFAs (up to 20%), PUFAs (up to 10%), carbohydrate (50–60%), and protein (≈15%) (Expert Panel on Detection, Evaluation, and Treatment of High Blood Cholesterol in Adults, 2001). Total calorie intake should be balanced with energy expenditure to maintain weight and prevent weight gain. The TLC program also recommends moderate physical activity to expend at least 200 kcal/day. The TLC diet can be achieved through a variety of dietary intake patterns and may be based on individual preferences. For the most part, the DASH diet, Mediterranean diets, and vegetarian diets all meet the TLC diet recommendations for saturated fat and dietary cholesterol intake.

When plant sterols (1 g/1000 kcal), viscous fiber (8.2 g/1000 kcal), and plant protein (≈25 g/1000 kcal) were incorporated into a diet already low in dietary cholesterol (99 mg/1000 kcal) and saturated fat (7.7% of energy), both normal and hyperlipidemic subjects had a significant decrease in total cholesterol (−22.3%), LDL-C (−29.0%), the total cholesterol: HDL-C ratio (−19.8%), and the LDL-C:HDL-C ratio (−26.5%) compared with baseline (Jenkins *et al.*, 2002). Based on these blood lipid results, the calculated CHD risk reduction of this Portfolio Diet is −30.0% (Jenkins *et al.*, 2002). In a community intervention trial, the TLC diet, in conjunction with lifestyle modifications such as stress management, smoking cessation, and physical activity, significantly decreased systolic (−6 mm Hg) and diastolic (−3 mm Hg) blood pressure in pre-hypertensive individuals (Bavikati *et al.*, 2008). The blood-pressure-lowering effect was greater in women than men and greater in normal and overweight individuals than in obese individuals; there were no racial differences in blood pressure change. The TLC diet can effectively contribute to the prevention and treatment of elevated cholesterol levels, and thereby lower CVD risk.

Functional Foods and Nutrition Labeling Terminology

Functional Foods

Functional foods have received much attention for their potential in disease risk reduction and optimal health promotion. Numerous definitions exist for the term "functional food," making it difficult to develop consistent terminology. The International Food Information Council defines functional food as any food or food component that may have health benefits beyond basic nutrition (Stevens *et al.*, 2008). In the case of CVD, foods such as fatty fish, flaxseed, oats, psyllium, grapes, garlic, and tea, as well as sterol/stanol-enhanced margarines, have been found to significantly modify CVD risk (Hasler *et al.*, 2000). Peer-reviewed evidence of their effectiveness in modifying CVD risk is ranked and interpreted for the development of appropriate food and nutrient recommendations.

The Academy of Nutrition and Dietetics (AND), formerly known as the American Dietetic Association (ADA) considers all foods functional at some biochemical level, but specifically classifies functional foods as those that provide additional health benefits beyond necessity (ADA, 2009). Functional foods are divided into four categories: conventional foods (i.e. whole foods), modified foods, medical foods (e.g. phenylketonuria formulas), and foods for special dietary use (e.g. hypo-allergenic foods) (ADA, 2009). Modified foods include subcategories of fortified, enriched, and enhanced food products. Fortified food products have additional nutrients incorporated during processing that do not naturally occur in the food, such as calcium-fortified orange juice. Enriched food products have naturally occurring nutrients reincorporated into the food that were lost during processing (e.g. folate-enriched breads), while enhanced food products are enhanced with bioactive nutrients (e.g. phytosterol-enhanced margarines) (ADA, 2009).

Food and Nutrition Recommendations

Health and governmental organizations, including the FDA and the AND, provide specific nutrient and food recommendations for reducing the risk of disease. The FDA bases unqualified Health Claims on significant scientific agreement that a food or nutrient decreases the risk of a specific disease (FDA, 2003). The FDA allows Qualified Health Claims when significant scientific agreement is not reached but emerging evidence suggests a favorable relationship between a food or nutrient and the risk of a specific disease (FDA, 2003). Since they are regulated by the FDA, unqualified and Qualified Health Claims can be used in food labeling when appropriate. The AND has a rating system based on strong, fair, weak, consensus, and insufficient evidence ratings to advise clinical practitioners on how to make recommendations for patients (ADA, 2004a). Conventional and modified foods that decrease the risk of CHD are listed in Table 48.10.

World Health Organization and Food and Agriculture Organization Summary on the Strength of the Evidence for Dietary and Lifestyle Factors for CVD Risk

The WHO Programme on CVD is focused on preventing, monitoring, and managing CVD globally. The main aims are to develop global approaches for lowering the rates of incidence, morbidity, and mortality due to CVD. The 2002 WHO report states that there is sufficient evidence that the mortality rates of CVD have been associated with behavioral risk factors such as poor dietary habits, increased tobacco use, and inadequate amounts of physical activity

TABLE 48.10 Strength of evidence for specific foods and nutrients associated with CHD risk reduction

Type of food	Bioactive component	Recommended amount	FDA health claim[a]	AND evidence[b]
Whole oats	β-glucan soluble fiber	3 g/day soluble fiber	Unqualified (A)	Strong (fiber)
Barley	β-glucan soluble fiber	3 g/day soluble fiber	Unqualified (A)	Strong (fiber)
Psyllium husk	Soluble fiber	7 g/day soluble fiber	Unqualified (A)	Strong (fiber)
Fortified margarines/ salad dressings	Plant sterols/ stanol esters	2 g/day sterols/ stanols	Unqualified (A)	Strong (stanols/ sterols)
Soy protein	Plant protein	25 g/day	Unqualified (A)	Fair (soy protein)
Nuts	Unsaturated fatty acids, vitamin E	1.5 oz/day	Qualified (B)	Fair (nuts)
Walnuts	Omega-3 fatty acids[c]	1.5 oz/day *or* 1 tbsp/day oil	Qualified (B)	Fair (nuts) Fair (omega-3 FA)
Fatty fish	Omega-3 fatty acids	8 oz/week	Qualified (B)	Fair (omega-3 FA)
Flaxseed	Omega-3 fatty acids[c]	0.5 tbsp/day *or* <1 tsp/day oil	Qualified (B)	Fair, (omega-3 FA)
Canola oil	Unsaturated fatty acids, omega-3 fatty acids[c]	1.5 tbsp/day	Qualified (C)	Fair (omega-3 FA)
Olive oil	Monounsaturated fatty acids	2 tbsp/day	Qualified (C)	N/A
Corn oil	Unsaturated fatty acids	1 tbsp/day	Qualified (D)	N/A

[a]FDA grading system indicating the strength of a claim.
[b]Information derived from ADA Disorders of Lipid Metabolism (Thornburg *et al.*, 1995).
[c]Derived from α-linolenic acid (ALA).
Adapted with permission from ADA (2004b).

(Cardiovascular Disease Programme, 2002). The biological factors contributing to increased CVD risk are being overweight, and having central obesity, elevated blood pressure, diabetes, and dyslipidemia (Cardiovascular Disease Programme, 2002). These are often coupled with increased intake of SFAs, refined carbohydrates and salt, and low intake of fruits and vegetables (Cardiovascular Disease Programme, 2002). In their joint report published in 2002, the WHO and the FAO of the United Nations summarized the strength of the evidence for the various dietary and lifestyle factors associated with CVD risk (Joint FAO/WHO Expert Consultation, 2002). An adaptation of this summary is given in Box 48.4.

Major Co-Morbidities of Cardiovascular Disease

Obesity

There is convincing evidence that being overweight or obese increases risk for CVD (Lloyd-Jones *et al.*, 2010). A shift towards more urbanized ways of life as well as increased industrialization in most countries has resulted in marked changes in diet, behavior, and lifestyle, with diet becoming more energy-dense and high in fat, and lifestyles trending towards being more sedentary. In countries going through an economic transition, the rising rates of obesity may occur alongside increased prevalence of chronic

> **BOX 48.4   Summary of the evidence on dietary and lifestyle factors associated with CVD risk (Joint WHO/FAO Expert Consultation, 2002)**
>
> | | | |
> |---|---|---|
> | **Convincing evidence** | Decreased risk | EPA and DHA, LA intake, vegetables and fruits (including berries), potassium, low to moderate alcohol intake, regular physical activity |
> | | Increased risk | *Trans* fatty acids, high sodium intake, myristic and palmitic acids, high alcohol intake, overweight |
> | | No relationship | Vitamin E supplementation |
> | **Probable evidence** | Decreased risk | ALA, oleic acid intake, dietary fiber, whole-grain cereals, nuts (unsalted), plant sterols/stanols, folate |
> | | Increased risk | Dietary cholesterol, unfiltered boiled coffee (this contains a terpenoid lipid known as cafestol that is found to raise total and LDL-cholesterol levels) |
> | | No relationship | Stearic acid |
> | **Possible evidence** | Decreased risk | Flavonoids, soy products |
> | | Increased risk | Fats rich in lauric acid, β-carotene supplements |
> | | No relationship | – |
> | **Insufficient evidence** | Decreased risk | Calcium, magnesium, vitamin C |
> | | Increased risk | Carbohydrates, iron |
> | | No relationship | – |

undernutrition (Joint FAO/WHO Expert Consultation, 2002). In low-income countries, obesity occurs in persons of higher-economic status, most likely due to a higher energy intake, whereas in higher-income countries obesity is widespread in lower socioeconomic groups (Joint FAO/WHO Expert Consultation, 2002), which may be related to the low relative cost of high-energy and nutrient-poor foods. However, this trend is expanding across groups in higher-income countries. Since the risk of hypertension, CVD, and diabetes are all associated with increased weight, the prevention of obesity plays a pivotal role in the prevention and management of several chronic diseases (Lloyd-Jones *et al.*, 2010). There is strong evidence to suggest that moderate to high fitness levels greatly reduce the risk of CVD, and all-cause mortality, regardless of BMI level, and results from epidemiological studies have shown that ongoing physical activity, regardless of body weight, is protective against chronic disease (Nocon *et al.*, 2008; Shiroma and Lee, 2010). Prevention of weight gain would therefore greatly decrease CVD risk and allow for better management of CVD with age.

Childhood Obesity

There is a worldwide trend towards increased prevalence of childhood obesity (Steyn *et al.*, 2005), which would play a significant role in children's nutritional and health outcomes as they enter adulthood. Strong associations between childhood obesity and early-onset hypertension, dyslipidemia, and insulin resistance have been reported (Raghuveer, 2010), and studies have shown that the childhood onset of obesity and the associated co-morbidities adversely affect the vasculature, resulting in premature onset and accelerated progression of atherosclerosis (Berenson *et al.*, 1998; Freedman *et al.*, 2008). Clinical manifestations of atherosclerotic cardiovascular disease have not been observed in obese children, and so assessment of subclinical markers is needed to evaluate disease risk, progression and monitoring of the effects of interventions implemented (Raghuveer, 2010). Our primary aim should be to prevent the premature onset of the disease before the development of clinical disease events (Balagopal *et al.*, 2011). Thus, efforts to curb the rate of incidence, as well as morbidity and mortality due to CVD, are needed at an early age.

Diabetes

The current global estimate for diabetes cases is 150 million, and this number is expected to double by the year 2025 (Joint FAO/WHO Expert Consultation, 2002). Type 2 diabetes, previously a disease of the middle- and older-aged, is now detected in all age groups including adolescents and children (Cardiovascular Disease Programme, 2002). Diabetes increases risk for stroke, peripheral vascular disease, and CHD (Grundy *et al.*, 1999; Goldberg, 2000). Similar numbers of people are thought to have impaired glucose tolerance, which is associated with a two- to three-fold increase in risk for vascular disease (Liao *et al.*, 2001; DECODA Study Group (International Diabetes Epidemiology Group), 2002). CVD is the most common complication of type 2 diabetes (Cardiovascular Disease Programme, 2002); diabetes is associated with an increased prevalence of hypertension and dyslipidemia (Grundy *et al.*, 1999; Goldberg, 2000). Efforts to curb the risk of mortality due to CHD or CVD may be therefore be thwarted by rapid increases in the incidence of diabetes (Cardiovascular Disease Programme, 2002). Also, overweight and obesity increase risk of diabetes, thus indicating a critical need for healthy dietary and lifestyle behaviors for preventing and reducing overweight and obesity, as well as CVD risk and the risk of type 2 diabetes (Cardiovascular Disease Programme, 2002). A summary of the recommendations for reducing diabetes risk given by the Joint WHO/FAO Expert Consultation on Diet, Nutrition and the Prevention of Chronic Diseases (2002) is presented in Box 48.5.

Healthy Lifestyle Behaviors

Behavioral patterns play significant roles in one's health status; unhealthy behaviors account for 40% of premature deaths (Schroeder, 2007). Physical activity recommenda-

---

BOX 48.5   Recommendations for reducing diabetes risk (Joint FAO/WHO Expert Consultation, 2002)

Prevention and treatment of overweight and obesity

Maintaining an optimum BMI ($21-23 \text{ kg/m}^2$) and avoiding weight gain (>5 kg) in adulthood

Voluntary weight reduction in the overweight and obese with impaired glucose tolerance

Participating in an endurance activity at moderate or greater level of intensity (e.g. brisk walking) for 1 hour or more per day on most days per week

Saturated fat intake <10% total energy with an intake of <7% for high-risk groups

Adequate dietary fiber intakes through regular consumption of fruits, vegetables, whole-grain cereals, and legumes. Minimum daily intake of 20 g

---

tions aim to reduce the risk of disease and increase overall health. The World Health Organization (WHO) recommends at least 30 minutes of moderate-intensity physical activity on most days to reduce CVD and other disease risks (Waxman, 2004). The US Department of Health and Human Services (USDHHS) recommends the equivalent, 150 minutes of moderate-intensity aerobic activity or 75 minutes of vigorous-intensity aerobic activity each week, for adults (Tay *et al.*, 2008). Evidence strongly suggests that adherence to these guidelines reduces CHD risk, via a decrease in triglycerides and LDL-C levels, as well as an increase in HDL-C levels (Thornburg *et al.*, 1995). Moreover, adherence to these recommendations lowers risk for chronic diseases such as CHD, stroke, metabolic syndrome, type 2 diabetes, and some cancers by allowing one to achieve appropriate energy balance, manage weight, lower blood pressure, achieve a favorable lipid profile, and prevent premature death (Office of Disease Prevention and Health Promotion, 2008). A summary of the physical activity recommendations provided in the WHO Global Strategy on Diet, Physical Activity and Health Report (WHO, 2004) is given in Table 48.11.

The recommendations for moderate-intensity physical activity refer to exercises that include brisk walking (>3 miles/hour), water aerobics, cycling (<10 miles/hour), and tennis (doubles); equivalent vigorous-intensity exercises include jogging or running, swimming laps, cycling (≥10 miles/hour), and tennis (singles) (Tay *et al.*, 2008). These aerobic activities should be done in addition to daily baseline activity, defined as the activity required for everyday living, and in at least 10-minute intervals to be considered physical activity for the purpose of improving health. If these recommendations are unattainable for physical or other reasons, health benefits are still gained with lesser amounts of activity; any amount of exercise is better than remaining inactive (Tay *et al.*, 2008). Additional benefits may be gained by exceeding these recommendations.

Additionally, the USDHHS recommendations include muscle strength training, which should be done at least two days of the week for all major muscle groups. Strength training provides additional health benefits beyond those obtained from aerobic exercise, including improvements in muscular tone and bone strength. Examples of strength exercises include weightlifting, calisthenics, push-ups, and sit-ups. Flexibility exercises such as stretching also are encouraged (Tay *et al.*, 2008).

The advantages of regular physical activity for children and older adults are similar to those for adults. Children

TABLE 48.11 Summary of the World Health Organization Physical Activity Recommendations (WHO, 2004)

Age group	Recommendation
Children 5–17 years	Accumulate at least 60 minutes of moderate- to vigorous-intensity physical activity daily: amounts greater than 60 minutes will provide additional health benefits. Most daily physical activity should be aerobic; vigorous intensity activities should also be incorporated, including those that strengthen muscle and bone at least 3 times per week: bone loading activities can be a part of playing games, running, turning or jumping.
Adults 18–64 years	Accumulate at least 150 minutes of moderate-intensity aerobic physical activity throughout the week or at least 75 minutes of vigorous-intensity aerobic physical activity during the week or an equivalent combination of moderate-and vigorous-intensity activity. Aerobic activity should be performed in bouts at least 10 minutes in length; additional health benefits can be achieved by increasing moderate-intensity aerobic physical activity to 300 minutes or to 150 minutes of vigorous-intensity aerobic physical activity per week, or an equivalent combination of moderate- and vigorous-intensity activity.
Adults >65 years	Be as physically active as possible with all abilities and health conditions; accumulate at least 150 minutes of moderate-intensity aerobic physical activity throughout the week or at least 75 minutes of vigorous-intensity aerobic physical activity during the week, or an equivalent combination of moderate- and vigorous-intensity activity. Aerobic activity should be performed in bouts at least 10 minutes in length; additional health benefits can be achieved by increasing moderate-intensity aerobic physical activity to 300 minutes or to 150 minutes of vigorous-intensity aerobic physical activity per week, or an equivalent combination of moderate- and vigorous-intensity activity. Older adults with poor mobility should perform physical activity to enhance balance and prevent falls on 3 or more days per week. Muscle strengthening activities involving major muscle groups should be performed on at least 2 or more days per week. Physical activity can include walking, dancing, gardening, hiking, swimming, cycling, household chores, play, games, sports, planned exercise, and occupational activity if the individual works.

should engage in at least 60 minutes of physical activity per day to promote health; the majority of activity should be aerobic, but also include muscle and bone-strengthening exercises (Tay *et al.*, 2008). Guidelines for older adults are equivalent to those for younger adults; however, older adults may experience obstacles due to physical limitations. Older adults can include exercises that improve balance to decrease the risk of falls. Those seeking to maintain or lose weight may require increased physical activity duration and/or intensity based on individual needs and abilities.

Another behavioral pattern found to increase CVD risk is sleep. Sleep deprivation (<7 hours per night) is associated with CVD, obesity, and type 2 diabetes; both short and long durations of sleep increase glucose intolerance,

obesity, and hypertension, all risk factors for CVD (Institute of Medicine, 2006). Obstructive sleep apnea (OSA), a sleep disorder that involves breathing pauses of >10 seconds due to obstruction of the airway during sleep, is associated with CVD and related risk factors (Institute of Medicine, 2006); OSA results in severe and intermittent oxygen loss and carbon dioxide retention during sleep (Somers *et al.*, 1993), and if repetitive can cause vasoconstriction of the peripheral blood vessels and a sharp increase in blood pressure (Somers *et al.*, 1989a,b, 1995). Additionally, CVD and diabetes are risk factors for OSA (Sin *et al.*, 1999). The National Sleep Foundation recommends 7–9 hours of sleep for adults and 8.5–9.25 hours of sleep for adolescents to achieve optimal health (National Sleep Foundation, 2011).

Diet and Lifestyle Interventions Complement Drug Therapy

Diet has significant additive effects on reducing CVD risk factors, particularly LDL-C and systolic blood pressure (SBP), especially when adopted early in life and maintained across the lifespan. Individually, each dietary recommendation may have a relatively small effect, but in combination can affect treatment options in terms of the drug therapy and dose needed. A combination of these recommendations has been shown to reduce LDL-C in amounts similar to those gained from standard, first-generation statins (National Cholesterol Education Program Expert Panel, 2002). For example, a diet with ≤30% total fat, <10% SFA, and <300 mg cholesterol per day lowered LDL-C levels by −8% compared with an average American diet (Yu-Poth et al., 1999). In Table 48.12 we see the estimated LDL-C-lowering effects of various diet recommendations and their estimated cumulative effect in the range of −20% to −30% (Jenkins et al., 2000).

For those individuals on drug therapy, there are additive benefits for also implementing a TLC diet (National Cholesterol Education Program Expert Panel, 2002). Hunninghake and colleagues (1993) found a further −5% reduction in LDL-C levels when diet therapy (SFA < 7%; cholesterol <200 mg/day) was used in combination with

lovastatin, 20 mg/day, an effect similar to that attained when the statin dose is doubled (National Cholesterol Education Program Expert Panel, 2002). Studies using plant sterols (3–5.1 g/day) as a part of diet therapy, in persons on statin treatment, showed between −17% and −20% reductions in LDL-C levels (Gylling et al., 1997; Blair et al., 2000). The combination of diet and drug therapy is preferred over increasing statin doses over time (National Cholesterol Education Program Expert Panel, 2002).

Hypertension is a major CVD risk factor; treatment of hypertension significantly reduces CVD morbidity and mortality (Chobanian et al., 2003). Several diet and lifestyle modifications have been shown to effectively reduce SBP, which is a strong indicator of CVD risk (Chobanian et al., 2003). These include reducing intake of sodium (Chobanian and Hill, 2000; Sacks et al., 2001; Vollmer et al., 2001); adopting a Dietary Approaches to Stop Hypertension (DASH) eating pattern that is high in fruits and vegetables and in potassium, and utilizes low-fat dairy products (Sacks et al., 2001); weight loss in overweight or obese individuals (Trials of Hypertension Prevention Collaborative Research Group, 1997; He et al., 2000); increased physical activity (Kelley and Kelley, 2000; Whelton et al., 2002); and moderation in alcohol consumption (Xin et al., 2001). Indeed, cessation of smoking is imperative for CVD risk reduction (DGAC, 2010a). The SBP-lowering effects of these recommendations are presented in Table 48.13. Combined diet and lifestyle interventions would significantly lower SBP, and allow for increased efficacy of anti-hypertensive drug therapy, and decrease CVD risk (Chobanian et al., 2003).

Possible additive effects of dietary strategies can be utilized in persons undergoing drug therapy. Persons at high risk for CVD due to increased LDL-C levels and hypertension, who are on drug regimens, may lower their recommended doses, prevent increases in doses over-time, and reduce occurrences of adverse side-effects of pharmacotherapy with recommended diet therapy. For example, LDL-C lowering by diet would decrease the dose of statin required and, in the case of n-3 fatty acids and phytosterols, also boost the pharmacokinetic action of these drugs (Bruckert and Rosenbaum, 2011). Reductions in sodium intake are manageable and can significantly decrease blood pressure (He et al., 2000), allowing for more effective management of hypertension. Physical activity also may decrease insulin resistance, preventing weight gain, increas-

TABLE 48.12 Approximate and cumulative LDL-cholesterol reductions achievable by dietary and lifestyle modifications

Dietary component	Recommendation	Approximate LDL reduction
Major:		
Saturated fat	<7% calories	8–10%
Dietary cholesterol	<200 mg/day	3–5%
Weight reduction	Lose 10 lb (4.5 kg)	5–8%
Other:		
Viscous fiber	5–10 g/day	3–5%
Plant sterol/stanol esters	2 g/day	6–15%
Cumulative estimate		20–30%

Adapted and reproduced from the Third Report of the National Cholesterol Education Program Expert Panel on Detection, Evaluation and Treatment of High Blood Cholesterol in Adults – Adult Treatment Panel III (National Cholesterol Education Program Expert Panel, 2002).

TABLE 48.13 Approximate systolic blood pressure (SBP) reductions achievable by diet and lifestyle modifications

Factor	Recommendation	Approximate SBP reduction range
Sodium intake	Reduce dietary sodium to no more than 2400 mg or 6 g of sodium chloride daily	2–8 mm Hg
Adopt DASH[a] eating plan	Consume a diet rich in fruits, vegetables, and low-fat dairy products with a reduced content of total and saturated fat	8–14 mm Hg 13–19 mm Hg*
Weight reduction	Achieve and maintain a normal body weight; BMI: 18.5–24.9 kg/m^2	5–20 mm Hg/ 10 kg weight loss
Physical activity	Achieve regular aerobic physical activity for at least 30 minutes each day, most days of the week	4–9 mm Hg
Alcohol consumption	Limit consumption to no more than 1 drink per day for women, and no more than 2 drinks per day for men	2–4 mm Hg

[a]Dietary Approaches to Stop Hypertension (Appel et al., 1997).
*Adherence to the DASH diet in combination with a weight management program may further reduce SBP levels (Blumenthal et al., 2010).
Adapted from National High Blood Pressure Education Program (2003).

ing HDL, and lowering total cholesterol levels, as well as managing blood pressure (He et al., 2000; Durstine et al., 2001; Whelton et al., 2002; Saris et al., 2003), and dyslipidemia (DGAC, 2010a). Given these findings, medical advice aimed at maximizing compliance to both diet and drug regimens would allow for significant reduction of CVD risk in the long term. Overall lifestyle modification, which includes healthful dietary patterns, smoking cessation, and physical activity for weight loss and manage-

ment, would be most beneficial for decreasing CVD incidence in high-risk individuals on drug therapy (Yu-Poth et al., 1999; Bruckert and Rosenbaum, 2011).

A Need for Population-Based Approaches

There have been major improvements in socioeconomic status and increased urbanization in many countries, coupled with distinct changes in lifestyle, including increased caloric and saturated fat intake, increased tobacco use, and reduced physical activity levels, all of which increase risk factors for CVD (Joint FAO/WHO Expert Consultation, 2002). Deaths due to CVD now account for between 35% and 65% of all deaths, and exceed deaths due to infections and malnutrition worldwide (Gersh et al., 2010). In the USA there has been a steady decrease in age-adjusted CHD (−2%) and in stroke mortality (−3%) per year, mainly attributable to the control of risk factors and the use of therapeutics (Ford and Capewell, 2007); management of CVD prevalence is attainable. However, with increased global prosperity and urbanization, epidemics of hypertension, obesity, and diabetes are more widespread (Balkau et al., 2007), and these factors in combination increase risk for CVD dramatically. Results from the INTERHEART study, a case-control study on 25 countries, showed that more than 90% of the attributable risk of myocardial infarction or heart attacks was due to nine modifiable risk factors: hypertension, diabetes, smoking, abdominal obesity, the apolipoprotein B/apolipoprotein AI ratio, fruit and vegetable intake, exercise, regular alcohol consumption, and a psychosocial index (Yusuf et al., 2004; Joshi et al., 2007; Anand et al., 2008; Teo et al., 2009). These results illuminate the value of a global risk assessment for an individual (Cardiovascular Disease Programme, 2002), which aims to look at the complement of factors contributing to development of the disease.

Epidemiological theory proposes that, for conditions of high risk and prevalence within the population, small improvements in the population distribution of risk would have a greater impact on disease reduction than the intensive, individual treatment of high-risk patients (Rose, 2001). Examples of these include decreasing the amount of salt used in food processing, removing certain fats from the food chain, or having a smoke-free environment.

Ideally, a combination of both high-risk and population-wide strategies would be the best approach for treatment and prevention (Mendis, 2001) versus the traditional, clinic-based strategy focused on high-risk groups (Gersh *et al.*, 2010); indeed, persons without elevated risk factors but with chronic disease would also benefit. However, the lack of resources in many areas, coupled with the burden of non-communicable diseases, pose a challenge for health-care delivery (Mayosi *et al.*, 2009). None the less, public health responses may utilize several combinations of the main components of prevention that include either individual level prevention, the use of an integrated health-care system, or policy and societal changes (Gersh *et al.*, 2010). Such population-based approaches are thought by many to be especially cost-effective and allow for a shift towards a more primary, preventive, and community-based form of health care.

Future Directions

Atherosclerotic cardiovascular disease is a leading cause of all global deaths, with a major proportion of these now occurring within the growing populations of low- and middle-income countries (WHO, 2011). Traditionally, the burden of CVD has been largely in the developed countries, but as developing countries achieve economic growth the emerging burden of this disease is evident in their vulnerable population groups (Novotny, 2005). The health inequalities already present in low- to middle-income countries may only amplify the impact of CVD among the population (Ezzati *et al.*, 2005) and early attempts should be made to address this possible public health challenge, as recommended by the WHO global strategy for diet, physical activity, and health (Ziraba *et al.*, 2009).

The search for targeted interventions aimed at both the prevention and treatment of CVD has focused on identifying healthy dietary and lifestyle practices. The evolution of new science will facilitate the identification of the best nutrition practices for preventing CVD. Globally, these are consistent dietary recommendations for reducing CVD risk. However, this chapter also has identified several areas for which there is scientific controversy about diets, nutrients, and supplements. In the future, it will be important to resolve these controversies to evolve better dietary recommendations and determine how these may be used with lifestyle modifications and pharmacological treatments. It is likely that dietary recommendations will be individualized even more in the future to accommodate genetic differences in diet responsiveness, as well as identifying approaches that can be followed and enjoyed for a lifetime. In addition, it will be essential to effectively translate nutrition messages to the public, and worldwide, to achieve current dietary recommendations and attain the associated public health benefits. It is evident that, to achieve these goals that result in marked changes in dietary patterns, there needs to be a broad-based effort that shifts the demand for foods that make up a heart-healthy diet.

Suggestions for Further Reading

Appel, L.J., Moore, T.J., Obarzanek, E., *et al.* (1997) A clinical trial of the effects of dietary patterns on blood pressure. DASH Collaborative Research Group. *N Engl J Med* **336**, 1117–1124.

Falk, E. (2006) Pathogenesis of atherosclerosis. *J Am Coll Cardiol* **47**(Suppl 1), C7–12.

FAO (Food and Agriculture Organization of the United Nations). *Food-Based Dietary Guidelines*. http://www.fao.org/ag/humannutrition/nutritioneducation/fbdg/en.

Gersh, B.J., Sliwa, K., Mayosi, B.M., *et al.* (2010) Novel therapeutic concepts: the epidemic of cardiovascular disease in the developing world: global implications. *Eur Heart J* **31**, 642–648.

Jenkins, D.J.A., Kendall, C.W.C., Marchie, A., *et al.* (2003). Effects of a dietary portfolio of cholesterol-lowering foods vs lovastatin on serum lipids and c-reactive protein. *JAMA* **290**, 502–510.

Joint FAO/WHO Expert Consultation (2002) Diet, Nutrition and the Prevention of Chronic Diseases: Report of a Joint WHO/FAO Expert Consultation. Geneva.

Katan, M.B., Brouwer, I.A., Clarke, R., *et al.* (2010) Saturated fat and heart disease. *Am J Clin Nutr* **92**, 459–460.

Kris-Etherton, P.M., Harris, W.S., and Appel, L.J. (2002) Fish consumption, fish oil, omega-3 fatty acids, and cardiovascular disease. *Circulation* **106**, 2747–2757.

Moore, K.J. and Tabas, I. (2011) Macrophages in the pathogenesis of atherosclerosis. *Cell* **145**, 341–355.

References

ADA (American Diabetes Association) (1999) Nutrition recommendations and principles for people with diabetes mellitus. *Diabetes Care* **22,** 542–545.

ADA (American Dietetics Association) (2004a) *The American Dietetic Association Evidence Analysis Library: Criteria for Recommendation Rating.* http://www.adaevidencelibrary.com/evidence.cfm?evidence_summary_id=250466.

ADA (American Dietetics Association) (2004b) Position of the American Dietetic Association: Functional Foods. *J Am Diet Assoc* **104,** 814–826.

ADA (American Dietetics Association) (2009) Position of the American Dietetic Association: Functional Foods. *J Am Diet Assoc* **109,** 735–746.

Adkins, Y. and Kelley, D.S. (2010) Mechanisms underlying the cardioprotective effects of omega-3 polyunsaturated fatty acids. *J Nutr Biochem* **21,** 781–792.

Agency for Healthcare Research and Quality (2004) *Effects of Omega-3 Fatty Acids on Cardiovascular Risk Factors and Intermediate Markers of Cardiovascular Disease.* US Department of Health and Human Services, Washington, DC.

AHA (American Heart Association), Council for High Blood Pressure Research Professional Education Committee, Council On Clinical Cardiology (2011) *My Life Check – Life's Simple 7.* http://mylifecheck.heart.org/Multitab.aspx?NavID=3.

Ahuja, K.D., Ashton, E.L., and Ball, M.J. (2003) Effects of two lipid-lowering, carotenoid-controlled diets on the oxidative modification of low-density lipoproteins in free-living humans. *Clin Sci (Lond)* **105,** 355–361.

Ajani, U.A., Ford, E.S., and Mokdad, A.H. (2004) Dietary fiber and C-reactive protein: findings from national health and nutrition examination survey data. *J Nutr* **134,** 1181–1185.

Albert, C.M., Oh, K., Whang, W., *et al.* (2005) Dietary alpha-linolenic acid intake and risk of sudden cardiac death and coronary heart disease. *Circulation* **112,** 3232–3238.

Alberti, K.G. and Zimmet, P.Z. (1998) Definition, diagnosis and classification of diabetes mellitus and its complications. Part 1: Diagnosis and classification of diabetes mellitus provisional report of a WHO consultation. *Diabet Med* **15,** 539–553.

Alpha-Tocopherol, Beta-Carotene Cancer Prevention Study Group (1994) The effect of vitamin E and beta carotene on the incidence of lung cancer and other cancers in male smokers. *N Engl J Med* **330,** 1029–1035.

Ambrozova, G., Pekarova, M., and Lojek, A. (2010) Effect of polyunsaturated fatty acids on the reactive oxygen and nitrogen species production by raw 264.7 macrophages. *Eur J Nutr* **49,** 133–139.

Anand, S.S., Islam, S., Rosengren, A., *et al.* (2008) Risk factors for myocardial infarction in women and men: insights from the INTERHEART study. *Eur Heart J* **29,** 932–940.

Appel, L.J., Moore, T.J., Obarzanek, E., *et al.* (1997) A clinical trial of the effects of dietary patterns on blood pressure. DASH Collaborative Research Group. *N Engl J Med* **336,** 1117–1124.

Appel, L.J., Sacks, F.M., Carey, V.J., *et al.* (2005) Effects of protein, monounsaturated fat, and carbohydrate intake on blood pressure and serum lipids: results of the OmniHeart randomized trial. *JAMA* **294,** 2455–2464.

Ascherio, A., Katan, M.B., Zock, P.L., *et al.* (1999) Trans fatty acids and coronary heart disease. *N Engl J Med* **340,** 1994–1998.

Ascherio, A., Rimm, E.B., Giovannucci, E.L., *et al.* (1992) A prospective study of nutritional factors and hypertension among US men. *Circulation* **86,** 1475–1484.

Ashton, E.L., Best, J.D., and Ball, M.J. (2001) Effects of monounsaturated enriched sunflower oil on CHD risk factors including LDL size and copper-induced LDL oxidation. *J Am Coll Nutr* **20,** 320–326.

Bagchi, D., Garg, A., Krohn, R.L., *et al.* (1997) Oxygen free radical scavenging abilities of vitamins C and E, and a grape seed proanthocyanidin extract in vitro. *Res Commun Mol Pathol Pharmacol* **95,** 179–189.

Balagopal, P.B., De Ferranti, S.D., Cook, S., *et al.* (2011) Nontraditional risk factors and biomarkers for cardiovascular disease: mechanistic, research, and clinical considerations for youth: a scientific statement from the American Heart Association. *Circulation* **123,** 2749–2769.

Balk, E., Chung, M., Chew, P., *et al.* (2005) Effects of soy on health outcomes. *Evidence Report/Technology Assessment No. 126.* Agency for Healthcare Research and Quality, Rockville, MD.

Balkau, B., Deanfield, J.E., Despres, J.P., *et al.* (2007) International Day for the Evaluation of Abdominal Obesity (IDEA): a study of waist circumference, cardiovascular disease, and diabetes mellitus in 168,000 primary care patients in 63 countries. *Circulation* **116,** 1942–1951.

Barcelo-Coblijn, G., Murphy, E.J., Othman, R., *et al.* (2008) Flaxseed oil and fish-oil capsule consumption alters human red blood cell n-3 fatty acid composition: a multiple-dosing trial comparing 2 sources of n-3 fatty acid. *Am J Clin Nutr* **88,** 801–809.

Bauman, D.E., Corl, B.A., and Peterson, D.G. (2003) The biology of conjugated linoleic acid in ruminants. In J. Sebedio, W.W. Christie, and R. Adolf (eds), *Advances in Conjugated Linoleic Acid Research.* AOCS Press, Champaign, IL, pp. 146–173.

Baumann, K.H., Hessel, F., Larass, I., *et al.* (1999) Dietary omega-3, omega-6, and omega-9 unsaturated fatty acids and growth factor and cytokine gene expression in unstimulated and stimulated monocytes. A randomized volunteer study. *Arterioscler Thromb Vasc Biol* **19,** 59–66.

Bavikati, V.V., Sperling, L.S., Salmon, R.D., *et al.* (2008) Effect of comprehensive therapeutic lifestyle changes on prehypertension. *Am J Cardiol* **102,** 1677–1680.

Beaton, G.H., Milner, J., Corey, P., *et al.* (1979) Sources of variance in 24-hour dietary recall data: implications for nutrition study design and interpretation. *Am J Clin Nutr* **32**, 2546–2559.

Berenson, G.S., Srinivasan, S.R., Bao, W., *et al.* (1998) Association between multiple cardiovascular risk factors and atherosclerosis in children and young adults. The Bogalusa Heart Study. *N Engl J Med* **338**, 1650–1656.

Berglund, L., Lefevre, M., Ginsberg, H.N., *et al.* (2007) Comparison of monounsaturated fat with carbohydrates as a replacement for saturated fat in subjects with a high metabolic risk profile: studies in the fasting and postprandial states. *Am J Clin Nutr* **86**, 1611–1620.

Beulens, J.W., De Bruijne, L.M., Stolk, R.P., *et al.* (2007) High dietary glycemic load and glycemic index increase risk of cardiovascular disease among middle-aged women: a population-based follow-up study. *J Am Coll Cardiol* **50**, 14–21.

Billman, G.E., Kang, J.X., and Leaf, A. (1999) Prevention of sudden cardiac death by dietary pure omega-3 polyunsaturated fatty acids in dogs. *Circulation* **99**, 2452–2457.

Bjelakovic, G., Nikolova, D., Gluud, L., *et al.* (2008) Antioxidant supplements for prevention of mortality in healthy participants and patients with various diseases. *Cochrane Database Syst Rev* (2) CD007176.

Blair, S.N., Capuzzi, D.M., Gottlieb, S.O., *et al.* (2000) Incremental reduction of serum total cholesterol and low-density lipoprotein cholesterol with the addition of plant stanol ester-containing spread to statin therapy. *Am J Cardiol* **86**, 46–52.

Blumenthal, J.A., Babyak, M.A., Hinderliter, A., *et al.* (2010) Effects of the DASH diet alone and in combination with exercise and weight loss on blood pressure and cardiovascular disease biomarkers in men and women with high blood pressure. *Arch Intern Med* **170**, 126–135.

Bolton-Smith, C. and Woodward, M. (1995) Antioxidant vitamin adequacy in relation to consumption of sugars. *Eur J Clin Nutr* **49**, 124–133.

Brandis, M., Keyes, J., and Windhager, E.E. (1972) Potassium-induced inhibition of proximal tubular fluid reabsorption in rats. *Am J Physiol* **222**, 421–427.

Brazier, M., Grados, F., Kamel, S., *et al.* (2005) Clinical and laboratory safety of one year's use of a combination calcium + vitamin D tablet in ambulatory elderly women with vitamin D insufficiency: results of a multicenter, randomized, double-blind, placebo-controlled study. *Clin Ther* **27**, 1885–1893.

Brenna, J.T. (2002) Efficiency of conversion of alpha-linolenic acid to long chain n-3 fatty acids in man. *Curr Opin Clin Nutr Metab Care* **5**, 127–132.

Brouwer, I.A., Wanders, A.J., and Katan, M.B. (2010) Effect of animal and industrial trans fatty acids on HDL and LDL cholesterol levels in humans–a quantitative review. *PLoS One* **5**, e9434.

Brown, B.G., Zhao, X.Q., Chait, A., *et al.* (2001) Simvastatin and niacin, antioxidant vitamins, or the combination for the prevention of coronary disease. *N Engl J Med* **345**, 1583–1592.

Brown, L., Rosner, B., Willett, W.W., *et al.* (1999) Cholesterol-lowering effects of dietary fiber: a meta-analysis. *Am J Clin Nutr* **69**, 30–42.

Bruckert, E. and Rosenbaum, D. (2011) Lowering LDL-cholesterol through diet: potential role in the statin era. *Curr Opin Lipidol* **22**, 43–48.

Burgess, J.W., Sinclair, P.A., Chretien, C.M., *et al.* (2006) Reverse cholesterol transport. In S.K. Cheema (ed.), *Biochemistry of Atherosclerosis.* Springer, New York, pp. 3–22.

Burr, M.L., Ashfield-Watt, P.A., Dunstan, F.D., *et al.* (2003) Lack of benefit of dietary advice to men with angina: results of a controlled trial. *Eur J Clin Nutr* **57**, 193–200.

Burr, M.L., Fehily, A.M., Gilbert, J.F., *et al.* (1989) Effects of changes in fat, fish, and fibre intakes on death and myocardial reinfarction: diet and reinfarction trial (DART). *Lancet* **2**, 757–761.

Calder, P.C. (2004) n-3 Fatty acids and cardiovascular disease: evidence explained and mechanisms explored. *Clin Sci (Lond)* **107**, 1–11.

Calzada, C., Colas, R., Guillot, N., *et al.* (2010) Subgram daily supplementation with docosahexaenoic acid protects low-density lipoproteins from oxidation in healthy men. *Atherosclerosis* **208**, 467–472.

Campbell, R.W., Murray, A., and Julian, D.G. (1981) Ventricular arrhythmias in first 12 hours of acute myocardial infarction. Natural history study. *Br Heart J* **46**, 351–357.

Canner, P.L., Berge, K.G., Wenger, N.K., *et al.* (1986) Fifteen year mortality in Coronary Drug Project patients: long-term benefit with niacin. *J Am Coll Cardiol* **8**, 1245–1255.

Cao, Y., Mauger, D.T., Pelkman, C.L., *et al.* (2009) Effects of moderate (MF) versus lower fat (LF) diets on lipids and lipoproteins: a meta-analysis of clinical trials in subjects with and without diabetes. *J Clin Lipidol* **3**, 19–32.

Cappuccio, F.P. and MacGregor, G.A. (1991) Does potassium supplementation lower blood pressure? A meta-analysis of published trials. *J Hypertens* **9**, 465–473.

Cappuccio, F.P., Markandu, N.D., Beynon, G.W., *et al.* (1985) Lack of effect of oral magnesium on high blood pressure: a double blind study. *Br Med J (Clin Res Ed)* **291**, 235–238.

Cardiovascular Disease Programme (2002) Integrated Management of Cardiovascular Risk. Report of a WHO meeting, 9–12 July, Geneva.

Carr, A.C. and Frei, B. (1999) Toward a new recommended dietary allowance for vitamin C based on antioxidant and health effects in humans. *Am J Clin Nutr* **69**, 1086–1107.

Carthy, E.P., Yamashita, W., Hsu, A., *et al.* (1989) 1,25-Dihydroxyvitamin D3 and rat vascular smooth muscle cell growth. *Hypertension* **13**, 954–959.

CDC (Centers for Disease Control and Prevention) (2010) *How Tobacco Smoke Causes Disease: The Biology and Behavioral Basis for Smoking-Attributable Disease: A Report of the Surgeon General.* US Department of Health and Human Services. National Center for Chronic Disease Prevention and Health Promotion, Office on Smoking and Health, Rockville, MD.

Chan, J.K., McDonald, B.E., Gerrard, J.M., *et al.* (1993) Effect of dietary alpha-linolenic acid and its ratio to linoleic acid on platelet and plasma fatty acids and thrombogenesis. *Lipids* **28**, 811–817.

Chapman, M.J., Redfern, J.S., McGovern, M.E., *et al.* (2010) Niacin and fibrates in atherogenic dyslipidemia: pharmacotherapy to reduce cardiovascular risk. *Pharmacol Ther* **126**, 314–345.

Chen, S.T., Maruthur, N.M., and Appel, L.J. (2010) The effect of dietary patterns on estimated coronary heart disease risk. *Circ Cardiovasc Qual Outcomes* **3**, 484–489.

Cheung, M.C., Zhao, X.-Q., Chait, A., *et al.* (2001) Antioxidant supplements block the response of HDL to simvastatin-niacin therapy in patients with coronary artery disease and low HDL. *Arterioscler Thromb Vasc Biol* **21**, 1320–1326.

Chinetti, G., Griglio, S., Antonucci, M., *et al.* (1998) Activation of proliferator-activated receptors alpha and gamma induces apoptosis of human monocyte-derived macrophages. *J Biol Chem* **273**, 25573–25580.

Chiu, K.C., Chu, A., Go, V.L., *et al.* (2004) Hypovitaminosis D is associated with insulin resistance and beta cell dysfunction. *Am J Clin Nutr* **79**, 820–825.

Chobanian, A.V., Bakris, G.L., Black, H.R., *et al.* (2003) The Seventh Report of the Joint National Committee on Prevention, Detection, Evaluation, and Treatment of High Blood Pressure: the JNC 7 report. *JAMA* **289**, 2560–2572.

Chobanian, A.V. and Hill, M. (2000) National Heart, Lung, and Blood Institute Workshop on Sodium and Blood Pressure : a critical review of current scientific evidence. *Hypertension* **35**, 858–863.

Christensen, J.H., Riahi, S., Schmidt, E.B., *et al.* (2005) n-3 Fatty acids and ventricular arrhythmias in patients with ischaemic heart disease and implantable cardioverter defibrillators. *Europace* **7**, 338–344.

Chu, Z.M., Yin, K., and Beilin, L.J. (1992) Fish oil feeding selectively attenuates contractile responses to noradrenaline and electrical stimulation in the perfused mesenteric resistance vessels of spontaneously hypertensive rats. *Clin Exp Pharmacol Physiol* **19**, 177–181.

Chung, B.H., Cho, B.H., Liang, P., *et al.* (2004) Contribution of postprandial lipemia to the dietary fat-mediated changes in endogenous lipoprotein-cholesterol concentrations in humans. *Am J Clin Nutr* **80**, 1145–1158.

Clarke, R., Frost, C., Collins, R., *et al.* (1997) Dietary lipids and blood cholesterol: quantitative meta-analysis of metabolic ward studies. *BMJ* **314**, 112–117.

Clifton, P., Keogh, J., and Noakes, M. (2008) Long-term effects of a high protein weight-loss diet. *Am J Clin Nutr* **87**, 23–29.

Cohen, H.W., Hailpern, S.M., and Alderman, M.H. (2008) Sodium intake and mortality follow-up in the Third National Health and Nutrition Examination Survey (NHANES III). *J Gen Intern Med* **23**, 1297–1302.

Colette, C., Percheron, C., Pares-Herbute, N., *et al.* (2003) Exchanging carbohydrates for monounsaturated fats in energy-restricted diets: effects on metabolic profile and other cardiovascular risk factors. *Int J Obesity Rel Metab Disord* **27**, 648–656.

Cuchel, M. and Rader, D.J. (2006) Macrophage reverse cholesterol transport: key to the regression of atherosclerosis? *Circulation* **113**, 2548–2555.

Cunningham, K.S. and Gotlieb, A.I. (2005) The role of shear stress in the pathogenesis of atherosclerosis. *Lab Invest* **85**, 9–23.

Cushing, S.D., Berliner, J.A., Valente, A.J., *et al.* (1990) Minimally modified low density lipoprotein induces monocyte chemotactic protein 1 in human endothelial cells and smooth muscle cells. *Proc Natl Acad Sci USA* **87**, 5134–5138.

Dansinger, M.L., Gleason, J.A., Griffith, J.L., *et al.* (2005) Comparison of the Atkins, Ornish, Weight Watchers, and Zone diets for weight loss and heart disease risk reduction. *JAMA* **293**, 43–53.

Davies, M.J., Woolf, N., Rowles, P.M., *et al.* (1988) Morphology of the endothelium over atherosclerotic plaques in human coronary arteries. *Br Heart J* **60**, 459–464.

DECODA Study Group (International Diabetes Epidemiology Group) (2002) Cardiovascular risk profile assessment in glucose-intolerant Asian individuals – an evaluation of the World Health Organization two-step strategy: the DECODA Study (Diabetes Epidemiology: Collaborative Analysis of Diagnostic Criteria in Asia). *Diabet Med* **19**, 549–557.

de Lorgeril, M., Salen, P., Martin, J.L., *et al.* (1999) Mediterranean diet, traditional risk factors, and the rate of cardiovascular complications after myocardial infarction: final report of the Lyon Diet Heart Study. *Circulation* **99**, 779–785.

De Moura, F.F., Lewis, K.D., and Falk, M.C. (2009) Applying the FDA definition of whole grains to the evidence for cardiovascular disease health claims. *J Nutr* **139**, 2220S–2226S.

De Roos, N.M., Schouten, E.G., and Katan, M.B. (2003) Trans fatty acids, HDL-cholesterol, and cardiovascular disease. Effects of dietary changes on vascular reactivity. *Eur J Med Res* **8**, 355–357.

DGAC (2010a) *Dietary Guidelines for Americans, 2010.* US Department of Agriculture, US Department of Health and Human Services (eds), 7th Edn. Washington, DC.

DGAC (2010b) *Report of the Dietary Guidelines Advisory Committee on the Dietary Guidelines for Americans.* US Department of Agriculture, US Department of Health and Human Services (eds). Washington, DC.

Djousse, L. and Gaziano, J.M. (2008a) Egg consumption and risk of heart failure in the Physicians' Health Study. *Circulation* **117**, 512–516.

Djousse, L. and Gaziano, J.M. (2008b) Egg consumption in relation to cardiovascular disease and mortality: the Physicians' Health Study. *Am J Clin Nutr* **87**, 964–969.

Dobnig, H., Pilz, S., Scharnagl, H., *et al.* (2008) Independent association of low serum 25-hydroxyvitamin D and 1,25-dihydroxyvitamin D levels with all-cause and cardiovascular mortality. *Arch Intern Med* **168**, 1340–1349.

Duo, L., Sinclair, A.J., Mann, N.J., *et al.* (2000) Selected micronutrient intake and status in men with differing meat intakes, vegetarians and vegans. *Asia Pac J Clin Nutr* **9**, 18–23.

Durstine, J.L., Grandjean, P.W., Davis, P.G., *et al.* (2001) Blood lipid and lipoprotein adaptations to exercise: a quantitative analysis. *Sports Med* **31**, 1033–1062.

Dyckner, T. and Wester, P.O. (1983) Effect of magnesium on blood pressure. *Br Med J (Clin Res Ed)* **286**, 1847–1849.

Dyerberg, J. and Bang, H.O. (1979) Lipid metabolism, atherogenesis, and haemostasis in Eskimos: the role of the prostaglandin-3 family. *Haemostasis* **8**, 227–233.

EFSA Panel on Dietetic Products Nutrition and Allergies (2010a) Scientific opinion on Dietary Reference Values for carbohydrates and dietary fibre. *EFSA J* **8**, 1462 [77pp].

EFSA Panel on Dietetic Products Nutrition and Allergies (2010b) Scientific opinion on Dietary Reference Values for fats, including saturated fatty acids, polyunsaturated fatty acids, monounsaturated fatty acids, trans fatty acids, and cholesterol. *EFSA J* **8**, 1461 [107pp].

Elmadfa, I. and Singer, I. (2009) Vitamin B-12 and homocysteine status among vegetarians: a global perspective. *Am J Clin Nutr* **89**, 1693S–1698S.

Englyst, K.N., Liu, S., and Englyst, H.N. (2007) Nutritional characterization and measurement of dietary carbohydrates. *Eur J Clin Nutr* **61**(Suppl 1), S19–S39.

Englyst, K.N., Vinoy, S., Englyst, H.N., *et al.* (2003) Glycaemic index of cereal products explained by their content of rapidly and slowly available glucose. *Br J Nutr* **89**, 329–340.

Estruch, R., Martínez-González, M.A., Corella, D., *et al.* (2006) Effects of a Mediterranean-style diet on cardiovascular risk factors. *Ann Intern Med* **145**, 1–11.

Expert Panel on Detection, Evaluation, and Treatment of High Blood Cholesterol in Adults (2001) Executive Summary of the Third Report of the National Cholesterol Education Program (NCEP) Expert Panel on Detection, Evaluation, and Treatment of High Blood Cholesterol in Adults (Adult Treatment Panel III). *JAMA* **285**, 2486–2497.

Ezzati, M., Van der Hoorn, S., Lawes, C.M., *et al.* (2005) Rethinking the "diseases of affluence" paradigm: global patterns of nutritional risks in relation to economic development. *PLoS Med* **2**, e133.

Falk, E. (2006) Pathogenesis of atherosclerosis. *J Am Coll Cardiol* **47**(Suppl 1), C7–12.

Falk, E., Shah, P.K., and Fuster, V. (2004) Atherothrombosis and thrombosis-prone plaques. In R.W. Alexander, R.A. O'Rourke, R. Roberts, *et al.* (eds), *Hurst's The Heart*, 11th Edn. McGraw-Hill, New York, pp. 1123–1139.

FDA (2003) Claims that can be made for conventional foods and dietary supplements. US Food and Drug Administration, Bethesda, Maryland. http://www.fda.gov/food/labeling nutrition/labelclaims/ucm111447.htm.

Feinman, R. and Fine, E. (2003) Thermodynamics and metabolic advantage of weight loss diets. *Metab Syndr Relat Disord* **1**, 209–219.

Ferdowsian, H.R. and Barnard, N.D. (2009) Effects of plant-based diets on plasma lipids. *Am J Cardiol* **104**, 947–956.

Ferrucci, L., Cherubini, A., Bandinelli, S., *et al.* (2006) Relationship of plasma polyunsaturated fatty acids to circulating inflammatory markers. *J Clin Endocrinol Metab* **91**, 439–446.

Finstad, H.S., Drevon, C.A., Kulseth, M.A., *et al.* (1998) Cell proliferation, apoptosis and accumulation of lipid droplets in U937-1 cells incubated with eicosapentaenoic acid. *Biochem J* **336**, 451–459.

Folsom, A.R., Nieto, F.J., McGovern, P.G., *et al.* (1998) Prospective study of coronary heart disease incidence in relation to fasting total homocysteine, related genetic polymorphisms, and B vitamins: the Atherosclerosis Risk in Communities (ARIC) study. *Circulation* **98**, 204–210.

Ford, E.S. and Capewell, S. (2007) Coronary heart disease mortality among young adults in the U.S. from 1980 through 2002: concealed leveling of mortality rates. *J Am Coll Cardiol* **50**, 2128–2132.

Fraser, G.E. (1999) Associations between diet and cancer, ischemic heart disease, and all-cause mortality in non-Hispanic white California Seventh-day Adventists. *Am J Clin Nutr* **70**, 532S–538S.

Fraser, G.E. (2009) Vegetarian diets: what do we know of their effects on common chronic diseases? *Am J Clin Nutr* **89**, 1607S–1612S.

Freedman, D.S., Patel, D.A., Srinivasan, S.R., *et al.* (2008) The contribution of childhood obesity to adult carotid intima-media thickness: the Bogalusa Heart Study. *Int J Obes (Lond)* **32**, 749–756.

Frikke-Schmidt, H. and Lykkesfeldt, J. (2009) Role of marginal vitamin C deficiency in atherogenesis: in vivo models and clinical studies. *Basic Clin Pharmacol Toxicol* **104**, 419–433.

Fung, T.T., Rexrode, K.M., Mantzoros, C.S., *et al.* (2009) Mediterranean diet and incidence of and mortality from coronary heart disease and stroke in women. *Circulation* **119**, 1093–1100.

Galan, P., Kesse-Guyot, E., Czernichow, S.B., *et al.* (2010) Effects of B vitamins and omega 3 fatty acids on cardiovascular diseases: a randomised placebo controlled trial. *BMJ* **341**, c6273.

Gardner, C.D., Fortmann, S.P., and Krauss, R.M. (1996) Association of small low-density lipoprotein particles with the incidence of coronary artery disease in men and women. *JAMA* **276**, 875–881.

Garg, A. (1998) High-monounsaturated-fat diets for patients with diabetes mellitus: a meta-analysis. *Am J Clin Nutr* **67**, 577S–582S.

Geleijnse, J.M., Giltay, E.J., Grobbee, D.E., *et al.* (2002) Blood pressure response to fish oil supplementation: metaregression analysis of randomized trials. *J Hypertens* **20**, 1493–1499.

Geleijnse, J.M., Kok, F.J., and Grobbee, D.E. (2003) Blood pressure response to changes in sodium and potassium intake: a metaregression analysis of randomised trials. *J Hum Hypertens* **17**, 471–480.

Geleijnse, J.M., Witteman, J.C., Bak, A.A., *et al.* (1994) Reduction in blood pressure with a low sodium, high potassium, high magnesium salt in older subjects with mild to moderate hypertension. *BMJ* **309**, 436–440.

Geng, Y.J. and Libby, P. (2002) Progression of atheroma: a struggle between death and procreation. *Arterioscler Thromb Vasc Biol* **22**, 1370–1380.

Gerhard, G.T. and Duell, P.B. (1999) Homocysteine and atherosclerosis. *Curr Opin Lipidol* **10**, 417–428.

Gersh, B.J., Sliwa, K., Mayosi, B.M., *et al.* (2010) Novel therapeutic concepts: the epidemic of cardiovascular disease in the developing world: global implications. *Eur Heart J* **31**, 642–648.

Giovannucci, E., Liu, Y., Hollis, B.W., *et al.* (2008) 25-Hydroxyvitamin D and risk of myocardial infarction in men: a prospective study. *Arch Intern Med* **168**, 1174–1180.

GISSI-Prevenzione Investigators (1999) Dietary supplementation with n-3 polyunsaturated fatty acids and vitamin E after myocardial infarction: results of the GISSI-Prevenzione trial. *Lancet* **354**, 447–455.

Glass, C.K. and Witztum, J.L. (2001) Atherosclerosis. The road ahead. *Cell* **104**, 503–516.

Gokce, N., Keaney, J.F., Jr, Frei, B., *et al.* (1999) Long-term ascorbic acid administration reverses endothelial vasomotor dysfunction in patients with coronary artery disease. *Circulation* **99**, 3234–3240.

Goldberg, R.B. (2000) Cardiovascular disease in diabetic patients. *Med Clin North Am* **84**, 81–93.

Goni, I., Garcia-Alonso, A., and Saura-Calixto, F. (1997) A starch hydrolysis procedure to estimate glycemic index. *Nutr Res* **17**, 427–437.

Goodnight, S.H., Jr, Harris, W.S., and Connor, W.E. (1981) The effects of dietary omega 3 fatty acids on platelet composition and function in man: a prospective, controlled study. *Blood* **58**, 880–885.

Goyens, P.L., Spilker, M.E., Zock, P.L., *et al.* (2006) Conversion of alpha-linolenic acid in humans is influenced by the absolute amounts of alpha-linolenic acid and linoleic acid in the diet and not by their ratio. *Am J Clin Nutr* **84**, 44–53.

Grimsgaard, S., Bonaa, K.H., Jacobsen, B.K., *et al.* (1999) Plasma saturated and linoleic fatty acids are independently associated with blood pressure. *Hypertension* **34**, 478–483.

Grundy, S.M., Benjamin, I.J., Burke, G.L., *et al.* (1999) Diabetes and cardiovascular disease: a statement for healthcare professionals from the American Heart Association. *Circulation* **100**, 1134–1146.

Grundy, S.M., Cleeman, J.I., Daniels, S.R., *et al.* (2005) Diagnosis and management of the metabolic syndrome: An American Heart Association/National Heart, Lung, and Blood Institute Scientific Statement. *Circulation* **112**, 2735–2752.

Grundy, S.M., Cleeman, J.I., Merz, C.N., *et al.* (2004) Implications of recent clinical trials for the National Cholesterol Education Program Adult Treatment Panel III guidelines. *Circulation* **110**, 227–239.

Guyton, J.R. and Capuzzi, D.M. (1998) Treatment of hyperlipidemia with combined niacin-statin regimens. *Am J Cardiol* **82**, 82U–84U.

Gylling, H., Radhakrishnan, R., and Miettinen, T.A. (1997) Reduction of serum cholesterol in postmenopausal women with previous myocardial infarction and cholesterol malabsorption induced by dietary sitostanol ester margarine: women and dietary sitostanol. *Circulation* **96**, 4226–4231.

Haddad, E.H., Berk, L.S., Kettering, J.D., *et al.* (1999) Dietary intake and biochemical, hematologic, and immune status of vegans compared with nonvegetarians. *Am J Clin Nutr* **70**, 586S–593S.

Halton, T.L., Willett, W.C., Liu, S., *et al.* (2006) Low-carbohydrate-diet score and the risk of coronary heart disease in women. *N Engl J Med* **355**, 1991–2002.

Hamilton, T.A., Ma, G.P., and Chisolm, G.M. (1990) Oxidized low density lipoprotein suppresses the expression of tumor necrosis factor-alpha mRNA in stimulated murine peritoneal macrophages. *J Immunol* **144**, 2343–2350.

Hansson, G.K. (2005) Inflammation, atherosclerosis, and coronary artery disease. *N Engl J Med* **352**, 1685–1695.

Hargrove, R.L., Etherton, T.D., Pearson, T.A., *et al.* (2001) Low fat and high monounsaturated fat diets decrease human low density lipoprotein oxidative susceptibility in vitro. *J Nutr* **131**, 1758–1763.

Harper, C.R., Edwards, M.J., Defilippis, A.P., *et al.* (2006) Flaxseed oil increases the plasma concentrations of cardioprotective (n-3) fatty acids in humans. *J Nutr* **136**, 83–87.

Harris, W.S. (2005) Alpha-linolenic acid: a gift from the land? *Circulation* **111**, 2872–2874.

Harris, W.S. (2006) The omega-6/omega-3 ratio and cardiovascular disease risk: uses and abuses. *Curr Atheroscler Rep* **8**, 453–459.

Harris, W.S. (2008) The omega-3 index as a risk factor for coronary heart disease. *Am J Clin Nutr* **87**, 1997S–2002S.

Harris, W.S., Miller, M., Tighe, A.P., *et al.* (2008) Omega-3 fatty acids and coronary heart disease risk: clinical and mechanistic perspectives. *Atherosclerosis* **197**, 12–24.

Harris, W.S., Mozaffarian, D., Rimm, E., *et al.* (2009) Omega-6 fatty acids and risk for cardiovascular disease: a science advisory from the American Heart Association Nutrition Subcommittee of the Council on Nutrition, Physical Activity, and Metabolism; Council on Cardiovascular Nursing; and Council on Epidemiology and Prevention. *Circulation* **119**, 902–907.

Hasler, C.M., Kundrat, S., and Wool, D. (2000) Functional foods and cardiovascular disease. *Curr Atheroscleros Rep* **2**, 467–475.

He, J., Whelton, P.K., Appel, L.J., *et al.* (2000) Long-term effects of weight loss and dietary sodium reduction on incidence of hypertension. *Hypertension* **35**, 544–549.

He, J., Wofford, M.R., Reynolds, K., *et al.* (2011) Effect of dietary protein supplementation on blood pressure: a randomized, controlled trial. *Circulation* **124**, 589–595.

He, K., Song, Y., Daviglus, M.L., *et al.* (2004a) Fish consumption and incidence of stroke: a meta-analysis of cohort studies. *Stroke* **35**, 1538–1542.

He, K., Song, Y., Daviglus, M.L., *et al.* (2004b) Accumulated evidence on fish consumption and coronary heart disease mortality: a meta-analysis of cohort studies. *Circulation* **109**, 2705–2711.

Health Canada (2010) Vitamin D and Calcium: Updated Reference Intakes. Health Canada. Ottawa. http://www.hc-sc.gc.ca/fn-an/nutrition/vitamin/vita-d-eng.php.

Hegsted, D.M., Ausman, L.M., Johnson, J.A., *et al.* (1993) Dietary fat and serum lipids: an evaluation of the experimental data. *Am J Clin Nutr* **57**, 875–883.

Hessler, J.R., Morel, D.W., Lewis, L.J., *et al.* (1983) Lipoprotein oxidation and lipoprotein-induced cytotoxicity. *Arteriosclerosis* **3**, 215–222.

Homocysteine Lowering Trialists (1998) Lowering blood homocysteine with folic acid based supplements: meta-analysis of randomised trials. *BMJ* **316**, 894–898.

Hooper, L., Thompson, R.L., Harrison, R.A., *et al.* (2004) Omega 3 fatty acids for prevention and treatment of cardiovascular disease. *Cochrane Database Syst Rev* CD003177.

Houston, M.C. (2010) The role of cellular micronutrient analysis, nutraceuticals, vitamins, antioxidants and minerals in the prevention and treatment of hypertension and cardiovascular disease. *Ther Adv Cardiovasc Dis* **4**, 165–183.

Houston, M.C. and Harper, K.J. (2008) Potassium, magnesium, and calcium: their role in both the cause and treatment of hypertension. *J Clin Hypertens (Greenwich)* **10**, 3–11.

Hsia, J., Heiss, G., Ren, H., *et al.* (2007) Calcium/vitamin D supplementation and cardiovascular events. *Circulation* **115**, 846–854.

Hu, F.B., Stampfer, M.J., Manson, J.E., *et al.* (1997) Dietary fat intake and the risk of coronary heart disease in women. *N Engl J Med* **337**, 1491–1499.

Hu, F.B., Stampfer, M.J., Rimm, E.B., *et al.* (1999) A prospective study of egg consumption and risk of cardiovascular disease in men and women. *JAMA* **281**, 1387–1394.

Hunninghake, D.B., Stein, E.A., Dujovne, C.A., *et al.* (1993) The efficacy of intensive dietary therapy alone or combined with lovastatin in outpatients with hypercholesterolemia. *N Engl J Med* **328**, 1213–1219.

Hunter, J. E., Zhang, J., and Kris-Etherton, P.M. (2010) Cardiovascular disease risk of dietary stearic acid compared with trans, other saturated, and unsaturated fatty acids: a systematic review. *Am J Clin Nutr* **91**, 46–63.

Hussein, N., Ah-Sing, E., Wilkinson, P., *et al.* (2005) Long-chain conversion of [13C]linoleic acid and alpha-linolenic acid in response to marked changes in their dietary intake in men. *J Lipid Res* **46**, 269–280.

Iestra, J.A., Kromhout, D., Van der Schouw, Y.T., *et al.* (2005) Effect size estimates of lifestyle and dietary changes on all-cause mortality in coronary artery disease patients: a systematic review. *Circulation* **112**, 924–934.

Iimura, O., Kijima, T., Kikuchi, K., *et al.* (1981) Studies on the hypotensive effect of high potassium intake in patients with essential hypertension. *Clin Sci (Lond)* **61**(Suppl 7), 77S–80S.

Institute of Medicine (1997) *Dietary Reference Intakes for Calcium, Phosphorus, Magnesium, Vitamin D and Fluoride.* National Academies Press, Washington, DC.

Institute of Medicine (1998) *Dietary Reference Intakes for Thiamin, Riboflavin, Niacin, Vitamin B6, Folate, Vitamin B12, Pantothenic Acid, Biotin, and Choline.* National Academies Press, Washington, DC.

Institute of Medicine (2000) *Dietary Reference Intakes for Vitamin C, Vitamin E, Selenium, and Carotenoids.* National Academies Press, Washington, DC.

Institute of Medicine (2002) *Dietary Reference Intakes for Energy, Carbohydrate, Fiber, Fat, Fatty Acids, Cholesterol, Protein, and Amino Acids.* National Academies Press, Washington, DC.

Institute of Medicine (2004) Sodium and chloride. In *Dietary Reference Intakes for Water, Potassium, Sodium, Chloride and Sulfate.* National Academies Press, Washington, DC.

Institute of Medicine (2005) *Dietary Reference Intakes for Energy, Carbohydrate, Fiber, Fat, Fatty Acids, Cholesterol, Protein, and*

Amino Acids (Macronutrients). National Academies Press, Washington, DC.

Institute of Medicine (2006) *Sleep Disorders and Sleep Deprivation: An Unmet Public Health Problem*. National Academies Press, Washington, DC.

Institute of Medicine (2010) *Dietary Reference Intakes for Calcium and Vitamin D*. National Academies Press, Washington, DC.

International Diabetes Federation (2006) *The IDF Consensus Worldwide Definition of the Metabolic Syndrome*. IDF Communications, Brussels. http://www.idf.org/webdata/docs/MetS_def_update2006.pdf.

Jacobs, D.R., Pereira, M.A., Meyer, K.A., *et al.* (2000) Fiber from whole grains, but not refined grains, is inversely associated with all-cause mortality in older women: the Iowa women's health study. *J Am Coll Nutr* **19,** 326S–330S.

Jakobsen, M.U., O'Reilly, E.J., Heitmann, B.L., *et al.* (2009) Major types of dietary fat and risk of coronary heart disease: a pooled analysis of 11 cohort studies. *Am J Clin Nutr* **89,** 1425–1432.

Jenkins, D.J., Kendall, C.W., Axelsen, M., *et al.* (2000) Viscous and nonviscous fibres, nonabsorbable and low glycaemic index carbohydrates, blood lipids and coronary heart disease. *Curr Opin Lipidol* **11,** 49–56.

Jenkins, D.J., Wolever, T.M., Taylor, R.H., *et al.* (1981) Glycemic index of foods: a physiological basis for carbohydrate exchange. *Am J Clin Nutr* **34,** 362–366.

Jenkins, D.J.A., Kendall, C.W.C., Faulkner, D., *et al.* (2002) A dietary portfolio approach to cholesterol reduction: combined effects of plant sterols, vegetable proteins, and viscous fibers in hypercholesterolemia. *Metabolism* **51,** 1596–1604.

Jenkins, D.J.A., Kendall, C.W.C., Marchie, A., *et al.* (2003) Effects of a dietary portfolio of cholesterol-lowering foods vs lovastatin on serum lipids and C-reactive protein. *JAMA* **290,** 502–510.

Jessup, M., Abraham, W.T., Casey, D.E., *et al.* (2009) 2009 focused update: ACCF/AHA Guidelines for the Diagnosis and Management of Heart Failure in Adults: a report of the American College of Cardiology Foundation/American Heart Association Task Force on Practice Guidelines: developed in collaboration with the International Society for Heart and Lung Transplantation. *Circulation* **119,** 1977–2016.

Joffres, M.R., Reed, D.M., and Yano, K. (1987) Relationship of magnesium intake and other dietary factors to blood pressure: the Honolulu heart study. *Am J Clin Nutr* **45,** 469–475.

Joint FAO/WHO Expert Consultation (2002) Diet, Nutrition and the Prevention of Chronic Diseases: Report of a Joint WHO/FAO Expert Consultation. Geneva.

Joint FAO/WHO Expert Consultation (2008) Fats and Fatty Acids in Human Nutrition: Report of an Expert Consultation. Food and Agriculture Organization of the United Nations.

Joshi, P., Islam, S., Pais, P., *et al.* (2007) Risk factors for early myocardial infarction in South Asians compared with individuals in other countries. *JAMA* **297,** 286–294.

Katan, M.B. (2006) The response of lipoproteins to dietary fat and cholesterol in lean and obese persons. *Curr Cardiol Rep* **8,** 446–451.

Katan, M.B., Beynen, A.C., De Vries, J.H., *et al.* (1986) Existence of consistent hypo- and hyperresponders to dietary cholesterol in man. *Am J Epidemiol* **123,** 221–234.

Katan, M.B., Brouwer, I.A., Clarke, R., *et al.* (2010) Saturated fat and heart disease. *Am J Clin Nutr* **92,** 459–460.

Kelley, G.A. and Kelley, K.S. (2000) Progressive resistance exercise and resting blood pressure: a meta-analysis of randomized controlled trials. *Hypertension* **35,** 838–843.

Key, T.J., Appleby, P.N., Spencer, E.A., *et al.* (2009) Mortality in British vegetarians: results from the European Prospective Investigation into Cancer and Nutrition (EPIC-Oxford). *Am J Clin Nutr* **89,** 1613S–1619S.

Key, T.J., Fraser, G.E., Thorogood, M., *et al.* (1999) Mortality in vegetarians and nonvegetarians: detailed findings from a collaborative analysis of 5 prospective studies. *Am J Clin Nutr* **70,** 516S–524S.

King, D.E., Egan, B.M., Woolson, R.F., *et al.* (2007) Effect of a high-fiber diet vs a fiber-supplemented diet on C-reactive protein level. *Arch Intern Med* **167,** 502–506.

Knekt, P., Ritz, J., Pereira, M.A., *et al.* (2004) Antioxidant vitamins and coronary heart disease risk: a pooled analysis of 9 cohorts. *Am J Clin Nutr* **80,** 1508–1520.

Kohls, K.J., Kies, C., and Fox, H.M. (1987) Blood serum lipid levels of humans given arginine, lysine and tryptophan supplements without food. *Nutr Rep Int* **35,** 5–11.

Kourlaba, G. and Panagiotakos, D.B. (2009) Dietary quality indices and human health: a review. *Maturitas* **62,** 1–8.

Kowey, P.R., Reiffel, J.A., Ellenbogen, K.A., *et al.* (2010) Efficacy and safety of prescription omega-3 fatty acids for the prevention of recurrent symptomatic atrial fibrillation. *JAMA* **304,** 2363–2372.

Kralova Lesna, I., Suchanek, P., Kovar, J., *et al.* (2008) Replacement of dietary saturated FAs by PUFAs in diet and reverse cholesterol transport. *J Lipid Res* **49,** 2414–2418.

Krauss, R.M., Blanche, P.J., Rawlings, R.S., *et al.* (2006) Separate effects of reduced carbohydrate intake and weight loss on atherogenic dyslipidemia. *Am J Clin Nutr* **83,** 1025–1031.

Kris-Etherton, P.M. and Harris, W.S. (2004) Adverse effect of fish oils in patients with angina? *Curr Atherosclerosis Rep* **6,** 413–414.

Kris-Etherton, P., Eckel, R.H., Howard, B.V., *et al.* (2001) AHA Science Advisory: Lyon Diet Heart Study: Benefits of a Mediterranean-Style, National Cholesterol Education

Program/American Heart Association Step I Dietary Pattern on Cardiovascular Disease. *Circulation* **103**, 1823–1825.

Kris-Etherton, P.M., Harris, W.S., and Appel, L.J. (2002) Fish consumption, fish oil, omega-3 fatty acids, and cardiovascular disease. *Circulation* **106**, 2747–2757.

Kritchevsky, S.B. and Kritchevsky, D. (2000) Egg consumption and coronary heart disease: an epidemiologic overview. *J Am Coll Nutr* **19**, 549S–555S.

Kromhout, D., Giltay, E.J., and Geleijnse, J.M. (2010) N-3 fatty acids and cardiovascular events after myocardial infarction. *N Engl J Med* **363**, 2015–2026.

Kusumoto, A., Ishikura, Y., Kawashima, H., *et al.* (2007) Effects of arachidonate-enriched triacylglycerol supplementation on serum fatty acids and platelet aggregation in healthy male subjects with a fish diet. *Br J Nutr* **98**, 626–635.

Lamarche, B., Tchernof, A., Moorjani, S., *et al.* (1997) Small, dense low-density lipoprotein particles as a predictor of the risk of ischemic heart disease in men. Prospective results from the Quebec Cardiovascular Study. *Circulation* **95**, 69–75.

Layman, D.K., Evans, E.M., Erickson, D., *et al.* (2009) A moderate-protein diet produces sustained weight loss and long-term changes in body composition and blood lipids in obese adults. *J Nutr* **139**, 514–521.

Leaf, A., Kang, J.X., Xiao, Y.F., *et al.* (2003) Clinical prevention of sudden cardiac death by n-3 polyunsaturated fatty acids and mechanism of prevention of arrhythmias by n-3 fish oils. *Circulation* **107**, 2646–2652.

Lee, K.N., Kritchevsky, D., and Pariza, M.W. (1994) Conjugated linoleic acid and atherosclerosis in rabbits. *Atherosclerosis* **108**, 19–25.

Lefebvre, P.J. and Scheen, A.J. (1998) The postprandial state and risk of cardiovascular disease. *Diabet Med* **15**, S63–S68.

Lemke, S.L., Vicini, J.L., Su, H., *et al.* (2010) Dietary intake of stearidonic acid-enriched soybean oil increases the omega-3 index: randomized, double-blind clinical study of efficacy and safety. *Am J Clin Nutr* **92**, 766–775.

Levin, A. and Li, Y.C. (2005) Vitamin D and its analogues: do they protect against cardiovascular disease in patients with kidney disease? *Kidney Int* **68**, 1973–1981.

Levitan, E.B., Mittleman, M.A., Håkansson, N., *et al.* (2007) Dietary glycemic index, dietary glycemic load, and cardiovascular disease in middle-aged and older Swedish men. *Am J Clin Nutr* **85**, 1521–1526.

Lewis, G.F. and Rader, D.J. (2005) New insights into the regulation of HDL metabolism and reverse cholesterol transport. *Circ Res* **96**, 1221–1232.

Li, D. (2011) Chemistry behind vegetarianism. *J Agric Food Chem* **59**, 777–784.

Li, D., Sinclair, A.J., Mann, N.J., *et al.* (2000) Selected micronutrient intake and status in men with differing meat intakes, vegetarians and vegans. *Asia Pac J Clin Nutr* **9**, 18–23.

Li, Y.C., Qiao, G., Uskokovic, M., *et al.* (2004) Vitamin D: a negative endocrine regulator of the renin-angiotensin system and blood pressure. *J Steroid Biochem Mol Biol* **89–90**, 387–392.

Liao, D., Shofer, J.B., Boyko, E.J., *et al.* (2001) Abnormal glucose tolerance and increased risk for cardiovascular disease in Japanese-Americans with normal fasting glucose. *Diabetes Care* **24**, 39–44.

Libby, P. (2002) Inflammation in atherosclerosis. *Nature* **420**, 868–874.

Libby, P. (2006) Inflammation and cardiovascular disease mechanisms. *Am J Clin Nutr* **83**, 456S–460S.

Lichtenstein, A.H., Appel, L.J., Brands, M., *et al.* (2006a) Diet and lifestyle recommendations revision 2006: a scientific statement from the American Heart Association Nutrition Committee. *Circulation* **114**, 82–96.

Lichtenstein, A.H., Matthan, N.R., Jalbert, S.M., *et al.* (2006b) Novel soybean oils with different fatty acid profiles alter cardiovascular disease risk factors in moderately hyperlipidemic subjects. *Am J Clin Nutr* **84**, 497–504.

Liou, Y.A., King, D.J., Zibrik, D., *et al.* (2007) Decreasing linoleic acid with constant alpha-linolenic acid in dietary fats increases (n-3) eicosapentaenoic acid in plasma phospholipids in healthy men. *J Nutr* **137**, 945–952.

Liu, S. and Willett, W.C. (2002) Dietary glycemic load and athero-thrombotic risk. *Curr Atheroscleros Rep* **4**, 454–461.

Liu, S., Willett, W.C., Stampfer, M.J., *et al.* (2000) A prospective study of dietary glycemic load, carbohydrate intake, and risk of coronary heart disease in US women. *Am J Clin Nutr* **71**, 1455–1461.

Lloyd-Jones, D.M., Hong, Y., Labarthe, D., *et al.* (2010) Defining and setting national goals for cardiovascular health promotion and disease reduction: the American Heart Association's Strategic Impact Goal through 2020 and beyond. *Circulation* **121**, 586–613.

Lock, A.L., Horne, C.A., Bauman, D.E., *et al.* (2005) Butter naturally enriched in conjugated linoleic acid and vaccenic acid alters tissue fatty acids and improves the plasma lipoprotein profile in cholesterol-fed hamsters. *J Nutr* **135**, 1934–1939.

Lopez-Garcia, E., Schulze, M.B., Manson, J.E., *et al.* (2004) Consumption of (n-3) fatty acids is related to plasma biomarkers of inflammation and endothelial activation in women. *J Nutr* **134**, 1806–1811.

Ludwig, D.S. (2002) The glycemic index: physiological mechanisms relating to obesity, diabetes, and cardiovascular disease. *JAMA* **287**, 2414–2423.

Ma, J., Folsom, A.R., Melnick, S.L., *et al.* (1995) Associations of serum and dietary magnesium with cardiovascular disease, hypertension, diabetes, insulin, and carotid arterial wall thickness: the ARIC study. Atherosclerosis Risk in Communities Study. *J Clin Epidemiol* **48**, 927–940.

Ma, Y., Griffith, J.A., Chasan-Taber, L., *et al.* (2006) Association between dietary fiber and serum C-reactive protein. *Am J Clin Nutr* **83**, 760–766.

Maestro, B., Campion, J., Davila, N., *et al.* (2000) Stimulation by 1,25-dihydroxyvitamin D3 of insulin receptor expression and insulin responsiveness for glucose transport in U-937 human promonocytic cells. *Endocr J* **47**, 383–391.

Marco, M.P., Craver, L., Betriu, A., *et al.* (2003) Higher impact of mineral metabolism on cardiovascular mortality in a European hemodialysis population. *Kidney Int Suppl* S111–S114.

Marti-Carvajal, A.J., Sola, I., Lathyris, D., *et al.* (2009) Homocysteine lowering interventions for preventing cardiovascular events. *Cochrane Database Syst Rev* CD006612.

Marx, N., Sukhova, G., Murphy, C., *et al.* (1998) Macrophages in human atheroma contain PPARgamma: differentiation-dependent peroxisomal proliferator-activated receptor gamma (PPARgamma) expression and reduction of MMP-9 activity through PPARgamma activation in mononuclear phagocytes in vitro. *Am J Pathol* **153**, 17–23.

Massaro, M., Basta, G., Lazzerini, G., *et al.* (2002) Quenching of intracellular ROS generation as a mechanism for oleate-induced reduction of endothelial activation and early atherogenesis. *Thromb Haemost* **88**, 335–344.

Matsuda, H. (1991a) Effects of external and internal K+ ions on magnesium block of inwardly rectifying K+ channels in guinea-pig heart cells. *J Physiol* **435**, 83–99.

Matsuda, H. (1991b) Magnesium gating of the inwardly rectifying K+ channel. *Annu Rev Physiol* **53**, 289–298.

Mayosi, B.M., Flisher, A.J., Lalloo, U.G., *et al.* (2009) The burden of non-communicable diseases in South Africa. *Lancet* **374**, 934–947.

McCarron, D.A. (1983) Calcium and magnesium nutrition in human hypertension. *Ann Intern Med* **98**, 800–805.

McCarron, D.A., Geerling, J.C., Kazaks, A.G., *et al.* (2009) Can dietary sodium intake be modified by public policy? *Clin J Am Soc Nephrol* **4**, 1878–1882.

McKeown, N.M. (2004) Whole grain intake and insulin sensitivity: evidence from observational studies. *Nutr Rev* **62**, 286–291.

McMurray, H.F., Parthasarathy, S., and Steinberg, D. (1993) Oxidatively modified low density lipoprotein is a chemoattractant for human T lymphocytes. *J Clin Invest* **92**, 1004–1008.

McVeigh, G.E., Brennan, G.M., Cohn, J.N., *et al.* (1994) Fish oil improves arterial compliance in non-insulin-dependent diabetes mellitus. *Arterioscler Thromb* **14**, 1425–1429.

Melamed, M.L., Michos, E.D., Post, W., *et al.* (2008) 25-Hydroxyvitamin D levels and the risk of mortality in the general population. *Arch Intern Med* **168**, 1629–1637.

Mendis, S. (2001) Epidemiology of coronary artery disease in Sri Lankans. In G.H.R. Rao and V.V. Kakkar (eds), *Coronary Artery Disease in South Asians*. Jaypee Medical Publishers, New Delhi.

Mensink, R.P. and Katan, M.B.(1992) Effect of dietary fatty acids on serum lipids and lipoproteins. A meta-analysis of 27 trials. *Arterioscler Thromb* **12**, 911–919.

Mensink, R.P., Zock, P.L., Kester, A.D., *et al.* (2003) Effects of dietary fatty acids and carbohydrates on the ratio of serum total to HDL cholesterol and on serum lipids and apolipoproteins: a meta-analysis of 60 controlled trials. *Am J Clin Nutr* **77**, 1146–1155.

Mente, A., De Koning, L., Shannon, H.S., *et al.* (2009) A systematic review of the evidence supporting a causal link between dietary factors and coronary heart disease. *Arch Intern Med* **169**, 659–669.

Mikkelsen, P., Toubro, S., and Astrup, A. (2000) The effect of fat-reduced diets on 24-h energy expenditure: comparisons between animal protein, vegetable protein, and carbohydrate. *Am J Clin Nutr* **72**, 1135–1141.

Moore, K.J., and Tabas, I. (2011) Macrophages in the pathogenesis of atherosclerosis. *Cell* **145**, 341–355.

Morgan, T., Myers, J., and Teow, B.H. (1984) The role of sodium and potassium in the control of blood pressure. *Aust N Z J Med* **14**, 458–462.

Mori, T.A. and Beilin, L.J. (2004) Omega-3 fatty acids and inflammation. *Curr Atheroscleros Rep* **6**, 461–467.

Morimoto, A., Uzu, T., Fujii, T., *et al.* (1997) Sodium sensitivity and cardiovascular events in patients with essential hypertension. *Lancet* **350**, 1734–1737.

Morris, R.C., Jr, Sebastian, A., Forman, A., *et al.* (1999) Normotensive salt sensitivity: effects of race and dietary potassium. *Hypertension* **33**, 18–23.

Morrow, D.A. and Gersh, B.J. (2007) Chronic coronary artery disease. In P. Libby, R.O. Bonow, D.L. Mann, *et al.* (eds), *Braunwald's Heart Disease: A Textbook of Cardiovascular Medicine*, 8th Edn. Saunders, Elsevier, Philadelphia, pp. 1353–1444.

Motoyama, T., Sano, H., and Fukuzaki, H. (1989) Oral magnesium supplementation in patients with essential hypertension. *Hypertension* **13**, 227–232.

Mozaffarian, D. and Ludwig, D.S. (2010) Dietary guidelines in the 21st century – a time for food. *JAMA* **304**, 681–682.

Mozaffarian, D., Aro, A., and Willett, W.C. (2009) Health effects of trans-fatty acids: experimental and observational evidence. *Eur J Clin Nutr* **63**(Suppl 2), S5–S21.

Mozaffarian, D., Ascherio, A., Hu, F.B., *et al.* (2005) Interplay between different polyunsaturated fatty acids and risk of coronary heart disease in men. *Circulation* **111**, 157–164.

Mozaffarian, D., Pischon, T., Hankinson, S.E., *et al.* (2004a) Dietary intake of trans fatty acids and systemic inflammation in women. *Am J Clin Nutr* **79**, 606–612.

Mozaffarian, D., Rimm, E.B., and Herrington, D.M. (2004b) Dietary fats, carbohydrate, and progression of coronary atherosclerosis in postmenopausal women. *Am J Clin Nutr* **80**, 1175–1184.

Naghavi, M., Libby, P., Falk, E., *et al.* (2003a) From vulnerable plaque to vulnerable patient: a call for new definitions and risk assessment strategies: Part I. *Circulation* **108**, 1664–1672.

Naghavi, M., Libby, P., Falk, E., *et al.* (2003b) From vulnerable plaque to vulnerable patient: a call for new definitions and risk assessment strategies: Part II. *Circulation* **108**, 1772–1778.

National Cholesterol Education Program Expert Panel (2002) Third Report of the National Cholesterol Education Program (NCEP) Expert Panel on Detection, Evaluation, and Treatment of High Blood Cholesterol in Adults (Adult Treatment Panel III). National Cholesterol Education Program, National Heart Lung and Blood Institute, National Institute of Health, Washington, DC.

National High Blood Pressure Education Program (2003) The JNC 7 Express: The Seventh Report of the Joint National Committee on Prevention, Detection, Evaluation, and Treatment of High Blood Pressure. http://www.nhlbi.nih.gov/guidelines/hypertension/jncintro.htm.

National Sleep Foundation (2011) *Sleep Apnea and Sleep.* NSF, Arlington, VA. http://www.sleepfoundation.org/article/sleep-related-problems/obstructive-sleep-apnea-and-sleep.

Natvig, H., Borchgrevink, C.F., Dedichen, J., *et al.* (1968) A controlled trial of the effect of linolenic acid on incidence of coronary heart disease. The Norwegian vegetable oil experiment of 1965–66. *Scand J Clin Lab Invest Suppl* **105**, 1–20.

Naves-Diaz, M., Alvarez-Hernandez, D., Passlick-Deetjen, J., *et al.* (2008) Oral active vitamin D is associated with improved survival in hemodialysis patients. *Kidney Int* **74**, 1070–1078.

Ness, A.R., Chee, D., and Elliott, P. (1997) Vitamin C and blood pressure – an overview. *J Hum Hypertens* **11**, 343–350.

Nestel, P.J. (2000) Fish oil and cardiovascular disease: lipids and arterial function. *Am J Clin Nutr* **71**, 228S–231S.

Nocon, M., Hiemann, T., Müller-Riemenschneider, F., *et al.* (2008) Association of physical activity with all-cause and cardiovascular mortality: a systematic review and meta-analysis. *J Cardiovasc Risk* **15**, 239–246.

Node, K., Huo, Y., Ruan, X., *et al.* (1999) Anti-inflammatory properties of cytochrome P450 epoxygenase-derived eicosanoids. *Science* **285**, 1276–1279.

Nordmann, A.J., Nordmann, A., Briel, M., *et al.* (2006) Effects of low-carbohydrate vs low-fat diets on weight loss and cardiovascular risk factors: a meta-analysis of randomized controlled trials. *Arch Intern Med* **166**, 285–293.

Novotny, T.E. (2005) Why we need to rethink the diseases of affluence. *PLoS Med* **2**, e104.

Obarzanek, E., Sacks, F.M., Vollmer, W.M., *et al.* (2001) Effects on blood lipids of a blood pressure-lowering diet: the Dietary Approaches to Stop Hypertension (DASH) trial. *Am J Clin Nutr* **74**, 80–89.

Office of Disease Prevention and Health Promotion (2008) *2008 Physical Activity Guidelines for Americans.* US Department of Health and Human Services, Washington, DC.

Oh, K., Hu, F.B., Cho, E., *et al.* (2005a) Carbohydrate intake, glycemic index, glycemic load, and dietary fiber in relation to risk of stroke in women. *Am J Epidemiol* **161**, 161–169.

Oh, K., Hu, F.B., Manson, J.E., *et al.* (2005b) Dietary fat intake and risk of coronary heart disease in women: 20 years of follow-up of the nurses' health study. *Am J Epidemiol* **161**, 672–679.

Ohgushi, M., Kugiyama, K., Fukunaga, K., *et al.* (1993) Protein kinase C inhibitors prevent impairment of endothelium-dependent relaxation by oxidatively modified LDL. *Arterioscler Thromb* **13**, 1525–1532.

Oomen, C.M., Ocke, M.C., Feskens, E.J., *et al.* (2001) Association between trans fatty acid intake and 10-year risk of coronary heart disease in the Zutphen Elderly Study: a prospective population-based study. *Lancet* **357**, 746–751.

Ornish, D., Brown, S.E., Billings, J.H., *et al.* (1990) Can lifestyle changes reverse coronary heart disease?: The Lifestyle Heart Trial. *Lancet* **336**, 129–133.

Ornish, D., Scherwitz, L.W., Billings, J.H., *et al.* (1998) Intensive lifestyle changes for reversal of coronary heart disease. *JAMA* **280**, 2001–2007.

Palinski, W., Rosenfeld, M.E., Yla-Herttuala, S., *et al.* (1989) Low density lipoprotein undergoes oxidative modification in vivo. *Proc Natl Acad Sci USA* **86**, 1372–1376.

Paolisso, G., Sgambato, S., Gambardella, A., *et al.* (1992) Daily magnesium supplements improve glucose handling in elderly subjects. *Am J Clin Nutr* **55**, 1161–1167.

Paolisso, G., Sgambato, S., Pizza, G., *et al.* (1989) Improved insulin response and action by chronic magnesium administration in aged NIDDM subjects. *Diabetes Care* **12**, 265–269.

Park, Y., Subar, A.F., Hollenbeck, A., *et al.* (2011) Dietary fiber intake and mortality in the NIH-AARP Diet and Health Study. *Arch Intern Med* **171**, 1061–1068.

Pereira, M.A., O'Reilly, E., Augustsson, K., *et al.* (2004) Dietary fiber and risk of coronary heart disease: a pooled analysis of cohort studies. *Arch Intern Med* **164**, 370–376.

Pilz, S., Dobnig, H., Fischer, J.E., *et al.* (2008) Low vitamin D levels predict stroke in patients referred to coronary angiography. *Stroke* **39**, 2611–2613.

Pischon, T., Hankinson, S.E., Hotamisligil, G.S., *et al.* (2003) Habitual dietary intake of n-3 and n-6 fatty acids in relation to inflammatory markers among US men and women. *Circulation* **108**, 155–160.

Plourde, M. and Cunnane, S.C. (2007) Extremely limited synthesis of long chain polyunsaturates in adults: implications for their dietary essentiality and use as supplements. *Appl Physiol Nutr Metab* **32,** 619–634.

Posner, B.M., Cobb, J.L., Belanger, A.J., *et al.* (1991) Dietary lipid predictors of coronary heart disease in men. The Framingham Study. *Arch Intern Med* **151,** 1181–1187.

Prince, R.L., Austin, N., Devine, A., *et al.* (2008) Effects of ergocalciferol added to calcium on the risk of falls in elderly high-risk women. *Arch Intern Med* **168,** 103–108.

Pyorala, M., Miettinen, H., Laakso, M., *et al.* (1998a) Hyperinsulinemia and the risk of stroke in healthy middle-aged men: the 22-year follow-up results of the Helsinki Policemen Study. *Stroke* **29,** 1860–1866.

Pyorala, M., Miettinen, H., Laakso, M., *et al.* (1998b) Hyperinsulinemia predicts coronary heart disease risk in healthy middle-aged men: the 22-year follow-up results of the Helsinki Policemen Study. *Circulation* **98,** 398–404.

Quinn, M.T., Parthasarathy, S., Fong, L.G., *et al.* (1987) Oxidatively modified low density lipoproteins: a potential role in recruitment and retention of monocyte/macrophages during atherogenesis. *Proc Natl Acad Sci USA* **84,** 2995–2998.

Raghuveer, G. (2010) Lifetime cardiovascular risk of childhood obesity. *Am J Clin Nutr* **91,** 1514S–1519.

Raitt, M.H., Connor, W.E., Morris, C., *et al.* (2005) Fish oil supplementation and risk of ventricular tachycardia and ventricular fibrillation in patients with implantable defibrillators: a randomized controlled trial. *JAMA* **293,** 2884–2891.

Rajavashisth, T.B., Andalibi, A., Territo, M.C., *et al.* (1990) Induction of endothelial cell expression of granulocyte and macrophage colony-stimulating factors by modified low-density lipoproteins. *Nature* **344,** 254–257.

Rammos, G., Tseke, P., and Ziakka, S. (2008) Vitamin D, the renin-angiotensin system, and insulin resistance. *Int J Urol Nephrol* **40,** 419–426.

Rauch, B., Schiele, R., Schneider, S., *et al.* (2010) OMEGA, a randomized, placebo-controlled trial to test the effect of highly purified omega-3 fatty acids on top of modern guideline-adjusted therapy after myocardial infarction. *Circulation* **122,** 2152–2159.

Richard, D., Kefi, K., Barbe, U., *et al.* (2008) Polyunsaturated fatty acids as antioxidants. *Pharmacol Res* **57,** 451–455.

Ridker, P.M., Brown, N.J., Vaughan, D.E., *et al.* (2004) Established and emerging plasma biomarkers in the prediction of first atherothrombotic events. *Circulation* **109**(Suppl IV)**,** IV6–IV19.

Roche, H.M. and Gibney, M.J. (1996) Postprandial triacylglycerolaemia: the effect of low-fat dietary treatment with and without fish oil supplementation. *Eur J Clin Nutr* **50,** 617–624.

Rose, G. (2001) Sick individuals and sick populations. *Int J Epidemiol* **30,** 427–432.

Rude, R.K. (1993) Magnesium metabolism and deficiency. *Endocrinol Metab Clin North Am* **22,** 377–395.

Rudel, L.L., Parks, J.S., Hedrick, C.C., *et al.* (1998) Lipoprotein and cholesterol metabolism in diet-induced coronary artery atherosclerosis in primates. Role of cholesterol and fatty acids. *Progr Lipid Res* **37,** 353–370.

Rudel, L.L., Parks, J.S., and Sawyer, J.K. (1995) Compared with dietary monounsaturated and saturated fat, polyunsaturated fat protects African green monkeys from coronary artery atherosclerosis. *Arterioscler Thromb Vasc Biol* **15,** 2101–2110.

Sacco, R.L. (2011) The new American Heart Association 2020 goal: achieving ideal cardiovascular health. *J Cardiovasc Med (Hagerstown)* **12,** 255–257.

Sacks, F.M., Bray, G.A., Carey, V.J., *et al.* (2009) Comparison of weight-loss diets with different compositions of fat, protein, and carbohydrates. *N Engl J Med* **360,** 859–873.

Sacks, F.M., Brown, L.E., Appel, L., *et al.* (1995) Combinations of potassium, calcium, and magnesium supplements in hypertension. *Hypertension* **26,** 950–956.

Sacks, F.M., Svetkey, L.P., Vollmer, W.M., *et al.* (2001) Effects on blood pressure of reduced dietary sodium and the Dietary Approaches to Stop Hypertension (DASH) diet. DASH-Sodium Collaborative Research Group. *N Engl J Med* **344,** 3–10.

Salas-Salvadó, J., Bulló, M., Babio, N., *et al.* (2011) Reduction in the incidence of type 2 diabetes with the Mediterranean diet: results of the PREDIMED-Reus nutrition intervention randomized trial. *Diabetes Care* **34,** 14–19.

Salmeron, J., Hu, F.B., Manson, J.E., *et al.* (2001) Dietary fat intake and risk of type 2 diabetes in women. *Am J Clin Nutr* **73,** 1019–1026.

Samaha, F.F., Iqbal, N., Seshadri, P., *et al.* (2003) A low-carbohydrate as compared with a low-fat diet in severe obesity. *N Engl J Med* **348,** 2074–2081.

Sanders, T.A., Vickers, M., and Haines, A.P. (1981) Effect on blood lipids and haemostasis of a supplement of cod-liver oil, rich in eicosapentaenoic and docosahexaenoic acids, in healthy young men. *Clin Sci (Lond)* **61,** 317–324.

Saris, W.H.M., Blair, S.N., Van Baak, M.A., *et al.* (2003) How much physical activity is enough to prevent unhealthy weight gain? Outcome of the IASO 1st Stock Conference and consensus statement. *Obesity Rev* **4,** 101–114.

Schaar, J.A., Muller, J.E., Falk, E., *et al.* (2004) Terminology for high-risk and vulnerable coronary artery plaques. Report of a meeting on the vulnerable plaque, June 17 and 18, 2003, Santorini, Greece. *Eur Heart J* **25,** 1077–1082.

Schmidlin, O., Forman, A., Tanaka, M., *et al.* (1999) NaCl-induced renal vasoconstriction in salt-sensitive African Americans: antipressor and hemodynamic effects of potassium bicarbonate. *Hypertension* **33,** 633–639.

Schrepf, R., Limmert, T., Claus Weber, P., et al. (2004) Immediate effects of n-3 fatty acid infusion on the induction of sustained ventricular tachycardia. Lancet 363, 1441–1442.

Schroeder, S.A. (2007) We can do better – improving the health of the American people. N Engl J Med 357, 1221–1228.

Serhan, C.N. (2005) Lipoxins and aspirin-triggered 15-epi-lipoxins are the first lipid mediators of endogenous anti-inflammation and resolution. Prostaglandins Leukot Essent Fatty Acids 73, 141–162.

Seshadri, P., Iqbal, N., Stern, L., et al. (2004) A randomized study comparing the effects of a low-carbohydrate diet and a conventional diet on lipoprotein subfractions and C-reactive protein levels in patients with severe obesity. Am J Med 117, 398–405.

Sesso, H.D., Buring, J.E., Christen, W.G., et al. (2008) Vitamins E and C in the prevention of cardiovascular disease in men: the Physicians' Health Study II randomized controlled trial. JAMA 300, 2123–2133.

Shai, I., Schwarzfuchs, D., Henkin, Y., et al. (2008) Weight loss with a low-carbohydrate, Mediterranean, or low-fat diet. N Engl J Med 359, 229–241.

Sharman, M.J., Gómez, A.L., Kraemer, W.J., et al. (2004) Very low-carbohydrate and low-fat diets affect fasting lipids and postprandial lipemia differently in overweight men. J Nutr 134, 880–885.

Sheng, H.-W. (2000) Sodium, chloride and potassium. In M. Stipanuk (ed.), Biochemical and Physiological Aspects of Human Nutrition. W.B. Saunders, Philadelphia, pp. 686–710.

Shimokawa, H. and Vanhoutte, P.M. (1989) Dietary omega 3 fatty acids and endothelium-dependent relaxations in porcine coronary arteries. Am J Physiol 256, H968–H973.

Shiroma, E.J. and Lee, I.M. (2010) Physical activity and cardiovascular health. Circulation 122, 743–752.

Shoji, T., Shinohara, K., Kimoto, E., et al. (2004) Lower risk for cardiovascular mortality in oral 1alpha-hydroxy vitamin D3 users in a haemodialysis population. Nephrol Dial Transplant 19, 179–184.

Simopoulos, A.P. (1999) Evolutionary aspects of omega-3 fatty acids in the food supply. Prostaglandins Leukot Essent Fatty Acids 60, 421–429.

Simopoulos, A.P., Leaf, A., and Salem, N., Jr (2000) Workshop statement on the essentiality of and recommended dietary intakes for omega-6 and omega-3 fatty acids. Prostaglandins Leukot Essent Fatty Acids 63, 119–121.

Sin, D.D., Fitzgerald, F., Parker, J.D., et al. (1999) Risk factors for central and obstructive sleep apnea in 450 men and women with congestive heart failure. Am J Resp Crit Care Med 160, 1101–1106.

Siri-Tarino, P.W., Sun, Q., Hu, F.B., et al. (2010) Saturated fat, carbohydrate, and cardiovascular disease. Am J Clin Nutr 91, 502–509.

Skeaff, C.M. and Miller, J. (2009) Dietary fat and coronary heart disease: summary of evidence from prospective cohort and randomised controlled trials. Ann Nutr Metab 55, 173–201.

Sofi, F., Abbate, R., Gensini, G.F., et al. (2010) Accruing evidence on benefits of adherence to the Mediterranean diet on health: an updated systematic review and meta-analysis. Am J Clin Nutr 92, 1189–1196.

Somers, V.K., Dyken, M.E., Clary, M.P., et al. (1995) Sympathetic neural mechanisms in obstructive sleep apnea. J Clin Invest 96, 1897–1904.

Somers, V.K., Dyken, M.E., Mark, A.L., et al. (1993) Sympathetic-nerve activity during sleep in normal subjects. N Engl J Med 328, 303–307.

Somers, V.K., Mark, A.L., Zavala, D.C., et al. (1989a) Contrasting effects of hypoxia and hypercapnia on ventilation and sympathetic activity in humans. J Appl Physiol 67, 2101–2106.

Somers, V.K., Mark, A.L., Zavala, D.C., et al. (1989b) Influence of ventilation and hypocapnia on sympathetic nerve responses to hypoxia in normal humans. J Appl Physiol 67, 2095–2100.

Spagnoli, L.G., Mauriello, A., Sangiorgi, G., et al. (2004) Extracranial thrombotically active carotid plaque as a risk factor for ischemic stroke. JAMA 292, 1845–1852.

St. Jeor, S.T., Howard, B.V., Prewitt, T.E., et al. (2001) Dietary protein and weight reduction: a statement for healthcare professionals from the Nutrition Committee of the Council on Nutrition, Physical Activity, and Metabolism of the American Heart Association. Circulation 104, 1869–1874.

Stampfer, M.J., Krauss, R.M., Ma, J., et al. (1996) A prospective study of triglyceride level, low-density lipoprotein particle diameter, and risk of myocardial infarction. JAMA 276, 882–888.

Stephens, N.G., Parsons, A., Schofield, P.M., et al. (1996) Randomised controlled trial of vitamin E in patients with coronary disease: Cambridge Heart Antioxidant Study (CHAOS). Lancet 347, 781–786.

Stevens, G.A., Dias, R.H., and Ezzati, M. (2008) The effects of 3 environmental risks on mortality disparities across Mexican communities. Proc Natl Acad Sci 105, 16860–16865.

Stevenson, W.G., Stevenson, L.W., Middlekauff, H.R., et al. (1993) Sudden death prevention in patients with advanced ventricular dysfunction. Circulation 88, 2953–2961.

Steyn, N.P., Labadarios, D., Maunder, E., et al. (2005) Secondary anthropometric data analysis of the National Food Consumption Survey in South Africa: the double burden. Nutrition 21, 4–13.

Stokes, J.B. (1982) Consequences of potassium recycling in the renal medulla. Effects of ion transport by the medullary thick ascending limb of Henle's loop. J Clin Invest 70, 219–229.

Strazzullo, P., D'Elia, L., Kandala, N.B., et al. (2009) Salt intake, stroke, and cardiovascular disease: meta-analysis of prospective studies. BMJ 339, b4567.

Streppel, M.T., Arends, L.R., Van't Veer, P., *et al.* (2005) Dietary fiber and blood pressure: a meta-analysis of randomized placebo-controlled trials. *Arch Intern Med* **165**, 150–156.

Summers, L.K., Fielding, B.A., Bradshaw, H.A., *et al.* (2002) Substituting dietary saturated fat with polyunsaturated fat changes abdominal fat distribution and improves insulin sensitivity. *Diabetologia* **45**, 369–377.

Tall, A.R., Jiang, X., Luo, Y., *et al.* (2000) 1999 George Lyman Duff memorial lecture: lipid transfer proteins, HDL metabolism, and atherogenesis. *Arterioscler Thromb Vasc Biol* **20**, 1185–1188.

Tanasescu, M., Cho, E., Manson, J.E., *et al.* (2004) Dietary fat and cholesterol and the risk of cardiovascular disease among women with type 2 diabetes. *Am J Clin Nutr* **79**, 999–1005.

Tavani, A., Bosetti, C., Negri, E., *et al.* (2003) Carbohydrates, dietary glycaemic load and glycaemic index, and risk of acute myocardial infarction. *Heart* **89**, 722–726.

Tay, J., Brinkworth, G.D., Noakes, M., *et al.* (2008) Metabolic effects of weight loss on a very-low-carbohydrate diet compared with an isocaloric high-carbohydrate diet in abdominally obese subjects. *J Am Coll Cardiol* **51**, 59–67.

Teng, M., Wolf, M., Ofsthun, M.N., *et al.* (2005) Activated injectable vitamin D and hemodialysis survival: a historical cohort study. *J Am Soc Nephrol* **16**, 1115–1125.

Teo, K.K., Liu, L., Chow, C.K., *et al.* (2009) Potentially modifiable risk factors associated with myocardial infarction in China: the INTERHEART China study. *Heart* **95**, 1857–1864.

Thies, F., Garry, J.M., Yaqoob, P., *et al.* (2003) Association of n-3 polyunsaturated fatty acids with stability of atherosclerotic plaques: a randomised controlled trial. *Lancet* **361**, 477–485.

Thomas, C.E., Jackson, R.L., Ohlweiler, D.F., *et al.* (1994) Multiple lipid oxidation products in low density lipoproteins induce interleukin-1 beta release from human blood mononuclear cells. *J Lipid Res* **35**, 417–427.

Thornburg, J.T., Parks, J.S., and Rudel, L.L. (1995) Dietary fatty acid modification of HDL phospholipid molecular species alters lecithin: cholesterol acyltransferase reactivity in cynomolgus monkeys. *J Lipid Res* **36**, 277–289.

Traber, M.G., Frei, B., and Beckman, J.S. (2008) Vitamin E revisited: do new data validate benefits for chronic disease prevention? *Curr Opin Lipidol* **19**, 30–38.

Trials of Hypertension Prevention Collaborative Research Group (1997) Effects of weight loss and sodium reduction intervention on blood pressure and hypertension incidence in overweight people with high-normal blood pressure: The Trials of Hypertension Prevention, Phase II. *Arch Intern Med* **157**, 657–667.

Trichopoulou, A., Costacou, T., Bamia, C., *et al.* (2003) Adherence to a Mediterranean diet and survival in a Greek population. *N Engl J Med* **348**, 2599–2608.

Tricon, S., Burdge, G.C., Jones, E.L., *et al.* (2006) Effects of dairy products naturally enriched with cis-9,trans-11 conjugated linoleic acid on the blood lipid profile in healthy middle-aged men. *Am J Clin Nutr* **83**, 744–753.

Trivedi, D.P., Doll, R., and Khaw, K.T. (2003) Effect of four monthly oral vitamin D3 (cholecalciferol) supplementation on fractures and mortality in men and women living in the community: randomised double blind controlled trial. *BMJ* **326**, 469.

Trumbo, P., Schlicker, S., Yates, A.A., *et al.* (2002) Dietary reference intakes for energy, carbohydrate, fiber, fat, fatty acids, cholesterol, protein and amino acids. *J Am Diet Assoc* **102**, 1621–1630.

Tsimikas, S., Philis-Tsimikas, A., Alexopoulos, S., *et al.* (1999) LDL isolated from Greek subjects on a typical diet or from American subjects on an oleate-supplemented diet induces less monocyte chemotaxis and adhesion when exposed to oxidative stress. *Arterioscler Thromb Vasc Biol* **19**, 122–130.

Van Buren, M., Rabelink, T.J., Van Rijn, H.J., *et al.* (1992) Effects of acute NaCl, KCl and KHCO3 loads on renal electrolyte excretion in humans. *Clin Sci (Lond)* **83**, 567–574.

Van Dam, R.M., Visscher, A.W., Feskens, E.J., *et al.* (2000) Dietary glycemic index in relation to metabolic risk factors and incidence of coronary heart disease: the Zutphen Elderly Study. *Eur J Clin Nutr* **54**, 726–731.

Vega-López, S., Ausman, L.M., Griffith, J.L., *et al.* (2007) Interindividual variability and intra-individual reproducibility of glycemic index values for commercial white bread. *Diabetes Care* **30**, 1412–1417.

Vega-López, S., Matthan, N.R., Ausman, L.M., *et al.* (2010) Altering dietary lysine:arginine ratio has little effect on cardiovascular risk factors and vascular reactivity in moderately hypercholesterolemic adults. *Atherosclerosis* **210**, 555–562.

Versari, D., Daghini, E., Virdis, A., *et al.* (2009) Endothelium-dependent contractions and endothelial dysfunction in human hypertension. *Br J Pharmacol* **157**, 527–536.

Volek, J.S., Fernandez, M.L., Feinman, R.D., *et al.* (2008) Dietary carbohydrate restriction induces a unique metabolic state positively affecting atherogenic dyslipidemia, fatty acid partitioning, and metabolic syndrome. *Progr Lipid Res* **47**, 307–318.

Volek, J.S., Phinney, S.D., Forsythe, C.E., *et al.* (2009) Carbohydrate restriction has a more favorable impact on the metabolic syndrome than a low fat diet. *Lipids* **44**, 297–309.

Vollmer, W.M., Sacks, F.M., Ard, J., *et al.* (2001) Effects of diet and sodium intake on blood pressure: subgroup analysis of the DASH-sodium trial. *Ann Intern Med* **135**, 1019–1028.

Von Schacky, C., Fischer, S., and Weber, P.C. (1985) Long-term effects of dietary marine omega-3 fatty acids upon plasma and cellular lipids, platelet function, and eicosanoid formation in humans. *J Clin Invest* **76**, 1626–1631.

Wallach, S. and Verch, R.L. (1986) Tissue magnesium in spontaneously hypertensive rats. *Magnesium* **5**, 33–38.

Wang, A.Y., Lam, C.W., Sanderson, J.E., *et al.* (2008a) Serum 25-hydroxyvitamin D status and cardiovascular outcomes in chronic peritoneal dialysis patients: a 3-y prospective cohort study. *Am J Clin Nutr* **87**, 1631–1638.

Wang, C., Harris, W.S., Chung, M., *et al.* (2006) n-3 Fatty acids from fish or fish-oil supplements, but not alpha-linolenic acid, benefit cardiovascular disease outcomes in primary- and secondary-prevention studies: a systematic review. *Am J Clin Nutr* **84**, 5–17.

Wang, L., Manson, J.E., Song, Y., *et al.* (2010) Systematic review: vitamin D and calcium supplementation in prevention of cardiovascular events. *Ann Intern Med* **152**, 315–323.

Wang, T.J., Pencina, M.J., Booth, S.L., *et al.* (2008b) Vitamin D deficiency and risk of cardiovascular disease. *Circulation* **117**, 503–511.

Ward, N.C., Hodgson, J.M., Croft, K.D., *et al.* (2005) The combination of vitamin C and grape-seed polyphenols increases blood pressure: a randomized, double-blind, placebo-controlled trial. *J Hypertens* **23**, 427–434.

Watts, G.F. and Karpe, F. (2011) Triglycerides and atherogenic dyslipidaemia: extending treatment beyond statins in the high-risk cardiovascular patient. *Heart* **97**, 350–356.

Waxman, A. (2004) WHO global strategy on diet, physical activity and health. *Food Nutr Bull* **25**, 292–302.

Weinberger, M.H. (1996) Salt sensitivity of blood pressure in humans. *Hypertension* **27**, 481–490.

Weinberger, M.H., Fineberg, N.S., Fineberg, S.E., *et al.* (2001) Salt sensitivity, pulse pressure, and death in normal and hypertensive humans. *Hypertension* **37**, 429–432.

Welch, A.A., Shakya-Shrestha, S., Lentjes, M.A., *et al.* (2010) Dietary intake and status of n-3 polyunsaturated fatty acids in a population of fish-eating and non-fish-eating meat-eaters, vegetarians, and vegans and the product-precursor ratio [corrected] of alpha-linolenic acid to long-chain n-3 polyunsaturated fatty acids: results from the EPIC-Norfolk cohort. *Am J Clin Nutr* **92**, 1040–1051.

Westerterp-Plantenga, M., Rolland, V., Wilson, S., *et al.* (1999) Satiety related to 24-h diet-induced thermogenesis during high protein/carbohydrate vs high fat diets measured in a respiratory chamber. *Eur J Clin Nutr* **53**, 495–502.

Whelton, P.K. and He, J. (1999) Potassium in preventing and treating high blood pressure. *Semin Nephrol* **19**, 494–499.

Whelton, P.K., He, J., Cutler, J.A., *et al.* (1997) Effects of oral potassium on blood pressure. Meta-analysis of randomized controlled clinical trials. *JAMA* **277**, 1624–1632.

Whelton, S.P., Chin, A., Xin, X., *et al.* (2002) Effect of aerobic exercise on blood pressure. *Ann Intern Med* **136**, 493–503.

Whelton, S.P., Hyre, A.D., Pedersen, B., *et al.* (2005) Effect of dietary fiber intake on blood pressure: a meta-analysis of randomized, controlled clinical trials. *J Hypertens* **23**, 475–481.

WHO (2004a) WHO Global Strategy on Diet, Physical Activity and Health. World Health Organization, Geneva. http://www.who.int/dietphysicalactivity/en/.

WHO (2004b) *The Atlas of Heart Disease and Stroke.* World Health Organization, Geneva. http://www.who.int/cardiovascular_diseases/en/cvd_atlas_01_types.pdf.

WHO (2011) *Cardiovascular Diseases (CVDs); Fact Sheet No. 317.* World Health Organization, Geneva. http://www.who.int/mediacentre/factsheets/fs317/en/index.html.

Widman, L., Wester, P.O., Stegmayr, B.K., *et al.* (1993) The dose-dependent reduction in blood pressure through administration of magnesium. A double blind placebo controlled cross-over study. *Am J Hypertens* **6**, 41–45.

Witteman, J.C., Grobbee, D.E., Derkx, F.H., *et al.* (1994) Reduction of blood pressure with oral magnesium supplementation in women with mild to moderate hypertension. *Am J Clin Nutr* **60**, 129–135.

Witteman, J.C., Willett, W.C., Stampfer, M.J., *et al.* (1989) A prospective study of nutritional factors and hypertension among US women. *Circulation* **80**, 1320–1327.

Wolf, M., Shah, A., Gutierrez, O., *et al.* (2007) Vitamin D levels and early mortality among incident hemodialysis patients. *Kidney Int* **72**, 1004–1013.

Wolfe, B.M. and Giovannetti, P.M. (1991) Short-term effects of substituting protein for carbohydrate in the diets of moderately hypercholesterolemic human subjects. *Metabolism* **40**, 338–343.

Wolk, A., Manson, J.E., Stampfer, M.J., *et al.* (1999) Long-term intake of dietary fiber and decreased risk of coronary heart disease among women. *JAMA* **281**, 1998–2004.

Xin, X., He, J., Frontini, M.G., *et al.* (2001) Effects of alcohol reduction on blood pressure: a meta-analysis of randomized controlled trials. *Hypertension* **38**, 1112–1117.

Xu, X.P., Meisel, S.R., Ong, J.M., *et al.* (1999) Oxidized low-density lipoprotein regulates matrix metalloproteinase-9 and its tissue inhibitor in human monocyte-derived macrophages. *Circulation* **99**, 993–998.

Yamamoto, M.E., Applegate, W.B., Klag, M.J., *et al.* (1995) Lack of blood pressure effect with calcium and magnesium supplementation in adults with high-normal blood pressure. Results from Phase I of the Trials of Hypertension Prevention (TOHP). Trials of Hypertension Prevention (TOHP) Collaborative Research Group. *Ann Epidemiol* **5**, 96–107.

Ye, Z. and Song, H. (2008) Antioxidant vitamins intake and the risk of coronary heart disease: meta-analysis of cohort studies. *Eur J Cardiovasc Prev Rehabil* **15**, 26–34.

Yin, K., Chu, Z.M., and Beilin, L.J. (1991) Blood pressure and vascular reactivity changes in spontaneously hypertensive rats fed fish oil. *Br J Pharmacol* **102**, 991–997.

Yokoyama, M., Origasa, H., Matsuzaki, M., *et al.* (2007) Effects of eicosapentaenoic acid on major coronary events in hypercholesterolaemic patients (JELIS): a randomised open-label, blinded endpoint analysis. *Lancet* **369**, 1090–1098.

Yoshida, H. and Kisugi, R. (2010) Mechanisms of LDL oxidation. *Clin Chim Acta* **411**, 1875–1882.

Young, I.S. and McEneny, J. (2001) Lipoprotein oxidation and atherosclerosis. *Biochem Soc Trans* **29**, 358–362.

Yu-Poth, S., Etherton, T.D., Reddy, C.C., *et al.* (2000) Lowering dietary saturated fat and total fat reduces the oxidative susceptibility of LDL in healthy men and women. *J Nutr* **130**, 2228–2237.

Yu-Poth, S., Zhao, G., Etherton, T., *et al.* (1999) Effects of the National Cholesterol Education Program's Step I and Step II dietary intervention programs on cardiovascular disease risk factors: a meta-analysis. *Am J Clin Nutr* **69**, 632–646.

Yusuf, S., Dagenais, G., Pogue, J., *et al.* (2000) Vitamin E supplementation and cardiovascular events in high-risk patients. The Heart Outcomes Prevention Evaluation Study Investigators. *N Engl J Med* **342**, 154–160.

Yusuf, S., Hawken, S., Ounpuu, S., *et al.* (2004) Effect of potentially modifiable risk factors associated with myocardial infarction in 52 countries (the INTERHEART study): case-control study. *Lancet* **364**, 937–952.

Zampelas, A., Panagiotakos, D.B., Pitsavos, C., *et al.* (2005) Fish consumption among healthy adults is associated with decreased levels of inflammatory markers related to cardiovascular disease: the ATTICA study. *J Am Coll Cardiol* **46**, 120–124.

Zemel, P.C., Zemel, M.B., Urberg, M., *et al.* (1990) Metabolic and hemodynamic effects of magnesium supplementation in patients with essential hypertension. *Am J Clin Nutr* **51**, 665–669.

Zhao, G., Etherton, T.D., Martin, K.R., *et al.* (2005) Anti-inflammatory effects of polyunsaturated fatty acids in THP-1 cells. *Biochem Biophys Res Commun* **336**, 909–917.

Zhao, G., Ford, E.S., Li, C., *et al.* (2010) Independent associations of serum concentrations of 25-hydroxyvitamin D and parathyroid hormone with blood pressure among US adults. *J Hypertens* **28**, 1821–1828.

Ziraba, A.K., Fotso, J.C., and Ochako, R. (2009) Overweight and obesity in urban Africa: a problem of the rich or the poor? *BMC Public Health* **9**, 46.

49

DIABETES

LINDSAY M. JAACKS[1], BS, JUDITH WYLIE-ROSETT[2], EDD, RD, AND ELIZABETH J. MAYER-DAVIS[3], MSPH, PhD, RD

[1]*UNC Gillings School of Global Public Health, Chapel Hill, North Carolina, USA*
[2]*Albert Einstein College of Medicine, Bronx, New York, USA*
[3]*UNC Gillings School of Global Public Health and School of Medicine, Chapel Hill, North Carolina, USA*

Summary

Glycemic control and reduction of cardiovascular disease risk are the major treatment goals for all types of diabetes. In addition to nutritional management (termed medical nutrition therapy [MNT] in the United States), these goals are accomplished through several modalities including a variety of pharmacological agents, close personal and laboratory monitoring, and care provided by a team of health professionals. All of these elements, integrated and coordinated, are essential in the management of diabetes.

There is not one diet for individuals with diabetes. Nutritional management should be based on individual assessment and development of an individualized treatment plan. The distribution of macronutrient intake may vary based on a number of factors, including matching insulin to lifestyle in type 1 diabetes (T1D) and weight loss in type 2 diabetes (T2D). Assessing micronutrient status is needed for patients in poor control, with complications, or with other evidence of being at risk.

This chapter will discuss the etiology, diagnosis, and attainment of glycemic control (with an emphasis on MNT) of T1D, T2D, and gestational diabetes (GDM). It will then discuss the role of nutrition in the prevention of complications and reduction of chronic disease risk factors for both T1D and T2D and the role of specific dietary components including herbal and other supplements and micronutrients in diabetes care. The chapter will conclude with a discussion of global public health issues relating to diabetes, and research needs and future direction of the role of nutrition in this complex disorder.

Introduction

According to the American Diabetes Association (ADA), diabetes is a group of metabolic disorders resulting from defects in insulin secretion, insulin action, or both, that results in hyperglycemia (American Diabetes Association, 2010a). Despite major advances in our understanding about and treatments for diabetes, this multifactorial condition continues to pose major challenges to individuals, families, communities, and nations throughout the world.

Present Knowledge in Nutrition, Tenth Edition. Edited by John W. Erdman Jr, Ian A. Macdonald and Steven H. Zeisel.
© 2012 International Life Sciences Institute. Published 2012 by John Wiley & Sons, Inc.

The present burden of diabetes, both in the United States and worldwide, is significant: an estimated 23.6 million people in the United States and 366 million people worldwide have diabetes (Centers for Disease Control and Prevention, 2008; International Diabetes Federation, 2011). Because of the growing public health burden of diabetes in the United States and throughout the world, three general approaches to reduce the burden of diabetes are now being considered: (1) *primary prevention* of diabetes in high-risk individuals through weight management and increasing physical activity; (2) *secondary prevention* of the onset and/or severity of complications (i.e. controlling metabolic disorders associated with diabetes); and (3) *tertiary prevention* of morbidity and mortality resulting from complications (US Department of Health and Human Services, 2010). Nutrition has a critical role to play at each level of prevention.

Four classes of diabetes are currently recognized by the ADA (American Diabetes Association, 2010a). *Type 1 diabetes (T1D)*, formerly known as insulin-dependent or juvenile diabetes, which represents approximately 5–10% of known cases of diabetes (American Diabetes Association, 2010a). *Type 2 diabetes (T2D)*, formerly known as non-insulin-dependent or adult-onset diabetes, which represents the majority (90–95%) of known cases of diabetes (American Diabetes Association, 2010a). *Gestational diabetes (GDM)*, which is defined as hyperglycemia identified during pregnancy (American Diabetes Association, 2010a). The last class of diabetes accounts for approximately 1–5% of known diabetes cases and includes diabetes resulting from genetic defects (monogenic diabetes) and diabetes that is secondary to other diseases or drug- or chemically induced diabetes (American Diabetes Association, 2010a). In some instances, the class of diabetes is not clear, but may become more apparent over time.

The overall goal of therapy for diabetes (T1D, T2D, and GDM) is to normalize macronutrient metabolism (particularly of carbohydrates and lipids) in order to prevent both acute (e.g. hyperglycemia and ketoacidosis) and chronic (e.g. microvascular, macrovascular, and neuropathic) complications. Results from clinical trials in individuals with both T1D and T2D indicate that improving metabolic control (glycemia, blood pressure, and lipids) greatly reduces the development and progression rates for microvascular, macrovascular, and neuropathic complications (Diabetes Control and Complications Trial Research Group, 1993; Harris and Eastman, 1998; UK Prospective Diabetes Study Group, 1998a,b,c). Despite

similarities in complications and risk factors, the primary prevention, underlying etiology, and treatment approaches differ among T1D, T2D, and GDM.

Type 1 Diabetes (T1D)

T1D is characterized by severe insulin deficiency requiring exogenous insulin to prevent ketoacidosis, coma, and death. Although T1D may occur at any age, onset usually occurs during childhood, adolescence, or early adulthood, with peak age of diagnosis at age 10 to 14 years. The SEARCH for Diabetes in Youth Study is a population-based, multicenter observational study of youth with clinically diagnosed diabetes in the United States (SEARCH for Diabetes in Youth Study Group, 2006). Based on data from 2002 to 2003, approximately 15 000 youth are newly diagnosed with T1D annually (SEARCH for Diabetes in Youth Study Group, 2006; Centers for Disease Control and Prevention, 2008). The incidence of T1D is higher in whites than in other ethnic/racial groups, with the greatest discrepancy at younger ages (SEARCH for Diabetes in Youth Study Group, 2006).

Prevention

Currently there are no established approaches for primary prevention of T1D; studies are ongoing to better understand environmental triggers as well as the potential role of immunosuppressive therapy and various other approaches.

Etiology and Diagnosis

T1D is characterized by T-cell-mediated autoimmune destruction of the beta-cells in the islets of Langerhans within the pancreas. Markers of this destruction include islet cell autoantibodies, autoantibodies to insulin, autoantibodies to GAD (GAD65), and autoantibodies to the tyrosine phosphatases IA-2 and IA-2β (American Diabetes Association, 2010a). Furthermore, T1D appears to be associated with particular histocompatibility leukocyte antigen (HLA) alleles (Atkinson, 2005). Often these antibodies can be found in the serum prior to the onset of clinical disease, and so it is important when considering the etiology of T1D to distinguish between the onset of autoimmunity, which can occur years before the onset of hyperglycemia, and the onset of the clinical disease (Atkinson, 2005; Muntoni and Muntoni, 2006). Testing for the presence of these antibodies can be used in a clinical setting to confirm a T1D diagnosis.

Although all immune-mediated forms of T1D share this common autoimmune destruction of beta-cells, the underlying etiology of this immune response involves a complex interaction of genetic and environmental factors, which is currently not well-established. For example, the factor(s) initiating autoimmunity are not clearly known (Atkinson, 2005) nor are the factor(s) influencing the rate of beta-cell destruction. Toxins or viral exposures have been suggested (Atkinson, 2005), but more recently the possibility of specific food ingredients at a critical time of life has been explored. Both the BABYDIAB and DAISY studies (Norris et al., 2003; Ziegler et al., 2003) suggested that there is a link between infant diet and the development of early autoimmunity against pancreatic beta-cells. Furthermore, the timing of this exposure (between 3 and 7 months) has been identified as a period of considerable vulnerability in the initiation of autoimmunity, particularly in so-called genetically high-risk individuals. Two particular types of food have been implicated: cow's milk (Mayer et al., 1988; Bodington et al., 1994; Norris and Scott, 1996; Norris et al., 1996; Virtanen et al., 1998; Vaarala et al., 1999) and gluten-containing cereals (Norris et al., 2003; Ziegler et al., 2003; Virtanen et al., 2006), including the timing of introduction of these and other complementary foods to infant diet.

Over the past several years, interesting hypotheses have been proposed regarding whether the absence of breastfeeding and/or early exposure to infant formula (i.e. a cow's milk protein) might be involved in the initiation of autoimmunity (Atkinson, 2005; Vaarala, 2005). Cross-sectional epidemiologic studies indicate a link between early introduction of cow's milk formula and development of T1D. Possible mechanisms suggested for this association include: (1) triggering autoantibody reactivity to the milk protein; and (2) almost by accident in an "innocent bystander" scenario in genetically susceptible individuals, a protein structure in the beta-cell with great similarity to the cow's milk protein is recognized as foreign and thus attacked. Equally important may be the absence of the immunoprotection of breastfeeding (Yoon and Jun, 2005).

One ecological study of the 37 world areas reporting a 3% yearly increase of T1D evaluated diabetes incidence in relation to dietary patterns using the Food and Agriculture Organization's Food Balance Sheets (Muntoni and Muntoni, 2006). The incidence of diabetes appeared to be related to the milk supply from 1961 to 2000. Several molecular, genetic, and clinical studies addressing the possible role of protein in cow's milk are ongoing, and a large-scale epidemiologic project called TRIGR is examining, on a population basis, a possible relationship between cow's milk and T1D (Akerblom et al., 2005; TRIGR Study Group, 2007). Should a relationship be established, it may be relevant only in persons with genetic susceptibility to autoimmunity, and thus broader versus targeted recommendations for breastfeeding would need to be resolved.

Several nutritional factors have been proposed as playing a role in beta-cell function including n-3 polyunsaturated fatty acids, vitamin D, and vitamin E. Genetically susceptible infants with higher intakes of n-3 fatty acids have been shown to have reduced risk of beta-cell autoimmunity (Norris et al., 2007). Maternal vitamin D consumption during pregnancy has also been associated with reduced beta-cell autoimmunity in infants (Fronczak et al., 2003). A prospective study looking at vitamin D supplementation during infancy found a reduced risk of diabetes in those infants receiving vitamin D (Hyppönen et al., 2001), further lending support to a potentially protective effect of vitamin D on the development of diabetes. Similar to vitamin D, vitamin E may also have a protective effect against T1D risk (Knekt et al., 1999; Costacou et al., 2008). The SEARCH Nutrition Ancillary Study (SNAS) will examine the effects of certain nutritional factors on sustaining beta-cell function in a large cohort of youth with clinically diagnosed T1D in the United States.

In addition to testing for the antibodies described previously, four criteria for the diagnosis of diabetes (both T1D and T2D) are currently used by the ADA: a hemoglobin A1c (A1C; World Health Organization, 2011) of at least 6.5% (when performed using a National Glycohemoglobin Standardization Program-certified and Diabetes Control and Complications Trial-standardized assay); a fasting plasma glucose (FPG) of at least 7.0 mmol/L (126 mg/dL); a 2-hour post-oral glucose tolerance test (2-h OGTT) plasma glucose of at least 11.1 mmol/L (200 mg/dL); or a random plasma glucose of at least 11.1 mmol/L (200 mg/dL) when accompanied by symptoms of diabetes (e.g. hyperglycemia) (American Diabetes Association, 2010b).

Screening of individuals for T1D is not currently recommended by the ADA, though testing for autoantibodies to identify individuals at risk of developing T1D is possible if other risk factors are present (such as prior transient hyperglycemia or relatives with T1D) (American Diabetes Association, 2010b).

Achieving Glycemic Control

Glycemic control and restoration of normal metabolism is the major treatment goal for all classes of diabetes. This task is accomplished using several modalities including a variety of pharmacological agents, close personal and laboratory monitoring (e.g. self-blood glucose testing, A1C, and renal function testing), and careful assessment by a variety of health professionals. All these elements, integrated and coordinated, are essential in the management of diabetes and are beyond the scope of this update on the nutritional dimensions of diabetes (Box 49.1). The reader is referred to ADA and European Association for the Study of Diabetes (EASD) publications to review specific recommendations (Rydén et al., 2007; American Diabetes Association, 2010b). This section will focus on nutritional aspects of glycemic control for individuals with T1D.

BOX 49.1   Summary of current American Diabetes Association (ADA) nutrition recommendations

- Achieve and maintain blood glucose as near to normal range as is safely possible by balancing dietary intake and physical activity with each other and with any antidiabetic medications.
- Achieve and maintain optimal serum lipid levels that reduce the risk of vascular disease.
- Achieve and maintain blood pressure as near to normal range as is safely possible.
- Provide adequate energy intake for achieving or maintaining a reasonable weight in adults, normal rate of growth and development in children and adolescents, and optimal nutrition during pregnancy and lactation or during recovery from catabolic illnesses.
- Prevent acute complications such as severe hypoglycemia or hyperglycemia.
- Prevent or treat long-term complications such as cardiovascular disease (including hypertension, dyslipidemia, and other risk factors), renal disease, and neuropathy (especially gastroparesis) by modifying dietary intake and physical activity.
- Consider personal and cultural preferences and willingness to change when addressing individual nutrition needs.
- Maintain pleasure of eating by limiting food choices only when supported by scientific evidence.

Adapted from American Diabetes Association (2008).

The Diabetes Control and Complications Trial (DCCT) was conducted in individuals with T1D to compare the effects of intensive versus standard glycemic control (Diabetes Control and Complications Trial Research Group, 1993). Intensive treatment reduced the mean A1C from 9% to 7.2%, and greater attention to dietary strategies accounted for almost one-fourth of the glycemic improvement (Diabetes Control and Complications Trial Research Group, 1988). The risk of development and progression of retinopathy, albuminuria, and neuropathy was reduced by between 50% and 75% over 8 years. Reduction in the risk of complications was linearly related to the reduction in A1C, indicating that risk reduction can be achieved by improving glycemic control, even if a perfect or normal metabolic state is not achieved (Diabetes Control and Complications Trial Research Group, 1988). These accomplishments, as well as efforts to attenuate the two- to three-fold increase in severe hypoglycemia and weight gain, were largely due to educational and nutritional strategies (Delahanty and Halford, 1993; Diabetes Control and Complications Trial Research Group, 1993).

Most recently, longer-term follow-up of the DCCT cohort in the Epidemiology of Diabetes Interventions and Complications (EDIC) study has documented a continued differential in the risk of microvascular (Genuth et al., 2005) and macrovascular (Nathan et al., 2005) complications, even though A1C levels in the two groups have been similar for approximately 8 years.

Medical Nutrition Therapy (MNT)

For all classes of diabetes, the first goal of MNT is to assist in the achievement and maintenance of metabolic normality, including blood glucose, lipid, and lipoprotein levels (Box 49.2). For T1D, this means coordinating an individual's insulin regimen with his/her food choices and physical activity (American Diabetes Association, 2008), as well as moment-to-moment measures of blood glucose levels throughout the day with self-blood-glucose monitoring. Multiple insulins are available (Table 49.1) and are often used in various combinations. A typical approach in terms of insulin use is a "basal-bolus" regimen, either via subcutaneous insulin infusion (SCII or pump therapy) or multiple daily injections (MDI) in which insulin is delivered as a bolus before meals in amounts matched to total carbohydrate intake, with basal insulin on board consistently over time. There are other approaches to MDI, which utilize different types of insulin. Patients can either vary their insulin dose to match the amount of food

BOX 49.2   Summary of medical nutrition therapy (MNT) implementation strategies by class of diabetes

Type 1 Diabetes (T1D)

- Assess usual lifestyle, focusing on eating and physical activity habits.
- Plan insulin therapy to match insulin action to lifestyle.
- Monitor blood glucose levels while keeping lifestyle consistent.
- Adjust insulin and lifestyle to achieve blood glucose levels in the target range.
- Create algorithms for adjusting insulin for lifestyle flexibility and to correct blood glucose levels that are not in the target range.

Type 2 Diabetes (T2D)

- If overweight, reduce calorie intake to achieve 5% to 10% weight loss.
- Increase physical activity.
- Monitor blood glucose approximately four times per day to assess pattern of glycemic control.
- If postprandial glucose level is high, spread food intake throughout the day (using five or six small meals/snacks rather than having fewer larger ones).
- Reduce and/or modify type of fat to achieve weight and lipid goals.

Gestational diabetes (GDM)

- Plan calorie intake to achieve desired weight gain based on desirable body weight.
- Balance carbohydrate intake throughout the day (usually 40–50% of calories).
- Monitor glucose approximately seven times per day; adjust intake to achieve glucose levels in target range.
- Add exogenous insulin if target glucose levels are not achieved by diet alone.

Secondary diabetes

- Assess interrelationship between primary disease(s) and secondary diabetes to establish treatment priorities.
- Institute diabetes treatment as needed to avoid short- and long-term complications.

Adapted from American Diabetes Association (2008).

TABLE 49.1   Insulin preparations: onset, peak, and duration of action

Insulin	Brand name	Onset of action	Peak action	Duration of action
Very rapid acting				
Insulin aspart analog	NovoLog	10–20 minutes	0.5–2.5 hours	3–5 hours
Insulin lispro analog	Humalog			
Regular insulin	Humulin R	30–40 minutes	2–4 hours	5–7 hours
	Novolin R			
Intermediate acting				
NPH insulin	Humulin N	1–3 hours	4–10 hours	14–24 hours
	Novolin N			
Lente insulin	Humulin L	2–4 hours	4–15 hours	16–24 hours
Long acting				
Ultralente insulin	Humulin U	3–4 hours	8–14 hours	18–24 hours
Insulin glargine	Lantus	1–2 hours	No peak	Approx. 24 hours
	Levemir			

Data from Wylie-Rosett *et al.* (2006).

consumed, with additional considerations for physical activity; or meals and physical activity can be held constant in order to match a constant dosing of insulin from day to day. Reduction of insulin dosage is the preferred method of preventing hypoglycemia during and/or after exercise, but this requires planning physical activity ahead of time. For unplanned exercise, increased carbohydrate intake may be needed (American Diabetes Association, 2008). Self-blood-glucose monitoring, education, and experience allow the individual to learn how to keep all of this in balance.

The approaches to nutritional interventions in the DCCT can be a powerful example of ideal nutrition counseling for patients with T1D. Dietary behaviors associated with better glycemic control in the intensively treated group included adherence to an overall meal plan (timing and amount of carbohydrate), appropriate treatment of hypoglycemia (avoiding excess consumption of carbohydrate to treat symptoms), prompt intervention for hyperglycemia (more insulin and/or less food), and consistent consumption of planned evening snacks (Delahanty and Halford, 1993). The mean level of weight gain in the intensively treated group was reduced by 50% after the intervention staff focused on strategies to control weight gain (e.g. avoiding excessive food consumption to prevent and treat hypoglycemia) (Diabetes Control and Complications Trial Research Group, 1988).

The American Dietetic Association has developed and evaluated MNT for patients with T1D (American Dietetic Association, 2002). In the randomized field test, specific guidelines for nutrition counseling were used by dietitians with 24 patients, and results were compared with those of 30 patients receiving "usual counseling" as the control treatment condition. The mean A1C in the guidelines-treated patient group was significantly reduced compared with the control group (1.0% vs. 0.3%) (American Dietetic Association, 2002).

The Dose Adjustment for Normal Eating (DAFNE) study saw improvements in A1C, quality of life, psychological well-being, and satisfaction with treatment in individuals with T1D who learned to use glucose testing to better match insulin to carbohydrate intake despite an increase in the number of daily glucose tests and insulin injections (DAFNE Study Group, 2002; American Diabetes Association, 2008). These quality-of-life results were well-maintained at approximately 4 years, though the glycemic control outcomes were maintained to a lesser extent (Speight et al., 2010).

The process of intensifying T1D management to improve glycemic control involves several stages and individualization of insulin, physical activity, monitoring, and nutrition therapy. The initial stage, usually lasting three or four visits, focuses on basic skills needed by newly diagnosed patients and those with little or no previous nutrition knowledge or a history of poor glycemic control. Nutrition counseling emphasizes consistency of carbohydrate intake and eating times. Blood glucose monitoring provides information about the patterns of response. Patients need to gain a basic understanding of the relationship between insulin action and lifestyle before moving on to more complex planning to achieve better glycemic control and a more flexible lifestyle. An initial bolus dose of insulin is often estimated to provide one unit per 15 g of carbohydrate. Gradually, algorithms are developed to adjust insulin for changes in carbohydrate intake or physical activity. After mastering insulin adjustment and supplementation, patients learn to adjust insulin for changes in food or activity using a ratio of carbohydrate intake to insulin dosage.

Specific Dietary Considerations

In addition to the ADA, several international societies have developed nutritional guidelines for the management of diabetes (Mann et al., 2004; American Diabetes Association, 2008; Canadian Diabetes Association Clinical Practice Guidelines Expert Committee, 2008). The conclusions drawn by these independent reviews are very similar and so this section will focus on the recent technical review and position statement of the ADA (American Diabetes Association, 2008). Where applicable, additional recommendations developed by the EASD will be presented (Mann et al., 2004).

Protein. Recommendations for protein intake in individuals with all classes of diabetes and normal renal function are based on the review for Daily Recommended Intakes by the Institute of Medicine, and are similar to recommendations for the general public: 15–20% of energy intake from protein (Institute of Medicine, 2005); EASD recommends 10–20% of energy intake from proteins in individuals with T1D or T2D and without established nephropathy (Mann et al., 2004). Protein intake needs to be adequate for normal growth, development, and maintenance of body functions. Individuals who may need more than 20% of energy intake from protein include those in a catabolic state, those with growth needs (children, adolescents, and pregnant women), and individuals on very-low-energy diets to achieve weight loss. In select patients with diabetes and micro- or macroalbuminuria (chronic kidney disease), the ADA recommends reducing protein intake to 0.8–1.0 g per kg body weight per day (American Diabetes Association, 2008) based on evidence that lowering protein intake is associated with improved renal function (urine albumin excretion rate and glomerular filtration rate) in select patients (Dullaart *et al.*, 1993; Pomerleau *et al.*, 1993; Narita *et al.*, 2001; Hansen *et al.*, 2002; Pijls *et al.*, 2002). The EASD recommends a reduction of protein intake to the lower end of this range (0.8 g per kg body weight per day) for individuals with T1D and established nephropathy (Mann *et al.*, 2004). Neither the ADA nor the EASD makes specific recommendations regarding the type of protein (Mann *et al.*, 2004; American Diabetes Association, 2008).

Fat. In considering the amount of fat in the diet, one must take into account postprandial glycemic excursions (American Dietetic Association, 2002; Sheard *et al.*, 2004; American Diabetes Association, 2010b). One recent case-control study of 652 individuals with T1D found that higher fat intake was associated with poor glycemic control (Snell-Bergeon *et al.*, 2009). However, whether or not *total* fat intake plays a role in postprandial glucose or overall glycemic control remains controversial. In contrast, it is now well-established that the *type* of fat consumed can influence long-term risk for chronic disease, and therefore the ADA recommends that all individuals with diabetes (T1D, T2D, and GDM) limit their saturated fat to less than 7% of total energy, minimize *trans* fat intake, and limit dietary cholesterol intake to less than 200 mg per day. In addition to these recommendations, the ADA also recommends consumption of two or more servings of fish per week in order to increase intake of n-3 fatty acids, which may contribute to improved cardiometabolic risk factor outcomes, a topic discussed later on in this chapter. Similar to the ADA, the EASD recommends limiting saturated and *trans* fat intakes (less than 10% of total energy intake, less than 8% if LDL cholesterol is elevated); limiting total fat intake to less than 35% of total energy intake (less than 30% if overweight or obese); limiting cholesterol intake (less than 300 mg/day); and consuming two to three servings of fish per week (Mann *et al.*, 2004).

Carbohydrates. Dietary carbohydrate is the major determinant of postprandial glucose concentration and is there-

fore integral to glycemic control. The ADA now recognizes *total* carbohydrate as the major determinant of postprandial glucose concentration with the type of carbohydrate as an additional determinant. The restriction of table sugar or sucrose is often used in an attempt to improve glycemic control. However, studies conducted in the 1970s and 1980s indicated that glycemic response to mono- and disaccharides ("table sugars") did not result in a higher postprandial glycemic response than polysaccharides ("starches") (Franz *et al.*, 2002). Although fructose has been shown to reduce postprandial hyperglycemia when it is substituted for sucrose or starch, the long-term consequences of high fructose intake on plasma lipids and other complications is unknown. A recent meta-analysis of 16 trials found that the effects of fructose intake on blood lipids in individuals with T2D are heterogeneous (Sievenpiper *et al.*, 2009), and therefore this substitution is not currently recommended by the ADA or EASD (Mann *et al.*, 2004; American Diabetes Association, 2008). The ADA's nutrition recommendations indicate that glycemic control is not contingent on restricting sucrose and suggest that the decision about sugar consumption should be based on overall nutrition considerations (Franz *et al.*, 2002; Sheard *et al.*, 2004; American Diabetes Association, 2010b). None the less, consumption of large quantities of sugars (e.g. high-fructose corn syrup in soft drinks and other beverages) is a major source of excess calories (Howard and Wylie-Rosett, 2002; Wylie-Rosett *et al.*, 2004).

The glycemic effect of carbohydrate-containing foods has been studied extensively and is the source of considerable debate with respect to the effects of a low-glycemic-index diet on glycemic control and weight (Franz *et al.*, 2002; Brand-Miller *et al.*, 2003; Sheard *et al.*, 2004; Wylie-Rosett *et al.*, 2004). The concept of *glycemic indexing* of food was developed to compare the effects of the quality of carbohydrate while keeping the amount of carbohydrate standardized. The estimated *glycemic load* of foods, meals, and dietary patterns is calculated by multiplying the glycemic index by the amount of carbohydrate in each food and then totaling for all of the foods in a meal or dietary pattern. The role of the glycemic index and/or glycemic load remains very controversial (Schulz *et al.*, 2005), although modifying the type as well as the amount of carbohydrate can improve glycemic control (Kripke, 2005). In a randomized study of a measured carbohydrate exchange diet versus a flexible low-glycemic-index diet, children with T1D on the low-glycemic diet had significant improvements in A1C and quality of life compared with children with T1D on the measured carbohydrate exchange diet (Gilbertson *et al.*, 2001). Recent results of randomized controlled trials in individuals with T2D have found mixed results: a 6-month trial found a moderate decrease in A1C (Jenkins *et al.*, 2008) while a 1-year trial found no improvements in A1C (Wolever *et al.*, 2008). A third trial found a decrease in A1C in both the low-glycemic diet group and the ADA diet education group at 1 year (Ma *et al.*, 2008). Meta-analysis results have also been mixed: a Cochrane review and a review by Brand-Miller *et al.* found significant decreases in A1C levels while on low-glycemic diets (Brand-Miller *et al.*, 2003; Thomas and Elliott, 2009) whereas Anderson *et al.* found no significant difference in A1C levels between a low- and a high-glycemic diet (Anderson *et al.*, 2004b). These inconsistent results may be due to the inclusion of studies of both T1D and T2D, the small number of included studies due to differences in outcome reporting (e.g. A1C vs. fructosamine vs. both), or other factors. Taking this evidence into account, the ADA and EASD recognize that considering the glycemic index of carbohydrates may provide additional benefit over considering total carbohydrate alone, provided that the overall attributes of the carbohydrate are taken into account (Mann *et al.*, 2004; American Diabetes Association, 2008). They therefore recommend dietary patterns including carbohydrates from whole-grain cereals, fruits, vegetables, legumes, and low-fat milk (Mann *et al.*, 2004; American Diabetes Association, 2008).

In further examining the effects of the amount and type of dietary carbohydrate in diabetes management, it has been documented that *intrinsic variables* can influence the degree of glucose excursions (Sheard *et al.*, 2004). These intrinsic variables include the physical form of the food (i.e. juice vs. whole fruit, mashed potato vs. whole potato), ripeness, degree of processing, type of starch (i.e. amylose vs. amylopectin), style of preparation (e.g. cooking method and time, amount of heat or moisture used), and the specific type (e.g. fettucine vs. macaroni) or variety (e.g. long-grain rice vs. short-grain rice) of the food. *Extrinsic variables* that may influence glucose response include fasting or preprandial glucose level, degree of insulin resistance, and the macronutrient distribution.

Findings from several randomized controlled trials (Jenkins *et al.*, 2002; Lu *et al.*, 2004; Cho *et al.*, 2005b; Tapola *et al.*, 2005; Ziai *et al.*, 2005; Clark *et al.*, 2006; Flammang *et al.*, 2006; Vuksan *et al.*, 2007; Magnoni

et al., 2008) indicate that fiber supplements (additional 4–19 g/day) do not improve glycemia or cardiovascular disease risk factors and therefore the recommended dietary intake for the general public is also recommended for people with diabetes: 14 g per 1000 kcal by the ADA and 20 g per 1000 kcal by the EASD (Mann *et al.*, 2004; American Diabetes Association, 2008). In essence, given the many factors that can affect glucose metabolism, including those beyond nutrition *per se* (e.g. medicines, activity), it is often problematic to predict the exact plasma glucose response to specific carbohydrate-containing foods. Certainly, blood-glucose self-monitoring and experience can help predict the glycemic effects of food products. Furthermore, a variety of methods can be used to estimate the nutrient content of meals, including carbohydrate counting, the exchange system, and experience. With emerging evidence of the relations among postprandial glycemia and cardiovascular disease (Tushuizen *et al.*, 2005), postprandial glucose levels are of increasing importance.

Several important dimensions of "carbohydrates and diabetes" deserve additional consideration.

First, because diabetes complications are associated with tissue-protein glycation, and because heated foods containing sugar can also form glycation end products (Howard and Wylie-Rosett, 2002; Vlassara *et al.*, 2002), concern has been expressed about the possible role of these ingested glycated products in the pathogenesis of diabetes complications. Although only about 10% of ingested advanced glycation end products enter the circulation, they are excreted slowly, especially in patients with diabetes. However, considerably more research is needed to determine whether such dietary components can alter the risk of diabetes complications.

The second consideration is the role of "carbohydrate substitutions." Fructose, mannitol, and sorbitol are often substituted for sucrose in "sugar-free" products. In experimental studies, these products can shift the balance from oxidation of fatty acids to esterification of fatty acids in the liver, which can in turn increase very-low-density lipoprotein synthesis (Franz *et al.*, 2002). Although the effects on serum lipids are inconsistent, susceptible individuals may have a worsening of dyslipidemia. These sweeteners appear to offer no documented advantage in the management of diabetes over other carbohydrate sources.

Third, reading dietary-product labeling about carbohydrates can be confusing. Many food products list the "net" or "impact" carbohydrate on the front of the label, a value considerably lower than the "total" carbohydrate listed in the nutrient facts panel. Fiber or fiber plus the sugar alcohols is usually subtracted to obtain the net or impact carbohydrate value, but there is no standardization. If patients with diabetes use these products, monitoring is needed to determine the effects on blood glucose (Wylie-Rosett *et al.*, 2004).

Fourth is the possible role of sugar or fat substitutes. "High-intensity sweeteners" are widely used as a replacement of various types of sugar in food and beverage products. Currently approved intense sweeteners include aspartame, saccharin, acesulfame K, and sucrolose. Patients with diabetes use products containing these sweeteners to control energy and carbohydrate intake (Franz *et al.*, 2002). Fat substitutes mimic one or more of the roles of fat in a food; they may be protein-based (usually from egg white or whey), carbohydrate-based (from modified starches, dextrins, or maltodextrins), or fat-based (from emulsifiers replacing triglycerides with mono- or disaccharides or from modification to achieve a partially absorbable or non-absorbable fat). Patients with diabetes may encounter difficulty eating fat substitutes if food products containing them are higher in energy density than the original product or when carbohydrate calculations are not adjusted (Franz *et al.*, 2002).

Fifth, alcohol consumption among persons with diabetes and the possible impact on both carbohydrate and fat metabolism needs to be considered. In general, the recommendations with regard to alcohol intake are similar to those for the general public, and moderate intake (the equivalent of two or fewer drinks) does not have a major effect on metabolic control (Franz *et al.*, 2002). However, alcohol can inhibit hepatic glucose production and cause hypoglycemia if consumed without food in patients taking insulin or sulfonylureas. Conversely, consuming large amounts of alcohol can raise blood glucose levels, especially in the presence of severe insulin deficiency. Finally, alcohol intake should be avoided or significantly limited by patients with pancreatitis, severe hypertriglyceridemia, severe neuropathy, myocardiopathy, or renal failure.

Gestational Diabetes (GDM)

Etiology and Diagnosis

In the past, GDM has been defined as glucose intolerance with onset during pregnancy (American Diabetes Association, 2010a). However, due to the high prevalence of T2D and undiagnosed diabetes, the ADA, in conjunc-

tion with the International Association of Diabetes and Pregnancy Study Groups (IADPSG), recommends that women diagnosed with diabetes at their first prenatal visit receive a diagnosis of overt diabetes (not GDM) and then only when the diabetes is resolved upon delivery should the diabetes be classified as gestational.

Approximately 7% of pregnancies are complicated by GDM. The ADA therefore recommends that risk assessment be carried out during the first prenatal visit for all women and that women deemed "very high risk" should be screened as soon as possible thereafter. Criteria for very high risk include: severe obesity, history of GDM or large-for-gestational-age neonate, presence of glycosuria, diagnosis of polycystic ovarian syndrome (PCOS), and strong family history of T2D (American Diabetes Association, 2010b). Women deemed "above low risk" at this visit should be tested at 24 to 28 weeks' gestation (American Diabetes Association, 2010b). According to the ADA, in order for a woman to be classified as "low risk" and therefore not require GDM screening, she must have *all* of the following characteristics: age less than 25 years, normal weight before pregnancy, member of racial/ethnic group with low diabetes prevalence, no known diabetes in first-degree relatives, no history of abnormal glucose tolerance, and no history of a poor obstetrical outcome (American Diabetes Association, 2010b).

The IADPSG now recommends that *all* women without prior diabetes undergo a 75 g oral glucose test between 24 and 28 weeks' gestation (American Diabetes Association, 2010b). In 2010 the ADA was planning on collaborating with obstetrical organizations in the United States to consider adopting these IADPSG guidelines. Though this change would result in a significant increase in prevalence of diagnosed GDM, it may be appropriate because evidence shows that treating even mild GDM reduces maternal and neonatal morbidity (Landon *et al.*, 2009). Diagnostic cut points for the fasting, 1-hour, and 2-hour post-glucose load tests were developed using data from the Hyperglycemia and Adverse Pregnancy Outcomes (HAPO) study (Leary *et al.*, 2010). In order to be diagnosed with GDM, a woman must have two of the following abnormal values: fasting of at least 5.3 mmol/L (95 mg/dL), 1-hour of at least 10.0 mmol/L (180 mg/dL), 2-hour of at least 8.6 mmol/L (155 mg/dL), and 3-hour of at least 7.8 mmol/L (140 mg/dL) (American Diabetes Association, 2010b). Importantly, it is now established that women with GDM are at very high risk for subsequent T2D after delivery. It is therefore recommended by the ADA that all women with

GDM receive a non-pregnant oral glucose tolerance test 6 to 12 weeks postpartum (American Diabetes Association, 2010b). The risk of developing T2D in women with GDM appears to be reduced by proper nutrition, activity, and possibly medication (Jovanovic and Pettit, 2004).

In addition to the adverse consequences for the mother, there appear to be important, long-term, adverse consequences to the child. Results from the HAPO study indicate that maternal glucose is significantly positively associated with neonatal adiposity, a relationship possibly mediated by neonatal hyperinsulinemia (HAPO Study Cooperative Research Group, 2009). Other results from the HAPO study indicate that maternal hyperglycemia is associated with increased levels of fetal umbilical cord blood C-peptide and increased risk of large for gestational age birth weight (HAPO Study Cooperative Research Group et al., 2008).

Achieving Glycemic Control

The goal of therapy in GDM is to achieve and maintain euglycemia in order to improve pregnancy outcomes; reduce risks to the fetus/baby, such as macrosomia and perinatal complications; and perhaps reduce chances of fetal malnutrition, with subsequent increased risk for adult chronic diseases. Women with GDM actually have nutrition requirements similar to those of other pregnant women but are much more likely to also be overweight. The Fourth International Workshop/Conference on Gestational Diabetes Mellitus recommended the following caloric intake per kilogram of present pregnant weight: 167 kJ (40 kcal)/kg if less than 80% desirable body weight (DBW); 126 kJ (30 kcal)/kg if 80–120% DBW; 100 kJ (24 kcal)/kg if 121–150% DBW; and 50 kJ (12 kcal)/kg if more than 150% DBW. A weight gain of 6.8 kg (15 lb) or less is recommended for women who are 150% or more DBW (Jovanovic, 1998). The recommendations addressed the effects of carbohydrate on the 1-hour postprandial glucose level, suggesting limiting carbohydrate to approximately 40% of energy intake and distributing intake across six feedings, with 10–15% for breakfast, 20–30% for lunch, 30–40% for dinner, and 10% for each of three between-meal snacks (Jovanovic 1998).

In addition to reducing caloric intake as described above, the euglycemic diet recommended for women with GDM (sometimes called the Jovanovic diet) also includes recommendations to restrict carbohydrate intake to less than 40% of calories (minimum of 175 g carbohydrate per day) and allows for 40% of calories to come from fat and 20% from protein. Another component of this diet is to have small breakfasts low in carbohydrates to counter the effects of cortisol (Jovanovic, 2000).

Although experiences with the above approaches to MNT during pregnancy among persons with GDM have stood the test of time, most clinicians and investigators feel strongly that randomized, controlled trials are needed to establish more valid guidelines with respect to dietary composition (amounts and types of carbohydrates and fats), weight gain, and energy and carbohydrate restriction.

Type 2 Diabetes (T2D)

Development of T2D is associated with insulin resistance and inadequate pancreatic beta-cell compensatory insulin production (American Diabetes Association, 2010a). Symptoms and signs associated with T2D are often related to the presence of complications and include poor wound healing, blurred vision, recurrent gum or bladder infections, and changes in hand or foot sensation. T2D may be present for several years before a clinical diagnosis is made (Harris et al., 1992). Many individuals are asymptomatic and their glucose elevation may be detected as the result of a routine blood test.

T2D is rare in children under the age of 10, but accounts for an increasing proportion of cases as age increases (SEARCH for Diabetes in Youth Study Group, 2006). Results from the SEARCH for Diabetes in Youth Study indicated that, in 2001, the prevalence (per 1000) of T2D was 0.01 in children less than 10 years of age and 0.42 in children 10–19 years of age (SEARCH for Diabetes in Youth Study Group, 2006).

Prevention

MNT plays a critical role in the primary prevention of T2D: the goal of MNT for individuals at high risk of developing T2D is to improve food choices and physical activity and achieve sustained weight loss and increased beta-cell sensitivity (Tuomilehto et al., 2001; Knowler et al., 2002). Over the past 10 years, studies have been conducted that establish the validity of efforts in primary prevention among those at high risk of developing T2D and the critical role of addressing overweight, obesity, and physical inactivity (Pan et al., 1997; Diabetes Prevention Program Research Group, 2002; Lindström et al., 2003; Uusitupa et al., 2003; Anderson et al., 2004a; Avenell *et al.*, 2004; Centers for Disease Control and Prevention Primary Prevention Working Group, 2004; Mayer-Davis *et al.*, 2004; Norris *et al.*, 2005; Orchard *et al.*, 2005; Uusitupa, 2005; Wylie-Rosett *et al.*, 2006).

The Da Quing Diabetes Prevention Study was a 6-year lifestyle intervention (diet, exercise, or diet plus exercise) in 577 adults with impaired glucose tolerance in China. The results of this study provided preliminary evidence that diet and exercise interventions can lower the conversion to overt diabetes (Pan *et al.*, 1997). The 20-year follow-up results showed that individuals in the combined intervention group had a 43% lower incidence of diabetes over the 20-year period and spent an average of 3.6 fewer years with diabetes compared with control-group participants (Li *et al.*, 2008).

The Finnish Diabetes Prevention Study (FDPS) was a randomized controlled trial in 522 individuals with impaired glucose tolerance randomized to one of two groups: lifestyle intervention or control (Tuomilehto *et al.*, 2001). The lifestyle intervention involved a low-fat (less than 30% of calories from fat; less than 10% of calories from saturated fat), high-fiber (at least 15 g/1000 kcal) diet in conjunction with moderate-intensity exercise for at least 30 minutes per day (Tuomilehto *et al.*, 2001). After an average follow-up of 3.2 years, results of the FDPS showed a 58% reduction in the incidence of T2D with lifestyle intervention (Lindström *et al.*, 2003; Uusitupa *et al.*, 2003; Uusitupa, 2005). There were small but significant reductions in total cholesterol, triglyceride, and systolic blood pressure and an increase in HDL cholesterol in the lifestyle intervention group but not in the control group, and PAI-1 (an inflammatory marker associated with increased cardiovascular disease risk) levels fell significantly in the lifestyle group in proportion to weight reduction (Uusitupa *et al.*, 2003). Studies from the FDPS of candidate genes affecting energy metabolism showed the importance of genetic polymorphisms in defining responses to lifestyle interventions (Uusitupa, 2005).

The Diabetes Prevention Program (DPP) was a randomized controlled trial conducted in 3234 individuals with impaired glucose tolerance randomized to one of three groups: standard lifestyle recommendations plus metformin, standard lifestyle recommendations plus placebo, or intensive lifestyle modification (Knowler *et al.*, 2002). The intensive lifestyle modification involved a healthy, low-calorie (subtracted 500 to 1000 calories from estimated amount of calories needed to maintain baseline weight), low-fat (25% of calories from fat) diet in conjunc-

tion with at least 150 minutes of moderate-intensity physical activity per week with an overall goal of achieving and maintaining a weight reduction of at least 7% of initial body weight (Diabetes Prevention Program Research Group, 2002; Knowler *et al.*, 2002). The program consisted of a 16-session core curriculum in which participants received individualized advice on how to reach their goals (Diabetes Prevention Program Research Group, 2002).

After an average follow-up period of 2.8 years, results of the DPP showed that the incidence of diabetes was reduced by 58% in the intensive lifestyle intervention group compared with only 31% in the metformin group (Diabetes Prevention Program Research Group, 2002; Centers for Disease Control and Prevention Primary Prevention Working Group, 2004; Mayer-Davis *et al.*, 2004; Wing *et al.*, 2004; Orchard *et al.*, 2005; Wylie-Rosett *et al.*, 2006). Further analysis revealed that weight loss was the dominant predictor of the observed reduced diabetes incidence: when adjusted for changes in diet and physical activity, each kilogram of weight loss resulted in a 16% reduction in diabetes risk (Hamman *et al.*, 2006). Furthermore, a lower percent of calories from fat and increased physical activity accounted for the weight loss, indicating that it was through these intermediates that the diabetes risk reduction was accomplished (Hamman *et al.*, 2006). Treatment effects did not differ by sex, race, or ethnic group. Recent 10-year follow-up of the DPP found that the cumulative incidence of diabetes remained the lowest in the intensive lifestyle intervention group (Gillis *et al.*, 2009).

Unlike the intensive lifestyle intervention, which was effective across the entire baseline body weight and fasting glucose ranges, metformin was ineffective in those with a BMI less than 30 kg/m^2 and minimally effective in those with a BMI less than 35 kg/m^2 or with a fasting glucose level less than 6.1 mmol/L (110 mg/dL). As in the FDPS, insulin sensitivity improved in the intensive lifestyle intervention group, with a smaller increase in the metformin group, but did not change in the placebo group. Insulin secretion decreased in all groups, but was associated with improved beta-cell function only in the intensive lifestyle intervention group. The intensive lifestyle intervention resulted in a lower prevalence and need for medical treatment of hypertension and dyslipidemia. It also lowered inflammatory biomarkers (CRP and PAI-1) associated with increased cardiovascular disease risk. In the placebo group, of the participants who did not have metabolic syndrome at baseline, 51% had developed it at the study's end. The lifestyle intervention reduced the prevalence by 33%; metformin reduced it by only 15%.

The simulated lifetime cumulative incidence of microvascular and macrovascular complications and life expectancy for the DPP indicated that, compared with placebo, the lifestyle intervention would reduce the cumulative incidence of blindness by 39%, end-stage renal disease by 38%, amputation by 35%, stroke by 9%, and coronary heart disease by 8%, and would increase life expectancy by 0.5 years (Wylie-Rosett *et al.*, 2006). Compared with the placebo intervention, the lifestyle intervention cost per quality-adjusted life-years would be approximately $1100 (Wylie-Rosett *et al.*, 2006). For metformin, the cost per quality-adjusted life-years was calculated using costs of the generic form of the drug as $1800 (Wylie-Rosett *et al.*, 2006).

Both the DPP and FDPS asked participants to self-monitor their food intake (Lindström *et al.*, 2003; Uusitupa *et al.*, 2003; Mayer-Davis *et al.*, 2004). In the FDPS, participants were asked to complete 3-day food records four times per year; in the DPP, participants were asked to self-monitor their activity, food intake, calories, and fat grams daily during the first 24 weeks and then at least 1 week per month thereafter. In the DPP, the frequency of dietary self-monitoring was related to success at achieving both the physical-activity goal and the weight-loss goal. Moreover, participants who were 65 or older were more likely to complete self-monitoring records, report a lower percentage of calories from fat, and meet the activity and weight-loss goals than those who were less than 45 years old (Mayer-Davis *et al.*, 2004). Thus, it is not surprising that older participants had a greater (71%) risk reduction in the development of diabetes with lifestyle intervention (Knowler *et al.*, 2002; Wing *et al.*, 2004). Lifestyle coaches in the DPP taught the participants to use a problem-solving approach to manage high-risk situations (stress, vacations, eating out) and used a toolbox approach to deal with barriers to lifestyle change (Diabetes Prevention Program Research Group, 2002).

Studies independent of the FDPS and DPP have found that an increase in fiber and whole-grain consumption may help prevent or delay the onset of diabetes (American Diabetes Association, 2008). Furthermore, the inclusion of an emphasis on increased fiber consumption in the FDPS and DPP lifestyle intervention groups lends support to a possible role of fiber consumption in the primary prevention of T2D.

Thus, current efficacy data from large randomized controlled trials (FDPS and DPP) support a moderately low-fat diet as part of a lifestyle intervention for weight loss and primary prevention of T2D. It is not unreasonable to consider other dietary strategies and distributions of macronutrients for achieving weight-loss goals (Davis *et al.*, 2009). A meta-analysis of randomized controlled trials that compared low-fat diets with non-energy-restricted low-carbohydrate diets found that the latter are effective and safe alternatives for weight loss (Nordmann *et al.*, 2006). Furthermore, a recent randomized trial (PREDIMED study) observed a lower 4-year incidence of diabetes in the two Mediterranean diet groups compared with the low-fat group in the absence of significant changes in weight (Salas-Salvado *et al.*, 2011).

The HEALTHY study was a randomized, controlled, multicenter study in middle-school-aged children in the United States, designed to reduce risk factors associated with T2D development (Gillis *et al.*, 2009). Preliminary results indicate that, although there was a decrease in the combined prevalence of overweight and obesity in schools (primary outcome), there were no differences between intervention and control schools. Intervention schools did, however, have significantly greater decreases in BMI z-scores, percentage of students with a waist circumference at or above the 90th percentile, fasting insulin levels, and obesity prevalence (HEALTHY Study Group *et al.*, 2010). The efficacy of the intervention in prevention of T2D will require additional participant follow-up and further testing.

Etiology and Diagnosis

The etiology of T2D, similar to T1D, is likely a complex interaction between environment and genetic predisposition, as indicated by the wide variability in the prevalence of T2D in cross-sectional and prospective studies (Permutt *et al.*, 2005; Roche *et al.*, 2005). Further complicating matters is the fact that, unlike T1D, the incidence of T2D shows strong social patterning due to differential exposure to obesogenic environments (Whiting *et al.*, 2010). Many indigenous populations are lean and have low rates of T2D, but the rates of diabetes and obesity dramatically increase with lifestyle or environmental changes (Wild *et al.*, 2004; Centers for Disease Control and Prevention, 2008).

Android fat distribution is associated with greater insulin resistance than gynoid fat distribution. Abdominal girth of at least 89 cm (35 in) in women and at least 102 cm

(40 in) in men is considered an indicator of increased insulin resistance, hypertension, and dyslipidemia (Obesity Education Initiative Expert Panel, 1998). Insulin resistance increases with age, and the incidence of diabetes rises sharply in the elderly (American Diabetes Association, 2010a).

In a few patients, genetic mutations appear to be associated with T2D (Roche *et al.*, 2005; American Diabetes Association, 2010a). For example, recent work using the DPP data has led to the identification of 27 single nucleotide polymorphisms (SNPs) in the SLC30A8 gene (codes for a protein that transports zinc molecules into insulin granules in beta-cells, which is essential for insulin storage and processing) that are associated with T2D (Billings *et al.*, 2010). A "thrifty genotype" that favors energy efficiency and could be maladaptive in an environment with an energy-dense food supply and low level of physical activity is another genetic concept being considered (Prentice *et al.*, 2005). Finally, metabolic adaptations in the fetus of a malnourished and/or hyperglycemic mother may be associated with a "thrifty phenotype" in the newborn and subsequent insulin resistance and increased risk for T2D (Bateson *et al.*, 2004).

There have been numerous studies examining the role of various nutritional (or activity) factors and the incidence of T2D. From the most general perspective, these studies can be divided into three categories: studies focusing on specific dietary components (examples include nuts, coffee, and fiber [Freeman, 2005; Lovejoy, 2005; Murakami *et al.*, 2005; van Dam and Hu, 2005]), studies examining total calories/weight loss (Pan *et al.*, 1997; Diabetes Prevention Program Research Group, 2002; Lindström *et al.*, 2003; Uusitupa *et al.*, 2003; Centers for Disease Control and Prevention Primary Prevention Working Group, 2004; Jack *et al.*, 2004; Mayer-Davis *et al.*, 2004; Wing *et al.*, 2004; Uusitupa, 2005; Orchard *et al.*, 2005; Wylie-Rosett *et al.*, 2006), and studies examining meal patterns (examples include Mediterranean diets [Karantonis *et al.*, 2006; Esposito *et al.*, 2009] and vegetarian diets [Barnard *et al.*, 2009]). In general, the studies that have identified specific food ingredients as related to T2D incidence have been large observational studies that particularly address the statistical significance of relative risk as the determinant of importance (Lovejoy, 2005; Murakami *et al.*, 2005; van Dam and Hu, 2005). The randomized trials that address total calories consumed along with accompanying increased physical activity and meal patterns address absolute risk and "numbers needed

to treat" as indicators of public health importance (Pan *et al.*, 1997; Diabetes Prevention Program Research Group, 2002; Lindström *et al.*, 2003; Uusitupa *et al.*, 2003; Centers for Disease Control and Prevention Primary Prevention Working Group, 2004; Jack *et al.*, 2004; Mayer-Davis *et al.*, 2004; Wing *et al.*, 2004; Orchard *et al.*, 2005; Uusitupa, 2005; Wylie-Rosett *et al.*, 2006).

Three categories of increased risk of developing diabetes are currently recognized by the ADA: an FPG between 5.6 and 6.9 mmol/L (100 and 125 mg/dL), defined as having impaired fasting glucose (IFG); a 2-h OGTT between 7.8 and 11 mmol/L (140 and 199 mg/dL), defined as having impaired glucose tolerance (IGT); an A1C between 5.7 and 6.4% with values between 6.0 and 6.4 considered very high risk (American Diabetes Association, 2010a).

It is estimated that approximately one-fourth of individuals with diabetes in the United States are currently undiagnosed. Therefore, it is recommended that all individuals, regardless of age, with a BMI ≥25 kg/m^2 and at least one other risk factor are tested for diabetes. Risk factors include physical inactivity, a first-degree relative with diabetes, hypertension (blood pressure of at least 140/90 mm Hg or on therapy for hypertension), a high-density lipoprotein (HDL) cholesterol level less than 35 mg/dL (0.90 mmol/L) and/or a triglyceride level greater than 250 mg/dL (2.82 mmol/L), an A1C of at least 5.7%, IFG, IGT, other clinical conditions associated with insulin resistance (e.g. acanthosis nigricans), a history of cardiovascular disease, women with PCOS, women who delivered a baby weighing more than 9 lb (4.1 kg) or who were diagnosed with GDM, and being a member of a high-risk ethnic population (e.g. African-American, Latino, Native American, Asian-American, Pacific Islander) (American Diabetes Association, 2010a). In the absence of any risk factors, it is recommended that testing begin at 45 years of age. If tests are normal, then testing should occur every 3 years. Testing should occur in a health-care setting and is equivalent to screening because the tests for diagnosis and for screening are the same.

Consistent with the guidelines for testing for T2D in adults, the ADA recommends testing overweight children (defined as BMI greater than the 85th percentile for age and sex, weight for height greater than the 85th percentile, or weight greater than 120% of ideal for height) who also have any two of the following risk factors: family history of T2D (first- or second-degree relative), maternal history of diabetes or GDM during child's gestation, member of high-risk race/ethnicity group (Native American, African-

American, Latino, Asian-American, Pacific Islander), or signs/symptoms associated with insulin resistance (e.g. acanthosis nigricans, hypertension, dyslipidemia, PCOS, small for gestational age birth weight) (American Diabetes Association, 2000).

Achieving Glycemic Control

The United Kingdom Prospective Diabetes Study (UKPDS) examined the benefit of metabolic control (glucose and blood pressure) in patients newly diagnosed with T2D (UK Prospective Diabetes Study Group, 1998a,b,c). Fundamentally, the UKPDS confirmed that the findings of the DCCT also applied to T2D. There was a reduction in macrovascular and microvascular complications, and the best results were achieved in those individuals who had both glucose and blood-pressure control. Similarly, there was a clear dose–response relationship between metabolic and blood-pressure control and the risk of diabetes complications.

The Lifestyle Over and Above Drugs in Diabetes (LOADD) randomized, controlled trial in New Zealand looked at the impact of intensive nutritional counseling over a period of 6 months in patients with T2D ($n = 93$). Significant reductions in the intervention group were observed in A1C, weight, BMI, and waist circumference compared with the control group (Coppell et al., 2010).

Medical Nutrition Therapy (MNT)

Similar to T1D, glycemic control and restoration of normal metabolism in T2D is accomplished using several modalities including a variety of pharmacological agents, close personal and laboratory monitoring, and careful assessment by a variety of health professionals. MNT for treatment of T2D progresses from prevention, primarily through weight loss, to improving insulin sensitivity, to improving metabolic control of glucose, lipids, and blood pressure. Among efforts to establish normal metabolism to prevent longer-term diabetes complications, reducing cardiovascular disease risk is a primary goal for MNT and the overall management of T2D, as well as T1D; a topic that will be discussed in more detail later on in this chapter (American Diabetes Association, 2010b). Diet and exercise are considered to be the first step to achieve euglycemia, with focus often on the health risks associated with overweight and obesity. However, medical care standards and experience with T2D indicate that, to reduce both cardiovascular and microvascular risk, patients often must take five or more medications to achieve blood glucose,

blood pressure, and cholesterol goals, as well as low-dose aspirin. Supporting the benefits of MNT, the amount of medication needed is likely to be less with a modest weight loss of 5–10% of body weight (Obesity Education Initiative Expert Panel, 1998; Norris et al., 2004; American Diabetes Association, 2010b). The impact of weight loss is most dramatically demonstrated by bariatric surgery, a procedure for selected patients with T2D and obesity. However, the effects of bariatric surgery appear to be largely independent of weight loss and may be due to changes in hormonal metabolism (Buchwald et al., 2004).

Guidelines for MNT in T2D, focusing particularly on controlling glycemia, dyslipidemia, and hypertension, have been validated and supported by a randomized trial (American Dietetic Association, 2002). Furthermore, the Look-AHEAD (Action for Health in Diabetes) Study, an ongoing multicenter, randomized controlled trial of an intensive lifestyle intervention in 5145 patients with T2D, found that a weight loss of 8.6% was associated with improved diabetes control, as indicated by reductions in diabetes medication use and A1C levels (Look AHEAD Research Group et al., 2007). Four-year results of the Look-AHEAD study indicate that the improvements in weight (loss of 6.15%), fitness, and A1C observed in the intensive lifestyle intervention group compared with the control group were sustained (Look AHEAD Research Group, 2010). When lifestyle changes or MNT do not achieve euglycemia, combinations of oral agents (Table 49.2) with or without concomitant insulin may be prescribed to improve insulin secretion and/or insulin sensitivity, with the starting medication typically metformin. Likewise, for both hypertension and hyperlipidemia a variety of agents exist and are increasingly being used in combination to treat T2D (American Diabetes Association, 2010b).

Dietary fat composition may require additional consideration in individuals with T2D. Decreasing dietary fat and increasing carbohydrate intake can potentially worsen the dyslipidemia of T2D by lowering HDL cholesterol levels and increasing the level of VLDL cholesterol, triglyceride, and LDL cholesterol – effects that can be ameliorated by weight loss (American Dietetic Association, 2002; Institute of Medicine, 2005). Studies that looked at the effect of supplementation of n-3 fatty acids in individuals with T2D have found mixed results: four randomized, controlled trials found that n-3 fatty acid supplementation increased fasting plasma glucose by a small (but significant) amount (Woodman et al., 2002; Pedersen et al., 2003; Mostad et al., 2006), whereas one

TABLE 49.2   Oral antidiabetic medications: mechanism of action and side-effects

Medication class and mechanism of action	Generic name	Brand name	Comments and side-effects
Sulfonylureas Stimulate the pancreatic beta-cells to secrete more insulin	Chlorpropamide (first-generation)	Diabinese	Hypoglycemia risk, especially when using Chlorpropamide and Glyburide compared with other sulfonylureas or in the elderly
	Glyburide (second-generation)	Micronase, Diabeta, Glynase Pres Tab	Weight gain (approximately 2 kg) upon treatment initiation common
	Glipizide (second-generation)	Glucotrol, Glucotrol XL	Higher doses should be avoided
	Glimepiride (third-generation)	Amaryl	
Meglitinides (glinides) Stimulate the pancreatic beta-cells to secrete more insulin	Repaglinide	Prandin	Must be administered more frequently than sulfonylureas
	Nateglinide	Starlix	Hypoglycemia risk, less than with sulfonylureas for Nateglinide Weight gain similar to sulfonylureas
Biguanides Reduce output of glucose from the liver	Metformin	Glucophage	May have gastrointestinal side-effects Interferes with B_{12} absorption but rarely associated with anemia Contraindicated in patients with renal dysfunction Check creatinine clearance if over 65 years of age
Alpha-glucosidase inhibitors Decrease rate of digestion of carbohydrate-containing foods	Acarbose	Precose	Reduced risk of hypoglycemia compared with other drug classes
	Miglitol	Glyset	Gastrointestinal side-effects, including gas and diarrhea
Thiazolidinediones Enhance insulin sensitivity	Rosiglitazone	Avandia	Fluid retention, which can lead to congestive heart failure in the elderly or other high-risk patients
	Pioglitazone	ACTOS	Contraindicated in liver disease. Check liver enzymes on an ongoing basis Weight gain
Dipeptidyl peptidase 4 inhibitors Prevent breakdown of GLP-1	Sitagliptin	Januvia	Do not cause hypoglycemia Upper respiratory tract infection risk

Data from Nathan *et al.* (2009).

small study found that supplementation significantly decreased A1C (Pooya *et al.*, 2010). A meta-analysis conducted using trials up to 2008 found no significant effect on glycemia or insulinemia in individuals receiving n-3 fatty acids vs. placebo supplements (Hartweg *et al.*, 2009).

Approaches to Reduce Complications of Chronic Disease Risk Factors in Type 1 and Type 2 Diabetes

Cardiovascular disease and its complications are by far the greatest cause of death in individuals with diabetes. Therefore, reduction in cardiovascular disease risk factors is a major treatment goal for all patients with diabetes.

Glycemic Control to Reduce Complications of Chronic Disease Risk Factors in T2D

The Action to Control Cardiovascular Risk in Diabetes (ACCORD) study was a randomized controlled trial that looked at the effects of intensive glycemic control (target A1C less than 6%) vs. standard glycemic control (target A1C between 7 and 7.9%) in 10 251 patients with extant diabetes on cardiovascular disease outcomes. The treatment arm receiving intensive control of blood pressure and lipids did not have a significant improvement over controls (Ismail-Beigi *et al.*, 2010). Results from two other large, randomized, controlled trials, the ADVANCE study and the Veterans Affairs Diabetes Trail (VADT), also found no significant reduction in cardiovascular disease risk with intensive glycemic control (ADVANCE Collaborative Group *et al.*, 2008; Duckworth *et al.*, 2009). The reader is referred to the ADA's position statement on intensive glycemic control and the prevention of cardiovascular events for more information on this topic (Skyler *et al.*, 2009). Together, the results of these three trials indicate that intensive treatment may not provide any additional benefit, at least in the time period of treatment and populations observed in these studies (Skyler *et al.*, 2009).

MNT to Reduce Complications of Chronic Disease Risk Factors in T1D and T2D

The Look-AHEAD Study also looked at the effect of achieving and maintaining weight loss on cardiovascular disease risk reduction. One-year results of the intervention indicated that the clinically significant weight loss (8.6%) was associated with reductions in cardiovascular disease risk factors as indicated by blood pressure, triglycerides, HDL cholesterol, and urine albumin-to-creatinine ratio

(Look AHEAD Research Group *et al.*, 2007). Reductions in C-reactive protein have also been observed (Belalcazar *et al.*, 2010). Four-year results of the study indicate that the improvements in systolic blood pressure and HDL cholesterol levels observed in the intensive lifestyle intervention group compared with the control group were sustained (Look AHEAD Research Group, 2010).

Results from a recent 2-year study of weight loss on a low-carbohydrate diet found significant increases in HDL cholesterol and significant decreases in total cholesterol in comparison with a low-fat diet (Shai *et al.*, 2008). This study also observed significant increases in insulin sensitivity in individuals with diabetes on a Mediterranean diet in comparison with a low-fat diet (Shai *et al.*, 2008).

Although MNT treatment guidelines focus on glycemic control, it is recognized that achieving an optimal lipid and lipoprotein profile and blood pressure level are also very important aspects of diabetes treatment. For the treatment and management of cardiovascular disease risk, the ADA recommends dietary patterns high in fruits, vegetables, whole grains, and nuts, low sodium intake (for patients with diabetes and symptomatic heart failure less than 2000 mg per day; in normotensive and hypertensive patients less than 2300 mg per day), and, for most individuals, a modest amount of weight loss (American Diabetes Association, 2008). To date, there are no large-scale randomized controlled trials of overall MNT recommendations and cardiovascular disease risk reduction in individuals with diabetes. However, improvements in glycemic control (as measured by A1C) in individuals with both T1D (DCCT) and T2D (UKPDS) have been associated with cardiovascular disease risk reduction (Stratton *et al.*, 2000; Nathan *et al.*, 2005).

Specific Dietary Components

Fat. There is little evidence to support suggestions that changing the percent of calories from fat (e.g. total fat intake) has any influence on cardiovascular disease risk factors in individuals with diabetes. However, as with glycemic control, the type of fat may play an important role. The ATP III guidelines classify most individuals with diabetes as being at high risk for cardiovascular disease within the next 10 years – that is, diabetes is a cardiovascular disease "risk factor equivalent" (Expert Panel on Detection, Evaluation, and Treatment of High Blood Cholesterol in Adults, 2001). Thus, the goals of treatment are lower than in the absence of diabetes: serum low-density lipoprotein level less than 2.6 mmol/L (100 mg/dL) and dietary goals with less than 7% of calories from saturated fat, minimal *trans* fat intake, and less than 200 mg of cholesterol per day.

Both monounsaturated and polyunsaturated fatty acids reduce LDL cholesterol levels, but they may differ with respect to their effect on HDL cholesterol levels. Reducing intake of total fat and saturated fatty acids in particular tends to further reduce a low HDL cholesterol level associated with insulin resistance and diabetes. However, weight loss may ameliorate this effect. In a meta-analysis of dietary intervention studies in patients with T2D, Garg (1998) reported that diets high in monounsaturated fats reduced the VLDL cholesterol and triglyceride levels by 22% and 19% respectively and did not adversely affect body weight.

Hydrogenation of the cis-isomer of fatty acids in oils creates *trans* isomers that function like more saturated fatty acids in food products and potentially in the human body. Epidemiological studies have linked *trans* fat consumption to increased cardiovascular disease risk, but to date there are no intervention studies that specifically address the extent to which *trans* fat intake may increase the risk of cardiovascular disease. Individuals with diabetes and/or other risk factors for cardiovascular disease should keep *trans* fat intake as low as possible (Christiansen *et al.*, 1997).

Considerable interest exists in the intake of fish and n-3 fatty acids (Connor, 2004). For example, the rates of diabetes and of cardiovascular disease are lower in population groups with a high fish intake, perhaps because fatty acids from fish and other sources that have the double bond in the n-3 position reduce triglyceride production (Nettleton and Katz, 2005). A recent meta-analysis of clinical trials of fish oils conducted in patients with T2D showed a 7% reduction in fasting triglyceride levels accompanied by a slight increase in LDL cholesterol (Hartweg *et al.*, 2009). Overall, the current evidence supports a possible role of n-3 fatty acid supplementation in decreasing triglyceride levels in individuals with diabetes, but a potential role in LDL and/or HDL levels is not clear.

Carbohydrates. The American Heart Association (AHA) recently released a scientific statement concerning the role of dietary sugar intake in cardiovascular health (Johnson *et al.*, 2009). Although clinical trial evidence linking additional consumption of sugars with adverse outcomes is missing, observational data indicate that increased intake of added sugars (the majority of which is in the form of sugar-sweetened beverages) is associated with increased energy intake and higher body weight along with decreased intake of essential vitamins. Based on this evidence and the fact that intake of added sugars greatly exceeds the 2005 United States Dietary Guidelines for discretionary calories (Institute of Medicine, 2005), the AHA now recommends limiting intake of added sugars to half discretionary calories, which equates to no more than 100 calories per day for women and no more than 150 calories per day for men (Johnson *et al.*, 2009). It is important to note that this recommendation is intended as a pragmatic way to limit caloric intake and is not based on a particular problem caused by carbohydrate or sugar intake.

Micronutrients and Supplements

The relations between diabetes and micronutrients are reciprocal: micronutrients can affect diabetes, and diabetes and its complications can alter the metabolism and impact of micronutrients. Poorly controlled diabetes can alter vitamin and mineral status, and micronutrients can affect glucose and overall energy homeostasis.

Studies indicate that many patients with diabetes consume supplements and do not alert their healthcare professionals about this use (Venters *et al.*, 2004). Consultation regarding the use of supplements should help patients with diabetes evaluate the potential risks and benefits of these products (Barringer *et al.*, 2003; Cefalu and Hu, 2004; Cicero *et al.*, 2004; Liu *et al.*, 2004; Narendhirakannan *et al.*, 2005; Schwartz *et al.*, 2005). One clinical study that evaluated the effects of a multivitamin supplement on quality of life and missed days of activity found some benefit for the subgroup with diabetes and those over 65 years of age (Barringer *et al.*, 2003). Although antioxidant nutrients appear to play a role in reducing oxidative stress and possibly in insulin sensitivity, there is insufficient evidence at present to warrant making any specific recommendation about use of the substances in diabetes management (American Diabetes Association, 2010b). This level of uncertainty has been raised by two large randomized controlled trials that failed to demonstrate a positive impact of antioxidant vitamins on cardiovascular disease, including patients with diabetes (Toole *et al.*, 2004; Lonn *et al.*, 2005). A survey of providers of alternative therapies used in diabetes found that the 10 most commonly recommended nutrient supplements were biotin, vanadium, chromium, vitamin B_6, vitamin C, vitamin E, zinc, selenium, alpha-lipoic acid, and fructo-oligosaccharides, and the 10 most commonly recommended herbal supplements were gymnema, psyllium, fenugreek, bilberry, garlic, Chinese ginseng, dandelion, burdock, prickly pear cactus, and bitter melon (Cicero *et al.*, 2004). Although these products may have some blood-glucose-lowering effects, a patient's use of these products is not generally evaluated as part of his or her medical or dietary history. Having an open dialog about the use of alternative therapies provides the opportunity to explore how they may interact with prescribed medications, either beneficially or harmfully (Cicero *et al.*, 2004).

Some of these supplements have received more attention – in the laboratory, clinical world, and media – than others. Although some research suggests that chromium supplementation may improve insulin sensitivity and glucose metabolism in patients with diabetes, research results are mixed. Limitations of the chromium studies to date include inadequate sample size, short duration, non-randomized design, lack of information about the pre-study chromium status of the study population, and different doses of chromium supplementation – all of which may account for the variability of the findings (Cefalu and Hu, 2004). Long-term clinical trials are needed to examine chromium in relation to diabetes using well-defined outcomes (e.g. T2D and cardiovascular disease) and metabolic parameters and to assess the safety of long-term chromium supplementation (Cefalu and Hu, 2004).

Magnesium modulates glucose transport across cell membranes, and poorly controlled diabetes can induce hypomagnesemia by increasing urinary excretion, with possible increased insulin resistance (Franz *et al.*, 2002). The clinical usefulness of supplementation, usually by intake of magnesium-based antacids, for patients with T2D and insulin resistance, is not, however, established. As another example of the present disconnect between laboratory and clinical studies, in laboratory experiments zinc and antioxidant requirements increase during wound healing (Franz *et al.*, 2002), but the need for supplementation for every patient postsurgery or with a foot ulcer remains to be confirmed (American Diabetes Association, 2010b).

Other inorganic trace elements such as vanadium, copper, iron, potassium, sodium, and nickel may play an important role in the maintenance of normoglycemia by activating the beta-cells of the pancreas. Sources of these elements are often contained in various alternative/complementary medications. For example, analysis of the mineral content of the leaves from four plants used in Asian traditional medicine (*Murraya koenigii*, *Mentha piperitae*, *Ocimum sanctum*, and *Aegle marmelos*) yielded moderate levels of copper, nickel, zinc, potassium, and sodium (which may account for the reported therapeutic benefit if the basic food supply is inadequate) (Narendhirakannan *et al.*, 2005). However, the need for this supplementation, should the nutrients in the dietary pattern recommended in the 2005 Dietary Guidelines be accomplished, is not apparent among persons with diabetes based on more valid clinical studies.

The B-vitamin group is a final category of "supplements" to consider, particularly thiamin, riboflavin, niacin, and vitamin B_6, all of which are involved in glucose metabolism. Among persons with poorly controlled diabetes and polyuria associated with hyperglycemia, requirements may be altered by excess excretion in the urine. Ironically, nicotinic acid itself can worsen glycemic control when it is used to treat hyperlipidemia; however, uncontrolled studies suggest that it may also help to protect beta-cell function from autoimmune destruction. Folate and vitamin B_{12} levels play a role in homocysteine metabolism, and plasma levels of these nutrients are inversely related to homocysteine levels. In patients with T2D, plasma homocysteine concentration is a significant predictor of cardiovascular events and death, perhaps due to worsening of endothelial dysfunction and/or structural vessel properties induced by oxidative stress (Huijberts *et al.*, 2005). Elevated fasting homocysteine levels appear to be a biomarker for subsequent development of T2D in women (Cho *et al.*, 2005a). However, to confirm that a particular measurement is actually a risk factor (versus a risk marker), it is desirable that a randomized, controlled trial be conducted to show that the alteration in the compound being measured is associated with benefits to patients. Such clinical trials are being completed, and results do not indicate a relationship between homocysteine perturbations and subsequent stroke or myocardial infarctions (Bønaa *et al.*, 2006; Lonn *et al.*, 2006).

Other Types of Diabetes

Monogenic Diabetes

Monogenic diabetes is a class of diabetes associated with genetic defects in beta-cell function. They are frequently associated with early onset of hyperglycemia (typically before 25 years of age). Three common forms of monogenic diabetes include maturity-onset diabetes of the young (MODY) and mutations in KIR6.2 (KCNJ11) and SUR1 (ABCC8). MODY is an autosomal dominant disorder associated with mutations on one of six common genetic loci. A mutation on chromosome 12 in the hepatocyte transcription factor, HNF-1α, is the most common form of the disorder. Individuals with MODY have impaired insulin secretion but normal insulin action. Mutations in the ATP-sensitive potassium transporter genes, KCNJ11 and ABCC8, are associated with glucose intolerance (van Dam *et al.*, 2005). In the majority of cases, these forms of diabetes are best managed with sulfonylureas rather than insulin, and glycemic control is typically not difficult to achieve.

Secondary Diabetes

Disorders directly affecting the pancreas can secondarily cause diabetes (American Diabetes Association, 2010a). Diabetes can also be secondary to endocrinopathies leading to increased counter-regulatory hormone production [e.g. acromegaly (excess growth hormone), Cushing's syndrome (excess cortisol), glucagonoma (excess glucagon), and phenochromocytoma (excess epinephrine)]. Pharmacological agents can also create insulin resistance or damage to the pancreatic beta-cells. Steroids and novel antipsychotic medications that increase insulin resistance and visceral fat may increase insulin requirements beyond endogenous capacity (American Diabetes Association, 2004, 2010a; Centers for Disease Control and Prevention, 2008).

Cystic fibrosis-related diabetes (CFRD) is the most common co-morbidity in people with CF. The addition of diabetes to CF is associated with poorer nutrition outcomes in addition to more severe inflammatory lung disease and greater mortality from respiratory failure, especially in women (American Diabetes Association, 2010b).

Global Public Health Issues

It is estimated that approximately 366 million people worldwide currently have diabetes (International Diabetes Federation, 2011). In 2011, approximately 4.6 million deaths were estimated to be attributable to diabetes (International Diabetes Federation, 2011). These high-prevalence and mortality estimates have led the International Diabetes Federation (IDF) to conclude that diabetes is "one of the most challenging health problems in the 21st century" (International Diabetes Federation, 2009). Approximately 70% of diabetic individuals live in low- and middle-income countries and it is now widely recognized that these countries carry the greatest diabetes

burden (International Diabetes Federation, 2009). It has been proposed that this heavy burden is the result of population aging, urbanization, and the resulting changes in diet and physical activity. However, there is growing evidence that, in some middle-income countries, especially including India and China, the prevalence in rural areas is approaching that in urban areas, perhaps related to mechanization (Yang *et al.*, 2010).

The estimated direct medical cost for prevention and treatment of diabetes worldwide was approximately US\$376 billion in 2010 and will exceed US\$490 billion by 2030 (Zhang *et al.*, 2010). Total costs are substantially higher due to loss of productive years of life, particularly in developing countries.

Achieving population-level impact in the primary, secondary, and tertiary prevention of diabetes is a complex task. Addressing nutrition issues at all three levels requires collaborations involving a wide variety of partners to ensure an appropriate balance between efforts to prevent and treat diabetes complications and efforts to prevent the onset of diabetes. Clearly, factors beyond what occurs in a doctor's office have a dramatic impact on both preventive and management strategies for chronic diseases, including all classes of diabetes. In the United States, insurance status, federal and state policies, opportunities for proper nutrition and activity at schools, reimbursement strategies, and federal deficits can all have a significant impact on the individual health provider and/or patient in terms of how well diabetes can be prevented and/or treated. Typically, these are not issues that are discussed in the office, but they must be included in larger efforts to address all aspects of nutrition and diabetes (Jack *et al.*, 2004; Ogilvie and Hamlet, 2005). The ability to capitalize on prevention opportunities requires a strong infrastructure to plan and support interventions, nurture partnerships, and monitor and evaluate progress. Much of the effort to date has targeted identifying individuals at risk for diabetes and also diabetes complications, and increasing public awareness of diabetes risks, especially in communities with populations at high risk of developing diabetes.

In the United States, many efforts within the voluntary, professional, academic, and private sectors address these challenges of diabetes. The National Diabetes Education Program (NDEP), a partnership of the National Institutes of Health and the Centers for Disease Control and Prevention (CDCP), tries to serve as a "coordinating entity" among more than 200 public and private organizations. In addition, the CDCP's Division of Diabetes

Translation is addressing community infrastructure and environmental issues to reduce the burden of diabetes, including public health surveillance systems for diabetes, applied translational research, state-based diabetes control programs, and public information (Murphy *et al.*, 2004). The National Institutes of Health has also expanded the focus of research to address how environmental factors and community infrastructure are related to obesity and the risk of diabetes and other chronic diseases. The ADA, an active member of NDEP, is partnering with the American Cancer Society and the American Heart Association to provide unified public messages and recommendations that address the role of nutrition in reducing chronic disease burden (Eyre *et al.*, 2004).

On an international scale, the World Health Organization has developed the Diabetes Programme, with the primary aims of setting international norms and standards, promoting surveillance, and encouraging prevention, especially in low- and middle-income communities and with a particular emphasis on developing countries. Advocacy work within this program has led to the development of Diabetes Action Now, a program in partnership with IDF that aims to increase awareness of diabetes and promote prevention in developing countries (World Health Organization and International Diabetes Federation, 2004).

With the growing awareness of the worldwide burden of diabetes, as well as the fact that scientific and economic studies, both in the care and prevention arenas, indicate that this burden does not have to occur, societal approaches need to be developed to complement clinical strategies to address diabetes in all of its complexities.

Future Directions

Understanding of gene–gene, gene–nutrient, and gene–nutrient–environment interactions can provide insights into the molecular basis of the metabolic dysregulation associated with diabetes (Permutt *et al.*, 2005; Roche *et al.*, 2005; Phillips *et al.*, 2008). This genetic heterogeneity is matched by clinical heterogeneity and the impact of various medications (e.g. steroids, novel antipsychotic agents) (American Diabetes Association *et al.*, 2004).

There is considerable evidence on the effectiveness of MNT and the role of nutrition in the primary and secondary prevention of diabetes and diabetes complications. However, additional research is needed to address environmental factors related to the rapid rise in the prevalence

of obesity and to develop effective techniques to reduce the obesity and physical inactivity epidemics – both of which are mutable (unlike age or race/ethnicity) and contribute to the increased prevalence of diabetes. Research is also needed to examine how nutritional factors other than energy balance may affect the risk of developing diabetes.

Current research will yield additional evidence to assess the long-term effectiveness of weight-loss lifestyle interventions in preventing diabetes and the development of diabetes complications. In the United States, not only is MNT an important component in the "ABCs" campaign to achieve goals for A1C, blood pressure, and cholesterol, but nutrition also is integral to current clinical trials addressing these risk factors.

Of particular practical need is a better understanding of how to both prevent and control weight gain. Evidence-based overweight and obesity guidelines were developed in 1998 by the National Heart, Lung, and Blood Institute (1998). Updates to these guidelines are currently being developed and will be released in the fall of 2011. Updates on progress can be found on the following website: http://www.nhlbi.nih.gov/guidelines/obesity/obesity2/index.htm. The guidelines recommend a comprehensive assessment that includes measuring and evaluating relative body weight or BMI, measuring body fat distribution (waist circumference as an index of visceral fat accumulation), evaluating overall risk status (for diabetes and related factors), and evaluating motivation to lose weight (National Heart, Lung, and Blood Institute, 1998). Although weight is frequently measured, BMI evaluation is often not recorded, and few practice settings measure waist circumference and assess weight-loss motivation. Research is needed to evaluate barriers to assessing weight, especially with respect to body-fat distribution and motivation. The more recent diabetes prevention trials strongly support a 5–10% weight loss in 6 months with a comprehensive approach that combines dietary, physical-activity, and behavioral interventions. Analysis from the DPP suggests that there may be a benefit of lifestyle changes even if no weight loss is achieved (Murphy *et al.*, 2004; Wing *et al.*, 2004; Wylie-Rosett *et al.*, 2006).

Another issue related to body weight is sustaining weight loss. A small, randomized trial of meal replacement in patients with T2D found a greater weight loss using a liquid-formula meal-replacement approach than with individualized meal planning. However, previous research suggests that providing menus may be as effective as providing food (Wing and Jeffery, 2001; Look AHEAD Research Group, 2003). Therefore, more research is needed to determine the extent to which being provided with a structure to avoid making food decisions facilitates achieving energy intake goals and weight loss. Further research on the short- and long-term effects of these formulas on metabolic parameters in individuals with diabetes is also needed.

Research needs to address how nutrition interacts with diabetes risk across the broad spectrum of this complex disorder to address primary prevention (how to curb the obesity epidemic and reduce the concomitant diabetes incidence), secondary prevention (how nutrition can help improve metabolic control and risks of developing complications), and tertiary prevention (how nutrition can help treat and control complications). These broad research needs will require multiple methods of research ranging from studies in nutrition–gene interaction and effects on cell metabolism to research that explores how community, state, national, and international policy may impact the prevalence of obesity and diabetes.

The long-term goal of MNT in diabetes is to prevent and/or delay complications by restoring metabolism as close to normal as possible. The focus for all classes of diabetes is on reducing cardiovascular risk factors such as hypertension and dyslipidemia. The distribution of macronutrient intake may vary based on a number of factors, including matching insulin to lifestyle in T1D and weight loss in T2D. Assessing micronutrient status is needed for patients in poor control, with complications, or with other evidence of being at risk.

There is no one diet for individuals with diabetes. MNT should be based on individual assessment and development of a treatment plan. Ideally, a registered dietitian who consults with the health-care team and the patient assesses the patient's needs and develops an individualized treatment plan that considers overall health needs in addition to ameliorating the metabolic effects of diabetes and its complications. Clearly, nutrition has and will continue to have a major role among persons with extant diabetes.

The importance of nutrition concepts and strategies has become even more important given the solid and convincing evidence of the ability to prevent T2D among high-risk individuals. The risk for developing diabetes is closely linked to lifestyle and obesity. Thus, the next great challenge for many will be to convert the important primary prevention science into active, practical, and widely available behavioral programs. These efforts will require more than just traditional nutrition science; they will also require the involvement of public health, industry, government, and society at large.

Suggestions for Further Reading

American Diabetes Association (2008) Position statement: nutrition recommendations and interventions for diabetes. *Diabetes Care* **31**, Suppl 1, S61–S78.

Franz, M.J., Powers, M.A., Leontos, C., *et al.* (2010) The evidence for medical nutrition therapy for type 1 and type 2 diabetes in adults. *J Am Diet Assoc* **110**, 1852–1889.

Mann, J.I., De Leeuw, I., Hermansen, K., *et al.* (2004) Evidence-based nutritional approaches to the treatment and prevention of diabetes mellitus. *Nutr Metab Cardiovasc Dis* **14**, 373–394.

Wylie-Rosett, J. and Vinicor, F. (2006) Diabetes mellitus In B.A. Bowman and R.M. Russell (eds), *Present Knowledge in Nutrition*, 9th Edn. International Life Sciences Institute, Washington, DC, pp. 669–686.

Wylie-Rosett, J., Albright, A.A., Apovian, C., *et al.* (2007) 2006–2007 American Diabetes Association Nutrition Recommendations: issues for practice translation. *J Am Diet Assoc* **107**, 1296–1304.

References

ADVANCE Collaborative Group, Patel, A., MacMahon, S., *et al.* (2008) Intensive blood glucose control and vascular outcomes in patients with type 2 diabetes. *N Engl J Med* **358**, 2560–2572.

Akerblom, H.K., Virtanen, S.M., Ilonen, J., *et al.* (2005) Dietary manipulation of beta cell autoimmunity in infants at increased risk of type 1 diabetes: a pilot study. *Diabetologia* **48**, 829–837.

American Diabetes Association (2000) Consensus Statement: Type 2 diabetes in children and adolescents. *Diabetes Care* **23**, 381–389.

American Diabetes Association (2008) Position statement: nutrition recommendations and interventions for diabetes. *Diabetes Care* **31**, Suppl 1, S61–S78.

American Diabetes Association (2010a) Position statement: diagnosis and classification of diabetes mellitus. *Diabetes Care* **33**, Suppl 1, S62–S69.

American Diabetes Association (2010b) Position statement: standards of medical care in diabetes. *Diabetes Care* **33**, Suppl 1, S11–S61.

American Diabetes Association, American Psychiatric Association, American Association of Clinical Endocrinologists, *et al.* (2004) Consensus development conference on antipsychotic drugs and obesity and diabetes. *Obes Res* **12**, 362–368.

American Dietetic Association (2002) *Nutrition Practice Guidelines for Type 1 and Type 2 Diabetes Mellitus (CD-ROM)*. American Dietetic Association, Chicago.

Anderson, J.W., Luan, J., and Høie, L.H. (2004a) Structured weight-loss programs: meta-analysis of weight loss at 24 weeks and assessment of effects of intervention intensity. *Adv Ther* **21**, 61–75.

Anderson, J.W., Randles, K.M., Kendall, C.W.C., *et al.* (2004b) Carbohydrate and fiber recommendations for individuals with diabetes: a quantitative assessment and meta-analysis of the evidence. *J Am Coll Nutr* **23**, 5–17.

Atkinson, M.A. (2005) ADA Outstanding Scientific Achievement Lecture 2004. Thirty years of investigating the autoimmune basis for type 1 diabetes: why can't we prevent or reverse this disease? *Diabetes* **54**, 1253–1263.

Avenell, A., Brown, T.J., McGee, M.A., *et al.* (2004) What are the long-term benefits of weight reducing diets in adults? A systematic review of randomized controlled trials. *J Hum Nutr Diet* **17**, 317–335.

Barnard, N.D., Cohen, J., Jenkins, D.J., *et al.* (2009) A low-fat vegan diet and a conventional diabetes diet in the treatment of type 2 diabetes: a randomized, controlled, 74-wk clinical trial. *Am J Clin Nutr* **89**, 1588S–1596S.

Barringer, T.A., Kirk, J.K., Santaniello, A.C., *et al.* (2003) Effect of a multivitamin and mineral supplement on infection and quality of life. *Ann Intern Med* **138**, 365–371.

Bateson, P., Barker, D., Clutton-Brock, T., *et al.* (2004) Developmental plasticity and human health. *Nature* **430**, 419–421.

Belalcazar, L.M., Reboussin, D.M., Haffner, S.M., *et al.* (2010) A one-year lifestyle intervention for weight loss in persons with type 2 diabetes reduces high C-reactive protein levels and identifies metabolic predictors of change, from the Look AHEAD (Action for Health in Diabetes) Study. *Diabetes Care* **33**, 2297–1303.

Billings, L.K., Fanelli, R.R., Taylor, A., *et al.* (2010) Discovery of novel variants in the SLC30A8 gene in the multiethnic cohort of the Diabetes Prevention Program (DPP). Poster session, 60th Annual Meeting, The American Society of Human Genetics, Washington, DC.

Bodington, M.J., McNally, P.G., and Burden, A.C. (1994) Cow's milk and type 1 childhood diabetes: no increase in risk. *Diabet Med* **11**, 663–665.

Bønaa, K.H., Njølstad, I., Ueland, P.M., *et al.* (2006) Homocysteine lowering and cardiovascular events after acute myocardial infarction. *N Engl J Med* **354**, 1578–1588.

Brand-Miller, J., Hayne, S., Petocz, P., *et al.* (2003) Low-glycemic index diets in the management of diabetes: a meta-analysis of randomized controlled trials. *Diabetes Care* **26**, 2261–2267.

Buchwald, H., Avidor, Y., Braunwald, E., *et al.* (2004) Bariatric surgery: a systematic review and meta-analysis. *JAMA* **292**, 1724–1737.

Canadian Diabetes Association Clinical Practice Guidelines Expert Committee. Canadian Diabetes Association (2008) Clinical practice guidelines for the prevention and management of diabetes in Canada. *Can J Diabetes* **32** (Suppl 1), S1–S201.

Cefalu, W.T. and Hu, F.B. (2004) Role of chromium in human health and in diabetes. *Diabetes Care* **27**, 2741–2751.

Centers for Disease Control and Prevention (2008) *National Diabetes Fact Sheet: General Information and National Estimates on Diabetes in the United States, 2007*. US Department of Health and Human Services, Centers for Disease Control and Prevention, Atlanta, GA.

Centers for Disease Control and Prevention Primary Prevention Working Group (2004) Primary prevention of type 2 diabetes mellitus by lifestyle intervention: implications for health policy. *Ann Intern Med* **140**, 951–957.

Cho, N.H., Lim, S., Jang, H.C., *et al.* (2005a) Elevated homocysteine as a risk factor for the development of diabetes in women with a previous history of gestational diabetes mellitus: a 4-year prospective study. *Diabetes Care* **28**, 2750–2755.

Cho, S.H., Kim, T.H., Lee, N.H., *et al.* (2005b) Effects of Cassia tora fiber supplement on serum lipids in Korean diabetic patients. *J Med Food* **8**, 311–318.

Christiansen, E., Schnider, S., Palmvig, B., *et al.* (1997) Intake of a diet high in trans monounsaturated fatty acids or saturated fatty acids. Effects on postprandial insulinemia and glycemia in obese patients with NIDDM. *Diabetes Care* **20**, 881–887.

Cicero, A.F., Derosa, G., and Gaddi, A. (2004) What do herbalists suggest to diabetic patients in order to improve glycemic control? Evaluation of scientific evidence and potential risks. *Acta Diabetol* **41**, 91–98.

Clark, C.A., Gardiner, J., McBurney, M.I., *et al.* (2006) Effects of breakfast meal composition on second meal metabolic responses in adults with type 2 diabetes mellitus. *Eur J Clin Nutr* **60**, 1122–1129.

Connor, W.E. (2004) Will the dietary intake of fish prevent atherosclerosis in diabetic women? *Am J Clin Nutr* **80**, 535–536.

Coppell, K.J., Kataoka, M., Williams, S.M., *et al.* (2010) Nutritional intervention in patients with type 2 diabetes who are hyperglycaemic despite optimised drug treatment – Lifestyle Over and Above Drugs in Diabetes (LOADD) study: randomised controlled trial. *Br Med J* **341**, c3393.

Costacou, T., Ma, B., King, I.B., *et al.* (2008) Plasma and dietary vitamin E in relation to insulin secretion and sensitivity. *Diabetes Obes Metab* **10**, 223–228.

DAFNE Study Group (2002) Training in flexible, intensive insulin management to enable dietary freedom in people with type 1 diabetes: dose adjustment for normal eating (DAFNE) randomised controlled trial. *Br Med J* **325**, 746.

Davis, N., Forbes, B., and Wylie-Rosett, J. (2009) Nutritional strategies in type 2 diabetes. *Mt Sinai J Med* **76**, 257–268.

Delahanty, L.M. and Halford, B.N. (1993) The role of diet behaviors in achieving improved glycemic control in intensively treated patients in the Diabetes Control and Complications Trial. *Diabetes Care* **16**, 1453–1458.

Diabetes Control and Complications Trial Research Group (1988) Weight gain associated with intensive therapy in the diabetes control and complications trial. The DCCT Research Group. *Diabetes Care* **11**, 567–573.

Diabetes Control and Complications Trial Research Group (1993) The effect of intensive treatment of diabetes on the development and progression of long-term complications in insulin-dependent diabetes mellitus. *N Engl J Med* **329**, 977–986.

Diabetes Prevention Program Research Group (2002) The Diabetes Prevention Program (DPP): description of lifestyle intervention. *Diabetes Care* **25**, 2165–2171.

Duckworth, W., Abraira, C., Moritz, T., *et al.* (2009) Glucose control and vascular complications in veterans with type 2 diabetes. *N Engl J Med* **360**, 129–139.

Dullaart, R.P., Beusekamp, B.J., Meijer, S., *et al.* (1993) Long-term effects of protein-restricted diet on albuminuria and renal function in IDDM patients without clinical nephropathy and hypertension. *Diabetes Care* **16**, 483–492.

Esposito, K., Maiorino, M.I., Ciotola, M., *et al.* (2009) Effects of a Mediterranean-style diet on the need for antihyperglycemic drug therapy in patients with newly diagnosed type 2 diabetes: a randomized trial. *Ann Intern Med* **151**, 306–314.

Expert Panel on Detection, Evaluation, and Treatment of High Blood Cholesterol in Adults (2001) Executive Summary of the Third Report of the National Cholesterol Education Program (NCEP) Expert Panel on Detection, Evaluation, and Treatment of High Blood Cholesterol in Adults (Adult Treatment Panel III). *JAMA* **285**, 2486–2497.

Eyre, H., Kahn, R., Robertson, R.M., *et al.* (2004) Preventing cancer, cardiovascular disease, and diabetes: a common agenda for the American Cancer Society, the American Diabetes Association, and the American Heart Association. *Circulation* **109**, 3244–3255.

Flammang, A.M., Kendall, D.M., Baumgartner, C.J., *et al.* (2006) Effect of a viscous fiber bar on postprandial glycemia in subjects with type 2 diabetes. *J Am Coll Nutr* **25**, 409–414.

Franz, M.J., Bantle, J.P., Beebe, C.A., *et al.* (2002) Nutrition principles for the management of diabetes and related complications (technical review). *Diabetes Care* **17**, 490–518.

Franz, M.J., Powers, M.A., Leontos, C., *et al.* (2010) The evidence for medical nutrition therapy for type 1 and type 2 diabetes in adults. *J Am Diet Assoc* **110**, 1852–1889.

Freeman, J. (2005) Healthy eating 101. Know your fats. Protect your heart by replacing harmful types with healthier ones. *Diabetes Forecast* **58**, 29–64.

Fronczak, C.M., Barón, A.E., Chase, H.P., *et al.* (2003) In utero dietary exposures and risk of islet autoimmunity in children. *Diabetes Care* **26**, 3237–3242.

Garg, A. (1998) High-monounsaturated-fat diets for patients with diabetes mellitus: a meta-analysis. *Am J Clin Nutr* **67**, 577S–582S.

Genuth, S., Sun, W., Cleary, P., *et al.* (2005) Glycation and carboxymethyllysine levels in skin collagen predict the risk of future 10-year progression of diabetic retinopathy and nephropathy in the diabetes control and complications trial and epidemiology of diabetes interventions and complications participants with type 1 diabetes. *Diabetes* **54**, 3103–3111.

Gilbertson, H.R., Brand-Miller, J.C., Thorburn, A.W., *et al.* (2001) The effect of flexible low glycemic index dietary advice versus measured carbohydrate exchange diets on glycemic control in children with type 1 diabetes. *Diabetes Care* **24**, 1137–1143.

Gillis, B., Mobley, C., Stadler, D.D., *et al.* (2009) Rationale, design and methods of the HEALTHY study nutrition intervention component. *Int. J Obes (Lond)* **33**, S29–S36.

Hamman, R.F., Wing, R.R., Edelstein, S.L., *et al.* (2006) Effect of weight loss with lifestyle intervention on risk of diabetes. *Diabetes Care* **29**, 2102–2107.

Hansen, H.P., Tauber-Lassen, E., Jensen, B.R., *et al.* (2002) Effect of dietary protein restriction on prognosis in patients with diabetic nephropathy. *Kidney Int* **62**, 220–228.

HAPO Study Cooperative Research Group (2009) Hyperglycemia and Adverse Pregnancy Outcome (HAPO) Study: associations with neonatal anthropometrics. *Diabetes* **58**, 453–459.

HAPO Study Cooperative Research Group, Metzger, B.E., Lowe, L.P., *et al.* (2008) Hyperglycemia and adverse pregnancy outcomes. *N Engl J Med* **358**, 1991–2002.

Harris, M.I. and Eastman, R.C. (1998) Is there a glycemic threshold for mortality risk? *Diabetes Care* **21**, 331–333.

Harris, M.I., Klein, R., Welborn, T.A., *et al.* (1992) Onset of NIDDM occurs at least 4–7 yr before clinical diagnosis. *Diabetes Care* **15**, 815–819.

Hartweg, J., Farmer, A.J., and Holman, R.R. (2009) Potential impact of omega-3 treatment on cardiovascular disease in type 2 diabetes. *Curr Opin Lipidol* **20**, 30–38.

HEALTHY Study Group, Foster, G.D., Linder, B., *et al.* (2010) A school-based intervention for diabetes risk reduction. *N Engl J Med* **363**, 443–453.

Howard, B.V. and Wylie-Rosett, J. (2002) Sugar and cardiovascular disease: a statement for healthcare professionals from the Committee on Nutrition of the Council on Nutrition, Physical Activity, and Metabolism of the American Heart Association. *Circulation* **106**, 523–527.

Huijberts, M.S.P., Becker, A., and Stehouwer, C.D.A. (2005) Homocysteine and vascular disease in diabetes: a double hit? *Clin Chem Lab Med* **43**, 993–1000.

Hyppönen, E., Läärä, E., Reunanen, A., *et al.* (2001) Intake of vitamin D and risk of type 1 diabetes: a birth-cohort study. *Lancet* **358**, 1500–1503.

Institute of Medicine (2005) *Dietary Reference Intakes for Energy, Carbohydrate, Fiber, Fat, Fatty Acids, Cholesterol, Protein, and Amino Acids*. National Academies Press, Washington, DC.

International Diabetes Federation (2011) *IDF Diabetes Atlas, 5th Ed.* International Diabetes Federation, Brussels.

Ismail-Beigi, F., Craven, T., Banerji, M.A., *et al.* (2010) Effect of intensive treatment of hyperglycaemia on microvascular outcomes in type 2 diabetes: an analysis of the ACCORD randomised trial. *Lancet* **376**, 419–430.

Jack, L., Jr, Liburd, L., Spencer, T., *et al.* (2004) Understanding the environmental issues in diabetes self-management education research: a reexamination of 8 studies in community-based settings. *Ann Intern Med* **140**, 964–971.

Jenkins, D.J., Kendall, C.W., Augustin, L.S., *et al.* (2002) Effect of wheat bran on glycemic control and risk factors for cardiovascular disease in type 2 diabetes. *Diabetes Care* **25**, 1522–1528.

Jenkins, D.J.A., Kendall, C.W.C., McKeown-Eyssen, G., *et al.* (2008) Effect of a low-glycemic index or a high-cereal fiber diet on type 2 diabetes. *JAMA* **300**, 2742–2753.

Johnson, R.K., Appel, L.J., Brands, M., *et al.* (2009) Dietary sugars intake and cardiovascular health: a scientific statement from the American Heart Association. *Circulation* **120**, 1011–1020.

Jovanovic, L. (1998) American Diabetes Association's Fourth International Workshop-Conference on Gestational Diabetes Mellitus: summary and discussion. Therapeutic interventions. *Diabetes Care* **21**, Suppl 2, B131–B137.

Jovanovic, L. (2000) Controversies in the diagnosis and treatment of gestational diabetes. *Cleve Clin J Med* **67**, 481–482.

Jovanovic, L. and Pettitt, D.J. (2001) Gestational diabetes mellitus. *JAMA* **286**, 2516–2518.

Karantonis, H.C., Fragopoulou, E., Antonopoulou, S., *et al.* (2006) Effect of fast-food Mediterranean-type diet on type 2 diabetics and healthy human subjects' platelet aggregation. *Diabetes Res Clin Pract* **72**, 33–41.

Knekt, P., Reunanen, A., Marniemi, J., *et al.* (1999) Low vitamin E status is a potential risk factor for insulin-dependent diabetes mellitus. *J Intern Med* **245**, 99–102.

Knowler, W.C., Barrett-Connor, E., Fowler, S.E., *et al.* (2002) Reduction in the incidence of type 2 diabetes with lifestyle intervention or metformin. *N Engl J Med* **346**, 393–403.

Kripke, C. (2005) Does a low glycemic index diet reduce CHD? *Am Fam Physician* **72**, 1224.

Landon, M.B., Spong, C.Y., Thom, E., *et al.* (2009) A multicenter, randomized trial of treatment for mild gestational diabetes. *N Engl J Med* **361**, 1339–1348.

Leary, J., Pettitt, D.J., and Jovanovič, L. (2010) Gestational diabetes guidelines in a HAPO world. *Best Practice and Research Clinical Endocrinology and Metabolism* **24**, 673–685.

Li, G., Zhang, P., Wang, J., *et al.* (2008) The long-term effect of lifestyle interventions to prevent diabetes in the China Da Qing Diabetes Prevention Study: a 20-year follow-up study. *Lancet* **371**, 1783–1789.

Lindström, J., Louheranta, A., Mannelin, M., *et al.* (2003) The Finnish Diabetes Prevention Study (DPS): Lifestyle intervention and 3-year results on diet and physical activity. *Diabetes Care* **26**, 3230–3236.

Liu, J.P., Zhang, M., Wang, W.Y., *et al.* (2004) Chinese herbal medicines for type 2 diabetes mellitus. *Cochrane Database Syst Rev* CD003642.

Lonn, E., Bosch, J., Yusuf, S., *et al.* (2005) Effects of long-term vitamin E supplementation on cardiovascular events and cancer: a randomized controlled trial. *JAMA* **293**, 1338–1347.

Lonn, E., Yusuf, S., Arnold, M.J., *et al.* (2006) Homocysteine lowering with folic acid and B vitamins in vascular disease. *N Engl J Med* **354**, 1567–1577.

Look AHEAD Research Group (2003) Look AHEAD (Action for Health in Diabetes): design and methods for a clinical trial of weight loss for the prevention of cardiovascular disease in type 2 diabetes. *Controlled Clin Trials* **24**, 610–628.

Look AHEAD Research Group (2010) Long-term effects of a lifestyle intervention on weight and cardiovascular risk factors in individuals with type 2 diabetes mellitus: four-year results of the Look AHEAD Trial. *Arch Intern Med* **170**, 1566–1575.

Look AHEAD Research Group, Pi-Sunyer, X., Blackburn, G., *et al.* (2007) Reduction in weight and cardiovascular disease risk factors in individuals with type 2 diabetes: one-year results of the look AHEAD trial. *Diabetes Care* **30**, 1374–1383.

Lovejoy, J.C. (2005) The impact of nuts on diabetes and diabetes risk. *Curr Diab Rep* **5**, 379–384.

Lu, Z.X., Walker, K.Z., Muir, J.G., *et al.* (2004) Arabinoxylan fibre improves metabolic control in people with Type II diabetes. *Eur J Clin Nutr* **58**, 621–628.

Ma, Y., Olendzki, B.C., Merriam, P.A., *et al.* (2008) A randomized clinical trial comparing low-glycemic index versus ADA dietary education among individuals with type 2 diabetes. *Nutrition* **24**, 45–56.

Magnoni, D., Rouws, C.H.F.C., Lansink, M., *et al.* (2008) Long-term use of a diabetes-specific oral nutritional supplement results in a low-postprandial glucose response in diabetes patients. *Diabetes Res Clin Pract* **80**, 75–82.

Mann, J.I., De Leeuw, I., Hermansen, K., *et al.* (2004) Evidence-based nutritional approaches to the treatment and prevention of diabetes mellitus. *Nutr Metab Cardiovasc Dis* **14**, 373–394.

Mayer, E.J., Hamman, R.F., Gay, E.C., *et al.* (1988) Reduced risk of IDDM among breast-fed children. The Colorado IDDM Registry. *Diabetes* **37**, 1625–1632.

Mayer-Davis, E.J., Sparks, K.C., Hirst, K., *et al.* (2004) Dietary intake in the Diabetes Prevention Program cohort: baseline and 1-year post-randomization. *Ann Epidemiol* **14**, 763–772.

Mostad, I.L., Bjerve, K.S., Bjorgaas, M.R., *et al.* (2006) Effects of n-3 fatty acids in subjects with type 2 diabetes: reduction of insulin sensitivity and time-dependent alteration from carbohydrate to fat oxidation. *Am J Clin Nutr* **84**, 540–550.

Muntoni, S. and Muntoni, S. (2006) Epidemiological association between some dietary habits and the increasing incidence of type 1 diabetes worldwide. *Ann Nutr Metab* **50**, 11–19.

Murakami, K., Okubo, H., and Sasaki, S. (2005) Effect of dietary factors on incidence of type 2 diabetes: a systematic review of cohort studies. *J Nutr Sci Vitaminol (Tokyo)* **51**, 292–310.

Murphy, D., Chapel, T., and Clark, C. (2004) Moving diabetes care from science to practice: The evolution of the National Diabetes Prevention and Control Program. *Ann Intern Med* **140**, 978–984.

Narendhirakannan, R.T., Subramanian, S., and Kandaswamy, M. (2005) Mineral content of some medicinal plants used in the treatment of diabetes mellitus. *Biol Trace Elem Res* **103**, 109–115.

Narita, T., Koshimura, J., Meguro, H., *et al.* (2001) Determination of optimal protein contents for a protein restriction diet in type 2 diabetic patients with microalbuminuria. *Tohoku J Exp Med* **193**, 45–55.

Nathan, D.M., Buse, J.B., Davidson, M.B., *et al.* (2009) Medical management of hyperglycemia in type 2 diabetes: a consensus algorithm for the initiation and adjustment of therapy: a consensus statement of the American Diabetes Association and the European Association for the Study of Diabetes. *Diabetes Care* **32**, 193–203.

Nathan, D.M., Cleary, P.A., Backlund, J.Y., *et al.* (2005) Intensive diabetes treatment and cardiovascular disease in patients with type 1 diabetes. *N Engl J Med* **353**, 2643–2653.

National Heart, Lung, and Blood Institute (1998) *Clinical Guidelines on the Identification, Evaluation, and Treatment of Overweight and Obesity in Adults: The Evidence Report.* National Institutes of Health, Bethesda, MD.

Nettleton, J.A. and Katz, R. (2005) n-3 long-chain polyunsaturated fatty acids in type 2 diabetes: A review. *J Am Diet Assoc* **105**, 428–440.

Nordmann, A.J., Nordmann, A., Briel, M., *et al.* (2006) Effects of low-carbohydrate vs low-fat diets on weight loss and cardiovascular risk factors: a meta-analysis of randomized controlled trials. *Arch Intern Med* **166**, 285–293.

Norris, J.M. and Scott, F.W. (1996) A meta-analysis of infant diet and insulin-dependent diabetes mellitus: do biases play a role? *Epidemiology* **7**, 87–92.

Norris, J.M., Barriga, K., Klingensmith, G., *et al.* (2003) Timing of initial cereal exposure in infancy and risk of islet autoimmunity. *JAMA* **290**, 1713–1720.

Norris, J.M., Beaty, B., Klingensmith, G., *et al.* (1996) Lack of association between early exposure to cow's milk protein and beta-cell autoimmunity. Diabetes Autoimmunity Study in the Young (DAISY). *JAMA* **276**, 609–614.

Norris, J.M., Yin, X., Lamb, M.M., *et al.* (2007) Omega-3 polyunsaturated fatty acid intake and islet autoimmunity in children at increased risk for type 1 diabetes. *JAMA* **298**, 1420–1428.

Norris, S.L., Zhang, X., Avenell, A., *et al.* (2004) Long-term effectiveness of lifestyle and behavioral weight loss interventions in adults with type 2 diabetes: a meta-analysis. *Am J Med* **117**, 762–774.

Norris, S.L., Zhang, X., Avenell, A., *et al.* (2005) Long-term effectiveness of weight-loss interventions in adults with pre-diabetes: a review. *Am J Prev Med* **28**, 126–139.

Obesity Education Initiative Expert Panel (1998) *Clinical Guidelines on the Identification, Evaluation, and Treatment of Overweight and Obesity in Adults: The Evidence Report.* US Department of Health and Human Services, Public Health Service, National Institutes of Health, National Heart, Lung, and Blood Institute.

Ogilvie, D. and Hamlet, N. (2005) Obesity: the elephant in the corner. *Br Med J* **331**, 1545–1548.

Orchard, T.J., Temprosa, M., Goldberg, R., *et al.* (2005) The effect of metformin and intensive lifestyle intervention on the metabolic syndrome: the Diabetes Prevention Program randomized trial. *Ann Intern Med* **142**, 611–619.

Pan, X.R., Li, G.W., Hu, Y.H., *et al.* (1997) Effects of diet and exercise in preventing NIDDM in people with impaired glucose tolerance. The Da Qing IGT and Diabetes Study. *Diabetes Care* **20**, 537–544.

Pedersen, H., Petersen, M., Major-Pedersen, A., *et al.* (2003) Influence of fish oil supplementation on in vivo and in vitro oxidation resistance of low-density lipoprotein in type 2 diabetes. *Eur J Clin Nutr* **57**, 713–720.

Permutt, M.A., Wasson, J., and Cox, N. (2005) Genetic epidemiology of diabetes. *J Clin Invest* **115**, 1431–1439.

Phillips, C.M., Tierney, A.C., and Roche, H.M. (2008) Gene–nutrient interactions in the metabolic syndrome. *J Nutrigenet Nutrigenomics* **1**, 136–151.

Pijls, L.T., de Vries, H., van Eijk, J.T., *et al.* (2002) Protein restriction, glomerular filtration rate and albuminuria in patients with type 2 diabetes mellitus: a randomized trial. *Eur J Clin Nutr* **56**, 1200–1207.

Pomerleau, J., Verdy, M., Garrel, D.R., *et al.* (1993) Effect of protein intake on glycaemic control and renal function in type 2 (non-insulin-dependent) diabetes mellitus. *Diabetologia* **36**, 829–834.

Pooya, S., Jalali, M.D., Jazayery, A.D., *et al.* (2010) The efficacy of omega-3 fatty acid supplementation on plasma homocysteine and malondialdehyde levels of type 2 diabetic patients. *Nutr Metab Cardiovasc Dis* **20**, 326–331.

Prentice, A.M., Rayco-Solon, P., and Moore, S.E. (2005) Insights from the developing world: thrifty genotypes and thrifty phenotypes. *Proc Nutr Soc* **64**, 153–161.

Roche, H.M., Phillips, C., and Gibney, M.J. (2005) The metabolic syndrome: the crossroads of diet and genetics. *Proc Nutr Soc* **64**, 371–377.

Rydén, L., Standl, E., Bartnik, M., *et al.* (2007) Guidelines on diabetes, pre-diabetes, and cardiovascular diseases: executive summary. The Task Force on Diabetes and Cardiovascular Diseases of the European Society of Cardiology (ESC) and of the European Association for the Study of Diabetes (EASD). *Eur Heart J* **28**, 88–136.

Salas-Salvado, J., Bullo, M., Babio, N., *et al.* (2011) Reduction in the incidence of type 2 diabetes with the Mediterranean diet. *Diabetes Care* **34**, 14–19.

Schulz, M., Liese, A.D., Mayer-Davis, E.J., *et al.* (2005) Nutritional correlates of dietary glycaemic index: new aspects from a population perspective. *Br J Nutr* **94**, 397–406.

Schwartz, J.R., Marsh, R.G., and Draelos, Z.D. (2005) Zinc and skin health: overview of physiology and pharmacology. *Dermatol Surg* **31**, 837–847.

SEARCH for Diabetes in Youth Study Group (2006) The burden of diabetes mellitus among US youth: prevalence estimates from the SEARCH for Diabetes in Youth Study. *Pediatrics* **118**, 1510–1518.

Shai, I., Schwarzfuchs, D., Henkin, Y., *et al.* (2008) Weight loss with a low-carbohydrate, Mediterranean, or low-fat diet. *N Engl J Med* **359**, 229–241.

Sheard, N.F., Clark, N.G., Brand-Miller, J.C., *et al.* (2004) Dietary carbohydrate (amount and type) in the prevention and management of diabetes: a statement by the American Diabetes Association. *Diabetes Care* **27**, 2266–2271.

Sievenpiper, J.L., Carleton, A.J., Chatha, S., *et al.* (2009) Heterogeneous effects of fructose on blood lipids in individuals with type 2 diabetes. *Diabetes Care* **32**, 1930–1937.

Skyler, J.S., Bergenstal, R., Bonow, R.O., *et al.* (2009) Intensive glycemic control and the prevention of cardiovascular events: Implications of the ACCORD, ADVANCE, and VA Diabetes Trials: A Position Statement of the American Diabetes Association and a Scientific Statement of the American College of Cardiology Foundation and the American Heart Association. *J Am Coll Cardiol* **53**, 298–304.

Snell-Bergeon, J.K., Chartier-Logan, C., Maahs, D.M., *et al.* (2009) Adults with type 1 diabetes eat a high-fat atherogenic diet that is associated with coronary artery calcium. *Diabetologia* **52**, 801–809.

Speight, J., Amiel, S.A., Bradley, C., *et al.* (2010) Long-term biomedical and psychosocial outcomes following DAFNE (Dose Adjustment For Normal Eating) structured education to promote intensive insulin therapy in adults with sub-optimally controlled Type 1 diabetes. *Diabetes Res Clin Pract* **89**, 22–29.

Stratton, I.M., Adler, A.I., Neil, H.A.W., *et al.* (2000) Association of glycaemia with macrovascular and microvascular complications of type 2 diabetes (UKPDS 35): prospective observational study. *Br Med J* **321**, 405–412.

Tapola, N., Karvonen, H., Niskanen, L., *et al.* (2005) Glycemic responses of oat bran products in type 2 diabetic patients. *Nutr Metab Cardiovasc Dis* **15**, 255–261.

Thomas, D. and Elliott, E.J. (2009) Low glycaemic index, or low glycaemic load, diets for diabetes mellitus. *Cochrane Database Syst Rev* CD006296.

Toole, J.F., Malinow, M.R., Chambless, L.E., *et al.* (2004) Lowering homocysteine in patients with ischemic stroke to prevent recurrent stroke, myocardial infarction, and death: the Vitamin Intervention for Stroke Prevention (VISP) randomized controlled trial. *JAMA* **291**, 565–575.

TRIGR Study Group (2007) Study design of the Trial to Reduce IDDM in the Genetically at Risk (TRIGR). *Pediatr Diabetes* **8**, 117–137.

Tuomilehto, J., Lindström, J., Eriksson, J.G., *et al.* (2001) Prevention of type 2 diabetes mellitus by changes in lifestyle among subjects with impaired glucose tolerance. *N Engl J Med* **344**, 1343–1350.

Tushuizen, M.E., Diamant, M., and Heine, R.J. (2005) Postprandial dysmetabolism and cardiovascular disease in type 2 diabetes. *Postgrad Med J* **81**, 1–6.

UK Prospective Diabetes Study Group (1998a) Effect of intensive blood-glucose control with metformin on complications in overweight patients with type 2 diabetes (UKPDS 34). *Lancet* **352**, 854–865.

UK Prospective Diabetes Study Group (1998b) Intensive blood-glucose control with sulphonylureas or insulin compared with conventional treatment and risk of complications in patients with type 2 diabetes (UKPDS 33). *Lancet* **352**, 837–853.

UK Prospective Diabetes Study Group (1998c) Tight blood pressure control and risk of macrovascular and microvascular complications in type 2 diabetes: UKPDS 38. *Br Med J* **317**, 703–713.

US Department of Health and Human Services (2010) *Diabetes Prevention and Control: A Public Health Imperative.* http://www.healthierus.gov/steps/summit/prevportfolio/strategies/reducing/diabetes/contents_diabetes.htm [2010, 08/17].

Uusitupa, M. (2005) Gene–diet interaction in relation to the prevention of obesity and type 2 diabetes: Evidence from the Finnish Diabetes Prevention Study. *Nutr Metab Cardiovasc Dis* **15**, 225–233.

Uusitupa, M., Lindi, V., Louheranta, A., *et al.* (2003) Long-term improvement in insulin sensitivity by changing lifestyles of people with impaired glucose tolerance: 4-year results from the Finnish Diabetes Prevention Study. *Diabetes* **52**, 2532–2538.

Vaarala, O. (2005) Is type 1 diabetes a disease of the gut immune system triggered by cow's milk insulin? *Adv Exp Med Biol* **569**, 151–156.

Vaarala, O., Knip, M., Paronen, J., *et al.* (1999) Cow's milk formula feeding induces primary immunization to insulin in infants at genetic risk for type 1 diabetes. *Diabetes* **48**, 1389–1394.

van Dam, R.M. and Hu, F.B. (2005) Coffee consumption and risk of type 2 diabetes: a systematic review. *JAMA* **294**, 97–104.

van Dam, R.M., Hoebee, B., Seidell, J.C., *et al.* (2005) Common variants in the ATP-sensitive K+ channel genes KCNJ11 (Kir6.2) and ABCC8 (SUR1) in relation to glucose intolerance: population-based studies and meta-analyses. *Diabet Med* **22**, 590–598.

Venters, J.Y., Hunt, A.E., Pope, J.F., *et al.* (2004) Are patients with diabetes receiving the same message from dietitians and nurses? *Diabetes Educ* **30**, 293–300.

Virtanen, S.M., Hyppönen, E., Läärä, E., *et al.* (1998) Cow's milk consumption, disease-associated autoantibodies and type 1 diabetes mellitus: a follow-up study in siblings of diabetic children. Childhood Diabetes in Finland Study Group. *Diabet Med* **15**, 730–738.

Virtanen, S.M., Kenward, M.G., Erkkola, M., *et al.* (2006) Age at introduction of new foods and advanced beta cell autoimmunity in young children with HLA-conferred susceptibility to type 1 diabetes. *Diabetologia* **49**, 1512–1521.

Vlassara, H., Cai, W., Crandall, J., *et al.* (2002) Inflammatory mediators are induced by dietary glycotoxins, a major risk factor for diabetic angiopathy. *Proc Natl Acad Sci USA* **99**, 15596–15601.

Vuksan, V., Whitham, D., Sievenpiper, J.L., *et al.* Supplementation of conventional therapy with the novel grain Salba (*Salvia hispanica* L.) improves major and emerging cardiovascular risk factors in type 2 diabetes: results of a randomized controlled trial. *Diabetes Care* **30**, 2804–2810.

Whiting, D., Unwin, N., and Roglic, G. (2010) Diabetes: equity and social determinants. In E. Blas and A.S. Kurup (eds), *Equity, Social Determinants and Public Health*. World Health Organization, Geneva, pp. 77–94.

Wild, S., Roglic, G., Green, A., *et al.* (2004) Global prevalence of diabetes: estimates for the year 2000 and projections for 2030. *Diabetes Care* **27**, 1047–1053.

Wing, R.R. and Jeffery, R.W. (2001) Food provision as a strategy to promote weight loss. *Obes Res* **9**, 271S–275S.

Wing, R.R., Hamman, R.F., Bray, G.A., *et al.* (2004) Achieving weight and activity goals among diabetes prevention program lifestyle participants. *Obes Res* **12**, 1426–1434.

Wolever, T.M., Gibbs, A.L., Mehling, C., *et al.* (2008) The Canadian Trial of Carbohydrates in Diabetes (CCD), a 1-y controlled trial of low-glycemic-index dietary carbohydrate in type 2 diabetes: no effect on glycated hemoglobin but reduction in C-reactive protein. *Am J Clin Nutr* **87**, 114–125.

Woodman, R.J., Mori, T.A., Burke, V., *et al.* (2002) Effects of purified eicosapentaenoic and docosahexaenoic acids on glycemic control, blood pressure, and serum lipids in type 2 diabetic patients with treated hypertension. *Am J Clin Nutr* **76**, 1007–1015.

World Health Organization (2011) Use of glycated haemoglobin (HbA1c) in the diagnosis of diabetes mellitus (WHO/NMH/CHP/CPM/11.1). World Health Organization, Geneva. http://www.who.int/diabetes/publications/report-hba1c_2011.pdf.

World Health Organization and International Diabetes Federation (2004) *Diabetes Action Now*. World Health Organization, Geneva.

Wylie-Rosett, J., Herman, W.H., and Goldberg, R.B. (2006) Lifestyle intervention to prevent diabetes: intensive and cost effective. *Curr Opin Lipidol* **17**, 37–44.

Wylie-Rosett, J., Segal-Isaacson, C.J., and Segal-Isaacson, A. (2004) Carbohydrates and increases in obesity: does the type of carbohydrate make a difference? *Obes Res* **12**, Suppl 2, 124S–129S.

Yang, W., Lu, J., Weng, J., *et al.* (2010) Prevalence of diabetes among men and women in China. *N Engl J Med* **362**, 1090–1101.

Yoon, J.W. and Jun, H.S. (2005) Autoimmune destruction of pancreatic beta cells. *Am J Ther* **12**, 580–591.

Zhang, P., Zhang, X., Brown, J., *et al.* (2010) Global healthcare expenditure on diabetes for 2010 and 2030. *Diabetes Res Clin Pract* **87**, 293–301.

Ziai, S.A., Larijani, B., Akhoondzadeh, S., *et al.* (2005) Psyllium decreased serum glucose and glycosylated hemoglobin significantly in diabetic outpatients. *J Ethnopharmacol* **102**, 202–207.

50

OSTEOPOROSIS

JOHN J.B. ANDERSON, PhD

University of North Carolina, Chapel Hill, North Carolina, USA

Summary

Advances in understanding of the roles of nutrient requirements for bone health in older populations have been achieved over the last decade. This chapter focuses on the nutritional requirements that impact on osteoporosis late in life. Calcium needs have been established as more critical than other single nutrients as determined by several meta-analyses of randomized controlled trials. Several other nutrients, including phosphorus, vitamin D, vitamin K, and protein, remain important for bone health and the prevention or delay of osteoporosis and fragility fractures. Healthy diets providing balanced intakes of all nutrients continue to be the preferred way to promote bone health of older adults along with other healthy lifestyles, such as participating in routine physical activities, not smoking, and consuming only moderate amounts of alcohol per day, if any. Physical activity helps maintain muscle mass, equilibrium/balance, and the general overall health of organ systems. Together, sound diet and regular activity help promote bone health and delay or prevent osteoporosis and associated fractures of elders.

Introduction

Early-life skeletal development is critical for late-life bone health. The individual bone models created by early-life events suggest that skeletal tissue is highly plastic until the early teens or even during the pre-teens in females, who are more developmentally advanced than males. The nutritional needs of growing children and adolescents required for the achievement of optimal bone mass and skeletal architecture remain, along with physical activity, the cornerstone for the prevention or delay of late-life osteoporosis (Weaver and Heaney, 2008).

Although osteoporosis usually manifests itself late in life, it is a disorder of bone growth greatly influenced by diet and lifestyle during the first two decades of life. The etiology of osteoporosis is complex and it is greatly affected by environmental factors, both dietary and usual lifestyle behaviors, as well as by genetic factors that are only recently being recognized. Osteoporosis is, therefore, a disease of multifactorial etiology, but not, strictly speaking, solely a disease of calcium deficiency.

Genetic analyses suggest that environmental factors contribute approximately 20% to the variance in bone density measurements (Ralston and Uitterlinden, 2010).

Present Knowledge in Nutrition, Tenth Edition. Edited by John W. Erdman Jr, Ian A. Macdonald and Steven H. Zeisel.
© 2012 International Life Sciences Institute. Published 2012 by John Wiley & Sons, Inc.

Diet and physical activity represent almost equal contributions to bone health. Therefore, the contribution of exercise needs to be factored into studies examining the effects of diet on skeletal development and maintenance. The functions of the musculoskeletal system in ambulation and other activities are critically linked in the maintenance of bone health during adult life and the elder years, perhaps even more so than dietary determinants.

The genetic determinants of bone health are significant, i.e. as much as approximately 80% of the variance in bone measurements is linked to heredity. Racial and ethnic differences in bone metabolism have been identified, but genetic factors governing mechanisms contributing to the metabolic differences have not been established. In fact, specific genes that govern bone tissue, both in development and in later maintenance, have remained elusive. Many genes are considered to be involved in orchestrating the functions of bone cells and, hence, bone tissue. Nutrient–gene interactions in the context of bone tissue are, however, poorly understood.

Definitions of Osteoporosis and Osteopenia

A combination of low bone mass and micro-architectural defects of both the organic matrix and mineral phases characterizes osteoporosis. Low bone mineral content (BMC) or low bone mineral density (BMD) are measured using dual-energy X-ray absorptiometry (DXA), whereas architectural defects are assessed by histomorphometry and physical tests of bone strength. Osteoporosis is distinguished from osteopenia by the degree of bone loss measured by DXA; the World Health Organization (WHO) cut-points below normal DXA bone scans of healthy young adults (20–29 years old) are listed in Table 50.1.

TABLE 50.1 World Health Organization bone mineral density cut-points below normal DXA scans of healthy young adults (20–29 years old)

Category of bone status	Individual BMD values compared to healthy young adult
Normal	>1 SD below mean for gender
Osteopenic	1–2.5 SDs below mean for gender
Osteoporotic	<2.5 SDs below mean for gender

BMD, bone mineral density; DXA, dual-energy X-ray absorptiometry; SD, standard deviation.

The public health costs of osteoporotic fractures are enormous: an estimated $17 billion a year was expended in the United States in 2005 (National Osteoporosis Foundation, 2010). Hip fractures represent the majority of this entire amount, as they typically require major medical care, hospitalization, and rehabilitation. Mortality of patients with hip fractures approaches an estimated 20% by 12 months post-fracture, an enormous toll. Spinal fractures, while much more common, generally require less medical care and cost, and mortality is very low.

Epidemiology of Osteoporosis

The epidemiology of osteoporosis is complicated by the definitions used.

DXA measurements classify osteoporosis of the lumbar spine and the proximal femur, two major sites of bone fractures, but not all osteoporotic subjects have fractures despite their low measurement values. Therefore, other factors not detected by DXA scans must contribute to prevent or to enhance fracture occurrence. Diet in the broadest sense may be one of these factors, and physical activity or musculoskeletal fitness is clearly a fracture-preventive factor. Other environmental factors, such as cigarette smoking and excessive alcohol consumption, are typically negative, as is early-life ovarian failure. The frequency of falls that may lead to fractures in older adults is another critical component impacting on osteoporotic subjects.

Incidence and Prevalence Rates

The statistics of osteoporosis are based on estimates of fractures, since relatively few bone measurements using DXA are made among older subjects. Prevalence rates in the United States of approximately two million older adults who have been hospitalized are estimated to be 70% hip fractures and 30% lumbar spinal and other fractures. However, most spinal fractures go unreported so that total fracture estimations are not accurate. New cases of hip fractures of older adults per year are much more accurate because nearly all patients are admitted to hospitals. The numbers of total (hip and other) fractures were reported in 2005 to be 300 000 in the United States (National Osteoporosis Foundation, 2008). Total US cases of osteoporosis were estimated to be 12 million by 2010 (National Osteoporosis Foundation, 2010) and the ratio is approximately four fractures in women to every one in men over age 50. In the developing world the rates are anticipated

TABLE 50.2 Selected nutritional risk factors for osteoporosis: deficient and excessive intakes of nutrients

Nutrient variable	Intake concern		Adverse skeletal consequences or effects
	Deficient	Excessive	
Calcium	X		Low bone mass, fracture
		X	Arterial calcification, renal stones
Phosphorus	X		Low bone mass, fracture
		X	Hyperparathyroidism, bone loss
Vitamin D	X		Osteomalacia, low bone mass
		X	Hypervitaminosis D, mineral deposits
Protein	X		Low bone matrix, poor mineralization
Animal		X	Increased acid load, bone loss (?)
Vitamin K	X		Low osteocalcin maturation, low bone mass
		X	Not established
Vitamin A	X		Decreased bone formation
		X	Increased bone resorption
Magnesium	X		Not established
		X	Not established
Fluoride	X		Low bone mass (?)
		X	Fluorosis

to increase even more as life expectancies continue to increase.

Environmental and Dietary Risk Factors

Many environmental risk factors for osteoporosis exist, such as inadequate physical activity throughout the life cycle. The nutritional risk factors are also numerous, and a few nutrients are briefly noted here (Table 50.2). Dietary macronutrients clearly are needed for healthy bone tissue, but a chronically excessive amount of acid-generating animal protein may have adverse effects on bone by promoting hypercalciuria (Kerstetter *et al.*, 2003), though this issue remains controversial. Adequate amounts of high-quality protein sources, however, are needed to maintain bone collagen and other matrix proteins and, hence, bone strength.

Insufficient calcium, phosphorus, and vitamin D intakes have been well established as major determinants of low bone mass and osteoporosis, but the metabolic relationships of these nutrients to bone are complex (see below under Pathophysiology of Osteoporosis). Too little protein in the diet, especially from high-quality sources, may have a negative impact on bone health in later life. An insufficiency of dietary vitamin K may also have an adverse effect on bone health, but only a few prospective trials have been reported on the linkage between vitamin K and bone

(Knapen *et al.*, 2007). Insufficiency of essential omega-3 fatty acids has also been suggested as contributing to suboptimal bone health, but this relationship has not yet been supported by clinical trials. The effects on bone health resulting from deficits of other nutrients are limited by a paucity of human investigations.

Pathophysiology of Osteoporosis

Functional declines of several organ systems contribute to the onset of osteoporosis, but the serum concentration of at least one hormone, i.e. parathyroid hormone (PTH), typically increases within the reference range late in life. Each of the major functional changes affecting bone tissue briefly described here increases with advancing age.

Declines in Estrogen and Androgen Production

Gender-related hormones generally decline in late life. Estrogens from the ovaries fall more precipitously beginning in the 40s and reach minimal levels by the early 50s, the typical onset of the postmenopausal period. Androgens, mainly testosterone, decline more gradually, beginning typically in the 60s. Each of these hormones has anabolic effects on the retention of bone mass. The decline or loss of these hormones hastens bone loss in the late decades of life.

Bone Tissue Changes: Declines in Mass and Organization

Bone turnover in late life favors bone resorption over bone formation, with the net result of gradual loss of both bone mass and microscopic architecture. This contributes to an increase in bone fragility and the risk of fracture, especially of trabecular or cancellous bone tissue (Figure 50.1A, B). The increase in the resorption rate and, hence, bone turnover, relates not only to diminished sex hormones, but also

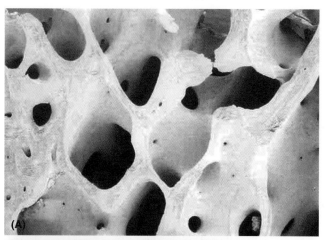

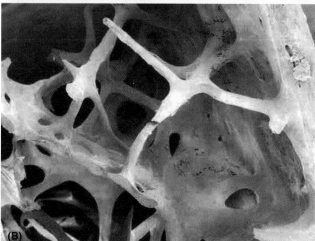

FIG. 50.1 Increased bone fragility and the risk of fracture, especially of trabecular or cancellous bone tissue, as shown by scanning electron micrographs. (A) Normal trabecular microarchitecture with health struts (cross-pieces) and vertical bars. (B) Osteoporotic trabecular bone with losses of connectivity as struts or bars have undergone resorption. Reproduced with permission. Copyright Dr David W. Dempster 2001.

to a chronic elevation of serum PTH concentration. An increase in dietary calcium intake will lower the PTH concentration within the normal reference range (McKane *et al.*, 1996), and it will have a beneficial effect in reducing the risk of fracture. (See later in this chapter.)

Declines in Intestinal Calcium Absorption

A steady decline in intestinal calcium absorption has been reported as starting in postmenopausal women without a decline in serum 25-hydroxyvitamin D (Nordin *et al.*, 2004). Whether the decline in intestinal calcium absorption results from a decrease in effectiveness of the vitamin D hormone, calcitriol, on the absorbing cell capacity for producing calcium-binding protein, or whether modification of other mechanisms, perhaps vitamin D-independent, might be responsible for this decline in calcium absorption, has not been established. Presumably, renal production of the calcitriol hormone from its precursor, calcidiol, remains optimal at late ages of life. Since renal function typically declines with age, the production of calcitriol would be expected to be compromised in those with renal deficits (see below).

Whereas calcium absorption may decline in efficiency in late life, no decline in phosphate absorption is thought to occur in older adults. Because of the delay in calcium absorption compared with phosphate entry into blood and the reduced calcium absorptive efficiency, the early postprandial PTH response is likely to be greater in older individuals (Anderson, 1991).

Declines in Renal Function

The major decline in renal function that may have a significant impact on bone is the lowering of the glomerular filtration rate (GFR), which may result in hyperphosphatemia and secondary hyperparathyroidism. An acute elevation in serum phosphate concentration helps lower serum calcium and it may also directly stimulate PTH secretion, as observed in younger adult and premenopausal women (Calvo *et al.*, 1990; Kemi *et al.*, 2009). Whether this phenomenon occurs in adults over 50 years has not been established. The net effect of this dietary excess of phosphorus is bone loss resulting from increased PTH-directed osteoclast-mediated resorption, especially in those with lowered GFR.

Increased Secretion of Parathyroid Hormone

PTH has a strong minute-to-minute regulatory role in maintaining the serum calcium concentration, really the

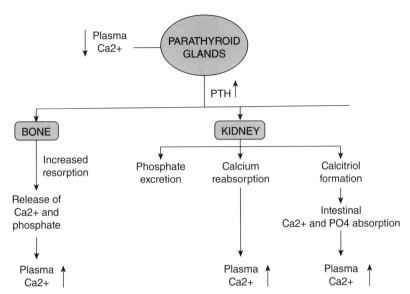

FIG. 50.2 Actions of parathyroid hormone that maintain homeostatic regulation of serum calcium ion concentration. Upward arrows represent increases and downward arrows represent decreases. Adapted from Ontjes, in Anderson et al. (2011).

ionic calcium concentration, at its physiological set concentration (1.25 mmol/L). When dietary calcium is low, serum calcium will decline and stimulate an increase in PTH secretion from parathyroid gland stores. Normocalcemia is restored by two PTH-mediated actions: calcium release from the bone envelope, including possibly also bone resorption, and increased renal tubular calcium reabsorption. In addition, serum phosphate ion concentrations are lowered by an increase in PTH. Figure 50.2 illustrates the actions of PTH on bone, kidney, and, indirectly, the small intestine. Reciprocal PTH effects occur in response to meals rich in calcium sources. Together these homeostatic changes result in tight regulation of the serum ionized calcium concentration.

Reduced Renal Formation of 1,25-Dihydroxyvitamin D

The second major adaptation operates more slowly to achieve appropriate calcium balance: positive in growing children and approximately zero balance in adults. During periods of low calcium intake (<500 mg/day), mild hypocalcemia leads to an increase in PTH secretion and then to an increase in calcitriol formation from its precursor, calcidiol. Higher serum concentrations of calcitriol, the hormonal form, act on intestinal absorbing cells to increase calcium absorption and reestablish calcium balance. This

genetic effect of the vitamin D hormone results in the intestinal cell synthesis of calcium-binding protein, which enhances calcium uptake in the blood. The renal capability of producing the calcitriol hormone remains fairly well intact in late life in individuals with normal renal function, i.e. normal GFR. Those with age- or disease-related declines in GFR have reduced synthesis of calcitriol in response to low calcium intakes.

Experimental Animal Model and In Vitro Studies of Nutritional Factors Affecting Bone

Many animal models have been studied in efforts to determine the effects of dietary components, especially calcium, on bone at various stages of the life cycle.

Rodent studies have been helpful in understanding bone concepts, but rodent bone metabolism differs too greatly from human bone tissue turnover to be useful for long-term studies. Unlike human bone, the skeletal growth of rodents continues throughout life. Rats and mice, therefore, are not useful models for the study of osteoporosis. Dog and swine models have served as more appropriate models for the study of bone metabolism, especially for short-term investigations. Their use as osteoporosis models, however, is limited.

Primate models have been utilized to investigate late-life bone loss following the loss of reproductive cycling in a few species of monkeys, but these models are not equivalent in most respects to human metabolism. Also, the great cost of these studies limits their use.

In summary, results of animal research on diet–bone relationships have been helpful, but they have not been overwhelmingly instructive for advancing human understanding of the metabolic aspects of osteoporosis development. In vitro studies are limited to the study of cell perturbations resulting from nutrient media content and hormones or factors that may have roles in osteoporosis.

Studies of Nutritional Factors Affecting Bone of Older Adults

Several nutrients have been shown to have important effects on bone health, but the emphasis in this chapter is placed on calcium, phosphorus, vitamin D, protein, and vitamin K. Other nutrients relating to bone health are briefly noted.

Observational Reports

Elderly female subjects who have been consuming recommended amounts of calcium on a daily basis have long been considered to have skeletal benefits, but the study designs were not sufficiently rigorous by current standards to be meaningful. For example, a report by Nordin (1960) suggested that calcium intakes of 800–1000 mg of calcium were optimal for bone health of practically all populations and that Asian diets containing 500 mg or so per day were grossly inadequate.

An instructive survey by Matkovic et al. (1979) supported the benefit of consuming a high-calcium diet based on milk and other dairy foods on bone mass compared with a non-dairy-consuming population in Yugoslavia. This study stimulated great increase in research on the calcium–bone linkage, but it essentially ignored the potential skeletal benefit of the higher-quality protein intake by the dairy consumers. Clinical investigations in fact support the enhancement of bone repair by elderly subjects supplemented with protein (Bonjour, 2005).

Randomized Controlled Trials (RCTs)

Many prospective investigations have been undertaken. A few examples of these RCTs are selected to demonstrate the effects of calcium plus vitamin D compared with calcium alone.

Calcium plus Vitamin D

A high-quality report that illustrates the positive effects of calcium supplements on bone is probably the largest study yet published. One arm of healthy postmenopausal subjects (62 years of age at initial screen) in the Women's Health Initiative (WHI) trial was administered calcium (1000 mg/day) plus vitamin D (400 IU/day) for an average period of 7 years (Jackson et al., 2006). (Both groups of women were quite health-conscious, and a large percentage were consuming adequate intakes of both calcium and vitamin D because of self-selection of supplements.) Compared with the placebo control group, the treated subjects did have at 7 years modestly greater BMD at the hip, but no reduction in hip fractures. No significant reductions were found in vertebral fractures or in fractures at other sites in the supplemented women. One adverse effect of the calcium and vitamin D treatment was an increase in the risk of renal stones.

Several other well-designed RCTs using calcium and vitamin D have been reported. An original study by Meunier's group based in Lyon, France, found that nonvertebral fractures were reduced following 1 year of therapy with daily calcium phosphate and vitamin D supplements in older women in nursing homes (Chapuy et al., 1992). The amounts of the each nutrient were 1000 mg for calcium, 600 mg for phosphorus, and 800 IU for vitamin D. A compliance rate of almost 100% was reported.

An additional investigation using this nutrient combination (with carbonate instead of phosphate as the anion) in Boston by Dawson-Hughes et al. (1997) provided similar results in both older women and men, but the reductions of fracture rates were not as impressive as in the Chapuy study. Numerous studies in other nations have arrived at similar conclusions.

Finally, a systematic review of trials of combined vitamin D and calcium supplementation supports the finding of skeletal gains when both nutrients are consumed at reasonable amounts, i.e. >300 IU of vitamin D and >1000 mg of calcium (Chung et al., 2009).

Calcium Alone

Trials using calcium alone have also been reported generally to improve BMD. Most of these have used supplements containing 1000 mg of calcium or more per day. Reid and colleagues (2006), who performed an RCT in postmenopausal women living in Auckland, New Zealand, used calcium supplementation (1000 mg/day as the citrate), which resulted in significant reductions of bone loss and turnover but no changes in fractures of the hip or other sites after 5 years. The authors stated in their conclusions that poor compliance reduced the effectiveness of the calcium supplements.

Riis and co-researchers in Denmark showed that calcium (1000 mg per day) supplementation helped slow bone loss in postmenopausal women, and they retained more bone mass than placebo-treated subjects (controls) over a period of 2 years (Riis *et al.*, 1987). Fractures were not significantly decreased in the calcium treatment group.

Similar studies by other investigators (Chevalley *et al.*, 1994; Recker *et al.*, 1996) have reported that calcium supplements prevented vertebral fractures in postmenopausal women. Reductions of fractures with calcium treatment alone, however, have not been supported by meta-analyses. (See next section.)

Meta-Analyses

A comprehensive meta-analysis of several trials examining calcium supplementation (>1200 mg/day) alone on fracture risk found that older subjects (>50 years) had the greatest reduction of fractures ($p < 0.05$) when they had low baseline calcium intake (<700 mg/day) and low serum 25-hydroxyvitamin D (<25 mmol/L), assuming good compliance (Tang *et al.*, 2007). This meta-analysis included data from 17 randomized trials that presented fractures.

Reid *et al.* (2008) first reported that elevated intakes of calcium alone (>800 mg/day) significantly lowered the risk of non-vertebral fractures. In a later analysis they showed that vitamin D supplementation alone was not beneficial in fracture reduction (Reid *et al.*, 2010a).

Two additional meta-analyses arrived at a similar conclusion that vitamin D alone did not reduce fracture risk or fractures in older women (Avenell *et al.*, 2010; DIPART analysis, 2010). Earlier vitamin D trials, however, were quite robust in supporting a beneficial effect of vitamin D supplementation on bone.

A meta-analysis of calcium plus vitamin D supplements by Boonen *et al.* (2007) found that both nutrients, calcium and vitamin D, were needed to reduce fracture risk in older women. This older analysis conflicts with the more recent analyses cited above, which suggest that calcium alone may be utilized by bone tissue for remodeling and that extra dietary vitamin D may be superfluous for bone formation when calcium intake and its absorption are both sufficient.

A previous Cochrane meta-analysis on the benefit of calcium supplementation alone for bone has been with-drawn (Shea *et al.*, 2002) and a new report of a revised meta-analysis by this group is awaited. The 2002 publication concluded that calcium was statistically beneficial, though weak in its quantitative effect on bone, and that fracture reduction was not demonstrated with statistical confidence. Bone strength is more related to the organic matrix, especially collagen, than it is to the hydroxyapatite mineral phase of bone, as measured by DXA. The lack of improvement in fracture rate by calcium/vitamin D supplementation alone may help explain this anomaly, since no appropriate measurement of the organic status of bone is readily available.

Interpretation of Human Studies

From a dietary perspective, calcium intakes may represent the single most important nutritional variable affecting bone health and preventing fractures. An adequate vitamin D status helps primarily in adaptation to low calcium intake and therefore to serum calcium concentrations at the low end of the normal range. Inadequate dietary phosphorus, although rare in the US population, may also contribute to osteoporosis. The major issue relating to phosphorus is that, at high chronic intakes typical in the United States, an elevated serum phosphate concentration exerts a lowering effect on serum calcium and thereby triggers the secretion of PTH which may adversely affect bone mass, even in premenopausal women with high calcium intakes (Kemi *et al.*, 2010). Except for phosphorus, other nutrients such as magnesium have not been sufficiently studied to suggest that their intakes are as critical for bone maintenance and health as calcium and vitamin D. Vitamin K clearly enhances the generation of the matrix protein, osteocalcin, but too few well designed trials have been reported.

Concern about excessive calcium supplementation in older subjects has arisen because of a report of increased risk of cardiovascular disease in a population of women in Auckland, New Zealand (Bolland *et al.*, 2008) and a meta-analysis on this association (Bolland *et al.*, 2010). Reid *et al.* (2010b) in their review of the adverse cardiovascular effects of long-term calcium supplementation have concluded that total calcium intakes from foods and supplements need to be more carefully monitored in efforts to both enhance bone status and reduce the risk of cardiovascular morbidity and mortality.

The latter reports raise the question of what should be reasonable intakes of calcium, i.e. total calcium from foods and supplements, in older subjects who are, because of age, low BMI, or other factors, at increased risk of fracture. The tolerable upper intake levels (ULs), i.e. presumably maximum safe calcium intakes, are set at 2500 mg/day across the life cycle (Institute of Medicine, 1997), but more recent data provided in the reports by Bolland (2008 and 2010) and Daly and Ebeling (2010) suggest that the UL may be safer when lowered to ~1500 mg/day. (A recent IOM report [Institute of Medicine, 2011] has reduced the UL for calcium in men and women 51 and older to 2000 mg/day.) The window of healthy calcium intakes would then range between ~800 and 1500 mg/day, slightly below the current adequate intakes for older adults of 1200 mg/day. Daily intakes of calcium above 1500 mg may increase the risk first of coronary artery calcification and then of cardiovascular morbidity and mortality.

A finding that older subjects who have high serum calcium concentrations are more likely to have increased carotid plaque thickness suggests that arterial calcification is occurring in many elderly individuals (Rubin *et al.*, 2006), but the mechanism(s) for the increase in carotid artery thickness or coronary artery calcification remain(s) elusive.

Future Directions

New RCTs are needed of postmenopausal women and elderly men that fine-tune our current understanding of the critical nutrients needed to support bone health in late life with or without concurrent physical activity programs (aerobic, etc.), and of diverse racial and ethnic groups. Most studies by far have included Caucasian subjects, but the nutrient requirements of other ethnic groups, especially African-Americans who have PTH responses to calcium challenges that differ from those of Caucasians (Cosman *et al.*, 2000) need greater understanding.

Several prospective RCT investigations of single nutrients or combinations of nutrients, beyond simply calcium and vitamin D, would advance understanding of the essential roles of these nutrients. For example, high phosphate intakes (and low calcium intakes) lasting 1–2 years would provide new information on the potentially chronic adverse effect of this altered diet ratio (by weight) on bone mass and density, and possibly rule in a major role of the phosphate regulatory hormone, fibroblast growth factor 23 (FGF23), in phosphate homeostasis.

Similarly, prospective RCTs of vitamin K in two or three different forms would help clarify the interchangeability of these molecules in the support of bone matrix proteins

Protein itself from high-quality sources rich in sulfates and phosphates needs to be examined in prospective RCTs to establish the beneficial effect of this macronutrient on matrix molecules and to rule out any adverse effect of a potential acid load generated by amino acid metabolism.

The role of magnesium in bone metabolism has been woefully underinvestigated, as only a very few prospective RCTs have been undertaken.

Finally, a combination of several nutrients, i.e. vitamin K and magnesium, provided as a supplement at modest doses of each nutrient along with calcium and vitamin D at RDA levels in a multi-arm prospective RCT would provide very useful data on older subjects, especially women, of all racial/ethnic groups. The study design would also benefit from incorporation of other arms receiving lesser amounts of supplemental calcium and vitamin D than 100% of the RDAs. Sources of calcium containing carbonate in some arms and phosphate in others would be desirable.

Advances in understanding of the roles of nutrient needs for bone health in older populations have been achieved over the last decade. Calcium needs have been established as being more critical for bone maintenance than other individual nutrients as determined by several meta-analyses of RCTs and other studies. Calcium supplementation, alone or with vitamin D, may also reduce fracture risk, but study results are inconsistent on this issue. Other nutrients, however, remain important for bone health and the prevention or delay of osteoporosis and fragility fractures. Further data from RCTs employing additional bone-related nutrients may help expand our understanding.

Healthy diets providing balanced intakes of all nutrients continue to be the optimal way to promote bone health along with other healthy lifestyles, such as participating in routine physical activities, not smoking, and consuming only moderate amounts of alcohol per day, if any.

Physical activity helps maintain muscle mass, equilibrium/balance, and the general overall health of organ systems. Together, sound diet and regular activity help promote good bone health and delay or prevent osteoporosis.

Suggestions for Further Reading

Anderson, J.J.B., Garner, S.C., and Klemmer, P.J. (eds) (2011) *Diet, Nutrients, and Bone Health*. Taylor & Francis, Boca Raton, FL.

Dawson-Hughes, B. (2008) Calcium and vitamin D. In C.J. Rosen (ed.), *Primer on the Metabolic Bone Diseases and Disorders of Mineral Metabolism*, 7th Edn. American Society for Bone and Mineral Research, Washington, DC, pp. 231–234.

Lanham-New, S.A. and Bonjour, J.-P. (2003) *Nutritional Aspects of Bone Health*. Royal Society of Chemistry, Cambridge, UK.

Weaver, C.M. and Heaney, R.P. (eds) (2006) *Calcium and Bone*. Humana Press, Totowa, NJ.

References

Anderson, J.J.B. (1991) Nutritional biochemistry of calcium and phosphorus. *J Nutr Biochem* **2**, 300–307.

Avenell, A., Gillespie, W.J., Gillespie, L.D., *et al.* (2009) Vitamin D and vitamin D analogues for preventing fractures associated with involutional and post-menopausal osteoporosis. *Cochrane Database Syst Rev* CD000227.

Bolland, M.J., Avenell, A., Baron, J., *et al.* (2010) Effect of calcium supplements on risk of myocardial infarction and cardiovascular events: meta-analysis. *BMJ* **341**, c3691.

Bolland, M.J., Barber, P., Doughty, R., *et al.* (2008) Vascular events in healthy older women receiving calcium supplementation: randomized controlled trial. *BMJ* **336**, 262–266.

Bonjour, J.-P. (2005) Dietary protein: an essential nutrient for bone health. *J Am Coll Nutr* **24**, 526S–536S.

Boonen, S., Lips, P., Bouillon, R., *et al.* (2007) Need for additional calcium to reduce the risk of hip fracture with vitamin D supplementation: evidence from a comparative meta-analysis of randomized controlled trials. *J Clin Endocrinol Metab* **92**, 1415–1423.

Calvo, M.S., Kumar, R., and Heath, H., III (1990) Persistently elevated parathyroid secretion and action in young women after four weeks of ingesting high phosphorus, low calcium diets. *J Clin Endocrinol Metab* **70**, 1334–1340.

Chapuy, M.C., Arlot, M.E., Duboeuf, F., *et al.* (1992) Vitamin D3 and calcium to prevent hip fractures in elderly women. *N Engl J Med* **327**, 1637–1642.

Chevalley, T., Rizzoli, R., Nydegger, V., *et al.* (1994) Effects of calcium supplements n femoral bone mineral density and vertebral fracture rate in vitamin-D-replete elderly patients. *Osteoporos Int* **4**, 245–252.

Chung, M., Balk, E.M., Brendel, M., *et al.* (2009) *Vitamin D and Calcium: A Systematic Review of Health Outcomes*. Evidence Report/Technology Assessment No. 183. AHRQ Publication No. 09-E015. [Also known as the Tufts AHRQ study.]

Cosman, F., Morgan, D.C., Nieves, J.W., *et al.* (1997) Resistance to bone resorbing effects of PTH in black women. *J Bone Min Res* **12**, 958–966.

Daly, R.M. and Ebeling, P.R. (2010) Is excess calcium harmful to health? *Nutrients* **2**, 505–522.

Dawson-Hughes, B., Harris, S.S., Krall, E.A., *et al.* (1997) Effect of calcium and vitamin D supplementation on bone density in men and women 65 years of age and older. *N Engl J Med* **337**, 670–676.

DIPART (Vitamin D Individual Patient Analysis of Randomized Trials) Group (2010) Patient level pooled analysis of 68500 patients from seven major vitamin D fracture trials in US and Europe. *BMJ* **340**, b5463.

Institute of Medicine (1997) *Dietary Reference Intakes: Calcium, Phosphorus, Magnesium, Vitamin D, and Fluoride*. National Academy Press, Washington, DC.

Institute of Medicine (2011) *Dietary Reference Intakes for Calcium and Vitamin D*. National Academies Press, Washington, DC.

Jackson, R.D., LaCroix, A.Z., Gass, M., *et al.* (2006) Calcium plus vitamin D supplementation and the risk of fractures. *N Engl J Med* **354**, 669–683.

Kemi, V.E., Karkkainen, M.U.M., Rita, H.J., *et al.* (2010) Low calcium: phosphorus ratio in habitual diets affects serum parathyroid hormone concentration and calcium metabolism in healthy women with adequate calcium intake. *Br J Nutr* **103**, 561–568.

Kemi, V., Rita, H.J., Karkkainen, M.U.M., *et al.* (2009) Habitual high phosphorus intakes and foods with phosphate additives negatively affect parathyroid hormone concentration: A cross-sectional study on healthy premenopausal women. *Public Health Nutr* **12**, 1886–1892.

Kerstetter, J.E., O'Brien, K.O., and Insogna, K.L. (2003) Dietary protein, calcium metabolism, and skeletal homeostasis revisited. *Am J Clin Nutr* **78**, 584S–592S.

Knapen, M.H.J., Schurgers, L.J., and Vermeer, C. (2007) Vitamin K2 supplementation improves bone geometry and bone strength indices in postmenopausal women. *Osteoporos Int* **18**, 963–972.

Matkovic, V., Kostial, K., Simonovic, I., *et al.* (1979) Bone status and fracture rates in two regions of Yugoslavia. *Am J Clin Nutr* **32**, 540–549.

McKane, W.R., Khosla, S., Egan, K.S., *et al.* (1996) Role of calcium intake in modulating age-related increases in parathyroid function and bone resorption. *J Clin Endocrinol Metab* **81**, 1699–1703.

National Osteoporosis Foundation (2008) *National Osteoporosis Foundation Fast Facts*. http://www.nof.org/node/40.

National Osteoporosis Foundation (2010) *National Osteoporosis Foundation Prevalence Report*. http://www.nof.org/advocacy/resources/prevalencereport.

Nordin, B.E.C. (1960) Osteomalacia, osteoporosis and calcium deficiency. *Clin Orthoped Relat Res* **17,** 235–258.

Nordin, B.E.C., Need, A.G., Morris, H.A., *et al.* (2004) Effect of age on calcium absorption in postmenopausal women. *Am J Clin Nutr* **80,** 998–1002.

Ontjes, D.A. (2011) Hormone actions in the regulation of calcium and phosphorus metabolism. In Anderson, J.J.B., Garner, S.C., and Klemmer, P.J. (Eds.) *Diet, Nutrients, and Bone Health*. CRC Press, Boca Raton, FL.

Ralston, S.H. and Uitterlinden, A.G. (2010) Genetics of osteoporosis. *Endocr Rev* **31,** 629–662.

Recker, R.R., Hinders, S., Davies, K.M., *et al.* (1996). Correcting calcium nutritional deficiency prevents spine fractures in elderly women. *J Bone Miner Res* **11,** 1961–1966.

Reid, I.R., Bolland, M., and Grey, A. (2008) Effect of calcium supplementation on hip fractures. *Osteoporos Int* **19,** 1119–1123.

Reid, I.R., Bolland, M., and Grey, A. (2010a) Vitamin D – let's get back to the evidence base. *IBMS Bone Key* **7,** 249–253.

Reid, I.R., Bolland, M., and Grey, A. (2010b) Does calcium supplementation increase cardiovascular risk? *Clin Endocrinol Oxf* **73,** 689–695.

Reid, I.R., Mason, B., Horne, A., *et al.* (2006) Randomized controlled trial of calcium in healthy older women. *Am J Med* **119,** 777–785.

Riis, B., Thomsen, K., and Christiansen, C. (1987) Does calcium supplementation prevent postmenopausal bone loss? A double-blind, controlled clinical trial. *N Engl J Med* **316,** 173–177.

Rubin, M.R., Rundek, T., McMahon, D.J., *et al.* (2006) Carotid artery plaque thickness is associated with increased serum calcium levels: The Northern Manhattan Study. *Atherosclerosis* **194,** 426–432.

Shea, B., Wells, G., Cranney, A., *et al.* (2002) Meta-analysis of calcium supplementation for the prevention of postmenopausal osteoporosis. VII. Meta-analysis of calcium supplementation for the prevention of postmenopausal osteoporosis. *Endocr Rev* **23,** 552–559.

Tang, B.M., Eslick, G.D., Nowson, C., *et al.* (2007) Use of calcium or calcium in combination with vitamin D supplementation to prevent fractures and bone loss in people aged 50 years and older: a meta-analysis. *Lancet* **370,** 657–666.

Weaver, C.M. and Heaney, R.P. (2008) Nutrition and osteoporosis. In C.J. Rosen (ed.), *Primer on the Metabolic Bone Diseases and Disorders of Mineral Metabolism*, 7th Edn. American Society for Bone and Mineral Research, Washington, DC, pp. 206–208.

51

CANCER

HOLLY NICASTRO, PhD AND JOHN A. MILNER, PhD

National Cancer Institute, Rockville, Maryland, USA

Summary

Evidence continues to mount that dietary habits can significantly influence one's cancer risk and/or tumor behavior. Experimental evidence using a variety of models substantiates the importance of multiple components in the diet that modify one or more cancer-related processes. Nevertheless, clinical intervention studies have been less compelling and make it difficult to draw firm conclusions about what adjustments in eating behaviors are needed. Inconsistencies in the literature may reflect individuality in response and therefore the need to better understand the quantity of the bioactive constituent needed to bring about a response, the timing of exposure for best response, and how genetics and biological insults including excessive energy and associated radicals, environmental contaminants, viruses and/or bacteria may modify the response. Regardless, exciting opportunities exist for identifying and validating biomarkers that can be used to identify who will benefit most or be placed at risk as a result of dietary change. While characterizing responsive individuals will not be easy, the societal benefits are enormous.

Introduction

Cancer is a collection of complex diseases characterized by abnormal cellular growth. Cancer cells exhibit several physiological hallmarks resulting from various genetic alterations that distinguish them from healthy cells: self-sufficiency in growth signals, insensitivity to growth-inhibitory signals, evasion of programmed cell death, limitless replicative potential, sustained angiogenesis, and tissue invasion and metastasis (Hanahan and Weinberg, 2000). Carcinogenesis is a multi-step process involving multiple genetic or epigenetic alterations that confer sur-

vival advantages to cells, usually over the course of many decades. The American Cancer Society estimated that there would be approximately 1596670 new cases of cancer and 571950 cancer deaths in the United States in 2011 (American Cancer Society, 2011). Worldwide, cancer accounts for 13% of all deaths, with that figure expected to increase.

Cancer is caused by endogenous and/or environmental factors. Endogenous factors, which account for a minority of cancers, include inherited germ-line mutations, inflammation, or hormones. Cancer also has several environmental causes, including radiation, viruses, bacteria, parasites,

Present Knowledge in Nutrition, Tenth Edition. Edited by John W. Erdman Jr, Ian A. Macdonald and Steven H. Zeisel.
© 2012 International Life Sciences Institute. Published 2012 by John Wiley & Sons, Inc.

tobacco use, and exposure to carcinogens, and/or improper diet. The majority of cancers are caused by environmental factors; this suggests that modifying environmental exposures such as diet could reduce the risk of developing cancer. The World Cancer Research Fund and American Institute for Cancer Research estimate that 34% of common cancers, and up to 70% of certain cancers including esophageal and endometrial cancers, are preventable if there is appropriate food, nutrition, physical activity, and body fatness (WCRF/AICR, 2007). Mounting evidence continues to highlight dietary change as an effective and cost-efficient approach for reducing cancer risk and for modifying the biological behavior of tumors. This chapter discusses the current knowledge on diet and cancer, current approaches to studying the relationship between food components and cancer development, and challenges and future directions in the field.

Studying Nutrition and Cancer

Intakes/Exposures

Diversity of Foods and Compounds

More than 25 000 different bioactive components are believed to occur in the foods that humans consume. At least 500 of these compounds have already been identified as possible modifiers of the cancer process, and others will likely surface with the use of high-throughput screening of natural products and improved detection methods. These bioactive food components may arise from plants (phytochemicals), animal sources (zoochemicals), fungi (fungochemicals), or the metabolism of food components by bacteria within the gastrointestinal tract (bacterochemicals) (Milner, 2006). This diverse array of dietary constituents may modify, either positively or negatively, cancer risk and tumor behavior (WCRF/AICR, 2007). Defining which food component is instrumental in bringing about a phenotypic change is exceedingly challenging because of the complexity of foods and the myriad of sites where food components may function. For example, some of the anticancer benefits of tomatoes and tomato products may be attributed not only to lycopene, but also to other carotenoids, flavonoids, vitamins, and minerals (Tan et al., 2010). Likewise, interactions among foods may influence the overall response. For example, combining vitamin D_3 and genistein was more effective in suppressing the growth of prostate cancer cells at biologically achievable concentrations than was either agent alone. This response appears to result from the ability of genistein to inhibit CYP 24

and thereby to increase the half-life of vitamin D_3 (Krishnan et al., 2007). It is likely that many other interactions among food constituents are occurring which have yet to be fully defined.

Methods of Assessing Exposure

Rapid, accurate, and inexpensive methods for assessing the intake of specific bioactive food components, both essential and non-essential nutrients, are fundamental to unraveling the relationship between dietary habits and cancer risks, yet represent a major methodological challenge. Errors in estimating food intakes and incomplete data about nutrient content or interactions among food components limit the usefulness of self-reported food consumption data. Because eating behaviors are exceedingly complex and may involve foods that are consumed intermittently and irregularly, self-reports are particularly prone to measurement error. Food frequency questionnaires (FFQ) are convenient, measure long-term behaviors and are relatively inexpensive, but they are limited by knowledge about particular foods and are hampered by the inability of individuals to accurately report their intakes retrospectively. A 24-hour recall, while providing more in-depth information about the types and amounts of foods consumed, provides a rather poor estimate of long-term usual intakes. Despite the increased subject burden and cost, a 7-day diary has been found to provide a far better estimate of exposure to dietary constituents including protein and potassium than found with the use of an FFQ (McKeown et al., 2001; Davis and Milner, 2007). However, these methods do not account for variables such as absorption, metabolism, distribution, or excretion that influence the amount of food components that reach target sites. Increasingly, the combined use of intake assessment and biomarker measurements is being employed to provide insight into individual responsiveness to individual and long-term exposures (Jenab et al., 2009).

The complexity of foods also presents challenges for analysis of intake. Reference standards for foods are not always available, and phytonutrient content of foods can vary considerably based on growth conditions, storage, or processing of the food. The genotype of plants may also be an important variable as evident in broccoli where glucoraphanin concentrations have been reported to vary more than 25-fold (Martin, 2007). In addition, the food matrix can have a profound effect on bioavailability of foods and dietary supplements (D'Archivio et al., 2010). Form or speciation is another factor which likely influences bioavailability. Overall, concentration in a food is only one factor that may influence the relationship between diet and cancer prevention.

Timing

Timing and duration of exposures are also important factors in determining the overall response to foods or supplements. In rats, the timing of exposure to dietary genistein exposure was determined to be exceedingly important in determining mammary cancer risk (Lamartiniere *et al.*, 2002). In this mammary model, treatment with genistein was protective after prepubertal and combined prepubertal and adult genistein treatments, but was not effective after prenatal- or adult-only treatment. Humans may also respond best with prolonged or early exposures, since, in a case-control study, an inverse relationship was observed between soy food intake in adolescents and breast-cancer incidence later in life; however, protection was not evident when intakes began later in life (Boyapati *et al.*, 2005). Admittedly, this is an area of investigation that deserves additional attention, especially as it might relate to fluctuations in epigenetic processes.

Data from the General Population Trial in Linxian, China, demonstrated that individuals who received a supplement containing β-carotene, vitamin E, and selenium, had a 13% reduction in cancer mortality. Post-intervention follow-up found that the beneficial effects of the supplement were evident and were magnified up to 10 years after termination of the supplementation program (Qiao *et al.*, 2009). The benefits were greater in individuals who were <55 years at the beginning of the intervention. Cancer risk appeared to increase in those who started supplements usage when beyond 55 years of age. These findings suggest that sustained exposure may not always be necessary to bring about a desired outcome. It is conceivable that the observed variation in risk as a function of age possibly reflected differences in the early-stage transformed cells.

The Women's Intervention Nutrition Study (WINS) provides evidence that long-term exposure may be needed to detect a biological response to dietary change (Chlebowski *et al.*, 2006). In this randomized, prospective, multicenter clinical trial the effect of a dietary intervention designed to reduce fat intake in women with resected, early-stage breast cancer receiving conventional cancer management was tested. This study provided evidence that approximately 4 years was required to detect a response to the reduced consumption of dietary fat. The hazard ratio of relapse events in the reduced fat intervention group compared with the control group was 0.76. Additionally, this study provided evidence that a subgroup of individuals, namely estrogen receptor (ER) negative individuals, were most responsive to a reduction in dietary fat. It should be noted that the Women's Health Initiative provided similar evidence that a reduction in fat (9%) was associated with a slight reduction in breast cancer risk (~24%) that was not observed until after more than 4 years.

Still other studies provide evidence of biological effects after short-term exposures, by monitoring changes in transcriptional mRNA expression (transcriptomics) by food components. Lin *et al.* (2007) have reported that consumption of a low-fat, low-glycemic-load diet can lead to marked changes in the expression of over 20 genes in human prostatic tissue for 6 weeks. These investigators suggest that a molecular approach to health and disease may help individualize appropriate interventions based on cellular signature changes brought about by diet. Significant changes in expression can occur within a few hours after consuming a food, as reported by van Erk *et al.* (2006). Breakfast cereals with different macronutrient profiles resulted in differential blood leukocyte gene expression in men after 2 hours. Thus, a bolus approach to a food or component may represent a relatively inexpensive approach to determine if a nutritional intervention strategy is appropriate, especially if the price of chips continues to decrease. A better understanding of temporal relationships will be needed if appropriate preemptive models are to be forthcoming.

Overall, time appears to be an important variable, yet the best time for intervention remains unresolved. Nevertheless, it does appear that several options are available for using dietary interventions to reduce cancer risk and modify tumor behavior (Table 51.1).

Interindividual Variability

In order to make specific recommendations to the public about nutrition and cancer prevention, research will need to focus on identifying responders and non-responders. Studying interindividual variability is fundamental to establishing which subpopulations and ideally individuals will derive benefits from dietary intervention and which will not. As important objective is the identification of those individuals who might be placed at risk as a result of dietary change. Since increasing evidence points to excess exposure to a wide array of food components including β-carotene, iron, zinc, selenium, vitamin D, indole-3

TABLE 51.1 Summary of current diet-related recommendations for cancer prevention from the 2007 WCRF/AICR Report

Category	Recommendations
Body fatness	Be as lean as possible within the normal range of body weight
Physical activity	Be physically active as part of everyday life
Food and drinks that promote weight gain	Limit consumption of energy-dense foods and avoid sugary drinks
Plant foods	Eat mostly foods of plant origin
Animal foods	Limit intake of red meat and avoid processed meat
Alcoholic drinks	Limit alcoholic drinks
Preservation, processing, preparation	Limit consumption of salt and avoid moldy grains or legumes
Dietary supplements	Aim to meet nutritional needs through diet alone (without dietary supplements)

Data from WCRF/AICR (2007).

carbinol, etc., to produce a "J-" or "U-" shaped response curve, it is extremely important that vulnerable subpopulations are also identified. Such knowledge will come from examining how diet-induced phenotypic responses depend on an individual's background (nutrigenetics), the expression of genes (epigenomics and transcriptomics), changes in the amounts and activities of proteins (proteomics), changes in small molecular weight compounds (metabolomics) or changes in the number or diversity of microbes in the gastrointestinal tract (the microbiome).

Epidemiological studies continue to provide important clues about the likely importance of multiple foods and components as deterrents to cancer. However, controlled-intervention studies, such as the Alpha-Tocopherol, Beta-Carotene (ATBC) study, the Polyp Prevention Trial, the Women's Healthy Eating and Living study (WHEL), etc., provide mixed messages about the physiological significance of dietary change (Wong *et al.*, 2003; Abrams *et al.*, 2005; Slattery *et al.*, 2007). For example, according to the 2008 World Cancer Research Report (WCRF/AICR 2007), there are 11 studies that have observed a decreased risk of colorectal cancer with increased intake of calcium, yet the response was statistically significant in only three

cases; furthermore, in one case, higher intake was linked with an increased risk in women but not in men. When meta-analysis was restricted to eight studies, a summary estimate was 0.95 per 200 mg/day with no evidence of heterogeneity (WCRF/AICR, 2007). Thus, while calcium was associated with protection, the overall response was relatively modest. While even a relative small change can have profound implications in a large population, it is possible that the change in risk is really a reflection of a large response in a subpopulation.

Nutrigenetics

Polymorphisms in genes may be one explanation for these modest responses in a large population but greater responses in a subpopulation. For example, inadequate calcium intake is associated with increased colorectal cancer risk in those with the Ff and ff genotypes for vitamin D receptor (VDR) FOK1 polymorphism (Wong *et al.*, 2003). A polymorphism in this receptor involving a T to C substitution at position 2 exon 2 has been identified with lower calcium accretion in children (Abrams *et al.*, 2005). The biological basis by which this polymorphism might influence cancer risk remains to be determined. Regardless, these data suggest that vulnerable individuals with inadequate calcium consumption may have an almost three-fold higher risk of developing colon cancer; again considerably greater than the roughly 20% reduction seen in population studies with greater calcium exposures. Recently, the association of VDR haplotypes has been examined in two large case-control studies (Slattery *et al.*, 2007). While the CDX2 polymorphism was not independently associated with colon or rectal cancer nor several dietary components, the bLFA haplotype (*Bsm*1 b, or B, poly(A) L, *Fok* F, and CDX2 A polymorphisms) was associated with an increased risk of colon cancer. It is important to recognize that the frequency of a polymorphism can vary markedly across populations as evident in a frequency of the A allele of the CDX2 polymorphism which occurred in 19% of non-Hispanic whites, 21% of Hispanics, 76% of African-Americans, and 47% of Asians. These data suggest that haplotype analysis that encompasses different domains of the VDR gene might further enhance understanding of the importance of dietary calcium as a deterrent to cancer. The use of polymorphism information may offer opportunities for identifying individuals who will benefit maximally or be placed at risk because of dietary change.

Polymorphisms may influence the metabolism and excretion of dietary cancer-preventive compounds and thereby alter their ability to induce or suppress metabolizing enzymes or transporters (El-Sohemy, 2007; Steck et al., 2007; Yu and Kong, 2007). Differential response to dietary cancer-preventive compounds may also relate to the variant of the enzyme being modified. For example, garlic appears to lead to an autocatalysis of CYP2E1, but does not appear to influence other CYP450s in the same manner (Davenport and Wargovich, 2005). Likewise, polymorphisms in the regulator region of metabolizing enzymes/transporters, such as AhR, CAR, and PXR, may also influence the overall response to bioactive food components (Okey et al., 2005; Yu and Kong, 2007).

Understanding gene constitution–nutrient interactions is further complicated by variations that can occur in copy number, either by deletion or amplification of large regions of specific chromosomes. Copy number is the most prevalent structural variation in the human genome, and may account for as much as 20% of the variation among individuals. Thus it may contribute significantly to genetic heterogeneity and may be a significant determinant of whether a diet is appropriate or not (Pinto et al., 2007). Variation in copy number has been reported for α-amylase, several cytochrome P450 genes, and Her2/Neu (Slamon et al., 1987; Ingelman-Sundberg et al., 2007; Perry et al., 2007) and likely occurs in many others. Typically, increases in copy number are associated with an increase in enzyme activity, and vice versa. This variation in enzymatic activity likely contributes significantly to some of the differential response to food components across individuals.

Epigenetics

Epigenetic modification regulates expression and activity of genes without modifying genomic sequences. Mechanisms include DNA methylation, histone modifications, gene silencing by microRNA, and chromosome stability. Genes involving cell cycle regulation, DNA repair, angiogenesis, and apoptosis can all be inactivated by the hypermethylation of their respective 5′ CpG islands. Key regulatory genes – including the cell cycle inhibitors $p21^{WAF1/CIP1}$ and $p16^{INK4a}$, pi-class glutathione S-transferase, the tumor suppressors cyclin-dependent kinase 2 (CDKN2) and PTEN – are all susceptible to control by DNA hypermethylation. The intake of multiple food components ranging from vitamin A to zinc may influence epigenetic processes. Actually, several non-essential and essential nutrients have been reported to influence DNA methylation patterns (Ross, 2003). Classical studies have demonstrated that methyl-deficient diets lead to marked changes in methylation patterns, at least some of which are consistent with alterations observed when a normal cell transforms to a neoplasm (Pogribny et al., 2006). Diets low in folate are linked with increased risk of several cancer types. This effect is believed to be due to abnormal DNA synthesis and methylation (Li and Tollefsbol, 2010). Restoring proper methylation may represent a fundamental process by which some bioactive food components may function to influence gene expression patterns. For example, (-)-epigallocatechin-3-gallate (EGCG) from green tea can reactivate methylation-silenced genes by inhibiting the enzymatic activity of DNA methyltransferase 1 (Fang et al., 2003).

Silencing and unsilencing of genes can also occur through modification of histones (Myzak and Dashwood, 2006; Glozak and Seto, 2007; Holloway and Oakford, 2007). In addition to factors that govern the overall recruitment and release of histones (histone occupancy); there is a complex interplay of reversible histone modifications that govern gene expression, including histone acetylation, methylation, phosphorylation, ubiquitination, and biotinylation. Modification of histone deacetylase (HDAC) has surfaced as one strategy for changing tumor behavior (Myzak and Dashwood, 2006; Glozak and Seto, 2007). Several food components including butyrate, diallyl disulfide, and sulforaphane have been reported to function as weak ligands for this enzyme and lead to reduced in vitro activity (Myzak and Dashwood, 2006; Dashwood and Ho, 2007). Addition of sulforaphane, an isothiocyanate found in cruciferous vegetables, to cell cultures leads to a concomitant increase in global and local histone acetylation status including the promoter regions of p21 and BAX genes. Most recently Dashwood and his research team have demonstrated that sulforaphane feeding markedly changes HDAC activity in humans (Dashwood and Ho, 2007). Impressively, these changes occurred within minutes after consumption of broccoli sprouts and persisted for a significant amount of time but within 24 hours returned to baseline values. How this temporal relationship is influenced by ingestion of multiple food components known to influence epigenetic process remains to be determined. Likewise, what impact these shifts in epigenetic regulation have on physiologically relevant processes in normal and cancerous cells remains to be clarified.

Transcriptomics

Transcriptomics is the study of the transcriptome, which represents the set of all cellular RNA molecules including mRNA, rRNA, tRNA, and other non-coding RNA. The transcriptome is roughly fixed for a given cell type, although mutations are recognized to influence the quantity of these molecules. A variety of environmental factors, including one's diet, can influence the transcriptome. Monitoring mRNA transcripts is increasingly being examined as a molecular biomarker for the detection of disease risk and/ or effectiveness of preventive or therapeutic agents, both dietary components and drugs. Such analyses offer the potential of earlier and more accurate prediction/diagnosis of disease and its progression. Since whole blood mRNA shares more than 80% of the transcriptome with major tissues, it appears to be a good surrogate tissue for predicting events in a target tissue (Liew *et al.*, 2006).

Transcriptomic profiling allows for a simultaneous monitoring of the expression of literally thousands of genes. While microarray technologies provide an important tool to discover expression changes influenced by diet and potentially the regulation of cellular processes, it must be remembered that any response may vary between healthy and diseased conditions. Studies using animals are beginning to identify specific sites of action of bioactive food components (Sunde, 2010). For example, the nuclear factor E2 p45-related factor 2 (Nrf2) and the Kelch domain-containing partner Keap1 are modified by sulforaphane (Cheung and Kong, 2010). Gene expression patterns from wild-type and Nrf2-deficient mice fed sulforaphane have highlighted several novel downstream events and thus clues about the true biological response to this food component. The up-regulation of glutathione S-transferase, nicotinamide adenine dinucleotide phosphate : quinone reductase, gamma-glutamylcysteine synthetase, and epoxide hydrolase, occurring because of release of Nrf2 from its cytosolic complex, likely helps explain the ability of sulforaphane to influence multiple processes including those involving xenobiotic metabolizing enzymes, antioxidants, and biosynthetic enzymes of the glutathione and glucuronidation conjugation pathways (Zhao *et al.*, 2010). Variation in nfr2 also appears to be involved in explaining the ability of caloric restriction to depress cancer risk (Martin-Montalvo *et al.*, 2011).

Mammals are known to adapt to excess exposure to foods and their components through shifts in absorption, metabolism or excretion. Thus, the quantity and duration of exposure to foods or their constituents must be considered when evaluating the response in gene expression patterns. Since microarray technologies provide only a single snapshot, over-interpretation of their physiological significance is possible. The cost of using mRNA microarray technologies has decreased and thus they have become more commonplace for analysis in population studies which are aimed at characterizing subjects and their response to agents including nutrients (Ornish *et al.*, 2008; Al Tamimi *et al.*, 2010). Transcriptomic technologies have been used to examine the relationship between diet and cancer risk among native Japanese and second-generation Japanese-American men as a function of consumption of animal fat and soy (Marks *et al.*, 2004). This technology was able to discriminate differences between those men with cancer and those who were cancer free. However, it should be noted that the number of clinical nutrition studies that incorporate transcriptomic technologies remain relatively sparse. Impressively van Erk *et al.* (2006) found that relatively short-term exposures were sufficient to cause significant changes in the human transcriptome, and suggested that this technology can be used to discriminate the effects of types of diets on gene patterns. Overall, it may be possible to use a bolus exposure to determine whether or not key cancer-related processes are responsive or not responsive to foods with proposed anti-cancer activity.

Recent discoveries of embryonic stem cell identity in poorly differentiated tumors suggest that cancer prediction using embryonic stem cell signatures may be an important direction for further research (Ben-Porath *et al.*, 2008; Zhu *et al.*, 2010). Increasing evidence points to the ability of several dietary components to influence stem cells (Trosko, 2008; Alexander *et al.*, 2010; Langelier *et al.*, 2010). The differential transcriptomic response between normal and cancer stem cells represents an exciting area of investigation that may ultimately have a major impact on our understanding of the food components that hold the greatest promise for retarding the recurrent of cancers.

Proteomics

Proteomics has been widely embraced by multiple biomedical disciplines including nutrition as a tool to identify biomarkers of health, disease and/or prevention/treatment responses (Thongboonkerd, 2007; Xiao *et al.*, 2009; Rahman *et al.*, 2010). High-throughput capabilities allow for the simultaneous examination of numerous proteins, and offer insights into subtle shifts in proteins in cells, tissues and/or biofluids. Unlike the genome, the proteome is dynamic and varies according to cell type and functional state of the cell, thus raising important issues about what biological specimens are best to monitor the response to foods or their components. It is interesting to note that gene expression patterns do not always correlate with protein expression patterns, and thus the examination of a protein profile may have particular physiological relevance to teasing apart responders from non-responders.

Proteomic studies are already beginning to provide valuable evidence about the pleiotropic effects of food components on cellular processes. For example, a proteomic study using F344 rats revealed that providing quercetin in the diet (10 g/kg for 11 weeks) markedly influenced the expression of proteins in the colon which are involved in energy metabolism, cytoskeleton organization, and apoptosis. (Dihal *et al.*, 2008). Evidence was provided that the response to quercetin shifted the balance from glycolysis towards fatty acid oxidation, possibly by reducing the expression of four proteins involved in glycolysis including fructose 1,6-biphosphate aldolase A(1,6-PAA), glyceraldehyde-3-phosphate dehydrogenase (GADPH), α-enolase, and pyruvate kinase isoenzyme M2 (PKM2). Resveratrol, which is found in grapes and peanuts, and genistein from soy have also been demonstrated to have a marked effect on multiple cellular networks (Cecconi *et al.*, 2008; Yan *et al.*, 2010). It is unclear if the response to these foods or food components reflects one or possibly a combination of changes in selected proteins.

Stable isotope labeling with amino acids in cell culture (SILAC) phosphoproteomic approaches have been used to investigate the specific effects of genistein on signaling pathways (Yan *et al.*, 2010). Remarkably, the tyrosine phosphorylation of 174 among 181 identified proteins was reduced by treatment with genistein. Other studies in leukemia HL-60 cells that investigated the proteomic response to genistein documented dose-dependent (50 μM >20 μM) inhibition of heterogeneous nuclear ribonucleo-proteins C1/C2 (hnRNP C), stathmin, and GTP-binding Ras-related protein-14, and activation of hnRNP H1 and Hsp70 protein-8. The expression of these proteins was also influenced by time of exposure, with levels of HnRNP C and Rab 14 protein decreasing, and those of HnRNP H1, Hsp70 protein-8, increasing from 24 to 72 hours after treatment with genistein (Zhang *et al.*, 2007). Additional studies are needed to determine if the shifts in a protein are due to changes in synthesis/degradation/modification and if these reflect a progressive (rheostat or off/on switch)

response and the compensatory mechanisms which come into play following more prolonged exposures.

A few human trials have begun to examine the impact of eating behaviors on proteomic profiles. For example, the effect of 300 g Brussels sprouts was examined on proteomic profiles of the white blood cells from five subjects (Hoelzl *et al.*, 2008). Up-regulation of manganese superoxide dismutase (MnSOD), which is induced by the transcription factor Nrf2, and repression of Hsp70, which inhibits apoptosis, were among the more significant findings. Proteomic investigations may be particularly useful for determining gene–nutrient interactions such as the intake of cruciferous vegetables and possibly other foods and better cancer-protective effect in GSTM1- and GSTT1-null individuals compared with those with a wild-type gene profile (Lampe, 2007).

Clinical proteomic studies also support the pleiotropic effects of food components. In a study with healthy postmenopausal women, soy isoflavones (50 mg for 8 weeks) reduced expression of four proteins including galectin-1, which is involved in cell-cycle progression, pleckstrin, an aconitase 2 precursor, and RNA polymerase III transcription initiation factor B in peripheral blood mononuclear cells (Fuchs *et al.*, 2007b). Conversely, genistein increased the level of 25 proteins including Hsp70 and filamin-A, which are known to suppress TNFα activity; 26S protease-8, which has been shown to inhibit NFkB activation; and cytosolic NADP$^+$-dependent isocitrate dehydrogenase, which influences overall mitochondria function (Fuchs *et al.*, 2007a). It is unclear if disease conditions will influence the proteomic profile that occurs following soy isoflavone exposure, but based on these finding such studies are warranted.

Proteomic studies may be useful for identifying processes which may influence overall cancer risk such as inflammation. Recently the anti-inflammatory properties of fish oils were examined as a modifier of proteins related to inflammation (de Roos *et al.*, 2008). The authors discovered a reduction of acute-phase proteins haptoglobin, haemopexin, and α-1-antitrypsin. A combination of two-dimensional and matrix-assisted laser desorption/ionization/time-of-flight mass spectrometric (MALDI TOF MS) technologies were able to identify haptoglobin α2 chain as an up-regulated serum protein in glioblastoma patients with levels of the protein increasing as the tumor grade increased (Kumar *et al.*, 2010). Since haptoglobin is known to be expressed in at least six phenotypes, proteomics may be useful for the systematic monitoring of isoforms and testing of efficacy of dietary interventions with fish oils or other interventions for specific subpopulations (Shah *et al.*, 2010).

While nutritional proteomics is in its infancy, it holds promise to provide a wealth of information for assessing how changes in dietary habits can influence critical cellular processes. Research in this area should allow for a greater understanding of the regulatory mechanisms for maintaining normal cellular homeostasis during normal, limited or excess exposures, and of the pathogenic mechanisms caused or modified by nutritional inadequacies; it should also help to define molecular targets of bioactive food components that can be used for predicting the response to diet. It will be important to characterize these proteins or groups of proteins that play a key part in cellular networks, define the physical boundaries (i.e. nuclear versus cytosolic) and establish their relationships with opposing biological processes (i.e. proliferation versus apoptosis). While biomarkers emanating from proteomic analyses cannot automatically be adopted for their clinical use, they are beginning to provide a biological base for predicting a response (Scott *et al.*, 2010).

Metabolomics

The metabolome refers to all of the low molecular weight compounds in a biological sample in a given context. The study of metabolomics has enormous potential for validating intake assessment methods or measuring biological changes in response to bioactive food components. Changes in amounts of metabolites generally appear more quickly than changes in amounts of DNA, RNA, or protein. This may allow researchers to detect changes early in the cancer process and determine any influence that dietary compounds have over the process (Kim and Maruvada, 2008). Measuring metabolites provides an additional advantage over measuring mRNA or protein, as a single metabolite may be a substrate of multiple enzymes with varying isoforms (Ellis *et al.*, 2007). Challenges of using metabolomics as a tool include the high number of metabolites and the decision of which metabolites are the most important to study. These can be addressed by measuring a metabolic fingerprint, or a subset of metabolites that provides a snapshot of the metabolome at a given time point.

Researchers have used metabolomic methods to profile cells at various stages in carcinogenesis based on shifts in glucose metabolism (Gatenby and Gillies, 2007). This has potential for allowing researchers to study how food com-

ponents influence these metabolic profiles, which could lead to information on molecular targets of compounds. Measuring metabolites may also assist in determining mechanism of action or bioavailability, as illustrated by a study which measured urinary metabolites in premenopausal women who consumed soy in the form of textured vegetable protein (conjugated isoflavone glucosides) or miso (unconjugated isoflavones). Changes in metabolites in response to miso were greater than those from textured vegetable protein, suggesting that composition of isoflavones may influence any biological effects (Solanky *et al.*, 2005).

Microbiomics

The microbiota in the human gastrointestinal tract consists of over 100 trillion microorganisms of over 500 bacterial species (Davis and Milner, 2009). Certain strains are associated with increased cancer risk, while others are associated with decreased risk. Therefore, it is important to identify dietary factors that promote the growth of beneficial bacteria while limiting the growth of harmful bacteria. Through metabolism of dietary components, the microbiota, depending on its composition, can form new bioactive compounds that influence cancer processes, either positively (hydrogen sulfide and secondary bile acids) or negatively (equol from soy isoflavones or urolithins from ellagic acid) (Larrosa *et al.*, 2006; O'Keefe *et al.*, 2009; Lampe, 2010).

The composition and activity of the microbiota can be modified by diet. Certain food compounds, particularly oligosaccharides found in vegetables, are not digested by humans, but rather by the microflora. These compounds, called prebiotics, promote selective growth or metabolic activity of beneficial bacteria such as lactobacilli and bifidobacteria. Probiotics, or live bacteria found in yogurts, cheeses, or functional foods and supplements, can colonize the gastrointestinal tract for short periods following consumption. Synbiotics include combinations of probiotics and prebiotics to enhance the survival and activity of the probiotic.

Physiological versus Pathological Conditions

A fundamental issue remains about the circumstances under which bioactive food components bring about their primary effect; namely, are they maintaining normal cellular function, influencing the transition of the normal to the neoplastic state, or altering the biological behavior of the neoplasm? Evidence exists that all three conditions can have importance in influencing cancer risk and tumor behavior, but that the biological mechanisms may be unique for each.

A wealth of evidence points to the ability of several bioactive food components to modify phase I and II enzymes and thereby help maintain normalcy in a cell (Milner, 2006; Yu and Kong, 2007). Modifying carcinogen metabolism and disposition is one of the major mechanisms by which dietary compounds can reduce cancer risk. The expression of phase I enzymes, which activate many carcinogens, is established by xenobiotic-sensing nuclear receptors such as AhR, CAR, PXR, and RXR. Phase II enzymes catalyze the conjugations of carcinogens and frequently are transcriptionally controlled by the Nrf2/ARE signaling pathways. Thus, the Nrf2/ARE signaling pathway likely represents a major target for several bioactive food components. The excretion of carcinogens and their metabolites is likely mediated by phase III transporters, which share common regulatory mechanisms with phase I/II enzymes. In addition to transcriptional regulation, the activities of phase I/II enzymes and phase III transporters could be directly activated or inhibited by dietary compounds.

There is limited evidence that bioactive food components can also influence the transition of normal to neoplastic cells. Classically, feeding a methyl-donor-deficient diet precipitates increased liver cancer, even in the absence of carcinogen exposure (Pogribny et al., 2006). More recently, studies have demonstrated that feeding a diet high in fat, but low in calcium and vitamin D and thus similar to that consumed as part of a Western diet, markedly increases colon cancer in rodents (Yang et al., 2007). It is unclear why there are few cases where deficiencies or inadequacies lead to cancer, but the paucity of cases may be related to the ability of the cell to adjust and survive through changes in autophagic homeostasis (Bergamini et al., 2004).

Multiple studies also indicate that several food components can alter cancer cell proliferation, as well as programmed cell death (apoptosis) (Enciso and Hirschi, 2007; Martin, 2007; Moriarty et al., 2007; Meeran and Katiyar, 2008). Key transitions in the cell cycle are known to be regulated by the activities of various protein kinase complexes composed of cyclin and cyclin-dependent kinases (CDK) molecules and to be influenced by multiple dietary components. Evidence that both essential and non-

essential dietary agents can modulate cell cycle checkpoints, and thus contribute to reduced tumor proliferation, continues to mount (Milner, 2006; Enciso and Hirschi, 2007; Moriarty et al., 2007; Meeran and Katiyar, 2008). Diverse agents such as apigenin (celery, parsley), curcumin (turmeric), (-)-epigallocatechin-3-gallate (green tea), resveratrol (red grape, peanuts, and berries), genistein (soybean), and allyl sulfur (garlic) have been shown to markedly influence the cell cycle, possibly by differing mechanisms. At least some of these changes may be associated with post-translational changes including shifts in the phosphorylation of key regulatory factors of cell division. (Knowles and Milner, 2003). Dietary components can modulate apoptosis through shifts in protein expression and function or mRNA expression, either directly or indirectly, to modulate gene expression in both the extrinsic and mitochondrial-mediated apoptotic pathways (Kim et al., 2007; Martin, 2007; Miyoshi et al., 2007). At least some bioactive components may cause apoptosis by enhancing free radical formation in the cell (Kim et al., 2007; Miyoshi et al., 2007). While there is evidence that multiple dietary components can induce apoptosis, the concentrations used in many of these studies are excessive and may not reflect any effects of more physiological exposures.

Sites of Action

Current information suggests that changes in multiple cellular processes may account for the response to bioactive food components and thus represent a pleiotropic response, unlike that which frequently occurs with drugs. Multiple processes including carcinogen metabolism, DNA repair, cell proliferation, programmed cell death, inflammation, differentiation, and angiogenesis are likely modified by bioactive food components (Figure 51.1) (Milner, 2006, 2008; Davis and Milner, 2007). Since multiple biological changes can occur simultaneously, it is difficult to determine which is most critical in dictating the overall response. The ability of multiple nutrients to influence the same process suggest synergistic, as well as antagonistic, interactions may occur depending on exposures.

The use of animal models, transgenic and knockout, will be fundamental to elucidating the specific site(s) of action of bioactive food components. Knockout mice have already assisted in identifying the nuclear factor E2 p45-related factor 2 (Nrf2) and the Kelch domain-containing partner Keap1 as the complex that is modified

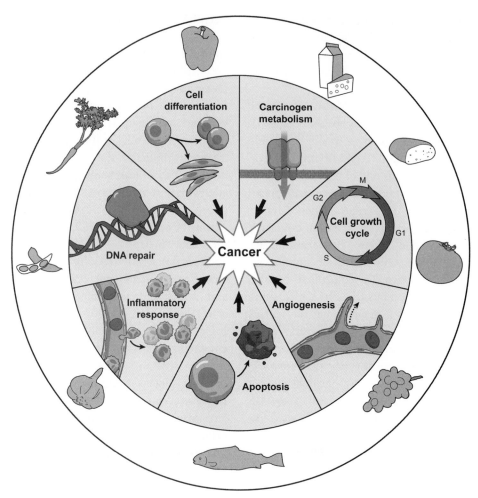

FIG. 51.1 Bioactive food components can influence multiple cancer processes. It remains unclear if the ability of food components to influence cancer relates to changes in one or a combination of effects on cellular processes.

by sulforaphane (Juge *et al.*, 2007; Yu and Kong, 2007). Gene expression profiles from wild-type and Nrf2-deficient mice fed sulforaphane have shown several novel downstream events and thus provided more clues about the true biological response to this food component. Another potential target for retarding cancer recurrence that has surfaced is the overexpressed human epidermal growth factor receptor 2 (HER-2/neu), which is treated by the monoclonal antibody Herceptin. Recent studies by Yee *et al.* (2005) suggest that fish oil may be as beneficial in retarding overexpression of Her2/neu as is Herceptin. These data suggest that copy number may also be an important determinant of the response to foods and their components.

Current Recommendations

The 2007 Report of the World Cancer Research Fund/American Institute for Cancer Research on Food, Nutrition, Physical Activity, and the Prevention of Cancer (WCRF/AICR, 2007) reviewed all relevant research on diet and cancer risk and provided recommendations for overall cancer prevention in the general public based on this research. The eight recommendations are summarized in Table 51.1. Because many foods and food components have been reported to have effects on particular cancers and not others, the report also includes summaries specific to cancer site. While reduced intake of red meat, processed meat, and alcohol are the only foods that have associations

TABLE 51.2 Summary of factors that modify the risk for colorectal cancers based on strength of evidence

Strength of evidence	Increases risk	Decreases risk
Convincing	Red meat Processed meat Alcoholic drinks (men) Body fatness Abdominal fatness Adult attained height	Physical activity
Probable	Alcoholic drinks (women)	Foods containing dietary fiber Garlic Milk Calcium
Limited, suggestive	Foods containing iron Cheese Foods containing animal fat Foods containing sugars	Non-starchy vegetables Fruits Foods containing folate Foods containing selenium Fish Foods containing vitamin D Selenium

Adapted from WCRF/AICR (2007).

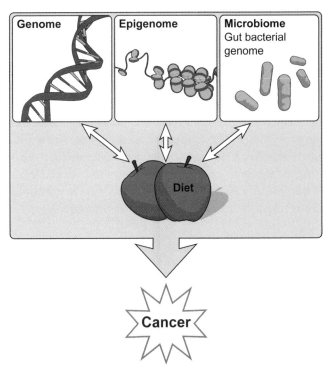

FIG. 51.2 An individual's genome, epigenome, and associated downstream events in transcriptomics, proteomics, and metabolomics, in concert with the microbiome, can markedly influence, either positively or negatively, the response to foods or food components. Three types of biomarkers are needed to adequately understand the role of diet in cancer prevention, namely (1) exposure, (2) effect (molecular target), and (3) susceptibility (genome–nutrient and nutrient–nutrient interactions).

with overall cancer prevention, there is sufficient data to draw further conclusions on the effects of foods and specific cancer sites, particularly cancers of the colon and rectum. Table 51.2 summarizes the findings of the report on food, nutrition, physical activity, and colorectal cancers. It is clear from a close examination of the available studies that there remains a dearth of controlled interventions to truly assess the ability of foods or their components to influence cancer risk and tumor behavior. It is also abundantly clear that considerable variability occurs in the literature. While current recommendations are appropriate, it is clear that not all individuals will respond identically to foods or food components. Additional research is needed to determine the best foods/components to consume and when during life to get maximum benefits. It is logical to assume that genetic and epigenetic events along with the microbiome will have a significant impact on the response to what is eaten (Figure 51.2).

Future Directions

It is becoming increasingly appreciated that the chances of developing cancer are significantly influenced by one's lifestyle. Since ancient times a host of food items have been touted for their medicinal value including the prevention of diseases such as cancer. A wealth of experimental evidence using a variety of models substantiates the importance of the diet in modifying cancer risk due to carcinogens or to genetic predisposition. The concept that foods and food components can serve as effective agents for cancer risk and tumor behavior has advanced the field markedly. Unfortunately, preclinical studies have not always been substantiated in clinical intervention studies. The reason for these inconsistencies remains elusive, but may relate to the quantity of the bioactive constituent consumed, the timing of exposure, genetics, and biological insults including excessive energy and associated radicals, environmental contaminants, viruses and/or bacteria. Exciting opportunities exist for identifying and validating biomarkers that can be used to identify the exposures, predict the molecular target needing modification, and identify those susceptible to the merits or risk associated with intervention (both genetic–nutrient and nutrient–nutrient interactions). While identification of those who will benefit most will not be easy, the societal benefits are enormous.

Suggestions for Further Reading

Davis, C.D., Emenaker, N.J., and Milner, J.A. (2010) Cellular proliferation, apoptosis and angiogenesis: molecular targets for nutritional preemption of cancer. *Semin Oncol* 37, 243–257.

Kussman, M., Krause, L., and Siffert, W. (2010) Nutrigenomics: where are we with genetic and epigenetic markers for disposition and susceptibility? *Nutr Rev* 68(Suppl 1), S38–47.

McCabe-Sellers, B., Lovera, D., Nuss, H., *et al.* (2008) Personalizing nutrigenomics research through community based participatory research and omics technologies. *OMICS* 12, 263–272.

References

Abrams, S.A., Griffin, I.J., Hawthorne, K.M., *et al.* (2005) Vitamin D receptor Fok1 polymorphisms affect calcium absorption, kinetics, and bone mineralization rates during puberty. *J Bone Miner Res* 20, 945–953.

Al Tamimi, D.M., Shawarby, M.A., Ahmed, A., *et al.* (2010) Protein expression profile and prevalence pattern of the molecular classes of breast cancer – a Saudi population based study. *BMC Cancer* 10, 223.

Alexander, L.S., Mahajan, A., Odle, J., *et al.* (2010) Dietary phosphate restriction decreases stem cell proliferation and subsequent growth potential in neonatal pigs. *J Nutr* 140, 477–482.

American Cancer Society (2011) *Cancer Facts and Figures 2011.* American Cancer Society, Atlanta, GA.

Ben-Porath, I., Thomson, M.W., Carey, V.J., *et al.* (2008) An embryonic stem cell-like gene expression signature in poorly differentiated aggressive human tumors. *Nat Genet* 40, 499–507.

Bergamini, E., Cavallini, G., Donati, A., *et al.* (2004) The role of macroautophagy in the ageing process, anti-ageing intervention and age-associated diseases. *Int J Biochem Cell Biol* 36, 2392–2404.

Boyapati, S.M., Shu, X.O., Ruan, Z.X., *et al.* (2005) Soyfood intake and breast cancer survival: a followup of the Shanghai Breast Cancer Study. *Breast Cancer Res Treat* 92, 11–17.

Cecconi, D., Zamo, A., Parisi, A., *et al.* (2008) Induction of apoptosis in Jeko-1 mantle cell lymphoma cell line by resveratrol: a proteomic analysis. *J Proteome Res* 7, 2670–2680.

Cheung, K.L. and Kong, A.N. (2010) Molecular targets of dietary phenethyl isothiocyanate and sulforaphane for cancer chemoprevention. *AAPS J* 12, 87–97.

Chlebowski, R.T., Blackburn, G.L., Thomson, C.A., *et al.* (2006) Dietary fat reduction and breast cancer outcome: interim efficacy results from the Women's Intervention Nutrition Study. *J Natl Cancer Inst* 98, 1767–1776.

D'Archivio, M., Filesi, C., Vari, R., *et al.* (2010) Bioavailability of the polyphenols: status and controversies. *Int J Mol Sci* 11, 1321–1342.

Dashwood, R.H. and Ho, E. (2007) Dietary histone deacetylase inhibitors: from cells to mice to man. *Semin Cancer Biol* 17, 363–369.

Davenport, D.M. and Wargovich, M.J. (2005) Modulation of cytochrome P450 enzymes by organosulfur compounds from garlic. *Food Chem Toxicol* 43, 1753–1762.

Davis, C.D. and Milner, J.A. (2007) Biomarkers for diet and cancer prevention research: potentials and challenges. *Acta Pharmacol Sin* 28, 1262–1273.

Davis, C.D. and Milner, J.A. (2009) Gastrointestinal microflora, food components and colon cancer prevention. *J Nutr Biochem* 20, 743–752.

De Roos, B., Geelen, A., Ross, K., *et al.* (2008) Identification of potential serum biomarkers of inflammation and lipid modulation that are altered by fish oil supplementation in healthy volunteers. *Proteomics* 8, 1965–1974.

Dihal, A.A., Van Der Woude, H., Hendriksen, P.J., *et al.* (2008) Transcriptome and proteome profiling of colon mucosa from quercetin fed F344 rats point to tumor preventive mechanisms, increased mitochondrial fatty acid degradation and decreased glycolysis. *Proteomics* 8, 45–61.

El-Sohemy, A. (2007) Nutrigenetics. *Forum Nutr* 60, 25–30.

Ellis, D.I., Dunn, W.B., Griffin, J.L., *et al.* (2007) Metabolic fingerprinting as a diagnostic tool. *Pharmacogenomics* 8, 1243–1266.

Enciso, J.M. and Hirschi, K.K. (2007) Nutrient regulation of tumor and vascular endothelial cell proliferation. *Curr Cancer Drug Targets* 7, 432–437.

Fang, M.Z., Wang, Y., Ai, N., *et al.* (2003) Tea polyphenol (-)-epigallocatechin-3-gallate inhibits DNA methyltransferase and reactivates methylation-silenced genes in cancer cell lines. *Cancer Res* **63**, 7563–7570.

Fuchs, D., Dirscherl, B., Schroot, J.H., *et al.* (2007a) Proteome analysis suggests that mitochondrial dysfunction in stressed endothelial cells is reversed by a soy extract and isolated isoflavones. *J Proteome Res* **6**, 2132–2142.

Fuchs, D., Vafeiadou, K., Hall, W.L., *et al.* (2007b) Proteomic biomarkers of peripheral blood mononuclear cells obtained from postmenopausal women undergoing an intervention with soy isoflavones. *Am J Clin Nutr* **86**, 1369–1375.

Gatenby, R.A. and Gillies, R.J. (2007) Glycolysis in cancer: a potential target for therapy. *Int J Biochem Cell Biol* **39**, 1358–1366.

Glozak, M.A. and Seto, E. (2007) Histone deacetylases and cancer. *Oncogene* **26**, 5420–5432.

Hanahan, D. and Weinberg, R.A. (2000) The hallmarks of cancer. *Cell* **100**, 57–70.

Hoelzl, C., Lorenz, O., Haudek, V., *et al.* (2008) Proteome alterations induced in human white blood cells by consumption of Brussels sprouts: results of a pilot intervention study. *Proteomics Clin Appl* **2**, 108–117.

Holloway, A.F. and Oakford, P.C. (2007) Targeting epigenetic modifiers in cancer. *Curr Med Chem* **14**, 2540–2547.

Ingelman-Sundberg, M., Sim, S.C., Gomez, A., *et al.* (2007) Influence of cytochrome P450 polymorphisms on drug therapies: pharmacogenetic, pharmacoepigenetic and clinical aspects. *Pharmacol Ther* **116**, 496–526.

Jenab, M., Slimani, N., Bictash, M., *et al.* (2009) Biomarkers in nutritional epidemiology: applications, needs and new horizons. *Hum Genet* **125**, 507–525.

Juge, N., Mithen, R.F., and Traka, M. (2007) Molecular basis for chemoprevention by sulforaphane: a comprehensive review. *Cell Mol Life Sci* **64**, 1105–1127.

Kim, Y.A., Xiao, D., Xiao, H., *et al.* (2007) Mitochondria-mediated apoptosis by diallyl trisulfide in human prostate cancer cells is associated with generation of reactive oxygen species and regulated by Bax/Bak. *Mol Cancer Ther* **6**, 1599–1609.

Kim, Y.S. and Maruvada, P. (2008) Frontiers in metabolomics for cancer research: proceedings of a National Cancer Institute workshop. *Metabolomics* **4**, 105–113.

Knowles, L.M. and Milner, J.A. (2003) Diallyl disulfide induces ERK phosphorylation and alters gene expression profiles in human colon tumor cells. *J Nutr* **133**, 2901–2906.

Krishnan, A.V., Swami, S., Moreno, J., *et al.* (2007) Potentiation of the growth-inhibitory effects of vitamin D in prostate cancer by genistein. *Nutr Rev* **65**, S121–123.

Kumar, D.M., Thota, B., Shinde, S.V., *et al.* (2010) Proteomic identification of haptoglobin alpha2 as a glioblastoma serum biomarker: implications in cancer cell migration and tumor growth. *J Proteome Res* **9**, 5557–5567.

Lamartiniere, C.A., Cotroneo, M.S., Fritz, W.A., *et al.* (2002) Genistein chemoprevention: timing and mechanisms of action in murine mammary and prostate. *J Nutr* **132**, 552S–558S.

Lampe, J.W. (2007) Diet, genetic polymorphisms, detoxification, and health risks. *Altern Ther Health Med* **13**, S108–111.

Lampe, J.W. (2010) Emerging research on equol and cancer. *J Nutr* **140**, 1369S–72S.

Langelier, B., Linard, A., Bordat, C., *et al.* (2010) Long chain-polyunsaturated fatty acids modulate membrane phospholipid composition and protein localization in lipid rafts of neural stem cell cultures. *J Cell Biochem* **110**, 1356–1364.

Larrosa, M., Gonzalez-Sarrias, A., Garcia-Conesa, M.T., *et al.* (2006) Urolithins, ellagic acid-derived metabolites produced by human colonic microflora, exhibit estrogenic and antiestrogenic activities. *J Agric Food Chem* **54**, 1611–1620.

Li, Y. and Tollefsbol, T.O. (2010) Impact on DNA methylation in cancer prevention and therapy by bioactive dietary components. *Curr Med Chem* **17**, 2141–2151.

Liew, C.C., Ma, J., Tang, H.C., *et al.* (2006) The peripheral blood transcriptome dynamically reflects system wide biology: a potential diagnostic tool. *J Lab Clin Med* **147**, 126–132.

Lin, D.W., Neuhouser, M.L., Schenk, J.M., *et al.* (2007) Low-fat, low-glycemic load diet and gene expression in human prostate epithelium: a feasibility study of using cDNA microarrays to assess the response to dietary intervention in target tissues. *Cancer Epidemiol Biomarkers Prev* **16**, 2150–2154.

Marks, L.S., Kojima, M., Demarzo, A., *et al.* (2004) Prostate cancer in native Japanese and Japanese-American men: effects of dietary differences on prostatic tissue. *Urology* **64**, 765–771.

Martin, K.R. (2007) Using nutrigenomics to evaluate apoptosis as a preemptive target in cancer prevention. *Curr Cancer Drug Targets* **7**, 438–446.

Martin-Montalvo, A., Villalba, J.M., Navas, P., *et al.* (2011) NRF2, cancer and calorie restriction. *Oncogene* **30**, 505–520.

McKeown, N.M., Day, N.E., Welch, A.A., *et al.* (2001) Use of biological markers to validate self-reported dietary intake in a random sample of the European Prospective Investigation into Cancer United Kingdom Norfolk cohort. *Am J Clin Nutr* **74**, 188–196.

Meeran, S.M. and Katiyar, S.K. (2008) Cell cycle control as a basis for cancer chemoprevention through dietary agents. *Front Biosci* **13**, 2191–2202.

Milner, J.A. (2006) Diet and cancer: facts and controversies. *Nutr Cancer* **56**, 216–224.

Milner, J.A. (2008) Nutrition and cancer: essential elements for a roadmap. *Cancer Lett* **269**, 189–198.

Miyoshi, N., Naniwa, K., Yamada, T., *et al.* (2007) Dietary flavonoid apigenin is a potential inducer of intracellular oxidative stress: the role in the interruptive apoptotic signal. *Arch Biochem Biophys* **466**, 274–282.

Moriarty, R.M., Naithani, R., and Surve, B. (2007) Organosulfur compounds in cancer chemoprevention. *Mini Rev Med Chem* **7**, 827–838.

Myzak, M.C. and Dashwood, R.H. (2006) Histone deacetylases as targets for dietary cancer preventive agents: lessons learned with butyrate, diallyl disulfide, and sulforaphane. *Curr Drug Targets* **7**, 443–452.

O'Keefe, S.J., Ou, J., Aufreiter, S., et al. (2009) Products of the colonic microbiota mediate the effects of diet on colon cancer risk. *J Nutr* **139**, 2044–2048.

Okey, A.B., Boutros, P.C., and Harper, P.A. (2005) Polymorphisms of human nuclear receptors that control expression of drug-metabolizing enzymes. *Pharmacogenet Genomics* **15**, 371–379.

Ornish, D., Magbanua, M.J., Weidner, G., et al. (2008) Changes in prostate gene expression in men undergoing an intensive nutrition and lifestyle intervention. *Proc Natl Acad Sci USA* **105**, 8369–8374.

Perry, G.H., Dominy, N.J., Claw, K.G., et al. (2007) Diet and the evolution of human amylase gene copy number variation. *Nat Genet* **39**, 1256–1260.

Pinto, D., Marshall, C., Feuk, L., et al. (2007) Copy-number variation in control population cohorts. *Hum Mol Genet,* **16** Spec No. 2, R168–73.

Pogribny, I.P., Ross, S.A., Wise, C., et al. (2006) Irreversible global DNA hypomethylation as a key step in hepatocarcinogenesis induced by dietary methyl deficiency. *Mutat Res* **593**, 80–87.

Qiao, Y.L., Dawsey, S.M., Kamangar, F., et al. (2009) Total and cancer mortality after supplementation with vitamins and minerals: follow-up of the Linxian General Population Nutrition Intervention Trial. *J Natl Cancer Inst* **101**, 507–518.

Rahman, M.A., Amin, A.R., and Shin, D.M. (2010) Chemopreventive potential of natural compounds in head and neck cancer. *Nutr Cancer* **62**, 973–987.

Ross, S.A. (2003) Diet and DNA methylation interactions in cancer prevention. *Ann NY Acad Sci* **983**, 197–207.

Scott, M.S., Boisvert, F.M., McDowall, M.D., et al. (2010) Characterization and prediction of protein nucleolar localization sequences. *Nucleic Acids Res* **38**, 7388–7399.

Shah, A., Singh, H., Sachdev, V., et al. (2010) Differential serum level of specific haptoglobin isoforms in small cell lung cancer. *Current Proteomics* **7**, 49–65.

Slamon, D.J., Clark, G.M., Wong, S.G., et al. (1987) Human-breast cancer – correlation of relapse and survival with amplification of the Her-2 Neu oncogene. *Science* **235**, 177–182.

Slattery, M.L., Herrick, J., Wolff, R.K., et al. (2007) CDX2 VDR polymorphism and colorectal cancer. *Cancer Epidemiol Biomarkers Prev* **16**, 2752–2755.

Solanky, K.S., Bailey, N.J., Beckwith-Hall, B.M., et al. (2005) Biofluid 1H NMR-based metabonomic techniques in nutrition research – metabolic effects of dietary isoflavones in humans. *J Nutr Biochem* **16**, 236–244.

Steck, S.E., Gammon, M.D., Hebert, J.R., et al. (2007) GSTM1, GSTT1, GSTP1, and GSTA1 polymorphisms and urinary isothiocyanate metabolites following broccoli consumption in humans. *J Nutr* **137**, 904–909.

Sunde, R.A. (2010) mRNA transcripts as molecular biomarkers in medicine and nutrition. *J Nutr Biochem* **21**, 665–670.

Tan, H.L., Thomas-Ahner, J.M., Grainger, E.M., et al. (2010) Tomato-based food products for prostate cancer prevention: what have we learned? *Cancer Metastasis Rev* **29**, 553–568.

Thongboonkerd, V. (2007) Proteomics. *Forum Nutr* **60**, 80–90.

Trosko, J.E. (2008) Role of diet and nutrition on the alteration of the quality and quantity of stem cells in human aging and the diseases of aging. *Curr Pharm Des* **14**, 2707–2718.

Van Erk, M.J., Blom, W.A., Van Ommen, B., et al. (2006) High-protein and high-carbohydrate breakfasts differentially change the transcriptome of human blood cells. *Am J Clin Nutr* **84**, 1233–1241.

WCRF/AICR (2007) *Food, Nutrition, Physical Activity, and the Prevention of Cancer: A Global Perspective.* American Institute for Cancer Research, Washington, DC.

Wong, H.L., Seow, A., Arakawa, K., et al. (2003) Vitamin D receptor start codon polymorphism and colorectal cancer risk: effect modification by dietary calcium and fat in Singapore Chinese. *Carcinogenesis* **24**, 1091–1095.

Xiao, Z., Blonder, J., Zhou, M., et al. (2009) Proteomic analysis of extracellular matrix and vesicles. *J Proteomics* **72**, 34–45.

Yan, G.R., Xiao, C.L., He, G.W., et al. (2010) Global phosphoproteomic effects of natural tyrosine kinase inhibitor, genistein, on signaling pathways. *Proteomics* **10**, 976–986.

Yang, K., Lipkin, M., Newmark, H., et al. (2007) Molecular targets of calcium and vitamin D in mouse genetic models of intestinal cancer. *Nutr Rev* **65**, S134–137.

Yee, L.D., Young, D.C., Rosol, T.J., et al. (2005) Dietary (n-3) polyunsaturated fatty acids inhibit HER-2/neu-induced breast cancer in mice independently of the PPARgamma ligand rosiglitazone. *J Nutr* **135**, 983–988.

Yu, S. and Kong, A.N. (2007) Targeting carcinogen metabolism by dietary cancer preventive compounds. *Curr Cancer Drug Targets* **7**, 416–424.

Zhang, D., Tai, Y.C., Wong, C.H., et al. (2007) Molecular response of leukemia HL-60 cells to genistein treatment, a proteomics study. *Leukemia Res* **31**, 75–82.

Zhao, C.R., Gao, Z.H., and Qu, X.J. (2010) Nrf2-ARE signaling pathway and natural products for cancer chemoprevention. *Cancer Epidemiol* **34**, 523–533.

Zhu, J., Ding, J., and Ding, F. (2010) Tumor stem cell, or its niche, which plays a primary role in tumorigenesis? *World J Gastrointest Oncol* **2**, 218–221.

52

NUTRITION AND GASTROINTESTINAL ILLNESS

ALAN L. BUCHMAN[1], MD, MSPH, FACP, FACG, FACN, AGAF AND
STEPHEN A. MCCLAVE[2], MD, AGAF

[1]Feinberg School of Medicine, Northwestern University, Chicago, Illinois, USA
[2]University of Louisville School of Medicine, Louisville, Kentucky, USA

Summary

The role of nutrition therapy has evolved to become a primary intervention in a number of disease states in the gastrointestinal system. Attention to nutrient agents that may ameliorate symptomatology and/or reverse pathophysiologic processes often serves to change the course of illness and hospitalization and improve patient outcomes.

Introduction

Nutritional issues, including development of macro- and micronutrient deficiencies as well as therapeutic nutrition, are important in a wide range of gastrointestinal disorders involving every organ of the gastrointestinal tract in addition to the liver and gallbladder. The role of disease-specific malnutrition in a variety of ailments as well as directed nutritional therapy is described below. This chapter is not meant to serve as a comprehensive encyclopedia of all the effects of nutrition and malnutrition on the gastrointestinal system. Nor do we do describe the important role of the digestive tract in the digestion, absorption, assimilation, and metabolism of nutrients,

which are covered elsewhere in this book. Rather, specific disease states for which nutrition has a profound role in medical and/or surgical management are used as examples. These include diseases that affect the esophagus (eosinophilic esophagitis and gastroesophageal reflux disease), the small intestine (celiac disease, inflammatory bowel disease, and intestinal failure), and the pancreas (acute and chronic pancreatitis). In some cases, nutrition may have a role in the pathogenesis and treatment of disease (eosinophilic esophagitis, gastroesophageal reflux disease, celiac disease, and Crohn's disease), and in others nutritional issues arise as a result of the disease (Crohn's disease, celiac disease, intestinal failure, and pancreatitis).

Esophagus

Eosinophilic Esophagitis

Eosinophilic esophagitis (EoE) is a relatively recently recognized disorder of the esophagus. Most subjects are male Caucasians who present with long-standing dysphagia or food impactions (Liacouras *et al.*, 2011). Many patients have evidence of atopy, including asthma, allergic rhinitis, eczema, abnormal skin testing or peripheral eosinophilia (Liacouras *et al.*, 2011). Histologically, tissue injury as well as the presence of eosinophils (>15–20 per high-powered field) in the squamous epithelium of the esophagus are observed; submucosal fibrosis may be evident. Environmental allergens, including food, have been implicated in the pathogenesis of EoE. The combination of skin prick and patch testing may be useful in the identification of offending food allergens in up to 70% of cases (Furuta *et al.*, 2007), although poor test standardization remains a limiting factor (Liacouras *et al.*, 2011). Although the mainstay of treatment in this evolving field has been topical corticosteroids (Liacouras *et al.*, 2011), dietary management through the use of a free amino acid-based "elemental" formula, generally delivered via a nasogastric tube because of poor taste (Markowitz *et al.*, 2003) has also been useful. More recently, Kagalwalla *et al.* (2006) proposed the use of food elimination diets; this has been successful in case series. In their series of 35 children, elimination of cow's milk protein, soy, wheat, eggs, peanuts, and seafood led to significant improvement in esophageal inflammation in 74%.

Gastroesophageal Reflux Disease

Gastroesophageal reflux disease (GERD) is perhaps the most common gastrointestinal disorder (Locke *et al.*, 1977). Transient relaxation of the lower esophageal sphincter (LES) is one of the mechanisms underlying the disorder's pathophysiology. This leads to reflux of acid into the esophagus where the mucosal lining may be damaged. Several foods have been associated with increased GERD symptoms. These include dietary fat, peppermint, coffee, caffeine, onions, citrus products, wine, and carbonated beverages because of relaxation of the LES. However, dietary modification has met with variable success for control of both GERD-like symptoms as well as objective evidence of pathology, and studies of specific food triggers have met with conflicting results (Karamanolis and Tack, 2006). High-fat-containing foods may, in addition to lowering the LES pressure, result in delayed gastric emptying

with a resultant enhancement of gastric acid secretion (Karamanolis and Tack, 2006). The incidence of GERD is also increased in obesity (Locke *et al.*, 1999; Ruhl and Everhardt, 1999), although this association has not been demonstrated in all studies (Lagergren *et al.*, 2000). The pathophysiology underlying this observation remains speculative, however. Factors including increased intra-abdominal pressure (Sugerman *et al.*, 1997) and increased basal and food-stimulated acid secretion (Mercer *et al.*, 1987; Wisen *et al.*, 1987) have been proposed. The role of weight loss in the management of GERD is currently undefined, although some studies have suggested an improvement in objective measures of GERD (Tolonen *et al.*, 2006).

Small Intestine

Celiac Disease

Better understanding of the disease prevalence, the nature of the immunologic responses, the long-term course, and the susceptibility to complications has contributed to improved management of the patient with celiac sprue (See and Murray, 2006; Green and Cellier, 2007). Celiac disease or sprue is a chronic disease in genetically predisposed individuals as a result of a potent immune response to the gluten protein contained in wheat, rye, and barley. Innate immune responses lead to the immediate reaction of increased permeability and release of inflammatory cytokines (interleukin, IL-15). Acquired responses promote further immune sensitivity, loss of tolerance, and development of chronic inflammation (See and Murray, 2006). The proinflammatory Th-1 response that characterizes celiac sprue perpetuates the elicitation of tumor necrosis factor and interferon-γ. The proximal small bowel is affected to a disproportionately greater degree than the distal small bowel and colon, as it sees the highest concentration of injurious peptides contained in the toxic grains. The extent of injury can involve from as little as 1% to as great as 100% of the length of the small bowel. The net effect of the chronic inflammation is a defect in the ability to absorb both micro- and macronutrients. Symptoms are fairly classic, with weight loss, diarrhea, steatorrhea, and, in children, failure to thrive. While patients are at risk for multiple micronutrient deficiencies (such as folate, B_{12}, and fat-soluble vitamins), iron deficiency is probably most common. Because of the variable involvement of the small bowel, however, there may be wide variation in symptomatology. It is not uncommon for patients who may even be obese or have no evidence of diarrhea to present with iron deficiency alone.

Extraintestinal manifestations of celiac sprue include infertility, peripheral neuropathy, ataxia and epilepsy, dermatitis herpetiformis, aphthous ulcers in the mouth, abnormalities of the dental enamel, and abnormalities of bone mineralization (See and Murray, 2006). Osteopenia is present in as many as 40% of newly diagnosed cases, with osteoporosis present in up to 26% of new cases (Mora et al., 2001). Patients with celiac disease are at increased risk for autoimmune disorders compared with the general population.

The diagnosis can be made through a serologic panel of antibodies and by biopsies of the small bowel. The most sensitive and specific antibodies are the anti-tissue transglutaminase and the anti-endomysial antibodies (See and Murray, 2006). Anti-gliadin IgG and IgA antibodies are not as sensitive or specific. Because an IgA deficiency can occur concomitantly in a small number of patients with celiac sprue, falsely normal levels of anti-tissue transglutaminase and anti-endomysial antibodies may be seen. Small bowel biopsy helps confirm the case in a patient on a regular diet who shows loss of villous height and evidence of an intense inflammatory infiltrate (especially plasma cells) in the lamina propria of the small bowel.

An interesting mnemonic, **"CELIAC,"** helps remind clinicians of the six key steps in the management of the patient with celiac sprue (James, 2005; See and Murray, 2006). The **C** stands for consult with a dietitian, the **E** for education about celiac disease, and the **L** for lifelong adherence to a gluten-free diet; **I** is for identification and treatment of nutrient deficiencies; **A** is for access to support groups; and the second **C** stands for continuous long-term support (James, 2005; See and Murray, 2006). Only dietary restriction of gluten and a gluten-free diet lead to resolution of symptoms and histology. However, non-compliance is a huge problem in management, an issue which is most often related to poor education.

In evaluating the patient on initial assessment, such factors as a dietary history, the support system and family situation, who prepares the food, and lifestyle travel and business responsibilities are all factors that need to be filtered into the management (See and Murray, 2006). Quantitation of the intake of gluten is not necessary. Patients should be encouraged to switch from grains which contain gluten (such as wheat, rye, barley, and bran) to gluten-free grains such as corn, oats, rice, soybeans, and potatoes. There is some concern about cross-contamination

with oats which is commonly stored with wheat on farms. A gluten-free diet focuses instead on plain meats, dairy, vegetables, fruits, and rice (James 2005; See and Murray, 2006).

General counseling for these patients includes recommendations that they avoid non-food sources of gluten such as toothpaste, mouthwash, and medication capsules. They should plan ahead when traveling or going to a friend's house for dinner. Celiac patients should avoid prepared foods and should be encouraged to "make foods from scratch." They should be educated about reading labels. When eating out, attendance at the same restaurants is to be encouraged in order to increase familiarity with the menu and avoid hidden sources of gluten. The highest risk of hidden gluten content occurs in sauces, seasoned food, and combination platters (Fine et al., 1997; See and Murray, 2006).

Patients should be reminded that non-compliance increases the chance of bone disease and the risk of lymphoma. Intestinal lymphoma may occur in as high as 10–15% of cases where patients are non-compliant (Catassi et al., 2002). If they are able to obtain lifelong compliance with a gluten-free diet, their risk for intestinal lymphoma should be no different from that of the general population. Finally, absence of symptoms does not guarantee that the patient is free from occult damage to the gastrointestinal tract occurring in response to exposure to gluten products.

Inflammatory Bowel Disease

Generalized protein-calorie malnutrition with weight loss is common in patients with Crohn's disease, albeit is less common in those with ulcerative colitis. Micronutrient deficiencies may also occur, generally because of decreased intake, malabsorption and/or increased losses, and, in some cases, increased requirements. Deficiencies of fat-soluble vitamin D are present in the vast majority of patients with Crohn's disease, even in those whose disease is in remission. Vitamin A deficiency is encountered less frequently, and vitamin E and K deficiencies are rare. Serum vitamin E concentration may be decreased, solely related to the decrease in serum total lipid concentration. Water-soluble vitamin deficiencies, with the exception of cobalamine (vitamin B_{12}) are rare. Vitamin B_{12} deficiency may develop in those patients with chronically active disease in their terminal ileum, or in those who have had resections of their terminal ileum totaling >60 cm (Behrend et al., 1995). The reduced bile-salt pool that occurs in conjunction with terminal ileal disease or resection leads to fat maldigestion and can result in deficiency of essential fatty acids and of fat-soluble vitamins (Bousvaros *et al.*, 1999). Vitamin K deficiency remains rare because the majority is synthesized by normal colonic flora, although this may be disrupted in patients with Crohn's colitis who receive antibiotic therapy. Bacterial overgrowth may also occur proximal to strictures, and the resultant bacteria compete with the enterocytes for nutrient absorption. Folate deficiency has been described in upwards of a third of patients with Crohn's disease (Elsbord and Larsen, 1979) and in those patients taking folic acid antagonists such as methotrexate or medications that decrease folic acid uptake (sulfasalazine). Folic acid's use in chemoprevention for colon cancer is controversial (Levine and Burakoff, 2007). Zinc deficiency may be observed in upwards of 40% of patients with Crohn's disease because of fecal loss of zinc in diarrhea (Valberg *et al.*, 1986). Deficiency can be difficult to determine based on measurement of serum zinc concentration because zinc is bound to albumin, other proteins, and amino acids, concentrations of which may be depressed in active Crohn's disease because of the presence of a protein-losing enteropathy. Similarly, conventional measures of iron deficiency may not be relevant in patients with active Crohn's disease or ulcerative colitis because ferritin, as an acute phase reactant, is often elevated in active disease, and the total iron binding capacity (TIBC) may be decreased.

In general, patients with Crohn's disease, in the absence of an intestinal obstruction, should consume a diet liberal in protein, and with sufficient energy to gain back lost weight, or to maintain a normal weight. There is no benefit to a low-carbohydrate or low-residual diet except in the presence of an intestinal obstruction. There is also no proven benefit from a diet with increased content of unrefined carbohydrate (Ritchie *et al.*, 1987). Potentially, diets high in complex carbohydrates and soluble fiber may be beneficial to patients with colitis because of the effects on colonic mucosa of short-chain fatty acids formed from the fermentation of dietary substrate, such as butyrate, acetate, and propionate. Data from studies using enteral nutritional support have suggested diets or formula high on long-chain triglycerides may be associated with an increased relapse risk in patients with Crohn's disease (Middleton *et al.*, 2005).

Dietary oxalate should be restricted in patients with steatorrhea from chronically active disease involving the terminal ileum or because of a terminal ileum resection.

Normally, dietary oxalate is bound by calcium. However, in the setting of steatorrhea, calcium binds preferentially to free fatty acids. Oxalate then passes into the colon where it is absorbed, possibly related to enhanced colonic permeability caused by the presence of bile salts which normally would have been reabsorbed in the terminal ileum. The oxalate is then filtered in the kidneys where it binds to calcium with the creation of calcium oxalate nephrolithiasis (Dobbins and Binder, 1977; Dharmsathaphorn *et al.*, 1982; Sangaletti *et al.*, 1989).

Exclusionary diets have been utilized in the management of Crohn's disease, although not ulcerative colitis. The concept of the exclusionary diet was based on patient reports of specific foods triggering relapse of their Crohn's disease. In studies by Jones *et al.* (1985), Persson *et al.* (1992), and Riordan *et al.* (1993), patients were made *nil per os* in a research setting, and each day an additional self-described food trigger was added to their diet. Wheat, dairy, and some cruciferous vegetables, as well as mustard greens were found to trigger diarrhea and other gastrointestinal complaints consistent with their symptoms of Crohn's disease. Similar foods were reported by Andresen (1942) to trigger the development of ulcerative colitis. Although wheat bran is an excellent water-holding and fecal bulking agent, dairy products can cause diarrhea and other symptoms in lactase-deficient individuals, and many vegetables have significant biomass, these products, as well as eggs, also contain relatively high concentrations of sulfur. In animal models, sulfur exerts toxic effects on colonocytes (Ohkusa, 1985; Roediger *et al.*, 1993). In one study, the percentage of patients with active Crohn's disease who maintained remission was greater in the exclusionary diet group than in those who received corticosteroids. One epidemiological study found a substantially greater likelihood of the development of Crohn's disease among individuals who consumed fast food at least twice weekly (Persson *et al.*, 1992).

Omega-3 fatty acids, named as such because of the double bond that exists between the third and fourth carbon atoms away from the fatty acid chain's methyl group ending, have been evaluated in several studies for the induction of remission and maintenance of remission in both Crohn's disease and ulcerative colitis. Current data taken in aggregate do not support the use of fish oils in the management of either disease (Lorenz-Meyer *et al.*, 1996; Feagan *et al.*, 2008). Similarly, several small studies in which glutamine was used as a therapy for Crohn's disease do not support its use as a therapeutic agent in irritable bowel disease (IBD); one rodent study suggested inflammation was worsened with glutamine supplementation (Shinozaki *et al.*, 1997; Akobeng *et al.*, 2000).

There are many small studies in which di- and tripeptide-based or free amino acid-based formulas have been used for nasoenteric feeding. The concept behind the use of these products arose because such non-protein-based products would decrease the antigenic load on the gut. However, studies with intact protein-based formulas showed equal efficacy. All of these enteral formulas were sterile, however, and may have resulted in a change in gut flora – perhaps species or total bacterial mass (Buchman, 2005). It must be understood, however, that, even if efficacy of enteral feeding as a primary treatment for Crohn's disease is inferior to treatment with corticosteroids or other pharmacologic interventions (Lochs *et al.*, 1991), enteral nutritional support (or parenteral, if indicated), is useful in the treatment and prevention of nutritional deficiencies and deficits and, in children, prevention and treatment of growth retardation.

The use of parenteral nutrition was based on the concept that so-called "bowel rest" would allow damaged mucosa to heal. Many studies were uncontrolled, and/or retrospective in disease, or used historic controls. Short-term remission rates approaching 64% after 3–6 weeks of therapy were achieved, which are better than with most medical therapies (Lashner *et al.*, 1989). However, long-term remission rates were less impressive and approached those following use of corticosteroids. Most studies have shown similar short- and long-term remission rates when enteral nutritional support was compared with the parenteral route. Although there is little data on the use of enteral nutritional support in the management of enterocutaneous fistulas, findings would suggest short-term closure rates are similar to that with infliximab, although long-term closure is rare (Afonso and Rombeau, 1990). There are certainly appropriate indications for parenteral nutrition in IBD: these include intestinal obstruction, bowel perforation, prolonged postoperative ileus, or use as part of a regimen to manage proximal entero-enteric or enterocutaneous fistulas.

Intestinal Failure

Nearly all macro- and micronutrient absorption occurs in the small intestine, with a lesser component absorbed in the colon. Intestinal failure results when nutrient and/or fluid intake and absorption are insufficient to meet basal requirements. Most commonly, intestinal failure results

---

BOX 52.1 Causes of short bowel syndrome and intestinal failure

In adults
Catastrophic vascular accidents
  Superior mesenteric venous thrombosis
  Superior mesenteric arterial embolism
  Superior mesenteric arterial thrombosis
Intestinal resection for tumor
Midgut volvulus
Multiple intestinal resections for Crohn's disease
Trauma
Radiation enteritis[a]
Refractory sprue*
Scleroderma and mixed connective tissue disease*
Chronic intestinal pseudo-obstruction*

In children
Congenital villus atrophy[a]
Extensive aganglionosis[a]
Microvillus inclusion disease
Gastroschisis
Jejunal or ileal atresia
Necrotizing enterocolitis
Midgut volvulus
Chronic intestinal pseudo-obstruction
Multiple intestinal resections for Crohn's disease
Trauma

*Functional short bowel syndrome may also occur in conditions associated with severe malabsorption, in which the bowel length is often intact.

---

from short bowel syndrome – an anatomic reduction in the length of functional intestine (Figure 52.1). Loss of bowel may occur congenitally, or may result from one of more surgical resections as a result of trauma or mesenteric vascular compromise (Box 52.1). Many although not all patients with short bowel syndrome will require parenteral infusion of nutrients, and/or fluid and electrolytes. Some patients with short bowel syndrome may remain nutritionally autonomous, or may be successfully weaned from parenteral support with proper medical and/or surgical management (Figure 52.2). Intestinal failure may also result from a "functional" short bowel syndrome because of severe malabsorption (Box 52.1).

Nutritional complications of intestinal failure include fluid and electrolyte depletion and acidosis, as well as macro- and micronutrient deficiencies (Table 52.1); supplementation may be required in large doses (Table 52.2).

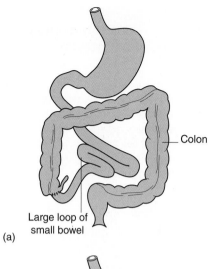

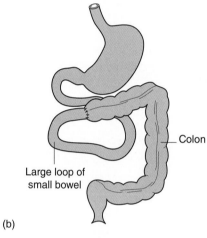

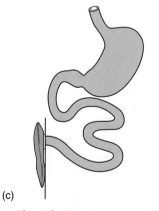

FIG. 52.1 The three common types of intestinal resection and anastomosis observed in patients with short bowel syndrome: ileocolonic anastomosis, jejunocolonic anastomosis, and end-jejunostomy.

TABLE 52.1 Daily stomal or fecal losses of electrolytes, minerals, and trace elements in severe short bowel syndrome[a]

Element	Concentration
Sodium	90–100 mEq/L
Potassium	10–20 mEq/L
Calcium	772 (591–950) mg/day
Magnesium	328 (263–419) mg/day
Iron	11 (7–15) mg/day
Zinc	12 (10–14) mg/day
Copper	1.5 (0.5–2.3) mg/day

[a]For sodium and potassium, the average concentration per liter of stomal effluent is given. The values for minerals and trace elements are mean 24-hour losses, with the range in parentheses.

TABLE 52.2 Vitamin and mineral requirements[a] in patients with a short bowel syndrome

Vitamin A	10 000–50 000 units daily[a]
Vitamin B$_{12}$	1000 µg SC monthly for patients with terminal ileal resection or disease
Vitamin C	200–500 mg daily
Vitamin D	50 000 units weekly to daily as 25 (OH$_2$)- or 1,25(OH$_2$)-D$_3$
Vitamin E	30 IU daily
Vitamin K	10 mg weekly; not always necessary if colon in continuity given bacterial synthesis
Calcium	1000–2000 mg daily
Magnesium	Variable – generally needs to be administered IV
Iron	As needed; absorbed in the duodenum, not always necessary
Selenium	60–150 µg daily
Zinc	220–440 mg daily (sulfate or gluconate form)
Bicarbonate	As needed

Note: the table lists rough guidelines only. Vitamin and mineral supplementation must be monitored routinely and tailored to the individual patient, because relative absorption and requirements may vary. Supplements may be taken orally unless otherwise indicated.
[a]Use cautiously in patients with cholestatic liver disease because of the potential for liver toxicity.

The goals of nutritional therapy are to treat and prevent these deficiencies, and to encourage intestinal adaptation, during which parenteral fluid and nutritional support are progressively weaned if possible. The first step towards nutritional autonomy involves maximization of residual intestinal absorptive function. This entails re-anastomosis

Management of Short Bowel Syndrome

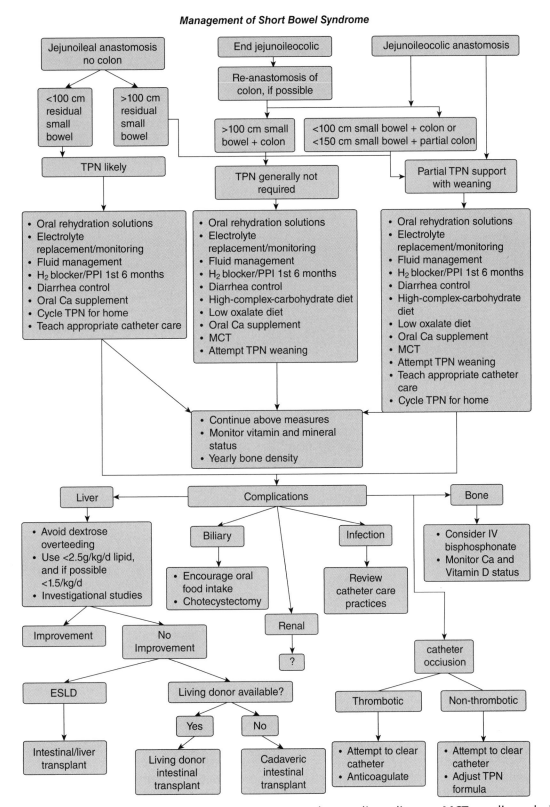

FIG. 52.2 Management of short bowel syndrome. ESLD, end-stage liver disease; MCT, medium-chain triglyceride; PPI, proton pump inhibitor; TPN, total parenteral nutrition. Reproduced with permission from Buchman *et al.* (2003).

of residual small bowel to colon in order to allow for carbohydrate salvage. Such salvage involves the bacterial fermentation of unabsorbed carbohydrates, including starches and soluble fibers, in the distal residual small intestine and colon (Figure 52.3). Byproducts of the fermentation process include short-chain fatty acids such as butyrate,

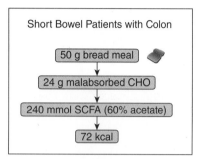

FIG. 52.3 Colonic absorption of malabsorbed carbohydrates (CHO) in a hypothetical patient with short bowel syndrome following ingestion of a 50-g bread meal. Unabsorbed carbohydrates, non-starch polysaccharides, and soluble fiber are fermented by colonic bacterial flora to hydrogen, methane, carbon dioxide, sulfides, and short-chain fatty acids (SCFAs), including acetate, butyrate, and propionate. By comparison, normal individuals absorb approximately 220–720 mmol SCFA from fermentation of 30–60 g nonstarch polysaccharides.

acetate, and propionate, which serve as energy substrates for colonocytes.

If dilated segments of small intestine are present, dysmotility often leads to bacterial overgrowth and decreased nutrient assimilation via maldigestion and impaired absorption. The dilated segments of intestine can be tapered using a STEP (serial transverse enteroplasty, Figure 52.4) or a Bianchi procedure. The intestine is lengthened, and although the absorptive surface area does not increase, absorption improves because the segment becomes more functional. Although residual intestinal absorptive capacity is the chief predictor of nutritional autonomy, in general a minimum of 100 cm of intestine, ending in an end ileostomy, or 40–60 cm of small bowel with colonic continuity, is required to achieve and maintain independence from parenteral nutrition requirements (Buchman et al., 2003). The ileocecal valve functions to decrease intestinal transit time and thereby increase nutrient–mucosa contact time, which in turn effects greater absorption but also helps prevent the translocation of colonic bacteria to the distal small bowel where they may compete with enterocytes for nutrient assimilation.

Regardless of the surgical approach to reconstruction of the gastrointestinal tract, enteral nutrient assimilation is needed, preferably via the oral route because of the salivary release of epidermal growth factor (EGF) (Piludu et al., 2003). Most nutrient absorption occurs within the initial

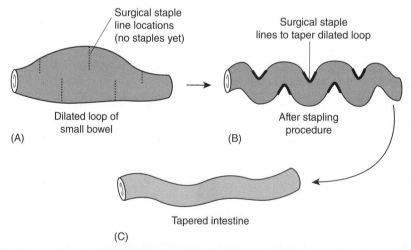

FIG. 52.4 Serial transverse enteroplasty (STEP), an intestinal tapering procedure that can be used to transform a dilated segment of intestine with little motility into a more functional segment with enhancement of fluid and nutrient absorption, most likely due to elimination of conditions favorable for bacterial overgrowth. (A) Diagrammatic depiction of a dilated intestinal segment, (B) staple line positions which lead to (C), a lengthened, but tapered and functionalized intestinal lumen.

100–150 cm of intestine (Borgstrom *et al.*, 1957). Notable exceptions include vitamin B$_{12}$ (absorbed in the terminal ileum), and water and sodium, which are absorbed throughout the small intestine and colon; iron and calcium are generally absorbed in the duodenum while some medium-chain triglyceride, calcium, and amino acid absorption may also occur in the colon. Although fat and fat-soluble vitamin A absorption occurs in the proximal jejunum, bile salt re-absorption in the terminal ileum is a necessary component of fat absorption. Bile salts, produced in the liver and stored in the gall bladder, are released into the bile duct in response to food, especially fatty foods. These bile salts mix with fat and create micelles, which serve to solubilize fat and lead to enhanced absorption. Although there is little data in humans because of the inability to study individuals prior to an intra-abdominal catastrophe or prior to the onset of inflammatory bowel disease, a plethora of animal studies have indicated that, during the adaptation process following resection, the intestine lengthens somewhat, but, more importantly, villus height and crypt depth increase, thereby increasing mucosal surface area and absorption. This process is largely complete by 6–12 months, or at most (in general) 24 months in humans (Cisler and Buchman, 2005).

Individuals who develop permanent intestinal failure will require long-term home parenteral nutrition. This nutritional therapy is typically provided in the form of an overnight infusion whereby the patient connects themselves to an intravenous infusion pump using a long-term indwelling central venous catheter. The parenteral nutrition solutions infuse overnight and the patient disconnects the following morning. Patients may require parenteral nutrition between 2 and 7 nights weekly.

The mainstay of medical treatment of short bowel syndrome, and, in some cases, non-short bowel intestinal failure, is control of diarrhea and maintenance of adequate hydration. Furthermore, oral intake needs to increase to 1.5–2 times pre-resection intake; this is termed *hyperphagia* (Crenn *et al.*, 2004). Although enteral supplementation with tube feeding may help achieve this goal, tube feeding presents additional challenges to the patient who already has to maintain themselves on parenteral nutrition. Not only does nutrient malabsorption occur in patients with intestinal failure, but medication malabsorption as well, and higher than conventional doses of medications may often be necessary. Furthermore, narcotics such as tincture of opium or codeine may be necessary to induce

a delay in gastrointestinal transit. Because of gastric hypersecretion for the initial 6 months following a massive enterectomy (Hyman *et al.*, 1986), high-dose proton pump inhibitor therapy is recommended to decrease gastric fluid losses. Increased gastric acid secretion that passes into the duodenum may acidify the normally alkaline duodenal fluid and lead to deconjugation of bile salts and inactivation of lipase, resulting in worsened carbohydrate maldigestion and fat malabsorption.

Recent studies have suggested a role for glucagon-like peptide II (GLP-II) in the enhancement of absorption of fluids and, to a lesser degree, nutrients, and studies have shown significantly enhanced fluid absorption in patients past the normal post-enterectomy adaptation phase with exogenous GLP-II administration (Jeppesen *et al.*, 2001, 2005). The data for growth hormone is less compelling, but does suggest that its use leads to enhanced fluid retention, although probably on the basis of enhanced renal tubular reabsorption of sodium (Byrne *et al.*, 2005).

Potential complications related to intestinal failure include hepatobiliary disease (steatohepatitis, cholestasis, calculous or non-calculous cholecystitis), metabolic bone disease, nephrolithiasis, and nephropathy. Additional complications related to therapy include catheter sepsis and other infections (exit site/subcutaneous cuff and tunnel); mechanical issues including catheter breakage and malpositioning; as well as catheter occlusion and/or occlusion of the vein through which parenteral solutions were infused (thrombotic/non-thrombotic) related to the indwelling catheter required for parenteral fluid administration (Buchman, 2001).

Successful intestinal transplantation was first successfully performed in 1989 (Hansmann *et al.*, 1989). It is currently approved for the treatment of patients with intestinal failure who have required parenteral nutrition but who have developed significant and potentially life-threatening complications, including, most frequently, intestinal failure-associated liver disease (IFALD), loss of venous catheter access, or recurrent infections or dehydration (Buchman *et al.*, 2003). As long-term survival improves, intestinal transplantation may become a viable option for patients with less severe complications of intestinal failure.

Patients who require only partial parenteral nutrition and/or fluid support should be encouraged to consume oral rehydration solutions. These solutions have high sodium concentration (90–100 mmol/L), which is designed to replace fecal sodium losses (Atia and Buchman,

Mechanism of Solute Coupled Na⁺ Co-Transport

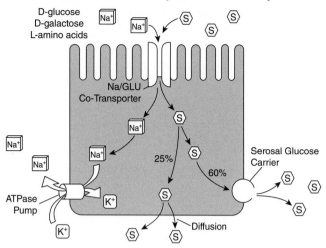

FIG. 52.5 Mechanism of solute-coupled Na⁺ co-transport. Sodium contained in oral rehydration solutions replaces diarrhea-associated Na⁺ losses and promotes water absorption by means of solvent drag. This schematic diagram illustrates the active, Na⁺-coupled co-transport of solute into the jejunal enterocyte, where the solute may be glucose (GLU), glucose polymers, galactose, oligopeptides, or L-amino acids. S, solute.

2009). They also contain substantial concentrations of glucose or similar sugars. Absorption of both sodium and glucose is an active process that occurs largely in the jejunum and utilizes the same transport mechanism (Banks and Farthing, 2002). As sodium and glucose enter the enterocyte, water passively diffuses, leading to enhanced fluid absorption and lessening the likelihood of dehydration (Figure 52.5).

It is also recommended that patients consume a high complex-carbohydrate diet if they have residual colon in continuity with small bowel (Buchman *et al.*, 2003; Atia *et al.*, 2011). In the absence of duodenal or proximal jejunal resections, lactose restriction is not necessary and deprives the patient of the major dietary calcium source. Micronutrient status, most notably the fat-soluble vitamins, essential fatty acids (linoleic) zinc and, to a lesser degree, selenium status, should be followed at regular intervals (at least twice yearly and more frequently if clinically indicated). Vitamin B$_{12}$ should be administered by the sublingual, intranasal, or intramuscular route if >60 cm of terminal ileum has been resected.

Pancreas

Acute Pancreatitis

Evolution in our understanding of the factors that contribute to the systemic inflammatory response syndrome (SIRS), which characterizes acute pancreatitis, has led to dramatic changes in management (McClave, in press). The sentinel acute pancreatis event (SAPE) hypothesis described by Schneider and Whitcomb (2002) suggests that an innocuous injury to the pancreatic acinar cells (such as high triglyceride levels, alcohol consumption, passage of a common bile-duct stone, or toxic drug) leads to a sentinel event. The sentinel event refers not to the injurious agent, but to the cascading, self-perpetuating, proinflammatory event that ensues. Increased vascular permeability, aggressive recruitment of neutrophils into the area of the pancreatic acinus, and elaboration of inflammatory cytokines, set up a vicious cycle of inflammation (the sentinel event) which leads to destruction of the acinar cells and autodigestion of the gland (Pandol *et al.*, 2007). This sentinel event represents a final common pathway of many different etiologic agents, with the difference between acute and chronic pancreatitis determined by whether the patient is able to resolve the injury and turn off the inflammation. Specific genetic defects (such as the SPINK-1 cystic fibrosis gene, and others) and the patient's overall antioxidant defense system are key factors in whether the sentinel event goes on to continuity, scar tissue, fibrosis, and chronic pancreatitis (Schneider and Whitcomb, 2002).

Nutritional therapy, primarily through delivery of early enteral nutrition (EN), improves the patient's capability for handling oxidative stress (McClave, in press). Providing early EN maintains gut integrity and prevents increases in gut permeability (Figure 52.6). Failure to provide luminal nutrients helps set up a gut–lung conduit of inflammation, where a cytokine storm produced at the level of the gut releases proinflammatory agents into lymphatic channels that pass directly up to the capillary system of the lungs (Alverdy *et al.*, 2003) (Figure 52.7). In this sense, EN actually protects the patient against acute respiratory distress syndrome (ARDS) and pneumonia. EN downregulates the systemic immune response by decreasing activation of macrophages and neutrophils of the innate system and stimulating a line of CD-4 Th-2 anti-inflammatory lymphocytes which emerge from the gut and pass out to distant sites throughout the body (Figure 52.6). EN also promotes the role of commensal bacteria,

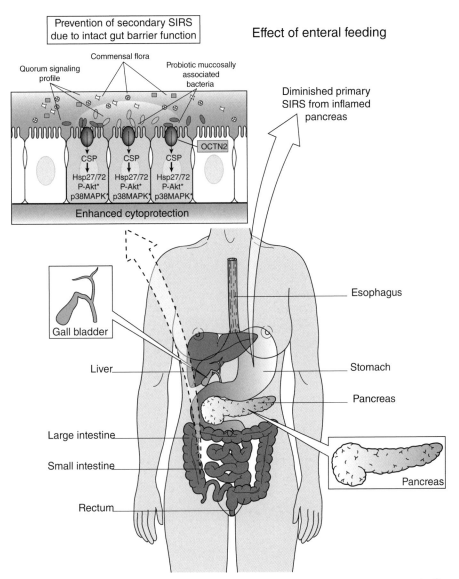

FIG. 52.6 Delivery of early enteral nutrition (EN) helps diminish the primary systemic inflammatory response syndrome (SIRS) caused by pancreatitis. EN maintains gut integrity, prevents increases in intestinal permeability, and exerts anti-inflammatory effects through stimulation and release of Th2 CD4 helper lymphocytes from the lamina propria. Both commensal and virulent organisms are present, but the overall effect is beneficial, stimulating heat shock proteins and maintaining tight junctions between epithelial cells.

which act on carbohydrate and fiber to produce short-chain fatty acids, which impact on butyrate receptors in the colon, exerting a further anti-inflammatory effect (Alverdy *et al.*, 2003; McClave, in press).

In fact the focus of management has shifted from being centered on pancreatic rest to maintaining gut integrity and modulating the immune response. The outcome ben-

efits from early EN are profound when compared with parenteral nutrition (PN), with significant decreases in infection, multiple organ failure, hospital length of stay, need for surgical intervention, and mortality (McClave *et al.*, 2006). These benefits cannot be attributed to a deleterious effect of PN, as early studies of EN vs. standard therapy (where no specialized nutritional therapy is

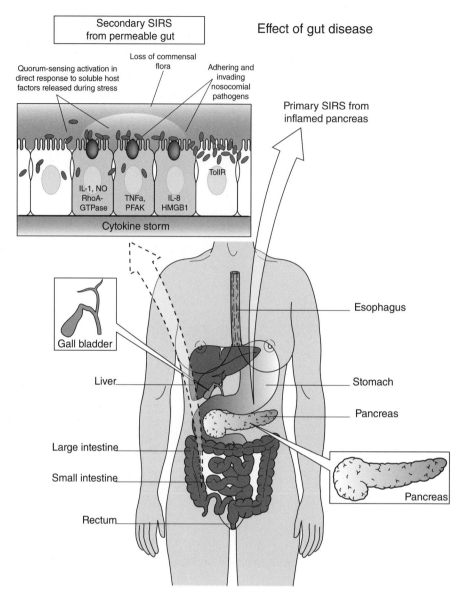

FIG. 52.7 Failure to utilize the gut in severe acute pancreatitis leads to disruption of intestinal barrier function and increased intestinal permeability. Quorum sensing by virulent organisms leads to their emergence and subsequent adherence to the gut wall. A cytokine "storm" results, with the release of inflammatory cytokines from the intestinal epithelial cells into lymphatic channels. The exit of pro-inflammatory Th1 CD4 helper lymphocytes from the lamina propria further up-regulates immune responses and leads to late complications via a subsequent secondary systematic inflammatory response syndrome (SIRS) response.

provided) have shown a potential mortality benefit when patients operated on for complications of pancreatitis are placed on tube feeding the day after surgery (McClave *et al.*, 2006).

PN clearly has a role in acute pancreatitis in patients for whom EN is not feasible. Results from two early studies

suggest that immediate initiation of PN may have an adverse effect (Sax *et al.*, 1987; Xian-Li *et al.*, 2004). Therefore, in an appropriate candidate, PN should be initiated 4–5 days after admission if EN is not feasible. After the first week of hospitalization, tolerance issues that result in hypocaloric enteral feeding insufficient to meet energy requirements may necessitate the addition of supplemental PN.

Candidates for early EN in acute pancreatitis are those patients who have a severe degree of illness as indicated by APACHE II scores of ≥8, the presence of three or more Ranson criteria, and/or evidence of pancreatic necrosis on computerized tomography (CT) scan (McClave and Ritchie, 2000). Deep jejunal access has been used most often for successful EN in these patients. Two studies now would suggest that gastric feeding is tolerated equally as well as jejunal feeding, particularly if it can be initiated within the first 48 hours of onset of disease. It is important to ensure full volume resuscitation before initiation of EN. A mean arterial pressure of ≥65 mm Hg, a central venous pressure of 8–12 mm Hg, urine output of >0.5 mL/kg/hour, and a mixed venous O_2 ≥65% would suggest that a patient is fully resuscitated and is thus a candidate for initiation of EN. The presence of pancreatic ascites, pseudocyst, necrosis, or fluid collection within the pancreas are not contraindications to EN. The only true contraindications would include documented intolerance (clear stimulation of the SIRS response to EN), fear of ischemia, or mechanical obstruction of the gastrointestinal (GI) tract. Early initiation of feeds within the first 48 hours helps minimize problems with ileus and delayed gastric emptying. Tolerance should be monitored closely for evidence of stimulation of the pancreas, the presence of which would necessitate shifting the level of infusion lower in the GI tract and possibly switching to a formula that has protein in the form of small peptides, and fat in the form of medium-chain triglycerides (MCTs). Serum amylase and lipase levels provide little prognostic information, but they may provide valuable feedback regarding evidence of stimulation of the inflamed pancreas. Variation in the serum levels from day to day should be expected with either pancreatic enzyme, but a steady rise in both enzymes in response to EN may indicate potential intolerance (McClave and Ritchie, 2000).

Three adverse scenarios may result from early EN in acute pancreatitis and include an asymptomatic stimulation of enzyme output, an uncomplicated exacerbation of symptoms (abdominal pain, nausea), and the more concerning increase in the SIRS response. Placing the level of infusion of formula lower in the GI tract (preferably below the ligament of Treitz), or switching to either a small-peptide/medium-chain triglyceride (MCT) oil formula or fat-free formula, usually resolves intolerance and allows the continuation of feeds.

For those patients identified to be appropriate candidates for PN, intravenous fat is tolerated well, but triglyceride levels of the blood should be followed closely. Triglyceride levels should be kept below 400 mg/dL. Moderate glucose control is important: the blood sugar should be kept between 80 and 150 mg/dL. These patients are at risk for refeeding syndrome, so the PN should be advanced slowly over several days, with close monitoring of serum potassium, phosphorus, and magnesium.

Chronic Pancreatitis

Issues related to nutritional therapy shift dramatically with the chronicity of fibrotic calcific pancreatitis. Factors develop over time which promote protein-energy malnutrition. These include maldigestion, food aversion, hypermetabolism, poor oral intake secondary to abdominal pain or nausea/vomiting, continued alcohol abuse, abnormalities of gastric emptying, and development of clinical diabetes mellitus (Scolapio et al., 1999). These same factors increase the risk for micronutrient deficiencies. The absence of pancreatic proteolytic enzymes to remove the B_{12}-binding R-factor leads to deficiencies of vitamin B_{12}. Chronic inflammation depletes the level of a patient's antioxidants, promoting deficiencies of selenium, β-carotene, lycopene, and vitamins A and E. Malabsorption of fat-soluble vitamins leads to a vitamin D deficiency and development of osteomalacia and osteoporosis. Vitamin K deficiencies occur less frequently (Petersoen and Forsmark, 2002).

Nutritional management of these patients necessitates abstinence from alcohol and control of abdominal pain. Control of abdominal pain alone stimulates appetite and promotes increases in oral intake. High-carbohydrate, low-fat, high-protein diets are best suited for the patient with chronic pancreatitis. Vegetable fat may be tolerated better than animal fat. Pancreatic enzymes should be taken with meals so that the enzymes and the food are present together in the lumen of the GI tract at the same time (Meier, 2002). Whereas non-enteric-coated pancreatic enzymes are better for controlling abdominal pain in chronic pancreatitis (due to feedback mechanisms in the duodenum), enteric-coated enzymes which are protected as they pass through the stomach are probably better suited to control the maldigestion seen with steatorrhea and chronic pancreatitis (Meier, 2002). Enteric-coated enzymes should not be used in the patient who requires acid suppression from proton pump inhibitors (due to interference with dissolution of the capsule encasing the enzymes). Enzyme supplements should provide 10% of the volume of enzyme output normally produced by the pancreas, such that approximately 30 000 IU of lipase are needed per meal (Meier, 2002). Enzymes with the highest trypsin content are required to control pain (>50 000 IU). Those patients most likely to respond to enzyme therapy and achieve pain relief are females with small-duct, less-advanced disease that is non-alcoholic in etiology. Fat restrictions in the diet may be needed in the patient for whom enzymes fail to control steatorrhea. Meals may be supplemented with oral small-peptide/MCT oil formulas. For the patient with recurrent pain, weight loss, continued steatorrhea, and frequent hospital admissions, a direct percutaneous endoscopic jejunostomy tube may be utilized to promote nutritional status, control pain, and reduce the number of hospital admissions per year. It is important to rule out small-bowel bacterial overgrowth, which can contribute to the diarrhea and be present in as many as one-third of patients with chronic pancreatitis. A daily antioxidant cocktail is valuable in minimizing the number of painful attacks and reducing the number of hospital admissions per year. Such cocktails should include vitamin E (270 IU/day), vitamin C (0.54 g/day), selenium (600 mg/day), β-carotene (9000 IU/day), and methionine (2 g/day) (De las Heras Castano et al., 2000).

Future Directions

Although the evidence of a role for dietary intake in the pathogenesis of IBD has been largely epidemiological, and studies of various nutritional programs to treat IBD have met with some, albeit not overwhelmingly positive results, new evidence suggests the possibility of a more substantial role for nutrition. That role is a more indirect one, and may be modulated through intestinal bacteria. Diet as well as specific nutrients may be determinant factors for the presence or absence of specific bacterial species, which themselves may have a causative effect on intestinal inflammation. Not limited to environmental factors, gastrointestinal disease is likely related to interactions between diet and genetics, as well as other environmental factors including toxins and proteins and what is probably a very complex relationship. This relationship becomes even more complex with the finding of single or multiple single nucleotide polymorphisms (SNPs) in the DNA sequence. Host genetic-based responses may be environmentally influenced, particularly by diet. Indeed, the burgeoning fields of "DNA-driven nutrition," nutrigenetics, and

nutrigenomics have suggested that gene expression may be influenced by diet. Similarly, a given nutritional therapy may be variably effective across a population, but more effective for a specific individual. These include cytoprotective, anti-inflammatory, and immunoregulatory effects. Indeed, nutrition and its interaction with other environmental factors as well as genetics may also play an important role in risk stratification as well as the pathogenesis of EoE and pancreatitis; the role in celiac disease is obvious. With regard to the latter, a more sophisticated understanding of the role of gluten and the development of inflammation has allowed for the development of novel therapies for celiac disease, although effectiveness of these therapies awaits completion of rigorous clinical trials. In pancreatitis, the emerging role of pharmaconutrient agents such as arginine to improve vasomotor abnormalities, glutamine to induce heat shock proteins, fish oil to reduce inflammation, and zinc to maintain gut integrity and promote antioxidant defenses all need to be investigated in a prospective randomized fashion.

Intestinal transplantation is also likely influenced by interactions between bacteria, diet, and other environmental factors, as well as genetic factors. Although short-term (i.e. 5-year) survival has improved dramatically in recent years, and rivals that of other organs, long-term survival (e.g. 10 years or more) has not improved substantially as a clear understanding of the pathogenesis of chronic rejection is not yet on the horizon. The potential influence of diet, intestinal bacterial flora, and genetics in development or prevention of chronic rejection cannot be underestimated.

Suggestion for Further Reading
Buchman, A.L. (2006) *Clinical Nutrition in Gastrointestinal Disease*. Slack, Thorofare, NJ.

References

Afonso, J.J. and Rombeau, J.L. (1990) Nutritional care for patients with Crohn's disease. *Hepatogastroenterology* **37**, 32–41.

Akobeng, A.K., Miller, V., Stanton, J., et al. (2000) Double-blind randomized controlled trial of glutamine-enriched polymeric diet in the treatment of active Crohn's disease. *J Pediatr Gastroenterol Nutr* **30**, 74–84.

Alverdy, J.C., Laughlin, R.S., and Wu, L. (2003) Influence of the critically ill state on host–pathogen interactions within the intestine: gut-derived sepsis redefined. *Crit Care Med* **31**, 598–607.

Andresen, A.F.R. (1942) Ulcerative colitis – an allergic phenomenon. *Am J Dig Dis* **9**, 91–98.

Atia, A.N. and Buchman, A.L. (2009) Oral rehydration solutions in non-cholera diarrhea: a review. *Am J Gastroenterol* **104**, 2596–2604.

Atia, A., Fernand, G.P., Hébuterne, X., *et al.* (2011) Pectin supplementation increases colonic short chain fatty acid (SCFA) production in patients with short bowel syndrome. *JPEN J Parenter Enteral Nutr* **35**, 229–240.

Banks, M.R. and Farthing, M.J. (2002) Fluid and electrolyte transport in the small intestine. *Curr Opin Gastroenterol* **18**, 176–181.

Behrend, C., Jeppesen, P.B., and Mortensen, P.B. (1995) Vitamin B12 absorption after ileorectal anastomosis for Crohn's disease: effect of ileal resection and time span after surgery. *Eur J Gastroenterol Hepatol* **7**, 397–400.

Borgstrom, B., Dahlqvist, A., Lundh, G., *et al.* (1957) Studies of intestinal digestion and absorption in the human. *J Clin Invest* **36**, 1521–1536.

Bousvaros, A., Zukakowski, D., Duggan, C., *et al.* (1999) Vitamins A and E serum levels in children and young adults with inflammatory bowel disease: effects of disease activity. *J Pediatr Gastroenterol Hepatol* **26**, 129–134.

Buchman, A.L. (2001) Complications of long-term home total parenteral nutrition: their identification, prevention, and treatment. *Dig Dis Sci* **46**, 1–18.

Buchman, A.L. (2005) Nutritional therapy for Crohn's disease. *Pract Gastroenterol* 17–28.

Buchman, A.L., Scolapio, S., and Fryer, J. (2003) AGA technical review on short bowel syndrome and intestinal transplantation. *Gastroenterology* **124**, 1111–1134.

Buchman, A.L., Iyer, K., Fryer, J. (2006) Parenteral nutrition-associated liver disease and the role for isolated intestine and intestine/liver transplantation. *Hepatology* **43**, 9–19.

Byrne, T.A., Wilmore, D.W., Iyer, K., *et al.* (2005) Growth hormone, glutamine, and an optimal diet reduce parenteral nutrition in patients with short bowel syndrome: a prospective, randomized, placebo-controlled, double-blind clinical trial. *Ann Surg* **242**, 655–661.

Catassi, C., Fabiani, E., Corrao, G., *et al.* (2002) Risk of non-Hodgkin lymphoma in celiac disease. *JAMA* **287**, 1413–1419.

Cisler, J.J. and Buchman, A.L. (2005) Intestinal adaptation in short bowel syndrome. *J Investig Med* **53**, 402–413.

Crenn, P., Morin, M.C., Joly, F., *et al.* (2004) Net digestive absorption and adaptive hyperphagia in adult short bowel patients. *Gut* **53**, 1279–1286.

De Las Heras Castano, G., Garcia de la Paz, A., Fernandez, M.D., *et al.* (2000) Use of antioxidants to treat pain in chronic pancreatitis. *Rev Esp Enferm Dig* **92**, 375–385.

Dharmsathaphorn, K., Freeman, D.H., Binder, H.J., *et al.* (1982) Increased risk of nephrolithiasis in patients with steatorrhea. *Dig Dis Sci* **27**, 401–405.

Dobbins, J.W. and Binder, H.J. (1977). Importance of the colon in enteric hyperoxaluria. *N Engl J Med* **296**, 298–301.

Elsborg, L. and Larsen, L. (1979) Folate deficiency in chronic inflammatory bowel diseases. *Scand J Gastroenterol* **14**, 1019–1024.

Feagan, B.G., Sandborn, W.J., Mittmann, U., *et al.* (2008). Omega-3 free fatty acids for the maintenance of remission in Crohn disease: the EPIC randomized controlled trials. *JAMA* **299**, 1690–1697.

Fine, K.D., Meyer, R.L., and Lee, E.L. (1997) The prevalence and causes of diarrhea in patients with celiac sprue treated with a gluten free diet. *Gastroenterology* **112**, 1830–1838.

Furuta, G.T., Liacouras, C.A., Collins, M.H., *et al.* (2007) Eosinophilic esophagitis in children and adults: a systematic review and consensus recommendations for diagnosis and treatment. *Gastroenterology* **133**, 1342–1363.

Green, P. and Cellier, C. (2007) Celiac disease. *N Engl J Med* **357**, 1731–1743.

Hansmann, M.L., Deltz, E., Gundlach, M., *et al.* (1989) Small bowel transplantation in a child. Morphologic, immunohistochemical, and clinical results. *Am J Clin Pathol* **92**, 686–692.

Hyman, P.E., Everett, S.L., and Harada, T. (1986) Gastric acid hypersecretion in short bowel syndrome in infants: association with extent of resection and enteral feeding. *J Pediatr Gastroenterol Nutr* **5**, 191–197.

James, S.P. (2005) National Institutes of Health consensus development conference statement on celiac disease, June 28–30, 2004. *Gastroenterology* **128**, S1–S9.

Jeppesen, P.B., Hartmann, B., Thulesen, J., *et al.* (2001) Glucagon-like peptide 2 improves nutrient absorption and nutritional status in short bowel patients with no colon. *Gastroenterology* **120**, 806–815.

Jeppesen, P.B., Sanguinetti, E.L., Buchman, A.L., *et al.* (2005) Teduglutide (ALX-0600), a dipeptidyl peptidase IV resistant glucagon-like peptide 2 analogue, improves intestinal function in short bowel syndrome patients. *Gut* **54**, 1224–1231.

Jones, V.A., Workman, E., Freeman, A.H., *et al.* (1985). Crohn's disease: maintenance of remission by diet. *Lancet* **ii**, 177–181.

Kagalwalla, A.F., Sentongo, T.A., Ritz, S., *et al.* (2006). Effect of six-food elimination diet on clinical and histologic outcomes in eosinophilic esophagitis. *Clin Gastroenterol Hepatol* **4**, 1097–1102.

Karamanolis, G. and Tack, J. (2006) Nutrition and motility disorders. *Best Pract Res Clin Gastroenterol* **20**, 485–505.

Lagergren, J., Bergström, R., and Nyrén, O. (2000) No relation between body mass and gastroesophageal reflux symptoms in a Swedish population based study. *Gut* **47**, 26–29.

Lashner, B.A., Evans, A.A., and Hanauer, S.B. (1989) Preoperative total parenteral nutrition for bowel resection in Crohn's disease. *Dig Dis Sci* **34**, 741–746.

Levine, J.S. and Burakoff, R. (2007) Chemoprophylaxis of colorectal cancer in inflammatory bowel disease: current concepts. *Inflamm Bowel Dis* **13**, 1293–1298.

Liacouras, C.A., Furuta, G.T., Hirano, I., *et al.* (2011) Eosinophilic esophagitis: updated consensus recommendations for children and adults. *J Allergy Clin Immunol* **128**, 3–20.

Lochs, H., Seinhardt, H.J., Klaus-Wentz, B., *et al.* (1991) Comparison of enteral nutrition and drug treatment in active Crohn's disease. Results of the European Cooperative Crohn's Disease Study. IV. *Gastroenterology* **101**, 881–888.

Locke, G.R., Talley, N.J., Felt, S.L., *et al.* (1977) Prevalence and clinical spectrum of gastroesophageal reflux: a population-based study in Olmsted County, Minnesota. *Gastroenterology* **112**, 1448–1456.

Locke, G.R., Talley, N.J., Fett, S.L., *et al.* (1999) Risk factors associated with symptoms of gastroesophageal reflux. *Am J Med* **106**, 642–649.

Lorenz-Meyer, H., Bauer, P., and Nicolay, C., *et al.* (1996) Omega-3 fatty acids and low carbohydrate diet for maintenance of remission in Crohn's disease. *Scand J Gastroenterol* **31**, 778–785.

Markowitz, J.E., Spergel, J.M., Ruchelli, E., *et al.* (2003) Elemental diet is an effective treatment for eosinophilic esophagitis in children and adolescents. *Am J Gastroenterol* **98**, 777–782.

McClave, S.A. (in press) Drivers of oxidative stress in acute pancreatitis: the role of nutrition therapy. *JPEN J Parenter Enteral Nutr*.

McClave, S.A. and Ritchie, C.S. (2000) Artificial nutrition in pancreatic disease: What lessons have we learned from the literature? *Clin Nutr* **19**, 1–6.

McClave, S.A., Chang, W.K., Dhaliwal, R., *et al.* (2006) Nutrition support in acute pancreatitis: a systematic review of the literature. *JPEN J Parenter Enteral Nutr* **30**, 143–156.

Meier, R. (2002) Nutrition in chronic pancreatitis. In M. Buchler, H. Friess, and W. Uhl (eds), *Chronic Pancreatitis*. Blackwell, Berlin, pp. 421–427.

Mercer, C.D., Wren, S.F., DaCosta, L.R., *et al.* (1987) Lower esophageal sphincter pressure and gastroesophageal pressure gradients in excessively obese patients. *J Med* **18**, 135–146.

Middleton, S.J., Rucker, J.T., Kirby, G.A., *et al.* (1995) Long-chain triglycerides reduce the efficacy of enteral feeds in patients with active Crohn's disease. *Clin Nutr* **14**, 229–236.

Mora, S., Barera, G., Beccio, S., *et al.* (2001) A prospective, longitudinal study of the long-term effect of treatment on bone density in children with celiac disease. *J Pediatr* **39**, 516–521.

Ohkusa, T. (1985) Production of experimental ulcerative colitis in hamsters by dextran sulfate sodium and change in intestinal microflora. *Jpn J Gastroenterol* **82**, 1337–1347.

Pandol, S.J., Saluja, A.K., Imrie, C.W., *et al.* (2007) Acute pancreatitis: bench to the bedside. *Gastroenterology* **132**, 1127–1151.

Persson, P.G., Ahlbom, A., and Hellers, G. (1992) Diet and inflammatory bowel disease: a case-control study. *Epidemiology* **3**, 47–52.

Petersoen, J.M. and Forsmark, C.E. (2002) Chronic pancreatitis and maldigestion. *Semin Gastrointest Dis* **13**, 191–199.

Piludu, M., Lantini, M.S., Isola, M., *et al.* (2003) Localisation of epidermal growth factor receptor in mucous cells of human salivary glands. *Eur J Morphol* **41**, 107–109.

Riordan, A.M., Hunter, J.O., Cowan, R.E., *et al.* (1993) Treatment of active Crohn's disease by exclusion diet: East Anglia multicentre controlled trial. *Lancet* **342**, 1131–1134.

Ritchie, J.K., Wadsworth, J., Lennard-Jones, J.E., *et al.* (1987) Controlled multicentre therapeutic trial of unrefined carbohydrate, fibre-rich diet in Crohn's disease. *Br Med J* **295**, 517–520.

Roediger, W.E.W., Duncan, A., Kapaniris, O., *et al.* (1993) Reducing sulfur compounds of the colon impairs colonocyte nutrition: implications for ulcerative colitis. *Gastroenterology* **104**, 802–809.

Ruhl, C.E. and Everhardt, J.E. (1999) Overweight, but not high dietary fat intake, increases risk of gastroesophageal reflux disease hospitalization: the NHANES I Epidemiologic Followup Study. First National Health and Nutrition Examination Survey. *Ann Epidemiol* **9**, 424–435.

Sax, H.C., Warner, B.W., Talamini, M.A., *et al.* (1987) Early total parenteral nutrition in acute pancreatitis: lack of beneficial effects. *Am J Surg* **153**, 117–124.

Sangaletti, O., Petrillo, M., and Bianchi Porro, G. (1989) Urinary oxalate recovery after oral oxalic load: an alternative method for the quantitative determination of stool fat for the diagnosis of lipid malabsorption. *J Int Med Res* **17**, 526–531.

Schneider, A. and Whitcomb, D.C. (2002) Hereditary pancreatitis: a model for inflammatory disease of the pancreas. *Best Pract Res Clin Gastroenterol* **16**, 347–363.

Scolapio, J.S., Malhi-Chowla, N., and Ukleja, A. (1999) Nutrition supplementation in patients with acute and chronic pancreatitis. *Gastroenterol Clin North Am* **28**, 695–707.

See, J. and Murray, J.A. (2006) Gluten-free diet: the medical and nutrition management of celiac disease. *Nutr Clin Pract* **21**, 1–15.

Shinozaki, M., Saito, H., and Muto, T. (1997) Excess glutamine exacerbates trinitrobenzenesulfonic acid-induced colitis in rats. *Dis Colon Rectum* **40,** S59–63.

Sugerman, H.J., DeMaria, E.J., Felton, W.L., III, *et al.* (1997) Increased intra-abdominal pressure and cardiac filling pressures in obesity-associated pseudotumor cerebri. *Neurology* **49,** 507–511.

Tolonen, P., Victorzon, M., Niemi, R., *et al.* (2006) Does gastric banding for morbid obesity reduce or increase gastroesophageal reflux? *Obes Surg* **16,** 1469–1474.

Valberg, L.S., Flanagan, P.R., Kertescz, A., *et al.* (1986) Zinc absorption in inflammatory bowel disease. *Dig Dis Sci* **31,** 724–731.

Wisen, O., Rossner, S., and Johansson, C. (1987) Gastric secretion in massive obesity. Evidence for abnormal response to vagal stimulation. *Dig Dis Sci* **32,** 968–972.

Xian-Li, H., Qing-Jiu, M., Jian-Guo, L., *et al.* (2004) Effect of total parenteral nutrition (TPN) with and without glutamine dipeptide supplementation on outcome in severe acute pancreatitis (SAP). *Clin Nutr Suppl* **1,** 43–47.

53

KIDNEY DISEASE

THIANE G. AXELSSON[1], RD, MSc, MICHAL CHMIELEWSKI[2], MD, PhD, AND
BENGT LINDHOLM[1], MD, PhD

[1]Karolinska Institutet, Stockholm, Sweden
[2]Medical University of Gdansk, Gdansk, Poland

Summary

Chronic kidney disease (CKD) is considered a worldwide public health threat (Levey *et al.*, 2007). In the United States alone, 9.6% of adults are likely to have some degree of CKD (Coresh *et al.*, 2005). Data from Europe, Australia, and Asia also confirm a similar high prevalence of CKD (Coresh *et al.*, 2005; Stevens *et al.*, 2006; Levey *et al.*, 2007). The increasing prevalence of CKD together with its numerous complications make CKD a growing burden in health-related, social, and economic terms all over the world (Hsu *et al.*, 2006; Rutkowski and Król, 2008). In the present review, we describe briefly the causes and consequences of metabolic abnormalities and nutritional deficiencies in CKD, and provide an overview of current therapies.

Introduction

The kidneys play a key role in maintaining fluid and electrolyte homeostasis, in excretion of metabolic waste products, and in the regulation of various hormonal and metabolic pathways. Even a slight reduction in renal function may therefore have metabolic and nutritional consequences.

Patients with manifest CKD consequently display a variety of metabolic and nutritional abnormalities, most prominently protein-energy wasting (PEW) (Young *et al.*, 1991; Qureshi *et al.*, 1998; Heimburger *et al.*, 2000). Metabolic and nutritional abnormalities arise in CKD from both pathophysiological (e.g. uremic toxicity, altered metabolism) and iatrogenic (e.g. polypharmacy and the

prescription of a low-protein diet to slow disease progression) causes. In the late stage of CKD, defined by the need to start renal replacement therapy (dialysis or kidney transplantation), some of these abnormalities are attenuated, while novel ones may occur (Figure 53.1).

Basic Kidney Physiology and Pathophysiology

Kidneys play a prominent role in the human organism, providing excretion of metabolic wastes, regulating water–electrolyte and acid–base balance, and secreting hormones. Their importance is reflected by the enormous amount of blood (about 1200 mL) flowing through the kidneys each minute.

Present Knowledge in Nutrition, Tenth Edition. Edited by John W. Erdman Jr, Ian A. Macdonald and Steven H. Zeisel.
© 2012 International Life Sciences Institute. Published 2012 by John Wiley & Sons, Inc.

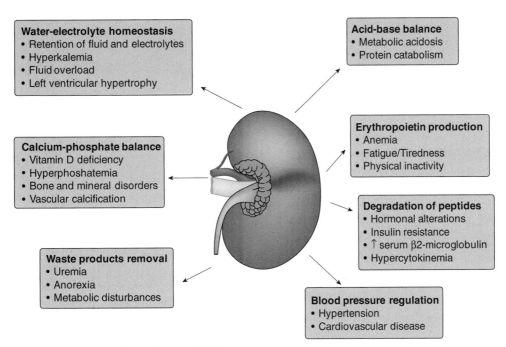

Water-electrolyte homeostasis
- Retention of fluid and electrolytes
- Hyperkalemia
- Fluid overload
- Left ventricular hypertrophy

Acid-base balance
- Metabolic acidosis
- Protein catabolism

Calcium-phosphate balance
- Vitamin D deficiency
- Hyperphoshatemia
- Bone and mineral disorders
- Vascular calcification

Erythropoietin production
- Anemia
- Fatigue/Tiredness
- Physical inactivity

Degradation of peptides
- Hormonal alterations
- Insulin resistance
- ↑ serum β2-microglobulin
- Hypercytokinemia

Waste products removal
- Uremia
- Anorexia
- Metabolic disturbances

Blood pressure regulation
- Hypertension
- Cardiovascular disease

FIG. 53.1 Major roles of the kidney in metabolic regulation.

As the physiological metabolic processes result in formation of numerous metabolites, kidney failure results in accumulation of compounds that are useless or even harmful to the organism. Whereas healthy kidneys remove these waste products by excreting them in the urine, renal insufficiency takes away this function and may also alter metabolic processes, resulting in a state of uremic intoxication. This process, being detrimental *per se*, has a significant impact on the patient's appetite and food intake. Accumulation of metabolic waste products also leads to a state of acidification, which is one of the major factors responsible for increased protein catabolism.

Apart from clearing metabolic wastes, kidneys are responsible for maintaining water–electrolyte balance. Deterioration of their function leads to altered potassium and sodium excretion. This can have a direct impact on cardiac function, and, in cases of severe hyperkalemia, may lead to cardiac arrest and sudden cardiac death, a common cause of death in patients with renal failure. Similarly, sodium removal may be decreased, leading to increased sodium load, and, consequently, to hypertension. The kidneys regulate blood pressure also through their secretory activities. They are the site of renin production, an enzyme involved in the renin–angiotensin–aldosterone system (RAAS). Alterations in RAAS activity are crucial for the development of hypertension. The secretory abilities of the kidneys are not limited to renin. Another major compound produced in the kidneys is erythropoietin. This hormone plays a major role in production of red blood cells. Therefore, anemia is a typical feature of chronic kidney insufficiency. Finally, the kidneys, by activating vitamin D and removing excess phosphate, regulate calcium–phosphate balance. CKD inevitably results in hypocalcemia, hyperphosphatemia, secondary hyperparathyroidism, and various forms of bone disorders or osteodystrophy.

CKD is often defined as a state of kidney damage and/or decreased glomerular filtration which lasts for at least 3 months. It can be caused by several illnesses, the most common being diabetes mellitus, hypertension, and primary glomerular diseases. CKD can be divided into five stages, depending on the presence of kidney damage, e.g. albuminuria, and on the glomerular filtration rate. CKD, regardless of the underlying pathology, is usually characterized by a progressive course with worsening of renal function, which may lead to stage 5 CKD, often described as end-stage renal disease (ESRD), which requires renal replacement therapy (RRT). There are two major kinds of RRT, dialysis and kidney transplantation. Dialysis is further divided into hemodialysis (HD) and peritoneal dialysis (PD).

As described above, kidneys have several functions that are crucial for the organism. Nutritional interventions play a pivotal role in diminishing metabolic and nutritional abnormalities associated with kidney insufficiency, both in patients treated with RRT, as well as in subjects in earlier stages of CKD.

Protein-Energy Wasting: Prevalence, Mechanisms and Significance

Among the complications of CKD, progressive loss of body protein mass and energy reserves is one of the most typical and detrimental. This loss has been termed protein-energy wasting (PEW) (Fouque *et al.*, 2008). It is most prevalent in patients with advanced stages of CKD, and may affect up to 75% of subjects with end-stage renal disease.

PEW is to a large extent caused by malnutrition, or, more precisely, by undernutrition. Impaired food intake is a consequence of several overlapping processes. A low-protein diet is advocated in CKD subjects as it has been shown to reduce uremic symptoms and retard the progression of the disease (Fouque and Laville, 2009). However, it may result in negative protein balance, especially in subjects not receiving amino acid and/or ketoacid supplementation. As CKD progresses, anorexia develops (Carrero *et al.*, 2008). This is due to uremic intoxication and hormonal derangements, including an increase in circulating levels of multiple anorexigens such as leptin and a decrease in some orexigens such as ghrelin. Finally, as patients progress towards end-stage renal disease, dialysis is introduced, complicated by significant losses of nutrients into the dialysate in both types of dialysis treatment.

However, malnutrition is not the only culprit for PEW occurrence. Chronic low-grade inflammation seems to be of equal importance (Stenvinkel *et al.*, 2000; Fouque *et al.*, 2008). This prevalent complication of CKD has been shown in several studies to decrease protein generation and to increase protein breakdown, resulting in a highly negative protein balance.

Several other disturbances predispose CKD patients to deteriorations of nutritional status. These include, for example, oxidative stress, acidosis, nutrient losses, social factors such as loneliness and poverty, and co-morbid conditions such as diabetes mellitus, cardiovascular disease, and infections, which are all highly prevalent in CKD patients (Fouque *et al.*, 2008). These and other potential causes of PEW are depicted in Figure 53.2.

It has to be remembered that obesity is a frequent finding in CKD, reflecting the growing prevalence of overweight and obesity in the general population. In fact, obesity is one of the most frequent risk factors for CKD progression (Zoccali, 2009) (also, see Chapter 45). However, PEW is equally frequent and equally detrimental in obese as it is in lean CKD subjects (Honda *et al.*, 2007).

PEW is a strong and independent predictor of cardiovascular and non-cardiovascular mortality in CKD patients. Decreased indices of nutritional status, as albumin, pre-albumin or cholesterol, have been associated with increased risk of death (Kovesdy and Kalantar-Zadeh, 2009). Similarly, decrease in muscle mass, and protein and energy intake, have been linked to worse outcome (Kovesdy and Kalantar-Zadeh, 2009). The importance of PEW as a determinant of poor outcome in the CKD population is reflected by the so-called "reverse epidemiology phenomenon". For example, in patients with advanced CKD, low (normal) cholesterol and low (normal) body mass index (BMI) predict poor outcome (Kalantar-Zadeh *et al.*, 2007). This stays in contrast to what is observed in the general population, with hypercholesterolemia and obesity being detrimental. Although many potential explanations have been proposed for these paradoxical associations, it seems that the most persuasive is the one in which PEW, resulting in low cholesterol and low BMI, leads to increase in mortality in CKD patients. This shows how crucial it is to prevent PEW in CKD subjects, to diagnose it as soon as it develops, and to treat it effectively.

Other Nutritional Aberrations in CKD

Acidosis

Although malnutrition is an important cause of PEW in CKD patients, other factors, including several hormonal and metabolic alterations related to loss of kidney function, can also predispose these patients to malnutrition. For example, metabolic acidosis, which is a common finding in CKD patients, induces increased protein catabolism with degradation of the essential, branched-chain amino acids and muscle protein. Moreover, metabolic acidosis is also known to suppress synthesis of proteins such as albumin (Ballmer and Imoberdorf, 1995).

Appetite

As mentioned above, loss of appetite, or anorexia, often resulting in insufficient intake of macronutrients and/or micronutrients, is also common in CKD and contributes

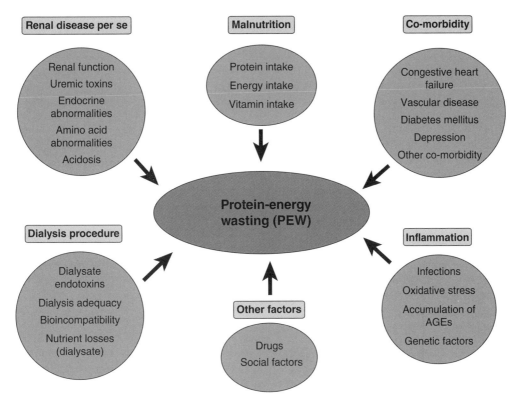

FIG. 53.2 Multiple causes of protein-energy wasting.
AGEs, advanced glycation end-products.

significantly to malnutrition (Kopple *et al.*, 1989). Anorexia commonly occurs when GFR is less than 10–15% of normal kidney function. One reasonable explanation for the often drastic decrease in appetite is the retention of toxic substances as a result of reduced renal clearance. In accordance with this, most patients improve their appetite when they start renal replacement therapy (RRT) (Bergstrom, 1999). Anorexia in CKD is associated with an increase in morbidity and mortality. Indeed both Kalantar-Zadeh *et al.* (2004) and Carrero *et al.* (2007) investigated maintenance hemodialysis (HD) patients and found that a decrease in appetite was related to greater risk of mortality.

The treatment of anorexia in dialysis patients should be based on a therapeutic strategy that includes several components. Increased dialysis treatment, for example in the form of daily dialysis sessions, and nutritional counseling as well as use of appetite stimulation and administration of nutritional supplements are often effective. Anorexia and nutritional status may be improved by normalization of plasma branched-chain amino acids through branched-chain amino acid supplementation (Bossola *et al.*, 2009). Megestrol acetate seems to improve anorexia and thereby the nutritional state in maintenance dialysis patients (Rammohan *et al.*, 2005). Subcutaneous ghrelin administration and melanocortin-receptor antagonists appear to be promising future therapeutic interventions.

Disorders in Vitamins and Trace Elements

Inadequate nutritional intake of macronutrients (protein, carbohydrates and fat) is not the only form of malnutrition that exists in CKD patients. They may also suffer from deficiencies of micronutrients, particularly vitamins and trace elements (Kalantar-Zadeh and Kopple, 2003). Inadequate dietary intakes, altered metabolism in uremia, and vitamin loss into the dialysate are likely to contribute to these deficiencies; dialysis treatment results in deficiencies of water-soluble vitamins (Boeschoten *et al.*, 1988; Gilmour *et al.*, 1993). The treatment of mineral and vitamin deficiencies will be discussed further in this chapter.

Insulin Resistance and Dyslipidemia

Diabetes mellitus is now the leading cause of CKD all over the world, accounting for up to 40% of cases of end-stage renal disease in some countries. However, insulin resistance is a typical finding in CKD, also in patients free from diabetes mellitus (also, see Chapter 47). Hypertriglyceridemia is another metabolic abnormality that typically appears as the renal function declines (Axelsson et al., 2004, 2006). While the mechanisms mediating this dysmetabolism remain unclear, it would appear that hypertriglyceridemia represents an early feature of renal failure, usually appearing together with albuminuria and often observed before an elevation of plasma creatinine can be seen (Sechi et al., 2002). Mechanistically, an accumulation of triglyceride-rich lipoproteins in CKD appears mainly to be a result of a decreased catabolism of lipids (Prinsen et al., 2003). As decreased insulin sensitivity occurs (commonly in patients with GFR <30 mL/min/1.73 m²), an overproduction of insulin-sensitive very-low-density lipoproteins (VLDL) is likely to contribute to hypertriglyceridemia in CKD patients. However, the role of an increased hepatic production of triglyceride-rich lipoproteins in the pathogenesis of renal dyslipidemia remains a subject of debate (Prinsen et al., 2003; Axelsson, 2008). As consequences of insulin resistance and dyslipidemia, CKD patients commonly suffer from muscle catabolism, cardiovascular disease, decreased appetite, and lipotoxicity.

Nutritional Assessment in CKD Patients

Many methods have been created to identify malnourished and wasted CKD patients, and to grade different degrees of PEW. Unfortunately, there is no single tool that can be used for this purpose; with so many concurrent metabolic and nutritional abnormalities, such a tool has remained elusive. The National Kidney Foundation Clinical Practice Guidelines for Nutrition in Chronic Renal Failure (Kidney Disease Outcomes Quality Initiative, 2000) thus recommend that nutritional status should not be evaluated with only a single measure alone, but instead using a combination of valid, complementary measures. These measures may include biological assessment of protein-energy status, subjective global assessment, dietary intake assessment, and anthropometry measurements.

Biomarkers

Biochemical parameters are routinely used to assess and monitor nutritional status in CKD patients. However, none of the currently favored biomarkers have been demonstrated to accurately reflect nutritional status in CKD (Ikizler et al., 1999; Stenvinkel et al., 2002; de Mutsert et al., 2009). Instead, strong associations between several biomarkers and mortality seem to derive, at least in part, from their close association with inflammation (de Mutsert et al., 2008), and in part from the important role of the kidney in metabolizing circulating peptides (Naseeb et al., 2008). However, as they are commonly used, we will shortly review the most common biomarkers: plasma concentrations of albumin, pre-albumin, and transferrin (Locatelli et al., 2002; Kamimura et al., 2005).

The amount of serum *albumin* is determined by its synthesis, breakdown, and volume of distribution (Klein, 1990; Jeejeebhoy, 2000). In CKD patients, factors such as overhydration, proteinuria and losses into the dialysate and urine may cause a decrease in plasma protein concentration. Counter-regulatory mechanisms may also influence the serum albumin concentration. Whereas, in the short term, protein deficiency decreases the rate of albumin synthesis (Rothschild et al., 1975), compensation in the long term may occur through a decrease in albumin breakdown and a shift of albumin from the extravascular to the intravascular space. Additionally, albumin has a relatively long half-life (approximately 20 days) and is present in large quantities (Kirsch et al., 1968), limiting the impact of a decreased protein intake on concentrations of albumin. Even in some extreme cases of malnutrition, such as marasmus, serum albumin levels in these patients remain normal (Whitehead and Alleyne, 1972). In kwashiorkor, on the contrary, serum albumin levels are usually low (Davies, 1948; Trowell et al., 1952). However, it is important to keep in mind that kwashiorkor is typically accompanied by infections (inflammatory state) and severe protein intake deficiency (which is usually not the case in the CKD population in most industrialized countries) (Rossouw, 1989; Friedman and Fadem, 2010). In a study by Kaysen et al. (2004) low serum albumin levels in dialysis patients were mainly associated with inflammation. Thus, it seems that hypoalbuminemia in CKD patients is rather associated with chronic inflammatory state than with insufficient food intake (Mak and Cheung, 2006). Like albumin, *pre-albumin* is mainly synthesized in the liver, and a reduced protein intake is associated with a decline in serum concentrations which are then restored by re-feeding (Kidney Disease Outcomes Quality Initiative, 1995), due to its lower concentration and shorter half-life (2–3 days) (Chertow et al., 2000; Neyra et al., 2000).

TABLE 53.1 Recommended values of biochemical parameters, limitations for assessment of nutritional status in CKD

Biomarkers[a]	Reference values	Limitations
Albumin	>4.0 g/dL	Affected by hypervolemia and inflammatory conditions
Pre-albumin	>30 mg/dL	Affected by inflammation, may be influenced by renal catabolism
Transferrin	Unknown	Affected by inflammation and iron metabolism

[a]Note that the relation between these biomarkers and nutritional status is weak or absent in CKD: see text.
Reproduced with permission from Kopple (2001).

However, serum pre-albumin levels are also greatly affected by inflammation (Ingenbleek *et al.*, 1972). In CKD, reduced renal catabolism also contributes to altered serum pre-albumin concentrations (Kopple, 2001). Lastly, *transferrin* is a visceral protein the main function of which is to transport iron in the circulation. Its concentration is affected by iron metabolism, much altered in CKD, and inflammation (Ferrari *et al.*, 2011). Thus, transferrin is not a reliable marker of nutritional status in CKD.

Despite the prevailing acceptance of these biomarkers in CKD, circulating levels of albumin and other proteins such as pre-albumin and transferrin are in fact *not* appropriate indicators of the nutritional status (Table 53.1).

Subjective Global Assessment (SGA)

With limited usefulness of current biomarkers, subjective global assessment (SGA) (Detsky *et al.*, 1987) has been proposed as a simple, inexpensive, and easy-to-apply subjective method of assessing nutritional status in this patient group. SGA is currently considered to be a reliable indicator of PEW in uremic patients (Kidney Disease Outcomes Quality Initiative, 2000; Toigo *et al.*, 2000). Furthermore, SGA uses scoring of a patient's medical history and physical examination to differentiate well-nourished, slightly malnourished, and severely malnourished patients. The attributes scored in the SGA evaluation include the following: gastrointestinal symptoms, dietary intake, body weight, disease state, and functional capacity.

Owing to its strong correlations with PEW (Cooper *et al.*, 2002) and outcomes (Yang *et al.*, 2007), SGA is

recommended as a component of longitudinal monitoring of chronic dialysis patients by, among others, K/DOQI, the National Kidney Foundation Kidney Disease/Dialysis Outcomes and Quality Initiative (2000). Although several studies show that SGA is a useful tool in CKD (Campbell *et al.*, 2007; Steiber *et al.*, 2007), it should be kept in mind that SGA is still a subjective score that may be biased by inter- and intrapersonal differences. As such, it is perhaps best employed in a longitudinal manner by the same trained investigator to follow patients over time.

Dietary Records

The estimation of dietary intake is of central importance in CKD patients. The most commonly used and easy ways to quantify individual intake of nutrients are the dietary interview, the 24-hour dietary recall, and the dietary record. These tools are especially useful for the estimation of macronutrient intake in the clinical setting. While under- or over-estimation of dietary intake is common using these methods, they have been successfully used in the CKD patient population. In HD patients, dietary protein intake assessed by 7-day food records correlated with intake estimated by normalized protein catabolic rate, and there were significant differences in diets between dialysis and non-dialysis days (Chauveau *et al.*, 2007). In a study investigating the accuracy of food records with regard to energy consumption, energy intake was evaluated using 4-day food diaries, and resting energy expenditure was measured by indirect calorimetry; energy intake based on 4-day food diaries was found to be underestimated (Avesani *et al.*, 2005).

Body Composition

Theoretically, body composition and the contents of fat, protein, and water should reflect long-term dietary intake and PEW (also, see Chapter 58). While several methods have been employed in CKD patients, they each suffer from the large variation of body water seen in this patient group.

Bioelectrical Impedance Analysis (BIA)

BIA and bioelectrical impedance spectrometry (BIS) have long been proposed as non-invasive, simple, and quick techniques for measuring body composition. BIA and BIS use measured variations in electrical currents of one or more frequencies passed through the body to estimate body water, fat, and fat-free mass. However, the problem of determining the amount and distribution of intra- and extracellular water in CKD patients limits the usefulness of this method for nutritional assessment.

Dual-Energy X-Ray Absorptiometry

A more reliable tool to estimate body composition is dual-energy X-ray absorptiometry (DEXA). DEXA passes low-energy X-rays through the body to measure fat mass, fat-free mass, and bone mineral density (Gotfredsen *et al.*, 1986). While DEXA is relatively good at measuring fat mass (Avesani *et al.*, 2004a), it is not used routinely in the clinical setting because of its high cost and its inaccuracy in severely overhydrated patients (Bhatla *et al.*, 1995). Furthermore, the amount of radiation, although small, is a concern in patients exposed to DEXA repeatedly over many years.

Anthropometrics

Skinfold thickness is an anthropometric tool widely used in clinical practice because of its low cost, simplicity, and non-invasive nature. It is used to estimate both fat mass and fat-free mass (Durnin and Womersley, 1974). However, skinfold thickness measurements suffer from a large intra- and inter-observer variability, and are only modestly reliable (Avesani *et al.*, 2004a). Another marker used to determine body fat mass is waist circumference. This is again a simple and easy method, which has been suggested to predict survival in CKD patients (Postorino *et al.*, 2009). However, as fat mass does not necessarily reflect PEW in CKD, waist circumference is likely not a good marker of the nutritional deficiencies associated with PEW (Table 53.2).

Treating Nutritional Deficiencies in CKD Patients

Renal Replacement Therapy

When patients reach end-stage renal disease, renal replacement therapy (RRT) is introduced. It improves indices of uremia to a different degree, depending on the RRT method applied. While renal transplantation is by far the best method of RRT, fully replacing native kidneys in the case of well-functioning grafts, dialysis has its drawbacks and limitations. Both the dialyzer membrane in HD and the peritoneal membrane in PD patients are far less selective than the kidney's glomerular barrier. Therefore, many essential nutrients are lost into the dialysate, and the dialysis procedure may cause a transitory inflammatory response stimulating protein catabolism. Nevertheless, dialysis has

TABLE 53.2   Advantages and disadvantages of nutritional assessment methods

Methods	Advantages	Disadvantages
Biomarkers	Widely accepted	Limited reliability, affected by inflammation
Subjective global assessment	Simple, inexpensive, easy to apply	Subjective; inter- and intrapersonal variability
Dietary records	Simple, inexpensive, easy to apply	Subjective; may easily be over- or underestimated
Body composition measurements		
Bioelectrical impedance analysis	Simple, non-invasive	Influenced by hydration status
Dual-energy X-ray absorptiometry	Reliable	Expensive, influenced by hydration status
Skinfold thickness	Simple, inexpensive, non-invasive	High intra- and inter-observer variability; useless in very obese patients

the capability of improving several indices of nutritional status. It has been demonstrated that adequate dialysis is a prerequisite for PEW prevention (Azar *et al.*, 2007). In patients in whom the dialysis dose does not meet their requirements, uremic intoxication and volume overload evolve. These factors play an important role in PEW development. In patients undergoing kidney transplantation, the immunosuppressive therapy, in particular corticosteroids, may lead to metabolic and nutritional alterations including metabolic syndrome and PEW (Ward, 2009).

Dietary Composition

Protein

The European Society of Parenteral and Enteral Nutrition (ESPEN) and the National Kidney Foundation (NKF) guidelines recommend that CKD patients stages 4–5 (GFR <30 mL/min) should keep a moderately reduced protein intake of 0.55–0.60 g/kg BW/day (Cano *et al.*, 2006). A very low protein diet with protein intake of 0.3–0.4 g/kg BW/day is also used in several countries, but patients receiving such a diet should be carefully monitored and supported by supplements with essential amino acids or keto acids to avoid a negative nitrogen balance (Cano *et al.*, 2006). (The progression of CKD may slow significantly when following a low–protein diet (Fouque *et al.*, 1992; Klahr *et al.*, 1994; Levey *et al.*, 1996; Pedrini *et al.*, 1996). A low-protein diet might have additional benefits in CKD patients, as it would lead to a decrease in hyperkalemia, hyperphosphatemia, and metabolic acidosis, as well as to the attenuation of other electrolyte disorders (Mitch and Remuzzi, 2004). Furthermore, many of the clinical and metabolic disturbances characteristic of uremia may be delayed or prevented by the reduction of nitrogenous wastes and inorganic ions (derived from a diet rich in protein).

When treating CKD patients, it must be kept in mind that the variation in protein requirements is much larger in these patients than in healthy subjects, as a result of additional sources of variability such as endocrine and biochemical abnormalities, anemia, drugs, physical inactivity, and co-morbid conditions. In addition, some non-essential amino acids become essential in CKD because of the loss of conversion in the kidney, and specific effects of the dialytic process may increase protein requirements, especially in HD patients (Bergstrom and Lindholm, 1993). Owing to these factors, it is currently recommended that CKD patients starting dialysis should discontinue a low-protein diet and instead have a protein intake of 1.2–1.3 g/kg BW/day, of which a large part should be of high biological value (Kopple, 2001). It is, however, interesting to note that recent findings suggest that a protein intake of 0.6–0.8 g of protein/kg BW/day may lead to improved preservation of residual renal function without adverse consequences in dialysis patients (Bergström *et al.*, 1993; Jiang *et al.*, 2009). Thus, whereas many patients may require less than 1.2 g/kg BW/day to maintain nitrogen equilibrium (Bergström *et al.*, 1993; Kopple *et al.*, 1995), some patients, e.g. those who develop PEW, may require higher amounts of protein (and energy). Indeed, studies have suggested that some patients may benefit from eating as much as 1.4–2.1 g protein/kg BW/day, especially during the initial months of dialysis treatment (Bergström *et al.*, 1993).

Fat

Fat is the most energy-dense macronutrient available and thus would seem to be likely to be beneficial to malnourished CKD patients, especially those on a low-protein diet. However, no studies exist that have explored the optimal amount of fat in the CKD diet. The ESPEN and NKF Kidney Disease Outcomes Quality Initiative Guidelines respectively for CKD patients recommend a total energy intake for adults that is similar to that of the general population, i.e. 35 kcal/kg/day, and for older adults (>60 years) 30–35 kcal/kg/day (Kent, 2005; Cano *et al.*, 2006).

For CKD patients at stages 1 to 3, the energy requirement is based on energy expenditure and depends on the nutritional status of the patient. Thus, those who are underweight need a higher calorie intake than patients who are of normal weight or overweight (Kent, 2005). Not only the quantity but also the quality of the dietary fat is important. In one study unsaturated fat supplementation (430 kcal, 47 g fat, 26.5 g monounsaturated fatty acids, and 3 g marine n-3 polyunsaturated fatty acids per day) in HD patients was associated with normalized blood lipids, reduced systemic inflammation, and improved nutritional status (Ewers *et al.*, 2009).

Carbohydrates

There is as yet no evidence that the energy requirements of CKD patients are systematically different from those of normal subjects. While most studies (Monteon *et al.*, 1986; Avesani *et al.*, 2004b) have shown normal resting energy expenditure (REE) in both early and late CKD, one study reported decreased REE in non-dialyzed CKD patients (Avesani *et al.*, 2004c). Thus, an energy intake of at least 35 kcal/kg body weight is currently recommended in CKD patients (Kopple, 2001). Importantly, studies show that most CKD patients have a much lower energy intake, and this may contribute to PEW (Avesani *et al.*, 2005). In dialysis patients, HD is mostly energy neutral, while PD patients may absorb about 60% of the daily dialysate glucose load (100–200 g glucose/24 hours) (Heimbürger *et al.*, 1992). See Table 53.3.

Vitamins

CKD patients commonly suffer from micronutrient deficiencies (Kalantar-Zadeh and Kopple, 2003). Of the

TABLE 53.3 Recommendation of protein and energy intake for CKD and ESRD patients

Patients	Protein intake	Energy intake[a]
CKD	0.60 g/kg/day	30–35 kcal/kg/day
ESRD	1.2 g/kg/day	30–35 kcal/kg/day

[a]Energy requirement may vary depending on patient's nutritional status and age (Kent, 2005).
ERSD, end-stage renal disease patients undergoing dialysis therapy.

water-soluble vitamins that have been studied, serum levels of ascorbic acid, thiamine (B$_1$), pyridoxine (B$_6$), and folic acid have all been reported to be low in dialysis patients (Gilmour et al., 1993). Thiamin deficiency with encephalopathy has been described in dialysis patients (Hung et al., 2001) and may be confounded by other neurologic diseases. A common dietary intake of 0.5 to 1.5 mg/day may be supplemented with a daily dose of 1–5 mg of thiamin hydrochloride. Vitamin B$_6$ coenzymes play a vital role in several aspects of amino acid utilization, and the need for vitamin B$_6$ is particularly critical if protein and amino acid intake is limited (Kopple et al., 1981). Indeed, changes in fasting plasma amino acid and serum high-density lipoprotein levels after correction of the vitamin B$_6$ deficiency in dialysis patients indicate its role in the pathogenesis of the abnormal amino acid and lipid metabolism of CKD (Kleiner et al., 1980). The daily requirement of pyridoxine may be higher in dialysis patients than in normal subjects, and dialysis patients should be supplemented with a minimum of 10 mg of vitamin B$_6$ per day (Kopple et al., 1981). As a water-soluble vitamin, folate is lost in dialysate. Because serum folate levels have been reported to be reduced in CKD, it is recommended to give 1 mg of folic acid daily. High doses of folic acid (5–10 mg/day) have been shown to reduce the markedly elevated plasma homocysteine levels in dialysis patients by about two-thirds, which is still above the normal range (Arnadottir et al., 1993). The question whether these high doses of folate should be prescribed in order to lower plasma homocysteine levels to reduce cardiovascular morbidity and mortality in CKD is still open, and prospective studies are needed in this area. Furthermore, while supplementation with vitamin C has also been recommended in CKD (Boeschoten et al., 1988), a high intake of vitamin C may aggravate hyperoxalemia in dialysis patients (Canavese et al., 2005) and controlled trials are lacking to support this recommendation.

Unlike water-soluble vitamins, supplementation of the fat-soluble vitamins A, D, E, and K is not recommended on a routine basis to CKD patients (Gilmour et al., 1993). Vitamin A tends to accumulate in CKD patients and can potentially have harmful effects. Vitamin D is converted in the kidneys from 25-hydroxyvitamin D to its active form, 1,25-dihydroxyvitamin D. Most patients with advanced CKD, especially CKD stages 4 and 5, are deficient in 1,25-dihydroxyvitamin D (and also in 25-hydroxyvitamin D), and supplementation of active vitamin D is often given on the basis of an evaluation of the bone metabolic status and taking the risks of hyper-phosphatemia and hypercalcemia into consideration (Jean et al., 2008). In most studies of uremic patients, blood levels of vitamin E have been found to be normal and stable (Clermont et al., 2000). As vitamin K$_2$ deficiency may play a role in the development of vascular calcification in CKD patients, it is possible that supplementation of vitamin K might be beneficial. Vitamin E is a strong antioxidant compound, and it has been proposed to reduce cardiovascular disease. This was tested in a randomized controlled trial with a high dose of vitamin E (800 IU α-tocopherol per day) supplementation (Boaz et al., 2000) in CKD patients with high cardiovascular risk. This study found a significant 50% decrease in cardiovascular incidents as compared with placebo.

Trace Elements

Dietary requirements for trace elements are not well defined in CKD patients (Kalantar-Zadeh and Kopple, 2003). Trace-element metabolism is frequently altered in CKD (Gilmour et al., 1993), and high levels of trace elements have been attributed to impaired renal elimination or contamination of dialysis fluids, while low levels of trace elements may occur as a result of inadequate dietary intake or loss of protein-bound trace elements into the dialysate (Gilmour et al., 1993). Zinc deficiency has been reported to be common in CKD (Rucker et al., 2010); however, it may be alleviated by zinc administration (Rashidi et al., 2009). Nevertheless, these results have not been generally confirmed and the role of zinc deficiency and requirements for extra zinc in CKD patients remain at present controversial (Gilmour et al., 1993).

Nutrition Counseling

The goal of nutritional management of CKD patients is to delay the need for dialysis by using low-protein diets while maintaining good nutritional status (Fouque and Aparicio, 2007). Thus, the specialized renal dietitian has a fundamental role in the assessment and treatment of CKD patients. In addition, dietary counseling should be offered as part of a multidisciplinary approach (Locatelli et al., 2002).

In CKD, both regular dietary counseling and protein-energy status assessment are of great importance. In order to avoid a decline in nutritional status during CKD progression, a regular schedule with follow-up evaluations by dietitians and nephrologists (Aparicio et al., 2001) is recommended. According to the Kidney Disease Outcomes Quality Initiative K/DOQI Recommendations for Nutritional Management guidelines (Kidney Disease Outcomes Quality Initiative, 2000), dietary interviews and counseling should be performed every 3 to 4 months. In addition, serum albumin level (although, as noted above, its value as a nutritional biomarker is questionable in CKD), together with body weight and SGA, should be monitored every 1 to 3 months. A key reason for monitoring protein-energy status is to adjust nutritional intakes to the patient's nutritional needs, to detect signs of PEW, and to identify patients requiring nutritional support.

Intradialytic Nutritional Support

In order to compensate for nutrient losses during dialysis and to further improve nutritional status of dialysis patients, intradialytic nutritional support can be used in the form of intravenous (in HD) and intraperitoneal (in PD) infusions. Intradialytic parenteral nutrition (IDPN) is an acknowledged method of protein and energy supplementation in HD patients. Typically composed of a mixture of amino acids, dextrose, and lipids, IDPN has been shown to increase protein synthesis and decrease protein degradation, resulting in a highly positive protein balance (Pupim et al., 2002). However, recent studies have demonstrated no clear additional benefit of IDPN over oral nutritional support (Cano et al., 2007). Therefore, current guidelines limit the use of IDPN to wasted subjects in whom oral nutritional support has turned out to be ineffective in improving nutritional status (Fouque et al., 2007).

Protein losses into the dialysate in PD patients are of even greater magnitude than those occurring in HD. Protein intake ought therefore to be increased in these subjects. Moreover, amino acid based peritoneal dialysis fluids have been developed. In this case, amino acids serve also as an osmotic factor (instead of the common osmotic agent, glucose), but, more importantly, they can improve protein balance of PD patients. One exchange with amino acid based fluid daily in wasted subjects treated with PD is usually enough to replace 24 hours of losses of protein and amino acids in PD patients.

Improving Appetite and Anabolic Interventions

As underlined earlier, nutrient losses into the dialysate are not the only culprit for poor nutritional status of dialysis patients. Decreased food ingestion, due to poor appetite, is also a common problem. Several factors are responsible, with inadequate dialysis, hormonal derangements, inflam-

mation, and co-morbidities being the major ones. Poor appetite has been shown to be a strong and independent predictor of mortality in dialysis patients. Therefore, several initiatives to improve ingestion have been introduced. These include: improving dialysis adequacy and treatment of co-morbidities, but also interventions that are targeted directly at improving appetite. Megestrol acetate, a progesterone derivative, has been shown to ameliorate anorexia and improve nutritional status in CKD patients (Monfared et al., 2009; Yeh et al., 2010). Some concerns have arisen with regard to side-effects caused by megestrol acetate (Bossola et al., 2005). However, it remains a useful tool in treating appetite disorders. Ghrelin, a small peptide produced in the stomach, strongly induces appetite. The concentration of its active, acylated form has been shown to be decreased in dialysis patients, especially in those with chronic inflammatory state (Mafra et al., 2010). Subcutaneous injections of ghrelin have been found to be effective in improving energy intake of wasted subjects on HD (Ashby et al., 2009). Similarly, anabolic interventions with growth hormone (GH), GH-releasing hormone, and insulin-like growth factor-1 (IGF-1) have been capable of improving protein and energy status in dialysis patients (Fouque et al., 2000; Feldt-Rasmussen et al., 2007; Niemczyk et al., 2010). However, the results so far should be interpreted with caution, as no large randomized clinical trials (RCTs) evaluating the impact of appetite improvement and/or anabolic intervention on survival have been performed. To date the only RCT to assess the role of GH in outcome in wasted HD subjects has been cancelled because of problems with patient recruitment (Kopple et al., 2008). A simplified algorithm for applying nutritional interventions is depicted in Figure 53.3.

Future Directions

Since the presence of PEW has been shown to be of considerable importance in determining clinical outcomes, trials should be designed to study the possibilities of effective PEW prevention and treatment in CKD patients. It is essential that nutritional requirements be met, but this may not be sufficient for prevention and treatment of PEW. One might assume that appropriate nutritional interventions would have an impact on patient outcome, but the evidence for such an impact is in fact scarce. One important reason is that "pure" malnutrition may not be the main determinant of PEW in CKD patients who suffer from so many other catabolic conditions, e.g. chronic systemic inflammation and co-morbidities, contributing

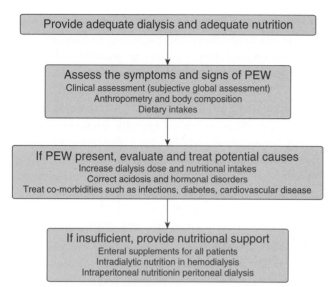

FIG. 53.3 Simplified algorithm for applying nutritional interventions in CKD.

to PEW and – by other mechanisms – to poor clinical outcomes. The number of adequately powered RCTs in this field is very limited. The studies that are available were usually of short duration and performed in small patient groups, and they rarely address "hard" end points such as survival. It seems, therefore, that there must be new trials in the future to verify the usefulness of nutritional initiatives in CKD patients. Such trials should aim at evaluating the impact of particular nutritional interventions, not only on nutrition indices but also on mortality of CKD patients.

Again one has to remember that PEW is a multifactorial process, with pure malnutrition being only one of the culprits. Therefore, it appears that only interventions targeted against several factors responsible for PEW could be expected to have a significant impact on patient outcomes. The future should hopefully provide us with such studies and with an answer to the issue of ideal nutritional support in patients with kidney diseases.

Suggestions for Further Reading

Byham-Gray, L.D., Burrowes, J.D., and Chertow, G.M. (2008) *Nutrition in Kidney Disease*. Humana Press, Totowa, NJ.

Kopple, J.D and Massry, S.G. (2004) *Kopple and Massry's Nutritional Management of Renal Disease*, 2nd Edn. Lippincott, Williams & Wilkins, Philadelphia.

Mitch, W.E. and Ikizler, T.A. (2009) *Handbook of Nutrition and the Kidney*, 6th Edn. Lippincott, Williams & Wilkins, Philadelphia.

Pereira, B.J., Sayegh, M.H., and Blake, P. (2005) *Chronic Kidney Disease, Dialysis, and Transplantation*, Elsevier Saunders, Philadelphia.

References

Aparicio, M., Chauveau, P., and Combe, C. (2001) Low protein diets and outcome of renal patients. *J Nephrol* **14,** 433–439.

Arnadottir, M., Brattstrom, L., Simonsen, O., et al. (1993) The effect of high-dose pyridoxine and folic acid supplementation on serum lipid and plasma homocysteine concentrations in dialysis patients. *Clin Nephrol* **40,** 236–240.

Ashby, D.R., Ford, H.E., Wynne, K.J., et al. (2009) Sustained appetite improvement in malnourished dialysis patients by daily ghrelin treatment. *Kidney Int* **76,** 199–206.

Avesani, C., Draibe, S., Kamimura, M., et al. (2004a) Assessment of body composition by dual energy X-ray absorptiometry, skinfold thickness and creatinine kinetics in chronic kidney disease patients. *Nephrol Dial Transplant* **19,** 2289–2295.

Avesani, C., Draibe, S., Kamimura, M., et al. (2004b) Resting energy expenditure of chronic kidney disease patients: influence of renal function and subclinical inflammation. *Am J Kidney Dis* **44,** 1008–1016.

Avesani, C.M., Draibe, S.A., Kamimura, M.A., et al. (2004c) Decreased resting energy expenditure in non-dialysed chronic kidney disease patients. *Nephrol Dial Transplant* **19,** 3091–3097.

Avesani, C., Kamimura, M., Draibe, S., et al. (2005) Is energy intake underestimated in nondialyzed chronic kidney disease patients? *J Ren Nutr* **15,** 159–165.

Axelsson, J. (2008) The emerging biology of adipose tissue in chronic kidney disease: from fat to facts. *Nephrol Dial Transplant* **23,** 3041–3046.

Axelsson, J., Bergsten, A., Qureshi, A.R., et al. (2006) Elevated resistin levels in chronic kidney disease are associated with decreased glomerular filtration rate and inflammation, but not with insulin resistance. *Kidney Int* **69,** 596–604.

Axelsson, J., Rashid Qureshi, A., Suliman, M.E., et al. (2004) Truncal fat mass as a contributor to inflammation in end-stage renal disease. *Am J Clin Nutr* **80,** 1222–1229.

Azar, A.T., Wahba, K., Mohamed, A.S., et al. (2007) Association between dialysis dose improvement and nutritional status among hemodialysis patients. *Am J Nephrol* **27,** 113–119.

Ballmer, P. and Imoberdorf, R. (1995) Influence of acidosis on protein metabolism. *Nutrition* **11**, 462–468; Discussion 470.

Bárány, P., Pettersson, E., Ahlberg, M., *et al.* (1991) Nutritional assessment in anemic hemodialysis patients treated with recombinant human erythropoietin. *Clin Nephrol* **35**, 270–279.

Bergström, J. (1999) Mechanisms of uremic suppression of appetite. *J Ren Nutr* **9**, 129–132.

Bergström, J. and Lindholm, B. (1993) Nutrition and adequacy of dialysis. How do hemodialysis and CAPD compare? *Kidney Int Suppl* **40**, S39–50.

Bergström, J., Fürst, P., Alvestrand, A., *et al.* (1993) Protein and energy intake, nitrogen balance and nitrogen losses in patients treated with continuous ambulatory peritoneal dialysis. *Kidney Int* **44**, 1048–1057.

Bhatla, B., Moore, H., Emerson, P., *et al.* (1995) Lean body mass estimation by creatinine kinetics, bioimpedance, and dual energy x-ray absorptiometry in patients on continuous ambulatory peritoneal dialysis. *ASAIO J* **41**, M442–446.

Boaz, M., Smetana, S., Weinstein, T., *et al.* (2000) Secondary prevention with antioxidants of cardiovascular disease in end stage renal disease (SPACE): randomised placebo-controlled trial. *Lancet* **356**, 1213–1218.

Boeschoten, E.W., Schrijver, J., Krediet, R.T., *et al.* (1988) Deficiencies of vitamins in CAPD patients: the effect of supplementation. *Nephrol Dial Transplant* **3**, 187–193.

Bossola, M., Muscaritoli, M., Tazza, L., *et al.* (2005) Malnutrition in hemodialysis patients: what therapy? *Am J Kidney Dis* **46**, 371–386.

Bossola, M., Tazza, L., and Luciani, G. (2009) Mechanisms and treatment of anorexia in end-stage renal disease patients on hemodialysis. *J Ren Nutr* **19**, 2–9.

Campbell, K., Ash, S., Bauer, J., *et al.* (2007) Evaluation of nutrition assessment tools compared with body cell mass for the assessment of malnutrition in chronic kidney disease. *J Ren Nutr* **17**, 189–195.

Canavese, C., Petrarulo, M., Massarenti, P., *et al.* (2005) Long-term, low-dose, intravenous vitamin C leads to plasma calcium oxalate supersaturation in hemodialysis patients. *Am J Kidney Dis* **45**, 540–549.

Cano, N., Fiaccadori, E., Tesinsky, P., *et al.* (2006) ESPEN guidelines on enteral nutrition: adult renal failure. *Clin Nutr* **25**, 295–310.

Cano, N.J., Fouque, D., Roth, H., *et al.* (2007) Intradialytic parenteral nutrition does not improve survival in malnourished hemodialysis patients: a 2-year multicenter, prospective, randomized study. *J Am Soc Nephrol* **18**, 2583–2591.

Carrero, J.J., Aguilera, A., Stenvinkel, P., *et al.* (2008) Appetite disorders in uremia. *J Ren Nutr* **18**, 107–113.

Carrero, J.J., Qureshi, A., Axelsson, J., *et al.* (2007) Comparison of nutritional and inflammatory markers in dialysis patients with reduced appetite. *Am J Clin Nutr* **85**, 695–701.

Chauveau, P., Grigaut, E., Kolko, A., *et al.* (2007) Evaluation of nutritional status in patients with kidney disease: usefulness of dietary recall. *J Ren Nutr* **17**, 88–92.

Chertow, G., Ackert, K., Lew, N., *et al.* (2000) Prealbumin is as important as albumin in the nutritional assessment of hemodialysis patients. *Kidney Int* **58**, 2512–2517.

Clermont, G., Lecour, S., Lahet, J., *et al.* (2000) Alteration in plasma antioxidant capacities in chronic renal failure and hemodialysis patients: a possible explanation for the increased cardiovascular risk in these patients. *Cardiovasc Res* **47**, 618–623.

Cooper, B., Bartlett, L., Aslani, A., *et al.* (2002) Validity of subjective global assessment as a nutritional marker in end-stage renal disease. *Am J Kidney Dis* **40**, 126–132.

Coresh, J., Byrd-Holt, D., Astor, B., *et al.* (2005) Chronic kidney disease awareness, prevalence, and trends among U.S. adults, 1999 to 2000. *J Am Soc Nephrol* **16**, 180–188.

Davies, J. (1948) The essential pathology of kwashiorkor. *Lancet* **1**, 317–320.

De Mutsert, R., Grootendorst, D., Axelsson, J., *et al.* (2008) Excess mortality due to interaction between protein-energy wasting, inflammation and cardiovascular disease in chronic dialysis patients. *Nephrol Dial Transplant* **23**, 2957–2964.

De Mutsert, R., Grootendorst, D., Indemans, F., *et al.* (2009) Association between serum albumin and mortality in dialysis patients is partly explained by inflammation, and not by malnutrition. *J Ren Nutr* **19**, 127–135.

Detsky, A., McLaughlin, J., Baker, J., *et al.* (1987) What is subjective global assessment of nutritional status? *JPEN J Parenter Enteral Nutr* **11**, 8–13.

Durnin, J. and Womersley, J. (1974) Body fat assessed from total body density and its estimation from skinfold thickness: measurements on 481 men and women aged from 16 to 72 years. *Br J Nutr* **32**, 77–97.

Ewers, B., Riserus, U., and Marckmann, P. (2009) Effects of unsaturated fat dietary supplements on blood lipids, and on markers of malnutrition and inflammation in hemodialysis patients. *J Ren Nutr* **19**, 401–411.

Feldt-Rasmussen, B., Lange, M., Sulowicz, W., *et al.* (2007) Growth hormone treatment during hemodialysis in a randomized trial improves nutrition, quality of life, and cardiovascular risk. *J Am Soc Nephrol* **18**, 2161–2171.

Ferrari, P., Kulkarni, H., Dheda, S., *et al.* (2010) Serum iron markers are inadequate for guiding iron repletion in chronic kidney disease. *Clin J Am Soc Nephrol* **6**, 77–83.

Fouque, D. and Aparicio, M. (2007) Eleven reasons to control the protein intake of patients with chronic kidney disease. *Nat Clin Pract Nephrol* **3**, 383–392.

Fouque, D. and Laville, M. (2009) Low protein diets for chronic kidney disease in non diabetic adults. *Cochrane Database Syst Rev* CD001892.

Fouque, D., Kalantar-Zadeh, K., Kopple, J., *et al.* (2008) A proposed nomenclature and diagnostic criteria for protein-energy wasting in acute and chronic kidney disease. *Kidney Int* **73**, 391–398.

Fouque, D., Laville, M., Boissel, J., *et al.* (1992) Controlled low protein diets in chronic renal insufficiency: meta-analysis. *BMJ* **304**, 216–220.

Fouque, D., Peng, S.C., Shamir, E., *et al.* (2000) Recombinant human insulin-like growth factor-1 induces an anabolic response in malnourished CAPD patients. *Kidney Int* **57**, 646–654.

Fouque, D., Vennegoor, M., Ter Wee, P., *et al.* (2007) EBPG guideline on nutrition. *Nephrol Dial Transplant* **22**(Suppl 2), ii45–87.

Friedman, A. and Fadem, S. (2010) Reassessment of albumin as a nutritional marker in kidney disease. *J Am Soc Nephrol* **21**, 223–230.

Gilmour, E.R., Hartley, G.H., and Goodship, T.H.J. (1993) Trace elements and vitamins in renal disease. In W.E. Mitch and S. Klahr (eds), *Nutrition and the Kidney*. Little, Brown and Co., Boston, pp. 114–127.

Gotfredsen, A., Jensen, J., Borg, J., *et al.* (1986) Measurement of lean body mass and total body fat using dual photon absorptiometry. *Metabolism* **35**, 88–93.

Heimburger, O., Qureshi, A.R., Blaner, W. S., *et al.* (2000) Handgrip muscle strength, lean body mass, and plasma proteins as markers of nutritional status in patients with chronic renal failure close to start of dialysis therapy. *Am J Kidney Dis* **36**, 1213–1225.

Heimbürger, O., Waniewski, J., Werynski, A., *et al.* (1992) A quantitative description of solute and fluid transport during peritoneal dialysis. *Kidney Int* **41**, 1320–1332.

Honda, H., Qureshi, A.R., Axelsson, J., *et al.* (2007) Obese sarcopenia in patients with end-stage renal disease is associated with inflammation and increased mortality. *Am J Clin Nutr* **86**, 633–638.

Hsu, C.C., Hwang, S.J., Wen, C.P., *et al.* (2006) High prevalence and low awareness of CKD in Taiwan: a study on the relationship between serum creatinine and awareness from a nationally representative survey. *Am J Kidney Dis* **48**, 727–738.

Hung, S.C., Hung, S.H., Tarng, D.C., *et al.* (2001) Thiamine deficiency and unexplained encephalopathy in hemodialysis and peritoneal dialysis patients. *Am J Kidney Dis* **38**, 941–947.

Ikizler, T., Wingard, R., Harvell, J., *et al.* (1999) Association of morbidity with markers of nutrition and inflammation in chronic hemodialysis patients: a prospective study. *Kidney Int* **55**, 1945–1951.

Ingenbleek, Y., De Visscher, M., and De Nayer, P. (1972) Measurement of prealbumin as index of protein-calorie malnutrition. *Lancet* **2**, 106–109.

Jean, G., Terrat, J., Vanel, T., *et al.* (2008) Daily oral 25-hydroxycholecalciferol supplementation for vitamin D deficiency in haemodialysis patients: effects on mineral metabolism and bone markers. *Nephrol Dial Transplant* **23**, 3670–3676.

Jeejeebhoy, K. (2000) Nutritional assessment. *Nutrition* **16**, 585–590.

Jiang, N., Qian, J., Sun, W., *et al.* (2009) Better preservation of residual renal function in peritoneal dialysis patients treated with a low-protein diet supplemented with keto acids: a prospective, randomized trial. *Nephrol Dial Transplant* **24**, 2551–2558.

Kalantar-Zadeh, K. and Kopple, J.D. (2003) Trace elements and vitamins in maintenance dialysis patients. *Adv Ren Replace Ther* **10**, 170–182.

Kalantar-Zadeh, K., Block, G., McAllister, C., *et al.* (2004) Appetite and inflammation, nutrition, anemia, and clinical outcome in hemodialysis patients. *Am J Clin Nutr* **80**, 299–307.

Kalantar-Zadeh, K., Horwich, T.B., Oreopoulos, A., *et al.* (2007) Risk factor paradox in wasting diseases. *Curr Opin Clin Nutr Metab Care* **10**, 433–442.

Kamimura, M., Majchrzak, K., Cuppari, L., *et al.* (2005) Protein and energy depletion in chronic hemodialysis patients: clinical applicability of diagnostic tools. *Nutr Clin Pract* **20**, 162–175.

Kaysen, G., Dubin, J., Müller, H., *et al.* (2004) Inflammation and reduced albumin synthesis associated with stable decline in serum albumin in hemodialysis patients. *Kidney Int* **65**, 1408–1415.

Kent, P.S. (2005) Integrating clinical nutrition practice guidelines in chronic kidney disease. *Nutr Clin Pract* **20**, 213–217.

Kidney Disease Outcomes Quality Initiative (1995) Measurement of visceral protein status in assessing protein and energy malnutrition: standard of care. Prealbumin in Nutritional Care Consensus Group. *Nutrition* **11**, 169–171.

Kidney Disease Outcomes Quality Initiative (2000) Clinical practice guidelines for nutrition in chronic renal failure. K/DOQI, National Kidney Foundation. *Am J Kidney Dis* **35**, S1–140.

Kirsch, R., Frith, L., Black, E., *et al.* (1968) Regulation of albumin synthesis and catabolism by alteration of dietary protein. *Nature* **217**, 578–579.

Klahr, S., Levey, A., Beck, G., *et al.* (1994) The effects of dietary protein restriction and blood-pressure control on the progression of chronic renal disease. Modification of Diet in Renal Disease Study Group. *N Engl J Med* **330**, 877–884.

Klein, S. (1990) The myth of serum albumin as a measure of nutritional status. *Gastroenterology* **99**, 1845–1846.

Kleiner, M.J., Tate, S.S., Sullivan, J.F., *et al.* (1980) Vitamin B6 deficiency in maintenance dialysis patients: metabolic effects of repletion. *Am J Clin Nutr* **33**, 1612–1619.

Kopple, J. (2001) National Kidney Foundation K/DOQI clinical practice guidelines for nutrition in chronic renal failure. *Am J Kidney Dis* **37**, S66–70.

Kopple, J., Berg, R., Houser, H., *et al.* (1989) Nutritional status of patients with different levels of chronic renal insufficiency. Modification of Diet in Renal Disease (MDRD) Study Group. *Kidney Int Suppl* **27**, S184–194.

Kopple, J., Bernard, D., Messana, J., *et al.* (1995) Treatment of malnourished CAPD patients with an amino acid based dialysate. *Kidney Int* **47**, 1148–1157.

Kopple, J.D., Cheung, A.K., Christiansen, J. S., *et al.* (2008) OPPORTUNITY: a randomized clinical trial of growth hormone on outcome in hemodialysis patients. *Clin J Am Soc Nephrol* **3**, 1741–1751.

Kopple, J.D., Mercurio, K., Blumenkrantz, M.J., *et al.* (1981) Daily requirement for pyridoxine supplements in chronic renal failure. *Kidney Int* **19**, 694–704.

Kovesdy, C.P. and Kalantar-Zadeh, K. (2009) Why is protein-energy wasting associated with mortality in chronic kidney disease? *Semin Nephrol* **29**, 3–14.

Levey, A., Adler, S., Caggiula, A., *et al.* (1996) Effects of dietary protein restriction on the progression of advanced renal disease in the Modification of Diet in Renal Disease Study. *Am J Kidney Dis* **27**, 652–663.

Levey, A., Atkins, R., Coresh, J., *et al.* (2007) Chronic kidney disease as a global public health problem: approaches and initiatives – a position statement from Kidney Disease Improving Global Outcomes. *Kidney Int* **72**, 247–259.

Locatelli, F., Fouque, D., Heimburger, O., *et al.* (2002) Nutritional status in dialysis patients: a European consensus. *Nephrol Dial Transplant* **17**, 563–572.

Mafra, D., Jolivot, A., Chauveau, P., *et al.* (2010) Are ghrelin and leptin involved in food intake and body mass index in maintenance hemodialysis? *J Ren Nutr* **20**, 151–157.

Mak, R. and Cheung, W. (2006) Energy homeostasis and cachexia in chronic kidney disease. *Pediatr Nephrol* **21**, 1807–1814.

Mitch, W. and Remuzzi, G. (2004) Diets for patients with chronic kidney disease, still worth prescribing. *J Am Soc Nephrol* **15**, 234–237.

Monfared, A., Heidarzadeh, A., Ghaffari, M., *et al.* (2009) Effect of megestrol acetate on serum albumin level in malnourished dialysis patients. *J Ren Nutr* **19**, 167–171.

Monteon, F., Laidlaw, S., Shaib, J., *et al.* (1986) Energy expenditure in patients with chronic renal failure. *Kidney Int* **30**, 741–747.

Naseeb, U., Shafqat, J., Jägerbrink, T., *et al.* (2008) Proteome patterns in uremic plasma. *Blood Purif* **26**, 561–568.

Neyra, N., Hakim, R., Shyr, Y., *et al.* (2000) Serum transferrin and serum prealbumin are early predictors of serum albumin in chronic hemodialysis patients. *J Ren Nutr* **10**, 184–190.

Niemczyk, S., Sikorska, H., Wiecek, A., *et al.* (2010) A super-agonist of growth hormone-releasing hormone causes rapid improvement of nutritional status in patients with chronic kidney disease. *Kidney Int* **77**, 450–458.

Pedrini, M., Levey, A., Lau, J., *et al.* (1996) The effect of dietary protein restriction on the progression of diabetic and nondiabetic renal diseases: a meta-analysis. *Ann Intern Med* **124**, 627–632.

Postorino, M., Marino, C., Tripepi, G., *et al.* (2009) Abdominal obesity and all-cause and cardiovascular mortality in end-stage renal disease. *J Am Coll Cardiol* **53**, 1265–1272.

Prinsen, B.H., De Sain-Van der Velden, M.G., De Koning, E.J., *et al.* (2003) Hypertriglyceridemia in patients with chronic renal failure: possible mechanisms. *Kidney Int Suppl* S121–124.

Pupim, L.B., Flakoll, P.J., Brouillette, J.R., *et al.* (2002) Intradialytic parenteral nutrition improves protein and energy homeostasis in chronic hemodialysis patients. *J Clin Invest* **110**, 483–492.

Qureshi, A.R., Alvestrand, A., Danielsson, A., *et al.* (1998) Factors predicting malnutrition in hemodialysis patients: a cross-sectional study. *Kidney Int* **53**, 773–782.

Rammohan, M., Kalantar-Zadeh, K., Liang, A., *et al.* (2005) Megestrol acetate in a moderate dose for the treatment of malnutrition–inflammation complex in maintenance dialysis patients. *J Ren Nutr* **15**, 345–355.

Rashidi, A., Salehi, M., Piroozmand, A., *et al.* (2009) Effects of zinc supplementation on serum zinc and C-reactive protein concentrations in hemodialysis patients. *J Ren Nutr* **19**, 475–478.

Rossouw, J. (1989) Kwashiorkor in North America. *Am J Clin Nutr* **49**, 588–592.

Rothschild, M., Oratz, M., and Schreiber, S. (1975) Regulation of albumin metabolism. *Annu Rev Med* **26**, 91–104.

Rucker, D., Thadhani, R., and Tonelli, M. (2010) Trace element status in hemodialysis patients. *Semin Dial* **23**, 389–395.

Rutkowski, B. and Król, E. (2008) Epidemiology of chronic kidney disease in central and eastern Europe. *Blood Purif* **26**, 381–385.

Sechi, L.A., Catena, C., Zingaro, L., *et al.* (2002) Abnormalities of glucose metabolism in patients with early renal failure. *Diabetes* **51**, 1226–1232.

Steiber, A., Leon, J., Secker, D., *et al.* (2007) Multicenter study of the validity and reliability of subjective global assessment in the hemodialysis population. *J Ren Nutr* **17**, 336–342.

Stenvinkel, P., Barany, P., Chung, S., *et al.* (2002) A comparative analysis of nutritional parameters as predictors of outcome in male and female ESRD patients. *Nephrol Dial Transplant* **17**, 1266–1274.

Stenvinkel, P., Heimburger, O., Lindholm, B., *et al.* (2000) Are there two types of malnutrition in chronic renal failure? Evidence for relationships between malnutrition, inflammation and atherosclerosis (MIA syndrome). *Nephrol Dial Transplant* **15**, 953–960.

Stevens, L., Coresh, J., Greene, T., *et al.* (2006) Assessing kidney function – measured and estimated glomerular filtration rate. *N Engl J Med* **354**, 2473–2483.

Toigo, G., Aparicio, M., Attman, P., *et al.* (2000) Expert Working Group report on nutrition in adult patients with renal insufficiency (part 1 of 2). *Clin Nutr* **19**, 197–207.

Trowell, H., Davies, J., and Dean, R. (1952) Kwashiorkor. II. Clinical picture, pathology, and differential diagnosis. *Br Med J* **2**, 798–801.

Ward, H. (2009) Nutritional and metabolic issues in solid organ transplantation: targets for future research. *J Ren Nutr* **19**, 111–122.

Whitehead, R. and Alleyne, G. (1972) Pathophysiological factors of importance in protein-calorie malnutrition. *Br Med Bull* **28**, 72–79.

Yang, F., Lee, R., Wang, C., *et al.* (2007) A cohort study of subjective global assessment and mortality in Taiwanese hemodialysis patients. *Ren Fail* **29**, 997–1001.

Yeh, S.S., Marandi, M., Thode, H.C., Jr, *et al.* (2010) Report of a pilot, double-blind, placebo-controlled study of megestrol acetate in elderly dialysis patients with cachexia. *J Ren Nutr* **20**, 52–62.

Young, G.A., Kopple, J.D., Lindholm, B., *et al.* (1991) Nutritional assessment of continuous ambulatory peritoneal dialysis patients: an international study. *Am J Kidney Dis* **17**, 462–471.

Zoccali, C. (2009) The obesity epidemics in ESRD: from wasting to waist? *Nephrol Dial Transplant* **24**, 376–380.

54

LIVER DISEASE

CRAIG J. MCCLAIN, MD, DANIELL B. HILL, MD, FACP, FAGA, AND
LUIS MARSANO, MD

University of Louisville, Louisville, Kentucky, USA

Summary

The liver is the largest and most complex metabolic organ of the body, with critical functions for anabolism, detoxification, and protection from gut-derived toxins; these functions are negatively affected in advanced liver disease. Malnutrition in liver disease is multifactorial, and its assessment is difficult because of the overlap of markers of liver disease with those of malnutrition. However, a subjective global assessment plus selective laboratory tests are usually adequate for identification of malnutrition. Advanced liver disease is strongly associated with malnutrition, and the severity of malnutrition correlates with the development of complications of liver disease, as well as mortality. Intense nutritional support can improve malnutrition in patients with liver disease, and may decrease infectious complications, improve cognitive function, and in some instances even decrease mortality.

Some individual nutrients used in high doses have shown beneficial effects in specific liver diseases, and others are promising. For example, vitamin E improved liver enzymes and histology in non-alcoholic steatohepatitis (NASH). Other therapeutic interventions which are considered "complementary and alternative medicine" may have some value, but need more study.

Obesity with insulin resistance is also a widespread problem and frequently leads to non-alcoholic fatty liver disease (NAFLD) and in some instances to NASH and cirrhosis. Indeed, NASH is now recognized as the major cause of cryptogenic cirrhosis. Excessive intake of some specific nutrients, such as n-6 fatty acids and fructose, has been implicated in the development of NASH. Dietary modifications with weight loss, increased physical activity, and bariatric surgery have all been shown to improve the hepatic steatosis.

In patients in need of liver transplantation, both undernutrition and obesity increase the rate of complications and length of stay after liver transplant. Correction of these problems is an important component of the pre-transplant management.

Introduction

The liver is the largest organ in the body, weighing approximately 1.5 kg in adults, and it is possibly the most complex organ in terms of metabolism. It has a unique dual blood supply, being perfused by both the portal vein and the hepatic artery, and comprises multiple cell types that have different functions. Hepatocytes make up over 80% of total liver mass and play a critical role in the metabolism of amino acids and ammonia, biochemical oxidation

Present Knowledge in Nutrition, Tenth Edition. Edited by John W. Erdman Jr, Ian A. Macdonald and Steven H. Zeisel.
© 2012 International Life Sciences Institute. Published 2012 by John Wiley & Sons, Inc.

reactions, and detoxification of a variety of drugs, vitamins, and hormones. Kupffer cells represent the largest reservoir of fixed macrophages in the body. They play a protective role against gut-derived toxins that have escaped into the portal circulation, and are a major producer of cytokines, which can markedly influence nutritional status. Hepatic stellate cells are the major storehouse for vitamin A in the body, and play an important role in collagen formation during liver injury. Other specific cell types also have unique functions (e.g., bile-duct epithelium in bile flow sinusoidal endothelial cells in adhesion molecule expression and endocytosis). The liver plays a vital role in protein, carbohydrate, and fat metabolism as well as in micronutrient metabolism. It synthesizes plasma proteins, non-essential amino acids, urea (for ammonia excretion), glycogen, and critical hormones such as the anabolic molecule, insulin-like growth factor-1. The liver is a major site for fatty acid metabolism, and bile from the liver is needed for fat absorption from the intestine. Thus, it seems obvious that the liver is important for proper nutrition.

A strong association exists between advanced liver disease and malnutrition. However, malnutrition is not always recognized in patients with liver disease, at least in part because weight loss in these patients can be masked by fluid retention. The loss of glycogen stores predisposes patients with advanced liver disease to enter a starvation state within a few hours of fasting that can lead to further protein catabolism and loss of function. Therefore, it is important to recognize malnutrition and initiate nutrition support early in these patients. Moreover, obesity and the metabolic syndrome are increasingly recognized as a major cause of abnormal liver enzymes and a spectrum of non-alcoholic fatty liver disease (NAFLD). Thus, both under-nutrition and obesity play important roles in liver disease.

This chapter begins with a discussion of the prevalence of malnutrition and nutritional assessment in patients with liver disease. Causes of malnutrition and cytokine-nutrient interactions are then discussed, followed by a review of nutritional support, including obesity, in liver disease, as well as nutrition and liver transplantation.

Assessment and Prevalence of Malnutrition

Malnutrition is widely present in liver disease, especially in more severe, chronic forms. When evaluating information concerning the prevalence of malnutrition in cirrhosis, it is important to use tests that accurately define nutritional status. Unfortunately, assessment of nutritional status in patients with liver disease is often quite difficult. Tests that are most frequently used include serum visceral protein concentrations, some assessment of immunity (total lymphocyte count or delayed hypersensitivity), anthropometry, percentage of ideal body weight, creatinine-height index, dietary history, subjective global assessment, and – in more sophisticated clinical settings – bioelectric impedance and body composition determinations. Unfortunately, almost all of these tests can be influenced either by underlying liver disease or by factors that may be causing the liver disease, such as chronic alcohol consumption or viral infection. Visceral protein concentrations are probably the tests most frequently used by nutritionists in evaluating nutritional status, especially protein malnutrition. The visceral proteins such as albumin, pre-albumin, and retinol-binding protein are all produced in the liver and correlate better with severity of underlying liver disease than with malnutrition (Merli et al., 1987). Alcohol and viral infection can influence immune function, and edema and ascites can influence anthropometry and bioelectric impedance (O'Keefe et al., 1980; Shronts et al., 1987; Shronts, 1988; Guglielmi et al., 1991; McCullough et al., 1991). Impaired renal function frequently occurs in more severe liver disease and influences indicators such as creatinine-height index (Pirlich et al., 1996). Thus, no ideal single indicator of malnutrition in liver disease exists and, often, subjective global assessment in conjunction with a combination of tests most appropriate for the particular patient will provide the best possible evaluation (Baker et al., 1982; Campillo, 2010). As an example, malnutrition is obvious by subjective global assessment in the alcoholic cirrhotic in Figure 54.1A, and malnutrition has markedly improved with two years of abstinence and appropriate nutrition in Figure 54.1B.

Probably the most extensive studies of nutritional status in patients with liver disease are in patients with alcoholic liver disease (ALD), and we will focus on abnormalities of ALD that can be extrapolated to other forms of liver disease. The best recent studies are two large studies in the Veterans Health Administration (VA) Cooperative Studies Program dealing with patients with alcoholic hepatitis (Mendenhall et al., 1984, 1986, 1993, 1995a,b). The first of these studies (#119) demonstrated that virtually every patient with alcoholic hepatitis had some degree of malnutrition (Mendenhall et al., 1984). Patients (284 with complete nutritional assessments) were divided into groups with mild, moderate, or severe alcoholic hepatitis based on

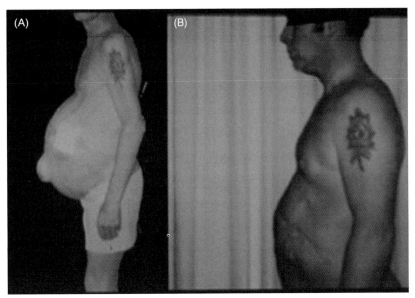

FIG. 54.1 Patient with alcoholic cirrhosis with severe PEM as determined by subjective global assessment with ascites and muscle wasting (A). This was corrected with abstinence (B).

TABLE 54.1 Nutritional status in alcoholic hepatitis

Initial laboratory test	Severity of liver disease		
	Mild	Moderate	Severe
Lymphocytes (1000–4000/ mm³)	2067 ± 14837	1598 ± 90	1366 ± 83
Albumin (35–51 g/L)	37 ± 1	27 ± 1	23 ± 1
Creatinine-height index (% of standard)	75.7 ± 2.84	62.9 ± 3.3	64.0 ± 4.65

Reproduced with permission from Elsevier (Mendenhall *et al.*, 1984). Copyright originally held by Excerpta Medica, Inc.

clinical and biochemical parameters. Patients had a mean alcohol consumption of 228 g/day (with almost 50% of energy intake coming from alcohol). The severity of liver disease was generally correlated with the severity of malnutrition (Table 54.1). Similar data were generated in a follow-up VA study on alcoholic hepatitis (#275) (Mendenhall *et al.*, 1993).

In both of these studies, patients were given a balanced 2500-kcal (10.5-MJ) hospital diet, monitored carefully by a dietitian, and encouraged to consume the diet. In the second study, patients in the therapy arm of the protocol also received an enteral nutritional support product high in branched-chain amino acids (BCAA), as well as the anabolic steroid oxandrolone (80 mg/day). In neither of these studies were patients fed by tube if voluntary oral intake was inadequate (probably a study design flaw in retrospect). Voluntary oral food intake correlated in a step-wise fashion with 6-month mortality data. Thus, patients who voluntarily consumed over 3000 kcal/day (12.6 MJ/ day) had virtually no mortality, whereas those consuming under 1000 kcal/day (4.2 MJ/day) had more than an 80% 6-month mortality (Figure 54.2) (Mendenhall *et al.*, 1995b).

Moreover, the degree of malnutrition correlated with the development of serious complications such as encephalopathy, ascites, and hepatorenal syndrome (Mendenhall *et al.*, 1995b). In the VA Cooperative Studies, the chronic alcohol-consuming control population without liver disease also frequently had some degree of protein-energy malnutrition. This is in contrast to many other studies in which only alcoholics with liver disease demonstrated significant protein-energy malnutrition (Antonow and McClain, 1985).

Because both of these VA studies evaluated patients with acute inflammatory response (hepatitis), it was important

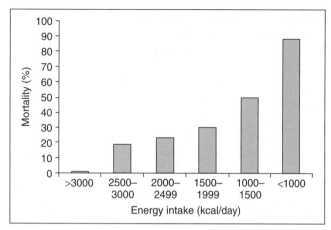

FIG. 54.2 A direct relationship was noted between voluntary caloric intake in Veterans Health Administration studies in patients with moderate and severe alcoholic hepatitis. It is not known whether providing enteral feeding to patients with inadequate caloric intake would have improved mortality. Reproduced with permission from Elsevier: Lolli *et al.* (1992). Copyright originally held by Editrice Gastroentrologica Italiana S.r.L.

to determine nutritional status in patients with stable ALD without alcoholic hepatitis. We evaluated patients with stable cirrhosis followed in an ascites clinic who were not actively drinking, were free of alcoholic hepatitis, and had bilirubin levels under 51 mmolL (3 mg/dL). They had indicators of malnutrition almost as severe as patients with alcoholic hepatitis (e.g. a creatinine-height index of 71%) (Antonow and McClain, 1985).

It could be argued that alcohol, rather than the underlying liver pathology, is the critical variable in malnutrition in liver disease. There have been several major studies evaluating patients having both alcoholic liver disease and non-alcoholic- (especially viral-) induced liver disease (DiCecco *et al.*, 1989; Lolli *et al.*, 1992; Thuluvath and Triger, 1994; Caregaro *et al.*, 1996; Sarin *et al.*, 1997).

Although the prevalence of malnutrition in liver disease varied somewhat in the different studies, there is a compelling, consistent observation that no difference in malnutrition occurred between alcohol- and non-alcohol-related causes of cirrhosis in the individual studies. In one of the most carefully designed studies, Sarin *et al.* (1997) demonstrated that protein-energy malnutrition was equally severe in alcoholic and non-alcoholic liver disease, and that dietary intake decreased equally in both diseases. Caregaro

et al. (1996) from Italy found that the prevalence, characteristics, and severity of protein-energy malnutrition were comparable in alcoholic and viral-induced cirrhosis. Malnutrition was correlated with the severity of the liver disease. Thus, multiple studies now document that the degree of liver injury, rather than the etiology, is critical in the development of nutritional disorders.

Causes of Malnutrition in Liver Disease

Multiple factors combine to cause malnutrition in patients with liver disease (Box 54.1). Poor nutritional intake can result from gastrointestinal disturbances, prolonged periods eating nothing during hospitalizations for complications of cirrhosis, and iatrogenic causes. Maldigestion and malabsorption can occur in liver disease and play an important role in causing malnutrition. Typical gastrointestinal disturbances in liver disease include dysgeusia, anorexia, nausea, and early satiety (Madden *et al.*, 1997). Although the exact pathophysiology of how liver dysfunction causes these manifestations is still debated, local and systemic neurohormonal mechanisms are likely involved in causing delayed gastric emptying, small-bowel dysmotility and bacterial overgrowth, and constipation (Thuluvath and Triger, 1989; Galati *et al.*, 1994, 1997; Isobe *et al.*, 1994; Quigley, 1996). Liver transplantation improves or reverses many of these gastrointestinal manifestations (Madrid *et al.*, 1997). Concomitant complications typical of liver disease, such as upper gastrointestinal bleeding, portal systemic encephalopathy, and sepsis, also cause prolonged periods of poor oral intake. Dietary management of fluid retention with salt and water restriction, dietary management of encephalopathy with protein

---

BOX 54.1   Major causes of malnutrition

Anorexia
Diarrhea and malabsorption
Nausea and vomiting
Poor food availability and quality
Metabolic disturbances (e.g. hypermetabolism and catabolism)
Cytokines
Liver complications (portal systemic encephalopathy, ascites, gastrointestinal bleed)
Unpalatable diets (low sodium, protein)
No feeding (nothing by mouth) for procedures

restriction, and carbohydrate and lipid restrictions used in patients with diabetes mellitus, chronic pancreatic insufficiency, and cholestatic liver disease can all affect diet palatability and can severely restrict patients' food choices.

Impaired lipid metabolism is also multifactorial in liver disease. Decreased intraluminal bile salts, small-bowel bacterial overgrowth, coexistent pancreatic insufficiency or intestinal disease (e.g., inflammatory bowel disease, sprue), and mucosal vascular hypertension and edema can worsen maldigestion and malabsorption. Cholestatic liver disorders are associated with decreased intraluminal concentration of bile salts, resulting in lipid and lipid-soluble-vitamin malabsorption (Vlahcevic et al., 1971). Impaired intestinal capacity for absorption of long-chain fatty acids, interference with lipid absorption by neomycin, binding of bile salts by cholestyramine, and exocrine pancreatic insufficiency may also contribute to lipid malabsorption (Thompson et al., 1971; Malagelada et al., 1974; Cabre et al., 1990). As a result, patients with liver disease may have decreased plasma levels of essential fatty acids and their polyunsaturated derivatives (McClain et al., 1999).

Low-grade endotoxemia facilitated by portal hypertension and gut bacterial translocation leads to a low-grade increase in proinflammatory cytokines that further affects nutrient management and overall metabolism (McClain et al., 1999) (Figure 54.3). Glycogen storage is impaired in cirrhotic livers partly because of hyperglucagonemia. This results in peripheral muscle proteolysis to provide amino acids for gluconeogenesis, thus contributing to protein malnutrition. Liver disease patients with portal hypertension and ascites are at increased risk of developing

a hypermetabolic state (resting energy expenditure >110% of its expected value), which contributes to overall malnutrition (John et al., 1989; Dols et al., 1991; Muller et al., 1992; Ksiazyk et al., 1996).

Healthcare providers must exert great care to improve nutritional status rather than inadvertently compounding the problem (e.g., long periods of fasting for procedures, unpalatable low-sodium diets). This concern is highlighted by the fact that 67% of patients in a VA Cooperative Study on alcoholic hepatitis did not consume the recommended 2500 kcal/day (10.5 MJ/day), even though these patients received expert care by nutritionists and hepatologists who knew that nutrition was a major outcome variable of the study (Mendenhall et al., 1995).

Cytokine–Nutrient Interactions

Dysregulated cytokine metabolism [with elevated proinflammatory cytokines such as tumor necrosis factor (TNF) and interleukin 8 (IL-8)] is well documented in many forms of liver disease; ALD has been studied in the greatest detail (McClain et al., 1999, 2004) (Figure 54.2). The cytokine interferon-a is used to treat both hepatitis B and C. Increased levels of cytokines have been postulated to cause many of the metabolic and nutritional abnormalities observed in liver disease, especially in more decompensated liver disease (McClain et al., 1999, 2004). Thus, abnormalities such as fever, anorexia, muscle breakdown and wasting, and altered mineral metabolism are likely to be at least partially cytokine mediated (Box 54.2). We will briefly review alterations in mineral metabolism, visceral proteins, hypermetabolism, and anorexia in relation to cytokines and liver disease.

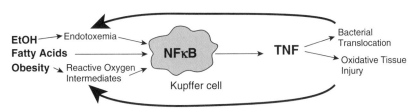

FIG. 54.3 Endotoxemia and oxidative stress occur in virtually all forms of liver disease, especially in alcoholic liver disease. Both endotoxin and reactive intermediates activate the critical redox-sensitive transcription factor NFκB in hepatic Kupffer cells, with subsequent cytokine production. Recent studies also show that certain free fatty acids can activate Toll receptors, with subsequent NFκB activation and inflammation. This activation will lead to further bacterial translocation with endotoxemia and further oxidative tissue injury. Antioxidants may have a role in blocking this cycle of tissue destruction.

BOX 54.2 Biological activities of cytokines

Cytokine effects	Metabolic complications of alcoholic hepatitis
Fever	Fever
Anorexia	Anorexia
Neutrophilia	Neutrophilia
Altered amino acids, decreased glutathione, catabolism with muscle wasting	Altered amino acids, decreased glutathione, catabolism with muscle wasting
Hypermetabolism	Hypermetabolism
Decreased serum zinc	Decreased serum zinc
Increased acute-phase reactants	Increased acute-phase reactants
Decreased bile flow	Cholestasis
Decreased albumin	Decreased albumin
Bone loss	Bone loss
Collagen deposition	Collagen deposition
Increased triacylglycerols	Triacyglycerols (Zieve's syndrome)
Increased endothelial permeability	Ascites and peripheral edema
Slow-wave sleep	Encephalopathy

Mineral Metabolism

Cytokines such as TNF and IL-1 generally cause a decrease in the serum zinc concentration and an internal redistribution of zinc, with zinc being sequestered in the liver and being lost from other tissues such as bone marrow and thymus (Gaetke *et al.*, 1997). This internal redistribution of zinc is thought to facilitate priority protein synthesis in the liver, and it also makes the plasma a less favorable environment for bacterial growth (zinc withholding) (Gaetke *et al.*, 1997). This zinc stress response can also be associated with loss of zinc from critical zinc finger proteins and loss of functional activity. We have shown that this plays a role in the increased gut permeability, endotoxemia, and fatty liver in ALD (Kang *et al.*, 2009; Zhong *et al.*, 2010a). There is frequently an increase in urinary zinc loss that can contribute to overall zinc deficits in patients with increased cytokine activity. Patients with liver disease regularly have decreased serum zinc concentrations and increased urinary zinc losses (McClain *et al.*, 1992). This zinc deficiency may play a role in the anorexia, sexual dysfunction, and immune impairment in liver disease. Although the serum and zinc concentrations are decreased with increased cytokine levels, the serum copper level generally increases, as does the binding protein for copper (ceruloplasmin) (McClain *et al.*, 1991). Increased copper can enhance hepatic oxidative stress and worsen liver injury.

Visceral Proteins

With increased cytokines, there is generally a depression in plasma proteins that are used as indicators of nutritional status, including albumin, transferrin, pre-albumin, and retinol-binding protein. This reduction in protein occurs initially because cytokines generally cause an increase in endothelial permeability, which then causes a decrease in these visceral proteins (Hennig *et al.*, 1988). Cytokines also generally decrease production (mRNA) of these visceral proteins, which partially accounts for long-term depression of the proteins (Boosalis *et al.*, 1989*)*. At the same time that these visceral proteins decrease, hepatic acute-phase proteins increase. Certain of these acute-phase reactants play a role in attenuating the ongoing toxic effects of cytokines (e.g. alpha-1 acid glycoprotein attenuates the toxic effects of TNF; Libert *et al.*, 1994).

Hypermetabolism and Hypercatabolism

Increased cytokine production can induce a hypermetabolic or hypercatabolic state. For example, TNF infusion into experimental animals causes a decrease in protein synthesis with an overall increase in net protein breakdown (Sakurai *et al.*, 1994). This may relate to the hypermetabolism and wasting seen in liver disease (John *et al.*, 1989).

Anorexia and Decreased Gastric Emptying

Cytokines frequently induce anorexia; indeed, TNF was initially termed cachectin (McClain *et al.*, 2004). Interferon is used as a therapeutic agent in certain forms of viral hepatitis, and it has anorexia and flu-like symptoms as major side-effects which generally improve as therapy progresses. Several cytokines such as IL-1 and TNF also impair gastric emptying, which occurs as a complication of liver disease (Suto *et al.*, 1994). Some patients will respond to prokinetic agents such as metoclopramide.

Nutrition Support

Interest in nutritional therapy in cirrhosis started when Patek *et al.* (1948) demonstrated that a nutritious diet improved the 5-year outcome of patients with cirrhosis compared with control subjects consuming an inadequate diet. These low-income patients had alcoholic cirrhosis. Several recent studies further support the concept of improved outcome with nutritional support in patients with cirrhosis. Hirsch *et al.* (1993) demonstrated that outpatients supplementing their diet with an enteral nutritional support product [1000 kcal (4.2 MJ), 34 g protein] had significantly improved protein intake and significantly fewer hospitalizations. These same investigators subsequently gave an enteral supplement to outpatients with alcoholic cirrhosis, and observed an improvement in nutritional status and immune function (Hirsch *et al.*, 1999*)*. In the VA Cooperative Study on nutritional support in ALD using both an anabolic steroid and an enteral nutritional supplement, improved mortality was seen with the combination of oxandrolone plus nutrition supplementation in patients who had moderate protein-energy malnutrition (Mendenhall *et al.*, 1995b). Those with severe malnutrition did not significantly benefit from therapy, possibly because their malnutrition was so advanced that no intervention, including nutrition, could help. Studies by Kearns *et al.* (1992) showed that patients with alcoholic liver disease hospitalized for treatment and given an enteral nutritional supplement via feeding tube had significantly improved serum bilirubin levels and liver function as assessed by antipyrine clearance. A multicenter randomized study of enteral nutrition versus steroids in patients with alcoholic hepatitis showed similar overall short-term results (Cabre *et al.*, 2000). Moreover, those receiving enteral nutrition (rich in BCAAs) had a better long-term outcome with fewer infectious deaths. Thus, traditional nutritional supplementation clearly improves nutritional status and, in some instances, hepatic function and other indicators of outcome in cirrhosis.

A defined approach is necessary to achieve appropriate nutritional support in patients with liver disease (Marsano and McClain, 1991, 1992; McCullough, 2000; Campillo *et al.*, 2003; Stickel *et al.*, 2003) (Box 54.3). For the patient who has been actively drinking alcohol, it is useful first to correct electrolyte imbalances and to treat and control withdrawal symptoms when present. (This will facilitate control of electrolyte disorders and decrease the risk of having a feeding tube or parenteral nutrition line pulled out.) An important component of the dietary management of the patient with advanced liver disease is to minimize periods without food intake because these patients rapidly enter into "starvation mode" with decreased glucose oxidation and increased protein and fat catabolism (Owen

---

BOX 54.3   Nutritional recommendations for patients with liver disease

Early nutrition assessment and regular follow-ups
Total energy: 1.2–1.4 × resting energy expenditure
Protein: 1.0–1.5 g/kg/day
Fat: 30–40% of non-protein energy
Formulate water and electrolyte intake to individual needs, renal function, diuretic sensitivity
Replace vitamins and minerals (avoid excessive iron and copper intake)
Complement daily requirements with enteral feedings (parenteral if enteral route otherwise contraindicated)

---

et al., 1983). To prevent this starvation, the diet should optimally be divided into three meals (the first early in the morning), three snacks, plus one bedtime supplement. The early breakfast improves cognitive function in patients with subclinical (minimal) hepatic encephalopathy (Vaisma *et al.*, 2010), and the bedtime supplement improves body protein stores. Importantly, an improvement in muscle mass with night-time supplements was demonstrated by Plank *et al.* (2008) who randomized 103 cirrhotic patients to receive two cans of Ensure Plus™ (710 kcal with 26 g of protein) or two cans of Diabetic Resource™ (500 kcal with 30 g of protein), either during the day or at bedtime, for a total of 12 months. Only the patients who received the supplements at bedtime gained lean muscle mass (2 kg) over 12 months (Plank *et al.*, 2008). This points out the great importance of late-night snacking in maintaining muscle mass. Unfortunately, there is a long tradition of protein restriction for patients with advanced liver disease who also have hepatic encephalopathy (HE). This tradition has no solid scientific basis, and recent studies do not support this approach. Cordoba *et al.* (2004), in a prospective randomized study, treated 30 cirrhotic patients who suffered episodic overt hepatic encephalopathy with either a low-protein enteral formula [with increased protein every 3 days (0 g, then 12 g, 24 g, and 48 g)] or a normal protein formula (1.2 g/kg/day) from the first day. Both formulas provided 30 kcal/kg/day. The outcome of hepatic encephalopathy was similar with both formulas (Cordoba *et al.*, 2004). In a second study, Gheorghe *et al.* (2005) treated 153 consecutive cirrhotic patients with overt HE with a diet providing 30 kcal/kg/day with 1.2 g protein/kg/day, divided into five "meals" from 8:00 a.m. to 10:00 p.m. Most patients improved their HE, with the best results seen in the more severe HE patients (Gheorghe *et al.*, 2005). The HE should be treated with lactulose and with rifaximin, if needed. If the HE persists despite maximal medical therapy and evaluation for other causes of changes in mentation, then protein intake can be decreased to the maximal tolerated, and a BCAA-enriched formula supplement can be administered to complete the nitrogen needs (see below).

BCAA-enriched diets were developed in an attempt to correct the abnormal ratios of BCAAs to aromatic amino acids observed in liver disease (<2.5 vs. 3.5–4 in normal subjects), with even greater disturbances in hepatic coma (0.8–1.2). Theoretical advantages of BCAA-enriched formulas include increased protein synthesis and decreased protein breakdown as a result of high leucine; use of BCAAs as an energy source for brain, muscle, and heart; better regulation of amino acid efflux from muscle during catabolism and hypoinsulinemia; improved ammonia metabolism by skeletal muscle; increased norepinephrine synthesis in brain; and decreased penetration of aromatic amino acids into the brain (BCAAs compete for the blood–brain amino acid transport system).

Because of the high cost of BCAA-enriched formulas and their limited role in hepatic encephalopathy, these formulas unfortunately are not generally considered cost effective in the United States. The major exception may be for the few patients who have chronic stable porto-systemic encephalopathy (PSE) who require multiple admissions to the hospital. In these patients, the enteral formula cost is more than offset by the savings of fewer hospitalizations. A large randomized trial of BCAA in advanced cirrhosis from Italy reported that BCAA supplementation attenuated progression of liver disease and improved markers of nutrition (Marchesini *et al.*, 2003). However, compliance was poor and use of this product remains limited in the United States, as noted above (Charlton, 2003; Marchesini *et al.*, 2003).

If the patient cannot take in adequate kilocalories and has a functioning gastrointestinal tract, then a feeding tube should be used and a standard enteral formula should be given following the guidelines already mentioned above. Enteral nutrition is desired over parenteral nutrition because of cost, risk of sepsis of the parenteral nutrition line, preservation of the integrity of the gut mucosa, and prevention of bacterial translocation and multiple organ failure. Moreover, total parenteral nutrition can, in some instances, cause liver disease as one of its complications. If enteral nutrition is not possible, then total parenteral nutrition (TPN) can be used with the knowledge that it is important to return to the enteral route as soon as the small bowel shows evidence of recovered function. Total parenteral nutrition (TPN) can be started with a standard amino acid formula in amounts that are increased until nitrogen needs are met. If the patients develop PSE, then standard therapy with lactulose, neomycin, or rifaximin must be given. If the patient is still unable to tolerate the amount of amino acids needed to satisfy nitrogen requirements, then the standard amino acids can be replaced by a BCAA-enriched solution specifically designed for liver disease (Charlton, 2003; Marchesini *et al.*, 2003). It is unusual to require either TPN or BCAA formulas, and the primary goal is always aggressive enteral support.

Individual Nutrients and Complementary and Alternative Medicine

A recent major thrust in therapy for liver disease has been supplementation with individual nutrients, or the use of complementary and alternative medicine (CAM) (Haas *et al.*, 2000; McClain *et al.*, 2003; Hanje *et al.*, 2006). A detailed discussion of CAM is necessary because it is estimated that >40% of the US population uses CAM, and patients with chronic disease processes such as cirrhosis are frequent users of CAM. Moreover, CAM use is frequently not reported to traditional physicians (McClain *et al.*, 2003). A variety of forms of CAM have been used effectively to treat or prevent liver injury in animal models, and preliminary data with some agents suggest efficacy in human liver disease. It is the responsibility of health-care workers to be aware of the potential benefits and toxicities of these agents and to demand well-designed randomized human trials on such products.

The specific CAM agents that will be reviewed in relation to liver disease include vitamin E, glutathione (GSH) pro-drugs and antioxidant cocktails, S-adenosylmethionine (SAM) and betaine, silymarin (milk thistle), and herbals.

Vitamin E

Vitamin E is a potent antioxidant that is widely used as a nutritional supplement. In patients with alcoholic liver disease and in experimental models of liver disease, depressed serum and hepatic levels of vitamin E have been documented. Vitamin E has been used extensively to protect against experimental models of liver injury, such as that induced by carbon tetrachloride. Zern's laboratory (Liu *et al.*, 1995) demonstrated that vitamin E inhibited hepatic activation of the oxidative-stress-sensitive transcription factor NFκB in the carbon tetrachloride model, and postulated that inhibition of this critical transcription factor for proinflammatory cytokine production (e.g., TNF) resulted in attenuation of liver injury. Hill *et al.* (1999) treated human peripheral blood monocytes and rat Kupffer cells in vitro with vitamin E, inhibiting both NFκB activation and TNF production. Vitamin E also inhibits activation of hepatic stellate cells and collagen production in vitro (Lee *et al.*, 1995).

Vitamin E was initially reported to have beneficial effects in some but not all studies of patients with fatty liver (non-alcoholic steatohepatitis, NASH) (Lavine, 2000; Hasegawa *et al.*, 2001; Sanyal *et al.*, 2010). A pilot study in children (Lavine, 2000) showed improvement in liver enzymes, and a study from Japan (Hasegawa *et al.*, 2001) showed that vitamin E not only improved liver enzymes but also decreased serum levels of the profibrotic cytokine, transforming growth factor beta. A study in alcoholic hepatitis patients showed improvement in hyaluronic acid (a marker of fibrosis) but no improvement in mortality (Mezey *et al.*, 2004). The most important and compelling vitamin E data are from a large multicenter NIH-funded trial which assigned 247 adults with NASH (without diabetes) to receive pioglitazone at a dose of 30 mg daily (80 subjects), vitamin E at a dose of 800 IU daily (84 subjects), or placebo (83 subjects) for 96 weeks (Sanyal *et al.*, 2010). Vitamin E therapy, as compared with placebo, was associated with a significantly higher rate of improvement in NASH (43% vs. 19%, $p = 0.001$). Serum alanine and aspartate aminotransferase levels were reduced with vitamin E and with pioglitazone, as compared with placebo ($p < 0.001$ for both comparisons). No treatment caused an improvement in fibrosis. Subjects who received pioglitazone gained more weight than did those who received vitamin E or placebo. In conclusion, vitamin E improved liver histology and liver enzymes and was not associated with the weight gain seen with pioglitazone, and 800 IU of vitamin E is probably the preferred "drug" therapy for NASH.

Glutathione Pro-Drugs and Combined Antioxidants

GSH is a tripeptide synthesized from glutamate, cysteine, and glycine. Glutathione, in its reduced form, is the main non-protein thiol in cells, and has an important role in detoxification of electrophiles and in protection against reactive oxygen toxicity. This includes protection against intracellular free radicals, reactive oxygen intermediates, and several endogenous and exogenous toxins (Lauterburg and Velez, 1988). GSH also protects against toxicity from certain drugs (e.g., acetaminophen). GSH cannot be taken up by hepatocytes, but a number of pharmacologic agents have been devised to enhance intracellular pools (e.g. N-acetylcysteine, 2-oxothiazolidine-4-carboxylic acid). There are two distinct intercellular GSH pools: cytosolic (approximately 80%) and mitochondrial (approximately 20%). Mitochondrial GSH detoxifies hydrogen peroxide and other organic peroxides produced in mitochondria. Chronic alcohol consumption has been reported to deplete GSH levels (Lauterburg and Velez, 1988). Moreover, alcohol causes a marked depletion of GSH in the mitochondrial pool, with at least part of that depletion attributed to its impaired transport from the cytosolic pool (Fernandez-Checa *et al.*, 1993). This depletion renders hepatocytes more vulnerable to oxidative stress. The molecular basis for the impaired GSH transport into mitochondria is unclear, but it has been reported that exogenous SAM – but not N-acetylcysteine or other pro-GSH molecules – restores mitochondrial functions, enhances mitochondrial transport, and corrects mitochondrial GSH deficiency.

GSH precursors also can regulate production of proinflammatory cytokines, such as TNF and IL-8, by Kupffer cells and monocytes, with increased GSH levels decreasing cytokine production (Pena *et al.*, 1999). This occurs at least in part, through inhibition of the oxidative-stress-sensitive transcription factor NFκB, which plays a central role in lipopolysaccharide (LPS)-stimulated TNF production.

The glutathione precursor N-acetylcysteine (NAC) has been used clinically for decades to treat acute acetaminophen overdose with good results if administered early (optimally within 12 hours of acetaminophen ingestion). A recent study evaluated the effects of intravenous NAC on transplant-free survival in patients with non-acetaminophen acute liver failure (Lee *et al.*, 2009). In the study, 173 patients received either NAC or placebo. In patients with early-stage non-acetaminophen-related acute liver failure, NAC improved transplant-free survival. This important study supports the use of intravenous NAC in patients with acute liver failure. Unfortunately, combined trials of antioxidants that not only increase glutathione but also provide other antioxidant effects have not shown efficacy in patients with chronic alcoholic liver disease (Phillips *et al.*, 2006). Thus, there is great scientific rationale for an antioxidant approach, but defining appropriate clinical populations, appropriate doses, and therapeutic intervals appear to be major challenges.

S-Adenosylmethionine (SAM)/Betaine

Elevated methionine and decreased methionine clearance represent a possible therapeutic target for liver disease, especially ALD. In animal models of liver injury, decreased levels of SAM and elevated levels of S-adenosylhomocysteine are regularly observed (Figure 54.4).

In human studies of alcoholic hepatitis and cirrhosis, abnormal hepatic gene expression in methionine and glutathione metabolism occurs and often contributes to decreased hepatic SAM, cysteine, and glutathione levels (Lee *et al.*, 2004). Rodent and primate studies demonstrate that SAM depletion occurred in the early stages of fatty liver infiltration in ALD, and decreased SAM concentration, liver injury and mitochondrial damage can be reversed with SAM supplementation (Lieber, 2002). S-Adenosylmethionine appears to attenuate oxidative stress and hepatic stellate cell activation in an ethanol–lipopolysaccharide-induced fibrotic rat model (Karaa

et al., 2008). Most importantly, a randomized double-blind trial was performed in 123 patients with alcoholic cirrhosis treated using SAM (1200 mg/day, orally) or placebo for two years (Mato *et al.*, 1999). When Child's C cirrhotics were excluded from the analysis, the overall mortality/liver transplantation rate was significantly greater in the placebo group than in the SAM group (20% vs. 12%), and differences between the 2-year survival curves of the two groups (defined as the time to death or liver transplantation) were also statistically significant. A subsequent Cochrane review of SAM and ALD could not find evidence supporting or refuting the use of SAM for patients with ALD (Rambaldi and Gluud, 2006) and the need for long-term, high-quality, randomized trials is clear.

Betaine (trimethylglycine) is a key nutrient in humans and is obtained from a variety of foods and nutritional supplements (Purohit *et al.*, 2007). In the liver, betaine can transfer one methyl group to homocysteine to form methionine. This process removes toxic metabolites (homocysteine and S-adenosylhomocysteine), restores SAM levels, reverses steatosis, prevents apoptosis, and reduces both damaged protein accumulation and oxidative stress (Purohit *et al.*, 2007; Kharbanda, 2009). Betaine also appears to attenuate alcoholic steatosis by restoring phosphatidylcholine generation via the phosphatidyleth-

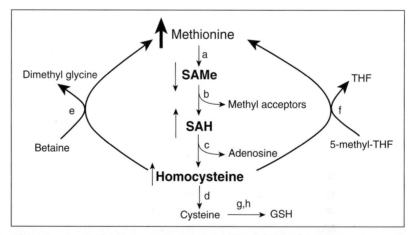

FIG. 54.4 Altered methionine metabolism pathway in ALD. (a) Methionine adenosyltransferase (MAT); (b) enzymes involved in transmethylation reactions, including phosphatidylethanolamine N-methyltransferase (PEMT); (c) S-adenosylhomocysteine (SAH) hydrolase; (d) cystathionine-β-synthase (CBS); (e) betaine homocysteine methyltransferase (BHMT); (f) methionine synthase (MS); (g) glutaminate-cysteine synthetase. ↑ ↓, effects of alcohol.

anolamine methytransferase pathway (Kharbanda *et al.*, 2007). Unfortunately, the most definitive human trial thus far (in NASH patients) showed limited benefit (Abdelmalek *et al.*, 2009).

Zinc

Zinc is an essential trace element that participates in cellular function through hundreds of zinc proteins, including zinc metalloenzymes and critical zinc transcription factors (McClain *et al.*, 1986, 1992). Altered zinc metabolism with zinc deficiency and decreased serum zinc is noted in most forms of clinical liver disease, especially ALD. Stress/inflammation caused by a variety of factors, including LPS/TNF, also causes an internal redistribution of zinc, with loss of zinc from some tissues (deficiency) and redirection to other tissues or organs such as the liver (redistribution). Importantly, zinc deficiency was recently shown to be induced by oxidative stress in which thiol oxidation of zinc-finger transcription factors causes zinc loss, leading to loss of DNA-binding activity (Zhou *et al.*, 2007; Kang *et al.*, 2009; Zhong *et al.*, 2010).

Recent studies from Kang *et al.* (2009) provide major new insights into the molecular mechanisms of altered zinc metabolism in the development and progression of experimental ALD, with important potential therapeutic implications for ALD and other forms of chronic liver disease. In both acute and chronic alcohol-induced hepatotoxicity, alcohol intake and oxidative stress disrupt tight junctions in the intestine, which leads to translocation of bacterial products such as endotoxin (Joshi *et al.*, 2009; Zhong *et al.*, 2010). Endotoxin activates TLR-4 and TNF production, with subsequent oxidative stress and liver injury. Endotoxin and TNF also play a critical role in liver fibrosis. Disruption of tight-junction proteins occurs not only in the intestine but also in the lung and likely at the blood–brain barrier, thus potentially predisposing to lung injury and hepatic encephalopathy (Joshi *et al.*, 2009). Zinc treatment in experimental animals with ALD attenuated the increased gut permeability, endotoxemia, TNF production, oxidative stress, and liver injury, while improving activity of key zinc transcription factors (Kang and Zhou, 2005; Joshi *et al.*, 2009; Kang *et al.*, 2009; Zhong *et al.*, 2010). Thus, zinc supplementation targets most postulated mechanisms for the development of ALD and certain other forms of chronic liver disease such as NAFLD.

A recent human pilot trial also suggests that zinc may stabilize or cause regression of hepatic fibrosis (Takahashi *et al.*, 2007). Polaprezinc, a synthetic zinc-containing compound with 34 mg of elemental zinc, was administered daily for 24 weeks to patients with chronic hepatitis or cirrhosis, and zinc-supplemented patients significantly improved their serum zinc levels and markers of fibrosis.

Silymarin

Silymarin, the active ingredient extracted from *Silybum marianum* (also known as milk thistle), was shown in experimental animals to protect against multiple types of liver injury, including that induced by carbon tetrachloride, acetaminophen, and iron overload and, very importantly, mushroom poisoning (Luper, 1998). Silymarin is probably the most widely used form of CAM in the treatment of liver disease. Clinically, it has been suggested to have hepatoprotective effects in various forms of toxic hepatitis, fatty liver, cirrhosis, ischemic injury, and viral-induced liver disease (Luper, 1998). It has antioxidant activities, protects against lipid peroxidation, and has anti-inflammatory and antifibrotic effects. Large controlled trials of silymarin performed in Europe have had variable results (Ferenci *et al.*, 1989; Pares *et al.*, 1998). Silymarin may be one of the most popular forms of CAM therapy for liver disease because it has a good safety profile, it has been extensively investigated in multiple forms of experimental liver injury in animals, and some positive results have been reported in humans.

Herbals

Herbals are widely used for a variety of chronic inflammatory processes such as rheumatoid arthritis, and the use of herbal products for liver disease has been extensively reviewed (Schuppan *et al.*, 1999; Haas *et al.*, 2000; McClain *et al.*, 2003; Hanje *et al.*, 2006). Green tea, green tea polyphenols, and grape-seed polyphenols were reported to have anti-inflammatory properties and to protect against certain forms of experimental liver injury (Yang *et al.*, 1998). Glycyrrhizin is an aqueous extract of the licorice root. It has antioxidant effects, inhibits collagen deposition in animal models of hepatic fibrosis, and decreases procollagen mRNA in hepatic stellate cells in vitro. However, it has aldosterone-like effects and can produce electrolyte abnormalities (McClain *et al.*, 2003) that limit its use. There are multiple herbal preparations that have been used extensively in Asia for hepatitis B and C. However, our understanding of these products is limited by inconsistencies in product preparation/composition and lack of strong randomized trials (Haas *et al.*, 2000; McClain *et al.*, 2003; Hanje *et al.*, 2006).

A major problem with herbals is that they are actually a combination of agents that have been poorly characterized and are not highly reproducible from one lot to the next. Moreover, some herbal compounds cause severe hepatotoxicity (Haas *et al.*, 2000; McClain *et al.*, 2003; Hanje *et al.*, 2006).

Potential Nutritional Toxicities in Liver Disease: Vitamin, Electrolyte, and Mineral Supplementation

Vitamins

In liver disease, vitamin deficiencies can occur not only because of decreased dietary intake, but also because of problems with malabsorption, especially of the fat-soluble vitamins. The use of antioxidant vitamins such as vitamin E has been proposed as therapy in some types of liver disease. However, supplementation, especially if large doses of specific vitamins such as vitamin A or niacin are used, can also cause liver toxicity or exacerbate the underlying liver disease.

Malabsorption of the fat-soluble vitamins A, D, E, and K is well described in patients with advanced cholestatic liver disease (Sokol, 1994). The malabsorption and deficiencies have been classically described in patients with primary biliary cirrhosis and primary sclerosing cholangitis. However, cholestasis can occur with advanced liver disease from other etiologies such as alcoholic or viral liver disease. Overt night blindness is unusual; however, sub-clinical vitamin A deficiency can be detected by testing a subject's dark adaptation (Russell, 2000). Because zinc deficiency can also affect dark adaptation, it must be corrected before the test is valid to test for vitamin A deficiency.

Fortunately, vitamin A deficiency in patients with cholestatic liver disease usually responds to dietary vitamin A supplements. However, parenteral vitamin A may be required for patients with night blindness. Caution must be used in giving vitamin A supplements to alcoholics and patients with alcoholic liver disease (Leo and Lieber, 1999). Vitamin A toxicity can occur even at the dosages of vitamin A present in some multivitamin preparations with the concomitant use of alcohol or with underlying cirrhosis. The stellate cell in the liver is the major storage site for vitamin A in the body.

Vitamin D deficiency can occur because of malabsorption of vitamin D and because the liver produces a metabolite of vitamin D, calcidiol, or 25-hydroxyvitamin D

(Sokol, 1994). Vitamin D deficiency in chronic liver disease is almost universal, with evidence of mild to severe vitamin D deficiency in more than 90% of patients independent of the cause of liver damage (Fisher and Fisher, 2007; Arteh *et al.*, 2010). Because vitamin D is an immunomodulator (von Essen *et al.*, 2010), the relation of vitamin D deficiency to severity of liver damage and response to therapy has been studied in viral chronic hepatitis C. Patients with chronic hepatitis C and low vitamin D levels have been found to have a lower response to interferon-based therapy and to have more liver fibrosis (Petta *et al.*, 2010; Lange *et al.*, 2011). Furthermore, vitamin D supplementation before interferon-based therapy may improve treatment response (Bitetto *et al.*, 2011). Metabolic bone disease is well documented in advanced liver disease, especially in primary biliary cirrhosis and primary sclerosing cholangitis (Bonkovsky *et al.*, 1990). Vitamin D and calcium supplements (discussed below) are frequently given to these patients, especially if there is evidence of osteoporosis. Patients with low plasma calcidiol levels should receive vitamin D supplementation (400–800 IU/day). If plasma calcidiol levels do not normalize on vitamin D, then calcidiol, which is more water soluble, can be given (Sokol, 1994). However, the effectiveness of this practice is not well documented.

Deficiencies in the antioxidant vitamin E may lead to lipid peroxidation and cell membrane instability. Decreased serum levels of vitamin E have been reported in advanced liver disease. If vitamin E is given to children with cholestatic liver disease before age 3 years, neurologic symptoms such as areflexia, ataxia, and sensory neuropathy can be improved (Sokol, 1994). Vitamin E supplementation in the range of 800 IU/day has generally been thought to be safe in liver disease, even long term; however, higher dosages may potentiate the effect of oral anticoagulants and interfere with platelet function. A meta-analysis of vitamin E therapy reported an increased mortality in patients (not liver disease patients) receiving high-dose vitamin E supplementation (Miller *et al.*, 2005). In spite of this concern, recent positive findings using 800 IU of vitamin E per day in NASH patients support its use and safety in liver disease (Sanyal *et al.*, 2010*)*.

Vitamin K malabsorption can occur in cholestatic liver disease and lead to prolongation of the prothrombin time because of deficiencies of vitamin K-dependent coagulation factors (Sokol, 1994). In patients with liver disease and a prolonged prothrombin time, vitamin K is often given parenterally to help determine whether the prolonged prothrombin time is due to vitamin K deficiency or malabsorption or to the severity of parenchymal liver disease itself.

Deficiencies of water-soluble vitamins can occur in liver disease. The best dietary sources for most water-soluble vitamins are fruits and vegetables. Patients with liver disease, especially advanced liver disease, can have problems with anorexia and develop dietary deficiencies of these vitamins. Deficiencies of vitamins related to alcohol usage per se can also occur in patients with liver disease. The intake of a daily multivitamin preparation is generally recommended in most patients with liver disease. In addition, we usually give folic acid (1 mg/day) for several months to replete dietary inadequacies. The amount of niacin contained in multivitamins (20 mg niacinamide) is unlikely to cause liver problems. When controlled-release niacin is used as a blood-lipid-lowering agent in dosages of 1 to 3 g/day, a dose-related increase in liver enzymes occurs (Gray *et al.*, 1994). Although hepatotoxicity is infrequent, it can occur with doses above 3 g/day and result in fulminant hepatic failure. Thus, the use of niacin as an antihyperlipidemic agent is contraindicated in patients with liver dysfunction.

The use of antioxidants, including antioxidant vitamins A, C, and E, has become popular because of the hypothesis that they can prevent cancer and slow the aging process by detoxifying toxic free radicals. The use of large doses of some of these agents should be avoided in patients known to have liver disease. As mentioned above, vitamin A toxicity can occur in patients with liver disease and other predisposed individuals. Excessive vitamin C supplementation should be avoided in patients with iron overload states, because vitamin C enhances iron uptake and potentiates free radical generation by transition metals (Sokol, 1996).

Electrolytes and Minerals

Sodium is the primary electrolyte present in body fluids outside cells, with only 5% of the sodium concentration of the body occurring intracellularly. This electrolyte, together with potassium, assists in maintaining the body's electrolyte and water balance. In addition, sodium and potassium play important roles in nerve conduction, muscle contraction, and transport of substances across membranes. Hyponatremia (low serum sodium) is a frequent complication of liver disease (Marsano and McClain, 1989). This usually occurs with normal or increased amounts of sodium being offset by greater increases in total water volume. The increased volume of water and

sodium is expressed as edema or ascites. Many factors contribute to decreased sodium concentrations, with two of the most important being impaired free water clearance and the use of diuretics. In patients with decompensated liver disease, the main way of treating hyponatremia is fluid restriction. Hypernatremia occurs much less frequently in liver disease, and it is usually due to medical interventions with agents such as diuretics or lactulose therapy.

Hypokalemia is frequently observed in liver disease (Marsano and McClain, 1989). Unlike sodium, potassium is predominantly an intracellular electrolyte. Hypokalemia may occur as a result of poor nutrition; losses because of nausea, vomiting, or diarrhea; or use of diuretics to control edema or ascites. Various metabolic factors (e.g., increased insulin levels and respiratory alkalosis) may shift potassium from the extracellular fluid into cells, thus decreasing the serum potassium concentration. Hypokalemia can produce a spectrum of consequences ranging from muscular weakness to cardiac arrhythmias and even cardiac arrest. Hyperkalemia is much less commonly observed in liver disease and usually accompanies renal failure and use of potassium-sparing diuretics. It is vital that patients not be placed on potassium-containing salt substitutes while on potassium-sparing diuretics because severe hyperkalemia can occur.

In liver disease, hypocalcemia can occur because of hypoalbuminemia. If hypocalcemia is due to hypoalbuminemia, there is a reduction in total serum calcium, but the ionized calcium remains normal and no treatment is necessary. However, hypocalcemic crisis due to transient hypoparathyroidism associated with magnesium deficiency has been reported in acute alcoholic fatty liver (Chiba *et al.*, 1987). This hypocalcemia improves with magnesium replacement and improvement in the acute liver disease.

Chronic calcium deficiencies also can occur with liver disease because of dietary insufficiencies and malabsorption. Reduced total and ionized plasma calcium levels can occur with vitamin D deficiency, such as that occurring with cholestatic liver disease, because calcium absorption is reduced with vitamin D deficiency. However, additional factors are thought to be involved in the low-turnover osteoporosis that can occur with cholestatic liver disease, because this osteoporosis can occur despite normal plasma vitamin D and calcium levels (Hay, 1995). Calcium supplementation at a dose of 1500 mg/day is usually given in cholestatic liver disease, although the effectiveness of such therapy is not well documented. This calcium supplementation is often given along with vitamin D supplementation, especially if plasma calcidiol levels are low.

Hypomagnesemia is frequently observed in liver disease, especially ALD (Flink, 1987). Major causes of the deficiency in liver disease include poor intake, impaired absorption, renal-related losses, and effects of drugs such as diuretics. Moreover, anti-rejection drugs such as cyclosporine and tacrolimus can cause a variety of metabolic and nutritional effects, including hypomagnesemia and hypophosphatemia, alterations in potassium, glucose intolerance, and hyperlipidemia. Hypophosphatemia may occur in very malnourished patients with liver disease and can be exacerbated by refeeding. Thus, serum levels need to be monitored, especially in aggressive refeeding of malnourished patients.

The role of trace elements in liver disease has been reviewed (McClain et al., 1991, 1992). Trace elements are present in the body in amounts equal to or less than those of iron, the most abundant trace metal. Iron overload is a well-documented cause of liver disease. Chronic iron overload can result in fibrosis, cirrhosis, and ultimately even hepatocellular carcinoma. Mechanisms for injury are thought to be multifactorial and most likely relate to oxidative stress and lipid peroxidation. The genetic basis for hereditary hemochromatosis has been identified, and genetic analysis for hemochromatosis is now clinically available (Bacon and Schilsky, 1999; Fleming et al., 2004). Iron deficiency can also occur in liver disease; it is usually caused by gastrointestinal bleeding, especially from esophageal varices or portal hypertensive gastropathy. Care must be taken with iron supplementation in patients with liver disease to avoid iron overload.

Zinc deficiency, as discussed previously, is well documented in liver disease. This is usually due to poor dietary zinc intake as well as increased losses, especially in the urine (McClain et al., 1991, 1992). Zinc deficiency in liver disease may present as neurosensory defects (with alterations in cognitive function, night vision, or appetite), skin lesions, hypogonadism, immune dysfunction, or altered protein metabolism. A major and frequently unrecognized complication of mineral deficiency in cirrhosis is severe muscle cramps. This is often associated with deficiencies of zinc and magnesium, and replacement with these two minerals often improves or corrects these disturbing symptoms.

Increased copper levels may cause hepatotoxicity, the classic example of which is Wilson disease (an autosomal recessive genetic disorder of copper overload) (Harris and Gitlin, 1996). Copper is excreted in the bile, and cholestatic liver diseases such as primary biliary cirrhosis and sclerosing cholangitis frequently have prominent copper overload. Interestingly, zinc has been used as a therapy for Wilson disease. Zinc blocks copper absorption by inducing intestinal metallothionein, thus preferentially reducing copper absorption at the intestinal level (Brewer, 1999).

Other trace metals of particular relevance to liver disease include selenium (potential antioxidant function), chromium (role in glucose tolerance), and manganese, which is excreted via the biliary route (McClain et al., 1991).

Obesity and Non-Alcoholic Steatohepatitis

In 1980, the term "NASH" (non-alcoholic steatohepatitis) was coined to describe a new syndrome occurring in patients who usually were obese females (often with type 2 diabetes) who had liver pathology consistent with alcoholic hepatitis but who denied alcohol use (Ludwig et al., 1980). The causes of this syndrome were unknown, and there was no defined therapy. Three decades later, this clinical syndrome is only a little better understood, and there is still no Food and Drug Administration-approved or even generally accepted drug therapy. Men are now proving to be equally affected, and terminology has been expanded to include NAFLD, which encompasses just fatty liver as well as fat plus inflammation/fibrosis (Neuschwander-Tetri and Caldwell, 2003; McClain et al., 2004; Cave et al., 2010). Patients with "primary" NASH typically have insulin resistance syndrome (synonymous with metabolic syndrome, syndrome X, etc.), which is characterized by obesity, type 2 diabetes, hyperlipidemia, hypertension, and, in some instances, other metabolic abnormalities such as polycystic ovary disease (Neuschwander-Tetri and Caldwell, 2003; McClain et al., 2004; Cave et al., 2010). "Secondary" NASH may be caused by drugs such as tamoxifen, certain industrial toxins, rapid weight loss, etc. (Cave et al., 2010). The etiology of NASH remains elusive, but most investigators agree that a baseline of steatosis requires a second "hit" capable of inducing inflammation, fibrosis, or necrosis to develop NASH. Second hits or insults that are thought to be etiologic in the development of NASH include oxidative stress, mitochondrial dysfunction, increased proinflammatory cytokines such as TNF, low levels of the anti-inflammatory adipokine adiponectin, and insulin resistance (McClain et al., 2004; Louthan et al., 2005).

The clinical features of NASH are generally non-specific. Patients are typically diagnosed in the fifth or sixth decade of life, although there is an increasing recognition of NASH in children. Most patients are asymptomatic, although some complain of fatigue and/or right upper quadrant discomfort. Many patients are diagnosed on routine physical examination (mild hepatomegaly) and laboratory evaluation (mild increase in aspartate aminotransferase and alanine aminotransferase <5 times normal). The aspartate aminotransferase/alanine aminotransferase ratio is usually less than 1 in NASH, thus helping to distinguish it from alcoholic steatohepatitis. The natural history of steatosis relates to histologic severity (Brunt, 2001). Fatty liver without inflammation has a relatively more benign course, while the presence of fibrosis and inflammation indicates a more ominous prognosis. Fat may decrease as NASH patients develop cirrhosis. NASH is a major cause of cryptogenic cirrhosis, an increasingly recognized cause of hepatomas, and an indicator for liver transplantation. Lastly, obesity can accelerate the course of other liver diseases such as ALD and hepatitis C (Naveau et al., 1994; Patton et al., 2004).

There is substantial evidence that specific dietary components play a role in the development/progression of NAFLD. As noted above, both steatosis and steatohepatitis appear to be triggered by mechanisms such as dys-regulated cytokines/adipokines, lipotoxicity, endotoxemia, alterations in gut microflora, and oxidative stress. These are all mechanisms that are associated with specific dietary habits (e.g. obesity, high-fat diets, excess fructose, diets low in n-3 fatty acids, etc.) (Musso et al., 2003). High-fat diets have frequently been implicated in NAFLD. Indeed, many animal models utilize such a diet (71% of energy from fat) to induce NAFLD (Lieber et al., 2004). These high-fat diets result in several of the metabolic derangements, including alterations in postprandial triglyceride metabolism, increased TNF-α, oxidative stress, circulating free fatty acids (FFA), and insulin resistance, that likely play an etiologic role in NAFLD. Not only is the amount of fat important in the development of NAFLD; the type and ratios of dietary fats also appear to be important. An increased fat intake with an excessive amount of n-6 fatty acids has been implicated in promoting necro-inflammation (Cortez-Pinto et al., 2006). On the other hand, a diet containing MCTs in the absence of LCTs has been reported to be hepatoprotective (Lieber et al., 2008). A large body of literature also exists regarding the role of fructose in the pathogenesis of NAFLD (Ouyang et al., 2008; Lim et al.,

2010). Specific sources of fructose, such as soft drinks, have also been implicated (Nseir et al., 2010). Recent animal studies have confirmed that diets containing 30% of fructose, either as free fructose and glucose or as sucrose, induce metabolic syndrome and intrahepatic accumulation of triglycerides. Fructose-induced NAFLD is associated with intestinal bacterial overgrowth and increased intestinal permeability, subsequently leading to an endotoxin-dependent activation of hepatic Kupffer cells and increased MCP-1 and TNF-α (Spruss et al., 2009; Sánchez-Lozada et al., 2010).

Current treatment recommendations for patients with NAFLD include both diet and physical activity for weight reduction and weight-loss surgery for extreme obesity. One year of intensive lifestyle intervention in patients with type 2 diabetes has been shown to reduce steatosis and incident NAFLD (Lazo et al., 2010). Studies examining the effects of dietary interventions reveal that caloric restriction can result in significant changes in both liver fat and volume within a few days (Yki-Järvinen, 2010). The use of low-carbohydrate diets in NAFLD is an area of increasing interest. A low-carbohydrate, ketogenic diet in patients with NASH led to significant weight loss and histologic improvement of fatty liver disease at 6 months (Tendler et al., 2007). Dietary avoidance of lipogenic, simple sugars (i.e., fructose) seems to be universally recommended (Yki-Järvinen, 2010). A reduction in the consumption of sweetened beverages can also lead to significant weight loss owing to a reduction in total calories consumed (Zivkovic et al., 2007). Vigorous exercise may be most beneficial, as it appears that exercise intensity may be more important than duration or total volume (Kistler et al., 2011). Weight loss by bariatric surgery attenuates both steatosis and steatohepatitis, but data supporting improvements in fibrosis are limited (Rafiq and Younossi, 2008). There remains no FDA-approved therapy for NAFLD. Pharmacologic therapies used in NAFLD mostly target components of the metabolic syndrome or oxidative stress associated with the pathogenesis of NASH (Rafiq and Younossi, 2008). As noted previously, a randomized, prospective trial involving adults without diabetes who had NASH reported that vitamin E therapy (800 IU, natural form, once daily) was associated with a significantly higher rate of histologic improvement over placebo (43% vs. 19%, $p = 0.001$) (Sanyal et al., 2010). For this reason, the use of vitamin E 800 IU daily has become standard practice ("drug therapy") in many areas of the country.

Nutrition and Liver Transplantation

Malnutrition in Liver Transplantation

Malnutrition is a risk factor for general post-operative morbidity (e.g., poor wound healing, infections, mortality), and this holds true for liver transplantation. In one study, malnutrition was the only variable of six studied that significantly affected outcome and that was potentially alterable and not completely dependent on underlying hepatic function (Shaw et al., 1985). In that study, a risk stratification scoring system, including encephalopathy, ascites, nutritional status, serum bilirubin, prothrombin time, age, and intraoperative blood loss, was used to assign patients a low, intermediate, or high risk for poor outcome following liver transplantation. The actuarial 1-year survival after liver transplantation was significantly poorer for high-risk patients than for intermediate- or low-risk patients (44.5%, 85.2%, and 90.5%, respectively) (Shaw et al., 1985). Moderately to severely malnourished patients had prolonged ventilator times, ICU lengths of stay, total hospital lengths of stay, and total hospitalization costs. Others have validated these data (Moukarzel et al., 1990; Pikul et al., 1994). Mortality increased 3.2-fold when significant loss in body cell mass was present preoperatively (Muller et al., 1992). Using a modified subjective global assessment of malnutrition, Pikul et al. (1994) found a 79% incidence of malnutrition in 68 adult liver transplant recipients; in those with moderate and severe malnutrition, they found a significant increase in the number of days requiring ventilatory support, number of days in the ICU and in hospital, and a higher incidence of tracheostomy. In this study, patients with moderate and severe malnutrition had a significantly higher mortality than did those with an adequate status or mild malnutrition. A universal component of chronic liver disease is the loss of muscle mass and strength, and these deficits are associated with impaired health-related quality of life which persists to a lesser degree after liver transplantation (Abbott et al., 2001; Pieber et al., 2006).

The pediatric literature presents similar information. In a study of 119 pediatric liver transplants, malnutrition (assessed as failure to grow in height) was also shown to predict post-operative complications (Moukarzel et al., 1990). Moreover, infants appear to be more susceptible to malnutrition associated with chronic liver disease than do older children; infants show both acute and chronic malnutrition with more severe reductions in weight and fat

body mass because their accelerated growth phase is affected (Roggero et al., 1997).

Nutritional Intervention Before Liver Transplantation

Dietary restrictions are necessary but often detrimental in maintaining adequate nutritional intake in patients with liver disease. Sodium restriction is probably the single most important restriction in the diet of patients with decompensated portal hypertension, but 1–2 g sodium diets are usually well tolerated and easily followed by well-coached patients. Fluid restriction is sometimes necessary to correct hyponatremia (Lowell, 1996). Restricting protein intake is commonly used to control hepatic encephalopathy, but current evidence does not support protein restriction (Cordoba et al., 2004; Gheorghe et al., 2005). Hepatic encephalopathy can be improved by interventions that include ensuring an adequate intestinal transit time; preventing small- and large-bowel bacterial overgrowth (by decreasing portal hypertension and using broad-spectrum antibiotics and lactulose); replacing electrolytes, vitamins, and minerals; and perhaps by adding casein or vegetable protein to the diet. Maintaining an adequate nutritional status might prevent proteolysis from providing substrate for gluconeogenesis. This would theoretically prevent excessive use of BCAAs for gluconeogenesis, and may prevent worsening hepatic encephalopathy. For example, early breakfast improves cognitive function in patients with covert (minimal) hepatic encephalopathy (Vaisma et al., 2010), and after each food intake alertness improves for a period of time, further supporting the use of frequent small meals in advanced liver disease. A large body of evidence has been accumulated on the use and safety of BCAA preparations in the management of overt hepatic encephalopathy. Some physicians and nutritionists have also extended the use of BCAA preparations to malnourished patients with cirrhosis in an attempt to improve nutritional states. One reviewer summarizes current data regarding that practice: "The cost to benefit ratio makes it impossible to justify the use of BCAA in every malnourished patient with cirrhosis" (Munoz, 1991).

Although a strong body of work suggests that malnutrition is a risk factor for morbidity and mortality after liver transplantation, limited data actually document the benefit of nutritional intervention before this surgery. One of the reasons for this lack of data is that, as the survival after liver transplantation improves, the number of patients needed for such studies grows, making it more difficult to perform them. Another reason is that, as we have discussed above, the reasons for malnutrition are multiple and vary from patient to patient. Nevertheless, nutritional intervention improves nutritional status in the pediatric population, and post-operative nutritional intervention decreases ICU and ventilatory-support days in adult liver transplant recipients (Reilly *et al.*, 1990; Charlton *et al.*, 1992). Similarly, aggressive bedtime nutrition support can minimize and reverse loss of muscle mass (Plank *et al.*, 2008).

When adequate oral intake cannot be maintained, nutritional goals should be supplemented by using nighttime enteral feedings via small-bore nasoenteric tubes. Only in rare instances when the enteral route fails or is contraindicated should total parenteral nutrition be used.

Nutrition Support After Liver Transplantation

Nutrition support after liver transplantation is generally simple because a patient's health improves remarkably rapidly after the surgery. Although increased protein catabolism and a negative nitrogen balance have been documented up to 4 weeks after transplantation, these have not been associated with a poor outcome (Plevak *et al.*, 1994). Immediate enteral feeding was well tolerated by 25 patients who were fed via a nasojejunal tube within 12 hours after liver transplantation. When compared with 24 control patients with a sham nasogastric tube, the only significant benefit seen was a decrease in viral infections (Hasse *et al.*, 1995). Nevertheless, nutrition support guidelines have been published for the post-transplant patient (Hasse, 1990). For patients who have a longer ICU stay after transplantation, the experience of Reilly *et al.* (1990) suggests that parenteral nutrition may reduce ICU length of stay (although a shortcoming of this study was that there were no patients fed enterally). Nutrition support will be needed in the minority of patients with complicated post-operative courses and prolonged hospital stays. The rule of using the gut whenever possible stands true in this setting as well.

Starting weeks to months after transplantation, patients are prone to develop hyperglycemia, hypertension, and hypercholesterolemia as drug-related side-effects and weight gain. Necessary traditional nutrition intervention is warranted in these circumstances. Certain foodstuffs may alter immunosuppressive medications (e.g., grapefruit juice increases tacrolimus blood levels), whereas others can cause disease (e.g., raw seafood can transmit bacteria and promote life-threatening infections in immunosuppressed individuals).

In addition, after liver transplantation, there is a period of accelerated loss of bone due to corticosteroid therapy and decreased patient mobility. After this period of accelerated bone loss, there is a progressive increase in bone mineral density that can continue for several years post-transplant (Porayko *et al.*, 1991). Calcium supplementation is important during the period of increased bone formation.

Conclusions

The liver is a unique metabolic organ that metabolizes and detoxifies nutrients, toxins, and drugs from the portal circulation and the arterial blood supply. It is responsible for the production of visceral proteins such as albumin, and anabolic hormones such as insulin-like growth factor-1, and it is the reservoir for the largest source (Kupffer cells) of fixed macrophages, which are responsible for clinical scavenging functions and cytokine production. When liver disease occurs, there are derangements in metabolic functions, with malnutrition being one critical consequence. The prevalence of malnutrition is high and correlates with the severity of liver disease, and the causes of malnutrition are multiple. It is important to initiate early assessment of nutritional status in patients with liver disease and to begin early nutritional support. Patients may have generalized protein calorie malnutrition or more selected depletion of individual nutrients (e.g., zinc, magnesium or folate deficiency). Nutritional supplementation has been shown to improve nutritional status, and in some situations improve liver function or clinical outcome in patients with chronic liver disease.

Future Directions

A vital future direction is a better understanding of the interactions and cross-talk between the liver and other organs/tissues (e.g., the gut–liver axis and liver–adipose tissue axis). The role of the gut microbiome in liver disease as well as obesity and systemic inflammation is a rapidly evolving area. How liver disease alters the gut microbiome, and whether changing the gut microbiome with probiotics/prebiotics attenuates or prevents liver disease, are important areas of active investigation. Clinical trials, including dose-finding studies and appropriate biomarkers, on the impact of nutritional support and individual nutrients (e.g. zinc) on hepatic outcome are needed. Nutrients can dramatically impact gene expression, and nutrient imbalance in diseases such as ALD may be a major contributor to dysregulated gene expression in liver injury. There is growing interest in the role of epigenetic changes, such as those induced by histone modifications and methylation reactions, that may markedly impact the development of a variety of types of liver disease. It is clear that nutrients and nutritional status may impact these epigenetic changes. Research into the above areas will markedly expand our understanding of mechanisms of various types of liver disease and potential nutritional interventions to prevent or treat liver disease.

Suggestions for Further Reading

Chen, Y., Yang, F., Lu, H., *et al.* (2011) Characterization of fecal microbial communities in patients with liver cirrhosis. *Hepatology* **54**, 562–572.

Delzenne, N.M. and Cani, P.D. (2011) Interaction between obesity and the gut microbiota: relevance in nutrition. *Annu Rev Nutr* **31**, 15–31.

Delzenne, N.M., Neyrinck, A.M., Bäckhed, F., *et al.* (2011) Targeting gut microbiota in obesity: effects of prebiotics and probiotics. *Nat Rev Endocrinol* **7**, 639–646.

Frazier, T.H., DiBaise, J.K., and McClain, C.J. (2011) Gut microbiota, intestinal permeability, obesity-induced inflammation, and liver injury. *JPEN J Parenter Enteral Nutr* **35**, 14S–20S.

Moghe, A., Joshi-Barve, S., Ghare, S., *et al.* (2011) Histone modifications and alcohol-induced liver disease: are altered nutrients the missing link? *World J Gastroenterol* **17**, 2465–2472.

References

Abbott, W.J., Thomson, A., Steadman, C., *et al.* (2001) Child-Pugh class, nutritional indicators and early liver transplant outcomes. *Hepatogastroenterology* **48**, 823–827.

Abdelmalek, M.F., Sanderson, S.O., Angulo, P., *et al.* (2009) Betaine for nonalcoholic fatty liver disease: results of a randomized placebo controlled trial. *Hepatology* **50**, 1818–1826.

Antonow, D.R. and McClain, C.J. (1985) Nutrition and alcoholism. In R.E. Tarter and D.H. Van Thiel (eds), *Alcohol and the Brain: Chronic Effects*. Plenum, New York, pp. 81–120.

Arteh, J., Narra, S., and Nair, S. (2010) Prevalence of vitamin D deficiency in chronic liver disease. *Dig Dis Sci* **55**, 2624–2628.

Bacon, B.R. and Schilsky, M.L. New knowledge of genetic pathogenesis of hemochromatosis and Wilson's disease. *Adv Intern Med* **44**, 91–116.

Baker, J.P., Detsky, A.S., Wesson, D.E., *et al.* (1982) Nutritional assessment: a comparison of clinical judgment and objective measurements. *N Engl J Med* **306**, 969–972.

Bitetto, D., Fabris, C., Fornasiere, E., *et al.* (2011) Vitamin D supplementation improves response to antiviral treatment for recurrent hepatitis C. *Transpl Int* **24**, 43–50.

Bonkovsky, H.L., Hawkins, M., Steinberg, K., *et al.* (1990) Prevalence and prediction of osteopenia in chronic liver disease. *Hepatology* **12**, 273–280.

Boosalis, M.G., Ott, L., Levine, A.S., *et al.* (1989) Relationship of visceral proteins to nutritional status in chronic and acute stress. *Crit Care Med* **17**, 741–747.

Brewer, G.J. (1999) Zinc therapy induction of intestinal metallothionein in Wilson's disease. *Am J Gastroenterol* **94**, 301–302.

Brunt, E.M. (2001) Nonalcoholic steatohepatitis: definition and pathology. *Semin Liver Dis* **21**, 3–16.

Cabre, E., Peraigo, J.L., Abad-Lucruz, A., *et al.* (1990) Plasma fatty acid profile in advanced cirrhosis: unsaturation deficit of lipid fractions. *Am J Gastroenterol* **85**, 1597–1604.

Cabre, E., Rodriguez-Iglesias, P., Caballeria, J., *et al.* (2000) Short- and long-term outcome of severe alcohol-induced hepatitis treated with steroids or enteral nutrition: a multicenter randomized trial. *Hepatology* **32**, 36–42.

Campillo, B. (2010) Assessment of nutritional status and diagnosis of malnutrition in patients with liver disease. In V.R. Preedy, R. Lakshman, R. Srirajaskanthan, *et al.* (eds), *Nutrition, Diet Therapy and the Liver*. CRC Press, Boca Raton, FL, pp. 22–46.

Campillo, B., Richardet, J.P., Scherman, E., *et al.* (2003) Evaluation of nutritional practice in hospitalized cirrhotic patients: results of a prospective study. *Nutrition* **19**, 515–521.

Caregaro, L., Alberino, F., Amodio, P., *et al.* (1996) Malnutrition in alcoholic and virus-related cirrhosis. *Am J Clin Nutr* **63**, 602–609.

Cave, M., Falkner, K.C., Ray, M., *et al.* (2010) Toxicant-associated steatohepatitis in vinyl chloride workers. *Hepatology* **51**, 474–481.

Charlton, C.P.J., Buchanan, E., Holden, C.E., *et al.* (1992) Intensive enteral feeding in advanced cirrhosis: reversal of malnutrition without precipitation of hepatic encephalopathy. *Arch Dis Child* **67**, 603–607.

Charlton, M. (2003) Branched-chain amino acid-enriched supplements as therapy for liver disease: Rasputin lives. *Gastroenterology* **124**, 1980–1982.

Chiba, T., Okimura, Y., Inatome, T., *et al.* (1987) Hypocalcemic crisis in alcoholic fatty liver: transient hypoparathyroidism due to magnesium deficiency. *Am J Gastroenterol* **82**, 1084–1087.

Cordoba, J., Lopez-Hellin, J., Planas, M., *et al.* (2004) Normal protein diet for episodic hepatic encephalopathy: results of a randomized study. *J Hepatol* **41**, 38–43.

Cortez-Pinto, H., Jesus, L., Barros, H., *et al.* (2006) How different is the dietary pattern in non-alcoholic steatohepatitis patients? *Clin Nutr* **25**, 816–823.

DiCecco, S.R., Wieners, E.J., Wiesner, R.H., *et al.* (1989) Assessment of nutritional status of patients with end-stage liver disease undergoing liver transplantation. *Mayo Clin Proc* **64**, 95–102.

Dolz, C., Raurich, J.M., Ibanez, J., *et al.* (1991) Ascites increases the resting energy expenditure in liver cirrhosis. *Gastroenterology* **100**, 738–744.

Ferenci, P., Dragosics, B., Dittrich, H., *et al.* (1989) Randomized controlled trial of silymarin treatment in patients with cirrhosis of the liver. *J Hepatol* **9**, 105–113.

Fernandez-Checa, J.C., Hirano, T., Tsukamoto, H., *et al.* (1993) Mitochondrial glutathione depletion in alcoholic liver disease. *Alcohol* **10**, 469–475.

Fisher, L. and Fisher, A. (2007) Vitamin D and parathyroid hormone in outpatients with noncholestatic chronic liver disease. *Clin Gastroenterol Hepatol* **5**, 513–520.

Fleming, R.E., Britton, R.S., Waheed, A., *et al.* (2004) Pathogenesis of hereditary hemochromatosis. *Clin Liver Dis* **8**, 755–773.

Flink, E.B. (1987) Magnesium deficiency: causes and effects. *Hosp Pract (Off Ed)* **22**, 116A–116P.

Gaetke, L., McClain, C.J., Talwalkar, R.T., *et al.* (1997) Effects of endotoxin on zinc metabolism in human volunteers. *Am J Physiol* **272**, E952–E956.

Galati, J.S., Holdeman, K.P., Bottjen, P.L., *et al.* (1997) Gastric emptying and orocecal transit in portal hypertension and end-stage chronic liver disease. *Liver Transpl Surg* **3**, 34–38.

Galati, J.S., Holdeman, K.P., Dalrymple, G.V., *et al.* (1994) Delayed gastric emptying of both the liquid and solid components of a meal in chronic liver disease. *Am J Gastroenterol* **89**, 708–711.

Gheorghe, L., Iacob, R., Vadam, R., *et al.* (2005) Improvement of hepatic encephalopathy using a modified high-calorie high-protein diet. *Romanian J Gastroenterol* **14**, 231–238.

Gray, D.R., Morgan, T., Chretien, S.D., *et al.* (1994) Efficacy and safety of controlled-release niacin in dyslipoproteinemic veterans. *Ann Intern Med* **121**, 252–258.

Guglielmi, F.W., Contento, F., Laddaga, L., *et al.* (1991) Bioelectric impedance analysis: experience with male patients with cirrhosis. *Hepatology* **13**, 892–895.

Haas, L., McClain, C.J., and Varilek, G. (2000) Complementary and alternative medicine and gastrointestinal diseases. *Curr Opin Gastroenterol* **16**, 188–196.

Hanje, A.J., Fortune, B., Song, M., *et al.* (2006) The use of selected nutritional supplements and complementary and alternative medicine in liver disease. *Nutr Clin Practice* **21**, 255–272.

Harris, Z.L. and Gitlin, J.D. (1996) Genetic molecular basis for copper toxicity. *Am J Clin Nutr* **63**, 836S–841S.

Hasegawa, T., Yoneda, M., Nakamura, K., *et al.* (2001) Plasma transforming growth factor-beta1 level and efficacy of alpha-tocopherol in patients with non-alcoholic steatohepatitis: a pilot study. *Aliment Pharmacol Ther* **15**, 1667–1672.

Hasse, J.M. (1990) Nutritional implications of liver transplantation. *Henry Ford Hosp Med J* **38**, 235–240.

Hasse, J.M., Blue, L.S., Liepa, G.U., *et al.* (1995) Early enteral nutrition support in patients undergoing liver transplantation. *JPEN J Parenter Enteral Nutr* **19**, 437–443.

Hay, J.E. (1995) Bone disease in cholestatic liver disease. *Gastroenterology* **108**, 276–283.

Hennig, B., Honchel, R., Goldblum, S.E., *et al.* (1988) Tumor necrosis factor-mediated hypoalbuminemia in rabbits. *J Nutr* **118**, 1586–1590.

Hill, D.B., Devalarja, R., Joshi-Barve, S., *et al.* (1999) Antioxidants attenuate nuclear factorkappa B activation and tumor necrosis factor-alpha production in alcoholic hepatitis patient monocytes and rat Kupffer cells, in vitro. *Clin Biochem* **32**, 563–570.

Hirsch, S., Bunout, D., de la Maza, P., *et al.* (1993) Controlled trial on nutrition supplementation in outpatients with symptomatic alcoholic cirrhosis. *JPEN J Parenter Enteral Nutr* **17**, 119–124.

Hirsch, S., de la Maza, M.P., Gattas, V., *et al.* (1999) Nutritional support in alcoholic cirrhotic patients improves host defenses. *J Am Coll Nutr* **18**, 434–441.

Isobe, H., Sakai, H., Satoh, M., *et al.* (1994) Delayed gastric emptying in patients with liver cirrhosis. *Dig Dis Sci* **39**, 983–987.

John, W.I., Phillips, R., Ott, L., *et al.* (1989) Resting energy expenditure in patients with alcoholic hepatitis. *JPEN J Parenter Enteral Nutr* **13**, 124–127.

Joshi, P.C., Mehta, A., Jabber, W.S., *et al.* (2009) Zinc deficiency mediates alcohol-induced alveolar epithelial and macrophage dysfunction in rats. *Am J Respir Cell Mol Biol* **41**, 207–216.

Kang, X., Liu, J., Zhong, W., *et al.* (2009) Zinc supplementation reverses alcohol-induced steatosis in mice through reactivating hepatocyte nuclear factor 4α and peroxisome proliferator-activated receptor-α. *Hepatology* **50**, 1241–1250.

Kang, Y.J. and Zhou, Z. (2005) Zinc prevention and treatment of alcoholic liver disease. *Mol Aspects Med* **26**, 391–404.

Karaa, A., Thompson, K.J., McKillop, I.H., *et al.* (2008) S-adenosyl-L-methionine attenuates oxidative stress and hepatic stellate cell activation in an ethanol-LPS-induced fibrotic rat model. *Shock* **30**, 197–205.

Kearns, P.J., Young, H., Garcia, G., *et al.* (1992) Accelerated improvement of alcoholic liver disease with enteral nutrition. *Gastroenterology* **102**, 200–205.

Kharbanda, K.K. (2009) Alcoholic liver disease and methionine metabolism. *Semin Liver Dis* **29**, 155–165.

Kharbanda, K.K., Mailliard, M.E., Baldwin, C.R., *et al.* (2007) Betaine attenuates alcoholic steatosis by restoring phosphatidylcholine generation via the phosphatidylethanolamine methyltransferase pathway. *J Hepatol* **46,** 314–321.

Kistler, K.D., Brunt, E.M., Clark, J.M., *et al.* (2011) Physical activity recommendations, exercise intensity, and histological severity of nonalcoholic fatty liver disease. *Am J Gastroenterol* **106,** 460–468.

Ksiazyk, J., Lyszkowska, M., and Kierkus, J. (1996) Energy metabolism in portal hypertension in children. *Nutrition* **12,** 469–474.

Lange, C.M., Bojunga, J., Ramos-Lopez, E., *et al.* (2011) Vitamin D deficiency and a CYP27B1-1260 promoter polymorphism are associated with chronic hepatitis C and poor response to interferon-alfa based therapy. *J Hepatol* **54,** 887–893.

Lauterburg, B.H. and Velez, M.E. (1988) Glutathione deficiency in alcoholics: risk factor for paracetamol hepatotoxicity. *Gut* **29,** 1153–1157.

Lavine, J.E. (2000) Vitamin E treatment of nonalcoholic steatohepatitis in children: a pilot study. *J Pediatr* **136,** 734–738.

Lazo, M., Solga, S.F., Horska, A., *et al.* (2010) Effect of a 12-month intensive lifestyle intervention on hepatic steatosis in adults with type 2 diabetes. *Diabetes Care* **33,** 2156–2163.

Lee, K.S., Buck, M., Houglum, K., *et al.* (1995) Activation of hepatic stellate cells by TGFalpha and collagen type I is mediated by oxidative stress through c-myb expression. *J Clin Invest* **96,** 2461–2468.

Lee, T.D., Sadda, M.R., Mendler, M.H., *et al.* (2004) Abnormal hepatic methionine and glutathione metabolism in patients with alcoholic hepatitis. *Alcohol Clin Exp Res* **28,** 173–181.

Lee, W.M., Hynan, L.S., Rossaro, L., *et al.* (2009) Intravenous N-acetylcysteine improves transplant-free survival in early stage non-acetaminophen acute liver failure. *Gastroenterology* **137,** 856–864.

Leo, M.A. and Lieber, C.S. (1999) Alcohol, vitamin A, and beta-carotene: adverse interactions, including hepatotoxicity and carcinogenicity. *Am J Clin Nutr* **69,** 1071–1085.

Libert, C., Brouckaert, P., and Fiers, W. (1994) Protection by alpha1-acid glycoprotein against tumor necrosis factor-induced lethality. *J Exp Med* **180,** 1571–1575.

Lieber, C.S. (2002) S-adenosyl-L-methionine and alcoholic liver disease in animal models: implications for early intervention in human beings. *Alcohol* **27,** 173–177.

Lieber, C.S., DeCarli, L.M., Leo, M.A., *et al.* (2008) Beneficial effects versus toxicity of medium-chain triacylglycerols in rats with NASH. *J Hepatol* **48,** 318–326.

Lieber, C.S., Leo, M.A., Mak, K.M., *et al.* (2004) Model of nonalcoholic steatohepatitis. *Am J Clin Nutr* **79,** 502–509.

Lim, J.S., Mietus-Snyder, M., Valente, A., *et al.* (2010) The role of fructose in the pathogenesis of NAFLD and the metabolic syndrome. *Nat Rev Gastroenterol Hepatol* **7,** 251–264.

Liu, S-L., Degli Esposti, S., Yao, T., *et al.* (1995) Vitamin E therapy of acute CC14-induced hepatic injury in mice is associated with inhibition of nuclear factor kappa B binding. *Hepatology* **22,** 1474–1481.

Lolli, R., Marchesini, G., Bianchi, G., *et al.* (1992) Anthropometric assessment of the nutritional status of patients with liver cirrhosis in the Italian population. *Ital J Gastroenterol* **24,** 429–435.

Louthan, M.V., Barve, S., McClain, C.J., *et al.* (2005) Decreased serum adiponectin: an early event in pediatric nonalcoholic fatty liver disease. *J Pediatr* **147,** 835–838.

Lowell, J.A. (1996) Nutritional assessment and therapy in patients requiring liver transplantation. *Liver Transpl Surg.* **2**(5 Suppl 11), 79–88.

Ludwig, J., Viggiano, T.R., McGill, D.B., *et al.* (1980) Nonalcoholic steatohepatitis: Mayo Clinic experiences with a hitherto unnamed disease. *Mayo Clin Proc* **55,** 434–438.

Luper, S. (1998) A review of plants used in the treatment of liver disease: Part 1. *Altern Med Rev* **3,** 410–421.

Madden, A.M., Bradbury, W., and Morgan, M.Y. (1997) Taste perception in cirrhosis: its relationship to circulating micronutrients and food preferences. *Hepatology* **26,** 40–48.

Madrid, A.M., Brahm, J., Buckel, E., *et al.* (1997) Orthotopic liver transplantation improves small bowel motility disorders in cirrhotic patients. *Am J Gastroenterol* **92,** 1044–1045.

Malagelada, J.R., Pihl, O., and Linscheer, W.G. (1974) Impaired absorption of molecular long-chain fatty acid in patients with alcoholic cirrhosis. *Am J Dig Dis* **19,** 1016–1020.

Marchesini, G., Bianchi, G., Merli, M., *et al.* (2003) Nutritional supplementation with branched-chain amino acids in advanced cirrhosis: a double-blind, randomized trial. *Gastroenterology* **124,** 1792–1801.

Marsano, L. and McClain, C.J. (1989) Effects of alcohol on electrolytes and minerals. *Alcohol Health Res World* **13,** 255–260.

Marsano, L. and McClain, C.J. (1991) Nutrition and alcoholic liver disease. *JPEN J Parenter Enteral Nutr* **15,** 337–344.

Marsano, L. and McClain, C.J. (1992) Nutritional support in alcoholic liver disease. In R.R. Watson and B. Watzl (eds), *Nutrition and Alcohol.* CRC Press, Boca Raton, FL, pp. 385–402.

Mato, J.M., Camara, J., Fernandez de Paz, J., *et al.* (1999) S-adenosylmethionine in alcoholic liver cirrhosis: a randomized, placebo-controlled, double-blind, multicenter clinical trial. *J Hepatol* **30,** 1081–1089.

McClain, C.J., Antonow, D.R., Cohen, D.A., *et al.* (1986) Zinc metabolism in alcoholic liver disease. *Alcohol Clin Exp Res* **10,** 582–589.

McClain, C.J., Barve, S., Deaciuc, I., *et al.* (1999) Cytokines in alcoholic liver disease. *Semin Liver Dis* **19**, 205–219.

McClain, C.J., Dryden, G., and Krueger, K. (2003) Complementary and alternative medicine in gastroenterology. In T. Yamada, N. Kaplowitz, L. Laine, *et al.* (eds), *Textbook of Gastroenterology*, 4th Edn. Lippincott Williams & Wilkins, Philadelphia, pp. 1135–1146.

McClain, C.J., Kasarskis, E.J., and Marsano, L. (1992) Zinc and alcohol. In R.R. Watson and B. Watzl (eds), *Nutrition and Alcohol*. CRC Press, Boca Raton, FL, pp. 281–307.

McClain, C.J., Marsano, L., Burk, R.F., *et al.* (1991) Trace metals in liver disease. *Semin Liver Dis* **11**, 321–339.

McClain, C.J., Mokshagundam, S.P.L., Barve, S.S., *et al.* (2004) Mechanisms of non-alcoholic steatohepatitis. *Alcohol* **34**, 1–13.

McClain, C.J., Song, Z., Barve, S.S., *et al.* (2004) Recent advances in alcoholic liver disease. IV. Dysregulated cytokine metabolism in alcoholic liver disease. *Am J Physiol Gastrointest Liver Physiol* **287**, G497–G502.

McCullough, A.J. (2000) Malnutrition in liver disease. *Liver Transpl* (**4** Suppl 1), S85–S96.

McCullough, A.J., Mullen, K.D., and Kalhan, S.C. (1991) Measurements of total body and extracellular water in patients with and without ascites. *Hepatology* **14**, 1102–1111.

Mendenhall, C.L., Anderson, S., Weesner, R.E., *et al.* (1984) Protein-calorie malnutrition associated with alcoholic hepatitis. *Am J Med* **76**, 211–222.

Mendenhall, C.L., Moritz, T.E., Roselle, G.A., *et al.* (1993) A study of oral nutritional support with oxandrolone in malnourished patients with alcoholic hepatitis: results of a Department of Veterans Affairs cooperative study. *Hepatology* **17**, 564–576.

Mendenhall, C.L., Moritz, T.E., Roselle, G.A., *et al.* (1995) Protein energy malnutrition in severe alcoholic hepatitis: diagnosis and response to treatment. The VA Cooperative Study Group #275. *JPEN J Parenter Enteral Nutr* **19**, 258–265.

Mendenhall, C., Roselle, G.A., Gartside, P., *et al.* (1995b) Relationship of protein calorie malnutrition to alcoholic liver disease: a reexamination of data from two Veterans Administration cooperative studies. *Alcohol Clin Exp Res* **19**, 635–641.

Mendenhall, C.L., Tosch, T., Weesner, R.E., *et al.* (1986) VA cooperative study on alcoholic hepatitis II: prognostic significance of protein-calorie malnutrition. *Am J Clin Nutr* **43**, 213–218.

Merli, M., Romiti, A., Riggio, O., *et al.* (1987) Optimal nutritional indexes in chronic liver disease. *JPEN J Parenter Enteral Nutr* **11**(Suppl), 130S–134S.

Mezey, E., Potter, J.J., Rennie-Tankersley, L., *et al.* (2004) A randomized placebo controlled trial of vitamin E for alcoholic hepatitis. *J Hepatol* **40**, 40–46.

Miller, E.R., 3rd, Pastor-Barriuso, R., Dalal, D., *et al.* (2005) Meta-analysis: high-dosage vitamin E supplementation may increase all-cause mortality. *Ann Intern Med* **142**, 37–46.

Moukarzel, A.A., Najm, I., Vargas, J., *et al.* (1990) Effect of nutritional status on outcome of orthotopic liver transplantation in pediatric patients. *Transplant Proc* **22**, 1560–1563.

Muller, M.J., Lautz, H.U., Plogmann, B., *et al.* (1992) Energy expenditure and substrate oxidation in patients with cirrhosis: the impact of cause, clinical staging and nutritional state. *Hepatology* **15**, 782–794.

Munoz, S.J. (1991) Nutritional therapies in liver disease. *Semin Liver Dis* **11**, 278–291.

Musso, G., Gambino, R., De Michieli, F., *et al.* (2003) Dietary habits and their relations to insulin resistance and postprandial lipemia in nonalcoholic steatohepatitis. *Hepatology* **37**, 909–916.

Naveau, S., Giraud, V., Borotto, E., *et al.* (1997) Excess weight risk factor for alcoholic liver disease. *Hepatology* **25**, 108–111.

Neuschwander-Tetri, B.A. and Caldwell, S.H. (2003) Nonalcoholic steatohepatitis: summary of an AASLD Single Topic Conference. *Hepatology* **37**, 1202–1219.

Nseir, W., Nassar, F., and Assy, N. (2010) Soft drinks consumption and nonalcoholic fatty liver disease. *World J Gastroenterol* **16**, 2579–2588.

O'Keefe, S.J., El-Zayadi, A.R., Carraher, T.E., *et al.* (1980) Malnutrition and immuno-incompetence in patients with liver disease. *Lancet* **2**, 615–617.

Ouyang, X., Cirillo, P., Sautin, Y., *et al.* (2008) Fructose consumption as a risk factor for non-alcoholic fatty liver disease. *J Hepatol* **48**, 993–939.

Owen, O.E., Trapp, V.E., Reichard, G.A., Jr, *et al.* (1983) Nature and quantity of fuels consumed in patients with alcoholic cirrhosis. *J Clin Invest* **72**, 1821–1832.

Pares, A., Planas, R., and Torres, M. (1998) Effects of silymarin in alcoholic patients with cirrhosis of the liver: results of a controlled, double-blind, randomized and multicenter trial. *J Hepatol* **28**, 615–621.

Patek, A.J., Jr, Post, J., Ralnoff, O.D., *et al.* (1948) Dietary treatment of cirrhosis of the liver. *JAMA* **139**, 543–549.

Patton, H.M., Patel, K., Behling, C., *et al.* (2004) The impact of steatosis on disease progression and early and sustained treatment response in chronic hepatitis C patients. *J Hepatol* **40**, 484–490.

Pena, L.R., Hill, D.B., and McClain, C.J. (1999) Treatment with glutathione precursor decreases cytokine activity. *JPEN J Parenter Enteral Nutr* **23**, 1–6.

Petta, S., Cammà, C., Scazzone, C., *et al.* (2010) Low vitamin D serum level is related to severe fibrosis and low responsiveness to interferon-based therapy in genotype 1 chronic hepatitis C. *Hepatology* **51**, 1158–1167.

Phillips, M., Curtis, H., Portmann, B., *et al.* (2006) Antioxidants versus corticosteroids in the treatment of severe alcoholic hepatitis–a randomised clinical trial. *J Hepatol* **44**, 784–790.

Pieber, K., Crevenna, R., Nuhr, M.J., *et al.* (2006) Aerobic capacity, muscle strength and health-related quality of life before and after orthotopic liver transplantation: preliminary data of an Austrian transplantation centre. *J Rehabil Med* **38**, 322–328.

Pikul, J., Sharpe, M.D., Lowndes, R., *et al.* (1994) Degree of preoperative malnutrition is predictive of postoperative morbidity and mortality in liver transplant recipients. *Transplantation* **57**, 469–472.

Pirlich, M., Selberg, O., Boker, K., *et al.* (1996) The creatinine approach to estimate skeletal muscle mass in patients with cirrhosis. *Hepatology* **24**, 1422–1427.

Plank, L.D., Gane, E.J., Peng, S., *et al.* (2008) Nocturnal nutritional supplementation improves total body protein status of patients with liver cirrhosis: a randomized 12-month trial. *Hepatology* **48**, 557–566.

Plevak, D.J., DiCecco, S.R., Wiesner, R.H., *et al.* (1994) Nutritional support for liver transplantation: identifying caloric and protein requirements. *Mayo Clin Proc* **69**, 225–230.

Porayko, M.K., Wiesner, R.H., Hay, J.E., *et al.* (1991) Bone disease in liver transplant recipients: incidence, timing, and risk factors. *Transplant Proc* **23**, 1462–1465.

Purohit, V., Abdelmalek, M.F., Barve, S., *et al.* (2007) Role of S-adenosylmethionine, folate, and betaine in the treatment of alcoholic liver disease: summary of a symposium. *Am J Clin Nutr* **86**, 14–24.

Quigley, E.M.M. (1996) Gastrointestinal dysfunction in liver disease and portal hypertension. Gut-liver interaction revisited. *Dig Dis Sci* **41**, 557–561.

Rafiq, N. and Younossi, Z.M. (2008) Effects of weight loss on nonalcoholic fatty liver disease. *Semin Liver Dis* **28**, 427–433.

Rambaldi, A. and Gluud, C. (2006) S-adenosyl-L-methionine for alcoholic liver diseases. *Cochrane Database Syst Rev* CD002235.

Reilly, J., Mehta, R., Teperman, L., *et al.* (1990) Nutritional support after liver transplantation: a randomized prospective study. *JPEN J Parenter Enteral Nutr* **14**, 386–391.

Roggero, P., Cataliotti, E., Ulla, L., *et al.* (1997) Factors influencing malnutrition in children waiting for liver transplants. *Am J Clin Nutr* **65**, 1852–1857.

Russell, R.M. (2000) The vitamin A spectrum: from deficiency to toxicity. *Am J Clin Nutr* **71**, 878–884.

Sakurai, Y., Zhang, X-J., and Wolfe, R.R. (1994) Effect of tumor necrosis factor on substrate and amino acid kinetics in conscious dogs. *Am J Physiol* **266**, E936–E945.

Sánchez-Lozada, L.G., Mu, W., Roncal, C., *et al.* (2010) Comparison of free fructose and glucose to sucrose in the ability to cause fatty liver. *Eur J Nutr* **49**, 1–9.

Sanyal, A.J., Chalasani, N., Kowdley, K.V., *et al.* (2010) Pioglitazone, vitamin E, or placebo for nonalcoholic steatohepatitis. *N Engl J Med* **62**, 1675–1685.

Sarin, S.K., Dhingra, N., Bansal, A., *et al.* (1997) Dietary and nutritional abnormalities in alcoholic liver disease: a comparison with chronic alcoholics without liver disease. *Am J Gastroenterol* **92**, 777–783.

Schuppan, D., Jia, J-D., Brinkhaus, B., *et al.* (1999) Herbal products for liver diseases: a therapeutic challenge for the new millennium. *Hepatology* **30**, 1099–1104.

Shaw, B.W., Jr, Wood, R.P., Gordon, R.D., *et al.* (1985) Influence of selected patient variables and operative blood loss on six-month survival following liver transplantation. *Semin Liver Dis* **5**, 385–393.

Shronts, E.P. (1983) Nutritional assessment of adults with end stage hepatic failure. *Nutr Clin Pract* **3**, 113–119.

Shronts, E.P., Teasley, K.M., Thoele, S.L., *et al.* (1987) Nutritional support of the adult liver transplant candidate. *J Am Diet Assoc* **87**, 441–451.

Sokol, R.J. (1994) Fat-soluble vitamins and their importance in patients with cholestatic liver diseases. *Gastroenterol Clin North Am* **23**, 673–705.

Sokol, R.J. (1996) Antioxidant defenses in metal-induced liver damage. *Semin Liver Dis* **16**, 39–46.

Spruss, A., Kanuri, G., Wagnerberger, S., *et al.* (2009) Toll-like receptor 4 is involved in the development of fructose-induced hepatic steatosis in mice. *Hepatology* **50**, 1094–1104.

Stickel, F., Hoehn, B., Schuppan, D., *et al.* (2003) Review article: Nutritional therapy in alcoholic liver disease. *Aliment Pharmacol Ther* **18**, 357–373.

Suto, G., Kiraly, A., and Tache, Y. (1994) Interleukin-1beta inhibits gastric emptying in rats: mediation through prostaglandin and corticotropin-releasing factor. *Gastroenterology* **106**, 1568–1575.

Takahashi, M., Saito, H., Higashimoto, M., *et al.* (2007) Possible inhibitory effect of oral zinc supplementation on hepatic fibrosis through downregulation of TIMP-1: a pilot study. *Hepatol Res* **37**, 405–409.

Tendler, D., Lin, S., Yancy, W.S., Jr, *et al.* (2007) The effect of a low-carbohydrate, ketogenic diet on nonalcoholic fatty liver disease: a pilot study. *Dig Dis Sci* **52**, 589–593.

Thompson, G.R., Barrowman, J., Gutierrez, L., *et al.* (1971) Actions of neomycin on the intraluminal phase of lipid absorption. *J Clin Invest* **50**, 321–323.

Thuluvath, P.J. and Triger, D.R. (1989) Autonomic neuropathy and chronic liver disease. *Q J Med* **72**, 737–747.

Thuluvath, P.J. and Triger, D.R. (1994) Evaluation of nutritional status by using anthropometry in adults with alcoholic and nonalcoholic liver disease. *Am J Clin Nutr* **60**, 269–273.

Vaisma, N., Katzman, H., Carmiel-Haggai, M., *et al.* (2010) Breakfast improves cognitive function in cirrhotic patients with cognitive impairment. *Am J Clin Nutr* **92,** 137–140.

Vlahcevic, Z.R., Buhac, I., Farrar, J.T., *et al.* (1971) Bile acid metabolism in patients with cirrhosis. 1. Kinetic aspects of cholic acid metabolism. *Gastroenterology* **60,** 491–498.

von Essen, M.R., Kongsbak, M., Schjerling, P., *et al.* (2010) Vitamin D controls T cell antigen receptor signaling and activation of human T cells. *Nat Immunol* **11,** 344–349.

Yang, F., de Villiers, W.J.S., McClain, C.J., *et al.* (1998) Green tea polyphenols block endotoxin-induced tumor necrosis factor-x production and lethality in a murine model. *J Nutr* **128,** 2334–2340.

Yki-Järvinen, H. (2010) Nutritional modulation of nonalcoholic fatty liver disease and insulin resistance: human data. *Curr Opin Clin Nutr Metab Care* **13,** 709–714.

Zhong, W., McClain, C.J., Cave, M., *et al.* (2010) The role of zinc deficiency in alcohol-induced intestinal barrier dysfunction. *Am J Physiol Gastrointest Liver Physiol* **298,** G625–G633.

Zhou, Z., Kang, X., Jiang, Y., *et al.* (2007) Preservation of hepatocyte nuclear factor-4 alpha is associated with zinc protection against TNF-alpha hepatotoxicity in mice. *Exp Biol Med (Maywood)* **232,** 622–628.

Zivkovic, A.M., German, J.B., and Sanyal, A.J. (2007) Comparative review of diets for the metabolic syndrome: implications for nonalcoholic fatty liver disease. *Am J Clin Nutr* **86,** 285–300.

55

ALCOHOL: ITS ROLE IN NUTRITION AND HEALTH

PAOLO M. SUTER, MD

University Hospital, Zurich, Switzerland

Summary

In view of the importance of alcoholic beverages in daily life as well as its absolute priority in metabolism, alcohol has considerable potential to affect the nutritional status and metabolism of all essential nutrients including the different energy sources. In view of the great variability among alcohol drinkers in patterns of drinking, amounts ingested, ingestion of other nutrients, metabolic characteristics, genetic factors, and lifestyle characteristics (such as exercise or smoking behavior), the effects of alcohol on nutritional status and disease risk are very heterogeneous. Alcohol-associated malnutrition includes both primary and secondary malnutrition. Because of the comparatively high energy content of alcohol, it displaces other energy sources and thus many essential nutrients in the diet, thereby lowering the intake of most nutrients (primary malnutrition). Gastrointestinal and metabolic complications of heavy alcohol intake (especially liver dysfunction) lead to so-called secondary malnutrition. Anorexia and vomiting from alcoholic gastritis further promote inadequate intakes of food. Malabsorption of nearly all nutrients can develop as a result of mucosal dysfunction, liver insufficiency, and pancreatic insufficiency. Alcoholic liver dysfunction causes a reduced capacity to transport nutrients in the blood, a reduced storage capacity, and an insufficient activation of nutrients such as vitamins. In addition, alcohol increases the excretion of nutrients in the urine and bile. In alcoholic patients, several mechanisms for the development of malnutrition usually occur simultaneously.

The effect of alcohol on morbidity and mortality is biphasic, and the relationship is J-shaped: low levels of ingestion are associated with reduced morbidity and mortality risks, whereas abstinence and higher levels of ingestion are associated with a higher mortality risk due to different cancers, alcoholic liver disease, and cardiovascular diseases such as arrhythmias, alcoholic cardiomyopathy, hypertension, and stroke. The reduced mortality risk at lower intakes is explained by the risk of coronary artery disease and a reduced risk of ischemic stroke. The amount of alcohol ingestion at the nadir of mortality risk is not known and varies from study to study and from one individual to another. The hallmark of excessive alcohol intake is metabolic and structural alterations at the level of the liver, and liver cirrhosis is the leading cause of death in heavy drinkers.

Often, both positive and negative effects occur. In view of the heterogeneity of responses for any given alcohol dose, the formulation of public health recommendations for safe consumption levels is becoming increasingly difficult. In any case, alcohol should not be recommended for health reasons or for health maintenance, especially as long as there are no specific, sensitive predictors for harmful alcohol use and abuse. In the setting of an overall healthy lifestyle with respect to nutrition and physical activity, light to moderate alcohol consumption may add to the quality of life; however, the benefits and risks are not equal for all.

Present Knowledge in Nutrition, Tenth Edition. Edited by John W. Erdman Jr, Ian A. Macdonald and Steven H. Zeisel.
© 2012 International Life Sciences Institute. Published 2012 by John Wiley & Sons, Inc.

Introduction

Alcohol is a major part of daily life globally, even in low-income countries. Presently, about 61% of US adults (67% of men and 55% of women) are current drinkers, about 14% are former drinkers, 24% of the adults are lifetime abstainers, and approximately 5% of the adults are classified as heavier drinkers (National Institute on Alcohol Abuse and Alcoholism (NIAAA), 2009; Schoenborn and Adams, 2010). Despite the wide acceptance of alcohol consumption in most societies, it remains an important cause and modulator of disease risk: worldwide, alcohol causes about 2.5 million (3.8% of total) deaths and 69.4 million (4.5% of total) of disability-adjusted life years (DALYs) (World Health Organization, 2010). Unintentional injuries alone account for about one-third of the 2.5 million deaths, whereas neuropsychiatric conditions account for close to 40% of the 69.4 million DALYs (WHO, 2010). With approximately 79 000 deaths per year attributable to excessive drinking, alcohol consumption represents the third leading cause of death after tobacco and poor diet/physical inactivity (Mokdad et al., 2004; NIAAA, 2009). Compared with other food items, alcohol has three characteristic features: depending on the absolute amount and frequency of consumption, it can be regarded as a nutrient, a toxin, or a psychoactive drug. Each consumer determines which aspect of alcohol will prevail for him- or herself.

The energy content of alcohol, compared with other energy sources, is rather high (1 g alcohol = 7.1 kcal = 29.7 kJ), and thus alcohol represents an important source of energy for many alcohol consumers. Alcohol energy contributes, depending on sex and age, to 1.3–5.5% of total energy intake of the US diet (mean for all adult men/women = 4.3%/2.4%), but in heavy drinkers it may contribute up to 50% of the daily energy intake. In view of the importance of alcoholic beverages as a source of energy, alcohol has a high potential to displace other essential nutrients.

Because of its potential toxicity and the inability of the body to store alcohol, it has to be eliminated as quickly as possible from the body. This absolute priority in metabolism is a major cause of the metabolic effects of alcohol on nearly all nutrients, on most if not all organ systems, and, consequently, on disease risks (Figure 55.1).

In view of the great variability among alcohol drinkers in patterns of drinking, amounts ingested, ingestion of other nutrients, and metabolic characteristics, as well as lifestyle characteristics (such as exercise or smoking behavior), the heterogeneous effects of alcohol on nutritional status and disease risk are not surprising. These effects are further complicated by genetically determined differences in alcohol metabolism (Higuchi et al., 2004; Druesne-Pecollo et al., 2009). For the purposes of this discussion, one "standard" drink corresponds to 0.6 fluid ounces or 14 g of alcohol, the amount contained in approximately 300 mL of beer, 150 mL of table wine (12% by volume), or 45 mL of liquor (40% by volume). A review of alcohol's effects on selected nutrients and on disease risk follows.

Alcohol Metabolism

Alcohol is rapidly absorbed from the stomach and the jejunum, and is distributed in the total water compartment of the body. Most of it is metabolized in the liver; however, a small amount may be metabolized in the stomach mucosa (i.e. during the first-pass metabolism) (Paton, 2005). The first-pass metabolism is higher in men than in women, declines with age, and is affected by different drugs such as aspirin, which decreases it. Alcohol can be metabolized via three different enzyme systems and, under usual conditions, depending on the dose and frequency of consumption, is metabolized by two major pathways: for light to moderate levels of intake, alcohol is metabolized in the alcohol dehydrogenase (ADH) pathway; for higher levels of intake, it is predominantly metabolized in the microsomal ethanol oxidizing system (MEOS) (Lieber and DeCarli, 1970). The oxidation of alcohol in both the ADH and the MEOS pathways leads to the production of acetaldehyde, which is further metabolized to acetate by acetaldehyde dehydrogenase (ALDH). Acetate is shuttled to the peripheral tissues and used as a source of energy. The metabolism of alcohol induces a change in the redox potential in the liver. This change contributes to different metabolic and clinical consequences and to functional abnormalities such as suppression of the Krebs cycle, with an increased transformation of pyruvate to lactate, impaired gluconeogenesis and hypoglycemia, greater fatty acid synthesis, reduced urate excretion, and hyperuricemia (Watson and Preedy, 2003).

These alcohol-induced metabolic perturbations depend on the dose of alcohol and the duration of consumption, but most metabolic, endocrine, and functional systems of the body are affected (Figure 55.1). The metabolic consequences of alcohol may be mediated directly or indirectly. Direct alcohol toxicity leads to an alteration in cellular

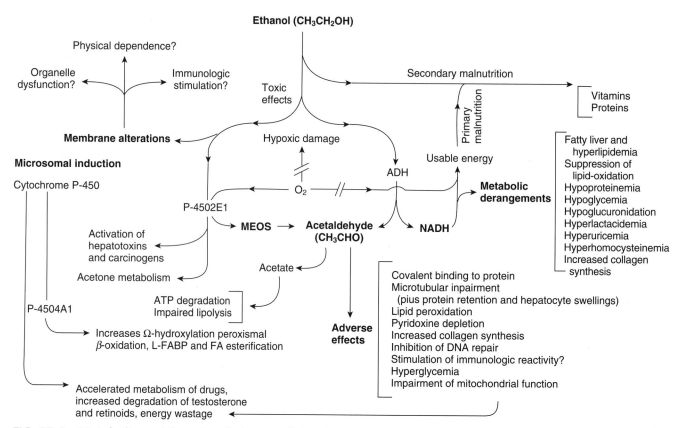

FIG. 55.1 Metabolic and functional abnormalities due to alcohol consumption. L-FABP, Liver-type fatty acid binding protein; MEOS, microsomal ethanol-oxidizing system. Reproduced with permission from Lieber (1995).

function resulting from alterations in membrane fluidity and in the intracellular redox potential, and acetaldehyde toxicity. Acetaldehyde elicits many different effects, such as increased free radical production and lipid peroxidation, inhibition of protein synthesis, and impaired vitamin metabolism (Niemelä, 2007; Guo and Ren, 2010).

The metabolism of alcohol shows a wide inter-individual variability that is modulated by different genotypes of the alcohol-metabolizing enzymes ADH and ALDH (Li, 2000; Druesne-Pecollo et al., 2009). Depending on the ADH genotype, higher maximal alcohol and acetaldehyde concentrations and slower elimination of alcohol are found, a situation that may lead to increased direct and indirect alcohol toxicity and thus a different alcohol-related disease pattern. In many people of Asian origin, the activity of ALDH may be low and thus cause a typical facial flushing reaction and headaches after ingestion of even small amounts of alcohol.

Although the capacity to metabolize alcohol varies widely, a healthy person metabolizes alcohol on average at 5 to 7g/hour. There is no useful and safe strategy (except a high fructose intake leading to a reduced nicotinamide adenine dinucleotide reoxidation) known to increase the rate of alcohol degradation.

The Nutritional Assessment of the Alcoholic Patient

Nutritional assessment of the alcoholic patient is a challenging task in either the clinical or community setting. The clinical signs of alcohol-related malnutrition depend on the stage of alcoholism, the level of socioeconomic integration, social and familial networks, associated alcohol- and non-alcohol-related diseases (especially liver disease), and concomitant medication intake of the patient (Santolaria-Fernandez et al., 1995). Socioeconomically integrated heavy drinkers, in the absence of any clinically manifested somatic diseases, rarely show signs of malnutrition (Salaspuro, 1993). With the progression of alcoholism, clinical signs from all organ systems and malnutrition may prevail. Different clinical signs of malnutrition may be found; for example, thin arms and legs due to muscle wasting (Urbano-Marquez and Fernandez-Sola, 2004; Fernandez-Solà *et al.*, 2007), edema (protein deficiency), glossitis (B-vitamin deficiency), and scaly, dry skin (zinc and essential fatty acid deficiency). Spider nevi and multiple hematomas due to easy bruising (vitamin C and K deficiency) may be found on the skin (Smith and Fenske, 2000). The parotid glands are often enlarged due to chronic parotitis. The patients may present with new bone fractures and several old costal fractures, and advanced osteoporosis (especially in men), attributable in part to impaired vitamin D nutriture and metabolism.

Alcohol-associated endocrine pathologies may manifest themselves as gynecomastia, testicular atrophy, and loss of body hair. Neurological signs may be limited to peripheral neuropathy (B-vitamin deficiency), different central nervous system impairments (see section on thiamin), or the full clinical picture of stroke. An impaired dark adaptation due to zinc deficiency is fairly common and should not be misinterpreted as vitamin A deficiency. In general, the nutritional assessment of the alcoholic patient is not different from the assessment of other patients. The biochemical assessment includes measurement of the conventional alcohol markers (i.e. liver transaminase levels and red blood cell mean cell volume) in combination with biochemical markers of nutritional status. Other newly developed biochemical markers for alcohol consumption [such as carbohydrate-deficient transferrin (CDT), fatty acid ethyl esters (FAEEs), or ethyl glucuronide (EtG)] may be helpful (Borucki *et al.*, 2005; Das *et al.*, 2008; Delanghe and De Buyzere, 2009; Mancinelli and Ceccanti, 2009). Chronic alcohol consumption in the range of 50–70 g/day induces hepatocytes to produce a transferrin molecule that is deficient in carbohydrates. The CDT is a marker for sustained and harmful alcohol consumption and returns slowly (the half-life of CDT is approximately 14 days) to normal upon cessation of alcohol intake. CDT measurements may be especially useful for the follow-up of patients in detoxification programs. Elevated levels of high-density lipoprotein (HDL) cholesterol, uric acid, and fasting triacylglycerol levels without other explanation may be signs of excessive alcohol intake.

The assessment of alcohol intake at either the population or individual level is very difficult, especially for drinking in the low to moderate range. Although heavy alcohol intake is detected sooner or later by typical clinical signs or laboratory test results, there is no reliable clinical sign or biochemical marker for the assessment of light to moderate alcohol intake. Intentional or unintentional underreporting and overreporting often lead to uncontrollable bias in epidemiological and clinical studies. The difficulty in assessing low to moderate levels of alcohol consumption represents probably one of the most important causes of inconsistency in research findings.

Alcohol and Nutrition

As a function of the amount of alcohol consumed, the duration of intake, and any associated diseases, drinking can impair the status of all nutrients. Alcohol-associated malnutrition includes both primary and secondary malnutrition. Because of the comparatively high energy content of alcohol, it displaces other energy sources and thus many essential nutrients in the diet, thereby lowering the intake of most nutrients (primary malnutrition). Gastrointestinal and metabolic complications of heavy alcohol intake (especially liver dysfunction) lead to so-called secondary malnutrition (Figure 55.1). Anorexia and vomiting from alcoholic gastritis further promote inadequate intakes of food. Malabsorption of nearly all nutrients can develop as a result of mucosal dysfunction, liver insufficiency, and pancreatic insufficiency (Seitz and Suter, 1994). Alcoholic liver dysfunction causes a reduced capacity to transport nutrients in the blood, a reduced storage capacity, and insufficient activation of nutrients such as vitamins. In addition, alcohol increases the excretion of nutrients in the urine and bile. In alcoholic patients, several mechanisms for the development of malnutrition usually occur simultaneously (Table 55.1) (Seitz and Suter, 1994). After gastric bypass surgery bariatric patients with a higher alcohol intake might elicit a higher risk of alcohol-induced nutritional disorders as well as higher alcohol toxicity due to an altered alcohol absorption kinetic, nutrient malabsorption as well as inadequate nutrient intake (Bal *et al.*, 2010; Maluenda *et al.*, 2010).

Effects of Alcohol on Energy Metabolism

In view of the increasing prevalence of obesity, the effects of alcohol on energy balance and energy metabolism are of great importance (Suter, 2005). Because alcohol is mostly devoid of other nutrients and ingestion is not regulated (in contrast to other substrates, there is no

TABLE 55.1　Alcohol and nutritional status: possible mechanisms of alcohol-mediated toxicity

Mechanism	Possible causes
Reduced dietary intake	Poverty
	Displacement of normal food
	Inappetance due to direct alcohol toxicity and secondarily due to disease (e.g. alcoholic gastritis)
	Anorexia due to medications
Impaired digestion	Alcoholic gastritis
	Impaired bile and pancreatic enzymes secretion
	Direct mucosal damage and impairment of mucosal enzymes (e.g. folyl conjugase)
	Altered gastrointestinal mobility
Malabsorption	Direct mucosal damage
	Indirect damage (e.g. due to folate deficiency)
	Motility changes including accelerated small intestinal transit time and diarrhea
	Pancreatic insufficiency
	Interactions with medications
Impaired transport in the circulation	Decreased synthesis of transport proteins due to liver damage
Impaired activation	Liver damage
	Inadequate supply of cofactors
Decreased storage	Liver pathology
	Alcoholic myopathy/sarcopenia/cachexia
Increased losses	Increased excretion in urine and bile
	Increased urinary losses due to medications
	Increased fecal losses
Increased requirements	Due to the above factors
	Increased metabolic rate

mechanism such as appetite regulation or hunger), alcohol's calories are unregulated, empty calories (Westerterp-Plantenga and Verwegen, 1999; Caton *et al.*, 2007). The importance of alcohol as a risk factor for weight gain and obesity is disputed (Liu *et al.*, 1994; Sakurai *et al.*, 1997; Suter, 2005). For weight maintenance, the energy balance has to be equilibrated, and alcohol has been reported to affect all components of the energy balance negatively, favoring a positive energy balance (Suter, 2005).

Because moderate drinkers generally add alcohol to their usual food intake, a positive energy balance with an increased risk of weight gain and obesity will result unless compensated for by other means. This risk is increased by the combination of a high-fat diet and even moderate alcohol intake because of the hyperphagic effect of alcohol (Yeomans, *et al.*, 1999). Alcohol substitution (i.e. the usual food energy sources are substituted by alcohol) is the typical feature of the heavy drinker and will result in malnutrition and weight loss (Figure 55.2).

Depending on the amount and frequency of consumption, alcohol leads to an increase in energy expenditure. In young, moderate drinkers, the addition and the substitution of 25% of their daily energy requirements by alcohol (corresponding to 96 ± 4 g alcohol) leads to an increased 24-hour energy expenditure of $7\% \pm 1\%$ and $4\% \pm 1\%$, respectively (Suter *et al.*, 1992). These increases of energy expenditure correspond to a thermic effect of 20–25% of the energy content of the ingested alcohol. Other studies (Suter *et al.*, 1994; Suter, 2005) reported a thermic effect of alcohol in healthy, moderate consumers in the range of 15–25%, which is rather high compared with other energy sources (e.g. the thermic effect of a mixed meal is approximately 12%).

Presently, it is not clear what fraction of the alcohol energy could be used for adenosine triphosphate (ATP) production. In their classical studies more than 100 years ago, Atwater and Benedict (1902) suggested that alcohol energy seems to be equivalent to the energy of carbohydrates or fat. However, subsequent studies revealed that, as a function of the pathway of the metabolic degradation of alcohol (i.e. ADH vs. MEOS), lower amounts of ATP are produced than theoretical calculations would suggest (Lieber, 1991). Nevertheless, epidemiological and experimental studies suggest that, despite some energy wastage, alcohol calories are largely a usable energy source in the moderate consumer.

Alcohol also affects the energy balance equation by its effects on substrate balance. Independently, whether alcohol is added to or substituted for usual food, lipid oxidation is suppressed approximately by a third (Suter *et al.*, 1992), producing a positive fat balance. The positive fat balance is not caused by a de novo lipogenesis from alcohol, but by acetate being used in the peripheral organs (mainly muscle) as a source of energy at the expense of a lower fat oxidation. Use of stable isotope mass spectrometry techniques has shown that most (98%) of the carbons of a moderate alcohol load (25 g) *are* transported as acetate to the peripheral tissues, and only a negligible amount of the ingested dose (<1%) is used for de novo lipogenesis (Siler *et al.*, 1999).

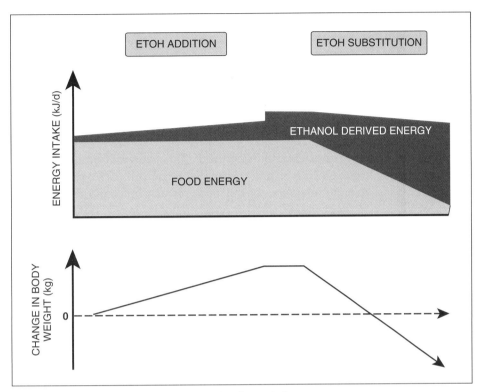

FIG. 55.2 Effect of alcohol on energy intake and body weight.

Despite these effects of alcohol on energy balance, some epidemiological and experimental studies were unable to identify moderate alcohol consumption as a risk factor for obesity (Liu *et al.*, 1994; Rohrer *et al.*, 2005; Wang *et al.*, 2010). Cross-sectional studies described positive or null associations between alcohol intake and body weight in men and inverse or null associations in women. There are only a few prospective studies about this association and they are equally controversial. Data from a 13-year follow-up in the Women's Health Study (Wang *et al.*, 2010) found that initially normal-weight light-to-moderate alcohol-consuming women gained less weight and had a lower risk of becoming overweight and/or obese as compared with non-drinking women. These controversial findings are not surprising in view of the difficulty in assessing alcohol intake and other lifestyle parameters that may compensate for some of the effects of alcohol. Furthermore socioeconomic factors determine alcohol consumption pattern and health behaviors (Schoenborn and Adams, 2010), including coping with factors affecting body-weight changes which explain the controversial outcomes in most if not all studies (Britton *et al.*, 2008). Because of the suppression of lipid oxidation and the resulting positive energy balance, even moderate amounts of alcohol have to be regarded as a risk factor for weight gain and obesity when not counterbalanced by other means (i.e. reduced energy intake and/or increased energy expenditure by physical activity). To counteract the effects of alcohol on fat oxidation, fat intake should be kept as low as possible and, whenever alcohol is consumed, fat intake has to be reduced, ideally in proportion to the amount of alcohol ingested to remain in substrate balance.

Alcohol enhances the abdominal deposition of fat (Dallongeville *et al.*, 1998), which is associated with several adverse health outcomes such as hypertension or dyslipidemia (Suter *et al.*, 1995; Sakurai *et al.*, 1997), and represents a typical feature of the metabolic syndrome. Again, the later relationship is complicated by epidemiologic findings reporting a lower prevalence of the typical features of the metabolic syndrome in mild to moderate alcohol consumers (Freiberg *et al.*, 2004; Alkerwi *et al.*, 2009).

Effects of Alcohol on Lipid Metabolism

As a function of the amount consumed, the frequency of drinking, and the presence of concomitant diseases (especially liver disease, overweight, and obesity), alcohol affects all lipoprotein fractions in the blood (Barona and Lieber, 1998; Brinton, 2010). The development of a fatty liver, a characteristic early sign of alcoholic liver disease, is partly caused by the alcohol-induced suppression of lipid oxidation in the liver, by an increased influx of fat from the peripheral tissues and by alcohol-induced alterations of transcriptional controls of lipid metabolism (Sozio and Crabb, 2008). These early changes are also associated with the typical signs of alcoholic hyperlipidemia, which include elevated serum triacylglycerol levels caused by an increased hepatic secretion of very-low-density lipoproteins (VLDL) and a diminished peripheral removal of the VLDLs resulting from impaired lipoprotein lipase. The rise in triacylglycerol levels is increased by the ingestion of a diet rich in fat. The effects of alcohol on triacylgylcerol levels are also seen during the postprandial phase; however, they can be partly counteracted by a concomitant reduction in fat intake and/or higher physical activity before or after the meal (Suter *et al.*, 1999). A recent study described a J-shaped relation between alcohol intake and plasma triacylglycerol levels, findings which are difficult to explain and which need to be confirmed in other studies (Tolstrup *et al.*, 2009). Obviously the response to alcohol might vary in certain subgroups of the population as a function of genetic and/or environmental factors.

The chronic moderate ingestion of alcohol leads to an increase in HDL cholesterol, which may be a major mechanism for the beneficial cardiovascular effects of alcohol (Manttari *et al.*, 1997). The alcohol-associated increase in HDL cholesterol may have multiple causes, including increased hepatic production and secretion of apoproteins, increased peripheral production due to lipid exchange within the different lipoprotein fractions, and decreased catabolism of the HDL particle caused by alcohol's effects on specific enzymes involved in lipid transfer or effects on postprandial lipemia (Sozio and Crabb, 2008). The HDL-raising effects of alcohol are nonlinear, showing a threshold effect on HDL cholesterol (Johansen *et al.*, 2003), and depend on different factors such as gender, body mass index, smoking habits, and genotype (e.g. ADH or apolipoprotein E genotype) (Lussier-Cacan *et al.*, 2002). One study (Lussier-Cacan *et al.*, 2002) reported that alcohol consumption intensifies the increase in low density lipoprotein (LDL) cholesterol and the decrease in HDL cholesterol associated with increasing BMI only in women with the apolipoprotein E genotype ε4/3. In this context, it should be remembered that obesity (besides physical

inactivity and smoking) represents one of the major causes of low HDL cholesterol.

The effects of alcohol on LDL cholesterol are only minor and less consistent than the effects on the other lipoprotein fractions. In animal studies, alcohol led to a decrease in LDL clearance due to a decreased hepatic LDL-receptor expression and specific effects on signaling pathways in lipid metabolism (Sozio and Crabb, 2008). Alcohol may unfavorably affect the size of the lipoprotein particles, especially LDL particles (Ayaori *et al.*, 1997). During the last few years, evidence has accumulated suggesting that lipoprotein subclass distributions according to particle size may be important modifiers of atherogenic risk. Individuals with a high concentration of small, dense LDL particles and their metabolic precursors, the large VLDL particles, have a higher cardiovascular risk than those with predominantly large LDL particles and small VLDL particles. The role of certain polyphenolic compounds of wine as modulators of LDL oxidation rates in vivo is uncertain (Fuhrman *et al.*, 1995), especially given the strong pro-oxidative effects of alcohol and the extremely variable bioavailability and bioefficacy of these compounds (Manach *et al.*, 2005; Ajmo *et al.*, 2008). The atherogenic lipoprotein(a) is lowered by alcohol consumption. A minor fraction of ethanol is metabolized by the formation of fatty acid ethyl esters (FAEEs) (Lange, 1982). Because these FAEEs accumulate in different tissues, they may be of pathophysiologic relevance in the development of alcohol-related pathologies (Petersen *et al.*, 2009), and they may represent useful markers of alcohol intake (Süße *et al.*, 2010).

Alcohol and Carbohydrate Metabolism

The effects of alcohol on glucose handling are multiple as a function of the dosage, duration of alcohol intake, and overall nutritional status. In healthy, moderate drinkers with normal food intake, alcohol's effects on carbohydrate metabolism are of hardly any clinical relevance. By contrast, excessive alcohol consumption may be associated with the typical clinical entity of alcoholic pancreatitis (Apte *et al.*, 2009), which results in exocrine pancreatic insufficiency with maldigestion and malabsorption. The reduced forms of nicotinamide-adenine dinucleotide (NADH) and acetate produced during alcohol metabolism represent major modulators of glucose metabolism.

The increased production of reducing equivalents caused by the oxidation of alcohol leads to a decrease in gluconeogenesis (Siler *et al.*, 1998). This decrease may bring about clinically dangerous and life-threatening hypoglycemia, especially in the heavy drinker with an overall inadequate diet and poor intake of carbohydrates (and thus low glycogen stores) (Flanagan *et al.*, 1998). This effect is being reinforced in people with diabetes by the ingestion of oral hypoglycemic agents, insulin, or both (Pedersen-Bjergaard *et al.*, 2005). The alcohol-induced reduction in gluconeogenesis also occurs in the fed state, but is usually compensated for by the glucose in the ingested food. The clinical features of hypoglycemia may share some of the signs of alcohol intoxication, and when it is misdiagnosed as simple alcohol intoxication deleterious health consequences may result. In addition, alcohol produces changes in the secretory response of different counter-regulatory hormones (such as epinephrine or growth hormone), thus resulting in the absence of the potential clinical warning signs of hypoglycemia (Pedersen-Bjergaard *et al.*, 2005). Alcohol also inhibits the storage of glycogen, further increasing the predisposition to hypoglycemia when carbohydrate intake is insufficient.

Light to moderate amounts of alcohol are inversely related to fasting and post-load insulin levels (Crandall *et al.*, 2009), which may represent an additional mechanistic factor for the cardioprotective effects of low-level alcohol consumption. In agreement with this, moderate alcohol intake has been associated with a reduction in coronary heart disease mortality in persons with type 2 diabetes mellitus (Valmadrid *et al.*, 1999) and with a lower risk for the development of the metabolic syndrome (Djousse *et al.*, 2004).

Effect of Alcohol on Fat-Soluble Vitamins

Vitamin A

Alcohol may interfere with the metabolism of all fat-soluble vitamins. Retinol (vitamin A), also an alcohol, shares some metabolic pathways with ethanol and thus has a high potential to be affected negatively by alcohol consumption. In light to moderate drinkers, vitamin A metabolism is not altered. Despite low intakes, frank vitamin A deficiency is rarely seen in alcoholics, probably because of the rather large hepatic stores of this vitamin. However, chronic alcohol consumption may lead to low levels of vitamin A in plasma, and, when alcoholic liver disease is present, decreased hepatic vitamin A levels are found. These lower levels are a result of an increased degradation

of the vitamin as a consequence of the induction of microsomal enzymes (Leo and Lieber, 1999) and the alcohol-induced decreased synthesis of retinol-binding protein (McClain *et al.*, 1979). This condition may lead to the prescription of vitamin A supplements; however, higher levels of vitamin A intake (independent of alcohol intake) are associated with considerable hepatotoxicity (Leo and Lieber, 1999), and alcohol represents one of the most important modulators of vitamin A toxicity – especially in the presence of liver disease. In the setting of chronic alcohol consumption, an increased production of polar retinol metabolites seems to be a central mechanism of hepatocellular damage (Dan *et al.*, 2005). A tissue-specific increase in endogenous all-*trans* retinoic acid may contribute to chronic ethanol toxicity (Kane *et al.*, 2010; Wolf, 2010). Further alcohol affects the expression and activation of retinoic acid receptors, thus impairing different signalling pathways (Kumar *et al.*, 2010).

Although the vitamin A precursor β-carotene is thought to bear no toxicity in humans, one epidemiological study reported an increased lung cancer rate in β-carotene-supplemented smokers, especially in those who were also drinking alcohol, an increase most likely due to alcohol-induced alterations in β-carotene metabolism (Albanes *et al.*, 1996). The negative effects of alcohol observed in this study were seen at rather low dosage levels, starting at ≥12.9 g/day. Although heavy drinkers (≥200 g/day) show lower β-carotene plasma concentrations than do control subjects, they show higher β-carotene serum levels than those drinking less (Ahmed *et al.*, 1994). These higher levels may be caused by an impaired utilization or excretion of β-carotene due to liver damage or a partial shift in the degradation of β-carotene from central cleavage to eccentric cleavage (Leo and Lieber, 1999). A recent rat study (Luvizotto *et al.*, 2010) showed that chronic alcohol intake up-regulates the hepatic expression of the carotenoid cleavage enzymes (15,15′-monooxygenase 1 (CMO1)). In view of the present evidence, it is not advisable to routinely prescribe either high-dose β-carotene, other carotenoids (Veeramachaneni *et al.*, 2008) or vitamin A supplements to heavy consumers of alcohol.

Vitamin E

Levels of vitamin E are reduced in chronic alcohol consumers independent of cirrhosis as a result of reduced intake and higher requirements (Bell *et al.*, 1992). Vitamin E supplementation has been reported to reduce alcohol-induced lipid peroxidation; however, vitamin E supplementation did not affect laboratory or clinical outcomes (de la Maza *et al.*, 1995; Sario *et al.*, 2007). Tocotrienol, an isoform of vitamin E, has been reported in a rat model to have protective effects on the development of alcoholic neuropathy (Tiwari *et al.*, 2009b) and neuroinflammation (Tiwari *et al.*, 2009a). If vitamin E supplements are given, an adequate vitamin K nutriture should be ensured, given that a high dose of vitamin E may lead to impairment of the vitamin K cycle and an increased tendency to bleed (Machlin, 1989).

Vitamin K

Data about the effect of alcohol on vitamin K nutriture is scarce. Acute and chronic alcohol consumption has been reported to lead to alterations in gamma-carboxylated molecules such as osteocalcin (Nyquist *et al.*, 1996). In the setting of alcoholic liver disease, vitamin K might have favorable effects on bone health (Shiomi *et al.*, 2002).

Vitamin D

Heavier alcohol consumption (with and without liver disease) may be associated with an increased fracture risk due to indirect and direct alcohol effects on bone metabolism and on vitamin D metabolism (Nyquist *et al.*, 1997; Alvisa-Negrín *et al.*, 2009; Guañabens and Parés, 2010). Heavier drinkers have a lower intake, absorption, and activation of vitamin D (Laitinen *et al.*, 1990). In addition, because of alcohol's effects on the target organs, tissue-specific vitamin D effects may be impaired. According to animal studies vitamin D deficiency may play a role in alcoholic myopathy (González-Reimers *et al.*, 2010).

Effects of Alcohol on Water-Soluble Vitamins

The metabolism of all water-soluble vitamins may be affected by the ingestion of alcohol. Alcohol's effects on water-soluble vitamin metabolism are dose dependent, and, in the range of light to moderate alcohol intake in healthy subjects eating a balanced diet, no adverse effects are expected. In heavy drinkers, a deficiency of several vitamins is usually present (Jamieson *et al.*, 1999), therefore the typical clinical signs of a *single* vitamin deficiency are not necessarily seen. In this section, alcohol's effects on a few selected water-soluble vitamins are summarized, but special attention is paid to thiamin and folic acid.

Thiamin

Excessive alcohol intake represents the major cause of thiamin deficiency in the US population, and alcohol intake has been identified as the major predictor of thiamin status (also, see Chapter 17). Up to 80% of heavy drinkers have impaired thiamin nutriture independent of the presence of liver disease. Insufficient dietary intake is the major cause of thiamin deficiency in alcoholics; in addition, the small amounts of ingested thiamin are malabsorbed (Tomasulo *et al.*, 1968). Low doses of thiamin are absorbed by a carrier-mediated active process or, at high concentrations, by passive diffusion. In the alcoholic, vitamin B_1 intake is generally low so that the vitamin is principally absorbed by the active process, which is, however, impaired by alcohol. The cellular transport of thiamin is mediated by two specific thiamin transporters (THTR1 and THTR2). Chronic alcohol consumption resulted in decreased carrier-mediated thiamin transport across the intestinal basolateral membranes and the renal brush border (Subramanian *et al.*, 2010; Subramanya *et al.*, 2010). Even in non-alcoholic subjects, active thiamin absorption is inhibited by an acute single dose of alcohol. Alcohol also induces a reduction in the activation of thiamin by phosphorylation and an increase in the dephosphorylation of phosphorylated thiamin. These effects are potentiated by the presence of liver disease. In addition, loss of the vitamin in urine may increase by alcohol intake due to a decreased and impaired transport of thiamin across the renal epithelia (Subramanian *et al.*, 2010). The thiamin storage capacity is reduced in the heavy drinker because of liver abnormalities and decreased muscle mass (Preedy *et al.*, 1999). Because of the reduced storage capacity of vitamin B_1 in general and especially in heavy drinkers for the aforementioned reasons, the vitamin has to be ingested regularly, on a more or less daily basis. Alcohol induces specific alterations of thiamin metabolism in the central nervous system (Hazell, 2009; Ke *et al.*, 2009), thereby producing the typical clinical symptoms of Wernicke–Korsakoff syndrome: encephalopathy, oculomotor dysfunction, and gait ataxia (Martin *et al.*, 2003; Harper, 2009; Pitel *et al.*, 2011). Wernicke–Korsakoff syndrome is probably the only medical emergency situation involving vitamin deficiencies: the neurological condition has to be treated immediately with parenteral thiamin (Donnino, *et al.*, 2007). Severe and/or insufficiently treated forms of thiamin deficiency could result in permanent amnesia and ataxia defining the Korsakoff syndrome. The syndrome shows typical clinical features including altered consciousness, ataxia, oculomotor abnormalities such as nystagmus and eye muscle paralysis, and psychosis. Up to 80% of heavy alcohol consumers show low circulating levels of vitamin B_1 due to low intakes, impaired absorption and storage, and reduced activation of the vitamin by phosphorylation. Autopsy data (reported prevalence of 0.8–2.8%) show that Wernicke's encephalopathy is underdiagnosed, i.e. it is often missed in clinical practice (prevalence based on clinical studies 0.04–0.13%) (Sechi and Serra, 2007). Different endogenous factors (e.g. transketolase enzyme variants with a decreased affinity for thiamin pyrophosphate, ApoE polymorphisms) and exogenous factors (thiamin intake, overall diet, amount of alcohol consumed) determine the risk for the development of a Wernicke–Korsakoff syndrome. During thiamin deficiency the metabolic and morphological changes occur within 10–14 days leading to irreversible structural lesions in the brain. The early diagnosis is thus of major importance; however, it is a very difficult task owing to the fact that classical symptoms are often lacking (Pitel et al., 2011). Therapy should be established also when there is only suspicion of the diagnosis. There is no consensus on the ideal dose, frequency, route of application or duration of the therapy. As an emergency therapy the application of ≥500 mg dissolved in 100 ml normal saline three times a day for 3 days could be envisioned (Sechi and Serra, 2007; Galvin et al., 2010). Because of the need of vitamin B_1 to metabolize glucose, no glucose infusions should be given to alcohol consumers except with the concomitant administration of thiamin. In view of the difficult diagnosis of Wernicke's encephalopathy and the high prevalence of thiamin deficiency, thiamin should be given to any heavy alcohol consumer independently from the clinical setting, i.e. also as a preventive strategy.

Although no prospective evidence supports the routine administration of several vitamins to alcoholic patients, present evidence suggest a high potential for a benefit of B-vitamin supplementation. Alcohol abstinence brings about an improvement of thiamin absorption (Holzbach, 1996). Research has shown that the neurotoxic effects of alcohol may be potentiated even in subclinical thiamin deficiency (Crowe and Kempton, 1997), and, accordingly, if alcohol abuse cannot be controlled, the preventive supplementation of thiamin and other B vitamins is indicated. Similarly, although controversial, the fortification of alcoholic beverages (e.g. beer) with thiamin might be considered as a mean to reduce the risk of a Wernicke–Korsakoff syndrome. Because of the interrelationship between thiamin and magnesium, an adequate supply of this

mineral should be ensured (McLean and Manchip, 1999). In the alcoholic patient (even when alcohol intake is reduced), thiamin deficiency may represent an important cause of heart failure, especially in combination with diuretics, which increase urinary thiamin losses (Suter and Vetter, 2000a; Keith et al., 2009).

Riboflavin

Riboflavin deficiency is common in the alcoholic patient and is due to low intakes and decreased bioavailability resulting from an alcohol-induced impairment of intraluminal hydrolysis of flavine adenine dinucleotide (FAD) in food sources (Pinto et al., 1987) (also, see Chapter 18). In addition, alcohol inhibits the transformation and activation of the vitamin not only at the level of absorption but also at the level of the peripheral tissues (Ono et al., 1987). Riboflavin is an essential cofactor in the conversion of vitamin B_6 and folate, and thus it represents an important modulator of the overall nutritional status of the B vitamins. Usually, riboflavin deficiency does not occur in isolation but in combination with a deficiency of other B-complex vitamins. Accordingly, the clinical entity is not typical. Because milk and milk products represent one of the major riboflavin sources, the low intake of this vitamin among heavy consumers of alcohol is not surprising.

Niacin

Light to moderate alcohol consumption does not interfere with niacin nutriture (also, see Chapter 19). A deficiency in niacin (vitamin B_3) is often found in the setting of chronic excessive alcohol consumption, usually together with deficiencies of other B-complex vitamins (Dastur et al., 1976) and other nutrients such as zinc. The prevalence of low plasma niacin levels in chronic alcohol consumers varies widely, probably because niacin can be obtained preformed from food and from synthesis in the liver from tryptophan. In chronic liver disease, the latter synthetic pathway is impaired (Rossouw et al., 1978). In excessive alcohol consumers, a low intake, decreased synthesis from tryptophan and increased urinary excretion, and an increased requirement might be of pathophysiological importance in the development of deficiency. The coenzyme forms of this vitamin (NAD and NADH) play an important role in alcohol metabolism (Hardman et al., 1991). In clinical practice, niacin deficiency symptoms (diarrhea, dermatitis, and dementia) might be confused with the Wernicke–Korsakoff syndrome (Cook et al., 1998). Niacin supplementation might lead to an increase in liver transaminase levels, which could be misinterpreted as an alcohol-induced increase in transaminase levels. Further pharmacological doses of niacin in the form of a supplement may exacerbate gastric ulcer disease and gout, both conditions that are often found in chronic alcohol consumers. Due to the multinutrient deficiency in excessive alcohol consumers, polyvitamin preparations should be used for therapeutic purposes (Pitsavas *et al.*, 2004) and should include trace elements such as zinc (Vannucchi and Moreno, 1989).

Vitamin B₆

Depending on liver function, between 50% and 90% of alcoholics show low pyridoxal-5'-phosphate (PLP) serum levels. The PLP content in liver tissue is reduced independent of the presence of liver disease. As for most nutrients, the pathogenesis of the impaired vitamin B₆ nutriture is multifactorial (also, see Chapter 20). The formation of the active vitamin (PLP) in the liver is reduced or even completely blocked by the ingestion of alcohol (Walsh *et al.*, 1966; Mitchell *et al.*, 1976). Acetaldehyde increases the degradation of the vitamin by displacing the vitamin from binding sites and this, in turn, leads to increased catabolism of the free vitamin and consecutively increased urinary loss (Pinto *et al.*, 1987). Because the vitamin has to be activated in a multi-step activation process at the level of the liver, supplementation of this vitamin does not necessarily lead to improved vitamin B₆ nutriture in alcoholics if they continue to ingest alcohol. A population-based cohort study and a recent meta-analysis (Larsson *et al.*, 2005, 2010) reported an inverse association between vitamin B₆ intake and the risk of colorectal cancer, especially in women consuming >30 g/week of alcohol. In agreement, in a meta-analysis the risk of colorectal cancer decreased by 49% for every 100-pmol/mL increase (approximately 2 SDs) in blood PLP levels (RR, 0.51; 95% CI, 0.38–0.69) (Larsson *et al.*, 2010).

Folic Acid

Folate deficiency is one of the most prevalent deficiencies in alcohol consumers (also, see Chapter 21). Up to 50% of heavy alcoholics show low concentrations of serum folate and/or low red blood cell folate (Gloria *et al.*, 1997). Beer consumers may show folate levels somewhat higher than these because of the folic acid content of this beverage. The clinical hallmark of folate deficiency is a megaloblastic anemia caused by damaged cell replication. It is found in all tissues, but especially in those with a high turnover rate, including the gastrointestinal mucosa (Halsted, 1995). The result is functional abnormalities and

clinical symptoms such as diarrhea. Accordingly, folate deficiency leads to a malabsorption of other nutrients, such as other water-soluble vitamins, and also folic acid itself. The malabsorption is further exacerbated by an abnormal enterohepatic circulation. The metabolic transformation to different active folate metabolites is impaired as a consequence of altered liver function and toxic alcohol and acetaldehyde effects on different enzymes. In addition, alcohol increases the urinary losses of this vitamin.

The impairment of absorption at the level of the gut and the kidney may be due to alcohol's effects on specific folate transporters in these tissues (Ross and McMartin, 1996). Because of an alcohol-induced rise in free radical production, the degradation of the vitamin is increased and may cause a tissue-specific deficiency. The alcohol-induced local impairment of folate metabolism may play a role in colorectal carcinogenesis (Hubner and Houlston, 2008). However, the alcohol-associated risk of colorectal carcinogenesis may vary in part according to the genetic polymorphisms of the 5,10-methylenetetrahydrofolate reductase (MTHFR) related to DNA methylation (Le Marchand *et al.*, 2005). The same may also apply to the process of carcinogenesis in other tissues such as oropharyngeal tissue (Capaccio *et al.*, 2005); however, the effects of folate might be also site specific (Duffy *et al.*, 2009). Recent data from the Nurses Health Study reported a lower alcohol-related risk for oral cancer in women with a higher folate intake (Shanmugham *et al.*, 2010). Several studies reported an inverse association between moderate alcohol intake and plasma homocysteine levels, whereas higher alcohol intake is consistently associated with increased plasma homocysteine levels, which are in part mediated by the alcohol-induced deficiency of folate, vitamin B₆ and also vitamin B₁₂. The pathophysiological relevance of the alcohol-induced increase of homocysteine is not known. How alcohol might modulate the biphasic effects (Sauer *et al.*, 2009) of folate nutriture on colon cancer risk (i.e. a moderate dietary increase of folate initiated before the establishment of neoplastic foci is protective, whereas excessive intake or increased intake once early lesions are established increases tumorigenesis) is not known (Schernhammer *et al.*, 2010).

Effects of Alcohol on Mineral and Trace Element Metabolism

Magnesium

Low serum and tissue levels of magnesium are a typical feature in heavy drinkers, and these alterations are more prevalent in the presence of liver disease (Kisters *et al.*, 1997). The magnesium nutriture is impaired as a result of reduced intake, malabsorption, increased urinary losses, secondary hyperaldosteronism, and increased fecal losses due to diarrhea (Romani, 2008). A reduction of alcohol intake is associated with an increase of the magnesium content of red blood cells (Kisters *et al.*, 1997; Romani, 2008). The decreased magnesium content of tissues may play a role in the development and progression of alcohol-associated pathologies (also, see Chapter 30). Magnesium content is especially decreased in heart tissue, a condition that may predispose to cardiac arrhythmias (a typical symptom in magnesium deficiency). Because of magnesium's effects in the maintenance of the membranes, a deficiency may exacerbate the development of organ damage, including liver damage. Magnesium plays a central role in over 300 biochemical reactions, one of them being thiamin phosphorylation. In view of the low toxicity of magnesium, this mineral should be replaced in the medical treatment of heavy drinkers (e.g. by supplementation with 200–300 mg elemental magnesium in chronic mild hypomagnesemia, where 1 mmol = 2 mEq = 24 mg elemental magnesium).

Zinc

Heavy alcohol consumption is associated with decreased serum zinc and lower hepatic zinc concentrations (Bode *et al.*, 1988) (also, see Chapter 34). The lower zinc levels are correlated with the degree of liver damage, but low zinc levels in serum are also found in less-advanced liver disease, such as fatty liver disease (Bode *et al.*, 1988; Stamoulis *et al.*, 2007). The deficient zinc status results from low intakes, reduced absorption, increased urinary excretion, and an alteration of zinc distribution. Usually, zinc deficiency in the alcoholic is multifactorial, but a low dietary intake is found in most heavy consumers of alcohol. The zinc malabsorption is caused by direct and indirect alcohol effects, such as mucosal damage (Zhong *et al.*, 2010a) and altered synthesis of zinc ligands (such as metallothionein) owing to alcohol-induced impaired protein synthesis. The presence and the degree of exocrine pancreatic insufficiency represent an additional modulator of zinc status. Alcoholic liver disease, especially alcoholic hepatitis, has been identified as the major predictor for metabolic perturbations in zinc nutriture (Stamoulis *et al.*, 2007). The increased urinary excretion of zinc correlates with the degree of liver damage (Rodriguez *et al.*, 1997) and is caused by decreased peripheral tissue zinc uptake and decreased serum levels of albumin. In patients with liver cirrhosis, the increased urinary zinc excretion persists even

after cessation of alcohol intake. The acute ingestion of alcohol among moderate drinkers causes increased urinary zinc excretion, a consequence that suggests direct effects of alcohol on zinc homeostasis at the level of the kidney (Rodriguez *et al.*, 1997). A disruption of the epithelial barrier in the distal small intestine plays an important role in alcohol-induced gut leakiness and consecutively also alcoholic endotoxemia and hepatitis. Zinc deficiency may interfere with the intestinal barrier function by a direct action on tight junction proteins or by sensitizing to the effects of alcohol (Zhong *et al.*, 2010a,b). In a mouse model, zinc supplementation reversed alcoholic steatosis by reactivation of the hepatocyte nuclear factor-4alpha (HHF-4α) and peroxisome proliferators activated receptor alpha (PPAR-α) as well as by the inhibition of oxidative stress (Kang *et al.*, 2009). Zinc deficiency has further been implicated in alcohol-induced alveolar-epithelial and macrophage dysfunction (Joshi and Guidot, 2007), and zinc supplementation might correct the dysfunction (Joshi *et al.*, 2009).

Malnutrition in combination with alcohol leads to a higher degree of zinc depletion. It has been suggested that alcohol-induced alterations in zinc metabolism may increase alcohol-associated carcinogenesis (Seitz *et al.*, 1998; Prasad *et al.*, 2009). In view of the multiple effects of zinc, clinical signs of zinc deficiency – abnormalities of taste and smell, hypogonadism, infertility, and an impaired dark adaptation – are often seen in alcoholics. Impaired dark adaptation is a characteristic symptom in alcohol consumers, one generally not caused by vitamin A deficiency but by zinc deficiency. Defective zinc nutriture may increase alcohol toxicity given that the rate-limiting enzyme in alcohol degradation, ADH, is a zinc metalloenzyme.

Alcohol and Mortality

The effect of alcohol on morbidity and mortality is biphasic, and the relationship is J-shaped: low levels of ingestion are associated with reduced morbidity and mortality risks, whereas abstinence and higher levels of ingestion are associated with a higher mortality risk due to different cancers, alcoholic liver disease, and cardiovascular diseases such as arrhythmias, alcoholic cardiomyopathy, hypertension, and stroke (Gaziano *et al.*, 2000; Hill, 2005; Kloner and Rezkalla, 2007; Djousse *et al.*, 2009; Sadakane *et al.*, 2009; Costanzo *et al.*, 2010; Klatsky, 2010; Mukamal *et al.*, 2010). The reduced mortality risk at lower intakes is explained by risk of coronary artery disease (Rimm *et al.*,

1996; Thun *et al.*, 1997; Gaziano *et al.*, 2000; Hill, 2005; Djousse *et al.*, 2009; Mukamal *et al.*, 2010) and reduced risk of ischemic stroke (Reynolds *et al.*, 2003). The amount of alcohol ingestion at the nadir of mortality risk is not known, and varies from study to study and from one individual to another. An analysis of data from 20 international cohort studies found a substantial variation in the nadir (the level of consumption at which mortality is least) (White, 1999). This meta-analysis estimated the nadir for US men to be 7.7 units of alcohol per week (95% confidence interval (CI) 6.4–9.1). In that study, 1 unit (1 drink) was considered to be 9 g alcohol for US men; 2.9 (95% CI 2.0–4.0) units per week for US women; and 12.9 (95% CI 10.8–15.1) units per week for UK men (White, 1999).

The J-shaped relationship has been reported in different studies, one of them being the American Cancer Society investigation (Thun *et al.*, 1997). In that study in men and in women, light alcohol intake was associated with a reduction in mortality risk because of a lower coronary artery disease risk. However, with increasing alcohol intake (even in the range of moderate intake), mortality risk rose, especially in women, whose risk of breast cancer also increased (Thun *et al.*, 1997).

The hallmark of excessive alcohol intake is metabolic and structural alterations at the level of the liver, and liver cirrhosis is the leading cause of death in heavy drinkers (Thun *et al.*, 1997; Harvey *et al.*, 2009; Rehm *et al.*, 2010). Age-adjusted death rates for liver cirrhosis have been reported as 12.6 and 6.0 per 100 000 for US men and women, respectively. In addition, approximately one-third of all traffic crash fatalities in the United States are alcohol related.

Alcohol and Cardiovascular Diseases

The protective effect of alcohol on coronary disease risk has been reported in men and women (Thun *et al.*, 1997; Rimm *et al.*, 1999; Hill, 2005; Kloner and Rezkalla, 2007; Sadakane *et al.*, 2009; Sun *et al.*, 2009; Costanzo *et al.*, 2010; Hvidtfeldt *et al.*, 2010; Mukamal *et al.*, 2010), with a risk reduction in the range of 20% to 40% (also, see Chapter 48). A recent study (Mukamal *et al.*, 2010) confirmed in a large US nationwide population the U-shaped relationship between light and moderate alcohol drinking and cardiovascular mortality: compared with lifetime abstainers the relative risk of cardiovascular mortality was 0.69 (95% CI 0.59–0.82) among light consumers (defined

as ≤3 drinks/week) and 0.62 (95% CI 0.50–0.77) among moderate drinkers (>3 to 7 drinks/week for women, >3 to 14 drinks/week for men). The magnitude of risk reduction was similar in subgroups of age, sex or even baseline health status. However, consumption above these limits led to an increased risk of cardiovascular and non-cardiovascular mortality. The intake levels related to the nadir of risk vary widely in different studies (White, 1999). It is important to recognize that several studies found the protective effects mainly in older people and/or those who do have one or more of the classical cardiovascular risk factors (Thun *et al.*, 1997; Snow *et al.*, 2009; Sun *et al.*, 2009; Hvidtfeldt *et al.*, 2010; Martin *et al.*, 2010). This finding suggests that alcohol may modulate the pathophysiological potential of some of the classic risk factors for coronary artery disease (Britton *et al.*, 2008). The pattern of drinking is an important modifier of the risk modulation. A recent study showed that the cardioprotective effect of moderate alcohol consumption disappears when, on average, light to moderate drinking is mixed with irregular heavy drinking occasions (Roerecke and Rehm, 2010).

The mechanisms of the cardioprotective effects of alcohol (Table 55.2) are not completely elucidated, and about 50% of the potential protection seems to be mediated by the alcohol-induced increase in HDL-cholesterol levels (Criqui, 1998). Favorable effects on fibrinolysis, thrombogenesis, coronary blood flow, postprandial metabolism, prostaglandin and thromboxane synthesis, arterial vasodilatation, other lipoprotein fractions than HDL-cholesterol, anti-inflammatory effects, antioxidative effects, ingestion of non-nutritive protective compounds, ischemic preconditioning, or behavioral aspects have also been suggested (Rimm *et al.*, 1999; Pagel *et al.*, 2004; Bertelli and Das, 2009; Collins *et al.*, 2009; Djousse *et al.*, 2009; Zheng *et al.*, 2010).

The protective effects of alcohol are independent of the beverage type (Rimm *et al.*, 1996; Spaak *et al.*, 2008, 2010; Brown *et al.*, 2009), although studies reported a higher protection in red wine consumers (Renaud *et al.*, 1999) because of its content of polyphenols and flavonoids (Opie and Lecour, 2007; Bertelli and Das, 2009). Red wine consumption may elicit a higher protection that is related to the personality traits (including lifestyle factors, risk control behavior, and socioeconomic factors) of the typical red-wine consumer and the ingestion of red wine mainly with a meal (Trevisan *et al.*, 1987; Mortensen *et al.*, 2001; Britton *et al.*, 2008; Hansel *et al.*, 2010).

TABLE 55.2 Summary and classification of possible cardioprotective mechanisms of alcohol

Cardioprotective mechanism	Effects
Lipid effects	Increase in HDL cholesterol
	Decrease in composition, size, and concentration of LDL cholesterol
	Decrease in lipoprotein(a)
	LDL-receptor effects
	Modified fatty acids
Blood coagulation	Modulation of coagulation factors
	Modulation of thrombogenesis
	Modulation of fibrinolysis
Endocrine effects	Insulin metabolism ("antidiabetic")
	Estrogen metabolism
	Steroid metabolism
Psychological effects	Control of type A behavior
	Anti-anxiety effects
	Stress control
Non-nutritive compounds	Polyphenolic compounds
	Phytoalexins (e.g. resveratrol)
Miscellaneous effects	Vasoreactivity
	Ischemic preconditioning
	Membrane fluidity
	Liver structure (liver sieve)
	Modulation of the metabolic syndrome
	Paraoxonase up-regulation

HDL, high-density lipoprotein; LDL, low-density lipoprotein.

If the cardioprotective effects of alcohol are really causal, then the central questions are, "How much is enough?" and "How much is too much?" A systematic review (using data from England and Wales) reported that the level of alcohol intake with the lowest mortality ranged from 0 units a week in men and women under 35 years of age to 3 units a week in women over 65 years of age and 8 units a week in men over 65 years of age (in this article, 1 unit was defined as 9 g of alcohol) (White *et al.*, 2002). Smoking is a major determinant of health, and the interaction between alcohol and smoking is of great importance. In a prospective cohort study of postmenopausal women (Ebbert *et al.*, 2005), alcohol ingestion among those who had never smoked was inversely associated with coronary heart disease mortality. Among current smokers, no association was found between alcohol ingestion and coronary heart disease mortality, but there was a positive association with cancer incidence among those consuming at least one drink daily. The combination of alcohol drinking and smoking is disadvantageous in any case (Taylor and Rehm,

2006), especially regarding carcinogenesis. Based on data from White *et al.* (2002) it can be concluded that the alcohol consumption levels with the greatest potential benefit are likely to be lower in the future due to a decline in coronary heart disease for reasons unrelated to alcohol intake. This also means that the cornerstone of coronary artery disease prevention remains in the control of the major classic cardiovascular risk factors (i.e. smoking, dyslipidemia, hypertension, and obesity). Despite the potentially favorable effects of alcohol on coronary artery disease risk, alcohol represents an important cause of hypertension (Suter and Vetter, 2000b; Taylor *et al.*, 2009), hemorrhagic stroke (Hillbom and Numminen, 1998; Patra *et al.*, 2010), alcoholic cardiomyopathy, heart insufficiency, and arrhythmias (Fogle *et al.*, 2010; Klatsky, 2010).

The protective effect of alcohol on coronary artery disease risk in the French population has been termed "The French Paradox." The French do indeed show a more than one-third lower mortality rate for ischemic heart disease than the Americans or British; however, the all-cause mortality rate in France is not much different and the mortality rate for some of the typical alcohol-associated diseases, such as oropharyngeal cancer or liver cirrhosis, is even higher in France than in other countries (Zureik and Ducimetière, 1996). Despite the many associations between alcohol and coronary artery disease mortality, recent data suggest that the protective effect of alcohol may be biased by "good habits" and not "just good wine" (Rimm, 1996), so that the drinker's habits become more important than the drink (Klatsky, 1999). Several studies reported that moderate alcohol drinkers or wine drinkers do show a healthier diet and behavior compared with other drinkers or abstainers (Klatsky *et al.*, 1990; Tjønneland *et al.*, 1999; Rouillier *et al.*, 2004; Ruidavets *et al.*, 2004). The cardioprotection may thus be mediated by synergistic effects of a low dose of alcohol in combination with health-prone behavior (Hansel *et al.*, 2010).

Alcohol and Type 2 Diabetes Mellitus

Most studies reported a J-shaped relationship between alcohol intake and the risk of type 2 diabetes in men and women (also, see Chapter 49). The lowest risk was seen in light to moderate consumers, whereas heavier alcohol consumption and binge drinking led to a higher risk for type 2 diabetes (Bantle *et al.*, 2008; Crandall *et al.*, 2009; Pietraszek *et al.*, 2010; Joosten *et al.*, 2011). Recent data from the Health Professionals Follow-up Study showed that a 7.5 g/day (about half a glass) increase in alcohol consumption over 4 years was associated with lower diabetes risk among initial non-drinkers (multivariable hazard ratio (HR) 0.78; 95% CI 0.60–1.00) and drinkers initially consuming <15 g/day (HR 0.89; 95% CI 0.83–0.96) but not among men initially drinking ≥15 g/day (HR 0.99; 95% CI 0.95–1.02; P (interaction) <0.01) (Joosten et al., 2011). Light to moderate amounts of alcohol increase insulin sensitivity for up to 24 hours and diminish the postprandial glucose excursion (Greenfield et al., 2005). The improved insulin sensitivity, effects on lipid metabolism and inflammation might play a causal role in the protection (Pietraszek et al., 2010). Some studies could not find a protective effect of alcohol, which may be in part explained by differences in the presence of the other risk factors, differences in the drinking pattern, beverage preference, or body composition and body weight (Pietraszek et al., 2010). In patients with sulfonylurea or insulin treatment, alcohol might increase the risk for hypoglycemia.

Alcohol and Hypertension

The first description of the relationship between alcohol and blood pressure was published by Lian in 1915. Cross-sectional, prospective, and interventional studies have reported an increase in systolic and diastolic blood pressure with increasing alcohol intake (Klatsky et al., 1977; Huntgeburth et al., 2005; Sesso et al., 2008). Most studies reported a dose–response relationship between alcohol intake and blood pressure without a threshold level of alcohol intake, and cessation of alcohol intake in moderate and heavy consumers led to a reduction in blood pressure (Grobbee et al., 1999). The decline in blood pressure upon cessation of excessive alcohol consumption shows wide variability. Based on a meta-analysis with the exclusive reduction of alcohol intake a significant reduction of mean systolic (2.52 to 4.10 mmHg) and of mean diastolic (1.49 to 2.58 mmHg) blood pressure was achieved (Xin et al., 2001). This decline in blood pressure would result in a 6% reduction of coronary heart disease risk and a 15% reduction in the risk of stroke or transient ischemic attacks (Xin et al., 2001). Blood pressure effects are more pronounced in daily alcohol consumers. Binge drinking may also lead to increased blood pressure. A recent study underlined the importance of the effect of the timing of blood pressure measurements after alcohol intake on the magnitude and direction of the blood pressure change (McFadden et al., 2005), and this may also be a reason for the inconsistent

effects of alcohol on blood pressure in epidemiological and some experimental studies. In one study, alcohol intake was associated with blood pressure and pulse pressure in older men not receiving therapy for hypertension but not in those receiving antihypertensive therapy (Wakabayashi, 2010). However, the potential cardioprotective effects of alcohol are also found in hypertensive subjects. The pathophysiologic mechanisms for the pressor effects of alcohol are not known exactly, and multiple mechanisms involving direct and indirect effects of alcohol on autonomic regulation, neurohumoral effects, effects on peripheral resistance vessels, calcium handling in the vascular smooth muscle cells, and altered stress perception have been suggested. Alterations in liver function may affect the metabolism of antihypertensive drugs. Heavier alcohol consumption is one of the most important reasons for resistant and difficult-to-treat hypertension (also, see Chapter 46).

Alcohol and Stroke

Alcohol has been identified as an independent risk factor for hemorrhagic stroke (Grobbee et al., 1999; Patra et al., 2010). The increased stroke risk is caused partly by the pressor effects of alcohol as well as by effects on cerebral vasculature (Hillbom and Numminen, 1998; Grobbee et al., 1999; Patra et al., 2010).

Because cardiovascular disease and ischemic stroke share some common pathophysiological features, alcohol may also have protective effects against ischemic stroke. In a study set in a multiethnic, urban society, moderate alcohol consumption (up to two drinks per day) had protective effects on ischemic stroke, with an odds ratio (OR) of 0.51, 95% CI 0.39–0.67) (Sacco et al., 1999). However, excessive drinking, considered to be 7 or more drinks per day (OR 2.96, 95% CI 1.05–8.29) and binge drinking were associated with a two- to four-fold increased risk of ischemic stroke. In addition, risk of ischemic stroke onset is transiently elevated in the hour after alcohol ingestion (Mostofsky et al., 2010). The cardioprotective effects of light alcohol consumption might also be present in stroke patients (Jackson et al., 2003). At present it is controversial as to whether light to moderate alcohol intake increases the risk of atrial fibrillation (Conen et al., 2008), an important risk factor for ischemic stroke. Data from the Health Professional Follow-up Study (Mukamal et al., 2005) reported that intake of two drinks or fewer per day was not associated with an increased risk for ischemic stroke, and that consuming red wine (not other beverages) was associated with a lower risk. Moderate alcohol consumption (especially wine consumption) is associated with a healthier lifestyle such as increased fruit and vegetable consumption (Klatsky *et al.*, 1990; Tjonneland *et al.*, 1999; Rouillier *et al.*, 2004), and an increased fruit and vegetable intake is associated with a reduced risk of stroke (Lock *et al.*, 2005; Mizrahi *et al.*, 2009). Accordingly a study from western New York showed that wine drinkers had a higher education, higher household incomes, a lower prevalence of smoking, and a higher vitamin intake (McCann *et al.*, 2003). Despite the rather high risk of a recurrent stroke, stroke patients modify their behavior and risk-factor profile insufficiently (Hornnes *et al.*, 2010).

Alcohol and Cognitive Function

Heavy alcohol consumption is one important cause for short- and long-term impairment of cognitive function. Alcohol elicits direct neurotoxicity and, if applied in large enough quantities for a long enough period, it leads to a multi-domain cognitive impairment that may further develop to ethanol-related dementia (which represents nearly 10% of all causes of dementia). Several studies reported that moderate alcohol consumption is associated with better cognitive functioning and a reduced risk of a cognitive decline with aging (Stampfer *et al.*, 2005; Brust, 2010). The data are controversial and vary according to, among other factors, the time point in life at which alcohol intake was practiced and the cognitive function (Panza *et al.*, 2009; Brust, 2010; Gross *et al.*, 2011). A protective level of consumption cannot be defined at present. Once again, it is not completely clear whether the light alcohol drinking or the behavior of the drinker is the protective principle.

Alcohol and Liver Disease

Alcoholic liver disease (ALD) includes a wide spectrum of injury, ranging from steatosis, through alcoholic hepatitis, to pathologies. Alcohol is one of the major causes of liver disease worldwide. The mechanisms of alcohol-induced liver injury are multiple and incompletely understood. One key mechanism is the induction of Cyp2E1 which leads to the generation of reactive oxygen species. The alcohol induction of Cyp2E1 predisposes further to xenobiotic induced liver damage due to enhanced biotransformation and increased production of toxic metabolites (Malhi *et al.*, 2010). Further alcohol enhances the genera-

tion of inflammatory cytokines (e.g. TNF-α, IL-1, or IL-6) with local as well as systemic effects (Malhi *et al.*, 2010).

There is a direct relationship between the per capita alcohol consumption (independent of the beverage type) and the death rate from liver cirrhosis. As with other alcohol-related pathologies, susceptibility to developing alcoholic cirrhosis varies from one individual to another as a function of the amount and duration of alcohol intake, gender, genetic predisposition, characteristics of alcohol metabolism, previous hepatitis B or C (Diehl, 2005), and potential nutritional factors (Halsted, 2004; O'Shea *et al.*, 2010). The quantity of alcohol consumed is the most important risk factor for ALD. The risk of developing ALD increases sharply with alcohol consumption over 40 g/day, and the risk for cirrhosis increases considerably in men consuming >60–80 g/day for ten years or longer, and >20 g/day in women (O'Shea *et al.*, 2010). The risk for ALD is higher for consumers of beer and spirits. For women, the threshold dose of alcohol is about half the threshold dosage of men, i.e. they are twice as sensitive to alcohol-induced hepatotoxicity. Further, women develop more severe ALD and within a shorter duration of alcohol exposure. The mechanisms of alcoholic liver damage are multiple, and include direct toxic effects of alcohol, acetaldehyde-mediated toxicity, increased oxygen requirements, and free radical damage. In addition, immune-mediated phenomena such as a proinflammatory state seem to be of central importance. In the development of alcoholic fatty liver, the altered redox potential (NADH/NAD+), impaired lipid oxidation, and increased lipogenesis seem to play a central role. The role of oxidative stress and injury in the pathogenesis of alcohol-induced hepatic injury is underlined by an inverse association between the serum alanine transaminase (ALT) and serum concentration of certain nutrients such as vitamin C, α- and β-carotene, and lutein/zeaxanthin. The nutritional deficiencies (ranging from protein energy malnutrition and multiple micronutrient deficiencies) described in this chapter are commonly found in alcoholic patients and should be corrected by a combination of normal food, targeted supplements and alcohol abstinence. Mortality in ALD increases directly proportional to the degree of malnutrition (Mendenhall *et al.*, 1995) (also, see Chapter 54).

Alcohol and Cancer

Alcohol consumption is related to an increased prevalence of oropharyngeal, esophageal, liver, colorectal, and female breast cancers (Seitz and Stickel, 2007). The combination of smoking and drinking increases the risk of the oropharyngeal cancers and of cancers in other locations. Alcohol per se has no direct carcinogenic properties, and the pathophysiologic bases of the alcohol-induced cancers are multiple and include effects of acetaldehyde or effects of alcohol on methyl-group and retinoic acid metabolism (Seitz and Stickel, 2007). A dose–response relationship between alcohol intake and cancer risk can often be found. The mechanisms of ethanol-induced carcinogenesis may vary according to location. Increased alcohol intake, in combination with a low micronutrient intake, increases cancer risk (e.g. colorectal cancer). Alcohol consumption is associated with an increased risk of breast cancer (especially hormone-sensitive cancer types) (Zhang *et al.*, 2007; Li *et al.*, 2010) and breast cancer recurrence, particularly among postmenopausal and overweight/obese women (Kwan *et al.*, 2010). A collaborative analysis (Hamajima *et al.*, 2002) of 53 studies reported that, compared with women who reported drinking no alcohol, the relative risk of breast cancer was 1.32 (1.19–1.45, $P < 0.00001$) for an alcohol intake of 35–44 g/day, and 1.46 (1.33–1.61, $P < 0.00001$) for ≥45 g/day. The relative risk of breast cancer increased by 7.1% (95% CI 5.5–8.7%; $P < 0.00001$) for each additional 10 g/day intake of alcohol, i.e. for each extra unit or drink of alcohol consumed on a daily basis (Hamajima *et al.*, 2002). Whether small amounts of alcohol intake are associated with an increased risk of breast cancer in women is not exactly known and is controversial. Alcohol has a high potential to modulate estrogen metabolism, leading to higher circulating estrogen levels (Onland-Moret *et al.*, 2005), so the potential detrimental effects of alcohol on estrogen-sensitive cancers is not surprising. Some of the controversy of the data can be explained by genetic factors and/or menopausal status or period of life with alcohol consumption. In view of the current evidence, light alcohol consumption seems to be safe for most women.

Individuals carrying the inactive aldehyde dehydrogenase 2*2 (ALDH 2*2) allele have an increased risk for alcohol-related oesophageal cancer. Carriers of other genetic variants (e.g. alcohol dehydrogenase 1C*1 (ADH1C*1) homozygotes or methylenetetrahydrofolate reductase (MTHFR) 677CT variants) also have a higher risk for alcohol-related cancers (Druesne-Pecollo *et al.*, 2009). Further lifestyle factors (e.g. smoking, poor oral hygiene, physical activity pattern), certain dietary deficien- cies (e.g. folate, vitamin B$_6$, methyl donors) or an excess of certain micronutrients (vitamin A/β-carotene) may potentiate the risk for alcohol-associated tumors (Seitz and Stickel, 2007) (also, see Chapter 51).

Alcohol and Bone and Muscle

The direct and indirect effects of alcohol on bone and muscle metabolism are multiple and depend on the amount, the duration of alcohol intake, the presence of liver disease, gender, genetic factors and concomitant factors (e.g. dietary factors including protein intake and resistance training). Light to moderate consumption may have favorable effects on bone health (Feskanich *et al.*, 1999; Venkat *et al.*, 2009; Jin *et al.*, 2010). A recent study (Tucker *et al.*, 2009) reported that moderate consumption of alcohol may be beneficial to bone in men and postmenopausal women. In men, high liquor intakes (>2 drinks/day) were associated with significantly lower bone mineral density (BMD), and stronger associations were found between BMD and beer or wine, relative to liquor (Tucker *et al.*, 2009).

In heavy drinkers, the calcium balance is negatively affected by low intakes and malabsorption of calcium due to direct mucosal damage, an impaired vitamin D nurite, and increased urinary calcium losses (Laitinen and Valimaki, 1993). In heavy drinkers, different structural and functional changes in the bone can be found. Low to moderate amounts of alcohol have no adverse effects on bone mass in postmenopausal women (Feskanich *et al.*, 1999) because of alcohol's effects on endogenous (and exogenous) estrogens (see above). Despite some controversial data that have been reported about the effects of alcohol on bone metabolism, in the clinical setting any unexplained fracture or osteoporosis (especially in men) may point to alcohol-related problems.

Alcohol consumption leads to a dose-dependent negative effect on skeletal muscle, leading to progressive functional and structural alterations of skeletal muscle cells with a concomitant decline in lean body mass (Nakahara *et al.*, 2003; Preedy *et al.*, 2003; Fernandez-Solà *et al.*, 2007). Alcoholic myopathy is a typical clinical feature of the heavy alcohol consumer (Preedy *et al.*, 2003). Importantly these effects are also seen at the level of the heart muscle in the form of alcoholic cardiomyopathy (Laonigro *et al.*, 2009).

Fetal Alcohol Syndrome

The teratogenic effects of alcohol have been known for centuries. It was not, however, until the late 1960s when it was first reported that heavy alcohol intake during pregnancy might be associated with fetal alcohol syndrome (FAS). FAS is characterized by typical physical and neurobehavioral features (Plant *et al.*, 1999; Calhoun and Warren, 2007; National Institute on Alcohol Abuse and Alcoholism (NIAAA), 2009). Children with FAS show a pre- and postnatal growth retardation, facial dysmorphy, and central nervous system dysfunctions that cause permanent cognitive impairment and learning disabilities (Hofer and Burd, 2009). FAS represents the severe endpoints of a vast spectrum of structural, behavioral, and neurodevelopmental abnormalities caused by exposure to alcohol in utero. Present evidence suggests that alcohol during pregnancy may lead to FAS or to a broader spectrum of defects which are now referred to as fetal alcohol spectrum disorders (FASDs) (NIAAA, 2009; Jones *et al.*, 2010; O'Leary *et al.*, 2010). FAS represents the most severe endpoint of the FASD spectrum. The pathogeneses of the FASDs are multiple and include epigenetic effects, fetal programming, and also the interference of alcohol with nutritional status (Ramsay, 2010). Despite knowledge of the relationship between alcohol and FAS/FASD, approximately 10% of pregnant women reported alcohol use in the past 30 days. Alcohol intake during pregnancy, but also during the week of conception increases the risk of early pregnancy loss. In view of the irreversible lifelong effects of alcohol drinking during pregnancy on the unborn child, pregnancy has to be a period of life during which alcohol intake should be avoided completely. Every woman of reproductive age has to remember that there is no safe amount of alcohol to drink while pregnant, no safe time to drink during pregnancy, and also no safe kind of alcoholic drink.

Outstanding Issues and Questions

Not only light and moderate but also heavier alcohol drinking is a global issue. Alcohol consumption has "global" effects on all cell and organ systems and should accordingly have "global health priority" at the national and international level (Beaglehole and Bonita, 2009). In addition to the existing tools for assessing hazardous alcohol intake (e.g. AUDIT, T-ACE, TWEAK: http://pubs.niaaa.nih.gov/publications/aa65/AA65.htm), more reliable biomarkers for quantifying alcohol intake should be developed. This would improve the quality of data in all fields of research from epidemiology to clinics. As this chapter has outlined, alcohol affects all nutrients as a function of the consumption pattern, genetic factors, age, and gender, as well as environmental factors. The interactions between these factors and potential positive and negative effects of alcohol on the risks of higher consumption are only incompletely understood. In agreement with recommendations from the NIAAA (2009), nutritional and metabolic aspects of alcohol consumption should be researched across the whole lifespan. Individual differences in benefit and risk should be assessed, and sensitive as well as specific markers and predictors for the differences should be identified. Light consumption may be associated with cardioprotective effects; however, there is nevertheless a need for a randomized trial as is done for any other health recommendation or drug. What are the key modifiers of the protective effects? Is the protection equal for women and men at all ages? What is the contribution of alcohol consumption to the global overweight and obesity pandemic? Strategies and tools to assess the predictive risk for susceptibility to problem drinking have to be researched. Another issue that needs clarification is whether nutritional effects of alcohol are mediators or modifiers of alcohol-related health problems. Furthermore an emerging field of potential high public-health relevance is the study of the interaction between epigenetic mechanisms and alcohol consumption as well as alcohol-associated diseases (Kaminen-Ahola *et al.*, 2010).

Future Directions

As a function of the amount of alcohol consumed and individual factors (genetic and environmental, including lifestyle and nutritional factors), the health and nutritional effects of alcohol may be positive or negative. Often, both positive and negative effects occur. In view of the heterogeneity of responses for any given alcohol dose, the formulation of public-health recommendations for safe consumption levels is becoming increasingly difficult. In today's world, the best approach to patient and public-health counseling about alcohol consumption is not to forbid it, but to try to formulate safe consumption levels for those wishing to drink. Alcohol should not be recommended for health reasons or for health maintenance, especially as long as there are no specific and sensitive predictors for harmful alcohol use and abuse.

Evidence suggests that the safe amount may vary considerably from one individual to another, even for those whose alcohol intake is in the light to moderate range. Identifying biochemical and genetic markers for risk assessment related to moderate alcohol consumption may help to formulate and implement specific individual recommendations. In addition, future research activities should focus on strategies for the implementation of safe drinking practices in combination with an overall healthy lifestyle with respect to nutrition and physical activity. In such a setting, light to moderate alcohol consumption may add to the quality of life; however, the benefit and risk are not equal for all.

Suggestions for Further Reading

Agarwal, D.P. and Seitz, H.K. (eds) (2001) *Alcohol in Health and Disease*. Marcel Dekker, New York.

Buglass, A.J. (ed.) (2011) *Handbook of Alcoholic Beverages: Technical, Analytical and Nutritional Aspects*. Wiley-Blackwell, Oxford.

Lieber, C. (1992) *Medical and Nutritional Complications of Alcoholism: Mechanisms and Management*. Kluwer Academic / Plenum Publishers, Amsterdam.

Mazzei, A. and D'Arco, A. (2009) *Alcoholic Beverage Consumption and Health*. Nova Science Publishers, Hauppage, NY.

Riley, E.P., Clarren, S., Weinberg, J., et al. (eds) (2010) *Fetal Alcohol Spectrum Disorder: Management and Policy Perspectives of FASD (Health Care and Disease Management)*. Wiley-Blackwell, Oxford.

Watson, R.R. and Preedy, V.R. (2004) *Nutrition and Alcohol: Linking Nutrient Interactions and Dietary Intake*. CRC Press, Boca Raton, FL.

Web Resources

Alcohol Policy UK: http://www.alcoholpolicy.net/

Australian Government website: http://www.alcohol.gov.au/

CDC Alcohol and Public Health: http://www.cdc.gov/alcohol/index.htm

National Health Service (NHS) UK website: http://www.nhs.uk/livewell/alcohol/Pages/Alcoholhome.aspx

National Institute on Alcohol Abuse and Alcoholism (NIAAA): http://www.niaaa.nih.gov/Pages/default.aspx

References

Ahmed, S., Leo, M.A., and Lieber, C.S. (1994) Interactions between alcohol and β-carotene in patients with alcoholic liver disease. *Am J Clin Nutr* **60**, 430–436.

Ajmo, J.M., Liang, X., Rogers, C.Q., *et al.* (2008) Resveratrol alleviates alcoholic fatty liver in mice. *Am J Physiol Gastrointest Liver Physiol* **295**, G833–842.

Albanes, D., Heinonen, O.P., Taylor, P.R., *et al.* (1996) α-Tocopherol and β-carotene supplements and lung cancer incidence in the Alpha-Tocopherol, Beta-Carotene Cancer Prevention Study: effects of base-line characteristics and study compliance. *J Natl Cancer Inst* **88**, 1560–1570.

Alkerwi, A.A., Boutsen, M., Vaillant, M., *et al.* (2009) Alcohol consumption and the prevalence of metabolic syndrome: a meta-analysis of observational studies. *Atherosclerosis* **204**, 624–635.

Alvisa-Negrín, J., González-Reimer, S.E., Santolaria-Fernández, F., *et al.* (2009) Osteopenia in alcoholics: effect of alcohol abstinence. *Alcohol Alcohol* **44**, 468–475.

Apte, M., Pirola, R., and Wilson, J. (2009) New insights into alcoholic pancreatitis and pancreatic cancer. *J Gastroenterol Hepatol* **24**, S51–S56.

Atwater, W.D. and Benedict, F.G. (1902) An experimental inquiry regarding the nutritive value of alcohol. *Mem Natl Acad Sci* **8**, 235–272.

Ayaori, M., Ishikawa, T., Yoshida, H., *et al.* (1997) Beneficial effects of alcohol withdrawal on LDL particle size distribution and oxidative susceptibility in subjects with alcohol-induced hypertriglyceridemia. *Arterioscler Thromb Vasc Biol* **17**, 2540–2547.

Bal, B., Koch, T.R., Finelli, F.C., *et al.* (2010) Managing medical and surgical disorders after divided Roux-en-Y gastric bypass surgery. *Nat Rev Gastroenterol Hepatol* **7**, 320–334.

Bantle, A.E., Thomas, W., and Bantle, J.P. (2008) Metabolic effects of alcohol in the form of wine in persons with type 2 diabetes mellitus. *Metabolism* **57**, 241–245.

Barona, E. and Lieber, C.S. (1998) Alcohol and lipids. In M. Galanter (ed.), *Recent Developments in Alcoholism, Vol. 14: Consequences of Alcoholism*. Plenum Press, New York, pp. 97–134.

Beaglehole, R. and Bonita, R. (2009) Alcohol: a global health priority. *Lancet* **373**, 2173–2174.

Bell, H., Bjorneboe, A., Eidsvoll, B., *et al.* (1992) Reduced concentration of hepatic α-tocopherol in patients with alcoholic liver cirrhosis. *Alcohol Alcohol* **27**, 39–46.

Bertelli, A.A. and Das, D.K. (2009) Grapes, wines, resveratrol, and heart health. *J Cardiovasc Pharmacol* **54**, 468–476.

Bode, J.C., Hanisch, P., Henning, H., *et al.* (1988) Hepatic zinc content in patients with various stages of alcoholic liver disease and in patients with chronic active and chronic persistent hepatitis. *Hepatology* **8**, 1605–1609.

Borucki, K., Schreiner, R., Dierkes, J., *et al.* (2005) Detection of recent ethanol intake with new markers: comparison of fatty acid ethyl esters in serum and of ethyl glucuronide and the ratio of 5-hydroxytryptophol to 5-hydroxyindole acetic acid in urine. *Alcohol Clin Exp Res* **29,** 781–787.

Brinton, E.A. (2010) Effects of ethanol intake on lipoproteins and atherosclerosis. *Curr Opin Lipidol* **21,** 346–351.

Britton, A., Marmot, M.G., and Shipley, M. (2008) Who benefits most from the cardioprotective properties of alcohol consumption – health freaks or couch potatoes? *J Epidemiol Community Health* **62,** 905–908.

Brown, L., Kroon, P.A., Das, D.K., *et al.* (2009) The biological responses to resveratrol and other polyphenols from alcoholic beverages. *Alcohol Clin Exp Res* **33,** 1513–1523.

Brust, J.C.M. (2010) Ethanol and cognition: indirect effects, neurotoxicity and neuroprotection: a review. *Int J Environ Res Public Health* **7,** 1540–1557.

Calhoun, F. and Warren, K. (2007) Fetal alcohol syndrome: historical perspectives. *Neurosci Biobehav Rev* **31,** 168–171.

Capaccio, P., Ottaviani, F., Cuccarini, V., *et al.* (2005) Association between methylenetetrahydrofolate reductase polymorphisms, alcohol intake and oropharyngolaryngeal carcinoma in northern Italy. *Laryngol Otol* **119,** 371–376.

Caton, S.J., Bate, L., and Hetherington, M.M. (2007) Acute effects of an alcoholic drink on food intake: aperitif versus co-ingestion. *Physiol Behav* **90,** 368–375.

Collins, M.A., Neafsey, E.J., Mukamal, K.J., *et al.* (2009) Alcohol in moderation, cardioprotection, and neuroprotection: epidemiological considerations and mechanistic studies. *Alcohol Clin Exp Res* **33,** 206–219.

Conen, D., Tedrow, U.B., Cook, N.R., *et al.* (2008) Alcohol consumption and risk of incident atrial fibrillation in women. *JAMA* **300,** 2489–2496.

Cook, C.C.H., Hallwood, P.M., and Thomson, A.D. (1998) B-Vitamin deficiency and neuropsychiatric syndromes in alcohol misuse. *Alcohol Alcohol* **33,** 317–336.

Costanzo, S., Di Castelnuovo, A., Donati, M.B., *et al.* (2010) Alcohol consumption and mortality in patients with cardiovascular disease: a meta-analysis. *J Am Coll Cardiol* **55,** 1339–1347.

Crandall, J.P., Polsky, S., Howard, A.A., *et al.* (2009) Alcohol consumption and diabetes risk in the Diabetes Prevention Program. *Am J Clin Nutr* **90,** 595–601.

Criqui, M.H. (1998) Do known cardiovascular risk factors mediate the effect of alcohol on cardiovascular disease? *Novartis Found Symp* **216,** 159–167.

Crowe, S.F. and Kempton, S. (1997) Both ethanol toxicity and thiamine deficiency are necessary to produce long-term memory deficits in the young chick. *Pharmacol Biochem Behav* **58,** 461–470.

Dallongeville, J., Marécaux, N., Ducimetière, P., *et al.* (1998) Influence of alcohol consumption and various beverages on waist girth and waist-to-hip ratio in a sample of French men and women. *Int J Obes Relat Metab Disord* **22,** 1778–1783.

Dan, Z., Popov, Y., Patsenker, E., *et al.* (2005) Hepatotoxicity of alcohol-induced polar retinol metabolites involves apoptosis via loss of mitochondrial membrane potential. *FASEB J* 845–847.

Das, S.K., Dhanya, L., and Vasudevan, D.M. (2008) Biomarkers of alcoholism: an updated review. *Scand J Clin Lab Invest* **68,** 81–92.

Dastur, D.K., Santhadevi, Q., and Quadros, E.V. (1976) The B-vitamins in malnutrition with alcoholism. *Br J Nutr* **36,** 143–159.

de la Maza, M.P., Petermann, M., Bunout, D., *et al.* (1995) Effects of long-term vitamin E supplementation in alcoholic cirrhotics. *J Am Coll Nutr* **14,** 192–196.

Delanghe, J.R. and De Buyzere, M.L. (2009) Carbohydrate deficient transferrin and forensic medicine. *Clin Chim Acta* **406,** 1–7.

Diehl, A.M. (2005) Recent events in alcoholic liver disease V. Effects of ethanol on liver regeneration. *Am J Physiol Gastrointest Liver Physiol* **288,** G1–6.

di Sario, A., Candelaresi, C., Omenetti, A., *et al.* (2007) Vitamin E in chronic liver diseases and liver fibrosis. In L. Gerald (ed.), *Vitamins and Hormones.* Academic Press, London, pp. 551–573.

Djousse, L., Arnett, D.K., Eckfeldt, J.H., *et al.* (2004) Alcohol consumption and metabolic syndrome: does the type of beverage matter? *Obes Res* **12,** 1375–1385.

Djousse, L., Lee, I.-M., Buring, J.E., *et al.* (2009) Alcohol consumption and risk of cardiovascular disease and death in women: potential mediating mechanisms. *Circulation* **120,** 237–244.

Donnino, M.W., Vega, J., Miller, J., *et al.* (2007) Myths and misconceptions of Wernicke's encephalopathy: what every emergency physician should know. *Ann Emerg Med* **50,** 715–721.

Druesne-Pecollo, N., Tehard, B., Mallet, Y., *et al.* (2009) Alcohol and genetic polymorphisms: effect on risk of alcohol-related cancer. *Lancet Oncology* **10,** 173–180.

Duffy, C., Assaf, A., Cyr, M., *et al.* (2009) Alcohol and folate intake and breast cancer risk in the WHI Observational Study. *Breast Cancer Res Treat* **116,** 551–562.

Ebbert, J.O., Janney, C.A., Sellers, T.A., *et al.* (2005) The association of alcohol consumption with coronary heart disease mortality and cancer incidence varies by smoking history. *J Gen Intern Med* **20,** 14–20.

Fernandez-Solà, J., Preedy, V.R., Lang, C.H., *et al.* (2007) Molecular and cellular events in alcohol-induced muscle disease. *Alcohol Clin Exp Res* **31,** 1953–1962.

Feskanich, D., Korrick, S.A., Greenspan, S.L., *et al.* (1999) Moderate alcohol consumption and bone density among postmenopausal women. *J Womens Health* **8**, 65–73.

Flanagan, D., Wood, P., Sherwin, R., *et al.* (1998) Gin and tonic and reactive hypoglycemia: what is important – the gin, the tonic, or both? *J Clin Endocrinol Metabol* **83**, 796–800.

Fogle, R.L., Lynch, C.J., Palopoli, M., *et al.* (2010) Impact of chronic alcohol ingestion on cardiac muscle protein expression. *Alcohol Clin Exp Res* **34**, 1226–1234.

Freiberg, M.S., Cabral, H.J., Heeren, T.C., *et al.* (2004) Alcohol consumption and the prevalence of the metabolic syndrome in the U.S.: a cross-sectional analysis of data from the Third National Health and Nutrition Examination Survey. *Diabetes Care* **27**, 2954–2959.

Fuhrman, B., Lavy, A., and Aviram, M. (1995) Consumption of red wine with meals reduces the susceptibility of human plasma and low-density-lipoprotein to lipid peroxidation. *Am J Clin Nutr* **61**, 549–554.

Galvin, R., Bråthen, G., Ivashynka, A., *et al.* (2010) EFNS guidelines for diagnosis, therapy and prevention of Wernicke encephalopathy. *Eur J Neurol* **17**, 1408–1418.

Gaziano, J.M., Gaziano, T.A., Glynn, R.J., *et al.* (2000) Light-to-moderate alcohol consumption and mortality in the physicians' health study enrollment cohort. *J Am Coll Cardiol* **35**, 96–105.

Gloria, L., Cravo, M., Camilo, M.E., *et al.* (1997) Nutritional deficiencies in chronic alcoholics: relation to dietary intake and alcohol consumption. *Am J Gastroenterol* **92**, 485–489.

González-Reimers, E., Durán-Castellón, M.C., López-Lirola, A., *et al.* (2010) Alcoholic myopathy: vitamin D deficiency is related to muscle fibre atrophy in a murine model. *Alcohol Alcohol* **45**, 223–230.

Greenfield, J.R., Samaras, K., Hayward, C.S., *et al.* (2005) Beneficial postprandial effect of a small amount of alcohol on diabetes and cardiovascular risk factors: modification by insulin resistance. *J Clin Endocrinol Metab* **90**, 661–672.

Grobbee, D.E., Rimm, E.B., Keil, U., *et al.* (1999) Alcohol and the cardiovascular system. In I. Macdonald (ed.), *Health Issues Related to Alcohol Consumption*. ILSI, Washington, DC, pp. 35–52.

Gross, A.L., Rebok, G.W., Ford, D.E., *et al.* (2011) Alcohol consumption and domain-specific cognitive function in older adults: longitudinal data from the Johns Hopkins Precursors Study. *J Gerontol B Psychol Sci Soc Sci* **66**, 39–47.

Guañabens, N. and Parés, A. (2010) Liver and bone. *Arch Biochem Biophys* **503**, 84–94.

Guo, R. and Ren, J. (2010) Alcohol and acetaldehyde in public health: from marvel to menace. *Int J Environ Res Public Health* **7**, 1285–1301.

Halsted, C.H. (1995) Alcohol and folate interactions: Clinical implications. In L.B. Bailey (ed.), *Folate in Health and Disease*. Marcel Dekker, New York, pp. 52–65.

Halsted, C.H. (2004) Nutrition and alcoholic liver disease. *Semin Liver Dis* **24**, 289–304.

Hamajima, N., Hirose, K., Tajima, K., *et al.* (2002) Alcohol, tobacco and breast cancer – collaborative reanalysis of individual data from 53 epidemiological studies, including 58 515 women with breast cancer and 95 067 women without the disease. *Br J Cancer* **87**, 1234–1245.

Hansel, B., Thomas, F., Pannier, B., *et al.* (2010) Relationship between alcohol intake, health and social status and cardiovascular risk factors in the urban Paris-Ile-de-France Cohort: is the cardioprotective action of alcohol a myth? *Eur J Clin Nutr* **64**, 561–568.

Hardman, M.J., Page, R.A., Wiseman, M.S., *et al.* (1991) Regulation of rates of ethanol metabolism and liver [NAD$^+$]/[NADH] ratio. In N.T. Palmer (ed.), *Alcoholism. A Molecular Perspective*. Plenum Press, New York, pp. 27–33.

Harper, C. (2009) The neuropathology of alcohol-related brain damage. *Alcohol Alcohol* **44**, 136–140.

Harvey, B.L., Anthony, R., and Matthew, C. (2009) Diagnosis and epidemiology of cirrhosis. *Med Clin North Am* **93**, 787–799.

Hazell, A.S. (2009) Astrocytes are a major target in thiamine deficiency and Wernicke's encephalopathy. *Neurochem Int* **55**, 129–135.

Higuchi, S., Matsushita, S., Masaki, T., *et al.* (2004) Influence of genetic variations of ethanol-metabolizing enzymes on phenotypes of alcohol-related disorders. *Ann NY Acad Sci* **1025**, 472–480.

Hill, J.A. (2005) In vino veritas: alcohol and heart disease. *Am J Med Sci* **329**, 124–135.

Hillbom, M. and Numminen, H. (1998) Alcohol and stroke: pathophysiologic mechanisms. *Neuroepidemiology* **17**, 281–287.

Hofer, R. and Burd, L. (2009) Review of published studies of kidney, liver, and gastrointestinal birth defects in fetal alcohol spectrum disorders. *Birth Defects Res A Clin Mol Teratol* **85**, 179–183.

Holzbach, E. (1996) Thiamin absorption in alcoholic delirium patients. *J Stud Alcohol* **57**, 581–584.

Hornnes, N., Larsen, K., and Boysen, G. (2010) Little change of modifiable risk factors 1 year after stroke: a pilot study. *Int J Stroke* **5**, 157–162.

Hubner, R.A. and Houlston, R.S. (2008) Folate and colorectal cancer prevention. *Br J Cancer* **100**, 233–239.

Huntgeburth, M., Ten-Freyhaus, H., and Rosenkranz, S. (2005) Alcohol consumption and hypertension. *Curr Hypertens Rep* **7**, 180–185.

Hvidtfeldt, U.A., Tolstrup, J.S., Jakobsen, M.U., et al. (2010) Alcohol intake and risk of coronary heart disease in younger, middle-aged, and older adults. *Circulation* **121**, 1589–1597.

Jackson, V., Sesso, H., Buring, J., et al. (2003) Alcohol consumption and mortality in men with preexisting cerebrovascular disease. *Arch Intern Med*, **163**, 1189–1193.

Jamieson, C.P., Obeid, O.A., and Powell-Tuck, J. (1999) The thiamin, riboflavin and pyridoxine status of patients on emergency admission to hospital. *Clin Nutr* **18**, 87–91.

Jin, L.H., Chang, S.J., Koh, S.B., et al. (2010) Association between alcohol consumption and bone strength in Korean adults: the Korean Genomic Rural Cohort Study. *Metabolism* **60**, 351–358.

Johansen, D., Andersen, P.K., Jensen, M.K., et al. (2003) Nonlinear relation between alcohol intake and high-density lipoprotein cholesterol level: results from the Copenhagen City Heart Study. *Alcohol Clin Exp Res* **27**, 1305–1309.

Jones, K.L., Hoyme, H.E., Robinson, L.K., et al. (2010) Fetal alcohol spectrum disorders: extending the range of structural defects. *Am J Med Genet Part A* **152A**, 2731–2735.

Joosten, M.M., Chiuve, S.E., Mukamal, K.J., et al. (2011) Changes in alcohol consumption and subsequent risk of type 2 diabetes in men. *Diabetes* **60**, 74–79.

Joshi, P.C. and Guidot, D.M. (2007) The alcoholic lung: epidemiology, pathophysiology, and potential therapies. *Am J Physiol Lung Cell Mol Physiol* **292**, L813–823.

Joshi, P.C., Mehta, A., Jabber, W.S., et al. (2009) Zinc deficiency mediates alcohol-induced alveolar epithelial and macrophage dysfunction in rats. *Am J Respir Cell Mol. Biol* **41**, 207–216.

Kaminen-Ahola, N., Ahola, A., Maga, M., et al. (2010) Maternal ethanol consumption alters the epigenotype and the phenotype of offspring in a mouse model. *PLoS Genet* **6**, e1000811.

Kane, M.A., Folias, A.E., Wang, C., et al. (2010) Ethanol elevates physiological all-*trans*-retinoic acid levels in select loci through altering retinoid metabolism in multiple loci: a potential mechanism of ethanol toxicity. *FASEB J* **24**, 823–832.

Kang, X., Zhong, W., Liu, J., et al. (2009) Zinc supplementation reverses alcohol-induced steatosis in mice through reactivating hepatocyte nuclear factor-4α and peroxisome proliferator-activated receptor-α. *Hepatology* **50**, 1241–1250.

Ke, Z.J., Wang, X., Fan, Z., et al. (2009) Ethanol promotes thiamine deficiency-induced neuronal death: involvement of double-stranded RNA-activated protein kinase. *Alcohol Clin Exp Res* **33**, 1097–1103.

Keith, M.E., Walsh, N.A., Darling, P.B., et al. (2009) B-vitamin deficiency in hospitalized patients with heart failure. *J Am Diet Assoc* **109**, 1406–1410.

Kisters, K., Schodjaian, K., Nguyen, S.Q., et al. (1997) Effect of alcohol on plasma and intracellular magnesium status in patients with steatosis or cirrhosis of the liver. *Med Sci Res* **25**, 805–806.

Klatsky, A.L. (1999) Is it the drink or the drinker? Circumstantial evidence only raises a probability. *Am J Clin Nutr* **69**, 2–3.

Klatsky, A.L. (2010) Alcohol and cardiovascular health. *Physiol Behav* **100**, 76–81.

Klatsky, A.L., Armstrong, M.A., and Kipp, H. (1990) Correlates of alcoholic beverage preference: traits of persons who choose wine, liquor or beer. *Br J Addict* **85**, 1279–1289.

Klatsky, A.L., Friedman, G.D., Siegelaub, A.B., et al. (1977) Alcohol consumption and blood pressure: Kaiser-Permanente multiphasic health examination data. *N Engl J Med* **296**, 1194–1200.

Kloner, R.A. and Rezkalla, S.H. (2007) To drink or not to drink? That is the question. *Circulation* **116**, 1306–1317.

Kumar, A., Singh, C.K., Dipette, D.D., et al. (2010) Ethanol impairs activation of retinoic acid receptors in cerebellar granule cells in a rodent model of fetal alcohol spectrum disorders. *Alcohol Clin Exp Res* **34**, 928–937.

Kwan, M.L., Kushi, L.H., Weltzien, E., et al. (2010) Alcohol consumption and breast cancer recurrence and survival among women with early-stage breast cancer: the Life After Cancer epidemiology study *J Clin Oncol* **28**, 4410–4416.

Laitinen, K. and Valimaki, M. (1993) Bone and the "comforts of life". *Ann Med* **25**, 413–425.

Laitinen, K., Valimaki, M., Lamberg-Allardt, C., et al. (1990) Deranged vitamin D metabolism but normal bone mineral density in Finnish noncirrhotic male alcoholics. *Alcohol Clin Exp Res* **14**, 551–556.

Lange, L.G. (1982) Nonoxidative ethanol metabolism: formation of fatty acid ethyl esters by cholesterol esterase. *Proc Natl Acad Sci USA* **79**, 3954–3957.

Laonigro, I., Correale, M., Di Biase, M., et al. (2009) Alcohol abuse and heart failure. *Eur J Heart Failure*, **11**, 453–462.

Larsson, S.C., Giovannucci, E., and Wolk, A. (2005) Vitamin B6 intake, alcohol consumption, and colorectal cancer: a longitudinal population-based cohort of women. *Gastroenterology* **128**, 1830–1837.

Larsson, S.C., Orsini, N., and Wolk, A. (2010) Vitamin B6 and risk of colorectal cancer: a meta-analysis of prospective studies. *JAMA* **303**, 1077–1083.

Le Marchand, L., Wilkens, L.R., Kolonel, L.N., et al. (2005) The MTHFR C677T polymorphism and colorectal cancer: the Multiethnic Cohort Study. *Cancer Epidemiol Biomarkers Prev* **14**, 1198–1203.

Leo, M.A. and Lieber, C.S. (1999) Alcohol, vitamin A, and beta-carotene: adverse interactions, including hepatotoxicity and carcinogenicity. *Am J Clin Nutr* **69**, 1071–1085.

Li, C.I., Chlebowski, R.T., Freiberg, M., et al. (2010) Alcohol consumption and risk of postmenopausal breast cancer by subtype: the women's health initiative observational study. *J Natl Cancer Inst* **102**, 1422–1431.

Li, T.K. (2000) Pharmacogenetics of responses to alcohol and genes that influence alcohol drinking. *J Stud Alcohol* **61**, 5–12.

Lieber, C.S. (1991) Perspectives: do alcohol calories count? *Am J Clin Nutr* **54**, 976–982.

Lieber, C.S. (1995) Medical disorders of alcoholism. *N Engl J Med* **333**, 1058–1065.

Lieber, C.S. and De Carli, L.M. (1970) Hepatic microsomal ethanol-oxidizing system: in vitro characteristics and adaptive properties in vivo. *J Biol Chem*, **245**, 2505–2512.

Liu, S., Serdula, M.K., Williamson, D.F., *et al.* (1994) A prospective study of alcohol intake and change in body weight among US adults. *Am J Epidemiol* **140**, 912–920.

Lock, K., Pomerleau, J., Causer, L., *et al.* (2005) The global burden of disease attributable to low consumption of fruit and vegetables: implications for the global strategy on diet. *Bull World Health Organ* **83**, 100–108.

Lussier-Cacan, S., Bolduc, A., Xhignesse, M., *et al.* (2002) Impact of alcohol intake on measures of lipid metabolism depends on context defined by gender, body mass index, cigarette smoking, and apolipoprotein E genotype. *Arterioscler Thromb Vasc Biol* **22**, 824–831.

Luvizotto, R.A.M., Nascimento, A.F., Veeramachaneni, S., *et al.* (2010) Chronic alcohol intake upregulates hepatic expression of carotenoid cleavage enzymes and PPAR in rats. *J Nutr* **140**, 1808–1814.

Machlin, L. (1989) Use and safety of elevated dosages of vitamin E in adults. *Int J Vitam Nutr Res* **30**(Suppl), 56–68.

Malhi, H., Guicciardi, M.E., and Gores, G.J. (2010) Hepatocyte death: a clear and present danger. *Physiol Rev* **90**, 1165–1194.

Maluenda, F., Csendes, A., De Aretxabala, X., *et al.* (2010) Alcohol absorption modification after a laparoscopic sleeve gastrectomy due to obesity. *Obes Surg* **20**, 744–748.

Manach, C., Williamson, G., Morand, C., *et al.* (2005) Bioavailability and bioefficacy of polyphenols in humans. I. Review of 97 bioavailability studies. *Am J Clin Nutr* **81**, 230S–242S.

Mancinelli, R. and Ceccanti, M. (2009) Biomarkers in alcohol misuse: their role in the prevention and detection of thiamine deficiency. *Alcohol Alcohol* **44**, 177–182.

Manttari, M., Tenkanen, L., Alikoski, T., *et al.* (1997) Alcohol and coronary heart disease: the roles of HDL-cholesterol and smoking. *J Intern Med* **214**, 157–163.

Martin, J., Barry, J., Goggin, D., *et al.* (2010) Alcohol-attributable mortality in Ireland. *Alcohol Alcohol* **45**, 379–386.

Martin, P.R., Singleton, C.K., and Hiller-Sturmhofel, S. (2003) The role of thiamine deficiency in alcoholic brain disease. *Alcohol Res Health* **27**, 134–142.

McCann, S.E., Sempos, C., Freudenheim, J.L., *et al.* (2003) Alcoholic beverage preference and characteristics of drinkers and nondrinkers in western New York (United States). *Nutr Metab Cardiovasc Dis* **13**, 2–11.

McClain, C.J., Van-Thiel, D.H., Parker, S., *et al.* (1979) Alteration in zinc, vitamin A and retinol-binding protein in chronic alcoholics: a possible mechanism for night blindness and hypogonadism. *Alcohol Clin Exp Res* **3**, 135–140.

McFadden, C.B., Brensinger, C.M., Berlin, J.A., *et al.* (2005) Systematic review of the effect of daily alcohol intake on blood pressure. *Am J Hypertens* **18**, 276–286.

McLean, J. and Manchip, S. (1999) Wernicke's encephalopathy induced by magnesium depletion. *Lancet* **353**, 1768.

Mendenhall, C., Roselle, G.A., Gartside, P., *et al.* (1995) Relationship of protein calorie malnutrition to alcoholic liver disease: a reexamination of data from two Veterans Administration cooperative studies. *Alcohol Clin Exp Res* **19**, 635–641.

Mitchell, D., Wagner, C., Stone, W.J., *et al.* (1976) Abnormal regulation of plasma pyridoxal-5′-phosphate in patients with liver disease. *Gastroenterology* **71**, 1043–1049.

Mizrahi, A., Knekt, P., Montonen, J., *et al.* (2009) Plant foods and the risk of cerebrovascular diseases: a potential protection of fruit consumption. *Br J Nutr* **102**, 1075–1083.

Mokdad, A.H., Marks, J.S., Stroup, D.F., *et al.* (2004) Actual causes of death in the United States, 2000. *JAMA* **291**, 1238–1245.

Mortensen, E.L., Jensen, H.H., Sanders, S.A., *et al.* (2001) Better psychological functioning and higher social status may largely explain the apparent health benefits of wine: a study of wine and beer drinking in young Danish adults. *Arch Intern Med* **161**, 1844–1848.

Mostofsky, E., Burger, M.R., Schlaug, G., *et al.* (2010) Alcohol and acute ischemic stroke onset: the Stroke Onset Study. *Stroke* **41**, 1845–1849.

Mukamal, K., Chung, H., Jenny, N., *et al.* (2005) Alcohol use and risk of ischemic stroke among older adults. The cardiovascular health study. *Stroke* **36**, 1830–1834.

Mukamal, K.J., Chen, C.M., Rao, S.R., *et al.* (2010) Alcohol consumption and cardiovascular mortality among U.S. adults, 1987 to 2002. *J Am Coll Cardiol* **55**, 1328–1335.

Nakahara, T., Hashimoto, K., Hirano, M., *et al.* (2003) Acute and chronic effects of alcohol exposure on skeletal muscle c-myc, p53, and Bcl-2 mRNA expression. *Am J Physiol Endocrinol Metab* **285**, E1273–1281.

National Institute on Alcohol Abuse and Alcoholism (NIAAA) (2009) Alcohol across the lifespan. Five Year Strategic Plan FY09-14. http://pubs.niaaa.nih.gov/publications/strategicplan/niaaastrategicplan.htm (accessed June 20, 2010).

Niemelä, O. (2007) Acetaldehyde adducts in circulation. *Novartis Found Symp* **285**, 183–192.

Nyquist, F., Karlsson, M.K., Obrant, K.J., *et al.* (1997) Osteopenia in alcoholics after tibia shaft fractures. *Alcohol Alcohol* **32**, 599–604.

Nyquist, F., Ljunghall, S., Berglund, M., *et al.* (1996) Biochemical markers of bone metabolism after short and long time ethanol withdrawal in alcoholics. *Bone* **19**, 51–54.

O'Leary, C.M., Nassar, N., Kurinczuk, J.J., *et al.* (2010) Prenatal alcohol exposure and risk of birth defects. *Pediatrics* **126**, e843–850.

Onland-Moret, N.C., Peeters, P.H.M., Van Der Schouw, Y.T., *et al.* (2005) Alcohol and endogenous sex steroid levels in postmenopausal women: a cross-sectional study. *J Clin Endocrinol Metab* **90**, 1414–1419.

Ono, S., Takahashi, H., and Hirano, H. (1987) Ethanol enhances the esterification of riboflavin in rat organ tissue. *Int J Vitam Nutr Res* **57**, 335.

Opie, L.H. and Lecour, S. (2007) The red wine hypothesis: from concepts to protective signalling molecules. *Eur Heart J* **28**, 1683–1693.

O'Shea, R.S., Dasarathy, S., and McCullough, A.J. (2010) Alcoholic liver disease. *Hepatology* **51**, 307–328.

Pagel, P.S., Kersten, J.R., and Warltier, D.C. (2004) Mechanisms of myocardial protection produced by chronic ethanol consumption. *Pathophysiology* **10**, 121–129.

Panza, F., Capurso, C., D'introno, A., *et al.* (2009) Alcohol drinking, cognitive functions in older age, predementia, and dementia syndromes. *J Alzheimers Dis* **17**, 7–31.

Paton, A. (2005) Alcohol in the body. *BMJ* **330**, 85–87.

Patra, J., Taylor, B., Irving, H., *et al.* (2010) Alcohol consumption and the risk of morbidity and mortality for different stroke types – a systematic review and meta-analysis. *BMC Public Health* **10**, 258.

Pedersen-Bjergaard, U., Reubsaet, J.L., Nielsen, S.L., *et al.* (2005) Psychoactive drugs, alcohol, and severe hypoglycemia in insulin-treated diabetes: analysis of 141 cases. *Am J Med Sci* **118**, 307–310.

Petersen, O.H., Tepikin, A.V., Gerasimenko, J.V., *et al.* (2009) Fatty acids, alcohol and fatty acid ethyl esters: toxic Ca2+ signal generation and pancreatitis. *Cell Calcium* **45**, 634–642.

Pietraszek, A., Gregersen, S., and Hermansen, K. (2010) Alcohol and type 2 diabetes. A review. *Nutr Metab Cardiovasc Dis* **20**, 366–375.

Pinto, J., Huang, Y.P., and Rivlin, R.S. (1987) Mechanisms underlying the differential effects of ethanol on the bioavailability of riboflavin and flavin adenine dinucleotide. *J Clin Invest* **79**, 1343–1348.

Pitel, A.-L., Zahr, N.M., Jackson, K., *et al.* (2011) Signs of preclinical Wernicke's encephalopathy and thiamine levels as predictors of neuropsychological deficits in alcoholism without Korsakoff's syndrome. *Neuropsychopharmacology* **36**, 580–588.

Pitsavas, S., Andreou, C., Bascialla, F., *et al.* (2004) Pellagra encephalopathy following B-complex vitamin treatment without niacin. *Int J Psychiatry Med* **34**, 91–95.

Plant, M.L., Abel, E.L., and Guerri, C. (1999) Alcohol and pregnancy. In I. Macdonald (ed.), *Health Issues Related to Alcohol Consumption*. ILSI, Washington, DC, pp. 182–213.

Prasad, A.S., Beck, F.W., Snell, D.C., *et al.* (2009) Zinc in cancer prevention. *Nutr Cancer* **61**, 879–887.

Preedy, V.R., Ohlendieck, K., Adachi, J., *et al.* (2003) The importance of alcohol-induced muscle disease. *J Muscle Res Motil* **24**, 55–63.

Preedy, V.R., Reilly, M.E., Patel, V.B., *et al.* (1999) Protein metabolism in alcoholism: effects on specific tissues and the whole body. *Nutrition* **15**, 604–608.

Ramsay, M. (2010) Genetic and epigenetic insights into fetal alcohol spectrum disorders. *Genome Medicine* **2**, 27.

Rehm, J., Taylor, B., Mohapatra, S., *et al.* (2010) Alcohol as a risk factor for liver cirrhosis: a systematic review and meta-analysis. *Drug Alcohol Rev* **29**, 437–445.

Renaud, S.C., Gueguen, R., Siest, G., *et al.* (1999) Wine, beer, and mortality in middle-aged men from eastern France. *Arch Intern Med* **159**, 1865–1870.

Reynolds, K., Lewis, L.B., Nolen, J.D.L., *et al.* (2003) Alcohol consumption and risk of stroke: a meta-analysis. *JAMA* **289**, 579–588.

Rimm, E.B. (1996) Alcohol consumption and coronary heart disease: good habits may be more important than just good wine. *Am J Epidemiol* **143**, 1089–1093.

Rimm, E.B., Klatsky, A., Grobbee, D., *et al.* (1996) Review of moderate alcohol consumption and reduced risk of coronary heart disease: is the effect due to beer, wine, or spirits? *BMJ* **312**, 731–736.

Rimm, E.B., Williams, P., Fosher, K., *et al.* (1999) Moderate alcohol intake and lower risk of coronary artery disease: meta-analysis of effects on lipids and haemostatic factors. *BMJ* **319**, 1523–1528.

Rodriguez, M.F., Gonzalez, R.E., Santolaria, F.F., *et al.* (1997) Zinc, copper, manganese, and iron in chronic alcoholic liver disease. *Alcohol* **14**, 39–44.

Roerecke, M. and Rehm, J. (2010) Irregular heavy drinking occasions and risk of ischemic heart disease: a systematic review and meta-analysis. *Am J Epidemiol* **171**, 633–644.

Rohrer, J.E., Rohland, B.M., Denison, A., *et al.* (2005) Frequency of alcohol use and obesity in community medicine patients. *BMC Fam Pract* **6**, 17.

Romani, A.M.P. (2008) Magnesium homeostasis and alcohol consumption. *Magnes Res* **21**, 197–204.

Ross, D.M. and McMartin, K.E. (1996) Effect of ethanol on folate binding by isolated rat renal brush border membranes. *Alcohol* **13**, 449–454.

Rossouw, J.E., Labadorios, D., Davis, M., *et al.* (1978) The degradation of tryptophan in severe liver disease. *Int J Vit Nutr Res* **48**, 281–289.

Rouillier, P., Boutron-Ruault, M.C., Bertrais, S., *et al.* (2004) Drinking patterns in French adult men – a cluster analysis of alcoholic beverages and relationship with lifestyle. *Eur J Nutr* **43**, 69–76.

Ruidavets, J.-B., Bataille, V., Dallongeville, J., *et al.* (2004) Alcohol intake and diet in France, the prominent role of lifestyle. *Eur Heart J* **25**, 1153–1162.

Sacco, R.L., Elkind, M., Boden-Albala, B., *et al.* (1999) The protective effect of moderate alcohol consumption on ischemic stroke. *JAMA* **281**, 53–60.

Sadakane, A., Gotoh, T., Ishikawa, S., *et al.* (2009) Amount and frequency of alcohol consumption and all-cause mortality in a Japanese population: the JMS Cohort Study. *J Epidemiol Community Health* **19**, 107–115.

Sakurai, Y., Umeda, T., Shinchi, K., *et al.* (1997) Relation of total and beverage-specific alcohol intake to body mass index and waist-to-hip ratio: a study of self-defense officials in Japan. *Eur J Epidemiol* **13**, 893–898.

Salaspuro, M. (1993) Nutrient intake and nutritional status in alcoholics. *Alcohol Alcohol* **28**, 85–88.

Santolaria-Fernandez, F.J., Gomez-Sirvent, J.L., Gonzalez-Reimers, C.E., *et al.* (1995) Nutritional assessment of drug addicts. *Drug Alcohol Depend* **38**, 11–18.

Sauer, J., Mason, J.B., and Choi, S.-W. (2009) Too much folate: a risk factor for cancer and cardiovascular disease? *Curr Opin Clin Nutr Metab Care* **12**, 30–36.

Schernhammer, E.S., Giovannucci, E., Kawasaki, T., *et al.* (2010) Dietary folate, alcohol and B vitamins in relation to LINE-1 hypomethylation in colon cancer. *Gut* **59**, 794–799.

Schoenborn, C.A. and Adams, P.E. (2010) Health behaviors of adults: United States, 2005–2007. *Vital Health Stat* **245**, 1–132.

Sechi, G. and Serra, A. (2007) Wernicke's encephalopathy: new clinical settings and recent advances in diagnosis and management. *Lancet Neurology* **6**, 442–455.

Seitz, H.K. and Stickel, F. (2007) Molecular mechanisms of alcohol-mediated carcinogenesis. *Nat Rev Cancer* **7**, 599–612.

Seitz, H.K. and Suter, P.M. (1994) Ethanol toxicity and the nutritional status. In F.N. Kotsonis, M. Mackey, and J. Hjelle (eds), *Nutritional Toxicology*. Raven Press, New York, pp. 95–116.

Seitz, H.K., Pöschl, G., and Simanowski, U.A. (1998) Alcohol and cancer. In M. Galanter (ed.), *Recent Advances in Alcoholism*. Plenum Press, New York, pp. 67–95.

Sesso, H.D., Cook, N.R., Buring, J.E., *et al.* (2008) Alcohol consumption and the risk of hypertension in women and men. *Hypertension* **51**, 1080–1087.

Shanmugham, J.R., Zavras, A.I., Rosner, B.A., *et al.* (2010) Alcohol–folate interactions in the risk of oral cancer in women: a prospective cohort study. *Cancer Epidemiol Biomarkers Prev* **19**, OF1–9.

Shiomi, S., Nishiguchi, S., Kubo, S., *et al.* (2002) Vitamin K2 (menatetrenone) for bone loss in patients with cirrhosis of the liver. *Am J Gastroenterol* **97**, 978–981.

Siler, S.Q., Neese, R.A., Christiansen, M.P., *et al.* (1998) The inhibition of gluconeogenesis following alcohol in humans. *Am J Physiol* **275**, E897–907.

Siler, S.Q., Neese, R.A., and Hellerstein, M.K. (1999) De novo lipogenesis, lipid kinetics, and whole-body lipid balances in humans after acute alcohol consumption. *Am J Clin Nutr* **70**, 928–936.

Smith, K.E. and Fenske, N.A. (2000) Cutaneous manifestations of alcohol abuse. *J Am Acad Dermatol*, **43**, 1–18.

Snow, W.M., Murray, R., Ekuma, O., *et al.* (2009) Alcohol use and cardiovascular health outcomes: a comparison across age and gender in the Winnipeg Health and Drinking Survey Cohort. *Age Ageing* **38**, 206–212.

Sozio, M. and Crabb, D.W. (2008) Alcohol and lipid metabolism. *Am J Physiol Endocrinol Metab* **295**, E10–16.

Spaak, J., Merlocco, A.C., Soleas, G.J., *et al.* (2008) Dose-related effects of red wine and alcohol on hemodynamics, sympathetic nerve activity, and arterial diameter. *Am J Physiol Heart Circ Physiol* **294**, H605–612.

Spaak, J., Tomlinson, G., McGowan, C.L., *et al.* (2010) Dose-related effects of red wine and alcohol on heart rate variability. *Am J Physiol Heart Circ Physiol* **298**, H2226–2231.

Stamoulis, I., Kouraklis, G., and Theocharis, S. (2007) Zinc and the liver: an active interaction. *Dig Dis Sci* **52**, 1595–1612.

Stampfer, M.J., Kang, J.H., Chen, J., *et al.* (2005) Effects of moderate alcohol consumption on cognitive function in women. *N Engl J Med* **352**, 245–253.

Subramanian, V.S., Subramanya, S.B., Tsukamoto, H., *et al.* (2010) Effect of chronic alcohol feeding on physiological and molecular parameters of renal thiamin transport. *Am J Physiol Renal Physiol* **299**, F28–34.

Subramanya, S.B., Subramanian, V.S., and Said, H.M. (2010) Chronic alcohol consumption and intestinal thiamin absorption: effects on physiological and molecular parameters of the uptake process. *Am J Physiol Gastrointest Liver Physiol* **299**, G23–31.

Sun, W., Schooling, C.M., Chan, W.M., *et al.* (2009) Moderate alcohol use, health status, and mortality in a prospective Chinese elderly cohort. *Ann Epidemiol* **19**, 396–403.

Süße, S., Selavka, C.M., Mieczkowski, T., *et al.* (2010) Fatty acid ethyl ester concentrations in hair and self-reported alcohol consumption in 644 cases from different origin. *Forensic Sci Int* **196**, 111–117.

Suter, P.M. (2005) Is alcohol consumption a risk factor for weight gain and obesity? *Crit Rev Clin Lab Sci* **42**, 1–31.

Suter, P.M., Gerritsen, M., Häsler, E., *et al.* (1999) Alcohol effects on postprandial lipemia with and without preprandial exercise. *FASEB J (Part I)*, **13**, A208.

Suter, P.M., Jéquier, E., and Schutz, Y. (1994) The effect of ethanol on energy expenditure. *Am J Physiol* **266**, R1204–R1212.

Suter, P.M., Maire, R., and Vetter, W. (1995) Is an increased waist:hip ratio the cause of alcohol-induced hypertension? The AIR94 study. *J Hypertens* **13**, 1857–1862.

Suter, P.M., Schutz, Y., and Jéquier, E. (1992) The effect of ethanol on fat storage in healthy subjects. *N Engl J Med* **326**, 983–987.

Suter, P.M. and Vetter, W. (2000a) Diuretics and vitamin B1: are diuretics a risk factor for thiamin malnutrition? *Nutr Rev* **58**, 319–323.

Suter, P.M. and Vetter, W. (2000b) The effect of alcohol on blood pressure. *Nutr Clin Care* **3**, 24–34.

Taylor, B., Irving, H.M., Baliunas, D., *et al.* (2009) Alcohol and hypertension: gender differences in dose–response relationships determined through systematic review and meta-analysis. *Addiction* **104**, 1981–1990.

Taylor, B. and Rehm, J. (2006) When risk factors combine: the interaction between alcohol and smoking for aerodigestive cancer, coronary heart disease, and traffic and fire injury. *Addictive Behav* **31**, 1522–1535.

Thun, M.J., Peto, R., Lopez, A.D., *et al.* (1997) Alcohol consumption and mortality among middle aged and elderly U.S. adults. *N Engl J Med* **337**, 1705–1714.

Tiwari, V., Kuhad, A., and Chopra, K. (2009a) Suppression of neuro-inflammatory signaling cascade by tocotrienol can prevent chronic alcohol-induced cognitive dysfunction in rats. *Behav Brain Res* **203**, 296–303.

Tiwari, V., Kuhad, A., and Chopra, K. (2009b) Tocotrienol ameliorates behavioral and biochemical alterations in the rat model of alcoholic neuropathy. *Pain* **145**, 129–135.

Tjonneland, A., Gronbæk, M., Stripp, C., *et al.* (1999) Wine intake and diet in a random sample of 48763 Danish men and women. *Am J Clin Nutr* **69**, 49–54.

Tolstrup, J., Grønbaek, M., and Nordestgaard, B.G. (2009) Alcohol intake, myocardial infarction, biochemical risk factors, and alcohol dehydrogenase genotypes. *Circ Cardiovasc Genet* 507–514.

Tomasulo, P.A., Kater, R.M.H., and Iber, F.L. (1968) Impairment of thiamine absorption in alcoholism. *Am J Clin Nutr* **21**, 1341–1344.

Trevisan, M., Krogh, V., and Farinaro, E. (1987) Alcohol consumption, drinking pattern and blood pressure: analysis of data from the Italian National Research Council Study. *Int J Epidemiol* **16**, 520–527.

Tucker, K.L., Jugdaohsingh, R., Powell, J.J., *et al.* (2009) Effects of beer, wine, and liquor intakes on bone mineral density in older men and women. *Am J Clin Nutr* **89**, 1188–1196.

Urbano-Marquez, A. and Fernandez-Sola, J. (2004) Effects of alcohol on skeletal and cardiac muscle. *Muscle Nerve* **30**, 689–707.

Valmadrid, C.T., Klein, R., Moss, S.E., *et al.* (1999) Alcohol intake and the risk of coronary heart disease mortality in persons with older-onset diabetes mellitus. *JAMA* **282**, 239–246.

Vannucchi, H. and Moreno, F.S. (1989) Interaction of niacin and zinc metabolism in patients with alcoholic pellagra. *Am J Clin Nutr* **50**, 364–369.

Veeramachaneni, S., Ausman, L.M., Choi, S.W., *et al.* (2008) High dose lycopene supplementation increases hepatic cytochrome P4502E1 protein and inflammation in alcohol-fed rats. *J Nutr* **138**, 1329–1335.

Venkat, K.K., Arora, M.M., Singh, P., *et al.* (2009) Effect of alcohol consumption on bone mineral density and hormonal parameters in physically active male soldiers. *Bone* **45**, 449–454.

Wakabayashi, I. (2010) History of antihypertensive therapy influences the relationships of alcohol with blood pressure and pulse pressure in older men. *Am J Hypertens* **23**, 633–638.

Walsh, M.P., Howorth, P.J.N., and Marks, V. (1966) Pyridoxine deficiency and tryptophan metabolism in chronic alcoholics. *Am J Clin Nutr* **19**, 379–383.

Wang, L., Lee, I.-M., Manson, J.E., *et al.* (2010) Alcohol consumption, weight gain, and risk of becoming overweight in middle-aged and older women. *Arch Intern Med* **170**, 453–461.

Watson, R.R. and Preedy, V.R. (2003) *Nutrition and Alcohol: Linking Nutrient Interactions and Dietary Intake.* CRC Press, Boca Raton, FL.

Westerterp-Plantenga, M.S. and Verwegen, C.R.T. (1999) The appetizing effect of an apéritif in overweight and normal-weight humans. *Am J Clin Nutr* **69**, 205–212.

White, I.R. (1999) The level of alcohol consumption at which all-cause mortality is least. *J Clin Epidemiol* **52**, 967–975.

White, I.R., Altmann, D.R., and Nanchahal, K. (2002) Alcohol consumption and mortality: modelling risks for men and women at different ages. *BMJ* **325**, 191.

Wolf, G. (2010) Tissue-specific increases in endogenous all-trans retinoic acid: possible contributing factor in ethanol toxicity. *Nutr Rev* **68**, 689–692.

World Health Organization (2010) Management of substance abuse: alcohol. http://www.who.int/substance_abuse/facts/alcohol/en/index.html (accessed August 5, 2010).

Xin, X., He, J., Frontini, M.G., *et al.* (2001) Effects of alcohol reduction on blood pressure. *Hypertension* **38**, 1112–1117.

Yeomans, M.R., Hails, N.J., and Nesic, J.S. (1999) Alcohol and the appetizer effect. *Behav Pharmacol* **10**, 151–161.

Zhang, S.M., Lee, I.M., Manson, J.E., *et al.* (2007) Alcohol consumption and breast cancer risk in the Women's Health Study. *Am J Epidemiol* **165**, 667–676.

Zheng, J.-P., Ju, D., Jiang, H., *et al.* (2010) Resveratrol induces p53 and suppresses myocardin-mediated vascular smooth muscle cell differentiation. *Toxicol Lett* **199**, 115–122.

Zhong, W., McClain, C.J., Cave, M., *et al.* (2010a) The role of zinc deficiency in alcohol-induced intestinal barrier dysfunction. *Am J Physiol Gastrointest Liver Physiol* **298**, G625–633.

Zhong, W., Zhao, Y., McClain, C.J., *et al.* (2010b) Inactivation of hepatocyte nuclear factor-4{alpha} mediates alcohol-induced downregulation of intestinal tight junction proteins. *Am J Physiol Gastrointest Liver Physiol* **299**, G643–651.

Zureik, M. and Ducimetière, P. (1996) High alcohol-related premature mortality in France: concordant estimates from a prospective cohort study and national mortality study. *Alcohol Clin Exp Res* **20**, 428–433.

56

EYE DISEASE

ROHINI VISHWANATHAN, PhD AND ELIZABETH J. JOHNSON, PhD

Tufts University, Boston, Massachusetts, USA

Summary

There is biological plausibility for a relationship between certain nutrients and certain eye diseases. This chapter discusses eye diseases and conditions and the beneficial nutrients. Even though evidence from epidemiological and intervention studies have at times yielded conflicting results, it is important to understand that nutrition can have a strong impact on eye diseases such as cataract, age-related macular degeneration (AMD), and retinitis pigmentosa (RP), which together account for ~60% of blindness worldwide. High dietary intake of vitamins C and E, starting early in life, may prevent the incidence of age-related nuclear cataracts as well as AMD. Lutein and zeaxanthin intake may protect against nuclear and posterior subcapsular cataract (PSC), while vitamins B_1, B_2, B_3, and folate may protect against nuclear and cortical cataract. Treatment with the Age-Related Eye Disease Study (AREDS) supplement (a combination of vitamins C and E, β-carotene, zinc, and copper) is beneficial for patients diagnosed with AMD. Apart from the AREDS vitamins, high doses of lutein and zeaxanthin have also been shown to benefit AMD patients. Lutein has also been found to improve visual function because of its role as macular pigment in healthy and also AMD-affected eyes. Among the B vitamins, B_6, B_{12}, and folate have shown some protective indications as a result of their ability to reduce hyperhomocysteinemia, a risk factor for AMD. Apart from increasing consumption of foods rich in the above vitamins and micronutrients, eating a healthy, well balanced diet is equally important in keeping the eyes healthy. Adhering to the Recommended Dietary Guidelines has been found to be associated with a reduced risk of nuclear cataract and advanced AMD. Greater intake of carbohydrates (≥200g/day) is also related to higher odds of cortical cataract. It is critical to eat not just the right amounts, but also the right types of carbohydrates, as high-glycemic-index foods are associated with an increased prevalence of AMD, and of nuclear and cortical cataract. Replacing refined carbohydrates with whole grains and limiting consumption of added sugars would be beneficial. Similarly, the types of fat in the diet could also influence the course of eye diseases. Intake of the omega-3 fatty acids, docosahexaenoic acid and arachidonic acid, is essential for visual development right from birth. Omega-3 fatty acids have also been shown to benefit AMD and RP patients. High intakes of omega-6 fatty acids can offset the omega-3 to omega-6 ratio, which has been shown to increase AMD risk. Adding one to two 3-ounce (85g) servings of omega-3 rich fatty fish per week to the diet can be beneficial. Omega-3 and omega-6 fatty acids and also antioxidant-rich oils ease dry-eye-related symptoms. RP patients may benefit from taking 15000IU/day of vitamin A in conjunction with a low vitamin E diet. Even though evidence for beneficial effects of anthocyanosides on visual function is minimal, adding anthocyanoside-rich foods like bilberries to the diet may be helpful because of their antioxidant potential. From the evidence presented in this chapter, it may be more practical to recommend consumption of foods rich in vitamins C and E, B vitamins, lutein and zeaxanthin, omega-3 fatty acids, and zinc, rather than consuming the nutrients in isolation, thus benefiting from the synergistic effects of all the components in the food.

Present Knowledge in Nutrition, Tenth Edition. Edited by John W. Erdman Jr, Ian A. Macdonald and Steven H. Zeisel.
© 2012 International Life Sciences Institute. Published 2012 by John Wiley & Sons, Inc.

Introduction

Nutrition has an essential role in the preservation and maintenance of vision . It has long been known that deficiencies of certain essential nutrients can result in visual impairment or blindness. The purpose of this chapter is to review the literature that evaluates the role of dietary components in the prevention of onset or progression of ocular diseases in humans. Figure 56.1 summarizes the nutrients that have been indicated to protect against such diseases, and that are needed in order to maintain normal visual function. Figure 56.2 shows the global causes of blindness. Of these the focus is on diseases for which there is strongest evidence for nutrition playing a role in the prevention and/or treatment. The diseases discussed at length are cataract, age-related macular degeneration, and retinitis pigmentosa. The nutrients of interest are vitamins C and E, carotenoids, B vitamins, omega-3 fatty acids, and zinc. In addition to the diseases of the eye, the possible role of certain nutrients and dietary components in the treatment of dry eye syndrome and visual function is also discussed.

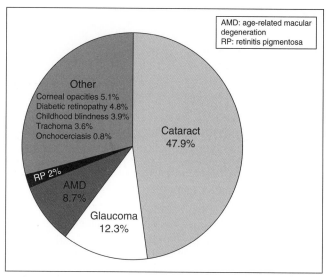

FIG. 56.2 The global causes of worldwide blindness as a percentage of total blindness. Data from Resnikoff *et al.* (2004).

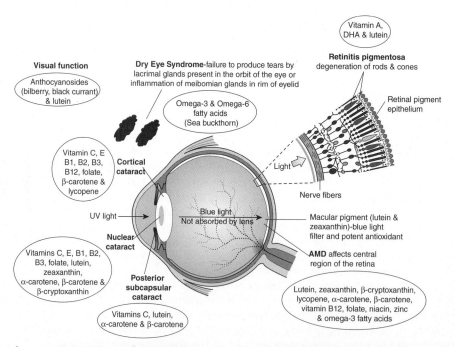

FIG. 56.1 Schematic representation of the different nutrients that have been indicated to protect against cataract, age-related macular degeneration (AMD), retinitis pigmentosa, and dry eye syndrome, and to maintain normal visual function. Reproduced with permission from Webvision.

Cataract

Age-related cataract is one of the major causes of visual impairment and blindness in the aging US population. Approximately 50% of the 30–50 million cases of worldwide blindness result from unoperated cataract (World Health Organization, 1991; Thylefors *et al.*, 1995). A clinically significant cataract is present in about 5% of Caucasian Americans aged 52–64 years and rises to 46% in those aged 75–85 years (Congdon *et al.*, 2004). In the United States, cataract extraction accompanied by ocular lens implant is the most common surgical procedure for the eye (Javitt, 1993). Lens implantation enables many to have reduced dependence on glasses. However, the procedure is costly, accounting for 12% of the Medicare budget and more than $3 billion in annual health expenditures (Javitt, 1993; Steinberg *et al.*, 1993). For these reasons, the prevention of cataract is a preferred alternative to surgery.

There are three types of cataract, defined by their location in the lens. Nuclear cataract occurs in the center, or nucleus, of the lens. Cortical cataract begins at the outer rim of the lens, which is referred to as the cortex, and progresses towards the center. Posterior subcapsular cataract (PSC) occurs in the central posterior cortex, just under the posterior capsule, the membrane that envelops the lens. Nuclear cataract is the most common type of cataract (Congdon *et al.*, 2004). It interferes with a person's ability to see distant objects and is usually the result of advancing age. Cortical cataract is most commonly seen in patients who have diabetes. PSC can be present in younger individuals and progresses more rapidly, resulting in glare and blurriness (Asbell *et al.*, 2005). This type of cataract is usually seen in patients who use steroids, or who suffer from diabetes or extreme nearsightedness. Figure 56.3(c) shows a scene viewed by a person affected by cataract.

There are various factors that may be involved in the development of cataracts, such as long-term light exposure, diabetes, smoking, alcohol use, and advancing age (Asbell *et al.*, 2005). Such factors can lead to aggregation

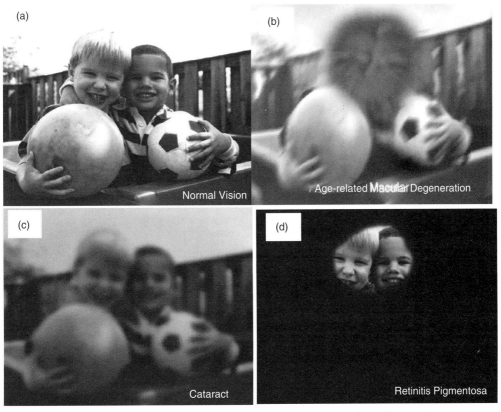

FIG. 56.3   A scene viewed by a person with (a) normal vision, (b) age-related macular degeneration, (c) cataract, and (d) retinitis pigmentosa. Photographs courtesy of National Eye Institute, National Institutes of Health.

of the lens proteins and osmotic damage, resulting in increased scattering of light and loss of transparency of the lens. Protein aggregation mainly occurs in the lens nucleus, and osmotic damage occurs in the lens cortex (Bunce *et al.*, 1990). Free radicals are generated in the lens during normal metabolic activities and also as a result of photo-oxidative reactions due to increased UVB exposure (related to cortical cataracts and PSC). These free radicals can also cause electrolyte imbalance and protein aggregation. Innate antioxidant defense mechanisms, enzymes such as superoxide dismutase and glutathione, and non-enzymatic molecules such as vitamins C and E, protect the lens from oxidative stress. Evidence related to nutrients that protect the lens from cataract development is discussed in the sections that follow. For each nutrient the probable mechanism of action, epidemiological evidence pertaining to both dietary intake and serum concentrations of the nutrient of interest, and finally randomized controlled trials, if any, are discussed. The observations are further divided based on the type of cataract (nuclear, cortical, or PSC) and the incidence of cataract extraction.

Vitamin C

The interest in studying vitamin C for cataract prevention and treatment results from that fact that its accumulation in the lens is 30- to 35-fold greater than in plasma. Not only is vitamin C a strong antioxidant but it also has the ability to absorb UV light (Bunce *et al.*, 1990). Several studies have found that a higher intake of vitamin C, from foods and supplements, was related to decreased risk of nuclear, cortical, PSC, or cataract extraction (Robertson *et al.*, 1989; Jacques and Chylack, 1991; Leske *et al.*, 1991; Hankinson *et al.*, 1992; Mares-Perlman *et al.*, 1995a, 2000; Jacques *et al.*, 1997, 2001; Taylor and Hobbs, 2001; Tan *et al.*, 2008a). The dose of supplementation, duration of either supplement use or intake from foods, age, type of cataract, and certain factors such as smoking, influence the effect of vitamin C on the incidence of cataract. Data from several epidemiological studies reporting a protective relationship have shown the mean range of daily vitamin C intake from diet and supplements to be 104–700 mg in the highest quintile groups, whereas the lowest quintile groups have intakes in the range 33–140 mg (Hankinson *et al.*, 1992; Mares-Perlman *et al.*, 1995a; Jacques *et al.*, 2001). In some studies even the lowest quintile groups had greater vitamin C intake than the RDA of 75 mg/day. On the other hand, intake of ~1000 mg of vitamin C was found to increase the risk of cataract in women aged ≥65

years from the Swedish Mammography cohort (Rautiainen *et al.*, 2010). Long-term vitamin C intake of ≥10 years was beneficial in reducing the incidence of cataract, lens opacities and also cataract extraction in all but one study, where the risk of cataract extraction was lower only in women <60 years and non-smokers (Hankinson *et al.*, 1992; Jacques *et al.*, 1997, 2001; Chasen-Taber *et al.*, 1999; Mares-Perlman *et al.*, 2000; Taylor *et al.*, 2002a; Tan *et al.*, 2008a). In epidemiological studies that had a <10-year follow-up, vitamin C intake did not have the same protective effect (Seddon *et al.*, 1994b; Leske *et al.*, 1998; Mares-Perlman *et al.*, 2000). Even with intakes of high doses of vitamin C, women aged ≥60 years were not protected from cortical cataract and cataract extraction (Leske *et al.*, 1998; Taylor *et al.*, 2002a; Gritz *et al.*, 2006). Summary of data from epidemiological studies on dietary intake of vitamin C is presented in Table 56.1.

Serum ascorbic acid concentrations have been reported to be inversely associated with the prevalence of cataract (Jacques and Chylack, 1991; Simon and Hudes, 1999; Valero *et al.*, 2002; Ferrigno *et al.*, 2005; Dherani *et al.*, 2008; Jalal *et al.*, 2009). Two studies found no association between plasma vitamin C and the risk of nuclear or cortical cataract (Vitale *et al.*, 1993; Nourmohammadi *et al.*, 2008). This may be because the plasma samples were analyzed 4 years prior to the lens examination in one study, and the population size was small in the second study. In contrast, the India–United States case-control study found an increased prevalence of PSC and nuclear cataracts with increased plasma vitamin C but this relationship became protective when vitamin C status was combined with other indices of antioxidant status such as glutathione peroxidase, vitamin E and glucose-6-phosphate dehydrogenase (Mohan *et al.*, 1989). A summary of data from epidemiological studies on serum concentrations of vitamin C is presented in Table 56.2.

There are no randomized control trials to date that have evaluated a vitamin C intervention alone on the incidence of cataract. Intervention studies using vitamin C in conjunction with other antioxidants and vitamins have yielded conflicting results, which are discussed later in the "Intervention Studies" section.

Epidemiologic evidence showed dietary vitamin C to be most beneficial towards nuclear cataract followed by cortical cataract, and lastly PSC (Leske *et al.*, 1991; Mares-Perlman *et al.*, 1995a; Gale *et al.*, 2001; Jacques *et al.*, 2001; Taylor *et al.*, 2002a; Tan *et al.*, 2008b). Vitamin C intake was also associated with reduced risk of cataract

TABLE 56.1 Dietary intake of vitamin C (from food and supplement) and risk of cataract

Study	Study design	Dietary intake	Study duration	OR/RR/HR[a] (95% confidence interval)	Result	Reference
Robertson et al.	Case-control	S	—	OR = 0.30 (0.12–0.75) P = 0.01	Vitamin C supplement intake was associated with 50% reduction in senile cataract	Robertson et al. (1989)
LOCCS	Case-control	F & S	—	OR = 0.48 (0.24–0.99) P ≥ 0.05(nuclear)	Significantly reduced odds of nuclear cataract were related to vitamin C intake	Leske et al. (1991)
Jacques and Chylack	Case-control	F & S	—	OR = 0.73 (0.31–1.73) (PSC) OR = 0.80 (0.50–1.29) (cortical) OR = 3.7, P < 0.10 (cortical) OR = 11.0, P < 0.05 (PSC)	Low vitamin C intake was associated with greater odds of cortical and PSC	Jacques and Chylack (1991)
NHS	Prospective	S	8 years	RR = 0.55 (0.32–0.96)	45% lower risk of cataract extraction associated with ≥10 years of supplementation	Hankinson et al. (1992)
PHS	Prospective	S	5 years	RR = 1.32 (0.85–2.04) P = 0.21	Vitamin C supplementation was not associated with decreased cataract risk	Seddon et al. (1994b)
BDES	Retrospective	F & S	—	OR = 0.62 (0.39–0.97) P = 0.09 (men)	Men in the highest quintile of vitamin C intake had reduced odds of nuclear opacity compared with the lowest quintile	Mares-Perlman et al. (1995a)
Tavani et al.	Case-control	F	—	OR = 0.8 (0.4–1.3)	Odds of cataract extraction in the highest quintile intake of vitamin C not different from the lowest quintile intake	Tavani et al. (1996)
NHS	Prospective	S	≥10 years	OR = 0.23 (0.09–0.60) P = 0.02 OR = 0.17 (0.03–0.85) P = 0.03	77% lower prevalence of early lens opacities in supplement users 83% lower prevalence of moderate lens opacities in supplement users	Jacques et al. (1997)
NHS	Prospective	S	12 years	RR = 0.95 (0.76–1.20) (>10 years)	Risk of cataract not reduced in supplement users vs. nonusers even for ≥10 years intake	Chasan-Taber et al. (1999)

(Continued)

TABLE 56.1 (Continued)

Study	Study design	Dietary intake	Study duration	OR/RR/HR[a] (95% confidence interval)	Result	Reference
				RR = 0.71 (0.47–1.08) (never smokers) RR = 0.72 (0.49–1.04) (women <60 years)	Risk of cataract extraction relatively lower in ≥10 years supplement users who never smoked and women aged <60 years	Mares-Perlman et al. (2000)
BDES	Prospective	S	5 years	OR = 0.4 (0.3–0.6) P < 0.001	Risk of any cataract was 60% lower with intake of any supplement containing vitamin C for >10 years	
NVP (NHS)	Prospective	F & S	13–15 years	OR = 0.31 (0.16–0.58) P = 0.003	Reduced prevalence of nuclear opacity in the highest quintile intake of vitamin C	Jacques et al. (2001)
		S		OR = 0.36 (0.18–0.72) P = 0.004	Reduced prevalence of nuclear opacity with ≥10 years intake of vitamin C relative to never intake	
NHS	Retrospective	F & S	13–15 years	OR = 0.43 (0.2–0.93) (women <60 years)	Vitamin C intake ≥362 mg/day was associated with 57% lower odds of developing cortical cataract than intake of <140 mg/day	Taylor et al. (2002a)
				OR = 0.40 (0.18–0.87) (≥10 years supplement use)	≥10 years supplement use was associated with 60% lower odds of cortical cataract	
BMES	Prospective	F & S	5–10 years	OR = 0.55 (0.36–0.86) P = 0.045	Reduced incidence of nuclear cataract in the highest quintile intake of vitamin C	Tan et al. (2008a)
SMS	Prospective	S	8.2 years	HR = 1.74 (1.24–2.46) (supplement)	In women aged ≥65 years vitamin C supplementation increased risk of cataract by 38%	Rautiainen et al. (2010)
				HR = 1.28 (0.94–1.73) (no supplement)		

[a]The OR/RR/HR values shown in the table are values obtained for the highest quintile/tertile/quartile group versus the lowest unless stated differently in the results. BDES, Beaver Dam Eye Study cohort; BMES, Blue Mountains Eye Study; F, food; HR, hazards ratio; LOCCS, Lens Opacities Case-Control Study; NHS, Nurses' Health Study cohort; NVP, Nutrition and Vision Project; OR, odds ratio; PHS, Physicians' Health Study; PSC, posterior subcapsular cataract; RR, relative risk; S, supplement; SMS, Swedish Mammography Study.

TABLE 56.2 Plasma vitamin C status and risk of cataract

Study	Study design	Study duration	OR/RR/HR[a] (95% confidence interval)	Result	Reference
IUCCS	Case-control	–	OR = 1.87 (1.29–2.69) (vitamin C) OR = 0.12 (0.03–0.56) (total antioxidants)	Risk of nuclear and PSC increased with high plasma vitamin C status, diminishes when combined with other antioxidants	Mohan et al. (1989)
Jacques et al.	Case-control	–	OR = 3.7 (P < 0.05) (cortical) OR = 11.3 (P < 0.10) (PSC)	Low plasma vitamin C was associated with increased risk of cortical cataract and PSC	Jacques and Chylack (1991)
BLS	Retrospective	4 years	OR = 1.21 (0.61–2.39) (middle vs. low quartile) OR = 1.01 (0.45–2.26) (high vs. low quartile)	High plasma vitamin C was not associated with reduced risk of nuclear or cortical cataracts	Vitale et al. (1993)
Valero et al.	Case-control	–	OR = 0.34 (0.23–0.50) P < 0.0001	Blood levels of vitamin C above 49 µmol/L were associated with 64% reduced odds of cataract	Valero et al. (2002)
INDEYE feasibility study	Cross-sectional	–	OR = 0.64 (0.48–0.85) P = 0.005	Reduced odds of cataract for the highest (≥15 µmol/L) vs. the lowest (<6.3 µmol/L) tertile of plasma vitamin C	Dherani et al. (2008)

[a]The OR/RR/HR values shown in the table are values obtained for the highest quintile/tertile/quartile group versus the lowest unless stated differently in the results.

BLS, Baltimore Longitudinal Study; HR, hazards ratio; IUCCS, India–US Case Control Study; OR, odds ratio; PSC, posterior subcapsular cataract; RR, relative risk.

extraction. In conclusion, long-term vitamin C intake for ≥10 years may provide protection against cataract, especially in adults <60 years of age. The optimal dose seems to be >140 mg/day with doses >300 mg/day providing no added benefit, possibly due to saturation of eye tissues (Hankinson *et al.*, 1992; Jacques *et al.*, 2001). Supplementation with especially high doses of >1 g/day may increase the risk of cataract.

Vitamin E

Vitamin E acts as a strong chain-breaking antioxidant in lipid peroxidation processes in vivo (Bunce *et al.*, 1990). Vitamin E may thus protect the lens from oxidative damage. Epidemiological studies that have evaluated the role of dietary vitamin E from food and supplements in the development and progression of cataracts have yielded mixed results (Table 56.3). Various factors such as supplement use, duration of supplementation, and age play a role in determining the relationship between vitamin E and the incidence of cataract. In the studies that reported a reduced incidence of nuclear cataract with high vitamin E intake, the effect was seen only with vitamin E supplement use for a duration of >10 years, except one study which showed an effect with >5 years' supplement use (Mares-Perlman *et al.*, 1995a, 2000; Leske *et al.*, 1998; Jacques *et al.*, 2001, 2005; Christen *et al.*, 2008). In the case of cortical cataract, no such trend was observed. Of the three studies that showed decreased risk of cortical cataract, one was a case-control study that assessed vitamin E intake from foods, the second study only included prior, not current, vitamin E supplement users, the majority of whom had doses of <10 mg/day, and the third study found an association with plasma vitamin E and not dietary vitamin E intake (Leske *et al.*, 1991; Rouhiainen *et al.*, 1996; Nadalin *et al.*, 1999). Two studies showed a decreased risk of cataract extraction with increased dietary intake of vitamin E from food and supplements (Robertson *et al.*, 1989; Tavani *et al.*, 1996). In studies that showed no relation between vitamin E intake and prevalence of nuclear or cortical cataract, PSC or cataract extraction, the duration of supplement use was <10 years (Hankinson *et al.*, 1992; Seddon *et al.*, 1994b; Lyle *et al.*, 1999), or the highest dose was <150 mg/day (Jacques and Chylack, 1991; Taylor *et al.*, 2002a), or the sample size was small (Jacques and Chylack, 1991), or the association was only marginally significant (Valero *et al.*, 2002). In studies that looked at highest versus lowest quintile of vitamin E intake from supplements, the mean vitamin E dose in the high quintile groups were in the

range 90–262 mg/day, whereas the range was 4–6 mg/day in the lowest quintile groups. One study found no significant difference in the prevalence of cataract between persons with vitamin E intake >35.7 mg/day and those with intakes <8.4 mg/day (Jacques and Chylack, 1991). The beneficial effects of vitamin E may be attributed to supplemental vitamin E and not to vitamin E from food sources alone.

In six of nine studies examining the relationship between plasma vitamin E and cataract (Table 56.4), increased plasma vitamin E was associated with decreased risk of cataract (Knekt *et al.*, 1992; Vitale *et al.*, 1993; Leske *et al.*, 1995; Rouhiainen *et al.*, 1996; Leske *et al.*, 1998; Nourmohammadi *et al.*, 2008). One study observed that cataract risk was not related to plasma vitamin E concentrations (Gale *et al.*, 2001). In contrast, Mares-Perlman *et al.* (1995c) found increased levels of plasma α-tocopherol to be a risk factor for nuclear cataract, and a study by Ferrigno *et al.* (2005) found that increased levels of vitamin E were related to increased prevalence of cortical cataract and PSC. A cross-sectional study that analyzed plasma, red blood cells, and lens vitamin E concentrations in cataract patients found no correlation between plasma or RBC-bound vitamin E and vitamin E in the lens (Krepler and Schmid, 2005). This suggests that plasma or RBC vitamin E concentration may not reflect vitamin E status of the lens and cannot be used as a clinically relevant marker to assess cataract risk.

In the only randomized, double-masked, placebo-controlled trial evaluating a vitamin E intervention, pharmacological doses of vitamin E (500 IU or 454 mg/day) for 4 years did not reduce the incidence or progression of nuclear, cortical, or PSC cataracts in subjects aged 55 to 80 years (McNeil *et al.*, 2004). Other intervention studies that evaluated vitamin E supplementation in conjunction with multivitamin or antioxidant supplementation are discussed in the section entitled "Intervention Studies". In conclusion, vitamin E supplementation may be beneficial when consumed for >10 years and at doses higher than the RDA of 15 mg/day but lower than pharmacologic levels (<300 mg/day). Associations were protective for nuclear and cortical cataracts and reduction in the incidence of cataract extraction, but not so much for PSC.

Carotenoids

The human lens contains significant amounts of lutein and zeaxanthin, but not β-carotene and lycopene, which are the dominant carotenoids in serum. Of the total lens

TABLE 56.3 Dietary intake of vitamin E (from food and supplement) and risk of cataract

Study	Study design	Dietary intake	Study duration	OR/RR/HR[a] (95% confidence interval)	Result	Reference
Robertson et al.	Case-control	S	–	OR = 0.44 (0.24–0.77) $P = 0.004$	Vitamin E supplementation was associated with a 50% reduction in risk of senile cataract	Robertson et al. (1989)
LOCCS	Case-control	F & S		OR = 0.59 (0.35–0.99) $P \leq 0.05$	High vitamin E intake was associated with reduced odds of cortical cataract	Leske et al. (1991)
NHS	Prospective	F & S	8 years	OR = 0.96 (0.72–1.29) $P = 0.88$	High vitamin E intake was not associated with cataract extraction	Hankinson et al. (1992)
BDES	Retrospective	F & S	–	OR = 0.67 (0.43–1.03) $P = 0.03$	High vitamin E intake was associated with decreased risk of nuclear sclerosis in men	Mares-Perlman et al. (1995a)
Tavani et al.	Case-control	F	–	OR = 0.5 (0.3–1.0)	Reduced risk of cataract extraction in the highest quintile intake of vitamin E compared with lowest quintile	Tavani et al. (1996)
TLSOC	Prospective	S	3–6 years	RR = 0.43 (0.19–0.99) $P < 0.05$	Risk of nuclear opacification reduced by half in vitamin E supplement users	Leske et al. (1998)
VECAT	Retrospective	S		OR = 0.44 (0.25–0.77)	Prior vitamin E supplementation was associated with absence of cortical cataract	Nadalin et al. (1999)
BDES	Prospective	F & S	5 years	OR = 0.5 (0.3–1.1) $P = 0.04$ (age >65 years) OR = 0.4 (0.2–1.1) $P = 0.02$ (hypertension)	Vitamin E was inversely associated with nuclear opacities only in persons who had some risk factors for cataract	Lyle et al. (1999)
BDES	Prospective	S	5 years	OR = 0.4 (0.3–0.6) $P < 0.001$	>10 years' use of vitamin E supplement was related to decreased incidence of cataract	Mares-Perlman et al. (2000)
NHS	Retrospective	S	13–15 years	OR = 0.49 (0.22–1.09) $P = 0.03$	Use of supplement for ≥10 years was associated with reduced odds of nuclear lens opacities	Jacques et al. (2001)
NHS	Retrospective	F & S	13–15 years	OR = 1.21 (0.75–1.95) (cortical) OR = 0.87 (0.39–1.92) (PSC)	Prevalence of cortical and PSC cataracts was not associated with dietary vitamin E	Taylor et al. (2002a)
WHS	Prospective RCT	F & S	10 years	RR = 0.86 (0.74–1.00) $P = 0.03$	Highest quintile intake of vitamin E from food and supplements was associated with reduced incidence of cataract	Christen et al. (2008)

[a]The OR/RR/HR values shown in the table are values obtained for the highest quintile/tertile/quartile group versus the lowest unless stated differently in the results.
BDES, Beaver Dam Eye Study; F, food; HR, hazards ratio; LOCCS, Lens Opacity Case-control Study; NHS, Nurses' Health Study cohort; OR, odds ratio; PSC, posterior subcapsular cataract; RCT, randomized controlled trial; RR, relative risk; S, supplement; TLSOC, The Longitudinal Study of Cataract; VECAT, Vitamin E and Cataract Prevention Study cohort; WHS, Women's Health Study cohort.

TABLE 56.4 Plasma vitamin E status and risk of cataract

Study	Study design	Study duration	OR/RR/HR[a] (95% confidence interval)	Result	Reference
BLS	Retrospective	4 years	OR = 0.52 (0.27–0.98)	High plasma levels of vitamin E were associated with a reduced risk of nuclear opacity	Vitale et al. (1993)
			OR = 0.57 (0.32–1.02)	Middle plasma levels of vitamin E, not high levels, were associated with reduced risk of cortical opacity	
LOCCS	Case-control	–	OR = 0.44 (0.21–0.90) $P < 0.05$	Risk of nuclear opacity reduced to half in persons with high α-tocopherol levels	Leske et al. (1995)
NFBDES	Cross-sectional	–	α-Tocopherol OR = 2.13 (1.05–4.34) $P = 0.05$ γ-Tocopherol: OR = 0.61 (0.32–1.19) $P = 0.04$	High plasma α-tocopherol was associated with increased risk of nuclear sclerosis; High plasma γ-tocopherol was associated with decreased risk of nuclear sclerosis	Mares-Perlman et al. (1995b)
KAPS	Prospective	3 years	RR = 3.7 (1.15–11.76) $P = 0.028$	Plasma vitamin E was inversely associated with progression of cortical lens opacity	Rouhiainen et al. (1996)
BDES	Prospective	5 years	OR = 0.4 (0.2–0.9) $P = 0.03$	Lower risk of cataract in third tertile of plasma vitamin E compared to first tertile	Lyle (1999)
TLSC	Prospective	3–6 years	RR = 0.58 (0.36–0.94) $P < 0.05$	Risk of nuclear opacification reduced by half in persons with higher levels of plasma vitamin E compared with lower	Leske et al. (1998)
Gale et al.	Cross-sectional	–	OR = 0.6 (0.3–1.3) $P = 0.667$ (nuclear) OR = 0.6 (0.3–1.1) $P = 0.18$ (cortical) OR = 0.7 (0.3–1.7) $P = 0.406$ (PSC)	No association between plasma vitamin E and nuclear, cortical and PSC cataracts	Gale et al. (2001)
CTNS report 2	Cross-sectional	–	OR = 1.99 (1.02–3.90) $P \leq 0.05$ (cortical) OR = 3.00 (1.22–7.37) (PSC)	High plasma vitamin E was associated with increased risk of cortical and PSC	Ferrigno et al. (2005)

[a]The OR/RR/HR values shown in the table are values obtained for the highest quintile/tertile/quartile group versus the lowest unless stated differently in the results. BDES, Beaver Dam Eye Study; BLS, Baltimore Longitudinal Study; CTNS, Clinical Trial of Nutritional Supplements and Age-related Cataract; KAPS, Kuopio Atherosclerosis Prevention Study cohort; LOCCS, Lens Opacity Case Control Study; NFBDES, Nutritional Factors in Beaver Dam Eye Study; OR, odds ratio; PSC, posterior subcapsular cataract; RR, relative risk; TLSC, The Longitudinal Study of Cataract.

lutein and zeaxanthin, 75% is present in the epithelium and cortex (Yeum *et al.*, 1999). Lutein and zeaxanthin, being potent antioxidants, may protect the lens from oxidative stress. Epidemiological studies have evaluated the relationships between intake of lutein/zeaxanthin and also other carotenoids and the incidence of cataract (Table 56.5). All the studies that looked at relations between carotenoid intake and cataract extraction found a significant reduction in the incidence of cataract extraction with higher intake of dietary lutein and zeaxanthin, and not β-cryptoxanthin, lycopene, or α- and β-carotene (Hankinson *et al.*, 1992; Brown *et al.*, 1999; Chasen-Taber *et al.*, 1999). Of the various carotenoid-rich foods, greens such as spinach, kale, and other cruciferous vegetables, which are rich in lutein, were associated with a decreased risk of cataract extraction rather than foods such as carrots, winter squash, and sweet potatoes (Tavani *et al.*, 1996; Chasen-Taber *et al.*, 1999). Risk of nuclear cataract was lower in the highest quintile intake groups of lutein, zeaxanthin, and β-carotene compared with the lowest quintile intake groups (Mares-Perlman *et al.*, 1995a; Lyle *et al.*, 1999; Jacques *et al.*, 2001). In one study high lutein and zeaxanthin intake was related to reduced prevalence of nuclear opacity but not 5-year change in lens opacity (Jacques *et al.*, 2005). However, this study analyzed data from a subset of the Nurses' Health Study cohort: analyses of the complete cohort showed that those with higher lutein and zeaxanthin intakes had a lower risk of nuclear cataract extraction (Chasen-Taber *et al.*, 1999). Two studies (Mares-Perlman *et al.*, 1995a; Jacques *et al.*, 2001) out of four found high dietary intake of β-carotene to be related to lower risk of nuclear cataract (Chasen-Taber *et al.*, 1999; Lyle *et al.*, 1999). With regard to plasma carotenoids, one study showed the risk of nuclear cataract to be the lowest in people with the highest plasma α- and β-carotene (Gale *et al.*, 2001), two studies showed no association with any of the measured carotenoids (Vitale *et al.*, 1993; Lyle, 1999), while one study showed increased risk of nuclear sclerosis in women (lutein and lycopene) but decreased risk (lutein, α-carotene, and β-cryptoxanthin) in men who smoked (Mares-Perlman *et al.*, 1995b).

Dietary intakes of plasma lutein, zeaxanthin, and β-carotene were not found to be related to cortical cataract risk (Vitale *et al.*, 1993; Gale *et al.*, 2001; Taylor *et al.*, 2002a) except in one study in which decreased risk was observed in men with high serum β-carotene whereas increased risk was observed in men with high serum lutein (Mares-Perlman *et al.*, 1995b). Risk of PSC was lower in women with the highest vs. lowest lutein/zeaxanthin intake and also in individuals with high plasma lutein/zeaxanthin concentrations (Chasen-Taber *et al.*, 1999; Gale *et al.*, 2001). Increased dietary intake of β-carotene (highest quintile group intake level was ~6.6 mg/day) was related to lowered risk of PSC only in women who never smoked (Taylor *et al.*, 2002a). Plasma β-carotene was not related to risk of PSC (Gale *et al.*, 2001). Other carotenoids such as β-cryptoxanthin and lycopene were not found to be related to any type of cataract or incidence of cataract extraction (Brown *et al.*, 1999; Chasen-Taber *et al.*, 1999; Gale *et al.*, 2001; Jacques *et al.*, 2001; Taylor *et al.*, 2002a), except in one study where cortical cataract was lowest in individuals with highest plasma lycopene (Gale *et al.*, 2001).

In a randomized, double-masked, placebo-controlled trial of β-carotene in US male physicians, no overall benefit or harm was observed with β-carotene supplementation (50 mg/day on alternate days) for 12 years to the incidence or extraction of cataract (Christen *et al.*, 2003). However, β-carotene supplementation appeared to lower the risk of cataract by about one-fourth in smokers. In a separate study, no effect was observed on the incidence of cataract extraction in male Finnish smokers supplemented with 20 mg/day of β-carotene (Teikari *et al.*, 1998b). In this study the cataract status at the start of the study was not known. Also, since the endpoint was cataract extraction, many cases of incident cataract that did not require surgery may have been excluded. Other intervention studies of β-carotene in combination with other antioxidants and vitamins are discussed in the "Intervention Studies" section.

In conclusion, there is strong evidence that long-term intake of dietary lutein and zeaxanthin may provide protection against the incidence of nuclear cataract, and to a lesser extent of PSC, but not cortical cataract. Most noteworthy is the fact that pharmacological doses are not necessary: an adequate amount is found in foods such as spinach, kale, and broccoli. The protective associations of β-carotene were strong only in non-smokers as smoking lowers the levels of β-carotene in serum and lens even with high dietary intake (Mosad *et al.*, 2010). Because of this fact, high doses of β-carotene supplements may have attenuated the risk of cataract in smokers (Christen *et al.*, 2003). The positive effects in this study should be interpreted with caution as two different studies have reported increased incidence of lung cancer in heavy smokers and in heavy smokers who were also exposed to asbestos

TABLE 56.5 Carotenoids (dietary intake from food and supplement and plasma status) and risk of cataract

Study	Study design	Dietary intake or plasma status	Study duration	OR/RR/HR[a] (95% confidence interval)	Result	Reference
NHS	Prospective	F	8 years	OR = 0.73 (0.55–0.97) $P < 0.001$	Women in the highest quintile intake of carotene had lower odds of cataract extraction compared with lowest quintile intake	Hankinson et al. (1992)
BDES	Retrospective	F	10 years	OR = 0.71 (0.46–1.10) $P = 0.064$ (β-carotene); OR = 0.29 (0.10–0.84) $P < 0.05$ (β-carotene in multivitamin user)	Men in the highest quintile intake for β-carotene who also used multivitamins had lower odds of severe nuclear sclerosis compared with men in the lowest quintile	Mares-Perlman et al. (1995a)
NF-EDSBD		P	–	OR = 2.80 (1.21–6.48) $P = 0.06$ (women); OR = 17.86 (1.47–217.16) $P = 0.04$ (women smokers); OR = 4.09 (1.67–10.03) $P = 0.006$ (lutein); OR = 2.26 (0.91–5.63) $P = 0.04$ (lycopene); OR = 0.27 (0.03–2.70) $P = 0.04$ (α-carotene); OR = 0.04 (0.00–0.41) $P = 0.03$ (β-cryptoxanthin); OR = 0.17 (0.01–1.91) $P = 0.05$ (lutein); OR = 0.28 (0.06–1.24) $P = 0.05$ (β-carotene); OR = 4.84 (0.83–28.1) $P = 0.03$ (lutein)	High plasma β-carotene increased the risk of nuclear sclerosis in women. This association was more significant in women who were present smokers; High plasma lutein and lycopene were associated with increased odds of nuclear sclerosis in women; High plasma α-carotene, β cryptoxanthin, and lutein were associated with reduced odds of nuclear sclerosis in men who smoked; Odds of cortical cataract were lower in men with high plasma β-carotene, not lutein	Mares-Perlman et al. (1995b)
BDES	Retrospective	F	10 years	OR = 0.5 (0.3–0.8) $P = 0.002$	Persons in the highest quintile of lutein intake in the distant past were half as likely to have an incident of nuclear cataract compared with persons in the lowest quintile of intake	Lyle et al. (1999)

Study	Design	Source	Duration	OR/RR (CI), P	Results	Reference
NHS	Prospective	F	12 years	RR = 0.88 (0.75–1.03) P = 0.04	Women in the highest quintile intake of lutein/zeaxanthin had a 22% decreased risk of cataract extraction than women in the lowest quintile intake	Chasen-Taber et al. (1999)
US-MHP	Prospective	F	8 years	RR = 0.81 (0.65–1.01) P = 0.03	Men in the highest quintile of lutein/zeaxanthin intake had a 19% lower risk of cataract relative to men in the lowest quintile	Brown et al. (1999)
NVP (NHS)	Prospective	F & S	13–15 years	OR = 0.52 (0.28–0.97) P = 0.04 (β-carotene) OR = 0.52 (0.29–0.91) P = 0.03 (lutein and zeaxanthin)	Women in the highest quintile intake of β-carotene and lutein/zeaxanthin had reduced odds of nuclear opacity compared with lowest quintile intake	Jacques et al. (2001)
Gale et al.	Cross-sectional	P	—	OR = 0.5 (0.3–0.9) P = 0.006 (α-carotene) OR = 0.7 (0.4–1.4) P = 0.033 (β-carotene) OR = 0.4 (0.2–0.7) P = 0.003 (lycopene) OR = 0.5 (0.2–1.0) P = 0.012 (lutein)	Risk of nuclear cataract was lowest in people with highest plasma α- and β-carotene. Risk of cortical cataract was lowest in people with highest plasma lycopene Risk of PSC was lowest in people with highest plasma lutein	Gale et al. (2001)
NHS	Retrospective	F & S	13–15 years	OR = 0.29 (0.08–1.05) P = 0.02 (α-carotene) OR = 0.28 (0.08–0.96) P = 0.02 (β-carotene) OR = 0.19 (0.05–0.68) P = 0.01 (total carotenoids)	In women who had never smoked, the odds of PSC in the highest quintile intake of α-carotene, β-carotene, and total carotenoids were lower than the lowest quintile intake	Taylor et al. (2002a)
WHS	Prospective	F	10 years	RR = 0.82 (0.71–0.95) P = 0.045	Women in the highest quintile intake of lutein/zeaxanthin had reduced risk of cataract compared with lowest quintile intake	Christen et al. (2008)

[a]The OR/RR/HR values shown in the table are values obtained for the highest quintile/tertile/quartile group versus the lowest unless stated differently in the results. BDES, Beaver Dam Eye Study; F, food; HR, hazards ratio; NF-EDSBD, Nutritional Factors in Eye Disease of Beaver Dam Eye; NHS, Nurses' Health Study cohort; NVP, Nutrition and Vision Project; OR, odds ratio; P, plasma; PSC, posterior subcapsular cataract; RR, relative risk; S, supplement; US-MHP, US Male Health Professionals Study; WHS, Women's Health Study cohort.

(Heinonen, 1994; Omenn *et al.*, 1996). The effect of supplementation with lutein and zeaxanthin, the only two carotenoids detected in the lens, on the incidence or progression of cataract has not been studied in a large-scale clinical setting. One study showed lutein supplementation (7 mg/day equivalent to lutein in ~100 g of spinach) improved visual acuity and glare sensitivity in people diagnosed with age-related cataract (Olmedilla *et al.*, 2003).

B Vitamins

Flavin dinucleotide (FAD), a cofactor for the enzyme glutathione reductase (GR), is derived from the B vitamin riboflavin. GR is necessary for maintaining the cellular pool of reduced glutathione, which is an important antioxidant that prevents the formation of protein disulfides and maintains transparency of the lens (Bunce *et al.*, 1990). Additionally, riboflavin deficiency has also been shown to interfere with the metabolism of folate, vitamins B_{12} and B_6 (Powers, 2003). A summary of studies evaluating B vitamins and cataracts can be found in Table 56.6. There is ample epidemiological data showing reduced prevalence of nuclear opacities with high dietary intake of either one or a combination of two or more B vitamins, which include riboflavin, folate, thiamin or niacin (Leske *et al.*, 1991; Mares-Perlman *et al.*, 1995a; Cumming *et al.*, 2000; Jacques *et al.*, 2001; Kuzniarz *et al.*, 2001; Jacques *et al.*, 2005). Riboflavin (3 mg/day) and niacin (40 mg/day) supplementation reduced the prevalence of nuclear cataract in a rural Chinese population, with the most benefit observed in people aged 65 to 74 years (Sperduto *et al.*, 1993). Riboflavin and niacin treatment in this study was found to have a deleterious effect on PSC, though the number of cases with PSC was small. In observational studies no association was observed between high intake of B vitamins and PSC (Leske *et al.*, 1991; Cumming *et al.*, 2000; Taylor *et al.*, 2002a). Reduced prevalence of cortical cataract was reported with the use of thiamin, riboflavin, niacin, folate, and B_{12} supplements in the cross-sectional Blue Mountains Eye Study. In the Lens Opacities Case-Control study, reduced prevalence was observed only with total intake from food and supplements of thiamin, riboflavin, and niacin (Leske *et al.*, 1991; Kuzniarz *et al.*, 2001). A null effect of dietary or supplemental intake of riboflavin on cataract extraction has also been reported (Hankinson *et al.*, 1992).

In most of the studies, the independent effects of the B vitamins, i.e. riboflavin, niacin, and thiamin by themselves, could not be determined as the nutrient intakes

were highly correlated (Sperduto *et al.*, 1993; Mares-Perlman *et al.*, 1995a; Cumming *et al.*, 2000; Jacques *et al.*, 2005). In all the epidemiological studies the doses of riboflavin (>1.3 mg/day), thiamin (>1.2 mg/day), and niacin (>16 mg/day) in the highest quintile groups were at levels much greater than the RDA. In conclusion, B vitamins, especially riboflavin, thiamin, niacin and also folate, from foods and supplements may provide protection against nuclear and cortical cataracts but not PSC.

Zinc

Zinc is a component of antioxidant enzymes such as superoxide dismutase, which is involved in the maintenance of structural integrity of the lens proteins (Flood *et al.*, 2002; Trumbo *et al.*, 2001). Zn^{2+} can also specifically interact with α-crystallin, a major lens protein and molecular chaperone, and enhance its ability to prevent protein aggregation and maintain lens transparency (Biswas and Das, 2007). However, compared with other antioxidants such as vitamins C and E and carotenoids, epidemiological data on zinc intake and cataract prevalence are minimal. The Blue Mountains eye follow-up study showed that above-median intakes of zinc in combination with vitamins C and E and β-carotene were associated with reduced incidence of nuclear cataract but not cortical or PSC cataract (Tan *et al.*, 2008a).

Some studies have suggested a deleterious effect of increased zinc concentrations in the lens and aqueous humor. Two studies reported significantly higher zinc content in the aqueous humor ($0.243 \pm 0.12 \mu g/mL$ vs. $0.154 \pm 0.56 \mu g/mL$, $P < 0.001$) and lens ($0.51 \pm 0.33 \mu mol/g$ vs. $0.32 \pm 0.20 \mu mol/g$, $P = 0.012$) of cataract patients vs. controls (Dawczynski *et al.*, 2002; Nourmohammadi *et al.*, 2006), while another study reported no significant difference (Aydin *et al.*, 2005). Based on this evidence it is unclear if high zinc concentration in the lens is a consequence of cataract or a factor that causes cataract (Nourmohammadi *et al.*, 2006). No positive conclusions of the protective effect of dietary zinc intake on cataract can thus be drawn.

Omega-3 Fatty Acids

The eye is rich in omega-3 fatty acids, especially docosahexaenoic acid (DHA), which is found in very high concentrations in the retina. Although there is no known biological rationale for the role of omega-3 fatty acids in the prevention of cataract, a few observational studies are presented (Hodge *et al.*, 2005). High intakes of dietary

TABLE 56.6 Dietary intake of B vitamins (from food and supplement) and risk of cataract

Study	Study design	Dietary intake	Study duration	OR/RR/RR/HR[a] (95% confidence interval)	Result	Reference
LOCCS	Case-control	F & S B$_1$	–	OR = 0.51 (0.30–0.86) (cortical)	Reduced prevalence of cortical and mixed cataracts was associated with higher dietary intake of vitamins B$_1$ and B$_3$	Leske et al. (1991)
		B$_3$		OR = 0.55 (0.34–0.91) (mixed) OR = 0.59 (0.34–1.00) (cortical) OR = 0.47 (0.30–0.76) (mixed) OR = 0.59 (0.36–0.97) (cortical)		
		B$_2$			In case of B$_2$, only prevalence of cortical cataract was reduced	
NHS	Prospective	B$_2$ (F & S)	8 years	$P \leq 0.05$ for above RR = 0.91 (0.69–1.20) P = 0.57 (F & S)	Dietary intake of riboflavin was not associated with cataract extraction	Hankinson et al. (1992)
Linxian cataract studies	RCT	B$_2$, B$_3$ (S)	5–6 years	RR = 0.78 (0.59–1.03) P = 0.06 (F only) OR = 0.45 (0.31–0.64) P < 0.001 (nuclear)	44% reduction in prevalence of nuclear cataract in people aged 65–74 years Negative effect on PSC and no effect on cortical cataract	Sperduto et al. (1993)
BDES	Retrospective	F & S B$_2$	10 years	OR = 2.64 (1.31–5.35) P = 0.007 (PSC) OR = 0.67 (0.46–0.98) P = 0.026 (women)	Men and women in the highest quintile intake of vitamin B$_2$ and folate had reduced odds of nuclear sclerosis	Mares-Perlman et al. (1995a)
		Folate		OR = 0.56 (0.36–0.87) P = 0.009 (men) OR = 0.63 (0.43–0.92) P = 0.04 (women) OR = 0.50 (0.32–0.79) P = 0.002 (men)		
		B$_1$		OR = 0.58 (0.38–0.91) P = 0.01 (men)	Reduced risk of nuclear sclerosis significant in men with a high intake of B$_1$. In case of B$_3$, the association was marginally significant	

(Continued)

TABLE 56.6 (*Continued*)

Study	Study design	Dietary intake	Study duration	OR/RR/HR[a] (95% confidence interval)	Result	Reference
BMES	Cross-sectional	F & S B$_3$	–	OR = 0.6 (0.4–0.9) P = 0.008	High intake of vitamins B$_1$, B$_2$ and B$_3$ was associated with reduced prevalence of nuclear cataract	Cumming et al. (2000)
		B$_1$		OR = 0.6 (0.4–0.9) P = 0.03		
		B$_2$		OR = 0.5 (0.3–0.9) P = 0.01		
NVP (NHS)	Retrospective	F & S B$_2$	13–15 years	OR = 0.37 (0.19–0.73) P = 0.03	Reduced prevalence of nuclear opacities in the highest quintile intake of B$_2$ and folate compared with lowest quintile intake	Jacques et al. (2001)
		Folate		OR = 0.44 (0.24–0.81) P = 0.005		
BMES	Cross-sectional	S			High intake of thiamin and folate was associated with reduced prevalence of nuclear and cortical cataract. High intake of vitamins B$_2$, B$_3$ and B$_{12}$ was associated with reduced prevalence of only cortical cataract	Kuzniarz et al. (2001)
		B$_1$		OR = 0.6 (0.4–1.0) P = 0.03 (nuclear) OR = 0.6 (0.3–0.9) P = 0.01 (cortical) OR = 0.7 (0.5–1.0) P = 0.02 (cortical)		
		Folate		OR = 0.4 (0.2–0.9) P = 0.03 (nuclear) OR = 0.6 (0.3–0.9) P = 0.01 (cortical)		
		B$_2$		OR = 0.7 (0.5–1.0) P = 0.07 (cortical)		
		B$_3$		OR = 0.6 (0.3–1.2) P = 0.06 (cortical)		
		B$_{12}$		OR = 0.6 (0.3–0.9) P = 0.02 (cortical)		

[a]The OR/RR/HR values shown in the table are values obtained for the highest quintile/tertile/quartile group versus the lowest unless stated differently in the results.
B$_1$, thiamin; B$_2$, riboflavin; B$_3$, niacin; BDES, Beaver Dam Eye Study cohort; BMES, Blue Mountains Eye Study; F, food; HR, hazards ratio; LOCCS, Lens Opacities Case-Control Study; NHS, Nurses' Health Study cohort; NVP, Nutrition and Vision Project; OR, odds ratio; PSC, posterior subcapsular cataract; RR, relative risk; S, supplement.

omega-3 polyunsaturated fatty acids were shown to reduce the incidence of nuclear cataract in the Blue Mountains Eye Study cohort (Townend *et al.*, 2007). A 16-year prospective study showed that women in the highest quintile intake of long-chain omega-3 fatty acids (0.21% of energy) had a 12% lower risk of cataract extraction compared with those in the lowest quintile intake (0.03% of energy) (Lu *et al.*, 2005). However, in a cohort of the Nurses' Health Study from the Boston, Massachusetts area, higher intake of α-linolenic acid (ALA) was associated with greater age-related change in lens nuclear density (Lu *et al.*, 2007). There is not enough evidence to conclude that omega-3 fatty acids are protective against cataract.

Intervention Studies

Based on the epidemiological evidence, several randomized controlled trials (RCTs) have evaluated whether a combination of the above mentioned nutrients can reduce the risk of cataract. The Age-Related Eye Disease Study (AREDS) reported that a combination of high-dose antioxidants (vitamin C, 500 mg; vitamin E, 400 IU; β-carotene, 15 mg) had no apparent effect on the 7-year risk of development or progression of age-related lens opacities or visual acuity loss (Age-Related Eye Disease Study Research, 2001a). The Antioxidants in the Prevention of Cataracts (APC) study also reported no effect of the exact same intervention on the 5-year progression of cataract in a population aged 35 to 50 years from south India (Gritz *et al.*, 2006). The Roche European American Cataract Trial (REACT), which used a similar intervention (vitamin C, 750 mg/day; vitamin E, 600 mg/day; β-carotene, 18 mg/day) found a significant reduction in the measure of lens opacity in the US population diagnosed with early age-related cataract after 3 years of treatment (*n* = 88 who completed 3 years of follow-up). The same effect was not observed in the UK population of this study due to differences in population characteristics (*n* = 70 who completed 3 years of follow-up). The UK cohort also included participants with more advanced cataract (Chylack *et al.*, 2002). Intervention with a supplement containing 14 different vitamins and 12 minerals, including vitamin C (180 mg/day), α-tocopherol (60 IU/day), and β-carotene (15 mg/day) reduced the prevalence of nuclear cataract by 36% in a rural Chinese population aged 65 to 74 years diagnosed with esophageal dysplasia (Sperduto *et al.*, 1993). In the Alpha-Tocopherol Beta-Carotene (ATBC) trial, α-tocopherol (50 mg/day) and β-carotene (20 mg/day) supplementation was not

found to lower the rates of cataract extraction in male Finnish smokers during a 5- to 8-year follow-up (Teikari *et al.*, 1997). Multivitamin/mineral supplementation (containing 100% RDA of B vitamins, vitamins C and E, no β-carotene) decreased the incidence of nuclear cataract events during a 9-year follow-up in an Italian population aged 55 to 75 years, who started the study with early or no cataract (Clinical Trial of Nutritional Supplements and Age-Related Cataract Study Group *et al.*, 2008). In the same study, the incidence of PSC actually increased with multivitamin/mineral supplementation.

The null findings of some studies could be caused by several factors such as age, nutritional status, overall health and geographic location, all of which influence the diet of study populations. In the case of AREDS, in addition to the multivitamin/mineral intervention, 66% of the population was taking a multivitamin Centrum without lutein (Age-Related Eye Disease Study Research Group, 2001a). Therefore, a majority of the population, whether in the control or treatment group, had an increase in their intake by approximately 100% of the RDA amounts of the nutrients of interest in addition to the study intervention. In the ATBC study, the population were all smokers, and also the true status of cataract at the start of the study was not known. The primary endpoint of the REACT study was change in percent pixels opaque (IPO) (Chylack *et al.*, 2002), which was different from the measures of lens opacity and visual acuity used in the other studies.

In conclusion, supplementation with multivitamins/minerals may reduce the incidence or progression of cataract in older adults with early or no cataract who generally consume diets with nutrients within 100% of the RDA amounts. However, more RCTs are needed to confirm these findings. Nutritional interventions seem to benefit nuclear cataract, which is more common in older adults, more than cortical cataract and PSC. With lutein and zeaxanthin being the major carotenoids found in the lens, more studies need to be done evaluating the effect of lutein and zeaxanthin interventions on cataract.

Age-Related Macular Degeneration (AMD)

AMD is the leading cause of blindness in adults aged 60 years and over in industrialized countries. The prevalence of AMD increases dramatically with age. Nearly 30% of Americans over the age of 75 years have early signs of AMD, and 7% have advanced AMD, whereas the respective prevalence is 8% and 0.1% in adults aged 43–54 years (Congdon *et al.*, 2004). None of the current treatment options can reverse the damage caused by AMD. As with cataracts, efforts are focused on preventing incidence and progression of the disease. Nutritional interventions are part of these efforts (Snodderly, 1995).

AMD is a disease that affects the posterior, central region of the retina, called the macula, which contains the densest concentration of photoreceptors and is responsible for sharp central vision. Figure 56.3(b) shows the loss of central vision that is found in AMD patients. Posterior to the photoreceptors is the retinal pigment epithelium (RPE), part of the blood–ocular barrier, which has several functions including phagocytosis of the photoreceptors (Jager *et al.*, 2008). The clinical hallmark and usually the first clinical signs of AMD is the presence of drusen. Drusen are extracellular deposits that accumulate between the RPE and the inner layer of the Bruch's membrane and appear as pale yellow spots on the retina (Abdelsalam *et al.*, 1999). They are formed as a result of the inability of the RPE to adequately perform its function of phagocytosis. Drusen can also be present in the normal aging eye. AMD can be classified into the following types based on the AREDS classification system: (1) early AMD – presence of few (<20) medium-sized drusen or retinal pigmentary abnormalities; (2) intermediate AMD – the presence of at least one large drusen, numerous medium-sized drusen, or geographic atrophy that does not extend to the center of the macula; (3) advanced or late AMD – can be either neovascular (wet, exudative) or non-neovascular (dry, atrophic, non-exudative). Advanced non-exudative is characterized by drusen and geographic atrophy that extends to the macula (Jager *et al.*, 2008). Advanced exudative is characterized by growth of new blood vessels under the RPE and sometimes into the sub-retinal space. The early stages of AMD are generally asymptomatic. In the later stages there may be distortion of vision or complete loss of visual function, especially central vision (Snodderly, 1995). Although specifics on the pathogenesis of AMD are not completely understood, the mechanisms of importance are chemical and light-induced oxidative stress, blue-light-induced damage to the RPE and photoreceptor rod cells, RPE dysfunction, hemodynamic processes, and also genetic factors. The retina is particularly susceptible to oxidative damage because of its high consumption of oxygen, its high concentration of polyunsaturated fatty acids, and its exposure to visible light (Nolan *et al.*, 2003). Depletion of macular pigment

(discussed in detail under "Carotenoids") is another predisposing risk factor for AMD that is responsive to nutritional intervention as it cannot be synthesized de novo. Since oxidative stress has been implicated in the etiology of AMD, various antioxidant nutrients will be examined for their role in protection against AMD in the sections below. The epidemiological evidence and intervention studies, if any, are organized based on dietary intake from food or supplement and plasma status of the nutrient of interest.

Vitamin C

Epidemiological evidence examining the relationship between dietary intake of vitamin C, from food and supplements, and plasma vitamin C with AMD is listed in Table 56.7. No protective association was reported between dietary vitamin C or plasma vitamin C concentration and AMD risk in any of the studies (Eye Disease Case-Control Study Group (EDCCSG), 1993; Seddon *et al.*, 1994a; West *et al.*, 1994; Christen *et al.*, 1999; Smith *et al.*, 1999; Cho *et al.*, 2004; Age-Related Eye Disease Study Research Group *et al.*, 2007). In one study, incidence of dry, exudative or non-exudative AMD over 8 years was reduced by 35% in individuals with above-median intake of vitamin C in combination with vitamin E, β-carotene, and zinc (van Leeuwen *et al.*, 2005). In the Blue Mountains Eye Study cohort, higher baseline intake of vitamin C was associated with an increased risk of incident early AMD during a 5-year follow-up period (Flood *et al.*, 2002). There is no conclusive evidence to state that dietary vitamin C in isolation can protect against AMD. Supplementation studies of vitamin C in combination with other antioxidant nutrients are discussed in the "Intervention Studies" section.

Vitamin E

Being a fat-soluble antioxidant, several studies looked at the relation between vitamin E and the incidence of AMD (Table 56.8). Increased dietary intake of vitamin E, from foods and supplements, was shown to reduce the incidence of AMD in only two studies (VandenLangenberg *et al.*, 1998; van Leeuwen *et al.*, 2005), whereas no such effect was reported in other epidemiological studies (Eye Disease Case-Control Study Group, 1993; Seddon *et al.*, 1994a; Mares-Perlman *et al.*, 1996; Christen *et al.*, 1999; Cho *et al.*, 2004). High plasma vitamin E concentration was associated with reduced prevalence of AMD in some studies (Eye Disease Case-Control Study Group, 1993;

TABLE 56.7 Vitamin C (dietary intake from food and supplements and plasma status) and risk of age-related macular degeneration (AMD)

Study	Study design	Dietary intake	Study duration	OR/RR/HR[a] (95% confidence interval)	Result	Reference
EDCCSG	Case-control	P	–	OR = 0.7 (0.5–1.2) $P = 0.27$	Plasma vitamin C was not associated with reduced odds of developing neovascular AMD	EDCCSG (1993)
EDCCSG	Case-control	F & S	–	OR = 1.01 (0.6–1.70) $P = 0.98$ (F & S); OR = 0.83 (0.52–1.33) $P = 0.22$ (F)	Highest quintile intake of vitamin C was not associated with advanced AMD	Seddon et al. (1994a)
BLSA	Case-control	P	–	OR = 0.55 (0.28–1.08) (AMD); OR = 0.17 (0.01–2.57) (severe AMD)	High plasma vitamin C was suggested to reduce the prevalence of AMD, but the effect was not significant	West et al. (1994)
BMES	Cross-sectional	F & S	–	OR = 1.3 (0.5–3.4) (late AMD); OR = 0.9 (0.5–1.4) (early AMD)	High intake of vitamin C was not associated with reduced odds of AMD	Smith et al. (1999)
PHS I	Prospective	S	7 years	RR = 1.03 (0.71–1.50)	Incidence of AMD was not reduced in vitamin C supplement users	Christen et al. (1999)
BMES	Prospective	F & S	5 years	OR = 2.3 (1.3–4.0) $P = 0.002$	Highest quintile of vitamin C intake was associated with increased risk of early AMD compared with lowest quintile intake	Flood et al. (2002)
NHS HPFS	Prospective	F & S	12–18 years	RR = 1.21 (0.88–1.67) $P = 0.18$ (early AMD); RR = 0.98 (0.58–1.66) $P = 0.52$ (late AMD)	Higher intake of vitamin C was not associated with reduced risk of AMD	Cho et al. (2004)
RS	Prospective	F & S	3–10 years	HR = 1.02 (0.94–1.10) $P = 0.04$ (vitamin C); HR = 0.65 (0.46–0.92) (combination)	High vitamin C intake was not associated with lower risk of AMD, but, in combination with vitamin E, β-carotene and zinc reduced risk by 35%	van Leeuwen et al. (2005)
AREDS report no. 22	Case-control	F	–	OR = 0.98 (0.67–1.43) $P = 0.39$ (neovascular AMD); OR = 1.14 (0.56–2.33) $P = 0.84$ (geographic atrophy)	Highest quintile intake of vitamin C was not associated with neovascular AMD and geographic atrophy	Age-Related Eye Disease Study Research Group et al. (2007)

[a]The OR/RR/HR values shown in the table are values obtained for the highest quintile/tertile/quartile group versus the lowest unless stated differently in the results. AREDS, Age-related Eye Disease Study; BLSA, Baltimore Longitudinal Study of Aging; BMES, Blue Mountains Eye Study; EDCCSG, Eye Disease Case-Control Study Group; F, food; HPFS, Health Professionals Follow-up Study; HR, hazards ratio; NHS, Nurses' Health Study; OR, odds ratio; P, plasma; PHS, Physicians' Health Study; PSC, posterior subcapsular cataract; RR, relative risk; RS, Rotterdam Study; S, supplement.

TABLE 56.8 Vitamin E (dietary intake from food and supplements and plasma status) and risk of age-related macular degeneration (AMD)

Study	Study design	Dietary intake	Study duration	OR/RR/HR[a] (95% confidence interval)	Result	Reference
EDCCSG	Case-control	P	–	OR = 0.6 (0.4–1.04) $P = 0.10$	Odds of developing neovascular AMD were not reduced with high plasma vitamin E status	EDCCSG (1993)
WHS	Prospective RCT	S 600IU/2 days	10 years	RR = 0.93 (0.72–1.19) $P = 0.54$	Risk of AMD was not significantly different in the vitamin E treatment group compared with placebo group	Seddon et al. (1994a)
BLSA	Case-control	P	–	OR = 0.43 (0.25–0.73) (AMD) OR = 0.31 (0.05–1.87) (severe AMD)	High plasma vitamin E was associated with reduced prevalence of AMD	West et al. (1994)
ATBC	Prospective RCT	S 50mg/day	5–8 years	OR = 1.13 (0.81–1.59)	Supplementation with vitamin E was not associated with reduced prevalence of AMD among smoking males	Teikari et al. (1998)
PHS I	Prospective	S	7 years	OR = 0.87 (0.53–1.43)	Vitamin E supplement users had a 13% non-significant reduced risk of AMD	Christen et al. (1999)
Taylor et al.	Prospective RCT	S 500IU/day	4 years	RR = 1.05 (0.69–1.61) RR = 1.36 (0.67–2.77)	Incidence of early AMD was 8.6% in vitamin E groups vs. 8.1% in placebo group Incidence of late AMD was 0.8% in vitamin E group vs. 0.6% in placebo group	Taylor et al. (2002)
NHS HPFS	Prospective	F & S	12–18 years	RR = 1.42 (1.01–1.99) $P = 0.55$ (early AMD) RR = 1.34 (0.92–1.96) $P = 0.32$ (late AMD)	Higher intake of vitamin E was not associated with reduced risk of AMD	Cho et al. (2004)
WHS	RCT	600IU every 2 days	10 years	RR = 0.90 (0.77–1.06) (AMD with or without vision loss)	Vitamin E supplementation did not reduce the incidence of AMD	Christen et al. (2010)

[a]The OR/RR/HR values shown in the table are values obtained for the highest quintile/tertile/quartile group versus the lowest unless stated differently in the results. ATBC, Alpha-Tocopherol Beta-Carotene Study; BLSA, Baltimore Longitudinal Study of Aging; EDCCSG, Eye Disease Case-Control Study Group; F, food; HPFS, Health Professionals' Follow up Study; HR, hazards ratio; NHS, Nurses' Health Study; OR, odds ratio; P, plasma; PHS, Physicians' Health Study; RCT, randomized controlled trial; RR, relative risk; S, supplement; WHS, Women's Health Study.

West *et al.*, 1994), but not in others (Sanders *et al.*, 1993; Mares-Perlman *et al.*, 1995c).

Three double-blind placebo-controlled primary prevention trials have been published that studied the effect of long-term vitamin E supplementation on the incidence or progression of AMD (Teikari *et al.*, 1998a; Taylor *et al.*, 2002b; Christen *et al.*, 2010). The risk of incidence or progression of AMD was not reduced in the vitamin E supplemented groups (doses were 50 mg/day or 75 IU/day, 500 IU/day and 600 IU/2 days) compared with the placebo groups in any of the studies. The doses of vitamin E used in these studies are well over the RDA for vitamin E. High doses of vitamin E ($\geq$400 IU/day) have been linked to increased risk of heart failure among people with diabetes or vascular disease (Lonn *et al.*, 2005). The hypothesis is that at such high doses vitamin E could act as a pro-oxidant and displace other fat-soluble antioxidants. In conclusion, there is no strong evidence to support the beneficial effect of vitamin E for the risk of AMD.

Vitamins C and E do not seem to have an independent protective effect on AMD as evidenced from the above reviewed literature. However, some studies have shown that, in combination with each other and with other antioxidants, vitamins C and E can reduce the risk of AMD. High dietary intake of a combination of vitamins C and E, β-carotene, and zinc was associated with a 35% reduced risk of AMD (van Leeuwen *et al.*, 2005). A similar observation was reported in three other studies. One of these looked at a combination of vitamins C and E, carotenoids, and selenium, the second at antioxidant intake, and the third at a combination of plasma vitamins C and E and β-carotene (Eye Disease Case-Control Study Group, 1993; West *et al.*, 1994; Snellen *et al.*, 2002). Studies that looked at supplementation with a combination of vitamins C and E are discussed in the "Intervention Studies" section.

Carotenoids

Among the carotenoids, lutein and zeaxanthin specifically accumulate in the macula, where they are referred to as macular pigment (Bone *et al.*, 1985). With a maximum absorption of 460 nm, macular pigment (MP) acts as an efficient filter, protecting the underlying photoreceptors and RPE from blue-light damage (Ahmed *et al.*, 2005). Concentrations of lutein and zeaxanthin in the retinas from AMD donors were found to be lower than in controls, suggesting that low MP density could be a risk factor for AMD (Bone *et al.*, 2001). Further evidence for this finding comes from studies that measured MP density in

vivo using a heterochromatic flicker photometer (Wooten *et al.*, 1999). Subjects with advanced AMD in one eye had significantly lower MP density in the fellow eye compared with healthy eyes of subjects without AMD (Beatty *et al.*, 2001). Another study found MP density in the eyes of AMD patients to be 32% lower than in normal disease-free eyes (Bernstein *et al.*, 2002). However, MP density was not related to intermediate AMD in a cross-sectional study of women participating in the Carotenoids in Age-related Eye Disease Study (CAREDS). After an exploratory analysis, the authors suggested that the observations may have been biased in older women, whose diets improved with age. The authors also suggested the possibility that low MP density could be the result, rather than the cause, of damage to the retina with AMD (LaRowe *et al.*, 2008). A similar observation was reported in a subset of the Rotterdam Eye Study, another cross-sectional study that examined MP density in subjects aged 55 years or older with or without AMD (Berendschot *et al.*, 2002). These conflicting observations may be due to the cross-sectional nature of the studies, as prospective data from another study found MP density to be reduced in subjects with late AMD (Schweitzer *et al.*, 2000).

Apart from their role as MP, lutein and zeaxanthin are strong antioxidants and can protect the retina from oxidative-stress-related damage. A number of studies have looked at the relationship between dietary intake of carotenoids, especially lutein and zeaxanthin, and the risk of AMD. High intake of carotenoids, particularly lutein and zeaxanthin, was related to a reduced risk of advanced neovascular AMD (Eye Disease Case-Control Study Group, 1993; Seddon *et al.*, 1994a; Snellen *et al.*, 2002). Cross-sectional data from the CAREDS showed high lutein and zeaxanthin intakes were related to a decreased risk of intermediate AMD in women <75 years, but not in women $\geq$75 years (Moeller *et al.*, 2006). Furthermore, the Blue Mountains Eye Study found that high intake of lutein/zeaxanthin reduced the risk of incident neovascular AMD and indistinct soft or reticular drusen during a 5- to 10-year follow-up (Tan *et al.*, 2008b). Lutein and zeaxanthin intake was also associated with a decreased risk of neovascular AMD and large or extensive intermediate drusen when comparing the highest to the lowest quintiles of intakes (Age-Related Eye Disease Study Research Group *et al.*, 2007). However, a nested case-control study of the Beaver Dam Eye Study cohort found no difference in serum lutein and zeaxanthin concentrations between early age-related macular degeneration and age-, sex-, and smoking-matched controls (Mares-Perlman *et al.*, 1995c). Serum concentrations are not a good measure of long-term dietary intake of lutein and zeaxanthin, which may have caused the null findings. A summary of studies on carotenoid intake and risk of AMD is shown in Table 56.9.

Based on the above observational findings, increased dietary intake of lutein and zeaxanthin, from either foods or supplements, would be a logical strategy in the prevention and/or treatment of AMD. Several studies have shown that increased consumption of lutein/zeaxanthin, from foods such spinach, corn, and egg yolks (Hammond *et al.*, 1997; Bone *et al.*, 2000; Wenzel *et al.*, 2006; Vishwanathan *et al.*, 2009), and from supplements (Landrum *et al.*, 1997; Bone *et al.*, 2003; Johnson *et al.*, 2008; Connolly *et al.*, 2010), can significantly improve MP density in healthy adults not diagnosed with AMD. In the Lutein Antioxidant Supplementation Trial (LAST), 10 mg/day of lutein for 1 year improved MP density, visual function and subjective results of Amsler grid testing in patients with atrophic AMD (Richer *et al.*, 2004).

In conclusion, lutein and zeaxanthin, because of their specific accumulation in the macula, are important nutrients that may be beneficial in the prevention and treatment of AMD. Studies that used lutein/zeaxanthin in combination with other vitamins and antioxidants as a treatment option are discussed in the "Intervention Studies" section.

B Vitamins

Vitamins B_{12} and B_6 and folate are essential for the transsulfuration and remethylation reactions in the metabolic pathway of homocysteine (Selhub and Miller, 1992). Low intakes and blood levels of vitamins B_{12} and B_6 and folate have been associated with hyperhomocysteinemia, i.e. increased plasma levels of homocysteine. Also, several observational studies have reported hyperhomocysteinemia to be associated with an increased risk of AMD (Heuberger *et al.*, 2002; Axer-Siegel *et al.*, 2004; Nowak *et al.*, 2005; Vine *et al.*, 2005; Coral *et al.*, 2006; Kamburoglu *et al.*, 2006; Rochtchina *et al.*, 2007; Krishnadev *et al.*, 2010). The mean plasma homocysteine levels were >15 μmol/L in AMD subjects in these studies. In the Blue Mountains Eye Study, in patients with serum homocysteine ≤15 μmol/L, low plasma B_{12} was associated with nearly four times higher odds of AMD (Rochtchina *et al.*, 2007). Low plasma vitamin B_{12} was also reported to be an independent risk factor for AMD in some studies (Kamburoglu *et al.*, 2006; Rochtchina *et al.*, 2007),

whereas other studies did not find any association (Heuberger *et al.*, 2002; Nowak *et al.*, 2005). The absence of an association of homocysteine with RBC folate and serum vitamin B_{12} in the Third National Health and Nutrition Examination Survey was attributed to limited information on changes in the diet and lifestyle of participants, exclusion of persons in an older age group due to missing data, and differences in fasting status at the time of blood draw (Heuberger *et al.*, 2002). However, an inverse association was observed between RBC folate and soft drusen in non-Hispanic Blacks in this study. Folate and vitamins B_6 and B_{12} have been explored as a treatment option for AMD as they are capable of reducing plasma homocysteine levels (Woodside *et al.*, 1998). The fact that vitamin B_{12} and folate may be independently related to incidence of AMD warrants their investigation in the treatment of AMD.

The Women's Antioxidant and Folic Acid Cardiovascular Study, a randomized, double-blinded, placebo-controlled study, showed that women at a high risk of cardiovascular disease supplemented with folic acid (2.5 mg/day), vitamin B_6 (50 mg/day), and vitamin B_{12} (1 mg/day) for an average of 7.3 years had a statistically significant 35–40% reduced risk of AMD (Christen *et al.*, 2009). After examining a subset of 300 participants for blood levels of homocysteine, the mechanism of action of supplementation was partly attributed to a significant reduction in plasma homocysteine concentrations. Since AMD diagnosis was self-reported and the population was women with a high risk of cardiovascular disease, the authors suggest caution when extrapolating the results to a general population. Other than vitamins B_6 and B_{12} and folate, two studies investigated the effect of niacin treatment in AMD patients. Niacin treatment caused vasodilatation of retinal arterioles in one study, and in another study niacin modified choroidal circulation (Metelitsina *et al.*, 2004; Barakat *et al.*, 2006). For a summary of the studies that have evaluated relationships between the B vitamins and AMD, see Table 56.10. In conclusion, vitamins B_{12} and B_6 and folate may be beneficial in reducing the risk of AMD, while niacin may help in the treatment of neovascular AMD. More RCTs are needed to confirm these findings.

Zinc

High concentrations of zinc are present in the photoreceptors and RPE compared with other tissues, suggesting that zinc may have an important role in protection against retinal diseases such as AMD (Newsome *et al.*, 1992). Zinc

TABLE 56.9 Carotenoids (dietary intake from food and supplement, plasma and retina status) and risk of age-related macular degeneration (AMD)

Study	Study design	Dietary intake	Study duration	OR/RR/HR[a] (95% confidence interval)	Result	Reference
EDCCSG	Case-control	P	—	OR = 0.3 (0.2–0.6) $P < 0.0001$ (total carotenoids)	High levels of total carotenoids in the blood were associated with reduced risk of NV AMD	Eye Disease Case-Control Study Group (1993)
				OR = 0.3 (0.2–0.6) $P = 0.0001$ (lutein/zeaxanthin)	High levels of individual carotenoids, except lycopene, were also associated with reduced risk of NV AMD	
				OR = 0.3 (0.2–0.5) $P < 0.0001$ (α-carotene) OR = 0.5 (0.3–0.8) $P = 0.003$ (β-carotene) OR = 0.4 (0.2–0.6) $P = 0.0001$ (cryptoxanthin) OR = 0.8 (0.5–1.3) $P = 0.40$ (lycopene)		
EDCCSG	Case-control	F	—	OR = 0.57 (0.35–0.92) $P = 0.02$ (total carotenoids)	Highest quintile intake of carotenoids was associated with a 43% lower risk for NV AMD	Seddon et al. (1994a)
				OR = 0.59 (0.4–0.96) $P = 0.03$ (β-carotene) OR = 0.43 (0.2–0.7) $P < 0.001$ (lutein/zeaxanthin)	Lutein and zeaxanthin were most strongly associated with a reduced risk for neovascular AMD	
BDES	Case-control	P	—	OR = 2.2 (1.1–4.5) (lycopene)	Low plasma lycopene was associated with increased likelihood of early AMD No association with lutein, zeaxanthin, β-cryptoxanthin, α- and β-carotene	Mares-Perlman et al. (1995c)
Bone RA et al.	Case-control	Retina	—	OR = 0.18 (0.05–0.64)	Highest quartile of retinal lutein/zeaxanthin was associated with an 82% lower risk of AMD compared with lowest quartile	Bone et al. (2001)
Snellen et al.	Case-control	F	—	OR = 2.4 (1.1–5.1)	Prevalence of NV AMD in subjects with low lutein intake was about twice as high as that in subjects with high intake	Snellen et al. (2002)
CAREDS	Cross-sectional	F & S	—	OR = 0.96 (0.75–1.23) (overall sample)	Prevalence of intermediate AMD was not statistically different between high and low lutein/zeaxanthin intake groups	Moeller et al. (2006)

(Continued)

TABLE 56.9 (*Continued*)

Study	Study design	Dietary intake	OR/RR/HR[a] (95% confidence interval)	Study duration	Result	Reference
			OR = 0.57 (0.34–0.95) (women <75 years at risk for diet changes) OR = 2.02 (0.88–4.62) (women ≥75 years at risk for diet changes)	—	Lower odds in women <75 years of age who are at risk for diet changes compared with women ≥75 years	Age-Related Eye Disease Study Research Group et al. (2007)
AREDS report no. 22	Case-control	F	OR = 0.65 (0.45–0.93) (neovascular AMD) OR = 0.45 (0.24–0.86) (geographic atrophy) OR = 0.73 (0.56–0.96) (large or extensive intermediate drusen) $P \leq 0.05$ (all of above)		Higher intake of lutein and zeaxanthin was associated with lower odds of neovascular AMD, geographic atrophy and large or extensive intermediate drusen	
BMES	Prospective	F	RR = 0.35 (0.13–0.92) $P = 0.033$ (NV AMD) RR = 0.66 (0.48–0.92) $P = 0.013$ (indistinct soft or reticular drusen)	5 and 10 years	Subjects in the top tertile (≥942 µg/day) of lutein and zeaxanthin intake were significantly less likely to develop NV AMD Subjects with above median (743 µg/day) intake were less likely to develop indistinct soft or reticular drusen	Tan et al. (2008b)
CAREDS	Cross-sectional	MPD	OR = 1.4 (0.9–2.1) $P = 0.16$ OR = 0.8 (0.5–1.2) OR = 0.5 (0.3–1.0) (women 54–69 years) OR = 1.0 (0.5–2.0) (women ≥70 years)	—	The odds for intermediate AMD among women in the highest quintile for MPOD were not significantly different from lowest quintile Odds reduced after excluding women at risk for diet change, but remained non-significant Middle-aged women (54–69 years) had marginally lower odds of AMD compared with women aged ≥70 years after adjusting for risk for diet change	LaRowe et al. (2008)

[a]The OR/RR/HR values shown in the table are values obtained for the highest quintile/tertile/quartile group versus the lowest unless stated differently in the result. AREDS, Age-related Eye Disease Study; BDES, Beaver Dam Eye Study; BMES, Blue Mountains Eye Study cohort; CAREDS, Carotenoids in Age-related Eye Disease Study; EDCCSG, Eye Disease Case-Control Study Group; F, food; HR, hazards ratio; MPOD, macular pigment density; NV, neovascular; OR, odds ratio; P, plasma; RR, relative risk; S, supplement.

TABLE 56.10 B vitamins (dietary intake from food and supplement and plasma status) and risk of age-related macular degeneration (AMD)

Study	Study design	Dietary intake	Study duration	OR/RR/HR[a] (95% confidence interval)	Result	Reference
NHANES III	Cross-sectional	RBC folate	–	OR = 0.8 (0.5–1.4) P = 0.40	RBC folate and plasma vitamin B₁₂ were not related to early and late AMD in the overall sample	Heuberger et al. (2002)
		Plasma B₁₂		OR = 0.7 (0.4–1.2) P = 0.11 OR = 0.7 (0.1–5.3) P = 0.78		
BMES	Cross-sectional	Serum B₁₂ Serum folate	–	OR = 2.30 (1.08–4.89) OR = 1.13 (0.58–2.22)	Subjects with low vitamin B₁₂ (<125 pmol/L) were twice as likely to have atrophic or NV AMD No such relation observed with folate	Rochtchina et al. (2007)
WAFCS	RCT	S	7.3 years	RR = 0.66 (0.47–0.93) P = 0.02 RR = 0.59 (0.36–0.95) P = 0.03	Combined supplementation with folic acid, vitamins B₆ and B₁₂ significantly lowered the risk of AMD	Christen et al. (2009)

[a]The OR/RR/HR values shown in the table are values obtained for the highest quintile/tertile/quartile group versus the lowest unless stated differently in the result.
BMES, Blue Mountains Eye Study; NHANES, National Health and Nutrition Examination Survey; P, plasma; RBC, red blood cells; RCT, randomized controlled trial; S, supplement containing folic acid (2.5 mg/day), vitamin B₆ (50 mg/day) and vitamin B₁₂ (1 mg/day); WAFCS, Women's Antioxidant and Folic Acid Cardiovascular Study.

functions as a cofactor for several ocular enzymes, including superoxide dismutase, a primary antioxidant used to regulate oxidative stress. Because oxidative stress in the retina is involved in the pathogenesis of AMD, the role of zinc in reducing the risk of AMD has been investigated. Further evidence for this hypothesis comes from a study in which zinc levels in the RPE and choroid were found to be significantly reduced by 24% in AMD eyes compared with normal eyes (Erie et al., 2009).

Prospective observational studies on zinc intake and incidence of AMD have reported conflicting results. In the Blue Mountains Eye Study, participants with higher intakes of zinc had relatively reduced incidence of AMD after 5 to 10 years of follow-up (Tan et al., 2008b). However, in the Nurses' Health Study and the Health Professionals Follow-up Study, zinc intake, either from food or as supplements, was not associated with a reduced risk of AMD (Cho et al., 2001b). No association was observed between zinc intake and prevalence of AMD-related drusen in the cohort of the Nurses' Health Study who also participated in the Nutrition and Vision Project (Morris et al., 2007).

Positive effects of zinc supplementation have been reported in RCTs. Zinc supplementation (100 mg as zinc sulfate) given to an elderly population with early stage AMD resulted in better maintenance of visual acuity than in the control population (Newsome et al., 1988). Supplementation with 50 mg/day of zinc monocysteine was found to significantly improve macular function in individuals with dry AMD (Newsome, 2008). The beneficial effect of zinc supplementation in this study may have been due to the presence of cysteine. Cysteine has the ability to be metabolized into other sulfur-containing compounds such as glutathione, an important antioxidant in the eye. No positive effect of supplementation with 200 mg/day of zinc for 2 years was observed in the healthy eye of patients diagnosed with drusen in one eye (Stur et al., 1996).

A study that tested zinc concentrations in post-mortem eyes found unexpectedly high concentrations of zinc in the sub-RPE deposits, with levels being especially high in eyes with AMD (Lengyel et al., 2007). The authors suggested that zinc may be involved in the formation of sub-RPE deposits and possibly in the development of AMD. However, the fact that zinc was associated with deposit formation does not prove that zinc caused the deposits. There could be a number of reasons for the presence of zinc in the deposits, the simplest being that they are made up of proteins, which may coincidentally, but not harmfully, bind zinc (Newsome and Brewer, 2008). The beneficial effects of zinc cannot be negated, based on the findings of this study. Another study suggested that zinc in low amounts may protect RPE but in high amounts can have the opposite effect based on cell culture data. The authors suggested that zinc supplementation may be beneficial in combination with other antioxidants and not in isolation (Wood and Osborne, 2003). However, clinical evidence would be required to confirm these experimental data on the potential negative effect of high-dose zinc supplementation. Based on data from RCTs, zinc supplementation may be beneficial in reducing the risk of AMD. Further evidence of the protective role of zinc supplementation in combination with other antioxidants and vitamins is described in the "Intervention Studies" section.

Omega-3 Fatty Acids

The rod outer segments of the retina have the highest concentration of DHA compared with any other neural subcellular component, about 30–65% of the total fatty acids (Neuringer et al., 1988). A recent study also suggested that omega-3 fatty acids in the retina have anti-inflammatory effects and, when converted to neuro-protectin, they protect against oxidation-induced apoptosis (Schweigert and Reimann, 2010). Findings from epidemiological studies that examined the relationship of fish intake, omega-3 fatty acids, DHA, and omega-6 fatty acids with incidence of early or late-stage AMD are presented (Table 56.11).

In a prospective 10- to 12-year follow-up of participants in the Nurses' Health Study and the Health Professionals Follow-up Study, consumption of >4 servings of fish per week was associated with a 35% lower risk of AMD compared with ≤3 servings per month (Cho et al., 2001a). Of the individual fish types examined in this study, a significant inverse association was found only with intake of tuna. Similar findings were reported in another prospective study where a 40% reduction in incidence of early AMD was associated with consumption of fish at least once a week, while consumption of fish at least three times a week reduced the incidence of late AMD (Chua et al., 2006). Three case-control studies and two cross-sectional studies also reported positive associations between fish intake and risk of AMD (Seddon et al., 2001, 2006; Age-Related Eye Disease Study Research Group, 2007; Delcourt et al., 2007; Augood et al., 2008). Two other cross-sectional studies failed to find any significant association between fish intake and AMD risk (Mares-Perlman et al., 1995d; Heuberger et al., 2001). The authors of the Beaver Dam Eye Study suggested that fish intakes were low and possibly not varied enough to detect a difference in the risk of AMD (Mares-Perlman et al., 1995d).

Several observational studies including the ones mentioned above also examined associations between omega-3 or omega-6 fatty acids and AMD risk. High dietary intake of omega-3 fatty acids was found to be protective against early and late AMD (Seddon et al., 2001, 2006; Chua et al., 2006; Age-Related Eye Disease Study Research Group, 2007; SanGiovanni et al., 2009). Higher intakes of DHA and eicosapentaenoic acid (EPA) were also associated with lowering the odds of neovascular AMD (Cho et al., 2001a; Augood et al., 2008). Surprisingly, intake of the omega-3 fatty acid, linolenic acid, was associated with

TABLE 56.11 Dietary intake of fish, long-chain polyunsaturated fatty acids and omega-3 fatty acids and risk of age-related macular degeneration (AMD)

Study	Study design	Dietary intake	Study duration	OR/RR/HR[a] (95% confidence interval)	Result	Reference
NHS HPFU	Prospective	Fish	5–10 years	RR = 0.7 (0.52–0.93) P = 0.05	Intake of >4 servings/week was associated with 35% reduced incidence of AMD compared with ≤3 servings/month	Cho et al. (2001a)
		Tuna		RR = 0.61 (0.45–0.83) P = 0.0007	Of all types of fish, significant association only with tuna	
		DHA		RR = 0.65 (0.46–0.91) P = 0.009	DHA intake had an inverse relation with AMD	
AREDS	Prospective	Omega-3	12 years	OR = 0.65 (0.45–0.92)	Highest intake was associated with 30% less likelihood of geographic and neovascular AMD	SanGiovanni et al. (2009)
EDCCS	Case-control	Fish (≤5.5 g linoleic acid)	–	OR = 0.60 (0.32–1.14) P = 0.05	High fish/DHA intake reduced risk of neovascular AMD only when intake of linoleic acid ≤5.5 g	Seddon et al. (2001)
		DHA and EPA (≤5.5 g linoleic acid)		OR = 0.75 (0.44–1.25) P = 0.05		
NHANES III	Cross-sectional	Fish	–	OR = 1.0 (0.7–1.4) P = 0.80; OR = 0.4 (0.2–1.2) P = 0.10	No association between fish intake and early or late AMD	Heuberger et al. (2001)
BMES	Prospective	Fish (low linoleic acid intake)	10 years	RR = 0.59 (0.36–0.99) P = 0.12	Increased intake of fish and omega-3 reduced incidence of early AMD only with below median levels of linoleic acid	Tan et al. (2009)
		Omega-3 (low linoleic acid intake)		RR = 0.48 (0.27–0.83) P = 0.01		
BMES	Prospective	Fish	5 years	OR = 0.58 (0.37–0.90)	At least 1 serving of fish associated with reduced risk of early AMD by 40%	Chua et al. (2006)
		Fish		OR = 0.25 (0.06–1.00)	At least 3 servings of fish caused significant reduction late AMD risk	
		Omega-3		OR = 0.41 (0.22–0.75)	High omega-3s reduced risk of incident early AMD	
EUREYE	Cross-sectional	DHA	–	OR = 0.32 (0.12–0.87) P = 0.03	Reduced odds of neovascular AMD with higher intake of DHA and EPA	Augood et al. (2008)
		EPA		OR = 0.29 (0.11–0.73) P = 0.02		
Seddon et al.	Prospective	Fish (<4.9 g/day linoleic acid)	–	RR = 0.36 (0.14–0.95) P = 0.045	>2 servings of fish reduced risk of late AMD in subjects consuming ≤4.9 g/day linoleic acid	Seddon et al. (2003)

[a]The OR/RR/HR values shown in the table are values obtained for the highest quintile/tertile/quartile group versus the lowest unless stated differently in the result.
AREDS, Age-related Eye Disease Study; BMES, Blue Mountains Eye Study; DHA, docosahexaenoic acid; EDCCS, Eye Disease Case-Control Study; EPA, eicosapentaenoic acid; NHANES, National Health and Nutrition Survey; NHS/HPFU, Nurses' Health Study/Health Professionals Follow-up Study.

a relative increase in risk of AMD in the Nurses' Health Study and the Health Professionals Follow-up Study cohort. However, the authors suggested that this could have been a chance finding as many individual fatty acids were assessed and also there is no specific biological mechanism for linolenic acid in the retina (Cho et al., 2001a).

Higher intake of omega-6 fatty acids seemed to negatively influence the protective effect of omega-3 fatty acids. In two prospective studies and one case-control study, reduced risk of early AMD or neovascular AMD associated with fish consumption was observed only among participants consuming low amounts of linoleic acid, an omega-6 fatty acid (Seddon et al., 2001, 2003; Tan et al., 2009). Higher consumption of linoleic acid was also independently associated with greater risk for AMD in the Eye Disease Case-control Study cohort (Seddon et al., 2001). When this study population was stratified by linoleic acid intake (≤5.5 or ≥5.6 g/day), the risk for AMD significantly decreased with high intake of omega-3 fatty acids only among those with low linoleic acid intake. A similar negative effect of above-median intake of linoleic acid on omega-3 fatty acids was reported in the US Twin Study of AMD (Seddon et al., 2006). A higher intake of arachidonic acid (ARA), another omega-6 fatty acid, was also associated with increased odds of neovascular AMD (Age-Related Eye Disease Study Research Group, 2007).

Based on observational findings, higher intake of omega-3 fatty acids, specifically DHA, may be beneficial in reducing the risk of early or late-stage AMD. Incorporating fatty fish in the diet can be a feasible way of increasing dietary omega-3 fatty acid intake. White fish are not rich in omega-3 fatty acids, and increased intake of white fish was not associated with reduced risk of AMD in the POLANUT cross-sectional study (Delcourt et al., 2007). The positive effects of omega-3 fatty acids seem to depend on the intake levels of omega-6 fatty acids. A healthy omega-6/omega-3 ratio (3:1 to 4:1) should be maintained in the diet to obtain protection against AMD (Simopoulos, 2002). The ongoing AREDS 2 study is evaluating the effect of an EPA and DHA intervention on the progression to late AMD.

Intervention Studies

Numerous studies that tested different combinations and doses of the above-mentioned nutrients on MP augmentation and AMD risk are discussed in this section. The AREDS intervention of vitamin C (500 mg), vitamin E (400 IU), β-carotene (15 mg), zinc (as zinc oxide, 80 mg), and copper (as copper oxide, 2 mg) was found to lower the risk of AMD by 25% in individuals who had intermediate or advanced AMD in one eye but not the other eye (Age-Related Eye Disease Study Research Group, 2001b). In the same high-risk group, these nutrients reduced the risk of vision loss caused by advance AMD by about 19%. For those subjects who had either no AMD or early AMD, the nutrients did not provide benefit. A daily supplement of 12 mg lutein, 1 mg zeaxanthin, 120 mg vitamin C, 17.6 mg vitamin E, 10 mg zinc, and 40 μg selenium for 6 months significantly increased MP density in an older adult population, of which 92.6% exhibited some features of AMD (Trieschmann et al., 2007). In the second treatment arm of the LAST, daily supplementation with 10 mg of lutein in combination with a broad spectrum of vitamins, minerals and other antioxidants for 12 months also improved MP density and visual function in patients with atrophic AMD (Richer et al., 2004). An RCT in individuals with non-advanced AMD in Italy, supplementation with 180 mg vitamin C, 30 mg vitamin E, 22.5 mg zinc, 1 mg copper, 10 mg lutein, 1 mg zeaxanthin, and 4 mg astaxanthin daily for 12 months improved a selective dysfunction in the central (0°–5°) retina (Parisi et al., 2008). In addition, two recent systematic reviews found that RCTs did not show that antioxidant supplements prevented early AMD (Chong et al., 2007; Evans and Henshaw, 2008). The AREDS 2 has begun and aims to refine the findings of AREDS by including lutein, zeaxanthin, and omega-3 fatty acids in the test formulation.

In conclusion, supplementation with a combination of vitamins C and E, β-carotene, zinc, and copper or the AREDS supplement may be beneficial in preventing progression of AMD and improving visual function in AMD patients. High doses of lutein/zeaxanthin supplements may also be beneficial as they increase MP density which may prevent further retinal damage in AMD patients. The ongoing AREDS 2 study is evaluating the effect of treatment with 10 mg lutein/2 mg zeaxanthin alone and in combination with omega-3 fatty acids in AMD patients.

Dietary Patterns, Cataracts, and AMD

The above sections focused primarily on the role of single nutrients or combinations of nutrients in the prevention and treatment of cataract and AMD. It is important to determine if adhering to the established Recommended Dietary Guidelines for all nutrients, including macronutrients, might have an impact on the prevention or progression of cataract and AMD. The Healthy Eating Index

(HEI) developed by the USDA is a single, summary measure of diet quality that can be used to monitor changes in dietary consumption patterns (Kennedy *et al.*, 1995). A strong inverse association was reported between adherence to Dietary Guidelines for Americans, measured as HEI score, and the prevalence of nuclear opacities in women from the Nurses' Health Study cohort (Moeller *et al.*, 2004). The same study also observed reduced prevalence of nuclear opacities in women in the highest quartile category of whole-grain intake. The strongest inverse associations were observed with overall HEI score, and not individual components of the diet, such as fruit or vegetable intake alone, stressing the importance of eating an overall well-balanced diet. The Women's Health Initiative also associated high HEI scores with lower prevalence of nuclear cataract (Mares *et al.*, 2010). Consumption of a high-quality diet, measured using an Alternate HEI, also reduced the odds of AMD in a case-control study of men and women diagnosed with advanced AMD (Montgomery *et al.*, 2010).

Dietary carbohydrates have a significant impact on the pathogenesis of both cataract and AMD. Hyperglycemia is thought to cause cataract through polyol pathway disruption, lipid peroxidation, glycation, and glycation-mediated oxidation that could all lead to increased oxidative stress in the lens and cause opacification (Schaumberg *et al.*, 2004; Chiu *et al.*, 2006b). The supply of blood and nutrients, including glucose, to the retina is high. However, glucose is efficiently metabolized as a result of which no glucose is stored in the retina. In cases of AMD, high concentrations of advanced glycation products accumulate in the drusen, probably as a result of impaired metabolism of glucose (Chiu *et al.*, 2006a). Glycemic index (GI), a physiologic measure of the glycemic quality of carbohydrate-containing foods, has also been implicated in the development of cataract and AMD (Jenkins *et al.*, 2002). Foods containing carbohydrates that break down most quickly during digestion have the highest glycemic index. Cross-sectional analysis of the baseline data of the non-diabetic population in the AREDS study showed high dietary GI and high dietary carbohydrate intake to be associated with higher prevalence of nuclear and cortical opacities, respectively (Chiu *et al.*, 2006b). High carbohydrate intake (≥200 g/day) was associated with higher odds of cortical but not nuclear opacities, compared with low carbohydrate intake (<185 g/day) in the Nurses' Health Study cohort (Chiu *et al.*, 2005). Total carbohydrate intake was also associated with pure cortical cataracts in the Melbourne

Visual Impairment project (Chiu *et al.*, 2010). In a prospective study with 12 to 14 years of follow-up, high dietary GI was not found to be related to higher incidence of cataract extraction (Schaumberg *et al.*, 2004).

In a study examining 1036 eyes of participants from the Nurses' Health Study cohort, dietary GI, and not total carbohydrate intake, was significantly related to AMD, specifically with abnormalities in the RPE. Neither total carbohydrate nor dietary GI was related to drusen. Dietary GI may thus be an independent risk factor for AMD (Chiu *et al.*, 2006a). High dietary GI was associated with a higher risk of large drusen, geographic atrophy, and neovascularization when baseline data of the AREDS population was analyzed. There was also a significant positive relation between dietary GI and severity of AMD (Chiu *et al.*, 2007).

In conclusion, adherence to the recommended dietary guidelines may prevent the incidence of cataract and AMD. Consumption of high-carbohydrate diets or high-GI foods could increase the risk of cataract, especially cortical cataract. The risk of AMD may also increase with consumption of high-GI foods.

Retinitis Pigmentosa

Retinitis pigmentosa (RP) is the leading cause of inherited blindness in the developed world, affecting 50 000 to 100 000 people in the United States and an estimated 1.5 million people worldwide (Berson, 2000; Delyfer *et al.*, 2004). RP refers to a group of inherited retinal disorders that result in the degeneration of rod and cone photoreceptors (Hartong *et al.*, 2006). The disease can be inherited as an autosomal-dominant (30–40% of cases), autosomal-recessive (50–60%), or X-linked (5–15%) trait (Hartong *et al.*, 2006). Mutations in the rhodopsin gene account for ~25% of dominant RP. Mutations in the *USH2A* gene may be the cause of ~20% of the recessive RP (Liu *et al.*, 2007). The *USH2A* gene encodes for the protein usherin and may be important for retinal development and maintaining homeostasis. Mutations in the GTPase regulator gene may account for ~70% of X-linked RP (Hartong *et al.*, 2006). These mutations cause ~30% of all cases of RP. Mutations have also been identified in other genes which include: enzymes of the phototransduction cascade (transducin α-subunit, guanylate cyclase, cGMP-dependent phosphodiesterase and arrestin); structural or trafficking proteins (peripherin/RD, ABCR); more rarely genes coding proteins involved in vitamin A metabolism (CRALBP, RPE 65) and phagocytosis of photoreceptor outer segments (McLaughlin *et al.*, 1993; Fuchs *et al.*, 1995; Dryja *et al.*, 1996, 1997; Perrault *et al.*, 1996; Marlhens *et al.*, 1997; Maw *et al.*, 1997; Allikmets, 2000; D'Cruz *et al.*, 2000). Mutations affecting proteins involved in specific biochemical pathways that transduce light can cause hyper-polarization and apoptosis of the rod photoreceptor cells. Clinically, rod cell death translates to night blindness which generally precedes defects in the peripheral visual field, i.e. tunnel vision (Figure 56.3d) by years or even decades. Cones are seldom directly affected by identified mutations. They degenerate secondarily to the rods as the disease progresses, which results in loss of central vision and complete blindness (Delyfer *et al.*, 2004). Many individuals with RP are not legally blind until their forties or fifties, and some even retain some sight throughout life. On the other hand, some RP patients go completely blind during childhood. Since RP affects rods and cones, nutrients that are essential in the normal functioning of these photoreceptor cells will be examined in detail as possible treatment options.

Vitamins A and E

Vitamins A and E are required for the maintenance of normal photoreceptor cell structure and function (Berson, 2000). Vitamin E deficiency results in a chain of oxidative reactions beginning with the highly reactive polyunsaturated fatty acids of the photoreceptor outer segments, followed by massive accumulation of lipofuscin in the RPE. In the absence of vitamin A, the damage resulting from vitamin E deficiency was found to increase (Robison *et al.*, 1979). Vitamin E also protects the stores of vitamin A in the retina from oxidation. Vitamin A deficiency results in loss of photoreceptor cells as the retina requires retinol, an essential structural component of the photoreceptor outer segment membranes (Robison *et al.*, 1980). Further interest in vitamins A and E was based on the observation that RP patients who happened to be taking supplements of vitamin A, vitamin E or both had slower declines in electroretinogram (ERG) amplitudes than those not taking supplements (Berson *et al.*, 1993).

A randomized, controlled, double-masked trial showed that RP patients given high-dose vitamin A (15 000 IU/day) had a significantly slower decline rate in cone ERG amplitude than patients given trace amounts of vitamin A or vitamin E alone. However, the results also suggested that the progression of the disease was faster among patients taking a daily supplement of 400 IU vitamin E versus those not taking this dose (Berson *et al.*, 1993). Serum vitamin A concentrations were found to be significantly lower in patients given 400 IU of vitamin E (Berson *et al.*, 1993). High vitamin E concentrations may reduce the amount of vitamin A reaching the eye, even though vitamin E may protect vitamin A reserves in the retina. In another study, supplementation of vitamin E (600 IU) in combination with taurine and diltiazem for 3 years decreased the rate of visual field loss in RP patients (Pasantes-Morales *et al.*, 2002). However, the authors attributed the positive effect on RP to taurine/diltiazem combination, while vitamin E was said to protect against any gastric mucosal injury that could be caused by diltiazem. Vitamin E supplementation has been shown to benefit patients with rare forms of RP, which are associated with diseases such as Bassen-Kornzweig disease (low plasma concentrations of apolipoprotein B) and familial isolated vitamin E deficiency (Bishara *et al.*, 1982; Yokota *et al.*, 1997).

Many clinicians recommend that adults with early or middle stages of RP take vitamin A supplementation of 15 000 IU/day and avoid high-dose vitamin E supplementation. No toxic effects were observed for this dose and duration of vitamin A supplementation (Berson *et al.*, 1993). It should be noted that doses of 25 000 IU or more over the long term are considered toxic and, because of the potential for birth defects, women who became pregnant were advised to not take vitamin A at such high doses (Institute of Medicine, 2001).

Omega-3 Fatty Acids

DHA is thought to be important for photoreceptor function since photoreceptor cell membranes containing rhodopsin and cone opsins have very high concentrations of this fatty acid (Fliesler and Anderson, 1983). Red blood cell membrane phosphatidylethanolamine (RBC PE) contents of DHA reflect the levels of DHA in the retina and are on an average lower in patients with RP than in unaffected individuals (Schaefer *et al.*, 1995; Hoffman *et al.*, 2004a). In a randomized, placebo-controlled study in individuals with X-linked RP (*n* = 44 males), DHA supplementation (400 mg/day) did not slow the progression of the disease. Similar results were obtained in another randomized, double-blind, controlled study of DHA supplementation (1200 mg/day) for 4 years in RP patients who were also given 15 000 IU/day of vitamin A (Berson *et al.*, 2004a). In the same study subgroups were created based on their use or non-use of vitamin A prior to entering the study. It was found that, in patients not on vitamin A prior to the study, addition of DHA slowed the course of the disease for the first 2 years. This was not, however, observed in the 3- or 4-year follow-up or in patients already on vitamin A prior to entering the study. Also, in the entire control group, those patients eating ≥0.2 g/day of omega-3-rich oily fish showed significantly less loss of central visual field sensitivity over 4 years (Berson et al., 2004b). The above studies also found that patients with low RBC PE DHA levels (<5% of total RBC PE fatty acids) had a faster rate of decline in visual field sensitivity than those with high RBC PE DHA levels (Berson et al., 2004b; Hoffman et al., 2004a). This observation has led to the recommendation that adults already taking vitamin A supplements should add one or two 3-oz (85-g) servings of omega-3-rich fish per week to their diet to maintain RBC PE DHA levels at 5% of RBC PE fatty acids. The authors estimated that the combination of vitamin A with an oily fish diet would, on average, provide a 60–70% slowing per year that would result in a total of almost 20 years of visual preservation for patients who start this regimen in their mid-30s. The proposed mechanism by which DHA may slow the progression of RP is through enhanced delivery of vitamin A to the remaining cones. Alternatively, vitamin A supplementation may facilitate incorporation of DHA into the retina. Adverse effects on retinal function were observed in RP patients on vitamin A prior to the study and taking 1200 mg/day of DHA for >2 years (Berson et al., 2004b). Therefore, recommendations have been made that patients with typical RP should not take 1200 mg of DHA by capsules for more than 2 years or eat too much oily fish while taking vitamin A supplements (Berson et al., 2004b).

Lutein

As described in the section on AMD, lutein, together with zeaxanthin, forms macular pigment in the posterior, central region of the retina called the macula. Since this region has the highest concentration of cones and is responsible for sharp, central vision, it was logical to examine the benefits of lutein in RP patients. In the vitamin A clinical trial described in the previous section (Berson et al., 1993), patients taking vitamin A who were also in the highest quintile intake of lutein (3.5–13 mg/day) had a slower rate of decline in the visual field area compared with those in the lower four quintiles (Berson et al., 2010). A beneficial trend was also seen when relating

ERG amplitude to quintile of lutein intake. In the first lutein intervention trial for RP, lutein supplementation (10 mg/day for 12 weeks followed by 30 mg/day for 12 weeks) improved central visual field in a randomized, cross-over, placebo-controlled, double-blind study design in a population of only 34 adults (Bahrami et al., 2006). In another double-blind RCT in 225 non-smoking RP patients aged 18 to 60 years, 4 years of supplementation with lutein (12 mg/day) in addition to vitamin A slowed the loss of mid-peripheral visual field sensitivity (Berson et al., 2010). Maximum slowing of mid-peripheral sensitivity also occurred among those with the highest serum lutein concentration and greatest increase in MP density. However, no significant effect of this intervention was observed on central field sensitivity. The detectable benefit of lutein supplementation preserving mid-peripheral function but not central function in RP may reflect an increased requirement for antioxidants in the photoreceptor outer segments, which are the most impaired. No toxic effects of lutein supplementation were observed in this study. Therefore, lutein supplementation may benefit non-smoking RP patients taking vitamin A. Follow-up of RP patients taking lutein and vitamin A (15 000 IU/day) along with a diet containing average amounts of omega-3 fatty acids (~0.2 g/day) is needed to confirm preservation of the mid-peripheral visual field (Berson et al., 2010).

Beyond Eye Disease

Dry Eye Syndrome

Dry eye syndrome (DES) is a condition where the eyes do not produce tears, or the tears are not of the correct consistency and evaporate too quickly. This produces dry eyes and increases the risk of inflammation. Published studies indicate that up to 20% of adults aged 45 years or more experience dry eye symptoms (Brewitt and Sistani, 2001). The incidence was observed to increase significantly with age and to be significantly higher in women (Moss et al., 2008). DES can be either evaporative or aqueous deficient, both of which can result in increased tear osmolarity. While the use of artificial tears is the main choice of treatment for DES and allows for temporary relief, it does not resolve the underlying cause.

Recent studies suggest that intake of omega-3 and omega-6 fatty acids may be effective in treating the underlying causes of DES. These fatty acids may improve the lipid layer of the tear film, thereby reducing evaporation. Furthermore, both omega-3 and omega-6 fatty acids are known to have anti-inflammatory properties (Simopoulos, 2000). In support of omega-3 fatty acids, intake of a high ratio of omega-3 to omega-6 fatty acids was reported to be related to a decrease in the incidence of DES in women (Miljanovic *et al.*, 2005). Pinna *et al.* (2007) evaluated the effect of daily supplementation with two omega-6 fatty acids, linoleic acid (28.5 mg) and γ-linolenic acid (15 mg), for 180 days on meibomian gland dysfunction (MGD), a common cause of DES (McCulley *et al.*, 1982; Driver and Lemp, 1997; Pinna *et al.*, 2007). Supplementation with linoleic acid and γ-linolenic acid caused significant reductions in secretion turbidity and meibomian gland obstruction. The same study also reported that eyelid hygiene alone caused significant reduction in eyelid edema, corneal staining, secretion turbidity, and meibomian gland obstruction. Eyelid hygiene combined with omega-6 fatty acid supplementation significantly reduced all of the above clinical symptoms. Supplementation with omega-6 fatty acids along with proper eyelid hygiene can have a significant positive impact on treating dry eye symptoms.

Sea buckthorn (SB) oil is rich in lipophilic antioxidants, such as vitamin E and carotenoids, while SB seed oil contains high proportions of omega-3 and omega-6 fatty acids (St. George and Cenkowski, 2007). In view of its antioxidant and essential fatty acid composition, the potential of SB oil to relieve DES symptoms was evaluated in a randomized, double-blinded, parallel trial in women and men aged 20 to 75 years with DES. SB oil (2 g/day for 3 months) attenuated the increase in tear-film osmolarity during the cold season and had a positive impact on symptoms of DES (Larmo *et al.*, 2010). The beneficial effect of SB oil can be attributed to the anti-inflammatory properties of the oils contained in SB. The only omega-6 fatty acid in SB oil used in this study was linoleic acid. All previous reports on beneficial effects of linoleic acid have been in combination with γ-linolenic acid (Barabino *et al.*, 2003; Macrì *et al.*, 2003; Pinna *et al.*, 2007). Also, the carotenoids and vitamin E in SB oil may protect the eye from oxidative damage, which leads to activation of inflammatory cascades. Antioxidant supplements containing vitamin E and carotenoids have previously been shown to benefit dry eye symptoms (Blades *et al.*, 2001; Peponis *et al.*, 2002).

In conclusion, omega-3 fatty acids, omega-6 fatty acids (linoleic and γ-linolenic acids), and antioxidant-rich oils such as SB oil may be beneficial in alleviating dry eye symptoms.

Visual Function
Phytonutrients

Bilberries and blackcurrants have been evaluated for their role in visual function as they contain high concentrations of phytonutrients. There is growing interest in studying bilberries to improve visual function after anecdotal reports stated that World War II pilots improved their night vision by eating bilberry jam. The medicinal property of bilberry (*Vaccinium myrtillus*) can be attributed to a class of plant pigments called anthocyanosides, which give purple coloration to fruits, leaves, and stems (Muth *et al.*, 2000; Canter and Ernst, 2004). Anthocyanosides are potent antioxidants that may slow the retinal angiopathy that occurs in AMD and diabetic retinopathy (Trevithick and Mitton, 1999). The possible mechanism of actions on visual apparatus may be the accelerated resynthesis of rhodopsin, modulation of retinal enzyme activity, and improved microcirculation (Canter and Ernst, 2004). In a systematic review of placebo-controlled trials evaluating the effects on night vision of anthocyanosides extracted from bilberry (Canter and Ernst, 2004), four RCTs found no effect (Levy and Glovinsky, 1998; Zadok *et al.*, 1999; Muth *et al.*, 2000; Mayser and Wilhelm, 2001). A fifth RCT and seven non-RCTs reported positive effects on outcome measures related to night vision (Canter and Ernst, 2004). One of the possible reasons for contradictory results could be the differences in the dose of anthocyanosides, which ranged from 36 mg to 2880 mg. Also, the composition of anthocyanosides in these studies was different as the bilberries were cultivated in different geographic locations. Eleven out of 12 studies enrolled subjects with normal or above average eyesight, which may have caused a ceiling effect resulting in no positive effect of the anthocyanosides intervention. The effects on subjects suffering impaired night vision due to pathological eye conditions have not been evaluated. A double-blind, placebo-controlled RCT of anthocyanosides extracted from blackcurrant (*Ribes nigrum*) reported a positive effect on visual fatigue associated with continuous viewing of computer monitors and other video display screens (Nakaishi *et al.*, 2000).

There is not enough data to positively conclude that anthocyanosides improve night vision. More controlled trials of bilberry anthocyanosides in subjects with impaired night vision will be necessary to confirm the positive effects. However, adding anthocyanoside-rich foods to the diet may be advisable as they have not been shown to have any harmful effects.

Lutein

The role of macular pigment in protecting the retina, and the beneficial effect of lutein supplementation in increasing MP density, are well established (see AMD section). Data are also accumulating that MP may improve visual function. There are two hypotheses that explain the mechanism by which MP improves visual function (Wooten and Hammond, 2002). The acuity hypothesis states that MP reduces the effect of chromatic aberration. The visibility hypothesis states that MP may improve vision through the atmosphere by preferentially absorbing blue haze (short-wave dominant air light that produces a veiling luminance when viewing objects at a distance). It has also been suggested that MP can improve glare disability and photostress recovery because of the light-filtering properties of MP (Stringham and Hammond, 2007). Some biological mechanisms, such as improvement in neuronal signaling efficiency in the eye, have also been suggested by which lutein and zeaxanthin may improve visual function (Stringham and Hammond, 2005). Since lutein intake has been shown to improve MP density, it has been suggested that lutein supplementation may improve visual function measures.

Six months of supplementation with 12 mg/day of lutein was shown to increase MP density in healthy subjects with a mean age of 23 years, and improved visual performance in glare function tests (Stringham and Hammond, 2008). Lutein has been reported to protect against the detrimental effects of long-term computer display light exposure in healthy subjects aged 22 to 30 years of age (Ma *et al.*, 2009). In this study, 12 weeks of supplementation with 12 mg/day of lutein was shown to improve contrast sensitivity. Lutein supplementation (5 mg) in combination with zeaxanthin (1 mg) and blackcurrant extract (200 mg) was also shown to reduce symptoms of visual fatigue associated with visual proof-reading tasks in healthy subjects aged 22 to 45 years (Yagi *et al.*, 2009).

The effect of lutein supplementation on visual performance has also been evaluated in patients with eye disease. In a double-blind, placebo-controlled study involving cataract patients ($n = 17$), supplementation with 15 mg lutein three times a week resulted in improved visual acuity and glare sensitivity (Olmedilla *et al.*, 2003). In patients with retinal degeneration, lutein supplementation (20–40 mg/day, 26 weeks) improved visual acuity and mean visual-field area, which began 2–4 weeks after the intervention but plateaued at 6–14 weeks (Dagnelie *et al.*, 2000). RCTs involving AMD patients have shown that lutein supplementation, ranging in dose from 8 mg to 15 mg, improved dark adaptation, visual acuity, foveal sensitivity, contrast sensitivity and glare recovery (Falsini *et al.*, 2003; Richer *et al.*, 2004; Cangemi, 2007). In conclusion, dietary intake of lutein seems to improve visual function.

DHA

Long-chain polyunsaturated fatty acids (LCPUFA) are essential for the normal development of vision (Neuringer *et al.*, 1984). The earliest evidence for the role of DHA in visual function was the observed improvement in visual acuity in preterm infants fed a formula supplemented with DHA (Carlson *et al.*, 1994). The photoreceptor outer segment membranes of the retina contain high concentrations of DHA, which is further reason to investigate the role of DHA in improving visual function (Fliesler and Anderson, 1983). Maternal DHA intake during the prenatal period was shown to play a critical role in the early development of the visual system in children well into the school-age years (Jacques *et al.*, 2011). A number of observational studies on lactating mothers and their infants found that high human milk and/or infant plasma DHA levels were associated with better visual acuity (Innis *et al.*, 2001; Innis, 2003; Jørgensen *et al.*, 2001). Similar associations were also observed in formula-fed infants (Jorgensen *et al.*, 1996; Birch *et al.*, 1998, 2005; Hoffman *et al.*, 2003).

Numerous RCTs have been done to evaluate the effects of supplementation with DHA, as well as ARA, another omega-3 fatty acid, on visual acuity in term infants (Hoffman *et al.*, 2009). A majority of the RCTs reported improved visual acuity in infants supplemented with DHA/ARA ($\geq 0.3\%/0.64\%$ of total fatty acids) starting near birth to 12 months in most studies (Makrides *et al.*, 1995; Birch *et al.*, 1998, 2002, 2010; Hoffman *et al.*, 2003, 2004b). No improvements in visual acuity were observed with DHA/ARA supplementation in other RCTs (Makrides *et al.*, 1995; Auestad *et al.*, 1997, 2001, 2003). The probable reasons for null effects of some RCTs could relate to the differences in the supplemented doses of DHA/ARA, the duration of supplementation, age of the infant at the time of assessment, the test method used, and the characteristics of the population studied. Trials that used supplemental doses of at least 0.32% DHA (close to the average amounts found in human milk) and at least 0.64% ARA were more likely to find positive outcomes. The timing of supplementation was also crucial, as DHA supplementation at 1.5, 4, 9, and 12 months improved visual acuity but not at 6 months. This was hypothesized to be due to this being an age at which visual development had temporarily plateaued (Birch *et al.*, 1998). A strong, positive, linear correlation was observed between the length of feeding DHA + ARA and visual function at 1 year of age.

Both DHA and ARA are extremely important for the development of vision in term infants. Several expert groups, such as the American Dietetic Association, the WHO Expert Panel, the European Food and Safety Authority, and the World Association of Perinatal Medicine, recommend that infants who cannot be breast-fed must receive formula supplemented with both DHA and ARA (Hoffman *et al.*, 2009). Infants should receive at least 0.32% fatty acids from DHA and 0.47% ARA, which are the average worldwide levels found in human milk (Brenna *et al.*, 2007).

Future Directions

Future research needs to take into consideration that a particular nutrient's benefit may be related to the stage at which the disease occurs. It is likely that some eye diseases, particularly those that are age-related, develop over many years and thus the timing of intervention may have a significant impact on the progression of the disease. Studies that evaluate nutritional interventions for prevention of eye disease and not treatment alone are also warranted. More studies are also needed to evaluate the impact of dietary patterns on eye diseases as nutrients are normally consumed as part of a diet and not in isolation. Dietary intervention studies that incorporate nutrient-rich foods rather than supplemental forms of the nutrients need to be done. The nutrient dosage is also a crucial factor in determining the effect on disease progression. At very high doses certain nutrients may have a negative effect. For example, ~1000 mg of vitamin C was related to increased risk of cataract; high intake of omega-6 fatty acids was related to increased risk of AMD; and high vitamin E supplementation was related to progression of RP. Intervention studies that evaluate nutrients at doses found in foods should also be done to determine the ideal beneficial levels. Research evaluating these factors may already be ongoing; in the meantime, eating a healthy diet rich in vitamins C and E, B vitamins, carotenoids, especially lutein and zeaxanthin, omega-3 fatty acids, and zinc is recommended to maintain visual health.

Suggestions for Further Reading

Chiu, C.J. and Taylor, A. (2007) Nutritional antioxidants and age-related cataract and maculopathy. *Exp Eye Res* **84**, 229–245.

Coleman, H. and Chew, E. (2007) Nutritional supplementation in age-related macular degeneration. *Curr Opin Ophthalmol* **18**, 220–223.

Evans, J.R. and Henshaw, E. (2008) Antioxidant vitamin and mineral supplements for preventing age-related macular degeneration *Cochrane Database Syst Rev* CD000253. [Update of *Cochrane Database Syst Rev.* 2000: CD000253.]

Fernandez, M.M. and Afshari, N.A. (2008) Nutrition and the prevention of cataracts. *Curr Opin Ophthalmol* **19**, 66–70.

Hartong, D.T., Berson, E.L., and Dryja, T.P. (2006) Retinitis pigmentosa. *Lancet* **368**, 1795–1809.

Krishnadev, N., Meleth, A.D., and Chew, E.Y. (2010) Nutritional supplements for age-related macular degeneration. *Curr Opin Ophthalmol* **21**, 184–189.

Roncone, M., Bartlett, H., and Eperjesi, F. (2010) Essential fatty acids for dry eye: a review. *Cont Lens Anterior Eye* **33**, 49–54.

References

Abdelsalam, A., Del Priore, L., and Zarbin, M.A. (1999) Drusen in age-related macular degeneration: pathogenesis, natural course, and laser photocoagulation-induced regression. *Surv Ophthalmol* **44**, 1–29.

Age-Related Eye Disease Study Research Group (2001a) A randomized, placebo-controlled, clinical trial of high-dose supplementation with vitamins C and E and beta carotene for age-related cataract and vision loss: AREDS report no. 9. [Erratum appears in *Arch Ophthalmol* 2008, **126**, 251.] *Arch Ophthalmol* **119**, 1439–1452.

Age-Related Eye Disease Study Research Group (2001b) A randomized, placebo-controlled, clinical trial of high-dose supplementation with vitamins C and E, beta carotene, and zinc for age-related macular degeneration and vision loss: AREDS report no. 8. [Erratum appears in *Arch Ophthalmol* 2008, 126, 1251.] *Arch Ophthalmol* **119**, 1417–1436.

Age-Related Eye Disease Study Research Group (2007) The relationship of dietary lipid intake and age-related macular degeneration in a case-control study: AREDS report no. 20. *Arch Ophthalmol* **125**, 671–679.

Age-Related Eye Disease Study Research Group, Sangiovanni, J.P., Chew, E.Y., et al. (2007) The relationship of dietary carotenoid and vitamin A, E, and C intake with age-related macular degeneration in a case-control study: AREDS report no. 22. [See Comment.] Arch Ophthalmol 125, 1225–1232.

Ahmed, S.S., Lott, M.N., and Marcus, D.M. (2005) The macular xanthophylls. Surv Ophthalmol 50, 183–193.

Allikmets, R. (2000) Simple and complex ABCR: genetic predisposition to retinal disease. Am J Hum Genet 67, 793–799.

Asbell, P.A., Dualan, I., Mindel, J., et al. (2005) Age-related cataract. Lancet 365, 599–609.

Auestad, N., Halter, R., Hall, R.T., et al. (2001) Growth and development in term infants fed long-chain polyunsaturated fatty acids: a double-masked, randomized, parallel, prospective, multivariate study. Pediatrics 108, 372–381.

Auestad, N., Montalto, M.B., Hall, R.T., et al. (1997) Visual acuity, erythrocyte fatty acid composition, and growth in term infants fed formulas with long chain polyunsaturated fatty acids for one year. Pediatr Res 41, 1–10.

Auestad, N., Scott, D.T., Janowsky, J.S., et al. (2003) Visual, cognitive, and language assessments at 39 months: a follow-up study of children fed formulas containing long-chain polyunsaturated fatty acids to 1 year of age. Pediatrics 112, e177–183.

Augood, C., Chakravarthy, U., Young, I., et al. (2008) Oily fish consumption, dietary docosahexaenoic acid and eicosapentanoic acid intakes, and associations with neovascular age-related macular degernation. Am J Clin Nutr 88, 398–406.

Axer-Siegel, R., Bourla, D., Ehrlich, R., et al. (2004) Association of neovascular age-related macular degeneration and hyperhomocysteinemia. Am J Ophthalmol 137, 84–89.

Aydin, E., Cumurcu, T., Özugurlu, F., et al. (2005) Levels of iron, zinc, and copper in aqueous humor, lens, and serum in nondiabetic and diabetic patients. Biol Trace Elem Res 108, 33–41.

Bahrami, H., Melia, M., and Dagnelie, G. (2006) Lutein supplementation in retinitis pigmentosa: PC-based vision assessment in a randomized double-masked placebo-controlled clinical trial [NCT00029289]. BMC Ophthalmology 6, 23.

Barabino, S., Rolando, M., Camicione, P., et al. (2003) Systemic linoleic and [gamma]-linolenic acid therapy in dry eye syndrome with an inflammatory component. Cornea 22, 97–101.

Barakat, M.R., Metelitsina, T.I., Dupont, J.C., et al. (2006) Effect of niacin on retinal vascular diameter in patients with age-related macular degeneration. Curr Eye Res 31, 629–634.

Beatty, S., Murray, I.J., Henson, D.B., et al. (2001) Macular pigment and risk for age-related macular degeneration in subjects from a Northern European population. Invest Ophthalmol Vis Sci 42, 439–446.

Berendschot, T.T.J.M., Willemse-Assink, J.J.M., Bastiaanse, M., et al. (2002) Macular pigment and melanin in age-related maculopathy in a general population. Invest Ophthalmol Vis Sci 43, 1928–1932.

Bernstein, P.S., Shao, D.-Y., and Wintch, S.W. (2002) Resonance Raman measurement of macular carotenoids in normal subjects and in age-related macular degeneration patients. Ophthalmology 109, 1780–1787.

Berson, E.L. (2000) Nutrition and retinal degenerations. Int Ophthalmol Clin 40, 93–111.

Berson, E.L., Rosner, B., Sandberg, M.A., et al. (1993) A randomized trial of vitamin A and vitamin E supplementation for retinitis pigmentosa. Arch Ophthalmol 111, 761–772.

Berson, E.L., Rosner, B., Sandberg, M.A., et al. (2004a) Clinical trial of docosahexaenoic acid in patients with retinitis pigmentosa receiving vitamin A treatment. Arch Ophthalmol 122, 1297–1305.

Berson, E.L., Rosner, B., Sandberg, M.A., et al. (2004b) Further evaluation of docosahexaenoic acid in patients with retinitis pigmentosa receiving vitamin A treatment: subgroup analyses. Arch Ophthalmol 122, 1306–1314.

Berson, E.L., Rosner, B., Sandberg, M.A., et al. (2010) Clinical trial of lutein in patients with retinitis pigmentosa receiving vitamin A. Arch Ophthalmol 128, 403–411.

Birch, E.E., Carlson, S.E., Hoffman, D.R., et al. (2010) The DIAMOND (DHA Intake And Measurement Of Neural Development) Study: a double-masked, randomized controlled clinical trial of the maturation of infant visual acuity as a function of the dietary level of docosahexaenoic acid. Am J Clin Nutr 91, 848–859.

Birch, E.E., Castañeda, Y.S., Wheaton, D.H., et al. (2005) Visual maturation of term infants fed long-chain polyunsaturated fatty acid–supplemented or control formula for 12 mo. Am J Clin Nutr 81, 871–879.

Birch, E.E., Hoffman, D.R., Castañeda, Y.S., et al. (2002) A randomized controlled trial of long-chain polyunsaturated fatty acid supplementation of formula in term infants after weaning at 6 wk of age. Am J Clin Nutr 75, 570–580.

Birch, E.E., Hoffman, D.R., Uauy, R., et al.(1998) Visual acuity and the essentiality of docosahexaenoic acid and arachidonic acid in the diet of term infants. Pediatr Res 44, 201–209.

Bishara, S., Merin, S., Cooper, M., et al. (1982) Combined vitamin A and E therapy prevents retinal electrophysiological deterioration in abetalipoproteinaemia. Br J Ophthalmol 66, 767–770.

Biswas, A. and Das, K.P. (2007) Zn2+ enhances the molecular chaperone function and stability of α-crystallin. Biochemistry 47, 804–816.

Blades, K.J., Patel, S., and Aidoo, K.E. (2001) Oral antioxidant therapy for marginal dry eye. Eur J Clin Nutr 55, 589.

Bone, R.A., Landrum, J.T., Dixon, Z., *et al.* (2000) Lutein and zeaxanthin in the eyes, serum and diet of human subjects. *Exp Eye Res* **71**, 239–245.

Bone, R.A., Landrum, J.T., Guerra, L.H., *et al.* (2003) Lutein and zeaxanthin dietary supplements raise macular pigment density and serum concentrations of these carotenoids in humans. *J Nutr* **133**, 992–998.

Bone, R.A., Landrum, J.T., Mayne, S.T., *et al.* (2001) Macular pigment in donor eyes with and without AMD: a case-control study. *Invest Ophthalmol Vis Sci* **42**, 235–240. [Erratum appears in *Invest Ophthalmol Vis Sci* 2001 **42**, 548.]

Bone, R.A., Landrum, J.T., and Tarsis, S.L. (1985) Preliminary identification of the human macular pigment. *Vision Res* **25**, 1531–1535.

Brenna, J.T., Varamini, B., Jensen, R.G., *et al.* (2007) Docosahexaenoic and arachidonic acid concentrations in human breast milk worldwide. *Am J Clin Nutr* **85**, 1457–1464.

Brewitt, H. and Sistani, F. (2001) Dry eye disease: the scale of the problem. *Surv Ophthalmol* **45**, S199–S202.

Brown, L., Rimm, E.B., Seddon, J.M., *et al.* (1999) A prospective study of carotenoid intake and risk of cataract extraction in US men. *Am J Clin Nutr* **70**, 517–524.

Bunce, G.E., Kinoshita, J., and Horwitz, J. (1990) Nutritional factors in cataract. *Annu Rev Nutr* **10**, 233–254.

Cangemi, F.E. (2007) TOZAL Study: an open case-control study of an oral antioxidant and omega-3 supplement for dry AMD. *BMC Ophthalmol* **7**, 3.

Canter, P.H. and Ernst, E. (2004) Anthocyanosides of *Vaccinium myrtillus* (bilberry) for night vision – a systematic review of placebo-controlled trials. *Surv Ophthalmol*, **49**, 38–50.

Carlson S.E., Werkman, S.H., Peeples, J.M., *et al.* (1994) Long-chain fatty acids and early visual and cognitive development of preterm infants. *Eur J Clin Nutr* **48**, S27–30.

Chasen-Taber, L., Willett, W.C., Seddon, J.M., *et al.* (1999) A prospective study of carotenoid and vitamin A intakes and risk of cataract extraction in US women. *Am J Clin Nutr* **70**, 517–524.

Chiu, C.-J., Hubbard, L.D., Armstrong, J., *et al.* (2006a) Dietary glycemic index and carbohydrate in relation to early age-related macular degeneration. *Am J Clin Nutr* **83**, 880–886.

Chiu, C.-J., Milton, R.C., Gensler, G., *et al.* (2006b) Dietary carbohydrate intake and glycemic index in relation to cortical and nuclear lens opacities in the Age-Related Eye Disease Study. *Am J Clin Nutr* **83**, 1177–1184.

Chiu, C.-J., Milton, R.C., Gensler, G., *et al.* (2007) Association between dietary glycemic index and age-related macular degeneration in nondiabetic participants in the Age-Related Eye Disease Study. *Am J Clin Nutr* **86**, 180–188.

Chiu, C.-J., Morris, M.S., Rogers, G., *et al.* (2005) Carbohydrate intake and glycemic index in relation to the odds of early cortical and nuclear lens opacities. *Am J Clin Nutr* **81**, 1411–1416.

Chiu, C.-J., Robman, L., McCarty, C.A., *et al.* (2010) Dietary carbohydrate in relation to cortical and nuclear lens opacities in the Melbourne visual impairment project. *Invest Ophthalmol Vis Sci* **51**, 2897–2905.

Cho, E., Hung, S., Willett, W.C., *et al.* (2001a) Prospective study of dietary fat and the risk of age-related macular degeneration. *Am J Clin Nutr* **73**, 209–218.

Cho, E., Seddon, J.M., Rosner B., *et al.* (2004) Prospective study on intake of fruits, vegetables, vitamins, and carotenoids and risk of age-related maculopathy. *Arch Ophthalmol* **122**, 883–892.

Cho, E., Stampfer, M.J., Seddon, J.M., *et al.* (2001b) Prospective study of zinc intake and the risk of age-related macular degeneration. *Ann Epidemiol* **11**, 328–336.

Chong, E.W.T., Wong, T.Y., Kreis, A.J., *et al.* (2007) Dietary antioxidants and primary prevention of age related macular degeneration: systematic review and meta-analysis [see Comment]. *BMJ* **335**, 755.

Christen, W.G., Ajani, U.A., Glynn, R.J., *et al.* (1999) Prospective cohort study of antioxidant vitamin supplement use and the risk of age-related maculopathy. *Am J Epidemiol* **149**, 476–484.

Christen, W.G., Glynn, R.J., Chew, E.Y., *et al.* (2009) Folic acid, pyridoxine, and cyanocobalamin combination treatment and age-related macular degeneration in women: the Women's Antioxidant and Folic Acid Cardiovascular Study. *Arch Intern Med* **169**, 335–341.

Christen, W.G., Glynn, R.J., Chew, E.Y., *et al.* (2010) Vitamin E and age-related macular degeneration in a randomized trial of women. *Ophthalmology* **117**, 1163–1168.

Christen, W.G., Liu, S., Glynn, R.J., *et al.* (2008) Dietary carotenoids, vitamins C and E, and risk of cataract in women: a prospective study. *Arch Ophthalmol* **126**, 102–109.

Christen, W.G., Manson, J.E., Glynn, R.J., *et al.* (2003) A randomized trial of beta carotene and age-related cataract in US physicians. *Arch Ophthalmol* **121**, 372–378.

Chua, B., Flood, V., Rochtchina, E., *et al.* (2006) Dietary fatty acids and the 5-year incidence of age-related maculopathy. *Arch Ophthalmol* **124**, 981–986.

Chylack, L.T., Brown, N.P., Bron, A., *et al.* (2002) The Roche European American Cataract Trial (REACT): a randomized clinical trial to investigate the efficacy of an oral antioxidant micronutrient mixture to slow progression of age-related cataract. *Ophthalmic Epidemiol* **9**, 49.

Clinical Trial of Nutritional Supplements and Age-Related Cataract Study Group, Maraini, G., Sperduto, R.D., *et al.*

(2008) A randomized, double-masked, placebo-controlled clinical trial of multivitamin supplementation for age-related lens opacities. Clinical trial of nutritional supplements and age-related cataract report no. 3. *Ophthalmology* **115,** 599–607.

Congdon, N., O'Colmain, B., Klaver, C.C.W., *et al.* (2004) Causes and prevalence of visual impairment among adults in the United States. *Arch Ophthalmol* **122,** 477–485.

Connolly, E.E., Beatty, S., Thurnham, D.I., *et al.* (2010) Augmentation of macular pigment following supplementation with all three macular carotenoids: an exploratory study. *Curr Eye Res* **35,** 335–351.

Coral, K., Raman, R., Rathi, S., *et al.* (2006) Plasma homocysteine and total thiol content in patients with exudative age-related macular degeneration. *Eye* **20,** 203–207.

Cumming, R.G., Mitchell, P., and Smith, W. (2000) Diet and cataract: the Blue Mountains Eye Study. *Ophthalmology* **107,** 450–456.

Dagnelie, G., Zorge, I.S., and McDonald, T.M. (2000) Lutein improves visual function in some patients with retinal regeneration: a pilot study via the internet. *Optometry* **71,** 147–164.

Dawczynski, J., Blum, M., Winnefeld, K., *et al.* (2002) Increased content of zinc and iron in human cataractous lenses. *Biol Trace Elem Res* **90,** 15–23.

D'Cruz, P.M., Yasumura, D., Weir, J., *et al.* (2000) Mutation of the receptor tyrosine kinase gene Mertk in the retinal dystrophic RCS rat. *Hum Mol Genet* **9,** 645–651.

Delcourt, C., Carriere, I., Cristol, J.P., *et al.* (2007) Dietary fat and the risk of age-related maculopathy: the POLANUT Study. *Eur J Clin Nutr* **61,** 1341–1344.

Delyfer, M.-N., Léveillard, T., Mohand-Saïd, S., *et al.* (2004) Inherited retinal degenerations: therapeutic prospects. *Biol Cell* **96,** 261–269.

Dherani, M., Murthy, G.V.S., Gupta, S.K., *et al.* (2008) Blood levels of vitamin C, carotenoids and retinol are inversely associated with cataract in a North Indian population. *Invest Ophthalmol Vis Sci* **49,** 3328–3335.

Driver, P. and Lemp, M.A. (1997) *Seborrhea and Meibomian Gland Dysfunction.* Mosby, St. Louis, MO.

Dryja, T.P., Hahn, L.B., Kajiwara, K., *et al.* (1997) Dominant and digenic mutations in the peripherin/RDS and ROM1 genes in retinitis pigmentosa. *Invest Ophthalmol Vis Sci* **38,** 1972–1982.

Dryja, T.P., Hahn, L.B., Reboul, T., *et al.* (1996) Missense mutation in the gene encoding the [alpha] subunit of rod transducin in the Nougaret form of congenital stationary night blindness. *Nat Genet* **13,** 358–360.

Erie, J.C., Good, J.A., Butz, J.A., and Pulido, J.S. (2009) Reduced zinc and copper in the retinal pigment epithelium and choroid in age-related macular degeneration. *Am J Ophthalmol* **147,** 276–282.

Evans, J.R. and Henshaw, K. (2008) Antioxidant vitamin and mineral supplements for preventing age-related macular degeneration. *Cochrane Database Syst Rev* CD000253. [Update of *Cochrane Database Syst Rev* (2000) CD000253.]

Eye Disease Case-Control Study Group (EDCCSG) (1993) Antioxidant status and neovascular age-related macular degeneration. *Arch Ophthalmol* **111,** 104–109.

Falsini, B., Piccardi, M., Iarossi, G., *et al.* (2003) Influence of short-term antioxidant supplementation on macular function in age-related maculopathy: a pilot study including electrophysiologic assessment. *Ophthalmology* **110,** 51–60. Discussion, 61.

Ferrigno, L., Aldigeri, R., Rosmini, F., *et al.* (2005) Associations between plasma levels of vitamins and cataract in the Italian-American Clinical Trial of Nutritional Supplements and Age-Related Cataract (CTNS): CTNS Report #2. *Ophthalmic Epidemiol* **12,** 71–80.

Fliesler, S.J. and Anderson, R.E. (1983) Chemistry and metabolism of lipids in the vertebrate retina. *Prog Lipid Res* **22,** 79–131.

Flood, V., Smith, W., Wang, J.J., *et al.* (2002) Dietary antioxidant intake and incidence of early age-related maculopathy: the Blue Mountains Eye Study. *Ophthalmology* **109,** 2272–2278.

Fuchs, S., Nakazawa, M., Maw, M., *et al.* (1995) A homozygous 1-base pair deletion in the arrestin gene is a frequent cause of Oguchi disease in Japanese. *Nat Genet* **10,** 360–362.

Gale, C.R., Hall, N.F., Phillips, D.I.K., *et al.* (2001) Plasma antioxidant vitamins and carotenoids and age-related cataract. *Ophthalmology* **108,** 1992–1998.

Gritz, D.C., Srinivasan, M., Smith, S.D., *et al.* (2006) The Antioxidants in Prevention of Cataracts Study: effects of antioxidant supplements on cataract progression in South India. *Br J Ophthalmol* **90,** 847–851.

Hammond, B., Johnson, E., Russell, R., *et al.* (1997) Dietary modification of human macular pigment density. *Invest Ophthalmol Vis Sci* **38,** 1795–1801.

Hankinson, S.E., Stampfer, M.J., Seddon, J.M., *et al.* (1992) Nutrient intake and cataract extraction in women: a prospective study. *BMJ* **305,** 244–251.

Hartong, D.T., Berson, E.L., and Dryja, T.P. (2006) Retinitis pigmentosa. *Lancet,* **368,** 1795–1809.

Heinonen, O.P. (1994) The effect of vitamin E and beta carotene on the incidence of lung cancer and other cancers in male smokers. *N Engl J Med* **330,** 1029–1035.

Heuberger, R.A., Fisher, A.I., Jacques, P.F., *et al.* (2002) Relation of blood homocysteine and its nutritional determinants to age-related maculopathy in the third National Health and Nutrition Examination Survey. *Am J Clin Nutr* **76,** 897–902.

Heuberger, R.A., Mares-Perlman, J.A., Klein, R., *et al.* (2001) Relationship of dietary fat to age-related maculopathy in the third National Health and Nutrition Examination Survey. *Arch Ophthalmol* **119**, 1833–1838.

Hodge, W., Barnes, D., Schachter H.M., *et al.* (2005) Effects of omega-3 fatty acids on eye health. *Evid Rep Technol Assess (Summ)* **(117)** 1–6.

Hoffman, D.R., Birch, E.E., Castañeda, Y.S., *et al.* (2003) Visual function in breast-fed term infants weaned to formula with or without long-chain polyunsaturates at 4 to 6 months: a randomized clinical trial. *J Pediatr* **142**, 669–677.

Hoffman, D.R., Boettcher, J.A., and Diersen-Schade, D.A. (2009) Toward optimizing vision and cognition in term infants by dietary docosahexaenoic and arachidonic acid supplementation: a review of randomized controlled trials. *Prostaglandins Leukot Essent Fatty Acids* **81**, 151–158.

Hoffman, D.R., Locke, K.G., Wheaton, D.H., *et al.* (2004a) A randomized placebo-controlled clinical trial of docosahexaenoic acid supplementation for X-linked retinitis pigmentosa. *Am J Ophthalmol* **137**, 704–718.

Hoffman, D.R., Theuer, R.C., Castañeda, Y.S., *et al.* (2004b) Maturation of visual acuity is accelerated in breast-fed term infants fed baby food containing DHA-enriched egg yolk. *J Nutr* **134**, 2307–2313.

Innis, S.M. (2003) Perinatal biochemistry and physiology of long-chain polyunsaturated fatty acids. *J Pediatr* **143**, 1–8.

Innis, S.M., Gilley, J., and Werker, J. (2001) Are human milk long-chain polyunsaturated fatty acids related to visual and neural development in breast-fed term infants? *J Pediatr* **139**, 532–538.

Institute of Medicine (2001) *Dietary Reference Intakes for Vitamin A, Vitamin K, Arsenic, Boron, Chromium, Copper, Iodine, Iron, Manganese, Molybdenum, Nickel, Silicon, Vanadium, and Zinc.* National Academy Press, Washington, DC.

Jacques, P.F. and Chylack, L.T., Jr (1991) Epidemiologic evidence of a role for the antioxidant vitamins and carotenoids in cataract prevention. *Am J Clin Nutr* **53**, 353S–355S.

Jacques, P.F., Chylack, L.T., Jr, Hankinson, S.E., *et al.* (2001) Long-term nutrient intake and early age-related nuclear lens opacities. *Arch Ophthalmol* **119**, 1009–1019.

Jacques, C., Levy, E., Muckle, G., *et al.* (2011) Long-term effects of prenatal omega-3 fatty acid intake on visual function in school-age children. *J Pediatr* **158**, 73–80.

Jacques, P.F., Taylor, A., Hankinson, S.E., *et al.* (1997) Long-term vitamin C supplement and prevalence of age-related opacities. *Am J Clin Nutr* **66**, 911–916.

Jacques, P.F., Taylor, A., Moeller, S., *et al.* (2005) Long-term nutrient intake and 5-year change in nuclear lens opacities. *Arch Ophthalmol* **123**, 517–526.

Jager, R.D., Mieler, W.F., and Miller, J.W. (2008) Age-related macular degeneration. *N Engl J Med* **358**, 2606–2617.

Jalal, D., Koorosh, F., and Fereidoun, H. (2009) Comparative study of plasma ascorbic acid levels in senile cataract patients and in normal individuals. *Curr Eye Res* **34**, 118–122.

Javitt, J.C. (1993) Who does cataract surgery in the United States? *Arch Ophthalmol* **111**, 1329.

Jenkins, D.J.A., Kendall, C.W.C., Augustin, L.S.A., *et al.* (2002) Glycemic index: overview of implications in health and disease. *Am J Clin Nutr* **76**, 266S–273S.

Johnson, E.J., Chung, H.-Y., Caldarella, S.M., *et al.* (2008) The influence of supplemental lutein and docosahexaenoic acid on serum, lipoproteins, and macular pigmentation. *Am J Clin Nutr* **87**, 1521–1529.

Jørgensen, M.H., Hernell, O., Hughes, E.L., *et al.* (2001) Is there a relation between docosahexaenoic acid concentration in mothers' milk and visual development in term infants? *J Pediatr Gastroenterol Nutr* **32**, 293–296.

Jørgensen, M.H., Hernell, O., Lund, P., *et al.* (1996) Visual acuity and erythrocyte docosahexaenoic acid status in breast-fed and formula-fed term infants during the first four months of life. *Lipids* **31**, 99–105.

Kamburoglu, G., Gumus, K., Kadayifcilar, S., *et al.* (2006) Plasma homocysteine, vitamin B12 and folate levels in age-related macular degeneration. *Graefes Arch Clin Exp Ophthalmol* **244**, 565–569.

Kennedy, E.T., Ohls, J., Carlson, S., *et al.* (1995) The Healthy Eating Index: design and applications. *J Am Diet Assoc* **95**, 1103–1108.

Knekt, P., Heliovaara, M., Rissenen, A., *et al.* (1992) Serum antioxidant vitamins and risk of cataract. *BMJ* **304**, 1392–1394.

Krepler, K. and Schmid, R. (2005) Alpha-tocopherol in plasma, red blood cells and lenses with and without cataract. *Am J Ophthalmol* **139**, 266–270.

Krishnadev, N., Meleth, A.D., and Chew, E.Y. (2010) Nutritional supplements for age-related macular degeneration. *Curr Opin Ophthalmol* **21**, 184–189.

Kuzniarz, M., Mitchell, P., Cumming, R.G., *et al.* (2001) Use of vitamin supplements and cataract: the Blue Mountains Eye Study. *Am J Ophthalmol* **132**, 19–26.

Landrum, J.T., Bone, R.A., Sprague, K., *et al.* (1997) A one-year study of supplementation with lutein on the macular pigment. *Exp Eye Res* **65**, 57–62.

Larmo, P.S., Jarvinen, R.L., Setala, N.L., *et al.* (2010) Oral sea buckthorn oil attenuates tear film osmolarity and symptoms in individuals with dry eye. *J Nutr* **140**, 1462–1468.

Larowe, T.L., Mares, J.A., Snodderly, D.M., *et al.* (2008) Macular pigment density and age-related maculopathy in the Carotenoids in Age-Related Eye Disease Study. An ancillary study of the Women's Health Initiative. *Ophthalmology* **115**, 876–883.

Lengyel, I., Flinn, J.M., Peto, T., *et al.* (2007) High concentration of zinc in sub-retinal pigment epithelial deposits. *Exp Eye Res* **84,** 772–780.

Leske, M.C., Chylack, L.T., He, Q., *et al.* (1998) Antioxidant vitamins and nuclear opacities: the longitudinal study of cataract. *Ophthalmology* **105,** 831–836.

Leske, M.C., Chylack, L.T., Jr, and Wu, S.Y. (1991) The Lens Opacities Case-Control Study. Risk factors for cataract. *Arch Ophthalmol* **109,** 244–251.

Leske, M.C., Wu, S.Y., Hyman, L., *et al.* (1995) Biochemical factors in the Lens Opacities Case-Control Study. *Arch Ophthalmol* **113,** 1113–1119.

Levy, Y. and Glovinsky, Y. (1998) The effect of anthocyanosides on night vision. *Eye* **12,** 967–969.

Liu, X., Bulgakov, O.V., Darrow, K.N., *et al.* (2007) Usherin is required for maintenance of retinal photoreceptors and normal development of cochlear hair cells. *Proc Natl Acad Sci USA* **104,** 4413–4418.

Lonn, E., Bosch, J., Yusuf, S., *et al.* (2005) Effects of long-term vitamin E supplementation on cardiovascular events and cancer. *JAMA* **293,** 1338–1347.

Lu, M., Cho, E., Taylor, A., *et al.* (2005) Prospective study of dietary fat and risk of cataract extraction among US women. *Am J Epidemiol* **161,** 948–959.

Lu, M., Taylor, A., Chylack, L.T., Jr, *et al.* (2007) Dietary linolenic acid intake is positively associated with five-year change in eye lens nuclear density. *J Am Coll Nutr* **26,** 133–140.

Lyle, B.J. (1999) Serum carotenoids and tocopherols and incidence of age-related nuclear cataract. *Am J Clin Nutr* **69,** 272–277.

Lyle, B.J., Mares-Perlman, J.A., Klein, B.E., *et al.* (1999) Antioxidant intake and risk of incident age-related nuclear cataracts in the Beaver Dam Eye Study. *Am J Epidemiol* **149,** 801–809.

Ma, L., Lin, X.-M., Zou, Z.-Y., *et al.* (2009) A 12-week lutein supplementation improves visual function in Chinese people with long-term computer display light exposure. *Br J Nutr* **102,** 186–190.

Macrì, A., Giuffrida, S., Amico, V., *et al.* (2003) Effect of linoleic acid and gamma-linolenic acid on tear production, tear clearance and on the ocular surface after photorefractive keratectomy. *Graefes Arch Clin Exp Ophthalmol* **241,** 561–566.

Makrides, M., Neumann, M., Simmer, K., *et al.* (1995) Are long-chain polyunsaturated fatty acids essential nutrients in infancy? *Lancet* **345,** 1463–1468.

Mares-Perlman, J.A., Brady, W.E., Klein, B.E., *et al.* (1995a) Diet and nuclear lens opacities. *Am J Epidemiol* **141,** 322–334.

Mares-Perlman, J.A., Brady, W.E., Klein, B.E., *et al.* (1995b) Serum carotenoids and tocopherols and severity of nuclear and cortical opacities. *Invest Ophthalmol Vis Sci* **36,** 276–288.

Mares-Perlman, J.A., Brady, W.E., Klein, B.E., *et al.* (1995c) Serum antioxidants and age-related macular degeneration in a population-based case-control study. *Arch Ophthalmol* **113,** 1518–1523.

Mares-Perlman, J.A., Brady, W.E., Klein, B.E., *et al.* (1995d) Dietary fat and age-related maculopathy. *Arch Ophthalmol* **113,** 743–748.

Mares-Perlman, J.A., Klein, R., Klein, B.E.K., *et al.* (1996) Association of zinc and antioxidant nutrients with age-related maculopathy. *Arch Ophthalmol* **114,** 991–997.

Mares-Perlman, J.A., Lyle, B.J., Klein, R., *et al.* (2000) Vitamin supplement use and incident cataracts in a population-based study. *Arch Ophthalmol* **118,** 1556–1563.

Mares, J.A., Voland, R., Adler, R., *et al.* (2010) Healthy diets and the subsequent prevalence of nuclear cataract in women. *Arch Ophthalmol* **128,** 738–749.

Marlhens, F., Bareil, C., Griffoin, J.M., *et al.* (1997) Mutations in RPE65 cause Leber's congenital amaurosis. *Nat Genet* **17,** 139–141.

Maw, M.A., Kennedy, B., Knight, A., *et al.* (1997) Mutation of the gene encoding cellular retinaldehyde-binding protein in autosomal recessive retinitis pigmentosa. *Nat Genet* **17,** 198–200.

Mayser, H.M. and Wilhelm, H. (2001) Effects of anthocyanosides on contrast vision [abstract]. *Invest. Ophthalmol Vis Sci* **42,** 63.

McCulley, J.P., Dougherty, J.M., and Denau, D.G. (1982) Classification of chronic blepharitis. *Ophthalmology* **89,** 1173–1180.

McLaughlin, M.E., Sandberg, M.A., Berson, E.L., *et al.* (1993) Recessive mutations in the gene encoding the [beta]-subunit of rod phosphodiesterase in patients with retinitis pigmentosa. *Nat Genet* **4,** 130–134.

McNeil, J.J., Robman, L., Tikellis, G., *et al.* (2004) Vitamin E supplementation and cataract: randomized controlled trial. *Ophthalmology* **111,** 75–84.

Metelitsina, T.I., Grunwald, J.E., Dupont, J.C., *et al.* (2004) Effect of niacin on the choroidal circulation of patients with age related macular degeneration. *Br J Ophthalmol* **88,** 1568–1572.

Miljanovic, B., Trivedi, K.A., Dana, R.M., *et al.* (2005) Relation between dietary n-3 and n-6 fatty acids and clinically diagnosed dry eye syndrome in women. *Am J Clin Nutr* **82,** 887–893.

Moeller, S.M., Parekh, N., Tinker, L., *et al.* (2006) Associations between intermediate age-related macular degeneration and lutein and zeaxanthin in the Carotenoids in Age-related Eye Disease Study (CAREDS): ancillary study of the Women's Health Initiative. *Arch Ophthalmol* **124,** 1151–1162.

Moeller, S.M., Taylor, R.A., Tucker, K.L., *et al.* (2004) Overall adherence to the dietary guidelines for Americans is associated with reduced prevalence of early age-related nuclear lens opacities in women. *J Nutr* **134,** 1812–1819.

Mohan, M., Sperduto, R.D., Angra, S.K., *et al.* (1989) Indian–US case-control study of age-related cataracts. India–US Case-Control Study Group. *Arch Ophthalmol* **107**, 670–676.

Montgomery, M.P., Kamel, F., Pericak-Vance, M.A., *et al.* (2010) Overall diet quality and age-related macular degeneration. *Ophthalmic Epidemiol* **17**, 58–65.

Morris, M.S., Jacques, P.F., Chylack, L.T., *et al.* (2007) Intake of zinc and antioxidant micronutrients and early age-related maculopathy lesions. *Ophthalmic Epidemiol* **14**, 288–298.

Mosad, S.M., Ghanem, A.A., El-Fallal, H.M., *et al.* (2010) Lens cadmium, lead, and serum vitamins C, E, and beta carotene in cataractous smoking patients. *Curr Eye Res* **35**, 23–30.

Moss, S.E., Klein, R., and Klein, B.E. (2008) Long-term incidence of dry eye in an older population. *Optom Vis Sci* **85**, 668–674.

Muth, E., Laurent, J., and Jasper, P. (2000) The effect of bilberry nutrition supplementation on night visual acuity and contrast sensitivity. *Altern Med Rev* **5**, 164–173.

Nadalin, G., Robman, L.D., McCarty, C.A., *et al.* (1999) The role of past intake of vitamin E in early cataract changes. *Ophthalmic Epidemiol* **6**, 105–112.

Nakaishi, H., Matsumoto, H., Tominanga, S., *et al.* (2000) Effects of black currant anthocyanoside intake on dark adaption and VDT work-induced transient refractive alteration in healthy humans. *Altern Med Rev* **5**, 553–562.

Neuringer, M., Anderson, G.J., and Connor, W.E. (1988) The essentiality of n-3 fatty acids for the development and function of the retina and brain. *Annu Rev Nutr* **8**, 517–541.

Neuringer, M., Connor, W.E., Van Petten, C., *et al.* (1984) Dietary omega-3 fatty acid deficiency and visual loss in infant rhesus monkeys. *J Clin Invest* **73**, 272–276.

Newsome, D. and Brewer, G.J. (2008) Comment on: "High concentration of zinc in sub-retinal pigment epithelial deposits" (Lengyel *et al.*, 2007) (*Exp Eye Res* **84**, 772–780). *Exp Eye Res* **86**, 860–861.

Newsome, D.A. (2008) A randomized, prospective, placebo-controlled clinical trial of a novel zinc-monocysteine compound in age-related macular degeneration. *Curr Eye Res* **33**, 591–598.

Newsome, D.A., Oliver, P.D., Deupree, D.M., *et al.* (1992) Zinc uptake by primate retinal pigment epithelium and choroid. *Curr Eye Res* **11**, 213–217.

Newsome, D.A., Schwartz, M., Leone, M.C., *et al.* (1988) Oral zinc in macular degeneration. *Arch Ophthalmol* **106**, 192–198.

Nolan, J., O'Donovan, O., and Beatty, S. (2003) The role of macular pigment in the defence against AMD. *AMD* **1**, 39–41.

Nourmohammadi, I., Modarress, M., Khanaki, K., *et al.* (2008) Association of serum alpha-tocopherol, retinol and ascorbic acid with the risk of cataract development. *Ann Nutr Metab* **52**, 296–298.

Nourmohammadi, I., Modarress, M., and Pakdel, F. (2006) Assessment of aqueous humor zinc status in human age-related cataract. *Ann Nutr Metab* **50**, 51–53.

Nowak, M., Swietochowska, E., Wielkoszynski, T., *et al.* (2005) Homocysteine, vitamin B12, and folic acid in age-related macular degeneration. *Eur J Ophthalmol* **15**, 764–767.

Olmedilla, B., Granado, F., Blanco, I., *et al.* (2003) Lutein, but not alpha-tocopherol, supplementation improves visual function in patients with age-related cataracts: a 2-y double-blind, placebo-controlled pilot study. *Nutrition* **19**, 21–24.

Omenn, G.S., Goodman, G.E., Thornquist, M.D., *et al.* (1996) Effects of a combination of beta-carotene and vitamin A on lung cancer and cardiovascular disease. *N Engl J Med* **334**, 1150–1155.

Parisi, V., Tedeschi, M., Gallinaro, G., *et al.* (2008) Carotenoids and antioxidants in age-related maculopathy Italian study: multifocal electroretinogram modifications after 1 year. *Ophthalmology* **115**, 324–333.

Pasantes-Morales, H., Quiroz, H., and Quesada, O. (2002) Treatment with taurine, diltiazem, and vitamin E retards the progressive visual field reduction in retinitis pigmentosa: a 3-year follow-up study. *Metab Brain Dis* **17**, 183–197.

Peponis, V., Papathanasiou, M., Kapranou, A., *et al.* (2002) Protective role of oral antioxidant supplementation in ocular surface of diabetic patients. *Br J Ophthalmol* **86**, 1369–1373.

Perrault, I., Rozet, J.M., Calvas, P., *et al.* (1996) Retinal-specific guanylate cyclase gene mutations in Leber's congenital amaurosis. *Nat Genet* **14**, 461–464.

Pinna, A., Piccinini, P., and Carta, F. (2007) Effect of oral linolein and gamma-linoleic acid on meibomian gland dysfunction. *Cornea* **26**, 260–264.

Powers, H.J. (2003) Riboflavin (vitamin B-2) and health. *Am J Clin Nutr* **77**, 1352–1360.

Rautiainen, S., Lindblad, B.E., Morgenstern, R., *et al.* (2010) Vitamin C supplements and the risk of age-related cataract: a population-based prospective cohort study in women. *Am J Clin Nutr* **91**, 487–493.

Resnikoff, S., Pascolini, D., Etya'ale, D., *et al.* (2004) Global data on visual impairment in the year 2002. *Bull World Health Organ* **82**, 844–851.

Richer, S., Stiles, W., Statkute, L., *et al.* (2004) Double masked, placebo-controlled, randomized trial of lutein and antioxidant supplementation in the intervention of atrophic age-related macular degeneration: the Veteran's LAST study (Lutein Antioxidant Supplementation Trial). *Optometry* **75**, 216–230.

Robertson, J.M., Donner, A.P., and Trevithick, J.R.(1989) Vitamin E intake and risk of cataracts in humans. *Ann NY Acad Sci* **570**, 372–382.

Robison, W.G., Kuwabara, T., and Bieri, J.G. (1979) Vitamin E deficiency and the retina: photoreceptor and pigment epithelial changes. *Invest Ophthalmol Vis Sci* **18**, 683–690.

Robison, W.G., Kuwabara, T., and Bieri, J.G. (1980) Deficiencies of vitamins E and A in the rat. Retinal damage and lipofuscin accumulation. *Invest Ophthalmol Vis Sci* **19**, 1030–1037.

Rochtchina, E., Wang, J.J., Flood, V.M., *et al.* (2007) Elevated serum homocysteine, low serum vitamin B12, folate, and age-related macular degeneration: the Blue Mountains Eye Study. *Am J Ophthalmol* **143**, 344–346.

Rouhiainen, P., Rouhiainen, H., and Saloneen, J.T. (1996) Association between low plasma vitamin E concentrations and progression of early cortical lens opacities. *Am J Epidemiol* **114**, 496–500.

Sanders, T.A.B., Haines, A.P., Wormald, R., *et al.* (1993) Essential fatty acids, plasma cholesterol, and fat-soluble vitamins in subjects with age-related maculopathy and matched control subjects. *Am J Clin Nutr* **57**, 428–433.

Sangiovanni, J.P., Agrón, E., Meleth, A.D., *et al.* (2009) ω-3 Long-chain polyunsaturated fatty acid intake and 12-y incidence of neovascular age-related macular degeneration and central geographic atrophy: AREDS report 30, a prospective cohort study from the Age-Related Eye Disease Study. *Am J Clin Nutr* **90**, 1601–1607.

Schaefer, E.J., Robins, S.J., Patton, G.M., *et al.* (1995) Red blood cell membrane phosphatidylethanolamine fatty acid content in various forms of retinitis pigmentosa. *J Lipid Res* **36**, 1427–1433.

Schaumberg, D.A., Liu, S., Seddon, J.M., *et al.* (2004) Dietary glycemic load and risk of age-related cataract.*Am J Clin Nutr* **80**, 489–495.

Schweigert, F.J. and Reimann, J. (2011) Micronutrients and their relevance for the eye–function of lutein, zeaxanthin and omega-3 fatty acids. *Klin Monbl Augenheilkd* **228**, 537–543.

Schweitzer, D., Lang, G.E., Remsch, H., *et al.* (2000) Age-related maculopathy. Comparative studies of patients, their children and healthy controls [German]. *Ophthalmologe* **97**, 84–90.

Seddon, J.M., Ajani, U.A., Sperduto, R.D., *et al.* (1994a) Dietary carotenoids, vitamins A, C, and E, and advanced age-related macular degeneration. Eye Disease Case-Control Study Group. *JAMA* **272**, 1413–1420.

Seddon, J.M., Christen, W.G., Manson, J.E., *et al.* (1994b) The use of vitamin supplements and the risk of cataract among US male physicians. *Am J Publ Health* **84**, 788–792.

Seddon, J.M., Cote, J., and Rosner, B. (2003) Progression of age-related macular degeneration. Association with dietary fat, trans unsaturated fat, nuts and fish intake. *Arch Ophthalmol* **121**, 1728–1737.

Seddon, J.M., George, S., and Rosner, B. (2006) Cigarette smoking, fish consumption, omega-3 fatty acid intake, and associations with age-related macular degeneration: The US Twin Study of Age-Related Macular Degeneration. *Arch Ophthalmol* **124**, 995–1001.

Seddon, J.M., Rosner, B., Sperduto, R.D., *et al.* (2001) Dietary fat and risk for advanced age-related macular degeneration. *Arch Ophthalmol* **119**, 1191–1199.

Selhub, J. and Miller, J. (1992) The pathogenesis of homocysteinemia: interruption of the coordinate regulation by S-adenosylmethionine of the remethylation and transsulfuration of homocysteine. *Am J Clin Nutr* **55**, 131–138.

Simon, J.A. and Hudes, E.S. (1999) Serum ascorbic acid and other correlates of self-reported cataract among older Americans. *J Clin Epidemiol* **52**, 1207–1211.

Simopoulos, A.P. (2000) Human requirement for n-3 polyunsaturated fatty acids. *Poult Sci* **79**, 961–970.

Simopoulos, A.P. (2002) The importance of the ratio of omega-6/omega-3 essential fatty acids. *Biomed Pharmacother* **56**, 365–379.

Smith, A., Clark, R., Nutt, D., *et al.* (1999) Anti-oxidant vitamins and mental performance of the elderly. *Hum Psychopharmacol* **14**, 459–471.

Snellen, E.L., Verbeek, A.L., Van den Hoogen, G.W., *et al.* (2002) Neovascular age-related macular degeneration and its relationship to antioxidant intake. *Acta Ophthalmol Scand* **80**, 368–371.

Snodderly, D.M. (1995) Evidence for protection against age-related macular degeneration by carotenoids and antioxidant vitamins. *Am J Clin Nutr* **62**, 1448S–1461S.

Sperduto, R.D., Hu, T.S., Milton, R.C., *et al.* (1993) The Linxian cataract studies. Two nutrition intervention trials. *Arch Ophthalmol* **111**, 1246–1253.

St George, S.D. and Cenkowski, S. (2007) Influence of harvest time on the quality of oil-based compounds in sea buckthorn (*Hippophae rhamnoides* L. ssp. *sinensis*) seed and fruit. *J Agric Food Chem* **55**, 8054–8061.

Steinberg, E.P., Javitt, J.C., Sharkey, P.D., *et al.* (1993) The content and cost of cataract surgery. *Arch Ophthalmol* **111**, 1041–1049.

Stringham, J.M. and Hammond, B.R. (2005) Dietary lutein and zeaxanthin: possible effects on visual function. *Nutr Rev* **63**, 59–64.

Stringham, J.M. and Hammond, B.R. (2007) The glare hypothesis for macular pigment function. *Optom Vis Sci* **84**, 859–864.

Stringham, J.M. and Hammond, B.R. (2008) Macular pigment and visual performance under glare conditions. *Optom Vis Sci* **85**, 82–88.

Stur, M., Tittl, M., Reitner, A., *et al.* (1996) Oral zinc and the second eye in age-related macular degeneration. *Invest Ophthalmol Vis Sci* **37**, 1225–1235.

Tan, A.G., Mitchell, P., Flood, V.M., *et al.* (2008a) Antioxidant nutrient intake and the long-term incidence of age-related cataract: the Blue Mountains Eye Study. *Am J Clin Nutr* **87**, 1899–1905.

Tan, J.S.L., Wang, J.J., Flood, V., *et al.* (2009) Dietary fatty acids and the 10-year incidence of age-related macular degeneration: the Blue Mountains Eye Study. *Arch Ophthalmol* **127**, 656–665.

Tan, J.S.L., Wang, J.J., Flood, V., *et al.* (2008b) Dietary antioxidants and the long-term incidence of age-related macular degeneration: the Blue Mountains Eye Study. *Ophthalmology* **115**, 334–341.

Tavani, A., Negri, E., and Laveccia, C. (1996) Food and nutrient intake and risk of cataract. *Ann Physiol* **6**, 41–46.

Taylor, A. and Hobbs, M. (2001) 2001 assessment of nutritional influences on risk for cataract. *Nutrition* **17**, 845–857.

Taylor, A., Jacques, P.F., Chylack, L.T., Jr, *et al.* (2002a) Long-term intake of vitamins and carotenoids and odds of early age-related cortical and posterior subcapsular lens opacities. *Am J Clin Nutr* **75**, 540–549.

Taylor, H.R., Tikellis, G., Robman, L.D., *et al.* (2002b) Vitamin E supplementation and macular degeneration: randomised controlled trial. *BMJ* **325**, 11.

Teikari, J.M., Laatikaineen, L., Virtamo, J., *et al.* (1998a) Six-year supplementation with alpha-tocopherol and beta-carotene and age-related maculopathy. *Acta Ophthalmol Scand* **76**, 224–229.

Teikari, J.M., Rautalahti, M., Haukka, J., *et al.* (1998b) Incidence of cataract operations in Finnish male smokers unaffected by alpha tocopherol or beta carotene supplements. *J Epidemiol Commun Health* **52**, 468–472.

Teikari, J.M., Virtamo, J., Rautalahti, M., *et al.* (1997) Long-term supplementation with alpha-tocopherol and beta-carotene and age-related cataract. *Acta Ophthalmol Scand* **75**, 634–640.

Thylefors, B., Negrel, A.D., Pararajasegaram, R., *et al.* (1995) Global data on blindness. *Bull World Health Organ* **69**, 115–121.

Townend, B.S., Townend, M.E., Flood, V., *et al.* (2007) Dietary macronutrient intake and five-year incident cataract: the Blue Mountains eye study. *Am J Ophthalmol* **143**, 932–939.

Trevithick, J.R. and Mitton, K.P. (1999) Antioxidants and diseases of the eye. In A.M. Pappas (ed.), *Antioxidant Status, Diet, Nutrition and Health*. CRC Press, Boca Raton, FL, pp. 545–565.

Trieschmann, M., Beatty, S., Nolan, J.M., *et al.* (2007) Changes in macular pigment optical density and serum concentrations of its constituent carotenoids following supplemental lutein and zeaxanthin: the LUNA study. *Exp Eye Res* **84**, 718–728.

Trumbo, P., Yates, A.A., Schlicker, S., *et al.* (2001) Dietary Reference Intakes: vitamin A, vitamin K, arsenic, boron, chromium, copper, iodine, iron, manganese, molybdenum, nickel, silicon, vanadium, and zinc. *J Am Diet Assoc* **101**, 294–301.

Valero, M.P., Fletcher, A.E., Destavola, B.L., *et al.* (2002) Vitamin C is associated with reduced risk of cataract in a Mediterranean population. *J Nutr* **132**, 1299–1306.

Vandenlangenberg, G.M., Mares-Perlman, J.A., Klein, R., *et al.* (1998) Associations between antioxidant and zinc intake and the 5-year incidence of early age-related maculopathy in the Beaver Dam Eye Study. *Am J Epidemiol* **148**, 204–214.

van Leeuwen, R., Boekhoorn, S., Vingerling, J.R., *et al.* (2005) Dietary intake of antioxidants and risk of age-related macular degeneration. *JAMA* **294**, 3101–3107.

Vine, A.K., Stader, J., Branham, K., *et al.* (2005) Biomarkers of cardiovascular disease as risk factors for age-related macular degeneration. *Ophthalmology* **112**, 2076–2080.

Vishwanathan, R., Goodrow-Kotyla, E.F., Wooten, B.R., *et al.* (2009) Consumption of 2 and 4 egg yolks/d for 5 wk increases macular pigment concentrations in older adults with low macular pigment taking cholesterol-lowering statins. *Am J Clin Nutr* **90**, 1272–1279.

Vitale, S., West, S., Hallfrisch, J., *et al.* (1993) Plasma antioxidants and risk of cortical and nuclear cataract. *Epidemiology* **4**, 195–203.

Wenzel, A.J., Gerweck, C., Barbato, D., *et al.* (2006) A 12-wk egg intervention increases serum zeaxanthin and macular pigment optical density in women. *J Nutr* **136**, 2568–2573.

West, S., Vitale, S., Hallfrisch, J., *et al.* (1994) Are antioxidants or supplements protective for age-related macular degeneration? *Arch Ophthalmol* **112**, 222–227.

Wood, J.P.M. and Osborne, N.N. (2003) Zinc and energy requirements in induction of oxidative stress to retinal pigmented epithelial cells. *Neurochem Res* **28**, 1525–1533.

Woodside, J., Yarnell, J., McMaster, D., *et al.* (1998) Effect of B-group vitamins and antioxidant vitamins on hyperhomocysteinemia: a double-blind, randomized, factorial-design, controlled trial. [Erratum appears in *Am J Clin Nutr* (1998) **68**, 758.] *Am J Clin Nutr* **67**, 858–866.

Wooten, B.R. and Hammond, B.R. (2002) Macular pigment: influences on visual acuity and visibility. *Progr Retinal Eye Res* **21**, 225–240.

Wooten, B.R., Hammond, B.R., Land, R.I., *et al.* (1999) A practical method for measuring macular pigment optical density. *Invest Ophthalmol Vis Sci* **40**, 2481–2489.

World Health Organization (1991) Use of intraocular lenses in cataract surgery in developing countries. *Bull World Health Organ* **69**, 657–666.

Yagi, A., Fujimoto, K., Michihiro, K., *et al.* (2009) The effect of lutein supplementation on visual fatigue: a psychophysiological analysis. *Appl Ergon* **40,** 1047–1054.

Yeum, K.-J., Shang, F., Schalch, W., *et al.* (1999) Fat-soluble nutrient concentrations in different layers of human cataractous lens. *Curr Eye Res* **19,** 502–505.

Yokota, T., Shiojiri, T., Gotoda, T., *et al.* (1997) Friedreich-like ataxia with retinitis pigmentosa caused by the His101Gln mutation of the alpha-tocopherol transfer protein gene. *Ann Neurol* **41,** 826–832.

Zadok, D., Levy, Y., and Glovinsky, Y. (1999) The effect of anthocyanosides in a multiple oral dose on night vision. *Eye* **13,** 734–736.

57

SPECIALIZED NUTRITION SUPPORT

VIVIAN M. ZHAO[1], PharmD AND THOMAS R. ZIEGLER[1, 2], MD

[1]*Emory University Hospital, Atlanta, Georgia, USA*
[2]*Emory University School of Medicine, Atlanta, Georgia, USA*

Summary

Malnutrition is common in hospitalized patients and is associated with adverse clinical outcomes. A variety of factors common in hospital patients contribute to protein-energy malnutrition and loss of essential vitamins, minerals, and electrolytes. Assessment of nutritional status requires a comprehensive evaluation and integration of medical and surgical history, current clinical and fluid status, dietary intake patterns, body weight changes, gastrointestinal symptoms, physical examination, and selected biochemical tests. Current guidelines suggest that goals for caloric intake between 20 and 25 kcal/kg/day and protein/amino acids between 1.2 and 1.5 g/kg/day are appropriate for most adult hospital patients. Adequate vitamins, minerals, electrolytes, essential amino acids, and essential fats must be provided based on recommended allowances for healthy individuals; however, true requirements in subtypes of hospital patients are unknown. The gastrointestinal (enteral) route should be the first choice for specialized feeding in the hospital setting, with parenteral nutrition modalities, via peripheral or central vein, reserved for those patients in whom adequate enteral nutrition is not possible. Metabolic, infectious, and mechanical complications can occur with both enteral and parenteral feeding modalities, which can be prevented or diminished with careful monitoring and adherence to current standards of practice. Relatively few rigorous, randomized controlled clinical trials (RCTs) have been conducted within the field of specialized feeding in the hospital setting, and many areas of uncertainty remain. However, numerous, large, multicenter RCTs are in progress and will help to define optimal use of these important adjunctive nutritional therapies over the next several years.

Introduction

The incidence and prevalence of malnutrition, which includes significant loss of lean body mass and/or depletion of essential vitamins and minerals, are quite high in hospitalized patients (Nathens *et al.*, 2002; Luo *et al.*, 2008; McClave *et al.*, 2009; Singer *et al.*, 2009; Barker *et al.*, 2011; De Luis *et al.*, 2011). Based on various observational studies of total hospital admissions and in intensive care unit (ICU) settings, malnutrition (depletion of essential micronutrients and/or loss of significant lean body mass or body weight) may occur in 20% to as high as 60% of patients (Giner *et al.*, 1996; Pirlich *et al.*, 2006; Barker *et al.*, 2011; De Luis *et al.*, 2011). Further, the

Present Knowledge in Nutrition, Tenth Edition. Edited by John W. Erdman Jr, Ian A. Macdonald and Steven H. Zeisel.
© 2012 International Life Sciences Institute. Published 2012 by John Wiley & Sons, Inc.

incidence of malnutrition worsens over time in patients requiring a prolonged hospital stay, in part due to inadequate ad libitum food intake and repeated catabolic insults (ASPEN Board of Directors and the Clinical Guidelines Task Force, 2002; Villet *et al.*, 2005; Pirlich *et al.*, 2006; Patel and Martin, 2008). Protein-energy malnutrition prior to and inadequate nutritional intake during hospitalization are each associated with higher rates of morbidity and mortality (ASPEN Board of Directors and the Clinical Guidelines Task Force, 2002; Schneider *et al.*, 2004; O'Brien *et al.*, 2006; Zaloga, 2006). The importance of adequate macro- and micronutrient intake for optimal cellular, immune, and organ function is outlined elsewhere in this volume. In highly catabolic ICU patients, protein-energy depletion has been associated with higher rates of hospital-acquired infection, poor wound healing, and skeletal muscle weakness (Schneider *et al.*, 2004; O'Brien *et al.*, 2006; Zaloga, 2006; McClave *et al.*, 2009; Singer *et al.*, 2009). Multiple pathophysiologic factors common in hospital patients put these individuals at risk for generalized protein-energy malnutrition and/or micronutrient depletion (Ziegler, 2009; see Box 57.1). The specialized enteral and parenteral nutrition support modalities that are currently available and that are the subject of this chapter have been developed to support vital cell and organ functions, muscle capacity and wound healing. Both enteral nutrition (EN) and parenteral nutrition (PN) formulations provide fluid, calories (as various carbohydrate, protein/amino acid, and fat sources), essential amino acids and fats, electrolytes, vitamins, and minerals, as outlined below.

Nutritional Assessment

Important aspects of comprehensive nutritional assessment, which involves integration of multiple factors, are outlined in Box 57.2 (Ziegler, 2009). There is currently no "gold standard" for nutritional assessment in hospital patients. For example, blood concentrations of albumin and pre-albumin, which may be useful in outpatient or epidemiologic settings, may be markedly decreased by inflammation, infection, decreased hepatic synthesis, and/or increased clearance from blood in hospital settings. Levels of these proteins in plasma may also be increased during fluid depletion or decreased with fluid overload. Blood concentrations of specific vitamins and minerals, as with blood electrolytes, are useful to follow in certain at-risk patients, but the possibility of changes due to fluid

---

> **BOX 57.1   Major pathophysiologic factors which contribute to malnutrition in hospital patients**
>
> - Decreased spontaneous food intake prior to or during hospitalization (e.g. due to anorexia, fatigue, gastrointestinal symptoms, NPO status).
> - Increased concentrations of catabolic hormones and cytokines (e.g. cortisol, catecholamines, tumor necrosis factor-α, interleukins).
> - Decreased blood levels of anabolic hormones (e.g. insulin-like growth factor-I, testosterone).
> - Resistance to anabolic hormones with consequent decreased substrate utilization (e.g. insulin resistance).
> - Abnormal nutrient losses (e.g. wounds, drainage tubes, renal replacement therapy, diarrhea, emesis, polyuria).
> - Decreased protein synthesis due to physical inactivity (e.g. bed rest, chemical paralysis).
> - Drug–nutrient interactions (e.g. diuretics, pressor effects, corticosteroids).
> - Increased energy, protein and/or specific micronutrient requirements (e.g. with infection, trauma, oxidative stress).
> - Iatrogenic factors (prolonged periods of inadequate enteral or parenteral nutrient provision in relation to metabolic requirements).
>
> NPO = *nil per os* (enteral food restriction due to diagnostic tests or therapeutic procedures).

---

status and inter-organ shifts necessitate serial monitoring to guide repletion strategies. Body weight often changes dramatically due to fluid status alterations.

A simple method to assess nutritional status, termed "subjective global assessment" (SGA), has been validated as a way to assess nutritional status and to predict clinical outcomes in stable patients without marked fluid shifts (Detsky *et al.*, 1987; Norman *et al.*, 2005). The SGA incorporates patient history regarding body weight loss, usual dietary intake, functional capacity, gastrointestinal symptoms, and physical-examination evidence of malnutrition (loss of muscle or fat mass, presence of edema) to classify patients as well nourished, moderately or suspected of being malnourished, or severely malnourished (Detsky *et al.*, 1987; Norman *et al.*, 2005). In Europe, a method of nutritional risk screening is commonly utilized in hospital settings, which involves scoring risk based on BMI, decrease in % of usual food intake, body weight changes,

BOX 57.2   Important steps in nutritional assessment of hospitalized patients

- Review past medical and surgical history, tempo of current illness and expected hospital course.
- Determine dietary intake pattern and previous use of specialized nutrition support.
- Obtain body weight history.
- Perform physical examination with attention to fluid status, organ functions, and evidence of protein-energy malnutrition or lesions consistent with vitamin/mineral deficiency.
- Evaluate gastrointestinal tract function to evaluate ability to tolerate enteral feeding.
- Determine ambulatory capacity, mental status.
- Measure or evaluate standard blood tests (organ function indices, electrolytes, pH, triglycerides, and selected vitamins and minerals if at risk for depletion.
- Estimate calorie and protein requirements.
- Evaluate enteral and parenteral access for nutrient delivery.

Patients with involuntary body weight loss of >5–10% of usual body weight in the previous several weeks or months, patients weighing less than 90% of their ideal body weight, or those with a body mass index (BMI) less than 18.5 kg/m² should be carefully evaluated for malnutrition.

age, and whether or not the patient is severely ill (Rasmussen *et al.*, 2010). More details regarding comprehensive nutritional assessment can be accessed in the online material from a review by Ziegler (2009).

Nutrient Intake Goals

Guidelines for energy and protein/amino acid intake in adult hospital patients have been outlined by major professional societies (Heyland *et al.*, 2003; Mirtallo *et al.*, 2004; Kreymann *et al.*, 2006; McClave *et al.*, 2009; Singer *et al.*, 2009). Specific approaches for pediatric patients are beyond the scope of this chapter, but have been recently published (Koletzko *et al.*, 2005; Mehta *et al.*, 2009). It is important to note that energy (calorie) needs in hospitalized patients, especially those who are critically ill, may vary considerably due to serial changes in clinical conditions (Kreymann *et al.*, 2006; McClave *et al.*, 2009; Singer *et al.*, 2009). Optimal caloric and protein/amino acid requirements in hospital patients are unknown due to a relative lack of rigorous, randomized, controlled clinical

trials (McClave *et al.*, 2009; Singer *et al.*, 2009; Yarandi *et al.*, 2011).

Resting energy expenditure (REE) can be determined using serial bedside metabolic cart measurements (indirect calorimetry), but technical issues can cause inaccuracies (Anderegg *et al.*, 2009; McClave *et al.*, 2009). REE can be estimated using standard predictive equations, most commonly the Harris-Benedict equation, which incorporates the patient's age, gender, weight, and height (McClave *et al.*, 2009; Ziegler, 2009). Unfortunately, this method may over- or underestimate REE in certain patients when clinical conditions are changing and/or with body weight changes due to changes in fluid status (Anderegg *et al.*, 2009; Ziegler, 2009). Recently published European and American clinical practice guidelines suggest that an adequate energy goal for most patients can be estimated at 20–25 kcal/kg/day, which is approximately equivalent to measured or estimated REE × 1.0–1.2. Ongoing RCTs are designed to better define caloric dosing guidelines in ICU patients, as data are particularly conflicting in these settings. Pre-hospital and pre-operative body weight should be used in energy intake estimates because measured body weight in the hospital (especially in the ICU) may reflect fluid status and is typically much higher than recent "dry" weight. An alternative is to use ideal body weight derived from routine tables or equations if recent dry weight is unavailable. In obese subjects, adjusted body weight should be used in the Harris-Benedict equation (Ziegler, 2009).

Studies conducted in the 1980s in ICU patients indicate that protein loads of more than 2.0 g/kg/day are not efficiently utilized for protein synthesis and the excess is oxidized and contributes to azotemia (Shaw *et al.*, 1987; Streat *et al.*, 1987). The commonly recommended protein/amino acid dose range is 1.2–1.5 g/kg/day for most individuals with normal renal and hepatic function (50–100% above the RDA of 0.8 g/kg/day); although some guidelines recommend higher doses (2.0–2.5 g/kg/day) in specific conditions such as burns and in patients requiring renal replacement therapy (McClave *et al.*, 2009; Singer *et al.*, 2009; Ziegler, 2009). The administered amino acid dose should be adjusted downward depending on the degree and tempo of azotemia (in the absence of renal replacement therapy). In patients with evidence of acute liver failure and encephalopathy (who are at risk for amino acid-induced increases in arterial blood ammonia levels), it may be prudent to provide lower doses of PN amino acids (0.6–1.2 g/kg/day), based on the degree of liver dysfunction, although protein restriction is not currently recommended in stable patients with chronic liver failure.

Enteral Nutrition Support

Whenever possible, enteral nutrition (EN) in hospital patients should consist of oral diets of regular foods as tolerated, supplemented as indicated with the wide variety of commercially available flavored oral liquid formulations or solid nutrient-rich products. Most hospital patients should also receive a complete multivitamin–mineral product to cover needs, although this recommendation is not evidence-based. Enteral tube feeding is the preferred route of nutritional delivery for patients who have a functional gastrointestinal (GI) tract but are unable to maintain adequate nutrient intake with oral diet alone.

EN is more physiologic, is associated with less severe infectious, metabolic, and mechanical complications, and is less costly than PN (ASPEN Board of Directors and the Clinical Guidelines Task Force, 2002; McClave et al., 2009). Specific indications for EN in adults and children are described in clinical practice guidelines (ASPEN Board of Directors and the Clinical Guidelines Task Force, 2002; Heyland et al., 2003; Mirtallo et al., 2004; Koletzko et al., 2005; Kreymann et al., 2006; ASPEN Board of Directors and Enteral Nutrition Practice Recommendations Task Force, 2009; McClave et al., 2009; Mehta et al., 2009; Singer et al., 2009). Although not evidence-based, common contraindications to EN include inability to gain access to the GI tract, mechanical or paralytic intestinal obstruction, intractable vomiting, severe diarrhea, diffuse peritonitis, paralytic ileus, bowel ischemia, and hemodynamic instability requiring mid- to high-dose vasopressors (ASPEN Board of Directors and the Clinical Guidelines Task Force, 2002; McClave et al., 2009; Singer et al., 2009; Ziegler, 2009).

EN administration must be individualized to each patient's specific needs. In order to determine the appropriate EN delivery method, GI tract integrity and functional capacity, presence and degree of malnutrition, underlying disease states, and patient tolerance must be assessed prior to and following the initiation of tube feeding. Gastrointestinal, mechanical, and metabolic complications, as well as pulmonary aspiration of feeds, can occur with enteral tube feeding. It is therefore essential to monitor enterally fed patients closely in order to identify potential complications (ASPEN Board of Directors and

Enteral Nutrition Practice Recommendations Task Force, 2009).

Routes for Enteral Tube Feeding

Successful enteral tube feeding is in part dependent upon careful selection of the appropriate enteral access device and placement technique. Understanding the indications, contraindications, advantages, and disadvantages of each different access device for enteral feedings will allow clinicians to select the best delivery method for patients (Table 57.3). Feeding tubes are usually made of polyurethane or silicone with various diameters, often designated as small-bore (5–12 French) or large-bore (≥14 French) (Minard, 1994). The tubes are typically classified according to insertion site (nasal, oral, percutaneous) and location of the terminal end of the enteral device (stomach, duodenum, proximal small bowel) (Table 57.1). Nasoenteral (NE) tubes are often inserted blindly at the bedside by experienced personnel or with the assistance of endoscopy or fluoroscopy. Gastrostomy and jejunostomy tubes can be placed endoscopically, fluoroscopically, laparoscopically, and percutaneously. Surgeons may also place the feeding tube intraoperatively when patients have pre-existing moderate or severe malnutrition and/or are anticipated to ingest inadequate amounts of oral dietary intake for a prolonged period of time after operation (Minard, 1994). Radiographic verification of correct placement of a blindly inserted small- or large-bore feeding tube is mandatory before administering feeding and medications (Minard, 1994; Metheny and Meert, 2004; Baskin, 2006; Metheny et al., 2007). Nasal or oral tubes are usually placed for short-term (<4–6 weeks) use, whereas tube enterostomies are typically placed for long-term (≥4 weeks) enteral nutrition support (Minard, 1994; Heyland et al., 2003; Metheny and Meert, 2004; Baskin, 2006; Metheny et al., 2007).

The selection of an enteral access route depends on patient-specific factors, including co-morbidities, GI anatomy with consideration of prior surgery, gastric and intestinal motility and function, risk of aspiration, and the anticipated duration of therapy (Minard, 1994; Heyland et al., 2003; Metheny and Meert, 2004; Baskin, 2006; Metheny et al., 2007; ASPEN Board of Directors and Enteral Nutrition Practice Recommendations Task Force, 2009). Gastric feedings generally require a functional stomach without delayed gastric emptying, obstruction, or fistula. Small bowel feedings are most appropriate for patients with gastroparesis, gastric outlet obstruction, pancreatitis, known esophageal reflux, and high aspiration

TABLE 57.1 Advantages and disadvantages of different enteral nutrition access routes

Route	Indications	Advantages	Disadvantages
Nasoenteric (NE) tube feeding (short term, <4 weeks)			
Nasogastric (NG)	Normal gastric emptying	Easy to place tube	Highest aspiration risk
	No esophageal reflux	Larger reservoir capacity in stomach	Tube displacement
Nasoduodenal (ND)	Gastroparesis	Lower aspiration risk than NG	May require endoscopic placement
	Impaired gastric emptying		Tube displacement
Nasojejunal (NJ)	Esophageal reflux	May initiate feedings immediately after injury or operation	Potential GI intolerance (bloating, cramping, diarrhea)
	See ND		
	Gastric dysfunction		Potential aspiration
	Pancreatitis	Lower aspiration risk than NG	
Tube enterostomy (long-term feeding required)			
Gastrostomy	See NG	Can be placed during GI surgery	Surgery is needed for surgical gastrostomies
Percutaneous[a] esophagostomy, gastrostomy (PEG)	No NE route available	No surgery needed for PEG	Requires stoma care
Operative laparoscopic[b] gastrostomy	Persistent dysphasia	PEG less costly than surgical gastrostomy	Potential complications: ○ aspiration risk ○ stoma site skin infection ○ skin excoriation at stoma site ○ fistula following tube removal
		Lower tube occlusion risk with large-bore tube	Requires stoma care
Jejunostomy	See NJ	Larger reservoir capacity Lower aspiration risk	
Percutaneous[a] endoscopic jejunostomy (PEJ)	High aspiration risk	Can be placed during GI surgery	Tube occlusion with small-bore tube or needle catheter
	Esophageal reflux	No surgery needed for PEJ	
Needle catheter jejunostomy (NCJ)	Inability to access upper GI tract (esophagus, stomach, duodenum)	PEJ less costly than surgical jejunostomy	Surgery required for jejunostomy placement
Operative laparoscopic jejunostomy		May initiate feeding immediately after operation	Potential complications: ○ GI intolerance ○ stoma site infection ○ skin excoriation at stoma site ○ fistula following tube removal

[a]Percutaneously placed tubes avoid risks of surgery and general anesthesia; however, may require endoscopy, abdominal ultrasound, or radiologic procedure with contrast media. Endoscopy may be difficult in the presence of a tumor or stricture, altered anatomy, or severe obesity.
[b]Laparoscopically or operatively placed tubes require general anesthesia; however, patients may be able to return home on the same day after the procedure.

risk. Although nasojejunal (NJ) feedings are not required unless patients have gastric feeding intolerance, small bowel feedings have been associated with a significant reduction in ventilator-associated pneumonia in some but not all studies (ASPEN Board of Directors and Enteral Nutrition Practice Recommendations Task Force, 2009). Combined gastro-jejunal tubes are indicated when gastric decompression is needed, but jejunal feeding is possible, as occurs in patients who have impaired gastric motility but normal small-bowel motility and absorption (Metheny and Meert, 2004; ASPEN Board of Directors and Enteral Nutrition Practice Recommendations Task Force, 2009).

Tube Feeding Formula Selection

Once an enteral route has been established for the initiation of tube feeding, an appropriate formula must be selected. There are numerous commercially available products, which fall into one of the following categories: standardized or polymeric, hydrolyzed, caloric dense, fiber-enriched, fat-modified, disease-specific, immune-modulated, and powdered formulas, to meet the various needs of most patients (Table 57.2). EN formulas vary in terms of caloric density, composition of macronutrients, macronutrient digestibility, viscosity, osmolarity, and cost. The polymeric formulas contain intact protein, complex carbohydrates, long- and medium-chain triglycerides, vitamins, minerals, and trace elements. All formulations are lactose- and gluten-free, and most are low residue as well as isotonic or slightly hypertonic, with a caloric content ranging from 1 to 2 kcal/mL.

Because of the variations between enteral formulas, a systematic comparison of the patient-specific variables and nutrient needs with the specific characteristics of the available formulas can be used to select an appropriate formula that will most approximate the individual's estimated requirements. Patient-specific variables include clinical status, nutritional status and requirements, metabolic abnormalities, digestive and absorptive capacity of the GI tract, disease state, expected outcomes, and possible routes available for administration. The simple correlation of a medical diagnosis with a specifically marketed formula can result in the administration of inappropriate nutrition support and an increased cost of nutrient provision.

Most hospital patients can be safely fed with standard, inexpensive, polymeric, enteral formulas (Table 57.2). The more calorically dense mixtures are useful for patients requiring fluid restriction. The addition of soluble fiber in enteral products is increasingly common in commercial formulas and may prevent constipation or control diarrhea. Available research in the role of fiber-enriched formulas in the management of diarrhea, however, has not demonstrated consistent benefit, probably because a myriad of factors can cause diarrhea in hospital patients (e.g. antibiotics) (Yang et al., 2005). The polymeric formulas are usually tolerated as well as, or better than, much more expensive hydrolyzed formulas (Ford et al., 1992; Mowatt-Larssen et al., 1992). Hydrolyzed formulas, which contain hydrolyzed casein or whey as the protein source (also known as oligomeric, semi-elemental, or peptide-based), are designed for patients with malabsorption and pancreatic insufficiency. Clinical data documenting the advantages of routine use of peptide-based formulas are limited; however, their use in patients with acute pancreatitis in one study showed a significantly shorter hospital length of stay when compared with polymeric formulas (Tiengou et al., 2006).

Commercial enteral formulas have been developed for use in disease-specific conditions such as diabetes, renal failure, pulmonary disease, and infection. Diabetes-specific formulas are developed with lower amounts of carbohydrate and higher amounts of fat as energy sources to improve glycemic control; some studies show that their use in hospitalized diabetic patients resulted in improved blood glucose control and decreased insulin requirements (Leon-Sanz et al., 2005; Pohl et al., 2005; Alish et al., 2010). Renal-specific products are available for patients with different degrees of renal failure (presence or absence of renal replacement therapy) (Table 57.2). Several RCTs suggest that formulas containing increased amounts of antioxidant nutrients (e.g. vitamins C and E) and anti-inflammatory lipids (e.g. eicosapentanoic acid, gamma-linolenic acid) result in improved clinical outcomes compared with standard EN formulations in patients with adult respiratory distress syndrome (ARDS) (Gadek et al., 1999; Singer et al., 2006), although results of a recent Phase II trial of omega-3 fatty acid enriched EN showed no benefit (Stapleton et al., 2011). A variety of so-called "immune-modulating" EN formulations are commercially available and are supplemented with, typically, a combination of glutamine, arginine, omega-3 fatty acids, probiotics, and or/antioxidants (ASPEN Board of Directors and Enteral Nutrition Practice Recommendations Task Force, 2009). Routine use of these designer formulations remains controversial because of inconsistent results (especially in ICU patients) and lack of effects on mortality (Marik and Zaloga, 2008; Dupertuis et al., 2009).

TABLE 57.2 Examples of commercially available enteral nutrition formulas in the United States

Categories	Potential indications	kcal (per mL)	Protein (g/L)	Fat (g/L)	Carbohydrate (g/L)	% water	Osmolality (mOsm/kg H₂O)
Polymeric							
Standard	Most patients	1.0	44	35	144	84	300
(e.g. Osmolite®;		1.2	56	39	158	82	360
Isocal®)		1.5	63	49	204	76	525
Caloric dense	Fluid- restricted	2.0	84	90	218	70	725
(e.g. TwoCal HN®)							
Fiber-enriched	Diarrhea	1.0	44	35	155	84	300
(e.g. Jevity®;		1.2	56	39	169	82	450
Ultracal®)		1.5	63	49	216	76	525
Hydrolyzed							
Semi-elemental/peptide-based	Pancreatitis, malabsorption	1.0	40–51	28–39	127–138	83–85	300–585
(e.g. Crucial®; Peptamen®)							
Disease-specific							
Immune-modulating (e.g. Impact with Glutamine®; Crucial®)	Immuno-suppressed, critical illness	1.3	78	43	150	81	630
Oxepa®	Adult respiratory distress syndrome	1.5	63	94	105	79	535
Nepro®	Renal failure, on dialysis	1.8	81	96	167	73	600
Suplena®	Renal failure, predialysis	1.8	45	96	202	73	600
Glucerna®	Diabetes	1.0	42	54	95.6	85	355
		1.2	60	60	114.5	81	720
		1.5	82	75	133.1	76	875
Promote®	Wound healing	1.0	62	26–28	130.0–138	84	340–380

This table does not constitute an all-inclusive list. Information provided by manufacturers.

However, meta-analyses in GI surgery patients suggest that use of these formulations results in lower rates of hospital total complications and infections and decreased length of hospital stay compared with standard EN products (Cerantola *et al.*, 2011).

Methods of Tube Feeding Administration

In the initial administration stages of tube feeding, diluting enteral formulas is not necessary. The practice of diluting formulas is more likely to promote microbial growth than full-strength formulations, and increases the risk of intolerance due to diarrhea secondary to microbial contamination (ASPEN Board of Directors and Enteral Nutrition Practice Recommendations Task Force, 2009). There is limited data to form strong recommendations for the best starting rate for enteral feeding at initiation. Enteral feedings can be administered as a continuous bolus, or using intermittent techniques, or via a combination of these methods (Table 57.3).

Continuous feedings are delivered slowly over 24 hours via gravity drip or with the assistance of an enteral infusion device (electronic feeding pump). Utilizing a feeding pump is more advantageous than gravity drip because it can enhance safety and accuracy in delivery by sustaining a constant infusion rate and making accidental bolus delivery unlikely to occur. Most commercially available formulas are well tolerated at full strength when delivered into the stomach or small intestine at 10 to 30 mL/hour. The infusion rate can generally be advanced in increments of 10 to 20 mL/hour every 8 to 12 hours as tolerated until goal rate is reached (ASPEN Board of Directors and Enteral Nutrition Practice Recommendations Task Force, 2009). Medically stable patients can tolerate a fairly rapid progression of infusion rate and achieve the established goal rate within 24 to 48 hours of initiation. There is also evidence to support starting EN at goal rates in stable adult patients (Rees *et al.*, 1985; Mentec *et al.*, 2001). Continuous administration is usually better tolerated, with lower incidence of GI intolerance and risk of aspiration than bolus tube feeds in hospital settings. Continuous infusion may be necessary for post-pyloric feedings because the small bowel cannot act as a reservoir for large feeding volumes over a short period of time. Hospitalized patients may initially benefit from a continuous infusion to establish tolerance and later transition to an intermittent or cyclic infusion schedule.

Bolus and intermittent feedings are the most physiologic feeding techniques because they mimic normal

TABLE 57.3 Methods of administration of enteral tube feeding

Method	Indications	Advantages	Disadvantages
Continuous	Initiation of feeding Critically ill patient Small bowel feeding Intermittent or bolus feeding intolerance	Pump-assisted Enhances tolerance Minimizes risk due to: ○ high gastric residual ○ aspiration ○ metabolic abnormalities	Restricts ambulation Increased cost due to equipment and supplies
Bolus – intermittent	Non-critically ill patient Home TF Rehabilitation patient Gastric feeding	Ease of administration No pump required) Short feeding time Most physiological	Highest aspiration risk Potential GI intolerance (nausea, vomiting, abdominal pain, diarrhea)
Cyclic – intermittent	Non-critically ill patient Home TF Rehabilitation patient Small bowel feeding	Physical and psychological freedom from pump Beneficial for transitioning TF to oral diet	Requires high infusion rate over short time (8–16 hours) May require formula with higher calorie and protein density to meet needs Potential GI intolerance

TF, tube feeding; GI, gastrointestinal.

dietary habits and allow bowel rest in between feedings (ASPEN Board of Directors and Enteral Nutrition Practice Recommendations Task Force, 2009; Table 57.3). These are the easiest to deliver and can be administered over a short period of time via syringe bolus or a feeding container by gravity drip with or without an enteral feeding pump (Lord and Harrington, 2005). Bolus feedings generally deliver the formula in less than 15 minutes, whereas intermittent feedings deliver it over 30–45 minutes. The feeding is initiated with full-strength formula three to eight times daily with increases of 60–120 mL every 8–12 hours as tolerated up to the goal volume of 250–500 mL per feeding, four to six times daily. Bolus and intermittent methods are primarily reserved for medically stable patients with gastric feeding tubes because the stomach can act as a reservoir to handle relatively large volumes within a short time. Feedings provided by this method may result in adverse GI effects due to the sudden delivery of a large, hyperosmolar formula (Lord and Harrington, 2005; ASPEN Board of Directors and Enteral Nutrition Practice Recommendations Task Force, 2009).

Cyclic feedings are defined as continuous infusion in an intermittent fashion, for which the formula is infused continuously over a set number of hours (i.e. 8–16 hours). Tube feedings can be cycled for patients with duodenal or jejunal feeding tubes, patients who are transitioning from tube to oral feeding (in which cycled feeding may stimulate appetite), or for those requiring eventual home EN. A cyclic feeding schedule allows bowel rest, free time off the pump, and flexibility to administer overnight and discontinue during the day to afford the patient greater mobility and an opportunity to eat oral food.

Regardless of the delivery technique, most patients on EN will require additional fluid to meet minimum fluid requirements (typically 30–40 mL/kg body weight). Supplemental fluid (i.e. sterile water or normal saline) is administered intermittently as flushes throughout the day (i.e. flush tube with at least 30 mL every 8 hours). To calculate additional fluid requirements, begin by determining the patient's total fluid needs. Then determine that amount of free water provided by the tube feeding formula by multiplying the percent free water content by the total volume of enteral formula to be administered daily (Table 57.2). Subtraction of the free water supplied by the formula from the calculated total free water requirement equals the remaining volume of free water required. The remaining volume is divided into three or four boluses per day.

Complications of Enteral Tube Feeding

While the administration of EN may appear less complex compared with PN, it is not without potential complications. Serious harm and death can result due to potential adverse events occurring throughout the process of ordering, administering, and monitoring. Complications include GI intolerance, mechanical tube complications, bronchopulmonary aspiration, enteral access device misplacement and displacement, metabolic abnormalities, and drug–nutrient interactions (Malone et al., 2007; Guenter et al., 2008; ASPEN Board of Directors and Enteral Nutrition Practice Recommendations Task Force, 2009). The acceptable ranges for gastric residual volumes at which to decrease tube feeding rates have been re-evaluated in recent years, and higher amounts than were previously routine have been advocated based on available data (Hurt and McClave, 2010). Many clinicians feel that if the gastric residual volume is ≥250 mL after two consecutive gastric residual checks, a promotility agent should be considered in adult patients. However, no adequately powered studies have to date demonstrated that elevated gastric residual volumes are reliable markers for increased risk of aspiration pneumonia (Hurt and McClave, 2010). Gastric residuals should be checked more frequently (i.e. every 4–6 hours for the first 48 hours) when gastric feedings are first initiated. After desired gastric feeding rate is established, gastric residual monitoring may be decreased to every 6–12 hours in the non-critically ill patients (Hurt and McClave, 2010). Patient positioning, use of post-pyloric continuous feeding, and judicious use of prokinetic agents (e.g. metoclopramide or erythromycin) have been advocated as important to prevent pulmonary aspiration of tube feeding in patients demonstrating intolerance (e.g. emesis, gastric distention) (Torres et al., 1992; McClave et al., 2002; Metheny et al., 2006). Patients should be monitored frequently for evidence of complications from enteral nutrition support. Table 57.4 lists common potential complications of tube feedings and suggested interventions.

Feeding tubes are prone to clogging for a variety of reasons, including use of small-bore feeding tubes, improper medication administration, and formula sediment accumulation in the lower segment of the tube, especially during slow administration rates of caloric-dense or fiber-enriched formulas (Lord, 2003). Most clogging can be prevented by use of a clean technique to minimize formula contamination, and adherence to protocols for proper flushing of tubes before and after each medication

TABLE 57.4 Complications of tube feeding

Complications	Possible causes	Possible management
Gastrointestinal		
Diarrhea (>4 bowel movements per day or large loose stool)	Medications (e.g.antibiotics) Formula intolerance Bacterial overgrowth Osmotic overload Decreased bulk *C. difficile*	Medication modifications: • Eliminate antibiotics, antacids, liquid formulations containing sorbitol. • Further dilute hypertonic medications. • Administer medications by intravenous route. • Administer bulking agents (e.g. psyllium). • Administer probiotics. • Administer antidiarrheal agents.[a] Stool culture for pathogens. Feeding modifications: • Change to a low-fat, high-fiber, or isotonic formula. • Decrease concentration of formula or rate.
Nausea or vomiting	Patient position Volume overload Delayed gastric emptying Nutrient intolerances GI tract obstruction Hyperglycemia	Elevate head of bed to 35–45 degrees. Position patient on right side to facilitate passage of gastric contents through pylorus. Medication modifications: • Consider reducing narcotic use. • Administer prokinetic agents (i.e. metoclopramide). • Consider antiemetic. Feeding modifications: • Decrease total volume or delivery rate. • Advance delivery rate slowly over 12–24 hours. • Stop feeding for 2 hours and check residuals. • Change to lactose-free or low-fat formula.
Constipation	Dehydration Decreased fiber GI obstruction	Change to fiber formula. Administer bulking agents. Tube flush with water. Stop feeding temporarily.
Mechanical		
Pulmonary aspiration	Supine position Impaired gag reflex Reflux Tube malposition or displacement Abnormal mental status	Elevate head of bed 30–45 degrees. Infuse feedings into duodenum or jejunum. Change to smaller bore tube. Radiographic confirmation for proper placement after insertion and after severe coughing, vomiting, or a seizure. Tape tube in place and mark with indelible ink at exit point for reference. Reconfirm placement prior to each feeding by checking residuals, ink mark.
Tube obstruction	Acid precipitation of formula Insufficient tube irrigation Medications	Flush tube before and after each medication, residual check, bolus feeding, and every 8 hours during continuous feeding, or whenever feeding is stopped. Infuse feedings into duodenum or jejunum. Do not mix medications with enteral formula. Adequately crush meds and mix powder with water. Use liquid meds where possible or administer via alternative route. Avoid administering bulk-forming agents via small bore tube.

[a]Begin antidiarrheal agent only when infectious and inflammatory etiologies and fecal impaction have been ruled out and causal medications have been changed or discontinued.

administration. Water is the preferred flush solution (e.g. every 4 hours during continuous feeding, before and after intermittent feedings, or after residual volume measurements in an adult patient [Lord, 2003; ASPEN Board of Directors and Enteral Nutrition Practice Recommendations Task Force, 2009]). Use sterile water for tube flushes in immunocompromised or critically ill patients, especially when the safety of tap water cannot be reasonably assumed (Lord, 2003). The recommended first-line method to unclog a tube is to instill warm water using slight manual pressure. Flushing with a combination of pancrealipase and sodium bicarbonate solution or with carbonated soda drink may dissolve the clog (Lord, 2003).

Metabolic complications of EN are similar to those that occur during PN, although the incidence and severity may be less (see below). As with PN, outlined below, prevention of refeeding syndrome and monitoring patient's tolerance of EN are essential for the safe delivery of EN (Stanga et al., 2008). Monitoring metabolic parameters prior to the initiation of enteral feedings and periodically during enteral therapy should be based on protocols and the patient's underlying disease state and length of therapy. Patients at risk of developing refeeding syndrome should be identified, and severe electrolyte abnormalities should be corrected prior to the initiation of nutrition support.

Parenteral Nutrition Support

As with enteral nutrition support, relatively few well-designed, adequately powered RCTs on PN efficacy in hospital settings have been published (Doig et al., 2005, 2009; Koretz, 2008, 2009; Casaer et al., 2011; Ziegler, 2011). Thus, current practices of PN use in hospital patients are largely based on guidelines from professional societies, which in turn are largely derived from observational studies, small clinical trials, and expert opinion (ASPEN Board of Directors and the Clinical Guidelines Task Force, 2002; Heyland et al., 2003; Mirtallo et al., 2004; Koletzko et al., 2005; Kreymann et al., 2006; McClave et al., 2009; Mehta et al., 2009; Singer et al., 2009). A caveat regarding efficacy of current PN modalities is that no rigorous RCT has featured an unfed or minimally fed control group. Such studies would be difficult to perform (and to recruit subjects for), particularly as the clinical effect of various durations of minimal or no feeding is essentially unknown in ICU and other hospital patients (Ziegler, 2011). Also, many of the earlier RCTs in nutrition support were conducted with excessive PN

caloric doses and liberal blood glucose control strategies compared with current practice. None the less, available data suggest that patients with moderate to severe generalized malnutrition benefit from PN in terms of overall morbidity and possibly mortality if EN is not possible (Ziegler, 2009).

Indications for Parenteral Nutrition

Although not evidence-based, commonly accepted indications for PN in hospital patients in settings when the enteral route is unavailable for feeding or when EN is not tolerated (especially in already malnourished patients) are as follows: (1) following massive small bowel ± colonic resection; (2) when there is a perforated small bowel or a proximal high-output fistula; (3) in other conditions associated with prolonged intolerance to EN (e.g. severe diarrhea or emesis, significant abdominal distention, partial or complete bowel obstruction, or acute gastrointestinal bleeding, severe hemodynamic instability) precluding adequate EN for >3–7 days (McClave et al., 2009; Singer et al., 2009; Ziegler, 2009). There are no data to support withholding of PN in patients with pre-existing protein-energy malnutrition who cannot tolerate EN. However, a recent large RCT from Belgium (4640 patients) explored the impact of timing of PN initiation in adult ICU patients receiving inadequate amounts of early enteral feeding (EN in all subjects began on day 2 of ICU admission) (Casaer et al., 2011). In the early-initiation group, supplemental PN to meet the caloric goal of 25–30 kcal/kg/day was started on ICU day 2, according to 2009 European clinical practice guidelines (Singer et al., 2009). In the late-initiation group, supplemental PN to meet the caloric goal of 25–30 kcal/kg/day was started on ICU day 7, according to 2009 American clinical practice guidelines (McClave et al., 2009). The early initiation of PN was associated with modestly increased ICU and hospital length of stay, infectious complications, indices of organ dysfunction, and total hospital costs (Casaer et al., 2011; Ziegler, 2011).

Contraindications for PN (largely not evidence-based) include: (1) when the GI tract is functional and access for enteral feeding is available; (2) if the patient cannot tolerate the intravenous fluid load required for PN, or has severe hyperglycemia or severe electrolyte abnormalities on the planned day of PN initiation; (3) when PN is unlikely to be required for >5–7 days; and (4) if new placement of an intravenous line solely for PN poses undue risks (McClave et al., 2009; Singer et al., 2009; Ziegler, 2009).

Parenteral Nutrition Administration

PN can be delivered as complete solutions given by either peripheral or central vein. A comparison of typical fluid, macronutrient and micronutrient content, and characteristics of peripheral and central vein PN is shown in Table 57.5. Because of the risk of phlebitis, peripheral vein PN provides low amounts of dextrose (5%; dextrose = 3.4 kcal/g) and amino acids (≤3.5%; 4 kcal/g) and a large proportion of the caloric content is given as fat emulsion (50–60% of total calories) (ASPEN Board of Directors and the Clinical Guidelines Task Force, 2002). Fluid restriction due to cardiac, hepatic, and/or renal dysfunction may be a contraindication to the use of large fluid volumes for PN; thus, peripheral vein PN is generally not indicated in ICU patients as larger volumes are required to meet energy and amino acid goals. Central venous PN allows concentrated dextrose and amino acid delivery via the superior vena cava. Adequate energy and amino acid intake in the vast majority of adults can thus be achieved with central venous volumes of 1 to 1.5 L/day (Table 57.5). Depending on fluid status, non-PN hydration fluid rate should be proportionally decreased when PN is infused (ASPEN Board of Directors and the Clinical Guidelines Task Force, 2002; McClave et al., 2009).

TABLE 57.5 Composition of typical parenteral nutrition formulations

Component	Peripheral vein PN	Central vein PN
Volume (L/day)	2–3	1–1.5
Dextrose (%)	5	10–25
Amino acids (%)	2.5–3.5	3–8
Lipid (%)	3.5–5.0	2.5–5.0
Sodium (meq/L)	50–150	50–150
Potassium (meq/L)	20–35	30–50
Phosphorus (mmol/L)	5–10	10–30
Magnesium (meq/L)	8–10	10–20
Calcium (meq/L)	2.5–5	2.5–5
Vitamins[a]		
Trace elements/minerals[b]		

[a]Vitamins typically added on a daily basis to peripheral vein and central vein PN are comprised of commercial mixtures of vitamins A, B_1 (thiamin), B_2 (riboflavin), B_3 (niacinamide), B_6 (pyridoxine), B_{12}, C, D, and E, biotin, folate, and pantothenic acid. Vitamin K is added on an individual basis (e.g. in patients with cirrhosis). Specific vitamins can also be supplemented individually.
[b]Trace elements/minerals typically added on a daily basis to peripheral vein and central vein PN are comprised of commercial mixtures of chromium, copper, manganese, selenium, and zinc. Minerals can also be supplemented individually.

PN electrolytes are adjusted as indicated to maintain serially measured serum levels within the normal range. With elevated blood levels, lower doses (or elimination) of specific electrolytes, as compared with the typical ranges outlined in Table 57.5, may be indicated until blood levels are within the normal range. Higher dextrose concentrations in central vein PN may increase potassium, magnesium, and phosphorus requirements. The relative percentage of sodium and potassium salts as chloride is increased to correct metabolic alkalosis, and the percentage of these salts as acetate is increased to correct metabolic acidosis. Tighter blood glucose control in ICU and other hospital patients is now the standard of care (<180 mg/dL) (NICE–SUGAR Study Investigators et al., 2009; Kavanagh and McCowen, 2010). To achieve these goals, regular insulin can be added to PN and/or the dextrose load can be reduced as needed (separate intravenous insulin infusions are commonly required with hyperglycemia in ICU settings) (Ziegler, 2009).

Conventional PN provides all essential nine amino acids and several non-essential amino acids, depending on the commercial amino acid formulation used (Yarandi et al., 2011). Although controversial, European guidelines recommend routine addition of glutamine as a conditionally essential amino acid in ICU patients, given the evidence that this amino acid may become conditionally essential in certain catabolic patients (Singer et al., 2009; Yarandi et al., 2011). The dose of amino acids is adjusted downwards or upwards in relation to goal amounts as a function of the degree of azotemia or hyperbilirubinemia in patients with acute renal and hepatic failure, respectively. Complete PN provides intravenous lipid emulsions as a source of both energy and essential linoleic and linolenic fatty acids. In the United States, the only commercially available lipid emulsion is soybean oil based; in Europe and other countries, intravenous soybean oil/medium-chain triglyceride mixtures, fish oil, olive oil/soybean oil mixtures, and combinations of these oils are approved for use in PN. Lipid is typically mixed with dextrose and amino acids in the same PN infusion bag ("all-in-one" solution) and given with PN over 16–24 hours. Lipid emulsion may also be infused separately from the main PN bag over 10–12 hours. The maximal recommended dose of lipid emulsion infusion is 1.0–1.3 g/kg/day, with monitoring of blood triglyceride levels at baseline and then approximately weekly and as indicated to assess clearance of intravenous fat (ASPEN Board of Directors and the Clinical Guidelines Task Force, 2002; Mirtallo et al., 2004; Ziegler, 2009).

> ## BOX 57.3   Clinical and metabolic complications of overfeeding and refeeding syndromes in patients receiving central venous parenteral nutrition
>
> - Intracellular shift of magnesium, phosphorus and/or potassium (excess dextrose infusion, refeeding hyperinsulinemia).
> - Immune cell dysfunction and infection (hyperglycemia).
> - Cardiac failure or arrhythmias (excess fluid, excess sodium and other electrolytes, refeeding-induced electrolyte shifts).
> - Neuromuscular dysfunction (thiamin depletion, refeeding-induced electrolyte shifts).
> - Azotemia (excess amino acid, inadequate energy provision in relation to amino acid dose).
> - Fluid retention (excess fluid, sodium, refeeding hyperinsulinemia).
> - Elevated liver function tests and/or hepatic steatosis (excess kilocalories, dextrose or fat).
> - Increased blood ammonia levels (excess amino acids with liver failure).
> - Hypercapnia (excess total kilocalories).
> - Respiratory insufficiency (refeeding-induced hypophosphatemia, excess fluid, kilocalories, carbohydrate or fat).
> - Hypertriglyceridemia (excess carbohydrate or fat).

Triglyceride levels should be maintained below 400–500 mg/dL by decreasing the amount of lipid infused to decrease risk of pancreatitis and diminished pulmonary diffusion capacity in patients with severe chronic obstructive lung disease (Box 57.3). In central venous PN, a reasonable initial guideline is to provide 60–70% of non-amino acid calories as dextrose and 30–40% of non-amino acid calories as fat emulsion (Mirtallo *et al.*, 2004; McClave *et al.*, 2009; Singer *et al.*, 2009; Ziegler, 2009).

Specific requirements for intravenous vitamins and minerals have not been rigorously defined in hospital patients (Mirtallo *et al.*, 2004; McClave *et al.*, 2009; Singer *et al.*, 2009; Ziegler, 2009, 2011). Therapy is therefore directed at meeting published recommended doses that maintain blood levels in the normal range in most stable patients using standardized intravenous preparations of combined vitamins and minerals (Table 57.5). However, several studies show that a significant proportion of ICU patients receiving conventional nutrition support variously exhibit low zinc, copper, selenium, vitamin C, vitamin E,

and vitamin D levels (Nathens *et al.*, 2002; Luo *et al.*, 2008). This may be due to pre-ICU depletion, increased ICU requirements (possibly secondary to oxidative stress), increased excretion, and/or tissue redistribution. Depletion of these essential nutrients may impair antioxidant capacity, immunity, wound healing and other important body functions. Thus, as with electrolytes, therapy is directed at maintaining normal blood levels, with serial measurements in blood as clinically and biochemically indicated.

PN formulations can be admixed under a sterile hood by trained pharmacists, but "premixed" off-the-shelf formulations are also available commercially. PN is administered by infusion pump to control delivery rates, and the infusion catheters incorporate an in-line filter to prevent microbial contamination.

Clinical Monitoring of Parenteral Nutrition

Monitoring of PN therapy in the hospital setting requires daily assessment of the multiple factors outlined in Boxes 57.1 and 57.2. Blood glucose should be monitored several times daily, and blood electrolytes and renal function tests should generally be determined daily. Blood triglyceride levels should be measured at baseline and then weekly until stable. Although guidelines are few, some centers routinely monitor periodic blood levels of copper, selenium, zinc, thiamin, vitamin B_6, vitamin C, and 25-hydroxyvitamin D (Ziegler, 2009). Liver function tests should be measured at least a few times weekly. pH should be monitored generally daily in ventilated patients when arterial blood gas pH measurements are available. Monitoring of blood glucose, electrolytes and organ function is routine in the ICU setting.

Adverse Effects of Parenteral Nutrition

Metabolic, infectious and mechanical complications may occur with PN (Solomon and Kirby, 1990; Mirtallo *et al.*, 2004; Grau *et al.*, 2007; Fallon *et al.*, 2010; Walshe *et al.*, 2010; Byrnes and Stangenes, 2011; Zeki *et al.*, 2011). Mechanical complications, particularly with insertion and use of central venous catheters, include pneumothorax, hemothorax, thrombosis, and bleeding. Catheter-related bloodstream infections can occur in PN patients and are not uncommon in these individuals, who typically have other risk factors for infection. For example, in a recent study of 1325 patients receiving PN in a tertiary-care hospital over a 12-year period, the catheter-related bloodstream infection rate was 10 to 13 per 1000 central venous catheter days, depending on the criteria used (Walshe *et al.*, 2010). Proper and safe administration of both peripheral and central vein PN requires strict catheter care and nursing care protocols, including use of dedicated catheter ports for PN administration and subclavian vein insertion sites for central venous PN (ASPEN Board of Directors and the Clinical Guidelines Task Force, 2002; Mirtallo *et al.*, 2004; Ziegler, 2009).

Potential metabolic and clinical consequences of overfeeding and refeeding syndrome during central venous PN in critically ill patients are shown in Box 57.3. High caloric, dextrose, amino acid, and fat loads ("hyperalimentation") are readily administered via a central vein. While not the standard of care per current guidelines, excess dextrose, fat, and overall calorie administration remains a common practice in some centers (ASPEN Board of Directors and the Clinical Guidelines Task Force, 2002; Mirtallo *et al.*, 2004). Risk factors for PN-associated hyperglycemia include: (1) use in obese, diabetic, and/or septic patients; (2) poorly controlled blood glucose at PN initiation; (3) initial use of high dextrose concentrations (>10%) or dextrose load (>150 g/day); (4) insufficient insulin administration and/or inadequate monitoring of blood glucose; and (5) concomitant administration of corticosteroids and pressor agents (Mirtallo *et al.*, 2004; McClave *et al.*, 2009).

Electrolyte administration requires careful monitoring and general day-to-day adjustment in PN to maintain normal blood levels. Overfeeding can induce several metabolic complications of varying degrees of severity affecting several organ systems (Box 57.3). A recent large study found that PN use *per se*, overfeeding, and sepsis were the major risk factors for liver dysfunction in critically ill patients (Grau *et al.*, 2007). Elevated transaminases and eventual PN-induced liver dysfunction that may lead to hepatic failure occur with PN administration, especially in individuals receiving chronic PN therapy (Mirtallo *et al.*, 2004). The mechanisms for PN-induced liver dysfunction remain unclear, but are probably multifactorial (Mirtallo *et al.*, 2004). Of interest, recent studies suggest that switching from conventional soybean-oil-based lipid emulsion to fish-oil-based lipid emulsion is associated with decreased PN-associated liver failure in children receiving chronic PN, but mechanisms remain obscure (Fallon *et al.* 2010). PN should be advanced carefully to goal rates and the composition adjusted as appropriate based on the results of close metabolic and clinical monitoring performed daily. The calories provided by dextrose present in non-PN intravenous fluids, the soybean oil lipid emulsion

carrier of propofol, a commonly used intravenous ICU sedative, and clevidipine, an intravenous calcium-channel blocker, as well as the nutrients provided in any administered EN, must be taken into account in the PN prescription to avoid overfeeding.

Refeeding syndrome is relatively common in at-risk patients (alcoholics, pre-existing malnutrition or electrolyte depletion, recent significant body weight loss, prolonged periods of intravenous hydration therapy alone, or administration of insulin or diuretics prior to refeeding) (Solomon and Kirby, 1990; Byrnes and Stangenes, 2011; Zeki *et al.*, 2011). In a recent study of at-risk hospital patients given EN, PN or both, 25% of 92 patients developed refeeding-induced hypophosphatemia (Zeki *et al.*, 2011). Refeeding syndrome is mediated by administration of excessive intravenous dextrose (>150–250 g or 1 L of PN with 15–25% dextrose). This markedly stimulates insulin release, which may rapidly decrease blood potassium, magnesium, and especially phosphorus concentrations due to intracellular shift and utilization in metabolic pathways (Solomon and Kirby, 1990; Byrnes and Stangenes, 2011; Zeki *et al.*, 2011). High doses of carbohydrate increase thiamin utilization and can precipitate symptoms of thiamin deficiency. Hyperinsulinemia may cause sodium and fluid retention by the kidney. This, together with decreased blood electrolytes (which can cause cardiac arrhythmias), can result in heart failure, especially in patients with pre-existing heart disease (Solomon and Kirby, 1990; Byrnes and Stangenes, 2011; Zeki *et al.*, 2011). Prevention of refeeding syndrome requires identification of at-risk patients, use of initially low PN dextrose (e.g. 1 L of PN with 10% dextrose), empiric provision of higher PN doses of potassium, magnesium, and phosphorus, based on blood levels and renal function, and supplemental PN thiamin (e.g. 100 mg/day for 3–5 days) (Stanga *et al.*, 2008; Ziegler, 2009; Zeki *et al.*, 2011).

Consultation with an experienced multidisciplinary nutrition support team for recommendations regarding the PN prescription is ideal when such personnel are available. Nutrition support team daily monitoring has been shown to reduce complications and costs, and to decrease inappropriate use of PN (Trujillo *et al.*, 1999; Kennedy and Nightingale, 2005).

Future Directions

Numerous areas of uncertainty remain with regard to administration of specialized EN and PN, despite routine use in hospitals and other settings (Ziegler, 2011). For example, the optimal timings for EN and PN initiation in hospital patients remain areas of uncertainty (Casaer *et al.*, 2011; Ziegler, 2011). Few prospective data are available on the clinical effects of minimal or no feeding over time (e.g. >7 days), and such data are unlikely to be forthcoming. Rigorous RCTs are needed to define optimal caloric and protein/amino acid dose regimens in subgroups of ICU and non-ICU patients (Ziegler, 2009, 2011). Some studies show that larger doses of standard soybean-oil-based intravenous fat emulsions induce pro-inflammatory and pro-oxidative effects and possibly immune suppression (Grau *et al.*, 2007). However, conflicting results of small RCTs comparing soybean-oil-based lipid emulsion with other types of lipid emulsion have not clarified optimal use (Waitzberg *et al.*, 2006). Available data suggest that glutamine may become a conditionally essential amino acid in ICU patients (Wischmeyer, 2008; Yarandi *et al.*, 2011). Glutamine serves as an important fuel for immune and gut mucosal cells, and has cytoprotective properties among other potentially beneficial functions. Several clinical trials have shown that glutamine-supplemented PN (0.2–0.5 g/kg/day as the L-amino acid or as glutamine dipeptides) has protein-anabolic effects, enhances indices of immunity, and decreases hospital infections (Wischmeyer, 2008; Yarandi *et al.*, 2011). Thus, some recent expert panels recommend that glutamine be routinely added to PN in ICU patients, if available (Heyland *et al.*, 2003; Singer *et al.*, 2009). Ongoing large, randomized controlled trials on glutamine-supplemented PN should provide the information that is needed. Phase III level, double-blind, intent-to-treat RCTs are needed in specific ICU patient subgroups to define clinically optimal calorie, protein/amino acid, and specific vitamin and mineral requirements, as well as to determine the efficacy of supplemental PN combined with EN to achieve caloric and protein/amino acid goals (McClave *et al.*, 2009; Singer *et al.*, 2009; Wischmeyer and Heyland, 2010; Cahill *et al.*, 2011). In addition, rigorous trials to verify proposed "pharmaconutrition" strategies (e.g. use of high doses of supplemental parenteral and enteral glutamine, vitamin C and other antioxidants, selenium, and/or zinc, etc.) are also needed (Wischmeyer and Heyland, 2010). Fortunately, numerous large, multicenter RCTs in this regard are in progress and will help to define optimal use of these important adjunctive nutritional therapies over the next several years.

Suggestions for Further Reading

ASPEN Board of Directors and Enteral Nutrition Practice Recommendations Task Force (2009) Enteral nutrition practice recommendations. *JPEN J Parenter Enteral Nutr* **33**, 122–167.

Doig, G.S., Simpson, F., and Sweetman, E.A. (2009) Evidence-based nutrition support in the intensive care unit: an update on reported trial quality. *Curr Opin Clin Nutr Metab Care* **12**, 201–206.

McClave, S.A., Martindale, R.G., Vanek, V.W., *et al.* (2009) Guidelines for the provision and assessment of nutrition support therapy in the adult critically ill patient: Society of Critical Care Medicine and American Society for Parenteral and Enteral Nutrition. *JPEN J Parenter Enteral Nutr* **33**, 277–316.

Singer, P., Berger, M.M., Van den Berghe, G., *et al.* (2009) ASPEN guidelines for parenteral nutrition: intensive care. *Clin Nutr* **28**, 387–400.

Ziegler, T.R. (2009) Parenteral nutrition in the critically ill patient. *N Engl J Med* **361**, 1088–1097.

References

Alish, C.J., Garvey, W.T., Maki, K.C., *et al.* (2010) A diabetes-specific enteral formula improves glycemic variability in patients with type 2 diabetes. *Diabetes Technol Ther* **12**, 419–425.

Anderegg, B.A., Worrall, C., Barbour, E., *et al.* (2009) Comparison of resting energy expenditure prediction methods with measured resting energy expenditure in obese, hospitalized adults. *JPEN J Parenter Enteral Nutr* **33**, 168–175.

ASPEN Board of Directors and Clinical Guidelines Task Force (2002) Guidelines for the use of parenteral and enteral nutrition in adult and pediatric patients. *JPEN J Parenter Enteral Nutr* **26**(1 Suppl), 1SA–138SA.

ASPEN Board of Directors and Enteral Nutrition Practice Recommendations Task Force (2009) Enteral Nutrition Practice Recommendations. *JPEN J Parenter Enteral Nutr* **33**, 122–167.

Barker, L.A., Gout, B.S., and Crowe, T.C. (2011) Hospital malnutrition: prevalence, identification and impact on patients and the healthcare system. *Int J Environ Res Public Health* **8**, 514–527.

Baskin, W.N. (2006) Acute complications associated with bedside placement of feeding tubes. *Nutr Clin Pract* **21**, 40–55.

Byrnes, M.C. and Stangenes, J. (2011) Refeeding in the ICU: an adult and pediatric problem. *Curr Opin Clin Nutr Metab Care* **14**, 186–192.

Cahill, N.E., Murch, L., Jeejeebhoy, K., *et al.* (2011) When early enteral feeding is not possible in critically ill patients: results of a multicenter observational study. *JPEN J Parenter Enteral Nutr* **35**, 160–168.

Casaer, M.P., Mesotten, D., Hermans, G., *et al.* (2011) Early versus late parenteral nutrition in critically ill adults. *N Engl J Med* **365**, 506–517.

Cerantola, Y., Hübner, M., Grass, F., *et al.* (2011) Immunonutrition in gastrointestinal surgery. *Br J Surg* **98**, 37–48.

De Luis, D.A., López Mongil, R., Gonzalez Sagrado, M., *et al.* (2011) Nutritional status in a multicenter study among institutionalized patients in Spain. *Eur Rev Med Pharmacol Sci* **15**, 259–265.

Detsky, A.S., McLaughlin, J.R., Baker, J.P., *et al.* (1987) What is subjective global assessment of nutritional status? *JPEN J Parenter Enteral Nutr* **11**, 8–13.

Doig, G.S., Simpson, F., and Delaney, A. (2005) A review of the true methodological quality of nutritional support trials conducted in the critically ill: time for improvement. *Anesth Analg* **100**, 527–533.

Doig, G.S., Simpson, F., and Sweetman, E.A. (2009) Evidence-based nutrition support in the intensive care unit: an update on reported trial quality. *Curr Opin Clin Nutr Metab Care* **12**, 201–206.

Dupertuis, Y.M., Meguid, M.M., and Pichard, C. (2009) Advancing from immunonutrition to pharmaconutrition: a gigantic challenge. *Curr Opin Clin Nutr Metab Care* **12**, 398–403.

Fallon, E.M., Le, H.D., and Puder, M. (2010) Prevention of parenteral nutrition-associated liver disease: role of omega-3 fish oil. *Curr Opin Organ Transplant* **15**, 334–340.

Ford, E., Hull, S., Jenning, L., *et al.* (1992) Clinical comparison of tolerance to elemental or polymeric enteral feedings in the postoperative patient. *J Am Coll Nutr* **11**, 11–16.

Gadek, J.E., DeMichele, S.J., Karlstad, M.D., *et al.* (1999) Effect of enteral feeding with eicosapentanoic acid, gamma-linolenic acid and antioxidants in patients with acute respiratory distress syndrome. Enteral Nutrition in ARDS Study Group. *Crit Care Med* **27**, 1409–1420.

Giner, M., Laviano, A., Meguid, M.M., *et al.* (1996) In 1995 a correlation between malnutrition and poor outcome in critically ill patients still exists. *Nutrition* **12**, 23–29.

Grau, T., Bonet, A., Rubio, M., *et al.* (2007) Liver dysfunction associated with artificial nutrition in critically ill patients. *Crit Care* **11**, R10.

Guenter, P., Hicks, R.W., Simmons, D., *et al.* (2008) Enteral feeding misconnections: a consortium position statement. *Jt Comm J Qual Patient Saf* **34**, 285–292.

Heyland, D.K., Drover, J.W., Dhaliwal, R., *et al.* (2002) Optimizing the benefits and minimizing the risks of enteral nutrition in the critically ill: role of small bowel feeding. *JPEN J Parenter Enteral Nutr* **26** (6 Suppl), S51–57.

Heyland, D.K., Dhaliwal, R., Drover, J.W., *et al.* (2003) Canadian clinical practice guidelines for nutrition support in mechanically ventilated, critically ill adult patients. *JPEN J Parenter Enteral Nutr* **27**, 355–373.

Hurt, R.T. and McClave, S.A. (2010) Gastric residual volumes in critical illness: what do they really mean? *Crit Care Clin* **26**, 481–490.

Kavanagh, B.P. and McCowen, K.C. (2010) Clinical practice. Glycemic control in the ICU. *N Engl J Med* **363**, 2540–2546.

Kennedy, J.F. and Nightingale, J.M. (2005) Cost savings of an adult hospital nutrition support team. *Nutrition* **21**, 1127–1133.

Koletzko, B., Agostoni, C., and Ball, P., *et al.* (2005) ESPEN/ESPGHAN guidelines on paediatric parenteral nutrition. *J Pediatr Gastroenterol Nutr* **41**, S1–S87.

Koretz, R.L. (2008) Parenteral nutrition and urban legends. *Curr Opin Gastroenterol* **24**, 210–214.

Koretz, R.L. (2009) Enteral nutrition: a hard look at some soft evidence. *Nutr Clin Pract* **24**, 316–324.

Kreymann, K.G., Berger, M.M., Deutz, N.E., *et al.* (2006) ESPEN guidelines on enteral nutrition: intensive care. *Clin Nutr* **25**, 210–223.

Leon-Sanz, M., Garcia-Luna, P.P., Planas, M., *et al.* (2005) Glycemic and lipid control in hospitalized type 2 diabetic patients: evaluation of 2 enteral nutrition formulas (low carbohydrate-high monosaturated fat vs. high carbohydrate). *JPEN J Parenter Enteral Nutr* **29**, 21–29.

Lord, L.M. (2003) Restoring and maintaining patency of enteral feeding tubes. *Nutr Clin Pract* **18**, 422–426.

Luo, M., Fernandez-Estivariz, C., Jones, D.P., *et al.* (2008) Depletion of plasma antioxidants in surgical intensive care unit patients requiring parenteral feeding: effects of parenteral nutrition with or without alanyl-glutamine dipeptide supplementation. *Nutrition* **24**, 37–44.

Malone, A.M., Seres, D.S., and Lord, L. (2007) Complications of enteral nutrition. In M.M. Gottschlich (ed.), *The ASPEN Nutrition Support Core Curriculum: A Case-Based Approach – The Adult Patient.* American Society of Parenteral and Enteral Nutrition, Silver Spring, MD, pp. 246–263.

Marik, P.E. and Zaloga, G.P. (2008) Immunonutrition in critically ill patients: a systematic review and analysis of the literature. *Intensive Care Med* **34**, 1980–1990.

McClave, S.A., DeMeo, M.T., DeLegge, M.H., *et al.* (2002) North American Summit on aspiration in the critically ill patient: consensus statement. *JPEN J Parenter Enteral Nutr* **26**(6 Suppl), S80–85.

McClave, S.A., Martindale, R.G., Vanek, V.W., *et al.* (2009) Guidelines for the provision and assessment of nutrition support therapy in the adult critically ill patient: Society of Critical Care Medicine and American Society for Parenteral and Enteral Nutrition. *JPEN J Parenter Enteral Nutr* **33**, 277–316.

Mehta, N.M., Compher, C., and ASPEN Board of Directors (2009) ASPEN Clinical Guidelines: nutrition support of the critically ill child. *JPEN J Parenter Enteral Nutr* **33**, 260–276.

Mentec, H., Dupont, H., Bocchetti, M., *et al.* (2001) Upper digestive intolerance during enteral nutrition in critically ill patients: frequency, risk, factors, and complications. *Crit Care Med* **29**, 1922–1961.

Metheny, N.A. and Meert, K.L. (2004) Monitoring feeding tube placement. *Nutr Clin Pract* **19**, 487–495.

Metheny, N.A., Clouse, R.E., Chang, Y.H., *et al.* (2006) Tracheobronchial aspiration of gastric contents in critically ill tube-fed patients: frequency, outcomes, and risk factors. *Crit Care Med* **34**, 1–9.

Metheny, N.A., Meert, K.L., and Clouse, R.E. (2007) Complications related to feeding tube placement. *Curr Opin Gastroenterol* **23**, 178–182.

Minard, G. (1994) Enteral access. *Nutr Clin Pract* **9**, 172–182.

Mirtallo, J., Canada, T., Johnson, D, *et al.* (2004) Safe practices for parenteral nutrition. *JPEN J Parenter Enteral Nutr* **28**, S39–70.

Mowatt-Larssen, C., Brown, R., Wojtysial, S., *et al.* (1992) Comparison of tolerance and nutritional outcome between a peptide and a standard formula in critically ill, hypoalbuminemic patients. *JPEN J Parenter Enteral Nutr* **16**, 20–24.

Nathens, A.B., Neff, M.J., Jurkovich, G.J., *et al.* (2002) Randomized, prospective trial of antioxidant supplementation in critically ill surgical patients. *Ann Surg* **236**, 814–822.

NICE–SUGAR Study Investigators, Finfer, S., Chittock, D.R., *et al.* (2009) Intensive versus conventional glucose control in critically ill patients. *N Engl J Med* **360**, 1283–1297.

Norman, K., Schütz, T., Kemps, M., *et al.* (2005) The Subjective Global Assessment reliably identifies malnutrition-related muscle dysfunction. *Clin Nutr* **24**, 143–150.

O'Brien, J.M., Jr, Phillips, G.S., and Ali, N.A. (2006) Body mass index is independently associated with hospital mortality in mechanically ventilated adults with acute lung injury. *Crit Care Med* **34**, 738–744.

Patel, M.D. and Martin, F.C. (2008) Why don't elderly hospital inpatients eat adequately? *J Nutr Health Aging* **12**, 227–231.

Pirlich, M., Schütz, T., Norman, K., *et al.* (2006) The German hospital malnutrition study. *Clin Nutr* **25**, 563–572.

Pohl, M., Mayr, P., Mertl-Roetzer, M., *et al.* (2005) Glycaemic control in type II diabetic tube-fed patients with a new enteral formula low in carbohydrates and high in monosaturated fatty acids: a randomized controlled trial. *Eur J Clin Nutr* **59**, 1121–1132.

Rasmussen, H.H., Holst, M., and Kondrup, J. (2010) Measuring nutritional risk in hospitals. *Clin Epidemiol* **2**, 209–216.

Rees, R.G., Keohane, P.P., Grimble, G.K., *et al.* (1985) Tolerance of elemental diet administered without starter regimen. *Br Med J* **290**, 1869–1870.

Schneider, S.M., Veyres, P., Pivot, X., *et al.* (2004) Malnutrition is an independent factor associated with nosocomial infections. *Br J Nutr* **92**, 105–111.

Shaw, J.H., Wildbore, M., and Wolfe, R.R. (1987) Whole body protein kinetics in severely septic patients. The response to glucose infusion and total parenteral nutrition. *Ann Surg* **205**, 288–294.

Singer, P., Berger, M.M., Van den Berghe, G., *et al.* (2009) ESPEN guidelines for parenteral nutrition: intensive care. *Clin Nutr* **28**, 387–400.

Singer, P., Theilla, M., Fisher, H., *et al.* (2006) Benefit of an enteral diet enriched with eicosapentaenoic acid and gamma-linolenic acid in ventilated patients with acute lung injury. *Crit Care Med* **34**, 1033–1038.

Solomon, S.M. and Kirby, D.F. (1990) The refeeding syndrome: a review. *JPEN J Parenter Enteral Nutr* **14**, 90–97.

Stanga, Z., Brunner, A., Leuenberger, M., *et al.* (2008) Nutrition in clinical practice–the refeeding syndrome: illustrative cases and guidelines for prevention and treatment. *Eur J Clin Nutr* **62**, 687–694.

Stapleton, R.D., Martin, T.R., Weiss, N.S., *et al.* (2011) A phase II randomized placebo-controlled trial of omega-3 fatty acids for the treatment of acute lung injury. *Crit Care Med* **39**, 1655–1662.

Streat, S.J., Beddoe, A.H., and Hill, G.L. (1987) Aggressive nutritional support does not prevent protein loss despite fat gain in septic intensive care patients. *J Trauma* **27**, 262–266.

Tiengou, L.E., Gloro, R., Pouzoulet, J., *et al.* (2006) Semi-elemental formula or polymeric formula: is there a better choice for enteral nutrition in acute pancreatitis? Randomized comparative study. *JPEN J Parenter Enteral Nutr* **30**, 1–5.

Torres, A., Serra-Batlles, J., Ros, E., *et al.* (1992) Pulmonary aspiration of gastric contents in patients receiving mechanical ventilation: the effect of the body position. *Ann Intern Med* **116**, 540–543.

Trujillo, E.B., Young, L.S., Chertow, G.M., *et al.* (1999) Metabolic and monetary costs of avoidable parenteral nutrition use. *JPEN J Parenter Enteral Nutr* **23**, 109–113.

Waitzberg, D.L., Torrinhas, R.S., and Jacintho, T.M. (2006) New parenteral lipid emulsions for clinical use. *JPEN J Parenter Enteral Nutr* **30**, 351–367.

Walshe, C.M., Boner, K.S., Bourke, J., *et al.* (2010) Diagnosis of catheter-related bloodstream infection in a total parenteral nutrition population: inclusion of sepsis defervescence after removal of culture-positive central venous catheter. *J Hosp Infect* **76,** 119–123.

Wischmeyer, P.E. (2008) Glutamine: role in critical illness and ongoing clinical trials. *Curr Opin Gastroenterol* **24,** 190–197.

Wischmeyer, P.E. and Heyland, D.K. (2010) The future of critical care nutrition therapy. *Crit Care Clin* **26,** 433–441.

Villet, S., Chiolero, R.L., Bollmann, M.D., *et al.* (2005) Negative impact of hypocaloric feeding and energy balance on clinical outcome in ICU patients. *Clin Nutr* **24,** 502–509.

Yang, G., Wu, X.T., Zhou, Y., *et al.* (2005) Application of dietary fiber in clinical enteral nutrition: a meta-analysis of randomized controlled trials. *World J Gastroenterol* **11,** 3935–3938.

Yarandi, S.S., Zhao, V.M., Hebbar, G., *et al.* (2011) Amino acid composition in parenteral nutrition: what is the evidence? *Curr Opin Clin Nutr Metab Care* **14,** 75–78.

Zaloga, G.P. (2006) Parenteral nutrition in adult inpatients with functioning gastrointestinal tracts: assessment of outcomes. *Lancet* **367,** 1101–1111.

Zeki, S., Culkin, A., Gabe, S.M., *et al.* (2011) Refeeding hypophosphataemia is more common in enteral than parenteral feeding in adult in patients. *Clin Nutr* **30,** 365–368.

Ziegler, T.R. (2009) Parenteral nutrition in the critically ill patient. *N Engl J Med* **361,** 1088–1097.

Ziegler, T.R. (2011) Nutrition support in critical illness – bridging the evidence gap. *N Engl J Med* **365,** 562–564.

58

BODY COMPOSITION EVALUATION

KRISTA CASAZZA, PhD, RD **AND TIM R. NAGY,** PhD

The University of Alabama at Birmingham, Birmingham, Alabama, USA

Summary

Body composition plays a critical role in the health of humans. This chapter focuses on a few of the more commonly used and/or available methodologies to determine body composition in human research, including anthropometry, bioelectrical impedance analysis (BIA), hydrodensitometry (HD), air displacement plethysmography (ADP), dual-energy X-ray absorptiometry (DXA), magnetic resonance imaging (MRI), and quantitative magnetic resonance (QMR). Because the emphasis of this chapter is to discuss research methods, we chose not to discuss any method that may pose harm to healthy research subjects, such as computed tomography with its associated radiation exposure.

Introduction

The methods of in vivo body composition analysis are based upon centuries-old mathematical, conductivity, and membrane permeability principles. However, recent technology has greatly enhanced the capacity to assess body composition using fairly precise and accurate methods.

Anthropometric procedures are often the most practical; however, the information that can be obtained from such measurements is limited. As such, anthropometric variables are often considered to be indices *related to* body composition, relying on the ability to categorize individuals usually for comparison with a reference population. Estimation using bioelectrical impedance allows for the assessment of body composition using the two-component model. This is because the water content of fat-free mass is relatively constant, and fat is an electrical resistor and, therefore, the lipid components of the membranes of the body cells behave as capacitors and reduce the flow of intracellular ions. Hydrodensitometry capitalizes on Archimedes' principle, where body volume of a subject immersed in water is equal to the loss in weight in water (weight in air minus weight in water) divided by the density of water. Similarly, air displacement plethysmography utilizes air pressure to determine volume, from which density and ultimately body composition can be determined. Dual-energy X-ray absorptiometry has rapidly become the method of choice for researchers conducting human studies that require information on body composition. Even with the potential pitfalls of DXA, it is clear

Present Knowledge in Nutrition, Tenth Edition. Edited by John W. Erdman Jr, Ian A. Macdonald and Steven H. Zeisel.
© 2012 International Life Sciences Institute. Published 2012 by John Wiley & Sons, Inc.

that this method for measuring body composition will continue to grow in popularity mainly due to its availability, ease of use with research subjects, and ability to quantify bone in addition to fat and lean tissue.

Some relatively newer methods have evolved in terms of body composition research. An important development in the field of body composition studies is the use of magnetic resonance imaging (MRI) to quantify adipose, lean, and bone tissue, as well as to provide information on the regional distribution, without exposure to ionizing radiation. Quantitative magnetic resonance (QMR) is a relatively new method for the determination of body composition. In this method, protons from different tissues are differentially affected by the instrument.

Ideally, a method for determining body composition in humans should be precise, accurate, readily accessible, inexpensive, rapid, non-invasive, and non-harmful; unfortunately, there are no such tests available. There are a vast number of variations (age sex, race, disease state) that influence body composition and must be considered. Which method one uses depends on the compartment of interest, availability of techniques, technical training of staff, condition of patient, and the location in which assessment will be done.

Anthropometric Indices

Anthropometry, the measurement of the human individual for the purposes of understanding physical variation, is useful for monitoring growth as well as for estimating risk factors for chronic disease and for nutritional assessment. Anthropometric instruments are generally portable and relatively inexpensive, procedures are non-invasive, and minimal training is required. However, information that can be obtained from such measurements is limited. Most notably, anthropometric assessment does not provide metric values for aspects of body composition. Therefore, rather than being seen as direct measurements, anthropometric variables are considered to be indices *related to* body composition. The primary use of anthropometric indices relies on the ability to categorize individuals usually for comparison with a reference population.

Body mass index (BMI) is the most commonly used primary outcome in both research and clinical practice. BMI is a global index for nutritional status, used to classify people as under- or overweight, but its relation to body composition per se is controversial (Wells and Fewtrell, 2006); BMI serves only as an anthropometric surrogate of adiposity, provides little information on fat-free components of weight, and has been shown to vary in its ability to predict body fat uniformly across all (heterogeneous) groups. Recent investigations indicate that current BMI categorization can identify a high prevalence of high adiposity in individuals with high BMI and a low prevalence of high adiposity in individuals with normal BMI, yet difficulties in the accurate assessment of adiposity among individuals with intermediate BMIs have been observed (Flegal *et al.*, 2010). Differences in BMI categorization and the relationship with adipose tissue mass between race/ethnic groups are an additional concern (Jackson *et al.*, 2009; Affuso *et al.*, 2010).

Body circumference at various sites is commonly used to provide information on body fat distribution and may be better able to predict adiposity relative to BMI. Waist circumference (WC, commonly measured at the level of the umbilicus or at the iliac crest) provides a simple measure of central fatness (Wells and Fewtrell, 2006) and has been used as a surrogate measure of abdominal adiposity, although there is no differentiation between intra-abdominal and subcutaneous adipose tissue compartments. A recent analysis of cross-sectional studies suggests that waist circumference or waist–hip ratio discriminate better in terms of adiposity and health outcomes as compared with BMI (Bosy-Westphal *et al.*, 2010; Qiao and Nyamdorj, 2010). In general, BMI, WC, and waist–hip ratio perform similarly as indicators of body fatness, and are more closely related to each other than to percentage body fat. Circumferences are often used for estimations of obesity, but they have also been proposed as measures of thinness, particularly low mid–upper arm circumference and low calf among older individuals (Wijnhoven *et al.*, 2010). Although there is support for use of circumference in addition to or in lieu of BMI, it should be recognized that the 95% confidence intervals for BMI and WC overlap in all comparison studies and the variations in observations among circumferences, as with BMI, are highly dependent upon age, gender, and race/ethnicity.

One of the simplest measurements for direct assessment of body fat is skinfold thickness, providing reasonable correlation with total percent body fat. Skinfold thickness is the double layer of skin and subcutaneous fat lifted as a fold and measured with standardized calipers and methodology at specific sites on the body. Understandably, because of the wide variation of subcutaneous fat across the body, multiple sites are required for sampling to provide accurate estimates. Values from various sites are incorporated into predictive equations, selection of which is based on characteristics of the cohort to be measured. The most widely applied method for calculating total body fat from measured skinfold was developed by Durnin and Womersley in 1974 (Braulio *et al.*, 2010). This uses the sum of four skinfold measurements to provide an estimation of the fat mass; subtracting this from total body weight gives an estimation of fat-free mass. Subsequently a vast number of prediction equations have been developed, many of which rely on values obtained from the reference population of Durnin and Womersley. Recent investigations suggest that the original values cannot be applied to individuals living today, and modification is required (Kagawa *et al.*, 2010). Moreover, skinfold thickness measurements for the assessment of non-fat tissue are likely to be ineffective because the thickness of adipose tissue and of muscle in limbs is essentially independent.

Bioelectrical Impedance Analysis

Bioelectrical impedance (BIA) capitalizes on the fact that each tissue of the body is characterized by a specific conductivity, which is directly related to the water and electrolyte content of the tissue. Within the tissue, the water is localized into two compartments, extracellular water (ECW) and intracellular water (ICW). BIA involves introduction of a small electric current to the body (Dehghan and Merchant, 2008). The impedance represents the whole resistivity of the tissues divided into resistive component (the opposition of the ECW component to the current) and the capacitive component, i.e. the current passes freely through the ECW, but penetration is reduced by the capacitance effect of cell membranes influencing passage through ICW. In terms of body composition estimation, the water content of fat-free mass is relatively constant: 0.732 L/kg (Leone *et al.*, 2000); thus in lean tissue, which is rich in water and electrolytes, the minimal impedance can be calculated from difference in conductivity. Conversely, fat is an electrical resistor and therefore the lipid components of the membranes of the body cells behave as capacitors and reduce the flow of intracellular ions, a fact not actually reflected by electrical data. The values of resistance and reactance depend on the frequency of the electric current. Mathematical modeling and theories on fluid resistivity are subsequently used to estimate the conductive path to ascertain total body water, fat-free mass (FFM), and body cell mass using

height, sex, age, and race. Total body percent fat mass can be defined as $[(wt - FFM_{TBM})/Weight] \times 100$.

BIA was initially designed using single-frequency impedance analyzers (usually 50 mHz). However, single-frequency BIA is limited in the ability to distinguish between fluid shifts and balance between ECW and ICW compartments. The overall effect in subjects who have a high ECW/ICW ratio and increased TBW would be an overestimation of FFM and underestimation of fat mass (FM) (Das *et al.*, 2003). Accordingly, multiple-frequency BIA (varying from 5 kHz to 1 MHz) has been developed. Mathematical modeling (e.g. Cole-Cole, Hanoi) produces estimates of theoretical resistance at zero frequency (reflecting purely ECW) and at an infinite frequency, reflecting passage through total body water space. This has not completely circumvented the issues associated with BIA, however. The human body is complex in shape, represented by not one but five heterogeneous cylinders with different resistivities, over which resistances are measured separately. Settle and colleagues (1980) observed that 85% of total body impedance was accounted for by the sum of the impedance of the arm and the leg although these segments only accounted for 35% of the total body volume. Thus, in an attempt to overcome the concerns with the assumption of the body as approximated by a single cylinder, a segmental approach was proposed in which the arm(s), leg(s), and trunk are determined separately and together with the length of these segments. Segmental BIA uses six electrodes instead of four (Mattsson and Thomas, 2006).

The accurate assessment of fluid status represents a major challenge. The determination of body fluid volumes by BIA is based on the assumption that electrical current at low frequencies cannot penetrate cell membranes and flows through the ECW only, whereas high-frequency current flows through ECW and ICW. Therefore the low and high frequencies are related to ECF, total body water, and BCM. However, the apparent resistivity is dependent upon the size of cells. For example, in overweight/obese states, greater lipid content would significantly change the path length around the cells, thereby limiting accuracy of measurement. Similarly, low hydration status or wasting would decrease the path.

Hydrodensitometry

Hydrodensitometry (HD), commonly referred to as underwater weighing (UWW), is a method of determining body composition based on the density of the body. Density is calculated as the ratio of the body's mass (M) and volume (V):

$$D_b = M / V$$

where body mass is estimated from the measurement of body weight and volume determined by underwater weighing. Using Archimedes' principle, body volume of a subject immersed in water is equal to the loss in weight in water (weight in air minus weight in water) divided by the density of water.

For human body composition measurements with HD, the body is considered a two-component model consisting of fat mass (FM) and FFM, and the density of the body is equal to the proportions and density of the two components (Going, 2005). The two most widely used models were developed by Siri (1956) and Brozek et al. (1963) more than 40 years ago. However, for these equations to accurately predict body composition, the densities of the components must be constant among individuals.

The density of fat mass is typically given at 0.9007 g/mL and seems to be fairly constant (Fidenza et al., 1953; Brozek et al., 1963). Fat-free mass consists of approximately 73.8% water (0.9937 g/mL), 19.4% protein (1.34 g/mL), and 6.8% mineral (3.038 g/mL), where the mineral is a combination of osseous (5.6%; 2.982 g/mL) and non-osseous (1.2%; 3.317 g/mL) (Brozek et al., 1963). However, these proportions, and therefore the density of FFM, can vary with age, sex, training, and race. This has led to the development of three- and four-component models in which total body water (by dilution techniques), and osseous mineral content (by DXA) are included in the calculation of percentage fat (Lohman, 1986; Going, 2005).

Notwithstanding its limitations, HD has long been considered the "gold standard" of body composition methodologies for humans. It is often used to gauge new methods for accuracy of measurements, and forms the basis for most multicomponent models.

Air-Displacement Plethysmography

Similar to HD, air-displacement plethysmography (ADP) calculates the density of the body, using mass and body volume to determine body composition. However, unlike UWW, volume is not determined by submersion in water.

Instead, ADP relies on the relationship between pressure and volume, that is, Boyle's law:

$$P_1 / P_2 = V_2 / V_1$$

where P_1 and V_1 are one condition and P_2 and V_2 are a second condition. Boyle's law is true only if temperature is kept constant within a closed system (i.e. isothermal conditions). However, under adiabatic conditions, the temperature of air does not remain constant and temperature changes with changes in volume. This situation is described as an isentropic process from:

$$P_1 / P_2 = (V_2 / V_1)^\gamma$$

where γ is the ratio of the specific heat capacity at constant pressure divided by the specific heat capacity at constant volume (C_P/C_V) (Van Wylen and Sonntag, 1965).

The Bod Pod plethysmograph (Life Measurement Instruments, Inc., Concord, CA) is one such instrument that can be used to determine the volume of the human body (Figure 58.1). The instrument consists of two

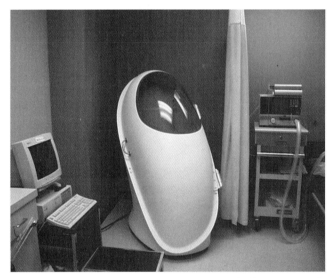

FIG. 58.1 An air-displacement plethysmograph located in the Department of Nutrition Sciences at the University of Alabama, Birmingham. Because the system measures pressure, it is important to house it in an area that does not experience rapid fluxes in air movement. This unit is housed in a room in which the room air circulation can be turned off during the measurement period, thereby decreasing measurement error.

chambers, a reference chamber that houses the electronics, and a test chamber for the subject. A diaphragm between the two chambers pulses to produce pressure changes within the chambers, thereby allowing for the determination of a change in volume in the test chamber. A complete review of the theory and mechanics can be found elsewhere (Fields *et al.*, 2002; Going, 2005).

A major advantage of ADP over UWW is ease of use, as the former does not require subjects to be immersed in water and to have the ability to hold their breath while underwater. This is particularly useful for studies involving children, the elderly, or disabled individuals. Our own personal experience from conducting ADP and UWW studies is that even normal healthy individuals are more relaxed and more likely to come back for repeat measurement when ADP rather than UWW is used. In addition, the technique is fairly rapid (8–12 minutes), and requires minimal compliance and a low degree of technical skill (Fields *et al.*, 2005).

Numerous studies have investigated the precision and accuracy of ADP (Fields *et al.*, 2002, 2005). Within-day variations (coefficients of variation; CVs) range between 1.7–4.5% and 2–2.3% between days and compare well with published reports from UWW (Fields *et al.*, 2002). Body fat determined from ADP has been shown to be within 1% and 2% compared with that measured by UWW and DXA respectively (Fields *et al.*, 2005).

Similar to UWW, APD relies on the consistency of body density to predict fat mass and therefore has the same issues that FFM can vary with age, sex, training status, and race. However, the ease of use makes ADP attractive for the determination of body composition in infants, children, and adults.

Dual-Energy X-Ray Absorptiometry

Dual-energy X-ray absorptiometry (DXA) allows for the determination of total and regional bone mineral (BM, g), total and regional bone mineral density (BMD, g/cm^2), fat mass (FM, g), bone mineral free lean tissue mass (LTM, g), and soft-tissue mass (STM, g; STM = FM + LTM) (Pietrobelli *et al.*, 1996; Nagy, 2001; Lohman and Chen, 2005). Even though DXA utilizes X-rays, the method is considered relatively safe since the radiation exposure is less than a person would receive on a transcontinental flight across the United States (4–6 mrem) (Lohman and Chen, 2005). However, some governing bodies do not approve of DXA use during pregnancy, thus necessitating

pregnancy testing in women of childbearing years. Repeated measurement of individuals and the testing of children have been questioned as well. However, where there is justification for their use, these procedures are typically approved.

The theory behind DXA has been reviewed in detail numerous times (Cullum *et al.*, 1989; Mazess *et al.*, 1990; Pietrobelli *et al.*, 1996), and will not be discussed here.

DXA has rapidly become the method of choice for researchers conducting human studies that require information on body composition. Numerous studies have validated the use of DXA by either analyzing large animals and comparing the DXA-derived values with chemical carcass analysis, or by measuring humans and comparing the results with those of other established techniques (underwater weighing or four-compartment model) (Brunton *et al.*, 1993; Ellis *et al.*, 1994; Pintauro *et al.*, 1996). Pintauro and colleagues (1996) utilized pigs within the pediatric weight range (15–37 kg) to validate the use of DXA in children. All pigs were scanned in duplicate to determine precision and then killed, and chemical carcass analysis was performed. The coefficients of variation ranged from a low of 0.9% for lean tissue to a high of 4.1% for fat mass. The relationship between fat and lean derived from carcass analysis and DXA was strong with r^2 >0.98. However, there was a significant difference in the absolute values between the two techniques. The authors then derived equations to correct the DXA-derived data to match that from chemical carcass analysis.

Wong *et al.* (2002) compared DXA measured values of body fat with values obtained from the four-compartment model in a group of girls and female adolescents. The four-compartment model utilizes data obtained from body density (obtained from underwater weighing or air-displacement plethysmography), body water (obtained from isotope dilution), and bone mineral content (obtained from DXA). By utilizing information from the various techniques, the models are typically able to account for more biological variability and are likely the most accurate methods for determining body composition (Wang *et al.*, 2005). Data from DXA was highly correlated with the four-compartment model ($r = 0.90$), however, an individual value for percentage fat mass could be over- or underestimated by 6.7% using DXA. Although the authors suggested that DXA was an appropriate method for determining body composition, it was not considered optimal.

In addition to questions concerning accuracy of the method, there are well-documented studies showing differences between instruments and well as among software versions on the same instrument (Huffman *et al.*, 2005; Lohman and Chen, 2005; Shypailo *et al.*, 2008). Huffman and co-workers (2005) assessed body composition on 106 apparently healthy subjects (34 males, 72 females; ages 8–72) using the Lunar DPX-L and Lunar Prodigy DXA. The results showed that, relative to the DPX-L, the Prodigy significantly overestimated body mass (percentage difference = 1.1%), total body bone mineral density (2.2%), total body bone mineral content (2.9%), fat mass (3.5%), and percentage fat (2.8%), but not lean tissue mass (−0.2%; $p = 0.35$). However, the two measures were well related and therefore corrections equations were published that allow comparison of the data between instruments.

More recently, Shypailo *et al.* (2008) evaluated 1384 pediatric scans (1.7 to 17.2 years of age) using two software versions (Hologic software V11.2 vs. V12.1). Their study showed that DXA-derived body composition values were not affected by subjects who weighed >40 kg. However, in subjects weighing <40 kg, body fat was greater and lean mass less on the latter software version, which had the effect of increasing the percentage body fat. The change was sufficiently different that 14% of girls and 10% of boys were reclassified from normal body fat to "at risk for obesity", and 7% and 5% were reclassified as obese. These studies suggest that data obtained from different software and/or instruments cannot necessarily be compared, and that users should be aware of software being utilized for their studies.

An important limitation of lean tissue measured by DXA is that it does include ECW as well as ICW, and so changes in hydration will be interpreted as change in lean tissue (Pietrobelli *et al.*, 1998).

Even with the potential pitfalls of DXA, it is clear that this method for measuring body composition will continue to grow in popularity mainly due to its availability, ease of use with research subjects, and ability to quantify bone in addition to fat and lean tissue. Figure 58.2 shows a typical bone and tissue image obtained from a DXA scan.

Magnetic Resonance Imaging

An important development in the field of body composition studies was the use of magnetic resonance imaging (MRI) to quantify body composition adipose, lean, and bone tissue as well as to provide information on the regional distribution without exposure to ionizing radia-

tion. By exploiting the particular characteristics of hydrogen protons, MRI can provide contrast between soft tissues (Bley *et al.*, 2009). MRI estimates the volume rather than the mass of tissue compartments.

Estimation of tissue volume by MRI is based upon the interaction between hydrogen protons abundant in all tissues and the magnetic fields generated by the MRI instrumentation. That is, when a strong magnetic field is applied to body tissues, the magnetic moments present in the nuclei of cells will align with the magnetic field. Although only a small number of protons become aligned, the number is sufficient to enable detection of a change when the field is removed or altered. Accordingly, the hydrogen protons absorb energy, which is released when the pulse is turned off. The time it takes for the nuclei to release and return to random orientation differs between fat and water (Ellis, 2000). This energy is integrated into cross-sectional imaging slices based on spatial variation in the phase and frequency of the energy absorbed and emitted, which can be summed to calculate regional tissue volumes (Wells and Fewtrell, 2006).

The classical approach of tissue density determination by MRI utilized chemical-shift-based water–fat separation, commonly known as Dixon water–fat separation. Dixon methods rely on the plane shifts created by fat–water resonance frequency between water and fat. Phase information is encoded by acquiring images at slightly different echo times. Dixon methods provide a fat-suppressed water-only image and a water-suppressed fat-only image. The two images are acquired at different echo times (TE) such that water and fat are in phase or out of phase. By adding and subtracting S_{in} and S_{out}, water and fat are easily separated.

Alternatives to the Dixon two-point method have been introduced in an effort to reduce inhomogeneities that resulted in water and fat swapping in the image (Costa *et al.*, 2008; Bley *et al.*, 2009). The Dixon method has evolved over the past 25 years, generating various modifications resulting in the three-point method and ultimately in IDEAL, the iterative decomposition of water and fat with echo asymmetry and least-squares estimation technique. Instead of collecting just two images, the IDEAL technique requires careful selection of echo times so that the reconstructed fat-only and water-only images have the maximum signal-to-noise ratio. IDEAL imaging provides uniform and reliable fat suppression throughout the body, with the potential to simplify MRI protocols (Hu *et al.*, 2010).

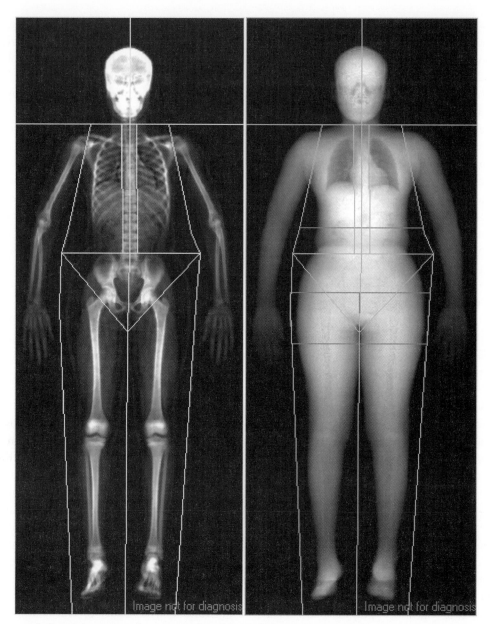

FIG. 58.2 Bone and tissue images of a research subject. The scans were obtained from a Lunar iDXA system. Segmentation lines are used to divide the body into regions of interest to provide data on specific areas.

Compartmental tissue measurements using MRI have shown excellent precision (Browning *et al.*, 2010; Thamer *et al.*, 2010). Comparisons of various body measures with MRI indicate that although, generally, there were significant correlations of all modalities with body fat content and mainly with subcutaneous fat, correlations with intra-abdominal fat were much weaker. If it is important to investigate fat distribution and especially the intra-abdominal adipose tissue, MRI cannot be substituted by simpler methods (Ludescher *et al.*, 2009). MRI has also broadened the scope of investigations into additional tissue depots. For example, brown adipose tissue, with its multilocular fat distribution and extensive mitochondrial, cytoplasm, and vascular supply, has a significantly lower fat signal, making its quantification difficult. However, the fat fraction metric from IDEAL–MRI has recently been demonstrated to be a sensitive and quantitative approach for noninvasively characterizing brown adipose tissue (Hu et al., 2010). Further, quantification of bone-marrow adipose tissue and its relation to loss of bone mineral content has led to investigations of the reciprocal relationship between fat and bone tissue compartments (Shen et al., 2007). Although there are obvious limitations in terms of finances, population and space requirements associated with MRI, techniques are likely to be of use in a variety of medical investigations (Muller et al., 2002).

Quantitative Magnetic Resonance

Quantitative magnetic resonance (QMR) is a relatively new method for the determination of body composition. Similar to MRI, QMR utilizes the measurement of hydrogen to determine fat and lean tissue, and total body water. Protons from different tissues are differentially affected by the instrument. Fat tissue produces a greater peak amplitude and has a greater rate of relaxation than lean because of a greater hydrogen density (40% more hydrogen per unit) (Taicher et al., 2003). A number of QMR instruments have now been validated, and used to determine body composition in mice, rats, pigs, and humans (Tinsley et al., 2004; Napolitano et al., 2008a; Johnson et al., 2009; Jones et al., 2009; Gallagher et al., 2010; Swe Myint et al., 2010).

The precision of QMR has been shown to be excellent. Gallagher et al. (2010) determined the coefficient of variation for fat to be 0.437% based on a standard deviation of 0.131 kg and an average fat value of 30.057 kg. Their results suggested that it may be possible to determine changes in fat mass of as little as 250 g, which is quite good compared with most methods. Similarly, Swe Myint and colleagues (2010) showed that QMR provides a benefit over other methods when the studies have a small standard deviation (0.5–1 kg) and a moderate difference among groups (1–2 kg). In this case, sample size can be reduced by up to 40% over conventional methods (DXA and/or the four-compartment method).

Although the precision of QMR is excellent, there are issues related to accuracy. Studies have demonstrated that QMR-measured fat, lean, and total body water in mice, rats, pigs, and humans differed significantly from other more established measures such as chemical carcass analysis and the four-compartment model (Napolitano et al.,

2008b; Johnson et al., 2009; Jones et al., 2009; Andres et al., 2010; Gallagher et al., 2010; Mitchell, 2010; Swe Myint et al., 2010). It is not clear at this time why the measures differ, but care should be taken when using QMR to determine absolute quantities of fat, lean or total body water. However, given QMR's excellent precision, it is extremely useful for measuring differences between groups, or within groups over time.

One of the major benefits of QMR is its non-invasive nature. Not only does the instrument not expose the subject to ionizing radiation; the method does not even require the subject to remain completely still, since it is not capturing an image per se. Clearly this is beneficial when studying a pediatric population or a potentially health-impaired population where involuntary movement cannot be helped. In addition, measurement times are on the order of minutes, which facilitates subject compliance and the ability to measure numerous subjects per unit time.

Assessment of Body Composition in Disease States

An important area of use of body composition techniques is in disease states. Due to the reliance on constant hydration of fat-free mass, which is not always the case in pathological processes, progressive involuntary weight loss or wasting presents a challenge in the accuracy of body composition assessment. Numerous studies have reported altered validity of BIA- and DXA-derived estimates with hydration status (Lohman et al., 2000; Testolin et al., 2000; Bredella et al., 2010). Accordingly, the clinical evaluation and monitoring of body composition across disease states is a concern. Assessments of body composition in individuals with body habitus varying from anorexia nervosa (Bredella et al., 2010) to those undergoing gastric bypass (Savastano et al., 2010) present added complexity. Further, disease states in which wasting is often a symptom (e.g. cancer, HIV) also impart validity issues. Inconsistencies have been reported in DXA, BIA, and MRI measurements in patients with HIV (Esposito et al., 2006; Scherzer et al., 2008), celiac disease (De Lorenzo et al., 1999), and short bowel disease (Carlsson et al., 2004). The limited agreement between methods prevents generalizability, particularly in comparisons across varying weight and disease states. It is important to recognize that, beyond the limitations of each assessment device, additional factors such as hydration may also influence validity.

TABLE 58.1 Major attributes of body composition methods

Method	Cost	Average test time	Accuracy[a]	Accessibility	Ease of use	Additional concerns
BMI	Low	<2 minutes	Low	High	Some training	Population-based differences
Body circumference	Low	<3 minutes	Low	High	Some training	Population-based differences
Skinfold	Low	5–10 minutes	Moderate	High	Some training	Population-based differences
BIA	Moderate	5–10 minutes	Moderate	Moderate	Some training	Hydration status
DXA	High	6–15 minutes	High	Low	Technician required	Radiation exposure
UWW	High	40–60 minutes		Low	Technician required	Breath hold
Air displacement plethysmography	High	8–12 minutes	Moderate	Moderate	Technician required	Air trapping/confinement
MRI	High	15–30 minutes	High	Low	Technician required	Space confinement
QMR	High	2–3 minutes	High	Low	Technician required	Space confinement

[a]As a measure of total adiposity, compared with UWW.

Future Directions

Ideally, a method for determining body composition in humans should be rapid, non-invasive and non-harmful, rapid, precise, accurate, readily accessible, and inexpensive. Unfortunately, there are no such tests available. Instead, those methods that are low cost and rapid have lower precision and accuracy and therefore are better suited for population-based studies (Table 58.1). Methods that have high precision and accuracy require expensive equipment with trained technicians, are not portable, and are costly, making them better suited for smaller studies. Practical considerations must be taken into account when choosing body composition methods.

Knowledge of the limitations of each method is critical for appropriate experimental design. For example, the use of UWW would not be ideal if the subject population to be studied varied dramatically in age, gender, training status, and race, because of differences in the density of FFM. Knowing the assumptions inherent in methods allows the researcher to choose the appropriate method or component model to minimize bias in the results.

There is still much to be done in the area of body composition methodology. Although many of the methods introduced in the chapter have been validated, many have not been validated in diverse groups. There is a critical need to increase the diversity of subject populations in validation studies so that future research is not hindered by the lack of adequate prediction equations.

Suggestions for Further Reading

Ellis, K. and Eastman, J. (1993) *Human Body Composition: In Vivo Methods, Models and Assessment*. Plenum, New York.

Heymsfield, S.B., Lohman, T.G., Wang, Z., *et al.* (2005) *Human Body Composition*, 2nd Edn. Human Kinetics, Champaign, IL.

Heyward, V.H. and Wagner, D.R. (2004) *Applied Body Composition Assessment*, 2nd Edn. Human Kinetics, Champaign, IL.

Lohman, T.G. (1992) *Advances in Body Composition Assessment*. Human Kinetics, Champaign, IL.

Speakman, J.R. (2001) *Body Composition Analysis of Animals: A Handbook of Non-Destructive Methods*. Cambridge University Press, Cambridge.

References

Affuso, O., Bray, M.S., Fernandez, J.R., *et al.* (2010) Standard obesity cut points based on BMI percentiles do not equally correspond to body fat percentage across racial/ethnic groups in a representative sample of children and adolescents. *Int J Body Comp Res* **8**, 117–122.

Andres, A., Mitchell, A.D., and Badger, T.M. (2010) QMR: validation of an infant and children body composition instrument using piglets against chemical analysis. *Int J Obesity* **34**, 775–780.

Bley, T.A., Wieben, O., and Uhl, M. (2009) Diffusion-weighted MR imaging in musculoskeletal radiology: applications in trauma, tumors, and inflammation. *Magn Reson Imaging Clin N Am* **17**, 263–275.

Bosy-Westphal, A., Booke, C.A., Blocker, T., *et al.* (2010) Measurement site for waist circumference affects its accuracy as an index of visceral and abdominal subcutaneous fat in a Caucasian population. *J Nutr* **140**, 954–961.

Braulio, V.B., Furtado, V.C., Silveira, M.G., *et al.* (2010) Comparison of body composition methods in overweight and obese Brazilian women. *Arq Bras Endocrinol Metabol* **54**, 398–405.

Bredella, M.A., Ghomi, R.H., Thomas, B.J., *et al.* (2010) Comparison of DXA and CT in the assessment of body composition in premenopausal women with obesity and anorexia nervosa. *Obesity (Silver Spring)* **18**, 2227–2233.

Browning, L.M., Mugridge, O., Chatfield, M.D., *et al.* (2010) Validity of a new abdominal bioelectrical impedance device to measure abdominal and visceral fat: comparison with MRI. *Obesity* **18**, 2385–2391.

Brozek, J., Grande., F., and Anderson, J.T. (1963) Densitometric analysis of body composition: revision of some quantitative assumptions. *Ann NY Acad Sci* **110**, 113–140.

Brunton, J.A., Bayley, H.S., and Atkinson, S.A. (1993) Validation and application of dual-energy x-ray absorptiometry to measure bone mass and body composition in small infants. *Am J Clin Nutr* **58**, 839–845.

Carlsson, E., Bosaeus, I., and Nordgren, S. (2004) Body composition in patients with short bowel syndrome: an assessment by bioelectric impedance spectroscopy (BIS) and dual-energy absorptiometry (DXA). *Eur J Clin Nutr* **58**, 853–859.

Costa, D.N., Pedrosa, I., McKenzie, C., *et al.* (2008) Body MRI using IDEAL. *Am J Roentgenol* **190**, 1076–1084.

Cullum, I.D., Ell, P.J., and Ryder, J.P. (1989) X-Ray dual photon absorptiometry: a new method for the measurement of bone density. *Br J Radiol* **62**, 587–592.

Das, S.K., Roberts, S.B., Kehayias, J.J., *et al.* (2003) Body composition assessment in extreme obesity and after massive weight loss induced by gastric bypass surgery. *Am J Physiol Endocrinol Metab* **284**, E1080–1088.

Dehghan, M. and Merchant, A.T. (2008) Is bioelectrical impedance accurate for use in large epidemiological studies? *Nutr J* **7**, 26.

De Lorenzo, A., Sorge, R.P., Candeloro, N., *et al.* (1999) New insights into body composition assessment in obese women. *Can J Physiol Pharmacol* **77**, 17–21.

Ellis, K.J. (2000) Human body composition: in vivo methods. *Physiol Rev* **80**, 649–680.

Ellis, K.J., Shypailo, R.J., Pratt, J.A., *et al.* (1994) Accuracy of dual-energy x-ray absorptiometry for body-composition measurements in children. *Am J Clin Nutr* **60**, 660–665.

Esposito, J.G.,Thomas, S.G., Kingdon,L., *et al.* (2006) Comparison of body composition assessment methods in patients with human immunodeficiency virus-associated wasting receiving growth hormone. *J Clin Endocrinol Metab* **91**, 2952–2959.

Fidenza, F.K., Keys, A., and Anderson, J.T. (1953) Density of body fat in man and other mammals. *J Appl Physiol* **6**, 252–256.

Fields, D., Goran, M.I., and McCrory, M.A. (2002) Body-composition assessment via air-displacement plethysmography in adults and children: a review. *Am J Clin Nutr* **75**, 453–467.

Fields, D.A., Higgins, P.B., and Radley, D (2005) Air-displacement plethysmography: here to stay. *Curr Opin Clin Nutr Metab Care* **8**, 624–629.

Flegal, K.M., Carroll, M.D., Ogden, C.L., *et al.* (2010) Prevalence and trends in obesity among US adults, 1999–2008. *JAMA* **303**, 235–241.

Gallagher, D., Thornton, J.C., He, Q., *et al.* (2010) Quantitative magnetic resonance fat measurements in humans correlate with established methods but are biased. *Obesity* **18**, 2047–2054.

Going, S.B. (2005) Hydrodensitometry and air displacement plethysmography. In S.B. Heymsfield, T.G. Lohman, Z. Wang, *et al.* (eds), *Human Body Composition*, 2nd Edn. Human Kinetics, Champaign, IL, pp. 17–33.

Hu, H.H., Smith, D.L., Jr, Nayak, K.S., *et al.* (2010) Identification of brown adipose tissue in mice with fat–water IDEAL–MRI. *J Magn Reson Imaging* **31**, 1195–1202.

Huffman, D.M., Landy, N.M., Potter, E., *et al.* (2005) Comparison of the Lunar DPX-L and Prodigy dual-energy X-ray absorptiometers for assessing total and regional body composition. *Int.J.Body Compos Res* **3**, 25–30.

Jackson, A.S.,Ellis, K.J., McFarlin, B.K., *et al.* (2009) Body mass index bias in defining obesity of diverse young adults: the Training Intervention and Genetics of Exercise Response (TIGER) study. *Br J Nutr* **102**, 1084–1090.

Johnson, M.S., Smith, D.L., Jr, and Nagy, T.R. (2009) Validation of quantitative magnetic resonance (QMR) for determination of body composition in rats. *Int J Body Comp Res* **7**, 99–107.

Jones, A.S., Johnson, M.S., and Nagy, T.R. (2009) Validation of quantitative magnetic resonance for the determination of body composition of mice. *Int J Body Comp Res* **7,** 67–72.

Kagawa, M., Uenishi, K., Mori, M., *et al.* (2010) Obesity screening for young Japanese males and females using skin fold measurements: the classification revisited. *Asia Pac J Clin Nutr* **19,** 289–293.

Leone, P.A., Gallagher, D., Wang, J., *et al.* (2000) Relative overhydration of fat-free mass in postobese versus never-obese subjects. *Ann NY Acad Sci* **904,** 514–519.

Lohman, T.G. (1986) Applicability of body composition techniques and constants for children and youth. *Exerc Sports Sci Rev* **14,** 325–357.

Lohman, T.G. and Chen, Z. (2005) Dual-energy X-ray absorptiometer. In S.B. Heymsfield, T.G. Lohman, Z. Wang, *et al.* (eds), *Human Body Composition*, 2nd Edn. Human Kinetics, Champaign, IL, pp. 63–77.

Lohman, T.G., Harris, M., Teixeira, P.J., *et al.* (2000) Assessing body composition and changes in body composition. Another look at dual-energy X-ray absorptiometry. *Ann NY Acad Sci* **904,** 45–54.

Ludescher, B., Machann, J., Eschweiler, G.W., *et al.* (2009) Correlation of fat distribution in whole body MRI with generally used anthropometric data. *Invest Radiol* **44,** 712–719.

Mattsson, S. and Thomas, B.J. (2006) Development of methods for body composition studies. *Phys Med Biol* **51,** R203–228.

Mazess, R.B., Barden, H.S., Bisek, J.P., *et al.* (1990) Dual-energy x-ray absorptiometry for total-body and regional bone-mineral and soft-tissue composition. *Am J Clin Nutr* **51,** 1106–1112.

Mitchell, A.D. (2011) Validation of quantitative magnetic resonance body composition analysis for infants using piglet model. *Pediatr Res* **69,** 330–335.

Muller, M.J., Bosy-Westphal, A., Kutzner, D., *et al.* (2002) Metabolically active components of fat-free mass and resting energy expenditure in humans: recent lessons from imaging technologies. *Obesity Rev* **3,** 113–122.

Nagy, T.R. (2001) The use of dual-energy X-ray absorptiometry for the measurement of body composition. In J.R. Speakman (ed.), *Body Composition Analysis of Animals: A Handbook of Non-Destructive Methods*. Cambridge University Press, Cambridge.

Napolitano, A., Miller, S.R., Murgatroyd, P.R., *et al.* (2008a) Validation of a quantitative magnetic resonance method for measuring human body composition. *Obesity* **16,** 191–198.

Napolitano, A., Miller, S.R., Murgatroyd, P.R., *et al.* (2008b) Validation of a quantitative magnetic resonance method for measuring human body composition. *Obesity* **16,** 191–198.

Pietrobelli, A., Formica, C., Wang, Z., *et al.* (1996) Dual-energy X-ray absorptiometry body composition model: review of physical concepts. *Am J Physiol* **271,** E941–E951.

Pietrobelli, A., Wang, Z., Formica, C., *et al.* (1998) Dual-energy X-ray absorptiometry: fat estimation errors due to variation in soft tissue hydration. *Am J Physiol Endocrinol Metab* **274,** E808–816.

Pintauro, S.J., Nagy, T.R., Duthie, C.M., *et al.* (1996) Cross-calibration of fat and lean measurements by dual-energy X-ray absorptiometry to pig carcass analysis in the pediatric body weight range. *Am J Clin Nutr* **63,** 293–298.

Qiao, Q. and Nyamdorj, R. (2010) The optimal cutoff values and their performance of waist circumference and waist-to-hip ratio for diagnosing type II diabetes. *Eur J Clin Nutr* **64,** 23–29.

Savastano, S., Belfiore, A., Di Somma, C., *et al.* (2009) Validity of bioelectrical impedance analysis to estimate body composition changes after bariatric surgery in premenopausal morbidly obese women. *Obes Surg* **20,** 332–339.

Scherzer, R., Shen, W., Bacchetti, P., *et al.* (2008) Comparison of dual-energy X-ray absorptiometry and magnetic resonance imaging-measured adipose tissue depots in HIV-infected and control subjects. Study of fat redistribution metabolic change in HIV infection. *Am J Clin Nutr* **88,** 1088–1096.

Settle, R.G., Foster, K.R., Epstein, B.R., *et al.* (1980) Nutritional assessment: whole body impedance and body fluid compartments. *Nutr Cancer* **2,** 72–80.

Shen, W., Chen, J., Punyanitya, M., *et al.* (2007) MRI-measured bone marrow adipose tissue is inversely related to DXA-measured bone mineral in Caucasian women. *Osteoporosis Int* **18,** 641–647.

Shypailo, R.J., Butte, N.F., and Ellis, K.J. (2008) DXA: can it be used as a criterion reference for body fat measurements in children? *Obesity(Silver Spring)* **16,** 457–462.

Siri, W.E. (1956) The gross composition of the body. *Adv Biol Med Phys* **4,** 239–280.

Swe Myint, K., Napolitano, A., Miller, S.R., *et al.* (2010) Quantitative magnetic resonance (QMR) for longitudinal evaluation of body composition changes with two dietary regimens. *Obesity* **18,** 391–396.

Taicher, G.Z., Tinsley, F.C., Reiderman, A., *et al.* (2003) Quantitative magnetic resonance (QMR) method for bone and whole-body-composition analysis. *Anal Bioanal Chem* **377,** 990–1002.

Testolin, C.G., Gore, R., Rivkin, T., *et al.* (2000) Dual-energy X-ray absorptiometry: analysis of pediatric fat estimate errors due to tissue hydration effects. *J Appl Physiol* **89,** 2365–2372.

Thamer, C., Machann, J., Staiger, H., *et al.* (2010) Interscapular fat is strongly associated with insulin resistance. *J Clin Endocrinol Metab* **95,** 4736–4742.

Tinsley, F.C., Taicher, G.Z., and Heiman, M.L. (2004) Evaluation of a quantitative magnetic resonance method for mouse whole body composition analysis. *Obes Res* **12**, 150–160.

Van Wylen, G.J. and Sonntag, R.E. (1965) *Fundamentals of Classical Thermodynamics*. Wiley, New York.

Wang, Z., Shen, W., Withers, R.T., *et al.* (2005) Multicomponent molecular-level models of body composition analysis. In S.B. Heymsfield, T.G. Lohman, Z. Wang, *et al.* (eds), *Human Body Composition*, 2nd Edn. Human Kinetics, Champaign, IL, pp. 163–176.

Wells, J.C. and Fewtrell, M.S. (2006) Measuring body composition. *Arch Dis Childhood* **91**, 612–617.

Wijnhoven, H. A., van Bokhorst-de van der Schueren, M.A., Heymans, M.W., *et al.* (2010) Low mid-upper arm circumference, calf circumference, and body mass index and mortality in older persons. *J Gerontol A Biol Sci Med Sci* **65**, 1107–1114.

Wong, W.W., Hergenroeder, A.C., Stuff, J.E., *et al.* (2002) Evaluation of body fat in girls and female adolescents: advantages and disadvantages of dual-energy X-ray absorptiometry. *Am J Clin Nutr* **76**, 384–389.

59

ESTIMATION OF DIETARY INTAKE

WIJA A. VAN STAVEREN[1], PhD, MARGA C. OCKÉ[2], PhD, AND
JEANNE H.M. DE VRIES[1], PhD

[1]Wageningen University, Wageningen, The Netherlands
[2]The National Institute for Public Health and Environment, Bilthoven, The Netherlands

Summary

In this chapter we describe the different dietary assessment methods, their strengths and weaknesses, and the importance of examining sources of error and variation. There is no best method for all purposes, and therefore the investigator has to select the method appropriate for the purpose and target group of the survey. In selecting a dietary assessment method, it is important to answer several basic questions, as follows. *Who:* Who are the subjects and is group-based or individual information wanted? *What:* What information is wanted on which foods, nutrients, or other food compounds? *When:* Is the focus usual or current diet? Are special times of the day, days of the week, or season of the year of interest? *Where:* Where food is consumed may sometimes be important–for example, whether the food was consumed at home or outside the home. *Why:* The aim of the study determines the type of information of interest, such as mean intakes of groups and distribution and characterization of individuals. It also determines how accurate data have to be to adequately answer the research question. This information plus consideration of practical issues such as available time, trained staff, computer facilities, and funding will direct a researcher to the most efficient method for answering specific research questions.

Introduction

Estimations of dietary intake always focus on food consumption of individuals or groups, but the underlying purpose may vary. For instance, metabolic studies are focused on the fate of nutrients in the body, and public health studies examine the adequacy of the diet and the relation between food consumption and health.

Various study designs exist for each objective, and the approaches are possible at different levels: national accounts of annual food availability per head of the population (food balance sheets), family budget and household consumption surveys, and individual food intake or dietary surveys. In the context of this book, we will concentrate on dietary methods. Several dietary assessment tools directed at the individual are available. They differ in the time frame used, the method of administration, assessment of the foods eaten, and conversion into food components. Moreover, the immediate goals (information on meals, food groups, and specific nutrients or compounds), underlying assumptions, and cognitive approaches to acquiring dietary intake information vary between dietary

Present Knowledge in Nutrition, Tenth Edition. Edited by John W. Erdman Jr, Ian A. Macdonald and Steven H. Zeisel.
© 2012 International Life Sciences Institute. Published 2012 by John Wiley & Sons, Inc.

TABLE 59.1 Dimensions in dietary survey methods

Assessment method	Dimension
Observation unit	Individual
	Household
	Other groups
Mode of administration	Double portion collection
	Record
	○ by mail, with or without check
	○ observation
	Interview
	○ telephone
	○ face to face
	○ computerized
	○ video
Time frame	Past intake
	○ recent past
	○ usual
	○ current
Measurement of amounts of foods	Weighing
	Estimation with/without models
Conversion into nutrients	Nutrient databases
	Direct chemical analyses

assessment methods (Table 59.1) (Cameron and van Staveren, 1988; Thompson *et al.*, 2010).

This chapter describes the main dietary assessment methods and the strengths and weaknesses of each. The concept of these methods has not changed much since the first edition of this book, but a wider range of suitable equipment and related resources for field use is available. More use is made of epidemiological studies, and the development and use of biomarkers have led to more information on sources of variation and errors inherent to these methods (Beaton *et al.*, 1994). These sources have to be taken into account in study design, data collection and treatment, and interpretation of results. Because the main causes of death are nutrition-related diseases (World Health Organization, 2003), obtaining more valid knowledge on dietary patterns is of the utmost importance.

Dietary Assessment Methods

In general, methods can be divided into two basic categories: those that record data at the time of eating (prospective methods consisting of weighed and estimated records) and those that collect data about diet eaten in the recent past or over a longer period of time (retrospective methods

consisting of 24-hour recalls, dietary history, and food frequency method).

Prospective methods may include several days of recording, sometimes accompanied by collecting duplicate samples for chemical analysis or performed by proxies, e.g. by observation. Retrospective methods may refer to recent diet (24-hour food recalls) or habitual diet (dietary history and food frequency method). The three methods differ in many aspects, but if they are performed as an interview some practical aspects are similar for all. Interviewers should have a thorough knowledge about the purpose of the method; dietary components of interest; nutrient database to be used; details of the standardized protocol, including a quality control system to minimize errors; and foods available in the marketplace (including prevalent ethnic foods) and preparation practices. The location and mode (written questionnaire, face-to-face or telephone interview, web-based application) of the assessment may affect respondents' willingness and ability to report their diet.

Also, in using face-to-face interviews, cognitive aspects should be taken into account, especially those that govern the interview process. Most important are the aspect of "relation," which makes the contribution relevant to the perceived aims of the conversation; the aspect of "quantity," which makes the interview informative but not overly elaborate; the aspect of "manner," which makes the interview clear rather than obscure; and finally the aspect of "quality," which holds the speakers not to say anything deemed false or that has insufficient basis (Greenfield and Kerr, 2008).

The success of the interview relies on the respondents' ability to remember and adequately describe their diet. Because memory of past events is based on a variety of cognitive processes, it is important to take advantage of what is known about how respondents interpret questions about their food consumption and how they remember dietary information, and how that information is retrieved, judged, and reported to the interviewer. Probing is useful, but the questions asked in an interview should be as neutral as possible.

In collaborative research all interviewers must have had the same training and must be visited regularly during fieldwork. Checks should be made to detect systematic differences among interviewers in data collecting and coding. Several aspects of the application of dietary assessment methodology may be facilitated by technology to help standardization of interviewers and to reduce costs of data collection and processing.

Dietary Records
Principles

In the weighed record technique, the subject is taught to weigh and record the food and its weight immediately before eating and to weigh any leftovers. In most surveys not all items are weighed. Where weighing would interfere with normal eating habits, describing the quantity of foods consumed is acceptable. For example, for meals eaten in a restaurant, the investigator will estimate weights from the description. The weighed method differs from the estimated record where subjects do not use a scale but keep records, in portion sizes, of all the foods they eat on one or more days. The portion sizes are described in natural units (household measures) by using the utensils commonly found in homes.

Practical Aspects

The number of days needed to record food intake depends on the aim of the survey and the expected between- and within-individual variation in intakes of the nutrients of interest. However, in practice no more than three or four consecutive days are included because of respondent fatigue. The form used to record intake is kept in a record book and may be closed or open (Nydahl *et al.*, 2009). A closed form is a precoded list of all of the commonly eaten foods in units of specified portion size. This list allows for rapid coding but could be less adequate because defined units may be unfamiliar to the subjects. A semi-open form may be meal-based and preconstructed with many foods and amount options listed, but including sufficient space for other foods. In general an open form is used more often. An optically readable food record has been tested, but a computerized record seems easier to handle.

If habitual diet is being assessed, it must be stressed that the subject must not use the opportunity to change intake. To avoid bias in response, it is advantageous not to disclose the nutrient being studied. Dietary records may be completed by someone other than the subject. For example, children <10 years old will not supply adequate records and the carer should help.

Respondents must be trained to record the level of detail needed to describe adequately the foods and amounts consumed, including the name of the food, preparation methods, and recipes. At the end of the recording period, the record should be checked in detail. The records should be coded for computer calculation as soon as possible so that the subject can be contacted again if necessary.

Strengths and Uses

Strengths include that two or more days of recording provide data on within- and between-individual variation in dietary intakes, which allows estimation of the population distribution of usual intake; multiple days of recording may allow individuals to be classified according to their usual intakes; and 2-day records kept intermittently over the year may provide an estimate of usual intake by an individual. Open-form records may provide data on less frequently eaten foods in a defined time period. Portions can be assessed or weighed to increase accuracy (Bingham *et al.*, 1995).

Weaknesses

In general, respondents must be literate and highly cooperative. This requirement may lead to response bias as a result of over-representation of more highly educated individuals who are interested in diet and health. Also, food consumed away from home may be less accurately reported, and the usual eating pattern may be influenced or changed by the recording process. In addition, since record keeping increases respondent burden, accuracy of records may decrease when the number of days increases. Finally, substantial under-reporting is suspected in specific subpopulations (e.g. obese persons) (Pietiläinen *et al.*, 2010).

Mobile telephones with an integrated camera to record food intake are new dietary record devices. It appears that adolescents readily adopt such technology, but, for valid assessment of food intake, improvements in the food-record design, the images, and the training of participants are required.

Twenty-Four-Hour Food Recall
Principles

An individual recalls actual food and beverage intake for the immediate past 24 or 48 hours or for the preceding days. The 24-hour food recall is the most common recall used. Food quantities are usually assessed by use of household measures, food models, or photographs.

Practical Aspects

The diet recall was traditionally conducted by a personal interview with open forms, precoded questionnaires or tape recorders, but computer-assisted interviews have become common (Slimani *et al.*, 1999; Conway *et al.*, 2003). More recently, self-administered computerized 24-hour diet recalls have been developed (Zimmerman *et al.*, 2009). In the case of interviews, training of the interviewers is crucial because diet is recalled by asking probing questions. Most commonly the recalled day is defined as from when the respondent gets up until the respondent gets up the next day. The 24-hour recall is often structured with specific probes to help the respondent to remember all foods consumed throughout the day. Sometimes at the end of the interview there is a checklist with foods or snacks that might be easily forgotten. For children (Baxter, 2009) and elderly people (Kumanyika *et al.*, 1997), specific adaptations to their cognitive processes can improve the recall process. For this purpose, computer-assisted 24-hour recalls usually consist of multiple steps (Conway *et al.*, 2003).

Because the recall method depends on subjects' ability to remember and adequately describe their diet, this method is not suitable for children younger than ≈7 years and many adults ≥75 years. The 24-hour recall method is appropriate for describing the mean intakes of groups of individuals. Days of the week must be equally represented. Two or more non-consecutive repeated 24-hour recalls in combination with statistical modeling allow estimation of the usual intake distribution of individuals. It is advised that no prior notification be given to the subjects about whether or when they will be interviewed about their food intake. Although notification could help the memory of some subjects, others might change their usual diet for the occasion (Cameron and van Staveren, 1988).

Strengths and Uses
The design of the method is appropriate for describing the mean intake of a group (Beaton *et al.*, 1979). Two or more days provide data on within- and between-individual variation, which allows for the estimation of the distribution of usual intake; open interviews provide data on less frequently eaten foods and are not culture specific, administration time can be short, the time period is well defined, and, in the event of interviewer administration, literacy is not required. Response rates are usually rather high for recalls. Administration by a dietician allows probing for incomplete information and requires fewer callbacks.

Weaknesses
Weaknesses are that respondents' recall depends on short-term memory and it is known that omission and intrusions occur; portion size is difficult to remember and might be misestimated; and intakes tend to be under-reported. A 1-day intake does not reflect usual dietary intake of an individual and does not provide information on within-individual variation. The method is vulnerable to variability between interviewers, and requires substantial staff time for interviewing, processing, and quality control. This is also the case for interviewer-administered computerized 24-hour recalls.

Dietary History
Principles
The dietary history assesses an individual's total daily food intake and usual meal pattern over varied periods of time. In practice the history usually covers the past month, 6 months, or 1 year. Originally, Burke (1947) developed the dietary history technique in three parts, including (1) an interview about the subject's usual daily pattern of food intake with quantities specified in household measures; (2) a cross-check using a detailed list of foods; and (3) a food diary in which the subject recorded food intake for 3 days. Today the diet history is applied in many ways. The meal pattern and the checklist of foods are considered as essential for the method, but the 3-day record is often omitted.

Practical Aspects
In an open interview the subject is questioned about a typical day's eating pattern or, alternatively, the interview may start with a 24-hour recall. The purpose of the study must be so well known to the interviewer that it is easy for him or her to judge how much detailed information should be collected for each food group. Usual portion sizes are estimated with standard household measures and may be checked by weighing.

Because a dietary history aims to record a food pattern, it is a more complex interview than the 24-hour recall which records only the food consumption of the day before the actual interview. This makes a diet history too difficult to administer for a non-nutritionist. Exceptions may be diet histories guided and controlled by a precoded interview form or computer software, especially if they are developed for self-administration.

The diet history is also more demanding for the subject. It is not appropriate for individuals with a large day-to-day variation in their diet, because the method asks for a habitual dietary pattern. A satisfactory history is not always obtained from young children (Waling and Larsson, 2009), people preoccupied with weight problems, and mentally retarded people.

A short version of this method with a limited checklist of foods is often used in the clinical setting for diagnosis and as a basis for therapeutic dietary guidelines.

Strengths and Uses

The dietary history is used for assessment of usual meal patterns and details of food intake. The data can be applied to classify in categories (e.g. quantiles) of intake and to assess the relative average intakes of groups of people and the distribution of intakes within these groups. Respondent literacy is not required for an interviewer-administered dietary history (Thompson and Subar, 2008)

Weaknesses

Respondents are asked to make many judgments about the usual food intake and the amounts of those foods, and the recall period is difficult to conceptualize accurately. Reports covering a longer period may be influenced by present consumption and reveal higher estimates. Respondents need to have a regular dietary pattern and a good memory, which may hamper getting a representative sample of the population. It may become even more difficult in future, because an increasing number of people snack throughout the day. Highly trained nutritionists with well-developed social skills are required to conduct the interview, and the interview is very liable to evoke socially desirable answers. Finally, because there is no standardized technique for conducting a diet history, the performance differs between studies.

Food Frequency Method
Principles

The first food frequency questionnaires were developed for large epidemiological studies, for instance on the relation between diet and chronic disease. In such studies the diet history puts too heavy a burden on subject and investigator.

The questionnaire is a pre-printed list of foods on which subjects are asked to estimate the frequency and very often also the amount of habitual consumption during a specified period. The types of foods vary between questionnaires depending on whether the researcher is interested in specific nutrients or the total diet. The list of foods on a food frequency questionnaire may be developed in several ways (Willett, 1998; Molag *et al.*, 2010). For epidemiological studies the best way is to select foods contributing most to the variance of intake from a recent food-consumption database of a similar population as the target population. A nutrient value must be assigned for each food item listed. The value is based most often on weight-

ing each food in an item by usage. The first questionnaires did not include quantitative estimates other than servings or portions per day, week, or month. The data from these questionnaires are based on the assumption that total intake is more determined by variation in consumption frequency than by variation in portion size, and that consumption frequency is unrelated to consumed quantities. Nevertheless, some investigators have built a quantitative aspect into the technique and called their method a semi-quantitative food frequency method. Not all investigators advocate inclusion of portion sizes, because errors made by the estimation may outweigh the variance in intake of most foods.

Practical Aspects

Food frequency questionnaires vary in the foods listed, the length of the reference period, response intervals for specifying frequency of use, procedure for estimating portion size, and manner of administration. Often there is a tension between the length of the questionnaire and the required detail of information. The longer the food list, the more detailed the information; however, the respondent may become tired and subsequently less precise in answering the questions. From a review by Molag *et al.* (2007) that investigated the characteristics of FFQs, it became clear that more accurate results were obtained with longer FFQs (200 vs. 100 items). However, longer FFQs have the risk that respondents do not complete the FFQ. The development of the food list is crucial to success and takes a lot of time, especially since a validation study has to be part of the development.

If the food frequency method is administered by an interviewer, all requirements mentioned for the diet history and 24-hour recall have to be taken into account but nutritionists are not necessarily required for the interview. The advantage of a food frequency method is that the food list can be completely standardized, which reduces between-interviewer variation. For the respondents it may be cognitively difficult to combine the intake of similar foods or mixed dishes over a longer period of time and to report about them in one question. Therefore separate questions might be introduced. A disadvantage is that these questions may lead to double counting. It is important to address the best time frame for the study objective, although it is questionable whether respondents can accurately report over a period longer than 2 months. Because the questionnaire is usually self-administered, the accompanying instructions are important. Web-based questionnaires have the advantage that they can easily give cognitive support and prevent respondents skipping questions.

Strengths and Uses

The food frequency method estimates the usual food (group) intake of an individual. When portion sizes are included or when certain assumptions are made, individuals can be ranked according to nutrient intake. A self-administered questionnaire may require little time to complete and to code; the response burden is generally low, and response rates, therefore, are high. The method can be automated easily and is not very costly.

Weaknesses

Weaknesses of this method include that memory of food use in the past is required and that the respondents' burden is governed by number and complexity of foods listed and quantification procedure. The listing of foods may be incomplete or missing details. The quantification of portion sizes might be less accurate than in records or recalls. Also, the development and testing of the food list will take much time; no information on day-to-day variation is provided; and the suitability is questionable for sub-populations who consume culture-specific foods not on the list. Longer food lists and longer reference periods often lead to overestimation of intake, and the cognitive process for answering questions about food frequency may be more complex than those about a daily food pattern. Because of these problems, relationships in epidemiological studies are attenuated and thus may obscure existing relationships.

Other Methods

Several brief dietary assessment methods have been developed. These instruments may be useful in clinical settings or for health promotion if only information of a part of the diet or qualitative information of the total intake is required. For example, a fat screener might be useful to increase awareness about unhealthy eating habits and in this way activate interest to alter consumption (Thompson and Subar, 2008). In addition, new technologies might allow so-called snapshot techniques, which collect detailed information on dietary practice at a specific point in time such as single meals or purchases rather than intake of a complete day (Illner *et al.*, 2010).

Combined Methods

Sometimes a combination of two or more methods provides greater accuracy. A combination might balance the shortcomings and strengths, as summarized in Table 59.2, of one method with those of another. For example, a 2-day record or 24-hour recalls combined with a food frequency list may provide valid absolute mean intakes of groups, including within- and between-individual variation as well as a classification of high-risk groups for low (e.g. iron) or high (e.g. cholesterol) intakes. The information from the records or recalls provides details about the type and amount of foods consumed and the FFQ provides information on the propensity of a person to consume the food, which is especially helpful if foods are consumed infrequently (Tucker, 2007). A combination of methods might be too expensive for small-scale studies but is often done in large multicenter studies (Kaaks *et al.*, 1994) or

TABLE 59.2 Sources of error in techniques for estimating food consumption

Sources of error	Weighed record	24-hour recall	Diet history	Food frequency
Variation with time	+	+	−	−
Response errors:				
omitting foods	+	+	+	
including foods	−	+	+	+
estimation of weight of foods	−	+	+	+
estimation of frequency of consumption of foods	n.a.	n.a.	+	+
changes in real diet	+	+/−	−	−
Errors in conversion into nutrient:				
FC tables	+	+	+	+
coding	+	+	+	−

+, error is likely; −, error is unlikely; n.a., not applicable.

TABLE 59.3 Estimation of time to be spent by the fieldworker for one interview on administration, coding, and checking

Method	Administration explanation (minutes)	Check completeness of interview (minutes)	Coding (minutes)
Weighted record 3 days *face-to-face* interview excluding travel time	30	30	60
24-hour recall	30	5–30	30
Diet history	45–90	–	60
Scannable FFQ	30–60	5	5–10 (scan)

nationwide surveys (Beaton *et al.*, 1997), often facilitated with automated methods. Another example is the 24-hour recall assisted by a food record. Lytle *et al.* (1993) concluded that this was a valid method for assessing the dietary intake of children. During interviews by trained staff the children used diaries to record their food intake and recalled their 24-hour food intakes using the diary as a memory prompt. Combined methods are more time consuming for respondents and fieldworkers, although computers have facilitated the blending of methods. Table 59.3 gives an estimation of the time required for fieldworkers for interviewing, checking, and coding.

Assessment of Specific Food Components and Dietary Supplements

Micronutrients and Bioactive Components

Knowledge of the validity of micronutrient status parameters as well as validity of intake measures is still limited, and further improvements in methods to assess micronutrient status are needed (Allen, 2009). The European Commission's EURopean micronutrient RECommendations Aligned Network of Excellence (EURRECA) reviewed the validity of dietary assessment methods for use in epidemiologic studies with a special focus on micronutrients (Serra Majem, 2009). Their findings support the value of current methods, when applied according the current rules. For many diseases, research interest has also shifted to the bioactive components of foods, such as flavonoids, glucosinolates, allyl compounds, and phytoestrogens. Dietary measurement tools often need to be adapted specifically to the bioactive component of interest. Moreover, assessment of these components requires good data about the content of the bioactive components in foods, which are often not available in food composition tables, necessitating chemical analyses in individual foods or replicate portions.

Dietary Supplements, Fortified Foods, and Functional Foods

Terms for dietary supplements, such as multivitamins or multiminerals, are widely used, but they have no standard scientific regulatory or marketplace definitions. Thus the composition and characteristics of these products vary. Also systematic information on the bioavailability and bioequivalence of vitamins and minerals in foods and other marketed products and on potential drug interactions is scarce. Collection of valid data on (components of) supplement use is therefore difficult (Yetley, 2007). This is problematic because, in Northern American and Western European populations, the use of dietary supplements, fortified foods, and functional foods is substantial. These products can contribute >50% of micronutrient intake for an individual. Failure to include such important sources of nutrient intake can result in estimates of intake that bear little relation to biochemical status, which is often the ultimate parameter of interest. Supplement users may take supplements irregularly. Therefore, to take a measure of supplement use on one or a few days as a proxy for long-term intake incorporates measurement error that attenuates measures of association with status parameters (Patterson *et al.*, 1998). The same conclusions will probably hold for fortified and functional foods.

In large-scale studies focusing on diet–disease relations, the frequency and number of supplements taken seem to be much more important than precision about content. Distinction between single and multiple vitamin supplements is essential; distinction between one-a-day and high-dose types is desirable. Within each of these subtypes the exact brand name or exact content does not seem to be necessary because assumptions about the amount will be approximately correct. For assessment of actual intake – in contrast to usual intake – and for quantitative assessment of the distribution of intake for a population, brand name and dose information are relevant.

An approach similar to that used for dietary supplements will probably work for foods marketed in a fortified or functional version as well as the ordinary version. Examples of such foods are milk products when calcium is the component of interest: consumers will probably know whether they buy the fortified version, and amounts of added calcium will not vary substantially. Usual intake of milk can then be questioned separately for calcium-fortified milk as a generic term. However, for many other types of functional foods, information at the brand-name level and subtype will be required. This may be the case because the consumer is unaware of consuming a fortified or functional product, the consumer does not know the specific content of the product, or the amounts of added components in some products vary enormously.

Alcohol

The assessment of alcohol intake should also be conducted carefully, because alcohol is not always considered a normal food substance. On a population level, alcohol intake might be assessed by using official data such as food balance sheets collected by the Food and Agriculture Organization of the United Nations or by using sales statistics. The advantage of such statistics is that the population is not aware of the registration, and socially desirable answers – a big problem in individual-based approaches – are thus avoided. However, these statistics do not provide data on manner and amount of alcohol consumption of specific groups or individuals, and are not very useful for epidemiological purposes. Most individual-based dietary assessment methods described here will include questions on alcohol intake. In addition, specific frequency questionnaires were developed to assess alcohol intake. Altogether, according to the literature, there are five main approaches (Feunekes *et al.*, 1999): the quantity frequency method (includes simple questions on intake of glasses of alcoholic drinks in a specific period), the extended quantity frequency (includes questions on specific drinks – wine, beer, liquor – and variability during the week and at weekends), prospective and retrospective diaries, and repeated 24-hour recall.

The mean level of alcohol intake may differ by 20% by applying various methods. Intake data yielded higher esti-mates for beer, wine, and liquor consumption than did sales information. Nevertheless, underestimation is common to all methods, and heavy drinkers will seldom participate in a survey on alcohol intake, which leads to selection bias. Ranking participants according to alcohol intake may distinguish those who consume small and large quantities sufficiently for epidemiological purposes.

There has been some discussion about including alcohol intake in research on estimating daily energy intake. On the one hand, if energy from alcohol is not included, the proportions of macronutrients contributing to the daily energy supply are incorrect. On the other hand, high alcohol intake may mask a relatively high fat intake contributing to the daily energy supply (Greenfield and Kerr, 2008).

Variation and Error

The choice of the most appropriate assessment tool depends on purpose and design, type of information required (such as means, medians, distribution), and practical issues (e.g. availability of funding, time, and skilled staff; characteristics of the subjects). In order to select the most appropriate dietary method to answer a research question, it is important to understand the potential sources of variation and error for each method and their effects on the results of the study.

Sources of Variation

At the level of the individual, dietary intake is characterized by daily variation superimposed on an underlying consistent pattern (Willett, 1998). Factors such as day of the week or season often contribute to daily variation in a systematic way whereas other aspects of dietary intake are random. Dietary data collected on multiple days incorporate these kinds of variation. In food frequency questionnaires and the dietary history method, participants are asked to filter out the underlying consistent dietary pattern themselves. It can easily be imagined that this is more difficult in the absence of a regular dietary pattern. All dietary data include variation that is due to measurement error, but measurement error can also result in the loss of some of the real variance. Measurement error usually consists of a random and a systematic component.

The degree of random and systematic variation in dietary data differs across nutrients. For example, total energy and macronutrient intake have relatively little random variation whereas intake of some nutrients such

TABLE 59.4 Within-subject (CV$_w$, %) and between-subject (CV$_b$, %) coefficients of variation in nutrient data collected by repeated 24-hour dietary recalls and food frequency questionnaires

Nutrient	24-hour dietary recalls				Food frequency questionnaires			
	Men		Women		Men		Women	
	CV$_w$	CV$_b$	CV$_w$	CV$_b$	CV$_w$	CV$_b$	CV$_w$	CV$_b$
Energy	26	18	24	18	12	23	11	20
Protein	27	16	26	17	13	20	12	18
Fat	38	26	37	24	16	28	14	25
Carbohydrates	26	24	22	22	14	27	12	25
Cholesterol	56	29	52	23	17	29	15	24
Retinol	259	35	155	44	32	41	41	50
Vitamin C	65	33	68	36	26	37	32	33
Calcium	40	29	32	31	24	32	18	31

Data are based on twelve 24-hour recalls and three food frequency questionnaires in 63 Dutch men and 59 Dutch women. Reproduced with permission from Ocké *et al.* (1997).

as retinol and marine fatty acids is characterized by large random variation resulting from the large variation in their daily intake. Within- and between-subject variation in nutrient intake is illustrated in Table 59.4 with data from a Dutch validation study for 24-hour recalls repeated 12 times and from food frequency questionnaires repeated three times (Ocké *et al.*, 1997). The findings are, however, culturally determined because they depend on dietary pattern.

Measurement Error

From a methodological point of view, four types of measurement error exist: random within-person error, systematic within-person error, random between-person error, and systematic between-person error (Willett, 1998). Systematic error is also called bias. The types and size of error vary with the particular dietary assessment method and probably also with the population in which it is applied. (See also Table 59.2.)

Random within-person error may be due to day-to-day variation in an individual's daily intake when habitual intake is estimated. Thus, error in this methodological sense is not a mistake in the data collection but rather a mismatch in time frame. Random within-person error also includes errors in the measurement of intake on any occasion that are not systematic. Examples of this type of error are foods that are omitted or included falsely in dietary records or recalls, portion sizes that are estimated inaccurately, and coding mistakes. When random within-person

error is the only type of error present, the precision of the estimated mean value for an individual depends on the within-subject variation and the number of replicate measurements, as shown in equation 1. This equation can also be rearranged to calculate the number of days required to estimate mean intake for an individual given the size of the random variation and the precision that is needed (Beaton *et al.*, 1979):

$$D_0 = Z_\alpha \frac{CV_w}{\sqrt{n}} \qquad (1)$$

where D_o is the greatest deviation from the mean (as a percentage of long-term true intake), Z_α is the normal deviate for the percentage of times the measured value should be within a specified limit (1.96 for 95% confidence), CV_w is the within-subject coefficient of variation, and n is the number of days for the person.

Systematic within-person error may be caused when a person consciously or unconsciously underestimates or exaggerates his food intake. An important food for an individual that is not included in a questionnaire or a question that is systematically misunderstood by an individual will also lead to systematic within-person error. If the dietary assessment method is repeatedly administered, the error will occur again. Consequently, the estimation of mean intake for an individual is not improved by repeated measurements and remains biased. Increasing evidence suggests that most dietary assessment methods, including those for recalls and records, are likely to be flawed with systematic person-specific biases (Kipnis *et al.*, 2003).

Random between-person errors may be due to random and systematic within-person errors if they are distributed randomly across individuals; an overestimation by some individuals is counterbalanced by an underestimation by others. The estimated mean intake is consequently not biased but the precision is affected and the distribution of measured intake is artificially widened. Estimates for the percentage of subjects below or above a certain cut-off level (e.g. estimated average requirement, EAR) are therefore not valid. Also, the validity of measures of associations with health parameters is hampered and for univariate association is attenuated. In equation 2 it is shown that the precision of the estimate of the mean group intake can be improved by increasing the number of subjects or the number of replicate measurements (Beaton *et al.*, 1979):

$$D_t = Z_\alpha \sqrt{\frac{CV_b^2}{g} + \frac{CV_w^2}{gn}} \qquad (2)$$

where D_t is the greatest deviation from the mean (as a percentage of long-term true intake), Z_α is the normal deviate for the percentage of times the measured value should be within a specified limit (1.96 for 95% confidence), CV_b is the between-subject coefficient of variation, CV_w is the within-subject coefficient of variation, g is the number of persons, and *n* is the number of days per person.

Systematic between-person error is caused by systematic within-person error that is not randomly distributed across individuals. The use of questionnaires that fail to include important foods for a population, or of incorrect standard portion sizes; people giving socially desirable answers; and recalls or records that do not include weekend days, will all result in systematic between-person error. As a result the mean intake is not estimated correctly, nor is the percentage of persons above or below a certain cut-off level. Testing whether an association with a health parameter exists is not affected by systematic between-person error that applies equally to all subjects. However, this error may be associated with a variable for which the relation to dietary intake is the topic of study, and a misleading conclusion might be drawn. An example is body mass index: subjects with a higher body mass index underreport their energy intake more than those with lower body mass index.

TABLE 59.5 The effects of random and systematic between-person error in dietary intake on parameters to be estimated

Parameter to be estimated	Type of between-person error	
	Random	Systematic
Mean intake	Precision ↓	Validity ↓
Distribution of intake	Validity ↓	No effect
% of subjects below RDA	Validity ↓	Validity ↓
Association with health outcome	Validity ↓	No effect

Prepared by Jan Burema.

The effects of random and systematic between-person measurement error on various parameters to be estimated are summarized in Table 59.5. Formulas and statistical models that correct for the effects of random measurement error are now available for many outcome measures such as the distribution of intake and measures of associations with other variables such as correlation coefficients, regression coefficients, and relative risks (Willett, 1998; Carroll *et al.*, 2006). Information on the size of random measurement error can be obtained from dietary reproducibility and validity studies. The former only gives information on part of the total random between-person error (i.e. not that based on systematic within-person error). In theory, validity studies supply information on the total error. However, in practice this is limited by the lack of a true gold standard, that is, dietary assessment methods without errors or with completely independent errors. The OPEN study (Kipnis *et al.*, 2003) is an example of a study that gives insight in the error matrix for 24-hour diet recalls and food frequency questionnaires.

Quality control checks can indicate systematic measurement error. An often-used check for underestimation is the ratio of energy intake to estimated basal metabolic rate. If this ratio is below a certain cut-off value, energy intake is very likely underreported (Willett, 1998; Livingstone and Black, 2003; Abbot *et al.*, 2008). Techniques for adjustments are not well developed for systematic measurement error associated with parameters of interest.

Assessment in Specific Situations

Clinical Settings

Diet might be assessed in a clinical setting for diagnostic purposes, as a screening tool for probable dietary risk, or as a basis for dietary advice. The required accuracy of the collected information depends on the purpose of the data collection. However, because dietary treatments should be evidence based rather than experience based, a reproducible estimate – standardized for specific purposes of the assessment – is required so that the results of treatment can be evaluated and compared. When current diet is the information of interest, structured questionnaires based on the meal pattern of the clinic may be efficient. This type of questionnaire can be computerized.

Geographic and Ethnic Differences

In remote areas food policy is more concerned than it is in the industrialized world with how people produce or otherwise obtain their food and how they deal with it. A method for collecting these data is food ethnography. This method is introduced by anthropologists with the aim of getting more insight into responses of populations to natural, social, cultural, and economic pressures. Food ethnography provides a descriptive analysis of the food system and food habits; it includes the ways in which individuals or groups choose, prepare, consume, and make use of available foods. The main deterrents to surveying remote areas are the cost and time involved in fielding survey teams. Mail, telephone, and internet services can be inexpensive alternatives to face-to-face interviewing. Special sampling techniques and procedures can be used to limit the geographical scatter of the sample selected from remote areas. Cluster sampling, for example, can reduce the number of such locations selected without affecting the representativeness of the sample, substantially reducing the logistic demands and operating costs of the survey (Cameron and van Staveren, 1988; Den Hartog et al., 2006).

Otherwise, for a quick insight in the adequacy of the diet, a food diversity score can give insight. It is well known that, in remote societies, diversity of available food can be very narrow. It is possible to survive and maintain health with narrow food diversity, if the foods are sufficiently nutrient dense and different in composition. Wahlqvist and Lee among others developed a food diversity score, which can be used as a kind of screening for the adequacy of food intake (Wahlqvist et al., 2009).

When an in-depth dietary assessment is required in minority groups with a strong ethnic identity, note that structured questionnaires or records need to be adapted. Employing interviewers with the same background if possible is a great help. Food composition databases should be checked for completeness regarding ethnic foods and recipes. Photo books are often necessary for identifying foods (Den Hartog et al., 2006).

Assessment in Specific Populations

Individuals with Disabilities

Disabilities affecting sight, hearing, speech, memory, or the ability to write are particular problems in the collection of all kinds of data, including dietary intake data from affected individuals. If only one faculty is affected, survey methods relying on other faculties will provide the solution needed. For example, carefully prepared, self-explanatory, written instructions and questionnaires are required when the subject of a study is deaf. The process can be helped by using printed instructions, questionnaires, and probing techniques or a sign-language interpreter. Replica models or pictures can help the identification of the foods and the quantity consumed. If speech is impaired, provision should be made for written responses.

When respondents are unable to answer, surrogate responders may be used. Individuals who are closest to the subject (e.g. carers) are assumed to be the best surrogate responders not only because they know the most about a subject's lifestyle but also because their commitment is probably greater (Den Hartog et al., 2006; Emmett, 2009). In institutionalized persons, e.g. care-dependent elderly, proxies may use an observation method, although it is not possible to apply such an intensive method to large numbers of residents (de Vries et al., 2009). Mean frequencies of food-group use reported by subjects and surrogates are more or less similar, depending on the type of food (e.g. frequencies are better for drinks than for other foods). Furthermore, although subjects reporting themselves at the extremes of the distribution seldom are reported by their surrogate to be at the other extreme, many are reported to be in the middle of the distribution. This limits the usefulness of surrogate information for analyses that rely on proper ranking of people. When surrogates are included in a study, analyses should also be conducted after the surrogates are excluded in order to examine the sensitivity of reported associations to possible biases in the surrogates' reports.

Another possibility is observation by interviewers. To adequately observe food habits, however, the interviewer needs to stay for one or more days in the home. The presence of an outsider may interfere with daily life. People may refrain from eating low-esteemed foods for reasons of dignity or vice versa, making the diet less varied and healthier. After some time subject and interviewer become used to one another, but this may take a lot of time.

Young Children

Young children up to the age of 7 years have insufficient ability to cooperate in dietary assessment procedures. Therefore parents or other carers have often functioned as surrogate respondents. Studies comparing direct observations with recalls by parents suggest that the latter are reliable reporters of food intake at home but not of consumption outside the home.

From the age of 8 years onwards there is a rapid increase in the ability to self-report food intake. Issues to take into account are limitations of memory, concept of time, attention span, and knowledge of foods and food preparation. Food preference and rapidly changing food habits affect the reliability of recall of food consumption. Of key importance in designing questionnaires is to understand how food-related information is organized in memory and subsequently retrieved in dietary recall. Domel *et al.* (1994) developed a model that showed that the most usual retrieval mechanism categories employed by children were: visual imagery (the color of foods and their shape); usual practice (familiarity with eating the food previously); behavior chaining (linking foods to other food items or activities during the meal) and food preference. In order to improve recall accuracy, the retention interval between intake and report must be minimized. For example, for a 24-hour recall interview it is preferable that no meals be consumed between the last meal to be reported and the start of the interview. Using photographs and technology, children were found to estimate food portion size with an accuracy approaching that of adults (Domel *et al.*, 1994). By adolescence, cognitive abilities should be fully developed; limiting problems in that age are issues of motivation and body image. Techniques including attractive technologies may improve reports because they may increase motivation, cooperation, and recognition of types of foods and portion sizes (Baxter, 2009).

The Elderly

When people become older the risk of disabilities increases. Ability of older adults to participate in dietary assessment studies requires careful consideration. Up to the age of 70 years, ability to participate will not differ seriously from that of younger adults. Accurate reporting by elderly people up to their 80s is regularly found, but older people may tend to report food habits from earlier in life. For these higher age groups, some techniques as reported above may help them to report reliably on their food intake. Because memory fades with age, surveying the elderly requires particular care. Adaptations of recording methods and diet histories have resulted in valid reports for older adults. As in adolescents a picture-sort technique including a cognitive processing approach helps elderly people to remember what they usually eat (Kumanyika *et al.*, 1997). With regard to 24-hour recalls and food frequency questionnaires, the possibility of cognitive decline needs to be borne in mind. For food frequency questionnaires, reviewing these with participants remains important in this group, especially in order to check that no answers to questions have been omitted. Therefore, testing the method of data collection is particularly important in this age group to ensure valid results. It may also be helpful to use a combination of different techniques, for example, a food record combined with dietary recall (de Vries *et al.*, 2009).

Equipment for Dietary Surveys

Mode of Administration and Survey Forms

Interviews may be conducted either face to face at home or in special settings, or by telephone. Also questions can be mailed, or computerized and asked via special websites. Each mode has advantages and disadvantages. For example, mailed and telephone interviews have lower costs, because no costs and time for traveling have to be included. However, the response rates are in general lower with these types of interview. Instructions with mailed questionnaires must be clear. Portion sizes, as in telephone interviews, may be difficult to assess (Cameron and van Staveren, 1988). Computerized interviews are highly standardized, and errors in coding are minimized, but the development is costly and takes time. Face-to-face interviews require highly skilled and trained interviewers. Survey forms should be clear, logical and easy to complete.

Several new technologies in the field of dietary assessment have become available in recent years or are under development. They address several aspects of the dietary methodology, including facilitation of interviews, estimation of portion sizes, and data processing. Examples of new technologies include mobile phones with cameras to identify the types and amounts of foods consumed, allowing real-time processing of dietary data (Weiss *et al.*, 2010); in addition automated 24-hour recalls have been developed that are self-administered and make use of photographs of portion sizes (Subar, 2010). Expected advantages of these innovative technologies are greater accuracy and cost reductions. Validation is, however, always necessary.

Scales and Models

The quantities consumed can be assessed in various ways although, as explained earlier, not all approaches are suitable for all purposes. Equipment for quantifying portion sizes is not always necessary because foods can be expressed in household measures, natural or commercial units, or typical serving sizes. Examples of this approach are the amount of coffee expressed as the number of cups of coffee, the quantity of egg by the number of eggs used, and the amount of green salad in the number of cups of standard salad. This approach is cognitively easier and preferable over estimation of rates; however, it is suitable for many but not all foods. It is, for example, less accurate for vegetables and meats. Information on the weight of the reported units and serving sizes and the volume of typical household measures is required for portions to be converted to weight.

Scales

If calibrated weighing scales of good quality are used, this method is most accurate for obtaining the quantity of a food. However, the weighed quantity does not necessarily represent the quantity that would have been eaten if the weighing process were not necessary. When scales are used, they should be robust, be accurate to at least 5 g, and weigh up to 1.5 kg so that a normal plate can be used when weighing the food to be eaten. The weights of foods need not be recorded by hand, but can be done verbally, for example by using a scale with an audiocassette or a scale that is directly connected to a computer.

Food Photographs

During the past decade food photographs have been used increasingly for estimating portion sizes. In most cases a series of photographs representing different quantities are offered to the subject, who is asked to identify the photograph that most resembles the quantity consumed. Sometimes only one photograph is available for each food, and the quantity is indicated as a fraction or multiple of the amount shown. This latter approach gives rise to larger systematic error than does a series of food photographs. Several studies have examined the validity of this type of portion size estimation or the added value of food photo-

graphs versus standard amounts. The angle at which the photographs are taken as well as the number and range of depicted quantities are important for the perception of the quantities shown.

Food Models

Food replicas are three-dimensional models representing specific foods. They are lifelike in size and color and are often made of plastic. Portion-size models are more abstract and represent sizes of portions (mounds, cubes, balls, etc.) rather than specific foods. Drawings are alternative ways to help in estimating amounts of foods. The validity of the various food models seems highly dependent on the specific model and the culture of the subject. It is important to check standard portion sizes regularly, because industry tends to increase the portion sizes of the foods they produce. More foods are now prepacked, and information about portion sizes from the manufacturer is often available. Technologies such as digital photography and more sophisticated approaches have the potential to improve the estimation of portion size in dietary assessment. Young people in particular are likely to respond positively to such technologies.

Computer Software

Today software is available for almost all dietary assessment methodologies. Many computer packages for developing food frequency questionnaires, data collecting and processing, and also for converting foods to nutrients, include a nutrient database as well as software to convert subjects' food consumption into intake of energy, nutrients, and other bioactive compounds. The quality of the databases, including nutrition survey data for selecting foods, food lists and food composition data, is critically important; the quality of the data for nutrients and other food components important for answering the research questions of the survey should therefore be checked and if necessary updated. Software should be chosen on the basis of the research needs and user-friendliness. Automation has been incorporated into dietary surveys to varying degrees, and changes quickly (Thompson et al., 2010).

Future Directions

What are the trends in dietary assessment methods and where are we going? The international conferences on dietary assessment methods have tried to answer this question every four years since 1992. Main conclusions are:

- There is not and never will be a method that can estimate dietary intake without error.
- Different types of error have different effects in analyses and in interpretation of data.
- The challenge is to develop methods for error structure of data sets and statistical approaches that take that error structure better into account.
- With the increasing number of foods marketed – including enriched products and supplements – the food list and consequently the interviews become very long and boring. Especially when more than one method has to be applied, this might affect the quality of the data collections.

Future developments in this respect may include improvements such as will enable:

- work with attractive computerized questionnaires, including pictures of foods and portion sizes;
- application of a cognitive approach in these questionnaires;
- researchers to make use of an internet approach and to use strip-codes on foods.

Suggestions for Further Reading

Den Hartog, A.P., van Staveren, W.A., and Brouwer, I.D. (2006) *Food Habits and Consumption in Developing Countries. Manual for Field Studies*. Wageningen Academic Publishers, Wageningen.

Journal of the American Dietetic Association 2010: the January volume, **110**(1), is a special issue on innovations in dietary assessment technology.

Serra-Majem, L., Ngo, J., and Roman Viñas, B. (2009) Micronutrient intake assessment in Europe: best evidence and practice. *Br J Nutr* **101**(Suppl 2), S1–S112.

Tucker, K.L. (2007) Assessment of usual dietary intake in population studies of gene–diet interaction. *Nutr Metab Cardiovasc Dis* **17**, 74–81.

References

Abbot, J.M., Thomson, C.A., and Ranger-Moore, J. (2008) Psychosocial and behavioral profile and predictors of self-reported energy underreporting in obese-middle-aged women. *J Am Diet Assoc* **108**, 114–119.

Allen, L.H. (2009) Limitations of current indicators of micronutrient status. *Nutr Rev* **67**, S21–23.

Baxter, S.D. (2009) Cognitive processes in children's dietary recalls: insight from methodological studies. *Eur J Clin Nutr* **63**(Suppl 10), S19–32.

Beaton, G.H. (1994) Approaches to analysis of dietary data: relationship between planned analyses and choice of methodology. *Am J Clin Nutr* **59**, 253S–261S.

Beaton, G.H., Burema, J., and Ritenbaugh, C. (1997) Errors in the interpretation of dietary assessments. *Am J Clin Nutr* **65**, 1100S–1107S.

Beaton, G.H., Milner, J., Corey, P. *et al.* (1979) Sources of variance in 24-hour dietary recall data: implications for nutrition study design and interpretation. *Am J Clin Nutr* **32**, 2546–2559.

Bingham, S.A., Cassidy, A., and Cole, J.T. (1995) Validation of weighed records and other methods of dietary assessment using the 24 h urine nitrogen technique and other biological markers. *Br J Nutr* **73**, 531–533.

Burke, B. (1947) The dietary history as a tool in research. *J Am Diet Assoc* **23**, 1041–1046.

Cameron, M.E. and van Staveren, W.A. (1988) *Manual on Methodology for Food Consumption Studies*. Oxford University Press, New York.

Carroll, R.J., Ruppert, D., Stefanski, L.A., *et al.* (2006) *Measurement Error in Nonlinear Models: A Modern Perspective*, 2nd Edn. Chapman & Hall, London.

Conway, J.M., Ingwersen, L.A., Vinyard, B.T., *et al.* (2003) Effectiveness of the US Department of Agriculture 5-step multiple-pass method in assessing food intake in obese and nonobese women. *Am J Clin Nutr* **77**, 1171–1178.

de Vries, J.H.M., de Groot, L.C.P.G.M., and van Staveren, W.A. (2009) Dietary assessment in elderly people: experiences gained from studies in the Netherlands. *Eur J Clin Nutr* **63**, S69–S74.

Den Hartog, A.P., van Staveren, W.A., and Brouwer, I.D. (2006) *Food Habits and Consumption in Developing Countries. Manual for Field Studies*. Wageningen Academic Publishers, Wageningen.

Domel, S.B., Thompson, W.O., Baranowski, T., *et al.* (1994) How children remember what they have eaten. *J Am Diet Assoc* **94**, 1267–1272.

Emmett, P. (2009) Workshop 2: The use of surrogate reporters in the assessment of dietary intake. *Eur J Clin Nutr* **63**, S78–S79.

Feunekes, G.I.J., van't Veer, P., van Staveren, W.A., *et al.* (1999) Alcohol intake assessments: the sober facts. *Am J Epidemiol* **150**, 105–112.

Greenfield, T.K. and Kerr, W.C. (2008) Alcohol measurement methodology in epidemiology: recent advances and opportunities. *Addiction* **103**, 1082–1099.

Illner, A., Nöthlings, U., Wagner, K., *et al.* (2010) The assessment of individual usual food intake in large-scale prospective studies. *Ann Nutr Metab* **56**, 99–105.

Kaaks, R., Plummer, M., Riboli, E., *et al.* (1994) Adjustment for bias due to error in exposure assessments in multicenter cohort studies on diet and cancer: a calibration approach. *Am J Clin Nutr* **59**, 245S–250S.

Kipnis, V., Subar, A.F., Midthune, D., *et al.* (2003) The structure of dietary measurement error: results of the OPEN biomarker study. *Am J Epidemiol* **158**, 14–21.

Kumanyika, .S.K., Tell, G.S., Shemanski, L., *et al.* (1997) Dietary assessment using a picture approach. *Am J Clin Nutr* **65**, 1123S–1129S.

Livingstone, M.B. and Black, A.E. (2003) Markers of the validity of reported energy intake. *J Nutr* **133**(Suppl 3), 895S–920S.

Lytle, L.A., Nichaman, M.Z., Obarzanek, E., *et al.* (1993) Validation of 24-hour recalls assisted by food records in third-grade children. *J Am Diet Assoc* **93**, 1431–1436.

Molag, M.L., de Vries, J.H., Duif, N., *et al.* (2010) Selecting informative food items for compiling food-frequency questionnaires: comparison of procedures. *Br J Nutr* **104**, 446–456.

Molag, M.L., de Vries, J.H., and Ocké, M.C. (2007) Design characteristics of food frequency questionnaires in relation to their validity. *Am J Epidemiol* **166**, 1468–1478.

Nydahl, M., Gustafsson, I.B., Mohsen, R., *et al.* (2009) Comparison between optical readable and open ended weighed food records. *Food Nutr Res* **53**. PMID 19262685.

Ocké, M.C., Bueno de Mesquita, H.B., Pols, M.A., *et al.* (1997) The Dutch EPIC food frequency questionnaire. II Relative validity and reproducibility for nutrients. *Int J Epidemiol* **26**, 49S–58S.

Patterson, R.E., Neuhouser, M.L., White, E., *et al.* (1998) Measurement error from assessing use of vitamin supplements at one point in time. *Epidemiology* **9**, 567–569.

Pietiläinen, K.H., Korkeila, M., Bogl, L.H., *et al.* (2010) Inaccuracies in food and physical activity diaries of obese subjects: complementary evidence from doubly labeled water and co-twin assessments. *Int J Obes (Lond)* **34**, 437–445.

Serra Majem, L. (ed.) (2009) Dietary assessment methods for micronutrient intake: a systematic review. *Br J Nutr* **102**(Suppl 1), S1–S149.

Slimani, N., Deharveng, G., Charrondiere, R.U., *et al.* (1999) Structure of the standardized computerized 24-h recall interview used as reference method in the 22 centres participating in the EPIC project. European Prospective Investigation into Cancer and Nutrition. *Comput Methods Programs Biomed* **58**, 251–266.

Subar, A.F. (2010) Assessment of the accuracy of portion size reports using computer-based food photographs aids in the development of an automated self-administered 24-hour recall. *J Am Diet Assoc* **110**, 55–64.

Thompson, F.E. and Subar, A.F. (2008) Dietary assessment methodology. In A. Coulston and C. Boushey (eds), *Nutrition in the Prevention and Treatment of Disease*, 2nd edn. Elsevier, Amsterdam.

Thompson, F.E., Subar, A.F., Loria, C.M., *et al.* (2010) Need for technological innovation in dietary assessment. *J Am Diet Assoc* **110**, 48–51.

Tucker, K.L. (2007) Assessment of usual dietary intake in population studies of gene–diet interaction. *Nutr Metab Cardiovasc Dis* **17**, 74–81.

Wahlqvist, M.L., Lee, M.S., and Kouris-Blazos, A. (2009) Demographic and cultural differences in older people's food choices and patterns. In M. Raats, L. de Groot, and W. van Staveren (eds), *Food for the Ageing Population*. Woodhead Publishing, Cambridge, pp. 20–43.

Waling, M.U. and Larsson, C.L. (2009) Energy intake of Swedish overweight and obese children is underestimated using a diet history interview *J Nutr* **139**, 522–527.

Weiss, R., Stumbo, P.J., and Divakaran, A. (2010) Automatic food documentation and volume computation using digital imaging and electronic transmission. *J Am Diet Assoc* **110**, 42–44.

Willett, W.C. (1998) *Nutritional Epidemiology*, 2nd Edn. Oxford University Press, New York.

World Health Organization (2003) Diet, nutrition and the prevention of chronic diseases. Report of a Joint WHO/FAO Expert Consultation. Technical Report Series 916. WHO, Geneva.

Yetley, E.A. (2007) Multivitamin and multimineral dietary supplements: definitions, characterization, bioavailability and drug interactions. *Am J Clin Nutr* **85**(Suppl), 269S–276S.

Zimmerman, T.P., Hull, S.G., and McNutt, S. (2009) Challenges in converting an interviewer-administered food probe database to self-administration in the National Cancer Institute Automated Self-administered 24-Hour Recall (ASA24). *J Food Comp Anal* **22**(Suppl 1), S48–S51.

60

TASTE AND FOOD CHOICES

ADAM DREWNOWSKI[1], PhD AND PABLO MONSIVAIS[2], PhD, MPH

[1]University of Washington Seattle, Washington, USA
[2]Centre for Diet and Activity Research, Cambridge, UK

Summary

The concept of "food taste" includes the sensations of taste, aroma, and texture, as well as the pleasure response to foods. Although taste is an important factor, food choices are complex decisions that are also guided by cost, convenience, and concerns about nutrition. While gustatory senses and olfaction mediate the perception of food attributes, the central nervous system determines the reward value associated with food consumption. Recent research has identified specific regions of the brain and pharmacological pathways that are involved in the hedonic response to foods. Taste preferences vary with age and gender, and can be modulated by anticipation as well as by nutritional and/or physical status. The notion that taste sensitivities and preferences alone determine dietary choices and therefore health outcomes is overly narrow and ignores the many intermediate steps between taste functioning, dietary choices, and health. Public health programs to improve population diets ought to consider age-specific food preferences and social norms of food consumption as well as a wide range of demographic and socioeconomic variables that mediate the link between taste preferences and food consumption.

Introduction

Taste is said to be the most important factor influencing food purchases (Glanz *et al.*, 1998), well ahead of cost, convenience, or consumer concerns with health, weight or dietary variety (Logue, 2004). The popular concept of "taste" is based on the physiologic sensations of taste, aroma, and texture (Drewnowski, 1997a) and on the sensory pleasure response to foods (Drewnowski, 1997a, 1998). This chapter will focus primarily on taste or gusta-tion, with the aim of understanding how taste sensations contribute to food liking and the patterns of food consumption.

Taste sensations are conventionally divided into five primary tastes: sweet, sour, salty and bitter, and the savory taste of umami. The mechanisms that underlie these five taste sensitivities can be broadly grouped into those that function as ion channels (salty and sour) and those that function via G-protein-coupled pathways (sweet, bitter, and umami). Tastants such as sucrose (sweet),

Present Knowledge in Nutrition, Tenth Edition. Edited by John W. Erdman Jr, Ian A. Macdonald and Steven H. Zeisel.
© 2012 International Life Sciences Institute. Published 2012 by John Wiley & Sons, Inc.

hydrochloric acid (sour), sodium chloride (salty), and quinine (bitter) need to be dissolved in water to stimulate the taste response. Two unique compounds, propylthiocarbamide (PTC) and 6-*n*-propylthiouracil, taste bitter to some people but are completely tasteless to others. Those compounds have long served as genetic markers for the perception of bitter taste.

Taste sensations can be measured using detection thresholds (lowest detectable amounts) or by scaling the perceived taste intensity of more concentrated taste solutions. Neither detection thresholds nor taste scaling can predict individual likes or dislikes for the tasted substance. In general, humans like sweet and dislike sour, salty, and bitter tastes; however, a great deal of individual variability in taste acuity or in hedonic response is observed.

Several lines of research have sought to link individual differences in taste response to food consumption patterns and chronic disease risk. The underlying assumption was that taste responses drove food-seeking behaviors, determined energy and nutrient intakes, and so affected chronic disease risk. In reality, food choices are influenced by a myriad of cultural, social, and economic variables in addition to taste.

In reality, there are multiple steps between an individual's gustatory profile and his or her food choices (Drewnowski, 1997a, 1998) and chronic disease risk. First, very few studies have examined taste responses, food preferences, and nutrient intakes in the same subject population. No direct association between taste function and health outcomes can be made, and in the absence of longitudinal data no causal pathways can be drawn. Secondly, population eating habits are influenced by age, gender, and energy needs, as well as by demographic and socioeconomic factors, making it difficult to link taste-related variables with particular health outcomes. Thirdly, there is new appreciation that taste responses are not static but can be modulated over the course of days and even hours, partly as a result of changes in nutritional status and partly as a result of activity in particular neuroendocrine systems.

The factors that influence taste and food preferences operate at multiple levels and can range from molecular biology to economics (Figure 60.1). Whereas the individual responsiveness to sugars or fat texture may depend on physiologic variables (Mattes, 2005), there is little doubt that the relatively low cost and accessibility of these nutrients in the modern food supply promotes their consumption (Drewnowski, 1998). Examining some of these

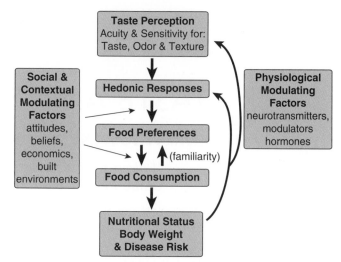

FIG. 60.1 Hypothesized chain of events between sensory perception and food consumption and nutritional status. At least three steps lie between sensitivity to taste stimuli and nutritional status, body weight, and disease risk. The strength of some links is modulated by various factors. Note that taste perception, hedonic responses, and food preferences receive feedback from a number of sources.

causal pathways linking taste with food selection is the topic of this review.

Measuring Taste Responses

Assessments of taste responsiveness measure taste perception as well as taste preferences. Taste perception includes taste acuity, determined using detection and recognition thresholds, and taste sensitivity, based on intensity scaling of more concentrated taste stimuli (Drewnowski, 2003). Most research in nutrition and taste psychophysics has focused on the detection and perception of four basic tastes: sweet, sour, salty and bitter. The typical stimuli were aqueous solutions of different simple sugars (sweet), sodium chloride (salty), citric or hydrochloric acid (sour), and either caffeine or quinine (bitter). The umami taste of glutamate was once considered to be a taste enhancer, but is now considered to be a distinct fifth taste (Beauchamp, 2009).

With the exception of bitter taste, the ability to detect extremely low concentrations of a given tastant does not predict preferences for that taste at above-threshold levels.

As a result, studies on taste and food choice have focused on intensity scaling of supra-threshold solutions (Bartoshuk, 1993) and on hedonic response profiles. Among the methods used for intensity scaling were 9-point category scales, visual analog scales (VAS), the labeled magnitude estimation scale (LMS), magnitude estimation, and other ratio scales (Mattes *et al.*, 2005). Intensity ratings recorded in taste psychophysics are on a logarithmic scale since taste, like other sensory systems, has sensitivity to stimulus concentrations that spans several orders of magnitude.

Measures of taste sensitivities are distinct from the hedonic response, a measure of the acceptability or pleasantness of a given taste stimulus. Intensity and hedonic ratings for the same taste stimuli follow different psychophysical curves. Laboratory studies have generally tested hedonic ratings for simple foods and beverages such as sugar solutions, sweetened lemonade, salted soups or tomato juice, or mixtures of milk, cream and sugar. Industry studies on the taste acceptability of more complex foods, conducted in commercial sensory evaluation laboratories, generally asked respondents to rate the acceptability of flavor, color, and texture, as well as the overall acceptability of the food product (Clydesdale, 1993). The key measure of liking has been the 9-point hedonic scale, commonly known as the hedonic preference scale (Drewnowski, 1997a).

The Taste Sensations

Taste responses, as measured by response thresholds, recognition thresholds, and hedonic responses, are both innate and acquired. Whereas much of the population's variation in response to sweetness is genetic (Keskitalo *et al.*, 2007), taste responses also evolve over the life course and can be altered by our dietary habits.

Growing children equate palatability with sweetness and selectively consume the sweetest and the most energy-dense foods (Birch, 1999). Sweetness signals food energy, and, at least for naturally sweet foods such as ripe fruits, also signals the presence of nutrients. Bitterness signals dietary danger (Drewnowski, 2001a), which is why bitter-tasting vegetables and fruits are often rejected by children and by pregnant women. Other tastes may signal other nutritional qualities. For instance, the savory umami taste, which is elicited by salts of the amino acid glutamate, may signal the protein content of foods.

Sweet Taste

Sweet foods and beverages are universally liked across all cultures and by all age groups (Drewnowski, 1997a, 1998). Hedonic response profiles for increasing concentrations of sugars are highly diverse and are strongly associated with age. While children typically show a monotonic rise in hedonic ratings with increasing sweetness, adults tend to show a non-monotonic pattern, where the degree of decline at highest sweetness levels is associated with age. For most adults, 10% of sugar in water is the ideal or optimal sweetness level. By contrast, young children aged 3–5 years did not show the characteristic hedonic optimum for sucrose, and selected the most intensely sweet solutions in the 20% range. The sweetness optimum declined during adolescence, and sweet taste preferences diminished further with age. Although taste functioning is still robust, sugar consumption among adults is less than half of what it is among younger age groups.

For children, sweetness is one of the most salient attributes of a food or beverage. Indeed young children categorized foods according to whether they were familiar or sweet (Birch, 1999). Children's preferences for intensely sweet foods and beverages have been attributed to the high energy needs of children, which increase the perceived reward value of consuming foods. This notion is rooted in a broader concept that the body's energy and nutrient requirements are dynamically manifested in taste sensitivities and preferences. Testing this concept, a number of influential studies attempted to link the taste preferences for sweetness with energy balance and body weight.

Despite many attempts, taste response profiles to increasing concentrations of sweet taste have never been linked to body weight or to body mass index (BMI = kg/m^2). Similarly, taste responses to sweetness have never been linked to dietary restraint, a measure of concern with dieting that was at one point said to measure the distance from the physiological set-point of body weight.

The suppression of taste preferences for sweetness following exposure to sweet solutions has been used as a measure of appetite control. Studies showing that obese persons did not reduce their preferences for sweet taste even after drinking 200 ml of sweet glucose solution (Cabanac and Duclaux, 1970) were used to support the argument that obese persons were hyper-responsive to sweet taste and incapable of judging whether they were hungry or not. However, the notion that obese persons failed to perceive or to respond to sweetness was abandoned as sensory studies demonstrated that taste sensitivity to sweetness of obese and lean persons was approximately the same (Thompson *et al.*, 1976). Studies using sucrose solutions, sweetened soft drinks, or chocolate milkshakes found no connection between preferences for sweetness and body weight. These studies, mostly conducted in the 1970s and 1980s, failed to make the case that a "sweet tooth" was the principal cause of human obesity.

More recent studies have shown that sweet taste can be modulated by hormones and other signaling molecules. Sweet taste receptors were found to have CB-1 cannabinoid receptors, and activation of CB-1 receptors by anandamide, an endocannabanoid, has been shown to increase the physiological response to sweetness (Yoshida *et al.*, 2010). Sweet taste threshold is also lowered by serotonin (Heath *et al.*, 2006). Countering this effect, sweet taste receptors also are responsive to leptin, a circulating peptide hormone produced by adipocytes. Leptin was found to reduce the response to sweetness by sweet taste receptors (Jyotaki *et al.*, 2010).

Bitter Taste

From birth, humans dislike and reject bitter tastes (Drewnowski, 1985, 2001a; Birch, 1999), which are a universal signal for potential dietary danger. The sensitivity to bitter taste is highest in infants, young children, and pregnant women, who would be the groups most vulnerable to bitter-tasting dietary toxins. The more intensely tasting bitter stimuli are most likely to be rejected (Drewnowski, 2001a). The acceptance of bitter taste, when present, has to be learned over time. Recent studies show that the newborn infant's rejection of sour and bitter solutions has changed to partial acceptance after the first year of life (Schwartz *et al.*, 2009). Even so, young children dislike bitter chocolate, preferring instead white chocolate, from which all bitter-tasting compounds have been removed. Adults learn to tolerate bitter taste later in life, especially when the bitter taste is accompanied by fat (chocolate), caffeine (coffee), or alcohol (beer) (Drewnowski, 2001a).

Genetic sensitivity to bitter tastes has been systematically explored using two bitter compounds: phenylthiocarbamide and 6-*n*-propylthiouracil (PROP). Individual taste sensitivity to these compounds is an inherited trait with an identified genetic basis (Kim *et al.*, 2003). The ability to taste phenylthiocarbamide/PROP has been associated with higher sensitivity to selected bitter compounds and with aversions to some bitter foods (Tepper, 2008).

Whether genetic PROP sensitivity, by affecting bitter taste, predicts food choices and dietary habits has been a topic of some debate (Duffy and Bartoshuk, 2000; Duffy, 2004; Drewnowski *et al.*, 2007; Tepper *et al.*, 2009).

Although plant-based diets, rich in cruciferous and other vegetables, may be protective against cancer, the active phytochemicals are almost always bitter, acrid, or astringent (Barratt-Fornell and Drewnowski, 2002; Drewnowski and Gomez-Carneros, 2002). Chemopreventive phenols, tannins, lignans, flavonoids, isoflavones, and glucosinolates impart a perceptible bitter taste to many vegetables and fruit (Drewnowski and Gomez-Carneros, 2002). Drewnowski and Rock (1995) first suggested that genetic taste markers might have an influence on the ability of cancer patients' compliance with therapeutic diets that were phytonutrient-rich, namely bitter-tasting vegetables and fruit. Based on previous research (Fischer *et al.*, 1963; Glanville and Kaplan, 1965), bitter brassica vegetables such as Brussels sprouts, cabbage, spinach, and kale are often disliked the most (Drewnowski and Gomez-Carneros, 2002).

While studies have been able to link PROP taster status taste responses to some bitter foods and some food preferences, no links were found to food consumption patterns or to disease risk. The argument that "supertasters" of PROP were at lower risk for heart disease because of their alleged dislike of the texture of dairy fat (Duffy, 2004) has not been supported by observational data on fat consumption in epidemiologic studies. A recent study of women found that, relative to PROP tasters, non-tasters did not consume more fat but did consume more calories overall at a buffet meal (Tepper *et al.*, 2011). However, another study of dietary patterns, biomarkers, and BMI of over 350 women found no link between PROP taster status and nutrition and health outcomes (Drewnowski *et al.*, 2007). The lack of consistent associations between PROP sensitivity and dietary habits suggests that many moderating and mediating factors are interposed between the taste acuity measures and food-seeking behavior (Tepper *et al.*, 2009). Moreover, being highly sensitive to PROP might also reflect heightened sensitivity to other taste and texture stimuli (Lim *et al.*, 2008; Reed, 2008).

Salt Taste

Sodium is essential for normal functioning of physiological processes. The taste for salty foods is partly a reflection of homeostatic requirements for sodium, which is continuously excreted into the environment. Taste responses to sodium chloride can be modified when dietary sodium intake is restricted. Research has shown that sodium depletion, achieved by medication or diet, can shift liking for salty stimuli to levels that would be aversive under normal, non-depleted conditions (Johnson, 2007). Depletion induced by drugs or exercise can also induce liking for salty foods (Beauchamp *et al.*, 1990) and can promote the development of novel flavor preferences that are linked to saltier tastes (Wald and Leshem, 2003). The liking for salty taste thus appears to be dynamic, in response to physiological demands.

In longer term experimental studies, limiting dietary sodium to 1600 mg/day led to an increase in the hedonic value of unsalted food and a decrease in the hedonic value of salted soups (Blais *et al.*, 1986). The same study showed that sodium restriction also led to a progressive reduction in the amount of table salt added to soup by the study participants. Such shifts in liking for salty taste can occur without changes in detection or recognition thresholds for salt stimuli (Blais *et al.*, 1986; Mattes, 1997; Lucas *et al.*, 2011).

A person's sensitivity and hedonic response to salty stimuli has implications for health. For instance, higher sodium recognition thresholds have been associated with hypertension and history of type-2 diabetes (Isezuo *et al.*, 2008; Michikawa *et al.*, 2009). However, sodium recognition thresholds are not consistently associated either with liking for salty taste or with the amounts of sodium consumed (Lucas *et al.*, 2011). Other studies have failed to support the claim that higher liking for salty taste was causally linked with a higher risk of hypertension (Mattes, 1997).

Observations that the liking for salty taste was flexible and could be modified by the levels of dietary sodium has led the 2010 Dietary Guidelines to suggest that a systematic and gradual reduction to the sodium content of processed foods was the best population-based approach to lowering sodium intake. Such a reduction would be part of a comprehensive population health program to control and prevent hypertension and other chronic diseases (Cook *et al.*, 2007; Dötsch *et al.*, 2009). The current 2010 Dietary Guidelines call for a reduction in sodium intakes down to 1500 mg per person per day. The Guidelines are to be implemented gradually over time, both to give the food industry time to formulate lower sodium foods and to allow the American public to adjust taste preferences to the lower level of sodium in the food supply.

Umami Taste

Together with salt taste, umami contributes to the savoriness of foods. For over 100 years, glutamate salts, including monosodium glutamate (MSG), have been used to evoke the umami taste, enhancing the sensory quality of certain savory foods (Bellisle, 1999). Only in the last 10 years was a g-protein-coupled receptor identified for this taste (Nelson *et al.*, 2002), establishing the umami sensation as a distinct taste pathway. Laboratory-based sensory studies have shown that MSG can potentiate the perceived savoriness of foods and improve hedonic response overall (Bellisle *et al.*, 1991; Roininen *et al.*, 1996; Okiyama and Beauchamp, 1998; Schiffman, 2000; Ball *et al.*, 2002; Carter *et al.*, 2011a).

The umami taste may be important for signaling nutritional characteristics of foods. Glutamate salts are related to glutamic acid, an amino acid integral to food proteins, but glutamic acid in protein does not have the umami taste. However, protein hydrolysis that occurs during fermentation and aging can release free glutamate. For example, free glutamate is found in abundance in soy sauces, aged cheeses, and even some fresh foods such as tomatoes and shellfish. Foods that are higher in protein or higher in free glutamate may be preferred by persons with greater sensitivity to MSG (Luscombe-Marsh *et al.*, 2008).

The flavor-enhancing effects of MSG and other glutamate salts could promote food consumption, but evidence that MSG is associated with excess energy intake is mixed. In short-term experimental studies, no significant differences in hunger ratings or differences in subsequent energy intake were observed following MSG supplementation (Rogers and Blundell, 1990). In other studies, adding MSG to foods led to a selective increase in the consumption of those foods but did not increase the total food energy consumed (Bellisle, 2008). In still other studies, the addition of MSG led to higher energy intakes at the next meal (Luscombe-Marsh *et al.*, 2009) or had no effect (Carter *et al.*, 2011b). More studies on MSG and body weight are clearly required. Whereas some have found a negative relation between MSG consumption and body weight (Essed *et al.*, 2007; Kondoh and Torii, 2008; Shi *et al.*, 2010), others have pointed to a link between MSG consumption and weight gain (Hirata *et al.*, 1997; Hermanussen *et al.*, 2006; He *et al.*, 2008).

Sour Taste

Sour stimuli and sour-tasting foods are, like bitterness, instinctively aversive (Desor *et al.*, 1975) and the ability to detect sourness has a strong genetic component (Wise et al., 2007). Sourness in foods is associated with acid content, which can be higher in foods that have spoiled. An aversion to sourness can therefore be viewed as a protective trait. However, fresh foods that are rich in essential nutrients can also be sour. Studies have linked greater sour preference in children to the consumption of fresh fruit (Liem et al., 2006). With obvious health benefits associated with greater acceptance of sour taste, researchers have explored means of increasing sour taste preference. While repeated exposure over a period of 8 days does not appear to increase the linking for sour beverages (Liem and de Graaf, 2004), adding sugar to sour solutions does appear to decrease the dislike toward sourness (Capaldi and Privitera, 2008). Other research indicates that, at least for children, a liking for very sour tastes may be part of a broader acceptance toward novel and intense stimuli (Liem et al., 2004).

Sensory Response to Fats

Fats endow foods with their characteristic taste and texture, and contribute to the overall palatability of the diet. The first sensory response to fat involves perception through the nose or mouth of fat-soluble volatile flavor molecules. Oral perception of fat content has been described as sensitivity to food texture as sensed by the oral cavity during chewing or swallowing. This form of fat perception is akin to somatosensation, mediated by nerve endings responsive to pressure or pain (Mattes et al., 2009). Other mechanisms of chemosensation have been implicated, involving g-protein-coupled receptors, lipid transporters and potassium channels inhibited by free polyunsaturated fatty acids (Gilbertson et al., 2005; Kahn and Besnard, 2009).

The orosensory experience evoked by fat depends on the food product. In dairy products, fat takes the form of emulsified globules that are perceived as smooth and creamy. Water binding qualities of fat account for the tenderness and juiciness of steaks and the moistness of cakes and other baked goods. Heat transfer at high temperature gives rise to food textures that are crisp, crunchy and brittle. Among textural qualities that depend on the fat content of foods are hard, soft, juicy, chewy, greasy, viscous, smooth, creamy, crunchy, crisp, and brittle. Generally, high fat content of foods has been a desirable sensory feature, and one that is often linked with higher product quality. As with salt preferences, self-reported preferences for fat in foods may be influenced to some extent by the amount of fat in the habitual diet (Cooling and Blundell, 1998).

Interactions between Fats and Sweetness

Fat potentiates the hedonic response to sweetness. A study using 20 different mixtures of dairy products of different fat content and sweetened with different amounts of sugar found evidence for hedonic synergy. Peak hedonic ratings were obtained for stimuli containing 20% fat wt/wt and 8% sucrose wt/wt, corresponding to whipping cream with sugar (Drewnowski. and Greenwood, 1983). These studies made use of response surface methodology and three-dimensional projections of the hedonic response surface. These findings of a hedonic synergy for sugar and fat mixtures were later extended to sweetened cream cheese, the French creamy white cheese fromage blanc, cake frostings, and ice cream.

Perceptual interactions between sugar and fat depend on sensory phenotypes. The perceived sweetness of sugared solutions is positively tied to the level of added sugar but also to the amount of fat. At a constant sugar concentration, increasing the percentage of fat by shifting the base solution from water to milk and to heavy cream increased sweetness ratings, and the effect was greatest for those who rated PROP as most bitter (Hayes and Duffy, 2007). More recently, the optimal combination of sugar–fat mixtures for liking was associated with oral and sensory phenotypes. While sweet, high-fat combinations of dairy and sugar are generally liked across all groups, persons who were most sensitive to the bitter taste of PROP and quinine tended to report greater creaminess of fat-containing stimuli and to have hedonic optima at lower levels of fat and sugar than the other groups (Hayes and Duffy, 2008).

Taste Preferences and Food Choices

Preferences for sweet taste, typically measured in the laboratory using sugar solutions, are thought to predict the liking and consumption of sweet foods and beverages in real life. However, studies have shown that taste preferences for sweet and salty tastes in aqueous solution were not a good predictor of self-reported liking for sweet or salty foods (Mattes et al., 2005). Of course, many studies of food likes and dislikes employed not actual foods but printed lists of food names. Such tools merely capture respondents' attitudes toward a verbal concept of a given food, since the food itself is never presented to the subject and is not available for consumption. Best correspondence between the two sets of ratings is obtained when the taste stimulus closely resembles the food product. For example, preferences for sugar solutions in water may predict the same subjects' preferences for cola or fruit juice. However, preferences for sugar solutions in water may not predict preferences for such foods as doughnuts or candy.

Taste preferences and food choices differ over the life course and in relation to our physical conditions. Preferences and aversions are modifiable by growth, maturation, and hormonal status. Both taste preferences and food choices are further shaped by prior experience and associative learning. Preferences for aversive tastes including bitter (caffeine), alcohol, and hot spices are all said to be the result of associating the often unpleasant taste with the desirable post-ingestive consequences (Logue, 2004). A previously neutral or even unpleasant taste can become preferred, provided it is linked with a suitable mechanism of reward.

Taste and Food Choices in Childhood

Studies of preschool children have shown that food preferences in early life are determined by two factors: familiarity and sweetness (Birch, 1999). Preferences for fat may be acquired early in life, as children learn to prefer those flavors that are associated with high energy density and fat content. Fat and sugar are the chief components of peanut butter and jelly sandwiches, chocolate candy, cookies, and ice cream.

Both sweet taste preference and sugar consumption decline between adolescence and adult life (Bowman, 1999). Whereas children's food preferences are often guided by taste alone (Birch, 1999), food choices of adults also tend to be influenced by nutritional beliefs and attitudes toward weight and dieting (Logue, 2004). However, all evidence is indirect, since no study examined taste preferences, diet-related attitudes, and food intakes in the same subject group. Other studies have shown that children's preferences for high-fat foods have a familial component. Studies on children aged 3–5 years later reported that both preferences for and the consumption of fats by children were linked to body mass indices of parents (Fisher and Birch, 1995; Wardle *et al.*, 2001).

Children also show an aversion to bitter foods (Drewnowski, 2001a; Logue, 2004). Typical food dislikes are based on taste (bitter), aversive trigeminal stimulation (sharp), and a variety of unpleasant food textures. Acquired preferences for coffee, beer, alcohol, and hot peppers are commonly cited as evidence that food preferences can be learned and modified with age.

Taste and Food Choices in Aging

Age-related deficits in taste and smell are reputed to decrease the enjoyment of food and reduce food consumption leading eventually to malnutrition and ill health (Morley, 2001; Hays and Roberts, 2006). However, the evidence supporting this view is mixed. While many elderly people suffer from a olfactory deficit and some suffer from taste deficits (Murphy, 2008), their impact on food choices, nutrition and health is not always clear. Older adults can also have a decline in sensory specific satiety (Rolls, 1999), which in theory would promote more homogeneous dietary habits. However, older adults often have diets that are as varied or even more varied than younger adults (Rolls, 1999).

Most studies on taste and aging have focused on taste acuity and sensitivity rather than on enjoyment, quantified through hedonic ratings. Early studies were guided by the hypothesis that elderly subjects suffering from taste losses would prefer sweeter and saltier stimuli and so consume more sugar and salt. Though some studies reported that hedonic ratings for solutions of sucrose, sodium chloride, and citric acid increased with age, other studies failed to confirm a broad age-related shift in hedonic response. Taste function is relatively robust, and whole-mouth tasting can be normal even into advanced old age. In at least one study, older adults showed no impairments in taste sensitivity and hedonic response profiles for sucrose and sodium chloride solutions (Drewnowski *et al.*, 1996). The same study showed that preference for salty stimuli had no impact on sodium consumption.

To promote food intake by the elderly, some have suggested flavor amplification (Rolls, 1999). Intervention studies using flavor enhancers in the foods consumed by elderly participants have shown both positive (Mathey *et al.*, 2001) and negative (Essed *et al.*, 2007) results. The diets of older persons can lack variety (Marshall *et al.*, 2001), but it is difficult to attribute these patterns to sensory limitations. Other factors such as poor dentition (Marshall *et al.*, 2002; Sahyoun *et al.*, 2003) and a host of psychosocial variables, including depression, loneliness, bereavement, and social support, all have a major impact on diet habits (Ahmed and Haboubi, 2010).

Taste and Food Choices in Obesity

Much research attention has focused on those taste responses in obesity that might contribute to unhealthful eating patterns and to weight gain. Perceptual and hedonic responses to sweet and fat tastes have received the greatest attention, in part because diets of obese persons tend to be energy dense and are relatively high in refined grains, added sugars, and fats (Miller *et al.*, 1990; Bolton-Smith and Woodward, 1994). Whereas the sources of sugar and fat can vary by continent and culture, the liking for good-tasting energy-dense foods is a universal human trait.

One line of research has examined taste acuity for sweetness and fat in obese children and adolescents (Pasquet *et al.*, 2007). While detection thresholds for sweetness were the same in lean and obese adults (Malcolm *et al.*, 1980), the linking for sugar and fat mixtures did differ.

Obese women selected fat-rich taste stimuli in sensory studies, and listed high-fat foods as their favorites on food preference checklists, including doughnuts, cake, cookies, ice cream, chocolate, pies, and other desserts. Conversely, anorectic women below normal body weight had lower preference ratings overall, tending to select stimuli that were relatively sweet but virtually fat-free (Drewnowski, 1989). Obese women and women who had recently lost weight gave the highest hedonic ratings to the energy-dense mixtures of sugar and fat (Drewnowski *et al.*, 1985). Those formerly obese patients were struggling at the time against weight regain. These findings are consistent with more recent studies showing that BMI was positively associated with dietary fat intake (Ahluwalia *et al.*, 2009).

Less is known regarding weight-related differences in perception or preference for savory or salty foods. Thresholds for salt were lower in obese adolescents (Pasquet *et al.*, 2007), and BMI of adults was positively associated with preference for salty and fatty foods (Keskitalo *et al.*, 2008). Obese women were less sensitive to the taste of MSG and preferred significantly higher levels in soup than normal-weight women (Pepino *et al.*, 2010). Obese men reported preferences for steaks, roasts, hamburgers, French fried potatoes, and pizza (Drewnowski, 1997a,b). These findings were consistent with intake data from studies showing that obese adults tend to over-consume energy-dense, salty foods (Cox *et al.*, 1999).

In some studies, taste preference profiles were linked to increased risk of weight gain. For example, a more favorable rating of sweetened, high-fat, dairy beverages was associated with weight gain in Pima Indians (Salbe *et al.*, 2004). Japanese adults who reported preferring rich and heavy foods (fat) and sweet foods also gained more weight than those who did not report such preferences (Matsushita *et al.*, 2009). Reducing body weight through surgery appears to lead to changes in taste perception and preferences. Obese patients who underwent bariatric surgery

showed increased sensitivity to sweet taste (Miras and le Roux, 2010). The surgery has also been shown to reduce obese adults' motivation to eat highly palatable foods (Schultes *et al.*, 2010).

Neurobiology of Taste and Appetite

Human beings eat for survival, maintaining energy balance and fulfilling their nutrient needs. The impulse to eat in response to an energy deficit is a powerful motivational drive that is controlled by several regions of the hypothalamus and pharmacological pathways of the brain (Kalra and Kalra, 2004; Wurst *et al.*, 2007). But eating is also one of life's greatest pleasures, and the taste senses mediate the enjoyment of food independent of hunger (Lowe and Butryn, 2007). The hedonic motivations to eat involve anticipation (wanting/craving) and reward (liking) associated with consuming palatable foods and beverages (Berridge, 1996; Barbano and Cador, 2007a), which can override homeostatic signals to promote excess energy intake and the development of obesity. While the neurobiological substrates and pharmacological pathways controlling hedonic motivations are to some extent shared with those involved in homeostatic regulation of appetite, some differences are apparent (Barbano and Cador, 2007b; Kenny, 2011).

Craving and Wanting

Studies of food cravings have implicated the serotonergic system, endogenous opiate peptides, and endocannabinoids. Serotonergic pathways were first linked to food cravings and intake from studies of clinically depressed individuals (Pelchat, 2002; Pelchat, 2009). Serotonin is primarily associated with cravings for carbohydrates in what is thought to be a homeostatic regulatory process: Low serotonin levels stimulate the ingestion of carbohydrates, which can increase levels of L-tryptophan, the metabolic precursor of serotonin (Pelchat, 2002; Yanovski, 2003).

Endogenous opiates or endorphins are implicated in food cravings for fats and sweets (Drewnowski *et al.*, 1995). Opiates act via the mu-type opioid receptor (Kelley *et al.*, 2002) to increase the response to sweet taste by humans and the intake of sweet solutions by rats (Pecina and Berridge, 2005). Fat consumption in rats was likewise increased by the opiate agonists morphine and butorphanol. Endogenous opiates also mediate the hedonic response to preferred foods (Levine *et al.*, 2003). Opiate antagonists such as naloxone, naltrexone or nalmefene appear to reduce food intakes by lowering preferences for selected foods. Whereas the consumption of non-preferred foods remained stable after naltrexone, rated pleasantness of a sweet solution declined (Hetherington, 2001). Similar results were obtained with another opiate antagonist, nalmefene (Yeomans and Wright, 1991).

Plant-derived or synthetic cannabinoids have long been used for alleviating nausea and promoting food intake in cancer and AIDS patients. The discovery of endocannabinoids in the 1990s fostered research on the natural function of these fatty acid-derived neurotransmitters. The orexigenic effect of endocannabinoids is thought to be localized to endocannabinoid receptors in the hypothalamus and limbic forebrain. Endocannabinoid levels are elevated with fasting. As mentioned in a previous section of this chapter, endocannabinoids also have a peripheral target that could also explain their orexigenic effects. Sweet taste receptors express CB-1 receptors, which, when activated, enhance the response to sweet stimuli (Jyotaki *et al.*, 2010; Yoshida *et al.*, 2010). Unlike opiate receptor blockade, pharmacological block of CB-1, an endocannabinoid receptor, reduces intake of all food, both preferred and non-preferred (Di Marzo and Matias, 2005). Such an intervention can lead to weight loss, which arises partly through a reduction in energy intake and partly through an increase in energy expenditure and fat oxidation (Addy *et al.*, 2008).

Food Liking and Reward

Eating is driven by brain circuitry that is linked to reward centers in the striatum (Stricker and Woods, 2004), where feeding is thought to be reinforced by dopaminergic projections from the midbrain (Wang *et al.*, 2001, 2004; Epstein and Leddy, 2006). Unlike opiates and endocannabinoids, dopamine's release is not tied to the reported hedonics of a food stimulus (Volkow *et al.*, 2002). Abnormalities in reward circuitry have been linked to obesity. Human brain imaging has shown an inverse relationship between levels of the D2-type dopamine receptor in the striatum and subjects' BMI (Wang *et al.*, 2001; Volkow *et al.*, 2008). More recent work using functional magnetic resonance brain imaging found that women who gained weight over a 6-month period showed a weaker pattern of activity in the striatum relative to weight-stable women (Stice *et al.*, 2010). The result led to the suggestion

that low sensitivity of the reward pathway could promote overconsumption of food, which in turn could weaken the responsiveness of the reward system further.

Recent research has found that food reward centers can be modulated by the pharmacological pathways involved in energy homeostasis. Animal studies indicate that two hormones involved in energy homeostasis, insulin and leptin, can influence the function of dopaminergic and opioid signaling in the midbrain (Figlewicz and Benoit, 2009). These experiments also show that insulin and leptin reduce food reward behaviors. Other studies have suggested that two gut peptides also involved in energy balance modulate brain areas involved in food reward (Fulton, 2010). Ghrelin receptors are found throughout the dopaminergic pathways of the brain, including ventral tegmental area (VTA) neurons of the midbrain (Guan *et al.*, 1997), where ghrelin can enhance the activity of dopaminergic neurons (Abizaid *et al.*, 2006). Imaging studies have shown that ghrelin enhances the response to visual food cues detected in the striatum and VTA of the midbrain (Malik *et al.*, 2008). Similarly, Peptide YY (PYY) administration appears to activate the VTA and ventral striatum, and when PYY levels are high (as after a meal), food intake appears to be correlated with activity in the orbitofrontal cortex (part of the circuitry involved in hedonic drive) rather than by hypothalamic centers involved in homeostatic eating (Batterham *et al.*, 2007).

Binge Eating and Food Addiction

Pathology of the neural circuits and pharmacological pathways described earlier in this chapter are thought to underlie binge eating, a phenomenon of disordered eating in humans characterized by bouts of excess food intake, particularly of palatable foods, that are not compensated by either purging (as with bulimia nervosa) or anorexia (Spitzer *et al.*, 1992). The concept has been invoked to explain unhealthy patterns of food consumption that may reflect disordered craving and reward (Pelchat, 2009). Parallels have been drawn between binge eating and drug addiction, since both behavioral syndromes involve cravings and loss of control. The drawing of this parallel has sparked debate as to whether binge eaters suffer from an "addiction to food" (Pelchat, 2009).

Pharmacologically, the parallel between drug and alcohol addiction and binge eating is consistent. Endogenous opiate peptides are thought to mediate alcohol cravings, and naltrexone, a long-lasting opiate antagonist, has been used to curb these cravings in alcoholics. Addictions to opiates such as morphine and methadone have been associated with an enhanced appetite for sweets, and opiate withdrawal is eased by ice cream and chocolate (Drewnowski et al., 1995). These effects are consistent with other studies showing that opioid antagonists reduce the hedonic response to palatable foods (Nathan and Bullmore, 2009).

Binge eating has implications for the dopaminergic pathways of the mesolimbic system. Animal studies indicate that binges of fat or sugar (both nutrients that are typically contained in palatable foods) can lead to excessive release of dopamine (Avena et al., 2009), which may lead to compensatory changes in dopamine receptors. Functional imaging studies have found a paucity of available D2-type dopamine receptors in both obese and drug-addicted subjects (Wang et al., 2004). Together, these findings suggest that these pathways provide a common anatomical substrate for behavioral responses to both food and drugs of abuse.

Palatability and Satiety

Satiety is one among many mechanisms regulating energy balance. Palatability and satiety have opposite effects on food intakes. While palatability increases appetite and therefore food consumption, satiety limits consumption by reducing meal size or by delaying the onset of the next meal. As such, both palatability and satiety help to adjust energy intakes to energy needs. However, in experimental studies, both palatability and satiety tend to be measured in terms of the amounts of food consumed. As a result, the foods that are overeaten are by definition the most palatable and the least satiating.

Standard measures of palatability include the perceived pleasantness of a given food, intent to eat, or the amount of food consumed. Among standard measures of satiety are reduced hunger, fullness, reduced intent to consume a meal or a snack, or the amount of food consumed. Some investigators have made a distinction between satiety and satiation (Mattes et al., 2005). Whereas satiation is responsible for the termination of a given meal and reduced meal size, satiety, defined as a state of internal repletion, delays the onset or reduces the size of the next meal. Increased satiety has also been measured in terms of reduced palatability. Sensory-specific satiety was specifically defined as reduced palatability of the just-consumed food relative to other foods.

The low satiating power of energy-dense, sweet and fat-rich foods has been singled out for special scrutiny (Holt et al., 1995; Erlanson-Albertsson, 2005). Some researchers have argued that the palatability of sugar overrode normal satiety signals, leading to overeating and overweight (Green et al., 1994). Others have noted that fat had low satiating power, judging by the "passive overeating" of fat-rich foods (Blundell et al., 1993). One question is whether palatable fat-rich foods are overeaten because of their high energy density or because of their fat content (Blundell et al., 1993). If satiety is macronutrient driven, fat may be overeaten because it affects satiety less than a corresponding amount (in kilocalories) of carbohydrate or protein. The creation of palatable and yet highly satiating foods, the avowed goal of the weight-loss industry, may represent a contradiction in terms.

Food Preferences and Habitual Food Intake

Food preferences are said to predict food consumption. However, people may have positive attitudes toward the foods they already eat so that food preferences may merely be a reflection of existing eating habits. For instance, a study of school children found that higher liking for vegetables and fruit was associated with higher consumption (Brug et al., 2008). It may be that higher consumption led to the reports of higher liking (Aldridge et al., 2009).

The association between food liking and food use has implications for dietary intake assessment. Food frequency questionnaires (FFQs), used to assess dietary intakes in large-scale survey studies, consist of a list of about 100 or more names of foods and food groups (Willett, 1998). Respondents are asked to report the usual frequency of consumption of each food using anchored 9-point category scales where the categories can range from "never or less than once per month" to "5+ per day" (Willett, 1998). The self-reported frequency of food use is thought to be a measure of past dietary behavior, based on a combination of memory and retrieval processes (Willett, 1998). Past efforts at improving FFQ instruments have focused on aided recall, cognitive interviewing and other ways to help the respondents' memory of past food use (Subar et al., 1995; Willett, 1998).

Yet the frequency of food use may be no more that a general attitude, positive or negative, toward a mental image of a given food. Food preference checklists are long lists of food names, with respondents asked to indicate the degree of liking using anchored 9-point category scales ranging from "1 = dislike extremely" to "9 = like extremely". Correlations between self-reported food preferences and frequencies of use have shown that dislikes were strongly associated with non-use (Drewnowski *et al.*, 2000). FFQ instruments performed no better than food preference checklists in assessing the fat content of a typical diet (Drewnowski, 2001b; Kristal *et al.*, 2005).

Economics of Food Choice Behavior

Consumer food choices are economic decisions made in response to taste, reward value, incomes, time constraints, and the perceived nutritional value of foods. Taste response or the liking for foods alone do not always predict purchase intent, or actual consumer behavior. Consumption patterns are also influenced by price, convenience, safety and nutritional concerns (Glanz *et al.*, 1998; Sobal and Bisogni, 2009). Other demographic, cultural and socioeconomic factors also modulate the connection between taste responsiveness and food choice.

Besides taste, the monetary cost of food is a dominant factor guiding food selection and is a major constraint on the diet quality of individuals, particularly those of lower socioeconomic position (Beydoun and Wang, 2008). Several economic studies have made the association between the declining monetary and time cost of food and rising obesity rates (Philipson, 2001; Lakdawalla and Philipson, 2009). Those studies pointed to the widespread availability of palatable energy-dense fast foods, the entry of women into the labor force, and lower physical activity associated with work (Philipson, 2001; Cutler *et al.*, 2003).

However, not all foods have become less expensive. There is a growing price disparity between the lower-cost, energy-dense foods based on refined grains, added sugars, and added fats and the more expensive nutrient-dense foods including lean meats, dairy products, whole grains, and fresh vegetables and fruit (Monsivais and Drewnowski, 2007; Monsivais *et al.*, 2010). Furthermore, healthier foods are not always available in economically disadvantaged areas (Jetter and Cassady, 2006; Larson *et al.*, 2009). Disparities in access to healthy foods, together with decreasing time devoted to food preparation and consumption, may help explain some of the observed disparities in health (Wiig and Smith, 2009; Davis and You, 2010).

The nature of the relation between diet quality and diet cost, at different socioeconomic levels, has important implications for the study of diets and disease risk. Whereas spending more money does not guarantee a healthier diet, reducing food costs below a certain limit virtually guarantees that the resulting diet will be nutrient-poor (Darmon *et al.*, 2002). One key question is whether palatable, low-cost, energy-dense diets are associated with higher energy consumption overall. In other words, can BMI values be linked directly to food prices and to diet costs, after adjusting for covariates? Although some studies have demonstrated this association (Powell and Bao, 2009; Sturm and Datar, 2008), the answers to all these questions are far from clear.

Future Directions

Public health and nutrition campaigns have focused on persuading consumers to replace palatable energy-dense foods with less palatable but arguably healthier options (Ashfield-Watt *et al.*, 2007). Nutritional education strategies aimed at improving diet quality have focused almost exclusively on the nutritional quality of foods, and not on taste or the pleasure response. Yet humans have an innate preference for good-tasting, energy-dense foods, which are available in an ever-expanding variety of attractive, palatable, convenient, and inexpensive forms. Taste preferences are also associated with a range of demographic, economic, social, and cultural variables. How these variables interact to produce individual and population-level patterns in food consumption is an important emerging area of research. The results of this research will be critical for informing the development of nutrition guidance and interventions that directly account for the role of taste in food choice.

Suggestions for Further Reading

Darmon, N. and Monsivais, P. (2010) Economic influences on food behaviour. In S.E. Colby (ed.), *Why We Eat What We Eat*. Kendall Hunt, Dubuque, IA, pp. 65–94.

Drewnowski, A. (2007) The real contribution of added sugars and fats to obesity. *Epidemiol Rev* **29**, 160–171.

Mattes, R.D. (2006) Orosensory considerations. *Obesity* **14**(Suppl 4), 164S–167S.

Reed, D.R., Tanaka, T., and McDaniel, A.H. (2006) Diverse tastes: genetics of sweet and bitter perception. *Physiol Behav* **88**, 215–226.

References

Abizaid, A., Liu, Z.W., Andrews, Z.B., *et al.* (2006) Ghrelin modulates the activity and synaptic input organization of midbrain dopamine neurons while promoting appetite. *J Clin Invest* **116**, 3229–3239.

Addy, C., Wright, H., Van Laere, K., *et al.* (2008) The acyclic CB1R inverse agonist taranabant mediates weight loss by increasing energy expenditure and decreasing caloric intake. *Cell Metab* **7**, 68–78.

Ahluwalia, N., Ferrières, J., Dallongeville, J., *et al.* (2009) Association of macronutrient intake patterns with being overweight in a population-based random sample of men in France. *Diabetes Metab* **35**, 129–136.

Ahmed, T. and Haboubi, N. (2010) Assessment and management of nutrition in older people and its importance to health. *Clin Interv Aging* **5**, 207–216.

Aldridge, V., Dovey, T.M., and Halford, J.C.G. (2009) The role of familiarity in dietary development. *Develop Rev* **29**, 32–44.

Andrieu, E., Darmon, N., and Drewnowski, A. (2006) Low-cost diets: more energy, fewer nutrients. *Eur J Clin Nutr* **60**, 434–436.

Ashfield-Watt, P.A., Welch, A.A., Godward, S., *et al.* (2007) Effect of a pilot community intervention on fruit and vegetable intakes: use of FACET (Five-a-day Community Evaluation Tool). *Public Health Nutr* **10**, 671–680.

Avena, N.M., Rada, P., and Hoebel, B.G. (2009) Sugar and fat bingeing have notable differences in addictive-like behavior. *J Nutr* 2 **139**, 623–628.

Ball, P., Woodward, D., Beard, T., *et al.* (2002) Calcium diglutamate improves taste characteristics of lower-salt soup. *Eur J Clin Nutr* **56**, 519–523.

Barbano, M.F. and Cador, M. (2007a) Opioids for hedonic experience and dopamine to get ready for it. *Psychopharmacology (Berl)* **191**, 497–506.

Barbano, M.F. and Cador, M. (2007b) Neurobiology of nutrition and obesity. *Nutr Rev*, **65**, 517–534.

Barratt-Fornell, A. and Drewnowski, A. (2002) The taste of health: nature's bitter gifts. *Nutr Today* **37**, 144–150.

Bartoshuk, L.M. (1993) The biological basis of food perception and acceptance. *Food Qual Pref* **4**, 21–32.

Batterham, R.L., Ffytche, D.H., Rosenthal, J.M., *et al.* (2007) PYY modulation of cortical and hypothalamic brain areas predicts feeding behaviour in humans. *Nature* **450**, 106–109.

Beauchamp, G.K. (2009) Sensory and receptor responses to umami: an overview of pioneering work. *Am J Clin Nutr* **90**, 723S–727S.

Beauchamp, G.K., Bertino, M., Burke, D., *et al.* (1990) Experimental sodium depletion and salt taste in normal human volunteers. *Am J Clin Nutr* **51**, 881–889.

Bellisle, F. (1999) Glutamate and the UMAMI taste: sensory, metabolic, nutritional and behavioural considerations. A review of the literature published in the last 10 years. *Neurosci Biobehav Rev* **23**, 423–438.

Bellisle, F. (2008) Experimental studies of food choices and palatability responses in European subjects exposed to the Umami taste. *Asia Pac J Clin Nutr* **17**(Suppl 1), 376–379.

Bellisle, F., Monneuse, M.O., Chabert, M., *et al.* (1991) Monosodium glutamate as a palatability enhancer in the European diet. *Physiol Behav* **49**, 869–873.

Berridge, K.C. (1996) Food reward: brain substrates of wanting and liking. *Neurosci Biobehav Rev.* **20**, 1–25.

Beydoun, M.A. and Wang, Y. (2008) How do socio-economic status, perceived economic barriers and nutritional benefits affect quality of dietary intake among US adults? *Eur J Clin Nutr* **62**, 303–313.

Birch, L.L. (1999) Development of food preferences. *Annu Rev Nutr* **19**, 41–62.

Blais, C.A., Pangborn, R.M., Borhani, N.O., *et al.* (1986) Effect of dietary sodium restriction on taste responses to sodium chloride: a longitudinal study. *Am J Clin Nutr* **44**, 232–243.

Blundell, J.E., Burley, V.J., Cotton, J.R., *et al.* (1993) Dietary fat and the control of energy intake: evaluating the effects of fat on meal size and postmeal satiety. *Am J Clin Nutr* **57**(5 Suppl), 772S–777S; Discussion 777S–778S.

Bolton-Smith, C. and Woodward M. (1994) Dietary composition and fat to sugar ratios in relation to obesity. *Int J Obes Relat Metab Disord* **18**, 820–828.

Bowman, S.A. (1999) Diets of individuals based on energy intakes from added sugars. *Family Econ Nutr Rev* **12**, 31–38.

Brug, J., Tak, N.I., te Velde, S.J., *et al.* (2008) Taste preferences, liking and other factors related to fruit and vegetable intakes among schoolchildren: results from observational studies. *Br J Nutr* **99**(Suppl 1), S7–S14.

Cabanac, M. and Duclaux, R. (1970) Obesity: absence of satiety aversion to sucrose. *Science* **168**, 496–497.

Capaldi, E.D. and Privitera, G.J. (2008) Decreasing dislike for sour and bitter in children and adults. *Appetite* **50**, 139–145.

Carter, B.E., Monsivais, P., and Drewnowski, A. (2011a) The sensory optimum of chicken broths supplemented with calcium di-glutamate: a possibility for reducing sodium while maintaining taste. *Food Qual Pref* **22**, 699–703.

Carter, B.E., Monsivais P., Perrigue, M.P., *et al.* (2011b) Supplementing chicken broth with monosodium glutamate reduces hunger and desire to snack but does not affect energy intake in women. *Br J Nutr* **106**, 1441–1448.

Clydesdale, F.M. (1993) Color as a factor in food choice. *Crit Rev Food Sci Nutr* **33**, 83–101.

Cook, N.R., Cutler, J.A., Obarzanek, E., *et al.* (2007) Long term effects of dietary sodium reduction on cardiovascular disease outcomes: observational follow-up of the trials of hypertension prevention (TOHP). *BMJ* **334**, 885.

Cooling, J. and Blundell, J. (1998) Are high-fat and low-fat consumers distinct phenotypes? Differences in the subjective and behavioural response to energy and nutrient challenges. *Eur J Clin Nutr* **52**, 193–201.

Cox, D.N., Perry, L., Moore, P.B., *et al.* (1999) Sensory and hedonic associations with macronutrient and energy intakes of lean and obese consumers. *Int J Obes Relat Metab Disord* **23**, 403–410.

Cutler, D.M., Glaeser, E.L., and Shapiro, J.M. (2003) Why have Americans become more obese? *J Econ Perspect* **17**, 93–118.

Darmon, N., Ferguson, E.L., and Briend, A. (2002) A cost constraint alone has adverse effects on food selection and nutrient density: an analysis of human diets by linear programming. *J Nutr.* **132**, 3764–3771.

Davis, G.C. and You, W. (2010) The Thrifty Food Plan is not thrifty when labor cost is considered. *J Nutr* **140**, 854–857.

Desor, J.A., Maller, O., and Andrews, K. (1975) Ingestive responses of human newborns to salty, sour, and bitter stimuli. *J Comp Physiol Psychol.* **89**, 966–970.

Di Marzo, V. and Matias, I. (2005) Endocannabinoid control of food intake and energy balance. *Nature Neurosci* **8**, 585–589.

Dötsch, M., Busch, J., Batenburg, M., *et al.* (2009) Strategies to reduce sodium consumption: a food industry perspective. *Crit Rev Food Sci Nutr* **49**, 841–851.

Drewnowski, A. (1989) Taste responsiveness in eating disorders. *Ann NY Acad Sci* **575**, 399–408; Discussion 408–409.

Drewnowski, A. (1997a) Taste preferences and food intake. *Annu Rev Nutr* **17**, 237–253.

Drewnowski, A. (1997b) Why do we like fat? *J Am Diet Assoc* **97**(7 Suppl), S58–62.

Drewnowski, A. (1998) Energy density, palatability, and satiety: implications for weight control. *Nutr Rev* **56**, 347–353.

Drewnowski, A. (2001a) The science and complexity of bitter taste. *Nutr Rev* **59**, 163–169.

Drewnowski, A. (2001b) Diet image: a new perspective on the food-frequency questionnaire. *Nutr Rev* **59**, 370–372.

Drewnowski, A. (2003) Genetics of human taste perception. In R.L. Doty (ed.), *Handbook of Olfaction and Gustation*, 2nd Edn. Marcel Dekker, New York, pp. 847–860.

Drewnowski, A. and Gomez-Carneros, C. (2000) Bitter taste, phytonutrients, and the consumer: a review. *Am J Clin Nutr* **72**, 1424–1435.

Drewnowski, A. and Greenwood, M.R. (1983) Cream and sugar: human preferences for high-fat foods. *Physiol Behav* **30**, 629–633.

Drewnowski, A. and Rock, C.L. (1995) The influence of genetic taste markers on food acceptance. *Am J Clin Nutr* **62**, 506–511.

Drewnowski, A. and Specter, S.E. (2004) Poverty and obesity: the role of energy density and energy costs. *Am J Clin Nutr* **79**, 6–16.

Drewnowski, A., Brunzell, J.D., Sande, K., *et al.* (1985) Sweet tooth reconsidered: taste responsiveness in human obesity. *Physiol Behav* **35**, 617–622.

Drewnowski, A., Hann, C., Henderson, S.A., *et al.* (2000) Both food preferences and food frequency scores predict fat intakes of women with breast cancer. *J Am Diet Assoc* **100**, 1325–1333.

Drewnowski, A., Henderson, S.A., and Cockroft, J.E. (2007) Genetic sensitivity to 6-n-propylthiouracil has no influence on dietary patterns, body mass indexes, or plasma lipid profiles of women. *J Am Diet Assoc* **107**, 1340–1348.

Drewnowski, A., Henderson, S.A., Driscoll, A., *et al.* (1996) Salt taste perceptions and preferences are unrelated to sodium consumption in healthy older adults. *J Am Diet Assoc* **96**, 471–474.

Drewnowski, A., Krahn, D.D., Demitrack, M.A., *et al.* (1995) Naloxone, an opiate blocker, reduces the consumption of sweet high-fat foods in obese and lean female binge eaters. *Am J Clin Nutr* **161**, 1206–1212.

Duffy, V.B. (2004) Associations between oral sensation, dietary behaviors and risk of cardiovascular disease (CVD). *Appetite* **43**, 5–9.

Duffy, V.B. and Bartoshuk, L.M. (2000) Food acceptance and genetic variation in taste. *J Am Diet Assoc* **100**, 647–655.

Erlanson-Albertsson, C. (2005) How palatable food disrupts appetite regulation. *Basic Clin Pharmacol Toxicol* **97**, 61–73.

Epstein, L.H. and Leddy, J.J. (2006) Food reinforcement. *Appetite.* **46**, 22–25.

Essed, N.H., van Staveren, W.A., Kok, F.J., *et al.* (2007) No effect of 16 weeks flavor enhancement on dietary intake and nutritional status of nursing home elderly. *Appetite* **48**, 29–36.

Figlewicz, D.P. and Benoit, S.C. (2009) Insulin, leptin, and food reward: update 2008. *Am J Physiol Regul Integr Comp Physiol* **296**, R9–R19.

Fischer, R., Griffin, F., and Kaplan, A.R. (1963) Taste thresholds, cigarette smoking, and food dislikes. *Med Exp Int J Exp Med* **9**, 151–167.

Fisher, J.O. and Birch, L.L. (1995) Fat preferences and fat consumption of 3- to 5-year-old children are related to parental adiposity. *J Am Diet Assoc* **95**, 759–764.

Fulton, S. (2010) Appetite and reward. *Front Neuroendocrinol* **31**(1), p. 85–103.

Gilbertson, T.A., Liu, L., Kim, I., *et al.* (2005) Fatty acid responses in taste cells from obesity-prone and -resistant rats. *Physiol Behav* **86**, 681–690.

Glanville, E.V. and Kaplan, A.R. (1965) Food preference and sensitivity of taste for bitter compounds. *Nature* **205**, 851–853.

Glanz, K., Basil, M., Maibach, E., *et al.* (1998) Why Americans eat what they do: taste, nutrition, cost, convenience, and weight control concerns as influences on food consumption. *J Am Diet Assoc* **98**, 1118–1126.

Green, S.M., Burley, V.J., and Blundell, J.E. (1994) Effect of fat- and sucrose-containing foods on the size of eating episodes and energy intake in lean males: potential for causing overconsumption. *Eur J Clin Nutr* **48**, 547–555.

Guan, X.-M., Yu, H., Palyha, O.C., *et al.* (1997) Distribution of mRNA encoding the growth hormone secretagogue receptor in brain and peripheral tissues. *Brain Res Mol Brain Res* **48**, 23–29.

Hayes, J.E. and Duffy, V.B. (2007) Revisiting sugar–fat mixtures: sweetness and creaminess vary with phenotypic markers of oral sensation. *Chem Senses* **32**, 225–236.

Hayes, J.E. and Duffy, V.B. (2008) Oral sensory phenotype identifies level of sugar and fat required for maximal liking. *Physiol Behav* **95**, 77–87.

Hays, N.P. and. Roberts, S.B (2006) The anorexia of aging in humans. *Physiol Behav.* **88**, 257–266.

He, K., Zhao, L., Daviglus, M.L., *et al.* (2008) Association of monosodium glutamate intake with overweight in Chinese adults: the INTERMAP Study. *Obesity (Silver Spring)* **16**, 1875–1680.

Heath, T.P., Melichar, J.K., Nutt, D.J., *et al.* (2006) Human taste thresholds are modulated by serotonin and noradrenaline. *J Neurosci* **26**, 12664–12671.

Hermanussen, M., García, A.P., Sunder, M., *et al.* (2006) Obesity, voracity, and short stature: the impact of glutamate on the regulation of appetite. *Eur J Clin Nutr* **60**, 25–31.

Hetherington, M.M. (2001) *Food Cravings and Addiction.* Leatherhead Food Research Association, Leatherhead.

Hirata, A.E., Andrade, I.S., Vaskevicius, P., *et al.* (1997) Monosodium glutamate (MSG)-obese rats develop glucose intolerance and insulin resistance to peripheral glucose uptake. *Braz J Med Biol Res.* **30**, 671–674.

Holt, S.H., Miller, J.C., Petocz, P., *et al.* (1995) A satiety index of common foods. *Eur J Clin Nutr* **49**, 675–690.

Isezuo, S.A., Saidu, Y., Anas, S., *et al.* (2008) Salt taste perception and relationship with blood pressure in type 2 diabetics. *J Hum Hypertens* **22**, 432–434.

Jetter, K.M. and Cassady, D.L. (2006) The availability and cost of healthier food alternatives. *Am J Prev Med* **30**, 38–44.

Johnson, A.K. (2007) The sensory psychobiology of thirst and salt appetite. *Med Sci Sports Exerc* **39**, 1388–1400.

Jyotaki, M., Shigemura, N., and Ninomiya, Y. (2010) Modulation of sweet taste sensitivity by orexigenic and anorexigenic factors. *Endocr J* **57**, 467–475.

Kalra, S.P. and Kalra, P.S. (2004) Overlapping and interactive pathways regulating appetite and craving. *J Addict Dis* **23**, 5–21.

Kelley, A.E., Bakshi, V.P., Haber, S.N., *et al.* (2002) Opioid modulation of taste hedonics within the ventral striatum. *Physiol Behav* **76**, 365–377.

Kenny, P.J. (2011) Reward mechanisms in obesity: new insights and future directions. *Neuron* **69**, 664–679.

Keskitalo, K., Tuorila, H., Spector, T.D., *et al.* (2007) Same genetic components underlie different measures of sweet taste preference. *Am J Clin Nutr* **86**, 1663–1669.

Keskitalo, K., Tuorila, H., Spector, T.D., *et al.* (2008) The Three-Factor Eating Questionnaire, body mass index, and responses to sweet and salty fatty foods: a twin study of genetic and environmental associations. *Am J Clin Nutr* **88**, 263–271.

Khan, N.A. and Besnard, P. (2009) Oro-sensory perception of dietary lipids: new insights into the fat taste transduction. *Biochim Biophys Acta* **1791**, 149–155.

Kim, U.K., Jorgenson, E., Coon, H., *et al.* (2003) Positional cloning of the human quantitative trait locus underlying taste sensitivity to phenylthiocarbamide. *Science* **299**, 1221–1225.

Kondoh, T. and Torii, K. (2008) MSG intake suppresses weight gain, fat deposition, and plasma leptin levels in male Sprague-Dawley rats. *Physiol Behav* **95**, 135–144.

Kristal, A.R., Peters, U., and Potter, J.D. (2005) Is it time to abandon the food frequency questionnaire? *Cancer Epidemiol Biomarkers Prev* **14**, 2826–2828.

Lakdawalla, D. and Philipson, T. (2009) The growth of obesity and technological change. *Econ Human Biol* **7**, 283–293.

Larson, N.I., Story, M.T., and Nelson, M.C. (2009) Neighborhood environments: disparities in access to healthy foods in the U.S. *Am J Prev Med* **36**, 74–81.

Levine, A.S., Kotz, C.M., and Gosnell, B.A. (2003) Sugars: hedonic aspects, neuroregulation, and energy balance. *Am J Clin Nutr* **78**, 834S–842S.

Liem, D.G. and de Graaf, C. (2004) Sweet and sour preferences in young children and adults: role of repeated exposure. *Physiol Behav* **83**, 421–429.

Liem, D.G., Bogers, R.P., Dagnelie, P.C., *et al.* (2006) Fruit consumption of boys (8–11 years) is related to preferences for sour taste. *Appetite* **46**, 93–96.

Liem, D.G., Westerbeek, A., Wolterink, S., *et al.* (2004) Sour taste preferences of children relate to preference for novel and intense stimuli. *Chem Senses* **29**, 713–720.

Lim, J., Urban, L., and Green. B.G. (2008) Measures of individual differences in taste and creaminess perception. *Chem Senses* **33**, 493–501.

Logue, A.W. (2004) *The Psychology of Eating and Drinking*. Brunner-Routledge, New York.

Lowe, M.R. and Butryn, M.L. (2007) Hedonic hunger: a new dimension of appetite? *Physiol Behav* **91**, 432–439.

Lucas, L., Riddell, L., Liem, G., *et al.* (2011) The influence of sodium on liking and consumption of salty food. *J Food Sci* **76**, S72–S76.

Luscombe-Marsh, N.D., Smeets, A.J., and Westerterp-Plantenga, M.S. (2008) Taste sensitivity for monosodium glutamate and an increased liking of dietary protein. *Br J Nutr* **99**, 904–908.

Luscombe-Marsh, N.D., Smeets, A.J., and Westerterp-Plantenga, M.S. (2009) The addition of monosodium glutamate and inosine monophosphate-5 to high-protein meals: effects on satiety, and energy and macronutrient intakes. *Br J Nutr* **102**, 1-9.

Malcolm, R., O'Neil, P.M., Hirsch, A.A., *et al.* (1980) Taste hedonics and thresholds in obesity. *Int J Obes* **4**, 203–212.

Malik, S., McGlone, F., Bedrossian, D., *et al.* (2008) Ghrelin modulates brain activity in areas that control appetitive behavior. *Cell Metab* **7**, 400–409.

Marshall, T.A., Stumbo, P.J., Warren, J.J., *et al.* (2001) Inadequate nutrient intakes are common and are associated with low diet variety in rural, community-dwelling elderly. *J Nutr* **131**, 2192–2196.

Marshall, T.A., Warren, J.J., Hand, J.S., *et al.* (2002) Oral health, nutrient intake and dietary quality in the very old. *J Am Dent Assoc* **133**, 1369–1379.

Mathey, M.F., Siebelink, E., de Graaf, C., *et al.* (2001) Flavor enhancement of food improves dietary intake and nutritional status of elderly nursing home residents. *J Gerontol A Biol Sci Med Sci* **56**, M200–M205.

Matsushita, Y., Mizoue, T., Takahashi, Y., *et al.* (2009) Taste preferences and body weight change in Japanese adults: the JPHC Study. *Int J Obes (Lond)* **33**, 1191–1197.

Mattes, R.D. (1997) The taste for salt in humans. *Am J Clin Nutr* **65**(2 Suppl), 692S–697S.

Mattes, R.D. (2005) Fat taste and lipid metabolism in humans. *Physiol Behav* **86**, 691–697.

Mattes, R.D. (2009) Is there a fatty acid taste? *Annu Rev Nutr* **29**, 305–327.

Mattes, R.D., Hollis, J., Hayes, D., *et al.* (2005) Appetite: measurement and manipulation misgivings. *J Am Diet Assoc* **105**(5 Suppl 1), S87–97.

Michikawa, T., Nishiwa, Y, Okamura, T., *et al.* (2009) The taste of salt measured by a simple test and blood pressure in Japanese women and men. *Hypertens Res* **32**, 399–403.

Miller, W.C., Lindeman, A.K., Wallace, J., *et al.* (1990) Diet composition, energy intake, and exercise in relation to body fat in men and women. *Am J Clin Nutr* **52**, 426–430.

Miras, A.D. and le Roux, C.W. (2010) Bariatric surgery and taste: novel mechanisms of weight loss. *Curr Opin Gastroenterol* **26**, 140–145

Monsivais, P. and Drewnowski, A. (2007) The rising cost of low-energy-density foods. *J Am Diet Assoc* **107**, 2071–2076.

Monsivais, P., McLain, J., and Drewnowski, A. (2010) The rising disparity in the price of healthful foods: 2004–2008. *Food Policy* **35**, 514–520.

Morley, J.E. (2001) Decreased food intake with aging. *J Gerontol A Biol Sci Med Sci* **56**, 81–88.

Murphy, C. (2008) The chemical senses and nutrition in older adults. *J Nutr Elder* **27**, 247–265.

Nathan, P.J. and Bullmore, E.T. (2009) From taste hedonics to motivational drive: central mu-opioid receptors and binge-eating behaviour. *Int J Neuropsychopharmacol* **12**, 995–1008.

Nelson, G., Chandrashekar, J., Hoon, M.A., *et al.* (2002) An amino-acid taste receptor. *Nature* **416**, 199–202.

Okiyama, A. and Beauchamp, G.K. (1998) Taste dimensions of monosodium glutamate (MSG) in a food system: role of glutamate in young American subjects. *Physiol Behav* **65**, 177–181.

Pasquet, P., Frelut, M.L., Simmen, B., *et al.* (2007) Taste perception in massively obese and in non-obese adolescents. *Int J Pediatr Obes* **2**, 242–248.

Pecina, S. and Berridge, K.C. (2005) Hedonic hot spot in nucleus accumbens shell: where do mu-opioids cause increased hedonic impact of sweetness? *J Neurosci* **25**, 11777–11786.

Pepino, M.Y., Finkbeiner, S., Beauchamp, G.K., *et al.* (2010) Obese women have lower monosodium glutamate taste sensitivity and prefer higher concentrations than do normal-weight women. *Obesity (Silver Spring)* **18**, 959–965.

Pelchat, M.L. (2002) Of human bondage: food craving, obsession, compulsion, and addiction. *Physiol Behav* **76**, 347–352.

Pelchat, M.L. (2009) Food addiction in humans. *J Nutr* **139**, 620–622.

Philipson, T. (2001) The world-wide growth in obesity: an economic research agenda. *Health Econ* **10**, 1–7.

Powell, L.M., Bao, Y. (2009) Food prices, access to food outlets and child weight. *Econ Hum Biol* **7**(1), 64–72.

Reed, D.R. (2008) Birth of a new breed of supertaster. *Chem Senses* **33**, 489–491.

Rogers, P.J. and Blundell, J.E. (1990) Umami and appetite: effects of monosodium glutamate on hunger and food intake in human subjects. *Physiol Behav* **48**, 801–804.

Roininen, K., Lahteenmaki, L., and Tuorila, H. (1996) Effect of umami taste on pleasantness of low-salt soups during repeated testing. *Physiol Behav* **60**, 953–958.

Rolls, B.J. (1999) Do chemosensory changes influence food intake in the elderly? *Physiol Behav* **66**, 193–197.

Rose, D. (2007) Food stamps, the Thrifty Food Plan, and meal preparation: The importance of the time dimension for US Nutrition Policy. *J Nutr Educ Behav* **39,** 226–232.

Sahyoun, N.R., Lin, C.-L., and Krall, E. (2003) Nutritional status of the older adult is associated with dentition status. *J Am Dent Assoc* **103,** 61–66.

Salbe, A.D., DelParigi, A., Pratley, R.E., *et al.* (2004) Taste preferences and body weight changes in an obesity-prone population. *Am J Clin Nutr* **79,** 372–378.

Schiffman, S.S. (2000) Intensification of sensory properties of foods for the elderly. *J Nutr* **130**(4S Suppl), 927S–930S.

Schultes, B., Ernst, B., Wilms, B., *et al.* (2010) Hedonic hunger is increased in severely obese patients and is reduced after gastric bypass surgery. *Am J Clin Nutr* **92,** 277–283.

Schwartz, C., Issanchou, S., and Nicklaus, S. (2009) Developmental changes in the acceptance of the five basic tastes in the first year of life. *Br J Nutr* **102,** 1375–1385.

Shi, Z., Luscombe-Marsh, N.D., Wittert, G.A., *et al.* (2010) Monosodium glutamate is not associated with obesity or a greater prevalence of weight gain over 5 years: findings from the Jiangsu Nutrition Study of Chinese adults. *Br J Nutr* **104,** 457–463.

Sobal, J. and Bisogni, C.A. (2009) Constructing food choice decisions. *Ann Behav Med* **38**(Suppl 1), S37–46.

Spitzer, R.L., Devlin, M., and Walsh, B.T. (1992) Binge eating disorder: A multisite field trial of the diagnostic criteria. *Int J Eating Dis* **11,** 191–203.

Stice, E., Yokum, S., Blum, K., *et al.* (2010) Weight gain is associated with reduced striatal response to palatable food. *J Neurosci* **30,** 13105–13109.

Stricker, E.M. and Woods, S.C. (2004) *Neurobiology of Food and Fluid Intake.* Available from http://libraries.ou.edu/access.aspx? url=http://dx.doi.org/10.1007/b111152.

Subar, A.F., Thompson, F.E., Smith, A.F., *et al.* (1995) Improving food frequency questionnaires–a qualitative approach using cognitive interviewing. *J Am Diet Assoc* **95,** 781–788.

Sturm, R. and Datar, A. (2008) Food prices and weight gain during elementary school: 5-year update. Public Health.

Tepper, B.J. (2008) Nutritional implications of genetic taste variation: the role of PROP sensitivity and other taste phenotypes. *Annu Rev Nutr* **28,** 367–388.

Tepper, B.J., Neilland, M., Ullrich, N.V., *et al.* (2011) Greater energy intake from a buffet meal in lean, young women is associated with the 6-n-propylthiouracil (PROP) non-taster phenotype. *Appetite* **56,** 104–110.

Tepper, B.J., White, E.A., Koelliker, Y., *et al.* (2009) Genetic variation in taste sensitivity to 6-n-propylthiouracil and its rela-

tionship to taste perception and food selection. *Ann NY Acad Sci* **1170,** 126–139.

Thompson, D.A., Moskowitz, H.R., and Campbell, R.G. (1976) Effects of body-weight and food-intake on pleasantness ratings for a sweet stimulus. *J Appl Physiol* **41,** 77–83.

Volkow, N.D., Wang, G.J., Fowler, J.S., *et al.* (2002) "Nonhedonic" food motivation in humans involves dopamine in the dorsal striatum and methylphenidate amplifies this effect. *Synapse* **244,** 175–180.

Volkow, N.D., Wang, G.J., Telang, F., *et al.* (2008) Low dopamine striatal D2 receptors are associated with prefrontal metabolism in obese subjects: Possible contributing factors. *Neuroimage* **42,** 1537–1543.

Wald, N. and Leshem, M. (2003) Salt conditions a flavor preference or aversion after exercise depending on NaCl dose and sweat loss. *Appetite* **40,** 277–284.

Wang, G.-J., Volkow, N.D., Logan, J., *et al.* (2001) Brain dopamine and obesity. *Lancet* **357,** 354–357.

Wang, G.J., Volkow, N.D., Thanos, P.K., *et al.* (2004) Similarity between obesity and drug addiction as assessed by neurofunctional imaging: a concept review. *J Addict Dis* **23,** 39–53.

Wardle, J., Guthrie, C., Sanderson, S., *et al.* (2001) Food and activity preferences in children of lean and obese parents. *Int J Obes Relat Metab Disord* **25,** 971–977.

Wiig, K. and Smith, C. (2009) The art of grocery shopping on a food stamp budget: factors influencing the food choices of low-income women as they try to make ends meet. *Public Health Nutr* **12**(10), 1726–1734.

Willett, W. (1998) *Nutritional Epidemiology,* 2nd Edn. Oxford University Press, New York.

Wise, P.M., Hansen, J.L., Reed, D.R., *et al.* (2007) Twin study of the heritability of recognition thresholds for sour and salty taste. *Chem Senses* **32,** 749–754.

Wurst, F.M., Rasmussen, D.D., Hillemacher, T., *et al.* (2007) Alcoholism, craving, and hormones: the role of leptin, ghrelin, prolactin, and the pro-opiomelanocortin system in modulating ethanol intake. *Alcohol Clin Exp Res* **31,** 1963–1967.

Yanovski, S. (2003) Sugar and fat: Cravings and aversions. *J Nutr* **133,** 835S–837S.

Yeomans, M.R. and Wright, P. (1991) Lower pleasantness of palatable foods in nalmefene-treated human volunteers. *Appetite* **16,** 249–259.

Yoshida, R., Ohkuri, T., Jyotaki, M., *et al.* (2010) Endocannabinoids selectively enhance sweet taste. *Proc Natl Acad Sci USA* **107,** 935–939.

61

ENERGY INTAKE, OBESITY, AND EATING BEHAVIOR

ALEXANDRA M. JOHNSTONE, PhD

Rowett Institute of Nutrition and Health, Aberdeen, UK

Summary

In the context of the rising obesity epidemic, understanding the role of eating patterns and diet composition in calorie intake and body weight is clearly important for the development of dietary strategies that encourage body weight control in adults. It is now accepted that there are many nutritional and non-nutritional factors that will influence energy intake (EI) and eating behavior. Non-nutritional factors include palatability of food, portion size, sensory variety, and meal patterns (e.g. snacking). It is accepted that these factors can contribute to passive overconsumption of calories, at least in the short term, and that these attributes make a major contribution to the reward value of food. The main nutritional factors are macronutrient composition and energy density (ED). People do not always eat in response to a physiological hunger cue, so common psychological influences on eating behavior are discussed. Future perspectives for developing our understanding of control of eating and energy intake within a multidisciplinary obesity team are discussed.

Introduction

With obesity growing as a major public-health concern, our eating environment is ever more in focus as a contributing factor to weight gain. We live in an "obesogenic environment" where lifestyle choices associated with eating behavior and physical activity contribute to the development of obesity. Definition and classification of obesity have been outlined in Chapter 45, "Obesity as a Health Risk." Reversing the effects of obesity is a huge challenge, and understanding the role of food, energy, and nutrients on eating behavior(s) is essential in order to develop dietary strategies for both the prevention and treatment of obesity.

This is complicated by the fact that eating and food choice are a social experience and the pleasure or reward value of feeding behavior(s) can override the physiological processes that control metabolism and body weight, at least in the short term.

The content of this chapter refers to work on adults, with some reference to work on children's eating preferences mentioned in Chapter 60, "Taste and Food Choices." Little directly comparable research has been conducted across the lifespan to include interventions in children, young people, adults, and the elderly, and this is an area for future research. Furthermore, energy intake is only one side of the energy balance equation and needs to be

Present Knowledge in Nutrition, Tenth Edition. Edited by John W. Erdman Jr, Ian A. Macdonald and Steven H. Zeisel.
© 2012 International Life Sciences Institute. Published 2012 by John Wiley & Sons, Inc.

considered in that context. The role of exercise in appetite control and body weight has recently been reviewed by Hopkins *et al.* (2010), who highlight the benefits of exercise but also the variable nature and diversity in weight-loss response.

Nutritional Influences on Energy Intake, Obesity and Eating Behavior

It is now accepted that both nutritional and non-nutritional factors influence food intake. The main nutritional factors are macronutrient composition and energy density (ED). How these influence eating behavior and calorie intake in the short and medium term are discussed.

Appetite Control Definitions

As much of the work within this chapter refers to appetite, commonly used terms relating to appetite are defined below. Appetite control and methodological aspects have recently been reviewed by Blundell *et al.* (2010) within the context of the evaluation of foods for health claims. A major mechanism by which feeding behavior is coupled to physiological (and other) events is the process of learning. To understand feeding behavior, hunger and satiety processes, the mechanism by which learning links feeding behavior to physiological, sensory, nutritional, situational, and other learning cues must be appreciated. A major form of learning in this regard is termed associative conditioning of preferences, appetites, and satieties (Blundell *et al.*, 2010).

Hunger is a motivational construct that describes the drive to eat, which is not directly measurable, and is, rather, inferred from objective conditions and conscious sensations reflecting the mental urge to eat. In simple terms, this is a cue that we learn to recognize as telling us to go to search for food and to eat. The hunger cue does not tell us what to eat, or how much, but simply to initiate eating. It is influenced by a number of internal physiological factors (e.g. declining blood glucose, hunger pangs in the stomach) and external non-physiological factors (e.g. time of day, social conditioning). Hunger has a large, learned, anticipatory component rather than being the direct consequence of unconditioned physiological signals *per se*.

Appetite is defined as "the disposition or desire to eat a specific food." This term is used in everyday language to express an appetite for "something sweet" or "something savoury." It has been argued that appetite is enhanced by sensory factors that influence palatability of food, such as taste, texture, or temperature. Appetite is *sensory specific* and has a large learned component. Appetite is not rigidly determined by physiological signals *per se*, although they may exert a considerable influence.

Blundell proposed the satiety cascade 20 years ago (Blundell, 1991), to provide a conceptual framework for examining the impacts of foods on satiation (processes that bring an eating episode to an end) and satiety (processes that inhibit further eating in the postprandial period). This is shown in Figure 61.1 (adapted from Blundell *et al.*, 2010).

Satiety is another motivational construct and typically used to refer to "a state of inhibition of eating." Simply, this can be considered as the inter-meal interval. This is mainly influenced by physiological postprandial and central nervous system effects. For example, early postingestive events include gastric distension and emptying and release of hormones, followed by postabsorptive events, including mechanisms arising from the action of glucose, fats and amino acids after absorption across the intestine into the bloodstream and interactions with the CNS. After a meal, we do not eat for a period of time and this reflects satiety.

Satiation is defined as "the process leading to the termination of an episode of eating." This describes the process of meal termination or stopping eating, and may be expressed as a feeling of fullness. Meal termination is affected by psychological events and behavior, as well as an early cephalic phase response. These are the sensory perceptions generated by smell, taste, temperature, and texture that inhibit eating in the short term. Cognitive beliefs that we hold about food may inhibit eating in the short term.

The Role of Diet Composition

Although there is a strong genetic component to obesity (Vimaleswaran and Loos, 2010), the fact that the incidence of this disease has dramatically increased over the past 20 years implicates an environmental and behavioral basis. Some workers have emphasized the increase in energy intake (Hill, 2006), whereas others attribute increasing weight gain to decreased energy expenditure because of an increasingly sedentary lifestyle (Levine, 2003). The mechanisms linking energy intake and expenditure are unclear, but it seems reasonable to believe that appetite (sensations that promote food ingestion or rejection) is central to the maintenance of energy balance and

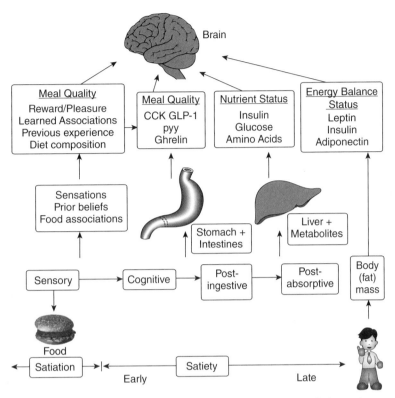

FIG. 61.1 Example of the "Satiety Cascade". Adapted from Blundell *et al.* (2010).

body weight. The role of micronutrients (vitamins, minerals and trace elements) and phytochemicals in appetite and food intake is an evolving field, but is not covered in this review.

The dietary macronutrients are those that provide energy, and are protein, fat, carbohydrate, and alcohol. It is generally accepted that diet composition strongly affects ad libitum energy intake under laboratory (Poppitt *et al.*, 1998) and free-living (de Castro, 2006) conditions, with protein highlighted as the most satiating macronutrient (Halton and Hu, 2004). Even when ingested at the same level of energy density, protein is the most satiating macronutrient (Johnstone *et al.*, 1996; Stubbs *et al.*, 1996). Under these conditions differences between carbohydrate and fat are less clear-cut.

Recent findings suggest that an elevated protein intake seems to play such a key role in body-weight management, through (1) increased satiety related to increased diet-induced thermogenesis, (2) its effect on thermogenesis, (3) body composition, and (4) decreased energy efficiency (Westerterp-Plantenga and Lejeune, 2005). Supported by these mechanisms, a relatively larger weight loss and stronger body-weight maintenance thereafter have been observed with protein-enriched diets. The safety and efficacy of high-protein diets for weight loss has been questioned, with Eisenstein *et al.* (2002) summarizing the experimental and epidemiological data. Protein-induced satiety has been shown acutely (within single meals that contain between 25% and 81% of energy from protein), with reductions in subsequent energy intake. It has been shown with high-protein ad libitum diets lasting from 14 days (Johnstone *et al.*, 2008) up to 6 months (Skov *et al.*, 1999).

Carbohydrate tends to exert a more acute effect on satiety than fat (Raben *et al.*, 1996). The role of carbohydrate in regulation of appetite and energy balance has attracted attention as a mediator of short-term appetite (Stubbs *et al.*, 2001), and has been reviewed by Mattes *et al.* (2005). Both the type and amount of carbohydrate consumed influence many ingestive processes. Hypotheses based on the glycemic index value of carbohydrate-containing foods suggest that both low and high insulin responses to foods promote hunger and energy intake (Flint *et al.*, 2007). The role of fuel oxidation in appetite control is discussed by Stubbs (1995), and suggests that the hierarchy in the oxidation of nutrients is linked to the potency of effect on appetite control, such that protein is more satiating than carbohydrate than fat.

Fat intake's association with energy balance has been reviewed by Westerterp-Plantenga (2004). A paradox becomes apparent when considering fat intake and satiety (Blundell *et al.*, 1995). Although the body appears to generate potent physiological responses that are triggered by fat ingestion, many studies have demonstrated that people who consume high-fat foods (either through personal choice or in experimental situations) tend to overconsume energy, a process termed passive overconsumption. Rodent studies suggest that fat delivered to the intestine (duodenum or jejunum) generates potent satiety signals. On the other hand, exposure to high-fat foods leads to a form of passive overconsumption that suggests that fat has a weak effect on satiety (poor fullness feedback). When human subjects are given a range of high-fat foods, they increase their EI and gain weight compared with subjects eating a medium- or low-fat diet (Blundell and Stubbs, 1999). This may be explained by the fact that fat consumed orally takes some time to reach the intestine, and its negative feedback action is likely to be diluted by other nutrients. Fat produces potent oral stimulation (positive feedback) that facilitates intake; high-fat foods normally have a high-energy density, which means that a large amount of fat energy can be consumed before fat-induced satiety signals become operative. The signals are apparently too delayed to prevent the intake of large amounts of this food (Blundell and Macdiarmid, 2006).

Alcohol is exceptional in that its ingestion can stimulate EI, and thereby induce counter-compensatory feeding behavior (Yeomans, 2010). Given that alcohol is also a drug with depressant effects on the central nervous system (CNS), this is not surprising. Whether there is an association between alcohol intake and obesity is controversial (Suter, 2005) although, in terms of overall energy contribution, significant consumption of alcohol-based beverages has the propensity to increase total EI and hence contribute to obesity. Alcohol may also promote increased snacking and EI, which is not compensated for.

The Role of Energy Density

Energy density (ED) is the amount of energy in a particular weight of food (kJ/g). Dietary ED tends to act as a constraint on feeding behavior (Rolls, 2009), influencing satiety or the feeling of fullness after eating. It is influenced by the moisture content of food (adding weight with no calories), fiber content (adding volume with limited calories), and macronutrient composition, mainly from fat content, because of its high energy content per gram. One classic experiment on how ED affects satiety and food intake is the provision of a soup-based preload before eating, which reduces EI at the next meal (Himaya and Louis-Sylvestre, 1998); interestingly, provision of a glass of water does not have the same effect on satiety as incorporating it into food to lower ED (Rolls *et al.*, 1999), which suggests a role for viscosity on gut responsiveness.

A diet that is low in ED will induce an energy deficit, determined by the rate (volume over time) at which low ED foods can be digested and absorbed. This might be a useful strategy to achieve weight loss. One dietary strategy to decrease ED is to increase the intake of water-rich foods such as fruit and vegetables, allowing a satisfying portion size whilst decreasing EI. Data from clinical trials suggest that substantial weight loss can be achieved with this approach (Yao and Roberts, 2001). Conversely, if a diet is too high in ED, overconsumption will tend to occur because the amount of food people eat tends to be conditioned and there is relatively weak defense against excess EI (Rolls, 2010). Consumption of foods with a high ED may increase the risk of passive overconsumption and weight gain. As a general rule, then, decreasing the fat content either of individual foods or the diet as a whole should decrease the ED of the diet. Studies performed in subjects who were fed a diet where the ED was varied while maintaining the macronutrient composition found that subjects ate a similar weight of food regardless of macronutrient composition, thus promoting energy overconsumption on diets with a high ED (Stubbs *et al.*, 1998a,b). Conversely, several studies have shown that, if the amount of fat in the diet was varied while keeping the ED constant, subjects consumed a similar weight of food and hence EI remained unchanged (Stubbs,1995; Bell *et al.*, 1998). These studies, however, involved diets that were highly constructed in terms of macronutrient composition and ED in order to create dissociations, and hence do not reflect typical population diets. What the studies suggest is that the overall ED of the diet is strongly influenced by fat content, and is probably a major contributor to total EI.

While many previous studies have focused on the link between ED and foods, beverages can also make a significant contribution to the total EI of an individual. In Australia, beverages contribute 16.3% of the total daily EI for all persons (McLennan and Podger, 1998); in the USA soft-drink consumption has increased by more than 60% between 1977 and 1998 (Economics Research Service, 1999). Of recent interest is the role of liquid carbohydrate intake as a contributing factor to the rise in obesity. Energy-containing drinks (fizzy, alcohol, milk, or juice) appear to increase daily intake in free-living adults aged 18–75 years in comparison with days when they are not consumed, suggesting these extra calories are not compensated for in subsequent eating (de Castro, 1993). This concurs with laboratory studies of Mattes and Campbell (2009), suggesting energy-containing beverages are less compensated for in the next eating episode compared with solid food. It has also been suggested that fructose, a major ingredient in sweetened beverages (often as high-fructose corn syrup), may promote appetite and food intake (Bray et al., 2004); this is thought to be associated with insufficient secretion of insulin and leptin and suppression of ghrelin (Melanson et al., 2008).

The Role of Dietary Fiber

There is much evidence that dietary fiber is a key component in the diet for prevention of chronic diseases such as cardiovascular disease (CVD), as shown by considerable research on glycemic index (GI) and glycemic load (GL), especially in subjects with impaired metabolic control (hyperlipidemia or diabetes). This can be achieved by altering the amount of available carbohydrate or type of carbohydrate. CVD risk profile may also be independently improved with whole-grain consumption, such as oats as it is suggested that they may have positive anti-inflammatory effects, possibly relating to beta-glucan content (Kallio et al., 2008). Fiber may be useful in the treatment of obesity by facilitating compliance to low EI (Rigaud et al., 1987; Astrup et al., 1990). It can impact on satiety in several ways: it increases food volume; decreases ED; increases gastric volume; retards gastric emptying, which maximizes early satiety signals; and influences satiety hormones in the gut. Increasing fiber intake during weight maintenance, however, has limited impact on body weight control (Aston et al., 2008).

Different types of fiber have been examined for their impact on satiety. Specifically, soluble fibers, which provide viscosity to a food, can increase its satiating effects (Dikeman and Fahey, 2006), with highly viscous fiber reducing subsequent food intake more than medium- or low-viscosity fiber (Vuksan et al., 2009) by forming a viscous gel matrix in the gut, believed to slow gastric emp-

tying and to lead to a greater feeling of fullness (Howarth et al., 2001; Hoad et al., 2004). Viscous fibers can slow absorption of glucose in the small intestine and lead to lower postprandial glycemic and insulinemic responses (Behall et al., 2006; Casiraghi et al., 2006). Both of these mechanisms are postulated to increase satiety. Insoluble fiber has limited effects on gastric emptying and absorption in the small intestine, but it may be partially fermented in the large intestine. Research on resistant starch (RS) and satiety is inconsistent (Raben et al., 1994; de Roos et al., 1995; Nilsson et al., 2008). It is possible that certain types or amounts of RS could improve satiety by increasing levels of the gut hormones glucagon-like peptide-1 (GLP1) or peptide YY (PYY). One study has reported that RS may mediate satiety by altering colonic fermentation and gastric emptying rate (Nilsson et al., 2008), with colonic fermentation (as measured by breath hydrogen) positively correlated with satiety and inversely correlated with gastric emptying.

Non-Nutritional Influences on Energy Intake, Obesity, and Eating Behavior

Examining the non-nutritional influences on eating behavior tends to focus on what we eat (food choice), whereas the physiological or metabolic aspects focus on how much we eat (calorie content or weight of food intake). The sensory (odor, texture, taste, appearance) aspects of a food or meal can significantly alter our choice, at least in the short term. These sensory or hedonic parameters influence the reward aspects of eating behavior, and much research focuses on assessing responses to changing single parameters. It is worth noting that Finlayson and co-workers have recently developed assessment techniques for quantifying "liking" and "wanting" foods. Liking is the hedonic evaluation (pleasantness, appreciation) of tasting a particular food, whereas wanting refers to the desire to actually ingest a particular food. Wanting has a much more direct effect on food intake than liking (Finlayson et al., 2007).

The Role of Palatability

The palatability of a food can be thought of as its sensory capacity to stimulate ingestion of that food (Mela and Rogers, 1998). This definition takes account of the fact that the palatability of the food is jointly determined by the nature of the food (odor, taste, texture, and state), the sensory capabilities and metabolic state of the subject, and the environment in which the food and subject interact.

Palatability is therefore not stable; indeed, the palatability of a food typically declines as its own ingestion proceeds, as described below. This has been called sensory-specific satiety (Le Magnen, 1971; Rolls *et al.*, 1981a). Satiety is said to be sensory specific in relation to foods because the palatability of a food declines as its ingestion proceeds whereas unsampled foods do not change in perceived pleasantness (O'Doherty and Rolls, 2000). This suggests that, once a given amount of a certain food has been ingested, its palatability will decline to a point where it is deemed less palatable than other foods. This in turn should promote subsequent selection of those other foods and so maintain a variety of foods ingested in a meal. In this context, it is important to ascertain exactly why the pleasantness of a specific food declines as its ingestion proceeds. The texture of foods can influence palatability and calorie intake. Both people and rodents can consume more ad libitum from liquid foods than they can consume in solid foods. This is related to rate of eating, which is higher for liquids when compared with semi-solids. For example, eating 500 g of apples takes about 17 minutes, whereas drinking the equivalent amount of apple juice can be done in 1.5 minutes (Flood-Obbagy and Rolls, 2009). However, it should be noted that slower eating does not necessarily lead to lower food intake.

Commercially available foods are largely designed to maximize both the sensory and dietary parameters, which make foods appealing to enhance consumer demand and repeat sales. These foods are likely to promote weight gain. However, the food industry produces the types of food that consumers demand. Further knowledge about the importance of palatability and food intake in the long term and how to alter food processing to maximize palatability of food during weight loss is likely to be a future research area.

The Role of Sensory Variety

In summary, short-term studies (within-day) have indicated that increasing sensory variety leads to an increase in food intake (Rolls *et al.*, 1981a,b). It has been shown that increased variety of foods made available either sequentially or simultaneously increases very short-term food intake (i.e. within a meal) (Bellisle and Le Magnen, 1981; Rolls *et al.*, 1981b; Rolls, 1985; Spiegel and Stellar, 1990). Changes in the variety of similar foods offered at a meal elevate EI, compared with one food offered throughout (Bellisle and Le Magnen, 1981; Rolls *et al.*, 1981b, Rolls, 1985). Spiegel and Stellar (1990) have shown this

to be the case in both lean and overweight women. They also found that simultaneous increases in the variety of foods offered elevates intake as compared with sequential increases in the variety of foods offered in a single meal. Rolls has reported that the greater the dissimilarity between different foods, the greater the variety-stimulating effect on the short-term intake of foods (Rolls, 1985). This is explained by the phenomenon of "sensory-specific satiety". This refers to the decline in reward value during consumption of a food because of repeated exposure to a particular sensory signal. This can be simply described as increased boredom with the taste of a particular product.

It has also been shown by Blundell's group that combinations of sensory attributes associated with mixtures of fat and sugar can have a large effect on EI at a specific feeding episode (Green and Blundell, 1996). This suggests that increases in EI will be promoted by the combination of sensory attributes of foods. More food is often consumed in the presence of other people, a phenomenon known as "social facilitation of energy intake" (de Castro, 1997), a feature of social eating.

One longer term study conducted over a week (Stubbs *et al.*, 2001b) assessed the effects of increasing the variety of nutritionally very similar but sensorially distinct foods available ad libitum in lean and overweight men. Offering 5, 10 or 15 food items per day led to a significant increase in food and EI in the lean men. These data indicate that increasing the variety of sensorially distinct but nutritionally similar foods increased food intake. This had a potent effect on EI and energy balance because subjects actively increased the amount of food they ingested in response to the variety offered. It is not clear if this effect would be maintained over a more prolonged period of time (weeks or months).

The Role of Eating Patterns – Snacking and Frequency of Eating

There is no strong relationship between eating frequency and obesity; obese people ingest more energy than non-obese people, therefore it might be reasonable to assume that meal size is a key factor in overconsumption in obesity. However, the combined contribution of meals and snacks to overeating is still debated within the research arena. There are two alternative hypotheses about how snacking may influence EI and body weight (Johnstone *et al.*, 2000): (1) snacking helps "fine tune" meal-time EIs to match intake with requirements; (2) habitual consumption of calorific drinks and snacks between meals is a major factor driving EI up and predisposing people to weight gain (Booth, 1988). For example, snackers report consuming more energy than non-snackers do (McCrory *et al.*, 2002), but these people may be more physically active and use snacking to modify EI. This is further complicated by the lack of a universal definition of a "snack", either by time of day (e.g. intermeal interval) or size ("small meal") or nutrient profile (food group) or structure (e.g. solid/liquid). The evidence in relation to meal patterns, appetite, EI, and body weight is indirect and fragmentary. Cross-sectional studies tend to support no or a negative relationship between meal frequency and body mass index (BMI) (Fábry *et al.*, 1964; Fábry and Tepperman, 1970). In contrast, increased snacking is associated with television viewing and the latter is associated with increased adiposity (Jackson *et al.*, 2009). Bellisle *et al.* (1997) argue that examinations of the relationship between snacking and energy balance in free-living subjects are extensively flawed by misreporting and misclassification of meals and snacks.

Snacking and commercially available snack foods are often believed to elevate EI (Drummond *et al.*, 1996; Gatenby, 1997; Grogan *et al.*, 1997). This does not mean that ingestion of commercially available foods (commonly termed snack foods) may not influence appetite and EI. Snack foods can differ from other foods in ED, orosensory characteristics which may influence the hedonics of eating, and macronutrient composition. There is some evidence that people who snack frequently exhibit a greater capacity to compensate for changes in the energy content of specific meals, relative to subjects who derive most of their EI from fewer, larger meals (Westerterp-Plantenga *et al.*, 1994). Few controlled laboratory studies have examined whether simply altering the number of small, intermeal "snack" events affects total daily food and EI, although less controlled interventions have been conducted (Fábry *et al.*, 1964). Whereas the inclusion of snack foods in short-term protocols may elevate EI at a given eating episode (Green and Blundell, 1996), data from a more real-life context (Lawton *et al.*, 1998) suggest that, over periods of several days, altering meal patterns *per se* does not drastically alter EI in lean young adults. These data suggest that altering the temporal distribution of EI in itself is not likely to lead to weight gain. However, different subjects may respond differently. Westerterp-Plantenga *et al.* (1994) have shown that habitual meal feeders do not compensate well for alterations in the ED of specific meals and habitual snackers compensate more accurately. It is probable that, just as diet composition and sensory characteristics can interact to affect EI, so can diet composition and ED, especially in certain groups of subjects.

Habitually skipping breakfast is associated with a higher BMI in observational studies in adults (Keski-Rahkonen *et al.*, 2003) and consuming breakfast is associated with achieving and maintaining weight loss (Wing and Phelan, 2005). However, targeting the importance of a single eating episode for intervention has proved largely unsuccessful for weight control (Giovannini *et al.*, 2010). Controlled laboratory studies have examined frequency of eating, using small-portion feeding regimes ("nibbling") with isocaloric, larger-portion feeding regimes ("gorging"), to assess eating frequency and regularity on energy and nutrient metabolism (e.g. Verboeket-van de Venne and Westerterp, 1993), and have reported no metabolic advantage of either regime.

The Role of Portion Size

Since the 1970s, the portion size of commercially available foods and beverages has increased, a trend observed in a variety of settings including restaurants, supermarkets, and also in the home environment (Rolls, 2010). Laboratory-based studies examining single-meal eating episodes have suggested increased portion size promotes increased EI. There is a clear relationship between amount served and amount consumed, even when participants serve themselves. The "bottomless soup bowl experiment", where subjects received tomato soup with a hidden self-filling tube, consumed 73% more soup (113 kcal), compared with when the bowl was refilled by a server (Wansink *et al.*, 2005). Other studies suggest this effect persists for up to 4 days (Kelly *et al.*, 2009), but this would have to be sustained over an extended period of time to contribute to weight gain. Studies in a more natural environment, such as a cafeteria-style restaurant or workplace, have also indicated that increasing the size of a meal portion by 50% increased intake with no apparent compensatory reduction, even when studied for a month (Diliberti *et al.*, 2004). Self-reports of food intake also suggest poor regulation with increased portion size (Bray *et al.*, 2004). One study reports men and women eating 19.4 MJ extra (a 16% increase in EI) over an 11-day period when provided with larger portions, which would equate to a 0.5-kg weight gain (Rolls *et al.*, 2007). This feature of modern eating behavior has, in particular, been the focus of media attention, with "supersize" portions being blamed for the rise in obesity in children and adults. Roughly 41% of Americans report consuming three or more commercially prepared meals a week in 1999–2000 (Kant and Graubard, 2003). The ready availability and low cost of large portions of energy-dense foods can contribute to a positive energy balance over a prolonged period. However, the data do not prove that portion size plays a role in the etiology of obesity, and there is little evidence that decreasing portion size is acceptable or effective for weight control. Reducing portion sizes or marketing of foods for dieting is not straightforward, since consumers equate large portions with good value and small portions with feeling deprived. Improving consumer awareness about nutritional information at point of sale and incentives for the food industry to offer a variety of portions are measures likely in the future to be considered by policy makers to control food provision within the "obesogenic" eating environment.

Psychological Influences on Energy Intake, Obesity, and Eating Behavior

There is a growing body of evidence that suggests that subjects behave differently in relation to various nutritional challenges. These are often termed "responders" and "non-responders" to interventions. The reasons for disparity in response may be physiological (e.g. body size or age), genetic (e.g. leptin resistance), phenotypic (gene–nutrient interaction), or psychological influences. There are a number of common categories of psychological influences on eating behavior, discussed below.

Restrained Eating Behavior

Dietary restraint refers to the tendency to restrict food intake in order to control body weight. Investigators commonly use a questionnaire such as the Dutch Eating Behavior Questionnaire (DEBQ, van Strien et al., 1986) or the three-factor eating inventory (TFEI, Stunkard and Messick, 1985) to classify subjects as restrained eaters. Dietary restraint can also be associated with "disinhibition," loss of control over eating resulting in binge eating. Examples from the literature in which dietary restraint can influence study results include two studies conducted by Westerterp-Plantenga et al. (1997, 1998) where restrained women responded to covert manipulations of meals by failing to compensate for dietary inclusion of the fat mimetic (Olestra) as an energy deficit whereas non-restrained lean women compensated EI by 44%. An additional difference in response was that the EIs of restrained women were actually (or were self-reported as) lower than those of their unrestrained counterparts.

Emotional and External Eating Behavior

The DEBQ and EI questionnaires can also identify the extent to which external environment and internal emotional aspects influence food intake. The *externality theory* of human obesity was developed by Schachter and co-workers in the 1960s (Schachter et al., 1968). They proposed that obese subjects are more reactive to external food-related cues and less sensitive to internal hunger and satiation cues than lean individuals. This relates to a scenario such as walking past a baker's shop and buying a nice cake or pastry to eat, with no prior plan to have a snack. Inter-individual differences in susceptibility to weight gain may be due, in part, to variability in responsiveness to environmental (external) triggers, particularly in an obesogenic environment. The phenomenon of food craving ("an irresistible urge to consume a specific food"), in particular for high-fat foods (Waters et al., 2001), has been implicated as an important factor influencing appetite control. Burton et al. (2007) identified an association between food craving and external eating scores among a mixed-age sample of both males and females. More specifically this was in relation to total food cravings and cravings for high-fat foods, with food craving accounting for approximately 8–20% of the variance in BMI. This area merits further investigation, since the link between eating behavior(s), externality, and food craving as a risk factor for obesity is not well understood.

Emotionality Theory

Food intake can have a remarkable effect on mood, and most individuals will have their own food-associated, mood-related habits, e.g. a cup of coffee to get going in the morning or eating sweet foods to reduce anxiety. Emotional states can have major effects on eating behavior, and result in either overeating or undereating. There have been several reviews of studies concerning emotional eating in relation to body weight (e.g. Allison and Heshka, 1993). These studies have almost always dealt with negative emotions such as depression or fear, comparing obese and normal-weight subjects, with results indicating relative overeating in obese individuals during negative emotional states. A psychosomatic interpretation has been that eating by obese individuals in response to negative emotions is a learned behavior to reduce the negative state (Kaplan and Kaplan, 1957). Geliebter and Aversa (2003) conducted a questionnaire study of underweight, normal-weight, and obese subjects and also similarly reported that the overweight group ate more than the other weight groups when experiencing negative emotions and situations, whereas underweight individuals reported eating more when experiencing positive emotions and situations. Most striking was the undereating by underweight individuals during negative emotions and situations, which may contribute to their being underweight. The relationship between mood and food will continue to be hotly debated at an individual and population level.

Stress and Eating Behavior

Stress is a fact of modern everyday life and the interaction between stress and eating is complex, with subgroups of the general population either increasing or decreasing their food intake during or after stress, depending on eating behavior profile and personality phenotype. There is a relationship between reported stress/daily hassles and increased consumption of high-fat and high-sugar foods between meals (snacking) (Wallis and Hetherington, 2009). The impact of stress on eating behavior varies with both the types of stress experienced and the personality and eating phenotype. For example, O'Connor et al. (2008) have reported that work-related, ego-threatening and interpersonal stresses were associated with increased snacking, whereas physical stressors were associated with decreased snacking. Accordingly, chronic stress may contribute to the obesity epidemic. Also, restrained or disinhibited eating will alter response to stress in terms of increasing and decreasing food intake (Haynes et al., 2003). The relationship between food intake and stress varies with gender, obesity, and eating behavior(s) (e.g. emotional eating, dietary restraint) (Wardle et al., 2000).

Physiological Influences on Energy Intake, Obesity, and Eating Behavior

When food is ingested, physiological and psychological responses are induced that depend on its energy and macronutrient content and structure. The macronutrient composition determines the caloric content, digestibility, and rate of passage of a meal through the gastrointestinal tract (the gut) and strongly influences the secretion of peptide hormones from the gut. These hormones in turn feedback to brain centers that control eating behavior, metabolism, and energy utilization. During meal processing, the gut secretes a number of newly identified hormones that signal to the brain to suppress future food intake. Physiological changes, such as gut peptide concentrations, are related to appetitive ratings or food intake,

and can be used as biomarkers of appetite. The regulation of appetite is, however, complex and it is not surprising that multiple control systems exist. A review of satiety and satiation bio-markers is detailed in de Graaf et al. (2004), with a summary of common plasma markers below.

Glucose has been central to many short-term appetite-regulation theories since the proposal of the glucostatic theory of eating in the 1950s (Mayer, 1995). This theory suggests, in part, that a spontaneous meal request is frequently preceded by a transient decline in blood glucose utilization (see Van Itallie, 1990, for a review). Thus, it has been proposed as an appetitive biomarker candidate. However, this may not be the case because glucose is not a robust measure of meal initiation since feeding occurs in the absence of transient declines in blood glucose. Indeed, changes in insulin concentration have also been identified as appetite markers in normal-weight subjects (Flint et al., 2007).

A more recently identified potential biomarker of meal initiation is the gut peptide, ghrelin. Data have suggested ghrelin to be a potent stimulator of ad libitum food intake when administered intravenously, with changes in concentration mirroring subjective ratings of hunger (Wren et al., 2001) in lean and obese subjects (Druce et al., 2005).

Cholecystokinin (CCK) has been the most extensively studied gut peptide associated with satiation, and is particularly linked to fat ingestion (see Moran, 2000, for a review). CCK is released from the gastrointestinal tract by the local action of digested food, and exerts various functions: stimulation of gall bladder contraction and exocrine pancreatic secretion, inhibition of gastric emptying, and inhibition of appetite. CCK acts as a positive feedback signal to stimulate digestive processes and as a negative feedback signal to limit the amount of food consumed during an individual meal (Beglinger and Degen, 2004).

Drugs that can be considered suitable candidates for appetite suppressants are agents that peripherally enhance satiety peptide systems include GLP-1 (Halford et al., 2010). *Glucagon-like peptide 1* (GLP-1) is released predominantly in the ileum and influences gastrointestinal motility and, through this mechanism, may moderate appetite (Holst, 2007). Because of these actions, GLP-1 or GLP-1 receptor agonists are being evaluated for the therapy of type 2 diabetes.

Peptide YY (PYY) is released primarily in the colon and acts as an agonist on a receptor in the hypothalamus. The studies of Batterham et al. (2002) suggest a differential expression in lean and obese subjects to suppress short-term food intake. Further work on different diet compositions and energy load are required to establish it as a novel biomarker.

Insulin is unlikely to be a biomarker of satiety since it is involved in long-term energy balance. In healthy subjects it stabilizes blood glucose by stimulating the uptake of glucose by peripheral tissues and by suppressing hepatic glucose production (de Graaf *et al.*, 2004). The role of insulin in metabolic health is discussed in more detail in Chapter 45, "Obesity as a Health Risk."

Leptin is a product of the ob gene, and is synthesized mainly by adipose tissue, providing information on the availability of fat stores to the hypothalamus. Thus, the effects of leptin as a biomarker are most potent when humans are not in energy balance, particularly when energy restricted. Leptin is not a sensitive marker of short-term satiety. The role of adipose tissue and expression of inflammatory markers is not covered by this chapter but is discussed elsewhere, for example, Chapter 45, "Obesity as a Health Risk."

Glucose-dependent insulinotropic polypeptide (GIP) is released in response to glucose and fat ingestion. Short-term (within-day) intervention studies in lean and obese subjects suggest that it has a poor relationship with appetite ratings and is therefore not a major biomarker of appetite.

Future Directions

Developing our understanding of control of eating, energy intake, and the development of obesity is likely to be best achieved by multidisciplinary groups of researchers working on large projects. The following are some that have attracted European Union funding streams that will provide novel data over the next 5 years:

Obesity and the Workplace

Since many adults spend a substantial amount of their time at work and consume at least one meal at work each day, a healthy workplace environment is important, particularly as jobs become more sedentary. An increased prevalence of obesity among employees can have indirect economic consequences for employers in terms of lost productivity through illness and absenteeism of employees. This will become an area of focus for policy makers, particularly in order to increase our understanding of stress-induced eating and its potential impact on body-weight regulation. There are currently limited initiatives

to reduce stress, particularly in the workplace. Shaping the work environment to reduce the incidence of disadvantageous eating patterns and promote healthier physical activity patterns in order to control calorie intake and body weight requires evidence-based research. In particular, research may focus on elucidating how typical stress situations in modern life trigger disadvantageous eating patterns and preferences for certain foods.

Food Addiction?

A key attribute of our modern environment is a plentiful supply of safe, energy-dense food. The shared giving and receiving of food is important in a social context, and the consumption of highly palatable food can be intensely rewarding. Public health strategies that fail to preserve this are doomed to failure through population non-compliance. The neuropsychology of food reward and food choice and the links between the appetite regulatory network, eating behavior, and food preference are not understood. Future research will likely focus on brain neuroanatomy and interactions with food to challenge whether food is indeed "addictive" and to investigate the pathways involved in the "rewarding" aspects of food and whether this experience can be replicated in healthier food-product alternatives so as to control body weight.

Gut–Brain Control of Energy Balance across the Lifespan

Hunger involves a complex interaction of psychological and physiological systems that link the gut (the gastrointestinal tract) and brain (Badman and Flier, 2005). There are three important elements to the regulation of EI: food – its nutrient, energy and physical composition; the gut – the origin of multiple feedback signals; and the brain. Together, these form the food–gut–brain axis, which is important in the common scenario of overconsumption. During early neonatal life, the developing hypothalamic projections are sensitive to peripheral hormonal signals, which may include the gut hormones, and this developmental programming may influence susceptibility to obesity and chronic disease in adult life. It is important to understand exactly how early life nutrition may affect subsequent eating behavior to inform appropriate recommendations and design foods targeted at the young. Towards the end of life, different problems arise: dysfunction of neural and neuroendocrine processes can result in loss of appetite, and consequent wasting adds to morbidity and impairs quality of life in the elderly. Here, the greater need may be to develop foods that stimulate appetite effectively in this population.

Understanding Mechanisms of Dietary-Induced Satiety for Weight Control

Dietary interventions based on caloric restriction or macronutrient manipulation can promote weight loss, as can exercise-induced energy deficit. In theory, weight loss is easy, whereby calorie intake is less than expenditure. However, in practice this is often difficult to achieve in the medium to long term by obese subjects. One of the main reasons for failure to adhere to a diet is feeling hungry. We do not understand the variability in psychological and behavioral parameters of hunger/satiety and food preference during energy deficit (exercise or diet induced) across the life course, and how these manipulations relate to gut hormones, neural activation, and energy metabolism. The psychological, behavioral, and endocrine/neurological bases of these effects and their applicability across age, gender, and phenotype remain to be determined.

Suggestions for Further Reading

Blundell, J., de Graaf, C., Hulshof, T., et al. (2010) Appetite control: methodological aspects of the evaluation of foods. *Obes Rev* **11**, 251–270.

de Graaf, C., Blom, W.A., Smeets, P.A., et al. (2004) Biomarkers of satiation and satiety. *Am J Clin Nutr* **79**, 946–961.

de Krom, M., Bauer, F., Collier, D., et al. (2009) Genetic variation and effects on human eating behavior. *Annu Rev Nutr* **29**, 283–304.

Delzenne, N., Blundell, J., Brouns, F., et al. (2010) Gastrointestinal targets of appetite regulation in humans. *Obes Rev* **11**, 234–250.

Hetherington, M.M. (2002) The physiological-psychological dichotomy in the study of food intake. *Proc Nutr Soc* **61**, 497–507.

Jebb, S.A. (2007) Dietary determinants of obesity. *Obes Rev* **8**(Suppl 1), 93–97.

References

Allison, D.B. and Heshka, S. (1993) Emotion and eating in obesity? A critical analysis. *Int J Eating Dis* **13**, 289–295.

Aston, L.M., Stokes, C.S., and Jebb, S.A. (2008) No effect of a diet with a reduced glycaemic index on satiety, energy intake and body weight in overweight and obese women. *Int J Obes (Lond)* **32**, 160–165.

Astrup, A., Vrist, E., and Quaade, F. (1990) Dietary fibre added to very low calorie diet reduces hunger and alleviates constipation. *Int J Obes* **14**, 105–112.

Badman, M.K. and Flier, J.S. (2005) The gut and energy balance: visceral allies in the obesity wars. *Science* **307**, 1909–1914.

Batterham R.L., Cowley M.A., Small C.J., et al. (2002) Gut hormone PYY(3–36) physiologically inhibits food intake. *Nature* **418**, 650–654.

Beglinger, C. and Degen, L. (2004) Fat in the intestine as a regulator of appetite – role of CCK. *Physiol Behav* **83**, 617–621.

Behall, K.M., Scholfield, D.J., Hallfrisch, J.G., et al. (2006) Consumption of both resistant starch and beta-glucan improves postprandial plasma glucose and insulin in women. *Diabetes Care* **29**, 976–981.

Bell, E.A., Castellanos, V.H., Pelkman, C.L., et al. (1998) Energy density of foods affects energy intake in normal-weight women. *Am J Clin Nutr* **67**, 412–420.

Bellisle, F. and Le Magnen, J. (1981) The structure of meals in humans: eating and drinking patterns in lean and obese subjects. *Physiol Behav* **27**, 649–658.

Bellisle, F., McDevitt, R., and Prentice, A.M. (1997) Meal frequency and energy balance. *Br J Nutr* **77**(Suppl 1), S57–70.

Blundell, J. (1991) Pharmacological approaches to appetite suppression. *Trends Pharmacol Sci* **12**, 147–157.

Blundell, J., de Graaf, C., Hulshof, T., et al. (2010) Appetite control: methodological aspects of the evaluation of foods. *Obes Rev* **11**, 251–270.

Blundell, J.E. and Macdiarmid, J.I. (1997) Passive overconsumption fat intake and short-term energy balance. *Ann NY Acad Sci* **827**, 392–407.

Blundell, J.E. and Stubbs, R.J. (1999) High and low carbohydrate and fat intakes: limits imposed by appetite and palatability and their implications for energy balance. *Eur J Clin Nutr* **53**(Suppl 1), S148–165.

Blundell, J.E., Cotton, J.R., Delargy, H., et al. (1995) The fat paradox: fat-induced satiety signals versus high fat overconsumption. *Int J Obes Relat Metab Disord* **19**, 832–835.

Booth, D.A. (1988) Mechanisms from models – actual effects from real life: the zero-calorie drink-break option. *Appetite* **11**(Suppl 1), 94–102.

Bray, G.A., Nielsen, S.J., and Popkin, B.M. (2004) Consumption of high-fructose corn syrup in beverages may play a role in the epidemic of obesity. *Am J Clin Nutr* **79**, 537–543.

Burton, P., Smit, H.J., and Lightowler, H.J. (2007) The influence of restrained and external eating patterns on overeating. *Appetite* **49**, 191–197.

Casiraghi, M.C., Garsetti, M., Testolin, G., et al. (2006) Postprandial responses to cereal products enriched with barley beta-glucan. *J Am Coll Nutr* **25**, 313–320.

De Castro, J.M. (1993) The effects of the spontaneous ingestion of particular foods or beverages on the meal pattern and overall nutrient intake of humans. *Physiol Behav* **53**, 1133–1144.

De Castro, J.M. (1997) Socio-cultural determinants of meal size and frequency. *Br J Nutr* **77**(Suppl 1), S39–54.

de Castro, J.M. (2006) Macronutrient and dietary energy density influences on the intake of free-living humans. *Appetite* **46**, 1–5.

de Graaf, C., Blom, W.A., Smeets, P.A., *et al.* (2004) Biomarkers of satiation and satiety. *Am J Clin Nutr* **79**, 946–961.

de Roos, N., Heijnen, M.L., de Graaf, C., *et al.* (1995) Resistant starch has little effect on appetite, food intake and insulin secretion of healthy young men. *Eur J Clin Nutr* **49**, 532–541.

Dikeman, C.L. and Fahey, G.C. (2006) Viscosity as related to dietary fiber: a review. *Crit Rev Food Sci Nutr* **46**, 649–663.

Diliberti, N., Bordi, P.L., Conklin, M.T., *et al.* (2004) Increased portion size leads to increased energy intake in a restaurant meal. *Obes Res* **12**, 562–568.

Druce, M.R., Wren, A.M., Park, A.J., *et al.* (2005) Ghrelin increases food intake in obese as well as lean subjects. *Int J Obes (Lond)* **29**, 1130–1136.

Drummond, S., Crombie, N., and Kirk, T. (1996) A critique of the effects of snacking on body weight status. *Eur J Clin Nutr* **50**, 779–783.

Economics Research Service, US Department of Agriculture (1999) *America's Eating Habits: Changes and Consequences.* USDA/ERS, Washington, DC.

Eisenstein, J., Roberts, S.B., Dallal, G., *et al.* (2002) High-protein weight-loss diets: are they safe and do they work? A review of the experimental and epidemiologic data. *Nutr Rev* **60**, 189–200.

Fábry, P. and Tepperman, J. (1970) Meal frequency – a possible factor in human pathology. *Am J Clin Nutr* **23**, 1059–1068.

Fábry, P., Hejl, Z., Fodor, J., *et al.* (1964) The frequency of meals. Its relation to overweight, hypercholesterolemia, and decreased glucose-tolerance. *Lancet* **2**, 614–615.

Finlayson, G., King, N., and Blundell, J.E. (2007) Liking vs. wanting food: importance for human appetite control and weight regulation. *Neurosci Biobehav Rev* **31**, 987–1002.

Flint, A., Gregersen, N.T., Gluud, L.L., *et al.* (2007) Associations between postprandial insulin and blood glucose responses, appetite sensations and energy intake in normal weight and overweight individuals: a meta-analysis of test meal studies. *Br J Nutr* **98**, 17–25.

Flood-Obbagy, J.E. and Rolls, B.J. (2009) The effect of fruit in different forms on energy intake and satiety at a meal. *Appetite* **52**, 416–422.

Gatenby, S.J. (1997) Eating frequency: methodological and dietary aspects. *Br J Nutr* **77**(Suppl 1), S7–20.

Geliebter, A. and Aversa, A. (2003) Emotional eating in overweight, normal weight, and underweight individuals. *Eating Behav* **3**, 341–347.

Giovannini, M., Agostoni, C., and Shamir, R. (2010) Symposium overview: Do we all eat breakfast and is it important? *Crit Rev Food Sci Nutr* **50**, 97–99.

Green, S.M. and Blundell, J.E. (1996) Effect of fat- and sucrose-containing foods on the size of eating episodes and energy intake in lean dietary restrained and unrestrained females: potential for causing overconsumption. *Eur J Clin Nutr* **50**, 625–635.

Grogan, S.C., Bell, R., and Conner, M. (1997) Eating sweet snacks: gender differences in attitudes and behaviour. *Appetite* **28**, 19–31.

Halford, J.C., Boyland, E.J., Blundell, J.E., *et al.* (2010) Pharmacological management of appetite expression in obesity. *Nat Rev Endocrinol* **6**, 255–269.

Halton, T.L. and Hu, F.B. (2004) The effects of high protein diets on thermogenesis, satiety and weight loss: a critical review. *J Am Coll Nutr* **23**, 373–385.

Haynes, C., Lee, M.D., and Yeomans, M.R. (2003) Interactive effects of stress, dietary restraint, and disinhibition on appetite. *Eat Behav* **4**, 369–383.

Hill, J.O. (2006) Understanding and addressing the epidemic of obesity: an energy balance perspective. *Endocr Rev* **27**, 750–761.

Himaya, A. and Louis-Sylvestre, J. (1998) The effect of soup on satiation. *Appetite* **30**, 199–210.

Hoad, C.L., Rayment, P., Spiller, R.C., *et al.* (2004) In vivo imaging of intragastric gelation and its effect on satiety in humans. *J Nutr* **134**, 2293–2300.

Holst, J.J. (2007) The physiology of glucagon-like peptide 1. *Physiol Rev* **87**, 1409–1439.

Hopkins, M., King. N.A., and Blundell, J.E. (2010) Acute and long-term effects of exercise on appetite control: is there any benefit for weight control? *Curr Opin Clin Nutr Metab Care* **13**, 635–640.

Howarth, N.C., Saltzman, E., and Roberts, S.B. (2001) Dietary fiber and weight regulation. *Nutr Rev* **59**, 129–139.

Jackson, D.M., Djafarian, K., Stewart, J., *et al.* (2009) Increased television viewing is associated with elevated body fatness but not with lower total energy expenditure in children. *Am J Clin Nutr* **89**, 1031–1036.

Johnstone, A.M., Horgan, G.W., Murison, S.D., *et al.* (2008) Effects of a high-protein ketogenic diet on hunger, appetite, and weight loss in obese men feeding ad libitum. *Am J Clin Nutr* **87**, 44–55.

Johnstone, A.M., Stubbs, R.J., and Harbron, C.G. (1996) Effect of overfeeding macronutrients on day-to-day food intake in man. *Eur J Clin Nutr* **50**, 418–430.

Kallio, P., Kolehmainen, M., Laaksonen, D.E., *et al.* (2008) Inflammation markers are modulated by responses to diets differing in postprandial insulin responses in individuals with the metabolic syndrome. *Am J Clin Nutr* **87,** 1497–1503.

Kant, A.K. and Graubard, B.I. (2003) Predictors of reported consumption of low-nutrient-density foods in a 24-h recall by 8–16 year old US children and adolescents. *Appetite* **41,** 175–180.

Kaplan, H.I. and Kaplan, H.S. (1957) The psychosomatic concept of obesity. *J Nerv Ment Dis* **125,** 181–201.

Kelly, M.T., Wallace, J.M., Robson, P.J., *et al.* (2009) Increased portion size leads to a sustained increase in energy intake over 4 d in normal-weight and overweight men and women. *Br J Nutr* **102,** 470–477.

Keski-Rahkonen, A., Kaprio, J., Rissanen, A., *et al.* (2003) Breakfast skipping and health-compromising behaviors in adolescents and adults. *Eur J Clin Nutr* **57,** 842–853.

Lawton, C.L., Delargy, H.J., Smith, F.C., *et al.* (1998) A medium-term intervention study on the impact of high- and low-fat snacks varying in sweetness and fat content: large shifts in daily fat intake but good compensation for daily energy intake. *Br J Nutr* **80,** 149–161.

Le Magnen, J. (1971) Advances in studies on the physiological control and regulation of food intake. In E. Stellar and J.M. Sprague (eds), *Progress in Physiological Psychology.* Academic Press, New York, pp. 203–261.

Levine, J.A. (2003) Non-exercise activity thermogenesis. *Proc Nutr Soc* **62,** 667–679.

Mattes, R.D. and Campbell, W.W. (2009) Effects of food form and timing of ingestion on appetite and energy intake in lean young adults and in young adults with obesity. *J Am Diet Assoc* **109,** 430–437.

Mattes, R.D., Hollis, J., Hayes, D., *et al.* (2005) Appetite: measurement and manipulation misgivings. *J Am Diet Assoc* **105**(Suppl 1), S87–97.

Mayer, J. (1955) Regulation of energy intake and the body weight: the glucostatic theory and the lipostatic hypothesis. *Ann NY Acad Sci* **63,** 15–43.

McCrory, M.A., Suen, V.M., and Roberts, S.B. (2002) Biobehavioral influences on energy intake and adult weight gain. *J Nutr* **132,** 3830S–3834S.

McLennan, W. and Podger, A. (1998) National Nutrition Survey. Nutrient Intakes and Physical Measurements Catalogue No. 4805.0. Australian Bureau of Statistics, Canberra.

Mela, D.J. and Rogers, P.J. (1998) *Food, Eating and Obesity. The Psychobiological Basis of Appetite and Weight Control.* Chapman & Hall, London

Melanson, K.J., Angelopoulos, T.J., Nguyen, V., *et al.* (2008) High-fructose corn syrup, energy intake, and appetite regulation. *Am J Clin Nutr* **88,** 1738S–1744S.

Moran, T.H. (2000) Cholecystokinin and satiety: current perspectives. *Nutrition* **16,** 858–865.

Nilsson, A.C., Ostman, E.M., Holst, J.J., *et al.* (2008) Including indigestible carbohydrates in the evening meal of healthy subjects improves glucose tolerance, lowers inflammatory markers, and increases satiety after a subsequent standardized breakfast. *J Nutr* **138,** 732–739.

O'Connor, D.B., Jones, F., Conner, M., *et al.* (2008) Effects of daily hassles and eating style on eating behavior. *Health Psychol* **27** (1 Suppl), S20–31.

O'Doherty, J. and Rolls, E.T. (2000) Sensory-specific satiety-related olfactory activation of the human orbitofrontal cortex. *NeuroReport* **11,** 399–403.

Poppitt, S.D., McCormack, D., and Buffenstein, R. (1998) Short-term effects of macronutrient preloads on appetite and energy intake in lean women. *Physiol Behav* **64,** 279–285.

Raben, A., Holst, J.J., Christensen, N.J., *et al.* (1996) Determinants of postprandial appetite sensations: macronutrient intake and glucose metabolism. *Int J Obes Relat Metab Disord* **20,** 161–169.

Raben, A., Tagliabue, A., Christensen, N.J., *et al.* (1994) Resistant starch: the effect on postprandial glycemia, hormonal response, and satiety. *Am J Clin Nutr* **60,** 544–551.

Rigaud, D., Ryttig, K.R., Leeds, A.R., *et al.* (1987) Effects of a moderate dietary fibre supplement on hunger rating, energy input and faecal energy output in young, healthy volunteers. A randomized, double-blind, cross-over trial. *Int J Obes* **11**(Suppl 1), 73–78.

Rolls, B.J. (1985) Experimental analyses of the effects of variety in a meal on human feeding. *Am J Clin Nutr* **42** (5 Suppl), 932–939.

Rolls, B.J. (2009) The relationship between dietary energy density and energy intake. *Physiol Behav* **97,** 609–615.

Rolls, B.J. (2010) Plenary lecture 1: Dietary strategies for the prevention and treatment of obesity. *Proc Nutr Soc* **69,** 70–79.

Rolls, B.J., Bell, E.A., and Thorwart, M.L. (1999) Water incorporated into a food but not served with a food decreases energy intake in lean women. *Am J Clin Nutr* **70,** 448–455.

Rolls, B.J., Rolls, E.T., Rowe, E.A., *et al.* (1981a) Sensory specific satiety in man. *Physiol Behav* **27,** 137–142.

Rolls, B.J., Rowe, E.A., Rolls, E.T., *et al.* (1981b) Variety in a meal enhances food intake in man. *Physiol Behav* **26,** 215–221.

Schachter, S., Goldman, R., and Gordon, A. (1968) Effects of fear, food deprivation and obesity on eating. *J Pers Soc Psychol* **10,** 91–97.

Skov, A.R., Toubro, S., Rønn, B., *et al.* (1999) Randomized trial on protein vs carbohydrate in ad libitum fat reduced diet for the treatment of obesity. *Int J Obes Relat Metab Disord* **23,** 528–536.

Spiegel, T.A. and Stellar, E. (1990) Effects of variety on food intake of underweight, normal-weight and overweight women. *Appetite* **15,** 47–61.

Stubbs, R.J. (1995) Macronutrient effects on appetite. *Int J Obes Relat Metab Disord* **19**(Suppl 5), S11–19.

Stubbs, R.J., Johnstone, A.M., Harbron, C.G., *et al.* (1998a) Covert manipulation of energy density of high carbohydrate diets in 'pseudo free-living' humans. *Int J Obes Relat Metab Disord* **22,** 885–892.

Stubbs, R.J., Johnstone, A.M., Mazlan, N., *et al.* (2001) Effect of altering the variety of sensorially distinct foods, of the same macronutrient content, on food intake and body weight in men. *Eur J Clin Nutr* **55,** 19–28.

Stubbs, R.J., Johnstone, A.M., O'Reilly, L.M., *et al.* (1998b) The effect of covertly manipulating the energy density of mixed diets on ad libitum food intake in 'pseudo free-living' humans. *Int J Obes Relat Metab Disord* **22,** 980–987.

Stubbs, R.J., van Wyk, M.C., Johnstone, A.M., *et al.* (1996) Breakfasts high in protein, fat or carbohydrate: effect on within-day appetite and energy balance. *Eur J Clin Nutr* **50,** 409–417.

Stunkard, A.J. and Messick, S. (1985) The three-factor eating questionnaire to measure dietary restraint, disinhibition and hunger. *J Psychosom Res* **29,** 71–83.

Suter, P.M. (2005) Is alcohol consumption a risk factor for weight gain and obesity? *Crit Rev ClinLab Sci* **42,** 197–227.

Van Itallie, T.B. (1990) The glucostatic theory 1953–1988: roots and branches. *Int J Obes* **14**(Suppl 3), 1–10.

van Strien, J.E., Frijters, J.E.R., Bergers, G.P.A., *et al.* (1986) The Dutch Eating Behaviour Questionnaire (DEBQ) for assessment of restrained, emotional, and external eating behavior. *Int J Eating Dis* **5,** 295–313.

Verboeket-van de Venne, W.P. and Westerterp, K.R. (1993) Frequency of feeding, weight reduction and energy metabolism. *Int J Obes Relat Metab Disord* **17,** 31–36.

Vimaleswaran, K.S. and Loos, R.J. (2010) Progress in the genetics of common obesity and type 2 diabetes. *Exp Rev Mol Med* **26.** PMID 20184785.

Vuksan, V.,Panahi, S., Lyon, M., *et al.* (2009) Viscosity of fiber preloads affects food intake in adolescents. *Nutr Metab Cardiovasc Dis* **19,** 498–503.

Wallis, D.J. and Hetherington, M.M. (2009) Emotions and eating. Self-reported and experimentally induced changes in food intake under stress. *Appetite* **52,** 355–362.

Wansink, B., Painter, J.E., and North, J. (2005) Bottomless bowls: why visual cues of portion size may influence intake. *Obes Res* **13,** 93–100.

Wardle, J., Steptoe, A., Oliver, G., *et al.* (2000) Stress, dietary restraint and food intake. *J Psychosom Res* **48,** 195–202.

Waters, A., Hill, A., and Waller, G. (2001) Bulimics' response to food cravings: is binge eating a product of hunger or emotional state? *Behav Res Ther* **39,** 866–877.

Westerterp-Plantenga, M.S. (2004) Fat intake and energy-balance effects. *Physiol Behav* **83,** 579–585.

Westerterp-Plantenga, M.S. and Lejeune, M.P. (2005) Protein intake and body-weight regulation. *Appetite* **45,** 187–190.

Westerterp-Plantenga, M.S., Wijckmans-Duijsens, N.E., ten Hoor, F., *et al.* (1997) Effect of replacement of fat by nonabsorbable fat (sucrose polyester) in meals or snacks as a function of dietary restraint. *Physiol Behav* **61,** 939–947.

Westerterp-Plantenga, M.S., Wijckmans-Duysens, N.A., and ten Hoor, F. (1994) Food intake in the daily environment after energy-reduced lunch, related to habitual meal frequency. *Appetite* **22,** 173–182.

Westerterp-Plantenga, M.S., Wijckmans-Duijsens, N.E.G., Verboeket-van de Venne, W.P.G., *et al.* (1998) Energy intake and body weight effects of six months' reduced or full fat diets, as a function of dietary restraint. *Int J Obes Relat Metab Disord* **22,** 14–22.

Wing, R.R. and Phelan, S. (2005) Long-term weight loss maintenance. *Am J Clin Nutr* **82** (1 Suppl), 222S–225S.

Wren, A.M., Seal, L.J., Cohen, M.A., *et al.* (2001) Ghrelin enhances appetite and increases food intake in humans. *J Clin Endocrinol Metab* **86,** 5992.

Yao, M. and Roberts, S.B. (2001) Dietary energy density and weight regulation. *Nutr Rev* **59,** 247–258.

Yeomans, M.R. (2010) Alcohol, appetite and energy balance: is alcohol intake a risk factor for obesity? *Physiol Behav* **100,** 82–89.

62

STRATEGIES FOR CHANGING EATING AND EXERCISE BEHAVIOR TO PROMOTE WEIGHT LOSS AND MAINTENANCE

RENA R. WING[1], PhD, AMY GORIN[2], PhD, AND DEBORAH F. TATE[3], PhD

[1]Brown University, Providence, Rhode Island, USA
[2]University of Connecticut, Storrs, Connecticut, USA
[3]University of North Carolina at Chapel Hill, North Carolina, USA

Summary

This chapter focuses on behavioral approaches for changing eating and exercise behaviors, with specific application to weight control. After reviewing the history of behavioral approaches and the core strategies that are taught in these programs, the chapter highlights research on the most effective ways to change dietary intake and physical activity, such as the recommended level of caloric intake and activity and strategies to promote adherence to these recommendations. The chapter also addresses newer directions in the field, focusing on strategies to promote social support, the use of media to cost-effectively disseminate programs, and the critical question of how best to maintain behavior changes long term.

Introduction

The leading causes of disease and death in the United States – coronary heart disease and cancer – are related to lifestyle factors. By changing eating and exercise habits and eliminating smoking, the prevalence of these diseases could be markedly reduced. The goal of this chapter is to provide readers with an overview of behavioral strategies that can be used to modify lifestyle behaviors. Although the behavioral principles are applicable to changing any type of health habit, this chapter will focus primarily on obesity, and will review strategies that may help in both the treatment and prevention of this disease.

History of Behavioral Weight Loss Programs

The underlying premise of a behavioral approach is the functional analysis of behavior, also known as the "A-B-C" model. A functional analysis involves identifying the

Present Knowledge in Nutrition, Tenth Edition. Edited by John W. Erdman Jr, Ian A. Macdonald and Steven H. Zeisel.
© 2012 International Life Sciences Institute. Published 2012 by John Wiley & Sons, Inc.

behaviors to be changed, which in the case of obesity would be eating and exercise behaviors, and the antecedent cues in the environment and the consequences or reinforcers that influence the behaviors. Behaviorists propose that, by changing the antecedents and consequences, it is possible to change the behavior.

$$\text{Antecedent} \rightarrow \text{Behavior} \leftarrow \text{Consequences}$$
$$\text{(Cues)} \qquad\qquad\qquad \text{(Reinforcers)}$$

The earliest application of behavioral principles to the problem of obesity occurred in the 1960s–1970s. With the notable exception of Stuart's initial study of eight overweight women (1967), these early behavioral weight-loss programs were typically conducted in groups with mildly overweight patients, and lasted about 10 weeks. The primary "behavior" that was targeted was a change in eating patterns (when and where food was eaten) rather than total calories. Similarly, participants were encouraged to change activity patterns by strategies such as using stairs instead of elevators, but no specific calorie goals for physical activity were prescribed. These early studies produced weight losses of 3.8 kg over an 8- to 10-week treatment program and were shown to be more effective than alternative approaches, such as nutrition education or psychotherapy.

The next generation of behavioral programs, conducted in the 1980s and 1990s, placed increasing emphasis on caloric intake and expenditure. Although moderate goals were initially prescribed for these behaviors, over time stricter dietary regimens and higher doses of activity were recommended. There was also increased attention given to changing cognitions, with introduction of concepts such as relapse prevention, and a gradual lengthening of treatment programs. By the end of the 1990s, average weight losses of 8.5–10 kg over approximately 24 weeks had become typical (Wing, 2008).

With these improvements in initial weight loss outcomes, attention shifted toward improving maintenance of the outcomes. As will be discussed later in the chapter, it quickly became apparent that, in order to reduce weight regain, a chronic disease model of obesity treatment was needed, and some type of ongoing therapy had to be provided. Programs were lengthened and various forms of ongoing treatment contact were provided. Thus, gradually, standard behavioral programs became longer, more intensive, and more effective. Figure 62.1 presents the weight losses achieved in behavioral treatment programs from

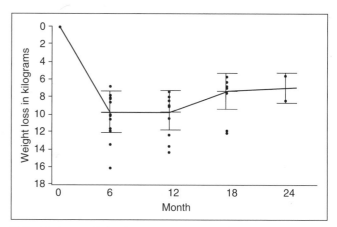

FIG. 62.1 Weight-loss outcomes in behavioral treatments from 1990 to 2000. Reproduced with permission from Wing, (2008).

1990 to 2000; weight losses in these trials averaged 10.37 kg at 6 months (12 studies), 10.35 kg at 12 months (eight studies), 8.2 kg at 18 months (seven studies), and 7.1 kg at 24 months (two studies).

Given the improvements in initial weight losses and longer-term maintenance, it also became possible to examine the role of weight loss in promoting health improvements. Several trials demonstrated that lifestyle interventions could successfully reduce the risk of developing hypertension and could also improve treatment outcomes for those with hypertension (Trials of Hypertension Prevention Collaborative Research Group, 1997; Whelton et al., 1998). In 2002, the Diabetes Prevention Program showed that lifestyle intervention could reduce the risk of developing diabetes by over 58% compared with placebo, and was twice as effective as metformin in preventing this disease (Knowler et al., 2002). More recently, behavioral weight loss interventions have been shown to reduce urinary incontinence in overweight/obese women (Subak et al., 2009), to improve non-alcoholic steatohepatitis (Promrat et al., 2010) and osteoarthritis (Christensen et al., 2007), and to improve glycemic control and cardiovascular risk factors in individuals with type 2 diabetes (Look AHEAD Research Group, 2007). Marked improvements in mood and quality of life also occur with these programs (Williamson et al., 2009).

Behavioral Strategies

This section provides a brief description of the key behavioral strategies used in weight-loss programs. These same basic strategies would be applicable to changing any type of nutrition behavior.

Identifying the Behaviors to Be Changed

The first step of a behavioral intervention is to clearly identify the specific behaviors to be modified. For example, for weight loss, the key behaviors that are targeted are those related to energy balance (calories consumed and calories expended). In applying behavioral principles to reduction of cholesterol levels, the key behaviors would include reductions in intakes of saturated fat and cholesterol. Similarly, in an intervention to reduce blood-pressure levels, reducing sodium intake would be an additional behavioral focus.

Setting Goals

In changing behaviors, it is helpful to set specific goals that can be achieved by the participant. Often both behavioral goals and physiological (outcome) goals are identified. For example, participants in weight-loss programs may aim to consume no more than 1200 kcal/day (5023 kJ/day), or to expend at least 1000 kcal/week (4186 kJ/week) in exercise; a weight-loss goal of 2 lb or 1 kg per week is often used. Short-term goals have been shown to be more effective than long-term goals in promoting behavior change (Bandura and Simon, 1977). Often behaviors are "shaped" by setting easier goals initially and then increasing the goal as the participant progresses. An example of shaping is seen in physical activity, where participants are first helped to increase their activity to 250 kcal/week (1046 kJ/week) or 500 kcal/week (2093 kJ/week) before attempting the 1000 kcal/week (4186 kJ/week) goal.

Self-Monitoring

A key strategy in the behavioral treatment of obesity is teaching participants to observe and record their own eating- and activity-related behavior, a technique known as self-monitoring. A variety of information can be recorded through self-monitoring, including the type and amount of food eaten, the number of calories in each food, the number of fat grams, and other eating-related items such as eating situation and pre-meal mood. Similarly, types and amounts of physical activity can be recorded in minutes or calories. Participants are instructed to record their intake daily and bring their self-monitoring books to group meetings, providing an opportunity for feedback from group leaders and other participants. Self-monitoring is usually done on a daily basis for the initial 6 months of treatment and then periodically during maintenance. Several studies support the utility of self-monitoring, suggesting a strong association between the completeness and consistency of self-monitoring and weight loss (Burke et al., 2008).

Technologies including internet and mobile devices (PDAs, smartphones, etc.) as well as objective activity monitors (accelerometers, pedometers, etc.) offer alternatives to the traditional paper-based diary and calorie books. Internet-based diaries allow the user to look up calories in a database and save those foods to an online record that is accessible from any internet-connected location. PDA and smartphone applications work in a similar fashion but offer the convenience of being portable so that monitoring can occur at the time a food is eaten. Recent studies show that self-monitoring intake using a Personal Digital Assistant (PDA) improves adherence to self-monitoring (Burke et al., 2008). For monitoring of physical activity, newer objective monitors are available that record acceleration or steps, and allow the user to upload the data to an internet site.

Stimulus Control

A central tenet of behavior modification is that an individual's behavior is influenced by his or her environment. Thus, by manipulating their surroundings, participants can change the likelihood of behavioral outcomes. Participants in behavioral treatment programs are taught to restructure their environment to decrease cues for inappropriate food consumption and increase cues for appropriate diet and exercise (Stuart, 1967). For example, participants are instructed to limit their purchases of high-fat foods and, if purchased, to store these foods out of sight. Conversely, participants are encouraged to purchase more fruits and vegetables and to increase the visibility of these items by storing them in prominent locations. To prompt physical activity, participants are encouraged to put items related to exercise in places where they will be seen on a frequent basis. Other stimulus-control strategies such as restricting eating to a designated place and eliminating the pairing of eating with other activities (e.g. watching television, reading) may also be effective means for altering antecedents that influence eating behavior. Stimulus-control techniques could be used to change other types of dietary behaviors; for example, individuals attempting to reduce their blood pressure might be instructed to remove the salt shakers from the table.

Problem Solving

When attempting to make permanent lifestyle changes, participants face many hurdles and obstacles. To help participants successfully navigate this process, training in problem-solving skills is included in behavioral treatment programs. Participants are taught to: (1) identify a specific problem that is hindering their weight-loss effort; (2) generate as many solutions as possible to the problem; (3) evaluate the possible solutions and select one; (4) implement the solution; and (5) evaluate the outcome and repeat the problem-solving process if necessary. Problem-solving techniques are used for individually identified problems; for example, one participant may have difficulty with overeating while preparing dinner while another may focus on the difficulty of eating out in restaurants. Perri and colleagues (2001) have demonstrated the importance of teaching problem solving during the maintenance phase of a behavioral weight-loss program.

Cognitive Restructuring

A more recent addition to behavioral weight-loss treatment is cognitive restructuring. Cognitive restructuring involves identifying and modifying maladaptive thoughts contributing to overeating and physical inactivity. These thoughts can take several forms such as dichotomous thinking (e.g. "If I can't exercise for 30 minutes, I might as well not do it all") and rationalization (e.g. "I've had a stressful day so I deserve a piece of cake"). Participants are often unaware of the impact thoughts have on behavior. Cognitive restructuring serves to highlight this process by having participants identify and challenge maladaptive thoughts and develop more positive self-statements to assist in behavior change.

Relapse Prevention

Helping participants prepare and plan for lapses in the weight-loss process is also included in behaviorally based programs. An extension of Marlatt and Gordon's work with addictions (1985), relapse prevention in behavioral weight-control programs involves teaching participants to anticipate problematic situations that might result in overeating and develop specific strategies for overcoming these lapses. Participants are encouraged to have a plan in place so that one overeating slip or lapse does not develop into a full-blown relapse.

Focusing on relapse prevention during the maintenance program has improved long-term outcomes in some

behavioral programs (Perri *et al.*, 1984) but not in others (Perri *et al.*, 2001).

Changing Eating Behavior

As noted above, the behaviors that must be targeted to produce weight loss are the behaviors related to energy balance. However, the best way to accomplish these changes remains unclear. In fact, there is little information about very basic aspects of these behaviors, e.g. the level of caloric intake that is best to prescribe, or the types of macronutrient composition in the diet that should be recommended. In the following sections, we will describe some of the behavioral research that has addressed these issues. Readers interested in more information about behavior changes to reduce intake of saturated fat or sodium or to increase intake of fiber, fruits, and vegetables are referred to the excellent review by Kumanyika *et al.* (2000).

Calorie Intake

Behavioral weight-loss programs typically utilize low-calorie diets of approximately 1200–1500 kcal/day (5023–6278 kJ/day) that are designed to produce weight losses of approximately 1–2 lb (0.5–1.0 g) per week. These regimens have been developed based on empirical studies comparing diets of different caloric levels. For example, in the 1980s and early 1990s, there was a great deal of interest in the use of very low calorie diets (VLCDs) during the initial phase of a behavioral program (Wadden and Stunkard, 1986; National Task Force on the Prevention and Treatment of Obesity, 1993). VLCDs are diets of 400–800 kcal/day (1674–3348 kJ/day), typically given as liquid formula or as lean meat, fish, and fowl. These regimens were found to produce large initial weight losses, averaging 20 kg over 12 weeks. However, since weight regain occurred when these diets were stopped, researchers suggested that it might be helpful to utilize VLCDs to increase initial weight loss, but to combine these diets with behavioral techniques to help maintain the weight loss long term. Several studies evaluated this combination (Wing *et al.*, 1991, 1994; Wadden *et al.*, 1994). Unfortunately the results consistently showed that participants rapidly regained their weight after completing the VLCDs, even if they had been taught behavioral strategies. Thus in the longer term, there was no advantage of these stricter calorie levels compared with the more modest degrees of calorie restriction, and consequently the field returned to the use of the 1200–2000 daily calorie level recommendations.

Macronutrient Composition

A second issue relates to the macronutrient composition of the diet. In the past, behavioral researchers focused primarily on calories and paid less attention to the types of foods consumed. However, based on epidemiological and metabolic studies showing an association between dietary fat intake and body weight (Tucker and Kano, 1992), researchers began to examine whether restricting fat intake would improve long-term weight-loss outcome. Behavioral weight-loss programs that taught patients to decrease calories and fat intake were found to be more effective than programs that focused on only calories or only fat, and thus the field began to adopt this approach (Schlundt et al., 1993; Jeffery et al., 1995; Pascale et al., 1995).

More recently there has been interest in low-carbohydrate diets (e.g. the Atkins or South Beach diets), some of which allow unlimited intake of protein and fat but drastically reduce carbohydrate intake. In the short term, these regimens appear to improve weight loss, but longer-term results have not been as supportive. For example, Dansinger and colleagues (2005) randomly assigned 160 overweight/obese participants to one of four dietary regimens: Atkins (low-carbohydrate diet), Zone (balanced diet), Weight Watchers (point-system diet that is low in fat), or Ornish (very low fat diet). There were no differences in weight loss at one year between the four groups (all groups lost 2.1–3.2 kg at 1 year). However, those who adhered best to whichever diet they had been prescribed had the best weight losses. This finding, stressing the importance of adherence rather than the actual macronutrient composition of the diet, has been confirmed in several other recent trials (Alhassan et al., 2008; Sacks et al., 2009).

Food Provision and Structured Meal Plans

Behaviorists have long recognized the importance of modifying the home environment as a means of influencing eating behaviors, and emphasized stimulus-control techniques to rearrange the home environment. Recently, behavioral researchers suggested that it might be possible to make even greater changes in the home environment by actually providing patients with the food they should eat in appropriate portion sizes. In a programmatic series of studies, Jeffery and Wing showed that participants who were actually provided with the foods they should eat had

better dietary adherence and greater weight losses than participants given the same calorie goals but left on their own to develop their meal plans (Jeffery et al., 1993; Wing et al., 1996). Positive results have also been obtained in several other studies where participants were given prepared meals (Pi-Sunyer et al., 1999) or where Slim-Fast™ (Ditschuneit et al., 1999) was used for one or two meals per day along with a healthy low-fat dinner meal. These studies suggest that simplifying eating, by providing individuals with structure and models of appropriate meals, may promote adherence to weight-loss regimens. Since, as described above, the most important factor in the dietary prescription is the level of adherence to the dietary prescription, techniques such as food provision may be critical in improving weight-loss outcomes.

Changing Exercise

The single best predictor of long-term maintenance of weight loss is physical activity (Pronk and Wing, 1994). Individuals who continue to exercise long term are the ones who are most successful at maintaining their weight loss. The challenge for behavioral researchers is to get overweight individuals to adopt and maintain an exercise program. Typically, behavioral weight-loss programs stress brisk walking or other similar moderate-intensity activities as the primary form of physical activity. Gradually increasing physical activity until reaching a goal of 200 minutes per week (40 minutes on 5 days per week) is encouraged.

Home Based versus Supervised

Having patients exercise under supervised condition allows researchers to better quantify the activity, to adjust the intensity or dose of activity over time, and to teach participants about warming up, cooling down, etc. However, traveling to a supervised site adds an extra burden for the participant and may discourage continued adherence. Several researchers have compared long-term participation and weight losses (Perri et al., 1997; Andersen et al., 1998) in supervised activity vs. home-based lifestyle activity programs. Andersen et al. (1998) compared a supervised exercise group that attended three aerobic dance classes per week with a lifestyle group whose members exercised on their own. Initial weight losses were comparable; there was, however, a trend for the lifestyle group to regain less weight during follow-up. Perri et al. (1997) also found similar initial weight losses between lifestyle vs. supervised exercise groups, but at month 15 the home-based program had an average weight loss of 11.65 kg whereas the supervised group had a mean weight loss of 7.01 kg, suggesting that home-based exercise may be more effective than supervised exercise for long-term weight-loss maintenance.

Short Bouts Versus Long Bouts

The supervised versus lifestyle programs described above may have differed not only in location but also in the way in which the activity occurred. In the studies cited above, participants in the supervised exercise conditions completed their activity in one bout on each of 3–5 days/week. The lifestyle conditions were told to "accumulate" 30 minutes of exercise each day. These participants may likewise have done this exercise in one bout, or alternatively completed several short bouts each day. Since lack of time is considered the greatest barrier to exercise, it may be easier for participants to exercise in multiple short bouts (four 10-minute bouts), rather than one 40-minute bout. To test this hypothesis, Jakicic and co-workers completed two weight-loss studies (1995, 1999) comparing programs which prescribed the same amount of lifestyle exercise in either one 40-minute bout or four 10-minute bouts 5 days per week. The first study found better exercise adherence over 6 months and somewhat greater weight losses in the short-bout condition (Jakicic et al., 1995). The second study (Jakicic et al., 1999) again found greater exercise participation in the short-bout group for the first several weeks of the study; however, from 6 to 18 months of the program, no differences between the short-bout and long-bout groups were observed. These two groups had comparable exercise participation, initial and long-term weight loss (–3.7 kg and –5.8 kg) and long-term improvements in fitness. Thus short-bout prescriptions of exercise may be particularly helpful during the initial phase of a weight-loss program; for long-term changes these two different types of exercise format appear to provide alternative, equally effective approaches to physical activity.

Providing Home Exercise Equipment

Another approach to promoting adherence to exercise is to provide patients with home exercise equipment. Although it is often noted anecdotally that such equipment receives little use over time, there has been little

empirical investigation of this strategy. Jakicic et al. (1997) observed a correlation between the number of pieces of activity equipment in the home and the activity level. Conceptually it would appear that providing exercise equipment to participants (like providing food) would help cue the appropriate behavior and reduce barriers related to access, cost, etc. Jakicic et al. (1999) examined this strategy in a study of overweight women participating in a behavioral weight-loss program, where one group was asked to complete their exercise in short bouts and another group was given the same exercise prescription and provided with a home treadmill. The group given the exercise equipment maintained a higher activity level from months 13–18 of the program and had significantly better weight loss over the 18-month study (–7.4 vs. –3.7 kg). Thus, this study supports the use of this strategy for improving long-term exercise adherence and weight loss.

Decreasing Sedentary Activities

Several studies have attempted to decrease sedentary activity, rather than increase exercise, as a way to influence overall activity level and either treat or prevent obesity. To date, this approach has been used primarily with children. Epstein and colleagues have studied various approaches to the treatment of obesity in children aged 8–12, and recently compared the effects of decreasing sedentary activities (TV, video games), increasing physical activity, versus the combination (Epstein et al., 1995). The group that focused on decreasing sedentary activities had the greatest decreases in percent overweight at 4 months and at 1 year (–18.7% in sedentary; –10.3% in combined, and –8.7% in the increased physical activity group). The group that was instructed to decrease sedentary activity also reported the greatest increases in their liking for vigorous activity. All groups showed comparable improvements in fitness level.

Reducing television viewing as a means to prevent obesity was also examined in a school-based study (Robinson, 1999) with 192 children (mean age 9 years). One school was randomly assigned to an 18-lesson, 6-month curriculum designed to decrease TV viewing. The children in that school self-monitored their television, video game, and videotape use and attempted a 10-day "turnoff" during which they watched no TV or video games. Subsequently, they attempted to decrease these sedentary activities to 7 hours per week. Electronic devices were attached to home television sets to monitor and budget viewing time. The control school received no intervention.

Children in the intervention school had statistically significant decreases in television viewing and meals eaten in front of the TV. The intervention children also had smaller increases in BMI (18.38 to 18.67) than the control children (18.10 to 18.81) over the 7-month study.

While reducing sedentary activity has demonstrated empirical support among children, only one small randomized controlled trial (RCT) has tested this approach among adults. Otten and colleagues (2009) recruited 36 adults who viewed 3 hours of TV per day or more, and randomized them to an intervention group with a goal of reducing TV viewing by 50% or to a control group. After 3 weeks, the TV reduction group showed significantly greater positive changes in energy expenditure per day (119 kcal/day vs. −95 kcal/day; $p<0.05$) and a trend toward improvements in energy intake relative to controls ($P = 0.07$), suggesting that this might also be a promising strategy for adults.

Amount of Physical Activity

Behavioral weight-loss programs have traditionally encouraged participants to gradually increase their physical activity until they achieve a 1000-kcal/week (4186 kJ/week) goal. (A 150-lb (68-kg) individual could achieve this caloric expenditure by walking 10 miles (16 km) per week or 2 miles (3.2 km) on each of 5 days in the week.) However, it was unclear whether this amount of activity was sufficient for weight loss and maintenance. The notion that higher levels of activity may be associated with better long-term weight-loss maintenance was first suggested by data collected in the National Weight Control Registry (Klem *et al.*, 1997). This registry is a database of over 6000 individuals who have lost at least 30 lb (13 kg; mean = 66 lb, 30 kg) and kept it off at least 1 year (mean = 6 years). Data from the first 784 subjects in the registry (629 women; 155 men) indicated that on average these individuals were expending 2829 kcal/week (11 841 kJ/week) in physical activity (Klem *et al.*, 1997). More recently this high level of physical activity in successful weight-loss maintainers was confirmed using accelerometers to provide an objective measure of physical activity (Phelan *et al.*, 2007).

Further evidence supporting the need for high levels of exercise for weight-loss maintenance emerged in post-hoc

analyses from a study of physical activity and weight loss (Jakicic *et al.*, 2008). Subjects ($n = 170$) were divided into categories according to their self-reported activity level. There was a strong association between physical activity and weight loss. Those participants who reported greater than 2000 kcal/week of activity had the best weight loss and maintenance.

Based on these data, Jeffery and colleagues conducted a randomized clinical trial comparing the weight-loss effects of a standard behavioral weight-loss program with a 1000-kcal/week (4186 kJ/week) exercise prescription, with a group prescribed a 2500 kcal/week (10 464 kJ/week) level of activity (Jeffery *et al.*, 2003). After 12–18 months, the group prescribed the higher dose of activity lost on average 3–4 kg more weight than the lower dose group. By follow-up at 30 months, most participants were no longer maintaining high levels of physical activity; thus, weight loss at 30 months did not differ between the randomized groups (Tate *et al.*, 2007). However, those who maintained their physical activity at the 2500 kcal/week level or greater showed greater weight losses than those who did less activity (12 kg vs. 0.8 kg).

Jakicic and colleagues (2008) recently examined a related and important question: what is the optimal amount and intensity of physical activity for weight loss and maintenance? In a 24-month randomized controlled trial, participants were assigned to one of four groups, with either a lower dose (1000 kcal/week) or a high dose (2000 kcal/week) of exercise, at either a moderate (50–65% maximal heart rate, HR_{max}) or vigorous (70–85% HR_{max}) intensity; all groups included standard energy restriction and a face-to-face behavioral weight-loss program. After 12 months there appeared to be no effect of either intensity level or dose. Similarly, at 24 months, all groups had regained weight, and the net weight losses were not different. Since the exercise was unsupervised, the authors speculate that participants did not adhere to the intensity prescription and over time the doses may have converged. However, as noted above, those who reported ≥2000 kcal/week of activity had the best weight loss and maintenance.

Support for Healthy Eating and Exercise Behavior

When changing eating and exercise habits, people are often influenced by the actions and words of those around them. Recent evidence suggests that both obesity and weight loss can spread in social networks (Christakis and Fowler, 2007; Gorin *et al.*, 2008). Several studies have evaluated the effects of including spouses, other family members, and friends in the treatment process with mixed results. A meta-analysis of this literature (Black *et al.*, 1990) suggested a small positive effect for spouse involvement, and a more recent review (McLean *et al.*, 2003) indicated that family involvement was modestly effective for both children and adults but less so for adolescents.

In a cleverly designed study, Wing and Jeffery (1999) evaluated two different approaches to social support. These investigators recruited participants for a weight-loss program and asked them to identify three overweight friends who would also like to be in the program and work with them as a team to lose weight. Individuals who identified three friends were compared with individuals who were unable or unwilling to identify three friends or were not asked to recruit others (i.e. this aspect of the study was not randomized). This natural social-support intervention was crossed with an experimental manipulation of social support in a 2×2 research design. The experimental manipulation of social support included intra-group cohesiveness activities and inter-group competitions in which participants competed for money that was returned contingent on maintenance of weight loss. Those participants who were recruited with friends and given the social-support manipulation had the best outcome. Whereas 95% of these individuals completed the 10-month study, only 76% of the standard behavioral group (those recruited alone and not given the social support intervention) completed the study. Moreover, 66% of participants recruited with others and given the social-support intervention maintained their weight loss in full from month 4 of the program to month 10; only 24% of the standard behavioral group maintained their weight loss in full over the same time frame.

Kumanyika and colleagues (2009) recently reported the results of the SHARE trial, a culturally specific intervention for African-American adults that utilized the same 2×2 research design as Wing and Jeffery's earlier work. No differences in weight loss were seen between the social support conditions. Post hoc analyses revealed that participating in weight-loss treatment with family members or friends was beneficial only if the support partners themselves were more engaged in treatment activities and lost weight. More research is needed to better understand how

to harness the power of social networks to influence healthy behavior change.

Media-Based Interventions for Weight Loss

Traditionally, behavioral weight-loss programs have been offered in face-to-face meetings with health professionals. However, because obesity is such a pervasive problem, research has focused on developing treatment approaches that involve little or no face-to-face contact and thus can be more easily disseminated.

Telephone calls have been used as part of traditional clinic-based programs. Phone calls enable therapists to maintain contact with participants but also gradually reduce the number of in-person contacts. Self-directed materials supplemented with telephone counseling were found to be superior to delayed controls (VanWormer *et al.*, 2009) and when delivered with weekly and then bi-weekly frequency can be similar to face-to-face interventions delivered with the same frequency and superior to lower frequency telephone calls (Digenio *et al.*, 2009).

Internet-based interventions have proliferated over the past decade and are now recognized as an alternative to deliver all or some of the components of face-to-face behavioral programs. The great potential of the internet is low-cost delivery of printed materials and the interactive nature of the communication. Early research showed that including behavioral components (self-monitoring, structured weekly guidance, feedback, etc.) with access to informational websites produces significantly better weight losses compared with informational websites alone (Tate *et al.*, 2001) and subsequent studies have shown that providing ongoing feedback and counseling support via e-mail or chat groups can enhance weight losses of internet programs (Tate *et al.*, 2003; Harvey-Berino *et al.*, 2004).

Tate and colleagues (2006) found that initial weight losses could be improved even by using computer-automated feedback. Participants were randomized to a self-directed internet program, an internet program supplemented with weekly computer-automated feedback about self-monitoring and weight-loss progress (automated e-counseling), or an internet program supplemented with weekly e-mail counseling advice provided by a human weight-loss counselor. After 3 months, the automated counseling group and the human e-counseling groups had achieved weight losses that were similar to each other and both were significantly better than the self-directed internet group. At 6 months, the human counseling group achieved the largest weight losses, but the automated counseling group produced average weight losses of about 5% of initial body weight, suggesting the approach may be an inexpensive way to provide ongoing feedback.

Though internet weight-control studies can produce weight losses of a magnitude that would achieve health benefits, the outcomes have been regarded as less than what can be produced using face-to-face counseling methods. Recently, a large RCT confirmed these speculations. Harvey-Berino and colleagues (2010) randomized 481 overweight adults to an internet-only program, an in-person program, or a hybrid program including the internet program plus monthly in-person meetings. Weight losses were significantly greater in the in-person condition compared with the other two internet groups. Interestingly, the hybrid condition that included periodic in-person visits did not improve weight losses compared with the internet-only condition. This finding replicates a prior study showing no additional benefit to adding monthly in-person visits to a comprehensive internet behavioral weight-loss program (Micco et al., 2007).

With the surge in adoption of cell-phone and mobile web-enabled devices, internet access no longer requires a laptop or large computer, allowing weight-loss programs and tools to be more portable. Though the body of research is still quite small, a few studies suggest the potential of delivering weight-loss programs via mobile technologies. A program consisting of an initial binder of print materials, daily tailored text messages (delivered two to five times per day) and a monthly phone call from a counselor showed a 3% average weight loss after 4 months compared with a 1% average weight loss among control participants who received monthly print materials (Patrick et al., 2009). Turner-McGrievy and colleagues (2009) conducted a randomized trial comparing available weight-control audio podcasts delivered twice each week to podcasts that were matched in frequency and duration but were designed using key concepts from social cognitive theory. The theoretically based podcasts produced about a 3% weight loss after 12 weeks compared with no weight loss with the other podcasts. Thus, as with internet-delivered programs, mobile programs that provide structure or tailored feedback, or are based on sound theoretical behavior-change

principles, appear superior to self-directed educational programs.

Maintenance of Initial Weight Loss

Despite the initial success of behavioral weight-loss programs, weight regain is common. It is often reported that 95% of individuals who lose weight will regain it within 3–5 years, raising doubts about whether successful weight-loss maintenance is possible and leading some to question whether weight loss is a futile treatment goal. The National Weight Control Registry, a database of over 6000 individuals who have lost at least 30 lb (13.6 kg) and kept it off for at least a year, provides evidence that weight loss can be maintained over the long run. On average, Registry members have maintained a weight loss of 72.8 lb (33 kg) for almost 6 years (Wing and Phelan, 2005). Key behavioral strategies used by Registry members are described in Box 62.1 (Klem et al., 1997; Wyatt et al., 2002; Gorin et al., 2004; Raynor et al., 2004, 2006; Phelan et al., 2006, 2007, 2009; Butryn et al., 2007). To maintain their weight losses, these individuals report continuing to consume a low-calorie, low-fat diet (Klem et al., 1997; Phelan et al., 2006). Most report eating breakfast every day (Wyatt et al., 2002), and they maintain a consistent diet (with low levels of dietary variety) across weekdays and weekends (Gorin et al., 2004). Registry members also report high levels of physical activity (Klem et al., 1997; Phelan et al., 2007; Catenacci et al., 2008). A key characteristic of these successful weight-loss maintainers is their ongoing vigilance about their diet, exercise, and body weight (Butryn et al., 2007). For example, 44%

> **BOX 62.1   Behaviors reported by National Weight Control Registry members**
>
> Consume a low-calorie, low-fat diet
> Engage in high levels of physical activity
> Limit TV viewing
> Daily self-weighing
> Maintain diet consistency across weekdays/weekends
> Limit dietary variety
> Eat breakfast daily
> Limit fast-food intake
> Use of fat and sugar modifiers in foods

report weighing themselves daily, and another 31% report weighing at least once weekly. Even within this highly successful group, however, small weight gains of just a few pounds are difficult to recover from (Phelan *et al.*, 2003), arguing for the need to adopt a chronic care model of obesity management and to provide continued support to facilitate weight control.

Interventions designed specifically for maintenance, not just extensions of the initial weight-loss phase, have recently been developed. In the STOP Regain trial (Wing *et al.*, 2006), participants were recruited after they had lost significant amounts of weight through any type of program on their own. To maintain this weight loss, participants were taught a self-regulation approach that involved daily weighing, comparison of their current weight with a goal weight (weight at the start of the maintenance program), and, depending on the discrepancy or correspondence between the two weights, making adjustments in eating and exercise behaviors or providing self-reinforcement. Weight, calories, and minutes of exercise were reported weekly via a telephone call-in or email, and, if successful at weight maintenance, participants were provided with a small monthly gift to reinforce their progress. The intervention was tested in two different delivery formats – via the internet or face to face – and compared with a newsletter control group. Over an 18-month period, only 46% and 52% of participants in the face-to-face and internet groups, respectively, regained 5 lb (2.3 kg) or more compared with 72% of control-group participants. The face-to-face group also reduced the magnitude of weight regain by almost 50% compared with the control group. In the active intervention groups, participants who weighed themselves daily had the most weight-loss maintenance success and were over 80% less likely to regain weight compared with those who weighed themselves less often.

A maintenance-specific treatment group that involved some face-to-face meetings was also successful in preventing weight regain in the Weight Loss Maintenance Trial (Svetkey *et al.*, 2008). Following an initial 6-month weight-loss induction phase, adults who had lost at least 4 kg were randomly assigned to a self-directed, minimal-contact control group, an interactive technology-based condition, or a personal-contact intervention. Contact for the technology-based group occurred via the internet, and participants were encouraged to log in to the study website once a week, enter their weight, and utilize interactive features including goal-setting and problem-solving

modules. The personal-contact group consisted of monthly telephone contacts with a case manager, with in-person visits every 4 months. At 30 months, the personal-contact group was superior, regaining 1.5 kg and 1.2 kg less than the self-directed and interactive technology-based groups, respectively. Taken together with findings from STOP Regain, it appears that some face-to-face contact over an extended period may facilitate weight-loss maintenance.

What the content of this extended contact should be remains unclear. In the recently published PRIDE study (West *et al.*, 2011), two different face-to-face maintenance interventions were compared: a standard skills-based group that focused on reviewing and refining behavioral skills, and a motivation-focused group that aimed to increase motivation to engage in healthy behaviors by strengthening satisfaction with progress, cultivating participants' identities as successful weight losers, eliciting personal motivations for engaging in long-term behavior change efforts and supporting autonomous self regulation, and increasing motivation to engage in non-food-related activities. Compared with an education control group, both active-treatment groups achieved comparable 18-month weight losses (–5.48% for motivation-focused vs. –5.55% in skill-based, $P = 0.98$), and both groups lost significantly more than controls (–1.51%; $P = 0.0012$ in motivation-focused and 0.0021 in skill-based). As the field moves forward, theoretical models that recognize the unique process of behavior-change maintenance, and not just initiation, will likely inform the development of more effective weight-loss maintenance approaches (Rothman, 2000).

Future Directions

Behavioral treatments have been shown to be effective in producing significant initial weight losses and improving health. Currently attention is focused on developing more effective weight-loss-maintenance interventions. While we know that changing both eating and exercise behaviors is critical for long-term weight control, we lack basic information regarding how to promote long-term adherence to these healthier behaviors. Given the epidemic of obesity, there is also a need to explore more cost-effective ways to deliver intervention. Finally, research related to the prevention of obesity is a high priority; such research will need to examine how eating and exercise behaviors are developed in young children, and the role of both the home and the outside environment in supporting these behaviors. A better understanding of the development and maintenance of healthy eating and exercise behaviors is critical, not only for combating the obesity epidemic but also for the treatment and prevention of hypertension, hyperlipidemia, and some forms of cancer.

Acknowledgment

Preparation of this chapter was supported in part by NIH grants DK056992 and HL090864 awarded to Dr Rena Wing.

Suggestions for Further Reading

Jakicic, J.M., Marcus, B.H., Lang, W., *et al.* (2008) Effect of exercise on 24-month weight loss maintenance in overweight women. *Arch Intern Med* **168**, 1550–1559; Discussion 1559–1560.

Knowler, W.C., Barrett-Connor, E., Fowler, S.E., *et al.* (2002) Reduction in the incidence of type 2 diabetes with lifestyle intervention or metformin. *N Engl J Med* **346**, 393–403.

Sacks, F.M., Bray, G.A., Carey, V.J., *et al.* (2009) Comparison of weight-loss diets with different compositions of fat, protein, and carbohydrates. *N Engl J Med* **360**, 859–873.

Wing, R.R. (2008) Behavioral approaches to the treatment of obesity. In G. Bray and C. Bouchard (eds), *Handbook of Obesity: Clinical Applications*, 3rd Edn. Informa Healthcare, New York, pp. 227–248.

Wing, R. and Phelan, S. (2005) Long-term weight loss maintenance. *Am J Clin Nutr* **82**, 222S–225S.

References

Alhassan, S., Kim, S., Bersamin, A., *et al.* (2008) Dietary adherence and weight loss success among overweight women: results from the A TO Z weight loss study. *Int J Obes (Lond)* **32**, 985–991.

Andersen, R., Frankowiak, S., Snyder, J., *et al.* (1998) Effects of lifestyle activity vs. structured aerobic exercise in obese women: a randomized trial. *JAMA* **281**, 335–340.

Bandura, A. and Simon K.M. (1977) The role of proximal intentions in self-regulation of refractory behavior. *Cog Therap Res* **1**, 177–193.

Black, D.R., Gleser, L.J., and Kooyers, K.J. (1990) A meta-analytic evaluation of couples weight-loss programs. *Health Psychol* **9**, 330–347.

Burke, L.E., Sereika, S.M., Music, E., *et al.* (2008) Using instrumented paper diaries to document self-monitoring patterns in weight loss. *Contemp Clin Trials* **29**, 182–193.

Butryn, M.L., Phelan, S., Hill, J.O., *et al.* (2007) Consistent self-monitoring of weight: a key component of successful weight loss maintenance. *Obesity (Silver Spring)* **15**, 3091–3096.

Catenacci, V.A., Ogden, L.G., Stuht, J., *et al.* (2008) Physical activity patterns in the National Weight Control Registry. *Obesity (Silver Spring)* **16**, 153–161.

Christakis, N.A. and Fowler, J.H. (2007) The spread of obesity in a large social network over 32 years. *N Engl J Med* **357**, 370–379.

Christensen, R., Bartels, E.M., Astrup, A., *et al.* (2007) Effect of weight reduction in obese patients diagnosed with knee osteoarthritis: a systematic review and meta-analysis. *Ann Rheum Dis* **66**, 433–439.

Dansinger, M.L., Gleason, J.A., Griffith, J.L., *et al.* (2005) Comparison of the Atkins, Ornish, Weight Watchers, and Zone diets for weight loss and heart disease risk reduction: a randomized trial. *JAMA* **293**, 43–53.

Digenio, A.G., Mancuso, J.P., Gerber, R.A., *et al.* (2009) Comparison of methods for delivering a lifestyle modification program for obese patients: a randomized trial. *Ann Intern Med* **150**, 255–262.

Ditschuneit, H.H., Flechtner-Mors, M., Johnson, T.D., *et al.* (1999) Metabolic and weight-loss effects of a long-term dietary intervention in obese patients. *Am J Clin Nutr* **69**, 198–204.

Epstein, L.H., Valoski, A.M., Vara, L.S., *et al.* (1995) Effects of decreasing sedentary behavior and increasing activity on weight change in obese children. *Health Psychol* **14**, 109–115.

Gorin, A.A., Phelan, S., Wing, R.R., *et al.* (2004) Promoting long-term weight control: does dietary consistency matter? *Int J Obes Relat Metab Disord* **28**, 278–281.

Gorin, A.A., Wing, R.R., Fava, J.L., *et al.* (2008) Weight loss treatment influences untreated spouses and the home environment: evidence of a ripple effect. *Int J Obes (Lond)* **32**, 1678–1684.

Harvey-Berino, J., Pintauro, S., Buzzell, P., *et al.* (2004) Effect of internet support on the long-term maintenance of weight loss. *Obes Res* **12**, 320–329.

Harvey-Berino, J., West, D., Krukowski, R., *et al.* (2010) Internet delivered behavioral obesity treatment. *Prev Med* **51**, 123–128.

Jakicic, J.M., Marcus, B.H., Lang, W., *et al.* (2008) Effect of exercise on 24-month weight loss maintenance in overweight women. *Arch Intern Med* **168,** 1550–1559; Discussion 1559–1560.

Jakicic, J.M., Wing, R.R., Butler, B.A., *et al.* (1995) Prescribing exercise in multiple short bouts versus one continuous bout: effects on adherence, cardiorespiratory fitness, and weight loss in overweight women. *Int J Obes Relat Metab Disord* **19,** 893–901.

Jakicic, J.M., Wing, R.R., Butler, B.A., *et al.* (1997) The relationship between presence of exercise equipment in the home and physical activity level. *Am J Health Promot* **11,** 363–365.

Jakicic, J., Wing, R., and Winters, C. (1999) Effects of intermittent exercise and use of home exercise equipment on adherence, weight loss, and fitness in overweight women. *JAMA* **282,** 1554–1560.

Jeffery, R.W., Hellerstedt, W.L., French, S., *et al.* (1995) A randomized trial of counseling for fat restriction versus calorie restriction in the treatment of obesity. *Int J Obes Relat Metab Disord* **19,** 132–137.

Jeffery, R.W., Wing, R.R., Sherwood, N.E., *et al.* (2003) Physical activity and weight loss: does prescribing higher physical activity goals improve outcome? *Am J Clin Nutr* **78,** 684–689.

Jeffery, R.W., Wing, R.R., Thornson, C., *et al.* (1993) Strengthening behavioral interventions for weight loss: a randomized trial of food provision and monetary incentives. *J Consult Clin Psychol* **61,** 1038–1045.

Klem, M.L., Wing, R.R., McGuire, M.T., *et al.* (1997) A descriptive study of individuals successful at long-term maintenance of substantial weight loss. *Am J Clin Nutr* **66,** 239–246.

Knowler, W.C., Barrett-Connor, E., Fowler, S.E., *et al.* (2002) Reduction in the incidence of type 2 diabetes with lifestyle intervention or metformin. *N Engl J Med* **346,** 393–403.

Kumanyika, S.K., Van Horn, L., Bowen, D., *et al.* (2000) Maintenance of dietary behavior change. *Health Psychol* **19,** 42–56.

Kumanyika, S.K., Wadden, T.A., Shults, J., *et al.* (2009) Trial of family and friend support for weight loss in African American adults. *Arch Intern Med* **169,** 1795–1804.

Look AHEAD Research Group (2007) Reduction in weight and cardiovascular disease risk factors in individuals with type 2 diabetes: one-year results of the look AHEAD trial. *Diabetes Care* **30,** 1374–1383.

Marlatt, G.A. and Gordon, J.R. (1985) *Relapse Prevention: Maintenance Strategies in Addictive Behavior Change.* Guilford, New York.

McLean, N., Griffin, S., Toney, K., *et al.* (2003) Family involvement in weight control, weight maintenance, and weight-loss inter-

ventions: a systematic review of randomized trials. *Int J Obes Relat Metab Disord* **27,** 987–1005.

Micco, N., Gold, B., Buzzell, P., *et al.* (2007) Minimal in-person support as an adjunct to internet obesity treatment. *Ann Behav Med* **33,** 49–56.

National Task Force on the Prevention and Treatment of Obesity (1993) Very-low-calorie diets. *JAMA* **270,** 967–974.

Otten, J.J., Jones, K.E., Littenberg, B., *et al.* (2009) Effects of television viewing reduction on energy intake and expenditure in overweight and obese adults: a randomized controlled trial. *Arch Int Med* **169,** 2109–2115.

Pascale, R.W., Wing, R.R., Butler, B.A., *et al.* (1995) Effects of a behavioral weight loss program stressing calorie restriction versus calorie plus fat restriction in obese individuals with NIDDM or a family history of diabetes. *Diabetes Care* **18,** 1241–1248.

Patrick, K., Raab, F., Adams, M.A., *et al.* (2009) A text message-based intervention for weight loss: randomized controlled trial. *J Med Internet Res* **11,** e1.

Perri, M.G., Martin, A.D., Leermakers, E.A., *et al.* (1997) Effects of group- versus home-based exercise in the treatment of obesity. *J Consult Clin Psychol* **65,** 278–285.

Perri, M.G., McKelvey, W.F., Renjilian, D.A., *et al.* (2001) Relapse prevention training and problem-solving therapy in the long-term management of obesity. *J Consult Clin Psychol* **69,** 722–726.

Perri, M.G., Shapiro, R.M., Ludwig, W.W., *et al.* (1984) Maintenance strategies for the treatment of obesity: an evaluation of relapse prevention training and posttreatment contact by mail and telephone. *J Consult Clin Psychol* **52,** 404–413.

Phelan, S., Hill, J.O., Lang, W., *et al.* (2003) Recovery from relapse among successful weight maintainers. *Am J Clin Nutr* **78,** 1079–1084.

Phelan, S., Lang, W., Jordan, D., *et al.* (2009) Use of artificial sweeteners and fat-modified foods in weight loss maintainers and always-normal weight individuals. *Int J Obes Relat Metab Disord (Lond)* **33,** 1183–1190.

Phelan, S., Roberts, M., Lang, W., *et al.* (2007) Empirical evaluation of physical activity recommendations for weight control in women. *Med Sci Sports Exerc* **39,** 1832–1836.

Phelan, S., Wyatt, H.R., Hill, J.O., *et al.* (2006) Are the eating and exercise habits of successful weight losers changing? *Obesity* **14,** 710–716.

Pi-Sunyer, F., Maggio, C., McCarron, D., *et al.* (1999) Multicenter randomized trial of a comprehensive prepared meal program in type 2 diabetes. *Diabetes Care* **22,** 191–197.

Promrat, K., Kleiner, D.E., Niemeier, H.M., *et al.* (2010) Randomized controlled trial testing the effects of weight loss on nonalcoholic steatohepatitis. *Hepatology* **51**, 121–129.

Pronk, N.P. and Wing, R.R. (1994) Physical activity and long-term maintenance of weight loss. *Obes Res* **2**, 587–599.

Raynor, D.A., Phelan, S., Hill, J.O., *et al.* (2006) Television viewing and long-term weight maintenance: results from the National Weight Control Registry. *Obesity* **14**, 1816–1824.

Raynor, H.A., Jeffery, R.W., and Wing, R.R. (2004) Relationship between changes in food group variety, dietary intake, and weight during obesity treatment. *Int J Obes Relat Metab Disord* **28**, 813–820.

Robinson, T. (1999) Reducing children's television viewing to prevent obesity. *JAMA* **282**, 1561–1567.

Rothman, A.J. (2000) Toward a theory-based analysis of behavioral maintenance. *Health Psychol* **19**(1 Suppl), 64–69.

Sacks, F.M., Bray, G.A., Carey, V.J., *et al.* (2009) Comparison of weight-loss diets with different compositions of fat, protein, and carbohydrates. *N Engl J Med* **360**, 859–873.

Schlundt, D.G., Hill, J.O., Pope-Cordle, J., *et al.* (1993) Randomized evaluation of a low fat ad libitum carbohydrate diet for weight reduction. *Int J Obes Relat Metab Disord* **17**, 623–629.

Stuart, R.B. (1967) Behavioral control of overeating. *Behav Res Ther* **5**, 357–365.

Subak, L.L., Wing, R., West, D.S., *et al.* (2009) Weight loss to treat urinary incontinence in overweight and obese women. *N Engl J Med* **360**, 481–490.

Svetkey, L.P., Stevens, V.J., Brantley, P.J., *et al.* (2008) Comparison of strategies for sustaining weight loss: the weight loss maintenance randomized controlled trial. *JAMA* **299**, 1139–1148.

Tate, D.F., Jackvony, E.H., and Wing, R.R. (2003) Effects of internet behavioral counseling on weight loss in adults at risk for type 2 diabetes. *JAMA* **289**, 1833–1836.

Tate, D.F., Jackvony, E.H., and Wing, R.R. (2006) A randomized trial comparing human e-mail counseling, computer-automated tailored counseling, and no counseling in an internet weight loss program. *Arch Int Med* **166**, 1620–1625.

Tate, D.F., Jeffery, R.W., Sherwood, N.E., *et al.* (2007) Long-term weight losses associated with prescription of higher physical activity goals. Are higher levels of physical activity protective against weight regain? *Am J Clin Nutr* **85**, 954–959.

Tate, D.F., Wing, R.R., and Winett, R.A. (2001) Using internet technology to deliver a behavioral weight loss program. *JAMA* **285**, 1172–1177.

Trials of Hypertension Prevention Collaborative Research Group (1997) Effects of weight loss and sodium reduction interven-tion on blood pressure and hypertension incidence in over-weight people with high-normal blood pressure: The Trials of Hypertension Prevention, Phase II. *Arch Intern Med* **157**, 657–667.

Tucker, L.A. and Kano, M.J. (1992) Dietary fat and body fat: a multivariate study of 205 adult females. *Am J Clin Nutr* **56**, 616–622.

Turner-McGrievy, G.M., Campbell, M.K., Tate, D.F., *et al.* (2009) Pounds Off Digitally study: a randomized podcasting weight-loss intervention. *Am J Prev Med* **37**, 263–269.

VanWormer, J.J., Martinez, A.M., Benson, G.A., *et al.* (2009) Telephone counseling and home telemonitoring: the Weigh by Day Trial. *Am J Health Behav* **33**, 445–454.

Wadden, T.A. and Stunkard, A.J. (1986) Controlled trial of very low calorie diet, behavior therapy, and their combination in the treatment of obesity. *J Consult Clin Psychol* **54**, 482–488.

Wadden, T.A., Foster, G.D., and Letizia, K.A. (1994) One-year behavioral treatment of obesity: comparison of moderate and severe caloric restriction and the effects of weight maintenance therapy. *J Consult Clin Psychol* **62**, 165–171.

West, D.S., Gorin, A.A., Subak, L.L., *et al.* (2011) Motivation-focused weight loss maintenance intervention is as effective as a behavioral skills-based approach. *Int J Obes Relat Metab Disord* **35**, 259–269.

Whelton, P.K., Appel, L.J., Espeland, M.A., *et al.* (1998) Sodium reduction and weight loss in the treatment of hypertension in older persons: a randomized controlled trial of nonpharmaco-logic interventions in the elderly (TONE). *JAMA* **279**, 839–846.

Williamson, D.A., Rejeski, J., Lang, W., *et al.* (2009) Impact of a weight management program on health-related quality of life in overweight adults with type 2 diabetes. *Arch Intern Med* **169**, 163–171.

Wing, R.R. (2008) Behavioral approaches to the treatment of obesity. In G. Bray and C. Bouchard (eds), *Handbook of Obesity: Clinical Applications.*, 3rd Edn. Informa Healthcare, New York, pp. 227–248.

Wing, R.R. and Jeffery, R. (1999) Benefits of recruiting par-ticipants with friends and increasing social support for weight loss and maintenance. *J Consult Clin Psychol* **67**, 132–138.

Wing, R.R. and Phelan, S. (2005) Long-term weight loss mainte-nance. *Am J Clin Nutr* **82**, 222S–225S.

Wing, R.R., Blair, E., Marcus, M., *et al.* (1994) Year-long weight loss treatment for obese patients with type II diabetes: does including of an intermittent very-low-calorie diet improve outcome? *Am J Med* **97**, 354–362.

Wing, R.R., Jeffery, R.W., Burton, L.R., *et al.* (1996) Food provision vs. structured meal plans in the behavioral treatment of obesity. *Int J Obes Relat Metab Disord* **20,** 56–62.

Wing, R.R., Marcus, M.D., Salata, R., *et al.* (1991) Effects of a very-low-calorie diet on long-term glycemic control in obese type 2 diabetic subjects. *Arch Int Med* **151,** 1334–1340.

Wing, R.R., Tate, D.F., Gorin, A.A., *et al.* (2006) A self-regulation program for maintenance of weight loss. *N Engl J Med* **355,** 1563–1571.

Wyatt, H.R., Grunwald, G.K., Mosca, C.L., *et al.* (2002) Long-term weight loss and breakfast in subjects in the National Weight Control Registry. *Obes Res* **10,** 78–82.

63

EPIDEMIOLOGIC APPROACHES TO EVALUATION OF NUTRITION AND HEALTH

SUSAN E. STECK, PhD, MPH, RD

University of South Carolina, Columbia, South Carolina, USA

Summary

Nutritional epidemiology encompasses a variety of endeavors, including monitoring the dietary intake and nutritional status of populations, contributing to the evidence for or against hypotheses related to nutrition and health outcomes, and designing interventions to promote healthy eating habits. When examining nutrition and health relationships with epidemiologic methods, there are a number of issues that must be considered because of unique features of dietary intake as a determinant of health. For example, diet is a complex exposure and populations often consume dietary factors within a narrow range of intake, creating challenges in our ability to observe associations owing to the limited contrasts available. The types of epidemiologic study designs used to examine nutrition and health, along with examples from the literature, are discussed in this chapter. Focus is given to the challenges and strengths of each study design, as well as to issues inherent in epidemiology such as bias, confounding, and external validity in interpretation of study results. One specific diet–disease relationship that has been studied with both observational studies and clinical trials will be discussed to illustrate some of the concepts presented in the chapter. Finally, suggestions for future directions for enhancing epidemiologic studies of nutrition and health are proffered.

Introduction

Epidemiology is defined as "the study of the occurrence and distribution of health-related states or events in a specified population, including the study of the determinants influencing such states, and the application of this knowledge to control the health problem" (Porta, 2008).

When applied to nutrition and health, there are a number of issues that must be considered in view of the unique features of dietary intake as a determinant of health. For example, diet is a complex exposure and one that is ubiquitous. For the majority of dietary factors of interest, most individuals are consuming some amount, and thus it is often impossible to compare absent exposure from present

Present Knowledge in Nutrition, Tenth Edition. Edited by John W. Erdman Jr, Ian A. Macdonald and Steven H. Zeisel.
© 2012 International Life Sciences Institute. Published 2012 by John Wiley & Sons, Inc.

exposure as is possible with other lifestyle factors such as cigarette smoking or use of non-steroidal anti-inflammatory drugs. Many dietary factors are correlated with one another, creating challenges in trying to determine the independent effects of a specific dietary factor. In addition, populations often consume dietary factors within a narrow range of intake, creating challenges in our ability to observe associations within a population being studied due to the limited contrasts available. Usually, relative risks of dietary factors determined from epidemiologic studies are modest (around 0.5 to 2.0), but, given the high prevalence of exposure, these can be quite meaningful from a public health point of view.

Nutritional epidemiology includes several activities, such as monitoring the dietary intake and nutritional status of populations, contributing to the evidence for or against hypotheses related to nutrition and health outcomes, and designing interventions to promote healthy eating habits. This chapter will focus on the study designs and methodologic considerations when evaluating nutrition and health outcomes using epidemiologic approaches. Because of inherent limitations in epidemiologic study designs and the possibility of biases, no one epidemiologic study alone can provide definitive evidence that a dietary factor causes or prevents a health outcome. The epidemiologic literature must be evaluated and taken in context with other epidemiologic studies, as well as with other lines of evidence, such as in vitro and animal model experimental studies, when determining the merit of a given exposure–disease relationship. There are various methods for dietary assessment in humans and these are an important component of nutritional epidemiologic studies but will be covered in more detail in another chapter of this book and not discussed here.

Diet can be investigated in epidemiologic studies at several different levels, anywhere from very broadly as dietary patterns to food group or individual food intake to more specifically as individual nutrient or phytochemical intake. For the estimation of nutrient or phytochemical intake, a food composition database is required to convert the reported food consumed into nutrients and phytochemicals. Thus, this adds an additional layer of potential measurement error given that the nutrient value for a given food in a food composition database may be very different from what was actually consumed by the study participant. Analyzing whole food intake or dietary patterns has the benefit of not having to rely on food composition databases, and thus eliminates that additional source of error.

There is ongoing debate comparing the attributes of the holistic approach (dietary patterns and food groups) with that of the reductionist approach (individual nutrients or phytochemicals) for studies of nutrition and health. The study of individual nutrients or phytochemicals lends itself better to understanding biologic mechanisms because associations that are observed in epidemiologic studies can be tested in the laboratory and in experimental models to identify the active agents in foods and their biologic properties. On the other hand, the study of food groups or dietary patterns has more potential for public health applicability given that the combination of individual nutrients and phytochemicals found in whole foods is likely to be most beneficial, and dietary patterns can be more easily translated into public health recommendations. Certainly, there is a need for multiple levels of analyses in improving our understanding of the role of nutrition in health.

Epidemiologic Study Designs

There are two broad types of epidemiology: (1) descriptive epidemiology, which describes distributions of disease by place, time or person and includes ecological and migrant studies, and (2) analytical epidemiology which tests specific hypotheses about exposure–disease relationships and includes case-control studies, cohort studies, clinical trials, and meta-analyses. The following sections will describe these major study designs, discuss strengths and weaknesses of each, and provide examples of their application to the investigation of nutrition and health.

Ecological or International Correlation Studies

Ecological studies are investigations into the relationship between an exposure and a disease outcome at the population level, rather than the individual level. In studies of nutrition and health, per capita intake of a given food can be estimated from national aggregate data and correlated with disease rates across various countries (or across regions within a country if differences in eating habits exist within the different subpopulations in the country). Several important hypotheses have been generated by studies that compare international rates of disease with country-specific dietary intake, for example the association between dietary fat and breast cancer and the association between meat intake and colorectal cancer (Willett, 1998).

One benefit of the ecological approach is that, because of the heterogeneity in diets across different countries and cultures, much larger contrasts in dietary intake can be examined than can be obtained in observational studies of a more homogeneous population. For example, intake of soy is high among Asian populations but not among the US population. Thus, studies of the association between soy intake and a given health outcome within the United States would be limited by the narrow range of intake within this population. In fact, if a higher level of intake is required before an effect can be observed, studies in the United States are likely to find null associations, as has been discussed for the relationship between soy intake and breast cancer risk (Gammon *et al.*, 2008). Another example where the narrow range in intake limits the ability to observe associations is that of fat and breast cancer (Hebert and Wynder, 1987), where ecological studies support a linear association, but the majority of observational studies within specific populations have found null associations. Narrow ranges in intake in studies of individuals' diets as well as different effects for different types of fat may partly explain these conflicting results.

Another advantage of ecological studies is that they can be performed relatively quickly and inexpensively compared with other types of epidemiologic studies. However, a major limitation of ecological studies is the lack of information on other variables that could confound the relationship between the dietary factor and the health outcome (for example, smoking, physical activity, and socioeconomic status which can be related to both dietary intake and disease outcomes, meeting the definition of a confounder). Without appropriate measurement and control for these potential confounders, a causal association may be erroneously attributed to the dietary factor when, in fact, the causal agent may be a different factor that is related to both the dietary factor and the disease outcome. For this reason, causality should not be inferred from ecological studies. Also, because ecological studies use national aggregrate data, the findings are impossible to reproduce in other studies. Replication and consistency of findings in epidemiologic studies are important components of establishing a causal link between an exposure and outcome. Thus, cross-national or cross-cultural comparisons can still play a role in advancing the science of nutrition and health, but the role is limited to that of hypothesis-generating and not inferring causality.

Migrant Studies

Migrant studies provide some of the most compelling evidence for a major role of diet and other environmental or lifestyle factors in disease etiology. For example, numer-ous studies have observed that, when populations migrate to a new country, very soon (within one or two generations) they will develop the cancer rates of the new host country. These relationships are striking, particularly when the disease rates of the host country and the country of origin are in sharp contrast with one another, for example stomach cancer rates have historically been much higher in Japan than in the United States. Japanese Americans who were born in Japan have similar stomach cancer rates to those from their host country, while second-generation Japanese Americans have stomach cancer rates similar to those of the US population (Tominaga, 1985; Kamineni *et al.*, 1999). These types of studies provide evidence that it is not only genetics or inherited susceptibility that is responsible for disease; lifestyle and environment are also very important. Thus, while migrant studies do not identify the specific dietary habits or biologic mechanisms involved, these studies contribute greatly to our knowledge about the relative importance of diet and other environmental factors in health outcomes.

Case-Control Studies

A case-control study is one type of observational study in epidemiology that collects data at the individual level and estimates risk of a disease or health outcome. In these studies, investigators recruit cases (individuals with the disease or health outcome) and controls (individuals without the disease or health outcome of interest from within the same population in which the cases arose), and make comparisons regarding exposures that may be associated with disease risk. For example, in a study of the association between cruciferous vegetable intake and breast cancer, investigators would identify women diagnosed with breast cancer (cases) and women without breast cancer (controls) and then ask them to recall their dietary intake over a certain period of time to assess intake of cruciferous vegetables. Using statistical methods, the investigators could then examine whether increased intake of cruciferous vegetables was associated with reduced risk of breast cancer within this population. Other factors that may be related to both cruciferous vegetable intake and breast cancer risk (i.e. potential confounders) would also be assessed and controlled for, either by matching the cases and controls on that factor (for example, matching on age is often performed in case-control studies), or by adjusting for those factors in the statistical models.

Case-control studies tend to dominate the epidemiologic literature because they are usually less expensive and time-consuming than other types of individual-level epidemiologic studies (e.g. cohort studies or clinical trials discussed below). Case-control studies also have the advantages of being able to study rare diseases more easily and being able to assess a number of different risk factors in a given study. As with cohort studies, data can be collected on potential confounding variables and these can be controlled for in the design of the study by matching or in the statistical analyses by using multivariate methods.

However, there are several potential biases associated with case-control studies that need to be considered in the interpretation of the results. These include selection bias and information bias. Selection bias refers to the act of choosing subjects in a way that alters the observed association between the exposure and disease of interest. There are several ways in which selection bias can enter a study. A classic example is the use of hospital controls, where control subjects are selected from the hospital from which cases were treated. If the exposure of interest is more likely to be present or absent in the hospital-based controls than in the general population (e.g. because it is also associated with their reason for hospitalization), then this can lead to distorted results.

Even when controls are selected from the general population, rather than from a hospital, selection bias is possible if controls are recruited using methods that would exclude certain participants with different socioeconomic status or health status. For example, recruiting controls via random-digit-dialing would exclude participants without telephones, which tends to be an indicator of low socioeconomic status (Langseth, 1996), or recruiting controls with drivers' licenses from the Department of Motor Vehicles would exclude individuals who do not drive, perhaps an indicator of low literacy or poor health. In addition, controls who volunteer for studies tend to be more health conscious than the general population, so, especially when participation rates among the control population are low, this could result in the diets of the control population being much healthier than the general population, causing erroneous findings. Thus, exclusion of certain groups in the control population may bias study results, pointing to the importance of trying to minimize these potential sources of bias when determining recruitment strategies and selection criteria for a given study.

Information bias is another potential limitation in case-control studies. Information bias occurs when data are collected differently in cases than in controls such that results may be misleading. One form of information bias

that is especially problematic in case-control studies of diet and disease is recall bias. Since cases are recruited after diagnosis, they are asked to recall their dietary intake prior to disease diagnosis. If the diagnosis of disease distorts their recall in a systematic way, then spurious associations may appear when in fact there is no causal association. Examples of this could be that women diagnosed with colon cancer recall consuming more red meat than they actually consumed because they think red meat is to blame for their disease status, or individuals diagnosed with diabetes change their diet soon after diagnosis and report their diet after diagnosis rather than prior to diagnosis, or perhaps symptoms of the disease itself force the individual to change their dietary habits in the months leading up to diagnosis, as could be the case in oral cancers, and the cases recall their more recent diet instead of that consumed prior to the onset of symptoms. Regardless of the reason, if cases recall their diet in a systematic way differently from controls, then recall bias can occur and cause misleading results.

Another type of information bias is interviewer bias, which can occur if the interviewer knows the disease status of the participant and conducts the interview differently because of that knowledge. Finally, even the use of objective biomarkers of nutrients as the exposure measurement can lead to information bias if the biomarker is affected by the disease process. Given the likelihood that relative risks for a given diet–disease relationship are relatively small, even minor measurement error caused by bias could affect results of case-control studies, and it is difficult to completely eliminate these potential sources of bias in each study (Willett, 1998). Because of these limitations, case-control studies of a given dietary factor and disease outcome can produce inconsistent results, and are at times in contrast to those obtained with cohort studies.

Cohort Studies

In a prospective cohort study, participants from a defined study population are recruited prior to the onset of disease and followed for a period of time to determine who is diagnosed with the disease of interest. Dietary intake assessment occurs at baseline, and in the majority of studies this is repeated at intervals during the follow-up period. In this way, the role of nutrition in the prevention or causation of disease can be determined prior to disease diagnosis by comparing the frequency of disease in individuals exposed to the frequency of disease in the non-exposed (or less exposed) individuals. Thus, many of the biases associated with case-control studies that are a consequence of the timing of exposure assessment occurring after disease diagnosis are eliminated or reduced in cohort studies, such as recall bias and interviewer bias. Another advantage is that cohort studies allow for measurement of diet over time, so that changes in diet can be assessed and examined in relation to disease etiology. In addition, cohort studies can examine a variety of disease outcomes in one study.

There are some disadvantages to cohort studies, however. Because some chronic diseases are rare, such as cancers of certain organ sites, a large number of participants (usually tens of thousands) have to be enrolled and followed for a long period of time in order to obtain enough disease outcomes to study the hypotheses of interest. Loss to follow-up can be a concern if participants who drop out of the study are different in important ways from those who stay in the study, and can lead to distorted associations. Thus, cohort studies require extensive retention efforts to maintain participation in the study. For these reasons, cohort studies are typically much more expensive and time-consuming than case-control studies.

Another concern in cohort studies is external validity. External validity refers to the ability to generalize the results of a given study to different populations or groups that did not take part in the study. Because cohort studies tend to recruit participants based on an exposure of interest (e.g. farmers exposed to pesticides) or by a defined study region, demographic or occupation (e.g. European Investigation in Nutrition and Cancer [Riboli and Kaaks, 1997], Women's Health Initiative [1998], or Nurses' Health Study [Colditz *et al.*, 1997]), rather than a disease of interest as in a case-control study, the generalizability of the results may be limited to a specific group of people. This can also limit the ability of the study to observe an association if the study population is very homogeneous with insufficient variation in dietary intake.

A special kind of case-control study called a nested case-control study can be performed within a cohort study, which is less costly and time-consuming than starting a brand new cohort, and can minimize bias as compared with a traditional case-control study. In a nested case-control study, investigators choose a subset of the entire cohort to examine a hypothesis of interest. As in a case-control study, individuals diagnosed with a given disease are chosen, and a subset of controls without the disease are chosen from the cohort for comparison. Frequencies of exposures (measured in the past prior to disease onset)

are then compared between cases and controls. This is especially advantageous for biomarker-based studies where it is less costly to conduct the laboratory measurements on a subset of the cohort rather than the entire cohort, and it minimizes information bias because the biologic specimens were collected prior to disease diagnosis. Thus, nested case-control studies can incorporate the advantages of both case-control and cohort studies while minimizing the disadvantages, thus improving efficiency of design.

Clinical Trials

Randomized controlled trials or interventions are often considered the gold standard of epidemiologic study designs because of their ability to control the exposure of interest rather than relying on dietary recall or laboratory measurement of exposures. In a randomized controlled trial, participants are randomly assigned to either a placebo (control) group or a treatment (intervention) group and are followed for a period of time to examine whether the intervention group has fewer disease outcomes than the control group. These can be double-blinded, in which neither the investigators nor the participants are aware of their study assignment, or single-blinded, where the participants are aware of their assignment but the study investigators are not. Clinical trials involving a single agent can often be double-blinded because the dietary factor can be put in a capsule form that can be made to look, smell, and taste exactly like a placebo capsule. However, for obvious logistical reasons, whole diet interventions cannot be double-blinded owing to the inability to blind the participants to a change in the foods they are consuming. While dietary supplements in capsule form are easy to administer, and allow for creating large contrasts between the intervention and control groups, they are at times not appropriate because the real interest is on whole foods or dietary patterns.

A major advantage of randomized controlled clinical trials is the ability to reduce confounding by other factors. Randomization, if done correctly, reduces the potential confounding effects of factors that may be related to diet and disease because the presence of these other factors is randomly distributed between intervention and control groups. Clinical trials are generally thought to be able to directly examine cause and effect for a given exposure and disease or health outcome. This study design is useful for studying rare exposures, and, in the case of a single agent supplement, can create larger contrasts between groups than might be available in observational studies.

However, particularly when diet is being studied, there are some disadvantages to randomized controlled trials that can restrict our ability to address hypotheses of interest with this study design because of ethical or logistical concerns. Clearly, only dietary factors that are thought to prevent rather than cause disease can be examined in an intervention as it would be unethical to randomize individuals to an exposure that is thought to increase risk of disease. In addition, the evidence that the intervention will work must be considerable enough to warrant the expense and effort of conducting the study, while at the same time not so substantial that it would be unethical to withhold the intervention from the control group.

For studies employing whole diet interventions (such as a low-fat diet or high fruit and vegetable diet intervention), it is often difficult to create large enough contrasts between the study arms to observe an effect on the disease of interest, and contamination of the control group is often a possibility especially when the dietary factor or dietary pattern being studied receives substantial media attention. Compliance with the intervention and control diets needs to be monitored carefully. Additionally, clinical trials are limited in that the effects of only one or a few dietary factors can be assessed in a given trial.

Many chronic diseases have long latency periods, so interventions must be administered for long periods of time. To try to minimize the length of the study, large trials of dietary factors have often enrolled high-risk subjects where the time to disease diagnosis would be much shorter, for example, smokers and asbestos workers in trials of β-carotene and lung cancer (Alpha-Tocopherol Beta Carotene Cancer Prevention Study Group, 1994; Omenn *et al.*, 1996), or have employed intermediate endpoints such as enrolling individuals with a previous polyp removed in studies of diet and polyp recurrence (Schatzkin *et al.*, 2000). These studies have frequently resulted in unexpected findings, i.e. either (most commonly) no effect or (more rarely) unexpected increased risk of the intervention on cancer incidence or mortality as in the case of the β-carotene lung cancer trials (reviewed in Lippman *et al.*, 1998; Byers, 1999; Davies *et al.*, 2006; Bjelakovic *et al.*, 2007). Many reasons for these unexpected results have been discussed (Forman *et al.*, 2004; Meyskens and Szabo, 2005; Prentice, 2007; Rock, 2007). Incorporating these lessons learned into new, innovative study designs is essential if we are to advance public health through diet. In many of the studies, most notably the β-carotene lung cancer trials, large doses of single agents as supplements

were used as the intervention, despite the fact that the epidemiologic evidence was in support of food-based sources of nutrients often at lower levels of intake than found in supplements (Mayne, 1996). More recently, large dietary intervention trials have shown no effect of increasing fruit and vegetable intakes, or reducing fat and increasing fiber intakes (or some combination of these) on cancer incidence, survival, or recurrence of precancerous lesions (Schatzkin *et al.*, 2000; Prentice *et al.*, 2006; Pierce *et al.*, 2007). Possible reasons for null effects of dietary interventions are discussed in detail in the Future Directions section.

Meta-Analyses and Pooling Studies

Given the challenges associated with each epidemiologic study design and the limitations previously noted regarding drawing conclusions from only one study or from only one population, the use of meta-analyses and pooling projects has increased in recent years (Smith-Warner *et al.*, 2006). Meta-analyses and pooling studies represent methods for combining data from multiple studies and multiple populations to summarize the effect of a dietary factor on a particular health outcome. A meta-analysis is a systematic review of the literature which combines the results from previous studies and determines a summary estimate of effect, in contrast to pooled studies where the actual study data from multiple studies are obtained and re-analyzed with the larger sample size (and presumably larger variation in dietary intake).

Meta-analyses provide a systematic way of reviewing and summarizing the literature, but are faced with challenges when it comes to nutrition data. Intake of a given dietary factor is often categorized into quantiles in epidemiologic studies, and the number of quantiles used (whether it be tertiles, quartiles, quintiles, etc.) varies from study to study, as do the cutpoints used to create those quantiles (and these cutpoints unfortunately are not always reported), and the confounding variables included in the models. Thus, the dose of the dietary factor that is associated with an effect is not readily apparent, and determining how to summarize the data is no trivial matter. Pooling projects, on the other hand, obtain the original data from multiple studies and can thus create new quantiles using all of the data and can standardize the covariates, outcome variables, and types of analyses. As with meta-analyses, pooling projects must deal with the fact that different studies use different dietary assessment methods and different food composition databases, resulting potentially in various units of intake that must be converted to a common unit, and varying accuracy in intake estimates for a given nutrient or dietary factor. Thus, while these types of studies have strength in numbers (number of studies or sample size of the population) and minimize some of the aforementioned issues related to narrow ranges in intake, external validity, and low power for uncommon exposures or rare diseases, the accuracy of results is still dependent on the quality of the data collection methods used in the studies that they are summarizing. An example of a large pooling project is the ongoing Pooling Project of Prospective Studies of Diet and Cancer, which began in 1991 and combines data from 16 prospective cohort studies(Smith-Warner et al., 2006). Multiple papers have been published using these data, and, in particular, the project has enabled the examination of associations between dietary factors and rare diseases such as pancreatic cancer, renal cell cancer, and ovarian cancer with more power than previous studies given the larger sample size (Koushik et al., 2005; Genkinger et al., 2009; Lee et al., 2009).

Example of Diet and Disease Relationship Studied with Multiple Epidemiologic Study Designs

Folate and Colorectal Cancer

There is no doubt that a true success story in nutritional epidemiology is the identification through numerous types of study designs that folic acid supplementation can reduce the incidence of neural tube defects (Wolff et al., 2009) (also, see Chapter 21). This conclusion led to the implementation of mandatory folic acid fortification in the United States and Canada in 1998, with many other countries following suit later, and a concomitant reduction in rates of neural tube defects has been reported in several countries (Honein et al., 2001; Ray et al., 2002; Chen and Rivera, 2004; Hertrampf and Cortes, 2004; De Wals et al., 2007). However, the effect of folic acid on colorectal cancer is not as clear (Ulrich and Potter, 2006; Kim, 2008).

In multiple observational studies, high folate intake is associated with reduced risk of colorectal cancer. Both case-control and cohort studies have supported this association (Giovannucci, 2002; Kim, 2008; Kim et al., 2010; Lee et al., 2011), with measurement of folate in the diet or as a biomarker measured in red blood cells, and a few small clinical trials have provided evidence that folic acid

supplementation reduces recurrence of adenomatous polyps (precursors to colorectal cancer) (Paspatis and Karamanolis, 1994; Jaszewski et al., 2008), while other trials have found no significant effect, either protective or adverse, on recurrent adenomas (Logan et al., 2008; Wu et al., 2009). However, an ecological study examining time trends in the United States and Canada found increased incidence of colorectal cancer in these countries following the initiation of mandatory fortification (Mason et al., 2007). While this does not prove causality due to the possibility of ecologic fallacy, one clinical trial has observed increased risk of advanced adenomas in individuals supplemented with folic acid compared with placebo (Cole et al., 2007). A possible explanation for this lies in our knowledge about the biologic mechanisms for folate's anti-cancer effects. Folate is involved in DNA synthesis and DNA methylation, and may have a protective role in preventing carcinogenesis but a potentiating role for pre-neoplastic lesions by supporting the proliferation of neoplastic cells. Thus, the evidence for health benefits of even a single dietary factor can be quite complex, and dietary factors that may be beneficial for one health outcome may turn out to be detrimental for another health outcome.

Future work in genetics and epigenetics may help to identify the most beneficial application of folic acid to the promotion of overall health. As an example, the gene that encodes an enzyme involved in folate metabolism, 5,10-methylenetetrahydrofolate reductase (MTHFR), is polymorphic, and a single nucleotide polymorphism (SNP) in MTHFR (C677T) results in a functional change to the enzyme (TT and CT genotype carriers have lower enzyme activity than CC genotype carriers) and has been consistently shown to be associated with colorectal cancer risk in meta-analyses of epidemiologic studies (Huang et al., 2007; Hubner and Houlston, 2007; Taioli et al., 2009). The association of candidate gene SNPs involved in nutrient metabolism with a human disease outcome can provide further evidence for a causal association between the nutrient and the disease.

In addition, the examination of gene–diet interactions can help to explain the inconsistent associations observed in epidemiologic studies of diet alone or of genes alone (Nowell et al., 2004; Hunter, 2005). Associations between specific dietary factors and disease may only become apparent in those individuals with certain genetic variants related to the disease process or related to the activity or metabolism of the dietary factor, thus providing some explanation for null associations observed in epidemiologic studies that do not take genetics into account, even in the presence of solid experimental data of a biologic effect for a given dietary factor. For the folate-*MTHFR* example, the effect of the *MTHFR TT* genotype appears to be modified by folate status, such that the beneficial effect disappears under low folate conditions (Bailey, 2003). Other genes and environmental factors are likely to influence these associations (e.g. alcohol can also modify the effect of folate on colorectal cancer risk and there are multiple other SNPs within *MTHFR* and other genes involved in one-carbon metabolism that may play a role [Bailey, 2003; Steck *et al.*, 2008]), so the ability to analyze large complex sets of data with multiple interactions (and the subsequent need for large sample sizes) is an ongoing challenge in the field of gene–diet interactions. Data from genome-wide association studies are now being combined with environmental exposure data to examine gene–environment interactions on an even larger scale. Beyond sequence changes to DNA, other heritable factors such as DNA methylation (in which folate is directly involved) and histone modification (i.e. epigenetic factors) are known to be important in disease etiology, are influenced by nutrition, and are beginning to be incorporated into epidemiologic studies of nutrition and health (Waterland and Michels, 2007; Ulrich and Grady, 2010).

Future Directions

As discussed here, clinical trials are often not feasible or ethical for examining diet and health relationships. In fact, several reasons may explain the absence of a dietary intervention effect when, in fact, an association between diet and the health outcome exists (Hebert and Miller, 1988; Jeffery and Keck, 2008). These include: (1) the distinction between the diets of the intervention and control groups in the trial was not great enough to observe a difference in disease incidence between the groups due either to (a) targeting the wrong foods or dietary patterns for the intervention, or (b) the fact that the control group was eating a diet too similar to the intervention group because of self-selection of health-conscious individuals into the trial, non-compliance by the intervention group, or compensatory change in the control group; (2) genetic heterogeneity, such that a true effect in susceptible subpopulations is masked when all individuals are grouped together in analyses; (3) the targeted timepoint for the intervention was not relevant to, or appropriate for, the disease process under study (e.g. the study population involved older adults when earlier-life interventions were needed, or the intervention period was too short to produce an effect); or (4) the intervention may work only in those individuals whose diets are deficient or insufficient to begin with, and these are not the typically health-conscious people who enroll in clinical trials. Given these limitations of clinical trials, observational studies will continue to be essential in providing evidence for or against diet–disease hypotheses, and finding ways to strengthen these studies is a critical future direction.

Enhancing dietary measurement is one such way to improve epidemiologic studies of nutrition and health. Developing technology for dietary assessment such as administration via the internet, PDAs or cell phones is underway and recognized as an important current need in nutritional epidemiology (Guillén *et al.*, 2009; Ngo *et al.*, 2009; Arab *et al.*, 2010; Six *et al.*, 2010; Subar *et al.*, 2010; Thompson *et al.*, 2010). In addition, as discussed above, insufficient variation in the diets of populations has been a limiting factor for many diet–disease relationships studied with epidemiologic methods. This is being addressed by pooling large cohort studies to obtain greater variation in diet and greater numbers of disease outcomes to investigate those hypotheses that have conflicting results in previous studies as discussed above (Smith-Warner *et al.*, 2001; Cho *et al.*, 2004; Smith-Warner *et al.*, 2006).

Additionally, timing of dietary exposure is recognized as crucial, particularly in diseases with long latencies such as cancer (Michels, 2003a; Steck *et al.*, 2007; Gammon *et al.*, 2008). Thus, finding ways to incorporate early life exposures or exposure assessment across the lifecourse in epidemiologic studies will contribute greatly to our understanding of diet–disease relationships (Michels, 2003b). Furthermore, new analytic methods for handling time-varying data, such as marginal structure models, are being employed in epidemiologic studies of diet and health (Robins *et al.*, 2000; Bodnar *et al.*, 2004). Marginal structure models allow for adjustment of time-dependent confounding, as in the case when a confounder is associated with outcome and with subsequent exposure, and when past exposure is associated with the level of the confounder. An example of this is the association between prenatal iron supplementation and anemia at delivery where dose of iron supplementation can change over time based on the time-dependent covariates of a subject's side-effects or biomarkers of iron status (Bodnar *et al.*, 2004). Depending on the analyses, the direction of the effect of iron supplementation on anemia can be reversed, from an adverse effect when using an ordinary logistic regression model, to an inverse association when using a marginal structure model, which highlights the importance of employing appropriate analytic methodology to obtain fitting interpretations of epidemiologic studies of diet and health.

Some of the limitations of clinical trials are logistically impossible to overcome in human studies, such as those related to the long latency period of chronic disease development, e.g. intervening early and following individuals to a bona fide health outcome is usually infeasible. Others, however, such as the idea that genetic susceptibility may be modifying effects of dietary factors, may be better understood by designing smaller, shorter-term intervention studies that utilize our increasing knowledge about biologic mechanisms of disease (Lampe, 2004; Prentice *et al.*, 2004). Applying what we know about the human genome and emerging "-omics" technologies (e.g. nutrigenomics, epigenomics, proteomics, metabonomics) in the field of nutrition (Stover, 2004; Zeisel *et al.*, 2005; Jenab *et al.*, 2009) should lead to innovative areas of research that will deepen our understanding of the biologic processes involved in diet and disease, and reconcile trial data with a preponderance of ecological, observational, and laboratory evidence that implicates certain foods in disease etiology. Such understanding has very practical implications for translating findings to individuals and communities in which the dietary factors will have a beneficial and substantial effect.

Suggestions for Further Reading

Langseth, L. (1996) *Nutritional Epidemiology: Possibilities and Limitations*. ILSI Europe Concise Monograph Series. International Life Sciences Institute, Washington, DC.

Mackerras, D. and Margetts, B.M. (2005) Nutritional epidemiology. In W. Ahrens and I. Pigeot (eds), *Handbook of Epidemiology*. Springer, Berlin, pp. 999–1042.

Margetts, B.M. and Nelson, M. (1997) *Design Concepts in Nutritional Epidemiology*. Oxford University Press, New York.

Willett, W. (1998) *Nutritional Epidemiology*. Oxford University Press, New York.

References

Alpha-Tocopherol Beta Carotene Cancer Prevention Study Group (1994) The effect of vitamin E and beta carotene on the incidence of lung cancer and other cancers in male smokers. *N Engl J Med* **330**, 1029–1035.

Arab, L., Wesseling-Perry, K., Jardack, P., *et al.* (2010) Eight self-administered 24-hour dietary recalls using the internet are feasible in African Americans and Whites: the Energetics Study. *J Am Diet Assoc* **110**, 857–864.

Bailey, L.B. (2003) Folate, methyl-related nutrients, alcohol, and the MTHFR 677C →T polymorphism affect cancer risk: intake recommendations. *J Nutr* **133**, 3748S–3753S.

Bjelakovic, G., Nikolova, D., Gluud, L.L., *et al.* (2007) Mortality in randomized trials of antioxidant supplements for primary and secondary prevention: systematic review and meta-analysis. *JAMA* **297**, 842–857.

Bodnar, L.M., Davidian, M., Siega-Riz, A.M., *et al.* (2004) Marginal structural models for analyzing causal effects of time-dependent treatments: an application in perinatal epidemiology. *Am J Epidemiol* **159**, 926–934.

Byers, T. (1999) What can randomized controlled trials tell us about nutrition and cancer prevention? *CA Cancer J Clin* **49**, 353–361.

Chen, L.T. and Rivera, M.A. (2004) The Costa Rican experience: reduction of neural tube defects following food fortification programs. *Nutr Rev* **62**, S40–43.

Cho, E., Smith-Warner, S.A., Spiegelman, D., *et al.* (2004) Dairy foods, calcium, and colorectal cancer: a pooled analysis of 10 cohort studies. *J Natl Cancer Inst* **96**, 1015–1022.

Colditz, G.A., Manson, J.E., and Hankinson, S.E. (1997) The Nurses' Health Study: 20-year contribution to the understanding of health among women. *J Womens Health* **6**, 49–62.

Cole, B.F., Baron, J.A., Sandler, R.S., *et al.* (2007) Folic acid for the prevention of colorectal adenomas. *JAMA* **297**, 2351–2359.

Davies, A.A., Davey Smith, G., Harbord, R., *et al.* (2006) Nutritional interventions and outcome in patients with cancer or preinvasive lesions: systematic review. *J Natl Cancer Inst* **98**, 961–973.

De Wals, P., Tairou, F., Van Allen, M.I., *et al.* (2007) Reduction in neural-tube defects after folic acid fortification in Canada. *N Engl J Med* **357**, 135–142.

Forman, M.R., Hursting, S.D., Umar, A., *et al.* (2004) Nutrition and cancer prevention: a multidisciplinary perspective on human trials. *Annu Rev Nutr* **24**, 223–254.

Gammon, M.D., Fink, B.N., Steck, S.E., *et al.* (2008) Soy intake and breast cancer: elucidation of an unanswered question. *Br J Cancer* **98**, 2–3.

Genkinger, J.M., Spiegelman, D., Anderson, K.E., *et al.* (2009) Alcohol intake and pancreatic cancer risk: a pooled analysis of fourteen cohort studies. *Cancer Epidemiol Biomarkers Prev* **18**, 765–776.

Giovannucci, E. (2002) Epidemiologic studies of folate and color-ectal neoplasia: a review. *J Nutr* **132**, 2350S–2355S.

Guillén, S., Sanna, A., Ngo, J., *et al.* (2009) New technologies for promoting a healthy diet and active living. *Nutr Rev* **67**, S107–S110.

Hebert, J.R. and Miller, D.R. (1988) Methodologic considerations for investigating the diet-cancer link. *Am J Clin Nutr* **47**, 1068–1077.

Hebert, J.R. and Wynder, E.L. (1987) Dietary fat and the risk of breast cancer. *N Engl J Med* **317**, 165–166.

Hertrampf, E. and Cortes, F. (2004) Folic acid fortification of wheat flour: Chile. *Nutr Rev* **62**, S44–48; Discussion, S49.

Honein, M.A., Paulozzi, L.J., Mathews, T.J., *et al.* (2001) Impact of folic acid fortification of the US food supply on the occur-rence of neural tube defects. *JAMA* **285**, 2981–2986.

Huang, Y., Han, S., Li, Y., *et al.* (2007) Different roles of MTHFR C677T and A1298C polymorphisms in colorectal adenoma and colorectal cancer: a meta-analysis. *J Hum Genet* **52**, 73–85.

Hubner, R.A. and Houlston, R.S. (2007) MTHFR C677T and colorectal cancer risk: a meta-analysis of 25 populations. *Int J Cancer* **120**, 1027–1035.

Hunter, D.J. (2005) Gene–environment interactions in human dis-eases. *Nat Rev Genet* **6**, 287–298.

Jaszewski, R., Misra, S., Tobi, M., *et al.* (2008) Folic acid supple-mentation inhibits recurrence of colorectal adenomas: a rand-omized chemoprevention trial. *World J Gastroenterol* **14**, 4492–4498.

Jeffery, E.H. and Keck, A.S. (2008) Translating knowledge gener-ated by epidemiological and in vitro studies into dietary cancer prevention. *Mol Nutr Food Res* **52**(Suppl 1), S7–17.

Jenab, M., Slimani, N., Bictash, M., *et al.* (2009) Biomarkers in nutritional epidemiology: applications, needs and new hori-zons. *Hum Genet* **125**, 507–525.

Kamineni, A., Williams, M.A., Schwartz, S.M., *et al.* (1999) The incidence of gastric carcinoma in Asian migrants to the United States and their descendants. *Cancer Causes Control* **10**, 77–83.

Kim, D.H., Smith-Warner, S.A., Spiegelman, D., *et al.* (2010) Pooled analyses of 13 prospective cohort studies on folate intake and colon cancer. *Cancer Causes Control* **21**,1919–1930.

Kim, Y.-I. (2008) Folic acid supplementation and cancer risk: point. *Cancer Epidemiol Biomarkers Prev* **17**, 2220–2225.

Koushik, A., Hunter, D.J., Spiegelman, D., *et al.* (2005) Fruits and vegetables and ovarian cancer risk in a pooled analysis of 12 cohort studies. *Cancer Epidemiol Biomarkers Prev* **14**, 2160–2167.

Lampe, J.W. (2004) Nutrition and cancer prevention: small-scale human studies for the 21st century. *Cancer Epidemiol Biomarkers Prev* **13**, 1987–1988.

Langseth, L. (1996) *Nutritional Epidemiology: Possibilities and Limitations*. ILSI Europe Concise Monograph Series. International Life Sciences Institute, Washington, DC.

Lee, J.E., Mannisto, S., Spiegelman, D., *et al.* (2009) Intakes of fruit, vegetables, and carotenoids and renal cell cancer risk: a pooled analysis of 13 prospective studies. *Cancer Epidemiol Biomarkers Prev* **18**, 1730–1739.

Lee, J.E., Willett, W.C., Fuchs, C.S., *et al.* (2011) Folate intake and risk of colorectal cancer and adenoma: modification by time. *Am J Clin Nutr* **93**, 817–825.

Lippman, S.M., Lee, J.J., and Sabichi, A.L. (1998) Cancer chemo-prevention: progress and promise. *J Natl Cancer Inst* **90**, 1514–1528.

Logan, R.F., Grainge, M.J., Shepherd, V.C., *et al.* (2008) Aspirin and folic acid for the prevention of recurrent colorectal adeno-mas. *Gastroenterology* **134**, 29–38.

Mason, J.B., Dickstein, A., Jacques, P.F., *et al.* (2007) A temporal association between folic acid fortification and an increase in colorectal cancer rates may be illuminating important biologi-cal principles: a hypothesis. *Cancer Epidemiol Biomarkers Prev* **16**, 1325–1329.

Mayne, S.T. (1996) Beta-carotene, carotenoids, and disease preven-tion in humans. *FASEB J* **10**, 690–701.

Meyskens, F.L., Jr and Szabo, E. (2005) Diet and cancer: the dis-connect between epidemiology and randomized clinical trials. *Cancer Epidemiol Biomarkers Prev* **14**, 1366–1369.

Michels, K.B. (2003a) Early life predictors of chronic disease. *J Womens Health (Larchmt)* **12**, 157–161.

Michels, K.B. (2003b) Nutritional epidemiology – past, present, future. *Int J Epidemiol* **32**, 486–488.

Ngo, J., Engelen, A., Molag, M., *et al.* (2009) A review of the use of information and communication technologies for dietary assessment. *Br J Nutr* **101**(Suppl S2), S102–S112.

Nowell, S.A., Ahn, J., and Ambrosone, C.B. (2004) Gene–nutrient interactions in cancer etiology. *Nutr Rev* **62**, 427–438.

Omenn, G.S., Goodman, G.E., Thornquist, M.D., *et al.* (1996) Effects of a combination of beta carotene and vitamin A on lung cancer and cardiovascular disease. *N Engl J Med* **334**, 1150–1155.

Paspatis, G.A. and Karamanolis, D.G. (1994) Folate supplementa-tion and adenomatous colonic polyps. *Dis Colon Rectum* **37**, 1340–1341.

Pierce, J.P., Natarajan, L., Caan, B.J., *et al.* (2007) Influence of a diet very high in vegetables, fruit, and fiber and low in fat on prognosis following treatment for breast cancer: the Women's

Healthy Eating and Living (WHEL) randomized trial. [See Comment]. *JAMA* **298**, 289–298.

Porta, M. (2008) *A Dictionary of Epidemiology*. Oxford University Press, New York.

Prentice, R.L. (2007) Observational studies, clinical trials, and the Women's Health Initiative. *Lifetime Data Anal* **13**, 449–462.

Prentice, R.L., Caan, B., Chlebowski, R.T., *et al.* (2006) Low-fat dietary pattern and risk of invasive breast cancer: the Women's Health Initiative Randomized Controlled Dietary Modification Trial. *JAMA* **295**, 629–642.

Prentice, R.L., Willett, W.C., Greenwald, P., *et al.* (2004) Nutrition and physical activity and chronic disease prevention: research strategies and recommendations. *J Natl Cancer Inst* **96**, 1276–1287.

Ray, J.G., Meier, C., Vermeulen, M.J., *et al.* (2002) Association of neural tube defects and folic acid food fortification in Canada. *Lancet* **360**, 2047–2048.

Riboli, E. and Kaaks, R. (1997) The EPIC Project: rationale and study design. European Prospective Investigation into Cancer and Nutrition. *Int J Epidemiol* **26**(Suppl 1), S6.

Robins, J.M., Hernan, M.A., and Brumback, B. (2000) Marginal structural models and causal inference in epidemiology. *Epidemiology* **11**, 550–560.

Rock, C.L. (2007) Primary dietary prevention: is the fiber story over? *Recent Results Cancer Res* **174**, 171–177.

Schatzkin, A., Lanza, E., Corle, D., *et al.* (2000) Lack of effect of a low-fat, high-fiber diet on the recurrence of colorectal adenomas. Polyp Prevention Trial Study Group. *N Engl J Med* **342**, 1149–1155.

Six, B.L., Schap, T.E., Zhu, F.M., *et al.* (2010) Evidence-based development of a mobile telephone food record. *J Am Diet Assoc* **110**, 74–79.

Smith-Warner, S.A., Spiegelman, D., Ritz, J., *et al.* (2006) Methods for pooling results of epidemiologic studies. *Am J Epidemiol* **163**, 1053–1064.

Smith-Warner, S.A., Spiegelman, D., Yaun, S.S., *et al.* (2001) Intake of fruits and vegetables and risk of breast cancer: a pooled analysis of cohort studies. *JAMA* **285**, 769–776.

Steck, S.E., Gaudet, M.M., Eng, S.M., *et al.* (2007) Cooked meat and risk of breast cancer–lifetime versus recent dietary intake. *Epidemiology* **18**, 373–382.

Steck, S.E., Keku, T., Butler, L.M., *et al.* (2008) Polymorphisms in methionine synthase, methionine synthase reductase and serine hydroxymethyltransferase, folate and alcohol intake, and colon cancer risk. *J Nutrigenet Nutrigenomics* **1**, 196–204.

Stover, P.J. (2004) Nutritional genomics. *Physiol Genomics* **16**, 161–165.

Subar, A.F., Crafts, J., Zimmerman, T.P., *et al.* (2010) Assessment of the accuracy of portion size reports using computer-based food photographs aids in the development of an automated self-administered 24-hour recall. *J Am Diet Assoc* **110**, 55–64.

Taioli, E., Garza, M.A., Ahn, Y.O., *et al.* (2009) Meta- and pooled analyses of the methylenetetrahydrofolate reductase (MTHFR) C677T polymorphism and colorectal cancer: a HuGE-GSEC review. *Am J Epidemiol* **170**, 1207–1221.

Thompson, F.E., Subar, A.F., Loria, C.M., *et al.* (2010) Need for technological innovation in dietary assessment. *J Am Diet Assoc* **110**, 48–51.

Tominaga, S. (1985) Cancer incidence in Japanese in Japan, Hawaii, and western United States. *Natl Cancer Inst Monogr* **69**, 83–92.

Ulrich, C.M. and Grady, W.M. (2010) Linking epidemiology to epigenomics – where are we today? *Cancer Prev Res* **3**, 1505–1508.

Ulrich, C.M. and Potter, J.D. (2006) Folate supplementation: too much of a good thing? *Cancer Epidemiol Biomarkers Prev* **15**, 189–193.

Waterland, R.A. and Michels, K.B. (2007) Epigenetic epidemiology of the developmental origins hypothesis. *Annu Rev Nutr* **27**, 363–388.

Willett, W. (1998) *Nutritional Epidemiology*. Oxford University Press, New York.

Wolff, T., Witkop, C.T., Miller, T., *et al.* (2009) Folic acid supplementation for the prevention of neural tube defects: an update of the evidence for the U.S. Preventive Services Task Force. *Ann Intern Med* **150**, 632–639.

Women's Health Initiative (1998) Design of the Women's Health Initiative clinical trial and observational study. The Women's Health Initiative Study Group. *Controlled Clin Trials* **19**, 61–109.

Wu, K., Platz, E.A., Willett, W.C., *et al.* (2009) A randomized trial on folic acid supplementation and risk of recurrent colorectal adenoma. *Am J Clin Nutr* **90**, 1623–1631.

Zeisel, S.H., Freake, H.C., Bauman, D.E., *et al.* (2005) The nutritional phenotype in the age of metabolomics. *J Nutr* **135**, 1613–1616.

64

NUTRITION MONITORING IN THE UNITED STATES

RONETTE R. BRIEFEL[1], DrPH, RD AND MARGARET A. MCDOWELL[2], PhD, MPH, RD

[1]*Mathematica Policy Research, Washington, DC, USA*
[2]*National Institute of Health, Bethesda, Maryland, USA*

Summary

The US nutrition monitoring program is comprised of national and state surveys of individuals and households, health record systems, and specialized databases on food and dietary supplement composition, environmental contaminants, and food availability. Although the continuous National Health and Nutrition Examination Survey (NHANES) still collects the most comprehensive health and nutrition data on the US population, a growing number of other federal and state surveys and databases also contribute information on diet and health knowledge, attitudes and behaviors, food consumption, nutrition, and health for the general population and subgroups at nutritional risk.

Since 2000 a growing array of data resources have come into use to monitor US trends in dietary intake, nutritional status, and nutrition-related health conditions (e.g. obesity, hypertension, diabetes, osteoporosis, and dental caries); to evaluate nutrition assistance programs, food fortification and food labeling policies, and food safety; and to conduct research on nutrition standards and diet and health relationships. Greater recognition of the role of the food environment (e.g. store proximity, food price structure, and community characteristics) in food choices and diet quality is evident today.

Introduction

Nutrition monitoring has been defined as "an on-going description of nutrition conditions in the population, with particular attention to subgroups defined in socioeconomic terms, for purposes of planning, analyzing the effects of policies and programs on nutrition problems, and predicting future trends" (Mason *et al.*, 1984). This chapter provides a brief history of the National Nutrition Monitoring and Related Research Program (NNMRRP) in the United States, uses of nutrition monitoring data, monitoring activities since 2000, and nutrition monitoring research to meet challenges in the future.

The NNMRRP is composed of interconnected federal and state activities that provide information about the dietary and nutritional status of the US population, condi-

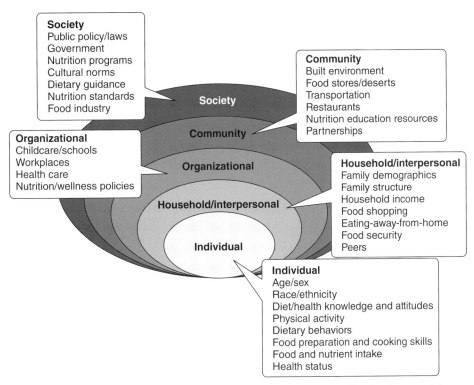

FIG. 64.1 Socio-ecologic model for nutrition and health monitoring. Individuals' nutrition and health status are influenced by interpersonal, organizational, community, and societal factors; a comprehensive nutrition monitoring program should assess the factors and levels shown in the socio-ecologic model for nutrition and health monitoring. Adapted from Centers for Disease Control and Prevention (2010).

tions existing in the US that affect the dietary and nutritional status of individuals, and relationships between diet and health (Briefel, 2006; Briefel and Bialostosky, 2008). Nutrition is one component of a broader socio-ecologic framework (Figure 64.1) in which individuals are influenced by their families, communities, and programs and policies at the federal, state, and local levels (Glanz *et al.*, 2005). A general conceptual model representing the relationship between food and health is presented in Figure 64.2. This figure aligns with the five NNMRRP measurement component areas described in past reports: (1) food supply determinations; (2) food and nutrient consumption; (3) food composition and nutrient databases; (4) knowledge, attitudes, and behavior assessments; and (5) nutrition and related health measurements (US Department of Health and Human Services (HHS) and US Department of Agriculture (USDA), 1993; Life Sciences Research Office (LSRO), 1995; Briefel, 2006). For this chapter update, a sixth measurement area on environmental factors was added to incorporate food access and the built envi-

ronment (Brownson *et al.*, 2009). The US nutrition monitoring program is a model for integrating national and state data from many sources to understand the relationship between food and health and to improve nutrition in the population.

History and Recent Accomplishments/ Activities

A nutrition monitoring system was first established with the passage of the Food and Agriculture Act (Pub. L. 95–113) in 1977. Major legislative efforts to increase federal efforts to coordinate nutrition surveys occurred in the late 1970s and 1980s and culminated in the passage of the National Nutrition Monitoring and Related Research Act 1990 (Pub. L. 101–445) in 1990 (US Congress, 1990). The Act established several mechanisms to ensure the collaboration and coordination of federal agencies as well as state and local governments involved in nutrition monitoring. These included the formation of an

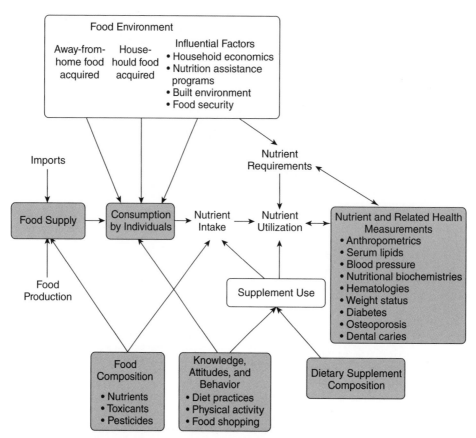

FIG. 64.2   Relationship of food to health. A comprehensive nutrition monitoring program should assess the characteristics of, and interactions between, the food environment; food supply; food and dietary supplement composition; and individuals' food consumption, nutrient intake, knowledge/attitudes/behaviors, and nutrition/health status. These components reflect the relationship of food to health. Adapted from Life Sciences Research Office (1995).

interagency board to coordinate annual budget reports, biennial reports on progress and policy implications of scientific findings, and periodic scientific reports to describe the nutritional and related health status of the US population. A National Nutrition Monitoring Advisory Council provided scientific and technical guidance to the board and made important contributions to improving information dissemination and focusing attention on issues such as the coverage of high-risk population subgroups, assessment of the needs of data users, and integration of federal, state, and private data needs.

The *Ten-Year Comprehensive Plan* guided federal actions for nutrition monitoring during the period 1992 to 2002 (US Department of Health and Human Services (HHS) and US Department of Agriculture, 1993). The plan identified three national objectives critical to the success of the overall goal of a coordinated, comprehensive nutrition-

monitoring program: (1) provide for a comprehensive program through continuous and coordinated data collection; (2) improve the comparability and quality of data across the program; and (3) improve the research base for nutrition monitoring. During the period 1992–1997, federal efforts were focused on improving survey coordination and survey methods, conducting research, and increasing nutrition information dissemination (Dwyer *et al.*, 2003a; Briefel, 2006). To meet one of the research objectives, an 18-item food security measure was developed to track the prevalence of hunger and food insecurity in the population and high-risk subgroups (Hamilton *et al.*, 1997). This measure is used in national surveys, evaluation studies of nutrition assistance programs, and other research studies on low-income groups.

Since 2000 the major activities and accomplishments were related to the integration of the two national nutrition surveys, the US Department of Health and Human Services' National Health and Nutrition Examination Survey (NHANES), and the US Department of Agriculture's Continuing Survey of Food Intakes by Individuals (CSFII) (Murphy, 2003; Woteki, 2003). An expanded array of diet and health information resources including specialized food and dietary supplement composition, food environment, food safety, and food supply databases were developed to support monitoring and research activities. Nutrition monitoring data were also used to support health-care-reform legislation, to expand child and adult feeding programs, and to improve school nutrition standards.

Nutrition monitoring has also been the focus of scientific and professional organizations. In 1999 the US National Academy of Sciences (NAS) sponsored a symposium on the future of nutrition monitoring in view of the fact that the 1990 legislation was up for reauthorization in 2002. The purpose of the meeting was to draw attention to the federal, research, industry, media, and consumer uses of NNMRRP data, and to discuss the future challenges for the program. Despite the NAS symposium, a report by the American Societies for Nutritional Sciences Working Group (Woteki *et al.*, 2002), and other efforts to gain support for reauthorization, the nutrition monitoring legislation was not renewed in 2002. Monitoring activities are continuing, but without the formal, coordinated guidance of an interagency board or legislative mandate. In 2002 a workshop was held with nutrition monitoring stakeholders to develop recommendations on how best to meet data needs for policy and research with the integrated survey (Dwyer *et al.*, 2003a,b,c,d). In 2004 a US National Research Council panel published a review of the infrastructure to support food and nutrition programs, research and decision making, and, in 2005, a report on recommendations to improve the data for such purposes (National Research Council (NRC), 2004, 2005). The 2005 report provides the most recent information on nutrition monitoring activities, but does not cover the entire program to the extent of the 2000 *Directory* more than a decade ago (Interagency Board for Nutrition Monitoring and Related Research (IBNMRR), 2000).

Since 2005 the major sources of nutrition monitoring data are individual federal and state government reports, journal articles, and special reports commissioned by the federal government to address specific topics and research needs. For example, a report by Logan *et al.* (2002) summarizes the types of data available from national surveys

and surveillance systems that can be used to assess the relationship between food assistance program participation and nutrition and health outcomes. The coordinated interagency reporting and data syntheses that occurred between 1984 and 2000 have been discontinued (LSRO, 1995; IBNMRR, 2000; Woteki *et al.*, 2002; Briefel, 2006). While these joint efforts served to improve coordination by increasing communication and standardization and reducing duplication of effort, they also require staff and other resources that can be labor intensive and political. In their place a broader range of research and reporting initiatives led by individual agencies have been undertaken. For example, the National Cancer Institute maintains a website that provides information on dietary methods, surveillance, and analysis approaches for assessing the diet, nutritional status, and physical activity of populations (http://riskfactor.cancer.gov/). There is a continued need for Congressional support to ensure that there is a sound NNMRRP in the future with steady financial resources for national nutrition monitoring (Woteki *et al.*, 2002; NRC, 2005).

Purposes and Uses of Nutrition Monitoring Data Today

Nutrition monitoring serves a vital role in health policy making and research (US Congress, 1990; LSRO, 1995; Office of Science and Technology Policy, 1996). Monitoring provides information and a database for establishing public policy and identifying research priorities. Nutrition research provides data for policy making and for identifying nutrition monitoring needs for data. Box 64.1 provides examples of uses of nutrition monitoring data for public policy and scientific research purposes. Monitoring provides information for public policy decisions related to nutrition education programs such as the *Dietary Guidelines for Americans* (USDA and HHS, 2010), MyPyramid (now called MyPlate) (USDA, 2011), and 5 A Day (CDC, 2008); public health programs such as the National Cholesterol Education Program (NCEP) (NCEP Expert Panel, 2002) and the National High Blood Pressure Education Program (National Heart, Lung, and Blood Institute, 2004); federally supported nutrition assistance programs such as school meals and the Special Supplemental Nutrition Program for Women, Infants, and Children (WIC) (Logan *et al.*, 2002; Woteki *et al.*, 2002; Fox *et al.*, 2004); the USDA Food Plans (Carlson *et al.*, 2007a,b);

BOX 64.1   Uses of nutrition monitoring data

Public Policy

Monitoring and surveillance

- Identify high-risk groups and geographical areas with nutrition-related problems to facilitate implementation of public health intervention programs and food assistance programs.
- Evaluate changes in agricultural policy that may affect the nutritional quality and healthfulness of the US food supply.
- Track trends in dietary behavior, nutritional status, and health to assess progress toward achieving the nutrition and health objectives in *Healthy People 2010* and the *Dietary Guidelines for Americans.*
- Recommend guidelines for prevention, detection, and management of nutrition and health conditions.
- Develop reference standards for nutritional status.
- Assess environmental exposures from food consumption.
- Monitor food production and marketing.

Regulatory

- Develop food labeling policies.
- Document the need for, and monitor, food fortification policies.
- Establish food safety guidelines.

Nutrition-related programs

- Develop nutrition education and dietary guidance (e.g. *Dietary Guidelines for Americans* and MyPlate).
- Plan and evaluate food assistance programs.
- Plan and assess nutrition intervention programs and public health programs.

Scientific Research

- Establish nutrient requirements through the lifecycle (e.g. *Dietary Reference Intakes*) and assess nutrient adequacy and excess.
- Study diet–health relationships and the relationship of knowledge and attitudes to diet and health behavior.
- Develop biomarkers of diet and health behaviors and nutritional status.
- Foster and conduct nutrition monitoring research – national and international.
- Conduct food composition analysis.
- Study the economic aspects of food consumption.
- Assess the contribution of dietary supplements to usual nutrient intake.

and food production and marketing such as the development of reduced-fat or reduced-calorie food products.

Monitoring data are used to evaluate progress towards achievement of long-term health objectives including the 2010 and 2020 Health Objectives for the Nation (US Department of Health and Human Services, 2000). The Healthy People findings are used to inform policy development, identify areas of future nutrition research, and evaluate diet and health guidance for the US population. NHANES data on heights and weights were used to develop growth charts to assess children's growth and weights status (Kuczmarski *et al.*, 2000).

Specific uses of the dietary intake and biomarker data collected during the NHANES include assessments of the population's dietary intakes and serum nutrient

levels to determine and evaluate the Dietary Reference Intakes recommended by expert groups convened by the Institute of Medicine (Institute of Medicine (IOM) 2000, 2010a,b); evaluations of fortification policies by the Food and Drug Administration (FDA) (Lewis *et al.*, 1999; Centers for Disease Control and Prevention (CDC), 2000; Woteki, 2003; Bailey *et al.*, 2010); use of dietary supplements by the US population (Heimbach, 2001); and dietary exposure estimation for nutrient and non-nutrient food components by the Environmental Protection Agency (EPA) (1997). The data have been used to establish reference ranges for dietary exposures in children and adults and to evaluate public health initiatives to the human health effects of environmental exposures (CDC, 2009).

Numerous private industries use nutrition monitoring data for marketing purposes and research. Food industry has used national food consumption data to assess brand-name loyalty, to target marketing practices, and to study the relationship of a particular food commodity such as soup or iron-fortified cereals to overall intake and nutritional status. Pharmaceutical companies have used NHANES data to estimate the proportion of the population taking a particular drug, to estimate treatment of various health conditions with drugs (Dodd *et al.*, 2009), and to conduct cost–benefit analysis of the use of cholesterol-lowering drugs and cardiovascular risk. National survey data on the population's use of dietary supplements have been used by trade associations to study the characteristics of users and the nutritional effects of supplements. Consumers and practitioners also use national nutrition data to learn about diet and health, the effects of supplements on diet, nutrition, and health, and the effectiveness of weight-loss practices.

Nutrition monitoring data have also been used to identify food and nutrition research priorities of significance to public health. The Institute of Medicine used NHANES dietary and biochemical data in its review of the Dietary Reference Intakes for calcium and vitamin D, and NHANES 2003–2006 hypertension and dietary data to recommend strategies to reduce sodium intake in the United States (Institute of Medicine, 2010a,b). Trends in energy and food and nutrient intake based on national dietary data have been used to understand the relationship between changes in dietary intake and the population's increase in overweight and health status (Logan *et al.*, 2002; Briefel and Johnson, 2004; Fox *et al.*, 2004; Briefel, 2007). State-level data have been used to plan health and nutrition education programs. For example, New York used Behavioral Risk Factor Surveillance System (BRFSS) data on the consumption of whole milk to plan a state campaign to encourage people to drink low-fat milk, and Arkansas used BRFSS data on physical activity and hypertension to design interventions and education programs to target African-American women.

Nutrition Monitoring Components in the United States

Background

The first national dietary surveys were carried out in the 1930s. Since then, more than 35 surveys, surveillance systems, and databases have been developed and evolved to meet the information needs of federal agencies, research-ers, and data users. Chronological listings of past nutrition monitoring surveys and activities have been published (US Department of Health and Human Services and US Department of Agriculture, 1993; LSRO, 1995; NRC, 2005; Briefel, 2006). This section of the chapter describes ongoing nutrition monitoring activities by the components shown in the food-to-health framework in Figure 64.2. Additionally, a new section on environmental data sources has been added to reflect growing interest in ecological factors that are related to food consumption patterns (French *et al.*, 2001; McKinnon *et al.*, 2009). Table 64.1 summarizes information on the federally sponsored surveys of households, individuals, and nutrition assistance program participants, and surveillance activities since 2000. Table 64.2 summarizes information on food supply and availability, environmental databases and the technical databases used in national nutrition monitoring. Website information links for each data source are included in Tables 64.1 and 64.2 and listed at the end of the chapter.

Food Supply and Food Availability (Per Capita) Data Systems

Annual per capita nutrient availability or national food supply estimates have been produced by the USDA Economic Research Service (ERS) since 1909 (Table 64.2). Food supply data reflect the amounts of foods and nutrients available for consumption and thus trends in food available for consumption rather than actual food intakes by individuals and households. Food supply data are often used to: (1) assess the potential of the US food supply to meet the nutritional needs of the population; (2) evaluate the effects of technological alterations and marketing changes on the food supply; (3) indicate the relationships between food and nutrient availability and nutrient–disease associations; and (4) facilitate management of federal marketing, food assistance, nutrition education, food enrichment and fortification policy. The Food Availability Data System has been expanded since the last edition of this chapter to include per capita loss-adjusted food availability (LAFA) information and nutrient availability information. The LAFA information adjusts the per capita food availability data for food spoilage and other losses to more closely approximate actual per capita intake, resulting in per capita estimates for each food commodity group: the number of calories per day and the number of MyPyramid equivalents per day (now called MyPlate) (USDA, 2011). Nutrient availability information provides estimates of the amounts per capita per day of food energy and 27 nutrients and dietary components (for example,

TABLE 64.1 Major federally sponsored nutrition monitoring surveys, surveillance systems, and activities (2000–2011)

Survey name	Federal department (agency)	Schedule (initial year)	Sample design (estimates)	US target group	Sample (size)	Survey content, measures, and link for further information
Individual-Level Data Collection and Reports						
National Health and Nutrition Examination Survey (NHANES)	HHS (CDC/ NCHS) "What We Eat in America" funded by USDA/ARS	Periodic 1971–1974, 1976–1980, 1982–1984, 1988–1994 Continuous, annual: 1999– present	Cross-sectional (national)	Civilian, household population; all ages since 1999	Annual sample: ~5000 persons interviewed and examined annually	Household interview, physical exam, and post-exam components. Dietary information: two dietary recalls per person since 2002; food security, supplement use, diet behavior, and health questionnaires. Exam includes measured height and weight; biomarker assessments; clinical tests (vary by survey) NHANES link: http://www.cdc.gov/ nchs/nhanes.htm USDA: "What We Eat in America (WWEIA)" tables: http:// www.ars.usda.gov/Services/ docs.htm?docid=13793
Flexible Consumer Behavior Survey (component of NHANES)	HHS (CDC/ NCHS) Funded by USDA/ERS	Special module (2005–2010)	Cross-sectional (national)	NHANES subsample 1+ years	In-person and telephone interview methods	Core questions asked in the NHANES household interview; post-exam phone interview. Family and individual level data Link:http://www.ers.usda.gov/ Briefing/DietQuality/flexible.htm
National Health Interview Survey (NHIS)	HHS (CDC/ NCHS)	Annual (1957)	Cross-sectional (national, selected state estimates with combined years combined)	Civilian, household population, all ages	All ages (sample sizes have varied) 2010 sample: 34329 households yielded 89976 individuals	In-person household interview. Content includes core questionnaire on basic health and demographic items and special modules on current health topics (content and topics vary) Link: http://www.cdc.gov/nchs/nhis/ about_nhis.htm
Health and Diet Survey (HDS)	HHS (FDA/ CFSAN)	Periodic since 1982	Cross-sectional	Random-digit-dialing (RDD) telephone survey	2008 sample: 2584 adults 18 years and over	Tracks consumer knowledge, attitudes, and practices related to foods and dietary supplements Link: http://www.fda.gov/ForConsumers/ ConsumerUpdates/ ucm202611.htm

Survey	Agency	Frequency (year started)	Design	Population/sampling	Sample size	Description
Behavioral Risk Factor Surveillance System (BRFSS)	HHS (CDC/NCCDPHP)	Annual (1984)	Cross-sectional (national and state)	Civilian, households with telephones; age 18+ years. Sampling frame: 50 states, DC, Puerto Rico, Virgin Islands, and Guam	In 2010, 451075 adults participated in BRFSS	Telephone interviews. Core questions and state-specific questions asked. Field operations are managed by state health departments that follow guidelines provided by the CDC. Link: http://www.cdc.gov/brfss/technical_infodata/surveydata/2010.htm
Youth Risk Behavior Surveillance System (YRBSS)	HHS (CDC/NCCDPHP)	Biennial (1991)	Cross-sectional (national and state)	Youth in school grades 9–12; ages 12–21 years	National school-based survey samples; 2009 data on 16410 persons 12–21 years based on 47 states, DC, and 20 local regions	Monitors priority health-risk behaviors and the prevalence of obesity and asthma among youth and young adults. Link: http://www.cdc.gov/HealthyYouth/yrbs/index.htm
National Immunization Survey (NIS)	HHS (CDC NCIRD and CDC/NCHS)	Annual and periodic surveys (1994)	Cross-sectional (national and state)	Annual surveys of children 19–35 months; add-on survey of teens 13–17 years since 2006 (NIS-Teen); adult survey conducted 2007	2010 NIS included 25948 children 19–35 months. 2008 NIS-Teen: surveyed 19257 teens	RDD telephone survey followed by mail survey to providers. Breastfeeding questions since 2001. Link: http://www.cdc.gov/breastfeeding/data/NIS_data/index.htm
State and Local Area Integrated Telephone Survey (SLAITS)	HHS (CDC/NCHS) with government agency and nonprofit organization support	Periodic (1997)	Cross-sectional (national and state)	RDD design; uses NIS sampling frame; children and adults have participated	Sample size varies. The 2007 National Survey of Children's Health (with HRSA) collected information on 91642 children birth–17 years	Health data on varied topics at the national, state, and local levels. The 2011 survey expects to collect information on 91800 children birth–17 years. Link: http://www.cdc.gov/nchs/slaits.htm

(Continued)

TABLE 64.1 (*Continued*)

Survey name	Federal department (agency)	Schedule (initial year)	Sample design (estimates)	US target group	Sample (size)	Survey content, measures, and link for further information
National Survey of Family Growth (NSFG)	HHS (CDC/ NCHS)	Periodic cycles (1973–2002) Continuous, annual surveys since 2006	Cross-sectional (national)	National samples of US household population	Target age: 15–44 years; ~4400 interviews/year	Information on family life, marriage and divorce, pregnancy, infertility, use of contraception, breastfeeding, and men's and women's health Link: http://www.cdc.gov/nchs/nsfg.htm
Pregnancy Risk Assessment Monitoring System (PRAMS)	HHS (CDC/ NCCDPHP)	Annual (1987)	Cross-sectional (state)	Women with recent live birth	Randomly sampled from birth certificates; 1300–1400 mothers from each participating state	Mixed mode (mail; phone if needed). Data used to monitor changes in maternal and child health indicators Link: http://www.cdc.gov/prams/
Infant Feeding Practices Survey (IFPS)	HHS (FDA/ CFSAN) with several federal partners	Periodic IFPS I: 1992–1993 IFPS II: 2005–2007	Longitudinal (nationally distributed)	Pregnant women and their infants; sampled from a large national consumer opinion panel	Pregnant women and their infants followed up to 12 months post-partum. ~4000 pregnant women identified and ~2000 mothers completed IFPS II	Brief phone interview and series of mail questionnaires on pre- and postnatal diet and health, infant feeding and health, child care, and WIC Link: http://www.cdc.gov/ifps/
Early Childhood Longitudinal Study Program (ECLS)	DoEd (NCES)	3 cohorts	Longitudinal	Children from birth through age 8 years	ECLS–Birth: 14000 children born in 2001 ECLS–Kindergarten class 1998–1999 Kindergarten class through 8th grade ECLS–Kindergarten class 2010–2011: Following through grade 5 (in progress)	Child development, school readiness, and early school experiences assessed; measured height and weight; food consumption questionnaire ascertained food consumption frequency (home and school) General Link: http://nces.ed.gov/ecls/ ECLS-K links: http://nces.ed.gov/ecls/kinderdataprocedure.asp Codebook: http:// sodapop.pop.psu.edu/codebooks/ecls/k5userpart1.pdf

Survey	Sponsor	Dates/Frequency	Design	Population	Sample	Content and Links
Current Population Survey (CPS) Food Security Supplement (FSS)	DOL (BLS) Conducted by the Census Bureau	Food Security Supplement (FSS) data collected since 1995	Cross-sectional (national)	Supplement to the monthly CPS sample: ~44 000 households surveyed in 2008	FSS ascertains food security, food expenditures, and use of food and nutrition assistance programs	CPS–FSS is the source of USDA's annual reports on household food security and state-level statistics on food insecurity Link: http://www.ers.usda.gov/Data/foodsecurity/cps/
American Time Use Survey (ATUS)-Eating and Health (EH) Module of the CPS	DOL (BLS) conducts CPS Bureau of the Census administers CPS EH module sponsored by USDA/ERS and NIH/NCI	3 EH modules released (2006–2008)	Cross-sectional (national)	National sample of individuals in households	Individuals 15+ years sampled from CPS households	Data uses: relationships among time use patterns and eating patterns, nutrition, and obesity; food and nutrition assistance programs; grocery shopping and meal preparation Links: http://www.bls.gov/tus/ehdatafiles_2008.htm and http://www.bls.gov/tus/ehmquestionnaire.pdf
Food Safety Survey	HHS (FDA) and USDA (FSIS)	Periodic 2006 (1988)	Cross-sectional (national)	Individuals sampled from households with telephones in 50 states and DC	RDD sample of 2275 individuals ages 18+ years	Food handling, food allergies, food-borne illnesses, consumption of potentially unsafe foods Link: http://www.fda.gov/Food/ScienceResearch/ResearchAreas/ConsumerResearch/ucm080374.htm

Surveys of Nutrition Assistance Programs and Program Participants

Survey	Sponsor	Dates/Frequency	Design	Population	Sample	Content and Links
Studies of Special Supplemental Nutrition Program for Women Infants and Children (WIC) participants	USDA (FNS)	Biennial since 1992 (multiple studies)	Cross-sectional	Participants in WIC	Varies by survey	Breastfeeding, food consumption, infant feeding practices, program practices, WIC food package Link: http://www.fns.usda.gov/oral/menu/Published/WIC/WIC.htm
Studies of Child and Adult Care Food Program (CACFP)	USDA (FNS)	Child Care Food Program began in 1968; name changed in 1990	Day-care programs with CACFP	Children and adults receiving day-care services in CACFP	Children to age 18 years and adults	CACFP provides reimbursement to qualified caregivers for meals and supplements (snacks) served to participants Link: http://www.fns.usda.gov/cnd/care/default.htm

(Continued)

TABLE 64.1 (*Continued*)

Survey name	Federal department (agency)	Schedule (initial year)	Sample design (estimates)	US target group	Sample (size)	Survey content, measures, and link for further information
School Nutrition Dietary Assessment Survey (SNDA)	USDA (FNS)	Periodic (1991–1992) SNDA-III: 2004–2005 SNDA-IV: 2010	Cross-sectional (national)	Nationally representative samples of districts, schools, and students (SNDA-III) Nationally representative samples of districts and schools (SNDA-IV)	SNDA-III national sample: 2314 public school students in grades 1–12 from 287 sampled schools SNDA-IV: ~600 school food authorities and 900 schools primarily through mail and web-based surveys	Data: interviews, dietary recall (usual nutrient intake), measured height and weight, and information on foods served on school menus and competitive foods available in school Nutrient content of school meals compared with USDA standards. Students' diets assessed using the Dietary Reference Intakes Link: http://www.fns.usda.gov/ora/menu/Published/CNP/cnp.htm
Evaluation studies of nutrition programs for older Americans	HHS (AOA)	2011 (1993–1995)	Cross-sectional (national)	Adults ages 60 years and older in group or home settings	~2000 in-person interviews with program participants and nonparticipants; ~100 Areas Agencies on Aging	Funded under Titles III-C of the Older Americans Act. Outcomes include nutrient intake based on 24-hour dietary recalls, health outcomes from Medicare records, and costs per program meal Links: http://www.aoa.gov/aoaroot/aoa_programs/hcltc/nutrition_services/index.aspx#purpose, and http://www.aoa.gov/AoARoot/Program_results/Program_Evaluation.aspx

Household-Level Data Collection and Reports

Consumer Expenditure Survey (CES)	DOL	Every 10 years (pre-1980); Annual since 1984	Cross-sectional (national)	2 national samples of US households: Quarterly interview and weekly diary samples Multiple visits for all sampled households	Sample sizes: 3200 households/quarter for diary survey 15 000 households/quarter for interview survey	Households and family expenditures, income, and household characteristics. Separate questionnaires for diary and interview surveys Link: http://www.bls.gov/cex/

National Household Food Acquisition and Purchase Survey (FoodAPS)	USDA (ERS)	2012	Cross-sectional (national)	National sample of Supplemental Nutrition Assistance Program (SNAP) and non-SNAP low-income households and non-SNAP higher income households	Sample sizes: 5000 households (3500 low-income and 1500 higher income households)	Households' acquisition and purchase/expenditures of all foods and beverages acquired over a 7-day period for all household members, shopping behavior and dietary quality Link: http://www.ers.usda.gov/Briefing/DietQuality/food_aps.htm
Records-Based Systems						
Pediatric Nutrition Surveillance System (PedNSS)[a]	HHS (CDC/NCCDPHP)	Annual since 1973	Surveillance records	Sample: low-income children	2009 sample: 46 states, US territories, 6 tribal organizations, and DC. ~9 million children under 5 years of age participated	Existing WIC, Early and Periodic Screening, Diagnosis, and Treatment (EPSDT) Program; and Maternal and Child Health (MCH) program data used. Birth weight, stature, weight status, anemia, and breastfeeding Link: http://www.cdc.gov/pednss/what_is/pednss/index.htm
Pregnancy Nutrition Surveillance System (PNSS)[a]	HHS (CDC/NCCDPHP)	Annual since 1979	Surveillance records	Sample: low-income pregnant women	2008 sample: 1.3 million records from 30 states, DC, and 6 tribal organizations	Public health surveillance system; monitors risk factors associated with infant mortality and poor birth outcomes among low-income pregnant women who participate in federally funded public health programs including WIC and MCH programs Uses existing data from WIC and Title V MCH Program Link: http://www.cdc.gov/pednss/what_is/pnss/

(Continued)

TABLE 64.1 (Continued)

Survey name	Federal department (agency)	Schedule (initial year)	Sample design (estimates)	US target group	Sample (size)	Survey content, measures, and link for further information
National Vital Statistics System (NVSS)	HHS (CDC/NCHS)	Annual (1915)	Records	US population	States cooperate with NCHS and use standard reporting forms	Federal law mandates national collection and publication of births and other vital statistics such as deaths (including fetal), marriages, and divorces Link: http://www.cdc.gov/nchs/nvss/about_nvss.htm
NCHS Linked Mortality Files	HHS (CDC/NCHS)		Records linkage			NCHS linked several surveys with death certificate records from the National Death Index Link to list: http://www.cdc.gov/nchs/data_access/data_linkage/mortality.htm

aCDC plans to stop data collection of PedNSS and PNSS in 2011. Instead, data will be tracked in the studies of WIC participants by USDA (see WIC entry under "Surveys of Nutrition Assistance Programs and Program Participants).
AOA, Administration on Aging; ARS, Agricultural Research Service; BLS, Bureau of Labor Statistics; CB, Census Bureau; CDC, Centers for Disease Control and Prevention; CFSAN, Center for Food Safety and Nutrition; DOC, Department of Commerce; DoEd, Department of Education; DOL, Department of Labor; ERS, Economic Research Service; FDA, Food and Drug Administration; FNS, Food and Nutrition Service; FSIS, Food Safety Inspection Service; HHS, Department of Health and Human Services; HRSA, Health Resources and Services Administration; NCCDPHP, National Center for Chronic Disease Prevention and Health Promotion; NCHS, National Center for Health Statistics; NCI, National Cancer Institute; NCIRD, National Center for Immunization and Respiratory Diseases; NIH, National Institutes of Health; USDA, US Department of Agriculture.

TABLE 64.2 Food supply measures and technical databases that support national nutrition monitoring

Database name	Department (agency)	Data release (year)	Description
Food Supply and Food Environment Databases			
Food Supply and Availability and Nutrient Availability (per capita) in the US	USDA (ERS)	Food availability tracked since 1909; tabulated through 2008 Loss-adjusted results available since 1970	Three distinct but related data series: Food supply per capita by commodity groupings; raw and loss-adjusted results; and nutrient availability per capita. The data serve as proxies for actual/individual consumption Link: http://www.ers.usda.gov/Data/FoodConsumption/
Fisheries Disappearance Data	DOC (NMFS)	Annual since 1910	Records data on domestic and imported fish and shellfish adjusted for exports; edible weight (lb) reported. 2009 Annual Report: Fisheries of the United States includes per capita consumption data Link: http://www.st.nmfs.noaa.gov/st1/fus/fus09/index.html
Food Environment Atlas	USDA (ERS)	Released 2010	Provides a spatial overview of access to healthy foods in communities. Statistics on food environment indicators linked to food choices and diet quality such as store and restaurant proximity, food prices, food and nutrition assistance programs, and community characteristics Link: http://www.ers.usda.gov/foodatlas/
Food Composition			
National Nutrient Database for Standard Reference (NNDSR)	USDA (ARS/NDL)	Release 22 (SR22) released 9/2009; data on 7538 food items and up to 143 nutrients and food components	NNDSR consists of several relational database files. Food composition values are the basis for FNDDS files and numerous other US food composition databases and tables. Data are updated regularly Link: http://www.ars.usda.gov/Services/docs.htm?docid=8964
Food and Nutrient Database System for Dietary Studies (FNDDS)	USDA (ARS/FSRG)	FNDDS v.4.1 applied to NHANES 2007–2008 data	Series of data files including nutrient values for foods and gram weights for typical food portions. The NNDSR files are used to process and report dietary interview data from NHANES/WWEIA. The base nutrient values are from the NNDSR Link http://www.ars.usda.gov/Services/docs.htm?docid=12089
MyPyramid Equivalents Database (MPED)	USDA (ARS/FSRG)	2008 MPED version 2 applied to NHANES 2003–2004 (2006 MPED version 1 applied to 1994–2002 USDA survey food codes)	Contains ounce and cup equivalents data for foods included in the USDA food coding databases to allow linkages to dietary intake data and estimates of MyPyramid equivalents. MPED 2.0 includes the number of MyPyramid equivalents of each of the 32 major groups and subgroups that are present in 100g of foods in the FNDDS 2.0 and for all foods and food modifications reported eaten in WWEIA, NHANES 2003–2004 Links: http://www.ars.usda.gov/Services/docs.htm?docid=8498 and http://www.ars.usda.gov/Services/docs.htm?docid=17558 *(Continued)*

TABLE 64.2 (Continued)

Database name	Department (agency)	Data release (year)	Description
Total Diet Study	HHS (FDA)	Ongoing since 1961	Market basket study: ~280 foods are sampled from around the US, prepared for consumption, and chemically analyzed; levels of radioactive contaminants, pesticide residues, industrial chemicals, and toxic and nutrient elements are measured Link: http://www.fda.gov/Food/FoodSafety/FoodContaminantsAdulteration/TotalDietStudy/default.htm
Food Label and Package Survey	HHS (FDA)	2006–2007 (periodic since 1976–1978)	Representative sample of 1227 processed, packaged food products (labels) from the retail food supply drawn from 2005 Nielsen database of US food stores. Data are combined with Nielsen sales data to estimate products with nutrition labeling, health claims, and food safety statements Link: http://www.fda.gov/Food/LabelingNutrition/ConsumerInformation/ucm122084.htm
Dietary Supplement Products			
Dietary Supplements Ingredient Database (DSID)	USDA (ARS/NDL)	Release 1 (2009)	Estimated levels of 18 vitamin and mineral ingredients derived from analytical data for 115 representative unspecified adult multivitamin and multimineral supplement (MVM) products Link: http://dietarysupplementdatabase.usda.nih.gov/
Dietary Supplement Labels Database	HHS (NIH/NLM)	Data reflect 2005–2009 label information compiled for the Dietary Supplements On-Line Database (DSOL) (©2005–2009 by DeLima Associates)	Label ingredient information on more than 4000 brands of dietary supplements Link: http://dietarysupplements.nlm.nih.gov/dietary/
Food Safety			
FoodNet	HHS (CDC, FDA), USDA, and 10 Emerging Infections Program sites around the US participate	Website lists products by year	Principal foodborne disease component of CDC's Emerging Infections Program (EIP). FoodNet is a collaborative project of the CDC, ten EIP sites, USDA, and FDA. Annual reports, MMWR articles, and tables produced Link: http://www.cdc.gov/foodnet/
OutbreakNet	HHS (CDC)	1998–2007 posted online	Most of the data consists of outbreaks reported to the National Outbreak Reporting System (NORS) by the state, local, territorial, or tribal health department that conducted the outbreak investigation Link: http://wwwn.cdc.gov/foodborneoutbreaks/

ARS, Agricultural Research Service; CDC, Centers for Disease Control and Prevention; DOC, Department of Commerce; ERS, Economic Research Service; FDA, Food and Drug Administration; FSRG, Food Surveys Research Group; HHS, Department of Health and Human Services; MMWR, Morbidity and Mortality Weekly Report; NDL, National Data Laboratory; NIH, National Institutes of Health; NLM, National Library of Medicine; NMFS, National Marine Fisheries Service; USDA, US Department of Agriculture.

protein, carbohydrates, fats, vitamins, and minerals) in the US food supply. Other sources of annual US per capita food availability information include fish availability data reported by the National Marine Fisheries Service (since 1910), consisting of annual estimates of per capita consumption of fish and shellfish based on "disappearance" in the food distribution system.

Environmental Factors: Macro Level Information on the Distribution and Determinants of Food Choices and Diet Quality

A number of environmental factors affect the distribution and availability of foods in the neighborhoods where people live. Persons living in lower-income communities may experience food deserts, or areas that lack access to affordable and healthy foods such as fresh fruits and vegetables or low-fat milk (Beaulac *et al.*, 2009). The National Household Food Acquisition and Purchase Survey (FoodAPS) is a new 2012 data collection funded by USDA's Economic Research Service to assess households' food acquisition and expenditures, and diet quality among low-income and higher-income households (Table 64.1). Data collection will include 7-day food diaries of foods purchased, home scanners of foods purchased from retailers, and interviews about shopping behaviors, household income, and participation in nutrition assistance programs.

Previous research on food expenditures and food shopping have relied on the Consumer Expenditure Survey (CES) and the availability of proprietary databases. Monthly and annual proprietary sales data purchased from A.C. Nielsen Company (since 1985) measure grocery-store sales of all scannable packaged food products (NRC, 2005). Nielsen supermarket scanner data (SCANTRACK) do not reflect fruits and vegetables or prepared foods from supermarkets, restaurants, or other food outlets. Another source of household purchase information is Nielsen's Homescan Consumer Panel data. Consumers transmit data on scanned purchases, including fresh foods, weekly through a telephone line. A number of other proprietary databases include scanner data, food prices, and household purchases, but are limited in that they include only foods purchased at retail stores, and not foods purchased at restaurants (NRC, 2004, 2005). The FoodAPS is intended to address these limitations by collecting scanner data for foods purchased at retail stores and recording all foods obtained and purchased from all sources, including school meals and restaurants.

Food Security

Since 1995 a special yearly supplement to the Current Population Survey (CPS) conducted by the United States Census Bureau has been devoted to measuring the extent of food insecurity and hunger among people living in low-income households (Hamilton *et al.*, 1997). The 18-item food security measure has been included in NHANES, the CPS, and the School Nutrition Dietary Assessment (SNDA) studies. In 2005 a National Research Council panel recommended additional research to address measurement issues related to item nonresponse and food insecurity labels used to assess households and individuals (NRC, 2006; Nord and Hopwood, 2007).

Estimating Food and Nutrient Consumption of Individuals

NHANES is the only nationally representative survey that collects dietary recall and dietary supplement intake information on children and adults. Dietary data collection was expanded in 2002 when the NHANES and USDA CSFII survey programs were integrated. Two dietary recalls are collected on all NHANES survey participants using in-person (Day 1) and telephone-interview (Day 2) modes (Murphy, 2003; Raper *et al.*, 2004). The USDA automated multiple-pass method (AMPM) and dietary interview system and USDA Survey Nutrient Databases used to collect and process NHANES dietary recall data were integrated into the 2002 NHANES (Dwyer *et al.*, 2003a,b; Moshfegh *et al.*, 2008). The NHANES diet and supplement intakes are related to health status in the same individuals, with emphasis on ethnic/racial determinants of health (Briefel, 2007).

Evaluations of USDA's nutrition and food assistance programs are also routinely conducted and provide information on the dietary intakes and nutrition and health behaviors of program participants, often low-income and/or disadvantaged populations (Logan *et al.*, 2002; Fox *et al.*, 2004) (Table 64.1). A series of studies have been conducted to evaluate the nutrition and health effects of participating in WIC and to provide current participant and program characteristics of the WIC program. The SNDA first assessed the diets of American schoolchildren and the contribution of the National School Lunch

Program to overall nutrient intake in 1992. The third study in 2005 measured schoolchildren's heights and weights, usual nutrient intake, and mean food intake, and collected information on school food service operations, the quality of meals offered, and foods and beverages available in vending machines, school stores and à la carte lines. Data from the SNDA studies have been instrumental in addressing changes to school meal regulations to increase dietary quality and reduce excess calories in light of childhood obesity (Institute of Medicine, 2005).

In addition to the national survey programs, periodic assessments of food and nutrient consumption of specific subgroups of the population not adequately covered in national surveys have been conducted for military populations, American Indians, children, low-income populations, and pregnant and lactating women. FDA's Infant Feeding Practices Survey II assesses the diets of pregnant women and new mothers and their infant feeding practices (Table 64.1).

Food Intake and Nutrients from Foods and Dietary Supplements

USDA/ARS, CDC/NCHS and many other groups report trends in mean and usual intakes of nutrients from foods, and total intakes from foods and dietary supplements (Dwyer *et al.*, 2003a,b; Murphy, 2003; Woteki, 2003; Briefel and Johnson, 2004; Bailey *et al.*, 2010). Results are used to examine the food and nutrient intakes of the non-breastfeeding general population and subgroups of the population as it relates to various socioeconomic factors (Logan *et al.*, 2002; Woteki, 2003). Improved statistical-analysis methodologies to estimate total usual food and nutrient intakes are readily accessible to NHANES data users, thus improving the quality and completeness of nutrient intake estimates (Carriquiry, 2003; Tooze *et al.*, 2006).

NHANES dietary results are also linked to other federal food and nutrition surveillance and reporting systems including the Food and Drug Administration's (FDA's) Total Diet Study, the Environmental Protection Agency's pesticides and environmental toxicants databases, and USDA's commodity databases (Table 64.2). Survey data linkages such as these illustrate the vital role that health and nutrition data play in health monitoring and surveillance. For example, national dietary data were used to estimate food exposure to pesticides and mercury (EPA, 1997; CDC, 2009).

Food Composition Databases Used to Estimate Nutrient Intakes from Foods

Since 1892, USDA has operated the National Nutrient Database for Standard Reference (NNDSR) for the purpose of deriving representative nutrient values for more than 6000 foods and up to 80 components consumed in the United States (Table 64.2). Data are obtained from the food industry, from USDA-initiated analytical contracts, and from the scientific literature, and are updated to reflect changes in the food supply as well as changes in analytical methodology (Dwyer *et al.*, 2003c). These values are used as the core of most nutrient databases developed in the United States for special purposes, such as those employed in the commercially available dietary analysis programs. USDA produces the Food and Nutrient Database for Dietary Studies, which contains data for energy and 60 nutrients/components for each food item for analysis of NHANES – What We Eat in America. A system is in place at USDA to periodically update this database with the most current information available from the National Nutrient Database (NNDB) and to retroactively apply revised or new food composition data to earlier food composition databases for tracking nutrient consumption patterns (Anderson *et al.*, 2001; Ahuja *et al.*, 2006). USDA also releases special interest databases (e.g. fluoride and choline).

FDA's Total Diet Study provides annual food composition analysis based on the foods consumed most frequently in NHANES. Representative foods are collected from retail markets, prepared for consumption, and analyzed individually for nutrients and other food components at the Total Diet Laboratory to estimate consumption of selected nutrients (e.g. folate) and organic and elemental contaminants such as pesticide residues. The Food Label and Package Survey is conducted to monitor labeling practices of US food manufacturers. The survey also includes a surveillance program to identify levels of accuracy of selected nutrient declarations compared with values obtained from nutrient analyses of products.

Dietary Supplement Composition Databases (Label and Analytical)

The National Institutes of Health Office of Dietary Supplements, USDA, and NCHS collaborate to support the development and maintenance of a dietary supplements food composition database (Dwyer *et al.*, 2003c). The Dietary Supplements Labels Database of the National

Library of Medicine is based on the Dietary Supplements On-Line Database ©2005–2009 by DeLima Associates. The database contains information on the ingredients of over 4000 products of dietary supplements sold in the United States; information in the database obtained from publicly available sources including product-specific labels and information from manufacturers' websites.

The USDA/ARS Nutrient Data Laboratory (NDL) worked with the HHS/NIH, Office of Dietary Supplements and other federal agencies to develop the Dietary Supplement Ingredient Databases (DSID) (see Chapter 73). DSID-1 provides information on analyzed levels of nutrients in adult multivitamin/minerals (MVMs). The DSID is intended primarily for research applications. Product data are grouped by nutrient levels rather than by product names. Statistical regression methods were used to estimate mean percent differences from label values and variability at specific nutrient levels for each of the eight vitamins and ten minerals analyzed. DSID data are appropriate for conducting population studies of nutrient intake, rather than for assessing individual products.

Assessing Nutrition and Diet Knowledge, Attitudes, and Behavior

National and state surveys that measure knowledge, attitudes, and behavior about diet and nutrition and how these relate to health were added to the nutrition monitoring program in the early 1980s and have expanded in scope and number over time. Surveys have addressed specific topics such as shopping behaviors, weight-loss practices, diet and health knowledge, infant feeding practices, food handling practices, and progress toward achieving nutrition-related national health objectives.

Consumer Behaviors

New surveys of consumer knowledge and behaviors conducted and/or funded by the USDA include the 2005–2010 Flexible Consumer Behavior Survey as an NHANES component and the FoodAPS (Table 64.1). The Flexible Consumer Behavior Survey collects information on household economics (e.g. income, nutrition program participation), the types of foods available at home, the frequency of eating away from home, and behaviors (e.g. food-label reading, grocery shopping practices). The FoodAPS study will collect information on consumers' shopping behaviors and eating away from home.

Adult Behaviors

The NHANES collects information on adults' health and nutrition behaviors including dietary supplement use, weight-loss practices, physical activity, breastfeeding, and smoking. Accelerometers were introduced to measure physical activity in the 2003–2004 NHANES (Tudor-Locke et al., 2010). The focus of the BRFSS, initiated in 1984 as a telephone survey of adults, is on personal health practices such as intake, physical activity, weight control practices, and health screening practices (Table 64.1). BRFSS data have been used by state health departments to plan, initiate, and guide health promotion and disease prevention programs, and to monitor their progress over time. BRFSS collects self-reported height and weight for estimates of overweight and obesity and includes optional modules on dietary habits that states can collect periodically. Topics include the consumption of fruits and vegetables and high fat and cholesterol foods, binge drinking, physical activity, and the use of supplements, particularly folic acid. In 2002, BRFSS data began to be used for prevalence estimates for metropolitan and micropolitan statistical areas, allowing CDC to make estimates for counties to assist local public health planners and program evaluators. In general, the focus of FDA's Health and Diet Survey is on people's awareness of relationships between diet and risk for chronic disease and on health-related knowledge and attitudes. The survey has studied consumer use of food labels, weight-loss practices, and the effectiveness of the National Cholesterol Education Program.

Youth Behaviors

The NHANES collects information on children's breast-feeding, infant-feeding practices, dietary intake, supplement use, weight-loss practices, physical activity, and smoking (Woteki, 2003; Briefel, 2007). In addition to answering survey questions about physical activity levels, respondents wore physical activity monitors in NHANES in 2003–2006. These monitors improved physical activity measurement, which has relied in the past on self-report or parental reports for children. The Youth Risk Behavior Surveillance System (YRBSS) includes national school-based surveys of high-school students as well as state, territorial and local school-based surveys conducted by health and education agencies. Information is collected on students' health risk behaviors that include smoking, dietary intake, weight-loss practices, and physical activity. Every two years, CDC conducts a national survey to produce data representative of students in grades 9–12 in the 50 states and the District of Columbia.

Maternal and Infant Health

CDC's Pregnancy Risk Assessment Monitoring System is used by 29 states to monitor selected maternal attitudes, behaviors, and experiences related to adverse maternal and infant outcomes. The second Infant Feeding Practices Survey assessed the diets of pregnant and new mothers and tracked breastfeeding and other infant-feeding practices. Information on breastfeeding is collected in several other studies, including the NHANES, the National Survey of Family Growth (NSFG), the National Immunization Survey (NIS), and state surveillance systems, the Pregnancy Nutrition Surveillance System and the Pediatric Nutrition Surveillance System (Table 64.1).

Food Safety

The FDA conducted a study to assess consumer food handling practices and awareness of microbiological hazards, and several studies to evaluate the Nutrition Facts Label features and usability by consumers (Table 64.1). The Food Safety Survey tracks consumers' knowledge, behaviors, and perceptions about food safety and consumption of potentially risky foods. FoodNet is a cooperative surveillance effort between CDC's Emerging Infections Program, FDA, and the Food Safety and Inspection Service, USDA, to monitor food-borne illness and to conduct epidemiologic research on illnesses attributable to food-borne pathogens (Table 64.2). FoodNet includes laboratory analysis and surveys of physicians and the population. Twelve-month cycles of the population survey are conducted to assess diarrheal disease and exposure.

Assessing the Nutritional Status and Health of the US Population

Nutrition and related health data support a wide variety of policy, research, health and nutrition education, and health care utilization and evaluation activities. Population and records-based surveys conducted by the CDC are used to assess population trends and to assess the health and nutritional status of individuals and population groups (Table 64.1). In addition to providing national population reference data obtained using health interview and examination methods, NHANES results are used to monitor national prevalence rates of diseases and risk factors, and trends in nutritional and health status over time. NHANES follow-up studies have explored the relationships of nutri-

tion and health to risk of death and disability. The continuous NHANES, which began in 1999, has a continuous, annual sample design. The design includes oversampling of Hispanics, African-Americans, older adults, and low-income white persons. Beginning in 2011, Asians are oversampled to produce reliable estimates for this growing population subgroup and for comparisons of health status and risk factors between race/ethnicity groups.

The National Health Interview Survey provides information about self-reported height, weight, and health conditions annually and about special nutrition and health topics periodically, such as vitamin/mineral supplement usage, youth risk behavior, aging, food program participation, diet and nutrition knowledge, cancer, and disability and food preparation (Table 64.1). Other special supplements relate to tracking progress in meeting national health objectives. Large sample sizes enable data to be reported for the major racial/ethnic subgroups in the US population in addition to age group, gender, and income level.

The State and Local Area Integrated Telephone Survey (SLAITS) was developed to supplement national data with state and regional data. SLAITS uses a telephone methodology and draws its sample from the same frame as the NIS. Previous topics included a national study on early childhood health in 2007 (Blumberg *et al.*, 2009).

A number of surveillance systems, primarily conducted by CDC, also contribute nutrition-related health information (height, weight, hemoglobin, and hematocrit), particularly for low-income pregnant women, infants, and children who participate in publicly funded health, nutrition, and food-assistance programs in participating states (Table 64.1). The Pregnancy Nutrition Surveillance System monitored nutrition-related problems and behavioral risk factors associated with low birth weight in high-risk prenatal populations, primarily drawn from the WIC program. The Pediatric Nutrition Surveillance System monitored key indicators of nutritional status in low-income infants and children. Information on anemia, weight status, birth weight, breastfeeding, and TV/video watching are collected primarily on children in the WIC program.

The National Center for Health Statistics conducts a number of records surveys, including tracking deaths due to nutrition-related conditions (Table 64.1). The National Survey of Family Growth collects information on subjects relating to maternal and child health such as breastfeeding and prenatal care. The surveys and surveillance systems that continuously collect nutrition and health measurements are important for monitoring trends over time, for tracking progress toward achieving national health objectives, and for generating reference distributions.

Data Availability

NNMRRP data are available in several formats. Many survey datasets and technical databases are posted on federal agency websites. Additionally, detailed survey documentation, brief reports and data tabulations, statistical guidelines, data analysis tutorials and guidelines, and questionnaires are also available online. Data users can subscribe to agency listservs to receive updates pertaining to data releases, stakeholder meetings, and data users' conferences. Articles published in the peer-reviewed literature are often cited in PubMed and can be located using search terms that identify the data source(s) of interest. The websites for the major surveys and surveillance systems have been included as references in this publication. A catalogue of existing surveillance systems that provide data relevant to childhood obesity research was established in 2001 by a collaborative led by the Robert Wood Johnson Foundation with CDC, the National Institutes of Health, and USDA (National Collaborative on Childhood Obesity Research, 2011).

Statistical Analysis Tools for Researchers

The internet postings for many survey programs include working papers on survey design and methodology, statistical guidelines and software recommendations for data analysis, and sample programs and tutorials to assist data users with data analysis planning, data file access, statistical analysis program data review and recoding, and more. A comprehensive web-based tutorial for NHANES surveys, including a separate dietary data analysis tutorial developed jointly by the National Cancer Institute (NCI), NCHS, and the USDA's, Agricultural Research Service, is available at CDC's website (http://www.cdc.gov/nchs/tutorials/Nhanes/). Additional information on dietary intake and physical activity measurement can be found on NCI's website (http://riskfactor.cancer.gov/studies/nhanes/).

Future Directions

A focused, comprehensive, nutrition-monitoring program includes improving methodologies for the collection and interpretation of data, timely processing and release of data, expanding coverage of population subgroups, and

conducting research to address current nutrition and public health issues. In the early 1990s the US President's Science Advisor identified the need for human nutrition research "that is ultimately aimed at promoting health, preventing disease, and reducing health care costs" (Office of Science Technology and Policy, 1996). To meet the expanding needs of the monitoring program, current nutrition monitoring research is aimed at (1) improving data collection, including population coverage and the use of technology; (2) the assessment of nutritional status using anthropometric, dietary, and laboratory approaches and biomarkers of diet and nutritional status; (3) understanding the behavioral and economic aspects of diet and health; and (4) conducting food composition analysis. Future directions are summarized below.

Population Subgroup Coverage

Many surveys of NNMRRP are designed to collect data on various subgroups of the population, such as low-income persons and minorities; however, data are still limited for select subgroups of the population such as the homeless and Native Americans. Special subnational studies are the most economical way to cover these and other minority groups. Research is also needed on appropriate methods (such as questionnaires, interviewing procedures, physical measures, and biological indicators) for subgroups at increased nutritional risk.

State and Local Monitoring

In addition to expanded coverage of population subgroups, improved geographic coverage is needed to provide nutrition data at state and local levels. National surveys provide data representative of the United States and major geographic regions, but cannot also provide data representative of states, counties, and cities. The CDC surveillance systems provide data for participating states that are complementary to national data, but there is increasing interest in collecting state and local data to address local health and welfare concerns. In 2004, the New York City Department of Health and Mental Hygiene conducted the New York City HANES with technical assistance from CDC (New York City Department of Health and Mental Hygiene, n.d.). National methods were adapted for use in a smaller scale examination. About 2000 New Yorkers were sampled to receive a health examination to estimate the prevalence of overweight, diabetes, high blood pressure, and high serum cholesterol; and exposure to tobacco, pesticides, and heavy metals; they were also interviewed to assess depression and risky behaviors. Statistics are accessible on the NYC HANES website.

Use of Technology

Researchers have been investigating the use of alternative data collection methods to augment in-person and telephone interviews. For example, an automated self-administered 24-hour dietary recall (ASA24™), adapted from the AMPM method used to collect dietary recalls in NHANES, was developed by the National Cancer Institute and made available to researchers and clinicians for public use (Subar *et al.*, 2007, 2010). Surveys such as NHANES have incorporated the use of self-administered computerized instruments for sensitive topics and adolescents. Research efforts should focus on the identification and development of methods and the utilization of computer technology that will enhance the monitoring of the nutritional status of the US population and support the timely interpretation and release of information to users. Improvements in standardizing data collection and analysis techniques to estimate total nutrient intake and usual food consumption have led to the NHANES tutorials and publications to inform researchers about issues in measuring diet at the population level (Carriquiry, 2003; Tooze *et al.*, 2006) and the use of available databases, e.g. MyPyramid equivalents database (see Table 64.2).

State and local monitoring systems should also take advantage of new technology for electronic data transfer. BRFSS is exploring the possibility of using web-based data collection in future surveys that would take advantage of technology and access to the Intranet. However, accommodations will still be needed to assess at-risk groups with no telephone or Intranet access.

Biomarkers

The development and applied use of biomarkers in surveys such as NHANES that collect biological samples (i.e. blood, urine, saliva, and hair) are an important research area for nutrition monitoring. Biomarkers are substances within individuals or tissue samples that can be related to exposure, susceptibility to disease, or health outcomes (NRC, 2008). Biochemical measures of long-term exposure or nutritional status are not subject to the same inaccuracies or bias as the reporting of long-term dietary intake, but the sensitivity and specificity of biomarkers need to be evaluated for their role in assessing exposure to foods and nutrients, and for identifying high-risk popula-

tion groups. For example, following the recommendations of an IOM panel on strategies to reduce sodium intake in the US, plans are underway to incorporate urinary sodium measures in future NHANES (Institute of Medicine, 2010a). Further research to develop better biological indicators of nutritional status and dietary intake as a means of studying nutrition and health is needed to maximize the usefulness of NNMRRP data for nutrition policy making. The ongoing evaluation of standards and laboratory methods is also important to interpret time trends (Yetley *et al.*, 2011).

Behavioral and Economic Aspects of Diet and Health

Research to develop and standardize questionnaires for valid and reliable estimators of knowledge, attitudes, and behavior will aid in the development of public health strategies at federal, state, and local levels to improve dietary status, promote health, and prevent nutrition-related disease. Adding questions on dietary or health behaviors to surveys designed to link socioeconomic factors can augment information on diet and health relationships. For example, the American Time Use Survey draws its sample from the CPS: respondents complete a time diary and report their height and weight. A food and eating module includes information on time spent snacking, TV watching, food shopping, and preparing food.

Nutrition Monitoring in Other Countries

Nutrition surveillance activities in developing and developed countries include the use of food balance sheets, household budget surveys, individual surveys of dietary intake, consumer expenditure surveys, and periodic assessments of the nutrition and health status of individuals in the population (World Health Organization, 2011b). Food balance sheets are commonly used for surveillance in developing countries since they are more available and less costly than other surveillance methods. In developed countries monitoring often includes nutritional status measures and biomonitoring of environmental chemicals and toxicants such as blood lead (Board on Environmental Studies and Toxicology, 2006). In addition to NHANES in the United States, biomedical samples have been included in nutrition and health surveys conducted in Australia, Canada, the United Kingdom, and New Zealand (Department of Health and Ageing, 2011). For example, the United Kingdom has collected weighed food records for dietary intake estimates, and blood and urine specimens, blood pressure, and anthropometric measures for the assessment of nutritional and health status. In 2001, the UK Expenditure and Food Survey was initiated in order to improve estimates of food eaten away from home, and improved the method used for dietary exposure in the National Food Survey (Rimmer, 2001). School nutrition policies have also been studied using similar methods to those used in the SNDA studies in the United States (Nelson et al., 2004).

Comparisons of data across countries have been facilitated by standardizing definitions of nutrition indicators and outcomes. Examples of worldwide monitoring of nutrition outcomes include the World Health Organization (WHO) body mass index database (WHO, 2011a), and the Food and Agriculture Organization (FAO) of the United Nations' assessment of food insecurity as a follow-up activity to the World Food Summit in 1996 (FAO, 2004).

Nutrition topics of international concern include micronutrient deficiencies (most notably iodine, vitamin A, folic acid, and iron), child growth and malnutrition, breastfeeding, and obesity and chronic disease prevention. The WHO provides technical and financial support to member states for developing, strengthening, and implementing their national nutrition plans of action (WHO, 2011a,b). Federal agencies in the US also provide technical consultation on nutrition survey data collection methodologies and interpretation of data to assist other countries' nutrition monitoring and surveillance efforts. For example, CDC provides support for preventing micronutrient deficiencies worldwide (CDC, 2011), and ARS/USDA has shared the dietary intake data collection method with Canada for use in the Community Health Survey. The NHANES staff have provided expert consultation on health and nutrition measures to health officials in New Zealand, Australia, Korea, Canada, and the European Union (CDC, 2009). These collaborations foster the standardization of data across countries and serve as an important avenue for the exchange of data and ideas internationally.

Public Health Implications

The primary goal of the *Ten-Year Comprehensive Plan* put forth in the early 1990s – to establish a comprehensive nutrition monitoring and related research program by collecting quality data that are continuous, coordinated, timely, and reliable, using comparable methods for data collection and reporting of results; conducting relevant research; and efficiently and effectively disseminating and exchanging information with data users – is still pertinent more than 20 years later. Given competing demands for limited national resources and resulting budget limitations, the goals for the NNMRRP will continue to be evaluated against other competing national needs at specific points in time. Efforts and resources are critical in order to continue progress and research to expand and strengthen the nutrition monitoring program in the United States in an efficient manner.

Nutrition monitoring data are needed to track progress in meeting the prevention agenda for the nation and addressing the obesity epidemic (Institute of Medicine, 2005). The nutrition monitoring program must be positioned to answer the major research and policy questions that are relevant in the 21st century: the relationship of diet and health habits (including physical activity) to the increasing prevalence of overweight and obesity; the chronic disease burden and disparities of health across racial–ethnic and socioeconomic groups; food security during an economic recession; consumer behavior; food safety especially for vulnerable groups (children, aging, and immune-compromised persons); nutrient–gene interactions; and biomarkers of nutrition and health status. The ability to meet the policy needs of the future will depend on research and the availability of reliable, current, national nutrition data.

Suggestions for Further Reading

Briefel, R.R. (2007) The changing consumption patterns and health and nutritional status in the United States: evidence from national surveys. In E. Kennedy and R. Deckelbaum (eds), *The Nation's Nutrition*. ILSI Press, Washington, DC, pp. 11–27.

Briefel, R.R. and Bialostosky, K. (2008) Interpretation and use of data from the National Nutrition Monitoring and Related Research Program. In E.R. Monsen and L. Van Horn (eds), *Research: Successful Approaches*, 3rd Edn. American Dietetic Association, Chicago, Chapter 10.

National Research Council (2005) Panel on Enhancing the Data Infrastructure in Support of Food and Nutrition Programs, Research, and Decision Making. Committee on National Statistics, Division of Behavioral and Social Sciences and Education.

Improving Data to Analyze Food and Nutrition Policies. National Academies Press. Washington, DC. National Research Council (2008) Committee on Advances in Collecting and Utilizing Biological Indicators and Genetic Information in Social Science Surveys. In M. Weinstein, J.W. Vaupel, and K.W. Wachter (eds), *Biosocial Surveys.* National Academies Press. Washington, DC.

Saelens, B.E. and Glanz, K. (2009) Work group I: Measures of the food and physical activity environment: instruments. *Am J Prev Med* **36**(4 Suppl), S166–170.

References

Ahuja, J., Goldman, J., and Perloff, B. (2006) The effect of improved food composition data on intake estimates in the United States of America. *J Food Comp Anal* **19**, S7–S13.

Anderson, E., Perloff, B., Ahuja, J.K.C., *et al.* (2001) Tracking nutrient changes for trends analysis in the United States. *J Food Comp Anal* **13**, 287–294.

Bailey, R., McDowell, M.A., Dodd, K.W., *et al.* (2010) Total folate and folic acid from foods and dietary supplements of US children aged 1–13 y. *Am J Clin Nutr* **92**, 353–358.

Beaulac, J., Kristjansson, E., and Cummins, S. (2009) A systematic review of food deserts, 1966–2007. *Prev Chronic Dis* **6**, A105.

Blumberg, S.J., Foster, E.B., Frasier, A.M., *et al.* (2009) Design and operation of the National Survey of Children's Health, 2007. National Center for Health Statistics, *Vital Health Stat* 1. <ftp://ftp.cdc.gov/pub/Health_Statistics/NCHS/slaits/nsch07/2_Methodology_Report/NSCH_Design_and_Operations_052109.pdf>

Board on Environmental Studies and Toxicology (2006) US and international biomonitoring efforts. *Human Biomonitoring for Environmental Chemicals.* National Academies Press, Washington, DC, Chapter 2

Briefel, R.R. (2006) Nutrition monitoring in the United States. In B. Bowman and R. Russell (eds), *Present Knowledge in Nutrition*, 9th Edn. ILSI Press, Washington, DC, pp. 838–858.

Briefel, R.R. (2007) The changing consumption patterns and health and nutritional status in the United States: evidence from national surveys. In E. Kennedy and R. Deckelbaum (eds), *The Nation's Nutrition.* ILSI Press, Washington, DC, pp. 11–27.

Briefel, R.R. and Bialostosky, K. (2008) Interpretation and use of data from the National Nutrition Monitoring and Related Research Program. In E.R. Monsen and L. Van Horn (eds), *Research: Successful Approaches*, 3rd Edn. American Dietetic Association, Chicago, Chapter 10.

Briefel, R.R. and Johnson, C.L. (2004) Secular trends in dietary intake in the United States. *Ann Rev Nutr* **24**, 401–431.

Brownson, R., Hoehner, C., Day, K., *et al.* (2009) Measuring the built environment for physical activity: state of the science. *Am J Prev Med* **36**, S99–S123.

Carlson, A., Lino, M., and Fungwe, T. (2007a) *The Low-cost, Moderate-cost, and Liberal Food Plans, 2007* (CNPP-20). US Department of Agriculture, Center for Nutrition Policy and Promotion, Alexandria, VA.

Carlson, A., Lino, M., Juan, W., *et al.* (2007b) *Thrifty Food Plan, 2006.* Center for Nutrition Policy and Promotion, US Department of Agriculture, Alexandria, VA.

Carriquiry, A.L. (2003) Estimation of usual intake distributions of nutrients and foods, *J Nutr* **133**, 601S–8S.

Centers for Disease Control and Prevention (2000) Folate status in women of childbearing age – United States, 1999, *Morb Mortal Wkly Rep* **49**, 962–925.

Centers for Disease Control and Prevention (2008) *5 A Day*, Centers for Disease Control and Prevention, Atlanta, GA. http://www.cdc.gov/nccdphp/dnpa/5aday/.

Centers for Disease Control and Prevention (2009) Report of the NHANES Review Panel to the NCHS Board of Scientific Counselors. http://www.cdc.gov/nchs/data/bsc/NHANES ReviewPanelReportrapril09.pdf.

Centers for Disease Control and Prevention (2010) The Social-Ecological Model: A Framework for Prevention http://www.cdc.gov/ncipc/dvp/social-ecological-model_dvp.htm.

Centers for Disease Control and Prevention (2011) IMMPaCT. International micronutrient malnutrition prevention and control program: projects and tools: CDCynergy for micronutrients. http://www.cdc.gov/immpact/.

Department of Health and Ageing (2011) National monitoring in public health nutrition, viewed 1 June 2011, http://www.health.gov.au/nutritionmonitoring.

Dodd, A.H., Colby, M., Boyd, K., *et al.* (2009) Treatment approach and HbA1c control among US adults with type 2 diabetes, NHANES 1999–2004, *Curr Med Res Opin* **25**, 1605–1613.

Dwyer, J., Picciano, M., and Raiten, D. (2003a) Future directions for the integrated CSFII-NHANES: What We Eat In America-NHANES, *J Nutr* **133**, 576S–581S.

Dwyer, J., Picciano, M.F., Raiten, D.J., *et al.* (2003b) Collection of food and dietary supplement intake data: What We Eat In America – NHANES, *J Nutr* **133**, 590S–600S.

Dwyer, J., Picciano, M.F., Raiten, D.J., *et al.* (2003c) Estimation of usual intakes: What We Eat In America – NHANES. *J Nutr* **133**, 609S–623S.

Dwyer, J., Picciano, M.F., Raiten, D.J., *et al.* (2003d) Food and dietary supplement databases for What We Eat In America-NHANES. *J Nutr* **133**, 624S–634S.

Environmental Protection Agency, Office of Air Quality Planning and Standards and Office of Research and Development (1997) *Mercury study report to Congress, EPA-452/R-97-003*, Environmental Protection Agency, Washington, DC.

Food and Agriculture Organization (2004) *Monitoring progress towards the World Food Summit and millennium development goals*. The state of food security in the world.: Food and Agriculture Organization, Rome. <http://www.fao.org/docrep/007/y5650e/y5650e00.htm>.

Fox, M.K., Hamilton, W., and Lin, B.-H. (2004) Effects of food assistance and nutrition programs on nutrition and health. Food Assistance and Nutrition Research Report No. 19-4. Economic Research Service, US Department of Agriculture, Washington, DC.

French, S.A., Story, M., and Jeffery, R.W. (2001) Environmental influences on eating and physical activity, *Annu Rev Public Health* **22**, 309–335.

Glanz, K., Sallis, J.F., Saelens, B.E., et al. (2005) Healthy nutrition environments: concepts and measures. *Am J Health Prom* **19**, 330–333.

Hamilton, W.L., Cook, J.T., Thompson, W.W., et al. (1997) *Household food security in the United States in 1995: summary report of the Food Security Measurement Project*. US Department of Agriculture, Food and Consumer Service, Alexandria, VA.

Heimbach, J.T. (2001) Using the National Nutrition Monitoring System to profile dietary supplement use. *J Nutr* **131**, 1335S–1338S.

Institute of Medicine (2000) *Dietary Reference Intakes: Applications in Dietary Assessment*. National Academy Press, Washington, DC.

Institute of Medicine (2005) *Preventing Childhood Obesity: Health in the Balance*. National Academies Press, Washington, DC.

Institute of Medicine (2010a) *Strategies to Reduce Sodium Intake in the United States, A Report of the Committee on Strategies to Reduce Sodium Intake*. National Academies Press, Washington, DC.

Institute of Medicine (2010b) *Dietary Reference Intakes for Vitamin D and Calcium*. Institute of Medicine, Washington, DC. <http://www.iom.edu/Activities/Nutrition/DRIVitDCalcium.aspx>.

Interagency Board for Nutrition Monitoring and Related Research (2000) *Nutrition Monitoring in the United States: The Directory of Federal and State Nutrition Monitoring and Related Research Activities* National Center for Health Statistics, Hyattsville, MD.

Kuczmarski, R.J., Ogden, C.L., Grummer-Strawn, L.M., et al. (2000) CDC growth charts: United States. *Adv Data* No. 314.

Lewis, C.J., Crane, N.T., Wilson, D.B., et al. (1999) Estimated folate intakes: data updated to reflect food fortification, increased bioavailability, and dietary supplement use. *Am J Clin Nutr* **70**, 198–207.

Life Sciences Research Office, Federation of American Societies for Experimental Biology (1995) *Third Report on Nutrition Monitoring in the United States*, vols 1 and 2. US Government Printing Office, Washington, DC.

Logan, C., Fox, M.K., and Lin, B.-H. (2002) Effects of food assistance and nutrition programs on nutrition and health, vol. 2, Food Assistance and Nutrition Research Report No. 19-2. US Department of Agriculture, Washington, DC.

Mason, J.B., Habicht, J.P., Tabatabai, H., et al. (1984) *Nutritional Surveillance*. WHO, Geneva.

McKinnon, R.A., Reedy, J., Morrissette, M.A., et al. (2009) Measures of the food environment: a compilation of the literature, 1990–2007. *Am J Prev Med* **36**, S124–133.

Moshfegh, A.J., Rhodes, D.G., Baer, D.J., et al. (2008) The US Department of Agriculture automated multiple-pass method reduces bias in the collection of energy intakes. *Am J Clin Nutr* **88**, 324–332.

Murphy, S.P. (2003) Collection and analysis of intake data from the integrated survey. *J Nutr* **133**, 585S–589S.

National Cholesterol Education Program (2002) Expert Panel on Detection, Evaluation, and Treatment of High Blood Cholesterol in Adults (Adult Treatment Panel III) Third Report of the National Cholesterol Education Program (NCEP) Expert Panel on Detection, Evaluation, and Treatment of High Blood Cholesterol in Adults (Adult Treatment Panel III). *Circulation*, vol. **106**, no. 25, pp. 3143–421.

National Collaborative on Childhood Obesity Research (2012) Catalogue of surveillance systems. <http://www.nccor.org/css.html>.

National Heart, Lung, and Blood Institute (2004) Seventh Report of the Joint National Committee on Prevention, Detection, Evaluation, and Treatment of High Blood Pressure (JNC 7). HHS Publication No. 04-5230, US Department of Health and Human Services, Washington, DC.

National Research Council, Committee on National Statistics (2004) In J. Casey and J.K. Scholz (eds), *Summary of Workshop on Food and Nutrition Data Needs*. National Academy Press, Washington, DC.

National Research Council Panel on Enhancing the Data Infrastructure in Support of Food and Nutrition Programs, Research, and Decision Making, Committee on National Statistics, Division of Behavioral and Social Sciences and Education (2005) *Improving Data to Analyze Food and Nutrition Policies*. National Academies Press, Washington, DC.

National Research Council, Committee on National Statistics, Panel to Review the US Department of Agriculture's Measurement of Food Insecurity and Hunger (2006) *Food*

Insecurity and Hunger in the United States: an Assessment of the Measure. National Academies Press, Washington, DC.

National Research Council, Committee on Advances in Collecting and Utilizing Biological Indicators and Genetic Information in Social Science Surveys (2008) In M. Weinstein, J.W. Vaupel, and K.W. Wachter (eds), *Biosocial Surveys.* The National Academies Press, Washington, DC.

Nelson, M., Bradbury, J., Poulter, J., *et al.* (2004) *School Meals in Secondary Schools in England.* Research Report 557. Department for Education and Skills, London.

New York City Department of Health and Mental Hygiene n.d., *New York City Health and Nutrition Examination Survey (NYC HANES)*, New York City Department of Health and Mental Hygiene, New York. <http://www.nyc.gov/html/doh/html/hanes/hanes.shtml>.

Nord, M. and Hopwood, H. (2007) Recent advances provide improved tools for measuring children's food security. *J Nutr* **137,** 533–536.

Office of Science and Technology Policy, Executive Office of the President (1996) *Meeting the Challenge: a Research Agenda for America's Health, Safety, and Food.* US Government Printing Office, Washington, DC.

Raper, N., Perloff, B., Ingwersen, L., *et al.* (2004) An overview of USDA's dietary intake data system, *J Food Comp Anal* **17,** 545–555.

Rimmer, D.J. (2001) An overview of food eaten outside the home in the United Kingdom National Food Survey and the new Expenditure and Food Survey. *Public Health Nutr* **4,** 1173–1175.

Subar, A.F., Crafts, J., Zimmerman, T.P., *et al.* (2010) Assessment of the accuracy of portion size reports using computer-based food photographs aids in the development of an automated self-administered 24-hour recall. *J Am Diet Assoc* **110,** 55–64.

Subar, A.F., Thompson, F.E., Potischman, N., *et al.* (2007) Formative research of a quick list for an automated self-administered 24-hour dietary recall. *J Am Diet Assoc* **107,** 1002–1007

Tooze, J.A., Midthune, D., Dodd, K.W., *et al.* (2006) A new method for estimating the usual intake of episodically-consumed foods with application to their distribution. *J Am Diet Assoc* **106,** 1575–1587.

Tudor-Locke, C., Brasher, M.M., Johnson, W.D., *et al.* (2010) Accelerometer profiles of physical activity and inactivity in normal weight, overweight, and obese US men and women. *Int J Behav Nutr Phys Act* **7,** 1–11.

US Congress (1990) *National Nutrition Monitoring and Related Research Act 1990.* US Department of Health and Human Services and US Department of Agriculture, Washington, DC.

US Department of Agriculture (2011) Choose MyPlate. <http://www.choosemyplate.gov/>.

US Department of Agriculture and US Department of Health and Human Services (2010) *Dietary Guidelines for Americans, 2010*, 7th Edn. US Government Printing Office, Washington, DC.

US Department of Health and Human Services (2000) *Healthy People 2010*, 2nd Edn. With *Understanding and Improving Health and Objectives for Improving Health*, 2 vols. US Government Printing Office, Washington, DC.

US Department of Health and Human Services and US Department of Agriculture (1993) Ten-year comprehensive plan for the National Nutrition Monitoring and Related Research Program. *Fed Reg* **58,** 32752–32806.

US Environmental Protection Agency, Office of Air Quality Planning and Standards and Office of Research and Development 1997, *Mercury study report to Congress, EPA-452/R-97-003*, Environmental Protection Agency, Washington, DC.

World Health Organization (2011a) Global database on body mass index. An interactive surveillance tool for monitoring nutrition transition. <http://apps.who.int/bmi/index.jsp

World Health Organization (2011b) Global database on national nutrition policies and programmes. <http://www.who.int/nutrition/databases/policies/en/index.html>.

Woteki, C.E. (2003) Integrated NHANES: uses in national policy. *J Nutr* **133,** 582S–584S.

Woteki, C.E., Briefel, R.R., Klein, C.J., *et al.* (2002) Nutrition monitoring: summary of a statement from an American Society for Nutritional Sciences Working Group. *J Nutr* **132,** 3782–3783.

Yetley, E.A., Coates, P.M., and Johnson, C.L. (2011) Overview of a roundtable on NHANES monitoring of biomarkers of folate and vitamin B-12 status: measurement procedure issues. *Am J Clin Nutr* **94,** 297S–302S.

Web Resources

Administration on Aging (2010) *AoA Program Evaluations and Related Reports*, Administration on Aging, Washington, DC, viewed 16 September 2010. <http://www.aoa.gov/AoARoot/Program_results/Program_Evaluation.aspx>.

Administration on Aging (2010) *Nutrition Services (OAA Title IIIC): the Purpose of the Program and How It Works*, Administration on Aging, Washington, DC, viewed 16 September 2010. <http://www.aoa.gov/aoaroot/aoa_programs/hcltc/nutrition_services/index.aspx#purpose>.

Agricultural Research Service (2009) *ARS Human Nutrition National Program: Food Composition and Nutrition Data Links*, US Department of Agriculture, Washington, DC, viewed 7 September 2010. <http://www.ars.usda.gov/Aboutus/docs.htm?docid=6300>.

Agricultural Research Service (2009) *FoodLink*, US Department of Agriculture, Washington, DC, viewed 16 September 2010. <http://www.ars.usda.gov/Services/docs.htm?docid=8498>.

Agricultural Research Service (2010) *Food and Nutrient Database for Dietary Studies*, US Department of Agriculture, Washington, DC, viewed 16 September 2010. <http://www.ars.usda.gov/Services/docs.htm?docid=12089>.

Agricultural Research Service (2010) *MPED*, US Department of Agriculture, Washington, DC, viewed 16 September 2010. <http://www.ars.usda.gov/Services/docs.htm?docid=17558>.

Agricultural Research Service (2010) *USDA National Nutrient Database for Standard Reference*, US Department of Agriculture, Washington, DC, viewed 16 September 2010. <http://www.ars.usda.gov/Services/docs.htm?docid=8964>.

Agricultural Research Service (2010) *What we Eat in America (WWEIA)*, US Department of Agriculture, Washington, DC, viewed 16 September 2010. <http://www.ars.usda.gov/Services/docs.htm?docid=13793>.

Center for Nutrition Policy and Promotion (2010) *Nutrient Content of the US Food Supply*, Center for Nutrition Policy and Promotion, Alexandria, VA, viewed 7 September 2010. <http://www.cnpp.usda.gov/USFoodSupply.htm>.

Centers for Disease Control and Prevention (2007) *The Social–Ecological Model: a Framework for Prevention*, Centers for Disease Control and Prevention, Atlanta, GA, viewed 14 September 2010. <http://www.cdc.gov/ncipc/dvp/social-ecological-model_dvp.htm>.

Centers for Disease Control and Prevention (2008) *5 A Day*, Centers for Disease Control and Prevention, Atlanta, GA, viewed 13 September 2010. <http://www.cdc.gov/nccdphp/dnpa/5aday/>.

Centers for Disease Control and Prevention (2009) *FoodNet Surveillance*, Centers for Disease Control and Prevention, Atlanta, GA, viewed 7 September 2010. <http://www.cdc.gov/foodnet/surveillance.htm>.

Centers for Disease Control and Prevention (2009) *Infant Feeding Practices Study II: introduction*, Centers for Disease Control and Prevention, Atlanta, GA, viewed 16 September 2010. <http://www.cdc.gov/ifps/>.

Centers for Disease Control and Prevention (2009) *Infant Feeding Practices Study II*, Centers for Disease Control and Prevention, Atlanta, GA, viewed 7 September (2010) <http://www.cdc.gov/breastfeeding/data/infant_feeding.htm>.

Centers for Disease Control and Prevention (2009) *National Health Interview Survey*, Centers for Disease Control and Prevention, Atlanta, GA, viewed 16 September 2010. <http://www.cdc.gov/nchs/nhis/about_nhis.htm>.

Centers for Disease Control and Prevention (2009) *NCHS Data Linked to Mortality Files*, Centers for Disease Control and Prevention, Atlanta, GA, viewed 16 September 2010. <http://www.cdc.gov/nchs/data_access/data_linkage/mortality.htm>.

Centers for Disease Control and Prevention (2009) *OutbreakNet—Foodborne Outbreak Online Database*, Centers for Disease Control and Prevention, Atlanta, GA, viewed 16 September 2010. <http://wwwn.cdc.gov/foodborneoutbreaks/>.

Centers for Disease Control and Prevention (2009) *What Is PedNSS?* Centers for Disease Control and Prevention, Atlanta, GA, viewed 16 September 2010. <http://www.cdc.gov/pednss/what_is/pednss/index.htm>.

Centers for Disease Control and Prevention (2010) *About the National Vital Statistics System*, Centers for Disease Control and Prevention, Atlanta, GA, viewed 16 September 2010. <http://www.cdc.gov/nchs/nvss/about_nvss.htm>.

Centers for Disease Control and Prevention (2010) *Behavioral Risk Factor Surveillance System: Turning Information into Health*, Centers for Disease Control and Prevention, Atlanta, GA, viewed 7 September 2010. <http://www.cdc.gov/brfss/>.

Centers for Disease Control and Prevention (2010) *Breastfeeding Among US Children Born 1999—-2007, CDC National Immunization Survey*, Centers for Disease Control and Prevention, Atlanta, GA, viewed 16 September 2010. <http://www.cdc.gov/breastfeeding/data/NIS_data/index.htm>.

Centers for Disease Control and Prevention (2010) *BRFSS Annual Survey Data*, Centers for Disease Control and Prevention, Atlanta, GA, viewed 16 September 2010. <http://www.cdc.gov/brfss/technical_infodata/surveydata/2009.htm>.

Centers for Disease Control and Prevention (2010) *FoodNet—Foodborne Diseases Active Surveillance Network*, Centers for Disease Control and Prevention, Atlanta, GA, viewed 16 September 2010. <http://www.cdc.gov/foodnet/>.

Centers for Disease Control and Prevention (2010) *National Health and Nutrition Examination Survey*, Centers for Disease Control and Prevention, Atlanta, GA, viewed 16 September 2010. <http://www.cdc.gov/nchs/nhanes.htm>.

Centers for Disease Control and Prevention (2010) *National Survey of Family Growth*, Centers for Disease Control and Prevention, Atlanta, GA, viewed 16 September 2010. <http://www.cdc.gov/nchs/nsfg.htm>.

Centers for Disease Control and Prevention (2010) *Pediatric and Pregnancy Nutrition Surveillance System*, Centers for Disease Control and Prevention, Atlanta, GA, viewed 7 September 2010. <http://www.cdc.gov/pednss/>.

Centers for Disease Control and Prevention (2010) *Pregnancy Risk Assessment Monitoring System (PRAMS): Home*, Centers for Disease Control and Prevention, Atlanta, GA, viewed 16 September 2010. <http://www.cdc.gov/prams/>.

Centers for Disease Control and Prevention (2010) *State and Local Area Integrated Telephone Survey*, Centers for Disease Control and Prevention, Atlanta, GA, viewed 16 September 2010. <http://www.cdc.gov/nchs/slaits.htm>.

Centers for Disease Control and Prevention (2010) *YRBSS: Youth Risk Behavior Surveillance System*, Centers for Disease Control and Prevention, Atlanta, GA, viewed 16 September 2010. <http://www.cdc.gov/HealthyYouth/yrbs/index.htm>.

Economic Research Service (2008) *Food Availability (Per Capita) Data System*, US Department of Agriculture, Washington, DC, viewed 16 September 2010. <http://www.ers.usda.gov/Data/FoodConsumption/>.

Economic Research Service (2009) *Diet Quality and Food Consumption: Flexible Consumer Behavior Survey (FCBS)*, US Department of Agriculture, Washington, DC, viewed 16 September 2010. <http://www.ers.usda.gov/Briefing/DietQuality/flexible.htm>.

Economic Research Service (2009) *Diet Quality and Food Consumption: the National Household Food Acquisition and Purchase Survey (FoodAPS)*, US Department of Agriculture, Washington, DC, viewed 16 September 2010. <http://www.ers.usda.gov/Briefing/DietQuality/food_aps.htm>.

Economic Research Service (2009) *Food Security in the United States: Current Population Survey Food Security Supplement (CPS-FSS)*, US Department of Agriculture, Washington, DC, viewed 16 September 2010. <http://www.ers.usda.gov/Data/foodsecurity/cps/>.

Economic Research Service (2009) *Food Security in the United States*, US Department of Agriculture, Washington, DC, viewed 7 September 2010. <http://www.ers.usda.gov/Briefing/FoodSecurity/>.

Economic Research Service (n.d.) *Your Food Environment Atlas*, US Department of Agriculture, Washington, DC, viewed 16 September 2010. <http://www.ers.usda.gov/foodatlas/>.

Food and Drug Administration (2008) *Total Diet Study*, Food and Drug Administration, Silver Spring, MD, viewed 16 September 2010. <http://www.fda.gov/Food/FoodSafety/FoodContaminantsAdulteration/TotalDietStudy/default.htm>.

Food and Drug Administration (2010) *Consumer Nutrition and Health Information: Food/Nutrition Research and Surveys*, Food and Drug Administration, Silver Spring, MD, viewed 13 September 2010. <http://www.fda.gov/Food/LabelingNutrition/ConsumerInformation/default.htm>.

Food and Drug Administration (2010) *Food Label and Package Survey 2006–2007*, Food and Drug Administration, Silver Spring, MD, viewed 16 September 2010. <http://www.fda.gov/Food/LabelingNutrition/ConsumerInformation/ucm122084.htm>.

Food and Drug Administration (2010) *Health and Diet Survey*, Food and Drug Administration, Silver Spring, MD, viewed 7 September 2010. <http://www.fda.gov/Food/LabelingNutrition/ucm202775.htm>.

Food and Drug Administration (2010) *Survey Shows Gains in Food-Label Use, Health/Diet Awareness*, Food and Drug Administration, Silver Spring, MD, viewed 16 September 2010. <http://www.fda.gov/ForConsumers/ConsumerUpdates/ucm202611.htm>.

Food and Nutrition Service (2010) *Child and Adult Care Program*, US Department of Agriculture, Washington, DC, viewed 16 September 2010. <http://www.fns.usda.gov/cnd/care/default.htm>.

Food and Nutrition Service (2010) *Child Nutrition*, US Department of Agriculture, Washington, DC, viewed 16 September 2010. <http://www.fns.usda.gov/ora/menu/Published/CNP/cnp.htm>.

Food and Nutrition Service (2010) *WIC Studies*, US Department of Agriculture, Washington, DC, viewed 16 September 2010. <http://www.fns.usda.gov/ora/menu/Published/WIC/WIC.htm>.

Lando, A. and Verrill, L. (2009) *2006 FDA/FSIS Food Safety Survey Topline Frequency Report*, Food and Drug Administration, Silver Spring, MD, viewed 16 September 2010. <http://www.fda.gov/Food/ScienceResearch/ResearchAreas/ConsumerResearch/ucm080374.htm>.

National Cancer Institute (2010) *Automated Self-Administered 24-Hour Dietary Eecall (ASA24Ô)*, National Cancer Institute, Rockville, MD, viewed 17 September 2010. <http://riskfactor.cancer.gov/tools/instruments/asa24/>

National Cancer Institute (2010) *Usual Dietary Intakes: Food Intakes, US Population, 2001–2004*, National Cancer Institute, Rockville, MD, viewed 15 September 2010. <http://riskfactor.cancer.gov/diet/usualintakes/pop/#results>.

National Center for Education Statistics (2006) *Combined User's Manual for the ECLS-K Fifth-Grade Data Files and Electronic Codebooks*, National Center for Education Statistics, Washington, DC, viewed 16 September 2010. <http://sodapop.pop.psu.edu/codebooks/ecls/k5userpart1.pdf>.

National Center for Education Statistics (n.d.) *Early Childhood Longitudinal Study (ECLS): Overview*, National Center for Education Statistics, Washington, DC, viewed 16 September 2010. <http://nces.ed.gov/ecls/>.

National Center for Education Statistics (n.d.) *Early Childhood Longitudinal Study (ECLS): Data Collection Procedures*, National Center for Education Statistics, Washington, DC, viewed 16 September 2010. <http://nces.ed.gov/ecls/kinderdataprocedure.asp>.

National Center for Health Statistics (2009) *National Health Interview Survey*, Centers for Disease Control and Prevention,

Atlanta, GA, viewed 7 September 2010. <http://www.cdc.gov/nchs/nhis/htm>.

National Center for Health Statistics (2010) *National Health and Nutrition Examination Survey*, Centers for Disease Prevention and Control, Atlanta, GA, viewed 7 September 2010. <http://cdc.gov/nchs/nhanes.htm>.

National Library of Medicine (2010) *Dietary Supplements Labels Database*, National Library of Medicine, Rockville, MD, viewed 16 September 2010. <http://dietarysupplements.nlm.nih.gov/dietary/>.

National Marine Fisheries Service, Office of Science and Technology (2009) *Fisheries of the United States—2009*, National Marine Fisheries Service, Silver Spring, MD, viewed 16 September 2010. <http://www.st.nmfs.noaa.gov/st1/fus/fus09/index.html>.

Nutrient Data Laboratory (2009) *Dietary Supplement Ingredient Database*, Nutrient Data Laboratory, Beltsville, MD, viewed 16 September 2010. <http://dietarysupplementdatabase.usda.nih.gov/>.

US Bureau of Labor Statistics (2009) *Consumer Expenditure Survey*, US Bureau of Labor Statistics, Washington, DC, viewed 16 September 2010. <http://www.bls.gov/cex/>.

US Bureau of Labor Statistics (2010) *2008 Eating and Health Module microdata files*, US Bureau of Labor Statistics, Washington, DC, viewed 16 September 2010. <http://www.bls.gov/tus/ehdatafiles_2008.htm>.

US Bureau of Labor Statistics (2010) *American Time Use Survey Eating and Health Module Questionnaire*, US Bureau of Labor Statistics, Washington, DC, viewed 16 September 2010. <http://www.bls.gov/tus/ehmquestionnaire.pdf>.

US Bureau of Labor Statistics (n.d.) *American Time Use Survey*, US Bureau of Labor Statistics, Washington, DC, viewed 7 September 2010. <http://www.bls.gov/tus/home.htm>.

65

DIETARY STANDARDS AND GUIDELINES: SIMILARITIES AND DIFFERENCES AMONG COUNTRIES

JOHANNA T. DWYER, DSc, RD

Tufts University, Boston, Massachusetts, and *National Institutes of Health, Bethesda Massachusetts, USA*

Summary

Nutrient reference values and dietary guidelines are two key dietary standards necessary for nutrition science and policy making. Nutrient reference values are dietary standards for nutrient requirements that all humans share, and that are usually quite similar from country to country. Dietary guidelines are evidence-based, country-specific recommendations for food patterns that promote healthy weights and good health while helping to prevent and reduce diet-related disease. They differ from country to country. Nutrient reference values should be and are gradually converging and being harmonized between countries. In contrast, dietary guidelines remain unique to each country because of differences in foodways, cuisines, customs, economics, and food production capacity. The reasons for the similarities and differences between these two standards across several countries are described, and likely future directions are suggested. The focus is on standards published in English that are used by governments of highly industrialized countries with Western eating patterns. Possible useful future directions for dietary reference values and dietary guidelines are summarized as the chapter concludes.

Introduction

Dietary reference intake values and dietary guidelines are two dietary standards that are essential nutrition policy tools. Their characteristics and purposes are quite different between countries. Therefore, in this increasingly global nutrition world, scientists and policy makers need to understand what they are, how they vary, and their proper use. Clarifications of the various meanings of the requirement estimates used in Western countries and provided in this chapter may be helpful in sorting out true differences between reference standards and expert groups, and differences arising simply as a result of semantics.

Dietary Reference Intakes

Definition

Dietary nutrient reference intake values describe and quantify universal human requirements for essential nutrients. The reason for developing dietary reference values is

Present Knowledge in Nutrition, Tenth Edition. Edited by John W. Erdman Jr, Ian A. Macdonald and Steven H. Zeisel.
© 2012 International Life Sciences Institute. Published 2012 by John Wiley & Sons, Inc.

to provide uniform, evidence-based, quantitative data on human nutrient needs. This information can be used for many purposes, including diagnosis or assessment of individual intakes, and in the examination and interpretation of nutrition surveys to provide an assessment of probable nutrient intake adequacy of populations. The reference standards are also used for planning of individual diets, food labeling, formulating criteria for food programs, institutional feeding, and other nutritional interventions. When reference values are used appropriately, they help to harmonize nutrient-based dietary assessment and planning, both within and between countries.

Nutrient Reference Values and Their Meanings
Table 65.1 presents a summary of the terms used in various countries for their nutrient reference standards. The reference values for nutrients used have various names in different countries, but generally the terms refer to similar concepts and use a similar framework for establishing them. Table 65.2 compares the terminology used by expert groups in different Western countries. In the future it is hoped that nutrient intake values can be better harmonized to improve the objectivity and transparency of values of recommendations and to smoothe the consideration of differences among them (King and Garza, 2007).

Similarities Across Countries
Today, methods for ascertaining nutrient requirements are becoming more widely accepted and harmonized between countries, with the result that values are converging more than ever before. The data on which dietary standards are based are generally similar from one country to another. They include relevant human clinical and experimental data (such as depletion–repletion studies, dose–response studies, and balance studies), epidemiological studies, and relevant animal studies. The methods used in formulating dietary standards generally involve a review of the literature and recommendations by expert scientists on the nutrient in question.

Most groups setting recommendations now provide values for classical nutrient requirements and newer sections on dietary factors that are relevant to the reduction in risk of diet-related diseases. These chronic disease risk reduction values are challenging since the causes of the diseases are multifactorial, including but not limited to one or more dietary constituents. When experimental studies are possible for studying chronic diseases, they are

usually of short duration with high doses and surrogate markers from which lower intakes over many years and chronic disease endpoints are inferred. Risk reduction values are therefore not usually determined experimentally; rather, they are based largely on observational epidemiology, with all the difficulties residual confounding creates for establishing causal inference.

There is variability in nutrient requirements even among individuals who are similar in age, sex, and life stage, and therefore statistical concepts are essential in the derivation and interpretation of nutrient requirement estimates. The use of probability models and statistical techniques is vital in the formulation of human nutrition requirements since human nutrient needs all have a probability distribution that must be dealt with by a probability approach (Rand, 1990). For individuals, the values are stated in probabilistic terms since an individual's nutrient requirements are never known with certainty.

Virtually all of the groups setting nutrient reference standards now use similar statistical approaches for determining the midpoint of the distribution of requirements for a given function for each nutrient, and for deriving an estimate of the standard deviation of the requirements. The standard setting groups also use probability theory to state a level that ensures health for most individuals at some point above the mean requirement, such as 2 standard deviations. Although data are often lacking at present, a second set of distributions of risk of excessive intakes is used as the basis for establishing the tolerable upper intake levels (ULs) of nutrients.

Most groups setting nutrient requirements base them on criteria that reflect a meaningful biomarker of a nutrient-related function (Yates, 2007). This is critical since the choice of the indicator or function chosen will determine the amount of the nutrient that is needed. Desirable criteria exhibit a dose–response function, are responsive to inadequacy or excess of a single nutrient, resist rapid day-to-day changes in response to inadequate, adequate, or excessive intakes, are easily measurable or assessable with non-invasive methods, and are unresponsive to environmental changes other than nutrient intakes (King and Garza, 2007). Although functional criteria that reflect chronic disease endpoints are often the most relevant, the data for using them are often not available (Trumbo, 2008).

Methods for using nutrient reference values in dietary assessment and planning are also becoming increasingly popular and uniform. One such use is in developing

TABLE 65.1   Glossary of terms used for describing nutrient reference values by various expert bodies

Term	Abbreviation	Description	Comments
Adequate intake	AI	Value estimated when an RDA or PRI cannot be established or determined	Term used by Institute of Medicine/Health Canada. EFSA defines the AI as the average observed daily level of intake by a population group that is assumed to be adequate
Acceptable macronutrient distribution range	AMDR		Term used by Institute of Medicine/Health Canada
Average nutrient requirement	ANR	Mean intake to meet the average physiological requirement	Term similar to Institute of Medicine/Health Canada EAR
Average requirement	AR		Term similar to Institute of Medicine/Health Canada EAR
Dietary reference intake	DRI		Term used by Institute of Medicine/Health Canada
Dietary reference value	DRV		Term used in UK
Estimated average requirement	EAR		Term used by Institute of Medicine/Health Canada
Estimated values		An experimentally supported value that provides appropriate information for adequate and safe intakes when human requirements for a nutrient cannot yet be determined with desirable accuracy	Used in the DACH countries in Europe
Guiding values		Aids for orientation if some regulation of intake is needed (e.g. a lower limit for intake of water, fluoride, dietary fiber, or an upper limit for fat, cholesterol, alcohol, and table salt) for health reasons	Used in the DACH countries in Europe
Individual nutrient level, x = percentile chosen	INL x		Term used by UNU/WHO/FAO
Lower reference nutrient intake	LRNL		Term used by UNU/WHO/FAO

TABLE 65.1 (*Continued*)

Term	Abbreviation	Description	Comments
Lower threshold intake	LTL	Intake below which nearly all individuals in the population or group will be unable to maintain metabolic integrity according to the criterion chosen (e.g. the 2.55th percentile; mean -2 SD)	Term suggested by the Scientific Committee on Food of the EU and EFSA
Nutrient intake value	NIV		
Population reference intake level	PRL	Intake that will meet the needs of nearly all healthy people in the population or group (the 97.5th percentile)	Term used by the Scientific Committee on Food of the EU
Recommended dietary allowance	RDA		Term used by Institute of Medicine/Health Canada
Recommendation		Average requirement increased by 2 SD, or lacking a normal distribution of values, the average requirement increased by 20–30% (assuming a coefficient of variation of 10–15%)	Term used in the DACH countries in Europe
Recommended intake		Intake of a nutrient representing the average requirement for a defined group of individuals (similar to the EAR)	Used in Nordic recommendation
Reference intake range for macronutrients	RI	The intake range for macronutrients, expressed as intakes that are adequate for maintaining health and associated with a low risk of selected chronic diseases	EFSA and EU definition
Reference nutrient intake	RNL		
Upper tolerable nutrient intake level	UL	ESA refers to this as the level of chronic daily intake of a nutrient from all sources judged to be unlikely to pose a risk of adverse effects	
Upper nutrient level	UNL		

dietary guidelines, which will be discussed later in the chapter.

Differences

In spite of the similarities noted above, there are still many differences between countries in the processes they use to set recommendations and in their estimates of nutrient requirements.

Although nutrient requirements are defined the same by most expert groups, there are still inconsistencies in the conceptual frameworks they use, which may lead the unwary to assume that differences in expert reports are

TABLE 65.2 Comparison of terminology used for describing dietary standard nutrient values by various groups

Terms used	UN University	USA/ Canada	UK	EU/EFSA	WHO/FAO	Australia/ NZ
Dietary reference intake	NIV	DRI	DRV			
Average requirement	ANR	EAR	EAR	AR		EAR
Recommended intake level for individuals	INL x	RDA	RNI	PRI	RNI	RDI
Lower reference nutrient intake			LRNI	LTI		
Safe intake		AI	Lower end of safe intake range	Lower end of safe intake range		AI
Upper level of safe intake	UNL	UL	Upper end of safe intake range	Upper end of safe intake range	UL	UL
Acceptable macronutrient distribution range		AMDR		RI minimum and maximum population ranges	Population mean intake goals	

AI, adequate intake; ADMR, acceptable macronutrient distribution range; ANR, average nutrient requirement; AR, average requirement; DRI, dietary reference intake; DRV, dietary reference value; EAR, estimated average requirement; INLx, individual nutrient level, x = percentile chosen; LRNI, lower reference nutrient intake; LTI, lower threshold intake; NIV, nutrient intake value; PRI, population reference intake; RDA, recommended dietary allowance; RDI, reference daily intake/recommended daily intake; RNI, reference nutrient intake; UL, tolerable upper intake level.
Modified with additions and adapted from King *et al.* (2007).

much greater than they actually are. The reasons for the differences in estimates of nutrient requirements include the relative emphasis given to different types of evidence (human epidemiological or experimental studies, and that from other species), and the functional criteria chosen; the literature available when the reviews were done also contributes to differences. Differences also exist as a result of variations in dietary composition (which affect nutrient absorption and bioavailability), in the anthropometric reference standards used (e.g. height, weight, body mass or growth rates of reference individuals), definitions of reference groups (by age, health status, occupation, income),

groups at risk (e.g. premature infants, the very old, smokers, etc.), and assumptions about the climate, altitude, and temperature. Reference values also vary according to the functional criteria chosen, underlying assumptions about nutrient bioavailability, and how values are extrapolated if evidence is unavailable for certain life-stage groups.

Countries also differ in the extent to which the standard setting process is reproducible and objective. In some countries systematic evidence-based reviews are used to support the development of their reference values in order to promote a transparent and rigorous process for reviewing the relevant data and that facilitates the update of reference

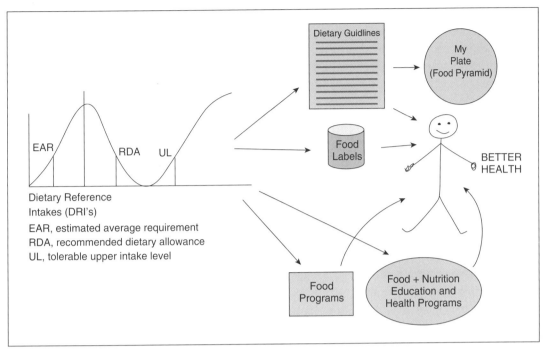

FIG. 65.1 Relationship between dietary standards, dietary guidelines, and associated interventions and health.

values as new evidence becomes available (Russell, 2008). Systematic reviews lend transparency to the process of developing dietary reference values, and clarify the process (Thuraisingam *et al.*, 2009). However, they require some modifications for this purpose (Lichtenstein *et al.*, 2008; Russell *et al.*, 2009). Challenges in applying systematic reviews for the development of dietary reference intakes include defining and prioritizing the key research questions, the quality of studies, and finding biomarkers or intermediate (surrogate) outcomes that can be used when there is a dearth of studies directly linking nutrient intakes to clinical or functional outcomes. Nevertheless, using vitamin A as an example, the process was judged to promise a greater degree of transparency and objectivity in setting nutrient reference values than not using it (Russell *et al.*, 2009). The US Institute of Medicine/Health Canada efforts on vitamin D and calcium incorporated a systematic evidence-based review in the process of updating nutrient reference values (Chung *et al.*, 2009, 2010). An independent panel of technical experts helped informatics experts to prioritize and select key questions and outcomes of interest; methods for using existing systematic reviews were refined for determining requirement-related questions; and quality assessment tools and methods for translating results from studies not designed to address the issues of interest were developed and applied (Chung *et al.*, 2010).

Methods for using nutrient requirements for planning and assessing nutrient intakes vary from one expert group to another. Since there is considerable variability in the intakes of similar individuals under similar circumstances that must be taken into account in dietary assessment and in planning, these procedures also require the application of statistics to adjust food consumption surveys for usual intakes. These methods are briefly described in a recent paper (Murphy and Vorster, 2007) and more extensively in volumes devoted to dietary assessment and planning (Institute of Medicine, 2000, 2003) (Figure 65.1).

Examples of Dietary Reference Intakes for Nutrients from Various Countries

Dietary Reference Intakes (DRIs) of the United States and Canada

The DRIs used in the United States and Canada are described in detail elsewhere and briefly below (Murphy, 2005; Barr, 2006b; Institute of Medicine, 2008). The key DRIs are defined as follows.

Estimated Average Requirement (EAR)

The EAR is the amount of a nutrient that meets the requirement for a specific criterion of adequacy for half of the individuals in the population of a given age, sex, and life stage or physiological condition (such as pregnancy or lactation). This is an average or median value since the amount of the nutrient needed to achieve adequacy varies from one individual to the next. Because nutrient requirements are usually distributed normally or can be transformed mathematically to achieve a normal distribution, this is a useful summary number. For most nutrients there are many different functional criteria that might be chosen for setting the requirement, and therefore it is important to justify the choice of a given criterion. Because the EAR is a mean requirement for a group, and because the variation around the mean is considerable, the EAR is not useful for estimating the nutrient adequacy of an individual's intake. At the EAR, half of the individuals in a group are below their requirement and half are above it. An individual whose usual intake is below the EAR has a risk of inadequacy between 50% and 100%. Dietary advice to the general public should attempt to promote distributions of intakes by individuals in which as many individuals as possible have usual intakes that are above the EAR and below the UL.

Recommended Dietary Allowance (RDA)

The RDA is the average daily dietary intake level that meets the nutrient requirements of nearly all (e.g. 97–98%) healthy persons of a specific sex, age, and life stage. It is the nutrient intake goal for planning the diets of individuals. In order to calculate the RDA, it is assumed that the requirement distribution is normal, and that the amount of the nutrient needed to cover virtually everyone in the population (defined statistically as 2 standard deviations about the EAR) is calculated. When no standard deviation is available, the coefficient of variation is used. It is usually assumed to be 10% (1.2 times the EAR) or 15% (1.3 times the EAR) on the basis of existing nutrient data. If an individual has an intake that is less than the RDA but more than the EAR, his risk of inadequacy would be between 2–3 % and 50%. As intakes fall further below the RDA, the risk but not the certainty of inadequacy rises. The RDA is an appropriate target to aim for in planning diets of individuals. However, it is not appropriate for assessing the diet of an individual since there are many whose intakes are below the RDA who may still be getting enough of the nutrient to be above their nutrient requirement levels. Because the RDA exceeds the actual needs of all but about 2–3% of the population, it is also overly generous as a standard for evaluating group intakes and should not be used for that purpose. An online interactive tool to help individuals find recommended intakes of nutrients and safe levels of nutrients is now available at http://ods.od.nih.gov/health_information/dietary_reference_intakes.aspx.

Adequate Intake (AI)

The EARs for some nutrients are not known for the particular functional criterion that is most relevant, and in this case it is not possible to apply statistical theory and derive an RDA. However, often there is enough information to make some quantitative recommendations about adequate and healthful nutrient intake levels. Under such circumstances an AI is set as a tentative goal or target for the nutrient intake of individuals until more information is available. Because knowledge is limited, it tends to be generous. The definitions vary somewhat, but it is often the average or median intake of a group of healthy people, all of whom are assumed to be meeting their nutrient needs. Therefore falling short of it does not signify deficiency since the AI is not a requirement. The most common use of AI is for young infants where it is based on the mean intakes of groups of healthy infants.

Acceptable Macronutrient Distribution Range (AMDR)

The AMDR is a range of acceptable macronutrient distributions for individuals, usually presented as a proportion of total dietary intake. Ranges are provided for protein, fat (omega-3 and omega-6 fatty acids), and carbohydrates. The values are estimates that are thought to minimize the potential for chronic disease over the long term, and that at the same time permit essential nutrients and energy to be consumed at adequate levels. For dietary cholesterol, *trans* fatty acids, and saturated fatty acid levels as low as possible while consuming a nutritionally adequate diet are recommended. For added sugars, the recommendation is to limit them to no more than 25% of energy intake. However, such a limit is likely to be appropriate only for very active individuals. For most Americans who are much more sedentary, their energy needs are so low that, after following the dietary patterns recommended by the 2005 and 2010 Dietary Guidelines for Americans and meeting their other nutrient needs, the percent of calories from added sugars would have to be far lower than 25% to stay in energy balance. Also, the American Heart Association has urged stricter upper limits based on their reviews of the evidence associating dietary sugars and cardiovascular health, and suggested a limit of closer to 13% of calories from added sugars (Johnson *et al.*, 2009).

Upper Intake Levels (UL)

A relatively recent innovation in dietary reference values for nutrients is the tolerable or safe upper intake level for a nutrient. Intakes far in excess of the RDA may also give rise to health problems. The UL is the highest level of chronic, usually daily, nutrient intakes that is likely to pose no risk of adverse effects on health to almost everyone in the population. As intake levels rise above the UL, adverse effects are increasingly likely. Usually the functional criterion used for setting the UL is that which is likely to harm health and for which sufficient data are available. Unfortunately, for many nutrients, so few data are available at present that ULs cannot be set. However, lack of a UL does not mean that the risk of adverse effects does not exist.

Estimated Energy Requirement (EER)

Small excesses in energy intake can, over time, result in weight gain. Also enough is known about energy output to permit quite exact calculations of energy output and intakes. The EAR and RDA do not apply for energy. Instead, energy needs are stated as minimal average requirements for individuals. The EER is derived from equations derived from experimental data on the energy need of individuals of normal weight with a healthy body mass index of between 18.5 and 25 for adults of a given sex, age, height, weight, and physical activity level. A calculator is available based on these data for EER and for the estimated energy requirement for those who want to lose weight at http://www.mypyramid.gov.

Total Energy Expenditure (TEE)

The TEE is an estimate of the total energy expenditure needed to maintain current body weight and activity levels.

Water Intake

Standard values for water are also provided, based on what is known about nutrient needs for water.

Reference Daily Intake or Recommended Daily Intake (RDI) and Daily Value (DV)

In addition to the dietary standards described above, in many countries additional standard values have been developed to facilitate various uses, such as food labeling. A few of these terms that are common in the United States and Canada are listed below. These terms are not DRIs but are related reference values. The RDI is the daily dietary intake level of a nutrient which was considered at the time they were defined to suffice to meet the requirements of nearly all (97–98%) of healthy individuals in each life stage and sex group. It is used to determine the Daily Value (DV), which is displayed on food labels in the United States, Canada, and Australia. Although newer DRIs are now available, some of these DVs are based on older RDAs of the United States dating from 1968. There is debate about whether the RDA or the EAR should be used in food labeling, but at present the RDA seems to be the better alternative (Murphy *et al.*, 2006a). There is also much agitation about whether and what nutrition information should be placed on the front of food packages, and whether, if such information is made available, it influences consumer purchasing decisions (Wartella *et al.*, 2010)

World Health Organization/Food and Agricultural Organization/United Nations University (WHO-FAO-UNU)

Dietary standards have been promulgated jointly by three United Nations organizations to provide energy and nutrient requirement values that can be used, with appropriate adjustments, in virtually all countries (Taylor *et al.*, 2005). Expert groups are convened to make recommendations on specific nutrient requirements and nutrient intakes. The quantitative estimates of nutrient requirements are usually published as individual monographs clustering similar nutrients together rather than in a single volume with all nutrients.

In 2007 the UN University proposed a uniform terminology and a generic framework for establishing recommended nutrient intake values, or NIVs (King and Garza, 2007; King *et al.*, 2007). These include the *average nutrient requirement* (ANR) that reflects the median requirement for a nutrient in a specific population. The *individual nutrient level* (INL) is the recommended level of nutrient intake for all healthy people in the population. It is set at a certain level above the mean requirement, such as 2 standard deviations above the mean requirements, thus covering the needs of 98% of the population and referred to as INL98. However, it could also be set at levels other than 2 standard deviations above the mean requirement if the decision was made to cover less than virtually the entire population's needs. Finally there is the *upper nutrient level* (UNL), which consists of the highest level of daily nutrient intake that is likely to pose no risk of adverse health effects for almost all individuals in a specific life-stage group.

Micronutrients reviewed by WHO/FAO focus on those most likely to present problems in human nutrition. Over the years they have included calcium, ascorbic acid, vitamin D, vitamin B_{12}, folate, iron, and the trace elements. In addressing requirements for vitamins A, iron, vitamin B_{12} and folate, and for trace elements, the expert groups initially used the term *basal requirements* as those sufficient to maintain all demonstrable functions of the nutrient. *Normative requirements* were defined as higher levels sufficient to maintain tissue stores or adaptive capacities that were judged to be desirable. The newer UNU recommended terminology is now gradually being adopted instead.

In the WHO/FAO system, energy requirements are based on energy expenditure, except in children. Energy needs are presented as average needs (so that half of a homogeneous population would have higher and half lower requirements).

There is universal agreement that the first goal of population nutrient intake goals is to ensure that all inhabitants of a country have access to affordable and available food that meets their nutritional needs. In the past decade, a WHO study group developed population nutrient intake goals that it judged to be both consistent with the maintenance of health and to include a low prevalence of diet-related disease in the population. The recommendations were designed to decrease risk factors for non-communicable diseases stemming from diet and physical activity, and to increase awareness of the influence of these factors on health. Nutrient intake goals for populations vary from country to country depending on the food supply and many other factors, and so they are generally best stated as ranges. The range of population nutrient intake goals recommended by WHO/FAO and other authoritative bodies is presented in Table 65.3. Since these ranges were published, several additional expert groups have met to further refine them.

Requirements for protein and macronutrients are presented as near the top end of the normal distribution of intakes or needs: a level termed "safe level of intake". Fats, oils and carbohydrates have also been reviewed. Nutrient requirements for essential fatty acids have been stated, but since there are also increased risks of chronic non-communicable diseases from fats, recommendations for ranges of population mean intakes that are thought to be consistent with good health have also been stated. The terms used are *estimated average requirement* (EAR), the *acceptable macronutrient distribution range* (AMDR) with *lower* (L-AMDR) and *upper* (U-AMDR) levels of the acceptable macronutrient distribution range that correspond to upper and lower bounds of confidence intervals. Finally there is the *upper level* (UL). For fatty acids the UL was used only with *trans* fatty acids. The UL is used to describe instances where biochemical indicators were needed to confirm adverse effects, measurable with a probability of occurrence. The latest recommendations include type and amount of fat, total carbohydrate, complex carbohydrates and free sugars, protein, dietary fiber, salt, and fruits and vegetables (which are viewed as sources of bioactive constituents that are seen as beneficial) (World Health Organization, 2003a).

Among the other more recent WHO/FAO/UNU technical reports are monographs reporting expert consultations on human energy requirements (Report of the Joint FAO/WHO/UNU Expert Consultation, 2004); diet in the prevention of chronic diseases (World Health Organization, 2003b); vitamin and mineral requirements (Joint FAO/WHO Expert Consultation on Human Vitamin and Mineral Requirements, 2004); protein and amino acid requirements (Joint WHO/FAO/UNU Expert Consultation, 2007); scientific updates on fat and fatty acid requirements for adults (Elmadfa and Komsteiner, 2009) and children (Uuay and Dangour, 2009; Uuay et al., 2009); criteria for applying estimates for fat in dietary guidelines (Smit, 2009); the health effects of *trans* fatty acids (Koletzko, 2008; Uauy et al., 2009); and an interim summary of conclusions and dietary recommendations on total fat and fatty acids from a Joint FAO/WHO Expert Consultation on Fats and Fatty Acids in Human Nutrition and carbohydrates (Mann et al., 2007; Nishida and Martinez Nocito, 2007). The UN University has also issued documents to assist in applying dietary reference values, including one on establishing upper levels of nutrient intakes (Joint FAO/WHO Technical Workshop on Nutrient Risk Assessment, 2006).

United Kingdom

Dietary reference values (DRV) are terms used in the UK to refer to recommended intakes which are set for energy and 33 nutrients by the Committee on Medical Aspects of Food Policy (COMA) (Panel on Dietary Reference Values of the Committee on Medical Aspects of Food Policy, 1991, 2006). The DRVs are provided as four values, all for population groups, not for individuals. *Estimated average requirement* (EAR) is the level at which 50% of the population's requirements are met. It is the average

TABLE 65.3 Selected recommended ranges of population nutrient intake goals as percent of calories unless otherwise stated from various authoritative bodies

Nutrient or dietary factor	WHO 2003 goals	EFSA 2010	USA/Canada 2002 (acceptable macronutrient distribution range)
Total fat	15–30%	20–35%	20–35%
Saturated fatty acids	<10%	As low as possible	As low as possible
Polyunsaturated fatty acids (PUFAs)	6–10%	Not stated	–
n-6 PUFAS	5–8%	4% linolenic and 0.5% α-linolenic	5–10% linoleic
n-3 PUFAs	1–2%	250 mg EPA+DHA	0.6–1.2%
Trans fatty acids	1%	As low as possible	As low as possible
Monounsaturated fatty acids (MUFAs)	By difference from others	Not stated	–
Total carbohydrate	55–75%	45–60%	45–65%
Free sugars (all mono- and disaccharides added to foods plus sugars naturally present in honey, syrups and fruit juices)	<10%	Not stated	<25%
Protein	10–15% of calories		10–35%
Cholesterol	<300 mg/day	Not stated	As low as possible
Sodium chloride (sodium)	<5 g/day (<2 g/day)	Not discussed	
Fruits and vegetables	>400 g/day	Not discussed	
Total dietary fiber	From foods	25 g	25–38 g (14 g/1000 kcal)
Non-starch polysaccharide (NSP)	From foods (fruits, vegetables, whole grains, etc)		
Sodium chloride (sodium) g/day	<5 (2)		

EFSA, European Food Safety Authority; WHO, World Health Organization. Reproduced with permission from Taylor (2005).

requirement for a particular nutrient or for energy. This is similar to the EAR value in the US/Canadian DRI. The *Reference nutrient intake* (RNI) is the amount of a nutrient that is sufficient for almost all individuals (97.5% of the population). The RNI is equivalent to the UK's previous recommended daily amount (RDA) value. It is similar to the recommended dietary allowance (RDA) of the US/Canadian standards. RNIs have been set for adults and children over the age of 5 years for vitamins A, B₁ (thiamin), B₂ (riboflavin), B₃ (niacin), C, D, folate, calcium, iron, phosphorus, magnesium, potassium, and zinc. The *lower reference nutrient intake* (LRNI) is the amount of a nutrient that is sufficient for only a few individuals (2.5% of the population's needs are met). Therefore most people need more than this. The *Safe Intake* is a range of intakes that is sufficient for almost all individuals' needs but not so high as to cause harmful effects. This level is given for nutrients for which there is insufficient information to set more precise levels. This value is somewhat like the AI in the DRIs. The DRVs in the United Kingdom also include a *High Intake* which is the upper level of intake for a nutrient above which there is no further benefit and effects may be harmful. This is similar to the UL in the DRI. DRVs for total fat, fatty acids, starch, sugars, and fiber (as non-starch polysaccharides, or NSP) have been set as a percentage of daily energy intake in addition to those for energy and some vitamins and minerals. Desirable intakes of total fat, saturated fats, sugars, and starches are expressed as a percentage of the EAR for energy. Energy estimates are based on resting energy expenditure during sleep or rest, plus the energy expended in physical activity. Separate energy requirements for pregnant and lactating mothers are also given in the report.

Other dietary standards exist in the UK for purposes other than defining requirements. The *Guideline Daily Amounts* (GDAs) are not DRVs, but the amounts of fat, saturated fat, and other nutrients as target values used in nutrient labels in the United Kingdom to help consumers make sense out of nutrient labeling and achieve nutrient goals for the population. The GDAs are set based on various dietary reference values used in the United Kingdom or other countries that use the term.

European Union (EU)

Early Efforts. Until recently, many of the countries in the EU set their own dietary standards, making assessments of dietary adequacy and planning between countries confusing and difficult. The various European reference values for children and their similarities and differences have recently been discussed (Prentice *et al.*, 2004). In 1993, the Scientific Committee on Food of the EU defined three reference levels. The five Scandinavian countries (Denmark, Finland, Iceland, Norway, and Sweden) have published Nordic Nutrition Recommendations jointly for many years (Becker *et al.*, 2004). The DACH consortium of the German-speaking countries of Europe, Austria, Germany, and Switzerland jointly published its recommendations (German Nutrition Society, 2000). The DACH has now expanded to include Hungary, Slovenia, and Czechoslovakia as well. In the DACH the term *recommendation* is used to refer to what the Institute of Medicine/Health Canada refer to as the RDI, and the *estimated value* for the AI in that system and *Guiding Values* correspond to the AMDR for macronutrients and alcohol. The RDA and EAR are used for fluoride, water, and dietary fiber.

EURECCA. Starting in 2006, nutrition scientists in the countries of the EU came together in a European Commission effort at better coordinating the setting and assessing of nutrient requirements in the Union (Pijls *et al.*, 2009). Harmonization had proven difficult because existing recommendations use different terminology and different age groups – particularly in childhood and adolescence, and there are differences in target values for assessing requirements for nutrients and in some cases local variations in dietary requirements (Pavlovic *et al.*, 2007). Although the concepts, definitions, and defined population groups were quite similar, differences between countries were evident in criteria for adequacy, assumptions made, and types of evidence used to establish micronutrient recommendations.

The differences between countries were summarized in a recent report from the EURECCA consortium (Doets *et al.*, 2008). For example, recommendations for vitamin D in 50-year-olds varied greatly; the median was 5 μg/day but the inter-quartile range was from 5 to 8 μg/day, with one country having no recommendations. For 70-year-olds, although the median was 10 μg/day, again the variability was great, ranging from 5 to 10 μg/day. Similarly for vitamin A, the median was 900 μg/day of retinol equivalents with an inter-quartile range of 700–1000 μg/day at both 50 and 70 years of age (Doets *et al.*, 2008). European experts also performed a systematic review of micronutrient intakes that showed that across Europe different methods were applied to estimate the adequacy of micronutrient intakes, leading to different prevalence estimates of micronutrient inadequacy (Tabacchi *et al.*, 2009). Few of the countries used the recommended average requirement cut-point method or the probability approach to estimating the prevalence of inadequacy. The resulting prevalence of folate inadequacy thus revealed about 25% of the adult females surveyed had inadequate intakes when judged against these various criteria, but, when compared against the estimated average requirement cut-point value of 320 μg/day, nearly 75% of the women would have inadequate intakes. Although the work of harmonization in Europe is still in progress, these results on adequacy of folic acid levels in the various European countries illustrate the need for uniform methods for setting requirements and estimating adequacy. In their absence, comparisons across countries are impossible. The European Food Safety Authority (EFSA) is the body in the European Union that sets dietary reference values. It recently published recommendations for carbohydrates, dietary fiber, fats, and water, and it is now addressing vitamins and minerals (European Food Safety Authority, 2008, 2010a,b; EFSA Panel on Dietetic Products, 2010b,c). Some examples of 2010 EFSA recommendations were provided in Table 65.3 (EFSA Panel on Dietetic Products, 2010a,b,c).

Australia and New Zealand

Australia and New Zealand jointly publish nutrient reference values which are derived in a manner similar to that used by the Institute of Medicine/Health Canada and the UK Ministry of Health (Australian National Health and Medical Research Council and New Zealand Ministry of Health, 2006). Because the populations and food ways (e.g. cultural, social, and economic practices relating to the production and consumption of food) are similar to those in English-speaking North America, their recommendations are particularly germane to users in these countries. An interesting feature of the Australia/New Zealand guidelines is the presentation of a summary of recommendations to reduce chronic disease risk based on these experts' reviews of the evidence. Suggested dietary targets are provided for vitamins A, C, E, folate, sodium, potassium, dietary fiber, and long-chain omega-3 fatty acids. Acceptable macronutrient distribution ranges are also provided that are designed to reduce chronic disease risk and ensure adequate micronutrient levels for protein, fat, linoleic acid, α-linolenic acid, and carbohydrate

Other Countries

Many countries in the developing world use WHO/FAO dietary standards or adopt the standards of nearby neighbors that have similar populations and circumstances. Affluent countries such as Japan, Korea, and Singapore have established their own values, based in part on data from their countries and in part on data from one or more of the countries discussed above. There are also efforts to harmonize values in regions such as Southeast Asia (Barba and Cabrera, 2008).

Dietary Guidelines

Definition

Dietary guidelines are evidence-based recommendations of foods and food patterns that will meet nutrient needs, promote healthy weight and good health, and assist in reducing risk of diet-related diseases. They are designed to assist policymakers and consumers within specific countries to implement this advice. They also form the basis for government nutrition initiatives and nutrition education and consumer outreach by industry and health professionals.

Dietary guidelines are needed because consumers think of eating in terms of food and dietary patterns, not of nutrients. Since people eat foods and not nutrients, recommendations about healthful levels of nutrients need to be translated into foods.

Nutrient Reference Values versus Dietary Guidelines

Nutrient reference standards differ from dietary guidelines in several ways. Nutrient standards are based on requirement estimates for specific nutrients but there are no human requirements for specific foods. Requirement levels are often lower than levels specified in dietary guidelines, which describe desirable and culturally acceptable dietary practices, which are often different from requirements (Hegsted, 1975). In addition to recommendations that cover or exceed nutrient requirements, and recommendations for ranges of population mean intakes of macronutrients thought to be consistent with good health and prevention of chronic disease, dietary guidelines have also included recommendations for type and amount of protein, fat, carbohydrate, salt, dietary fiber, types of fruits and vegetables, dairy products, protein-rich foods, and grains. Epidemiological evidence is used to a much greater extent in setting dietary guidelines than in setting nutrient requirements. Also, while nutrient requirements are generally the same for virtually all human beings, dietary guidelines are culture specific. Finally, national authorities are in a better position to establish dietary guidelines for their populations than are international groups. Certainly some aspects of dietary guidelines that reflect universal nutrient needs are similar across countries (Smitasiri and Uauy, 2007). However, country-specific dietary guidelines are probably more feasible and practical because countries differ so much in environmental circumstances, including the types of foods that are available, their nutritional content, and accessibility. In addition there are vast differences in food cultures, lifestyles, public health priorities, economics and challenges of a cultural, social, political, and communications nature between countries. Translating dietary and nutrient standards into food-based dietary guidelines is therefore primarily a local endeavor because food and food patterns are so deeply rooted in culture, and because social and cultural sensibilities are so important.

Development of Dietary Guidelines

The WHO and FAO led a worldwide effort in the 1990s to transform quantitative recommendations for nutrient intakes into general advice about dietary choices at the country level through the development of food-based dietary guidelines (Taylor, 2005). Thanks to that effort, many countries have updated and refined their country-specific food-based dietary guidelines. The process of food-based dietary guidelines development uses a stepwise approach which is summarized in Box 65.1 and described elsewhere in greater detail (World Health Organization, 2003a; Ashwell *et al.*, 2008). Guidelines that work well generally are well integrated with other nutrition information and education tools. For example, they consider not only eating and energy inputs, but also energy output and physical activity. Model dietary patterns and nutrient profiles are easy for nutritionists to create, but they are not easy to meet with common foods. Successful dietary guidelines take into account the fact that changes in food composition and availability may be needed. Without such changes many people will find the guidelines too difficult to follow.

Similarities of Dietary Guidelines Among Countries

Some characteristics of food-based dietary guidelines are common in most countries. These include maintenance of a healthy weight, promotion of consumption of a variety of foods, and increased consumption of fruits and vegetables. Most guidelines also encourage physical activity and lowering consumption of salt and sugar. In addition, depending on the country, some specify consumption of certain types of fats (monounsaturates and polyunsaturates) and discourage consumption of others (saturated/*trans* fats and cholesterol); specify types of carbohydrates ("complex" vs. total or "added" sugars), protein sources

> **BOX 65.1   Main steps in the process of developing dietary guidelines**
>
> *Identify:*
>
> - *Diet–health relationships* – Evidence on diet – health relationships is available from reviews that are carried out regularly by national and international agencies.
> - *Country-specific diet-related problems* – Specific diet-related health patterns, disease and mortality rates should be reviewed to identify and prioritize nutrition problems of public health significance.
> - *Nutrients of public-health importance* – Nutrient imbalances in the population (groups) should be identified by comparing habitual intake from dietary surveys with dietary reference values, and by using anthropometric and available biochemical indicators of nutritional status.
> - *Foods relevant for food-based dietary guidelines (FBDG)* – Food groups that are sources of nutrients of public health importance and foods for which intakes explain differences between groups who do and do not achieve target nutrient recommendations should be identified from observed patterns of dietary intake. Intake of food groups with established relationships to health (e.g. fruit and vegetables) should also be estimated.
> - *Food consumption patterns* - Food consumption patterns in the population that are consistent with achievement of recommended intakes of nutrients should be identified. In addition it is important to identify population characteristics for each pattern. Recommendations for FBDG should be made, taking into account specific needs of population groups.

(plant vs. animal origin), and grains (processed vs. whole grains), and give guidelines for water and alcohol consumption. Some also mention specific nutrients, or deal with specific problems such as inadequate intakes of iron, vitamin A, or iodine. Others mention food safety. Recommendations sometimes include statements to encourage positive behaviors that have an indirect effect on nutrition and health, such as considering meals as social occasions, enjoying food, emphasizing the role of family life and well-being, and stressing consumption of traditional or local foods (Taylor, 2005). However, only a few guidelines mention these latter recommendations.

Differences in Dietary Guidelines Among Countries

The FAO has developed an excellent website that provides detailed information on dietary guidelines from the various countries in the world. It is accessible at: http://www.fao.org/ag/agn/nutrition/education_guidelines_country_en.stm. Note that at the very time that dietary standards are increasingly being harmonized across countries, dietary guidelines are becoming more country-specific. The reasons for this relate to the more extensive use of population-based surveys of dietary intakes and health status within countries, permitting better recognition of specific nutritional problems. Also governments are increasingly aware that the cultural and economic context in which dietary recommendations are made is very country-specific.

Examples of Dietary Guidelines

Dietary Guidelines for Americans

The Dietary Guidelines for Americans are part of the core of federal dietary guidance and nutrition-related public health efforts in the United States (Dietary Guidelines Advisory Committee, 2005; Murphy, 2005; US Department of Health and Human Services and US Department of Agriculture, 2005; Dietary Guidelines Advisory Committee on the Dietary Guidelines for Americans, 2011). The policy document that incorporates them serves as a cornerstone upon which all Federal nutrition policy, education and food-assistance programs are based. In addition, all Federal dietary guidance for the public is required to be consistent with the evidence-based Dietary Guidelines so that the government speaks in a consistent and uniform manner. Consumer-focused outreach and educational materials based on the Dietary Guidelines are now widely available at http://www.healthierus.gov/dietaryguidelines.

The advisory committee for the 2010 version of the Dietary Guidelines for Americans used the USDA's new Nutrition Evidence Library for a systematic review process to review, synthesize, and analyze the latest science relevant to questions arising during guidelines development. The systematic reviews were used more extensively than was possible in earlier editions of the guidelines. The 2010 Dietary Guidelines Advisory Committee Report's overall theme was the challenge of the obesity epidemic in the United States, particularly that among children, since the prevalence of obesity has tripled in the past 30 years. It recommended four major priorities for action which are summarized below (Dietary Guidelines Advisory Committee on the Dietary Guidelines for Americans, 2011):

1. Reduce overweight and obesity by reducing overall calorie intake and increasing physical activity.
2. Shift food intake patterns to a more plant-based diet that emphasizes vegetables, cooked dry beans and peas, fruits, whole grains, nuts, and seeds. In addition increase the intake of seafood and fat-free and low-fat milk and milk products while consuming only moderate amounts of lean meats, poultry, and eggs.
3. Significantly reduce intake of foods containing added sugars and solid fats because these dietary components contribute excess calories and few, if any, nutrients. Reduce sodium. Eat fewer refined grains, especially those in foods with added sugar, solid fat, and sodium.
4. Meet the 2008 Physical Activity Guidelines for Americans (Office of Disease Prevention and Health Promotion, 2008).

MyPyramid

This is the latest version of an icon to educate consumers about diet and lifestyle that is consistent with the Dietary Guidelines for Americans. It replaces the previous food-group pyramid with a new icon that stresses physical activity, moderation, and the proper balance between food groups in the diet. Its development has been described (Britten *et al.*, 2006), and details of its construction have been outlined (Murphy, 2005). The pyramid contains six food groups, a variety of which are needed each day for health. The food groups are: vegetables, emphasizing dark green and orange vegetables, and dry beans and peas; fruits, emphasizing variety and de-emphasizing fruit juices; milk and milk-based products; meat and beans, emphasizing low-fat and lean meats such as fish as well as more beans, peas, nuts, and seeds; grains (of which at least half should be whole grains); and oils, with an emphasis on vegetable, nut, and fish sources. In addition, the top of the pyramid includes discretionary calories, including items such as candy, alcohol, and additional foods from any other group. The widths of the bands in the pyramid food group suggest proportionality and how much of the food group a person should choose. The narrowing of the food-group band from the bottom to the top represents moderation. The base of the pyramid where the band is wider stands for foods with little or no solid fats, added sugars or other caloric sweeteners, suggesting that these should be selected more often since they are the most nutrient dense. The current pyramid has 12 sets of possible patterns based on energy needs, with the appropriate guide for each individual based on sex, age group, and physical activity level. The current pyramid version and many other tools are available in personalized versions at http://www.MyPyramid.gov.

DASH

An alternative eating pattern suggested as appropriate in the Dietary Guidelines for Americans is the Dietary Approaches to Stop Hypertension (DASH) diet, which is reduced in sodium. This eating plan is also rich in fruits, vegetables, whole grains, and low-fat dairy foods, including meat, fish, poultry, nuts, and beans, and is limited in sugar-sweetened foods and beverages, red meat, and added fats. The DASH diet is based on clinical studies that show that it reduces both systolic and diastolic blood pressure (Appel et al., 1997; Sacks et al., 2001).

Disease-Specific Guidelines of Professional Associations in the USA

In North America and elsewhere in the world over the past several decades, many different disease-oriented associations have published guidelines devoted to preventing or curing various chronic diseases. The disease-specific guidelines are similar in most respects to the recommendations embodied in MyPyramid (Krebs-Smith and Kris-Etherton, 2007). Although the guidelines have no direct influence on government programs, they may influence both individuals and the policies of professional associations. Usually a group of experts on the disease in question chosen by the convening group is gathered to review the literature and provide their expert opinion. The objectivity of the group varies, as does the thoroughness of the reviews, which can vary from extremely extensive to quite cursory. The more extensive reviews include systematic evidence-based literature reviews to help ensure that all relevant information is obtained and that all of the relevant data are presented. Consortia such as the Cochrane Collaborative, the Agency for Health Research and Quality of the US Department of Health and Human Services have websites which summarize recent reviews that may be useful. The degree of specificity of topics chosen also varies greatly. For example, the American Institute of Cancer Research (AICR)/World Cancer Research Foundation conducted extensive evidence-based systematic reviews on various cancer sites before promulgating its guidelines (World

Cancer Research Foundation and American Institute for Cancer Research, 2009). Other expert groups limit their work to reviews based on more cursory analysis of the literature and expert opinion (American Heart Association Nutrition Committee et al., 2006; Gidding et al., 2006, 2009; Kushi et al., 2006; Johnson et al., 2009). The disease guidelines are largely focused on reducing risks of a specific disease and contain specific recommendations that are thought to reduce risk of the specific disease in question. Among the other organizations producing such guidelines are the American Diabetes Association (American Diabetes Association, 2008, 2010), the American Cancer Society (Kushi et al., 2006), and the American Heart Association (American Heart Association Nutrition Committee et al., 2006; Gidding et al., 2006, 2009; Johnson et al., 2009). At present there are no data that show that adhering to these guidelines actually does reduce the risk of chronic degenerative diseases any more than would adherence to the more general guidelines

Canada's Food Guide

Canada's Guidelines for Healthy Eating are clear, simple messages intended to promote healthy eating (Katamay et al., 2007), which are summarized in Box 65.2. The Canadian food guide was extensively revised in 2007 and is an integral part of Canadian health policy (Bush et al., 2007; Health Canada, 2007; Tarasuk, 2010). It employs six food groups: vegetables and fruit, grain products, milk (Barr, 2006b; Bush et al., 2007) and alternatives, meat and alternatives, oils and fats, and beverages. It also includes advice on physical activity and specific advice for individuals of different ages (children, men and women over age 50 years) and stages (women of childbearing age).

Note that the North American guidelines from the United States and Canada are similar in their basic messages because the populations, cultures, and economic and environmental conditions are alike in the two countries. They both recommend a food-based approach to eating, and the same foods/constituents to eat and to avoid. The differences are largely in the style of their presentation, language (Canadian guidelines are published in both French and English), timing (Canada's last update was in 2007 while the USA's was in 2010), and graphics used to convey the gist of the recommendations (rainbow in the Canadian guidelines vs. the US pyramid). For determining food patterns, the modeling process and foods chosen differ somewhat between the US and Canadian guidelines but again the final result is basically similar. Neither coun-

BOX 65.2 Canada's Guidelines for Healthy Eating

1. Enjoy a variety of foods.
2. Emphasize cereals, breads, other grain products, vegetables, and fruits.
3. Choose lower-fat dairy products, leaner meats and foods prepared with little or no fat.
4. Achieve and maintain a healthy body weight by enjoying regular physical activity and healthy eating.
5. Limit salt, alcohol, and caffeine.

Health Canada also endorses these specific messages about the Canadian diet:

- provide energy consistent with the maintenance of body weight within the recommended range;
- include essential nutrients in amounts specified in the recommended nutrient intakes (RNIs);
- include no more than 30% of energy as fat (33 g/1000 kcal or 39 g/5000 kJ) and no more than 10% as saturated fat (11 g/1000 kcal or 13 g/5000 kJ);
- provide 55% of energy as carbohydrate (138 g/1000 kcal or 165 g/5000 kJ) from a variety of sources;
- be reduced in sodium content;
- include no more than 5% of total energy as alcohol, or 2 drinks daily, whichever is less;
- contain no more caffeine than the equivalent of 4 cups of regular coffee per day;
- ensure that community water supplies containing less than 1 mg/L fluoride should be fluoridated to that level.

Data from Katamay *et al.* (2007).

try's planners appear to have modeled the effect of use of dietary supplements into guideline recommendations.

World Health Organization/Food and Agricultural Organization Recommendations for Food-Based Dietary Guidelines

In the 1990s the WHO/FAO undertook a major project to help countries develop food-based dietary guidelines (FAO/WHO, 2006). The methods for developing country-specific guidelines were outlined, and workshops were held to facilitate the process. At the same time, generic dietary guidelines were issued that the international organizations asserted belonged in all countries. However, since the year 2000, the WHO/FAO efforts have led a large number of countries to develop their own set of dietary guidelines

(Food and Agriculture Organization of the United Nations, 2009). They differ most markedly because of the different problems the various countries face, the resources available to deal with them, and the affluence of the various country populations.

United Kingdom

The food-based dietary guidelines developed by the UK's Food Standards Agency for all healthy individuals are summarized in Box 65.3 (Food Standards Agency, 2006). They reflect recommendations for nutrient intake that are based on advice from the UK's Committee on Medical Aspects of Food and Nutrition Policy (COMA) and the Scientific Advisory Committee on Nutrition (SACN). The Department of Health's 1991 report on Dietary Reference Values (DRVs) was used in devising the guidelines. The UK's national food guide was subjected to consumer testing before it was issued (Hunt, 2007; Hunt *et al.*, 2007). *The Balance of Good Health* is the UK's pictorial representation of the proportion that different food groups should make up in the diets of older children and adults in the UK.

Australia/New Zealand

Box 65.4 shows the dietary guidelines for Australia and New Zealand. They were developed in 2003 in a process that included systematic reviews and grading of the evidence (Baghurst, 2003; Australian National Health and Medical Research Council and New Zealand Ministry of Health, 2006).

European Union

In the year 2000, the EU issued a countrywide integrated non-communicable disease intervention strategy (World Health Organization, 2000). It included an emphasis on physical activity and a 12-point guide to eating patterns provided in Box 65.5. This was a beginning, but many European countries preferred to formulate their own dietary guidelines since food habits and food availability differed so much between countries (World Health Organization, 2003a; EFSA Panel on Dietetic Products, 2010a). The European Food Information Council (EUFIC) has compiled a comprehensive compendium of dietary guidelines and graphics for most of the European countries (European Food Information Council, 2009). The WHO's European office has provided a report on food-based dietary guidelines in Europe (World Health

BOX 65.3 Food-based dietary guidelines for the United Kingdom issued by the Food Standards Agency

All healthy individuals should consume:

- Plenty of starchy foods such as rice, bread, pasta, and potatoes (choosing whole-grain varieties when possible).
- Plenty (at least 5 portions) of a variety of fruit and vegetables each day.
- Moderate amounts of protein-rich foods such as meat, fish, eggs, and alternatives such as nuts and pulses.
- Moderate amounts of milk and dairy, choosing reduced fat versions, or eating smaller amounts of full-fat versions, or eating them less often.
- Less saturated fat, salt, and sugar. A special report issued by the Scientific Advisory Committee on Nutrition in 2003 recommended no more than 6 g salt daily.
- The UK guidelines recognize that, although most individuals should be able to get all the nutrients they need from following a healthy balanced diet, certain groups within the population may need to take dietary supplements, including the following:
  - Pregnant women and those women who may become pregnant should take 400 micrograms (µg) of folic acid daily until the 12th week of pregnancy, and folate-rich foods such as green vegetables, brown rice, and fortified breakfast cereals.
  - Pregnant and breastfeeding women should also take a daily 10-µg supplement of vitamin D.
  - Children under the age of 5 years who are not good eaters may need to take a supplement containing vitamins A, D, and C. Children who have a good appetite and eat a wide variety of foods, including fruit and vegetables, may not need them.
  - Individuals should consider taking a daily 10-µg vitamin D supplement if they are of Asian origin, rarely get outdoors or are housebound, wear clothes that cover all the skin when outdoors, or eat no meat or oily fish.

BOX 65.4 Dietary guidelines for Australia and New Zealand

Enjoy a wide variety of nutritious foods:

- Eat plenty of vegetables, legumes, and fruits.
- Eat plenty of cereals (including breads, rice, pasta, and noodles), preferably whole grain.
- Include lean meat, fish, poultry, and/or alternatives.
- Include milks, yoghurts, cheeses, and/or alternatives. Reduced-fat varieties should be chosen where possible.
- Drink plenty of water.

Take care to:

- Limit saturated fat and moderate total fat intake.
- Choose foods low in salt.
- Limit your alcohol intake if you choose to drink.
- Consume only moderate amounts of sugars and foods containing added sugars.

Prevent weight gain: be physically active and eat according to your energy needs.

- Care for your food: prepare and store it safely.
- Encourage and support breastfeeding.

Future Directions

Dietary Reference Values

Reconcile Differences in Reference Values and Speed Harmonization Efforts

Harmonization by the Institute of Medicine/Health Canada, WHO/FAO, EURECCA, the German-speaking countries of continental Europe, and Australia/New Zealand is gaining traction. Over the next decade it is to be hoped that even more consultation and collaboration will occur between these various bodies to avoid over-duplication. Ongoing efforts on harmonization include efforts of the United Nations University/WHO/FAO, EURECCA (European Recommendations Combined), fledgling efforts in Southeast Asia, the United States and Health Canada, the Nordic countries, and German-speaking countries in continental Europe.

Refine and Improve Concepts Such as the UL, the AI, and Models for Non-Nutrient Bioactives

The ULs are currently set on the basis of relatively scanty data, with functional criteria that are sometimes not clini-

Organization, 2003a). Recently the European Food Safety Authority (EFSA) issued a scientific opinion endorsing the development of food-based dietary guidelines in Europe (European Food Safety Authority, 2008, 2010b; EFSA Panel on Dietetic Products, 2010a).

BOX 65.5 European Union Twelve-Point Guide to Eating Patterns (part of the European Union's countrywide integrated non-communicable disease intervention strategy)

1. Eat a nutritious diet based on a variety of foods originating mainly from plants rather than animals.
2. Eat bread, grains, pasta, rice, or potatoes, several times a day.
3. Eat a variety of vegetables and fruits, preferably fresh and local, several times a day (at least 400 g/day).
4. Maintain body weight between the recommended limits (a BMI of 20–25) by taking moderate levels of physical activity, preferably daily.
5. Control fat intake (not more than 30% of daily energy) and replace most saturated fats with unsaturated vegetable oils or soft margarines.
6. Replace fatty meat and meat products with beans, legumes, lentils, fish, and poultry or lean meat.
7. Use milk and dairy products (kefir, sour milk, yoghurt, and cheese) that are low in both fat and salt.
8. Select foods that are low in sugar, and eat refined sugar sparingly, limiting the frequency of sugary drinks and sweets.
9. Choose a low-salt diet. Total salt intake should not be more than one teaspoon (6 g) per day, including the salt in bread and processed, cured and preserved foods. (Salt iodization should be universal where iodine deficiency is endemic.)
10. If alcohol is consumed, limit intake to no more than 2 drinks (each containing 10 g of alcohol) per day.
11. Prepare food in a safe and hygienic way. Steam, bake, boil or microwave to help reduce the amount of added fat.
12. Promote exclusive breastfeeding and the introduction of safe and adequate complementary foods from the age of about 6 months, but not before 4 months, while breastfeeding continues.

cally meaningful, and they are difficult to manipulate statistically. A model for nutrient risk assessment that would deal with ULs has been proposed by a joint WHO/FAO committee shows promise (Aggett, 2007). A conceptual framework for developing recommendations for non-

nutrient bioactive components in food such as polyphenolics is also needed.

Refine Population Nutrient Intake Goal Use
The quantitative intake goals for a population and those for individuals are not the same, because the target for the population depends on the distribution of intakes within the population. For example, if the goal is a mean population intake of 30% of calories from fat, individual goals must be much lower since some will surely not adhere to the targets completely and thus their intakes will exceed the mean population intake. This fact is widely misunderstood in formulating guidelines and targets, and needs to be addressed.

Clarify the Influence on Nutrient Requirements of Diet and Host-Related Factors that Vary from Country to Country
Habitual diets differ greatly from one country to another and affect the bioavailability of many micronutrients including calcium, magnesium, iron, zinc, protein, folate, vitamin A, and carotenoids. Host-related factors that may also vary from one country to the next and affect bioavailability and thus nutrient requirements are intestinal factors (e.g. secretion of hydrochloric acid, gastric acid, or intrinsic factor, other alterations in the permeability of the intestinal mucosa), and systemic factors (host, age, sex, ethnicity, genotype, and life stages such as pregnancy and lactation, as well as chronic and acute infections). These factors all may influence estimates of dietary requirements and may necessitate country-specific recommendations that take them into account (Gibson, 2007)

Fill Data Gaps Needed to Refine Requirements
Gaps in requirement data are quite large for some ages and life stages, especially for very young infants, weanlings, and the very old. Dose-response data also often do not exist for these and other age/sex/life-stage groups. When data are lacking, extrapolation and interpolation must be used, introducing further uncertainty. Although the needs for further research are usually mentioned in committee recommendations, once reports are issued, the research agenda tends to be neglected. When the time comes to update recommendations, the relevant research is then unavailable. Efforts now being made to synthesize research needs in a systematic way, and to call the attention of

researchers to them, should help to move the process forward in the future (Suitor and Meyers, 2007).

Adopt Meaningful Triggers for Revising and Updating Nutrient Reference Values

Until recently, countries usually updated the dietary standards for all nutrients simultaneously. This was an expensive, time-consuming process which meant that only a few experts could be engaged to deal with each nutrient. Recently, selective updating has become popular. It is triggered by indicators that a substantial amount of new data exists that may affect requirements. Selective updating permits greater focus on nutrients of public-health significance at a given time. Focusing on only a few nutrients makes it possible to have more expertise on targeted nutrients on scientific advisory committees, and permits the preparation of systematic evidence-based reviews that would be too costly to do for many nutrients all at once.

Refine Procedures for Setting Dietary Reference Intakes

The process currently used by the Institute of Medicine/Health Canada for setting DRIs relies heavily on funders asking critical questions which are then addressed by systematic evidence-based reviews of the literature. Systematic reviews are expensive and time consuming, and yet, to improve the quality of dietary reference values and guidelines, they must be funded by the public sector since the questions are not of interest to other sectors. The reviews are done by informatics experts who ensure the completeness of the search and who are assisted by content experts. The systematic reviews are then provided to an expert committee that reviews the data and other evidence, and sets the final values. Further refinements in the DRI process have been summarized (Institute of Medicine, 2008).

Find Functional Criteria Involving Chronic Disease

There is great interest in using chronic-disease endpoints as functional criteria for setting requirements, but there are so many data gaps that it has not proven possible to do so for any micronutrients, including calcium (Trumbo, 2008). The AMDRs have been set using chronic-disease endpoints derived from epidemiological data, but they are not based on experimentally determined data, nor can they ever be. Thus the standards of evidence for setting the AMDRs are far less than that used for estimating micronutrient needs.

Link Personalized Nutrition and Functional Criteria Using New Genetic Findings

The idea of establishing nutrient requirements and dietary guidelines based on an individual's nutrient needs generated by profiling the different single nucleotide polymorphisms (SNPs) involved in nutrient metabolism has been proposed for minimizing DNA damage and to maximize genomic and ultimately human health. Also of interest is whether single nucleotide polymorphisms that create metabolic inefficiencies are distributed by race and ethnicity so that certain large populations are differentially affected. If so, it is possible that needs for certain nutrients and dietary reference intakes for specific population groups might be quite different. While it may be possible to know if this is the case in a decade or two, at present there is little consensus on the nutrient needs and chronic-disease-related implications of various SNPs. Also, the measures of DNA damage and methods for minimizing these using nutrients are not yet standardized or reliable enough to permit their use (Fenech, 2010).

Make Appropriate Applications in Dietary Assessment and Planning

Over the past decade techniques for estimating usual intakes and using DRI for assessment and planning have become available (Barr, 2006a). They have been put to use in many studies of dietary adequacy in the United States, Canada, and elsewhere. Because the methods are relatively new, those who apply them need to be wary of pitfalls that can occur in assessing individuals and groups (Murphy, 2008; Murphy and Vorster, 2007; Murphy et al., 2006b). It is important that editorial boards of scientific journals refine their publication standards to insist that appropriate statistical analytic methods be used for dietary assessment and planning. The quality of surveys used for assessing nutrient adequacy varies, and this may affect the results obtained (Garcia-Alvarez et al., 2009). One problem is in determining whether the dietary reference value is flawed or if a true deficiency exists. For example, in the United States, most individuals are deficient in vitamin E according to intake data from the National Health and Nutrition Examination Survey, and yet no known adverse clinical or functional effect seems to have resulted. Such findings should trigger additional study of the reference standard to determine whether or not adjustments need to be made.

Dietary Guidelines

Use Systematic Evidence-Based Reviews in Dietary Guideline Formulation

Many of the questions that arise in formulating dietary guidelines require the daunting and time-consuming task of collecting and synthesizing a large body of literature if systematic reviews are to be used. Nevertheless, the evidence-based approach for establishing dietary guidelines proved useful in the United States in 2005 (Dietary Guidelines Advisory Committee, 2005; King and Dietary Guidelines Advisory Committee, 2007) and it has now been institutionalized in producing the Dietary Guidelines for Americans. However, much of the literature is not directed to the questions of greatest interest in formulating guidelines, and the quality of the evidence available is sometimes poor (Marantz *et al.*, 2008), signaling the need for more studies that directly approach the questions of importance to guideline formation.

Consider Topics to Include in Dietary Guidelines

There is ongoing debate over how several topics should be dealt with in guidelines. Fortified foods are often not dealt with at all or only very briefly. Food-based dietary guidelines often fail to mention dietary supplements although in many countries nutrient-containing supplements contribute large amounts to the intakes of some nutrients among groups at certain life stages. Moreover, in modeling efforts to assess shortfalls in current diets, the contributions of nutrient-containing supplements are not usually included. Yet it is well known that in some cases, such as with vitamin B_{12} among older adults, or folic acid in some women in the pre-conceptional period who are eating poor diets, intakes from food alone may not suffice to meet nutrient needs. These issues need to be recognized and dealt with. "Processed" and "organic" and "whole" foods are another controversial topic. They are viewed by some as less desirable than "unprocessed" foods, although the definitions and meanings of such terms are vague. These need to be defined, and clear rationales given, if available, for the statements made. In fact food processing has a positive role to play in improving food safety and decreasing waste (Frisch and Elmadfa, 2007). Also it is essential that the food production sector be engaged in aligning products available with the dietary guidelines (Roodenburg *et al.*, 2008). Other challenges are whether recommendations about "biotech" or genetically modified foods, foods from cloned animals such as cloned salmon, and nanotechnological applications in foods belong in dietary guidelines. Current evidence suggests that they do not pose health and safety concerns and that they are rather matters of individual preference. Alcohol is a problematic topic because it is both a food and a drug, and because its use is regarded as a moral issue by significant segments of the population in many countries. Also, some individuals simply are unable to tolerate even small amounts of alcohol without suffering adverse behavioral effects. Although alcohol produces health benefits in some individuals, such as increased HDL cholesterol levels that are clear from moderate consumption, others accrue health risks, such as increased risk of breast cancer. Thus guidance about alcohol needs to be carefully crafted by advisory committees.

Consider the Costs of Adhering to Dietary Guideline Patterns

It is important that the dietary patterns recommended in dietary guidelines be economically realistic for the population they are directed to. Low-energy-density foods can be expensive (Cassady *et al.*, 2007; Monsivais and Drewnowski, 2007) and people with low BMI have more expensive diets (Schroder *et al.*, 2006). Feasibility testing of guidelines needs to take this into account, and food policy must be considered as well.

Strengthen Links between Guidelines and the Production, Agriculture, Health, and Education Sectors

The feasibility of implementing guidelines in light of the country's existing commodities and food supplies must be taken into account, if for no other reason than to identify gaps and shortfalls and to make plans to remedy them (Duxbury and Welch, 1999). Unfortunately, most dietary guidelines are used primarily by the health sector, with little attention paid to food and agricultural sectors and in education, or in setting policies that cut across sectors (Albert, 2007).

Tailor Dietary Guidelines to Individuals

How best to develop more personalized guidelines will continue to be an issue. Dietary guidelines may need to be adapted for individuals in special groups at risk such as pregnant women or the very old and frail. Other groups call for tailoring because of their unconventional eating habits, such as vegetarians (Jacobs *et al.*, 2009). Using modern communications technology, it is now possible for consumers and health professionals to tailor and then download gender- and age-specific dietary guidelines from on-line web-based applications; such tools are available now in several countries (Stehle, 2007). In the United States one can create a personalized eating plan at http://www.MyPyramid.gov.

Integrate Dietary Guidelines with Other Community Efforts

Dietary guidelines must fit into the broader context of activities devoted to nutrition. Dietary guidelines are only one of a number of nutrition information and education tools. Harmonization of the guidelines with nutrition labels and other aids is important to increase their effectiveness.

Some experts have called for greater attention to issues such as sustainability of food resources, and the "carbon footprint" of foods suggested in guidelines. These issues are increasingly important parts of government policies (Yeatman, 2008).

Communicate Dietary Guidelines Better

One of the greatest challenges in dietary guidelines development is to ensure that messages motivate changes in behavior, which they often do not. Some messages, such as guidance to eat higher-nutrient-density, lower-caloric-density foods, are difficult to communicate, although they may be scientifically appropriate (Miller *et al.*, 2009). There is also the danger of over-medicalizing eating and implying that dietary changes can accomplish more than is realistic to expect (Fitzpatrick, 2006). The guidelines need to be communicated more widely both to consumers and to relevant policy makers (Albert, 2007). The assistance of professional communicators and dietitians can help to ensure that this is done (Brown, 2005).

Measure Adherence to Dietary Guidelines

There are several indices of dietary quality to assess adherence to dietary guidelines or other recommendations, of which the best known is the Healthy Eating Index or HEI (Guenther *et al.*, 2007; Fransen and Ocke, 2008). Indices of dietary quality have been criticized because energy intake is often not taken into account, components are scored in an arbitrary manner, and it is not clear how or if they relate to health outcomes. Alternative measures are available but it is not clear that they perform better than the HEI itself (Fogli-Cawley *et al.*, 2006). The latest version of the Healthy Eating Index and scoring information can be accessed at http://www.cnpp.usda.gov/

HealthyEatingIndex.htm. Unfortunately in spite of years of dietary guidance, the healthfulness of the US food supply has not increased dramatically (Krebs-Smith *et al.*, 2010).

Measure Guideline Effectiveness

The effectiveness of dietary guidelines has been measured in a number of ways. In the United States, dietary guidelines have become one of the major policy tools for government and are used to assess the advisability of many government programs as well as serving as nutrition education tools for communicating to consumers. While it is to be hoped that consumers will follow the guidelines and improve their health, there is little evidence that this is happening. Several efforts have been made to evaluate whether those individuals with "guideline-like" diets in post-hoc modeling of cohorts in epidemiological studies fare better health-wise than those whose diets did not conform to them.

Develop Triggers for Guideline Revision

In many countries such as the United States, dietary guidelines are revised on a regular basis every 5 or 10 years. There may be a need for the development of other criteria for revising guidelines. This has been done for the DRI, and perhaps it would be useful to do so for dietary guidelines as well.

Suggestions for Further Reading

Ashwell, M., Lambert, J.P., Alles, M.S., *et al.* (2008) How we will produce the evidence-based EURECCA toolkit to support nutrition and food policy. *Eur J Nutr* **47**(Suppl 1), 16.

Bermudez, O.K., Dwyer, J.T., Yu, W., *et al.* (2007) Dietary guidelines in three regions of the world. In C Berdanier and J.T. Dwyer (eds), *Handbook of Food and Nutrition*, 2nd Edn. CRC Press, Boca Raton, FL, pp. 429–450.

Dietary Reference Intakes of the Institute of Medicine/Health Canada can be accessed at http://fnic.nal.usda.gov.

Dwyer, J. (2005) Dietary Guidelines–National Perspectives. In Shils, M.E. *et al.* (ed.), *Modern Nutrition in Health and Disease*. Lippincott, Williams and Wilkins, Philadelphia, pp. 1673–1686.

European Food Based Dietary Guidelines, including an historical and developmental overview and a table of all countries and graphics from EU member states, are available from http://www.eufic.org/article/en/expid/food-based-dietary-guidelines-in-europe.(European Food Information Council, 2009).

Miraglia, M.L. and Dwyer, J.T (2011) New dietary guidelines and physical activity guidelines for Americans. *Am J Lifestyle Med* **5**, 144–155.

References

Aggett, P.J. (2007) Nutrient risk assessment: setting upper levels and an opportunity for harmonization. *Food Nutr Bull* **28**, S27–37.

Albert, J. (2007) Global patterns and country experiences with the formulation and implementation of food-based dietary guidelines. *Ann Nutr Metab* **51**, 2–7.

American Diabetes Association (2008) Nutrition recommendations and interventions for diabetes: a position statement of the American Diabetes Association. *Diabetes Care* **31**, S61–S78.

American Diabetes Association (2010) Executive summary: standards of medical care in diabetes – 2010. *Diabetes Care* **33**, S4–S10.

American Heart Association Nutrition Committee, Lichtenstein, A.H., Appel, L.J., *et al.* (2006) Diet and lifestyle recommendations revision 2006: a scientific statement from the American Heart Association Nutrition Committee. *Circulation* **114**, 82–96.

Appel, L., Moore, T., Obarzanek, E., *et al.* (1997) A clinical trial of the effects of dietary patterns on blood pressure. *N Engl J Med* **336**, 1117–1124.

Ashwell, M., Lambert, J.P., Alles, M.S., *et al.* (2008) How we will produce the evidence-based EURRECA toolkit to support nutrition and food policy. *Eur J Nutr* **47**(Suppl 1), 2–16.

Australian National Health and Medical Research Council and New Zealand Ministry of Health (2006) *Nutrient Reference Values for Australia and New Zealand Including Recommended Dietary Intakes.* http://www.nhmrc.gov.au/_files_nhmrc/file/publications/synopses/n35.pdf

Baghurst, K.I. (2003) Dietary guidelines: the development process in Australia and New Zealand. *J Am Diet Assoc* **103**, S17–21.

Barba, C.V. and Cabrera, M.I. (2008) Recommended dietary allowances harmonization in Southeast Asia. *Asia Pac J Clin Nutr* **17**(Suppl 2), 405–408.

Barr, S.I. (2006a) Applications of Dietary Reference Intakes in dietary assessment and planning. *Appl Physiol Nutr Metab* **31**, 66–73.

Barr, S.I. (2006b) Introduction to dietary reference intakes. *Appl Physiol Nutr Metab* **31**, 61–65.

Becker, W., Lyhne, N., Pedersen, A.N., *et al.* (2004) Nordic nutrition recommendations 2004 – integrating nutrition and physical activity. *Scand J Nutr* **48**, 178–187.

Britten, P.L., Weaver, J., Kris-Etherton, C., *et al.* (2006) MyPyramid food intake pattern modeling for the Dietary Guidelines Advisory Committee. *J Nutr Educ Behav* **38**, S143–S152.

Brown, D. (2005) New dietary guidelines need dietetic interpretation. *J Am Diet Assoc* **105**, 1356–1357.

Bush, M., Martineau, C., Pronk, J.A., *et al.* (2007) Eating Well with Canada's Food Guide: "A tool for the times". *Can J Diet Pract Res* **68**, 92–96.

Cassady, D., Jetter, K.M., and Culp, J. (2007) Is price a barrier to eating more fruits and vegetables for low-income families? *J Am Diet Assoc* **107**, 1909–1915.

Chung, M., Balk, E.M., and Brendel, M.E.A. (2009) Vitamin D and calcium: a systematic review of health outcomes. *Evidence Report No. 183, AHRQ publication no. 09-E105.* Agency for Healthcare Research and Quality, Rockville, MD.

Chung, M., Balk, E.M., Ip, S., *et al.* (2010) Systematic review to support the development of nutrient reference intake values: challenges and solutions. *Am J Clin Nutr* **92**, 273–276.

Dietary Guidelines Advisory Committee(2005) *The Report of the Dietary Guidelines Advisory Committee on Dietary Guidelines for Americans, 2005.* http://www.health.gov/dietaryguidelines/dga2005/report/default.htm.

Dietary Guidelines Advisory Committee on the Dietary Guidelines for Americans (2011) *Report of the Dietary Guidelines Advisory Committee on the Dietary Guidelines for Americans, 2010,* Washington, DC.

Doets, E.L., De Wit, L. S., Dhonukshe-Rutten, R.A., *et al.* (2008) Current micronutrient recommendations in Europe: towards understanding their differences and similarities. *Eur J Nutr* **47**(Suppl 1), 17–40.

Duxbury, A.J. and Welch, R.M. (1999) Agriculture and dietary guidelines. *Food Policy* **24**, 197–209.

EFSA Panel on Dietetic Products, Nutrition, and Allergies (2010a) Scientific Opinion on establishing food-based dietary guidelines. *EFSA J* **8**, 1460. http://www.efsa.europa.eu/en/efsajournal/scdoc/1460.htm.

EFSA Panel on Dietetic Products, Nutrition, and Allergies (2010b) Scientific Opinion on Dietary Reference Values for fats, including saturated fatty acids, polyunsaturated fatty acids, monounsaturated fatty acids, trans fatty acids and cholesterol. *EFSA J* **8**, 1461. http://www.efsa.europa.eu/de/efsajournal/pub/1461.htm.

EFSA Panel on Dietetic Products, Nutrition, and Allergies (2010c) Scientific Opinion on Dietary Reference Values for carbohydrates and dietary fiber. *EFSA J* **8**, 1462. http://www.efsa.europa.eu/en/efsajournal/pub/1462.htm.

Elmadfa, I. and Komsteiner, M. (2009) Fats and fatty acid requirements for adults. *Ann Nutr Metab* **55**, 56–75.

European Food Information Council (2009) *EUFIC Review 10/2009: Food-Based Dietary Guidelines in Europe.* http://www.eufic.org/article/en/expid/food-based-dietary-guidelines-in-europe/.

European Food Safety Authority (2008) *Public Consultation of the Scientific Panel on Dietetic Products, Nutrition and Allergies on a Draft Opinion Related to Food-Based Dietary Guidelines.* http://www.efsa.europa.eu/EFSA/efsa_locale-1178620753812_1211902045161.htm.

European Food Safety Authority (2010a) EFSA sets European dietary reference values for nutrient intakes. http://www.efsa.europa.eu/en/press/news/nda100326.htm.

European Food Safety Authority (2010b) Outcome of the Public Consultation on the Draft Opinion of the Scientific Panel on Dietetic Products, Nutrition, and Allergies (NDA) on Establishing Food-Based Dietary Guidelines *EFSA Journal* **8**, 1506. www.efsa.europa.eu/en/scdocs/scdoc/1506.htm.

FAO/WHO (2006) *FAO/WHO Technical Consultation on National Food-based Dietary Guidelines report.* FAO, Cairo.

Fenech, M.F. (2010) Dietary reference values of individual micronutrients and nutriomes for genome damage prevention: current status and a road map to the future. *Am J Clin Nutr* **91**, 1438S–1454S.

Fitzpatrick, M. (2006) Dietary dogma. *Br J Gen Pract* **56**, 63.

Fogli-Cawley, J., Dwyer, J., Saltzman, E., *et al.* (2006) The 2005 Dietary Guidelines for Americans Adherence Index: development and application. *J Nutr* **136**, 2908–2915.

Food and Agriculture Organization of the United Nations (2009) *Food-Based Dietary Guidelines: Food Guidelines by Country.* http://www.fao.org/ag/humannutrition/nutritioneducation/fbdg/en/.

Food Standards Agency (2006) *FSA Nutrient and Food Based Guidelines for UK Institutes.* Food Standards Agency, London.

Fransen, H.P. and Ocke, M.C. (2008) Indices of diet quality. *Curr Opin Clin Nutr Metab Care* **11**, 559–565.

Frisch, G. and Elmadfa, I. (2007) Impact of food processing on the implementation of dietary guidelines. *Ann Nutr Metab* **51**, 50–53.

Garcia-Alvarez, A., Blanquer, M., Ribas-Barba, L., *et al.* (2009) How does the quality of surveys for nutrient intake adequacy assessment compare across Europe? A scoring system to rate the quality of data in such surveys. *Br J Nutr* **101**(Suppl 2), S51–63.

German Nutrition Society, Austrian Nutrition Society, Swiss Society for Nutrition Research, *et al.* (2000) *Reference Values for Nutrient Intake (D-A-CH).* Umshau/Braus, Frankfurt am Main.

Gibson, R. (2007) The role of diet- and host-related factors in nutrient bioavailability and thus in nutrient-based dietary requirement estimates. *Food Nutr Bull* **28**, S 77–S100.

Gidding, S.S., Dennison, B.A., Birch, L.L., *et al.* (2006) Dietary recommendations for children and adolescents: a guide for practitioners. *Pediatrics* **117**, 544–559.

Gidding, S.S., Lichtenstein, A.H., Faith, M.S., *et al.* (2009) Implementing American Heart Association pediatric and adult nutrition guidelines: a scientific statement from the American Heart Association Nutrition Committee of the Council on Nutrition, Physical Activity and Metabolism, Council on Cardiovascular Disease in the Young, Council on Arteriosclerosis, Thrombosis and Vascular Biology, Council on Cardiovascular Nursing, Council on Epidemiology and Prevention, and Council for High Blood Pressure Research. *Circulation* **119**, 1161–1175.

Guenther, M., Reedy, J., Krebs-Smith, S., *et al.* (2007) *Development and Evaluation of the Healthy Eating Index – 2005: Technical Report.* Center for Nutrition Policy and Promotion, US Department of Agriculture, Washington, DC.

Health Canada (2007) *Eating Well with Canada's Food Guide: A Resource for Educators and Communicators.* Health Canada, Ottawa.

Hegsted, D.M. (1975) Dietary standards. *J Am Diet Assoc* **66**, 13–21.

Hunt, P. (2007) Commentary on Hunt, P., Gatenby, S. and Rayner, M. (1995) The format for the National Food Guide: performance and preference studies. *J Human Nutr Diet* **8**, 335–351. *J Hum Nutr Diet* **20**, 227–228.

Hunt, P., Gatenby, S., and Raynert, M. (2007) The format for the National Food Guide: performance and preference studies. *J Hum Nutr Diet* **20**, 210–226.

Institute of Medicine (2000) *Dietary Reference Intakes: Applications in Dietary Assessment.* National Academy Press, Washington, DC.

Institute of Medicine (2003) *Dietary Reference Intakes: Applications in Dietary Planning.* National Academies Press, Washington, DC.

Institute of Medicine (2008) *The Development of DRIs 1994–2004: Lessons Learned and New Challenges – Workshop Summary.* National Academies Press. Washington, DC.

Jacobs, D.R., Jr, Haddad, E.H., Lanou, A.J., *et al.* (2009) Food, plant food, and vegetarian diets in the US dietary guidelines: conclusions of an expert panel. *Am J Clin Nutr* **89**, 1549S–1552S.

Johnson, R.K., Appel, L.J., Brands, M., *et al.* (2009) Dietary sugars intake and cardiovascular health: a scientific statement from the American Heart Association. *Circulation* **120**, 1011–1020.

Joint WHO/FAO/UNU Expert Consultation (2007) Protein and amino acid requirements in human nutrition. *World Health Organization Tech Rep Ser* 1–265.

Joint FAO/WHO Expert Consultation on Human Vitamin and Mineral Requirements (2004) *Vitamin and Mineral Requirements in Human Nutrition*, 2nd Edn. Report of a Joint FAO/WHO Expert Consultation, Bangkok, Thailand, 21–30 September 1998. World Health Organization, Geneva.

Joint FAO/WHO Technical Workshop on Nutrient Risk Assessment (2006) *A Model for Establishing Upper Levels of Intake for Nurients and Related Substances*. World Health Organization, Geneva.

Katamay, S.W., Esslinger, K.A., Vigneault, M., *et al.* (2007) Eating well with Canada's Food Guide (2007): development of the food intake pattern. *Nutr Rev* **65**, 155–166.

King, J.C. and Dietary Guidelines Advisory Committee (2007) An evidence-based approach for establishing dietary guidelines. *J Nutr* **137**, 480–483.

King, J.C. and Garza, C. (2007) Harmonization of nutrient intake values. *Food Nutr Bull* **28**, S3–12.

King, J.C., Vorster, H.H., and Tome, D.G. (2007) Nutrient intake values (NIVs): a recommended terminology and framework for the derivation of values. *Food Nutr Bull* **28**, S16–S26.

Krebs-Smith, S.M. and Kris-Etherton, P. (2007) How does MyPyramid compare to other population-based recommendations for controlling chronic disease? *J Am Diet Assoc* **107**, 830–837.

Krebs-Smith, S.M., Reedy, J., and Bosire, C. (2010) Healthfulness of the U.S. food supply: little improvement despite decades of dietary guidance. *Am J Prev Med* **38**, 472–477.

Kushi, L.H., Byers, T., Doyle, C., *et al.* (2006) American Cancer Society Guidelines on Nutrition and Physical Activity for cancer prevention: reducing the risk of cancer with healthy food choices and physical activity. *CA Cancer J Clin* **56**, 254–281; Quiz 313–314.

Lichtenstein, A.H., Yetley, E.A., and Lau, J. (2008) Application of systematic review methodology to the field of nutrition. *J Nutr* **138**, 2297–2306.

Mann, J., Cummings, J.H., Englyst, H.N., *et al.* (2007) FAP/WHO scientific update on carbohydrates in human nutrition: conclusions. *Eur J Clin Nutr* **61**(Suppl 1), S132–S137.

Marantz, P.R., Bird, E.D., and Alderman, M.H. (2008) A call for higher standards of evidence for dietary guidelines. *Am J Prev Med* **34**, 234–240.

Miller, G.D., Drewnowski, A., Fulgoni, V., *et al.* (2009) It is time for a positive approach to dietary guidance using nutrient density as a basic principle. *J Nutr* **139**, 1198–1202.

Monsivais, P. and Drewnowski, A. (2007) The rising cost of low-energy-density foods. *J Am Diet Assoc* **107**, 2071–2076.

Mozaffarian, D., Aro, A., and Willett, W.C. (2009) Health effects of trans-fatty acids: experimental and observational evidence. *Eur J Clin Nutr* **63**, S5–S21.

Murphy, S.P. (2005) Dietary standards in the United States. In B.A. Bowman and R.M. Russell (eds), *Present Knowledge in Nutrition*, 9th Edn. ILSI Press, Washington, DC.

Murphy, S.P. (2008) Using DRIs for dietary assessment. *Asia Pac J Clin Nutr* **17**(Suppl 1), 299–301.

Murphy, S.P. and Vorster, H.H. (2007) Methods for using nutrient intake values (NIVs) to assess or plan nutrient intakes. *Food Nutr Bull* **28**, S51–S60.

Murphy, S.P., Barr, S.I., and Yates, A.A. (2006a) The Recommended Dietary Allowance (RDA) should not be abandoned: an individual is both an individual and a member of a group. *Nutr Rev* **64**, 313–315; Discussion 315–318.

Murphy, S.P., Guenther, P.M., and Kretsch, M.J. (2006b) Using the dietary reference intakes to assess intakes of groups: pitfalls to avoid. *J Am Diet Assoc* **106**, 1550–1553.

Nishida, C. and Martinez Nocito, F. (2007) FAO/WHO scientific update on carbohydrates in human nutrition: introduction. *Eur J Clin Nutr* **61**, S1–14.

Office of Disease Prevention and Health Promotion (2008) *Physical Activity Guidelines for Americans*. US Department of Health and Human Services, Washington, DC.

Panel on Dietary Reference Values of the Committee on Medical Aspects of Food Policy (1991) *Dietary Reference Values for Food Energy and Nutrients for the United Kingdom*. HMSO, London.

Panel on Dietary Reference Values of the Committee on Medical Aspects of Food Policy. (2006) *Dietary Reference Values for Food Energy and Nutrients for the United Kingdom*. Department of Health, London.

Pavlovic, M., Prentice, A., Thorsdottir, I., *et al.* (2007) Challenges in harmonizing energy and nutrient recommendations in Europe. *Ann Nutr Metab* **51**, 108–114.

Pijls, L., Ashwell, M., and Lambert, J. (2009) EURRECA – a Network of Excellence to align European micronutrient recommendations. *Food Chem* **113**, 748–753.

Prentice, A., Branca, F., Decsi, T., *et al.* (2004) Energy and nutrient dietary reference values for children in Europe: methodological approaches and current nturitional recommendations. *Br J Nutr* **92**(Suppl 2), S83–S146.

Rand, W.M. (1990) The probability approach to nutrient requirements. *Food Nutr Bull* **12**, 1–8.

Report of the Joint FAO/WHO/UNU Expert Consultation (2004) *Human Energy Requirements*. United National University, World Health Organization, Food and Agriculture Organization of the United Nations, Rome.

Roodenburg, A.J.C., Feunekes, G.I.J., Leenen, R., *et al.* (2008) Food products and dietary guidelines: how to align? *Trends Food Sci Technol* **19**, 165–170.

Russell, R., Chung, M., Balk, E.M., *et al.* (2009) Opportunities and challenges in conducting systematic reviews to support the development of nutrient reference values: vitamin A as an example. *Am J Clin Nutr* **89**, 728–733.

Russell, R.M. (2008) Current framework for DRI development: what are the pros and cons? *Nutr Rev* **66**, 455–458.

Sacks, F.M., Svetkey, L.P., Vollmer, W.M., *et al.* (2001) Effects on blood pressure of reduced dietary sodium and the Dietary Approaches to Stop Hypertension (DASH) diet. *N Engl J Med* **344**, 3–10.

Schroder, H., Marrugat, J., and Covas, M.I. (2006) High monetary costs of dietary patterns associated with lower body mass index: a population-based study. *Int J Obes (Lond)* **30**, 1574–1579.

Smit, L.A., Mozaffarian, D., and Willett, W. (2009) Review of fat and fatty acid requirements and criteria for developing dietary guidelines. *Ann Nutr Metab* **55**, 44–55.

Smitasiri, S. and Uauy, R. (2007) Beyond recommendations: implementing food-based dietary guidelines for healthier populations. *Food Nutr Bull* **28**, S141–151.

Stehle, P. (2007) Dissemination of nutritional knowledge in Germany – nutrition circle, 3D food pyramid and 10 nutrition guidelines. *Ann Nutr Metab* **51**, 21–25.

Suitor, C. and Meyers, L. (2007) *Dietary Reference Intakes: Research Synthesis Workshop Summary*. National Academies Press, Washington, DC.

Tabacchi, G., Wijnhoven, T.M., Branca, F., *et al.* (2009) How is the adequacy of micronutrient intake assessed across Europe? A systematic literature review. *Br J Nutr* **101**(Suppl 2), S29–36.

Tarasuk, V. (2010) Policy directions to promote healthy dietary patterns in Canada. *Appl Physiol Nutr Metab* **35**, 229–233.

Taylor, C.L., Albert, J., Weisel,L.R., *et al.* (2005) International Dietary Standards: FAO and WHO. In B.A. Bowman and R.M. Russell (eds), *Present Knowledge in Nutrition*, 9th Edn. ILSI Press, Washington, DC.

Thuraisingam, S., Riddell, L., Cook, K., *et al.* (2009) The politics of developing reference standards for nutrient intakes: the case of Australia and New Zealand. *Public Health Nutr* **12**, 1531–1539.

Trumbo, P.R. (2008) Challenges with using chronic disease endpoints in setting dietary reference intakes. *Nutr Rev* **66**, 459–464.

US Department of Health and Human Services and US Department of Agriculture (2005) *Dietary Guidelines for Americans, 2005*. US Government Printing Office. Washington, DC. http://www.health.gov/dietaryguidelines/dga2005/document/default.htm.

Uuay, R. and Dangour, A.D. (2009) Fat and fatty acid requirements and recommendations for infants of 0–2 years and children of 2–18 years. *Ann Nutr Metab* **55**, 76–96.

Uuay, R., Aro, A., Clarke, R., *et al.* (2009) WHO Scientific Update on *trans* fatty acids: summary and conclusions. *Eur J Clin Nutr*, **63**, S68–S75.

Wartella, E, Lichtenstein, A.H., and Boon, C.S. (eds) (2010) *Examination of Front of Package Nutrition Rating Systems and Symbols: Phase 1 Report*. National Academies Press, Washington, DC.

World Cancer Research Foundation and American Institute for Cancer Research (2009) *Food, Nutrition, Physical Activity and the Prevention of Cancer: a Global Perspective*. http://www.dietandcancerreport.org/.

World Health Organization (2000) *CINDI (Countrywide Integrated Noncommunicable Disease Intervention) Dietary Guide - EUR/00/5018028*. http://www.paho.org/english/AD/DPC/NC/cindi-diet.pdf.

World Health Organization (2003a) *Food-Based Dietary Guidelines in the WHO European Region*. WHO Regional Office for Europe, Copenhagen.

World Health Organization (2003b) *Diet, Nutrition and the Prevention of Chronic Diseases. Report of a Joint WHO/FAO Expert Consultation*. World Health Organization, Geneva.

Yates, A.A. (2007) Using criteria to establish nutrient intake values (NIVs). *Food Nutr Bull* **28**, S38–S50.

Yeatman, H. (2008) Window of opportunity – positioning food and nutrition policy within a sustainability agenda. *Aust N Z J Public Health* **32**, 107–109.

66

THE ROLE OF UNITED NATIONS AGENCIES IN ESTABLISHING INTERNATIONAL DIETARY STANDARDS*

ROBERT WEISELL, PhD AND JANICE ALBERT, PhD

Food and Agriculture Organization of the United Nations, Rome, Italy

Summary

Information about human nutrient requirements is essential for ensuring the adequacy of food supplies and preventing food/nutrient deficiencies. This information is also required for preventing excessive consumption of some nutrient substances. Food-based dietary guidelines are examples of national policies that make use of nutrient requirement dietary standards.

In this chapter, the work of the Food and Agriculture Organization and the World Health Organization related to nutrient requirements is explained. The recommended levels of intake for essential nutrients produced by these UN agencies take into consideration the diversity of situations in countries, and are used to promote actions to encourage healthy eating patterns. The work of the Codex Alimentarius Commission in providing guidelines for the presentation of specific nutrition information on the label of food products is discussed. Over time, there has been an evolution in the types and quality of data available as well as the efforts to strengthen the process of decision-making regarding scientific advice.

Introduction

In its most pragmatic sense, knowledge of human nutrient requirements is essential for assessing whether food supplies are adequate to meet a population's nutritional needs.

The views expressed are those of the authors and do not necessarily reflect the views of the Food and Agriculture Organization of the United Nations.

*Authors' note: This chapter is an update of Chapter 64 in the 9th edition publication. Thus, while there is new information included, some of the information given in the earlier edition remains accurate and important.

In turn, this information can contribute to the estimation of the numbers of persons globally, regionally or nationally who may be food/nutrient deficient or at nutritional risk. Such knowledge also underpins the ability to plan for food production to meet nutritional needs and for nutrition interventions such as food fortification. More recently, interest has expanded to include concerns about excess consumption of nutrient substances as well as dietary choices that may contribute to reducing the risk of some diseases. Food-based dietary guidelines and efforts to provide nutrition information on food labels are examples of national policies that are designed both to assist consumers in making better food choices and in turn to

Present Knowledge in Nutrition, Tenth Edition. Edited by John W. Erdman Jr, Ian A. Macdonald and Steven H. Zeisel.
© 2012 International Life Sciences Institute. Published 2012 by John Wiley & Sons, Inc.

support the implementation of nutrition-related health programs. These nutrition interventions are based on nutrient recommendations.

This chapter explains the United Nations' work related to nutrient requirements and some of their practical applications. Primary emphasis is given to the Food and Agriculture Organization (FAO) and the World Health Organization (WHO), although in some instances the collaborative work has extended to other UN organizations such as the United Nations University (UNU) and the International Agency for Atomic Energy (IAEA). The activities relate primarily to the normative work and complementary mandates of the FAO and WHO in their efforts to periodically quantify and, in turn, recommend levels of intake for essential nutrients which take into consideration the diversity of situations in countries, and to promote actions to encourage practical guidance for healthy eating patterns. In addition it highlights the work of the Joint FAO/WHO Food Standards Programme (commonly known as the Codex Alimentarius Commission[1]) in providing guidelines for the presentation of specific nutrition information on the labels of food products. Although the activities are listed as distinct and separate entities, it should be remembered that they actually form an interrelated mosaic of initiatives with continual and frequent overlapping.

Attention is drawn to the range of terms used to refer to various review processes, e.g. Expert Committee, Expert Consultation, Technical Workshop, and Scientific Update; each type of review has its own protocol and rules of procedures; these rules continually change. Together, these procedures lead to a variety of forums for carrying out the Organizations' work.

Experts from academia and research institutes have always been the central players and contributors to the reviews. In addition, the reports of national agencies have often been part of the background documentation of the meetings. At times the recommendations from these reports became in full or in part the UN reports' recommendations after careful consideration and debate. One

important development in recent reports and also in current work is the more systematic application of criteria to describe the strength of evidence and to draw conclusions from the scientific review of the totality of the evidence. Thus, over time, there have been improvements in the types and quality of data available as well as the efforts to strengthen the process of decision making in relation to scientific advice.

Recommended Nutrient Intakes

Throughout history, human societies have observed relationships between the consumption of certain foods and the preservation of good health or the avoidance of disease. However, today's concept of nutrition that human health requires a steady intake of a variety of specific dietary substances in defined amounts is less than 200 years old. During the 20th century a number of countries established expert committees to provide scientific advice on topics related to nutrient requirements and other information important to consumers in order to address the public-health needs of their respective populations.

International efforts to address food and nutrition issues were a component of the work of the League of Nations during the 1930s (League of Nations, 1936), and the United Nations took up this task during its earliest days in 1948 when the Standing Advisory Committee to the newly formed FAO considered that "the problem of assessing the calorie and nutrient requirements of human beings, with the greatest possible degree of accuracy, is of basic importance to FAO" (FAO, 1950). Over time, scientific and technical recommendations about nutrient requirements have been made by expert groups established by the FAO and WHO. In 1949, when FAO and WHO began their collaborative efforts on nutrition, the FAO/WHO Expert Committee on Nutrition was formed to provide technical advice to the Director-Generals of the two organizations in all areas of nutrition on a regular basis (WHO, 1950). The outcomes of these discussions have been widely used internationally.

Energy and Protein

Although a range of nutrition topics have been covered by expert groups convened by the FAO and WHO, macronutrients and in particular energy and protein have received the most attention over the years. This is because of the considerable concern about hunger and food insufficiency

---

[1] The Codex Alimentarius Commission and its committees deal with a wide range of food quality, food safety, and trade topics. The nutrition work described in this chapter relates primarily to food quality. In recent years, a transition has begun with a shift from trade-based standards to consumer-based standards and guidelines. (See Randell, 2010, and CAC, 2006.)

that predates the 1950s and continues through to the present. More recently, micronutrients and concerns for overnutrition (notably energy intake) have received increasing attention. In the past, no defined process existed for selecting a particular nutrient for investigation, and the decision had been based largely on the immediate concern at that particular moment.

Reports focusing solely on energy requirements, or "calorie needs," the original term used, were issued in 1950, 1957, and 2004 (FAO, 1950, 1957a, 2004). Reports concerning protein requirements were made available in 1957, 1964/1965, and 2007 (FAO, 1957b, 1964; WHO, 1965, 2007). There have been several instances when FAO and WHO published the report of a joint meeting under their respective publication series and at times not in the same year. Such was the case for FAO (1964) and WHO (1965); FAO (1973) and WHO (1973a); FAO (2002) and WHO (2004b). Energy and protein intake recommendations were considered together in reports published in 1973 and 1985 (FAO, 1973; WHO, 1973a, 1985). Owing to a number of issues following the 1973 report, two "informal" gatherings of experts took place in 1975 and 1979 to discuss the issues that were emerging (FAO, 1975; WHO, 1979) and to prepare for the next expert consultation which occurred in 1981, and the report was issued in 1985.

Many of the considerations outlined by these first expert meetings are still pertinent today. They noted that requirements set by experts were intended for groups of persons rather than individuals, and they specified that an average requirement can never be compared directly with an individual requirement.

Energy

In the 1981 meeting report (WHO, 1985), the experts corrected some of the information in the 1973 report (FAO, 1973; WHO, 1973a) and rejected the concept of a reference man or woman as too restrictive and not reflective of the wide range of both body size and patterns of physical activity. The use of a reference man or woman was replaced by actual body weights, which were increasingly available as well as the set of ideal body weights.

For energy a new methodology for calculating requirements was presented. It was based on total energy expenditure (TEE) values for various activities and lifestyles, representative body weights for various populations throughout the world, and a set of equations for calculating basal metabolic rate (BMR) values. The approach specified that estimates for energy requirements should be based, as much as possible, on estimates of TEE since the prevailing method of determination – from observed intakes of food energy – was and still is problematic and at the same time served to support a circular argument that access to food determined energy needs. The experts were, however, aware of the limited data on energy expenditures, particularly among children, and they acknowledged that no reliable and widely usable method was available to collect such data from the range of population groups worldwide. They encouraged immediate work to address this data gap. Moreover, in specifying the importance of the BMR in expressing energy requirements, they indicated that research was needed to obtain a database of BMR values, an activity that began immediately after the consultation (Schofield et al., 1985).

By 2000, scientific understanding related to energy requirements and protein as well as amino acids had advanced to a stage that they required independent deliberations. To facilitate two expert meetings, one on energy and one on protein, a series of working groups were tasked with addressing key issues and presenting their results as background papers.

An expert consultation on energy requirements was convened in 2001, and its report (FAO, 2004) contains a considerable level of new information including requirements based on improved data for TEE, most notably for infants and the elderly. Among the most important new concepts and recommendations are the following.

- The calculations of energy requirements for all ages are based on measurements and estimates of total daily energy expenditure, and on the energy needs for growth, pregnancy, and lactation.
- The requirements and dietary energy recommendations for infants/children and adolescents have been modified in the light of new data and correct previous overestimations for the former group and underestimations for the latter.
- Starting as early as 6 years of age, proposals are made for differentiating the requirements for populations with lifestyles that involve different levels of habitual physical activity.
- Reassessment of energy requirements for adults based on energy-expenditure estimates expressed as multiples of basal metabolism.

- A classification of physical activity levels based on the degree of habitual activity was devised that is consistent with long-term good health, the reduced risk of diseases associated with sedentary lifestyles and the maintenance of a healthy body weight.
- The energy needs of pregnancy and lactation were based on newly developed factorial estimates.
- The total additional dietary energy needs during pregnancy should be distributed within the two last trimesters.

Following this consultation, a technical workshop was held to discuss the specific issue of "food energy" since recommendations for optimal energy requirements become practical only when they are related to foods that provide the energy to meet these requirements. The gains in understanding of the digestion and metabolism of food and the increasing sophistication of analytical techniques meant that the various options available to express the energy value of foods needed to be standardized and harmonized. The recommendations of this workshop were published in 2003 (FAO, 2003).

Carbohydrates

Recommendations concerning carbohydrates in human nutrition were first issued in 1980 (FAO, 1980). A second expert meeting was held and a report issued in 1998 (FAO, 1998). The latter report continued the discussions begun in 1980, but also focused on the role of carbohydrates in the maintenance of health and in reducing the risk of chronic diseases. Further, it included a section on goals and guidelines for carbohydrate food choices.

Several key points from the 1998 report are listed in Table 66.1. The report specified terminology and classification nomenclature for carbohydrate components, and encouraged the production and consumption of root crops and pulses. Discussions focused not only on the maintenance of health and reduction of disease risk, but also on glycemic index, which was regarded as a potentially useful indicator of the impact of foods on the blood glucose response. Further, the report text indicates there is no evidence of a direct involvement of sucrose, other sugars and starch in the etiology of lifestyle-related diseases.

Following the 1997 Expert Consultation, discussions were initiated to determine the best approach to update

TABLE 66.1 Highlights of the recommendations on carbohydrate from the 1997 Joint Expert Consultation FAO

Issue	Recommendation
Definition of carbohydrate	Carbohydrates are polyhydroxy aldehydes, ketones, alcohols, acids, their simple derivatives and their polymers having linkages of the acetal type. They may be classified according to their degree of polymerization and may be divided initially into three principal groups, namely sugars, oligosaccharides, and polysaccharides.
Role in maintenance of health	Optimum diet of at least 55% of total energy from a variety of carbohydrate sources for all ages except for children under the age of 2 years. Fat should not be specifically restricted below the age of 2 years. Optimum diet should be gradually introduced beginning at 2 years of age.
Role in disease risk reduction	The bulk of carbohydrate-containing foods consumed should be those rich in non-starch polysaccharides and with a low glycemic index. Appropriately processed cereals, vegetables, legumes, and fruits are particularly good food choices. Excess energy intake in any form will cause body fat accumulation, so that excess consumption of low-fat foods, while not as obesity-producing as excess consumption of high-fat products, will lead to obesity if energy expenditure is not increased. Excessive intakes of sugars which compromise micronutrient density should be avoided.

Adapted from FAO (1998).

the recommendations on carbohydrates. This was considered necessary given the developments and other relevant recommendations made during the intervening period, including those from the 2002 Joint WHO/FAO Expert Consultation on Diet, Nutrition and the Prevention of Chronic Diseases (WHO, 2003). As a result the FAO and WHO agreed to undertake a scientific update on some of the key issues related to carbohydrates in human nutrition. The issues identified included terminology and classification, measurement, physiology, carbohydrates and associated diseases such as obesity, diabetes mellitus, cardiovascular diseases, and cancer, as well as the roles of glycemic index and glycemic load (Nishida et al., 2007).

The Scientific Update drew a number of conclusions, some of which endorsed those from the 1997 Expert Consultation. An improvement in the definition of dietary fiber was noted, and the experts recommended that it be based on well-established health benefits and the ability to fulfill regulatory requirements. The experts went further and proposed that dietary fiber be defined as intrinsic plant cell wall polysaccharides and thus the methods of analysis should be such as to accommodate this definition. The scientific update endorsed the recommendation of the 2002 Joint WHO/FAO Expert Consultation (WHO, 2003) concerning the restriction of beverages high in free sugars and the limitation of total intake of free sugars to reduce the risk of overweight and obesity; this recommendation was considerably more emphatic than that from the 1997 Expert Consultation (FAO, 1998). Whereas the 1997 Expert Consultation recommended the use of a particular food's low glycemic index as a guide to the quality of a carbohydrate-containing food, the Scientific Update urged caution in relying on it as a sole determinant. The scientific update closed with a call for research and discussion in a number of scientific areas which would hopefully lead to a subsequent expert consultation on carbohydrates.

Protein and Amino Acids

The most recent meeting on protein requirements was held in 2002, and the subsequent report was issued in 2007 (WHO, 2007). Within that report, as was the case in its predecessor (WHO, 1985), the dietary requirements for protein and amino acids are based on an intake which balances all losses observed in a healthy, weight-stable subject. In using nitrogen equilibrium as the proxy measure of protein intake and losses, the minimum protein requirement (MPR) is determined as the intake resulting in zero

balance. The intake for nitrogen equilibrium was derived from a meta-analysis of nitrogen balance studies by linear regression for each individual studied (Rand et al., 2003).

The 2007 report differs from previous reports in distinguishing between safe intakes for individuals and for populations. For an individual, as in previous reports, the safe individual intake is defined as the 97.5th percentile of the distribution of individual requirements, nominally the average + 1.96 SD. However, for a population, a safe intake (<2.5% risk of deficiency) must also account for the distribution of individual intakes as well as requirements, which is accomplished via an algorithm. In almost all circumstances the safe population intake is greater than the safe individual intake. The approximate deficiency prevalence is the proportion of the population with intakes below the mean requirement. A tolerable upper limit (TUL) is not identified although the report reviews the evidence of harm or toxicity from very high protein diets and concludes that, because intakes of three to four times the safe individual intakes are consumed without obvious harm, the TUL may be much higher than the value of twice the safe intake assumed in previous reports.

Table 66.2 summarizes all protein requirement values identified in the report, shown in terms of the method adopted and the components of the requirement values: i.e. the metabolic demand and efficiency of utilization used to calculate the average requirement; the requirement coefficient of variation (CV) and safe intake for individuals.

Although it adopted the nitrogen balance method, the 2007 report reviewed extensively its main limitations, noting both the difficulties of making the appropriate measurements with sufficient accuracy, and those associated with the interpretation of the results. Of primary concern was the fact that the shape of the observed balance response curve does not conform to the predicted balance responses of well-nourished adults fed varying intakes of high-quality protein. Some deviation from this theoretical curve might be expected, but few reported balance studies conform to the theoretical response in any way and the individual variation in balance studies is very large with individual requirement values ranging from 0.34 to 2.8 g/kg protein per day.

In addition, concerns about nitrogen balance extend to the possible overestimation of requirements through use of efficiency values for dietary protein utilization, which are too low in the factorial models adopted for children and pregnancy. While the overestimation of requirements

TABLE 66.2 Protein requirements for various population groups from the 2002 Joint Expert Consultation

Population group	Method	Demand g protein/kg/day	Efficiency	Mean requirement g/kg/day	CV %	Safe level g/kg/day
Infants (0–6 months)	Factorial: maintenance plus growth; maintenance from N-balance studies with milk and egg (0.58g protein/kg/day); growth from TBK measurements of body composition.	0.385 + deposition	0.66: maintenance and growth	1.41–0.98	8–13%	1.77–1.14
Children (6 months–18 years)	Factorial: maintenance plus growth; adult maintenance value (0.66g protein/kg/day), plus growth costs from TBK studies of protein gain adjusted with efficiency value (0.58), from N balance studies on children 6 months to 12 years.	0.30 + deposition	0.47: maintenance; 0.58: growth	1.12–0.66(f) 1.12–0.69(m)	8.9–12%	1.31–0.82(f) 1.31–0.85(m)
Adults, all ages, men and women	N-balance(meta-analysis): linear regression: n=235 individual multilevel studies; demand = median intercept, efficiency = median slope.	0.30 (−48.1 mg N/kg)	0.47	0.654	>12%	0.83
Pregnancy	Factorial: demand from increased maintenance costs associated with increased body weight (0.5, 3.2, 7.3g/day), plus mean protein deposition estimated from TBK accretion in normal healthy pregnant women gaining 13.8kg (0, 1.9, 7.4g/day). Efficiency from N balance studies in primiparous teenagers.	Trimester/time period		g/day		g/day
		1st 0.5+0		0.5	12%	0.7
		2nd 3.2+1.9	0.42: deposition	7.7	12%	9.6
		3rd 7.3+7.4	0.42: deposition	24.9	12%	31.2
Lactation	Factorial: demand from mean milk protein output (total N less non-protein nitrogen), by well-nourished women exclusively breastfeeding (first 6 months postpartum) and partially breastfeeding (second 6 months). Efficiency from N balance studies in non-lactating adults.	0–6 months 6.79–7.60	0.47: milk protein production	14.3–16.2	12%	17.9–20.2
		6–12 months 4.69	0.47: milk protein production	10	12%	12.5

Adapted from WHO (2007).

for infants and children is unlikely to result in harm, the report reviews evidence that excessive protein intakes in pregnancy can have adverse effects on pregnancy outcomes, and advises that any additional protein during pregnancy should consist of additional normal food rather than high-protein supplements.

The magnitude of *amino acid* requirements has been a major controversy since the 1985 report (WHO, 1985), especially that of lysine, the limiting amino acid in wheat and other cereals. The 1985 report defined amino acid requirement patterns from nitrogen balance studies, which had been extensively reviewed in the 1971 Expert Consultation (FAO, 1973; WHO, 1973a) and recommended that the protein quality of protein sources and diets be assessed in terms of digestibility and amino acid score, subsequently defined as the protein digestibility corrected amino acid score (PDCAAS) method (FAO, 1991). The 1985 report adopted an adult scoring pattern with very low levels of indispensable amino acids so that protein quality ceased to be an issue for adults apart from digestibility. A considerable body of new stable-isotope studies together with a re-evaluation of the older nitrogen balance studies was examined in the new report, enabling the development of a new amino acid scoring pattern for adult maintenance. The cogent feature of this new pattern is the considerably higher values of all indispensable amino acids (IAA). With the exception of histidine, the sulphur amino acids, and tryptophan, this resulted in all values being close to twice as high as the values in the 1985 report (WHO, 1985). Scoring patterns for all the age groups less than 18 years of age were devised from the adult maintenance pattern and the amino acid pattern of tissue protein.

Implications of the 2007 Recommendations

As an initial reaction, the new lower protein requirements for infants and preschool children could relax the concern for this group including those in developing countries. However, because no long-term studies have been reported at these new requirement intakes, caution is advisable.

The impact of the 10% increase in protein requirements for adults is difficult to assess. A risk assessment study of protein deficiency described in the report (WHO, 2007) identified a significant problem of inadequate protein quantity and quality which is most serious for the typical diet of a developing country, but is also identified within some groups consuming vegetarian diets typical of developed countries, and even to a limited extent a typical omnivore diet. However, because of assumptions and uncertainties in the risk assessment, the report is cautious in its consideration of risk management in terms of increasing supplies of animal protein as has been suggested (Young *et al.*, 1998). The main uncertainty relates to the adaptive metabolic demands model of the protein requirement within which protein intakes and requirements are correlated and thus would markedly reduce the risk of deficiency (Millward and Jackson, 2004). Given the considerable impact which the underlying assumptions about the protein requirement carry for policy formulation, the report calls for continuing research into processes and mechanisms which enable health to be achieved on protein intakes as habitually consumed.

Fats (and Oils) and Fatty Acids

Nutritional needs for dietary fats, oils and fatty acids were addressed during meetings in 1977 (FAO, 1977), 1993 (FAO, 1994), and 2008 (FAO, 2010). All expert groups found it necessary to develop recommendations that take into consideration poorer populations whose diets may lack sufficient fat and more affluent populations that may experience health risks related to excessive consumption of fat.

The most recent consultation in 2008 was prompted by the recognition of the dramatic changes in diets and lifestyles occurring in the period since the 1994 report. These changes have been caused partly but not exclusively by enhanced industrialization, urbanization, economic development, and market globalization, particularly in the developing countries where major socioeconomic changes are occurring. Unhealthy dietary patterns and insufficient physical activity have also increased, resulting in greater prevalence of diet-related chronic diseases in all socioeconomic groups; these conditions now represent the main cause of global deaths and disability (WHO, 2011).

In addition there have been a number of major developments in this field, resulting in the need for an update. Primary among these developments is the large number of population-based cohort studies and randomized control trials conducted and addressing the impact of fats and specifically of different fatty acids on health. There is an enhanced knowledge of the role of particular fatty acids in determining health and nutritional well-being. More is known about how they are metabolized in the body, how they control gene transcription and expression, and how they interact with each other. In addition, fat and fatty acids are now recognized to be key nutrients that affect early growth and development as well as nutrition-related chronic disease later in life. The health consequences of these nutrients go well beyond their role as fuels; specific n-3 and n-6 fatty acids are essential nutrients while others affect the prevalence and severity of cardiovascular disease, diabetes, cancer, and age-related functional decline. This makes the process of defining requirements and recommendations more complex, and thus there is a need to focus on the role of individual fatty acids and on how needs vary with age and physiological status.

With respect to the recommendations in the previous 1993 Consultation (FAO, 1994), the 2008 Consultation placed more emphasis on the role of certain fatty acid categories, an example being the convincing role of long-chain polyunsaturated fatty acids in neonatal and infant mental development as well as a beneficial role in the maintenance of long-term health and prevention of some chronic diseases. A high intake of saturated fatty acids and to an even greater extent *trans* fatty acids contributes substantially to adverse blood lipid changes and the development of the cardiovascular diseases that claim many lives in affluent societies and that are now also the main cause of adult death in developed and developing countries. The 2008 Consultation also recognized that the entities n-3 PUFA or n-6 PUFA include more than one fatty acid, each with its individual properties, and the umbrella term lacks precision, particularly in the area of food labeling. A summary of the Report's recommendations for adults is given in Table 66.3, and those for infants and children are summarized in Table 66.4.

Trans Fatty Acids

A WHO Scientific Update on *trans* fatty acids (TFAs) (Nishida and Uauy, 2009) was conducted during in late October 2007, a year before the 2008 Expert Consultation on Fats and Fatty Acids in Human Nutrition. The conclusions of this scientific update contributed substantially to the deliberations of the 2008 Expert Consultation.

Earlier gatherings such as the 1993 Joint FAO/WHO Expert Consultation on Fats and Oils in Human Nutrition (FAO, 1994), the WHO Expert Consultation on Obesity: Preventing and Managing the Global Epidemic (WHO, 2000), and the Joint WHO/FAO Expert Consultation on Diet, Nutrition and the Prevention of Chronic Diseases (WHO, 2003) had expressed alarm concerning the growing evidence of harm from the consumption of *trans* fatty acids. It was decided that, by 2007, sufficient new data were available to conduct a review and update. The Scientific Update concluded as follows:

TABLE 66.3 Recommended dietary intakes from the 2008 Joint Expert Consultation for total fat and fatty acid intake: adults

Fat/FA	Measure (Explanations of the abbreviations are listed below Table 66.4)	Numeric amount
Total fat	AMDR	20–35%E
	U-AMDR	35%E
	L-AMDR	15%E
SFA	U-AMDR	10%E
MUFA	AMDR	By difference[a,b]
Total PUFA	AMDR (LA + ALA + EPA + DHA)	6–11%E
		11%E
	U-AMDR	6%E
	L-AMDR	2.5–3.5%E
	AI	
n-6 PUFA	AMDR (LA)	2.5–9%E
	EAR	2%E (SD of 0.5%)
	AI	2–3%E
n-3 PUFA	AMDR (n-3[c])	0.5–2%E
	L-AMDR (ALA)	≥ 0.5%E
	AMDR (EPA + DHA)	0. 250–2[d] g/day
TFA	UL (total TFA from ruminant and industrially produced sources)	<1%E

[a]Total fat [%E] – SFA [%E] – PUFA [%E] – TFA [%E].
[b]Can be up to 15–20%E, according to total fat intake.
[c](ALA + n-3 long-chain PUFA.)
[d]For secondary prevention of CHD.
Adapted from FAO (2010).

- The evidence on the effects of TFAs and disease outcomes strongly supports the need to remove partially hydrogenated vegetable oil (PHVO) from the human food supply.
- The evidence available from controlled trials and observational studies indicates that TFA consumption from PHVO adversely affects multiple cardiovascular risk factors and contributes significantly to increased risk of CHD events.
- Controlled studies and observational studies suggest that TFA may worsen insulin resistance, particularly among predisposed individuals with risk factors, e.g. pre-existing insulin resistance, visceral adiposity, or lower physical activity.
- Further studies are needed to confirm the apparent effects of TFA on weight gain and diabetes incidence in humans.

TABLE 66.4 Recommended dietary intakes from the 2008 Joint Expert Consultation for total fat and fatty acid intake: infants (0–24 months) and children (2–18 years)

Fat/FA	Age group	Measure	Numeric amount
Total fat	0–6 months	AMDR	40–60%E
		AI	Based on composition % of total fat in HM
	6–24 months	AMDR	Gradual reduction, depending on physical activity, to 35%E[a]
	2–18 years	AMDR	25–35%E
SFA	2–18 years	U-AMDR	8%E
			Children from families with evidence of familial dyslipidemia (high LDL cholesterol) should receive lower SFA but not reduce total fat intake
MUFA	2–18 years	AMDR	Total fat [%E] – SFA [%E] – PUFA [%E] – TFA [%E]
Total PUFA	6–24 months	U-AMDR	<15%E
	2–18 years	U-AMDR	11%E
LA and ALA	0–24 months	Comment	Essential and indispensable
n-6 PUFA	0–6 months	AI	0.2–0.3%E
AA	0–6 months	AI	HM composition as %E of total fat
LA	6–12 months	AI	3.0–4.5%E
	6–12 months	U-AMDR	<10%E
	12–24 months	AI	3.0–4.5%E
	12–24 months	U-AMDR	<10%E
n-3 PUFA			
ALA			
	0–6 months	AI	0.2–0.3%E
	6–12 months	AI	0.4–0.6%E
	6–12 months	U-AMDR	<3%E
	12–24 months	AI	0.4–0.6%E
DHA	12–24 months	U-AMDR	<3%E
	0–6 months	AI	0.1–0.18%E
	0–6 months	U-AMDR	No upper value within the HM range up to 0.75%E
	0–6 months	Comment	Conditionally essential due to limited synthesis from ALA
	6–12 months	AI	10–12 mg/kg
EPA+DHA	12–24 months	AI	10–12 mg/kg
	0–24 months	Comment	Critical role in retinal and brain development
	2–4 years	AI	100–150 mg (age adjusted for chronic disease prevention)
TFA	4–6 years	AI	150–200 mg (bridged from an infant value of 10 mg/kg
	6–10 years	AI	200–250 mg to the adult value assigned at age 10 years)
	2–18 years	UL	<1%E (total TFA – from ruminants and industrially produced sources)

[a]For infants 6–12 months, the proposed fat intake as a %E is lower than those recommended in the 1994 report. The primary reasons are the concern over increased obesity rates and the redefined growth standards based on human milk-fed infants, associated with leaner growth in later infancy (WHO MGRS, 2006).

%E, percent of energy; AI, adequate intake (expressed as a range); EAR, estimated average requirement; AMDR, acceptable macronutrient distribution range; L-AMDR, lower level of acceptable macronutrient distribution range; U-AMDR, upper level of acceptable macronutrient distribution range; UL, upper level; this term was developed for instances where biochemical indicators are needed to confirm any adverse effects, measurable with a probability of occurrence. In the case of FA this only applies to TFA.

L-AMDR and U-AMDR refer to the upper and lower range of the AMDR, very much similar to the use of UCI and LCI for the upper and lower bounds of confidence intervals.

Adapted from FAO (2010).

- Although TFAs from ruminant sources and industrial partially hydrogenated oils appear to be not dissimilar in their detrimental health effects, to date there is no conclusive evidence supporting an association of the former with coronary heart disease (CHD) risk due to the amounts usually consumed.
- TFAs produced by partial hydrogenation of fats and oils should be considered industrial food additives having no demonstrable health benefits and clear risks to human health. The result would be a substantial health gain for the population at large, with greatest health benefits obtained when replacement oils are rich in n-3 and n-6 polyunsaturated fatty acids (PUFA) and in monounsaturated fatty acids (MUFA).

Based on the above, the participating experts at the Scientific Update acknowledged the need to review the current recommendation that the mean population intake of TFAs, i.e. partially hydrogenated oils and fats, should be less than 1% of daily energy intake. There is sufficient epidemiological and experimental evidence to support revising this recommendation so that it encompasses the great majority of the population, and not just the population mean, to protect large subgroups from having high intakes. This could be accomplished (and has been in some countries and cities) by the virtual elimination of PHVO in the human food supply. The outcomes of this Scientific Update provide the evidence and scientific bases to promote discussions in the international scientific community involved in nutrition and health as well as agriculture and food production, and among relevant health professionals, national and international food regulatory agencies, civil society, and the private sector in order to achieve this goal.

Vitamins and Minerals

The human requirements for vitamins, minerals, and trace elements have been the subject of several FAO/WHO expert meetings. Calcium was reviewed in 1961 (FAO, 1962). Later, an expert meeting was held in 1965 on vitamin A, thiamin, riboflavin, and niacin (FAO, 1967) and was followed in 1969 by a meeting focused on ascorbic acid, vitamin D, vitamin B_{12}, folic acid, and iron (FAO, 1970). Vitamin A, iron, folate, and vitamin B_{12} were reviewed again in 1985 (FAO, 1988), the first two because they were major nutritional public health problems and the latter two because of their close association with anemia.

The WHO convened the first expert group on trace elements in 1973 (WHO, 1973b). By 1990, additional information regarding the role and importance of many trace elements had come to light, and a second expert consultation on trace elements was held under the auspices of the FAO and WHO as well as the International Atomic Energy Agency (IAEA) (WHO, 1996). This group attempted to ensure a reasonable degree of uniformity in the analysis and presentation of the many nutrients considered. A notable conclusion was that trace element requirements can change according to the type and amount of food consumed, interrelationships with other nutrients, and the nutritional status of the individual.

In 1998 a joint FAO/WHO expert consultation on human vitamin and mineral requirements was held (FAO, 2002; WHO, 2004b). This expert group met to deliberate on all vitamins and minerals in the human diet and to derive recommendations about levels of intake that were specified as recommended nutrient intakes or RNIs. These values were based on the available scientific evidence, although, as is often the case, difficulties in data interpretation resulted in some issues being left unresolved.

Further, the meeting report highlights the question as to whether changes in recommended intakes for vitamins and minerals are the result of better scientific knowledge and understanding of the biochemical role of the nutrients, or whether the criteria for setting the levels of the requirements have changed. The report also suggests that, while RNIs for vitamins and minerals were initially established on the understanding that they are meant to meet the basic nutritional needs of over 97% of the population, a fundamental criterion in industrialized countries has become the presumptive roles these nutrients may play in "prevention" against an increasing range of disease conditions that characterize these populations. The latter approach implies the notion of "optimal nutrition" relative to recommended intakes. Further, the report notes that questions have been raised as to whether some of the developments in approaches to establishing recommended intakes are applicable to developing country populations. and acknowledges that, from an international perspective, the RNIs for several if not many micronutrients such as folate, vitamin A, and selenium will need to be re-evaluated as soon as significant additional data become available.

The tables listing the RNIs for minerals and for water-fat-soluble vitamins issued as a result of this meeting, as well as estimated average requirements (EARs) for several nutrients, can be found in the meeting reports (FAO, 2002; WHO, 2004b).

The FAO and WHO continue work to update the requirements for vitamins and minerals. In 2002, the FAO provided a report to the Codex Committee on Nutrition and Foods for Special Dietary Uses (CAC, 2003). This committee works under the mandate of the Codex Alimentarius, an international foods-standards-setting organization. The report responds to an earlier communication from the Commission of the Codex Alimentarius on behalf of the Committee, requesting that the FAO and WHO, under their mandate to provide scientific advice to Codex committees, work to include upper levels of intake for vitamins and minerals in their future efforts to develop recommended nutrient intakes. The FAO report specifies the intent to produce a general technical document outlining the principles to be adopted in addressing the topic of upper levels of intake and the safety of specific vitamins and minerals.

Upper Levels of Intake for Nutrients and Related Substances

In 2004, the FAO and WHO responded to the request from Codex by announcing a joint effort to develop a framework for establishing upper levels of intake of nutrients and related substances (WHO, 2006). The workshop participants were asked to develop an internationally applicable approach (or "model") intended to specify the scientific process of nutrient risk assessment. Such a model can be used in the future to identify upper levels of intake for nutrients and related substances. The workshop tasks did not include identifying such levels of intake, but rather focused on the important first step of establishing a scientifically sound approach for assessing the risk, if any, associated with nutrients and related substances. The workshop addressed the scientific decisions relating to the nutrient risk assessment process; nutrient risk management decisions and policy-setting activities were considered outside its scope.

Harmonization of Nutrient Intake Values

The United Nations University's Food and Nutrition Program, in collaboration with the FAO, WHO, and UNICEF, convened in December 2005 a group of international experts to review the harmonization of approaches for developing nutrient-based dietary standards. The group did not address the setting of numeric values for any nutrient but instead the development of a theoretical framework for setting nutrient intake values. The report was published in the *Food and Nutrition Bulletin* (King and Garza, 2007). The recommended terminology coming from this meeting is summarized below.

- **Nutrient intake values (NIV)** is the umbrella term for the full set of recommendations. *(Analogous to DRI [US] or DRV [UK]).*
- **Average nutrient requirement (ANR)** is the average or median requirement estimated from a statistical distribution of requirements for a specific criterion and for a particular age- and sex-specific group. *(Analogous to EAR [US and UK]).*
- **Individual nutrient level (INLx)** is the recommended level for all healthy individuals in a specific population and will cover the needs of most (x) individuals where x refers to the percentile chosen for setting the INL, based on the CV of the requirements. *(Analogous to RDA [US] and RNI [UK]).*
- **Upper nutrient level (UNL)** is the highest level of habitual nutrient intake that is likely to pose no risk of adverse health effects in almost all individuals in the general population. *(Analogous to UL [US] upper end of safe intake range [UK]).*

Public Health Applications of Nutrient Recommendations

FAO and WHO recommendations have always aimed to inform government authorities in their activities to improve public health. In this section, two public health endeavors that are commonly led by national authorities, dietary guidelines and nutrition labeling, are discussed. While this chapter focuses on these two strategies, it should be noted that there is extensive debate about innovative approaches to improve consumer information to enable consumers to select foods that will enable them to create healthier diets. Other forms of consumer information are emerging that may augment food-based dietary guidelines and nutrition labels.

Food-Based Dietary Guidelines

Quantitative recommendations for the intake of nutrient substances provide the nutritional goals needed to ensure the health of populations. It is, however, difficult for consumers to apply this information when selecting foods and planning meals. There is a need to "transform" such quantitative recommendations into general advice about dietary choices.

While international recommendations on nutrient needs provide critical information for the development of dietary guidelines, an international set of such guidelines is neither feasible nor practical. The types of foods available differ among regions and countries, and foods vary in their nutritional content. The vast differences in food availability and accessibility coupled with differences in lifestyles, cultures, and public-health priorities mean that national authorities are in the best position to establish dietary guidelines suitable for their population and for their food supply. For this reason, international organizations such as the FAO and WHO have as their goal the support of national and regional efforts to develop food-based dietary guidelines (FBDGs). The discussion here focuses on guidelines targeted at the general public, but separate dietary guidelines are at times developed for segments of the population with specific nutritional needs such as infants and young children, as well as for persons with disease conditions such as autoimmune deficiency, hypertension, and diabetes.

In brief, the purpose of FBDGs is to assist the targeted population in implementing nutrition and related-health recommendations. Such guidelines present information using language and symbols that the public can easily understand. They usually focus on common foods, portion sizes, and behaviors. A complementary objective of developing FBDGs is to provide a tool for nutrition education to be used by health providers, teachers, journalists, extension agents, and others working directly with the public.

The FAO and WHO have promoted the concept of FBDG for nearly two decades. In 1992, the International Conference on Nutrition (ICN) was held. During this high-level intergovernmental meeting, 159 nations endorsed the "World Declaration and Plan of Action for Nutrition" which called upon governments to promote appropriate diets and healthy lifestyles (FAO/WHO, 1992). In 1995, the FAO and WHO sponsored an Expert Consultation on the Preparation and Use of Food-Based Dietary Guidelines in Cyprus (WHO, 1998) which reviewed experiences and elaborated a process for developing FBDG. Following the consultation, FAO and WHO promoted the development of FBDG through their regional offices and institutions and technical cooperation projects.

Main Features of FBDGs

Although FBDGs from different countries often appear to be similar, they have usually been developed to meet the specific needs of a nation's population and to suit the cultural, social, and economic contexts. The food graphics associated with FBDG are highly promoted and may become important symbols in a nation's nutrition communication and education strategy.

Existing FBDGs from countries throughout the world share certain commonalities. These are as follows:

- All promote consumption of a variety of foods.
- All promote maintenance of a healthy weight.
- All encourage increased consumption of fruits and vegetables.
- Most encourage lowering consumption of salt or sodium.
- Most encourage lowering consumption of sugar.
- Most encourage physical activity.
- Some specify types of fats and discourage consumption of saturated fats.
- Some specify carbohydrates and encourage consumption of whole-grain products.
- Some encourage increased consumption of water.
- Some mention specific nutrients.

In countries where deficiencies in iron, vitamin A, and/or iodine are common, the guidelines may address these nutritional problems. FBDGs in some countries contain recommendations that reflect societal values and may be intended to motivate positive behaviors that have an indirect impact on diets and health. For example, some FBDG encourage meals being regarded as social occasions. Some promote the consumption of local and/or traditional foods. Many FBDGs contain negative messages such as discouragement of smoking. It is common for FBDGs to encourage moderation in alcohol consumption. Some guidelines contain information about food preparation and food safety.

Whereas the importance of consuming a variety of foods is easily appreciated by nutritionists, the concept of variety is often misunderstood by consumers. Many countries have used an illustration as part of FBDG to convey the concept of variety. The graphics attempt to specify types of foods, proportions of foods, and portion sizes organized according to cultural perceptions of foods. Examples of FBDG graphics can be found on the FAO Food and Nutrition website, http://www.fao.org/ag/humannutrition/nutritioneducation/49741/en/

As appropriate, the graphics take different forms and usually have social significance for the population; for example, national symbols may be used. Although the text and graphics are designed to be used together, some FBDG graphics appear alone on packages and posters. Therefore, consumer testing should be carried out to ensure that the graphic is interpreted accurately.

Process for Developing FBDGs

FBDGs are usually created through a comprehensive process that includes methods to ensure that the recommendations are understood and feasible for the average consumer and widely supported by the various government agencies, professional societies, and food-industry and consumer associations. The development of FBDG follows a series of steps, each of which requires different types of activities and expertise. The process of developing FBDGs may take several years and should include the following activities:

- Planning with multisectoral committee;
- Characterization of target group(s);
- Setting nutrition and health objectives;
- Preparing technical guidelines;
- Testing feasibility of recommendations;
- Preparing FBDG;
- Validation of recommendations and food graphic;
- Implementation;
- Evaluation.

Nutrition Labeling of Packaged Foods and Codex

Nutrition labeling is intended to assist consumers to select food products according to their specific health needs and preferences. In terms of food policies, nutrition labeling is considered to be less restrictive than regulations that would require that a product have specific nutritional qualities. Through the market, nutrition labeling can motivate food producers to increase the availability of food products that possess the nutritional qualities that are desired by consumers. For instance, consumers who wish to avoid sodium, sugar, or saturated fats are provided with the information they need to select products; at the same time, products that are high in sodium, sugar, or saturated fats are available for consumers who desire them.

During the past 20 years, nutrition labeling has been evolving rapidly, with complex debates ongoing in a number of countries. After the United States implemented the Nutrition Labeling and Education Act of 1990, which required that the vast majority of packaged foods carry a nutrition fact label, a number of other countries (e.g. Canada, Australia, New Zealand, Brazil, Chile, Uruguay, and Malaysia) implemented similar policies requiring panels containing nutrient information on the side or back of packages (Hawkes, 2010). Other types of nutrition labels, which feature simple graphics and could appear on the front of the package, are under discussion in a number

of countries. In addition to information on food packages, there is consideration of the provision of nutrition information at the point of sale in retail food outlets.

Regardless of whether a label is voluntary or mandatory, governments seek to prevent nutrition labeling that could mislead consumers. Fraudulent labels are unfair to other producers, and undermine consumer confidence in food products. Governments and private organizations establish standard formats for labeling nutrients to ensure that consumers can read the labels and compare products.

The WHO Global Strategy on Diet, Physical Activity and Health provides an example of the linkages between scientific recommendations about nutrition and United Nations initiatives to stimulate governments and other societal actors to implement measures to improve public health. The WHO issued the World Health Report 2002: Reducing Risks, Promoting Healthy Life (WHO, 2002) which describes how, in most countries, a few major risk factors account for much of the morbidity and mortality. The report notes that unhealthy diets and physical inactivity are among the leading causes of three of the major non-communicable diseases (cardiovascular diseases, diabetes, and some cancers). In response to a request from member states through a resolution (WHA 55.23) of the World Health Assembly held in 2002, the WHO developed the Global Strategy on Diet, Physical Activity and Health. It was endorsed through Resolution 57.17 by the World Health Assembly in 2004 (WHO, 2004a).

The Strategy specifies recommendations for populations and individuals intended to (1) assist in reducing the risk factors for non-communicable diseases stemming from diet and physical activity; (2) increase awareness of the influences of diet and physical activity on health; (3) encourage development of appropriate policies; and (4) monitor scientific data and influences on diet and physical activity. In the WHO strategy, the Codex Alimentarius Commission (CAC) was identified as having a role to play in achieving the aims of reducing the risk of diet-related chronic diseases. Through work on food standards, there can be positive effects on the nutritional qualities of foods and consumers' abilities to make informed food choices. The FAO and WHO proposed specific actions that the CAC could take in support of the WHO Global Strategy, and improvements in nutrition labeling were among the proposals that were accepted.

The Codex Committee on Food Labelling (CCFL) and the Codex Committee on Nutrition and Foods for Special Dietary Uses (CCNFSDU) have been the main committees through which Codex is addressing nutrition- and diet-related chronic diseases. After these committees have carried out their technical work, their recommendations will be deliberated by the CAC at large. Changes in the Codex standards could influence the nutritional qualities of foods worldwide.

At the 38th session of the CCFL in 2010, the Committee made proposals to amend the current Codex guidelines on nutrition labeling. The Committee decided that nutrient declarations that constitute the mandatory declaration – that is, declarations that should be present when a nutritional claim is made – should include saturated fat, total sugars, and sodium/salt, in addition to the energy value, amounts of protein, available carbohydrate, and fat that were required previously (CAC, 2010a). The Committee also established "Principles and Criteria for Legibility of Nutrition Labelling" (CAC, 2010a) that address issues of format, numerical presentation and design elements.

The current Codex guidelines for labeling indicate that vitamins and minerals may be listed when recommended intakes have been established and/or when they are of nutritional importance in the country concerned. It specifies that, when nutrient declarations occur, only those vitamins and minerals that are present in significant amounts should be listed (a footnote is included to indicate that, as a rule, 5% of the recommended intake constitutes a significant amount). Numerical information on vitamins and minerals is to be expressed in metric units and/or as a percentage of the Nutrient Reference Value (NRV). The existing NRVs are listed within the guidelines and include values for: protein, vitamin A, vitamin D, vitamin C, thiamin, riboflavin, niacin, vitamin B_6, folic acid, vitamin B_{12}, calcium, magnesium, iron, zinc, and iodine. However, the CCNFSDU is currently reviewing the guideline NRVs for the purposes of nutrition labeling of foods for the general population (CAC, 2010b).

Future Directions

In the 21st century, the world is considerably different from when FAO and WHO were created just over 60 years ago. A number of countries, mainly in Africa and Asia, were not independent nations; the member states belonging to FAO and WHO numbered about 50 and most were from the developed world. The populations of each country still consumed what was considered a national diet. The volume and variety of food that was traded was less, and there was less dissemination of scientific information about nutrition.

The *modus operandi* within FAO and WHO was also different from today. In the area of scientific reviews and establishing standards, recommendations, and codes, the process was largely an internal process. The Director-Generals of each organization would confer with the member states, usually through the ministries of agriculture for the FAO and ministries of health for the WHO. Studies and meetings would then be initiated, very often consisting of outside experts who would advise the agency heads on a particular subject in their personal capacities. Whereas the reports of these studies were of interest to many outside the organizations, they aimed primarily to assist the organizations in carrying out their work. Further, the UN system was smaller and less complex as agencies such as UNICEF and the World Food Programme did not exist; today these agencies play important roles in relation to undernutrition.

Increasingly the nutrition community has become larger while the similarities among countries make the world seem smaller. The range of parties interested in the work of the FAO and WHO has expanded, and these parties seek to be included in that work. Originally the contact of the FAO and WHO with the world was only through its member states; now non-governmental organizations (NGOs), consumer advocates, and industry expect to be included, and some may be able to play large roles. There is an increased call for transparency in how the organizations function, including how they develop scientific recommendations. National regulations are being influenced by international standards and agreements. In this regard, the impact of FAO and WHO scientific recommendations on nutrition will no doubt become more far-reaching and significant.

Acknowledgment

The authors would like to acknowledge the contribution from D.J. Millward to the section on Protein and Amino Acids.

Suggestions for Further Reading

Readers are directed to the References for recommended reading.

Recent FAO/WHO reports on human nutrient requirements and listings of past and upcoming FAO/WHO expert meetings are available on both organizations' websites (http://www.fao.org/ag/humannutrition/nutrition/en).

References

CAC (Codex Alimentarius Commission) (2003) *Report of the 24th Session of the Codex Committee on Nutrition and Foods for Special Dietary Uses*, 26th Session of the Joint FAO/WHO Food Standards Programme Codex Alimentarius Commission. ALINORM 03/26A, Rome. http://www.codexalimentarius. net/web/archives.jsp?year=03; select Alinorm 3/26A at paragraph 119. Accessed September 17, 2010.

CAC (Codex Alimentarius Commission) (2006) *Understanding the Codex Alimentarius*, 3rd Edn. WHO and FAO, Rome. ftp://ftp.fao.org/codex/Publications/understanding/ Understanding_EN.pdf. Accessed May 2, 2011.

CAC (Codex Alimentarius Commission) (2010a) *Report of the 38th Session of the Codex Committee on Food Labelling, Quebec City, Canada, 3–7 May 2010.* Joint FAO/WHO Food Standards Programme Codex Alimentarius Commission, Thirty-third Session, Geneva, 5–9 July 2010. ALINORM 10/33/22.

CAC (Codex Alimentarius Commission) (2010b) *Report of the 31st Session of the Codex Committee on Nutrition and Foods for Special Dietary Uses, Dusseldorf, Germany, 2–6 November 2009.* Joint FAO/WHO Food Standards Programme Codex Alimentarius Commission, 33rd Session, Geneva, 5–9 July 2010. ALINORM 10/33/26.

FAO (1950) *Calorie Requirements: Report of the Committee on Calorie Requirements.* FAO Nutritional Studies No. 5. Food and Agriculture Organization, Rome.

FAO (1957a) *Calorie Requirements: Report of the Second Committee on Calorie Requirements.* FAO Nutritional Studies No. 15. Food and Agriculture Organization, Rome.

FAO (1957b) *Protein Requirements: Report of the FAO Committee.* FAO Nutritional Series No 16. Food and Agriculture Organization, Rome.

FAO (1962) *Calcium Requirements: Report of an FAO/WHO Expert Group.* FAO Nutrition Meetings Report Series No. 30. Food and Agriculture Organization, Rome.

FAO (1964) *Protein Requirements: Report of a Joint FAO/WHO Expert Group.* FAO Nutrition Meeting Report Series No. 37. Food and Agriculture Organization, Rome.

FAO (1967) *Requirements of Vitamin A, Thiamine, Riboflavin and Niacin: Report of a Joint FAO/WHO Expert Group.* FAO Nutrition Meetings Report Series No. 41. Food and Agriculture Organization, Rome.

FAO (1970) *Requirements of Ascorbic Acid, Vitamin D, Vitamin B12, Folic Acid and Iron: Report of a Joint FAO/WHO Expert Group.* FAO Nutrition Meeting Report Series No. 47. Food and Agriculture Organization, Rome.

FAO (1973) *Energy and Protein Requirements; Report of the Joint FAO/WHO Ad Hoc Expert Committee.* FAO Nutrition Meeting Report Series No. 52. Food and Agriculture Organization, Rome.

FAO (1975) Energy and protein requirements: recommendations by a joint FAO/WHO informal gathering of experts. *Food Nutr* **1**, 11–19.

FAO (1977) *Dietary Fats and Oils in Human Nutrition: a Joint FAO/ WHO Report.* FAO Food and Nutrition Paper 3. Food and Agriculture Organization, Rome.

FAO (1980) *Carbohydrates in Human Nutrition: Joint FAO/WHO Report.* FAO Food and Nutrition Paper 15. Food and Agriculture Organization, Rome.

FAO (1988) *Requirements of Vitamin A, Iron, Folate and Vitamin B_{12}: Report of a Joint FAO/WHO Expert Consultation.* FAO Food and Nutrition Series No. 23. Food and Agriculture Organization, Rome.

FAO (1991) *Protein Quality Evaluation in Human Diets: Report of a Joint FAO/WHO Expert Consultation.* FAO Food and Nutrition Paper No. 51, Food and Agriculture Organization, Rome.

FAO (1994) *Fats and Oils in Human Nutrition: Report of a Joint Expert Consultation.* FAO Food and Nutrition Paper 57. Food and Agriculture Organization, Rome.

FAO (1998) *Carbohydrates in Human Nutrition: Report of the Joint FAO/WHO Expert Consultation.* FAO Food and Nutrition Paper 66. Food and Agriculture Organization, Rome.

FAO (2002) *Human Vitamin and Mineral Requirements: Report of a Joint FAO/WHO Expert Consultation.* FAO/WHO nonseries publication. Food and Agriculture Organization, Rome.

FAO (2003) *Food Energy – Methods of Analysis and Conversion Factors: Report of a Technical Workshop.* FAO Food and Nutrition Paper 77. Food and Agriculture Organization, Rome.

FAO (2004) *Human Energy Requirements: Report of a Joint FAO/ WHO/UNU Expert Consultation.* FAO Food and Nutrition Technical Report Series No. 1, Food and Agriculture Organization, Rome.

FAO (2010) *Fats and Fatty Acids in Human Nutrition: Report of a Joint FAO/WHO Expert Consultation.* FAO Food and Nutrition Paper 91. Food and Agriculture Organization, Rome.

FAO/WHO (1992) *World Declaration on Nutrition and Plan of Action for Nutrition; Final Report of the International Conference on Nutrition.* Food and Agriculture Organization, Rome.

Hawkes, C. (2010) Government and voluntary policies on nutrition labeling: a global overview. In J. Albert (ed.), *Innovations in Food Labelling*. Food and Agriculture Organization of the United Nations, Rome, and Woodhead Publishing Limited, Oxford, pp. 37–58.

King, J.C. and Garza, C. (2007) Harmonization of nutrient intake values. *Food Nutr Bull* **28**, S1–S153.

League of Nations (1936) *The Problem of Nutrition*, Vol. **2**. Technical Commission on Nutrition, League of Nations, Geneva.

Millward, D.J. and Jackson, A. (2004) Protein:energy ratios of current diets in developed and developing countries compared with a safe protein:energy ratio: implications for recommended protein and amino acid intakes. *Public Health Nutr* **7**, 387–405.

Nishida, C., Martinez Nocito, F., and Mann, J. (2007) Joint FAO/WHO scientific update on carbohydrates in human nutrition. *Eur J Clin Nutr* **61**(Suppl. 1), S1–S137.

Nishida, C. and Uauy, R. (2009) WHO scientific update on trans fatty acids (TFA). *Eur J Clin Nutr* **63**(Suppl 2), S1–S75. Please also look at the remainder of the supplement S5–S75.

Rand, W.M., Pellett, P.L., and Young, V.R. (2003) Meta-analysis of nitrogen balance studies for estimating protein requirements in healthy adults. *Am J Clin Nutr* **77**, 109–127.

Randell, A. (2010) The Codex Alimentarius and Food Labelling: delivering consumer protection. In J. Albert (ed.), *Innovations in Food Labelling*. Food and Agriculture Organization of the United Nations, Rome, and Woodhead Publishing, Oxford, pp. 5–16.

Schofield, W.N., Schofield, C., and James, W.P.T. (1985) Basal metabolic rate – review and prediction, together with an annotated bibliography of source material. *Human Nutr Clin Nutr* **39C**(Suppl 1), 5–96.

WHO (1950) *Report of the First Joint FAO/WHO Expert Committee on Nutrition*. World Health Organization, Geneva.

WHO (1965) *Protein Requirements: Report of a Joint FAO/WHO Expert Group*. WHO Technical Report Series No. 301. World Health Organization, Geneva.

WHO (1973a) *Energy and Protein Requirements: Report of the Joint FAO/WHO Ad Hoc Expert Committee*. WHO Technical Report Series No. 522, World Health Organization, Geneva.

WHO (1973b) *Trace Elements in Human Nutrition: Report of a WHO Expert Committee*. WHO Technical Report Series No. 532, World Health Organization, Geneva.

WHO (1979) Protein and Energy Requirements: A Joint FAO/WHO Memorandum. *Bull World Health Organ* **57**, 65–79.

WHO (1985) *Energy and Protein Requirements: Report of a Joint FAO/WHO/UNU Expert Consultation*. WHO Technical Report Series 724. World Health Organization, Geneva.

WHO (1996) *Trace Elements in Human Nutrition: A Report of a Joint FAO/WHO/IAEA Expert Consultation*. WHO Technical Report Series. World Health Organization, Geneva.

WHO (1998) *Preparation and Use of Food-based Dietary Guidelines: Report of a Joint FAO/WHO Consultation*. WHO Technical Report Series 880. World Health Organization, Geneva.

WHO (2000) *Obesity: Preventing and Managing the Global Epidemic: Report of a WHO Expert Consultation*. World Health Organization Technical Report Series 894. World Health Organization, Geneva.

WHO (2002) *The World Health Report 2002 – Reducing Risks, Promoting Healthy Life*. World Health Organization, Geneva. http://www.who.int/whr/2002/en/. Accessed September 17, 2010.

WHO (2003) *Diet, Nutrition and the Prevention of Chronic Diseases: Report of a Joint WHO/FAO Expert Consultation*. World Health Organization Technical Report Series 916. World Health Organization, Geneva.

WHO (2004a) WHA 57. 17 Global Strategy on Diet, Physical Activity and Health. Fifty-Seventh World Health Assembly, Resolutions and Decisions Annexes. 17–22 May 2004, pp. 38–55. http://www.who.int/dietphysicalactivity/strategy/eb11344/strategy_english_web.pdf. Accessed 17 September 2010.

WHO (2004b) *Human Vitamin and Mineral Requirements: Report of a Joint FAO/WHO Expert Consultation*, 2nd Edn. FAO/WHO Non-series Publication. World Health Organization, Geneva. http://whqlibdoc.who.int/publications/2004/9241546123.pdf. Accessed September 17, 2010.

WHO (2006) *A Model for Establishing Upper Levels of Intake for Nutrients and Related Substances: Report of a Joint FAO/WHO Technical Workshop on Food Nutrient Risk Assessment*. World Health Organization, Geneva. http://www.who.int/ipcs/methods/nra/en/index.html. Accessed 17 September 2010.

WHO (2007) *Protein and Amino Acid Requirements in Human Nutrition: Report of a Joint FAO/WHO/UNU Expert Consultation*. WHO Technical Report Series No. 935. World Health Organization, Geneva.

WHO (2011) *Global Status Report on Noncommunicable Diseases*. World Health Organization, Geneva.

Young, V.R., Scrimshaw, N.S., and Pellett, P.L. (1998) Significance of dietary protein source in human nutrition: animal and/or plant proteins? In J.C. Waterlow, D.G. Armstrong, L. Fowden, et al. (eds), *Feeding a World Population of More than Eight Billion People: A Challenge to Science*. Oxford University Press, New York, pp. 205–221.

67

EMERGENCE OF DIET-RELATED CHRONIC DISEASES IN DEVELOPING COUNTRIES

BARRY M. POPKIN, PhD

University of North Carolina at Chapel Hill, Chapel Hill, North Carolina, USA

Summary

Over the past 20 years the way individuals eat, drink, and move has changed remarkably across the globe. Related to this has been an increase in energy imbalance and obesity throughout the world. The changes in diets, activity, and obesity have been linked with major increases in hypertension and diabetes (best documented) as well as other dimensions of cardiovascular disease and most cancers. Key points discussed in this chapter include the following.

- The underlying causes are shifts in use and availability of technology, major changes in the processing, distribution and marketing of food and drinks, and mass media changes.
- The technological changes that have affected movement and food are discussed. Prime examples relate to edible oils, added caloric sweeteners, access to supermarkets and their role in the entire vertical chain from production to consumer purchases. Later in the chapter examples of key changes are presented.
- The influence of multinational companies is discussed and shown to have evolved within a much more complex economic environment with many local clones and options.
- The biological mismatch between our preferences and the mechanisms related to hunger and thirst and satiation as contrasted with the vast shifts linked to modern technology in options for eating, drinking, and moving are discussed.
- Global dynamics of obesity are examined. The prevalence of overweight and obesity status are presented, as are other statistics related to age and social class burden.

Examples of the chronic disease burden estimates are presented, especially for well-measured examples.

Introduction

In the past two decades there has been a remarkable global transformation in the way individuals eat, drink, and move. A consequence of this has been not only a marked increase in positive energy imbalance and weight gain but also a large shift in the nature of diets that is having profound effects on the patterns of chronic diseases. This chapter will focus mainly on changes that have occurred in what we have often termed developing countries. This includes the very poorest, such as Haiti and sub-Saharan African countries, and also transitional economies that in many cases are emerging as global superpowers, such as Brazil, China, and India. We will exclude the former Soviet

Present Knowledge in Nutrition, Tenth Edition. Edited by John W. Erdman Jr, Ian A. Macdonald and Steven H. Zeisel.
© 2012 International Life Sciences Institute. Published 2012 by John Wiley & Sons, Inc.

Union, as it represents a unique case of countries with very poor diets and high levels of nutrition-related noncommunicable diseases (NR-NCDs).

The transformation in how people eat, drink, and move has been going on for many millennia; however, the changes in the stages of the nutrition transition in the past 20 to 25 years in the developing world are unprecedented (Popkin, 2002, 2006a). Billions of people live in countries that have essentially conquered undernutrition and famine and have only pockets of malnutrition while experiencing major shifts toward positive energy balance. The dietary and activity pattern shifts associated with these changes have led to rapid increases in NR-NCDs, while at times they have also led to rapid inequality in access to new technologies and food-and-drink options. The complex phenomena of the double burden of malnutrition and obesity have arisen at the household and national levels in many countries, whereas other countries have shifted more rapidly toward minimal malnutrition.

This chapter explores all of these issues, discussing first the next social, technological, and economic forces underlying dietary shifts. It then examines some of the major issues that have led to a profound mismatch between biology and the technology that provides food and drink and reduces physical movement and exertion.

The Major Global Forces Underlying Dietary Shifts: Globalization of Economic, Demographic, Social, and Technological Forces

Dietary shifts are not a case of McDonald's, Pepsi, and Walmart changing how the world eats and drinks. Rather, the major factors include: (a) the worldwide trade of technology innovations that affect energy expenditures during leisure, transportation, and work; (b) the globalization of modern food processing, marketing, and distribution techniques (most frequently linked with Westernization of the world's diet); (c) the vast expansion of the global mass media; and (d) other changes that constitute the rubric of impacts resulting from an increased opening up of the world economy (Popkin, 2006b). Globalization has certainly enhanced the interconnectedness of the world in terms of the trade in goods, technology, and services and the spread of the modern mass media. These changes began in the last half of the twentieth century and were accelerated by a push from higher-income countries for more open markets for their goods, services, and technologies. During this period, international agencies (e.g. the International Monetary Fund (IMF) and the World Bank) and most higher-income countries promoted a "free trade" agenda as the panacea for the ills of the developing world. This chapter does not focus on the exact linkages among aspects of globalization and how each affects the increased trade in services, commodities, processed products, technology, and investments; rather, the focus is on understanding how technological and other shifts are linked to and affect diet, activity, and obesity throughout the world. It is impossible at this time, with the available databases, to fully link each aspect of globalization exactly to each one of these elements; we can, however, document many threads of change that clearly relate to their global shifts.

In the post-World War II period, urbanization and major demographic changes began to occur as societies, first in Asia, then in Latin America and the Middle East, and finally in sub-Saharan Africa, began the demographic transition toward increased child spacing, later ages at marriage, and ultimately reduced total fertility. At the same time, economic and social pressures began the inexorable shift in population to urban areas. These changes occurred very unevenly across the developing world and have been carefully documented by demographers, first by Kingsley and later by a great many other scholars (Davis, 1945).

An equally profound epidemiological transition accompanied these demographic changes in a complex weaving of shifts in fertility, morbidity, and mortality (Omran, 1971). Jointly these led to major shifts in population age distribution, and they were linked to a demographic set of changes unprecedented in human history.

Urbanization, linked to these changes but also equally linked to social, economic, and technological forces that created excess food in rural areas to feed urban populations, provided opportunities for improved education, and economic welfare moved rapidly across the developing world. These changes, which mirrored those in Europe one to two centuries earlier, occurred quite rapidly (United Nations, 2002). The underlying economic, technological, and social transformations that were complexly intertwined with these demographic shifts are critical for understanding how we eat, drink, and move.

Technology of Movement

Since the 1980s the pervasive shifts in technological innovations related to all dimensions of movement and energy expenditure at work in urban areas have become omnipresent, and similar shifts are rapidly reaching all rural areas. While several major shifts are occurring, including a global increase in the proportion of service-sector jobs and a reduction in the effort required by each job, it is the change of energy expended in each occupation that appears to be most important (Popkin, 2008b). We have also documented important shifts in home technology and the resulting reduced energy expenditures, and the same is true for leisure movement.

Food Systems

Some might call this the McDonaldization or Coca-colonization of the world; however, this is the trivial tip of the iceberg of changes and is not as important as many would argue. Far before Walmart or Coke or Kentucky Fried Chicken appeared in the developing world in any meaningful way, a number of diet-related revolutions were occurring. They included the following.

The Edible Oils Story

The edible vegetable oils story is particularly important, as its effects have been quite profound. Until the decade following World War II, the majority of fats available for human consumption were animal fats, milk, butter, and meat. Subsequently, a revolution in the production and processing of oilseed-based fats occurred. The principal vegetable oils include soybean, sunflower, rapeseed, palm, and peanut. Technological breakthroughs in the development of high-yield oilseeds and in the refining of high-quality vegetable oils greatly reduced the cost of baking and frying fats, margarine, butter-like spreads, salad oils, and cooking oils in relation to animal-based products (Williams, 1984). Worldwide demand for vegetable fats was fueled by health concerns regarding the consumption of animal fats and cholesterol. Furthermore, a number of major economic and political initiatives led to the development of oil crops, not only in Europe and the United States but also in Southeast Asia (palm oils) and in Brazil and Argentina (soybean oil). The net effect was that from 1945 to 1965 there was an almost fourfold increase in US production of vegetable oils, while animal fat production increased by only 11% (US Department of Agriculture, 1966).

In developing nations one of the earliest shifts toward a higher-fat diet began with major increases in domestic production and imports of oilseeds and vegetable oils rather than increased imports of meat and milk. At this stage, vegetable oils contributed far more energy to the human food supply than meat or animal fats (Morgan, 1993). With the exception of peanut oil, global availability of vegetable oils (soybean, sunflower, rapeseed, and palm) approximately tripled between 1961 and 1990. Soybeans now account for the bulk of vegetable oil consumption worldwide. It is also important to note that many of these processed oils are not regulated well, and some of the new edible oils or other foods are highly pathogenic (Wallingford, 2004).

The Added Sugar Revolution

It is difficult to understand quite how the global sweetening of the food supply occurred. During this same period, however, all processed food companies began to put increased types and amounts of added sugars from many food sources into processed food, and sugar became an increasingly cheap global product (Popkin and Nielsen, 2003).

The Animal Source Food Revolution

Delgado and others have documented the profound shift in global production and consumption of beef, pork, poultry, and dairy products and to a much lesser extent seafood and fish (Delgado, 2003a). Many agricultural scholars have shown how this shift grew out of an approach to diet and agriculture developed in the United States and Europe that globally influenced the increased subsidization of all components related to the production of animal source foods (Gardner, 2002). Elsewhere I have provided discussions of this history and its impact on US and global prices and consumption patterns of animal source foods (Popkin, 2008b, 2011).

Food Systems Changes

Simultaneously to the changes just outlined, there have been major revolutions in the way food is processed, distributed, and marketed. One of the primary influences is the modern food distribution system, personified by Walmart and the modern mass media.

An important change in the global food system is occurring in food distribution. No research to date has provided any analysis of the consequences of these food distribution shifts for dietary intake patterns. Fresh markets ("wet" or open public markets) are disappearing as the major source of food supplies in the developing world. They are being replaced by large, multinational, regional, and local supermarkets, usually part of global chains (e.g. Carrefour,

Tesco, or Walmart). In some countries, such as South Africa and China, domestic chains have been patterned to function and look like the global chains and have even grown into global giants. Megastores are increasingly encountered. For example, in Latin America, the supermarkets' share of all retail food sales increased from 15% in 1990 to 60% by 2000 (Balsevich *et al.*, 2003). In comparison, 80% of retail food sales in the United States in 2000 occurred in supermarkets. In one decade the role of supermarkets in Latin America expanded equivalent to about a half-century of expansion in the United States. Supermarket use has spread across both large and small countries, from capital cities to rural villages, and from upper- and middle-class families to the working class (Hu *et al.*, 2004). This same process is also occurring at varying rates and stages in Asia, Eastern Europe, and Africa (Minten and Reardon, 2008).

Many factors are causing this food system phenomenon (Wilkinson, 2004). Consumer demand for processed and safer foods is on the rise in developing countries. Additionally, as countries modernize, the opportunity cost of women's time has grown, and building a market for time-saving prepared foods has become more important. Transportation and access to technology such as refrigerators have also played a role in the demand for and access to supermarkets. Other factors include the liberalization of direct foreign investment, loosening trade restrictions, and the saturation of Western markets that has pushed growing companies into other locales. Furthermore, improvements in supermarkets' logistics and procurement systems have allowed them to compete on cost with the more typical outlets in developing countries: the small "mom-and-pop" stores and wet markets for fruits, vegetables, and other products.

Supermarkets are large providers of processed, higher-fat, added-sugar, and salt-laden foods in developing countries, but they have also been the purveyors of some good. For example, supermarkets were instrumental (a) in developing the ultraheat treatment (UHT) that gives milk a long shelf life, thereby providing a safe source of milk for all income groups; and (b) in establishing food safety standards (Balsevich *et al.*, 2003). Most importantly, supermarkets have solved the cold chain for animal source foods (dairy, beef, pork, poultry, and fish/seafood) to keep them sanitary.

It remains to be understood how the shift in marketing to these mega-supermarkets will affect the structure of diets and the total amount of food consumed (Minten and

Reardon, 2008). Research is needed into the ways in which these new food markets affect overall prices as well as the relative prices of different food-group categories. Other research needs to address how the new food markets change the consumption of refined versus complex carbohydrates, calorically sweetened foods, animal source foods, and fruits and vegetables, among other key issues.

Mass Media Changes

One of the least discussed and least understood areas of change affecting dietary and physical activity patterns is the role of the modern mass media. Throughout the developing world, there has been a profound increase in the ownership of television sets accompanied by the penetration of modern television programming and advertising. More recently the media have penetrated via computers and cell phones. This has been accompanied by a proliferation of modern magazines and ready access to DVDs of Western movies. The health implications of this phenomenon are not understood. Examples from China are used to illustrate this set of changes. Many scholars directly attribute responsibility for child obesity to television viewing, both as a result of its effect on energy expenditure and because of the direct marketing of food on television. This remains to be studied in most developing countries in a rigorous causal manner.

Do Coca-Cola and McDonald's Have Any Responsibility?

There is a view among some researchers that the US fast-food sector and soft-drink industry have led to the decline of healthy diets throughout the developing world (Zimmet, 2000; Lobstein *et al.*, 2004). American food companies have certainly spread across the globe. Coca-Cola is sold in more than 200 countries, and more than half of McDonald's sales are made outside the United States. Many other examples can be found to show that McDonald's, Pizza Hut, and Kentucky Fried Chicken restaurants are rapidly spreading across the globe. They are quickly followed or even preceded by local food chains that imitate their models, even to the point of serving the same dishes and being equally hygienic and efficient (Popkin, 2008b).

Major questions include: What are these companies doing to impact diets in the developing world? Are they leading people away from their healthy traditional diets to higher-fat and added-sugar-laden food products prepared away from home? Are they leading to increased portion sizes worldwide, as they have in the United States? The answer might be "yes" or "no" depending on which country one studies and how one examines the data. We have shown in one study of four countries a huge variance in the proportions of food consumed from away-from-home and fast-food sources (Adair and Popkin, 2005).

Biological Mismatch

Many scholars, including this author, have discussed one or more ways in which our evolved biology is mismatched with modern food and drink and the technologies of marketing and distribution (Trevantham, 1999; Gluckman and Hanson, 2004). This perspective in many ways argues that fatness and not thinness is self-selected and that obesity is a selective adaptation that was critical to earlier survival. However, the components noted below are critical to energy imbalance. In my work I identify four major domains where this mismatch between modern food-and-drink consumption and energy expenditure clashes with our evolved biology and profoundly affects overall energy imbalance.

Our Evolved Biology	*Modern Technology*
• sweet preferences	• cheap caloric sweeteners, use of sugars in food processing
• thirst and hunger vs. satiety mechanisms are not linked	• caloric beverage revolution
• fatty food preference	• edible oils revolution, cheap edible oils
• desire to reduce exertion	• technology in all phases of movement and exertion

The area most discussed recently is the issue of beverage compensation. Richard Mattes and others have led a revolution in our understanding of the way the body deals differentially with food and beverages of any composition (DiMeglio and Mattes, 2000; DellaValle *et al.*, 2005; Flood *et al.*, 2006; Mattes, 2006; Mourao *et al.*, 2007). In the history of beverages, only recently have we shifted from water to caloric beverages (Wolf *et al.*, 2008). We do not fully understand why we do not compensate for sugar-sweetened and any other caloric beverages by reducing food intake, but it has been shown that we do not. As a result of modern production and marketing of sugar-

sweetened beverages (SSBs), juices, and other fatty and/or sweet drinks, an increase in consumption of high-calorie beverages is occurring globally.

The other areas are documented by scholars in the field and are not addressed in this paper (Eaton and Konner, 1985; Eaton *et al.*, 1988, 1997; Trevantham, 1999; Cordain *et al.*, 2000, 2002, 2005; Gluckman and Hanson, 2004; Jönsson *et al.*, 2006; Power and Schulkin, 2009).

Major Global Dietary and Eating Behavior Shifts

Globally, the overall diet appears to have become increasingly energy dense and sweeter. At the same time, high-fiber foods are being replaced by processed versions. There is enormous variability in eating patterns worldwide, but the broad themes seem to fit most countries. The studies and literature on dietary shifts in low- and middle-income countries are very sparse. The lack of data, the lack of scientists skilled in going beyond simple descriptive analyses of major nutrient and food-group patterns, and the lack of rigorous work on trends cause major gaps.

The global shifts in the energy density of diets are difficult to document. Yet one can document large increases in the consumption of edible oils and animal source foods for selected countries with the help of well-collected, repeated 24-hour recall measures of dietary intake (Du *et al.*, 2002; Popkin and Du, 2003). However, in general most research has had to rely on food disappearance data from the Food and Agricultural Organization (Popkin and Drewnowski, 1997). These data, which do not accurately pick up small shifts in consumption and waste (Crane *et al.*, 1992), demonstrate that shifts in edible oil intake are universal. One set of analyses that compared edible oil intake patterns in the 1960s with those in the 1990s based on food disappearance data shows large increases in the edible oils available for intake, particularly in lower-income countries (Guo *et al.*, 2000). Looking at daily average intake in a country such as China, where we have measured the intake with recall plus direct measures of daily household consumption, we find very high levels of intake. For example, average individual edible oils consumption for all Chinese age 2 years and older was about 12.9% of the caloric intake in 2006 (Popkin, 2008a).

Animal source food changes are equally dramatic (Delgado *et al.*, 2001; Delgado, 2003b; Catelo *et al.*, 2008). In China, for example, we have documented very large increases in animal source food intake (Popkin and

Du, 2003; Popkin, 2008a). Egg, poultry, beef, and pork consumption have increased rapidly in China, and milk intake has recently begun to rise. Today the average Chinese adult consumes more than 1300 kcal/day of pork, poultry, beef, mutton, fish, eggs, and dairy. As we have shown elsewhere, the structure of consumption shifts in China is such that, for each additional increase in income, adults proportionally increase their intake of animal source foods (Guo *et al.*, 2000; Popkin and Du, 2003; Du *et al.*, 2004).

Concurrent shifts are occurring in the use of caloric sweeteners. Only a few countries have published studies on the exact foods in which added caloric sweeteners are found; the United States and South Africa are two of these (Steyn *et al.*, 2003; Duffey *et al.*, 2007; Popkin, 2010). In the United States, calorically sweetened beverages (e.g. soft drinks and fruit drinks) account for more than half of the increase in added-calorie sweeteners in the past several decades; the pattern is much broader in South Africa and Mexico (Barquera *et al.*, 2008).

The studies on fiber intake and other changes toward processed foodstuffs are much less complete to date. Since the issue of reduced fiber intake in the Western diet was first discussed as a source of major health concerns, there have been few systematic studies of shifts in fiber intake throughout the world. There is documentation of specific shifts in diet from coarse grains to refined grains in a few countries.

Similarly, studies on fruit and vegetable intake indicate declines in many countries and regions of the world, but again the declines have not been systematically studied (Popkin *et al.*, 2001a,b). There are also selected countries where fruit and vegetable intakes remain very high (e.g. Spain, Greece, and South Korea) (Kim *et al.*, 2000; Lee *et al.*, 2002; Moreno *et al.*, 2002).

Minimal research has examined frequency of food consumption and snacking and the relation to the types of processing and cooking. Carlos Monteiro and his colleagues are working to document a trend he calls disturbing: the increased shift toward consumption of ultraprocessed foods as contrasted with partly processed foods (Monteiro, 2009).

Snacking and eating frequency have been studied for a few countries. For China we found the emergence of these phenomena among a population that previously had eaten only two or three meals and nothing between meals except tea or water. In unpublished data on China we found a tripling of snacking events between 2004 and 2006, and expect the 2009 data to reveal a further increase. We found

this shift in all income groups and in both urban and rural areas.

A second shift we documented in China is a major increase in fried-food consumption and preparation (Wang *et al.*, 2008). There is no research on this topic for other countries; however, in China the vast increase in the consumption of edible oils seems to have led to this large shift toward frying food instead of boiling or baking.

Global Obesity Dynamics

UNC scholars have completed a major project that analyzed 44 developing countries in nationally representative surveys of women of childbearing age. All women aged 20–49 were weighed and measured with the same equipment and same methods to obtain the measure of overweight status ($25 \text{ kg/m}^2 \leq \text{BMI}$) (Popkin *et al.*, 2011).

The surveys were repeated two to five times for each country during the past two decades (Jones-Smith *et al.*, 2011) and represent a set of surveys conducted with identical sampling and protocol for collection of directly measured weight and height, date of birth, gender, and other sociodemographic data. These data provide a current, highly controlled set of measurements that are comparable in collection methodology, sampling, weighting for national representation, and analysis.

Prevalence

Figure 67.1 provides the current data on each country ranked by the country's per capita gross national product (GNP). These are mainly from the past 3 to 5 years and represent the most up-to-date, accurate assessment possible. In urban areas only four of these countries (Vietnam at 10.7%, Cambodia at 15.7%, Madagascar at 13.9%, and Ethiopia at 15.9%) are below the 20.0% level of prevalence for overweight and obesity. Another eight countries have a prevalence between 20% and 29%, and all the rest have a higher prevalence.

In rural areas a large number of countries have lower levels. Eighteen countries have overweight plus obesity levels over 20%, and a number of large countries have levels that are far higher. These results are presented in more detail elsewhere and represent a set of surveys conducted with identical sampling and protocol for collection of directly measured weight and height, date of birth, gender, and other sociodemographic data (Jones-Smith *et al.*, 2011).

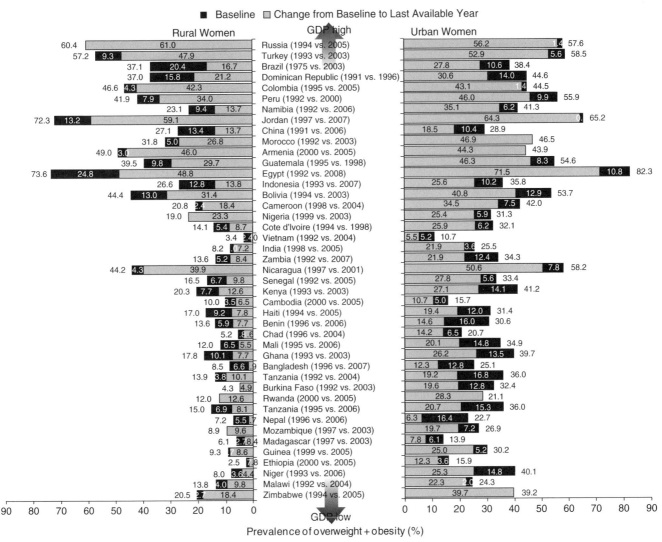

FIG. 67.1 The prevalence of overweight and obesity (BMI ≥25) among women in rural and urban areas of 42 countries by region. Data from Jones-Smith *et al.* (2011) and Popkin *et al.* (2012).

There are too few countries with data for children aged 6–18 for us to systematically discuss child and adolescent overweight status. Elsewhere we have reviewed the trends and levels of child overweight for a small number of developing countries (Popkin *et al.*, 2006). There are studies on preschoolers, however, in which the authors use weight-for-height z-scores above 1 as a criterion (Martorell *et al.*, 2000). We have data for a few countries, including China (13.0% prevalence in ages 6–18 in 2006), Vietnam (1.2% prevalence in ages 6–18 in 2002), Bangladesh (4.4% in ages 10–17 in 2007), and Zambia (9.6% in ages 10–17 in 2007). All used International Obesity Task Force (IOTF) standards (Cole *et al.*, 2000).

Trends for Adults

The absolute change in prevalence between two points in time is divided by the length of time in years to create the absolute annual rate of change in prevalence (expressed in percentage points). The annualized rate of change in prevalence is particularly useful in handling issues where initial prevalence rates are much lower for adults. The results are presented in Figure 67.2 for all countries. As can be seen, in urban areas only Rwanda and in rural areas only Nigeria, Burkino Faso, Rwanda, and Mozambique experienced a decline in overweight plus obesity prevalence. Overall the results show in urban areas an average change in the prevalence of obesity and overweight of about 1.0%. In rural

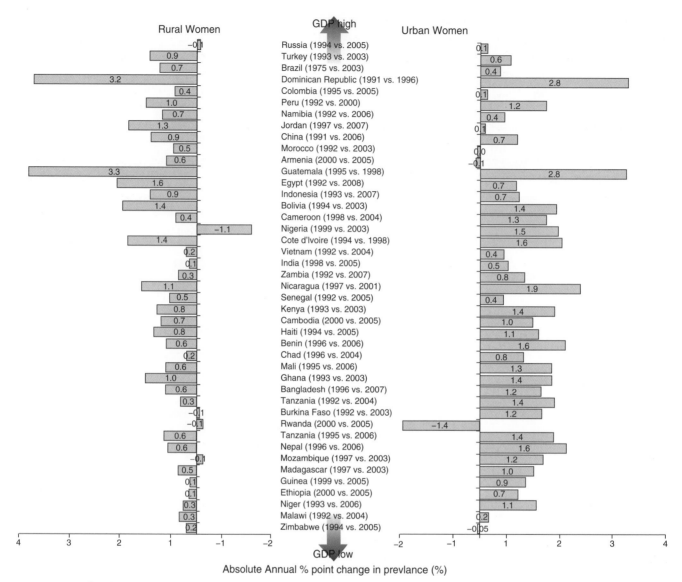

FIG. 67.2   Absolute annual % point change in prevalence in women in 42 developing countries ranked by gross domestic product (GDP) per capita in 2009 US dollars. Data from Jones-Smith *et al.* (2011) and Popkin *et al.* (2012).

areas there is much greater variability, but the overall average is about 0.9%.

Shifting the Burden Toward the Poor

A cross-sectional study of 38 countries found that countries with GNPs above $2500 per capita, plus half the poorer countries, had a higher prevalence of overweight among the poor than among the rich (Monteiro *et al.*, 2002, 2004a,b, 2007). The work of Monteiro and col-

leagues in Brazil was important, but focused mainly on cross-sectional snapshots. It did not tell us whether the rich reduce excessive weight gain relative to the poor as a country or an individual gains GNP per capita or income per capita.

A new set of studies (Jones-Smith *et al.*, 2011) explored the same issue of higher prevalence of obesity and overweight status for higher versus lower socioeconomic status (SES) groups. In this work, trends for the same countries were examined. Forty-one countries provided two to five nationally represented cross-sectional surveys for a sample of women aged 18–49 ($n = 556\,352$). In the majority of country-years, the groups with the highest wealth and education still had the highest age-standardized prevalence of overweight and obesity (97 out of 111 total country-years). However, in approximately half of the countries (21 out of 41), the increases in prevalence over time were greater in the lowest SES group compared with the highest SES group (Jones-Smith *et al.*, 2011).

The Double Burden of Under- and Overnutrition

A phenomenon first explored by Doak and later by others is the double burden of obesity and concurrent undernutrition within the same household (Doak *et al.*, 2002, 2005; Garrett and Ruel, 2005; Custodio *et al.*, 2010; Motlagh *et al.*, 2011). These papers show that, as very poor countries added income and new technologies, the proportion of households with individuals who were both acutely malnourished and overweight (based on body mass index for both measures) increased before being reduced. Doak *et al.* (2005) presented data for seven countries and found that the proportions of dual-burden households were largest in Kyrgyzstan (15.5%) and Indonesia (11.0%), which were then low- to middle-GNP countries based on a GNP comparison of the seven countries. The lowest prevalence of dual-burden households occurs at both ends of the per capita GNP comparison, in Vietnam (3.7%) and the United States (5.4%), respectively (Doak *et al.*, 2005). Ruel and colleagues extended this work to chronically malnourished (stunted) children as one component of the pair and overweight mothers as the other (Garrett and Ruel, 2005).

In many ways these initial studies were part of a broader phenomenon that has now been studied in depth, namely countries with large coexisting undernourished and overweight populations. This is the broader social and health problem. One of the earliest studies on this much more prevalent and important topic was conducted in India (Griffiths and Bentley, 2001).

This issue of populations with large proportions that are malnourished and increasing segments that are becoming overweight is of great concern. In an earlier paper we documented that across the developing world, in both urban and rural areas, the occurrence of maternal obesity was greater than that of maternal underweight (Mendez

et al., 2005). As shown in Figures 67.1 and 67.2, overweight has grown in prevalence in all of these countries, yet, in Haiti, India, and most of the sub-Saharan African countries, large proportions of preschoolers and smaller proportions of other children, adolescents, adults, and the elderly are also undernourished.

This represents a major global problem. Consider India, home to probably half of the world's malnourished children and low-weight infants and a quarter or more of its adults with BMIs below 17. At the same time diabetes, heart disease, and many co-morbidities are caused by excessive visceral fatness and other metabolic issues associated with relatively low BMIs of 22 to 24 (Shetty, 2002; Yajnik *et al.*, 2002; Yajnik, 2004; Ghosh, 2005). Reddy, in a vast number of publications, has critically documented this topic for India (e.g. Reddy, 2002, 2004; Chow *et al.*, 2007).

For governments, the complications of having to focus on undernutrition while addressing emerging obesity and all other NR-NCDs are great. Furthermore, the politics of addressing hunger are appealing, while those of addressing obesity are not.

Hypertension, Diabetes, Cardiovascular Disease Mortality, and Cancers

A vast number of studies document the growing threat of diabetes and hypertension across the developing world and in turn the growing burden of cardiovascular disease and an array of cancers. In the cancer area, the World Cancer Research Foundation (WCRF) and the American Institute for Cancer Research completed a thorough study of the increases in the array of cancers across the developing world and the ever-growing role of obesity and abdominal fat in the incidence and prevalence of cancers and cancer survivorship (WCRF, 2007). In the cardiovascular area, a new Institute of Medicine volume has examined this issue (Fuster *et al.*, 2010; Institute of Medicine, 2010). Many other papers document hypertension increases (Gu *et al.*, 2005; Kearney *et al.*, 2005) or diabetes increases (Zimmet *et al.*, 1997; King *et al.*, 1998; Wild *et al.*, 2004). For instance, about 6.6% of adults have diabetes, and another 7.9% have impaired glucose tolerance. There are no global studies with the new guidelines for measurement of diabetes yet.

These same studies note that India and China already exceed all the new cases of diabetes in all other countries. They also show that, among the top ten countries with adult diabetes, Brazil, Pakistan, Indonesia, and Mexico are also in the top ten in terms of prevalence, along with India and China.

There are a number of critical dimensions to this rapid increase in chronic diseases. Foremost is what appears to be a much greater susceptibility at much lower BMI levels across Asian, Middle Eastern, and Latin American populations. In one or two cases, such as Pacific Islanders, it appears that a much higher BMI level is associated with the same risk of the chronic diseases that we find at lower BMI levels for non-Hispanic whites in the United States (WHO Expert Consultation, 2004). In most situations, however, higher levels of visceral fat are found for the same BMI levels among these populations. There also appear to be some populations more susceptible to diabetes (South Asians) and others more susceptible to hypertension and stroke (East Asians) (Carter *et al.*, 1996; Eastern Stroke and Coronary Heart Disease Collaborative Research Group, 1998; Ramachandran *et al.*, 2001, Lee *et al.*, 2007).

We do not fully understand the genetic or epigenetic dimensions of this phenomenon. One potential key to the much higher visceral fat levels among the South Asian population may be the fact that South Asian women with BMIs of 16.5 or 17.0 can reproduce successfully, whereas it might take a much higher BMI level in other societies to achieve reproductive success.

For whatever reasons, we are seeing very rapid increases in the risk of type 2 diabetes in Mexico and other South American countries, remarkably rapid increases in hypertension in China, and equally rapid increases in diabetes in India and the Middle East. The epicenter for cardiovascular disease and cancer has shifted toward these low- and middle-income countries.

Conservative estimates of diabetes show a global estimate of 6.6% and an additional 7.9% with impaired glucose tolerance in 2010 from the WHO. More importantly, both the WHO and the World Diabetes Federation show that, of the top ten countries with diabetes among individuals ages 20–79, the United States is ranked third, with 36 million cases. India and China, with 87.0 and 62.6 million cases, respectively, are numbers one and two, and Pakistan, Brazil, Indonesia, Mexico, Bangladesh, Russia, and Egypt round out the top ten.

When we shift from just diabetes to all the nutrition-related non-communicable diseases, diet and obesity emerge as major causes of most cancers and cardiovascular disease, both new cases and consequent deaths from, in the low- and middle-income countries. In China we have documented an increased rate of adult mortality, and the causes are mainly cancers and cardiovascular disease (Popkin, 2008a). In China, after decades of very rapid declines in mortality from infectious diseases, smoking, poor diet, and obesity represent the major causal factors in this huge increase among men and women. For India, the discussion is focused mainly on the 100 million cases of diabetes that will emerge over the next several decades, but the cardiovascular burden from this has been noted to be very large (Institute of Medicine, 2010).

Future Directions

The low- and middle-income world is not prepared for the large shift in causes of disability, morbidity, and mortality from NR-NCDs. Some basic scientific questions need to be understood, and there are many programmatic and policy issues as well.

Foremost from a scientific point of view is the need for a greater understanding of susceptibility as it varies across racial and ethnic national and regional subpopulations. Why do South Asians gain excessive visceral fat at BMI levels of 20–22 and become so susceptible to diabetes? Are there issues in their dietary and activity patterns that can explain this? Is this the result of a unique shared history in that subcontinent of intergenerational malnutrition and stunting and all the other issues often discussed in research into the developmental origins of disease research? Similarly, why are East Asians more susceptible to hypertension and stroke? Is this a dietary issue, or are there other explanations that can be evaluated to reduce this risk? There are many related questions for Hispanics and persons from the Middle East, the Arabian Gulf states, and sub-Saharan Africa.

The double burden of under- and overnutrition poses a major set of research issues heretofore not fully explored. When malnutrition becomes a small and focused problem, as in Chile and Mexico, it can be managed through targeted programs. However, when both under- and overnutrition have large public health impacts and reach 10–40% of the population, targeting does not work. What, then, are the major program and policy options for addressing both problems while not exacerbating one or the other?

Resource constraints force most of these countries to develop prevention activities. What are they? Just what can we do to reduce caloric intake while also promoting a healthier eating and activity pattern? There is literally no case study at the national level of effective prevention options. Are there price policy, regulatory, and other macro options that will work? And where does public education fit in?

Underlying the program and policy research needs is an almost total lack of detailed data on individual dietary intake. At a time when household food consumption and food purchases are becoming less relevant for the diets of many individuals of different age–gender subgroupings, only one or two countries even collect systematically detailed dietary intake data episodically. For these countries, few individuals are skilled in analyzing the data at the disaggregated food level necessary to understand dynamic shifts, the causes of these shifts, and the program options. Furthermore, up-to-date food composition tables are not available. What are the low-cost options for updating these food composition tables? Are there user fee options? How do we develop the resources to train the next generation of scholars needed for public policy research? Only India, which is investing in a new generation of public health schools, has begun to address this topic nationally.

In addition to issues unique to each country and region, there are of course the same basic scientific questions. However, the nutrition community, which does not have the extensive national and multinational institutions available to agriculture, urgently needs not only basic science but also ways to adapt to the unique environments and genetics of each country.

Suggestions for Further Reading

There are few broad-based data-driven studies and books exploring diet-related chronic diseases in the low- and middle-income world. In general, aside from small case studies and explorations of changes within each country, only Carlos Monteiro and Barry Popkin have examined issues across a range of countries. One collection of articles and two books provide handy overviews. Other than these publications, the reader should consult the references from this volume to study this topic.

Caballero, B. and Popkin, B.M. (eds) (2002) *The Nutrition Transition: Diet and Disease in the Developing World*. Academic Press, London.

Popkin, B.M. (2008) *The World Is Fat: The Fads, Trends, Policies, and Products That Are Fattening the Human Race*. Avery-Penguin, New York.

Public Health Nutrition 5(Suppl) (2002) Includes a series of case studies and broad articles.

References

Adair, L.S. and Popkin, B.M. (2005) Are child eating patterns being transformed globally? *Obes Res* **13**, 1281–1299.

Balsevich, F., Berdegue, J.A., Flores, L., *et al.* (2003) Supermarkets and produce quality and safety standards in Latin America. *Am J Agric Econ* **85**, 1147–1154.

Barquera, S., Hernandez-Barrera, L., Tolentino, M.L., *et al.* (2008) Energy intake from beverages is increasing among Mexican adolescents and adults. *J Nutr* **138**, 2454–2461.

Carter, J.S., Pugh, J.A., and Monterrosa, A. (1996) Non-insulin-dependent diabetes mellitus in minorities in the United States [Comment]. *Ann Intern Med* **125**, 221–232.

Catelo, M.A.O., Narrod, C.A., and Tiongco, M. (2008) *Structural Changes in the Philippine Pig Industry and Their Environmental Implications*. IFPRI, Washington, DC.

Chow, C., Cardona, M., Raju, P.K., *et al.* (2007) Cardiovascular disease and risk factors among 345 adults in rural India – the Andhra Pradesh Rural Health Initiative. *Int J Cardiol* **116**, 180–185.

Cole, T.J., Bellizz, M.C., Flegal, K.M., *et al.* (2000) Establishing a standard definition for child overweight and obesity worldwide: international survey. *BMJ* **320**, 1240–1243.

Cordain, L., Eaton, S.B., Miller, J.B., *et al.* (2002) The paradoxical nature of hunter-gatherer diets: meat-based, yet non-atherogenic. *Eur J Clin Nutr* **56**, S42–S52.

Cordain, L., Eaton, S.B., Sebastian, A. *et al.* (2005) Origins and evolution of the Western diet: health implications for the 21st century. *Am J Clin Nutr* **81**, 341–354.

Cordain, L., Miller, J.B., Eaton, S.B., *et al.* (2000) Plant–animal subsistence ratios and macronutrient energy estimations in worldwide hunter–gatherer diets. *Am J Clin Nutr* **71**, 682–692.

Crane, N., Lewis, C., and Yetley, E. (1992) Do time trends in food supply levels of macronutrients reflect survey estimates of macronutrient intake? *Am J Publ Health* **82**, 862–866.

Custodio, E., Descalzo, M.A., Roche, J., *et al.* (2010) The economic and nutrition transition in Equatorial Guinea coincided with a double burden of over- and under nutrition. *Econ Hum Biol* **8**, 80–87.

Davis, K. (1945) The world demographic transition. *Ann Am Acad Polit Soc Sci* **237**, 1–11.

Delgado, C.L. (2003a) A food revolution: rising consumption of meat and milk in developing countries. *J Nutr* **133**, 3907S–3910S.

Delgado, C.L. (2003b) Rising consumption of meat and milk in developing countries has created a new food revolution. *J Nutr* **133**, 3907S–3910S.

Delgado, C.L., Rosegrant, M.W., and Meijer, S. (2001) Livestock to 2020: the revolution continues. *Paper presented at the annual meetings of the International Agricultural Trade Research Consortium (IATRC)*. Auckland.

DellaValle, D.M., Roe, L.S., and Rolls, B.J. (2005) Does the consumption of caloric and non-caloric beverages with a meal affect energy intake? *Appetite* **44,** 187–193.

DiMeglio, D.P. and Mattes, R.D. (2000) Liquid versus solid carbohydrate: effects on food intake and body weight. *Int J Obes Rel Metab Dis* **24,** 794–800.

Doak, C., Adair, L., Bentley, M., *et al.* (2002) The underweight/overweight household: an exploration of household sociodemographic and dietary factors in China. *Publ Health Nutr* **5,** 215–221.

Doak, C.M., Adair, L.S., Bentley, M., *et al.* (2005) The dual burden household and the nutrition transition paradox. *Int J Obes* **29,** 129–136.

Drenowski, A. and Popkin, B. (1997) The nutrition transition: new trends in the global diet. *Nutr Rev* **55,** 31–43.

Duffey, K. and Popkin, B.M. (2007) Shifts in patterns and consumption of beverages between 1965 and 2002. *Obesity* **15,** 2739–2747.

Duffey, K.J., Gordon-Larsen, P., Jacobs D.R., Jr, *et al.* (2007) Beverage intake patterns and the metabolic syndrome: a 20-year CARDIA study. Chapel Hill.

Du, S., Lu, B., Zhai, F., *et al.* (2002) A new stage of the nutrition transition in China. *Publ Health Nutr* **5,** 169–174.

Du, S., Mroz, T.A., Zhai, F., *et al.* (2004) Rapid income growth adversely affects diet quality in China – particularly for the poor! *Soc Sci Med* **59,** 1505–1515.

Eastern Stroke and Coronary Heart Disease Collaborative Research Group (1998) Blood pressure, cholesterol, and stroke in eastern Asia. *Lancet* **352,** 1801–1807.

Eaton, S.B. and Konner, M. (1985) Paleolithic nutrition: a consideration on its nature and current implications. *N Engl J Med* **312,** 283–289.

Eaton, S.B., Eaton, S.B., 3rd, and Konner, M.J. (1997) Paleolithic nutrition revisited: a twelve-year retrospective on its nature and implications. *Eur J Clin Nutr* **51,** 207–216.

Eaton, S.B., Shostak, M., and Konner, M. (1988) *The Paleolithic Prescription: a Program of Diet and Exercise and a Design for Living.* Harper & Row, New York.

Flood, J., Roe, L., and Rolls, B. (2006) The effect of increased beverage portion size on energy intake at a meal. *J Am Diet Assoc* **106,** 1984–1990.

Fuster, V., Chockalingam, A., De Quadros, C.A., *et al.* (2010) *Promoting Cardiovascular Health in the Developing World: A Critical Challenge to Achieve Global Health.* National Academies Press, Washington, DC.

Gardner, B.L. (2002) *American Agriculture in the Twentieth Century: How It Flourished and What It Cost.* Harvard University Press, Cambridge, MA.

Garrett, J.L. and Ruel, M.T. (2005) Stunted child-overweight mother pairs: prevalence and association with economic development and urbanization. *Food Nutr Bull* **26,** 209–221.

Ghosh, A. (2005) Factor analysis of metabolic syndrome among the middle-aged Bengalee Hindu men of Calcutta, India. *Diabetes Metab Res Rev* **21,** 58–64.

Gluckman, P.D. and Hanson, M.A. (2004) Living with the past: evolution, development, and patterns of disease. *Science* **305,** 1733–1736.

Griffiths, P.L. and Bentley, M.E. (2001) The nutrition transition is underway in India. *J Nutr* **131,** 2692–2700.

Gu, D., Reynolds, K., Wu, X., *et al.* (2005) Prevalence of the metabolic syndrome and overweight among adults in China. *Lancet,* **365,** 1398–1405.

Guo, X.G., Mroz, T.A., Popkin, B.M., *et al.* (2000) Structural change in the impact of income on food consumption in China, 1989–1993. *Econ Devel Cult Change* **48,** 737–760.

Hu, D., Reardon, T., Rozelle, S., *et al.* (2004) The emergence of supermarkets with Chinese characteristics: challenges and opportunities for China's agricultural development. *Devel Policy Rev* **22,** 557–586.

Institute of Medicine (2010) *Promoting Cardiovascular Health in the Developing World: A Critical Challenge to Achieve Global Health.* National Academies Press, Washington, DC.

Jones-Smith, J.C., Gordon-Larsen, P., Siddiqi, A., *et al.* (2011) Is the Burden of Overweight Shifting to the Poor Across the Globe? Time Trends Among Women in 39 low- and middle-income countries (1991–2008). *Int J Obes.* DOI: 10.1038/ijo.2011.179.

Jones-Smith, J., Gordon-Larsen, P., Siddiqi, A., *et al.* (2011) Cross-national comparisons of time trends in overweight inequality by socioeconomic status among women using repeated cross-sectional surveys from 37 developing countries (1989–2007). *Am J Epidemiol* **173,** 667–675.

Jönsson, T., Ahren, B., Pacini, G., *et al.* (2006) A Paleolithic diet confers higher insulin sensitivity, lower C-reactive protein and lower blood pressure than a cereal-based diet in domestic pigs. *Nutr Metab (Lond)* **3,** 39.

Kearney, P.M., Whelton, M., Reynolds, K., *et al.* (2005) Global burden of hypertension: analysis of worldwide data. *Lancet* **365,** 217–223.

Kim, S., Moon, S., and Popkin, B.M. (2000) The nutrition transition in South Korea. *Am J Clin Nutr* **71,** 44–53.

King, H., Aubert, R.E., and Herman, W.H. (1998) Global burden of diabetes, 1995–2025: prevalence, numerical estimates, and projections. *Diabetes Care* **21,** 1414–1431.

Lee, C.M., Huxley, R.R., Lam, T.H., *et al.* (2007) Prevalence of diabetes mellitus and population attributable fractions for coronary heart disease and stroke mortality in the WHO South-East Asia and Western Pacific regions. *Asia Pac J Clin Nutr* **16,** 187–192.

Lee, M.J., Popkin, B.M., and Kim, S. (2002) The unique aspects of the nutrition transition in South Korea: the retention of healthful elements in their traditional diet. *Public Health Nutr* **5**, 197–203.

Lobstein, T., Baur, L., and Uauy, R. (2004) Obesity in children and young people: a crisis in public health. *Obes Rev* **5**(Suppl 1), 4–104.

Martorell, R., Kettel Khan, L.K., Hughes, M.L., *et al.* (2000) Overweight and obesity in preschool children from developing countries. *Int J Obes Relat Metab Disord* **24**, 959–967.

Mattes, R. (2006) Fluid calories and energy balance: the good, the bad, and the uncertain. *Physiol Behav* **89**, 66–70.

Mendez, M.A., Monteiro, C.A., and Popkin, B.M. (2005) Overweight exceeds underweight among women in most developing countries. *Am J Clin Nutr* **81**, 714–721.

Minten, B. and Reardon, T. (2008) Food prices, quality, and quality's pricing in supermarkets versus traditional markets in developing countries. *Appl Econ Perspect Policy* **30**, 480–490.

Monteiro, C.A. (2009) Nutrition and health. The issue is not food, nor nutrients, so much as processing. *Publ Health Nutr* **12**, 729–731.

Monteiro, C.A., Conde, W.L., Lu, B., *et al.* (2004a) Obesity and inequities in health in the developing world. *Int J Obes Rel Metab Dis* **28**, 1181–1186.

Monteiro, C.A., Conde, W.L., and Popkin, B.M. (2002) Is obesity replacing or adding to undernutrition? Evidence from different social classes in Brazil. *Public Health Nutr* **5**, 105–112.

Monteiro, C.A., Conde, W.L., and Popkin, B.M. (2007) Income-specific trends in obesity in Brazil: 1975–2003. *Am J Publ Health* **97**, 1808–1812.

Monteiro, C.A., Moura, E.C., Conde, W.L., *et al.* (2004b) Socioeconomic status and obesity in adult populations of developing countries: a review. *Bull World Health Organ* **82**, 940–946.

Moreno, L.A., Sarria, A., and Popkin, B.M. (2002) The nutrition transition in Spain: a European Mediterranean country. *Eur J Clin Nutr* **56**, 992–1003.

Morgan, N. (1993) World vegetable oil consumption expands and diversifies. *Food Rev* **16**, 26–30.

Motlagh, M.E., Kelishadi, R., Amirkhani, M.A., *et al.* (2011) Double burden of nutritional disorders in young Iranian children: findings of a nationwide screening survey. *Public Health Nutr* **14**, 605–610.

Mourao, D., Bressan, J., Campbell, W. *et al.* (2007) Effects of food form on appetite and energy intake in lean and obese young adults. *Int J Obes (Lond)* **31**, 1688–1695.

Omran, A.R. (1971) The epidemiologic transition. A theory of the epidemiology of population change. *Milbank Mem Fund Quart* **49**, 509–538.

Popkin, B.M. (2002) An overview on the nutrition transition and its health implications: the Bellagio meeting. *Public Health Nutr* **5**, 93–103.

Popkin, B.M. (2006a) Global nutrition dynamics: the world is shifting rapidly toward a diet linked with noncommunicable diseases. *Am J Clin Nutr* **84**, 289–298.

Popkin, B.M. (2006b) Technology, transport, globalization and the nutrition transition. *Food Policy* **31**, 554–569.

Popkin, B.M. (2008a) Will China's nutrition transition overwhelm its health care system and slow economic growth? *Health Affairs (Millwood)* **27**, 1064–1076.

Popkin, B.M. (2008b) *The World Is Fat – The Fads, Trends, Policies, and Products That Are Fattening the Human Race.* Avery-Penguin Group, New York.

Popkin, B.M. (2010) Patterns of beverage use across the lifecycle. *Physiol Behav* **100**, 4–9.

Popkin, B.M. (2011) Agricultural policies, food and public health. *EMBO Rep* **12**, 11–18.

Popkin, B.M. and Du, S. (2003) Dynamics of the nutrition transition toward the animal foods sector in China and its implications: a worried perspective. *J Nutr* **133**, 3898S–3906S.

Popkin, B.M. and Nielsen, S.J. (2003) The sweetening of the world's diet. *Obes Res* **11**, 1325–1332.

Popkin, B.M., Adair, L.S., and Ng, S.W. (2011) Then and now: global nutrition transition and the pandemic of obesity in developing countries. *Nutr Rev* **70**, 3–21.

Popkin, B.M., Adair, L.S., and Ng, S.W. (2012) Global nutrition transition and the pandemic of obesity in developing countries. *Nutr Rev* **70**(1): 3–21.

Popkin, B.M., Conde, W., Hou, N., *et al.* (2006) Is there a lag globally in overweight trends for children compared with adults? *Obesity (Silver Spring)* **14**, 1846–1853.

Popkin, B.M., Horton, S., and Kim, S. (2001b) The nutrition transition and prevention of diet-related chronic diseases in Asia and the Pacific. *Food Nutr Bull* **22**, 1–58.

Popkin, B.M., Horton, S., Kim, S.W., *et al.* (2001a) Trends in diet, nutritional status, and diet-related noncommunicable diseases in China and India: the economic costs of the nutrition transition. *Nutr Rev* **59**, 379–390.

Power, M.L. and Schulkin, J. (2009) *The Evolution of Obesity.* Johns Hopkins University Press, Baltimore, MD.

Ramachandran, A., Snehalatha, C., Kapur, A., *et al.* (2001) High prevalence of diabetes and impaired glucose tolerance in India: National Urban Diabetes Survey. *Diabetologia* **44**, 1094–1101.

Reddy, K.S. (2002) Cardiovascular diseases in the developing countries: dimensions, determinants, dynamics and directions for public health action. *Public Health Nutr* **5**, 231–237.

Reddy, K.S. (2004) Cardiovascular disease in non-Western countries. *N Engl J Med* **350**, 2438–2440.

Shetty, P.S. (2002) Nutrition transition in India. *Public Health Nutr* **5,** 175–182.

Steyn, N.P., Myburgh, N.G., and Nel, J.H. (2003) Evidence to support a food-based dietary guideline on sugar consumption in South Africa. *Bull World Health Organ* **81,** 599–608.

Trevantham, W., Smith, E.O., and McKenna, J.J. (eds) (1999) *Evolutionary Medicine*. Oxford University Press, New York.

US Department of Agriculture (1966) 1996 US fats and oils statistics. *US Department of Agriculture Statistical Bulletin No. 376.* ERS, Washington, DC.

United Nations (2002) *World Urbanization Prospects, 2001.* United Nations, New York.

Wallingford, J.C., Yuhas, R., Du, S., *et al.* (2004) Fatty acids in Chinese edible oils: evidence for unexpected impact in changing diet. *Food Nutr Bull* **25,** 330–336.

Wang, Z., Zhai, F., Shufa, D. *et al.* (2008) Dynamic shifts in Chinese eating behaviors. *Asia Pac J Clin Nutr* **17,** 123–130.

WCRF (2007) *Food, Nutrition, Physical Activity and the Prevention of Cancer: a Global Perspective*. Washington DC World Cancer Research Fund in association with the American Institute for Cancer Research, Washington, DC.

WHO Expert Consultation (2004) Appropriate body-mass index for Asian populations and its implications for policy and intervention strategies. *Lancet* **363,** 157–163.

Wild, S., Roglic, G., Green, A., *et al.* (2004) Global prevalence of diabetes: estimates for the year 2000 and projections for 2030. *Diabetes Care* **27,** 1047–1053.

Wilkinson, J. (2004) Globalisation, food processing and developing countries: driving forces and the impact on small farms and firms. *Electr J Agric Devel Econ* **1,** 184–201.

Williams, G. (1984) Development and future direction of the world soybean market. *Q J Int Agric* **23,** 319–337.

Wolf, A., Bray, G.A., and Popkin, B.M. (2008) A short history of beverages and how our body treats them. *Obes Rev* **9,** 151–164.

Yajnik, C.S. (2004) Obesity epidemic in India: intrauterine origins? *Proc Nutr Soc* **63,** 387–396.

Yajnik, C.S., Lubree, H.G., Rege, S.S., *et al.* (2002) Adiposity and hyperinsulinemia in Indians are present at birth. *J Clin Endocrinol Metab* **87,** 5575–5580.

Zimmet, P. (2000) Globalization, coca-colonization and the chronic disease epidemic: can the Doomsday scenario be averted? *J Intern Med* **247,** 301–310.

Zimmet, P.Z., McCarty, D.J., and De Courten, M.P. (1997) The global epidemiology of non-insulin-dependent diabetes mellitus and the metabolic syndrome. *J Diabetes Complications* **11,** 60–68.

68

FOOD INSECURITY, HUNGER, AND UNDERNUTRITION

DAVID L. PELLETIER[1], PhD, CHRISTINE M. OLSON[1], PhD, AND
EDWARD A. FRONGILLO[2], PhD

[1]*Cornell University, Ithaca, New York, USA*
[2]*University of South Carolina, Columbia, South Carolina, USA*

Summary

Food insecurity, hunger, and undernutrition are poverty-related problems that affect all of the world's population to varying extents. The United Nations estimated that nearly 925 million people (16%) in developing countries were "undernourished" in 2010, but this method does not yield an accurate measure of food security at the household or individual level. Chronic undernutrition (stunting) is found in 33% of preschoolers in developing countries, and underweight is found in 19% of this age group. The United States uses definitions and methods very different from those used in low-income countries, but in 2009 it was estimated that 14.7% of US households were food insecure and about one-third of these (5.7%) had very low food security. Despite decades of research and an increasing level of attention by national governments and international organizations, the exact relationships among these problems and the most effective policy, programmatic and political means for eliminating them remain elusive. Doing so is becoming even more challenging in light of the emergence of nutrition-related chronic diseases in these same countries and population groups.

Introduction

Recent decades have witnessed some fundamental changes in the way food insecurity, hunger, and undernutrition are understood within scientific and policy communities. In previous eras these three problems typically were viewed as a causal or chronological continuum, with food insecurity representing a situation of inadequate access to food owing to social and economic circumstances, hunger representing the immediate physiological manifestation of inadequate intake, and undernutrition representing the physical consequences of chronically or acutely inadequate intake. Such a view has a variety of distorting effects on how each is measured and on notions of their prevalence, causes, consequences, and appropriate policy responses. This chapter describes the current understanding of the nature of each of these problems, their relationships with each other, what is known about prevalence, causes and consequences, and policy implications. For convenience the food-security situation in

Present Knowledge in Nutrition, Tenth Edition. Edited by John W. Erdman Jr, Ian A. Macdonald and Steven H. Zeisel.
© 2012 International Life Sciences Institute. Published 2012 by John Wiley & Sons, Inc.

developed and developing countries is described in separate sections.

Food Insecurity and Hunger in Food-Rich Countries: The United States as a Case Example

Nature of the Problem

Though food insecurity and hunger have long been nutrition concerns among poorer countries of the world, these problems have re-emerged as nutrition concerns for food-rich countries such as the United States. This section of the chapter will briefly describe food insecurity, its measurement, and prevalence in the United States, and then review its consequences.

In 1989 an expert panel convened by the American Institute of Nutrition for the Life Sciences Research Organization identified food insecurity and hunger as core indicators of an individual's nutritional state (Anderson, 1990). This group put forth the initial consensus definitions of food insecurity and hunger. Food insecurity is the "limited or uncertain availability of nutritionally adequate and safe foods or limited or uncertain ability to acquire acceptable foods in socially acceptable ways." Hunger, a narrower and more severe form of deprivation, is "the painful or uneasy sensation caused by a lack of food, the recurrent and involuntary lack of food." Hunger can result in malnutrition over time and is a potential, although not necessary, consequence of food insecurity (Anderson, 1990). Food insecurity is experienced primarily at two different levels of social organization: the household or family eating unit, and the individual level. Hunger is generally used to describe an experience of food deprivation at the individual level.

In early research to define the concept and components of food insecurity, Radimer and colleagues (1992) described food insecurity and hunger as a managed process. The household food manager, generally a woman in US society, has some control over the sequence in which the various components of food insecurity are experienced and who in the household experiences them. Adults and children in the same household experience different components of food insecurity at different times and to different degrees. None the less, there is a general sequence to the phenomenon: household-level food insecurity with the depletion of household food supplies and anxiety are generally experienced first; the quantity and quality of women's food intake, as well as the quality of the household food supply, are affected next; and finally the quantity and quality of children's food intake are affected. This basic understanding of the sequenced nature of the phenomenon has been incorporated into instruments for measuring the problem.

In 2004, the US Department of Agriculture requested the Committee on National Statistics (CNSTAT) of the National Academies to convene a panel of experts to review the concepts and methodology for measuring food insecurity and hunger in the United States. One particular conceptual issue included in the charge to the panel was "the appropriateness of identifying hunger as a severe range of food insecurity" (National Research Council, 2006, p. 2). The panel concluded: "hunger is a concept distinct from food insecurity, which is an indicator and possible consequence of food insecurity, that can be useful in characterizing the severity of food insecurity. Hunger itself is an important concept, but should be measured at the individual level distinct from, but in the context of food insecurity" (Wunderlich and Norwood, 2006). The CNSTAT panel indicated that hunger is more than the painful and uneasy sensation caused by the lack of food. It is the result of prolonged, involuntary lack of food and should result in physiological symptoms such as discomfort, illness, weakness, or severe pain. In addition, the panel recommended that USDA use alternative labels for the more severe levels of food insecurity, particularly food insecurity with hunger. Table 68.1 shows the revised labels used by USDA to describe the range of food security.

Measurement

The 10-year comprehensive plan for the National Nutritional Monitoring and Related Research Program set in motion a series of collaborative efforts across government agencies, academia, and the private sector to create a measure of food insecurity and hunger that could be used annually to assess the prevalence of food insecurity and hunger in the US population (US Department of Health and Human Services, 1993; Food and Consumer Service, 1995). The process of developing this measure is well described in the nutrition literature (Carlson et al., 1999). The development and testing of questionnaire items by two groups, the Community Childhood Hunger Identification Project sponsored by the Food Research and Action Center (Wehler et al., 1992) and the Division of Nutritional Sciences at Cornell University (Kendall et al., 1995), were of critical importance to this effort. In April

TABLE 68.1 Old and new labels for describing the ranges of food security

General categories (old and new labels are the same)	Detailed categories		
	Old label	New label	Description of conditions in the household
Food security	Food security	High food security	No reported indications of food-access problems or limitations
		Marginal food security	One or two reported indications – typically of anxiety over food sufficiency or shortage of food in the house. Little or no indication of changes in diets or food intake
Food insecurity	Food insecurity without hunger	Low food security	Reports of reduced quality, variety, or desirability of diet. Little or no indication of reduced food intake
	Food insecurity with hunger	Very low food security	Reports of multiple indications of disrupted eating patterns and reduced food intake

1995, the US Bureau of the Census administered the 18-item food-security scale to 45 000 households in its regular Current Population Survey. With data from this survey and methods from item-response theory (Rasch modeling), the scale was further refined, cut-points in the scale for differentiating levels of severity of the phenomena were defined, and categories of responses representing different levels of food insecurity were created (Carlson *et al.*, 1999).

The US Household Food Security Survey Module is an 18-item scale with a 12-month time reference (Bickel *et al.*, 2000). The scale has been shown to have good reliability, with a reliability coefficient of 0.81 for households with children and 0.74 for all households (extreme values that would inflate the reliability coefficient were omitted) (Hamilton *et al.*, 1997). In addition, responses to the Current Population Survey items follow a similar pattern across samples from diverse populations including racial and ethnic minorities (Frongillo, 1999). Scale scores are significantly related to the poverty income ratio (income relative to the poverty line) and weekly food expenditures in the expected ways, thus indicating validity (Hamilton *et al.*, 1997).

The Household Food Security Survey Module has now been administered to participants in the Current Population Survey conducted by the US Census Bureau for 14 years (1995–2008). The CNSTAT panel confirmed the importance of continuing to measure food insecurity in the US population and recommended that: "USDA should con-

tinue to measure and monitor food insecurity regularly in a household survey" (Wunderlich and Norwood, 2006, p. 49). The panel made several additional recommendations concerning measurement issues with the survey, item response theory, and other potential survey vehicles that could be used in measuring food insecurity in the population.

Other advances that have been made in the measurement of food insecurity are described in the Food Security Briefing Room of the USDA Economic Research Service web site (www.ers.usda.gov/Briefing/FoodSecurity). One particularly noteworthy advance has been the development of the Children's Food Security Scale (Nord and Hopwood, 2007).

Prevalence

In 2009, 14.7% of US households were food insecure. About one-third of food-insecure households or 5.4% had very low food security (Nord *et al.*, 2010). About 50 million persons including 17.1 million children lived in food-insecure households. Households with very low food security generally experienced the condition for 7 months of the year, for a few days in each month.

Food insecurity varies by household characteristics in expected ways. In 2009, households with incomes below the official poverty line had a prevalence of 43.0%, nearly three times the national average. Households with children had a rate (23.1%) that is nearly twice the rate of those without children (11.4%). Black and Hispanic households had a prevalence of 24.9% and 26.9%, and 36.6% of households headed by a single woman with children were food insecure.

From 1995 through 2000, there was a downward trend in the prevalence of household-level food insecurity in the United States. From 2000 to 2004 there was a gradual increase from 10.1% to 11.9% in the prevalence of food insecurity, a drop to 11% in 2005, and then a near level prevalence until 2008. The 2009 prevalence of food insecurity was the highest observed since the food security surveys began in 1995 (Nord *et al.*, 2010).

Consequences

The early research of Radimer *et al.* (1992) suggests that individual household members experience food insecurity differently, with adults experiencing negative changes in diet quality and quantity before children. Available research supports this hypothesis, specifically that mothers compromise their own nutritional status to feed their children (Rose and Olivera, 1997; McIntyre *et al.*, 2003; Olson, 2005).

While there is a large research literature on the adverse consequences of food insecurity in food-rich countries, most studies are cross-sectional and thus are constrained in specifying the direction of causality. In recent years, a few longitudinal studies have investigated the relationship between food insecurity and a variety of different outcomes. Since these types of studies are more supportive of making causal inferences, only longitudinal studies concerning consequences will be discussed here. Reviews of cross-sectional studies will be cited.

Several reviews, including an earlier version of this chapter in the ninth edition of *Present Knowledge in Nutrition*, show that adults living in food-insecure households consume diets that are low in essential nutrients and some food groups, particularly fruits and vegetables (Olson, 2005; Holben, 2006; Pelletier *et al.*, 2006). In addition, adults in food-insecure household are more likely to have poorer health and functional status, as well as being at greater risk for chronic health conditions and compromised management of these conditions. There are few longitudinal studies with adults to support causal inferences of food insecurity resulting in poorer health, although knowledge of how these factors are related certainly makes such inferences plausible.

The noted exception to the generalization above is with the health outcomes of weight gain and obesity. Three different longitudinal studies of adult women, one using a national sample of US women and one each with urban and rural samples of women, found no significant relationship between initial food insecurity status and weight gain or risk of becoming obese over follow-up periods of about two years (Jones and Frongillo, 2007; Whitaker and Sarin, 2007; Olson and Strawderman, 2008). However, Olson and Strawderman (2008) found an interaction between initial obesity and food insecurity, with women who were both obese and food insecure in early pregnancy at the greatest risk of major weight gain at 2 years postpartum, pointing to the possibility of a third factor associated with both constructs. None the less, these authors found stronger support for obesity leading to food insecurity than food insecurity leading to obesity. In a national sample, Jones and Frongillo (2007) found that, among overweight women who were on a weight-gain trajectory, those who were food insecure gained significantly less. This relationship was not observed in healthy-weight or obese women. Finally, again in a national sample of women, Jones and Frongillo (2006) found persistently food-insecure women gained less weight across time, but full participation in the Food Stamp Program offset this weight change. Taken together, these studies do not support a strong causal inference of food insecurity leading to major weight gain or obesity in adult women.

In 2008, 22.5% of children in the United States lived in food-insecure households and 1.5% of children lived in households with very low food security among children, a statistic from the children's measure of food insecurity (Nord *et al.*, 2010). These statistics indicate that a large proportion of US children are potentially affected by exposure to food insecurity. Cross-sectional as well as a small number of short-term longitudinal studies described in several reviews indicate that household insecurity and children's food insecurity are associated with poorer nutritional status, as well as poorer growth, health, mental and psychological functioning, and cognitive and academic achievement (Ashiabi and O'Neal, 2008; Cook and Frank, 2008; Kursmark and Weitzman, 2009).

Three different longitudinal studies from three different countries, the United States, Canada, and the United Kingdom, found adverse health and developmental outcomes associated with food insecurity in children ranging in age from the preschool years to adolescence (Jyoti *et al.*, 2005; Belsky *et al.*, 2010; Kirkpatrick *et al.*, 2010). Using data from the Early Childhood Longitudinal Study–Kindergarten Cohort, Jyoti *et al.* (2005) found that children who lived in marginally food-insecure households during their kindergarten years had significantly lower social and mathematics skills in third grade. Using data from the Canadian National Longitudinal Survey of Children and Youth that followed children for 10 years, hunger measured using one question was associated with a 2.5-fold increased risk of overall poor health among children who entered the cohort as preschoolers (Kirkpatrick et al., 2010). Among these children, no significant relationships between hunger and being diagnosed with one of six chronic health conditions or asthma were found, nor were any significant relationships found in the cohort of older youth. Among the younger cohort, the experience of two or more episodes of hunger was associated with nearly a five-fold increase in risk of poorer general health. Belsky and colleagues (2010) studied children from a cohort of 1116 families with twins from the United Kingdom called the Environmental Risk Longitudinal Twin Study (E-Risk). Food insecurity was measured using seven items from the USDA Household Food Security Survey Module when the children were 7 to 10 years old, with food insecurity defined as two or more positive responses. Child development outcomes were measured when the children were 12 years old. Children from food-insecure households had lower IQs and higher levels of behavioral and emotional problems. But when differences in household income, mothers' personalities, and household organization were accounted for, the only outcome for which food insecurity remained a significant predictor was emotional outcomes. Cognitive development outcomes were totally accounted for by household income, and behavior outcomes were accounted for by maternal personalities and household organization around the children's needs. Concerning their finding on emotional outcomes, the authors conclude, "This finding . . . constitutes the strongest evidence to date that food insecurity, and not just impoverished, chaotic, and neglectful households prone to disrupted food situations, can influence children's mental health" (Belsky et al., 2010, p. 5). Thus there is reasonably strong evidence from longitudinal studies that food insecurity influences children's physical and emotional health.

Four different longitudinal studies have examined the relationship of food insecurity and weight outcomes in children (Jyoti et al., 2005; Rose and Bodor, 2006; Bronte-Tinkew et al., 2007; Bhargava et al., 2008). Three have used data from the US Early Longitudinal Study – Kindergarten Cohort with follow-up periods of 1 to 5 years and several different measures of the weight outcomes (Jyoti et al., 2005; Rose and Bodor, 2006; Bhargava et al., 2008). Food insecurity was measured using the US Household Food Security Scale and operationalized as ≥ 1 positive response, ≥ 3 positive responses and as a continuous scale score. No consistent results emerged from these three studies: One study found a positive association, one a negative association and one no association. The fourth study used data from the US Early Childhood Longitudinal Study-Birth Cohort, 9- and 24-month surveys (Bronte-Tinkew et al., 2007). Using structural equation modeling to examine the direct and indirect associations between food insecurity and toddlers' overweight, investigators found the food insecurity did not directly affect overweight. Food insecurity worked through parenting practices and infant feeding to indirectly influence overweight. Overall, the evidence does not support a strong causal inference that food insecurity in households causes overweight in children.

Substantial progress has been made in the last several years in research on food insecurity and hunger in food-rich countries. A major review of the concept, measure, and measurement processes used in national surveillance and research has affirmed the validity and utility of food insecurity, while suggesting that additional research is needed on more severe food insecurity that previously had been called hunger. In addition, substantial progress has been made in uncovering the mechanisms through which food insecurity affects health and development. Much less has been accomplished in understanding the causes of food insecurity, and few, if any, major intervention studies have been conducted on preventing food insecurity. These are fruitful areas for further research.

Food Insecurity and Hunger in Poor Countries

Nature of the Problem

The concept of food security gained international prominence with the World Food Conference of 1974 (Maxwell, D., 1996). The most commonly cited definition is "access by all people at all times to enough food for an active, healthy life" (World Bank, 1986). This definition emphasizes that food security is relevant for individuals, implies each individual's entitlement and right to food, requires sufficient and sustainable access to food, and has consequences. The complexity of food security (Maxwell and

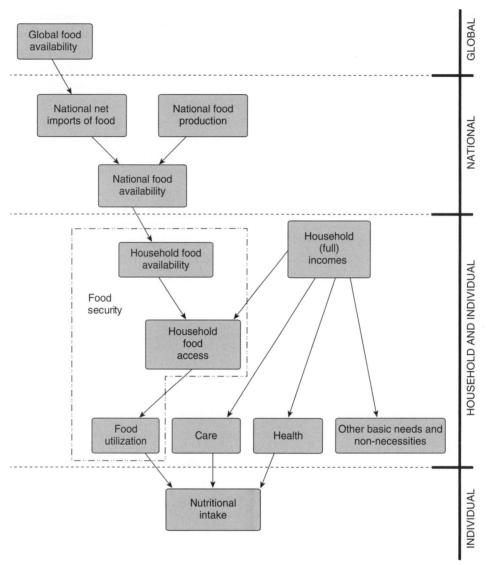

FIG. 68.1 Simplified conceptual framework for food security from the global and the national to the household and the individual. Adapted from Smith (1998).

Frankenberger, 1992) is reflected in three significant shifts in thinking about food security over the past 30 years: (a) from global and national levels to household and individual levels, (b) from a food-first to a livelihood perspective, and (c) from objective to subjective understandings (Maxwell, D., 1996).

Food security is salient at global, regional, national, provincial, community, household, and individual levels (Figure 68.1). At the global and national levels, food security concerns the overall availability of food, and at the national level results from importing and producing food.

At the household level, food security concerns the availability and access to food by the household, which results from household production and availability from the market or others in the community. At the individual level, food security concerns the utilization or consumption of food, which results from its availability to and access by the household and also the distribution within the household (Riely *et al.*, 1997). "An individual person is food secure when his or her consumption of food is sufficient, certain (not vulnerable to consumption shortfalls), and sustainable" (Smith, 1998).

Food is a fundamental need in that each individual must have access to necessary nutrients to survive and to participate actively in society. But, food is only one of the needs that people must attempt to meet. The term "livelihood security" captures the understanding that households often make trade-offs to ensure their long-term viability as productive and reproductive units (Maxwell, D., 1996). Livelihood security refers to the stocks and flows of assets and cash to meet basic needs, offset risk, ease shocks, and meet contingencies (Maxwell and Frankenberger, 1992; Davies, 1996). People may go hungry in the present to preserve assets and future ability to make their living. They may forgo eating now to preserve seed for future planting or to save an animal for future use (Maxwell, D., 1996). Livelihood security implies other trade-offs as well, such as forgoing some food to be able to buy medication to treat illness.

Food insecurity is a form of deprivation, and one can refer to both the conditions and feelings of deprivation (Maxwell, S., 1996). Whereas previously the tendency was to consider food security solely as referring to the adequacy of food or nutrients in objective terms, the understanding now is that the subjective experience of individuals is central. From this understanding, which is consistent with that discussed in the previous section on the United States, the relevant food security is that which is actually perceived by a household or individual rather than that which is decided on by researchers or policy makers, given that households will behave according to their perception and not according to indicators defined by outsiders (Maxwell, S., 1996). Important categories of behaviors potentially influenced by one's perceptions of food insecurity are investment (e.g. in productive assets, education, and children), risk avoidance (e.g. regarding adoption of new agricultural technologies or management practices), and survival strategies (e.g. rural–urban migration, diversification of livelihood strategies).

These three shifts in thinking about food security shape our current understanding of its nature in poor countries. This understanding has important implications for how food security is assessed and for efforts to improve food security.

Measurement

At the global and national levels, food security has primarily been measured by estimating "the number of people whose food intake does not provide enough calories to meet their basic energy requirements" (Food and Agriculture Organization, 1999). The FAO refers to these people as the undernourished. The FAO method largely reflects national food availability, and does not adequately reflect people's ability to access food (Smith, 1998). Therefore, this method yields a direct measure of food security at the national level if it is defined in terms of national food availability (see Figure 68.1). But the FAO method does not yield an accurate measure of food security at the household or individual level because it does not adequately reflect access to and utilization of food.

The Food Insecurity and Vulnerability Information and Mapping System at FAO provides information about global and national food security. The system draws on existing information, such as crop forecasting and early warning systems, household food security and nutritional information systems, and vulnerability assessment and mapping systems (Food and Agriculture Organization, 1999; Anon., 2000).

At the household and individual levels, food security has been measured in various ways, often indirectly. Food security affects dietary intake and ultimately nutritional status and physical well-being, as well as other outcomes. While measures of dietary intake of individuals can assess some aspects of food security such as energy insufficiency and nutrient inadequacy, they do not assess the cognitive and affective components of uncertainty (expressed as anxiety), unacceptability, or unsustainability. For example, current intake may be adequate but food insecurity still may be experienced because of concern over future intake. Alternatively, intake may be inadequate, but only temporarily so as to protect supplies and prevent future food insecurity. Growth status is also used as an indicator, but again does not assess most of the components of food security and depends on factors such as health and child care.

Food security is related to available economic and social resources. Precursors such as income or total expenditure are correlated with energy sufficiency, but they only capture this component of food insecurity and are indirect (Haas et al., 1992). Food-related management or "coping" strategies have also been used to assess food insecurity (Maxwell, D., 1996; Maxwell, et al., 1999). Management strategies both result from and affect the experience of food insecurity and may be useful as early indications of future food insecurity. The presence or absence of particular management strategies, however, often is not indicative of food security, and measures of management strategies do not include all components of the experience of food insecurity.

Because the more directly linked a measure is to the phenomenon of interest, the more accurate that measure will be, it is important to measure the experience of food insecurity itself, including whatever its key components are in a given location (Frongillo, 1999). This experience could be objectively and definitively measured by observing in detail a household over time (Frongillo, 1999; Hamelin *et al.*, 1999). Because such an approach is not feasible for a large number of households, this experience can instead be measured subjectively by assessing not only aspects of the availability of, access to, and utilization of food, but also how a person feels about it (e.g. anxiety, worry) and what a person thinks about it (e.g. perceptions, social acceptability). Because these manifestations are overt, we can tap into these to directly measure the experience of food insecurity in a comprehensive manner.

One way to develop direct measures that include these components and can complement existing measures is to base them on an in-depth understanding of the experience of food insecurity at the household level (Eilerts, 1999; Wolfe and Frongillo, 2000). This approach was first used in the United States but has now been used in many low- and middle-income countries (Studdert *et al.*, 2001; Frongillo *et al.*, 2003; Pérez-Escamilla *et al.*, 2004; Coates *et al.*, 2006b; Frongillo and Nanama, 2006; Melgar-Quinonez *et al.*, 2006; González *et al.*, 2008). Furthermore, the Food and Nutrition Technical Assistance Project has developed technical guides for developing new measures (Frongillo *et al.*, 2004) and for adapting a generic questionnaire developed and tested through consensus of international experts (Coates *et al.*, 2007). This research demonstrates that (1) experience-based measures are valid for differentiating households both at a given time and with changes over time, (2) developing such measures is feasible in programmatic settings, and (3) many, but not all, aspects of the experience of food insecurity are common across locations and cultures (Coates *et al.*, 2006a).

Prevalence

Information about the prevalence of food insecurity at the global, regional, and national levels is primarily available from FAO estimates of undernourishment. According to these estimates, nearly 925 million people or 16% of people in developing countries are undernourished (Table 68.2; http://www.fao.org/publications/sofi/en/). Because of its large population, Asia has by far the largest number

TABLE 68.2 Prevalence of undernourishment in developing countries

Region	Undernourished in total population (2010)	
	Number (millions)	Prevalence (%)
Asia and Pacific	578	16
Latin America and Caribbean	53	8[a]
Near East and North Africa	37	8[a]
Sub-Saharan Africa	239	30
All developing countries	925	16

[a]Provisional.
Data from Food and Agricultural Organization of the United Nations (2010).

of undernourished people. Sub-Saharan Africa has by far the largest prevalence of undernourishment at 30%. As explained earlier, these estimates are likely to be an accurate reflection of food availability at the global, regional, and national levels, but not of food security at the household or individual levels.

Consequences

Food insecurity adversely affects well-being in many ways. Mechanisms that bring about such effects may be biological, acting through decreased nutrient intake, or social and behavioral. In the latter case this may act through, for example, compromised time, energy, and attention for care of self and dependents. Some adverse effects of food insecurity include infants with low birth weight and high risk of mortality, children with impaired cognitive and neurological development that leads to reduced learning capacity and school performance, and adults with low work productivity and capacity to be food secure. The cycle is completed as these adults have children (Tweeten *et al.*, 1992). Other consequences are a range of behavioral responses to uncertainty (including investment, risk avoidance, and survival strategies); the experience of stress, alienation, deprivation, and adverse family and social interactions (Hamelin *et al.*, 2002); and those conditions described earlier in relation to the United States which are presumed also to affect children in poor countries.

Undernutrition

Nature of the Problem

Scientific understanding of the nature, causes, and solutions related to undernutrition in developing countries has shifted significantly in the last 50 years as a result of new evidence, experience, disciplinary perspectives, and ideology (Jonsson, 2010). From mid-century through the 1960s, the major focus was on protein deficiency. Based on the earlier description of kwashiorkor by Williams (1933) and the prevailing nutrient-deficiency paradigm then current in nutritional sciences, attention was directed toward estimating human requirements for protein and individual amino acids under varying physiological states and conditions of health and disease prevalent in developing countries. Simultaneously, a variety of other disciplines (e.g. animal and agricultural sciences, food science), development agencies, and governments sought to develop and implement technological and food-based means for increasing animal protein or essential amino acids in the food supplies and diets in developing countries. This protein era came to an unusually rapid end in the 1970s, at least in the expert communities, with the downward revision of estimated protein requirements (World Health Organization, 1973), but the protein focus continues to influence thinking and food and nutrition policy in many countries even today. This episode also has negatively affected nutrition's image within scientific and development communities, an impact that reverberates to this day, resulting from the perception that nutritionists directed attention to protein deficiency and then changed their mind after many other scientists and institutions had redirected their work to help close the protein gap.

Further shifts in thinking have involved the era of the energy gap in the 1960s and 1970s (Food and Agriculture Organization, 1969; Reutlinger and Selowsky, 1976), multisectoral nutrition planning, applied nutrition programs, and nutrition surveillance in the 1970s and 1980s (Levinson, 1995), and micronutrient deficiencies in the 1990s to the present (World Bank, 1994; Micronutrient Initiative, 2009). Since the 1990s the discourse in international nutrition has included a wide array of problems and causes (e.g. growth faltering, low birth weight, maternal undernutrition, iodine, vitamin A, iron and zinc deficiencies, diarrhea, human immunodeficiency virus (HIV) and other infectious diseases, inadequate infant and child feeding practices, female time constraints, limited household income and agricultural production, food insecurity, environmental degradation, and urbanization), and a wide array of partial solutions (e.g. growth monitoring, supplementary feeding, exclusive breastfeeding, complementary feeding, nutrition education, behavior-change communications, oral rehydration, child spacing, fortification, vitamin A, iron and multiple micronutrient supplementation, income generation, food aid, home gardening, and agricultural intensification). In more recent years, the field has experienced yet another controversial shift, with the interest in the potential for ready-to-use foods (RUF), fortified complementary foods, lipid-based supplements, and other formulations to be used at community rather than clinic level, to address severe acute malnutrition and possibly mild and moderate undernutrition (Briend *et al.*, 2006; Nackers *et al.*, 2010).

These diverse perspectives on nutrition, exacerbated by institutional interests and rivalries, have contributed to the perception among many policy makers and donors that the nutrition problem is too complicated, it has created a fragmentation of effort across international and government agencies, and it has inhibited the development of a consensus about priority problems, actions, and strategies (Morris *et al.*, 2008; Pelletier, 2008b). In an effort to respond to this situation in the early 1990s, the nutrition section of the United Nations Children's Fund (UNICEF) developed and promoted an inclusive conceptual framework for organizing scientific knowledge and experience, fostering a common understanding and developing coherent strategies for addressing them (Figure 68.2). The framework explicitly recognizes that the relative importance of the three underlying causes of malnutrition (food, health, and care) can vary widely across households, communities, and countries. This context specificity implies that universal causes and solutions do not exist and that the binding constraints must be assessed and acted upon in each national or local setting. The potential impact of such an approach has been documented by the Iringa Nutrition Program in Tanzania, which gave rise to the UNICEF strategy, and was repeated in Thailand, Indonesia, and Vietnam (United Nations Standing Committee on Nutrition, 1996; Sternin *et al.*, 1999). Much work is still required, however, to counter the tendency for specialized scientists, professionals, and institutions to single out and promote that part of the framework that suits their particular interests and agendas even when the context suggests that other actions may be more appropriate (Pelletier, 2000; Morris *et al.*, 2008).

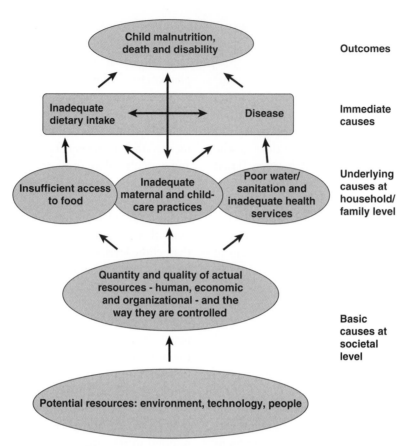

FIG. 68.2 United Nations Children's Fund (UNICEF) conceptual framework for the causes of malnutrition. Adapted from UNICEF (1991).

Measurement and Prevalence

In contrast to the diversity in perspectives about causes and solutions, there has been a long-standing agreement that anthropometric indicators represent a satisfactory basis for estimating the prevalence and trends in general undernutrition among preschool children at global, national and local levels (WHO, 1995). These indicators include: height for age, which indicates the cumulative effects of malnutrition in the life of the child; weight for height, which indicates recent nutritional experiences (typically weeks or months); and weight for age, which reflects the combined effects of recent and longer-term conditions. These indicators are considered to be sensitive to the immediate and underlying causes of malnutrition as depicted in Figure 68.2, although they are not specific to any particular cause such as food insecurity, infectious disease, or inappropriate child care and feeding.

For the developing world as a whole, 19.3% of preschoolers were estimated to be underweight in 2007 (low

weight for age, Table 68.3) and 32.5% were stunted (low height for age, Table 68.4). In Sub-Saharan Africa the prevalence of underweight (19.6%) and stunting (38.5%) in 2007 has remained virtually unchanged since 1990. Asia and its sub-regions have experienced greater improvements, eliminating about one-third of the underweight and stunting that was present in 1990. However, the overall levels remained high in 2007 in the populous South-Central region (32.5% underweight and 30.6% stunted). The overall prevalence of stunting in Latin American and the Caribbean was 23.7 in 1990 and had reduced to 15.7 in 2007.

Consequences

An impressive body of evidence suggests that undernutrition has pervasive effects on human performance, health, and survival (United Nations Standing Committee on Nutrition, 2002; World Bank, 2006). This includes effects on morbidity (Lanata and Black, 2001), mortality (Pelletier

TABLE 68.3 Prevalence (%) of underweight[a] among preschool children[b] by region, 1990–2007

United Nations regions	1990	1995	2000	2007
All of Africa	21.5	21.1	20.5	19.6
North Africa	10.8	10.0	9.2	8.2
East Africa	25.6	24.6	23.6	22.3
West Africa	25.1	24.4	23.6	22.5
Middle Africa	24.3	23.3	22.3	21.0
Southern Africa	11.7	12.1	12.5	13.2
All of Asia	33.8	30.0	26.4	21.6
East Asia	16.2	11.5	8.1	4.8
South-Central Asia	49.9	44.6	39.4	32.5
Southeast Asia	30.6	26.5	22.9	18.3
Western Asia	12.8	10.7	9.0	7.0
Latin America and Caribbean	7.5	6.2	5.0	3.8
All	28.7	25.7	22.8	19.3

[a]Underweight is defined as a weight for age ≤2 standard deviations of the median value of the World Health Organization international growth reference.
[b]Ages 0–5 years.
Data from United Nations Standing Committee on Nutrition (2010).

TABLE 68.4 Prevalence (%) of stunting[a] among preschool children[b] by region, 1990–2007

United Nations Regions	1990	1995	2000	2007
All of Africa	40.3	39.8	39.3	38.5
North Africa	29.4	27.4	25.5	23.0
East Africa	48.1	47.4	46.7	45.7
West Africa	38.1	38.1	38.1	38.1
Middle Africa	45.3	43.8	42.3	40.3
Southern Africa	35.4	34.7	34.1	33.3
All of Asia	48.6	43.1	37.7	30.6
East Asia	35.9	28.2	21.7	14.4
South-Central Asia	60.7	54.6	48.4	39.9
Southeast Asia	47.0	41.5	36.2	29.4
Western Asia	28.2	25.9	23.7	20.9
Latin America and Caribbean	23.7	20.9	18.1	14.8
All	44.4	40.1	36.1	32.5

[a]Stunting is defined as a height for age ≤2 standard deviations of the median value of the World Health Organization international growth reference.
[b]Ages 0–5 years.
Data from United Nations Standing Committee on Nutrition (2010).

et al., 1993, 1995), intrauterine growth (Kramer, 1987), cognitive and social development (Pollitt et al., 1993; Grantham-McGregor, 1995), schooling (Victoria et al., 2008), adult physical work capacity (Haas et al., 1996), adult-onset chronic diseases (Victoria et al., 2008), economic productivity (Haddad and Bouis, 1990; Victoria et al., 2008), and economic growth (Fogel, 1994). It is estimated that undernutrition is responsible for 35% of all deaths to children under 5 years in developing countries (Black et al., 2008) and increases cause-specific mortality due to neonatal disorders, diarrhea, pneumonia, and malaria (Caulfield et al., 2004).

Recent Policy Developments

Since the turn of the millennium a series of significant events have converged that present major opportunities for addressing food insecurity and malnutrition in developing countries. These include the prominent role given to these issues in the Millennium Development Goals (United Nations Development Programme, 2003), a set of eight development goals advanced by the United Nations in 2000 and since ratified by over 190 UN member states; the conclusions of the Copenhagen Consensus (Lomborg, 2007) that nutrition interventions represent one of the most cost-effective investments in all of international development; the publication of the high-profile Lancet Child Survival Series (Black *et al.*, 2003) and Child Nutrition Series (Black *et al.*, 2008) documenting the profound impacts of malnutrition; the greater attention to nutrition paid by the World Bank (World Bank, 2006); the Global Food Security Initiative endorsed by the G8 Nations after the world food crisis in 2008 (L'Aquila Food Security Initiative, 2009); and the convergence on a framework for action by major multilateral, bilateral, and private organizations (Bezanson and Isenman, 2010). These events and initiatives have generated unprecedented attention and resources for addressing food insecurity and malnutrition, representing important key steps in the policy process, but the ultimate success of these will depend upon the level of commitment, convergence, and capacity-building that occurs as they are implemented at country level (Pelletier *et al.*, 2011).

Future Directions

This chapter has attempted to illustrate some of the similarities and common themes among hunger, food insecurity, and undernutrition as they occur in developed and developing countries. The reality, however, is that research, policies, and programs have tended to neglect the potentially important commonalities among them. This section highlights some of these and suggests that our scientific understanding of these problems and our ability to address them through policies and programs would be enhanced by focusing on these and other commonalities.

In developed and developing countries, undernutrition and food insecurity often coexist in the same populations with obesity and chronic disease. There are multiple biological, social, and behavioral causes for this coexistence that operate through life-course, intergenerational, genetic, and epigenetic mechanisms. For example, undernutrition in gestation brings greater biological risk for obesity and chronic disease, either through changing the sensitivity of the hypothalamic–pituitary–adrenal axis, which in turn alters appetite and physical activity, or through the action of components of the maternal diet on gene expression (Victoria *et al.*, 2008). Undernutrition and food insecurity may also increase risk of obesity and chronic disease because of compromised dietary quality or quantity, or because of psychological stress that affects behavior (Jyoti *et al.*, 2005). This coexistence suggests a need for two types of research. One is to better understand the factors, conditions, and processes that produce this "dual burden" at household, community, and national levels. The other is to develop and evaluate policy and programmatic strategies that address both problems simultaneously and/or that address one problem (e.g. food insecurity or undernutrition) while not inadvertently exacerbating the other (e.g. obesity). There has been some conceptual treatment of this issue (Hamm and Bellows, 2003; Rayner *et al.*, 2006; Dixon *et al.*, 2007), but the feasibility and effectiveness of various proposals have yet to be examined. This requires research at multiple levels of analysis (individual, household, community, and national) because the causes and the intervention options vary across these levels.

Integrative or cross-boundary research and theory development should also be done to advance the translation of scientific knowledge into effective large-scale action, in settings as diverse as the mega-cities, towns and rural areas of Sub-Saharan Africa, South Latin America, Europe, the United States, and all other regions of the developed and developing world. Each of the problems discussed here, from hunger to obesity and from undernutrition to chronic disease, is complex in its etiology and suffers from major gaps in the scientific knowledge of "what works." This is true on a small scale and even more so on a large scale. Superimposed upon this is enormous sociocultural, ecological, economic, and political diversity, as well as wide variation in the administrative and organizational capacities to implement effective action on a large scale. A large number of theories and frameworks exist in political and policy sciences, management sciences, sociology, and other fields that could guide efforts to develop and implement effective actions in these varied contexts (Parsons, 1995; Sibeon, 1997; Vasu *et al.*, 1998; Clark, 2002). However, it is still uncommon for these to be applied in research and policy related to the focal problems in this chapter and public health more broadly (Walt and Gilson, 1994; Pelletier, 2008a; Breton and de Leeuw, 2010). The application and further development of these theories and frameworks for the purpose of improving population health are important opportunities and challenges as the field of nutrition matures from its current status as a largely bench, clinical, and epidemiological science.

The emergent interest in implementation sciences has the potential to stimulate this maturation of the field (Alegria, 2009; Satterfield *et al.*, 2009) As yet there is not a widely shared understanding of the boundaries and content of "implementation sciences," and related terms such as translational research, operations research, knowledge translation, and health systems research. A broad definition useful for present purposes is the study of the social, cultural, behavioral, economic, management, and political factors that can facilitate or inhibit the adoption, adaptation, and use of evidence-based interventions, practice guidelines, scientific knowledge and real-world experience into the process of policy formulation, the implementation of policies and programs, and efforts to enhance the quality and effectiveness of implementation. This definition is useful for the problems discussed in this chapter because it acknowledges the importance of varied contextual factors, is relevant at multiple scales (clinical, community, national, and global), acknowledges that policy formulation and implementation pose distinctive challenges, and can be applied to policies and interventions outside of health care such as community health, agriculture, social protection, education, and so on. The conceptual development and real-world application of implementation sciences, as a fundamentally integrative and transdisciplinary endeavor (Satterfield *et al.*, 2009), constitute an urgent priority for understanding and addressing food insecurity, undernutrition, obesity, and nutrition-related chronic disease in the coming years.

Finally, while the above research topics are important for informing the design of effective interventions, programs, and policies specifically aiming to address food insecurity, undernutrition, and obesity, it is also important to consider the impact of macro-level forces on these problems. The forces include climate change; global food and economic crises; maldistribution of water and arable land; the growing influence of transnational food companies; the sustainability of food systems, health-care systems, and social protection programs; and the weak state of national and global governance systems for addressing these issues. Individually and collectively, these forces pose urgent threats to the food security and nutritional status of populations, can undermine the impact of the more direct nutrition interventions, and are likely to become more severe in the coming years. The nutrition community can play important roles by partnering with other organizations in research, advocacy, and policy development related to these issues.

Suggestions for Further Reading

Bezanson, K. and Isenman, P. (2010) Scaling up nutrition: a framework for action. *Food Nutr Bull* **31**, 178–186.

Coates, J., Frongillo, E.A., Houser, R., *et al.* (2006) Commonalities in the experience of household food insecurity across cultures: what are measures missing? *J Nutr* **136**, 1438S–1448S.

Dinour, L.M., Bergen, D., and Yeh, M.C. (2007) The food insecurity–obesity paradox: a review of the literature and the role food stamps may play. *J Am Diet Assoc* **107**, 1952–1961.

Hamelin, A.M., Beaudry, M., and Habicht, J.P. (2002) Characterization of household food insecurity in Quebec: food and feelings. *Social Sci Med* **54**, 119–132.

Jonsson, U. (2010) The rise and fall of paradigms in public health nutrition [Commentary]. *World Nutr* **1**, 128–158.

Larson, N.I. and Story, M.T. (2011) Food insecurity and weight status among U.S. children and families: a review of the literature. *Am J Prev Med* **40**, 166–173.

Maxwell, S. (1996) Food security: a post-modern perspective. *Food Policy* **21**, 155–170.

Melchior, M., Caspi, A., Howard, L.M., *et al.* (2009) Mental health context of food insecurity: a representative cohort of families with young children. *Pediatrics* **124**, e564–e572.

World Bank (2006) *Repositioning Nutrition as Central to Development: A Strategy for Large Scale Action.* World Bank, Washington, DC.

References

Alegria, M. (2009) AcademyHealth 25th Annual Research Meeting chair address: From a science of recommendation to a science of implementation. *Health Serv Res* **45**, 5–14.

Anderson, S. (1990) Core indicators of nutritional status for difficult-to-sample populations. *J Nutr Educ* **120**, 1559–1600.

Anon. (2000) Food Insecurity and Vulnerability Mapping System. http://www.fivims.net/.

Ashiabi, G.S. and O'Neal, K.K. (2008) A framework for understanding the association between food insecurity and children's developmental outcomes. *Child Development Perspectives* **2**, 71–77.

Belsky, D.W., Moffitt, T.E., Arseneault, L., *et al.* (2010) Context and sequelae of food insecurity in children's development. *Am J Epidemiol* **1**, 809–818.

Bezanson, K. and Isenman, P. (2010) Scaling up nutrition: a framework for action. *Food Nutr Bull* **31**, 178–186.

Bhargava, A., Joliffe, D., and Howard, L.L. (2008) Socio-economic, behavioural and environmental factors predicted body weight and household insecurity scores in the Early Childhood Longitudinal Study-Kindergarten. *Br J Nutr* **100**, 438–444.

Bickel, G., Nord, M., Price, C., *et al.* (2000) *Guide to Measuring Household Food Security*. USDA Food and Nutrition Service, Alexandria VA.

Black, R.E., Allen, L.H., Bhutta, Z.A., *et al.* (2008) Maternal and child undernutrition: global and regional exposures and health consequences. *Lancet* **371**, 243–260.

Black, R.E., Morris, S., and Bryce, J. (2003) Where and why are 10 million children dying each year? *Lancet* **361**, 2–10.

Breton, E. and de Leeuw, E. (2010) Theories of the policy process in health promotion research: a review. *Health Promot Int* **26**, 82–90.

Briend, A., Prudhon, C., Weise Prinzo, Z., *et al.* (2006) Putting the management of severe malnutrition back on the international health agenda. *Food Nutr Bull* **27**(Suppl), S3–S6.

Bronte-Tinkew, J., Zaslow, M., Capps, R., *et al.* (2007) Food insecurity works through depression, parenting and infant feeding to influence overweight and health in toddlers. *J Nutr* **137**, 2160–2165.

Carlson, S.J., Andrews, M.S., and Bickel, G.W. (1999) Measuring food insecurity and hunger in the United States: development of a national benchmark measure and prevalence estimates. *J Nutr Educ* **129**, 510S–516S.

Caulfield, L., de Onis, M., Blössner, M., and Black, R. (2004) Undernutrition as an underlying cause of child deaths associated with diarrhea, pneumonia, malaria, and measles. *Am J Clin Nutr* **80**, 193–198.

Clark, T.W. (2002) *The Policy Process: A Practical Guide for Natural Resource Professionals*. Yale University Press, New Haven, CT.

Coates, J., Frongillo, E.A., Houser, R., *et al.* (2006a) Commonalities in the experience of household food insecurity across cultures: What are measures missing? *J Nutr* **136**, 1438S–1448S.

Coates, J., Swindale, A., and Bilinsky, P. (2007) Household Food Insecurity Access Scale (HFIAS) for Measurement of Household Food Access: Indicator Guide (v. 3), Food and Nutrition Technical Assistance Project, Academy for Educational Development, Washington, DC.

Coates, J., Wilde, P.E., Webb, P., *et al.* (2006b) Comparison of a qualitative and a quantitative approach to developing a household food insecurity scale for Bangladesh. *J Nutr* **136**, 1420S–1430S.

Cook, J.T. and Frank, D.A. (2008) Food security, poverty, and human development in the United States. *Ann NY Acad Sci* **1136**, 193–209.

Davies, S. (1996) *Adaptable Livelihoods: Coping with Food Insecurity in the Malian Sahel*. Macmillan Press, London.

Dixon, J., Omwega, A., Friel, S., *et al.* (2007) The health equity dimensions of urban food systems. *J Urban Health* **84**, 118–129.

Eilerts, G. (1999) Food security measurement in the United States: new ideas for third-world assessments? Food Insecurity and Vulnerability Information and Mapping Systems, Food and Agriculture Organization, United Nations, Rome.

Fogel, R. (1994) Economic growth, population theory, and physiology: the bearing of long-term processes on the making of economic policy. *Am Econ Rev* **84**, 369–395.

Food and Agriculture Organization (1969) *Manual on Food and Nutrition Policy*. FAO, Rome.

Food and Agriculture Organization (2010) *State of Food Insecurity in the World*. FAO, Rome.

Food and Consumer Service and National Center for Health Statistics (1995) Papers and proceedings. In *Conference on Food Security Measurement and Research*. USDA, Alexandria, VA.

Frongillo, E.A., Jr (1999) Validation of measures of food insecurity and hunger. *J Nutr Educ* **129**(2 Suppl), 506S–509S.

Frongillo, E.A. and Nanama, S. (2006) Development and validation of an experience based measure of household food insecurity within and across seasons in northern Burkina Faso. *J Nutr* **136**, 1409S–1419S.

Frongillo, E.A., Chowdhury, N., Ekström, E.C., *et al.* (2003) Understanding the experience of household food insecurity in rural Bangladesh leads to a measure different from that used in other countries. *J Nutr* **133**, 4158–4162.

Frongillo, E.A., Nanama, S., and Wolfe, W.S. (2004) Technical guide to developing a direct, experience based measurement tool for household food insecurity. Food and Nutrition Technical Assistance, Academy for Educational Development.

González, W., Jiménez, A., Madrigal, G., *et al.* (2008) Development and validation of measure of household food insecurity in urban Costa Rica confirms proposed generic questionnaire. *J Nutr* **138**, 587–592.

Grantham-McGregor, S. (1995) A review of the studies of the effect of severe malnutrition on mental development. *J Nutr Educ* **125**, 2233S–2238S.

Haas, J.D., Murdoch, S., Rivera, J.M.R., *et al.* (1996) Early nutrition and later physical work capacity. *Nutr Rev* **54**, S41–48.

Haas, J.W., Sypher, B.D., and Sypher, H.E. (1992) Do shared goals really make a difference? *Manage Comm Q* **6**, 166–179.

Haddad, L. and Bouis, H. (1990) The impact of nutritional status on agricultural productivity: wage evidence from the Philippines. *Oxf Bull Econ Stat* **53**, 45–68.

Hamelin, A.M., Beaudry, M., and Habicht, J.P. (2002) Characterization of household food insecurity in Quebec: food and feelings. *Social Sci Med* **54**, 119–132.

Hamelin, A.M., Habicht, J.P., and Beaudry, M. (1999) Food insecurity: consequences for the household and broader social implications. *J Nutr Educ* **129**, 525S–528S.

Hamilton, W.L., Cook, J.T., and Thompson, W.W. (1997) Household food insecurity in the United States in 1995: summary report of the Food Security Measurement Project. Food and Consumer Service, USDA, Alexandria, VA.

Hamm, M.W. and Bellows, A.C. (2003) Community food security and nutrition educators. *J Nutr Educ Behav* **35**, 37–43.

Holben, D.H. (2006) Position of the American Dietetic Association: food insecurity and hunger in the United States. *J Am Diet Assoc* **106**, 446–458.

Jones, S.J. and Frongillo, E.A. (2006) The modifying effects of Food Stamp Program participation on the relation between food insecurity and weight change in women. *J Nutr* **136**, 1091–1094.

Jones, S.J. and Frongillo, E.A. (2007) Food insecurity and subsequent weight gain in women. *Public Health Nutr* **10**, 145–151.

Jonsson, U. (2010) The rise and fall of paradigms in public health nutrition [Commentary]. *World Nutr* **1**, 128–158.

Jyoti, D.F., Frongillo, E.A., and Jones, S.J. (2005) Food insecurity affects school children's academic performance, weight gain, and social skills. *J Nutr* **135**, 2831–2839.

Kendall, A., Olson, C.M., and Frongillo, E.A.J. (1995) Validation of the Radimer/Cornell measures of hunger and food insecurity *J Nutr Educ* **125**, 2793–2801.

Kirkpatrick, S.I., McIntyre, L., and Potestio, M.L. (2010) Child hunger and long-term adverse consequences for health. *Arch Pediatr Adolesc Med* **164**, 754–762.

Kramer, A. (1987) Determinants of low birth weight: methodological assessment and meta-analysis. *Bull World Health Organ* **65**, 663–737.

Kursmark, M. and Weitzman, M. (2009) Recent findings concerning childhood food insecurity. *Curr Opin Clin Nutr Metab Care* **12**, 310–316.

Lanata, C.F. and Black, R.E. (2001) Diarrheal and respiratory diseases. In R. Semba and M. Bloem (eds), *Nutrition and Health in Developing Countries*. Humana Press, Totowa, NJ, pp. 93–129.

L'Aquila Food Security Initiative (2009) http://www.g8italia2009.it/static/G8_Allegato/LAquila_Joint_Statement_on_Global_Food_Security%5B1%5D,0.pdf.

Levinson, J. (1995) Multisectoral nutrition planning: a synthesis of experience. In P. Pinstrup-Andersen, D.L. Pelletier, and H. Alderman (eds), *Enhancing Child Nutrition: An Agenda for Action*. Cornell University Press, Ithaca, NY.

Lomborg, B.E. (2007) *Solutions for the World's Biggest Problems*. Cambridge University Press, Cambridge.

Maxwell, D. (1996) Measuring food insecurity: the frequency and severity of "coping strategies." *Food Policy* **21**, 291–303.

Maxwell, D., Ahiadeke, C., and Levin, C. (1999) Alternative food-security indicators: revisiting the frequency and severity of "coping strategies." *Food Policy* **24**, 411–429.

Maxwell, S. (1996) Food security: a post-modern perspective. *Food Policy* **21**, 155–170.

Maxwell, S. and Frankenberger, T. (1992) *Household Food Security: Concepts, Indicators, Measurements. A Technical Review*. United Nations Children's Fund and International Fund for Agricultural Development, New York.

McIntyre, L., Glanville, N.T., Raine, K.D., *et al.* (2003) Do low-income lone mothers compromise their nutrition to feed their children? *CMAJ* **168**, 686–691.

Melgar-Quinonez, H.R., Zubieta, A.C., MkNelly, B., *et al.* (2006) Household food insecurity and food expenditure in Bolivia, Burkina Faso, and the Philippines. *J Nutr* **136**, 1431S–1437S.

Micronutrient Initiative (2009) *A United Call to Action on Vitamin and Mineral Deficiencies: Global Report 2009*. Micronutrient Initiative, Ottawa.

Morris, S.S., Cogill, B., and Uauy, R. (2008) Effective international action against undernutrition: why has it proven so difficult and what can be done to accelerate progress? *Lancet* **371**, 608–621.

Nackers, F., Broillet, F., Oumarou, D., *et al.* (2010) Effectiveness of ready-to-use therapeutic food compared to a corn/soy-blend-based pre-mix for the treatment of childhood moderate acute malnutrition in Niger. *J Trop Pediatr* **56**, 407–413.

Nord, M. and Hopwood, H. (2007) Recent advances provide tools for measuring children's food security. *J Nutr* **137**, 533–536.

Nord, M., Coleman-Jensen, A., Andrews, M., *et al.* (2010). *Household Food Security in the United States, 2009*. USDA/ERS Economic Research Report No. 108. USDA Research Service, Washington, DC.

Olson, C.M. (2005) Food insecurity in women: a recipe for unhealthy trade-offs. *Top Clin Nutr* **20**, 321–328.

Olson, C.M. and Strawderman, M.S. (2008) The relationship between food insecurity and obesity in rural childbearing women. *J Rural Health* **24**, 60–66.

Parsons, W. (1995) *Public Policy: An Introduction to the Theory and Practice of Policy Analysis*. Edward Elgar Publishing, Aldershot.

Pelletier, D.L. (2000) Toward a common understanding of malnutrition: assessing the contributions of the UNICEF conceptual framework. In *World Bank/UNICEF Assessment of Contributions to Nutrition Policy*. World Bank, Washington.

Pelletier, D.L. (2008a) Beyond partial analysis. In R.D. Semba and M.W. Bloem (eds), *Nutrition and Health in Developing Countries*, 2nd Edn. Humana Press, Totowa, NJ.

Pelletier, D.L. (2008b) Commitment, consensus and capacity: an evidence-based agenda. Paper presented to the 36th Session of the UN Standing Committee on Nutrition, Hanoi.

Pelletier, D., Frongillo, E., Gervais, S., *et al.* (2011) Nutrition agenda setting, policy formulation and implementation: lessons from the mainstreaming nutrition initiative. *Health Policy Plan* PMID 21292709.

Pelletier, D.L., Frongillo, E.A., Jr, and Habicht, J-P. (1993) Epidemiologic evidence for a potentiating effect of malnutrition on mortality. *Am J Public Health* **83**, 1130–1133.

Pelletier, D.L., Frongillo, E.A., Jr, Schroeder, D.G., *et al.* (1995) The effects of malnutrition on child mortality in developing countries. *Bull World Health Organ* **73**, 443–448.

Pelletier, D.L., Olson, C.M., and Frongillo, E.A. (2006) Food insecurity, hunger, and undernutrition. In B.A. Bowman and R.M. Russell (eds), *Present Knowledge in Nutrition*, 9th Edn. International Life Sciences Institute, Washington, DC, pp. 906–922.

Pérez-Escamilla, R., Segall-Corrêa, A.M., Kurdian Maranha, L., *et al.* (2004) An adapted version of the U.S. Department of Agriculture food insecurity module is a valid tool for assessing household food insecurity in Campinas, Brazil. *J Nutr* **134**, 1923–1928.

Pollitt, E., Gorman, K.S., and Engle, P.L. (1993) Early supplementary feeding and cognition. *Monogr Soc Res Child Dev* **58**, 1–122.

Radimer, K.L., Olson, C.M., and Greene, J.C. (1992) Understanding hunger and developing indicators to assess it in women and children *J Nutr Educ* **24**(Suppl), 36S–45S.

Rayner, G., Hawkes, C., Lang, T., *et al.* (2006) Trade liberalization and the diet transition: a public health response. *Health Promot Int* **21**, 67S–74S.

Reutlinger, S. and Selowsky, M. (1976) Malnutrition and poverty: magnitude and policy options. World Bank staff occasional papers. Johns Hopkins University Press, Baltimore, MD.

Riely, F., Mock, N., and Cogill, B. (1997) Food security indicators and framework for use in the monitoring and evaluation of food aid programs Food Security and Nutrition Monitoring (IMPACT) Project, for the US Agency for International Development, Arlington, VA.

Rose, D. and Bodor, J.N. (2006) Household food insecurity and overweight status in young school children: results from the Early Childhood Longitudinal Study. *Pediatrics* **117**, 464–473.

Rose, D. and Oliveira, V. (1997) Nutrient intakes of individuals from food-insufficient households in the United States. *Am J Public Health* **87**, 1956–1961.

Satterfield, J.M., Spring, B., Brownson, R.C., *et al.* (2009) Toward a transdisciplinary model of evidence-based practice. *Milbank Q* **87**, 368–390.

Sibeon, R. (1997) *Contemporary Sociology and Policy Analysis*. Tudor Business Publishing, San Diego.

Smith, L. (1998) Can FAO's measure of chronic undernourishment be strengthened? *Food Policy* **23**, 425–445.

Sternin, M., Sternin, J., and Marsh, D. (1999) Scaling up a poverty alleviation and nutrition program in Vietnam. In T.J. Marchione (ed.), *Scaling Up, Scaling Down: Overcoming Malnutrition in Developing Countries*. Gordon and Breach Publishers, Singapore.

Studdert, L.J., Frongillo, E., and Valois, P. (2001) Measuring household food insecurity in Java during Indonesia's economic crisis. *J Nutr* **131**, 2685–2691.

Tweeten, L., Mellor, J., Reutlinger, S., *et al.* (1992) Food security discussion paper. Prepared for US Agency for International Development International Science and Technology Institute, Washington, DC.

UNICEF (1991) Strategy for improved nutrition of children and women in developing countries. UNICEF Policy Review. http://www.ceecis.org/iodine/01_global/01_pl/01_01_other_1992_unicef.pdf.

United Nations Development Programme (2003) *Human Development Report, 2003. Millenium Development Goals: A Compact among Nations to End Human Poverty*. Oxford University Press, New York.

United Nations Standing Committee on Nutrition (1996) How nutrition improves. United Nations Administrative Committee on Coordination, Subcommittee on Nutrition (ACC/SCN), Geneva.

United Nations Standing Committee on Nutrition (2002) *Nutrition: A Foundation for Development*. United Nations SCN, Geneva.

United Nations Standing Committee on Nutrition (2010) *Sixth Report on the World Nutrition Situation*. United Nations SCN, Geneva.

US Department of Health and Human Services, US Department of Agriculture (1993) Ten year comprehensive plan for the National Nutrition Monitoring and Related Research Program. *Federal Register* **58**, 322–772.

Vasu, M.L., Stewart, D.W., and Garson, G.D. (1998) *Organizational Behavior and Public Management*. Marcel Dekker, New York.

Victoria, C.G., Adair, L., Fall, C., *et al.* (2008) Maternal and child undernutrition: consequences for adult health and human capital. *Lancet* **371**, 340–357.

Walt, G. and Gilson, L. (1994) Reforming the health sector in developing countries: the central role of policy analysis. *Health Policy Plan* **9**, 353–370.

Wehler, C.A., Scott, R.I., and Anderson, J.J. (1992) The Community Childhood Hunger Identification Project: a model of domestic hunger demonstration project in Seattle, Washington. *J Nutr Educ* **24**, 29S–35S.

Whitaker, R.C. and Sarin, A. (2007) Change in food security status and change in weight are not associated in urban women with preschool children. *J Nutr* **137**, 2134–2139.

Williams, C. (1933) A nutritional disease of childhood associated with a maize diet. *Arch Dis Child* **8**, 423–433.

Wolfe, W.S. and Frongillo, E.A.J. (2000) Building household food security measurement tools from the ground up. Food and Nutrition Technical Assistance (FANta) Project, Academy for Educational Development, Washington, DC.

World Bank (1986) *Poverty and Hunger: Issues and Options for Food Security in Developing Countries*. World Bank, Washington, DC.

World Bank (1994) *Enriching Lives: Overcoming Vitamin and Mineral Malnutrition in Developing Countries*. World Bank, Washington, DC.

World Bank (2006) *Repositioning Nutrition as Central to Development: A Strategy for Large Scale Action*. World Bank, Washington, DC.

World Health Organization (1973) Energy and protein requirements Report of a Joint FAO/WHO Ad Hoc Expert Committee. WHO Technical Report 522. FAO/WHO, Geneva.

World Health Organization (1995) The use and interpretation of anthropometry. WHO Technical Report 854. FAO/WHO, Geneva.

Wunderlich, G.S. and Norwood, J.L. (2006) *Food Insecurity and Hunger in the United States, An Assessment of the Measure*. (p. 48) Panel to Review the US Department of Agriculture's Measurement of Food Insecurity and Hunger, Committee on National Statistics, Division of Behavioral and Social Sciences and Education, National Research Council of the National Academies of Science. National Academies Press, Washington, DC.

69

PUBLIC NUTRITION IN HUMANITARIAN CRISES

HELEN YOUNG[1], PhD, KATE SADLER[1], PhD, AND ANNALIES BORREL[2], MSc

[1]*Tufts University, Medford, Massachusetts, USA*
[2]*UNICEF Office of Emergency Programmes – Humanitarian Policy and Advocacy, New York, USA*

Summary

Populations affected by humanitarian crises are prone to increases in nutritional risk, malnutrition, and micronutrient deficiency diseases. Nutrition in humanitarian crises is usually both a public-health and food-security priority, and requires a multi-sectoral response to reduce the nutritional risks and treat malnutrition directly.

This chapter describes five broad categories of public nutrition interventions, including strategies that:

- Address the nutritional needs of populations, including food security and livelihoods programs, general food distribution, and public health programs.
- Address the needs of the nutritionally vulnerable.
- Prevent and treat micronutrient deficiency diseases.
- Prevent and treat moderate acute malnutrition.
- Treat severe acute malnutrition.

The objectives, program design, and target groups for each of these are described, and remaining challenges are discussed. The importance of this sector has increased markedly as reflected by commitments in the broader policy environment and an increasing body of relevant policies and best practices. Significant progress has been made in a range of areas, and, for the future, improved evidence about what works will serve to further strengthen policy and program guidance.

Introduction

Emergencies capture news headlines, ranging from sudden-onset floods in Pakistan to the frequent occurrence of drought-related food insecurity in Niger (Gronewold, 2010; Khristof, 2010). News coverage is patchy, focusing on high-profile visible emergencies while ignoring the more chronic, protracted crises, which are less well documented and have been termed "silent disasters" (Eriksson, 2007).

This chapter provides an overview of the characteristic nutritional problems that occur in natural disasters and complex emergencies, and the progress and challenges for defining and assessing these. It then reviews the core public nutrition interventions in emergencies, emphasizing the important role of a *public nutrition* approach[1].

Many emergency contexts are associated with fragile and conflict-affected states, and war and conflict are consistently the main causes of famine (United Nations ESC/ECA, 2009). At the same time, trends over the past 30 years show an increase in the number and frequency of natural disasters[2] (EM-DAT, 2009), the effects of which may be exacerbated by conflict and insecurity, or political and economic instability. The number of African countries facing food crises and requiring emergency assistance annually has climbed from 15 before 2001, to more than 25 since then (UN ESC/ECA, 2009). Populations affected by crises include those displaced across international borders (refugees living in camp situations and or integrated with host populations[3]), those internally displaced within their own countries, as well as those remaining in their places of origin who are affected by war or drought or a combination of both.

International emergency response is often referred to as international "humanitarian action," which includes both the provision of humanitarian assistance to meet material needs, and also humanitarian protection – which means ensuring safety from acute harm and broader protection considerations of protecting and upholding rights. Humanitarian action has strong legal foundations in international humanitarian law, and the core humanitarian principles of humanity, impartiality, neutrality, and independence that are derived from this (IASC, 2002).

Within the context of climate change, disaster management is also increasingly becoming encapsulated by the newer concept of disaster risk reduction, which is concerned with the development of policies and practices that will reduce risk and vulnerabilities throughout society. It has been widely adopted by the UN system and has its own global platform and initiatives (Schipper and Pelling, 2006). Increasing attention has been given over recent years to early recovery in conflict settings as part of a broader stabilization policy agenda that is aimed at building foundations for transition and recovery and includes a strong capacity-development component (Bailey and Pavanello, 2009). In the short term the humanitarian imperative may need to take priority, but should build upon and strengthen local systems where possible. Irrespective of the nature of the natural disaster or complex emergency, the overall approach to nutrition in emergencies described in this paper will apply, and is reflected in the wider body of best practice and literature referenced here.

Malnutrition in Emergencies

An elevated prevalence of acute malnutrition, as measured by the weight-for-height z-score of children under 5 years of age, is the most widely used indicator to gauge the severity of an emergency and plan for an adequate response. Generally higher rates of acute malnutrition have been recorded in emergencies in East Africa and countries bordering the Sahara, with relatively lower rates in southern Africa and Asia. There are, however, always exceptions, with high rates of acute malnutrition reported in Bangladesh and Nepal. Recent examples are shown in Table 69.1. Extreme crises, usually associated with conflict, forced displacement and insecurity, have produced prevalence rates exceeding 50%, for example in southern Sudan during the 1998 famine (Borrel and Salama, 1999). In the past decade, similar extreme rates have not been reported. This may be indicative of a more effective and efficient international response (there have been a number of acute crises, including Darfur, Niger, and Pakistan), but could also be a result of a relative lack of data characteristic of protracted and "silent emergencies."

The prevalence cut-off point used by the World Health Organization to indicate an emergency is 15% (WHO, 2000), although prevalence of acute malnutrition varies widely on a seasonal basis, intra-annually and also geographically (Young and Jaspars, 2009). In some protracted crises, global acute malnutrition (GAM) may appear to

---

[1] Public nutrition is a broad-based, problem-solving approach to addressing malnutrition in complex emergencies that combines analysis of nutritional risk and vulnerability with action-oriented strategies, including policies, programs, and capacity development (Young et al., 2004a).

[2] A natural hazard may be classified as either "slow onset" (e.g. drought) or "sudden onset" such as floods, tropical cyclones, tsunamis and strong wind, storm surges, forest fires, landslides, and sand- or dust storms.

[3] A refugee is a person who: "owing to well-founded fear of being persecuted . . . is outside his country of nationality" (1951 Refugee Convention, http://www.unhcr.org/pages/49da0e466.html). In contrast an internally displaced person (IDP) has been forced to migrate within their own country.

TABLE 69.1 Examples of prevalence of acute malnutrition and other indicators from recent emergencies

Country	Region	Date	Context	GAM	Remarks
SE Ethiopia	Metta Woreda, East Hararghe zone	10/2009	Chronic food insecurity is a problem	11.4 (8.6–14/2)[a]	Stunting: 26.5% (20.6–32.4)
NE Kenya	Mandera East and West Districts	03/2009	Residents recovering from drought – surveys done before long rainy season	Ranges from 20.5% (16.6–24.4) to 32.3% (28.2–36.4)[a]	Low dietary diversity also reported
Somalia	Countrywide problems of drought and conflict-related insecurity	2010	South and central most affected	National average GAM 16%[a]	42% of the population in need of assistance
Sudan	North Darfur State	05–07/2009	Displaced and residents	Ranges from 16.9% to 34.5%[b]	Conflict- and drought-related food insecurity
Democratic Republic of Congo	Lubunga, Oriental Province	2009	Displaced by Lord's Resistance Army attacks	8.7% (6.1–11.4)[a]	Large numbers of abandoned illegitimate children
Uganda	West Nile, Northern Region	08/2009	Refugee settlements	<5%[a]	Anemia rates (children 6–59 months and women of reproductive age) ranged between 54% and 79%
Afghanistan	Jawsan province	05/2009	Residents	6.8 (5.2–8.8)[a]	Prevalence of stunting 55.3% (50.8–59.7)
Haiti	Port-au-Prince and nearby cities	2009	Earthquake 01/2010	Pre-crisis GAM 4.5%	Increase in GAM expected

[a]WHO growth standards.
[b]NCHS reference population.
GAM, global acute malnutrition.
Reproduced with permission from SCN NICS, (2010).

remain at unacceptably high levels for several years if not decades after the original emergency occurred. For example, Table 69.1 shows the range in rates in North Darfur in mid-2009 which all exceeded the emergency threshold. Increasing emphasis is being placed on context-specific trends, especially where the baseline prevalence is low to start with and therefore would have to rise dramatically to reach the emergency threshold.

Not all emergencies are characterized by increases in acute malnutrition, and in some situations micronutrient deficiency diseases (MDDs) may be a greater public health priority than acute malnutrition. For example, among refugees in northern Uganda the level of acute malnutrition remained well below 5%, although rates of anemia were between 54% and 79% (Table 69.1). Dye (2007) reviewed prevalence of micronutrient deficiencies in refugee settings worldwide and concluded that significant micronutrient deficiency continues to occur with regularity. Comparatively few studies have documented prevalence of micronutrient deficiencies in emergencies compared with assessments of acute malnutrition (Dye, 2007; Seal and Prudhon, 2007; Seal et al., 2007).

Nutritional Risk and Causes of Malnutrition in Emergencies

As a result of most emergencies there is likely to be increased nutritional risk associated with forced displacement, overcrowding, inadequate supplies of clean water, and poor sanitation. These all contribute to increased incidence of infectious disease. At the same time vulnerability is heightened by food insecurity, reliance on limited food rations, and social disruption that negatively affects child-caring behaviors. This represents a worsening of all three clusters of underlying causes of malnutrition, which relate to food, health, and care. UNICEF's original conceptual framework for the analysis of the underlying causes of malnutrition as part of its "triple A" approach (UNICEF, 1990) has been widely adopted in policies and good-practice guidelines for emergencies. It has been used to help decision-makers recognize and understand the principal causes of malnutrition (Young and Jaspars, 2006). In the most severe emergencies, a sudden deterioration in all three groups of underlying causes accounts for the extremely high prevalence and occurrence of "hotspots" (Young and Jaspars, 2006), although in less severe situations there are frequently debates between sectors as to the priority problem: food, health or care. In some protracted crises there are no obvious external shocks or hazards that have precipitated the emergency; rather, it is the combination of economic and political crises, and possibly conflict and insecurity, which undermines nutrition.

Assessment and Analysis of Nutrition in Emergencies

Assessing Nutritional Status of Children

Weight-for-height is the preferred nutritional index in emergency contexts as it reflects recent nutrition and wasting, and does not require the exact estimation of age, which might be difficult. The weight-for-height z-score of an individual child is calculated by comparing their measurements with an international reference or standard. In 2006, the WHO introduced a set of child growth standards which are now gradually replacing the 1977 NCHS/WHO growth reference for weight-for-height in surveys (Seal and Kerac, 2007; SCN, 2009). The growth standards are based on prescriptive criteria, which seek to define how children should grow. This involves value or normative judgments (de Onis et al., 2007a).

Categories of severe acute malnutrition (SAM) include less than −3 z-scores for severe acute malnutrition (SAM) or nutritional edema. The category of GAM includes less than −2 z-scores and nutritional edema. Children classified as suffering from moderate acute malnutrition (MAM) fall between the two, i.e. >−2 and <−3 z-scores with no nutritional edema.

The switch from the NCHS reference to the WHO standards has implications for prevalence estimates and numbers admitted into feeding programs. Studies indicate that the overall prevalence of GAM (wasting and/or edema) changes relatively little, but there is a significant increase in the prevalence of SAM. In turn this means an increase in the number of children eligible for admission into therapeutic feeding programs (Seal and Kerac, 2007; SCN, 2009). To allow comparisons, information systems such as SCN NICS report results in relation to both the NCHS reference and WHO standards.

The measurement of mid-upper-arm circumference (MUAC) for children aged between 1 and 5 years is a tool used for nutritional screening and increasingly for admission criteria for therapeutic and supplementary feeding programs. The arm circumference of infants and young children increases on average 1 to 2 cm up to 5 years of age. This means proportionally more younger children will be eligible for therapeutic feeding if a standard cut-off of 11.5 cm is used (WHO and UNICEF, 2009). This may be desirable as younger children tend to suffer higher mortality rates. MUAC may be used in surveys to estimate numbers of children eligible for therapeutic feeding programs, but is not useful for overall estimates of GAM as the results are not comparable with weight-for-height estimates (Myatt *et al.*, 2009).

Assessing Nutritional Status of Adults and Adolescents

Underweight among adults, often referred to as chronic undernutrition, has been reported as a public health problem in emergencies, for example in Somalia in 1992 (Collins and Myatt, 2000), Ethiopia in 2000 (Salama *et al.*, 2001), and South Sudan in 1998 (Borrel and Salama, 1999). Debate continues over the indices that should be used (MUAC vs. BMI), cut-off points and interpretation. A recent review recommended that low BMI (<18.5) among non-pregnant women aged 15 to 49 years, as used by WHO and WFP and in recent global meta-analyses (Black *et al.*, 2008), should be included as an indicator for monitoring food security and humanitarian crises (Young and Jaspars, 2009). Several issues affect interpretation of BMI data, including the need to adjust for body shape (sitting height to standing height ratio), the decline in height with older age, adaptation, and seasonal fluctuations (Young and Jaspars, 2006). The adjustments for body shape can be made using the Cormic Index (Collins, 2001), although this is not routine practice (Busolo, 2002).

There is no universally agreed definition of acute malnutrition in older people. If anthropometric measurement such as MUAC is used, HelpAge International recommends the WHO standard cut-off points in conjunction with the contextual, social, and clinical criteria and risk factors which are the key determinants of nutritional vulnerability among older people (Wells, 2005). Arm span and knee height can be used as proxies for height among the elderly, although their relationship to height for different ethnic groups has not been established (Busolo, 2002).

MUAC, in conjunction with clinical criteria (ability to stand, edema, and dehydration), has been used as a tool for rapid assessment of adults and older people, although the functional outcomes of different MUAC cut-offs are unknown. While child acute malnutrition is a composite indicator of poor health, lack of food, poor caring practices, etc., chronic undernutrition of adults at the population level is more intuitively a direct outcome of food insecurity and therefore potentially useful in emergencies.

However, the HIV epidemic does mean that there are increasing numbers of severely wasted adults, particularly in parts of Africa.

For adolescents, the variable age for the onset of puberty complicates measures of nutritional status. WHO has published the WHO 2007 Reference for school-aged children and adolescents, comprising BMI-for-age and height-for-age, for 5–19 years, and weight-for-age for 5–10 years (de Onis *et al.*, 2007b). In emergencies the WHO recommends that BMI-for-age be used by programs that target this group.

Assessing Nutritional Status of Populations

In emergencies, the two-stage 30-cluster nutrition survey is a well established and standardized tool for estimating the prevalence of acute malnutrition among children less than 5 years of age (SCF UK, 2004). While this approach has acceptable levels of precision for most contexts, in some cases a context-specific sample size is calculated (Kaiser *et al.*, 2006; Bilukha, 2008).

Nutrition surveys may include other nutrition and health indicators including crude mortality rate (CMR) and under-five mortality rates (Cairns *et al.*, 2009). Other useful indicators include vaccination coverage, vitamin A distribution coverage, or access to safe water sources. Food security indicators include receipt of rations, food frequency, and dietary diversity (Coates *et al.*, 2007), although these are usually collected as part of a broader household survey.

Interpretation; Classification Systems and Decision-Making Frameworks

The standardization of survey methods and analysis over the past decade has resulted in more reliable data. Challenges, however, remain with interpretation and in reaching valid conclusions. Two approaches and sets of tools have been developed for the interpretation of nutrition indicators. The first relates to the use of benchmarks as part of classification systems intended to monitor the severity of a humanitarian emergency or food security situation (see Case Study 1). The second are the decision-making frameworks designed to assist in prioritizing the most appropriate direct nutrition interventions.

Selective-feeding decision-making frameworks that combine benchmarks of nutritional status with "aggravating factors" (such as mortality, morbidity, and access to food) have been proposed and used to advise practitioners on the most appropriate intervention. However, the utility

Case Study 1   Nutritional surveillance as part of the Integrated Food Security Phase Classification System for classifying the severity of food insecurity and humanitarian crisis

Nutrition indicators have been used to gauge the severity of famine and complex emergencies for nearly half a century. There have been considerable efforts to standardize their use, including reaching agreement on reference levels that correspond to particular stages of food insecurity and humanitarian crises. A partnership of UN agencies, NGOs, and donor agencies has jointly developed a globally applicable food security severity scale, known as the Integrated Food Security Phase Classification (IPC, http://www.ipcinfo.org/). The IPC aims to provide a common technical approach to classify food security according to reference outcomes that are based on recognized international indicators. Indicators of wasting, chronic malnutrition, and mortality have been included in the IPC as "key reference outcome indicators" since its inception in 2004. Reference levels for each indicator (thresholds) have been attributed to each of the five phases of the classification (from generally food secure to famine/humanitarian catastrophe). For example, Phase 5 Humanitarian Catastrophe/Famine corresponds to a prevalence of acute malnutrition >30%; while Phase 4 Humanitarian Emergency corresponds to >15%, or GAM greater than usual and increasing. Such a scale facilitates comparisons between countries and over time, for decision-making about appropriate policies, programs, and resource allocation. The IPC has been introduced in several countries in Africa and Asia, and continues to gain momentum among governments, the UN, NGOs, and donors.

warning and intervention, resource allocation and targeting, and program monitoring. In emergencies, usually one or more of the following three methodological approaches are used. These include: representative nutrition surveys conducted every 2–12 months (Johnecheck and Holland, 2007), clinic-based surveillance data (based on existing growth monitoring data), and a purposively selected sentinel-site food security and nutritional surveillance system (Myatt, 2009). These approaches all have advantages and drawbacks. Regularly conducted nutrition surveys are relatively resource intensive but do provide valid and reliable data. Clinic-based surveillance potentially strengthens the capacity of existing clinics although the data may not be representative or timely. Sentinel-site surveillance provides timely and relevant data but it cannot be extrapolated to the wider population.

Nutritional status is limited as an early warning indicator since it is generally considered to be a late indicator for the deterioration in the nutritional situation. None the less, an analysis of trends can reveal deviations from normal patterns.

Internationally, there are a number of systems designed to monitor nutrition in emergencies. These include regular bulletins from the Nutrition Information in Crisis Situations [formerly the Refugee Nutrition Information System (RNIS), available on http://www.unscn.org/en/publications/nics/]; the Health and Nutrition Tracking System [Health and Nutrition Tracking Service (HNTS), 2009]; and the CRED (CE DAT, 2010).

of this framework may be limited in some contexts. For example, the prevalence of acute malnutrition may remain consistently higher than the benchmark (see, for example, Darfur in Table 69.1). A further limitation of this decision-making framework is that it is prescriptive and does not allow for possible non-food interventions that may positively affect population nutritional status or encourage more innovative interventions tailored for the context.

Nutritional Surveillance and International Tracking Systems

Nutritional surveillance monitors changes in malnutrition and population nutritional status over time for the purposes of problem identification and advocacy, timely

Food Security and Livelihood Assessments

Assessments of food insecurity and the impact of emergencies on livelihoods are assessed using specific approaches and methods (Seaman et al., 2000; Young et al., 2001; WFP/VAM, 2005). Many food security assessment approaches share the same conceptual understanding of food security and use similar data collection tools, although methods tend to be less standardized than nutrition survey tools. In general, they identify and disaggregate information using different livelihood or food economy groups and use qualitative methods to investigate the food security situation. Components of food security that are considered include access to food, food availability, and, in some situations, food utilization. An analysis of trends and recent changes in food security and livelihoods is crucial for understanding the situation and for designing the appropriate response.

Addressing the General Nutritional Needs of Populations

A range of intervention strategies are required to address the multiple nutritional risks that occur in emergencies, the choice of which is based on a process of assessment, analysis and prioritization and, in most cases, will be unique for a given situation.

Food Security Interventions and Protection of Livelihoods

Addressing food insecurity and protecting livelihoods has become a recognized component of a nutritional response in complex emergencies (Sphere Project, 2004; Jaspars, 2006) since these are critical for protecting and supporting nutrition albeit through indirect pathways. Increasingly a

range of food security interventions are applied that help people meet their food needs, earn income, and protect their assets, and these are summarized in Box 69.1 (Maxwell *et al.*, 2010). For example, recognizing the importance of livestock for maintaining the nutritional status of children in pastoralist areas across the developing world has long been recognized (Sadler *et al.*, 2009) and there is now an increasing interest in using emergency livestock-related interventions to protect primary resources during drought, to maintain access to milk and animal products for nutritionally vulnerable groups, and to improve the cost-benefit of drought-based interventions (Catley, 2008; Catley *et al.*, 2009).

Different contexts will determine which types of strategies are required. For non-displaced populations whose livelihoods are relatively intact, the interventions described

---

BOX 69.1   Examples of food security projects in emergency contexts

Definition: Food security exists when all people at all times have physical and economic access to sufficient, safe and nutritious food for a healthy and active life (World Food Summit Plan of Action, paragraph 1, 1996: FAO, 1996).

Agricultural production
1. Distribution of seeds, tools, and fertilizer.
2. Seed vouchers and fairs: bring together sellers and buyers.
3. Training and education in relevant skills.
4. Livestock interventions: animal health services; emergency destocking; restocking of livestock; distribution of livestock fodder and nutritional supplementation; and provision of alternative water sources.
5. Distribution of fishing nets and gear, or hunting implements.
6. Promotion of food processing, milling, and fortification.
7. Local agricultural extension and veterinary services.

Safety nets
8. Cash or Food-for-Work (CFW) provides food-insecure households with opportunities for paid work that at the same time produce outputs of benefit to themselves and the community
9. Income generating schemes allow people to diversify their sources of income in small-scale, self-employment business schemes.

Market interventions
10. Support of market infrastructure, e.g. transportation to allow producers to take advantage of distant markets.
11. Destocking: livestock purchase usually from pastoralists in times of drought.
12. Fair-price shops: sale of goods at controlled or subsidized prices.
13. Vouchers: which can be used to purchase or "redeem" a specified and predetermined range of goods and services.
14. Cash transfers: the provision of cash, which can either be unconditional or tied to a particular type of expenditure.

Microfinance projects
15. Credit and saving schemes: grants, loans, cattle or other livestock banks; cooperative savings accounts.

Case Study 2   Understanding the impact of livestock interventions on milk production and child nutrition

A recent study in the Shinile and Liben zones of Somali Region, Ethiopia, in 2009 documented the large contribution of animal milk to the dietary intake of young pastoralist children. When available, mothers added milk to most complementary foods. During a normal wet season, the average milk intake of a 1-year-old was estimated to provide about two-thirds of the mean energy required and 100% of the protein required by a child of this age. During a drought year, mothers estimated that milk intake by young children declined to negligible amounts and, in all cases, was replaced by cereal grain cooked and consumed with little else but water. Such a severe reduction in milk intake had a serious impact on dietary quality by reducing the amount of high quality protein, fatty acids, and micronutrients that young children consumed.

In a separate program in Ethiopia in 2008, Save the Children USA implemented an animal supplementary feeding project in Borana zone. Two of the feeding centers were evaluated and 48.6% (191/393) of cows either returned to milk production or began milk production following the birth of calves while in the feeding centers. These results were compared with the performance of cows outside the feeding centers, where lactation ceased. In one center the mean daily milk yield was 0.7 L/day (95% CI 0.44, 0.97; $n = 46$) and the estimated total milk production was 2276 L while cows were fed in the feeding center. In the other feeding center the mean daily milk yield was 0.9 L/day (95% CI 0.64, 1.22; $n = 63$) and the estimated total milk production was 3364 L while cows were fed in the feeding center. Informants stated that this milk was fed to children.

Studies such as these have shown that pastoralists themselves make logical associations between livestock health and production, milk supply, and human health and nutrition. However, there remain many opportunities for livelihoods projects in emergencies to design livestock interventions through a child-nutrition lens. Documentation of the impact of such projects would go some way to providing a better understanding of the most appropriate and effective responses in pastoral areas to protect the nutritional status of children.

Adapted from Bekele and Tsehay (2008) and Sadler and Catley (2009).

in Box 69.1 may be appropriate. In contrast, for populations displaced to camps, both refugees and IDPs, the opportunities for such innovative interventions may be limited as a consequence of lack of land or employment opportunities and the absence of markets that function. The process of prioritizing different interventions is a balance between relatively top-down short-term responses intended to save lives and reduce mortality (such as provision of general food assistance), and longer-term solutions that protect and support people's livelihoods and in so doing indirectly save lives and preserve people's dignity. This concept, and the challenges linked to it, are illustrated well by the international response to the ongoing crisis in Darfur (Young, 2007).

The Food Assistance Toolbox

General food distribution is the provision of dry food rations to those households deemed in need of food assistance. It has long been the most common strategy for ensuring that the nutritional needs of an emergency-affected population are met, and it remains the biggest single category of emergency response (Harvey *et al.*, 2010b). More recently there has been considerable debate about what types of intervention fit within the food assistance toolbox, with a particular focus on the use of vouchers and cash transfers as an appropriate alternative or complement to food aid for the protection and/or improvement of a population's food security and nutritional status. This is reflected in revised policy positions by, for example, WFP: "Food assistance refers to the set of instruments used to address the food needs of vulnerable people. The instruments generally include in-kind food aid, vouchers and cash transfers" (WFP, 2008b), and in practice, where the use of cash in responding to disasters is growing (Harvey, 2007).

General Food Distribution

A well-established body of best practice exists for the planning, distribution, and targeting of nutritionally adequate food rations including for populations suffering high levels of HIV (UNHCR *et al.*, 2002; WFP, 2002; FANTA/WFP, 2007). A nutritionally adequate ration is calculated on an average per capita energy requirement basis. An initial planning figure of 2100 kcal (8.8 MJ) per person per day is used, which is adjusted to suit specific conditions of the crisis; for example, the ambient temperature, demographic profile, activity levels, and the health status of the population. The recommended amount of total fat and protein in the ration is calculated based on percent of energy that each provides; 10–12% of energy should be obtained from protein and 17% of energy from fat.

Nutritionally adequate rations must also provide a source of micronutrients (see later in this chapter). In addition, general food rations should be culturally acceptable and safe for human consumption, comprise a variety of foods, be digestible for children, be fuel efficient, and be easy to store and prepare.

To fulfil these criteria, rations typically consist of a cereal such as sorghum, maize, wheat, or rice, a legume or pulse, and some oil or fat. These commodities are supplied in bulk, which facilitates the logistics and their distribution. High-profile acute crises continue to attract donations of foodstuffs unsuitable for emergency responses, which present challenges as to their practical use or their disposal, for example, US military ready-to-eat ration packs (MREs), high-protein biscuits, and infant food.

It is the policy of WFP and UNHCR either to provide the cereal grain in the form of milled flour, or to supply milling equipment during the initial response to a crisis. Milling greatly improves the digestibility of cereal grain for young children and older persons and the fuel efficiency of the cooking process. Where prevention of malnutrition in vulnerable groups such as children and pregnant or lactating women is a priority, a fortified blended food (FBF) is usually provided. The US government developed FBFs in the 1960s to serve as a protein-rich, micronutrient-dense food supplement appropriate for preschool-aged children in developing countries. Recent review has suggested that the formulation of these foods could be optimized to better meet the nutritional requirements for different vulnerable groups (de Pee and Bloem, 2009; Fleige *et al.*, 2010). In addition, they are likely to be increasingly used with other highly fortified foods such as the new lipid-based nutrient supplements (LNS) which are being considered for use in rations for groups with particularly high nutritional requirements (such as young children and pregnant and lactating women) (Chaparro and Dewey, 2009). Frequently, ration commodities may be sold or exchanged in order to obtain cooking fuel, to pay for milling costs, or to access a range of food items not provided in the ration.

Targeting strategies and distribution mechanisms are planned to ensure that the food ration reaches the affected communities in the most efficient and effective way. Targeting is closely linked with the assessment process, which identifies the worst affected geographical areas and/or the worst affected population groups within these areas. Identifying and reaching these groups is often challenging, particularly in areas where geographical access is limited;

a common characteristic of complex emergencies (see Case Study 3).

Case Study 3   From an acute to a protracted crisis: shifts in programming approach in the Darfur context, 2010

In the 7 years since the eruption of the civil war and mass forced displacement that triggered the Darfur complex emergency, there has been little evidence of significant permanent returns of the displaced to their places of origin. Instead conflict and insecurity continue to restrict mobility and access, and the long-term displaced have sought to adapt their livelihoods to their new settings, which includes some seasonal returns to their farms. But despite these adaptations the long-term displaced remain chronically vulnerable, and emergency levels of global acute malnutrition are common. Food assistance remains the single largest sector reaching, at the time of writing, up to 3 million conflict-affected people.

The World Food Programme and their operational partners have taken several strategic steps to tailor their programs to the changing context. First they have replaced their annual food security and nutrition assessments with a more appropriate sentinel-site food-security monitoring system. In their food distribution programs they have sought to reduce "errors of inclusion," i.e. to ensure food does not flow to those who do not need it, by further targeting the food-insecure. The mode of distribution has also changed from distributing to individual households to group distribution, which is managed by a community-based Food Relief Committee (FRC) comprising community-nominated representatives. The FRCs are intended to promote more community participation in the actual distribution and targeting of food aid in line with WFP policies. The introduction of the FRCs took place prior to the government expulsion of 13 INGOs in 2009, and their presence enabled WFP to continue food distributions throughout this difficult period.

In 2009, to complement the ongoing general food distribution program, WFP introduced a safety-net program (distribution of fortified blended food) to all households with children under 5 years of age in those areas with emergency levels of acute malnutrition. At the same time, on a trial basis, they introduced a voucher scheme to be scaled up in 2010. Such initiatives reflect a transition from emergency programming in an acute crisis to an approach that is better suited to a protracted emergency, although capacity to respond to acute humanitarian crises needs to be maintained.

Adapted from Young and Maxwell (2009).

Cash and Vouchers

Despite the relatively recent experience of cash and voucher schemes, numerous best practice guidelines and policy documents already exist (Creti and Jaspars, 2006; ACF, 2007; WFP, 2008b; Harvey *et al.*, 2010a). The most common interventions in this category used to address the nutritional needs of a population affected by crisis are:

- Cash transfers: the provision of cash, which can be either unconditional or tied to a particular type of expenditure.
- Vouchers: which can be used to purchase or "redeem" a specified and predetermined range of goods and services.

Generally cash transfers appear to be most suited to stable or peaceful contexts, where strong and accessible markets and banking systems exist. These conditions most often apply to later stages of a crisis (Harvey, 2007). Vouchers require that traders in targeted areas be identified and agreements set up with them for exchange. There is limited evidence to date that documents the direct impact of either cash or vouchers on the nutritional status of a population, but the evidence that does exist suggests that vouchers may be more effective than cash in meeting particular nutritional objectives (WFP, 2008b). This may be due to the greater control that women generally have over food and vouchers as opposed to cash resources, and to the fact that cash may be used for meeting needs that are not directly related to nutrition. Cash and vouchers can be productively combined with food transfers to mutually reinforce objectives that relate to addressing food insecurity and malnutrition.

Public Health Interventions

Malnutrition may be caused or exacerbated by disease, therefore a range of public health strategies are required to promote and protect health. In the emergency phase the priorities include initial assessment, public health surveillance, control of communicable diseases and epidemics (diarrheal diseases, measles, acute respiratory infections, and malaria), water and sanitation, and shelter and site planning (Salama and Roberts, 2005). Other specific issues of direct relevance to nutrition include curative health care, child health care, HIV/AIDS, and psychosocial and mental health services. The prevailing HIV/AIDS epidemic in southern Africa is undermining the ability of communities to recover from famine, as it directly affects able-bodied adults who are the most productive in terms

of food security (de Waal and Whiteside, 2003). Despite great advances in knowledge around the basic interventions that should be prioritized in emergencies, reviews of the global relief system suggest an ongoing failure to deliver (Checchi *et al.*, 2007). This reflects the huge challenges to delivery often seen in humanitarian emergencies, including very large geographic areas, extremely poor infrastructure, and conflict.

Reaching the Physiologically At-Risk Groups

Nutritional vulnerability in humanitarian crises is often exacerbated for certain groups because of their particular nutritional requirements or because of the physiological risks that they face. Examples include infants and young children, older people, women of reproductive age, and people with specific health conditions such as HIV/AIDS. Often referred to as nutritionally vulnerable groups, their specific needs may be met by additional programs including, for example, those targeted at specific population groups, or the adaptation of broad-based safety-net programs. Targeting individuals within a population requires a system for identifying and registering those who will then benefit from the intervention. This type of parallel program is not always cost-effective or feasible, although it is attractive as it potentially reduces the likelihood of resources reaching those who are not at greatest risk.

Adapting Broad-Based Safety-Net Programs

Safety-net programs seek to protect the vulnerable and prevent them from falling further into poverty or food insecurity by providing safety-net transfers such as food stamps or vouchers, subsidies, cash transfers, public works, etc. Broad-based safety-net programs can be adapted to better meet the needs of the nutritionally vulnerable, which mitigates the need for additional parallel programs targeting these groups. For example, the International Committee of the Red Cross (ICRC) has for many years implemented a policy whereby the general ration has been increased above that of other international agencies (2400 kcal per person per day, as opposed to the 2100 kcal recommended by other agencies) in order to obviate the need for a separate nutrition program (Navarro-Colorado *et al.*, 2008). Cash transfers, rather than food assistance, are increasingly being considered as a means to support the vulnerable, particularly in protracted humanitarian crises. While cash transfers are targeted on the basis of socioeconomic criteria, when combined with targeting of women of reproductive age and implemented with nutrition education, these programs enable women to meet their own and their children's additional requirements through the additional household income received. Monitoring of intra-household food distribution and/or nutrition education and awareness may be necessary to ensure that the most physiologically vulnerable do benefit.

Targeting Specific Age Groups with Nutrition Interventions

Exclusive breastfeeding for a duration of 6 months reduces morbidity and mortality among children (WHO, 2002). Humanitarian crises present additional risks for infants who are not breastfed. Poor sanitation and overcrowding, high prevalence of infectious diseases, a lack of access to clean water and cooking fuel for safe preparation of breast-milk substitutes (BMS), and a lack of a regular supply of BMS imply even greater risks associated with not breastfeeding (Kelly, 1993). Adherence to World Health Assembly legislation is frequently compromised, and unsolicited donations of BMS are often reported (Borrel *et al.*, 2001), including in the recent catastrophe in China (Coutsoudis *et al.*, 2009). A number of inter-agency and agency-specific policies and guidelines address the protection, promotion, and support for exclusive breastfeeding in humanitarian crises (Seal *et al.*, 2001). However, the application of these policies in practice is often poor, constrained by a lack of institutional memory and available expertise as well as a failure in agency leadership and coordination (Borrel *et al.*, 2001).

There are well-recognized challenges associated with designing effective programs and policies in countries which have pre-existing poor breastfeeding practices. For example, changes in practice brought about through individual counseling may not always be possible in humanitarian crises because of a loss of skilled community health workers and poorer access to the population. Recent evidence from Zimbabwe has highlighted the importance of ensuring that women receive support from their husbands, mothers-in-law, and other influential community members. Positive attitude change among family members can be achieved through innovative, feasible, and effective interventions such as road shows that reach a high proportion of the population (Jenkins, 2011). The increase in prevalence of HIV/AIDS has brought new challenges, and the absence of clear and consistent guidance for HIV-positive women in the past may have had a negative impact and undermined exclusive breastfeeding practices in the broader population. It is now recommended that mothers known to be HIV-infected should exclusively breastfeed their infants for the first 6 months of life, introducing appropriate complementary foods thereafter, and continue breastfeeding for the first 12 months of life (WHO, 2009). For women known to be HIV-positive and intending to breastfeed, extended antiretroviral prophylaxis for mother and infant throughout the breastfeeding period is recommended. Mothers known to be HIV-infected may consider expressing and heat-treating breast milk as an *interim feeding strategy*. For mothers whose status is not known, which is common in humanitarian crises, exclusive breastfeeding for 6 months is promoted and it is recommended that mothers are counseled for testing (Leyenaar, 2004).

The nutritional requirements for women during pregnancy and lactation are higher than the population average (WHO, 2000). Consequently, macronutrient (food) and micronutrient (iron and folic acid) supplements are usually provided to all pregnant and lactating women during pregnancy and for the first 6 months of breastfeeding, through emergency supplementary feeding programs (SFPs) or mother-and-child health clinics. If food resources are scarce, only some pregnant and lactating women are targeted, those with a MUAC of less than 21–23 cm (WHO, 1995). Evidence of the impact of providing macronutrient and micronutrient supplements to women for this short period is limited. Poor impact may be as a result of intra-household distribution patterns, ambiguity of the outcomes to be measured, a lack of opportunity to improve pre-pregnancy nutritional status, and limited possibilities for integrating nutrition interventions with other public health programs.

The nutritional risks that older people normally face are likely to be exacerbated in humanitarian crises because of the loss of support systems as a result of family separations or the disruption of informal and formal social networks. Furthermore, their needs may extend well beyond the acute crisis. For example, following the cyclone in Myanmar, older people received adequate food assistance, but equal emphasis needed to be placed on their longer-term food security needs (HelpAge International, 2009). Increased nutritional risk for older people may be as a result of lack of access to health care, exposure to the cold, psychological stress, and constraints on food preparation (Vespa and Watson, 1995), and a lack of mobility, limited employment opportunities, lack of access to land, food, and basic services, and psychosocial trauma (Pieterse and

Ismail, 2003). However, older people are still seldom involved in nutritional assessments, in decision-making about food aid requirements or in program design. As a result, programs often do not include them, or reflect their needs.

Populations Affected by Disabilities and Chronic Illnesses such as HIV and Tuberculosis

Food supplements are frequently targeted to individuals with disabilities, those with chronic illness, those receiving TB treatment, and, increasingly, persons with HIV/AIDS. The objectives of nutrition in this context are usually multiple, including strengthening household food security, meeting specific additional requirements, facilitating recovery from secondary acute malnutrition, and improving compliance with treatment regimes. While humanitarian crises do not necessarily cause an increase in HIV prevalence (Samuels, 2009), regional and national food insecurity is frequently associated with epidemics of HIV/AIDS. At the individual level, malnutrition and HIV/AIDS are inextricably linked. Malnutrition, reduced food intakes, and micronutrient deficiencies are associated with more rapid disease progression of HIV/AIDS. Nutrition interventions potentially have a wide range of benefits for HIV-related outcomes; however, their impact depends on the type of intervention, the duration for which it is given, and the underlying vulnerability of the infected person. Interventions range from support for appropriate breast-feeding regimes, nutrition-relevant education, micro- or macronutrient supplements, referral for treatment of secondary acute malnutrition, and interventions to strengthen household food security. HIV-affected persons should consume 20–100% above normal energy intakes depending on whether the individual is an adult or child, asymptomatic or symptomatic, and experiencing weight loss or no weight loss (Ivers et al., 2009). Furthermore, multi-micronutrient supplements have been shown to have beneficial effects on morbidity and other outcomes for HIV-affected children and adults, and have been recommended as interventions complementary to treatment regimes (Fawzi et al., 2005). Nutrition supplements alone are, however, insufficient, and need to be combined with other interventions such as treatment, counseling, care, and food security. There is increasing evidence to show that HIV-positive children who are malnourished respond well to adapted treatment protocols in regular community-based management of acute malnutrition (CMAM) programs, which can also be an opportunity to strengthen the

referral system for these children for ART treatment (Fergusson, 2009). In the absence of testing and treatment of HIV/AIDS, the targeting of these combined interventions remains problematic. While there is an increase in the available guidance on food assistance in the context of HIV/AIDS (FANTA/WFP, 2007; World Bank, 2007; WFP, 2008a), documentation and institutional experience of effective strategies are limited.

In conclusion, in most humanitarian crises there is a need to consider how nutrition programs can reach those with additional nutritional requirements, through both broad-based approaches and parallel programs targeting specific groups. In chronic protracted crises, it becomes increasingly important to adapt broad-based safety-net programs.

Preventing and Treating Micronutrient Deficiency Diseases

There are several risk factors common to emergency-affected populations that precipitate micronutrient deficiency diseases (MDDs). These include a reliance on general food rations; reduced access to markets or livelihood systems that would normally support access to a diverse range of foods; and increased exposure to infectious diseases such as diarrhea due to a poor public health environment. Consequently, micronutrient deficiencies have been reported for years in emergency settings, particularly among refugees, where they are most frequently assessed (Seal and Prudhon, 2007). MDDs most commonly reported include those that are endemic across the developing world such as vitamin A, iron, and iodine deficiency disorders as well as other MDDs that are specific to the emergency context including pellagra, scurvy, and beriberi (Cheung et al., 2003; Seal et al., 2005, 2007).

As a result of these outbreaks, the last two decades have seen increasing acknowledgment by UN agencies and NGOs that the nutrient content of a ration should not only meet minimum energy needs but should also help to prevent micronutrient deficiencies (Webb et al., 2009b). This is particularly important for nutritionally vulnerable groups such as young children and pregnant and lactating women, who have increased requirements. To achieve this and, where necessary, to treat MDDs, a range of strategies are used. These include improving access to foods rich in micronutrients, the provision of fortified food commodities, and supplementation.

Improving Access to Foods Rich in Micronutrients

A diverse diet is the most preferred method to ensure consumption of sufficient micronutrients to meet requirements. Although the provision of a fresh food commodity in the general food ration that is rich in one or more micronutrient(s), such as pulses, groundnuts, red palm oil, fruits, and vegetables, can be a strategy to prevent one or more deficiencies (Malfait *et al.*, 1993), it is costly and logistically difficult and is therefore rarely implemented. The move by WFP to increase the use of vouchers and cash transfers in place of direct food assistance was discussed earlier. In the right context, where markets are functioning and accessible and food supply is stable, evidence has shown that both types of intervention can improve households' access to nutrient-dense foods without the high costs of including fresh commodities in the food basket (WFP, 2008b). The use of livestock interventions is also a means to improve access to micronutrient-rich animal source foods for emergency-affected populations. Documented evidence of the impact of these interventions on nutritional status is, however, scarce.

Food Fortification

Food fortification in emergencies is most commonly applied through the provision of fortified food commodities or through community-based fortification of grain. WFP policy stipulates several food-aid commodities that must be fortified for use in the food-aid basket including vegetable oil with vitamin A, salt with iodine, and fortified, blended flours with multiple micronutrients (WFP, 2004). More recently, efforts have been made to fortify cereals using custom-designed milling and fortification equipment at refugee-camp level. There is some evidence to show that this is feasible and can improve the micronutrient status of some groups (Seal *et al.*, 2008). See Case Study 4 below. However, even where fortified grain and/or flour are provided, the micronutrient needs of some groups with high nutritional requirements may not be met (Chaparro and Dewey, 2010). For these groups, and where the provision of FBF is not possible, the provision of home-based fortificants and lipid-based nutrient supplements (or ready-to-use foods) is becoming more common.

Home-based fortificants (such as Sprinkles™) come in the form of single-dose sachets containing micronutrients in a powdered form, which are easily sprinkled on to foods prepared in the household. There is evidence that these products can impact the micronutrient status of vulnerable

---

Case Study 4   Fortification of food at refugee camp level in Zambia

In 2002, World Food Programme, CARE-Zambia, and Micronutrient Initiative (MI) established a pilot program for on-site milling, using mobile milling and fortication units (MFUs) in a remote refugee camp in Zambia. The aim of the program was to assess the feasibility of such an intervention and to assess the impact on the micronutrient status of the population.

At the outset, a task force was established comprising representatives from UNHCR, WFP, the government of Zambia, and two NGOs. They agreed that the new MFUs would need to have an output level sufficient to meet needs, produce a quality product in terms of acceptability and standards, and be easily maintained. A nutritional survey including assessment of micronutrient deficiencies was conducted as well as a community assessment with the refuges. The latter highlighted considerable skepticism toward the use of mills (previous experience had seen mills frequently breaking down) and to the fortification process. Consequently, a significant investment was made in sensitizing the population, which included supporting a visit to an established fortification program elsewhere in the country and the development of extensive education and communication materials to be used by community development workers.

The benefits of the fortification process were quickly evident. The fortified maize flour was widely accepted in terms of texture and taste. Refugees no longer had to wait for prolonged periods to mill their flour. Investment was made in training and providing new skills to those supervising and managing the installed MFUs. A follow-up survey showed that anemia had decreased from 47.7% to 24.3% and vitamin A deficiency had decreased from 46.3% to 20.3%. In general, the refugee population perceived that their health status had improved significantly since the program began.

This program demonstrated that on-site fortification using MFUs was a feasible intervention with a positive impact on nutritional status, particularly micronutrient status. With relatively small investment costs at the outset and even smaller recurring costs (forticants and maintenance), this approach was considered a feasible approach for fortifying rations, especially in isolated camps.

Adapted from van den Briel *et al.* (2006).

---

groups and reduce the prevalence of MDDs such as anemia (Zlotkin *et al.*, 2005) and that they are a feasible intervention in humanitarian emergencies (De Pee *et al.*, 2007).

"Lipid-based nutrient supplement" (LNS) refers generically to a range of highly fortified, lipid-based foods that includes products such as ready-to-use therapeutic food (RUTF), which has been widely adopted for the outpatient treatment of severe acute malnutrition (see below). There is currently considerable interest in using smaller doses of LNS to help meet the recommended nutrient intakes (both macro- and micro-) for nutritionally vulnerable groups such as young children in combination with other foods provided in the general ration (Chaparro and Dewey, 2010).

Supplementation

The distribution of micronutrient supplements is necessary to treat MDD outbreaks in an emergency-affected population and can be used to meet high requirements and prevent MDDs in vulnerable sub-groups in the short term (WHO/UNHCR, 1999a,b; Cheung et al., 2003). WHO, WFP, and UNICEF now recommend that, because of their particular nutritional vulnerability, all pregnant and lactating women and young children affected by emergencies receive a daily multiple micronutrient supplement until the emergency is over and access to nutrient-rich foods is restored (WHO et al., 2007). Vitamin A supplementation is routinely provided every 4 to 6 months for all children aged 6 to 59 months to prevent vitamin A deficiency and is known to be particularly important in humanitarian emergencies to reduce the risk of mortality and other complications of measles (Salama and Roberts, 2005). Vitamin A supplementation is often conducted in conjunction with measles or other vaccination campaigns.

Preventing and Treating Moderate Acute Malnutrition

Supplementary feeding programs (SFPs) are a standard emergency response strategy usually established to address high or increasing prevalence of GAM. They are designed to provide a good quality food supplement that is in addition to the normal diet. To be effective, the extra food provided must be additional to, and not a substitute for, the base diet (Sphere Project, 2004).

Types and Objectives of SFPs

There are two main types of SFP: targeted and blanket programs. Targeted SFPs typically aim to rehabilitate individuals suffering from MAM, particularly those from nutri-tionally vulnerable groups such as children or pregnant and lactating women, and to prevent an increase in the number of individuals suffering from severe acute malnutrition. They also commonly aim to reduce GAM and reduce or prevent excess mortality. A blanket SFP provides a food supplement to all individuals within a defined vulnerable group. This type of SFP is usually implemented where GAM levels are high, or where the general food ration is not yet well established. Where SFPs are used as a "holding operation" to prevent the deterioration of nutritional status of vulnerable groups until wider food security can be secured, advocacy for general nutritional support should be a key element of the program (Sphere Project, 2004)

Program Design

Implementation of an SFP usually requires multiple decentralized program sites, which might take advantage of existing structures and services such as health centers. Most commonly, dry take-home rations are provided weekly or fortnightly, and are taken home for preparation and consumption. Wet on-site feeding requires daily attendance and requires one to four prepared meals daily to be consumed "on-site". The former are preferable in most circumstances because they are less resource intensive, hold fewer opportunity costs for program beneficiaries, and reduce the risk of communicable disease transmission (WHO, 2000). Most guidance, including that published by the WHO, recommends that a supplementary ration should provide 500–700 kcal per beneficiary per day and should include 15–25 g of protein. They also recommend that these amounts should be doubled for dry take-home feeding with the assumption that some of the supplement will be shared with other family members. The foods distributed in SFPs vary, but almost always include FBFs such as corn–soy blend (CSB).

Challenges and Alternative Designs

Doubts about the efficacy of supplementary feeding programs using fortified blended flours have been raised repeatedly over the past 25 years (Briend and Prinzo, 2009). Many reasons have been put forward for the apparent poor performance of these programs, including inappropriate design (i.e. opportunity costs to participants that outweigh the perceived benefit of program attendance), poor acceptability of the treatment offered, and questionable effectiveness of FBFs for the treatment of wasting. Such supplements often have a nutritional profile (high protein, low fat, and high dietary fiber and anti-nutrient content) that does not seem the best adapted to promote rapid growth of malnourished children (de Pee and Bloem, 2009). Recent studies and programs that have compared the use of FBFs with new lipid-based nutrient supplements (LNSs) for the treatment of MAM have generally shown that LNSs hold potential for improving rates of weight gain and recovery in SFPs (Matilsky *et al.*, 2009; Nackers *et al.*, 2010). Use of these new commodities is also moving into the realm of programs that aim to *prevent* malnutrition in vulnerable groups, particularly in areas that experience very high levels of child wasting every year. Médecins Sans Frontières (MSF), for example, found that the distribution of a small dose of RUTF to all children for 3 months prior to the hungry season in one area of Niger considerably reduced the prevalence and incidence of acute malnutrition compared with previous years (Defourny *et al.*, 2009). However, there remain questions around the costs of this approach and its benefits vs. other child-survival interventions that also hold potential to prevent MAM and severe acute malnutrition (SAM) in some contexts (Schaetzel and Nyaku, 2010).

Treating Severe Acute Malnutrition

Therapeutic feeding programs (TFPs) are usually established when there are large numbers of children suffering from severe acute malnutrition (SAM). These children have a significantly increased risk of mortality (compared with well nourished individuals).

Types and Objectives of TFPs

Until recently, treatment of SAM in emergencies was restricted to in-patient management in therapeutic feeding centers (TFCs) or hospital units (WHO, 1999). This approach ignored the many barriers to accessing treatment that exist for poor people in the developing world (Collins, 2001) and, as a result, such programs were associated with poor coverage and late presentation of individuals with SAM. Individuals who present late are more likely to suffer from the many complications often associated with SAM such as hypoglycemia, hypothermia, severe infection, and refeeding syndrome, and these make the condition much more difficult to treat successfully. Evidence published over the last decade has shown that, by reducing barriers to access and supporting earlier presentation, large numbers of children with SAM can be treated from out-patient facilities without being admitted to in-patient units (Collins *et al.*, 2006b). This treatment approach, now

known as community-based management of severe acute malnutrition (CMAM), is supported by the WHO, the WFP, the UN SCN, and UNICEF as the most appropriate strategy for the treatment of SAM in emergencies and beyond (WHO/WFP/UN SCN/UNICEF, 2007) and can achieve both high coverage of children suffering from SAM in emergencies and high rates of recovery (Collins *et al.*, 2006a; Sadler *et al.*, 2007).

A typical objective of a TFP (whether delivered through a TFC or a CMAM program) is to treat severe acute malnutrition in the targeted group and to prevent excess mortality.

Program Design

CMAM programs focus on finding and treating SAM early in the progression of the condition, before metabolic and immunological status becomes severely compromised and requires in-patient treatment. To achieve this, and to ensure that individuals can stay in treatment with few costs to them or to their families, programs are designed to minimize barriers to access. Treatment services are decentralized close to where the target population lives and where possible provided from the same sites as those delivering supplementary feeding. Ideally, programs also ensure that target communities understand the services available to them and participate in design and implementation of programs. This helps to sustain early presentation and high coverage (Guerrero *et al.*, 2010).

Once identified, children are classified according to the severity of their clinical condition. Those suffering from SAM with medical complications require admission to in-patient facilities such as TFCs, and are treated according to WHO protocols with formula milks known as F75 and F100 (WHO, 1999). Discharge from the TFC to an out-patient treatment happens as soon as appetite returns. This takes an average of 2–5 days after admission to an in-patient facility. Ready-to-use therapeutic food (RUTF) is designed to be nutritionally equivalent to the F100 milk, and studies have shown that it is effective at rehabilitating severely malnourished children and promotes faster weight gain than F100 (Diop *et al.*, 2003). This food has made feasible the safe treatment of severely malnourished patients at home. In out-patient treatment RUTF is given in quantities that provide 150–220 kcal/kg/day. Those suffering from SAM with no medical complications do not require admission to in-patient facilities and are treated directly in out-patient treatment according to CMAM protocol (Valid International/Concern Worldwide, 2006).

Case Study 5 Integrating CMAM into national service delivery in Ethiopia

Because of the chronically high levels of acute malnutrition in many parts of Ethiopia, Concern's National CMAM (N-CMAM) program focused on supporting the Ministry of Health (MoH) to provide services to treat SAM as part of routine health delivery. Previously, the vertical nature of emergency programming meant that it was often difficult for the MoH to assume responsibility for a program that had not been "theirs" in the first place.

The N-CMAM program was implemented using a partnership approach, with the focus firmly on "ownership" by the MoH. The aim was for the program to establish a much needed service during "normal" times, and also to provide a base of capacity from which services could be rapidly scaled-up at times of crisis. The program provided a package of "minimal support" to the MoH, which consisted of training (set-up, on-the-job and training-of-trainers), joint supervision, workshops, experience-sharing visits, and community mobilization support. The program emphasized learning and innovation, in order to regularly refine and adapt the approach. Considerable support was also provided to the MoH at Federal level for the development of National SAM guidelines and a CMAM component in the National Nutrition Program Strategy.

While the minimal support package was important, the most crucial aspect of the program was the *nature* of the dialogue between the partners. Concern found the right balance between providing the support that was required and ensuring that the MoH were in the driving-seat at all times. In this way a strong partnership developed with all levels of the MoH steadily gaining confidence in their ability to offer quality CMAM services. When the food crisis of 2008 hit across much of the country, the MoH (with support from UNICEF) were able to rapidly scale-up decentralized CMAM services and implement the required policy changes. To date, approximately 30% of health facilities are offering CMAM services, a huge achievement in a vast country.

This case study demonstrates many of the key aspects involved in creating an enabling environment for the integration of nutrition services into national health systems. These include support for MoH technical leadership and coordination; the development of National Guidelines which are a powerful tool for promoting, strengthening, and maintaining harmonized services; and a long-term commitment by donors and INGO partners for capacity development and supplies.

Contribution by Emily Mates, Health and Nutrition Advisor, Concern Worldwide Ethiopia.

Special Groups

There is increasing evidence to show that infants and adults suffering from SAM can also respond well to treatment although there are more challenges linked to these groups. A recent review of the management of acutely malnourished infants <6 months old in emergency programs highlighted a general lack of guidance and wide variation in treatment approaches across programs (Kerac et al., 2010). Strategies with potential to improve inpatient outcomes of infants with SAM include implementation of routine kangaroo care, breastfeeding "corners" with skilled breastfeeding support including support for the "supplementary suckling technique,"[4] and tailored psychosocial stimulation/support of infants under 6 months. Strategies with potential for effective out-patient-based care of infants under 6 months with MAM or SAM include community-based breastfeeding support, psychosocial support programs, and women's group programs. Good recovery rates have been reported for severely malnourished adults in therapeutic feeding programs in Sudan, Somalia, and Angola, despite challenges such as relatively poorer compliance, increased risk of population displacement, and higher rates of underlying chronic illnesses such as HIV (Collins et al., 1998; Bahwere et al., 2009). There are opportunities for better integration of programs that treat SAM with HIV testing, treatment, and prevention of mother-to-child transmission (PMTCT) programs since SAM is closely linked to HIV, particularly in these groups.

Policy Development, Best Practices, and Capacity Development

Over the past two decades, positive shifts in the broader policy environment have influenced and strengthened the emergency nutrition sector. The nutrition sector as a whole has enjoyed higher visibility and profile, largely as a result of the global commitment to the Millennium Development Goals (MDGs) where reducing undernutrition is widely recognized as central to achieving MDG 1 and malnutrition is a key factor underpinning many of the other MDGs. Furthermore, a comprehensive review series recently published in *The Lancet* described a number of high-impact evidence-based nutrition interventions (Bhutta et al., 2008; Bryce et al., 2008). This series of

---

[4] This aims to simultaneously treat infants with SAM and maintain or re-establish breastfeeding where it has stopped.

publications and others have also highlighted the health implications and economic costs of not addressing undernutrition (World Bank, 2006; Black *et al.*, 2008; Victora *et al.*, 2008). This has led to a greater commitment to the nutrition sector by a number of agencies including the World Bank to identify the challenges and implement solutions (Horton *et al.*, 2008).

Secondly, building on the UN agencies' public commitments to address nutrition in humanitarian crises, agency accountability for nutrition has been further defined. For example, UNICEF's recently revised Core Commitments for Children in Humanitarian Action (UNICEF, 2010) refer to their commitment to facilitate co-ordination mechanisms, rapid assessments, provision of vitamin A supplements, support for infant and young-child feeding, and treatment for severe acute malnutrition using explicit results-based interventions. Similarly WFP has reaffirmed the role of nutrition within their food aid assistance responses, including the role of fortification for addressing micronutrient deficiencies (WFP, 2004). The humanitarian reform agenda, which was led by the Inter-Agency Standing Committee (IASC) and launched in 1995, aims to improve the impact in humanitarian responses through greater accountability, improved preparedness, development of standards and best practice, including monitoring mechanisms, as well as strengthening the sector's skilled human resource capacity (IASC Global Nutrition Cluster, 2010). In particular, the humanitarian reform presents an opportunity to ensure that there is a more coherent and shared process for planning and prioritization among all partners, leading to greater results within the sector. The nutrition cluster, led by UNICEF, has made efforts to further consolidate and strengthen the emergency nutrition sector. For example, it has undertaken activities aimed at improving nutritional assessment and in-country coordination, improving timeliness and deployment of skilled professionals, and bringing about the merging of guidelines, and a longer-term approach to capacity development. However, some challenges remain, for example a lack of a defined, coherent, and long-term vision for the nutrition cluster and short-term funding, which limit commitments to short-term time-bound projects rather than longer-term institutional change initiatives.

Thirdly, there are further efforts and mechanisms established now to bridge the prevailing divide between the humanitarian and development sectors. This is reflected by policies, commitments, and actions that explicitly reflect efforts to support early recovery of the sectors (including nutrition) from the outset of the humanitarian response. In practice this is leading to a greater emphasis being placed on strengthening national policies, systems, and capacities, and not just the delivery of life-saving services. For example, in Mozambique, the cluster "transformed" after the acute flooding crisis to focus more specifically on preparedness and capacity development, particularly in line with government priorities. In some countries, however, this remains challenging to implement in practice, particularly in fragile states in the context of ongoing conflict and insecurity as found in parts of Sudan.

Fourthly, building on the Sphere Project initiative which mobilized the international humanitarian community to develop a set of Minimum Standards for Disaster Response (Sphere Project, 2004) (see Case Study 6), results-based monitoring is increasingly reflected in donor and agency policies and guidelines which are being revised to reflect the highest standards of accountability and quality management (HAP, 2010; UNICEF, 2010).

Fifthly, the global architecture of nutrition is also evolving, albeit slowly, towards a multi-sectoral approach that explicitly links the sectors of nutrition food security as well as other sectors. A recent high-level UN Task Force and inter-agency initiative, which arose out of the recent global food crisis, has reaffirmed the need for a multi-sectoral approach to nutrition[5]. The inter-agency initiative, with broad ownership, has recommended that national nutrition strategies and key national stakeholders in nutrition should apply the "Three Ones" including "one agreed framework that provides the basis for co-ordinating the work of all partners; one national coordinating authority, with a broad multi-sectoral mandate; and one agreed national monitoring and evaluation system" (Bezanson and Isenman, 2010). Although as yet this policy shift has had limited impact, this emerging architecture may create new potential opportunities for emergency nutrition to have greater accountability within the broader sector and likewise to have better ownership by different sectors – particularly in the context of protracted and persistent crises such as climate change, HIV/AIDS, and the ongoing global economic crisis.

Humanitarian crises can present valuable opportunities to positively influence the development of new national legislation and policy, such as in Afghanistan (Islamic

---

[5] This multi-sectoral approach is also reinforced by specific donor policies such as DFID's: see DIFD, 2010.

Republic of Afghanistan: MOPH, 2008), or to revise earlier policies such as in Iraq (Tolvanen and Kumar, 2003) or reinforce existing policies such as following the cyclone in Bangladesh (Bangladesh Breastfeeding Foundation, 2007).

Operational practice in the emergency nutrition sector has also significantly influenced policy development and application (Heikens *et al.*, 2008). For example, community-based management of severe malnutrition, which developed based on the well-researched experiences of large-scale humanitarian nutrition programs, has influenced international policies. Furthermore, community-based treatment of severe malnutrition is increasingly institutionalized within national structures and government policies.

Other examples of best practice influencing policy include the standardization of nutrition surveys and the use of MUAC as admission criteria based on risk of mortality. Despite the wide array of best practice and policies that do exist, there are, however, inconsistencies in the application and adherence to these policies for a number of reasons. This includes some ambiguity and discrepancies that exist between the different agency-specific guidelines, a general lack of awareness of policies because of a rapid agency staff turnover, lack of systematic mechanisms that ensure adherence to policies and standards, and a failure to invest in national capacities.

It is widely recognized that capacity development is much broader than just training. While there is still no overarching capacity development framework that encompasses the broader institutional change initiatives necessary to strengthen the emergency nutrition sector as a whole, there are some efforts to embrace a more comprehensive approach. For example, the IASC cluster recognizes complementary strategies for capacity development, namely preparedness, strengthening the foundation of nutrition, and real-time learning (IASC Global Nutrition Cluster, 2007). Important training initiatives in emergency nutrition are being scaled up and are beginning to address the major challenges that continue to exist (NutritionWorks, 2010). The first of these challenges is that training continues to be *ad hoc* and, when undertaken, is overly focused on strengthening technical skills rather than on addressing the functional and core skills critical for effective leadership and change in nutrition. Furthermore, the training continues to focus on health and nutrition professionals rather than on professionals among multiple sectors. A second challenge is that the academic curricula for professional nutritionists frequently do not include the relevant skills and knowledge that are considered necessary to function effectively in humanitarian crises, such as the ability to design nutritional surveys, to develop food aid interventions, and to carry out Community-Based Management of Acute Malnutrition (CMAM). Professional training initiatives can no longer be left to ad hoc training initiatives within the operational agencies themselves, but need to be systematically incorporated into academic curricula, particularly within the national training and academic institutions located in crisis-affected countries themselves.

Case Study 6   Sphere Project: Minimum Standards in Food Security, Food Aid, and Nutrition

An important inter-agency initiative that has contributed to improved practice in humanitarian response over the past decade is the Sphere Project. Through a global consultative process, the Sphere Project has developed a set of Minimum Standards and related key indicators for different sectors including Food Security, Nutrition, Food Aid, Health, Water, and Shelter, plus common standards on Participation, Targeting, etc. The cornerstone of the Sphere Project is the Humanitarian Charter, which is based on the principles and provisions of international humanitarian law, international human rights law, and refugee law. The Humanitarian Charter reasserts the rights of emergency-affected populations to life with dignity. The Minimum Standards and their related indicators are considered by some to be a practical interpretation of what these rights mean in the context of humanitarian response, i.e. it aims to link human rights with standards for operation. The current version of the Sphere Project (2004) attempts to incorporate relevant human rights principles and values into the Sphere Standards as reflected in the Humanitarian Charter, including the right to life with dignity, non-discrimination, impartiality and participation. Although the Minimum Standards potentially establish a mechanism for transparency and accountability, ensuring their implementation will require more reflection on the precise modes and mechanisms of accountability (Young et al., 2004b). The Sphere Project is currently being updated to reflect the evolving challenges of humanitarian crisis (Sphere Project, 2011).

Future Directions

The speed in development of new nutrition supplements during the last decade has been phenomenal. Policy and clear program guidance have lagged behind and, as a result, there is a polarization of views on the "for" and "against" use of these products. Use of these new products will continue to grow in future programming. Building consensus among a broad range of stakeholders for evidence-based guidance will be important for both program design and resource allocation.

Concentration on the nutritional quality of food assistance, and the large number of new nutrition supplements on the market, have served to narrow the focus on nutrition as a clinical condition, and have swung attention toward a more medicalized model of treatment of individuals rather than having a broader public-nutrition approach of addressing problems at the population level, including causal analysis, risk reduction and prevention. The pendulum is just now beginning to swing toward increasing concerns for the broader nutrition problems of society, and to a broader view of the interventions needed to impact nutrition as part of a more integrated approach.

Progress has been accomplished within the sector in terms of maintaining and developing a body of best practice and a considerable degree of standardization internationally. With the advent of the IASC Nutrition Cluster, and earlier ongoing efforts to improve quality such as the Sphere and FANTA projects, etc., and renewed commitments to nutrition in emergencies by UN agencies, there is now greater consensus, awareness, and application of tried and tested tools and approaches.

A crucial and continuing challenge remains the lack of documented evidence on impact and outcomes. This knowledge gap is a big challenge linked to every type of intervention, and a major hindrance to further advances. Improved documentary evidence about what works will serve to strengthen this sector for the future.

While acute malnutrition among children was widely recognized as the most common characteristic of complex emergencies in the past, other forms of malnutrition (stunting, underweight, and MDDs) and nutritional risk among other age groups are increasingly recognized as important. Consequently, analytical frameworks need to broaden their concept of nutritional vulnerability and risk to incorporate all three groups of underlying causes that require both qualitative studies as well as epidemiological data. Furthermore, as a result of the multi-causal nature of malnutrition, direct nutrition interventions as described in this chapter should rarely be implemented in isolation of integrated health and food security programs.

The design and delivery of food and nutrition interventions in complex emergencies are frequently constrained by the characteristic breakdown of local infrastructure, including government, civil society, and community networks. Humanitarian agencies also face difficulties in identifying and accessing the most vulnerable groups, particularly in contexts where vulnerability is influenced by a complex number of determinants, not just physiological. Poor security and lack of access to the affected populations, rapidly changing situations, and a lack of timely and representative information for appropriate decision-making, are all critical challenges for designing appropriate nutrition responses.

The promotion and support to national capacity and to developing professional leadership in the countries directly affected by crises, within both the technical and policy domains, will be critical toward achieving more effective responses in future nutritional crises.

Acknowledgment

With acknowledgment of contributions by Emily Mates, Concern Worldwide Ethiopia and Lena Nguyen, Tufts University.

Suggestions for Further Reading

Field Exchange, Emergency Nutrition Network, http://www.ennonline.net/.
One Response, The Global Nutrition Cluster. http://oneresponse.info/GlobalClusters/Nutrition/Pages/default.aspx.
SCN NICS (2010) *Nutrition Information in Crisis Situations*. United Nations System Sub-Committee on Nutrition, Geneva.

References

ACF (2007) *Implementing Cash Based Interventions: a Guideline for Aid Workers*. Action Contre la Faim, Paris.

Bahwere, P., Sadler, K., and Collins, S. (2009) Acceptability and effectiveness of chickpea sesame-based ready-to-use therapeutic food in malnourished HIV-positive adults. *Patient Prefer Adherence* **3**, 67–75.

Bailey, S. and Pavanello, S. (2009) Untangling early recovery. *HPG Policy Brief*. Humanitarian Policy Group, London.

Bangladesh Breastfeeding Foundation (2007) Breastfeeding protects children in emergencies. Joint statement by BFF, UNICEF and WHO. http://www.ennonline.net/pool/files/ife/bangladesh-infant-feeding-in-emergencies-statement-dec-07.pdf.

Bekele, G. and Tsehay, A. (2008) Livelihoods-based drought response in Ethiopia: Impact Assessment of Livestock Feed

Supplementation. Pastoralist Livelihoods Initiative. Addis Ababa: Feinstein International Center, Tufts University, and Save the Children USA.

Bezanson, K. and Isenman, P. (2010) Policy brief. Scaling up nutrition: a framework for action. *Food Nutr Bull* **31,** 178–186.

Bhutta, Z.A., Ahmed, T., Black, R.E., *et al.*, 2008. What works? Interventions for maternal and child undernutrition and survival. *Lancet* **371,** 417–440.

Bilukha, O. (2008) Old and new cluster designs in emergency field surveys: in search of a one-fits all solution. *Emerg Themes Epidemiol* **5,** 7.

Black, R., Allen, L., Bhutta, Z., *et al.* (2008) Maternal and child undernutrition: global and regional exposures and health consequences. *Lancet* **371,** 243–260.

Borrel, A. and Salama, P. (1999) Public nutrition from an approach to a discipline: Concern's nutrition case studies in complex emergencies. *Disasters* **23,** 326–342.

Borrel, A., Taylor, A., McGrath, M., *et al.* (2001) From policy to practice: challenges in infant feeding in emergencies during the Balkan crisis. *Disasters* **25,** 149–163.

Briend, A. and Prinzo, Z.W. (2009) Dietary management of moderate malnutrition: time for a change. *Food Nutr Bull* **30,** S265–266.

Bryce, J., Coitinho, D., Darnton-Hill, I., *et al.* (2008) Maternal and child undernutrition: effective action at national level *Lancet* **371,** 510–526.

Busolo, D. (2002) Assessment of adults and older people in emergencies: approaches, issues and priorities. *USAID SMART Workshop.* HelpAge International, Washington, DC.

Cairns, L., Woodruff, B., Myatt, M., *et al.* (2009) Cross-sectional survey methods to assess retrospectively mortality in humanitarian emergencies. *Disasters* **33,** 503–521.

Catley, A. (2008) Livelihoods, Drought and Pastoralism: the Costs of Late Response. Feinstein International Center of Tufts University, Addis Ababa.

Catley, A., Abebe, D., Admassu, B., *et al.* (2009) Impact of drought-related vaccination on livestock mortality in pastoralist areas of Ethiopia. *Disasters* **33,** 665–685.

CE DAT (2010) CE DAT Complex Emergency Database [online]. Center for Research and the Epidemiology of Disasters (CRED). Available from http://www.cedat.be/.

Chaparro, C. and Dewey, K. (2009) Use of lipid-based nutrient supplements (LNS) to improve the nutrient adequacy of general food distribution rations for vulnerable sub-groups in emergency settings. FANTA-2, Washington, DC.

Chaparro, C.M. and Dewey, K.G. (2010) Use of lipid-based nutrient supplements (LNS) to improve the nutrient adequacy of general food distribution rations for vulnerable sub-groups in emergency settings. *Matern Child Nutr* **6**(Suppl 1), 1–69.

Checchi, F., Gayer, M., Grais, R., *et al.* (2007) Public health in crisis-affected populations. A practical guide for decision-makers. *HPG Report No. 61.* Humanitarian Policy Group, Overseas Development Institute, London.

Cheung, E., Mutahar, R., Assefa, F., *et al.* (2003) An epidemic of scurvy in Afghanistan: assessment and response *Food Nutr Bull* **24,** 247–255.

Coates, J., Rogers, B., Maxwell, D., *et al.* (2007) Dietary diversity measures in emergencies. Report submitted to The Strengthening Emergency Needs Assessment Capacity (SENAC) Project. World Food Programme, Rome.

Collins, S. (2001) Changing the way we address severe malnutrition during famine. *Lancet* **358,** 498–501.

Collins, S. and Myatt, M. (2000) Short-term prognosis in severe adult and adolescent malnutrition during famine. *JAMA* **284,** 621–626.

Collins, S., Dent, N., Binns, P., *et al.* (2006a) Management of severe acute malnutrition in children. *Lancet* **368,** 1992–2000.

Collins, S., Myatt, M., and Golden, B. (1998) The dietary treatment of severe malnutrition in adults. *Am J Clin Nutr* **68,** 193–199.

Collins, S., Sadler, K., Dent, N., *et al.* (2006b) Key issues in the success of community-based management of severe malnutrition. *Food Nutr.Bull* **27,** S49–S82.

Coutsoudis, A., Coovadia, H., and King, J. (2009) The breastmilk brand: promotion of child survival in the face of formula-milk marketing. *Lancet* **374,** 423–425.

Creti, P. and Jaspars, S. (2006) *Cash-Transfer Programming in Emergencies: a Practical Guide.* Oxfam, Oxford.

de Onis, M., Garza, C., Onyango, A., *et al.* (2007a) Comparison of the WHO child growth standards and the CDC 2000 growth charts. *J Nutr* **137,** 144–148.

de Onis, M., Onyango, A.W., Borghi, E., *et al.* (2007b) Development of a WHO growth reference for school-aged children and adolescents. *Bull World Health Organ* **85,** 660–667.

de Pee, S. and Bloem, M.W. (2009) Current and potential role of specially formulated foods and food supplements for preventing malnutrition among 6- to 23-month-old children and for treating moderate malnutrition among 6- to 59-month-old children. *Food Nutr Bull* **30,** S434–463.

de Pee, S., Moench-Pfanner, R., Martini, E., *et al.* (2007) Home fortification in emergency response and transition programming: experiences in Aceh and Nias, Indonesia. *Food Nutr Bull* **24,** 247–255.

de Waal, A. and Whiteside, A. (2003) New variant famine: AIDS and food crisis in Southern Africa. *Lancet* **362,** 1234–1237.

Defourny, I., Minetti, A., Harczi, G., *et al.* (2009) A large-scale distribution of milk-based fortified spreads: evidence for a new approach in regions with high burden of acute malnutrition. *PLos One* **4,** e5455.

DFID (2010) *The Neglected Crisis of Undernutrition.* DFID's strategy. http://www.parliament.uk/deposits/depositedpapers/2010/DEP2010-0651.pdf.

Diop, E., Dossou, N., Ndour, M., *et al.* (2003) Comparison of the efficacy of a solid ready-to-use food and a liquid, milk-based diet for the rehabilitation of severely malnourished children: a randomized tria. *Am J Clin Nutr* **78**, 302–307.

Dye, T.D. (2007) Contemporary prevalence and prevention of micronutrient deficiencies in refugee settings worldwide. *J Refugee Studies* **20**, 108–119.

EM-DAT (2009) *Natural Disaster Trends 1975–2009*. Université Catholique de Louvain Brussels. www.emdat.be.

Eriksson, A. (2007) Special report: silent disasters. *Nursing Health Sci* **9**, 243–245.

FANTA/WFP (2007). *Food Assistance Programming in the Context of HIV*. FANTA/AED, Washington, DC.

FAO (1996) Report on the World Food Summit, 13–17 November 1996. WFS 96/REP. http://www.fao.org/righttofood/kc/downloads/vl/en/details/214905.htm.

Fawzi, W., Msamanga, G., Spiegelman, D., *et al.* (2005) Studies of vitamins and minerals and HIV transmission and disease progression. *J Nutr* **135**, 938–944.

Fergusson, P. (2009) Improving survival of children with severe acute malnutrition in HIV-prevalent settings. *Int Health* **1**, 10–16.

Fleige, L.E., Moore, W.R., Garlick, P.J., *et al.* (2010) Recommendations for optimization of fortified and blended food aid products from the United States. *Nutr Rev* **68**, 290–315.

Gronewold, N. (2010) Flood disaster may require largest aid effort in modern history. *New York Times* August 20.

Guerrero, S., Myatt, M., and Collins, S. (2010) Determinants of coverage in community-based therapeutic care programs: towards a joint quantitative and qualitative analysis. *Disasters* **34**, 571–585.

HAP (2010) The 2010 HAP Standard in Accountability and Quality Management. Humanitarian Accountability Partnership, Geneva. http://www.hapinternational.org/pool/files/2010-hap-standard-in-accountability.pdf.

Harvey, P. (2007) Cash-based responses in emergencies. HPG Report No. 24. Humanitarian Policy Group, Overseas Development Institute, London.

Harvey, P., Haver, K., Hoffman, J., *et al.* (2010a) Delivering Money: Cash Transfer Mechanisms in Emergencies. Cash Learning Partnership, London.

Harvey, P., Proudlock, K., Clay, E., *et al.* (2010b) Food aid and food assistance in emergency and transitional contexts: a review of current thinking. Humanitarian Policy Group, London.

Health and Nutrition Tracking Service (2009) Main Conclusions of the First Expert Reference Group (ERG) Meeting: Meeting Minutes. World Health Organization, Geneva.

Heikens, G., Amadi, B., Manary, M., *et al.* (2008) Nutrition interventions need improved operational capacity. *Lancet* **371**, 181–182.

HelpAge International (2009) The situation of older people in cyclone-affected Myanmar: nine months after the disaster. HelpAge International, London.

Horton, S., Alderman, H., and Rivera, J. (2008) *Hunger and Malnutrition*. Copenhagen Consensus Center, Copenhagen.

IASC (2002) *Growing the Sheltering Tree: Protecting Rights Through Humanitarian Aciton*. IASC, Geneva.

IASC Global Nutrition Cluster (2007) *Capacity Development for Nutrition in Emergencies – An IASC Nutrition Cluster Strategy*. IASC Global Nutrition Cluster, Rome.

IASC Global Nutrition Cluster (2010) *Nutrition Cluster Overview*. http://oneresponse.info/globalclusters/nutrition/Pages/default.aspx.

Islamic Republic of Afghanistan MOPH (2008) National Infant and Young Child Feeding Policy 2009–2013. Ministry of Public Health, Kabul.

Ivers, L., Cullen, K., Freedberg, K., *et al.* (2009) HIV/AIDS, undernutrition, and food insecurity. *Clin Infect Dis* **49**, 1096–1102.

Jaspars, S. (2006) From food crisis to fair trade: livelihoods analysis, protection and support in emergencies. *ENN Special Supplement Series*. Emergency Nutrition Network, Oxford.

Jenkins, A.L., Tavengwa, N.V., Chasekwa, B., *et al.* (2011) Addressing social barriers and closing the gender knowledge gap: exposure to road shows is associated with more knowledge and more positive beliefs, attitudes and social norms regarding exclusive breastfeeding in rural Zimbabwe. *Matern Child Nutr* PMID 21972843.

Johnecheck, W. and Holland, D. (2007) Nutritional status in postconflict Afghanistan: evidence from the National Surveillance System Pilot and National Risk and Vulnerability Assessment. *Food Nutr Bull* **28**, 3–17.

Kaiser, R., Woodruff, B., Bilukha, O., *et al.* (2006) Using design effects from previous cluster surveys to guide sample size calculation in emergency settings. *Disasters* **30**, 199–211.

Kelly, M. (1993) Infant feeding in emergencies. *Disasters* **17**, 110–121.

Kerac, M., McGrath, M., and Seal, A. (2010) *Management of Acute Malnutrition in Infants (MAMI) Project*. Technical Review, Centre for International Health and Development and the Emergency Nutrition Network, University College London, London

Khristof, N.D. (2010) A famine looms in Niger. *New York Times* August 9.

Leyenaar, J. (2004) Human immuno-deficiency virus and infant feeding in complex humanitarian emergencies: priorities and policy considerations. *Disasters* **28**, 1–15.

Malfait, P., Moren, A., Dillon, J., *et al.* (1993) An outbreak of pellagra related to changes in dietary niacin among Mozambican refugees in Malawi. *Int J Epidemiol* **22**, 504–511.

Matilsky, D.K., Maleta, K., Castleman, T., et al. (2009) Supplementary feeding with fortified spreads results in higher recovery rates than with a corn/soy blend in moderately wasted children. J Nutr 139, 773–778.

Maxwell, D., Webb, P., Coates, J., et al. (2010) Fit for purpose? Rethinking food security responses in protracted humanitarian crises. Food Policy 35, 91–97.

Myatt, M. (2009) Guidelines for a sentinel-site surveillance system for monitoring growth, dietary diversity, and meal frequency in children aged between six and twenty-four months using small cohorts. Draft v 0.3.

Myatt, M., Duffield, A., Seal, A., et al. (2009) The effect of body shape on weight-for-height and mid-upper arm circumference based case definitions of acute malnutrition in Ethiopian children. Ann Hum Biol 36, 5–20.

Nackers, F., Broillet, F., Oumarou, D., et al. (2010) Effectiveness of ready-to-use therapeutic food compared to a corn/soy-blend-based pre-mix for the treatment of childhood moderate acute malnutrition in Niger J Trop Pediatr 56, 407–413.

Navarro-Colorado, C., Mason, F., and Shoham, J. (2008) Measuring the effectiveness of Supplementary Feeding Programs in emergencies. Network Paper 63. Humanitarian Policy Network, Overseas Development Institute, London.

NutritionWorks (2010) Pilot project to strengthen emergency nutrition training in preservice and in-service training courses. NutritionWorks/ENN, Kenya.

Pieterse, S. and Ismail, S. (2003) Nutritional risk factors for older refugees. Disasters 27, 16–36.

Sadler, K. and Catley, A. (2009) Milk matters: the role and value of milk in the diets of Somali pastoralist children in Liben and Shinile, Ethiopia. Feinstein International Center of Tufts University, Addis Ababa.

Sadler, K., Kerven, C., Calo, M., et al. (2009) Milk matters: a literature review of pastoralist nutrition and programming responses. Feinstein International Center, Medford, MA.

Sadler, K., Myatt, M., Feleke, T., et al. (2007) A comparison of the programme coverage of two therapeutic feeding interventions implemented in neighbouring districts of Malawi. Public Health Nutr 10, 907–913.

Salama, P. and Roberts, L. (2005) Evidence-based interventions in complex emergencies. Lancet 365, 1848.

Salama, P., Assefa, F., Talley, L., et al. (2001) Malnutrition, measles, mortality, and the humanitarian response during a famine in Ethiopia. JAMA 286, 563–571.

Samuels, F. (2009) HIV and emergencies: one size does not fit all. ODI Briefing Papers 50. Overseas Development Institute, London.

SCF UK (2004) Emergency Nutrition Assessment: Guidelines for Field Workers. Save the Children UK, London.

Schaetzel, T. and Nyaku, A. (2010) The Case for Preventing Malnutrition through Improved Infant Feeding and Management of Childhood Illness: Infant and Young Child Nutrition Project. http://www.path.org/files/IYCN_the_case_prev_mal.pdf.

Schipper, L. and Pelling, M. (2006) Disaster risk, climate change and international development: scope for, and challenges to, integration. Disasters 30, 19–38.

SCN (2009) Fact sheet on the implementation of 2006 WHO Child Growth Standards for emergency nutrition programs for children aged 6–59 months. IASC Global Nutrition Cluster and Standing Committee on Nutrition (SCN) Task Force on Assessment, Monitoring, and Evaluation, Washington, DC.

SCN NICS (2010) Nutrition Information in Crisis Situations. United Nations System Sub-Committee on Nutrition. Geneva.

Seal, A. and Kerac, M. (2007) Operational implications of using 2006 World Health Organization growth standards in nutrition programs: secondary data analysis. BMJ 334, 733.

Seal, A. and Prudhon, C. (2007) Assessing micronutrient deficiencies in emergencies: current practice and future directions. Nutrition Information in Crisis Situations. UN Standing Committee on Nutrition, Geneva.

Seal, A., Kafwembe, E., Kassim, I.A., et al. (2008) Maize meal fortification is associated with improved vitamin A and iron status in adolescents and reduced childhood anaemia in a food aid-dependent refugee population. Public Health Nutr 11, 720–728.

Seal, A., Taylor, A., and Gostelow, L. (2001) Review of policies and guidelines on infant feeding in emergencies: common ground and gaps. Disasters 25, 136–148.

Seal, A.J., Creeke, P.I., Dibari,F., et al. (2007) Low and deficient niacin status and pellagra are endemic in postwar Angola. Am J Clin Nutr 85, 218–224.

Seal, A.J., Creeke, P.I., Mirghani, Z., et al. (2005) Iron and vitamin A deficiency in long-term African refugees. J Nutr 135, 808–813.

Seaman, J., Clark, P., Boudreau, T., et al. (2000) The Household Economy Approach: A Resource Manual for Practitioners. Save the Children, London.

Sphere Project (2004) Humanitarian Charter and Minimum Standards in Disaster Response. Sphere Project, Geneva.

Sphere Project (2011) Humanitarian Charter and Minimum Standards in Humanitarian Response, 2011 Edition. Sphere Project, Geneva.

Tolvanen, M. and Kumar, S. (2003) Policy on the use of infant formula in Iraq. Nutrition Co-ordination Sector for Iraq, Baghdad.

UN ESC/ECA (2009) The status of food security in Africa. United Nations Economic and Security Council. Economic

Commission for Africa. Committee on Food Security and Sustainable Development Sixth Session. E/ECA/CFSSD/6/4.

UNHCR, UNICEF, WFP, et al. (2002) *Food and Nutrition Needs in Emergencies*. United Nations High Commissioner for Refugees, United Nations Children's Fund, World Food Programme, and World Health Organization, Geneva.

UNICEF (1990) *Strategy for Improved Nutrition of Children and Women in Developing Countries*. UNICEF, New York

UNICEF (2010) *Core Commitments for Children in Humanitarian Action*. UNICEF, New York.

Valid International/Concern Worldwide (2006) *Community-based Therapeutic Care (CTC): A Field Manual*. Valid International/Concern Worldwide, Oxford.

van den Briel, T., Cheung, E., Zewari, J., et al. (2006) Fortifying food in the field to boost nutrition: case studies from Afghanistan, Angola and Zambia. Occasional Paper 16. World Food Programme.

Vespa, J. and Watson, F. (1995) Who is nutritionally vulnerable in Bosnia-Hercegovina? *BMJ* **311**, 652–654.

Victora, C., Adair, L., Fall, C., et al. (2008) Maternal and child undernutrition: consequences for adult health and human capital. *Lancet* **371**, 340–357.

Webb, P. (2009)How nutrition is framed in the Consolidated Appeals Process (CAP): a review of 1992 to 2009. Report Prepared for the Inter Agency Standing Committee's Global Cluster on Nutrition. http://oneresponse.info/GlobalClusters/Nutrition/Documents/CAP%20review%20FINAL%20%28Webb%20%20May%207%202009%29.pdf.

Webb, P., Darnton-Hill, I., Harvey, P.W.J., et al. (2005) Micronutrient deficiencies and gender: social and economic costs. *Am J Clin Nutr* **81**, 1198S–1205S.

Wells, J. (2005) Protecting and assisting older people in emergencies. Network Paper 53. Humanitarian Policy Network, Overseas Development Institute, London.

WFP (2002) *Emergency Field Operations Pocketbook*. World Food Programme, Rome.

WFP (2004) *Micronutrient Fortification: WFP Experiences and Ways Forward. Policy Issues*. WFP, Rome.

WFP (2008a) *Food Assistance in the Context of HIV: Ration Design Guide*. WFP, Rome.

WFP (2008b) *Vouchers and Cash Transfers as Food Assistance Instruments: Opportunities and Challenges*. WFP, Rome.

WFP/VAM (2005) *Emergency Food Security Assessment Handbook*, 2nd Edn. WFP/VAM, Rome.

WHO (1995) Maternal anthropometry and pregnancy outcomes. A WHO Collaborative Study. *Bulletin WHO* **73**(Suppl).

WHO (1999) *Management of Severe Malnutrition, A Manual for Physicians and Other Senior Health Workers*, World Health Organization, Geneva.

WHO (2000) *The Management of Nutrition in Major Emergencies*. World Health Organization, United Nations High Commissioner for Refugees, International Federation of Red Cross and Red Crescent Societies, World Food Programme, Geneva.

WHO (2002) *Infant And Young Child Nutrition: Global Strategy on Infant and Young Child Feeding*. 55th World Health Assembly. WHO, Geneva.

WHO (2009) *Rapid Advice: HIV and Infant Feeding – Revised Principles and Recommendations*. WHO, Geneva.

WHO and UNICEF (2009) WHO child growth standards and the identifications of severe acute malnutrition in infants and children: a joint statement by the World Health Organization and the United Nations Children's Fund. WHO and UNICEF, Geneva.

WHO, WFP, and UNICEF (2007) Preventing and controlling micronutrient deficiencies in populations affected by an emergency: joint statement by the World Health Organization, the World Food Programme and the United Nations Children's Fund. World Health Organization, Geneva.

WHO/UNHCR (1999a) *Pellagra and Its Prevention and Control in Emergencies*. World Health Organization, Geneva.

WHO/UNHCR (1999b) *Thiamine Deficiency and Its Prevention and Control in Major Emergencies*. World Health Organization, Geneva.

WHO/WFP/UN SCN/UNICEF (2007) Community-based management of severe acute malnutrition: a joint statement by the World Health Organization, the World Food Program, the United Nations Standing Committee on Nutrition and the United Nations Children's Fund. World Health Organization, Geneva.

World Bank (2006) *Repositioning Nutrition as Central to Development: A Strategy for Large-Scale Action*. World Bank, Washington, DC.

World Bank (2007) *HIV/AIDs, Nutrition, and Food Security: What Can We Do? A Synthesis of International Guidance*. World Bank, Washington, DC.

Young, H. (2007) Looking beyond food aid to livelihoods, protection and partnerships: strategies for WFP in the Darfur states. *Disasters* **31**(Suppl 1), S40–56.

Young, H. and Jaspars, S. (2006) *The Meaning and Measurement of Acute Malnutrition in Emergencies: a Primer for Decision-Makers*. Humanitarian Policy Network, Overseas Development Institute, London.

Young, H. and Jaspars, S. (2009) Review of Nutrition and Mortality Indicators for the Integrated Food Security Phase Classification (IPC) Reference Levels and Decision-Making. A study commissioned by the SCN Task Force on Assessment, Monitoring and Evaluation, and the Integrated Food Security Phase Classification (IPC) Global Partners, Rome. http://www.

ipcinfo.org/attachments/IPC_NutMortalityIndicatorsReview.
pdf.

Young, H. and Maxwell, D. (2009) *Targeting and Distribution: Darfur Case-Study*. Feinstein International Center of Tufts University, Medford, MA.

Young, H., Borrel, A., Holland, D., *et al.* (2004a) Public nutrition in complex emergencies. *Lancet* **365,** 1899.

Young, H., Jaspars, S., Brown, R., *et al.* (2001) Food-security assessments in emergencies: a livelihoods approach. Humanitarian Policy Network, Overseas Development Institute, London.

Young, H., Taylor, A., Way, S.-A., *et al.* (2004b) Linking rights and standards: the process of developing "rights-based" minimum standards on food security, nutrition and food aid. *Disasters* **28,** 142–159.

Zlotkin, S.H., Schauer, C., Christofides, A., *et al.* (2005) Micronutrient sprinkles to control childhood anaemia. *PLoS Med* **2,** e1.

70

FOODBORNE INFECTIONS AND FOOD SAFETY

ROBERT V. TAUXE[1], MD, MPH AND MARGUERITE A. NEILL[2], MD

[1]National Center for Emerging and Zoonotic Infectious Diseases, Atlanta, Georgia, USA
[2]Brown University, Providence, Rhode Island, USA

Summary

Our food supply comes from millions of farms around the world, is processed in many thousands of packing sheds, slaughter plants, and canneries, and is prepared in millions of kitchens. It is a dynamic system, as changing foods, food sources, cuisines, and processing technologies lead to new food safety challenges. Along the way, the foods and food ingredients can be contaminated with a variety of pathogens, which can harm the final consumer. Infections caused by eating contaminated foods are common. They have been estimated to cause 48 million illnesses each year in the United States, with 128000 hospitalizations and 3000 deaths. A wide array of pathogens can be foodborne, which can cause a variety of syndromes. Some have reservoirs in the animals we eat, and contaminate the foods that are made from those animals. Others are present in the environment, and can contaminate foods in a number of ways. Still others have a human reservoir, and can contaminate food indirectly through sewage or by direct contact with an infected person. Though some level of contamination may be inevitable, much foodborne illness can be prevented. Preventing foodborne disease depends on measures taken from farm to table, which provide a series of hurdles that lower the risk. Taking care at each step of the food chain to prevent contamination can make food safer. For the riskiest foods and pathogens, definitive pathogen reduction steps such as heat-process canning and pasteurization have long been used to prevent serious harm. The many members of the food industry, the regulators and public health authorities, and the consumers themselves all have important roles to play in making food safer.

Introduction

Foodborne diseases caused by foods contaminated with microbes and their toxins have long complicated the search for a safe and nourishing food supply. For most of these microbes, the human is an accidental host, made ill by the chance presence of microbes that circulate in the animals we eat, or in the environments in which we raise and harvest our foods. For some microbes, such as those that cause typhoid fever, cholera, and bacillary dysentery, we humans are a primary reservoir, and contaminated food and water have been primary routes by which they move

Present Knowledge in Nutrition, Tenth Edition. Edited by John W. Erdman Jr, Ian A. Macdonald and Steven H. Zeisel.
© 2012 International Life Sciences Institute. Published 2012 by John Wiley & Sons, Inc.

from one host to the next. In general, the transmission of foodborne organisms has probably intensified over the centuries as humans have crowded together in cities, as animal husbandry has intensified, and as the distance from farm to plate has lengthened. The safety of foods has also changed significantly. Early in the 20th century, efforts to improve urban drinking water and sewage treatment systems largely controlled typhoid fever and cholera, and more recent disease-control efforts on farms and routine pasteurization have largely eliminated trichinosis from pork, and brucellosis and bovine tuberculosis transmitted through milk, and better slaughter practices have decreased the frequency of *E. coli* O157 infections. We are, however, left with a substantial burden of infections that still contaminate the foods we eat. The globalization of food supplies, the changing food habits of consumers and the mutation of microbes mean that newer challenges have emerged even as some of the longstanding ones have been controlled. This review summarizes the clinical and public-health perspective on foodborne diseases.

The concept that food can cause human illness dates back to antiquity. The germ theory of disease and, since the late 1800s, the microbiological identification of predominantly bacterial agents, laid the groundwork for the concept that food could be made safer by interventions limiting pathogen growth and survival. Improved water sanitation, better animal husbandry practices, the pasteurization of milk, and the widespread use of refrigeration have contributed to the steep decline in foodborne illnesses such as bovine tuberculosis, dysentery, and typhoid fever during the 20th century in the United States and other industrialized nations (CDC, 1999; Tauxe and Esteban, 2006) (Figure 70.1).

On the heels of these achievements, however, has come a very different set of issues in food safety during the last three decades. A far broader array of agents have come to be recognized as significant contributors to foodborne disease, including newly emergent bacterial pathogens and previously undescribed viruses and parasites. Several non-diarrheal human illnesses have been shown to have an infectious etiology that is foodborne in origin. In the natural evolution of analyses of food safety, their conceptual framework has become more dynamic, and at present the aim of such assessments is to define acceptable levels of risk.

This chapter will focus on newer developments in foodborne illness, including the expanded spectrum of human disease, recently described causative agents, changes in the

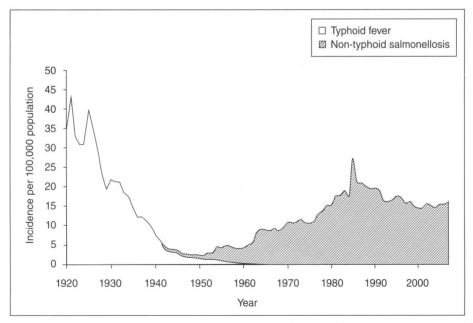

FIG. 70.1 The fall and rise of reported *Salmonella* infections, due to *Salmonella* serotype Typhi (typhoid fever) and non-typhoidal *Salmonella* serotypes (salmonellosis), United States, 1920–2007. Nationally reportable disease surveillance (Bureau of the Census, 1976; CDC, 2009a). Reproduced from Centers for Disease Control and Prevention (2009a), public domain.

TABLE 70.1 Classification of etiologic agents of foodborne disease

Infectious
  Bacteria
  Viruses
  Parasites
  Prions
Non-infectious
  Non-bacterial toxins
  Chemicals
  Poisonous mushrooms
  Heavy metals

epidemiology of foodborne disease, and current progress in prevention. It is beyond the scope of this chapter to include a comprehensive description of clinical manifestations, diagnosis, and treatment, and the reader is referred elsewhere (Butterton and Calderwood, 2008; Sodha *et al.*, 2010).

Causative Agents

Diverse etiologic agents are capable of causing diarrhea or other forms of foodborne disease in humans (Table 70.1). Infectious agents include bacteria, viruses, and parasites, each with its own ecological niche in nature. These agents may be normal inhabitants of animal gastrointestinal tracts, soil, or water ecosystems. For some the primary host is human, and for many others the reservoir is in other animals. Their pathogenic properties for humans may often be the accidental result of evolutionary changes conferring selective survival advantages in the host animal or environment.

Prions (proteinaceous infectious particles) are novel transmissible agents that do not contain any nucleic acids. Prions cause a group of diseases known as the transmissible spongiform encephalopathies (TSEs); in animals TSEs can be transmitted following oral inoculation with a species-specific prion protein. An epidemic in Great Britain of bovine spongiform encephalopathy (BSE, "mad cow disease") has been followed by an increase in humans of a fatal degenerative neurological disease, new variant Creutzfeld-Jacob disease (nvCJD), most probably related to consumption of BSE-contaminated foods.

In addition to infectious microorganisms, other entities are capable of causing foodborne disease. Non-bacterial toxins produced by dinoflagellates can cause paralytic shellfish poisoning and ciguatera. Chemical causes of foodborne illness include histamine, the causative agent of scombroid fish poisoning. Serious clinical illness can result from consumption of poisonous mushrooms, and clinical manifestations range from delirium to gastroenteritis with hepatorenal failure. Species of mushrooms that produce amatoxins and phallotoxins are causes of the latter form of illness. Heavy metals, including copper, zinc, tin, and cadmium, have caused acute nausea, vomiting, and abdominal cramps within 1 hour of consuming contaminated food.

Unfortunately, there is no 1:1 correspondence of an etiologic agent to a specific clinical scenario, and there can be considerable overlap among the categories in considering the etiologies of a patient's illness. The usefulness of this classification is to remind clinicians of all causes of a clinical illness with a possible foodborne etiology in order to ensure that appropriate questions are asked of the patient to ascertain whether significant exposures have occurred.

Types of Illness

Diarrhea and vomiting are most often considered the main manifestations of foodborne disease, but it is now recognized that a much wider range of human illness can be seen. Foodborne disease can present as an acute illness whose main manifestation is vomiting, diarrhea, sepsis, jaundice, or paralysis, or as a chronic illness with persistent diarrhea, neurological findings, or chronic anemia (Table 70.2). Common among these different forms of illness is an initial step in pathogenesis that takes place at the mucosal surface of the gastrointestinal tract. This may range from adherence and colonization by a bacterial pathogen, to viral replication within the cells that form the wall of the intestine, to absorption of a non-bacterial toxin.

The features of acute enteric illness following ingestion of contaminated food may be quite varied. Clues to the diagnosis are to discern the types of symptom and their relative predominance in the context of the illness as well as their intensity. Patients who experience nausea and vomiting with onset within 1–6 hours of a meal have likely ingested foods contaminated with a preformed toxin from either *Staphylococcus aureus* or *Bacillus cereus*. The vomiting is abrupt in onset and is intense, lasting for a few hours and resolving within a day with no specific therapy. Diarrhea is a less common component. Staphylococcal food poisoning was a major form of foodborne disease recognized during the middle of the 20th century.

TABLE 70.2 Clinical spectrum of illness in foodborne disease and examples of common causative agents

Type of Illness	Examples of Causative Agents
Acute enteric illness	
Nausea and vomiting within 6 hours	*Staphylococcus aureus, Bacillus cereus*
Vomiting and diarrhea	Rotavirus, norovirus
Diarrhea and abdominal cramping	ETEC, EPEC, *Clostridium perfringens*
Diarrhea and fever	Non-typhoidal Salmonellae, Vibrio
Bloody diarrhea	*Escherichia coli* 0157:H7, *Campylobacter jejuni, Shigella* spp *Vibrio parahemolyticus*
Enteric fever	*Salmonella* Typhi, *Brucella*
Acute sepsis	*V. vulnificus*
Acute hepatitis	Hepatitis A virus
Acute pseudoappendicitis	*Yersinia enterocolitica, Y. pyseudotuberculosis*
Acute neurologic illness	
Paralysis	Botulism, Paralytic shellfish poisoning, Guillain-Barré syndrome
Paresthesias	Scombroid, ciguatera
Meningitis	*Listeria monocytogenes*
Encephalitis	*Cronobacter sakazakii*
Chronic enteric illness	
Diarrhea >3 weeks	*Giardia, Crypstosporidium, Cyclospora*, Brainerd diarrheal syndrome
Chronic neurologic illness	
Seizures (neurocysticercosis)	*Taenia solium*
Congenital abnormalities	*Toxoplasma gondii*
Encephalitis (AIDS patients)	*T. gondii*
Chronic anemia	Hookworm
Vitamin B$_{12}$ deficiency	*Diphyllobothrium latum*

An illness consisting of vomiting and diarrhea without abdominal cramping is usually due to norovirus or rotavirus. Rotavirus occurs commonly in young children but may affect adults as well. Community-wide outbreaks of norovirus infections have been a particular challenge in wintertime.

Watery diarrhea accompanied by abdominal cramping, typically but not invariably without fever, may be due to specific types of diarrheagenic *Escherichia coli* (Nataro and Kaper, 1998) [enterotoxigenic *E. coli* (ETEC), enteropath-

ogenic *E. coli* (EPEC) or *Clostridium perfringens*]. ETEC are a major cause of diarrhea worldwide and are the most frequently implicated pathogen in travelers' diarrhea. EPEC were originally described as causative agents of nursery outbreaks in the 1940s and are relatively uncommon in the developed world today. In the developing world, they are a significant cause of diarrhea in infants, particularly at the time of weaning.

Fever accompanying abdominal cramps and diarrhea suggests an inflammatory or invasive diarrhea. When the diarrhea is non-bloody, in the developed world this is most commonly associated with the non-typhoidal salmonellae (Goldberg and Rubin, 1988). Bloody diarrhea accompanied by moderately severe cramping and/or abdominal pain indicates a serious infection, and should be treated as a medical emergency. In the developed world, causative agents include *Campylobacter jejuni* (Allos and Blaser, 1995) and *E. coli* O157:H7 (Tarr *et al.*, 2005). *Vibrio parahemolyticus* infection is common in Japan and along coasts of the United States (Daniels *et al.*, 2000). In the developing world, other infectious causes of bloody diarrhea include *Shigella flexneri* and *Shigella dysenteriae*, and *Entamoeba histolytica*.

Enteric fever is the designation for an illness characterized by fever for several days with headache, malaise, anemia, and splenomegaly. When the causative agent is *Salmonella* serotype Typhi, the illness is referred to as typhoid fever. *Brucella* can cause a similar syndrome. Typhoid fever is extremely uncommon in the United States today, but remains common in the developing world, and most currently reported cases are acquired through overseas travel. Some non-typhoidal *Salmonella* serotypes can cause a similar illness in immunocompromised persons (Levine *et al.*, 1991).

Sepsis (fever, chills, hypotension) is a very infrequent form of foodborne disease. A specific association exists with sepsis from *Vibrio vulnificus* infection in persons with underlying liver disease, particularly alcoholic cirrhosis.

Jaundice with nausea and anorexia can be the manifestation of acute infectious hepatitis. As a foodborne illness, this may be due to hepatitis A virus infection. The overall incidence of hepatitis A in the developed world is considerably lower than that in the developing world or in countries whose economies are in transition, and is decreasing rapidly where immunization is routine (CDC, 2009a). Infection early in childhood is often asymptomatic or unaccompanied by jaundice, and confers life-long immunity. Infection in adulthood is more frequently clinically symptomatic and is usually more serious. Hepatitis A is the most common travel-related illness that is vaccine preventable.

Focal abdominal pain and fever, mimicking appendicitis, is often how infections with *Yersinia enterocolitica* or *Y. pseudotuberculosis* present; though rare in the United States, they have been more commonly described in Europe (Ostroff *et al.*, 1992; Nuorti *et al.*, 2003; Long *et al.*, 2010).

A variety of acute neurological illnesses may be manifestations of a foodborne infection. Muscle weakness leading to frank paralysis may be due to botulism or paralytic shellfish poisoning (Underman and Leedom, 1993); Guillain-Barré syndrome has a similar presentation. This latter entity is now recognized in many cases as being a postinfectious complication of antecedent *Campylobacter jejuni* infection (Mishu *et al.*, 1993). Paresthesias (a tingling sensation in the skin) can occur in scombroid poisoning (histamine fish poisoning). Paresthesias occurring several hours after fish consumption and accompanied by reversal of hot and cold sensation in the mouth, and abdominal cramps, vomiting, and diarrhea is suggestive of ciguatera (Underman and Leedom, 1993). A distinctive feature of this illness is the propensity for pain in the extremities to persist for months to years after the acute illness.

Acute meningitis (fever, headache, stiff neck, and photophobia) can be a manifestation of foodborne disease when the causative illness is *Listeria monocytogenes* (Lorber, 1997). In contrast to many of the microorganisms already mentioned, *L. monocytogenes* is an opportunistic pathogen, mainly affecting those with a compromised immune system. Such immune compromise can be physiologic (associated with pregnancy), age related (infancy, the elderly), due to an underlying malignancy (that is either diagnosed and being treated or not yet diagnosed), or due to human immunodeficiency virus (HIV) infection. A febrile diarrheal illness in normal individuals has been noted in several listeriosis outbreaks; however, the overall frequency of *Listeria* as a cause of diarrhea is not yet known. *Cronobacter sakazakii* (formerly known as *Enterobacter sakazakii*) causes a devastating encephalitis in newborns; some cases have been linked to powdered infant formula (Bowen and Braden, 2006).

Chronic forms of enteric illness, such as diarrhea for more than 3 weeks, can be a form of foodborne disease from particular pathogens. In addition to *Giardia*, two other parasites, *Cryptosporidium* and *Cyclospora*, cause chronic diarrhea in previously healthy persons (Guerrant

and Bobak, 1991; Herwaldt, 2000). The prolonged diarrheal illness known as Brainerd diarrhea, associated once with drinking raw milk and more often with drinking untreated water, remains of unknown etiology, but causes a distinctive debilitating illness (Mintz, 2003).

Chronic neurologic illness can result from foodborne infection, often months to years after the initial infection. Seizures can result from the cyst forms of the pork tapeworm, *Taenia solium*, in the central nervous system. Neurocysticercosis is the most common cause of seizures worldwide (Carpio, 2002). A variety of congenital abnormalities (e.g. blindness, microcephaly, mental retardation) are associated with congenital toxoplasmosis. A form of encephalitis has been seen in AIDS patients as a consequence of reactivation of the latent cyst forms of *T. gondii*.

Pathogenic Mechanisms

The mechanisms by which foodborne illness develops are best characterized for bacterial causes. Presently four main mechanisms are recognized by which bacterial enteric pathogens cause disease, and recent progress has suggested a fifth mechanism (Table 70.3). Some organisms produce illness after a period of growth in food during which a toxin is elaborated. Ingestion of this preformed toxin can produce excessive vomiting shortly after consumption, such as from *S. aureus* or *B. cereus* contamination, or frank paralysis, as in botulism. Other ingested pathogens may secrete a toxin following attachment to and colonization of a particular section of the gastrointestinal tract. ETEC produce a toxin closely related to cholera toxin from *Vibrio*

TABLE 70.3 Pathogenic mechanisms in bacterial foodborne disease

Mechanism	Organism
Preformed toxin	*Staphylococcus aureus*
	Bacillus cereus
	Clostridium botulinum
Toxin secretion within the GI tract	*Escherichia coli* 0157:H7 and other Shiga-toxin producing *E. coli*
	Enterotoxigenic *Escherichia coli*
	Vibrio cholerae O1, O139
Cell penetration	*Campylobacter jejuni*
	Salmonella
Cell invasion	*Shigella*
	Yersinia enterocolitica
Adherence and signal transduction	Enteropathogenic *E. coli*

cholerae; both toxins cause a net secretion of water and electrolytes, resulting in watery diarrhea. By contrast, *E. coli* O157:H7 produces a Shiga toxin (closely related to that produced by *Shigella dysenteriae* type 1), which causes cell death and results in bloody diarrhea.

Apart from toxin production, two other mechanisms of disease induction are well recognized. Both *Salmonella* and *C. jejuni* can penetrate the mucosal layer of the gastrointestinal tract without causing cell death. Pathogens that invade the mucosal layer and cause cell death include *Shigella* and *Yersinia enterocolitica*. Bloody diarrhea is more common among pathogens with this latter mechanism of action.

Recent work to elucidate the pathogenic basis for EPEC-associated diarrhea has suggested a mechanism distinct from those already described. EPEC have been shown to produce certain attachment factors, including several secreted proteins. The interaction of these proteins with the cell surface receptor appears to initiate a series of events involving signal transduction. This in turn leads to changes in cellular ion fluxes, with subsequent secretion of water and electrolytes into the lumen of the gastrointestinal tract.

Some bacterial pathogens have overlapping mechanisms of pathogenicity, and not all members of a genus may have the same mechanism of causing diarrhea. Grouping organisms by their mechanism of action none the less serves a number of purposes: first, to function as an existing framework for classifying new pathogens; secondly, to discern genetic relationships among diverse bacterial species; and, thirdly, to use as a basis to predict the therapeutic usefulness of new therapies.

Epidemiology

The epidemiology of foodborne disease is a complex interplay of the expression of a pathogen's virulence traits, host susceptibility, physical characteristics of the contaminated food, geographic location, and season of the year. Some pathogens have a predilection for particular foods, usually resulting from an overlap between their ecological niche and the harvest and/or processing environment for the food (Table 70.4). Raw meat, raw poultry, and shellfish are typically contaminated with the pathogens that have animal reservoirs, including *Salmonella*, *Campylobacter*, *E. coli* O157:H7, vibrios, and *Toxoplasma*, which can cause illness if the food is inadequately cooked, or if other foods are secondarily contaminated through direct or indirect

contact with the meat and poultry. Processed foods such as peanut butter, salami, and commercial pot pies can be contaminated with organisms that persist in dry ingredients or in the processing environment itself, such as *Salmonella* and *Listeria monocytogenes*. Foods that are handled extensively before eating without an intervening kill step, such as salads and sandwiches, can transmit pathogens for which humans are the main reservoir, from foodhandlers infected with norovirus, hepatitis A or *Shigella*.

Substantial changes have occurred in the epidemiology of foodborne disease in the United States in the last half of the 20th century. In the early 1900s, milk-borne tuberculosis, staphylococcal food poisoning, and typhoid fever were the main forms of foodborne disease (Tauxe and Esteban, 2006). Today the spectrum of causative organisms, the risk factors for enteric infection, and the type of foods involved are vastly different (Hedberg *et al.*, 1994; Tauxe, 2002). Use of antimicrobials in food animals has selected for increasingly resistant strains of *Campylobacter* and *Salmonella* (Anderson *et al.*, 2003). Changes in diet in the United States have occurred because of recognition of the relationship between diets rich in saturated fat and subsequent cardiovascular disease. This has led some Americans away from the traditional meat and potatoes diet of the 1950s to a diet that emphasizes fresh fruits and vegetables, grains, and fish and poultry consumption. Changes in food distribution systems have led to an end of seasonality for many fresh fruits and vegetables. Commodities formerly considered exotic are now routinely available in most grocery stores in the United States, and they are likely to have arrived within several days of harvest or production elsewhere in the world. Consumption of prepared, preprocessed, or ready-to-eat foods from commercial establishments has increased, providing a context in which transmission from food handlers has been seen with some frequency, particularly with norovirus, and of cold food items requiring hand contact. Substantial demographic changes also have occurred, with increases in populations with an increased susceptibility to particular pathogens.

Surveillance

The purpose of surveillance for foodborne disease is to monitor disease trends over time, to implement and monitor the effectiveness of interventions for control, and to detect outbreaks. Disease reporting is usually laboratory based, with the isolation or detection of a pathogen in the

TABLE 70.4 Etiology of foodborne disease outbreaks by food, season, and geographic predilection

Etiology	Foods	Season	Geographic predilection
Bacterial			
Salmonella	Beef, poultry, eggs, dairy products, produce, processed foods	Summer, fall	None
Staphylococcus aureus	Ham, poultry, egg salads, pastries	Summer	None
Campylobacter jejuni	Poultry, raw milk	Spring, summer	Higher in California and Hawaii
Clostridium botulinum	Vegetables, fruits, fish, honey (infants)	Summer, fall	None
Clostridium perfringens	Beef, poultry, gravy, Mexican food	Fall, winter, spring	None
Shigella	Egg salads, lettuce	Summer	None
Vibrio parahemolyticus	Shellfish	Spring, summer, fall	Coastal states
Bacillus cereus	Fried rice, meats, vegetables	Year-round	None
Yersinia enterocolitica	Milk, tofu, pork chitterlings	Winter	Unknown
Vibrio cholerae O1	Shellfish	Variable	Tropical, Gulf Coast, Latin America
V. cholerae non-O1	Shellfish	Unknown	Tropical, Gulf Coast
Shiga toxin-producing Escherichia coli	Beef, raw milk, fresh produce	Summer, fall	Northern states
Viral			
Norwalk-like agents	Shellfish, salads	Year-round	None
Chemical			
Ciguatera	Barracuda, snapper, amberjack grouper	Spring, summer (in Florida)	Tropical reefs
Histamine fish poisoning (scombroid)	Tuna, mackerel, bonito, skipjack, mahi-mahi	Year-round	Coastal
Mushroom poisoning	Mushrooms	Spring, fall	Temperate
Heavy metals	Acidic beverages	Year-round	None
Monosodium-L-glutamate	Chinese food	Year-round	None
Paralytic shellfish poisoning	Shellfish	Summer, fall	Temperate coastal zones
Neurotoxic shellfish poisoning	Shellfish	Spring, fall	Subtropical

Adapted with permission from Fry et al. (2005)[3].

clinical microbiology laboratory. In general, only a small fraction of actual illnesses are reported, but this can vary considerably among pathogens according to the severity of illness and the ease and access to laboratory testing (Hedberg *et al.*, 1994). For *Salmonella*, this has been estimated directly from FoodNet surveys of populations and laboratories; an estimated 38 illnesses occur for every one that is diagnosed and reported (Voetsch *et al.*, 2004). Some pathogens are transmitted exclusively through food (e.g. *Trichinella spiralis*), whereas others may be transmitted most often through water (e.g. *Giardia*) or by person-to-person spread (e.g. *Shigella*), and only occasionally through food. In 2010, an analysis took many of these aspects into consideration in developing estimates of the burden of foodborne disease on health in the United States (Scallan *et al.*, 2011a,b). In that estimate, approximately one in 46 persons in the United States were estimated to have a foodborne illness each year, of which 3000 died. *Salmonella, Listeria*, norovirus, and *Toxoplasma* were responsible for 82% of deaths from known pathogens. A provocative estimate from this analysis, described in Scallan *et al.* (2011a), was that the 31 pathogens in the estimate did not account for the majority of illnesses nor of deaths. These disease estimates were based on data from several sources, and contained a number of assumptions, including estimates

of the total number of illnesses for each pathogen, the proportion of pathogen transmission that is foodborne, and the incidence of acute gastroenteritis with unknown agents. Continued refinements in surveillance will test the validity of these assumptions. FoodNet, the sentinel-site network for active surveillance of foodborne infections [a program of the Centers for Disease Control and Prevention (Scallan, 2007)], develops population-based estimates of incidence and tracks the trends of known foodborne pathogens. The FoodNet sites now have nearly 14% of the US population within the surveillance network, and important trends are emerging in the 14 years since FoodNet's inception in 1996 (Scallan, 2007; CDC, 2010). *Campylobacter*, initially the highest-incidence pathogen, varies markedly among the participating sites. The most recent data for 2010 (CDC, 2011) show a decline in incidence of *Campylobacter* infection by 27% since 1996 to below that for *Salmonella*, as well as a decline in *E. coli* O157 infections to 0.9/100 000, which reached the 2010 national goal. The incidence of *Listeria* and *Yersinia enterocolitica* infections has also declined during the surveillance period. These declines may indicate the success of current disease prevention efforts aimed at multiple points along the "farm to fork" continuum (Figure 70.2). Most of the declines occurred in the first decade; there has been

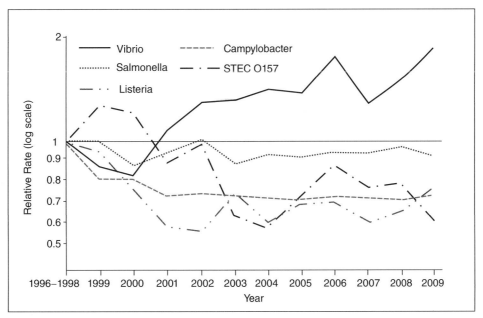

FIG. 70.2 Relative incidence of five infections as tracked in FoodNet from baseline in 1996–1998 through 2010. A decrease to 0.5 represents a 50% decrease in modeled incidence relative to the baseline period. Numbers for 2010 are preliminary. Reproduced from Centers for Disease Control and Prevention (2011), public domain.

little change in recent years, and the salmonellosis has not declined at all, so more efforts are clearly needed to reach even lower goals for 2020 (CDC, 2011). Since 1996–98, *Vibrio* infections increased, indicating the need for more prevention efforts focused on the risks associated with raw shellfish. Limitations to the FoodNet data include how well the population under surveillance captures the variety of the US population in terms of demographics and risk factors, and the fact that the system can only gather information on persons for whom diagnostic specimens were submitted and on pathogens which are routinely identified in clinical laboratories. However, FoodNet represents a significant advance over traditional public health surveillance in providing comparable information from different states, and provides more reliable estimates of the disease burden from particular foodborne pathogens.

PulseNet, developed under the auspices of the Centers for Disease Control and Prevention, is a system of laboratory-based electronic surveillance of foodborne bacterial infections that was also introduced in 1996 (Gerner-Smidt *et al.*, 2006). After *E. coli* O157, *Listeria* or *Salmonella* is isolated from an ill patient, the bacterial strain is sent to state public health laboratories, where a pulsed-field gel electrophoresis (PFGE) analysis is done. The PFGE "fingerprint" of that bacterial strain is stored, analyzed, and compared electronically with a national database of such "fingerprints." In this manner, PulseNet has been instrumental in identifying and investigating many geographically dispersed outbreaks. Because the typical interval between specimen collection and PFGE analysis is 14–16 days or more (Hedberg *et al.*, 2008), PulseNet operates with some delay, but this system has proven extraordinarily useful in detecting outbreaks that would otherwise have been missed until they were much bigger, and in facilitating epidemiological investigations of them (Tauxe, 2006). Food testing laboratories in the Food and Drug Administration (FDA) and Department of Agriculture (USDA) have joined the network, making it possible to link patterns isolated from ill people with those of isolates from foods. Adoption of the same laboratory protocols in Canada, Europe, Japan, and other regions is making it easier to identify and investigate international outbreaks (Swaminathan *et al.*, 2006).

Surveillance based on laboratory subtyping has greatly increased the recognition of outbreaks that are geographically dispersed. Large multi-state outbreaks have in recent years been traced to bagged baby spinach, to shredded lettuce served in fast-food tacos, and to raw cookie dough

(Grant *et al.*, 2008; CDC, 2009c; Sodha *et al.*, 2011). Large nationwide outbreaks of salmonellosis have been linked to peanut butter, other peanut-flavored products, broccoli flakes used on a vegetarian snack marketed at children, imported hot peppers, and fresh tomatoes (CDC, 2007a,b, 2008a, 2009b; Gupta *et al.*, 2007). Many of these outbreaks would not have been identified or successfully investigated without PulseNet (Tauxe, 2006). With molecular subtyping it has also become possible to find outbreaks that recur over time from the same source. In 2000 an outbreak of listeriosis was caused by the same strain, and traced to the same turkey-processing plant as a fatal case that had occurred 12 years before (Olsen *et al.*, 2005). In 2007, an outbreak of dry-cereal-associated infections was caused by the same strain of *Salmonella* serotype Agona as an outbreak in 1998, and linked to the same factory (CDC, 2008b). Recurrent outbreaks of *Salmonella* serotype Newport infection were linked to tomatoes from the eastern shore of Virginia in 2002 and 2005 (Greene *et al.*, 2008). All of these illustrate the important challenge of persistence of the organism in reservoirs and microniches that would not be clear without subtyping.

CDC also gathers reports of outbreak investigations from local and state health departments in order to track trends and better understand the sources of foodborne outbreaks. About 1200 foodborne outbreaks, with 20 000 to 40 000 associated cases, are reported each year (CDC, 2006). The great majority of these are investigated by local health departments.

Another, albeit sobering aspect of surveillance is that it needs to be viewed as the first line of defense in a bioterrorist event. Food processing today has increasingly centralized production and wide geographic distribution, which may have economic advantages but which make the food supply more vulnerable. Discussions of bioterrorism preparedness have often focused on airborne agents (e.g. anthrax), but consideration has also been given to scenarios involving the food supply. An unheralded attack may well resemble an unintentional outbreak, and is very likely to be identified and investigated with standard public-health procedures. Agricultural biosecurity will also need to be a component of the bioterrorism preparedness portfolio. A strong public-health infrastructure with efficient surveillance systems is likely to be the most effective defense against both naturally occurring epidemic disease and bioterrorism-related events. The importance of robust public-health surveillance in supporting both the public-health and national-security interests cannot be overemphasized.

TABLE 70.5 Populations at increased risk of infection and clinical illness from foodborne pathogens

Infants
Pregnant women
Persons over age 60 years
Persons with HIV infection
Alcoholics
Transplant recipients (bone marrow, solid organ)
Persons receiving cancer chemotherapy
Persons receiving immunosuppressive drugs, including
  steroids

The Challenges of Special Populations

As epidemiological investigations of outbreaks have delineated new and/or emerging pathogens as causative agents of foodborne disease, so too have new risk factors been defined for the acquisition of infection. The identification of groups with an increased risk for clinical illness following exposure is one of the most notable trends in foodborne disease epidemiology (Table 70.5). The magnitude of increased risk and the spectrum of pathogens differ among these groups. Young infants are particularly at risk for enteric infections, though they do not eat the foods that adults eat. *Yersinia enterocolitica* infections may offer a model for how indirect exposure can happen; bottle-fed infants get this infection when their caregiver is also cleaning pig intestines, and likely transfers the organism to the infant's bottle via their unwashed hands (Lee *et al.*, 1990). Persons over 60 years of age may have an increased susceptibility to infection irrespective of other risk factors such as malignancy. Older women seem to be particularly susceptible to salmonellosis (Reller *et al.*, 2008). The aging of the US population along with that in Western Europe and several other countries has clear-cut public health implications in underscoring the need to ensure a safe food supply. Advances in clinical medicine have created populations that never previously existed, for example, transplant recipients and those receiving immunosuppressive drugs. The epidemic of HIV infection has irrevocably changed modern society in numerous ways. With respect to foodborne pathogen exposures, HIV-infected patients are more likely to become ill, to have a more severe illness, and to have extraintestinal or unusual clinical manifestations.

These at-risk populations were previously estimated to constitute 10–20% of the population (CAST, 1994), but today the proportion is thought to be even higher. Many persons within these categories have no or only limited perception of their increased risk for foodborne disease. Although educational efforts seem a logical approach to disease prevention, this is often easier said than done. Some educational efforts, even when specifically targeted and culturally appropriate, have had disappointing results (Mouzin *et al.*, 1997). Because educational efforts alone may be insufficient to reduce risk, and because for some populations even one organism may represent an infective dose, additional measures of protection will need to be built into the food supply. Making food safe from farm to table is a joint responsibility of the food industry, the regulators, and the consumers. Technological interventions such as pasteurization of milk and retort canning of vegetables have long played a critical role in making food safer. Irradiation and high-pressure treatment are examples of new supplemental intervention to enhance food safety (Osterholm and Potter, 1997; Tauxe, 2001; Torres and Velazquez, 2005).

New Infectious Agents

Several infectious agents were added to the list of foodborne pathogens during the closing decades of the 20th century. Common to their "discoveries" was the magic combination of astute recognition of clinical illness and dogged epidemiological investigation backed up by intensive laboratory investigation. The yield from this combined approach ranged from new information for an "old" pathogen (the foodborne nature of *Listeria* transmission) to the discovery of a truly new pathogen (e.g. *E. coli* O157:H7).

Escherichia coli O157:H7 was first discovered as a human pathogen in 1982. It is now recognized as the most common cause of bloody diarrhea in North America and Western Europe, and has caused outbreaks on an unprecedented scale that have strained clinical and public health resources (Tarr *et al.*, 2005). Hemolytic uremic syndrome (HUS) may develop as a complication of this infection, and HUS caused by *E. coli* O157:H7 is the most common cause of acute renal failure in childhood. Diverse food vehicles, including undercooked ground beef, alfalfa sprouts, unpasteurized juice, unpasteurized milk, and lettuce, have transmitted this infection (Rangel *et al.*, 2005).

Salmonella has appeared in a variety of forms and foods. In the 1980s a worldwide pandemic of *Salmonella* serotype Enteritidis infections began that continues today. This pandemic is related particularly to eggs, as this type of *Salmonella* colonizes the ovaries of hens so that the internal contents of the eggs they lay are contaminated with it (Braden, 2006). In the late 1990s, two highly resistant strains of *Salmonella*, *Salmonella* serotype Typhimurium defined type 104 (DT104) and *Salmonella* serotype Newport with the multi-drug resistant AmpC gene (MDR AmpC) appeared in the United States, in cattle and in people. While they have been transmitted through various foods, they are most strongly associated with dairy cattle and with foods derived from them such as lean ground beef and unpasteurized milk (Glynn *et al.*, 1998; Gupta *et al.*, 2003). These two strains now represent 11% of human salmonellosis in the United States, and are not controlled by current measures.

Two newly described parasitic causes of foodborne disease include *Cryptosporidium* and *Cyclospora*. Originally considered a veterinary pathogen, *Cryptosporidium* had only on rare occasions been described as a human pathogen prior to 1980. This changed considerably with the advent of the HIV epidemic, in which HIV-infected patients, mainly those with extremely low CD4 lymphocyte counts, developed severe and unremitting watery diarrhea from *Cryptosporidium*. Contaminated water accounts for a larger proportion of transmission of this pathogen than contaminated foods (Roy *et al.*, 2004). A waterborne outbreak in Milwaukee in 1993 affected more than 400 000 persons and illustrated the vulnerability of some municipal water supplies (MacKenzie *et al.*, 1994).

Contaminated raspberries from Guatemala were the source for numerous outbreaks of diarrhea in 1996 in both the United States and Canada. Recognition of outbreaks was facilitated by extremely high attack rates (often greater than 80%) and a notably severe diarrheal illness. Yet these aspects were at odds with the largely negative diagnostic testing of stool samples. More intensive laboratory investigation ultimately identified *Cyclospora* as the causative agent (Herwaldt, 2000).

Novel foodborne diseases have been described for which there is as yet incomplete understanding of the pathogenic agent. Brainerd diarrhea is the designation for a chronic diarrhea syndrome that originally occurred in Brainerd, Minnesota. Illness was associated with raw milk consumption and was both severe and long lasting, with diarrhea for more than 1 year in many patients (Mintz, 2003).

New variant Creutzfeld–Jacob disease (nvCJD) is a dementing, ultimately fatal illness that occurred in otherwise healthy young and middle-aged adults, mainly in the United Kingdom in the late 1990s (Will *et al.*, 2000). Pathological changes in the brains of these patients and characterization of the prion in them indicates that nvCJD is a form of BSE (Bruce *et al.*, 1997). The human nvCJD cases were recognized after an epidemic of BSE in the United Kingdom that had occurred approximately 6 years earlier. It is likely that changes in rendering practices allowed meat and bonemeal to remain infectious with the BSE prion agent and that subsequent foodborne transmission to cattle ensued when these were used in feeds. The link is thought to be that the BSE agent crossed the species barrier and the human nvCJD cases resulted from acquisition of infection through consumption of BSE-contaminated beef or beef-derived products (Brown *et al.*, 2001).

Different Risks in Food Production

There are marked differences in food production practices today compared with those earlier in the 20th century. Agricultural products and food animals were raised in smaller groupings, and food products were usually only seasonally available to a population in the immediate vicinity of the harvest. Food technologies that are now commonplace (e.g. aquaculture, extended-shelf-life products) did not even exist. Today the scale of production within the food industry has markedly increased; for example, hamburger may be ground in lots of several thousand kilograms. Finished products are distributed over a much broader geographic region, and even raw materials may be transported in bulk over considerable distances. A large-scale outbreak of salmonellosis was the result of a tanker truck being used to transport pasteurized ice cream premix immediately after it had transported raw eggs contaminated with *Salmonella*. The subsequently contaminated ice cream product was distributed over the entire continental United States (Hennessy *et al.*, 1996). When an ingredient is contaminated, the resulting outbreak can be large and complex. In 2009, peanut butter and peanut paste from one small factory contaminated with *Salmonella* led to a large nationwide outbreak, and the recall of 3900 products (CDC, 2009b).

Foodborne outbreaks due to fresh produce have increased markedly in the last three decades as the consumption of fresh produce increased and as produce imported from around the world became available (Sivapalasingham *et al.*, 2004). This means that the health of the consumer in the United States is now linked directly to the sanitary conditions of field workers and the food safety systems of many countries.

Low-level contamination of a foodstuff may cause outbreaks that are difficult to detect because there may be a relatively small number of cases dispersed over a broad geographic area. New food and ingredient sources may introduce pathogens that were previously rare or geographically restricted. Pathogens that survive in low moisture environments or that multiply at refrigerator temperatures may persist in niches in the processing environment. New harvest and processing technologies may be implemented without full regard for the microbiological implications, leading to new opportunities for contamination. Efforts to enhance food safety must have built-in mechanisms that enable them to continually evolve, because challenges from new pathogens, new vehicles of transmission, and new risk factors will undoubtedly continue to arise.

Vaccine Prospects

Of the microbial agents commonly recognized as being transmitted by food, only three have an effective, licensed, human vaccine for prevention: hepatitis A, *Salmonella* serotype Typhi, and *Vibrio cholerae* O1. Typhoid and cholera occur at such exceedingly low rates in the United States that vaccination is not warranted; travelers to high-risk countries are advised to get typhoid immunization. Hepatitis A vaccination is increasingly being used to control local outbreaks or more broadly in states with high case rates. Some institutions and commercial establishments have chosen to provide hepatitis A vaccine for food handlers and others involved in food preparation.

An experimental human vaccine for *E. coli* O157:H7 has been developed that induces antibody to the O157 lipopolysaccharide. Vaccine constructs have been developed for *Shigella* and *Salmonella* that have been tested in animal models. Considerable work remains to be done to demonstrate their safety and efficacy.

Another avenue of pursuit in vaccine development has been the development of animal vaccines. Many foodborne pathogens are colonizers of animal digestive tracts. These include *E. coli* O157:H7 and ETEC in cattle and *Salmonella* and *Campylobacter* in poultry. *Salmonella* vaccines for chickens played an important part in the dramatic reduction of *Salmonella* serotype Enteritidis in egg-laying chicken flocks in Great Britain, and increasingly are used in the United States. Two commercial cattle vaccines are now licensed for use against *E. coli* O157. The optimum use of these vaccines and how best to combine them with other on-farm ("pre-harvest") control measures are areas of active investigation. Whether for humans or animals, the ultimate success of a vaccine will rest with defining the target group to be immunized, accessing that group consistently, and ensuring high vaccination rates.

Prevention

Surveillance for foodborne disease has become the ultimate cornerstone for preventive efforts. In recent years the major focus of outbreak investigations triggered by surveillance has been to ascertain a root cause for how a food became contaminated, whether as a raw product, during processing, or afterward. The findings are then used to devise control strategies to reduce or eliminate the problem of pathogen contamination. In the eyes of most public-health authorities, surveillance has been transformed from a slow, paper-pushing effort to one that is dynamic, interactive, and increasingly web-based.

Similarly, the field of prevention has seen rapid progress in recent years as the food industry has embraced the need to reduce the contamination of foods before they reach the final consumer. Food processing equipment manufacturers now routinely consider microbiological outcomes in their designs, and the processes themselves are being overhauled to produce a product that is microbiologically safer, as well as tasty, nutritious, and economically sound.

Much foodborne disease can be prevented by using multiple steps to reduce contamination from farm to fork. Much of the prevention of foodborne diseases occurs before the food is prepared and served. Minimizing contamination starts in the farm, field or fishery, where good practices may reduce the likelihood of contamination even before harvest. After harvest, our industrialized food supply offers many points at which contamination can be prevented or eliminated. A safety engineering approach that identifies those points, and sets controls in place to guarantee that they are effectively used, has become the new standard for much of the food industry. This approach, the Hazard Analysis and Critical Control Point (HACCP) approach, is geared to prevent contamination before it occurs rather than to inspect for contamination that has already occurred (Doores, 1999). An HACCP program depends on continuous monitoring of steps in food processing that are critical in preventing the introduction, survival, or outgrowth of pathogens, such as heating or acidification, as well as those that reduce the pathogen burden, such as retort canning, pasteurization, high-pressure treatment or irradiation. It is essential that documentation of the measurements of the parameter considered critical for control be recorded. Deviation from the accepted parameters for process control requires corrective action, which must also be documented. HACCP is well established for processed foods exposed to an adequate kill step. HACCP has been implemented in meat and poultry and seafood processing plants. The FDA Food Safety Modernization Act, which was signed January 4, 2011, mandates that similar approaches be implemented for other foods, among many other important changes (Government Printing Office, 2011).

Food-handling errors in the kitchen can lead to illness, and educating food handlers and consumers about food safety at the point of preparation can help prevent the occurrence of such mistakes. In a study comparing restaurants that had outbreaks with those that did not, the presence of a food service manager certified in food safety was significantly associated with not having an outbreak (Hedberg et al., 2006). Some jurisdictions are requiring restaurants to have such a manager on staff, in addition to passing standard restaurant inspections. In the kitchen at home, careful attention to the precepts of "Cook, Clean, Chill, and Separate" can reduce the risk of foodborne illness (www.fightbac.org/safe-food-handling, accessed February 28, 2011). This means: using a thermometer to be sure that meat and poultry are adequately cooked; washing hands and food preparation surfaces frequently; prompt refrigeration of leftovers in a refrigerator that is below 40°F (4.4°C); and keeping raw and cooked foods separate during purchase, storage, and preparation with careful attention to avoid cross-contaminating other foods with the utensils or hands that have touched raw meat and poultry.

Future Directions

Unpredictably but reliably, new foodborne diseases will continue to emerge. The constantly changing food supply will continue to offer opportunities for pathogens to infect us through new and unsuspected routes. Enhanced public-health vigilance, investigation of outbreaks, and microbiological and food science research will continue to be critical components of food safety. The globalization of the food supply will need to be matched by the expanded collaborative surveillance networks around the world, and by a commitment in many countries to address the identified hazards. Surveillance will increasingly include monitoring the circulation of human pathogens among animals and plants, and those present in foods, to provide an integrated view of the ecologies that drive them. The inappropriate uses of antibiotics in agriculture to promote growth and prevent disease will diminish, and with it the threat of antimicrobial-resistant strains of food-associated pathogens should decrease. The growing science of probiotics, at both the animal and human level, offers the hope of broad-scale prevention of infection by bolstering the resistance of gut flora to colonization by external pathogens.

The future of food safety lies in the joint efforts of consumers, food producers, public health authorities, and government. One major step in this direction is the recognition of a "farm to fork" continuum. Ensuring a safe food supply depends on efforts all along that continuum. Improved consumer education is needed that targets specific populations and/or food practices, and that results in consistent and long-lasting behavioral change, but by itself is insufficient. Safer processing is critical at animal slaughter and food-fabrication plants, and more critical pathogen control technologies, such as pasteurization, irradiation, and pressure treatment, will be needed for foods likely to be contaminated with deadly pathogens. Introducing safer practices in animal husbandry, fresh vegetable production, and shellfish harvesting will have long-term benefits for public health. Introducing safety specifications into purchase contracts can rapidly make the concerns of consumers and retailers heard all the way back at the primary producers. The food industry and governmental authorities need to adapt to both the global marketplace and to pathogens, for which national boundaries are irrelevant. Because much of the burden of foodborne disease is preventable, it is a reasonable expectation that scientifically based efforts can significantly reduce that burden and improve human health.

Suggestions for Further Reading

Morris, J.G., Jr (2011) How safe is our food? *Emerg Infect Dis* **17**, 127–128.

Scallan, E., Griffin, P.M., Angulo, F.J., *et al.* (2011) Foodborne illness acquired in the United States – unspecified pathogens. *Emerg Infect Dis* **17**, 16–22.

Scallan, E., Hoekstra, R.M., Angulo, F.J., *et al.* (2011) Foodborne illness acquired in the United States – major pathogens. *Emerg Infect Dis* **17**, 8–15.

Tauxe, R.V. (2006) Molecular subtyping and the transformation of public health. *Foodborne Pathog Dis* **3**, 4–7.

Tauxe, R.V. and Esteban, E. (2006) Advances in food safety to prevent foodborne diseases in the United States. In J.W. Ward and C. Warren (eds), *Silent Victories: The Practice of Public Health in Twentieth Century America*. Oxford University Press, Oxford, pp. 18–43.

References

Allos, B.M. and Blaser, M.J. (1995) *Campylobacter jejuni* and the expanding spectrum of related infections. *Clin Infect Dis* **20**, 1092–1101.

Anderson, A.D., Nelson, J.M., Rossiter, S., *et al.* (2003) Public health consequences of use of antimicrobial agents in food animals in the United States. *Microb Drug Resist* **9**, 373–379.

Bowen, A.B. and Braden, C.R. (2006) *Enterobacter sakazakii* infection in infants. *Emerg Infect Dis* **12**, 1185–1189.

Braden, C.R. (2006) *Salmonella enterica* serotype Enteritidis: A national epidemic in the United States. *Clin Infect Dis* **43**, 512–517.

Brown, P., Will, R.G., Bradley, R., *et al.* (2001) Bovine spongiform encephalopathy and variant Creutzfeldt-Jakob disease: background, evolution, and current concerns. *Emerg Infect Dis* **7**, 6–16.

Bruce, M.E., Will, R.G., Ironside, J.W., *et al.* (1997) Transmissions to mice indicate that "new variant" CJD is caused by the BSE agent. *Nature* **389**, 498–501.

Bureau of the Census (1976) *Historical Statistics of the United States: Colonial Times to 1970. Bicentennial Edition*, Vol. 1. US Government Printing Office, Washington, DC.

Butterton, J.R. and Calderwood, S.B. (2008) Acute infectious diarrheal diseases and bacterial food poisoning. In A.S. Fauci, E. Braunwald, D.L. Kasper, *et al.* (eds), *Harrison's Principles of Internal Medicine*, 17th Edn. McGraw-Hill, New York, pp. 813–818.

Carpio, A. (2002) Neurocysticercosis: an update. *Lancet Infect Dis* **2**, 751–762.

CAST (1994) *Foodborne Pathogens: Risks and Consequences: Task Force Report*. Council for Agricultural Science and Technology, Ames, IA.

CDC (1999) Safer and healthier foods. *Morb Mortal Wkly Rep* **48**, 905–913.

CDC (2006) Surveillance for foodborne disease outbreaks – United States, 2006. *Morb Mortal Wkly Rep* **58**, 609–615.

CDC (2007a) Salmonellosis outbreak – February 2007. Posted on March 7, 2007, at www.cdc.gov/ncidod/dbmd/diseaseinfo/salmonellosis_2007/030707_outbreak_notice.htm. Accessed May 9, 2010.

CDC (2007b) *Salmonella* Wandsworth outbreak investigation, June–July 2007. Posted July 18, 2007, at http://www.cdc.gov/salmonella/wandsworth.htm. Accessed May 9, 2010.

CDC (2008a) Outbreak of *Salmonella* Saintpaul infections associated with eating multiple produce items–United States, 2008. *Morb Mortal Wkly Rep* **57**, 929–934

CDC (2008b) Investigation of outbreak caused by *Salmonella* Agona. Posted on May 14, 2008, at www.cdc.gov/salmonella/agona/. Accessed May 9, 2010.

CDC (2009a) Centers for Diseases Control and Prevention. Summary of Notifiable Diseases – United States, 2007. *Morb Mortal Wkly Rep* **56**, 1–94

CDC (2009b) Investigation update: outbreak of *Salmonella* typhimurium infections 2008–2009. Posted on March 17, 2009, at http://www.cdc.gov/salmonella/typhimurium/update.html. Accessed May 9, 2010.

CDC (2009c) Multistate outbreak of *E. coli* O157:H7 infections linked to eating raw refrigerated, prepackaged cookie dough. Posted June 20, 2009, at www.cdc.gov/ecoli/2009/0630.html. Accessed May 9, 2010.

CDC (2010) Preliminary FoodNet data on incidence of pathogens commonly transmitted through foods – 10 sites, United States, 2009. *Morb Mortal Wkly Rep* **59**, 418–422.

CDC (2011) Vital signs: incidence and trends of infection with pathogens transmitted commonly through food – Foodborne Diseases Active Surveillance Network,10 U.S. Sites, 1996–2010. *Morb Mortal Wkly Rep* **60**, 749–755.

Daniels, N.A., MacKinnon, L., Bishop, R., *et al.* (2000) *Vibrio parahaemolyticus* in the United States, 1973–1998. *J Infect Dis* **181**, 1661–1666.

Doores, S. (1999) *Food Safety: Current Status and Future Needs*. American Society for Microbiology Press, Washington, DC, pp. 1–28.

Gerner-Smidt, P., Hise, K., Kincaid, J., *et al.* (2006) PulseNet USA: a five-year update. *Foodborne Pathog Dis* **3**, 9–19.

Glynn, M., Bopp, C., Dewitt, W., *et al.* (1998) The emergence of multidrug resistant *Salmonella enterica* serotype Typhimurium DT104 infections in the United States. *N Engl J Med* **328**, 1333–1338.

Goldberg, M.B. and Rubin, R.H. (1988) The spectrum of *Salmonella* infections. *Infect Dis Clin North Am* **2**, 571–598.

Government Printing Office (2011) FDA Food Safety Modernization Act. Public Law 111-353. Accessed February 28, 2011, at http://www.gpo.gov/fdsys/pkg/PLAW-111publ353/pdf/PLAW-111publ353.pdf.

Grant, J., Wendleboe, A.M., Wendel, A., *et al.* (2008) Spinach-associated *Escherichia coli* O157:H7 outbreak, Utah and New Mexico. *Emerg Infect Dis* **14**, 1633–1636.

Greene, S.K., Daly, E.R., Talbot, E.A., *et al.* (2008) Recurrent multistate outbreak of *Salmonella* Newport associated with tomatoes from contaminated fields, 2005. *Epidemiol Infect* **136**, 157–165.

Guerrant, R.L. and Bobak, D.A. (1991) Bacterial and protozoal gastroenteritis. *N Engl J Med* **325**, 327–340.

Gupta, A., Fontana, J., Crowe, C., *et al.* (2003) The emergence of multidrug-resistant *Salmonella enterica* serotype Newport resistant to expanded-spectrum cephalosporins in the United States. *J Infect Dis* **188**, 1707–1716.

Gupta, S.K., Nalluswami, K., Snider, C., *et al.* (2007) Outbreak of *Salmonella* Braenderup infections associated with Roma tomatoes, northeastern United States, 2004: a useful method for subtyping exposures in field investigations. *Epidemiol Infect* **135**, 1165–1173.

Hedberg, C.W., MacDonald, K.L., and Osterhom, M.T. (1994) Changing epidemiology of foodborne disease: a Minnesota perspective. *Clin Infect Dis* **18**, 671–682.

Hedberg, C.W., Smith, J.S., Kirkland, E., *et al.* (2006) Systematic environmental evaluations to identify food safety differences between outbreak and nonoutbreak restaurants. *J Food Prot* **69**, 2697–2702.

Hedberg, C.W., Greenblatt, J.F., Matyas, B., *et al.* (2008) Timeliness of enteric disease surveillance in 6 US states. *Emerg Infect Dis* **14**, 311–313.

Hennessy, T.W., Hedberg, C.W., Slutsker, L., *et al.* (1996) A national outbreak of *Salmonella enteritidis* infections from ice cream. *N Engl J Med* **334**, 1281–1286.

Herwaldt, B.L. (2000) *Cyclospora cayetanensis*: a review, focusing on the outbreaks of cyclosporiasis in the 1990s. *Clin Infect Dis* **31**, 1040–1057.

Lee, L.A., Gerber, A.R., Longsway, D.R., *et al.* (1990) *Yersinia enterocolitica* O:3 infections in infants and children, associated with the household preparation of chitterlings. *New Engl J Med* **322**, 984–987.

Levine, W.C., Buehler, J.W., Bean, N.H., *et al.* (1991) Epidemiology of nontyphoidal *Salmonella* bacteremia during the human immunodeficiency virus epidemic. *J Infect Dis* **164**, 81–87.

Long, C., Jones, T.F., Vugia, D.J., *et al.* (2010) *Yersinia pseudotuberculosis* and *Y. enterocolitica* infections, FoodNet 1996–2007. *Emerg Infect Dis* **16**, 566–567.

Lorber, B. (1997) Listeriosis. *Clin Infect Dis* **24**, 1–11.

MacKenzie, W.R., Hoxie, N.J., Proctor, M.E., *et al.* (1994) A massive outbreak in Milwaukee of *Cryptosporidium* infection transmitted through the public water supply. *N Engl J Med* **331**, 161–167.

Mintz, E.D. (2003) Brainerd diarrhea turns 20: a riddle wrapped in a mystery inside an enigma. *Lancet* **362**, 2037–2038.

Mishu, B., Ilyas, A.A., Kosli, C.L., *et al.* (1993) Serologic evidence of previous *Campylobacter jejuni* infections in patients with the Guillain Barré syndrome. *Ann Intern Med* **118**, 947–953.

Mouzin, E., Mascola, L., Tormey, M.P., *et al.* (1997) Prevention of *Vibrio vulnificus* infections: assessment of regulatory educational strategies. *JAMA* **278**, 576–578.

Nataro, J.P. and Kaper, J.B. (1998) Diarrheagenic *Escherichia coli*. *Clin Microbiol Rev* **11**, 142–201.

Nuorti, P.J., Niskanen, T., Hallanvuo, S., *et al.* (2003) A widespread outbreak of *Yersinia pseudotuberculosis* O:3 infection from iceberg lettuce. *J Infect Dis* **189**, 766–774.

Olsen, S.J., Patrick, M., Hunter, S.B., *et al.* (2005) Multistate outbreak of *Listeria monocytogenes* infection linked to delicatessen turkey meat. *Clin Infect Dis* **40**, 962–967.

Osterholm, M.T. and Potter, M.E. (1997) Irradiation pasteurization of solid foods: taking food safety to the next level. *Emerg Infect Dis* **3**, 575–577.

Ostroff, S.M., Kapperud, G., Lassen, J., *et al.* (1992) Clinical features of *Yersinia enterocolitica* infections in Norway. *J Infect Dis* **166**, 812–817.

Rangel, J.M., Sparling, P.H., Crowe, C., *et al.* (2005) Epidemiology of *Escherichia coli* O157:H7 outbreaks in the United States, 1982–2002. *Emerg Infect Dis* **11**, 603–609.

Reller, M.E., Tauxe, R.V., Kalish, L.A., *et al.* (2008) Excess salmonellosis in women in the United States: 1968–2000. *Epidemiol Infect* **136**, 1109–1117.

Roy, S.L., Delong, S.M., and Stenzel, S.A. (2004) Risk factors for sporadic cryptosporidiosis among immunocompetent persons in the United States from 1999 to 2001. *Clin Infect Dis* **42**, 2944–2951.

Scallan, E. (2007) Activities, achievements and lessons learned during the first 10 years of the Foodborne Diseases Active Surveillance Network, 1996–2005. *Clin Infect Dis* **44**, 318–325.

Scallan, E., Griffin, P.M., Angulo, F.J., *et al.* (2011a) Foodborne illness acquired in the United States – unspecified agents. *Emerg Infect Dis* **17**, 16–22.

Scallan, E., Hoekstra, R., Angulo, F.J., *et al.* (2011b) Foodborne illness acquired in the United States – major pathogens. *Emerg Infect Dis* **17**, 7–15.

Sivapalasingam, S., Friedman, C.R., Cohen, L., *et al.* (2004) Fresh produce: a growing cause of outbreaks of foodborne illness in the United States. *J Food Prot* **67**, 2342–2353.

Sodha, S.V., Griffin, P.M., and Hughes, J.M. (2010) Foodborne disease. In G.L. Mandell, J.E. Bennett, and R. Dolin (eds), *Principles and Practice of Infectious Diseases*, 7th Edn. Churchill-Livingstone, Philadelphia, pp. 1413–1427.

Sodha, S.V., Lynch, M., Wannemuehler, K., *et al.* (2011) Multistate outbreak of *Escherichia coli* O157:H7 infections associated with a national fast-food chain, 2006: a study incorporating epidemiological and food source traceback results. *Epidemiol Infect* **139**, 309–316.

Swaminathan, B., Gerner-Smidt, P., and Ng, L-K. (2006) Building PulseNet International: an interconnected system of laboratory networks to facilitate timely public health recognition and response to foodborne disease outbreaks and emerging foodborne diseases. *Foodborne Pathog Dis* **3**, 36–50.

Tarr, P.I., Gordon, C.A., and Chandler, W.L. (2005) Shiga-toxin-producing *Escherichia coli* and haemolytic uraemic syndrome. *Lancet* **365**, 1073–1086.

Tauxe, R.V. (2001) Food safety and irradiation: protecting the public from foodborne infections. *Emerg Infect Dis* **7**(Suppl 7), 516–521.

Tauxe, R.V. (2002) Emerging foodborne pathogens. *Int J Food Microbiol* **78**, 31–41.

Tauxe, R.V. (2006) Molecular subtyping and the transformation of public health. *Foodborne Pathog Dis* **3**, 4–8.

Tauxe, R.V. and Esteban, E.J. (2006) Advances in food safety and the prevention of foodborne diseases in the United States. In J.W. Ward and C. Warren (eds), *Silent Victories: The Practice of Public Health in Twentieth Century America*. Oxford University Press, Oxford, pp. 18–43.

Torres, J.A. and Velazquez, G. (2005) Commercial opportunities and research challenges in the high pressure processing of foods. *J Food Eng* **67**, 95–112.

Underman, A.E. and Leedom, J.M. (1993) Fish and shellfish poisoning. *Curr Clin Top Infect Dis* **13**, 203–225.

Voetsch, A.C., Van Gilder, J., Angulo, F.J., *et al.* (2004) FoodNet estimate of the burden of illness caused by nontyphoidal *Salmonella* infections in the United States. *Clin Infect Dis* **38**(Suppl 3), S127–S134.

Will, R.G., Zeidler, M., Stewart, G.E., *et al.* (2000) Diagnosis of new variant Creutzfeldt-Jakob disease. *Ann Neurol* **47**, 575–582.

71

FOOD ALLERGIES AND INTOLERANCES

STEVE L. TAYLOR, PhD AND JOSEPH L. BAUMERT, PhD

University of Nebraska, Lincoln, Nebraska, USA

Summary

Food allergies and intolerances affect a small but significant portion of the population. Symptoms can range from mildly annoying to severe and life-threatening. The true food allergies present the biggest risk because symptoms can occasionally be quite severe and the threshold dose of the offending food needed to provoke a reaction is quite small. The only management strategy for individuals with food allergies and intolerances is the specific avoidance of the offending food. Development of safe and effective avoidance diets can be quite difficult for individuals with true food allergies.

Introduction

Centuries ago, Lucretius stated, "What is food to one is bitter poison to another." Food allergies and sensitivities can be collectively referred to as *individualistic* adverse reactions to foods because these illnesses affected only certain individuals within the population. Although these diseases are often grouped together under the general heading of "food allergy," a variety of different types of illnesses are involved. The existence of several different types of adverse reactions to foods with varied symptoms, severity, prevalence, and causative factors is not recognized by some physicians. Consumers are even more likely to be confused regarding the definition and classification of adverse reactions to foods. Consumers perceive that "food allergies" are quite common (Sloan and Powers, 1986), but many self-diagnosed cases of "food allergy" incorrectly associate foods with a particular malady or ascribe various mild forms of postprandial eating discomfort to this category of illness.

Classification

Table 71.1 provides a classification scheme for the different types of illnesses that are known to occur in association with food ingestion and that only involve certain individuals in the population. Two major groups of individualistic adverse reactions to foods are known: true food allergies and food intolerances. The true food allergies involve abnormal immunological mechanisms whereas the food intolerances do not. Knowing and recognizing the difference between immunological food allergies and non-immunological food intolerances is crucial. True food allergies can be provoked in some cases by very low doses of the offending foods while those with intolerances can often tolerate larger doses of the offending food. A food allergy is an abnormal immunological response to a food or food component, usually a naturally occurring protein (Taylor and Hefle, 2001). Two different types of abnormal immunological responses are known to occur. Immediate

Present Knowledge in Nutrition, Tenth Edition. Edited by John W. Erdman Jr, Ian A. Macdonald and Steven H. Zeisel.

hypersensitivity reactions are antibody-mediated, whereas delayed hypersensitivity reactions are cell-mediated.

In contrast, food intolerances do not involve abnormal responses of the immune system (Taylor and Hefle, 2001). Three major categories of food intolerances are recognized: anaphylactoid reactions, metabolic food disorders, and food idiosyncrasies.

TABLE 71.1 Classification of individualistic adverse reactions to foods

Classification	Example
True food allergies	
Antibody-mediated food allergies	IgE-mediated food allergies (peanut, cows' milk, etc.)
	Exercise-associated food allergies
Cell-mediated food allergies	Celiac disease
	Other types of delayed hypersensitivity
Food intolerances	
Anaphylactoid reactions	
Metabolic food disorders	Lactose intolerance
Idiosyncratic reactions	Sulfite-induced asthma

IgE-Mediated Food Allergy

Mechanism

Immediate hypersensitivity reactions are mediated by allergen-specific IgE antibodies (Figure 71.1). In IgE-mediated food allergies, allergen-specific IgE antibodies are produced by B cells in response to the immunological stimulus created by exposure of the immune system to the allergen (Burks and Ballmer-Weber, 2006). Food allergens are usually naturally occurring proteins present in the food (Breiteneder and Mills, 2008). The allergen-specific IgE antibodies bind to the surfaces of mast cells in the tissues and basophils in the blood. This is the sensitization phase of the allergic response. The sensitization phase is asymptomatic. On subsequent exposure to the specific allergenic food, the allergens cross-link two or more of the IgE-antibodies affixed to the surfaces of mast cells or basophils. This interaction triggers the degranulation of the mast cell or basophil membrane and the release of a variety of potent physiologically active mediators into the bloodstream and tissues. The granules within mast cells and basophils contain many of the important mediators of the allergic reaction. These potent mediators are actually responsible for the symptoms of immediate hypersensitivity reactions. Histamine is perhaps the most important of the mediators

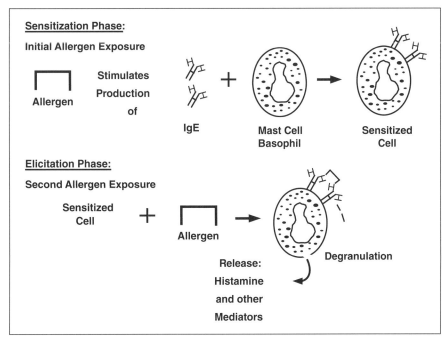

FIG. 71.1 Mechanism of IgE-mediated food allergy.

released from mast cells and basophils in an allergic reaction. It can elicit inflammation, pruritus, and contraction of the smooth muscles in the blood vessels, gastrointestinal tract, and respiratory tract (Taylor and Hefle, 2001). Other important mediators include various leukotrienes and prostaglandins. The leukotrienes are associated with some of the symptoms that develop more slowly in IgE-mediated food allergies, such as late-phase asthmatic reactions. This same type of IgE-mediated reaction is also responsible for allergic reactions to other environmental substances such as pollens, mold spores, animal danders, and bee venoms; only the source of the allergen is different.

During the sensitization phase, an individual forms allergen-specific IgE antibodies after exposure to a specific food protein. However, even among individuals predisposed to allergies, exposure to food proteins does not usually result in the formation of IgE antibodies. In normal individuals, exposure to a food protein in the gastrointestinal tract results in oral tolerance through either the formation of protein-specific IgG, IgM, or IgA antibodies or no immunological response whatsoever (clonal anergy) (Ko and Mayer, 2005). Heredity and other physiological factors are important in predisposing individuals to the development of IgE-mediated allergies including food allergies (Hourihane *et al.*, 1996). Studies with monozygotic and dizygotic twins demonstrate that genetics is an extremely important parameter and that identical twins may even inherit the likelihood of responding to the same allergenic food, e.g. peanuts (Sicherer *et al.*, 2000). Approximately 65% of patients with clinically documented allergy have first-degree relatives with allergic disease (Hourihane *et al.*, 1996). Conditions that increase the permeability of the small intestinal mucosa to proteins such as viral gastroenteritis, premature birth, and cystic fibrosis also seem to increase the risk of development of food allergy.

Symptoms

The onset time for these reactions ranges from a few minutes to several hours after the consumption of the offending food. IgE-mediated food allergies involve numerous symptoms ranging from mild and annoying to severe and life-threatening (Table 71.2). No individual with IgE-mediated food allergy suffers from all of the symptoms noted in Table 71.2. Furthermore, the symptoms are not necessarily consistent from one episode to another for an individual. The nature and severity of symptoms can also vary as a result of the amount of the

TABLE 71.2 Symptoms associated with IgE-mediated food allergy

Type	Symptom
Gastrointestinal	Nausea
	Vomiting
	Diarrhea
	Abdominal cramping
Cutaneous	Urticaria
	Dermatitis or eczema
	Angioedema
	Pruritus
Respiratory	Rhinitis
	Asthma
	Laryngeal edema
Generalized	Anaphylactic shock

offending food that has been ingested and the length of time since the previous exposure. An individual who experiences only mild symptoms on ingestion of a specific food, e.g. oral pruritus, may develop more serious manifestations on subsequent occasions, especially if avoidance of the offending food is not routinely practiced.

Gastrointestinal and cutaneous symptoms are among the more common manifestations of IgE-mediated food allergies. Respiratory symptoms are less commonly encountered but can be severe and life-threatening. Mild respiratory symptoms such as rhinitis and rhinoconjunctivitis are more likely to be encountered with exposure to environmental allergens such as directly inhaled airborne pollens or animal danders. However, respiratory reactions associated with food allergies can occasionally be severe (asthma and laryngeal edema). Those few food-allergic individuals who experience severe respiratory reactions in connection with the inadvertent ingestion of the offending food are most likely to be at risk for life-threatening episodes (Sampson *et al.*, 1992). Of the many symptoms involved in IgE-mediated food allergies, systemic anaphylaxis is the most severe manifestation. Systemic anaphylaxis, also sometimes referred to as anaphylactic shock, involves multiple organ systems and numerous symptoms. The symptoms can involve the gastrointestinal tract, respiratory tract, skin, and cardiovascular system. Death can occur from severe hypotension coupled with respiratory and cardiovascular complications. Anaphylactic shock is the most common cause of death in the occasional fatalities associated with IgE-mediated food allergies (Yunginger *et al.*, 1988; Sampson *et al.*, 1992; Bock *et al.*, 2007; Pumphrey and Gowland, 2007). The number of deaths occurring from IgE-mediated food allergies is not recorded in most countries, but more than 100 deaths are thought to occur in the United States each year (Sampson, 2003).

Oral Allergy Syndrome

Oral allergy syndrome is one of the more common and most mild forms of IgE-mediated food allergy (Wang, 2008). In this syndrome, ingestion of the offending foods – often fresh fruits and vegetables – elicits mild oropharyngeal symptoms: pruritus, urticaria, and angioedema. Fresh fruits and vegetables contain comparatively low quantities of the protein allergens, but oral allergy syndrome is an IgE-mediated response involving reactions to certain specific proteins (Wang, 2008). Apparently, the allergens in these fresh fruits and vegetables are rapidly digested by the proteases of the gastrointestinal tract (Taylor and Lehrer, 1996), and systemic reactions are rarely encountered. The allergens are also apparently heat labile (Taylor and Lehrer, 1996) because heat-processing eliminates their effects. Individuals with oral allergy syndrome are initially sensitized to one or more environmental pollens, frequently from birch or mugwort (Wang et al., 2008). Once sensitized to the pollen allergens, these individuals are reactive to proteins that exist in foods, which cross-react with these allergens.

Exercise-Induced Food Allergies

Exercise-induced food allergies are a subset of the immediate hypersensitivity reactions to foods. They involve allergen-specific IgE antibodies, but occur only when the food is eaten in conjunction with exercise (Williams and Simon, 2008). Numerous foods have been implicated, including shellfish, wheat, celery, and peach. The symptoms are as individualistic and variable as those for other food allergies. Exercise-induced allergies can also exist without any role for food intake (Williams and Simon, 2008). The mechanism of this illness is not well understood but the involvement of IgE antibodies is clear. With the recent national emphasis on increased physical activity, reports of this condition may increase.

Prevalence

The overall prevalence of IgE-mediated food allergies for all age groups is likely in the range of 3.5–4.0% for the United States. A recent analysis of the prevalence of food allergies revealed that the evidence basis was remarkably weak (Rona et al., 2007). For example, few epidemiologi-cal investigations involving clinical confirmation of IgE-mediated food allergies have been conducted using representative groups of adults. Most clinical investigations on the prevalence of IgE-mediated food allergies among adults have involved groups of patients seen at allergy clinics. Such selected groups of adults are unlikely to represent the entire population, and the prevalence rates for these groups are likely to be higher than for the general population. A large-scale epidemiological investigation of the prevalence of IgE-mediated food allergy was conducted in The Netherlands (Neistijl Jansen et al., 1994). This study revealed that although >10% of Dutch adults believed that they had adverse reactions to foods, the prevalence of these reactions was ~2% when clinical histories were confirmed by blinded food challenges (Neistijl Jansen et al., 1994). The prevalence rate for IgE-mediated food allergies among infants and young children is more clearly defined and is likely considerably higher than for adults (Sampson, 1990). Clinical trials among groups of unselected infants suggest that the prevalence of IgE-mediated food allergies is in the range of 4–8% (Bock et al., 1978; Sampson, 2004). Despite the lack of clinical epidemiological trials among adults, recent surveys conducted in the United States, Canada, and England indicate that the self-perceived prevalence of peanut allergy alone is 0.5–0.8% among all age groups (Emmett et al., 1999; Ben-Shoshan et al., 2010; Sicherer et al., 2010). Surveys in the United States of the self-perceived prevalence of tree nut, fish, and crustacean shellfish allergies indicate that 0.5%, 0.4%, and 1.9%, respectively, believe that they have these particular food allergies (Sicherer et al., 2004, 2010). These surveys did not include clinical investigations to confirm that peanut, tree nut, fish, or crustacean shellfish allergies truly existed in these individuals. Because these food allergies are often rather profound, overestimates associated with reliance on self-diagnosis are probably minimal. If the prevalence of these four food allergies is estimated at 3.4% and the prevalence of all food allergies among infants is 4–8%, then an overall estimate for IgE-mediated food allergies of 3.5–4.0% seems reasonable.

Persistence

Many food-allergic infants outgrow their food allergies within a few months to several years after the onset of the sensitivity (Sampson, 1996). Allergies to certain foods, such as cows' milk, are more commonly outgrown than are allergies to certain other foods such as peanut. Allergies to peanuts were considered to be a lifelong affliction until recently when clinical researchers have demonstrated that peanut allergy, especially when acquired very early in life, can be outgrown (Skolnick *et al.*, 2001), although that does not seem to be a frequent occurrence. While milk and egg allergy are more frequently outgrown than peanut allergy, recent studies have documented that these allergies are increasingly persistent in a sub-group of patients with milk and egg allergy (Savage *et al.*, 2007; Skripak *et al.*, 2007). The mechanisms involved in the loss of sensitivity to specific foods are not precisely known, but the development of immunological tolerance is definitely involved (Ko and Mayer, 2005).

Prevention of Sensitization

IgE-mediated food allergies are most likely to develop in high-risk infants – those born to parents with histories of allergic disease of any type (pollens, mold spores, animal danders, bee venoms, food, etc.). Preventing the development of food allergies in such infants has been a subject of great interest. Various strategies have been investigated. The restriction of the diet of the mother during pregnancy (excluding commonly allergenic foods such as peanuts) does not appear to help prevent allergy in the infant (Lack and Du Toit, 2008). These observations suggest that sensitization does not occur in utero. Breastfeeding for extended periods of time appears to delay but may not prevent the development of IgE-mediated food allergies (Zeiger and Heller, 1995), and infants can be sensitized to allergenic foods through exposure to the allergens in breast milk (Van Asperen *et al.*, 1983). Apparently, allergenic food proteins can resist digestion, can be absorbed at least to a small extent from the small intestine, and can be secreted in breast milk, leading to sensitization. The exclusion of certain commonly allergenic foods from the maternal diet during the lactation period will help to prevent sensitization through breast milk. The elimination of peanuts from the diet of lactating women with high-risk infants is often recommended, but milk and eggs are usually considered to be too important nutritionally to exclude from the diets of lactating women. The use of probiotics during lactation may also help to lessen the likelihood of allergic sensitization (Kirjavainen *et al.*, 1999). Hypoallergenic infant formula may also prevent the development of food allergies in high-risk infants (Businco *et al.*, 1993), although these formulas are more often used to prevent reactions after sensitization has already occurred. The use of partial whey hydrolysate

formula has been advocated because the partial hydrolysate is more likely to prevent sensitization than a formula based on whole milk (Vandenplas *et al.*, 1995). High-risk infants may still develop food allergies once solid foods are introduced into the diet (Zeiger and Heller, 1995).

Common Allergenic Foods and International Lists

Eight foods or food groups – milk, eggs, fish, Crustacea (shrimp, crab, lobster, etc.), peanuts, soybeans, tree nuts (walnuts, almonds, hazelnuts, etc.), and wheat – are responsible for the vast majority of IgE-mediated food allergies worldwide (FAO, 1995), but regional differences exist. Examples of food allergies that occur more frequently in certain parts of the world than in others would include celery allergy in Europe (Wuthrich *et al.*, 1990), sesame seed allergy in several areas of the world (Kanny *et al.*, 1996; Sporik and Hill, 1996), and buckwheat allergy in Japan (Ebisawa *et al.*, 2003). These regional differences likely relate to food preferences in those areas and sometimes to coexistent pollen allergies (e.g. celery allergy in individuals sensitized to mugwort pollen). Beyond the eight major foods or food groups, >160 other foods have been documented to cause IgE-mediated food allergies (Hefle *et al.*, 1996). Because food allergens are proteins, any food that contains protein is likely to elicit allergic sensitization on at least rare occasions. The eight most commonly allergenic foods or food groups contain comparatively high amounts of protein and are commonly consumed in the diet. However, several other commonly consumed foods with high protein contents, such as beef, pork, chicken, and turkey, are rarely allergenic.

Ingredients derived from the commonly allergenic foods will also be allergenic if they contain sufficient residual protein from the source material. The most common questions concerning food ingredients involve edible oils, protein hydrolysates, lecithin, flavors, gelatin, spices, and colors. The passage of the Food Allergen Labeling and Consumer Protection Act of 2004 (FALCPA) mandates source labeling of ingredients derived from commonly allergenic sources with few exceptions (highly refined oils and ingredients that become exempt through notifications or petitions that must be approved by the US Food and Drug Administration). Similar ingredient labeling regulations exist in other parts of the world including the European Union, Canada, Australia, and New Zealand, although differences do occur in the lists of commonly allergenic foods among different countries or regions.

When edible oils are highly refined through a process that involves hot solvent extraction with bleaching and deodorizing, virtually all of the protein is removed from the source material. Clinical challenge trials have shown that highly refined oils from peanut, soybean, and sunflower seed are safe for ingestion by individuals allergic to the source material through use of clinical challenge trials (Crevel *et al.*, 2000). Oils from other sources such as sesame seed and tree nuts may receive less processing and contain allergenic residues (Kanny *et al.*, 1996; Teuber *et al.*, 1997). Cold-pressed oils may also contain allergenic residues (Hoffman and Collins-Williams, 1994).

Protein hydrolysates are often obtained from commonly allergenic sources: soybean, wheat, milk, and peanuts. Several processes, including acid hydrolysis and enzymatic hydrolysis, are used to obtain these hydrolysates. The degree of hydrolysis of the proteins in hydrolysates varies according to the functional use, source, and method of hydrolysis. If the proteins are only partially hydrolyzed, they are likely to retain their allergenicity. If they are extensively hydrolyzed, they may be safe for most individuals allergic to the source material. However, even extensively hydrolyzed casein in hypoallergenic infant formula has triggered allergic reactions in some infants exquisitely sensitive to milk (Nilsson *et al.*, 1999). Infant formulas based upon partial whey hydrolysates are even more likely to elicit allergic reactions in infants allergic to milk (Businco *et al.*, 1989).

Lecithin can be derived from soybean, egg, rice, or sunflower seed, although soybean is by far the most common source. Commercial soy lecithin contains trace residues of soy proteins. The soy protein residues in lecithin include IgE-binding proteins (Müller *et al.*, 1998), but the levels may be insufficient to elicit allergic reactions in most soybean-allergic individuals. Many soybean-allergic individuals do not avoid lecithin.

Most flavoring formulations do not contain protein, and few formulations contain any components derived from allergenic sources (Taylor and Dormedy, 1998). Flavoring has only rarely caused well documented allergic reactions (Gern *et al.*, 1991; Taylor and Dormedy, 1998).

Gelatin is most frequently derived from beef and pork and is generally not considered allergenic when ingested. Gelatin can also be derived from fish, but fish gelatin is unlikely to elicit reactions in fish-allergic individuals (Hansen *et al.*, 2004).

Spices are rare causes of allergic reactions (Niinimaki *et al.*, 1989). A few spices have been occasionally implicated in allergic reactions including mustard (Rance *et al.*, 2001) and fenugreek, a common component of curry (Faeste *et al.*, 2009). Avoidance of specific spices in the diet can be quite difficult.

None of the colorants used in foods are derived from commonly allergenic sources. However, the natural colorants, carmine and annatto, contain protein residues, and both have been implicated in rare allergic reactions (Lucas *et al.*, 2001).

Many other food ingredients are derived from commonly allergenic sources, e.g. phytosterols, vitamin E, and isoflavones from soybean, lactose, butter acid and butter esters from milk, and isinglass and fish oil from fish. FALCPA and similar legislation or regulation in other countries mandates the source labeling of all of these ingredients. Many of these ingredients are not known to pose hazards to individuals allergic to the source food, although clinical evidence of the lack of allergenicity is typically not available. Source labeling of these ingredients will further restrict the dietary choices for food-allergic consumers.

Food Allergens

Food allergens are almost always naturally occurring proteins (Breiteneder and Mills, 2008). Foods contain hundreds of thousands of different proteins, and only a small percentage are known allergens. The major allergens have been identified, purified, and characterized for most of the commonly allergenic foods (Breiteneder and Mills, 2008). Multiple allergenic proteins exist in some commonly allergenic foods. Foods may contain both major and minor allergens. Major allergens are defined as proteins that bind to serum IgE antibodies from >50% of patients with a specific food allergy. For example, milk contains three major allergens: casein, β-lactoglobulin, and α-lactalbumin (Wal, 2002). These also happen to be the major milk proteins. Milk may also contain several minor allergens, e.g. bovine serum albumin, although the level of evidence for clinical relevance is less convincing for these minor allergens (Baldo, 1984). Peanuts contain at least three major allergens, named *Ara h* 1, *Ara h* 2, and *Ara h* 3 (Breiteneder and Mills, 2008). Peanuts also contain numerous minor allergens (Bannon *et al.*, 2000). In contrast, codfish (*Gad c* 1), Brazil nut (*Ber e* 1), and shrimp (*Pen a* 1) contain primarily one major allergenic protein (Breiteneder and Mills, 2008).

Treatment – Pharmacological, Immunotherapy, and Avoidance Diets

Pharmacological approaches (epinephrine and antihistamines) are available for treating the symptoms of an allergic reaction (Wang and Sampson, 2007). Antihistamines are often used to treat the symptoms of mild to moderate food allergy reactions. However, epinephrine is the drug of choice to treat severe anaphylactic reactions to foods. Immunotherapeutic approaches are under development, show some promise, but remain experimental. The first of the immunotherapeutic approaches involved administration of anti-IgE antibodies (Leung *et al.*, 2003). More recently, oral and sublingual immunotherapies have shown initial promise (Burks *et al.*, 2008). However, at present, avoidance diets remain as the mainstay approach for preventing allergic reactions to foods (Taylor *et al.*, 1999). For example, if allergic to peanuts, simply avoid peanuts in all forms.

Threshold Doses

Practical experience demonstrates that exposure to trace levels of the offending food can elicit adverse reactions. Anecdotal reports suggest that reactions could occur from exposure to the small quantities through using shared utensils or containers, kissing the lips of someone who has eaten the offending food, opening packages of the offending food, or inhalation of vapors from the offending food. Although these situations are not well documented, the amount of the offending food that would be ingested from such occurrences would be quite low. Other episodes have been more thoroughly documented. Allergic reactions have occurred to peanut protein in sunflower seed butter prepared on equipment used for peanut butter (Yunginger *et al.*, 1983), milk protein in sorbet manufactured with equipment also used for ice cream (Laoprasert *et al.*, 1998), and milk protein in tofutti manufactured with equipment also used for ice cream (Gern *et al.*, 1991). Although complete avoidance must be maintained, threshold doses do exist below which allergic individuals will not experience adverse reactions (Taylor *et al.*, 2002, 2010). Recent evidence suggests that the threshold dose for peanuts is in the low milligram range with an ED_{10} (minimal eliciting dose for 10% of peanut-allergic subjects) of 14.4 mg of whole peanuts (Taylor *et al.*, 2010). The most sensitive individuals reacted to as little as 0.4 mg of whole peanuts, and individual peanut thresholds varied over several orders of magnitude (Taylor *et al.*, 2010). The possibility exists that the threshold doses will not be the same for every allergenic food, but this remains to be fully elucidated.

Cross-Reactions

In the construction of safe and effective avoidance diets, questions often arise regarding the need to avoid closely related foods. For some foods, cross-reactions do seem to occur with closely related foods. For example, shrimp-allergic individuals will also typically be sensitive to other crustaceans including crab and lobster (Daul *et al.*, 1993). Similarly, cross-reactions commonly occur between different species of avian eggs (Langeland, 1983) and between milk from cows and goats (Bernard *et al.*, 1999). In contrast, some peanut-allergic individuals are allergic to other legumes such as soybean (Herian *et al.*, 1990), but this is not common. Clinical hypersensitivity to one legume, such as peanuts or soybeans, does not warrant exclusion of the entire legume family from the diet unless allergy to each individual legume is confirmed by clinical challenge trials (Bernhisel-Broadbent and Sampson, 1989). However, there are a few instances with legumes where cross-reactions become a more serious concern. The best example would be cross-reactions between lupine and peanut (Moneret-Vautrin *et al.*, 1999).

Cross-reactions are also known to occur between certain types of pollens and foods. Examples would include ragweed pollen and melons, mugwort pollen and celery, mugwort pollen and hazelnut, and birch pollen and various foods including carrots, apples, hazelnuts, and potatoes (Van Ree, 2004).

Cross-reactions are also known to occur between allergies to natural rubber latex and banana, chestnut, avocado, and kiwi among others (Blanco *et al.*, 1994).

Effect of Processing on Allergenicity

Allergenic food proteins are remarkably stable to food processing conditions (Taylor and Lehrer, 1996; Mills and Mackie, 2008). As noted earlier, proteins can be removed from products derived from allergenic sources; the highly refined edible oils are the best example. Most allergenic food proteins are quite stable to heat so that typical heat processing conditions do not affect the allergenicity of the resulting products (Taylor and Lehrer, 1996). Some exceptions are certain fruit and vegetable allergens that are sensitive to heat (Jankiewicz *et al.*, 1997), and fish allergens, which may be destroyed by canning but not other heat processes (Bernhisel-Broadbent *et al.*, 1992). Food allergens also tend to be resistant to proteolysis (Bannon *et al.*,

2002), which allows them to survive digestive processes and arrive in the intestine in immunologically active form. The resistance to proteolysis means that these allergens may survive, in whole or in part, the acid and enzymatic hydrolysis methods used to prepare protein hydrolysates (Taylor and Lehrer, 1996).

Impact of Agricultural Biotechnology

Concerns have arisen regarding the possible allergenicity of foods developed through agricultural biotechnology (Goodman *et al.*, 2005). Genetic modifications result in the transfer of one or more genes from one biological source to another. These genes code for specific proteins. Because food allergens are usually proteins, these novel proteins have some potential to be or become allergens. Millions of proteins exist in nature, including many in foods, and only a small percentage are allergens, so the probability of transferring a protein with allergenic potential into a transgenic food is quite small. Several strategies have been developed to assess the likelihood of allergenicity of these novel proteins from genetically modified foods (Goodman *et al.*, 2005). Certainly, the probability of transferring an allergen is enhanced if the gene is derived from a known allergenic source. The reliability of allergy assessment strategies was documented with the discovery that a gene from Brazil nuts cloned into soybeans to enhance the methionine content of soybeans coded for the major allergen from Brazil nuts, *Ber e* 1 (Nordlee *et al.*, 1996); commercialization of that transgenic variety of soybeans was immediately halted.

Cell-Mediated Allergy

Delayed hypersensitivities are cell-mediated allergic reactions and involve tissue-bound T lymphocytes that are sensitized to a specific foodborne substance that triggers the reaction (Taylor and Hefle, 2001). These reactions often result in localized tissue inflammation. In such reactions, symptoms begin to appear 6–24 hours after consumption of the offending food.

Celiac Disease

Celiac disease – also known as celiac sprue, non-tropical sprue, or gluten-sensitive enteropathy – is a malabsorption syndrome occurring in sensitive individuals upon the consumption of wheat, rye, barley, triticale, spelt, and kamut (Taylor and Hefle, 2001; Rubio-Tapia and Murray, 2008).

Celiac disease is characterized by mucosal damage in the small intestine resulting from consumption of the offending grains or protein-containing products derived from those grains (Rubio-Tapia and Murray, 2008). This mucosal damage leads to nutrient malabsorption. The loss of absorptive function along with the ongoing inflammatory process results in diarrhea, bloating, weight loss, anemia, bone pain, chronic fatigue, weakness, muscle cramps, and, in children, failure to gain weight and growth retardation (Taylor and Hefle, 2001). Evidence suggests that intraepithelial T cells in the small intestine are involved in the inflammatory mechanism occurring with celiac disease (Maiuri *et al.*, 1996). The precise role of the intestinal T cells in celiac disease remains to be defined.

Celiac disease is an inherited trait, although its inheritance is complex (Taylor and Hefle, 2001). It occurs in ~5% of first-degree relatives of celiac patients, and ~75% of monozygotic twin pairs are concordant for it (Holtmeier *et al.*, 1997). Histocompatibility locus antigen (HLA) class II genes are the major genes associated with celiac disease, but concordance for celiac disease is only 25–40% in siblings who are identical for one or both HLA haplotypes. Thus, genes outside of the HLA locus likely have some as yet undefined role in disease susceptibility.

The exact prevalence of celiac disease is a matter of some debate. Prevalence estimates from different parts of the world are complicated by use of different diagnostic approaches. Celiac disease appears to be latent or asymptomatic in some individuals whose symptoms only appear occasionally (Duggan, 1997; Rubio-Tapia and Murray, 2008). The prevalence of celiac disease appears to be highest in certain European regions and in Australia (Logan, 1992), occurring in about 1 in every 250 people. Even within European populations, considerable variability is observed in the prevalence of celiac disease (Logan, 1992). In the United States, symptomatic celiac disease occurs in about 1 of every 3000 individuals (Taylor and Hefle, 2001), but 1 in every 133 individuals may be at risk for development of symptoms (Fasano *et al.*, 2001). Recently, gluten-free foods have become quite popular in the United States, leading to the widespread belief that the prevalence of celiac disease is increasing. Many consumers of gluten-free foods are selecting these foods without a confirmed diagnosis of celiac disease or a serological indication that they may be at risk for development of celiac disease. In reality, the prevalence may not have changed but both awareness and diagnostic confirmation have increased.

Celiac disease is associated with the ingestion of gliadin from wheat and related prolamin proteins from other grains (Taylor and Hefle, 2001). The prolamin fraction of wheat is known as gluten; hence celiac disease is sometimes called gluten-sensitive enteropathy. A defect in mucosal processing of gliadin in celiac patients provokes the generation of toxic peptides that contribute to the abnormal T-cell response and the subsequent inflammatory reaction (Inman-Felton, 1999). The mechanism involved in celiac disease and the exact role of gliadin remain to be determined.

The tolerance for wheat, rye, barley, and related grains among celiac sufferers is unknown. Clearly, the threshold dose may vary from one individual to another because, in latent forms of celiac disease, normal dietary quantities of the offending grains seem to cause little problem. Many celiac sufferers attempt to avoid all sources of these grains, including a wide variety of common food ingredients derived from these grains (Taylor, 2009). Most of these individuals also avoid oats, although the role of oats in the elicitation of celiac disease was refuted (Janatuinen *et al.*, 1995). Because oats are often contaminated with wheat in commerce, some caution may still be necessary. Although evidence is scant, spelt and kamut, which are basically varieties of wheat, are likely to trigger celiac disease in susceptible individuals.

The risk of death as a direct result of celiac disease is low (Corrao *et al.*, 2001), but individuals suffering from celiac disease for prolonged periods are at increased risk for development of T-cell lymphoma (Meijer *et al.*, 2004). Celiac patients also appear more likely to have various other autoimmune diseases including dermatitis herpetiformis, thyroid diseases, Addison's disease, pernicious anemia, autoimmune thrombocytopenia, sarcoidosis, insulin-dependent diabetes mellitus, and IgA nephropathy (McGough and Cummings, 2005; Rubio-Tapia and Murray, 2008).

Food Intolerances

In contrast to true food allergies, food intolerances involve one of several non-immunological mechanisms. The distinction between food allergies and intolerances is important with respect to treatment as well as mechanism. Individuals with various types of food intolerances are typically able to tolerate some amount of the offending substance in their diet. In contrast, the threshold doses for the offending food with true food allergies are quite small.

Thus, the management of food intolerances is much easier. With a few very notable exceptions, little research has been conducted on food intolerances. In many cases, the cause-and-effect relationship between ingestion of the offending food or food ingredient and the adverse reaction has not been carefully established.

Anaphylactoid Reactions
Anaphylactoid reactions are a non-IgE-mediated release of mediators from mast cells and basophils (Taylor and Hefle, 2001). Because the same mediators are involved as in true IgE-mediated food allergies, the symptoms are quite similar. Although anaphylactoid reactions are documented with adverse reactions to drugs, no proof exists that anaphylactoid reactions occur with foods.

Metabolic Food Disorders
Metabolic food disorders occur as the result of genetically determined metabolic deficiencies that either affect the ability to metabolize a specific substance in foods or heighten sensitivity to a particular foodborne chemical (Taylor and Hefle, 2001). Lactose intolerance is an example of a metabolic food disorder (Taylor and Hefle, 2001). Inborn errors of metabolism such as phenylketonuria could be discussed within this context as some of them do respond to dietary restrictions. Conditions such as phenylketonuria are much more serious than lactose intolerance and involve special clinical oversight. They will not be discussed further in this chapter.

Lactose intolerance is associated with a deficiency of the enzyme, β-galactosidase (lactase), in the intestinal tract that leads to an inability to metabolize lactose from milk and other dairy products (Suarez and Savaiano, 1997). The symptoms of lactose intolerance are mild and are confined to the gastrointestinal tract, and include abdominal discomfort, flatulence, and frothy diarrhea (Suarez and Savaiano, 1997). Lactose intolerance affects a large number of people worldwide with a frequency as high as 60–90% among blacks, Native Americans, Hispanics, Asians, Jews, and Arabs (Taylor and Hefle, 2001). In contrast, the prevalence among North American Caucasians is ~6–12% (Taylor and Hefle, 2001). The usual treatment for lactose intolerance is the avoidance of dairy products containing lactose, but lactose-intolerant individuals can tolerate some lactose in their diets (Taylor and Hefle, 2001) and most have virtually no symptoms on consumption of the amount of lactose in 235 mL (1 cup) of milk (Taylor and Hefle, 2001). Additionally, some dairy products (e.g. yogurt, acidophilus milk) are better tolerated than others, apparently because they contain bacteria with β-galactosidase (Taylor and Hefle, 2001). Thus, lactose intolerance is a manageable condition.

Food Idiosyncrasies

Food idiosyncrasies are adverse reactions to foods or food ingredients that occur through unknown mechanisms. The best example of an idiosyncratic reaction is sulfite-induced asthma (Taylor *et al.*, 2008). Cause and effect are well established for sulfite-induced asthma but have not been well established in other types of food idiosyncrasies. Psychosomatic illnesses are also included in this category.

Sulfites are common food additives that also occur naturally in certain foods, especially fermented foods, usually in small amounts (Taylor *et al.*, 2008). Although asthma is the only well established symptom associated with sulfite sensitivity, only a small percentage of asthmatics are sulfite sensitive (Taylor *et al.*, 2008). Individuals with severe asthma who require steroids for control of symptoms are the primary risk group for sulfite sensitivity, but only ~5% of these are sulfite sensitive (Taylor *et al.*, 2008). Sulfite-induced asthma can be quite severe, and deaths have been documented (Taylor *et al.*, 2008). Sulfites added to foods must be declared on product labels so avoidance diets are reasonably easy to develop (Taylor *et al.*, 2008). Sulfite-sensitive individuals with asthma can tolerate the ingestion of small quantities of sulfite, especially when the sulfites are incorporated in certain types of foods (Taylor *et al.*, 1988). Although sulfite-induced asthma poses a considerable risk to sensitive individuals, this condition is manageable once it is recognized.

Many of the other idiosyncratic reactions also involve various food additives. Examples include tartrazine (a commonly used food colorant also known as FD&C Yellow 5) in asthma and/or chronic urticaria, other food colors in chronic urticaria, monosodium glutamate (a commonly used flavor enhancer) in asthma and monosodium glutamate symptom complex, and aspartame in migraine headache and urticaria (Bush and Taylor, 2009). Although tartrazine has been implicated in the elicitation of asthma and chronic urticaria for several decades, criticisms have arisen regarding the design of the clinical studies (Bush and Taylor, 2009). Both asthma and chronic urticaria are chronic conditions that are likely to flare at unpredicted times in susceptible individuals, many of whom take various medications continually to control symptoms. In the clinical studies, medications were withdrawn from the patients for variable periods before the challenges, which were often not blinded. When the symptoms were exacerbated, the investigators concluded that tartrazine was responsible. However, the alternative explanation might be that the symptoms flared simply because critical medications were withdrawn. In studies where some of the medications were continued, tartrazine challenges had no effect on similar patients (Bush and Taylor, 2009).

Monosodium glutamate symptom complex, a mild subjective illness, has not been confirmed by double-blind, placebo-controlled food challenges (Kenny, 1986; Bush and Taylor, 2009), and a national panel concluded that the role of monosodium glutamate in the elicitation of the complex was not proven, especially at doses <3 g (Raiten *et al.*, 1995). Monosodium glutamate has also been implicated as a causative factor in asthma, but the clinical studies linking it to asthma are subject to the same criticisms as mentioned for tartrazine (Bush and Taylor, 2009).

Future Directions

Although research on food allergies has increased in recent years, much uncertainty remains. The prevalence of true food allergies is not well understood in many countries including the United States, although a recently completed EU project called EuroPrevall holds considerable promise to improve the understanding of prevalence in that part of the world. The factors involved in sensitization certainly merit more attention. Oral tolerance to food proteins is the norm but we do not yet understand why tolerance does not develop in certain individuals, why certain proteins are more likely to become allergens, and the role of dietary practices in preventing sensitization. If IgE-mediated food allergies are increasing in prevalence as appearances indicate, that increases the importance of understanding the factors involved in the increase. The minimal threshold doses needed to provoke an adverse reaction in individuals with IgE-mediated food allergies need better understanding. Considerable variation exists among individuals with respect to individual threshold doses, and differences may also exist between different allergenic foods. A more complete understanding of individual and population threshold doses is needed to provide clear guidance for the protection of food-allergic consumers. The identity of many food allergens is known, but improved methods are needed to determine whether or not novel proteins introduced into the diet as part of novel foods, including genetically modified foods, have the potential to become new allergens. With respect to food intolerances, basic information such as the mechanism of sulfite-induced asthma is not available, and the cause-and-effect relationship between various food additives and possible food intolerances requires better elucidation.

Suggestions for Further Reading

Adkinson, N.F., Busse, W.W., Bochner, B.S., *et al.* (eds) (2009) *Middleton's Allergy – Principles and Practice*, 7th Edn. Mosby, St. Louis, MO.

Freeman, H.J., Chopra, A., Clandinin, M.T., *et al.* (2011) Recent advances in celiac disease. *World J Gastroenterol* 17, 2259–2272.

Metcalfe, D.D., Sampson, H.A., and Simon, R.A. (eds) (2008) *Food Allergy – Adverse Reactions to Foods and Food Additives*, 4th Edn. Blackwell Science, Malden, MA.

References

Baldo, B.A. (1984) Milk allergies. *Aust J Dairy Technol* **39**, 120–128.

Bannon, G.A., Besler, M., Hefle, S.L., *et al.* (2008) Peanut (*Arachis hypogaea*). *Int Symp Food Allergens* **2**, 87–122.

Bannon, G.A., Goodman, R.E., Leach, J.N., *et al.* (2002) Digestive stability in the context of assessing the potential allergenicity of food proteins. *Comments Toxicol* **8**, 271–275.

Ben-Shoshan, M., Harrington, D.W., Soller, L., *et al.* (2010) A population-based study on peanut, tree nut, fish, shellfish, and sesame allergy prevalence in Canada. *J Allergy Clin Immunol* **125**, 1327–1335.

Bernard, H., Creminon, C., Negroni, L., *et al.* (1999) IgE cross-reactivity with caseins from different species in humans allergic to cows' milk. *Food Agric Immunol* **11**, 101–111.

Bernhisel-Broadbent, J. and Sampson, H.A. (1989) Cross-allergenicity in the legume botanical family in children with food hypersensitivity. *J Allergy Clin Immunol* **83**, 435–440.

Bernhisel-Broadbent, J., Strause, D., and Sampson, H.A. (1992) Fish hypersensitivity. II. Clinical relevance of altered fish allergenicity caused by various preparation methods. *J Allergy Clin Immunol* **90**, 622–629.

Blanco, C., Carrillo, T., Castillo, R., *et al.* (1994) Latex allergy: clinical features and cross-reactivity with fruits. *Ann Allergy* **73**, 309–314.

Bock, S.A., Lee, W.Y., Remigio, L.K., *et al.* (1978) Studies of hypersensitivity reactions to foods in infants and children. *J Allergy Clin Immunol* **62**, 327–334.

Bock, S.A., Munoz-Furlong, A., and Sampson, H.A. (2007) Further fatalities caused by anaphylactic shock, 2001–2006. *J Allergy Clin Immunol* **119**, 1016–1018.

Breiteneder, H. and Mills, E.N.C. (2008) Food allergens: molecular and immunological characteristics. In D.D. Metcalfe, H.A. Sampson, and R.A. Simon (eds), *Food Allergy: Adverse Reactions to Foods and Food Additives*, 4th Edn. Blackwell Publishing, Malden, MA, pp. 43–61.

Burks, W. and Ballmer-Weber, B.K. (2006) Food allergy. *Mol Nutr Food Res* **50**, 595–603.

Burks, A.W., Laubach, S., and Jones, S.M. (2008) Oral tolerance, food allergy, and immunotherapy: implications for future treatments. *J Allergy Clin Immunol* **121**, 1344–1350.

Bush, R.K. and Taylor, S.L. (2009) Adverse reactions to food and drug additives. In N.F. Adkinson, W.W. Busse, B.S. Bochner, *et al.* (eds), *Middleton's Allergy: Principles and Practice*, Vol. 2, 7th Edn. Mosby, St. Louis, MO, pp. 1169–1187.

Businco, L., Cantani, A., Longhi, M., *et al.* (1989) Anaphylactic reactions to a cow milk whey protein hydrolysate (Alfa-Re Nestlé) in infants with cow's milk allergy. *Ann Allergy* **62**, 333–335.

Businco, L., Dreborg, S., Einarsson, R., *et al.* (1993) Hydrolysed cow's milk formulae. Allergenicity and use in treatment and prevention. An ESPACI position paper. *Pediatr Allergy Immunol* **4**, 101–111.

Corrao, G., Corazza, G.R., Bagnardi, V., *et al.* (2001) Mortality in patients with celiac disease and their relatives: a cohort study. *Lancet* **358**, 356–361.

Crevel, R.W.R., Kerkhoff, M.A.T., and Koning, M.M.G. (2000) Allergenicity of refined vegetable oil. *Food Chem Toxicol* **38**, 385–393.

Daul, C.B., Morgan, J.E., and Lehrer, S.B. (1993) Hypersensitivity reactions to crustacea and mollusks. *Clin Rev Allergy* **11**, 201–222.

Duggan, J.M. (1997) Recent developments in our understanding of adult coeliac disease. *Med J Aust* **166**, 312–315.

Ebisawa, M., Ikematsu, K., Imai, T., *et al.* (2003) Food allergy in Japan. *Allergy Clin Immunol Int* **15**, 214–217.

Emmett, S.E., Angus, F.J., Fry, J.S., *et al.* (1999) Perceived prevalence of peanut allergy in Great Britain and its association with other atopic conditions and with peanut allergy in other household members. *Allergy* **54**, 380–385.

Faeste, C.K., Namork, E., and Lindvik, H. (2009) Allergenicity and antigenicity of fenugreek (*Trigonella foenum-graecum*) proteins in foods. *J Allergy Clin Immunol* **123**, 187–194.

Fasano, A., Berti, I., Gerarduzzi, T., *et al.* (2001) Prevalence of celiac disease in at-risk and not-at-risk groups in the United States. *Arch Intern Med* **163**, 286–292.

Food and Agricultural Organization of the United Nations (1995) *Report of the FAO Technical Consultation on Food Allergies*. FAO, Rome, November 13–14.

Gern, J.E., Yang, E., Evrard, H.M., *et al.* (1991) Allergic reactions to milk-contaminated "non-dairy" products. *N Engl J Med* **324**, 976–979.

Goodman, R.E., Hefle, S.L., Taylor, S.L., *et al.* (2005) Assessing genetically modified crops to minimize the risk of increased food allergy: a review. *Int Arch Allergy Immunol* **137**, 153–166.

Hansen, T.K., Poulsen, L.K., Skov, P., *et al.* (2004) A randomized, double-blind, placebo-controlled oral challenge study to evaluate the allergenicity of commercial, food-grade fish gelatin. *Food Chem Toxicol* **42**, 2037–2044.

Hefle, S.L., Nordlee, J.A., and Taylor, S.L. (1996) Allergenic foods. *Crit Rev Food Sci Nutr* **36**, S69–S89.

Herian, A.M., Taylor, S.L., and Bush, R.K. (1990) Identification of soybean allergens by immunoblotting with sera from soy-allergic adults. *Int Arch Allergy Appl Immunol* **92**, 193–198.

Hoffman, D.R. and Collins-Williams, C. (1994) Cold-pressed peanut oils may contain peanut allergen. *J Allergy Clin Immunol* **93**, 801–802.

Holtmeier, W., Rowell, D.L., Nyberg, A., *et al.* (1997) Distinct δ T cell receptor repertoires in monozygotic twins concordant for coeliac disease. *Clin Exp Immunol* **107**, 148–157.

Hourihane, J.O'B., Dean, T.P., and Warner, J.O. (1996) Peanut allergy in relation to heredity, maternal diet, and other atopic diseases: results of a questionnaire survey, skin prick testing, and food challenge. *BMJ* **313**, 518–521.

Inman-Felton, A.E. (1999) Overview of gluten sensitive enteropathy (celiac sprue). *J Am Diet Assoc* **99**, 352–362.

Janatuinen, E.K., Pikkarainen, P.H., Kemppainen, T.A., *et al.* (1995) A comparison of diets with and without oats in adults with celiac disease. *N Engl J Med* **333**, 1033–1037.

Jankiewicz, A., Baltes, W., Bogl, K., *et al.* (1997) Influence of food processing on the immunochemical stability of celery allergens. *J Sci Food Agric* **75**, 357–370.

Kanny, G., de Hauteclocque, C., and Moneret-Vautrin, D.A. (1996) Sesame seed and sesame seed oil contain masked allergens of growing importance. *Allergy* **51**, 952–957.

Kenney, R.A. (1986) The Chinese restaurant syndrome: an anecdote revisited. *Food Chem Toxicol* **24**, 351–354.

Kirjavainen, P.V., Apostolou, E., Salminen, S.J., *et al.* (1999) New aspects of probiotics – a novel approach in the management of food allergy. *Allergy* **54**, 909–915.

Ko, J. and Mayer, L. (2005) Oral tolerance: lessons on treatment of food allergy. *Eur J Gastroenterol Hepatol* **17**, 1299–1303.

Lack, G. and Du Toit, G. (2008) Prevention of food allergy. In D.D. Metcalfe, H.A. Sampson, and R.A. Simon (eds), *Food Allergy: Adverse Reactions to Foods and Food Additives*, 4th Edn. Blackwell Publishing, Malden, MA, pp. 470–481.

Langeland, T. (1983) A clinical and immunological study of allergy to hen's egg white. VI. Occurrence of proteins cross-reacting with allergens in hen's egg white as studied in egg white from turkey, duck, goose, seagull, and in hen egg yolk, and hen and chicken sera and flesh. *Allergy* **39**, 339–412.

Laoprasert, N., Wallen, N.D., Jones, R.T., *et al.* (1998) Anaphylaxis in a milk-allergic child following ingestion of lemon sorbet containing trace quantities of milk. *J Food Prot* **61**, 1522–1524.

Leung, D.Y.M., Sampson, H.A., Yunginger, J.W., *et al.* (2003) Effect of anti-IgE therapy in patients with peanut allergy. *N Engl J Med* **348**, 986–993.

Logan, R.F.A. (1992) Descriptive epidemiology of celiac disease. In D. Branksi, P. Rozen, and M.F. Kagnoff (eds), *Gluten-Sensitive Enteropathy, Frontiers in Gastrointestinal Research*, Vol. 19. Karger, Basel, pp. 1–14.

Lucas, C.D., Taylor, S.L., and Hallagan, J.B. (2001) The role of natural color additives in food allergy. *Adv Food Nutr Res* **43**, 195–216.

Maiuri, L., Picarella, A., Boirivant, M., *et al.* (1996) Definition of the initial immunologic modifications upon in vitro gliadin challenge in the small intestine of celiac patients. *Gastroenterology* **110**, 1368–1378.

McGough, N. and Cummings, J.H. (2005) Coeliac disease: a diverse clinical syndrome caused by intolerance to wheat, barley, and rye. *Proc Nutr Soc* **64**, 434–450.

Meijer, J.W., Mulder, C.J., Goerres, M.G., *et al.* (2004) Coeliac disease and (extra)intestinal T-cell lymphomas: definition, diagnosis, and treatment. *Scand J Gastroenterol Suppl* **241**, 78–84.

Mills, E.N.C. and Mackie, A.R. (2008) The impact of processing on allergenicity of food. *Curr Opin Allergy Clin Immunol* **8**, 249–253.

Moneret-Vautrin, D.A., Guerin, L., Kanny, G., *et al.* (1999) Cross-allergenicity of peanut and lupine: the risk of lupine allergy in patients allergic to peanut. *J Allergy Clin Immunol* **104**, 883–888.

Müller, U., Weber, W., Hoffmann, A., *et al.* (1998) Commercial soybean lecithins: a source of hidden allergens? *Z Lebensm Unters Forsch* **207**, 341–351.

Neistijl Jansen, J.J., Kardinaal, A.F.M., Huijbers, G., *et al.* (1994) Prevalence of food allergy and intolerance in the adult Dutch population. *J Allergy Clin Immunol* **93**, 446–456.

Niinimaki, A., Bjorksten, F., Puukka, M., *et al.* (1989) Spice allergy: results of skin prick tests and RAST with spice extracts. *Allergy* **44**, 60–65.

Nilsson, C., Oman, H., Hallden, G., *et al.* (1999) A case of allergy to cow's milk hydrolysate. *Allergy* **54**, 1322–1326.

Nordlee, J.A., Taylor, S.L., Townsend, J.A., *et al.* (1996) Identification of Brazil nut allergen in transgenic soybeans. *N Engl J Med* **334**, 688–692.

Pumphrey, R.S.H. and Gowland, H. (2007) Further fatal allergic reactions to foods in the United Kingdom, 1999–2006. *J Allergy Clin Immunol* **119**, 1018–1019.

Raiten, D.J., Talbot, J.M., and Fisher, K.D. (1995) *Analysis of Adverse Reactions to Monosodium Glutamate (MSG)*. Life Sciences Research Office, Federation of American Societies for Experimental Biology, Bethesda, MD.

Rance, F., Abbal, M., and Dutau, G. (2001) Mustard allergy in children. *Pediatr Pulmonol* **23**, 44–45.

Rona, R.J., Keil, T., Summers, C., *et al.* (2007) The prevalence of food allergy: a meta analysis. *J Allergy Clin Immunol* **120**, 638–646.

Rubio-Tapia, A. and Murray, J.A. (2008) Gluten-sensitive enteropathy. In D.D. Metcalfe, H.A. Sampson and R.A. Simon (eds), *Food Allergy: Adverse Reactions to Foods and Food Additives*, 4th Edn. Blackwell Publishing, Malden, MA, pp. 211–222.

Sampson, H.A. (1990) Food allergy. *Curr Opin Immunol* **2**, 542–547.

Sampson, H.A. (1996) Epidemiology of food allergy. *Pediatric Allergy and Immunol* **7**(Suppl 9), 42–50.

Sampson, H.A. (2003) Anaphylaxis and emergency treatment. *Pediatrics* **111**, 1601–1608.

Sampson, H.A. (2004) Update on food allergy. *J Allergy Clin Immunol* **113**, 805–819.

Sampson, H.A., Mendelson, L., and Rosen, J. (1992) Fatal and near-fatal anaphylactic reactions to foods in children and adolescents. *N Engl J Med* **327**, 380–384.

Savage, J.H., Matsui, E.C., Skripak, J.M., *et al.* (2007) The natural history of egg allergy. *J Allergy Clin Immunol* **120**, 1413–1417.

Sicherer, S.H., Furlong, T.J., Maes, H.H., *et al.* (2000) Genetics of peanut allergy: twin study. *J Allergy Clin Immunol* **106**, 53–56.

Sicherer, S.H., Munoz-Furlong, A., Godbold, J.H., *et al.* (2010) US prevalence of self-reported peanut, tree nut, and sesame allergy: 11-year follow-up. *J Allergy Clin Immunol* **125**, 1322–1326.

Sicherer, S.H., Munoz-Furlong, A., and Sampson, H.A. (2004) Prevalence of seafood allergy in the United States by a random telephone survey. *J Allergy Clin Immunol* **114**, 159–165.

Skolnick, H., Conover Walker, M.K., Barnes-Koerner, C, *et al.* (2001) The natural history of peanut allergy. *J Allergy Clin Immunol* **107**, 367–374.

Skripak, J.M., Matsui, E.C., Mudd, K., *et al.* (2007) The natural history of IgE-mediated cow's milk allergy. *J Allergy Clin Immunol* **120**, 1172–1177.

Sloan, A.E. and Powers, M.E. (1986) A perspective on popular perceptions of adverse reactions to foods. *J Allergy Clin Immunol* **78**, 127–133.

Sporik, R. and Hill, D. (1996) Allergy to peanuts, nuts, and sesame seed in Australian children. *BMJ* **313**, 1477–1478.

Suarez, F.L. and Savaiano, D.A. (1997) Diet, genetics, and lactose intolerance. *Food Technol* **51**, 74–76.

Taylor, S.L. (2009) Gluten-free ingredients. In E.K. Arendt and F. Dal Bello (eds), *The Science of Gluten-Free Foods and Beverages*. American Association. of Cereal Chemists International, St. Paul, MN, pp. 83–87.

Taylor, S.L. and Dormedy, E.S. (1998) The role of flavoring substances in food allergy and intolerance. *Adv Food Nutr Res* **42**, 1–44.

Taylor, S.L. and Hefle, S.L. (2001) Food allergies and other food sensitivities. *Food Technol* **55**, 68–83.

Taylor, S.L. and Lehrer, S.B. (1996) Principles and characteristics of food allergens. *Crit Rev Food Sci Nutr* **36**, S91–118.

Taylor, S.L., Bush, R.K., and Nordlee, J.A. (2008) Sulfites. In D.D. Metcalfe, H.A. Sampson, and R.A. Simon (eds), *Food Allergy: Adverse Reactions to Foods and Food Additives*, 4th Edn. Blackwell Publishing, Malden, MA, pp. 353–368.

Taylor, S.L., Bush, R.K., Selner, J.C., *et al.* (1988) Sensitivity to sulfited foods among sulfite-sensitive asthmatics. *J Allergy Clin Immunol* **81**, 1159–1167.

Taylor, S.L., Hefle, S.L., Bindslev-Jensen, C., *et al.* (2002) Factors affecting determination of threshold doses for allergenic foods: how much is too much? *J Allergy Clin Immunol* **109**, 24–30.

Taylor, S.L., Hefle, S.L., and Munoz-Furlong, A. (1999) Food allergies and avoidance diets. *Nutr Today* **34**, 15–22.

Taylor, S.L., Moneret-Vautrin, D.A., Crevel, R.W.R., *et al.* (2010) Threshold dose for peanut: risk characterization based upon diagnostic oral challenges of a series of 286 peanut-allergic individuals. *Food Chem Toxicol* **48**, 814–819.

Teuber, S.S., Brown, R.L., and Haapanen, L.A.D. (1997) Allergenicity of gourmet nut oils processed by different methods. *J Allergy Clin Immunol* **99**, 502–507.

Van Asperen, P.P., Kemp, A.S., and Mellis, C.M. (1983) Immediate food hypersensitivity reactions on the first known exposure to food. *Arch Dis Child* **58**, 253–256.

Van Ree, R. (2004) Clinical importance of cross-reactivity in food allergy. *Curr Opin Allergy Clin Immunol* **4**, 235–240.

Vandenplas, Y., Hauser, B., Van den Borre, C., *et al.* (1995) The long-term effect of a partial whey hydrolysate formula on the prophylaxis of atopic disease. *Eur J Pediatr* **154**, 488–494.

Wal, J.M. (2002) Cows' milk proteins/allergens. *Ann Allergy Asthma Immunol* **89**(Suppl), 3–10.

Wang, J. (2008) Oral allergy syndrome. In D.D. Metcalfe, H.A. Sampson, and R.A. Simon (eds), *Food Allergy: Adverse Reactions to Foods and Food Additives*, 4th Edn. Blackwell Publishing, Malden, MA, pp. 133–143.

Wang, J. and Sampson, H.A. (2007) Food anaphylaxis. *Clin Exp Allergy* **37**, 651–660.

Williams, A.N. and Simon, R.A. (2008) Food-dependent exercise- and pressure-induced syndromes. In D.D. Metcalfe, H.A. Sampson, and R.A. Simon (eds), *Food Allergy: Adverse Reactions to Foods and Food Additives*, 4th Edn. Blackwell Publishing, Malden, MA, pp. 584–595.

Wuthrich, B., Stager, J., and Johansson, S.G.O. (1990) Celery allergy associated with birch and mugwort pollenosis. *Allergy* **45,** 566–571.

Yunginger, J.W., Gauerke, M.B., Jones, R.T., *et al.* (1983) Use of radioimmunoassay to determine the nature, quantity and source of allergenic contamination of sunflower butter. *J Food Prot* **46,** 625–628.

Yunginger, J.W., Sweeney, K.G., Sturner, W.Q., *et al.* (1988) Fatal food-induced anaphylaxis. *JAMA* **260,** 1450–1452.

Zeiger, R.S. and Heller, S. (1995) The development and prediction of atopy in high-risk children: follow-up at seven years in a prospective randomized study of combined maternal and infant food allergy avoidance. *J Allergy Clin Immunol* **95,** 1179–1190.

72

FOOD BIOFORTIFICATION: BREEDING AND BIOTECHNOLOGY APPROACHES TO IMPROVE NUTRIENTS IN VEGETABLES AND OIL QUALITY IN SOYBEAN

PRASAD BELLUR[1], PhD, SHANTALA LAKKANNA[1], MSc, JAYA JOSHI[1], PhD, JOSEPH CORNELIUS[2], PhD, FEDERICO TRIPODI[2], PhD, AND SEKHAR BODDUPALLI[3], PhD

[1]*Monsanto Research Centre, Bangalore, India*
[2]*Monsanto Company, St Louis, Missouri, USA*
[3]*Monsanto Vegetable Seeds, Woodland, California, USA*

Summary

During the past 20 years there has been a dramatic increase in obesity and diabetes across the globe. Escalation in prevalence and progression of this global, diet-linked epidemic is generally attributed to caloric-rich, nutrient-poor diets, increase in the aging population, and a sedentary lifestyle. Significant scientific support exists that increased consumption of vegetables is associated with lower risk of chronic diet-linked diseases. In spite of the inherent nutritive value and need for enhanced consumption, there is not enough consumption of vegetables because of their perceived poor taste, appearance appeal, and convenience. Enhancing the levels of precursors to essential nutrients and phytonutrients in vegetables would have a favorable impact on consumer sensory appeal, at the same time delivering higher nutritional value. Significant opportunity exists to integrate advances in breeding, biotechnology, high-throughput analytical, and molecular nutrition tools to address unmet consumer need and meet global demands for agricultural productivity. Germplasm diversity for various consumer and agronomic traits along with whole-genome sequence information, molecular markers, biochemical pathway insights, and high-throughput phenotyping enable rapid innovation of new crop varieties for enhancing consumption and ensuring crop productivity. In this chapter we have attempted to review the genetic and biotechnology approaches to enhance a few essential nutrients and bioactive phytonutrients in vegetables that are associated with nutritive value and consumer appeal. Progress in improving soybean oil quality with reduced saturated fat, improved shelf life, and elevated beneficial omega-3 fatty acids is also briefly discussed.

Present Knowledge in Nutrition, Tenth Edition. Edited by John W. Erdman Jr, Ian A. Macdonald and Steven H. Zeisel.
© 2012 International Life Sciences Institute. Published 2012 by John Wiley & Sons, Inc.

Introduction

Epidemiological studies suggest that consumption of diets rich in fruits and vegetables is associated with a reduction in diet- and age-related chronic illness. Per capita consumption of fruits and vegetables is very low compared with that recommended across the globe. USDA estimates that 90–97% of the US population have an inadequate intake of well-recognized nutrients such as dietary fiber, vitamin E, potassium, etc. As the human population is predicted to be nearly 9 billion by 2050, sufficient quantities of nutritious crops need to be produced. Hence, there is an urgent need and growing interest in the development of nutritionally fortified crop varieties with higher yield to alleviate the global obesity epidemic and address malnutrition that still persists in developing countries (Connolly, 2008).

Essential nutrients are generally perceived to be dietary substances that impact growth and survival of an organism. Recent studies suggest that essential nutrients play a role beyond these basic needs, and impact biological processes associated with chronic illnesses due to systemic inflammation and oxidative stress. Folates, for example, are crucial for nucleotide biosynthesis and amino acid metabolism in human cells (Bassett *et al.*, 2005; Rébeillé *et al.*, 2006). The repercussions of insufficient dietary folate include perturbation of one-carbon (C1) metabolism, which contributes to reduced turnover of erythrocytes (megaloblastic anemia), birth defects (neural tube defects [NTD]), as well as elevated plasma homocysteine levels (an emerging risk factor for vascular diseases) (Scott *et al.*, 2000; Jang *et al.*, 2005). In addition to dietary fortification, biofortification in staple crops and vegetables would meet the demand for higher consumption of this essential nutrient from fresh foods.

Along similar lines, calcium deficiency is a significant problem globally because of the growth in aging populations. Prolonged calcium deficiency leads to reductions in bone mass and disability due to osteoporosis. Biofortification of calcium in fruits and vegetables would not only increase dietary levels but also deliver other synergistic phytonutrients in crops that impact bioavailability and bone metabolism.

Chronic oxidative stress and inflammation are implicated in the incidence and progression of illnesses such as cardiovascular disease, neurological disorders, cancer, cataracts, inflammatory diseases, and age-related macular degeneration (Bramley *et al.*, 2000). α-Tocopherol is commonly recognized as the antioxidant, vitamin E. Emerging scientific evidence suggests that γ-tocopherol, which is naturally abundant in soy and corn, possesses predominantly anti-inflammatory activity and lower antioxidant activity compared with α-tocopherol. Significant progress has been made in altering both the quality and quantity of these vitamin E congeners in crops using both biotechnology and breeding approaches.

Not only are vegetables rich sources of essential nutrients but they also contain several bioactive phytonutrients such as lycopene, anthocyanins, and beneficial glucosinolates. Several of these components have been studied in isolation for their putative health benefits. In new and emerging research, epidemiologic, cell-based, and preclinical animal studies reveal the role of anthocyanins in lowering the risk of cardiovascular disease, diabetes, arthritis, and cancer, as a result of their antioxidant and anti-inflammatory activities (Middleton, 1998). Thus, it is conceivable that the primary mode of action of these phytonutrients or bioactive dietary components may be to reduce the rate of age-related increases in inflammation, which predisposes tissues to a range of chronic conditions. This hypothesis is supported by mechanistic studies in animal models and, to a lesser extent, by human intervention studies. Development of plant varieties with a combination of phytonutrients along with the essential nutrients, using breeding and biotechnology tools, would enable evaluation of their effects on human health and wellness in a whole-diet context rather than in isolation.

In addition to nutrition and health, some of these nutrients and phytonutrients, such as β-carotene, lycopene, flavonoids, and anthocyanins, bring about enhanced consumer appeal owing to their color (appearance) and their impact on taste and flavor. Carotenoid-derived volatiles are implicated in the production of the favorable aroma that is associated with fruits. There is also significant opportunity to remove unfavorable flavor components in dark-green leafy and cruciferous vegetables. For example, Iceberg lettuce is one of the most frequently consumed vegetables, but it has poor levels of such nutrients as vitamins A and C. Improving the nutritional content of this lettuce variety while maintaining its flavor could contribute significantly to public health. In contrast, bitter components in nutrient-rich Romaine lettuce varieties limit their consumption. Diets rich in brassica vegetables such as broccoli have been associated with health, and in particular the lower incidence of certain cancers. Broccoli accumulates significant amounts of the phytonutrient glucoraphanin, which is the dietary source of sulforaphane. There is significant scientific evidence that sulforaphane is a potent inducer of phase II antioxidant enzymes, which help reduce damage from oxidative stress and inflammation. Considerable biochemical evidence exists for a role of the antioxidant enzymes in potentiating or maintaining the activity of vitamins A, C, and E. Significant progress has been made in developing broccoli varieties that have higher levels of glucoraphanin, using genetic markers, without impacting broccoli taste. Hence, advanced metabolomics tools, combined with molecular marker tools, offer opportunities to discover and develop fruits and vegetables enhanced for both essential nutrients and phytonutrients in conjunction with improving their taste and appearance.

Biofortification refers to the nutritional enhancement of plants through conventional breeding, molecular breeding, and/or transgenic approaches (Figure 72.1). Access to a diversified germplasm coupled with robust and high-

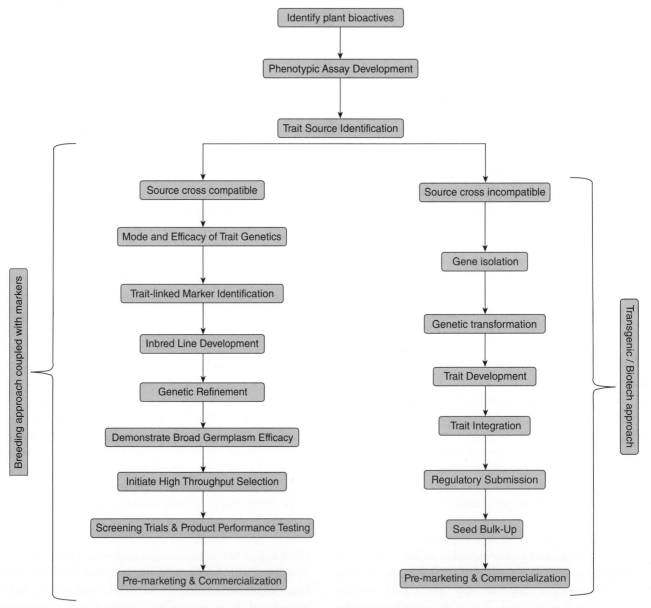

FIG. 72.1 Overview of approaches for enhancement of plant-derived bioactive compounds.

throughput crop-analytics methods form the basis for biofortification. Once the germplasm sources with desired attributes are identified, appropriate breeding strategies are employed to derive advanced breeding lines having acceptable agronomic and improved consumer benefits. Selecting for multiple traits by conventional plant breeding methods is difficult and quite time consuming. Modern plant breeding strategies that deploy marker-assisted breeding and high-throughput phenotyping tools accelerate the plant breeding process. Product development using breeding technologies is often limited by lack of availability of germplasm with a diversity of traits. In such cases, biotechnology approaches coupled with recent advances in genome sequencing, and in our understanding of biosynthetic pathways and detailed functionality of candidate genes, enable incorporation of novel traits into crops.

In this review we have attempted to describe progress in understanding the biosynthetic pathways and genetic regulation of nutrients such as folate, vitamin E, calcium, and bioactive phytonutrients such as anthocyanins, lycopene, and glucoraphanin. In addition to these micronutrients, which are abundant in vegetables, macronutrients such as edible oils have a major impact on overall health and wellness of consumers. Significant progress has been made in deploying biotechnology and breeding to decrease saturated fatty acids and incorporate stearidonic acid (SDA), a precursor to healthful omega-3 fatty acids, in soybean. Specific examples of progress in the development and commercializing of soybean-oil quality traits are also reviewed.

Biofortification of Crops with Essential Nutrients

Folate

Folate (vitamin B_9) is a generic term representing a family of molecules derived from tetrahydrofolate (THF) (also, see Chapter 21). THF and its derivatives or "folates" are essential cofactors for one-carbon transfer reactions, such as those crucial for nucleotide biosynthesis and amino acid metabolism (Bassett *et al.*, 2005; Rébeillé *et al.*, 2006). Folates are synthesized in plants and microorganisms. Hence, humans and animals depend for folates on the dietary supply (Scott *et al.*, 2000). The recommended dietary allowance (RDA) for folate is 400 μg/day for adults and 600 μg/day for pregnant women (DellaPenna, 2007). Clinical and epidemiological evidence shows that folate intake is suboptimal in most populations of the world. Insufficient dietary folate intake perturbs C1 metabolism,

which contributes to reduced turnover of erythrocytes (megaloblastic anemia), elevated plasma homocysteine levels (a risk factor for vascular diseases), birth defects (neural tube defects), increased risk of cardiovascular disease, aberrant DNA-methylation patterns (Scott *et al.*, 2000; Jang *et al.*, 2005), and several neurodegenerative disorders (Stover, 2004).

Folate is a complex molecule assembled from three different components: pteridine, para-aminobenzoic acid (PABA), and glutamate. In bacteria, folate synthesis takes place in the cytosol, whereas in plants, in addition to the cytosol, plastids and mitochondria are involved in this process. The pteridine moiety of folate is formed from guanosine triphosphate (GTP) in the cytosol, and the PABA moiety is formed from chorismate in plastids. Pteridine and PABA are then transported to the mitochondria, where they are coupled together, glutamylated and reduced to produce THF. THF with one glutamine (THF-Glu1), synthesized in the mitochondria, is exported to other cell compartments through folate transporters. A short chain of γ-linked glutamates is then added in mitochondria, plastids or cytosol, yielding folate polyglutamates (THFGlun). In *Arabidopsis*, three genes have been identified encoding folylpolyglutamate synthase (FPGS) isoforms located in the mitochondria, the cytosol, and the chloroplasts, respectively (Ravanel *et al.*, 2001).

No information is available in the literature on mapping of folate biosynthetic genes in crop plants. Transgenic approaches for folate enhancement in vegetables are summarized in Table 72.1. GTP–cyclohydrolase 1 (GCH-1) from a mammal and aminodeoxychorismate synthase (ADCS) from *Arabidopsis* were overexpressed in tomato under the control of E8, a fruit-specific promoter. Transgenic tomatoes with the mammalian gene showed a two-fold increase in folate levels whereas there was no change in folate levels with the *Arabidopsis* gene. Plants obtained by crossing *GCHI+/AtADCS* (double transgenics) accumulated up to 25-fold more folate than wild-type plants. The folate levels in these double transgenics were comparable to those in leafy vegetables and sufficient to provide the recommended dietary allowance of folate for a pregnant woman. Similarly, lettuce overexpressing GCH1 from chicken showed an 8.5-fold increase in folate levels. These results support the success of a transgenic approach for folate enhancement in vegetables.

Vitamin E

Vitamin E is the common name for eight naturally occurring compounds possessing α-tocopherol activity,

TABLE 72.1 Transgenic over-expression studies for enhancement of folate in selected vegetables

Crop	Gene(s)	Gene source	Promoter	Magnitude of increase	Reference
Tomato	GCH-1	Mammal	Fruit specific (E8)	Fruit folate increased by twofold	Díaz de la Garza et al. (2004); Garza et al. (2007)
	ADCS	Arabidopsis	Fruit specific (E8)	No difference	Garza et al. (2007)
	ADCS and GCH1	Cross between ADCS from Arabidopsis and GCH1 from mammal	Fruit specific (E8)	25-fold increase	Garza et al. (2007)
Lettuce	folE (GCH1)	Chicken	35S CaMV promoter	2.1- to 8.5-fold increase	Nunes et al. (2009)

representing lipid-soluble vitamins synthesized exclusively by plants and other oxygenic, photosynthetic organisms (Bramley et al., 2000) (also, see Chapter 14). Tocopherols and tocotrienols have four derivatives, namely alpha (α), beta (β), delta (δ), and gamma (γ), which differ in the number and location of ring methyl groups. They play important roles in the oxidative stability of vegetable oils and in the nutritional quality of crop plants. Natural α-tocopherol has a higher biological activity than synthetic tocopherols; however, all tocopherols have the ability to quench free radicals in cell membranes and to protect polyunsaturated fatty acids (Brigelius-Flohe and Traber, 1999; Hunter and Cahoon, 2007). Oxidized LDL levels are increased in atherosclerosis, and higher levels predict cardiovascular events. Vitamin E is shown to inhibit LDL oxidation both in vivo and by supplementation to people. Free radical tissue damage is related to cardiovascular disease, neurological disorders, cancer, cataracts, inflammatory diseases, and age-related macular degeneration (Bramley et al., 2000). Among vegetables, broccoli (Brassica oleracea var italica) stem tissues contain a higher tocopherol content than flowers and leaves (Guo et al., 2001). Regular consumption of broccoli at recommended dietary levels increases serum concentrations of γ-tocopherol (and lutein) without affecting α-tocopherol (or β-carotene) status in serum (Granado et al., 2006).

The tocopherol biosynthetic pathway in plants utilizes cytosolic aromatic amino acid metabolism for synthesis of the tocopherol head group, homogentisic acid (HGA), and the plastidic deoxyxylulose-5-phosphate pathway for synthesis of the hydrophobic tail. The biosynthetic pathway can be divided into upstream reactions that are important for flux regulation, and downstream reactions that control the composition. The first potential flux control points involve hydroxyphenyl pyruvate dioxygenase (HPPD) and geranyl geranyl diphosphate reductase (GGDPR), which synthesize the aromatic head group precursor HGA and the prenyl tail precursor phytyl-diphosphate (PDP), respectively. Another important flux-regulating enzyme is homogentisate phytyltransferase (HPT, also referred to as VTE2). This enzyme catalyzes the condensation of HGA and PDP to form the first prenylquinone intermediate, methylphytylbenzoquinone (MPBQ). MPBQ is further converted to DMPBQ (2,3-dimethyl-6-phytyl-1,4-benzoquinol) by the action of 2-methyl-6-phytyl-1,4-benzoquinol methyltransferase (VTE3). DMPBQ is converted to γ-tocopherol by tocopherol cyclase (VTE1). VTE1 also converts MPBQ to δ-tocopherol. Finally, VTE4 (γ-tocopherol methyltransferase) converts δ-tocopherol to β-tocopherol and γ-tocopherol to α-tocopherol (Bergmüller et al., 2003; Ajjawi and Shintani, 2004) depending upon the substrate.

Vitamin E has been enhanced in both model plants and commercial crops through breeding and biotechnological approaches. In the model plant Arabidopsis, QTLs have been identified for tocopherol levels in seeds using recom-

TABLE 72.2 Transgenic over-expression studies for enhancement of vitamin E in selected vegetables

Crop	Gene(s)	Gene source	Promoter	Magnitude of increase	Reference
Lettuce	HPT/VTE2 and tocopherol cyclase (TC/VTE1)	*Arabidopsis*	CaMV 35S promoter	>Twofold	Lee *et al.* (2007)
Lettuce	γ-TMT	*Arabidopsis*	CaMV 35S promoter	Twofold	Cho *et al.* (2005)
Potato	HPPD, HPT	*Arabidopsis*	Constitutively over-expressed	Twofold	Crowell *et al.* (2008)

binant inbred lines (RIL) developed from Landsberg *erecta* (Ler) and Columbia (Col) or Cape Verde Islands (Cvi) accessions (Gilliland *et al.*, 2006). VTE4 is also mapped to QVE3, a quantitative trait locus (QTL) for vitamin E. Vitamin E is enhanced in some plants through breeding but not in vegetables.

Vitamin E has been enhanced in some vegetables by a transgenic approach (Table 72.2). Seed-specific over-expression of VTE4 in *Arabidopsis* led to an 80-fold increase in seed α-tocopherol content and a corresponding decrease in its substrate, γ-tocopherol (Shintani and DellaPenna, 1998). Increased HPPD expression in *Arabidopsis* resulted in an increase of up to 37% in leaf tocopherol levels and a 28% increase in seed tocopherol levels relative to control plants (Tsegaye *et al.*, 2002). Hence, the allelic variations in VTE4 and HPPD could potentially impact α-tocopherol levels. The variation in the levels of vitamin E depended mainly on its accumulation in different plant organs, the highest level being in the seeds. Also, promoter choice is important for generating transgenics with enhanced vitamin E.

Calcium

Most fruits and vegetables are relatively poor sources of bioavailable calcium (Morris *et al.*, 2007). About 70% of dietary calcium comes from milk and dairy products. Only a few green vegetables and dried fruits are good sources of calcium whereas drinking water, including mineral water, provides 6–7% of the required daily dietary calcium (Guéguen and Pointillart, 2000). While there is no question of the nutritional effectiveness of the calcium provided by milk, debate still exists about whether milk provides biologically better calcium than other sources.

Calcium deficiency is a significant problem in human populations worldwide (also, see Chapter 28). Prolonged calcium deficiency leads to reductions in bone mass and osteoporosis. The Dietary Reference Intake (DRI) for calcium is set at levels associated with desirable retention of body calcium. Since high bone density decreases the incidence of bone fractures and the chances of osteoporosis, 1300 mg/day of calcium per person is recommended. Although osteoporosis affects both men and women, the incidence is higher in women. One important factor in achieving high bone density is maintaining a maximal level of calcium through absorption and retention. Enhancing the concentration of bioavailable calcium in fruits and vegetables could boost calcium uptake and thus reduce calcium-deficiency-related disorders.

In plants, calcium/H^+ antiporters are high-capacity, low-affinity transporters that efficiently sequester large amounts of calcium when cytosolic calcium concentrations are elevated during a signaling event (Hirschi, 2001). After the cytosolic calcium burst, plant vacuolar and plasma membrane transporters rigorously reset the cytosolic calcium level. The level of intracellular calcium is regulated in part by active efflux transporters that remove calcium from the cytosol. P-type calcium-ATPases perform a variety of roles, which include the restoration of the cytosolic calcium concentration to its resting level after a signal transduction event, replenishment of internal calcium stores, and resistance to toxic concentrations of calcium (Sanders *et al.*, 1999; Sze *et al.*, 1999).

Arabidopsis is reported to have up to 12 other putative cation/H^+ antiporters, termed CAX (**CA**lcium e**X**changer) genes. *Arabidopsis* CAX1 and CAX2 have proven functionality in suppressing calcium hypersensitivity in yeast mutants (*vcx1 pmc1*) (Hirschi *et al.*, 1996). *Arabidopsis*

TABLE 72.3 Transgenic studies for enhancing calcium in vegetables using *Arabidopsis* CAX genes

Crop	Gene(s)	Promoter	Magnitude of increase	Reference
Carrot	sCAX1	35S CaMV CDC	1.4- to 1.6-fold in roots	Park *et al.* (2004); Morris *et al.* (2008)
Potato	sCAX1	35S CaMV CDC	1.5- to 3.0-fold in tubers and 1.2- to 1.7-fold in leaves	Park *et al.* (2005b)
Tomato	sCAX1 CAX4	35S CaMV CDC	1.2- to 1.5-fold in fruits	Park *et al.* (2005a)
Lettuce	sCAX1	35S CaMV CDC	1.27- to 1.29-fold in leaves	Park *et al.* (2009)
Tomato	sCAX2A	35S CaMV	~1.5-fold in fruits	Chung *et al.* (2010)

CAX genes sCAX1 (shorter variant of CAX1), sCAX2A (shorter variant of CAX2A), and CAX4 have been expressed in different crop plants (tomato, lettuce, carrot, and potato). Among these, sCAX1 has been the most studied (Table 72.3) and its expression in carrot shows increased bioavailable calcium. In addition to increasing calcium levels, CAX genes are also reported to provide additional advantages such as reducing blossom-end rot and increasing shelf life in tomatoes.

Biofortification of Crops with Phytonutrients

Anthocyanins

Anthocyanins are vacuolar, water-soluble pigments that impart a red, purple, or blue color depending on the pH. They belong to a class of molecules called flavonoids. Generally, anthocyanins have a carbohydrate molecule (sugar, usually glucose) esterified at the 3-position of the aglycone anthocyanidins. About 17 anthocyanidins are found in nature and are classified according to functional groups. Of these, six anthocyanidins, namely cyanidin (Cy), delphinidin (Dp), petunidin (Pt), peonidin (Pn), pelargonidin (Pg), and malvidin (Mv), are ubiquitous. The antioxidant activity of anthocyanidins is mainly attributed to delphinidin, followed by cyanidin, pelargonidin, kuromanin, and callistephin. The aglycones such as cyanidin and delphinidin are the most abundant anthocyanins in daily foods and may possess the ability to inhibit the growth of human tumor cells in vitro in micromolar concentrations (Meiers, 2001). Epidemiologic studies have revealed the role of anthocyanins in lowering the risk of cardiovascular diseases, diabetes, arthritis, and cancer as a result of their antioxidant and anti-inflammatory activities (Middleton, 1998).

Anthocyanins are derivatives of the phenylpropanoid pathway. They are derived from a branch of the flavonoid pathway, for which chalcone synthase (CHS) provides the first committed step by condensing one molecule of *p*-coumaroyl-CoA with three molecules of malonyl-CoA to produce tetrahydroxychalcone. The closure of the C-ring to form flavanones is carried out by chalcone isomerase (CHI). Flavanones provide a central branch point in the flavonoid pathway and can serve as substrates for enzymes that introduce –OH groups at the 3′ and 5′ positions of the B-ring, or for the hydroxylation of the C-ring by flavanone 3-hydroxylase (F3H), a soluble di-oxygenase. Dihydroflavonol 4-reductase (DFR) provides one entry step to the biosynthesis of anthocyanins. It can utilize as a substrate either one or all three of the possible dihydro-flavonols (dihydromyricetin, dihydrokaempferol, or dihydroquercetin). This results in the formation of the corresponding leucoanthocyanidins, providing structure to the anthocyanin biosynthetic grid. The leucoanthocyanidins are converted into the corresponding anthocyanidins by the action of a leucoanthocyanidin dioxygenase/anthocyanidin synthase (LDOX/ANS) (Grotewald, 2006). Anthocyanidins also serve as substrates for anthocyanidin reductases, key enzymes in the formation of proanthocyanidins (Xie *et al.*, 2003). The next step in the anthocyanin pathway is catalyzed by ANS. ANS is similar to F3H, flavone synthase I (FNSI), and flavonol synthase (FLS). It is a member of the non-heme ferrous and 2-oxoglutarate-(2OG)-dependent family of oxygenases, which convert leucoanthocyanidin to the corresponding anthocyanidin (Nakajima *et al.*, 2001; Grotewald, 2006).

Tomatoes with enhanced anthocyanins have been produced through breeding (Willits *et al.*, 2005) as well as genetic engineering efforts (Mol *et al.*, 1998; Brown *et al.*, 2003; Jones *et al.*, 2003; Koes *et al.*, 2005; Torres *et al.*, 2005; Willits *et al.*, 2005; Mes *et al.*, 2008). Several studies indicate that R2R3 MYB-type and bHLH-type transcription factors (TFs) are involved in anthocyanin production (Goff *et al.*, 1992; Borevitz *et al.*, 2000; Ramsey and Glover, 2005; Tohge *et al.*, 2005; Gonzali *et al.*, 2009).

Heterologous expression of Petunia CHI in tomato resulted in higher levels of quercetin glycosides in their fruit peel (Muir *et al.*, 2001). Regulated expression of endogenous regulatory genes, ANT1 (Aintegumenta 1) (Matthews *et al.*, 2003) and DET1(*DE-ETIOLATED1*) (Davuluri *et al.*, *2005*), resulted in purple fruits in tomato. Expression of snapdragon TFs, Del (Delila, a bHLH TF) and Ros1 (Rosea 1, an R2R3 MYB-type TF), under the control of a fruit-specific E8 promoter resulted in tomato fruits enriched with anthocyanin (Butelli *et al.*, 2008). *Del* and *Ros1* stimulated the transcription of most of the structural genes involved in the biosynthetic pathway, including phenylalanine ammonia-lyase (PAL), CHI, and flavonoid 3050-hydroxylase (F3050H), which are necessary for the accumulation of anthocyanin (Table 72.4). Although there was anthocyanin accumulation, the levels of carotenoids remained unchanged. A group of cancer-susceptible mice that were fed with a diet supplemented with these high-anthocyanin tomatoes showed a significant extension of their average lifespan compared with those that were fed a diet supplemented with normal tomatoes (Butelli *et al.*, 2008).

In red and green cabbages, a comparative transcription analysis revealed the up-regulation of BoMYB2 and BoTT8 (Transparent Testa 8) genes and down-regulation of BoMYB3 expression in red cabbage. Hence, these were identified as probable candidate genes for anthocyanin biosynthesis in cabbage (Yuan *et al.*, 2009).

Lycopene

Lycopene is a natural, red, fat-soluble carotenoid synthesized by plants and microorganisms, but not by animals. It is an acyclic isomer of β-carotene, without provitamin A activity. It is a highly unsaturated, straight-chain hydrocarbon containing 11 conjugated and two non-conjugated double bonds. It undergoes *cis–trans* isomerization that is induced by light, thermal energy, or chemical reactions. In addition to its antioxidant properties, lycopene shows cardioprotective, anti-inflammatory, antimutagenic, anticarcinogenic, and chemopreventive activities (Bhuvaneswari and Nagini, 2005).

Lycopene is mainly available from fruits and vegetables such as tomatoes, carrots, watermelons, pink grapefruits, apricots, papaya, and pink guavas. Dietary intake of tomatoes and tomato products containing lycopene has been shown to be associated with a decreased risk of chronic diseases such as cancer and cardiovascular disease. Positive effects are also hypothesized for osteoporosis,

TABLE 72.4 Transgenic approaches for enhancement of anthocyanins in tomato

Gene	Source	Promoter	Strategy	Magnitude of increase	Reference
DET1	Tomato	Fruit-specific (P119, 2A11 and TFM7)	Suppression (RNAi)	~Threefold	Davuluri *et al.* (2005b)
Del and Ros1	Snapdragon	Fruit-specific promoter(E8)	Over-expression	Threefold	Butelli *et al.* (2008)
Lc and C1 (TFs)	Maize	Fruit-specific promoter (E8)	Over-expression	Two- to threefold increase	Bovy *et al.* (2002)
CHI	Petunia	CaMV double 35S promoter	Over-expression	78-fold in fruit peel	Muir *et al.* (2001)
ANT1	Tomato	Constitutive promoter	Over-expression	500-fold increase	Mathews *et al.* (2003)
Del	Antirrhinum	35S promoter	Over-expression	10-fold increase	Mooney *et al.* (1995)

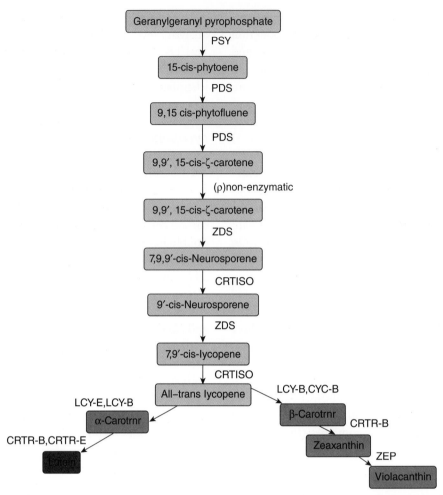

FIG. 72.2 Pathway of carotenoid biosynthesis. PSY, phytoene synthase; PDS, phytotene desaturase; ZDS, ζ-carotene desaturase; CRTISO, carotene isomerase; LCY-E, lycopene ε-cyclase; CRTR-B+CRTR-E, ε-ring hydroxylase; LCY-B,CYCB, lycopene β-cyclase; CRTR-B, β-ring hydroxylase; ZEP, zeaxanthin epoxidase.

neurodegenerative diseases, and hypertension (Bánhegyi, 2005). Carotenoids are biosynthesized in the plastids; chloroplasts in photosynthetic tissues, and chromoplasts in ripe fruits and flowers. Carotenoid biosynthesis (Figure 72.2) and its regulation in tomato are reviewed by Fraser *et al.* (2009). Geranyl geranyl pyrophosphate (GGPP) is a ubiquitous isoprenoid precursor in the formation of carotenoids. Two molecules of GGPP are condensed to form phytoene by phytoene synthase. Phytoene, a 15-*cis* geometric isomer, possesses three conjugated double bonds. Phytoene desaturase introduces a double bond at the 9′ of the phytoene molecule to create 15,9′-di-*cis*-phytofluene. Another double bond is then introduced at position 9, forming 9,15,9′-tri-*cis*-ζ-carotene. This molecule, with

seven conjugated double bonds, has a yellow/green coloration. The involvement of an enzymatic reaction for further desaturation and isomerization to yield 9,9′-di-*cis*-ζ-carotene needs to be investigated. Following the formation of 9,9′-di-*cis*-ζ-carotene, desaturation to 7,9,7′,9′-tetra-*cis*-lycopene (prolycopene) via 7,9,9′-tri-*cis*-neurosporene is catalyzed by ζ-carotene desaturase (Isaacson *et al.*, 2004). Cyclization of lycopene forms either β- or α-carotene via β- and ε-cyclase, respectively.

In tomato, 16 quantitative trait loci (QTLs) that modify the intensity of the red color in ripe fruits were identified (Liu *et al.*, 2003). Mutants with high pigment levels (hp1 and hp2) are also well characterized (Mustilli *et al.*, 1999; *Liu et al.*, 2004), but, as some of these mutants have weak stems and poor vigor, they were unsuitable for commercial exploitation (Liu *et al.*, 2004; Kolotilin *et al.*, 2007). In carrots, 24 genes involved in the carotenoid biosynthesis pathway were cloned and mapped over eight linkage groups (Santos and Simon, 2002; Just *et al.*, 2007). In watermelon, the sequence comparison of full-length cDNA of *LCYB* (lycopene b-cyclase) identified three single nucleotide polymorphisms (SNPs) in the coding region of *LCYB* between canary yellow and red. These SNPs showed perfect co-segregation with flesh-color phenotypes. One of the SNPs introduces an amino acid replacement of evolutionarily conserved Phe226 to Val, which may impair the catalytic function of *LCYB*. This SNP was used to develop a cleaved amplified polymorphic sequence (CAPS) marker, which perfectly co-segregated with flesh-color phenotypes (Clotault *et al.*, 2008).

In addition to regulation of lycopene through breeding, transgenic efforts have been made to regulate lycopene in several vegetables. Carotenoid genes from bacteria, yeast, *Arabidopsis*, pepper, and tomato were expressed to obtain transgenic tomato and carrot with varied levels of carotenoids (Table 72.5).

In addition to the potential health benefits, lycopene is a precursor in the production of volatiles that are responsible for aroma in tomato (Vogel *et al.*, 2010). Thus, altering lycopene levels impacts not only color appeal but also the sensory perception and liking of tomatoes.

Glucoraphanin (Sulforaphane Precursor)

Glucosinolates (GSLs) are S- and N-containing secondary metabolites found in Capparales and a few other families. GSLs are a group of ~120 anionic plant metabolites with a core structure comprising a sulfonated oxime, a β-thioglucose residue and a variable side chain. Both glycone and aglycone moieties are important in mediating herbivore interactions (Giamoustaris and Mithen, 1996). In humans they are important as progenitors of taste and flavor compounds of cruciferous vegetables. Following tissue damage, aliphatic GSLs are hydrolysed by myrosinases to give a complex mixture of products, of which glucose, sulphate, and isothiocyanates are major components. Although approximately 120 kinds of GSL have been identified in plants, each plant species has only a few major GSLs. *Brassica* species predominantly contain aliphatic (derived from methionine) and indolyl (derived from tryptophan) GSLs (Li and Quiros, 2003).

The formation of GSLs can be divided into three phases. First, certain aliphatic and aromatic amino acids are elon-

gated by inserting methylene groups into their side chains, followed by reconfiguration of the amino acid moiety to the core structure of the GSL. This is followed by formation of secondary transformations of the GSL. The biochemistry and biosynthesis of glucosinolates have been reviewed by Halkier and Gershenzon (2006).

MAM (methylthioalkylmalate synthase) genes are involved in the amino acid chain elongation in GSL biosynthesis (Kroymann *et al.*, 2001). Four MAM genes (MAM1, MAM2/MAML, MAML3, and MAML4) have been reported in *Arabidopsis*. The biosynthesis of the core glucosinolate structure involves the *conversion* of amino acids to aldoximes, aldoximes to thiohydroximic acids, and thiohydroximic acids to GSL. Conversion of amino acids to aldoximes involves cytochrome P450 genes (Hansen *et al.*, 2001; Kroymann *et al.*, 2001; Reintanz *et al.*, 2001; Wittstock and Halkier, 2002; Li and Quiros, 2003) whereas formation of thiohydroximic acids involves CYP83B1 (Barlier *et al.*, 2000; Bak *et al.*, 2001; Hansen *et al.*, 2001; Smolen and Bender, 2002), CYP83A1 (Bak and Feyereisen, 2001; Hemm *et al.*, 2003; Naur *et al.*, 2003), *C-S* lyase (Mikkelsen *et al.*, 2004), and UGT74B1 and AtST5a (Grubb *et al.*, 2004). Some of the genes involved in secondary transformations are *AOP2*, *AOP3* (Li *et al.*, 2001; Gao *et al.*, 2004), 2-ODD (2-oxoglutarate-dependent dioxygenase) (Hall *et al.*, 2001) and FMO (flavin-monooxygenase) (Hansen *et al.*, 2007). In addition, upstream regulators of the aliphatic glucosinolate pathway (MYB28, MYB29 and MYB76) have also been identified (Gigolashvili *et al.*, 2007a,b; Hirai *et al.*, 2007). Based on the homology to *Arabidopsis* gene sequences, GSL biosynthetic genes have been isolated from vegetable species such as broccoli and cauliflower (Mithen *et al.*, 1995; Li and Quiros, 2002).

Genetic and functional epistasis between the genes in the GSL biosynthetic pathway has been demonstrated in *Arabidopsis* (Kliebenstein, 2009). Six QTLs controlling GSL accumulation showed genetic epistasis (Kliebenstein *et al.*, 2005). The GSL desaturation gene, *BoGLS-ALK*, was successfully mapped on the L1 linkage group at 1.4 cM from the marker SRAP133 (Li and Quiros, 2001).

Metabolic engineering of glucosinolate profiles has included altering the expression of one or more CYP79 enzymes (Mikkelsen *et al.*, 2000). GSL biosynthetic genes of *Arabidopsis* have been overexpressed in different crops. Among vegetables, Chinese cabbage overexpressing *Arabidopsis* MAM1, CYP79F1, and CYP83A1 with CaMV 35S promoter resulted in significant enhancement of

TABLE 72.5   Summary of carotenoid enhancement through genetic engineering in selected vegetables

Gene	Source	Promoter	Strategy	Magnitude of increase	Reference
Tomato					
Dxs (1-deoxy-D-xylulose-5-phosphate synthase)	*E. coli*	CaMV 35S and fibrillin from pepper	Over-expression	2-fold increased phytoene and other carotenoids	Enfissi *et al.* (2005)
CrtB	*Erwinia uredovora*	Polygalacturonase (PG) from tomato	Over-expression	>2-fold increase in phytoene, lycopene and β-carotene	Fraser *et al.* (2009)
PSY-1	Tomato	CaMV 35S	Over-expression	1.5-fold increase of β-carotene	Fray *et al.* (1995), Fraser *et al.* (2007)
Crtl (phytoene desaturase)	*Erwinia uredovora*	CaMV 35S	Over-expression	3-fold increase β-carotene but reduction in lycopene and phytoene	Römer *et al.* (2000)
LCYB	*Erwinia herbicola* and from daffodil	PDS from tomato cyclase	Over-expression	50% increase in carotenoids	Apel and Bock (2009)
LCY-B	*Arabidopsis thaliana*	Pds from tomato	Over-expression	7-fold β-carotene without lycopene reduction	Rosati *et al.* (2000)
LCY-B	Tomato	CaMV 35S	Over-expression	31.7-fold β-carotene with reduced lycopene	D'Ambrosio *et al.* (2004)
CrtY	Tomato	Plastid atpI promoter	Over-expression	4-fold β-carotene without lycopene reduction	Wurbs *et al.* (2007)
LCY-B	Tomato	Pds from tomato	Anti-sense	1.3 fold lycopene	Rosati *et al.* (2000)
CYC-B	Tomato	CaMV35S	Anti-sense	Increased lycopene	Ronen *et al.* (2000)
LCY-B and CHY-B	*Arabidopsis* and pepper	Pds from tomato	Over-expression	12-fold β-carotene increase	Dharmapuri *et al.* (2002)
CRY-2	Tomato	CaMV35S		2-fold carotenoids	Giliberto *et al.* (2005)
DET-1	Tomato	Ripening enhanced promoters (P119, TFM7 and 2A11)	RNAi	2-fold increase lycopene, 10-fold β-carotene	Davuluri *et al.* (2005)
COP1LIKE	Tomato	CaMV35S	Over-expression	2-fold increase in carotenoids	Liu *et al.* (2004)
CUL4	Tomato	Ripening enhanced (TFM7)	Over-expression	2-fold carotenoids	Wang *et al.* (2008)
ySAMdc	Yeast	E8, fruit-specific ripening enhanced	Over-expression	3-fold lycopene	Mehta *et al.* (2002)
Fibrillin	Tomato	Tomato fibrillin		2-fold carotenoids	Simkin *et al.* (2007)
Carrot					
Crt	*Erwinia herbicola*	CaMV 35S	Over-expression	2- to 5-fold increase in carotenoids	Hauptmann *et al.* (1997)

gluconapin and glucobrassicanapin, leading to enhanced glucosinolates (Zang *et al.*, 2008).

Broccoli is one of the healthiest vegetables. In addition to being a good/excellent source of vitamins A, C, folate, and fiber, broccoli is also the major dietary source for sulforaphane (metabolite of precursor glucosinolate, glucoraphanin). Increasing scientific evidence indicates that sulforaphane naturally enhances enzymes that help protect the body from oxidative stress and inflammation caused by the harmful effects of free radicals and environmental pollutants. Sarikamis *et al.* (2006) developed hybrid broccoli with enhanced levels of glucoraphanin and glucoiberin, by introgression of genomic segments from the wild ancestor, *Brassica villosa*. The total level of glucoraphanin and glucoiberin is predominantly dependent upon the presence of *B. villosa* alleles at QTL1, but the ratio of these GSLs is dependent upon genotype at both QTL1 and QTL2 located on chromosomes 2 and 5. Figure 72.3 shows the biosynthesis pathway of aliphatic glucosinolates.

Clinical studies with the high-glucoraphanin broccoli varieties indicate higher blood levels of sulforaphane as well as a higher level of expression of phase II antioxidant enzymes compared with regular broccoli (Mithen *et al.*, 2003; Traka *et al.*, 2005). Antioxidant enzymes are involved in detoxification of environmental pollutants and are implicated in recycling of antioxidant vitamins A, C, and E. Effect of broccoli varieties with various levels of aliphatic glucosinolates on perception of taste is reported. Higher levels of glucoraphanin in cooked broccoli were not associated with liking (Baik *et al.*, 2003).

Biotechnology-Derived Soybean Traits

Biotechnology efforts concerning soybeans continue to focus on enhancing yield potential and improving the nutritive composition for use in food and feed products to help address growing global food and feed demands. Since 1996, agricultural biotechnology has had a major impact on soybean production globally; more than 90% of the soybeans in the United States and more than 70% of the soybeans grown globally today include a modified biotechnology component, in particular, herbicide-resistant Roundup Ready® soybeans.

Nutritionally enhanced soybean products present opportunities to bring direct benefits to consumers by enhancing the nutritional value of oils and fats. The 2009 global demand for vegetable oil in food was approximately

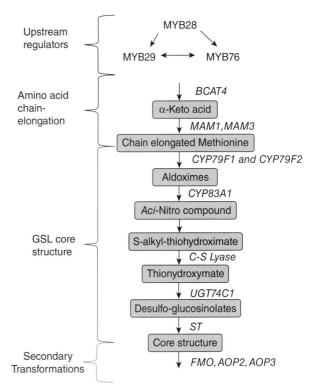

FIG. 72.3 Biosynthesis pathway of aliphatic glucosinolates. Upstream regulators, transcription factors involved in regulation of aliphatic glucosinolates. Amino acid chain elongation, elongation of aliphatic and aromatic amino acids by inserting methylene groups into their side chains. Glucosinolate core structure, reconfiguration of amino acid moiety to form core structure of glucosinolates. Secondary transformations, modification of initially formed glucosinolates.

110 MMT and is forecasted to grow to over 170 MMT by 2020. Soybean oil represents approximately 30% of the total vegetable oil produced worldwide, with the highest consumption of vegetable oils occurring in China, India, the European Union, and the United States (Goldbitz, 2005–2008; Mielke, 2006; USDA, 2009). Fat is the most concentrated source of energy in the diet. Structure and function of the fatty acids in oils impact human health, shelf stability, and taste (International Food Information Council, 2006).

It is recommended that healthy people consume less than 10% of calories from saturated fats daily. Replacing saturated fats with unsaturated fats in foods helps reduce the levels of low-density lipoprotein (LDL) cholesterol, a risk factor for heart disease. The *Dietary Guidelines for*

Americans (DHHS and USDA, 2005) recommend keeping total fat intake between 20% and 35% of calories, with most fats coming from sources of polyunsaturated and monounsaturated fatty acids such as fish, nuts, and vegetable oils. Hydrogenated oils contribute important textural and stability properties in food. However, hydrogenation results in the formation of *trans* fatty acids. The National Academy of Sciences' Institute of Medicine concluded that *trans* fatty acids are similar to saturated fats and dietary cholesterol with regard to their effect on blood LDL cholesterol, which is considered bad for heart health. In addition, some studies suggest that increased intake of *trans* fats may lower high-density lipoprotein (HDL) or good cholesterol. The Institute of Medicine recommends that the intake of *trans* fatty acid be as low as possible. In 2006 the US Food and Drug Administration required mandatory *trans* fat labeling on consumer packages. This resulted in the reformulation of many food products. Several municipalities and states followed with *trans* fat bans, resulting in quick adoption of *trans* fat alternatives in the food service industry (International Food Information Council, 2009). The median intake of total fat in the United States ranges from about 32% to 34% of total calories. Saturated fats provide approximately 11–12% of calories in adult diets in the United States.

Omega-3 fatty acids are considered essential fatty acids, meaning they are essential to human health but cannot be manufactured by the body. Some researchers (e.g. Burr *et al.* [1989] and GISSI-Prevenzione Investigators [1999]) found that, when long-chain omega-3s are incorporated in the diet, there is a dramatic reduction in overall and cardiac mortality in heart-attack patients. The American Heart Association (AHA) recommends long-chain, omega-3 intake of 1 g/day for heart patients and the incorporation of two servings of fatty fish per week for healthy individuals (which equates to approximately 500 mg/day, depending on the fish source). Unfortunately, current intake of long-chain omega-3 in most people's diets is well below these recommendations (Harris *et al.*, 2008).

Long-chain omega-3 fatty acids play an important role in maintaining health, including heart health. Currently, long-chain omega-3s can be found in fish, but, unfortunately, many consumers find it difficult or too expensive to incorporate fatty fish in the diet on a regular basis. Others are concerned about levels of heavy metals and pressure on natural resources. Recently, commercial efforts have resulted in the development of omega-3 enhanced soybeans containing stearidonic acid (SDA) that represent a renewable land-based source of essential omega-3 fatty acids. Common sources of omega-3 fatty acids include ALA (α-linolenic acid) found in canola, soybean and other vegetable oils, flax, walnuts, fatty fish, and algae. Studies have shown that the conversion of ALA to the more desirable long-chain forms of EPA (eicosapentaenoic acid) and DHA (docosahexaenoic acid) present in fatty fish, fish oils, and algal oils is inefficient because of the lack of the delta-6-desaturase enzyme in human bodies (Burdge *et al.*, 2002, 2003; Whelan, 2009). Studies have shown that, as a result, it can take a minimum of 14–20 g of ALA to get the same level of tissue enrichment as 1 g of EPA (Harris *et al.*, 2008).

SDA is an intermediate between ALA and EPA on the biosynthetic pathway and does not require the delta-6-desaturase for conversion to EPA. As a result, conversion of SDA to EPA is much more efficient than conversion of ALA to EPA. Using plant and fungal sources for the genes encoding these key enzymes, soybeans have been modified to express SDA which is not typically found in soybeans. The oil from these soybeans contains 20% SDA. SDA has been incorporated in several human clinical studies. James *et al.* (2003) found that, by incorporating SDA in the diet at 1500 mg/day, EPA levels in red blood cells could be increased significantly. SDA was approximately one-third as efficient as EPA in that study. In a human clinical study using SDA soybean oil over a 16-week period, Harris *et al.* (2008) found that there was a significant increase in red blood cell EPA levels whereas none was observed for participants using only conventional soybean oil, containing ALA as the omega-3 source at levels higher than adequate intake recommendations. These results were confirmed in a larger trial of 252 healthy volunteers (Lemke *et al.*, 2010).

Incorporation of SDA-enriched soybean oil using conventional processing methods resulted in acceptable flavor. Studies have been completed in a range of everyday food applications that incorporate SDA-enriched soybean oil in foods to determine impact on shelf life and consumer liking. In many foods, such as granola bars, spreads, baked goods, crackers, confectionery products, dressings, soups, and mayonnaise, flavor attributes are similar to those of control products throughout the shelf life.

Future Directions

Edible crops such as vegetables and oil seeds are the fundamental source of macro- and essential micronutrients and phytonutrients. Considerable progress has been made in understanding the basis for usefulness and enhancement of these beneficial dietary components. A majority of studies report the effects of dietary components in isolation that overlook the important aspect of interaction of these nutrients and dietary components as it relates to relative bioavailability, absorption, metabolism, and benefit. Lack of such knowledge leads to conflicting data between consumption and intervention studies with components in isolation. Availability of crops with or without modified levels of (phyto)nutrients enables well-designed dietary intervention studies to evaluate the effects of biofortified crops in comparison with conventional varieties. Examples of such products that are reviewed in this chapter include high-glucoraphanin broccoli and SDA-enhanced soybean. Advances in both molecular breeding and biotechnology coupled with understanding of biosynthetic pathways and "omics" tools enable rapid discovery and development of such crop varieties. Product development using conventional breeding approaches along with molecular breeding and phenotyping tools offers the advantages of speed to market and low cost. Biotechnology offers the advantage of introducing novel traits that are not limited by germplasm diversity and compatibility of trait sources. In addition, identification and validation of candidate biosynthetic genes and their regulation in crop plants could herald opportunities for marker-assisted breeding. With the scale and speed of generation of transgenic model crops, biotechnology tools provide excellent leverage for validating the candidate genes, highlighted by the examples of folate and calcium enhancement in vegetables reviewed in this chapter. Literature is insufficient on vitamin E enhancement in vegetables. As biosynthetic pathways and target genes are identified in model plants, application of breeding/biotechnology approaches could offer more possibilities for vitamin E enhancement. Among the emerging nutrients, there is compelling evidence for enhancement of anthocyanins using a transgenic approach. However, commercial viability of these varieties would be limited by consumer acceptance of overtly different-looking varieties coupled with the need for regulatory approval. Several studies report on enhancement of lycopene in tomatoes by breeding and transgenic approaches. Elevating lycopene levels by molecular breeding would increase consumption of tomatoes as a result of higher consumer appeal in flavor and appearance along with the potential nutritive value.

New and exciting products will be commercialized in the near future as a result of this knowledge, which will provide significant benefits to the consumer and the food industry. In the coming decades, the intersection between biology, agriculture, and human nutrition should continue to create new solutions to enhance the nutritional value and appeal of crops to consumers.

Acknowledgments

The authors gratefully acknowledge Dr Don James, Monsanto Vegetables Division, and Drs Padmini Sudarshana and Vijay Paranjape, Monsanto Research Centre, Bangalore, for their critical reviews of and inputs to the manuscript.

> ### Suggestions for Further Reading
> Readers are directed to the References for recommended reading.

References

Ajjawi, D. and Shintani, D. (2004) Engineered plants with elevated vitamin E: a nutraceutical success story. *Trends Biotechnol* **22**, 104–107.

Apel, W. and Bock, R. (2009) Enhancement of carotenoid biosynthesis in transplastomic tomatoes by induced lycopene-to-provitamin A conversion. *Plant Physiol* **151**, 59–66.

Baik, H.Y., Juvik, J., Jeffery, E.H., *et al.* (2003) Relating glucosinolate content and flavor of broccoli cultivars. *J Food Sci* **68**, 1043–1050.

Bak, S. and Feyereisen, R. (2001) The involvement of two P450 enzymes, CYP83B1 and CYP83A1, in auxin homeostasis and glucosinolate biosynthesis. *Plant Physiol* **127**, 108–118.

Bak, S.F., Tax, E., Feldmann, K.A., *et al.* (2001) CYP83B1, a cytochrome P450 at the metabolic branch point in auxin and indole glucosinolate biosynthesis in *Arabidopsis*. *Plant Cell* **13**, 101–111.

Bánhegyi, G. (2005) Lycopene – a natural antioxidant. *OrvHetil* **146**, 1621–1624.

Barlier, I., Kowalczyk, M., Marchant, A, *et al.* (2000) The SUR2 gene of *Arabidopsis thaliana* encodes the cytochrome P450 CYP83B1, a modulator of auxin homeostasis. *Proc Natl Acad Sci USA* **97**, 14819–14824.

Basset, G.J.C., Quinlivan, E.P., Gregory, J.F., III, *et al.* (2005) Folate synthesis and metabolism in plants and prospects for biofortification. *Crop Sci* **45**, 449–453.

Bergmüller, E., Porfirova, S., and Dörmann, P. (2003) Characterization of an *Arabidopsis* mutant deficient in gamma-tocopherol methyltransferase. *Plant Mol Biol* **52**, 1181–1190.

Bhuvaneswari, V. and Nagini, S. (2005) Lycopene: a review of its potential as an anticancer agent. *Curr Med Chem-Anti-Cancer Agents* **5**, 627–635.

Borevitz, J.O., Xia, Y., Blount, J., *et al.* (2000) Activation tagging identifies a conserved MYB regulator of phenylpropanoid biosynthesis. *Plant Cell* **12**, 2383–2394.

Bovy, A., de Vos, R., Kemper, M., *et al.* (2002) High-flavonol tomatoes resulting from the heterologous expression of the maize transcription factor genes LC and C1. *Plant Cell* **14**, 2509–2526.

Bramley, P.M., Elmadfa, I., Kafatos, A., *et al.* (2000) Vitamin E. *J Sci Food Agric* **80**, 913–938.

Brigelius-Flohe, R.M. and Traber, G. (1999) Vitamin E: function and metabolism. *FASEB J* **13**, 1145–1155.

Brown, C., Wrolstad, R., Durst, R., *et al.* (2003) Breeding studies in potatoes containing high concentrations of anthocyanins. *Am J Potato Res* **80**, 241–249

Burdge, G.C., Finnegan, Y.E., Minihane, A.M., *et al.* (2003) Effect of altered dietary n-3 fatty acid intake upon plasma lipid fatty acid composition, conversion of [13C]alpha-linolenic acid to longer-chain fatty acids and partitioning towards beta-oxidation in older men. *Br J Nutr* **90**, 311–321.

Burdge, G.C., Jones, A.E., and Wootton, S.A. (2002) Eicosapentaenoic and docosapentaenoic acids are the principal products of alpha-linolenic acid metabolism in young men. *Br J Nutr* **88**, 355–363.

Burr, M.L., Fehily, A.M., Gilbert, J.F., *et al.* (1989) Effects of changes in fat, fish, and fibre intakes on death and myocardial reinfarction: diet and reinfarction trial (DART). *Lancet* **334**, 757–761.

Butelli, E., Titta, L., Giorgio, M., *et al.* (2008) Enrichment of tomato fruit with health-promoting anthocyanins by expression of select transcription factors. *Nat Biotechnol* **26**, 1301–1308.

Cho, E.A., Lee, C.A., Kim, Y.S., *et al.* (2005) Expression of g-tocopherol methyltransferase transgene improves tocopherol composition in lettuce (*Lactuca sativa* L.). *Mol Cells* **19**, 16–22.

Chung, M., Han, J.S., Giovannoni, J., *et al.* (2010) Modest calcium increase in tomatoes expressing a variant of *Arabidopsis* cation/H+ antiporter. *Plant Biotechnol Rep* **4**, 15–21.

Clotault, J., Peltier, D., Berruyer, R., *et al.* (2008) Expression of carotenoid biosynthesis genes during carrot root development. *J Exp Bot* **59**, 3563–3573.

Connolly, E.L. (2008) Raising the bar for biofortification: enhanced levels of bioavailable calcium in carrots. *Trends Biotechnol* **26**, 401–403.

Crowell, E., McGrath, J., and Douches, D. (2008) Accumulation of vitamin E in potato (*Solanum tuberosum*) tubers. *Transgenic Res* **17**, 205–208.

D'Ambrosio, C., Giorio, G., Marino, I., *et al.* (2004) Virtually complete conversion of lycopene into β-carotene in fruits of tomato plants transformed with the tomato *lycopene β-cyclase* (t*lcy-b*) cDNA. *Plant Sci* **166**, 207–214.

Davuluri, G.R., van Tuinen, A., Fraser, P.D., *et al.* (2005) Fruit-specific RNAi-mediated suppression of DET1 enhances carotenoid and flavonoid content in tomatoes. *Nat Biotechnol* **23**, 890–895.

DellaPenna, D. (2007) Biofortification of plant-based food: enhancing folate levels by metabolic engineering. *Proc Natl Acad Sci* **104**, 3675–3676.

Dharmapuri, S., Rosati, C., Pallara, P., *et al.* (2002) Metabolic engineering of xanthophyll content in tomato fruits. *FEBS Lett* **519**, 30–34.

DHSS and USDA (2005) *Dietary Guidelines for Americans, 2005*, 6th Edn. US Government Printing Office, Washington, DC. http://www.health.gov/dietaryguidelines/dga2005/document/default.htm.

Díaz de la Garza, R., Quinlivan, E.P., Klaus, S.M., *et al.* (2004) Folate biofortification in tomatoes by engineering the pteridine branch of folate synthesis. *Proc Natl Acad Sci USA* **101**, 13720–13725.

Enfissi, E.M., Fraser, P.D., Lois, L.M., *et al.* (2005) Metabolic engineering of the mevalonate and non-mevalonate isopentenyl diphosphate-forming pathways for the production of health-promoting isoprenoids in tomato. *Plant Biotechnol J* **3**, 17–27.

Fraser, P.D., Enfissi, E.M.A., and Bramley, P.M. (2009) Genetic engineering of carotenoid formation in tomato fruit and the potential application of systems and synthetic biology approaches. *Arch Biochem Biophys* **483**, 196–204.

Fraser, P.D., Enfissi, E.M., Halket, J.M., *et al.* (2007) Manipulation of phytoene levels in tomato fruit: effects on isoprenoids, plastids, and intermediary metabolism. *Plant Cell* **19**, 3194–3211.

Fray, R.G., Wallace, A., and Fraser, P.D., *et al.* (1995) Constitutive expression of a fruit phytoene synthase gene in transgenic tomatoes causes dwarfism by redirecting metabolites from the gibberellin pathway. *Plant J* **8**, 693–701.

Gao, M., Li, G., Yang, B., *et al.* (2004) Comparative analysis of a *Brassica* BAC clone containing several major aliphatic glucosinolate genes with its corresponding *Arabidopsis* sequence. *Genome* **47**, 666–679.

Garza, J.F., Gregory, A.D., and Hanson, A.D. (2007) Folate biofortification of tomato fruit. *Proc Natl Acad Sci* **104**, 4218–4222.

Giamoustaris, A. and Mithen, R. (1996) Genetics of aliphatic glucosinolates. IV. Side-chain modification in *Brassica oleracea*. *Theor Appl Genet* **93**, 1006–1010.

Gigolashvili, T., Berger, B., Mock, H.P., *et al.* (2007a) The transcription factor HIG1/MYB51 regulates indolic glucosinolate biosynthesis in *Arabidopsis thaliana*. *Plant J* **50**, 886–901.

Gigolashvili, T., Yatusevich, R., Berger, B., *et al.* (2007b) The R2R3-MYB transcription factor HAG1/MYB28 is a regulator of methionine-derived glucosinolate biosynthesis in *Arabidopsis thaliana*. *Plant J* **51**, 247–261.

Giliberto, L., Perrotta, G., Pallara, P., *et al.* (2005) Manipulation of the blue light photoreceptor cryptochrome 2 in tomato affects vegetative development, flowering time, and fruit antioxidant content. *Plant Physiol* **137**, 199–208.

Gilliland, L.U., Magallanes-Lundback, M., Hemming, C., *et al.* (2006) Genetic basis for natural variation in seed vitamin E levels in *Arabidopsis thaliana*. *Proc Natl Acad Sci USA* **103**, 18834–18841.

GISSI Investigators (1999) Dietary supplementation with n-3 polyunsaturated fatty acids and vitamin E after myocardial infarction: results of the GISSI-Prevenzione trial. *Lancet* **354**, 447–455.

Goff, S.A., Cone, K.C., and Chandler, V.L. (1992) Functional analysis of the transcriptional activator encoded by the maize B gene: evidence for a direct functional interaction between two classes of regulatory proteins. *Genes Devel* **6**, 864–875.

Goldbitz, P. (ed.) (2005–2008) Statistics. In *Soya and Oilseed Bluebook 2005*. Soyatech, Manitoba, p. 335.

Gonzali, S., Mazzucato, A., and Perata, P. (2009) Purple as a tomato: towards high anthocyanin tomatoes. *Trends Plant Sci* **14**, 237–41.

Granado, F., Olmedilla, B., Herrero, C., *et al.* (2006) Bioavailability of carotenoids and tocopherols from broccoli: in vivo and in vitro assessment. *Exp Biol Med* **231**, 1733–1738.

Grotewold, E. (2006) The genetics and biochemistry of floral pigments. *Annu Rev Plant Biol* **57**, 761–780.

Grubb, C.D., Zipp, B.J., Ludwig-Müller, J., *et al.* (2004) *Arabidopsis* glucosyltransferase UGT74B1 functions in glucosinolate biosynthesis and auxin homeostasis. *Plant J* **40**, 893–908.

Guéguen, L. and Pointillart, A. (2000) The bioavailability of dietary calcium. *J Am Coll Nutr* **19**, 119S–136S

Guo, J.T., Lee, H.L., Chiang S.H., *et al.* (2001) Antioxidant properties of the extracts from different parts of broccoli in Taiwan. *J Food Drug Anal* **9**, 96–101.

Halkier, B.A. and Gershenzon, J. (2006) Biology and biochemistry of glucosinolates. *Annu Rev Plant Biol* **57**, 303–333.

Hall, C., McCallum, D., Prescott, A., *et al.* (2001) Biochemical genetics of glucosinolate modification in *Arabidopsis* and *Brassica*. *Theor Appl Genet* **102**, 369–374.

Hansen, B.G., Kliebenstein, D.J., and Halkier, B.A. (2007) Identification of a flavin-monooxygenase as the S-oxygenating enzyme in aliphatic glucosinolate biosynthesis in *Arabidopsis*. *Plant J* **50**, 902–910.

Hansen, C.H., Wittstock, U., Olsen, C.E., *et al.* (2001) Cytochrome P450 CYP79F1 from *Arabidopsis* catalyzes the conversion of dihomomethionine and trihomomethionine to the corresponding aldoximes in the biosynthesis of aliphatic glucosinolates. *J Biol Chem* **276**, 11078–11085

Harris, W., Lemke, S.L., Hansen, S.N., *et al.* (2008) Stearidonic acid-enriched soybean oil increased the omega-3 index, an emerging cardiovascular risk marker. *Lipids* **43**, 805–811.

Hauptmann, R., Eschenfeldt, W.H., English, J., *et al.* (1997) Enhanced carotenoid accumulation in storage organs of genetically engineered plants. *US Patent* 5618988.

Hemm, M.R., Ruegger, M.O., and Chapple, C. (2003) The *Arabidopsis* ref2 mutant is defective in the gene encoding CYP83A1 and shows both phenylpropanoid and glucosinolate phenotypes. *Plant Cell* **15**, 179–194.

Hirai, M.Y., Sugiyama, K., Sawada, Y., *et al.* (2007) Omics-based identification of *Arabidopsis* Myb transcription factors regulating aliphatic glucosinolate biosynthesis. *Proc Natl Acad Sci* **104**, 6478–6483.

Hirschi, K.D. (2001) Vacuolar H+/Ca2+ transport: who's directing the traffic? *Trends Plant Sci* **6**, 100–104.

Hirschi, K.D., Zhen, R.G., Cunningham, K.W., *et al.* (1996) CAX1, an H+/Ca2+ antiporter from *Arabidopsis*. *Proc Natl Acad Sci USA* **93**, 8782–8786.

Hunter, S.C. and Cahoon, E.B. (2007) Enhancing vitamin E in oilseeds: unraveling tocopherol and tocotrienol biosynthesis. *Lipids* **42**, 97–108.

International Food Information Council (2006) Dietary fats and fat replacers backgrounder. In *Foundation Media Guide on Food Safety and Nutrition*. http://ific.org/nutrition/fats/index.cfm.

International Food Information Council (2009) *2009 Food and Health Survey: Consumer Attitudes Toward Food, Nutrition and Health*. IFIC, Washington, DC.

Isaacson, T., Ohad, I., Beyer, P., *et al.* (2004) Analysis in vitro of the enzyme CRTISO establishes a poly-cis-carotenoid biosynthesis pathway in plants. *Plant Physiol* **136**, 4246–4255.

James, M.J., Ursin, V.M., and Cleland, L.G. (2003) Metabolism of stearidonic acid in human subjects: comparison with the metabolism of other n-3 fatty acids. *Am J Clin Nutr* **77**, 1140–1145.

Jang, H., Mason, J.B., and Choi, S.-W. (2005) Genetic and epigenetic interactions between folate and aging in carcinogenesis. *J Nutr* **135**, 2967S–2971S.

Jones, C.M., Mes, P., and Myers, J.R. (2003) Characterization and inheritance of the anthocyanin fruit (Aft) tomato. *J Hered* **94**, 449–456.

Just, B., Santos, C.A., Fonseca, M.E., *et al.* (2007) Carotenoid biosynthesis structural genes in carrot (*Daucus carota*): isolation, sequence-characterization, single nucleotide polymorphism (SNP) markers and genome mapping. *Theor Appl Genet* **114**, 693–704.

Kliebenstein, D. (2009) Advancing genetic theory and application by metabolic quantitative trait loci analysis. *Plant Cell* **21**, 1637–1646.

Kliebenstein, D.J., Kroymann, J., and Mitchell-Olds, T. (2005) The glucosinolate–myrosinase system in an ecological and evolutionary context. *Curr Opin Plant Biol* **8**, 264–271.

Koes, R., Verweij, W., and Quattrocchio, F. (2005) Flavonoids: a colorful model for the regulation and evolution of biochemical pathways. *Trends Plant Sci* **10**, 236–242.

Kolotilin, I., Koltai, H., Tadmor, Y., *et al.* (2007) Transcriptional profiling of high pigment-2dg tomato mutant links early fruit plastid biogenesis with its overproduction of phytonutrients. *Plant Physiol* **145**, 389–401.

Kroymann, J., Textor, S., Tokuhisa, J.G., *et al.* (2001) A gene controlling variation in *Arabidopsis* glucosinolate composition is part of the methionine chain elongation pathway. *Plant Physiol* **127**, 1077–1088.

Lee, K., Lee, S.M., Park, S.-Y., *et al.* (2007) Overexpression of *Arabidopsis* homogentisate phytyltransferase or tocopherol cyclase elevates vitamin E content by increasing gamma-tocopherol level in lettuce (*Lactuca sativa* L.). *Mol Cells* **24**, 301–306.

Lemke, S.L., Vicini, J.L., Su, H., *et al.* (2010) Dietary intake of stearidonic acid-enriched soybean oil increases the omega-3 index: randomized, double-blind clinical study of efficacy and safety. *Am J Clin Nutr* **92**, 766–775.

Li, G. and Quiros, C.F. (2001) Sequence-related amplified polymorphism (SRAP), a new marker system based on a simple PCR reaction: its application to mapping and gene tagging in *Brassica*. *Theor Appl Genet* **103**, 455–461.

Li, G. and Quiros, C.F. (2002) Genetic analysis, expression and molecular characterization of BoGSL-ELONG, a major gene involved in the aliphatic glucosinolate pathway of Brassica species. *Genetics* **162**, 1937–1943.

Li, G. and Quiros, C.F. (2003) In planta side-chain glucosinolate modification in *Arabidopsis* by introduction of dioxygenase *Brassica* homolog BoGSL-ALK. *Theor Appl Genet* **106**, 1116–1121.

Li, G., Riaz, A., Goyal, S., *et al.* (2001) Inheritance of three major genes involved in the synthesis of aliphatic glucosinolates in *Brassica oleracea*. *J Am Soc Hort Sci* **126**, 427–431.

Liu, Y.-S., Gur, A., Ronen, G., *et al.* (2003) There is more to tomato fruit colour than candidate carotenoid genes. *Plant Biotechnol J* **1**, 195–207.

Liu, Y., Roof, S., Ye, Z., *et al.* (2004) Manipulation of light signal transduction as a means of modifying fruit nutritional quality in tomato. *Proc Natl Acad Sci USA* **101**, 9897–9902.

Mathews, H., Clendennen, S.K., Caldwell, C.G., *et al.* (2003) Activation tagging in tomato identifies a transcriptional regulator of anthocyanin biosynthesis, modification, and transport. *Plant Cell* **15**, 1689–1703.

Mehta, R.A., Cassol, T., Li, N., *et al.* (2002) Engineered polyamine accumulation in tomato enhances phytonutrient content, juice quality, and vine life. *Nat Biotechnol* **20**, 613–618.

Meiers, S. (2001) The anthocyanidins cyanidin and delphinidin are potent inhibitors of the epidermal growth-factor receptor. *J Agric Food Chem* **19**, 958–962.

Mes, P.J., Boches, P., Myers, J.R., *et al.* (2008) Characterization of tomatoes expressing anthocyanin in the fruit. *J Am Soc Hort Sci* **133**, 262–269.

Middleton, E., Jr (1998) Effect of plant flavonoids on immune and inflammatory cell function. *Adv Exp Med Biol* **439**, 175–182.

Mielke, T. (2006) Ten oilseeds. *Oil World Annual*. ISTA Mielke, Hamburg.

Mikkelsen, M.D., Hansen, C.H., Wittstock, U., *et al.* (2000) Cytochrome P450 CYP79B2 from *Arabidopsis* catalyzes the conversion of tryptophan to indole-3-acetaldoxime, a precursor of indole glucosinolates and indole-3-acetic acid. *J Biol Chem* **275**, 33712–33717.

Mikkelsen, M.D., Naur, P., and Halkier, B.A. (2004) *Arabidopsis* mutants in the C–S lyase of glucosinolate biosynthesis establish a critical role for indole-3-acetaldoxime in auxin homeostasis. *Plant J* **37**, 770–777.

Mithen, R., Clarke, J., Lister, C., *et al.* (1995) Genetics of aliphatic glucosinolates. III. Side chain structure of aliphatic glucosinolates in *Arabidopsis thaliana*. *Heredity* **74**, 210–215.

Mithen, R., Faulkner, K., Magrath, R., *et al.* (2003) Development of isothiocyanate-enriched broccoli, and its enhanced ability to induce phase 2 detoxification enzymes in mammalian cells. *Theor Appl Genet* **106**, 727–734.

Mol, J., Grotewold, E., and Koes, R. (1998) How genes paint flowers and seeds. *Trends Plant Sci* **3**, 212–217.

Mooney, M., Desnos, T., Harrison, K., *et al.* (1995) Altered regulation of tomato and tobacco pigmentation genes caused by the *delila* gene of *Antirrhinum*. *Plant J* **7**, 333–339.

Morris, J., Hawthorne, K., Hotze, M.T., *et al.* (2008) Nutritional impact of elevated calcium transport activity in carrots. *Proc Natl Acad Sci USA* **105**, 1431–1435.

Morris, J., Nakata, P., McConn, M., *et al.* (2007) Increased calcium bioavailability in mice fed genetically engineered plants lacking calcium oxalate. *Plant Mol Biol* **64**, 613–618.

Muir, S.R., Collins, G.J., Robinson, S., *et al.* (2001) Overexpression of petunia chalcone isomerase in tomato results in fruit containing increased levels of flavonols. *Nature Biotechnol* **19**, 470–474.

Mustilli, A.C., Fenzi, F., and Ciliento, R. (1999) Phenotype of the tomato high pigment-2 mutant is caused by a mutation in the tomato homolog of DEETIOLATED1. *Plant Cell* **11**, 145–157.

Nakajima, J.-I., Tanaka, Y., Yamazaki, M., *et al.* (2001) Reaction mechanism from leucoanthocyanidin to anthocyanidin 3-glucoside, a key reaction for coloring in anthocyanin biosynthesis. *J Biol Chem* **276**, 25797–25803.

Naur, P., Petersen, B.L., Mikkelsen, M.D., *et al.* (2003) CYP83A1 and CYP83B1, two nonredundant cytochrome P450 enzymes metabolizing oximes in the biosynthesis of glucosinolates in *Arabidopsis*. *Plant Physiol* **133**, 63–72.

Nunes, A.C., Kalkmann, D.C., and Aragão, F.J. (2009) Folate biofortification of lettuce by expression of a codon optimized chicken GTP cyclohydrolase I gene. *Transgenic Res* **18**, 661–669.

Park, S., Cheng, N.H., Pittman, J.K., *et al.* (2005a) Increased calcium levels and prolonged shelf life in tomatoes expressing *Arabidopsis* H+/Ca2+ transporters. *Plant Physiol* **139**, 1194–1206.

Park, S., Elless, M.P., Park, J., *et al.* (2009) Sensory analysis of calcium-biofortified lettuce. *Plant Biotechnol J* **7**, 106–117.

Park, S., Kang, T.S., Kim,C.K., *et al.* (2005b) Genetic manipulation for enhancing calcium content in potato tuber. *J Agric Food Chem* **53**, 5598–5603.

Park, S.H., Kim, C.-K., Pike, L.M., *et al.* (2004) Increased calcium in carrots by expression of an *Arabidopsis* H+/Ca2+ transporter. *Mol Breed* **14**, 275–282.

Ramsay, N.A. and Glover, B.J. (2005) MYB-bHLH-WD40 protein complex and the evolution of cellular diversity. *Trends Plant Sci* **10**, 63–70.

Ravanel, S., Cherest, H., Jabrin, S., *et al.* (2001) Tetrahydrofolate biosynthesis in plants: molecular and functional characterization of dihydrofolate synthetase and three isoforms of folylpolyglutamate synthetase in *Arabidopsis thaliana*. *Proc Natl Acad Sci USA* **98**, 15360–15365.

Rébeillé, F., Ravanel, S., Jabrin, S., *et al.* (2006) Folates in plants: biosynthesis, distribution, and enhancement. *Physiol Plant* **126**, 330–342.

Reintanz, B., Lehnen, M., Reichelt, M., *et al.* (2001) bus, a bushy *Arabidopsis* CYP79F1 knockout mutant with abolished synthesis of short-chain aliphatic glucosinolates. *Plant Cell* **13**, 351–367.

Römer, S., Fraser, P.D., Kiano, J.W., *et al.* (2000) Elevation of the provitamin A content of transgenic tomato plants. *Nature Biotechnol* **18**, 666–669.

Ronen, G., Carmel-Goren, L., Zamir, D., *et al.* (2000) An alternative pathway to β-carotene formation in plant chromoplasts discovered by map-based cloning of beta and old-gold color mutations in tomato. *Proc Natl Acad Sci USA* **97**, 11102–11107.

Rosati, C., Aquilani, R., Dharmapuri, S., *et al.* (2000) Metabolic engineering of beta-carotene and lycopene content in tomato fruit. *Plant J* **24**, 413–419.

Sanders, D., Brownlee, C., and Harper, J.F. (1999) Communicating with calcium. *Plant Cell* **11**, 691–706.

Santos, C. and Simon, P.W. (2002) QTL analyses reveal clustered loci for accumulation of major provitamin A carotenes and lycopene in carrot roots. *Mol Genet Genomics* **268**, 122–129.

Sarikamis, G., Marquez, J., MacCormack, R., *et al.* (2006) High glucosinolate broccoli: a delivery system for sulforaphane. *Molec Breeding* **18**, 219–228.

Scott, J., Rébeillé, F., and Fletcher, J. (2000) Folic acid and folates: the feasibility for nutritional enhancement in plant foods. *J Sci Food Agric* **80**, 795–824.

Shintani, D. and DellaPenna, D. (1998) Elevating the vitamin E content of plants through metabolic engineering. *Science* **282**, 2098–2011.

Simkin, A.J., Gaffé, J., Alcaraz, J.P., *et al.* (2007) Fibrillin influence on plastid ultrastructure and pigment content in tomato fruit. *Phytochemistry* **68**, 1545–1556.

Smolen, G. and Bender, J. (2002) *Arabidopsis* cytochrome P450 cyp83B1 mutations activate the tryptophan biosynthetic pathway. *Genetics* **160**, 323–332.

Stover, P. (2004) Physiology of folate and vitamin B12 in health and disease. *Nutr Rev* **62**, S3–12.

Sze, H., Li, X., and Palmgren, M.G. (1999) Energization of plant cell membranes by H+ pumping ATPases: regulation and biosynthesis. *Plant Cell* **11**, 677–690

Tohge, T., Nishiyama, Y., and Hirai, M.Y., *et al.* (2005) Functional genomics by integrated analysis of metabolome and transcriptome of *Arabidopsis* plants over-expressing an MYB transcription factor. *Plant J* **42**, 218–235.

Torres, C.A., Davies, N.M., Yañez, J.A., *et al.* (2005) Disposition of selected flavonoids in fruit tissues of various tomato (*Lycopersicon esculentum* Mill.) genotypes. *J Agric Food Chem* **53**, 9536–9543.

Traka, M., Gasper, A.V., Smith, J.A., *et al.* (2005) Transcriptome analysis of human colon Caco-2 cells exposed to sulforaphane. *J Nutr* **135**, 1865–1872.

Tsegaye, D., Shintani, K., and DellaPenna, D. (2002) Overexpression of the enzyme p-hydroxyphenolpyruvate dioxygenase in

Arabidopsis and its relation to tocopherol biosynthesis. *Plant Physiol Biochem* **40,** 913–920.

USDA (2009) USDA Projections to 2018. Long-term Projections Report OCE-2009-1. http://www.ers.usda.gov/Publications/OCE091/OCE091.pdf.

Vogel, J.T., Tieman, D.M., Sims, C.A., *et al.* (2010) Carotenoid content impacts flavor acceptability in tomato (*Solanum lycopersicum*). *J Sci Food Agric* **90,** 2233–2240

Wang, S., Liu, J., Feng, Y., *et al.* (2008) Altered plastid levels and potential for improved fruit nutrient content by downregulation of the tomato DDB1-interacting protein CUL4. *Plant J* **55,** 89–103.

Whelan, J. (2009) Dietary stearidonic acid is a long chain (n-3) polyunsaturated fatty acid with potential health benefits. *J Nutr* **139,** 5–10.

Willits, M.G., Kramer, C.M., Prata, R.T., *et al.* (2005) Utilization of the genetic resources of wild species to create a nontransgenic high flavonoid tomato. *J Agric Food Chem* **53,** 1231–1236.

Wittstock, U. and Halkier, B.A. (2002) Glucosinolate research in the *Arabidopsis* era. *Trends Plant Sci* **7,** 263–270

Wurbs, D., Ruf, S., and Bock, R. (2007) Contained metabolic engineering in tomatoes by expression of carotenoid biosynthesis genes from the plastid genome. *Plant J* **49,** 276–288.

Xie, D.-Y., Sharma, S.B., Paiva, N.L., *et al.* (2003) Role of anthocyanidin reductase, encoded by BANYULS in plant flavonoid biosynthesis. *Science* **299,** 396–399.

Yuan, Y., Chiu, L.-W., and Li, L. (2009) Transcriptional regulation of anthocyanin biosynthesis in red cabbage. *Planta* **230,** 1141–1153.

Zang, Y.X., Kim, J.H., Park, Y.D., *et al.* (2008) Metabolic engineering of aliphatic glucosinolates in Chinese cabbage plants expressing *Arabidopsis* MAM1, CYP79F1, and CYP83A1. *BMC Reports* **41,** 472–478.

73

BIOACTIVE COMPONENTS IN FOODS AND SUPPLEMENTS FOR HEALTH PROMOTION

PAUL M. COATES[1], PhD, HOLLY NICASTRO[2], PhD, AND JOHN A. MILNER[2], PhD

[1]*National Institutes of Health, Bethesda, Maryland, USA*
[2]*National Cancer Institute, Rockville, Maryland, USA*

Disclaimer: The opinions expressed are those of the authors and do not constitute official policy of the National Institutes of Health.

Summary

Linkages among dietary habits, supplement use, and overall health emanate from a multitude of epidemiological, preclinical, and clinical studies. Unfortunately, inconsistencies arising from these investigations raise serious concerns about the factors that contribute to a response and about whether or not the available evidence is appropriate for public health – much less personalized – recommendations. These inconsistencies result in part from variations in experimental designs that have been used to address nutritional interventions for health outcomes, but they also reflect the multifactorial and complex nature of health and the specificity and interactions among dietary constituents when they are consumed in foods or individually as dietary supplements. The challenge of defining the best intervention strategy is underscored by the numerous and diverse agents which may alter cellular processes that are linked with growth, development, and disease resistance. The explosion of information about the interrelationships among genomics, proteomics, metabolomics, and dietary components is beginning to shed light on why variation in response may arise. Greater attention to these variables, along with a better understanding about the quantity and speciation of bioactive food components required to bring about a desired response, will surely help distinguish responders from non-responders. Ultimately, this will guide future research that will provide a sounder basis for dietary recommendations.

Introduction

Belief in the medicinal powers of foods and its components is not a new concept but has been handed down from generation to generation. Almost 2500 years ago, Hippocrates suggested, "Let food be thy medicine and medicine be thy food." Today consumers are bombarded by claims about the ability of foods and their constituents to modify health and/or the risk of chronic disease. Undeniably, strategies that utilize foods and dietary supplements to optimize nutrition for achieving one's "genetic potential," for improving physical and cognitive performance, and for reducing the risk of chronic diseases, are highly commendable and appropriate, particularly in this

Present Knowledge in Nutrition, Tenth Edition. Edited by John W. Erdman Jr, Ian A. Macdonald and Steven H. Zeisel.
© 2012 International Life Sciences Institute. Published 2012 by John Wiley & Sons, Inc.

era of mounting health-care costs. Defining the most effective use of foods or their isolated components will not be simple, but there is mounting scientific evidence to believe that such a personalized approach is feasible.

Why Foods and Dietary Supplements?

The putative health-promoting effects of bioactive components are often first identified by observational or ecologic studies in populations with certain food preferences. Examples of this include the observations that populations consuming large quantities of oily fish have lower population burdens of cardiovascular disease, or that populations consuming large quantities of soy have lower rates of certain cancers. These observations have usually led to investigation and characterization of the bioactive principles responsible for these effects in vitro or in animal models – in the examples above, long-chain polyunsaturated fatty acids and isoflavones, respectively (Sarkar and Li, 2003; Schmidt *et al.*, 2005). Frequently, these components have been isolated and characterized and then studied in various pre-clinical models in attempts to better understand their mechanisms of action outside the food matrix. Many of these isolated components are marketed as dietary supplements. In the United States, for example, the prevalence of use of dietary supplements is very high, with more than 50% of Americans consuming dietary supplements on a regular basis. By far the largest component of the US dietary supplement market comprises vitamins, minerals, and other nutrient supplements, although botanical dietary supplements (e.g. echinacea, ginseng, and ginkgo) are also commonly consumed.

In some instances, the health effects of individual components as part of foods have been borne out when single ingredients have been used as dietary supplements; in other cases, however, such as with tomatoes, it is the presence of the multiple components of the food matrix that is important in bringing about the desired response (Kim *et al.*, 2004). It is possible – but not automatically true – that the health benefit of a food component will be realized by consuming it as a supplement with one or more active components. Generally speaking, when consumers opt for a food-based and/or supplement-based choice for promoting health or for reducing the risk of chronic disease, they expect several features to be in place: the products are known to be safe, since they have been in use in the human diet for long periods; there are proven benefits; and there is reasonable consistency in the products from batch to

batch and over time. Research on all of these issues is needed, particularly as it relates to dietary supplements.

An Evidence-Based Approach to the Literature

Several questions arise about how to document the health benefits and risks of nutrients. Are ecological studies, in which particular patterns of food intake are associated with health benefits and low apparent risk for harm, sufficient to enable people to make informed decisions for proposing dietary change to populations or individuals? Are randomized, controlled, double-blind clinical trials most appropriate? Since genomics is increasingly recognized as modifying the response to food components, would haplotype-specific trials rather than randomized trials be a better way to evaluate health effects? Do we have reliable biomarkers of disease progression or surrogate endpoints for chronic diseases? The goal of an evidence-based approach is to sift through the relevant, available literature in a systematic fashion (Figure 73.1) and, based on the totality of the evidence, to assist researchers, policy-makers, clinicians, and ultimately consumers to make decisions about the role of bioactive food components in health promotion. For example, evidence-based reviews have

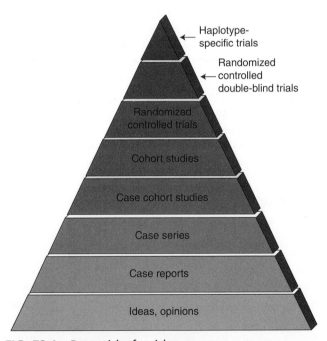

FIG. 73.1 Pyramid of evidence.

been used to assess the efficacy and safety of the probiotic supplement *Saccharomyces boulardii* for treatment of several types of diarrhea (McFarland, 2010) and to evaluate the potential cardioprotective effects of α-linolenic acid (Geleijnse *et al.*, 2010).

Dietary Modifiers and Biological Responses

Numerous reviews extolling the merits and possible risks associated with bioactive food components have surfaced in recent years (Kim *et al.*, 2009; Astrup *et al.*, 2010; Davis *et al.*, 2010; Messina, 2010). An estimated 25 000 phytochemicals exist, and approximately 5000 have been identified while many more remain unknown (Liu, 2003; Heber, 2004). Collectively, more than 500 dietary compounds have been recognized as potential modifiers of human health. Both essential and non-essential allelochemicals arising from plants, along with zoochemicals occurring in animal products, fungochemicals from mushrooms, and bacterochemicals from bacteria may be physiologically relevant modifiers of health. Compounds encompassing such diverse categories as minerals, amino acids, carbohydrates, fatty acids, carotenoids, dithiolthiones, flavonoids, glucosinolates, isothiocyanates, and allyl sulfurs may influence multiple pathways associated with growth, development, and disease resistance. For example, garlic (*Allium sativum*) has been valued for its medicinal properties for centuries. It has been suggested that garlic can reduce the risk of heart disease and cancer (Khanum *et al.*, 2004; Blomhoff, 2005), serve as a source of antioxidants and thereby reduce tissue damage (Banerjee *et al.*, 2003), and influence immunocompetence (Kyo *et al.*, 2001) and possibly mental function (Yamada *et al.*, 2004). Such data suggest that the health implications of bioactive food components may be extremely widespread and are likely not explained by a single cellular mechanism.

Population and Personalized Experimental Designs

The study of nutritional genomics has the potential to identify definitively which components in foods bring about either positive or negative consequences, and to clarify their relevant mechanisms of action and most importantly when they can be manipulated to optimize growth and development and reduce disease risk (Davis and Milner, 2004). Knowledge about how diet-induced

phenotypic responses depend on an individual's genetic background (nutrigenetics), the expression of genes (epigenomics and transcriptomics), changes in the amounts and activities of proteins (proteomics), shifts in small molecular weight compounds (metabolomics), and the diversity of the microbial flora of the gastrointestinal tract (microbiomics) – collectively referred to as "-omics" – will be key to distinguishing responders from non-responders.

Polymorphisms

It is now recognized that close to 21 000 protein-coding genes are found in the human genome (HUPO, 2010). Single nucleotide polymorphisms (SNPs) occurring in a gene coding sequence are of particular interest because they may cause an amino acid substitution and hence alter the biological function of a protein. For example, a SNP in the human gene encoding the low-density lipoprotein receptor results in a A370T codon substitution that leads to asparagine being replaced by serine; this change is associated with higher plasma cholesterol levels and an increased risk of developing cardiovascular disease. Polymorphisms occur at approximately one in every 1200 bases of DNA, with over 10 million SNPs estimated in the human genome. Genomic data for human and mouse (including SNPs, expressed sequence tags, gene expression patterns, and cluster assemblies) and cytogenetic information are increasingly available through a number of databases; these provide opportunities to evaluate genomics as a factor in explaining variation in response to food components in terms of human growth, development, performance, and health. Examples of websites that manage such databases include: hapmap.ncbi.nlm.nih.gov; www.gmod.org; www.genome.gov; www.ebi.ac.uk; and www.nugo.org.

Increasingly, genetic polymorphisms are thought to have a role in determining the response to foods and their components. Unfortunately, while this area is receiving increased attention, it remains unclear whether these polymorphisms are directly linked to outcome. Nevertheless, it is certainly plausible that polymorphic differences have contributed to the inconsistencies among studies of the health effects of dietary components. In a random sample of participants in the Alpha-Tocopherol, Beta-Carotene Cancer Prevention Study (ATBC Study), for example, the low prevalence of polymorphisms in genes coding for activation (phase I) enzymes CYP1A1 (0.07) and CYP2E1 (0.02) and the high prevalence in genes coding for detoxification (phase II) enzymes GSTM1 (0.40) and NQO1

(0.20) (Woodson *et al.*, 1999) may have influenced the outcomes and conclusions of the study. Further, in a nested case-control study within the ATBC Study, glutathione peroxidase 1 (hGPX1), a selenium-dependent enzyme involved in detoxification of hydrogen peroxide, was found to have a polymorphism exhibiting a proline to leucine replacement at codon 198. This polymorphism conferred a relative risk for lung cancer of 1.8 for heterozygotes and 2.3 for homozygous variants compared with homozygote wild types (Ratnasinghe *et al.*, 2000).

Several common genetic polymorphisms may also modulate cancer and cardiovascular disease risk through their influence on folate metabolism, including polymorphisms of the methylenetetrahydrofolate reductase (*MTHFR*) gene. Substituting C for T at nucleotide 677 in the MTHFR gene (C677T) results in reduced conversion of 5,10-methylenetetrahydrofolate to 5-methylenetetrahydrofolate, the form of folate that circulates in plasma. Women with the TT genotype have been reported to be at increased risk of squamous cell carcinoma when they have low plasma folate concentrations (Han *et al.*, 2007). Another common polymorphism is an A-to-C transition at nucleotide 1298 (A1298C), which leads to the replacement of glutamine by alanine and results in mild hyperhomocysteinemia and increased plasma folate levels compared with levels of carriers of the wild type (Boccia *et al.*, 2009). The MTHFR SNP A1298C is associated with increased risk of cardiovascular disease in patients with rheumatoid arthritis (Palomino-Morales *et al.*, 2010). These and other polymorphisms in MTHFR may be associated with risk of various cancers, including breast and colorectal cancer, although results have been mixed (Hazra *et al.*, 2010). Part of the inconsistency in results may relate not just to intake of folate, but also to intake of other vitamins, methyl donors, or other factors that influence DNA stability.

Polymorphisms in the vitamin D receptor (VDR) gene have been linked to bone health as well as the risk of some types of cancer. Common polymorphisms include BsmI, TaqI in intron 8 and exon 9, and a poly-A site in the 3′ end of the gene. The femoral and vertebral bone mineral density was greater in children with the homozygous recessive (bb) version of the VDR polymorphism BsmI compared with those with the dominant genotype (BB). Likewise, BsmI B and short poly-A polymorphisms in the 3′ end of the VDR gene have been associated with increased breast cancer risk, with a trend for increasing risk with increasing number of BsmI B alleles or short (S) poly-A

alleles (Ingles *et al.*, 2000). Using data from two large case-control studies, investigators found that the CDX2 polymorphism was not independently associated with colon or rectal cancer. However, the bLFA haplotype was associated with an increased risk of colon cancer, the BSfG haplotype was associated with an increased risk of rectal cancer, and the BSFA haplotype was associated with a decreased risk of rectal cancer, where A or G of the haplotype designations indicate the CDCX2 allele (Slattery *et al.*, 2007).

Literally millions of SNPs occur within the human genome, making it unlikely that a single base change will be found that is sufficient to account for a number of chronic diseases. However, since genetic variants are often inherited together in segments of DNA called haplotypes which are shared by a majority of the human population, they may be useful in deciphering the genetic differences that make some people more susceptible to disease than others, and likewise in determining how diet will impact their susceptibility. The International HapMap Project (http://www.hapmap.org/) and genome-wide association studies (GWAS) (Ferguson, 2010) may be particularly useful in teasing out genetic differences that determine the response to specific foods and their components. GWAS allow scanning of the entire genome covering over 1 million polymorphisms potentially associated with disease states, eliminating the bias that stems from choosing candidate genes. Recent GWAS have begun to take diet into account. When using a GWAS model that includes meat, fish, and milk intake, and work and leisure physical activity, investigators were able to identify novel susceptibility loci in the SLC2A1 and HP genes that are associated with total cholesterol levels (Igl *et al.*, 2010). In another study, investigators confirmed prior candidates and identified new candidate SNPs associated with plasma homocysteine, vitamin B_{12}, and vitamin B_6 (Hazra *et al.*, 2009).

Epigenomics and Dietary Exposure

Epigenomic modifications regulate expression and activity of genes without modifying genomic sequences. Mechanisms include DNA methylation, histone modifications, gene silencing by microRNA, and chromosome stability (Davis and Milner, 2007; Davis and Ross, 2007, 2008). Evidence already exists that the transcriptional silencing of genes by DNA methylation plays a crucial role in a number of disease states (Ross, 2003). Genes involving cell cycle regulation, DNA repair, angiogenesis, and apoptosis are all inactivated by the hypermethylation of their respective 5′ CpG islands. Key regulatory genes – including E-cadherin, pi-class glutathione S-transferase, the tumor suppressors cyclin-dependent kinases (CDKN2) and phosphatase gene (PTEN), and insulin-like growth factor (IGF-II) targeted histone acetylation and deacetylation – are influenced by DNA hypermethylation. While folate intake is recognized to influence DNA methylation patterns, other nutrients such as selenium can also have an impact (Davis and Uthus, 2003). Restoring proper methylation may represent a fundamental process by which selected nutrients are able to influence gene expression. Several recent studies have provided evidence that genistein, epigallocatechin gallate (EGCG), or potentially other bioactive food components can reverse hypermethylation and reactivate methylation-silenced genes in various tissue types (Fang et al., 2005; King-Batoon et al., 2008; Li and Tollefsbol, 2010).

Covalent modifications of histone tails, including phosphorylation, acetylation, methylation, ubiquitination, or biotinylation, regulate gene expression by changing the structure of chromatin. MicroRNAs inhibit the expression of target genes by binding to complementary sequences on mRNA. These epigenetic modifications are also subject to regulation by dietary components. Butyrate, sulforaphane from cruciferous vegetables, and diallyl disulfide from garlic function as histone deacetylase (HDAC) inhibitors (Myzak and Dashwood, 2006; Myzak et al., 2006). This disrupts the cell cycle by derepressing the cell cycle inhibitor P21 and induces apoptosis by depressing the pro-apoptotic BAX. Folate is a potential modulator of microRNA expression. In patients with head and neck squamous cell carcinoma, the oncogenic microRNA miR-222 is overexpressed in those with the lowest folate intake compared with those with the highest folate intake (Marsit et al., 2006). Further research is necessary to determine the extent to which dietary compounds regulate histone modifications and microRNA expression, and how such regulation modulates disease processes.

Bioactive Components and Transcriptomics

A fundamental action of several bioactive food components is that they serve as regulators of gene expression and/or modulate gene products. Typically, increasing intensity and duration of the exposure increases the number of gene expressions that are influenced (Prima et al., 2004; El-Bayoumy and Sinha, 2005). Thus, dose and duration of exposure become fundamental considerations in interpreting findings from microarray studies. Lin et al. (2007) have used a transcriptomics approach to determine changes in gene expression resulting from a low-fat/low-glycemic load diet in patients undergoing radical prostatectomy. Expression of 23 cDNAs in the experimental group versus none in the control group was significantly changed at the end of the intervention. While most studies are simple snapshots of genomic expression changes that can help identify important possible targets, they must be interpreted cautiously because of inherent biological variability (Barnes, 2008).

Molecular Targets

The era of molecular nutrition holds promise not only for increasing our understanding of the specific site(s) of action of food components but also for the development of a "nutritional preemption" strategy that will incorporate bioactive food components at points of initiation and progression of pathways that lead to unhealthy or lethal conditions. Success with this strategy will depend on early predictors of the response to food components rather than gross phenotypic changes. Similar to the USDA pyramid for dietary guidance, it is likely that the early predictive biomarkers will not be at the apex because of the lateness of the observation but will be focused at the base where they will be more specific and timelier for preemptive strategies. Molecular biomarkers (the "-omics" approach) will likely offer the sensitivity and reliability to evaluate dietary exposures and to provide invaluable insights into behaviors of specific molecular targets and predictors of individual responsiveness to dietary change (Milner, 2004). These biomarkers must be readily accessible, easily and reliably assayed, differentially expressed in normal and diseased conditions, directly associated with disease progression, modifiable, and – most importantly – predictive (Figure 73.2). The future of biomarkers of nutritional exposures, effect and susceptibility likely resides in the enhanced use of molecular technologies to help distinguish responders from non-responders.

Complementary and overlapping mechanisms appear to account for the response to bioactive food components in foods or dietary supplements (Figure 73.3). These biological responses encompass such diverse functions as serving as an antioxidant, promoting the activity of detoxification enzymes, shifting hormonal homeostasis, influencing cellular energetics, regulating cell division, and cellular differentiation. Since the responses may occur simultaneously, it is difficult to determine which is most important in dictating the change in health. Figure 73.3 demonstrates

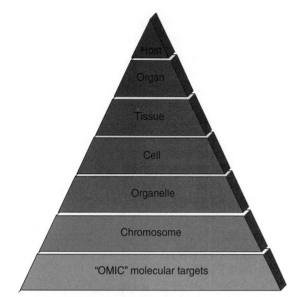

FIG. 73.2 Predictive biomarkers of response to bioactive components.

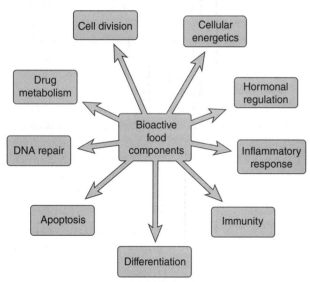

FIG. 73.3 Diet may influence several health-related processes.

some of the plausible processes by which dietary components may influence health outcomes. The ability of several nutrients to influence the same or multiple biological processes raises issues about possible synergy – as well as antagonistic interactions – that may occur within and among foods (Kensler *et al.*, 2000; Ikeda *et al.*, 2003).

DNA Instability

A host of factors can contribute to DNA instability and ultimately to cellular proliferation. Endogenous agents, including methylating species and reactive oxygen species arising during normal cellular respiration, can lead to DNA damage. Some nutrients such as unsaturated fatty acids and iron may influence this process by promoting the formation of the damaging agents, while other components (such as some flavonoids and folate) may function to enhance endogenous repair mechanisms (Fenech, 2005). Support for this comes from the observation that an aqueous fraction of Fushimi sweet pepper increases repair against UV-induced cyclobutane pyrimidine dimers in human fibroblasts (Nakamura *et al.*, 2000). Other data point to the essentiality of folate in maintaining normal DNA synthesis and repair (Beetstra *et al.*, 2005; Friso and Choi, 2005). Multiple studies suggest that berries and their individual components such as anthocyanins prevent DNA damage by scavenging free radicals, chelating damage-inducing metals, and increasing the expression of DNA repair genes (Duthie, 2007; Aiyer *et al.*, 2008). Some dietary components may also retard repair, as has been suggested following exposure to alcohol, the metabolites of which can form adducts with DNA repair enzymes (McKillop and Schrum, 2009). Unquestionably, DNA replication is central to cell growth, development, and generation of tissues and organs. Recent advances in understanding replication machinery have revealed striking conservation of components involved in the DNA replication processes from yeast to humans, thus raising the possibility of using various models to test the site of action of nutrients (Mathers, 2004).

Cellular Proliferation and Death

Cell homeostasis is regulated by a delicate balance among proliferation, growth arrest, differentiation, and apoptosis (programmed cell death). While vitamin A has been repeatedly linked to differentiation, other nutrients such as vitamin D may also be involved (Dong *et al.*, 2005). Numerous foods and dietary components inhibit or promote cell cycle progression by varied mechanisms. For example, indole-3-carbinol from *Brassica* vegetables inhibits elastase, which results in decreased cleavage of cyclin E to a low-molecular-mass form associated with increased proliferation (Nguyen *et al.*, 2008). Dysregulation of apoptosis frequently accompanies a wide array of conditions including cancer, neurodegeneration, autoimmunity, and heart disease. Diverse nutrients, including plant sterols, selenium, and even butyrate arising from fermentable fibers may promote apoptosis (Awad and Fink, 2000; McEligot *et al.*, 2005).

Inflammation and Immunonutrition

The immune system represents a primary defense against invading pathogens, non-self components, and cancer cells. Inflammation is a basic process by which the body reacts to infection, irritations, or other injuries, and is recognized as a type of non-specific immune response. The inflammatory processes, including the release of pro-inflammatory cytokines and formation of reactive oxygen and nitrogen species, are critical factors driving this process and can be influenced by several dietary components. Although pro-inflammatory actions are usually followed almost immediately by anti-inflammatory responses, excessive production of pro-inflammatory cytokines may lead to chronic inflammation. The ability of bioactive food components including zinc, epigallocatechin gallate, and omega-3 fatty acids appears to be mediated through unique molecular targets (Li *et al.*, 2004; Philpott and Ferguson, 2004; Calder, 2005; Cunningham-Rundles *et al.*, 2005).

The immune system protects against infection by producing specific antibodies in response to antigens. Vaccine-specific serum antibody production, delayed-type hypersensitivity response, vaccine-specific or total secretory IgA in saliva, and the response to attenuated pathogens are classic markers which can be influenced by dietary habits. Markers including natural killer cell cytotoxicity, oxidative burst of phagocytes, lymphocyte proliferation, and the cytokine pattern produced have also surfaced as potential predictors of immunocompetence. Since no single marker permits firm conclusions about the ability of diet to modulate the entire immune system, combining markers appears to be a suitable strategy. It is also clear that excesses of some nutrients can enhance the immune system while other food components can have detrimental effects (Calder and Kew, 2002).

Angiogenesis

The availability of nutrients can also influence angiogenesis. In adipose tissue, vascular endothelial cells provide oxygen and nutrients to the growing mass of adipocytes. In fact, the formation of new blood vessels from existing ones often precedes adipogenesis. Insights into how food components alter angiogenesis may be particularly useful in combating the growing global incidence of obesity. Likewise, the importance of angiogenesis in tumor growth

and metastasis serves as additional justification for examining the impact of diet on this process. It is known that vascular endothelial cell proliferation, migration, and capillary formation can be stimulated by several angiogenic growth factors as well by as eicosanoids synthesized from omega-6 fatty acids (Rose and Connolly, 2000). Lipoxygenase and cyclooxygenase products of omega-6 fatty acid metabolism are angiogenic in in-vitro assays. The activity of both of these enzymes can be suppressed by the consumption of resveratrol found in grapes or omega-3 fatty acids occurring in fish (Rose and Connolly, 2000; Kaga *et al.*, 2005). Likewise, genistein, selenium, curcumin, and green tea polyphenols have been reported to influence angiogenesis (Bhat and Singh, 2008).

Summary of Molecular Targets

Collectively, overwhelming evidence demonstrates that a variety of nutrients can influence a number of key intracellular targets. Determining which one of these targets is most important in altering tumor growth will not be a simple task. Likewise, unraveling the multitude of interactions among nutrients and other food components with these key events makes the challenge even more daunting. Finally, inter-individual differences probably reflecting genetic polymorphisms can mask the response to a compound and thereby complicate this undertaking to an even greater extent. Nevertheless, deciphering the role of diet is fundamental to optimizing health. Access to this information should help resolve the inconsistencies within the literature and provide clues to strategies that may be developed to assist individuals to improve their health.

Biomarkers and Long-Term Intervention

Scientifically sound intervention studies must be viewed as the cornerstone for establishing nutrition guidance. Unfortunately, the number of long-term intervention studies that would be needed to adequately define the needs for bioactive food components is likely impractical in terms of speed of discovery and cost. Alternative procedures that utilize validated and sensitive biological markers will need to be developed to assist in determining who might benefit most and who might be placed at risk, and the minimum quality of the food and/or component needed to bring about the intended response. The Biomarkers Consortium, a partnership between United States government agencies and private industry, was launched in 2006 with the aim of identifying and validating quantitative biomarkers. To date, the consortium has studied potential biomarkers for cancer, cardiovascular disease, rheumatoid arthritis, Alzheimer's disease, diabetes, and other chronic conditions. Their work has led to the identification of adiponectin as a predictive biomarker for type 2 diabetes (Wagner *et al.*, 2009).

In order to assess whether a food or its constituent has a physiological effect, it is imperative that stringent experimental design characteristics be followed, including: appropriateness of controls, randomization of subjects, blinding, statistical power of study, presence of bias, attrition rates, recognition and control of confounding factors (e.g. weight change or nutrition status), and appropriateness of statistical tests and comparisons. Each of these factors must become the mainstay for all clinical investigations. These same factors must also be considered in the conduct of preclinical investigations.

The question arises as to whether typical intakes of these dietary components are sufficient to bring about these effects and how frequently these food components must be consumed. Combs and Gray (1998) emphasized that the responses in antioxidant status, drug metabolism, and cell proliferation to a bioactive food component – in this case, selenium – was highly dependent on total intakes/exposures. Therefore, the development of "intended use" models represents a logical approach for determining the quantity of a food component needed for health promotion within specific segments of society, while building on the belief that not every individual will benefit from the same type of nutritional preemption strategies. There is also evidence that individuals do acclimate and accommodate to inadequacies in the food supply, and therefore the biological response cannot be considered constant (Young *et al.*, 1987). It is known that drug resistance frequently involves an induction mechanism thereby reducing or eliminating the response (Kohno *et al.*, 2005). Since bioactive food components have molecular targets, at least some of which are identical to those of specific drugs, it is logical to assume there is adjustment to their biological consequences as well.

Increasing the consumption of a wide variety of fruits, vegetables, and whole grains daily continues to be advocated as a practical strategy for consumers to optimize health and to reduce the risk of chronic diseases. The superiority of food blends is evident from the enhanced antioxidant potential achieved by combining multiple fruits rather than simply providing individual portions (Liu, 2004). Exposure to food blends may also result in

synergistic response by modifying multiple biological processes. For example, since quercetin and genistein block different phases of the cell cycle, their combined use is more effective in inhibiting the growth of human ovarian carcinoma cells than either provided alone (Shen and Weber, 1997). This has significance for dietary supplements, where the effects of individual constituents, as well as combinations of them, outside the food matrix will need to be carefully studied.

Omega-3 Fatty Acids as an Example

For more than 25 years, clinical studies have provided data on the potential health benefits of consuming polyunsaturated fatty acids (PUFAs) and particularly omega-3 fatty acids. Dietary omega-3 fatty acids may come from fish and fish oils [chiefly eicosapentaenoic acid (EPA) and docosahexaenoic acid (DHA)], plant sources such as canola oil, walnuts, soybeans, and flaxseed primarily as α-linolenic acid (ALA), and most recently some novel genetically modified plants with exaggerated amounts of EPA and DHA (Miller *et al.*, 2008).

Results of several studies have suggested that long-chain omega-3 fatty acid intake is associated with reduced risk of numerous diseases, including cardiovascular disease (CVD), stroke, certain cancers, immune disorders, asthma, and neurological disorders; rarely, however, has causality been established. Recently a series of evidence-based reports about the health effects of omega-3 fatty acids were developed by scientists in the Evidence-Based Practice Centers at Tufts–New England Medical Center, RAND–Southern California, and the University of Ottawa (summarized on http://ods.od.nih.gov/FactSheets/Omega3 FattyAcidsandHealth.asp#ref). The primary goal of these reports was to assess the nature and quality of the evidence relating omega-3 consumption from foods and supplements to health outcomes such as CVD prevention and treatment. The reports systematically reviewed the evidence from numerous lines of inquiry. Systematic review of the randomized controlled trials of the effects of omega-3 fatty acids on CVD risk factors (Balk *et al.*, 2004; Jordan *et al.*, 2004; Wang *et al.*, 2004) showed that there is considerable heterogeneity in treatment effects. It is apparent from these and other reports that the speciation of the bioactive components must be considered along with the multiple interactions with other dietary/environmental factors that may influence the overall response. For example, it is recognized that omega-3 fatty acids are not all equivalent in bringing about a biological response, and that confounders such as the total omega-6 fatty acid intake may influence the magnitude of the response (Luan *et al.*, 2001; Gago-Dominguez *et al.*, 2003; Leitzmann *et al.*, 2004).

Which Risk Factor Is Most Important?

There was a strong, consistent, dose-dependent beneficial effect on plasma triglyceride levels (10–30% lowering) that was generally significant across studies (Balk *et al.*, 2004). In addition, there was a small but significant beneficial effect on systolic and diastolic blood pressure (about 2 mm Hg decrease). There were possible beneficial effects on coronary artery restenosis after angioplasty, on exercise capacity in patients with coronary atherosclerosis, and on heart rate variability, especially in patients with recent myocardial infarction. There were non-significant increases in LDL- and HDL-cholesterol, and no consistent effects on carotid intima-medial thickness, on blood levels of apolipoproteins, lipoprotein(a), hemoglobin A1c, glucose, insulin, or C-reactive protein, or on any measures of hemostasis. A conclusion from these analyses is that if CVD benefits of omega-3 fatty acids exist, they are not well explained by their effects on the CVD risk factors examined, unless the overall benefit is due to the accumulation of small effects on several of them (e.g. triglycerides, blood pressure, etc.). Furthermore, it is obvious that, whatever criteria are used, all individuals do not respond identically to the same intervention strategy.

Generalizing Information for Prevention and Treatment

A fundamental question remains: do pathologic evaluations reflect what occurs normally (Prentice *et al.*, 2004)? Is it appropriate to extrapolate information about omega-3 fatty acids in the prevention of cardiovascular disease in unselected populations (primary prevention) from data obtained on prevention in patients with previous disease events (secondary prevention)? To date there is strong evidence that omega-3 fatty acid consumption in patients who have suffered myocardial infarction can reduce the risk of subsequent cardiovascular events and all-cause mortality, although the data regarding primary prevention in otherwise unselected subjects are less secure.

Likewise, information about the potential role of omega-3 fatty acids in one condition may not be sufficient for judging their importance in another condition. For example, in type 2 diabetes mellitus, omega-3 fatty acids

reduce serum triglycerides, but have no effect on total cholesterol, high-density lipoprotein cholesterol, or low-density lipoprotein cholesterol; there is insufficient evidence to draw conclusions regarding their role in altering insulin resistance. In rheumatoid arthritis, one measure (tender joint count) appears to be improved, but there is no obvious effect on other clinical outcomes. For most of the other indications in which omega-3 fatty acids have been suggested to have benefits (such as inflammatory bowel disease, renal disease, bone density or fractures, need for anti-inflammatory or immunosuppressive drugs), there are insufficient data to draw firm conclusions (MacLean *et al.*, 2004).

Questions also remain about the generalizability of information across various populations with different genetic backgrounds. Recent studies suggest that polymorphisms in genes involved in essential fatty acid metabolism can determine whether or not an individual will respond favorably or negatively to changes in intake of omega-3 fatty acids (Simopoulos, 2010). For example, intake of marine omega-3 fatty acids in individuals with two variant 5-lipoxygenase alleles is inversely associated with intima-medial thickness of the carotid artery, an indicator of atherosclerosis (Dwyer *et al.*, 2004). The highest and lowest intakes of monounsaturated fatty acids are associated with increased intima-medial thickness, although this finding was not statistically significant. These associations are not observed in individuals with the common allele. Such nutrient–gene interactions, the number of which is unknown, can account for variability in randomized, controlled trials on the efficacy of omega-3 fatty acids on disease prevention and treatment. Therefore, it is difficult to make recommendations on fatty acid intake that apply to broad populations.

Health Consequences of Omega-3 Fatty Acids as a Model

The example of omega-3 fatty acids illustrates the challenges in documenting health effects of bioactive food components. Overall, there is considerable potential for the role of omega-3 fatty acids in fish or in dietary supplements to reduce the risk of CVD events in previously affected patients, but the data are less certain in the context of primary prevention. Even though for some treatment effects the results were positive, there was considerable heterogeneity in the data. This undoubtedly reflects differences in experimental design (background diets, form and dose of intervention, duration of exposure, inclusion/

exclusion criteria for subjects, etc.), but it also reflects genetic differences among subjects, a topic dealt with earlier in this chapter. In any event, the evidence-based approach will allow us to more clearly delineate research directions and strategies for the future. In the case of omega-3 fatty acids, for example, more research is needed in well-designed primary prevention settings to determine the form (i.e. food vs. supplements), dose, duration, and subject selection where health effects can be assessed. The effects of omega-3 fatty acids in other settings need much more investigation. This does not mean that omega-3 fatty acids are without effect in these settings, but it does mean that the data are insufficient to make firm recommendations.

The same issues discussed with omega-3 fatty acids could reasonably apply to other nutrients and bioactive food components. Detailed discussion of each compound is beyond the scope of this chapter, but many of these compounds, including carotenoids, vitamin D, and flavonoids, are discussed in great detail in other chapters (Chapters 12, 13, and 27, respectively).

Future Directions

In the setting of health effects of bioactive components of foods and dietary supplements, it is important to remember that the effect sizes are very likely to be small and perhaps only realized over a long period of time. This could explain why it has been difficult in intervention trials to document the putative benefits of food-based ingredients (such as omega-3 fatty acids) found in epidemiologic studies. Most reports included a small number of subjects who were studied for only short periods of time. There was considerable heterogeneity in the interventions that were used and the outcomes that were measured. There was little indication, however, of serious adverse events, although these studies may not have been sufficiently powered to detect rare events. Systematic review of the literature, using appropriate analytical tools, can be valuable in judging the state of science, detecting modest effects (both positive and negative), and leading to the development of recommendations. Recommendations may include what further research is necessary and what research designs are most appropriate to pursue; they may also include messages for the public about health-promoting dietary habits or supplementation.

Research in nutrition and health must give greater attention to studies aimed at understanding the basic molecular mechanisms by which bioactive components influence cellular processes. Well-coordinated, multidisciplinary efforts among scientists – including nutrition scientists, molecular biologists, geneticists, statisticians, and clinical cancer researchers – will be needed to advance this molecular approach to nutrition and health. Many research questions and issues will need to be addressed for this approach to become a reality. For example, can the impact of a nutrient be evaluated by the use of a single molecular target, or do multiple targets need to be evaluated simultaneously to predict a response? What interactions are critical in modifying the response to bioactive food components? Additional attention to the importance of the time and duration of exposures for the overall response is needed. Key to moving this science forward will be the identification and validation of biomarkers that can be used to assess intake, effect, and susceptibility.

The development and implementation of a successful multidisciplinary effort that emphasizes a molecular approach to nutrition and health will take motivation, dedication, and specialized training. The challenges to this research are enormous, but so also are the potential rewards in terms of improving health.

Suggestions for Further Reading

Balk, E., Horsley, T., Newberry, S., *et al.* (2007) A collaborative effort to apply the evidence-based review process to the field of nutrition: challenges, benefits, and lessons learned. *Am J Clin Nutr* **85**, 1448–1456.

Institute of Medicine (2010) *Evaluation of Biomarkers and Surrogate Endpoints in Chronic Disease*. May 12. National Academy of Sciences, Washington, DC.

Kussman, M., Krause, L., and Siffert, W. (2010) Nutrigenomics: where are we with genetic and epigenetic markers for disposition and susceptibility? *Nutr Rev* **68**(Suppl 1), S38–47.

Simopoulos, A.P. (2010) Genetic variants in the metabolism of omega-6 and omega-3 fatty acids: their role in the determination of nutritional requirements and chronic disease risk. *Exp Biol Med (Maywood)* **235**, 785–795.

References

Aiyer, H.S., Vadhanam, M.V., Stoyanova, R., *et al.* (2008) Dietary berries and ellagic acid prevent oxidative DNA damage and modulate expression of DNA repair genes. *Int J Mol Sci* **9**, 327–341.

Astrup, A., Kristensen, M., Gregersen, N.T., *et al.* (2010) Can bioactive foods affect obesity? *Ann NY Acad Sci* **1190**, 25–41.

Awad, A.B. and Fink, C.S. (2000) Phytosterols as anticancer dietary components: evidence and mechanism of action. *J Nutr* **130**, 2127–2130.

Balk, E., Chung, M., Lichtenstein, A., *et al.* (2004) Effects of omega-3 fatty acids on cardiovascular risk factors and intermediate markers of cardiovascular disease. *Evid Rep Technol Assess (Summ)*, 1–6.

Banerjee, S.K., Mukherjee, P.K., and Maulik, S.K. (2003) Garlic as an antioxidant: the good, the bad and the ugly. *Phytother Res* **17**, 97–106.

Barnes, S. (2008) Nutritional genomics, polyphenols, diets, and their impact on dietetics. *J Am Diet Assoc* **108**, 1888–1895.

Beetstra, S., Thomas, P., Salisbury, C., *et al.* (2005) Folic acid deficiency increases chromosomal instability, chromosome 21 aneuploidy and sensitivity to radiation-induced micronuclei. *Mutat Res* **578**, 317–326.

Bhat, T.A. and Singh, R.P. (2008) Tumor angiogenesis – a potential target in cancer chemoprevention. *Food Chem Toxicol* **46**, 1334–1345.

Blomhoff, R. (2005) Dietary antioxidants and cardiovascular disease. *Curr Opin Lipidol* **16**, 47–54.

Boccia, S., Boffetta, P., Brennan, P., *et al.* (2009) Meta-analyses of the methylenetetrahydrofolate reductase C677T and A1298C polymorphisms and risk of head and neck and lung cancer. *Cancer Lett* **273**, 55–61.

Calder, P.C. (2005) Polyunsaturated fatty acids and inflammation. *Biochem Soc Trans* **33**, 423–427.

Calder, P.C. and Kew, S. (2002) The immune system: a target for functional foods? *Br J Nutr* **88**(Suppl 2), S165–177.

Combs, G.F. Jr and Gray, W.P. (1998) Chemopreventive agents: selenium. *Pharmacol Ther* **79**, 179–192.

Cunningham-Rundles, S., McNeeley, D.F., and Moon, A. (2005) Mechanisms of nutrient modulation of the immune response. *J Allergy Clin Immunol* **115**, 1119–1128; quiz, 1129.

Davis, C.D. and Milner, J. (2004) Frontiers in nutrigenomics, proteomics, metabolomics and cancer prevention. *Mutat Res* **551**, 51–64.

Davis, C.D. and Milner, J.A. (2007) Biomarkers for diet and cancer prevention research: potentials and challenges. *Acta Pharmacol Sin* **28**, 1262–1273.

Davis, C.D. and Ross, S.A. (2007) Dietary components impact histone modifications and cancer risk. *Nutr Rev* **65**, 88–94.

Davis, C.D. and Ross, S.A. (2008) Evidence for dietary regulation of microRNA expression in cancer cells. *Nutr Rev* **66**, 477–482.

Davis, C.D. and Uthus, E.O. (2003) Dietary folate and selenium affect dimethylhydrazine-induced aberrant crypt formation, global DNA methylation and one-carbon metabolism in rats. *J Nutr* **133**, 2907–2914.

Davis, C.D., Emenaker, N.J., and Milner, J.A. (2010) Cellular proliferation, apoptosis and angiogenesis: molecular targets for nutritional preemption of cancer. *Semin Oncol* **37**, 243–257.

Dong, X., Lutz, W., Schroeder, T.M., *et al.* (2005) Regulation of relB in dendritic cells by means of modulated association of vitamin D receptor and histone deacetylase 3 with the promoter. *Proc Natl Acad Sci USA* **102**, 16007–16012.

Duthie, S.J. (2007) Berry phytochemicals, genomic stability and cancer: evidence for chemoprotection at several stages in the carcinogenic process. *Mol Nutr Food Res* **51**, 665–674.

Dwyer, J.H., Allayee, H., Dwyer, K.M., *et al.* (2004) Arachidonate 5-lipoxygenase promoter genotype, dietary arachidonic acid, and atherosclerosis. *N Engl J Med* **350**, 29–37.

El-Bayoumy, K. and Sinha, R. (2005) Molecular chemoprevention by selenium: a genomic approach. *Mutat Res* **591**, 224–236.

Fang, M.Z., Chen, D., Sun, Y., *et al.* (2005) Reversal of hypermethylation and reactivation of p16INK4a, RARbeta, and MGMT genes by genistein and other isoflavones from soy. *Clin Cancer Res* **11**, 7033–7041.

Fenech, M. (2005) The Genome Health Clinic and Genome Health Nutrigenomics concepts: diagnosis and nutritional treatment of genome and epigenome damage on an individual basis. *Mutagenesis* **20**, 255–269.

Ferguson, L.R. (2010) Genome-wide association studies and diet. *World Rev Nutr Diet* **101**, 8–14.

Friso, S. and Choi, S.W. (2005) Gene–nutrient interactions in one-carbon metabolism. *Curr Drug Metab* **6**, 37–46.

Gago-Dominguez, M., Yuan, J.M., Sun, C.L., *et al.* (2003) Opposing effects of dietary n-3 and n-6 fatty acids on mammary carcinogenesis: The Singapore Chinese Health Study. *Br J Cancer* **89**, 1686–1692.

Geleijnse, J.M., De Goede, J., and Brouwer, I.A. (2010) Alpha-linolenic acid: is it essential to cardiovascular health? *Curr Atheroscler Rep* **12**, 359–367.

Han, J., Colditz, G.A., and Hunter, D.J. (2007) Polymorphisms in the MTHFR and VDR genes and skin cancer risk. *Carcinogenesis* **28**, 390–397.

Hazra, A., Fuchs, C.S., Kawasaki, T., *et al.* (2010) Germline polymorphisms in the one-carbon metabolism pathway and DNA methylation in colorectal cancer. *Cancer Causes Control* **21**, 331–345.

Hazra, A., Kraft, P., Lazarus, R., *et al.* (2009) Genome-wide significant predictors of metabolites in the one-carbon metabolism pathway. *Hum Mol Genet* **18**, 4677–4687.

Heber, D. (2004) Vegetables, fruits and phytoestrogens in the prevention of diseases. *J Postgrad Med* **50**, 145–149.

HUPO (2010) A gene-centric human proteome project: HUPO–the Human Proteome organization. *Mol Cell Proteomics* **9**,

427–429. http://www.mcponline.org/content/9/2/427.full.pdf+html?sid=7940440d-5566-48a1-ad41-8148d526687d.

Igl, W., Johansson, A., Wilson, J.F., *et al.* (2010) Modeling of environmental effects in genome-wide association studies identifies SLC2A2 and HP as novel loci influencing serum cholesterol levels. *PLoS Genet* **6,** e1000798.

Ikeda, N., Uemura, H., Ishiguro, H., *et al.* (2003) Combination treatment with 1alpha,25-dihydroxyvitamin D3 and 9-cis-retinoic acid directly inhibits human telomerase reverse transcriptase transcription in prostate cancer cells. *Mol Cancer Ther* **2,** 739–746.

Ingles, S.A., Garcia, D.G., Wang, W., *et al.* (2000) Vitamin D receptor genotype and breast cancer in Latinas (United States). *Cancer Causes Control* **11,** 25–30.

Jordan, H., Matthan, N., Chung, M., *et al.* (2004) Effects of omega-3 fatty acids on arrhythmogenic mechanisms in animal and isolated organ/cell culture studies. *Evid Rep Technol Assess (Summ)*, 1–8.

Kaga, S., Zhan, L., Matsumoto, M., *et al.* (2005) Resveratrol enhances neovascularization in the infarcted rat myocardium through the induction of thioredoxin-1, heme oxygenase-1 and vascular endothelial growth factor. *J Mol Cell Cardiol* **39,** 813–822.

Kensler, T.W., Curphey, T.J., Maxiutenko, Y., *et al.* (2000) Chemoprotection by organosulfur inducers of phase 2 enzymes: dithiolethiones and dithiins. *Drug Metabol Drug Interact* **17,** 3–22.

Khanum, F., Anilakumar, K.R., and Viswanathan, K.R. (2004) Anticarcinogenic properties of garlic: a review. *Crit Rev Food Sci Nutr* **44,** 479–488.

Kim, Y., DiSilvestro, R., and Clinton, S. (2004) Effects of lycopene-beadlet or tomato-powder feeding on carbon tetrachloride-induced hepatotoxicity in rats. *Phytomedicine* **11,** 152–156.

Kim, Y.S., Young, M.R., Bobe, G., *et al.* (2009) Bioactive food components, inflammatory targets, and cancer prevention. *Cancer Prev Res (Phila)* **2,** 200–208.

King-Batoon, A., Leszczynska, J.M., and Klein, C.B. (2008) Modulation of gene methylation by genistein or lycopene in breast cancer cells. *Environ Mol Mutagen* **49,** 36–45.

Kohno, K., Uchiumi, T., Niina, I., *et al.* (2005) Transcription factors and drug resistance. *Eur J Cancer* **41,** 2577–2586.

Kyo, E., Uda, N., Kasuga, S., *et al.* (2001) Immunomodulatory effects of aged garlic extract. *J Nutr* **131,** 1075S–1079S.

Leitzmann, M.F., Stampfer, M.J., Michaud, D.S., *et al.* (2004) Dietary intake of n-3 and n-6 fatty acids and the risk of prostate cancer. *Am J Clin Nutr* **80,** 204–216.

Li, R., Huang, Y.G., Fang, D., *et al.* (2004) (-)-Epigallocatechin gallate inhibits lipopolysaccharide-induced microglial activation and protects against inflammation-mediated dopaminergic neuronal injury. *J Neurosci Res* **78,** 723–731.

Li, Y. and Tollefsbol, T.O. (2010) Impact on DNA methylation in cancer prevention and therapy by bioactive dietary components. *Curr Med Chem* **17,** 2141–2151.

Lin, D.W., Neuhouser, M.L., Schenk, J.M., *et al.* (2007) Low-fat, low-glycemic load diet and gene expression in human prostate epithelium: a feasibility study of using cDNA microarrays to assess the response to dietary intervention in target tissues. *Cancer Epidemiol Biomarkers Prev* **16,** 2150–2154.

Liu, R.H. (2003) Health benefits of fruit and vegetables are from additive and synergistic combinations of phytochemicals. *Am J Clin Nutr* **78,** 517S–520S.

Liu, R.H. (2004) Potential synergy of phytochemicals in cancer prevention: mechanism of action. *J Nutr* **134,** 3479S–3485S.

Luan, J., Browne, P.O., Harding, A.H., *et al.* (2001) Evidence for gene–nutrient interaction at the PPARgamma locus. *Diabetes* **50,** 686–689.

MacLean, C.H., Mojica, W.A., Morton, S.C., *et al.* (2004) Effects of omega-3 fatty acids on lipids and glycemic control in type II diabetes and the metabolic syndrome and on inflammatory bowel disease, rheumatoid arthritis, renal disease, systemic lupus erythematosus, and osteoporosis. *Evid Rep Technol Assess (Summ)*, 1–4.

Marsit, C.J., Eddy, K., and Kelsey, K.T. (2006) MicroRNA responses to cellular stress. *Cancer Res* **66,** 10843–10848.

Mathers, J.C. (2004) The biological revolution – towards a mechanistic understanding of the impact of diet on cancer risk. *Mutat Res* **551,** 43–49.

McEligot, A.J., Yang, S., and Meyskens, F.L., Jr (2005) Redox regulation by intrinsic species and extrinsic nutrients in normal and cancer cells. *Annu Rev Nutr* **25,** 261–295.

McFarland, L.V. (2010) Systematic review and meta-analysis of *Saccharomyces boulardii* in adult patients. *World J Gastroenterol* **16,** 2202–2222.

McKillop, I.H. and Schrum, L.W. (2009) Role of alcohol in liver carcinogenesis. *Semin Liver Dis* **29,** 222–232.

Messina, M. (2010) A brief historical overview of the past two decades of soy and isoflavone research. *J Nutr* **140,** 1350S–1354S.

Miller, M.R., Nichols, P.D., and Carter, C.G. (2008) n-3 Oil sources for use in aquaculture–alternatives to the unsustainable harvest of wild fish. *Nutr Res Rev* **21,** 85–96.

Milner, J.A. (2004) Molecular targets for bioactive food components. *J Nutr* **134,** 2492S–2498S.

Myzak, M.C. and Dashwood, R.H. (2006) Histone deacetylases as targets for dietary cancer preventive agents: lessons learned with butyrate, diallyl disulfide, and sulforaphane. *Curr Drug Targets* **7,** 443–452.

Myzak, M.C., Dashwood, W.M., Orner, G.A., *et al.* (2006) Sulforaphane inhibits histone deacetylase in vivo and suppresses tumorigenesis in Apc-minus mice. *FASEB J* **20,** 506–508.

Nakamura, Y., Tomokane, I., Mori, T., *et al.* (2000) DNA repair effect of traditional sweet pepper Fushimi-togarashi: seen in suppression of UV-induced cyclobutane pyrimidine dimer in human fibroblast. *Biosci Biotechnol Biochem* **64,** 2575–2580.

Nguyen, H.H., Aronchik, I., Brar, G.A., *et al.* (2008) The dietary phytochemical indole-3-carbinol is a natural elastase enzymatic inhibitor that disrupts cyclin E protein processing. *Proc Natl Acad Sci USA* **105,** 19750–19755.

Palomino-Morales, R., Gonzalez-Juanatey, C., Vazquez-Rodriguez, T.R., *et al.* (2010) A1298C polymorphism in the MTHFR gene predisposes to cardiovascular risk in rheumatoid arthritis. *Arthritis Res Ther* **12,** R71.

Philpott, M. and Ferguson, L.R. (2004) Immunonutrition and cancer. *Mutat Res* **551,** 29–42.

Prentice, R.L., Willett, W.C., Greenwald, P., *et al.* (2004) Nutrition and physical activity and chronic disease prevention: research strategies and recommendations. *J Natl Cancer Inst* **96,** 1276–1287.

Prima, V., Tennant, M., Gorbatyuk, O.S., *et al.* (2004) Differential modulation of energy balance by leptin, ciliary neurotrophic factor, and leukemia inhibitory factor gene delivery: microarray deoxyribonucleic acid-chip analysis of gene expression. *Endocrinology* **145,** 2035–2045.

Ratnasinghe, D., Tangrea, J.A., Andersen, M.R., *et al.* (2000) Glutathione peroxidase codon 198 polymorphism variant increases lung cancer risk. *Cancer Res* **60,** 6381–6383.

Rose, D.P. and Connolly, J.M. (2000) Regulation of tumor angiogenesis by dietary fatty acids and eicosanoids. *Nutr Cancer* **37,** 119–127.

Ross, S.A. (2003) Diet and DNA methylation interactions in cancer prevention. *Ann NY Acad Sci* **983,** 197–207.

Sarkar, F.H. and Li, Y. (2003) Soy isoflavones and cancer prevention. *Cancer Invest* **21,** 744–757.

Schmidt, E.B., Arnesen, H., De Caterina, R., *et al.* (2005) Marine n-3 polyunsaturated fatty acids and coronary heart disease. Part I. Background, epidemiology, animal data, effects on risk factors and safety. *Thromb Res* **115,** 163–170.

Shen, F. and Weber, G. (1997) Synergistic action of quercetin and genistein in human ovarian carcinoma cells. *Oncol Res* **9,** 597–602.

Simopoulos, A.P. (2010) Genetic variants in the metabolism of omega-6 and omega-3 fatty acids: their role in the determination of nutritional requirements and chronic disease risk. *Exp Biol Med (Maywood)* **235,** 785–795.

Slattery, M.L., Herrick, J., Wolff, R.K., *et al.* (2007) CDX2 VDR polymorphism and colorectal cancer. *Cancer Epidemiol Biomarkers Prev* **16,** 2752–2755.

Wagner, J.A., Wright, E.C., Ennis, M.M., *et al.* (2009) Utility of adiponectin as a biomarker predictive of glycemic efficacy is demonstrated by collaborative pooling of data from clinical trials conducted by multiple sponsors. *Clin Pharmacol Ther* **86,** 619–625.

Wang, C., Chung, M., Lichtenstein, A., *et al.* (2004) Effects of omega-3 fatty acids on cardiovascular disease. *Evid Rep Technol Assess (Summ)*, 1–8.

Woodson, K., Ratnasinghe, D., Bhat, N.K., *et al.* (1999) Prevalence of disease-related DNA polymorphisms among participants in a large cancer prevention trial. *Eur J Cancer Prev* **8,** 441–447.

Yamada, N., Hattori, A., Hayashi, T., *et al.* (2004) Improvement of scopolamine-induced memory impairment by Z-ajoene in the water maze in mice. *Pharmacol Biochem Behav* **78,** 787–791.

Young, V.R., Gucalp, C., Rand, W.M., *et al.* (1987) Leucine kinetics during three weeks at submaintenance-to-maintenance intakes of leucine in men: adaptation and accommodation. *Hum Nutr Clin Nutr* **41,** 1–18.

Index

Note: page numbers in *italics* refer to figures; those in **bold** to tables or boxes. Prefixes are ignored in the alphabetical sequence – thus *S*-adenosylhomocysteine will be found below adenosine triphosphate.

Present Knowledge in Nutrition, Tenth Edition. Edited by John W. Erdman Jr, Ian A. Macdonald and Steven H. Zeisel.
© 2012 International Life Sciences Institute. Published 2012 by John Wiley & Sons, Inc.